Success in the Classroom, in Clinicals, and on t... SO-CFR-265

Classroom

- Detailed lecture notes organized by learning outcome
- Suggestions for classroom activities
- Guide to relevant additional resources
- Comprehensive PowerPoint™ presentations integrating lecture, images, animations, and videos
- Classroom Response questions
- Image Gallery
- Video and Animation Gallery
- Online course management systems complete with instructor tools and student activities available in a variety of formats

PEARSON mynursinglab™

- Saves instructors time by providing quality feedback, ongoing formative assessments and customized remediation for students.
- Provides easy, one-stop access to a wealth of teaching resources, such as test item files, PowerPoint™ slides, and video suggestions.
- A built-in electronic gradebook tracks students' progress on assessment and remediation activities.

Clinical

- Suggestions for Clinical Activities and other clinical resources organized by learning outcome

Real Nursing Simulations Facilitator's Guide: Institutional Edition

- 25 simulation scenarios that span the nursing curriculum
- Consistent format includes learning objectives, case flow, instructions for set up, student debriefing questions and more!
- Companion online course cartridge with student exercises, activities, videos, skill checklists, and reflective questions also available for adoption

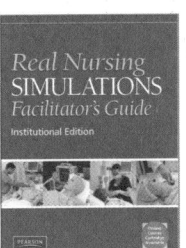

NCLEX-RN®

- Test Item Files with NCLEX®-style questions and complete rationales for correct and incorrect answers mapped to learning outcomes. *available in TestGen, Par Test, and MS Word*

Instructor Resources

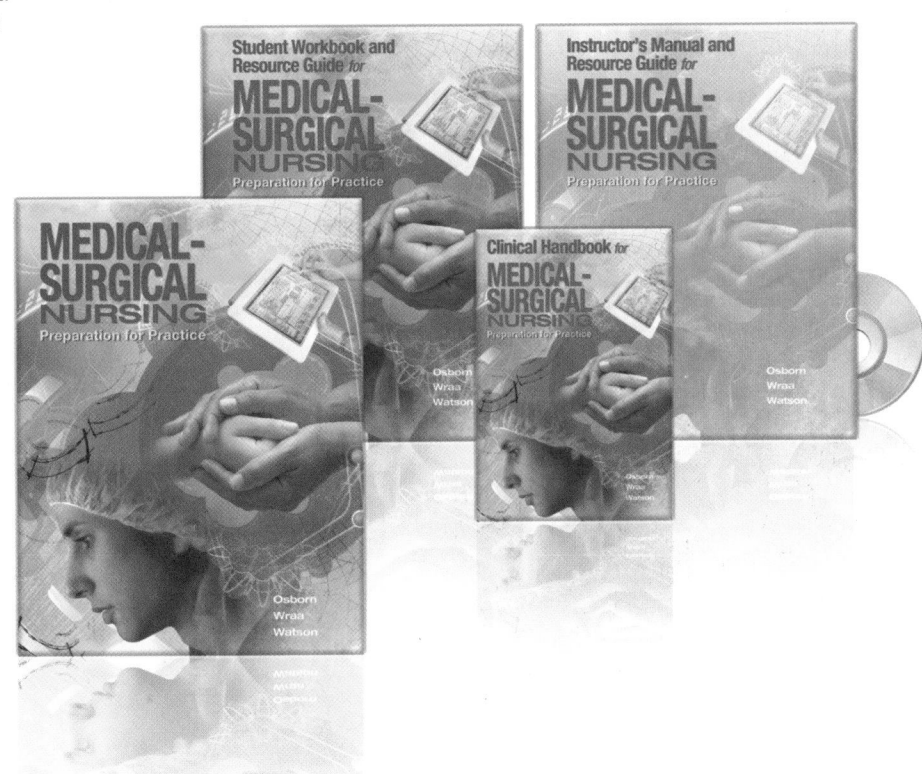

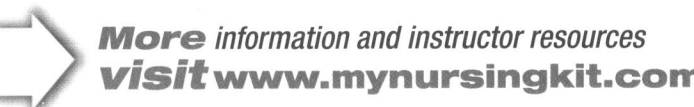

More information and instructor resources
visit www.mynursingkit.com

BRIEF CONTENTS

MEDICAL-SURGICAL NURSING
Preparation for Practice

Volume 2

Kathleen S. Osborn, RN, MS, EdD
California State University
Sacramento, California

Cheryl E. Wraa, RN, MSN
University of California, Davis Medical Center
California State University
Sacramento, California

Annita B. Watson, RN, MS, DNSc
California State University
Sacramento, California

Pearson
Boston   Columbus   Indianapolis   New York   San Francisco   Upper Saddle River
Amsterdam   Cape Town   Dubai   London   Madrid   Milan   Munich   Paris   Montreal   Toronto
Delhi   Mexico City   Sao Paulo   Sydney   Hong Kong   Seoul   Singapore   Taipei   Tokyo

Library of Congress Cataloging-in-Publication Data

Osborn, Kathleen S.

Medical-surgical nursing: preparation for practice/Kathleen S. Osborn, Cheryl E. Wraa, Annita B. Watson.

p. ; cm.

Includes bibliographical references and index.

ISBN-13: 978-0-13-178102-3

ISBN-10: 0-13-178102-2

1. Nursing. 2. Surgical nursing. I. Wraa, Cheryl E. II. Watson, Annita B., III. Title.

[DNLM: 1. Perioperative Nursing—methods. 2. Nurse's Role. 3. Nursing Care—methods. WY 161 081m 2010]

RT41.068 2010

610.73—dc22

2009002926

Publisher: Julie Levin Alexander
Publisher's Assistant: Regina Bruno
Editor-in-Chief: Maura Connor
Executive Acquisitions Editor: Pamela Fuller
Development Editor: iD8 Publishing Services, Marion Waldman
Editorial Assistant: Jennifer Aranda
Managing Production Editor: Patrick Walsh
Production Liaison: Cathy O'Connell
Production Editor: Emily Bush, S4Carlisle Publishing Services
Manufacturing Manager: Ilene Sanford
Creative Director: John Christiana, Design Development Services
Interior and Cover Design: Mary Siener, Design Development Services
Cover and Interior Illustration: A.k.A., Anthony Robinson
Director of Marketing: Karen Allman
Senior Marketing Manager: Francisco Del Castillo
Marketing Specialist: Michael Sirinides
Marketing Assistant: Crystal Gonzalez
Digital Media Product Manager: Travis Moses-Westphal
Media Project Manager: Deb O'Connell, All Things Media
Media Project Manager: Rachel Collett
Manager, Rights and Permissions: Zina Arabia
Manager, Visual Research: Beth Brenzel
Image Permission Coordinator: Fran Toepfer
Composition: S4Carlisle Publishing Services
Printer/Binder: Courier/Kendallville
Cover Printer: Lehigh-Phoenix Color/Hagerstown
Cover Photos: A.k.A., Anthony Robinson, Shayle Keating

Notice: Care has been taken to confirm the accuracy of information presented in this book. The authors, editors, and the publisher, however, cannot accept any responsibility for errors or omissions or for consequences from application of the information in this book and make no warranty, express or implied, with respect to its contents.

The authors and publisher have exerted every effort to ensure that drug selections and dosages set forth in this text are in accord with current recommendations and practice at time of publication. However, in view of ongoing research, changes in government regulations, and the constant flow of information relating to drug therapy and drug reactions, the reader is urged to check the package inserts of all drugs for any change in indications of dosage and for added warnings and precautions. This is particularly important when the recommended agent is a new and/or infrequently employed drug.

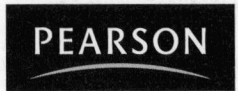

www.pearsonhighered.com

10 9 8 7 6 5 4 3 2
ISBN-10:   0-13-615738-6
ISBN-13:   978-0-13-615738-0

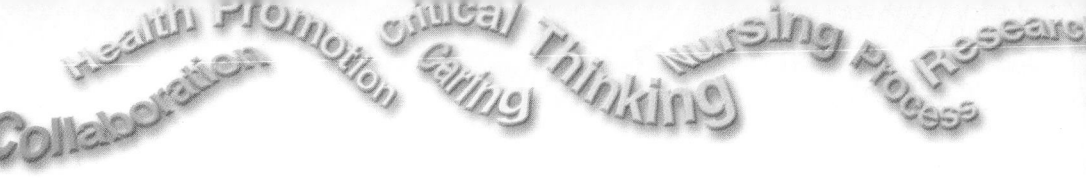

ABOUT THE AUTHORS

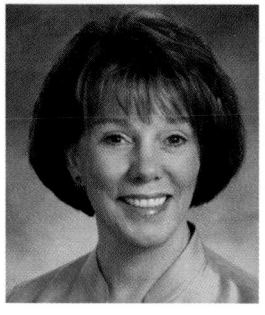

KATHLEEN S. OSBORN

Dr. Kathleen Osborn was first introduced to the profession of nursing at St. Francis School of Nursing in San Francisco, where she received her diploma. She went on to obtain a bachelor's degree in nursing from Sacramento State University, a master of science degree from the University of California, San Francisco, and a doctorate in educational leadership from the University of Southern California. Her clinical practice is in critical care, including cardiac, burn, neurological, and respiratory specialties. She has more than 29 years of experience teaching bachelor and master's degree students, as well as teaching nurses in hospital in-service and continuing education programs. Dr. Osborn's expertise includes program and course development, didactic lecturing, and clinical supervision of undergraduate and graduate students. She also has been actively involved in nursing research and publication throughout her clinical and teaching career. Since 1999, Dr. Osborn has participated as a nurse educator on humanitarian surgical missions to Laos, Africa, Vietnam, Honduras, Bangladesh, and Ecuador. She received the "Heroes in Healthcare" Community Service Award for her humanitarian work from the Coalition for Excellence in Healthcare, a division of the Health Communication Research Institute of Northern California. She also received the Community Service Award from Sacramento State University for her humanitarian work and her service to student development. In 1995, a perpetual faculty award was begun in her honor by the graduating class: The Guiding Light Award for Outstanding Performance by a Nursing Faculty.

This book is dedicated to the important people in my life. I want to thank my husband John for his devotion, patience, and understanding during this project. I also want to thank our children, Christopher and his wife Toni, Patrick, Staci, and Mike for their ongoing understanding of my time away from them. Finally, I want to thank all of the nursing students whom I have had the pleasure of teaching and the patients around the world that I have cared for. You have made my career fulfilling and happy.

—Kathleen Osborn

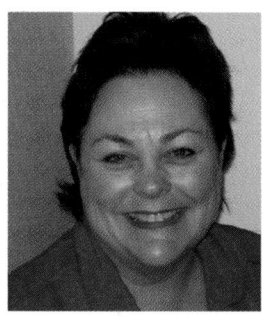

CHERYL E. WRAA

Cheryl Wraa received her nursing diploma from the Kaiser Foundation School of Nursing in Oakland, California. She went on to obtain a bachelor's degree, and master of science degree in nursing from California State University, Sacramento. Her clinical career has focused on critical care nursing, leadership, and education. Ms. Wraa's clinical practice includes the medical intensive care unit, emergency department, and flight nursing. She is currently the trauma program manager at a level 1 trauma center and clinical faculty for advanced medical–surgical nursing students in a baccalaureate program. Ms. Wraa is also an educator for Interplast and has participated on surgical missions to Vietnam, Bangladesh, and Ghana. She has been active in education and publication throughout her career and is currently a senior clinical editor for the *Journal of Emergency Nursing*. She is past president of the Air and Surface Transport Nurses Association, and president-elect of the Trauma Managers Association of California. Ms. Wraa received the Barbara A. Hess Award for her contributions to education in the air medical and ground transport field.

I dedicate this book to my parents for sharing their incredible faith, zest for life, and unconditional love— I miss you. To my mentors for sharing their wisdom— I would not be where I am without you. To my students for keeping the thirst for knowledge alive and, most importantly, to my family and friends for their unending support and love—I would not have survived this without you.

—Cheryl Wraa

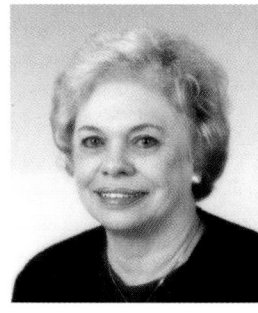

ANNITA B. WATSON

Dr. Annita Watson began her nursing career in Jamestown, New York, at WCA Hospital School of Nursing. She completed her bachelor's degree at Teachers College, Columbia University, and her master's and doctorate in nursing at the University of California, San Francisco. Her graduate focus was medical–surgical nursing and leadership and administration in the service and educational settings. Dr. Watson began her teaching career in 1970 at California State University, Sacramento, where she currently teaches at both the undergraduate and graduate levels. Her areas of practice include medical–surgical nursing, intensive care, long-term care, and community health. Throughout her career, she has served as a national consultant to health care agencies and educational programs on topics related to development of management systems, quality improvement of patient care, curriculum development and evaluation, and implementation of accreditation processes. She has published in like areas, and made numerous professional preparations. Research interests focus on measurement of patient and student outcomes. Currently Dr. Watson assumes a leadership role on several local and regional community boards, focusing on health services for vulnerable populations, for example, children, the elderly, and people who have been abused. Nationally, she serves as an accreditation site evaluator for the Commission on Collegiate Nursing Education. In 2008, she was awarded the Life Time Achievement Award for community service by California State University, Sacramento, recognizing her contributions to the health of the community and her ability to foster community-based learning experiences for students.

To my family, friends, colleagues, and students who supported me in completing this project. Thank you for your existence, endurance, and encouragement. I could not have completed this project without you. Your inspiration and guidance remain in my thoughts and prayers.

—Annita Watson

We extend a heartfelt thanks to our contributors, who gave their time, effort, and expertise so tirelessly to the development and writing of chapters and resources that helped foster our goal of preparing student nurses for evidence-based practice.

Text Contributors

Jaynce Agruss, PhD, APN/CNP
Coordinator, Family Nurse Practitioner Program
Rush University Medical Center
Chicago, Illinois
Chapter 62

Mary Alexander, MA, RN, CRNI, CAE
Chief Executive Officer
Education Manager
Infusion Nurses Society
Norwood, Massachusetts
Chapter 22

Nancy Ames, RN, MSN, CCRN
Critical Care Clinical Specialist
National Institutes of Health, Clinical Center
Nursing and Patient Care Services
Bethesda, Maryland
Chapter 36

Sue Apple, RN, DNSc
Assistant Professor
School of Nursing and Health Studies
Georgetown University
Washington, D.C.
Chapter 39

Jane Ashley, PhD, RN
Associate Professor
Connell School of Nursing
Boston College
Boston, Massachusetts
Chapters 25 and 27

Laurie Baker, RN, MS, APRN, BC, ANP
Coordinator, Barrow Neurosurgical Spine Assessment Clinic
Barrow Neurosurgical Associates
Phoenix, Arizona
Chapter 34

Patricia Baker, RN
Skills Lab Coordinator
School of Nursing and Health Studies
Georgetown University
Washington, D.C.
Chapters 24 and 32

Doris Ballard-Ferguson, RN, PhD
Professor
School of Nursing
Florida A&M University
Tallahassee, Florida
Chapter 7

Karen Bawel Brinkley, RN, PhD
Associate Professor
Chair, Advanced Medical-Surgical Nursing
School of Nursing
San Jose State University
San Jose, California
Chapter 55

Patricia Benner, RN, PhD, FAAN
Thelma Shobe Endowed Chair in Ethics and Spirituality in Nursing
University of California San Francisco
San Francisco, California
Chapter 2
The Foreword

Deborah Benvenuto, BS, CRNI
Education Manager
Infusion Nurses Society
Norwood, Massachusetts
Chapter 22

Debra Brady, DNP, RN, CNS
Assistant Professor of Nursing
California State University Sacramento
Sacramento, California
Chapters 59 and 60

Krista Margaret Brecht, RN, MSc(A)N
Nurse Specialist
Pain Programs
McGill University Health Centre
Montreal General Hospital
Montreal, QC
Chapter 26

Claudia Campbell, RN, BSN, CCRN
Manager of Pain Services LDS Hospital
Intermountain Healthcare
Salt Lake City, Utah
Chapter 15

Ann Cashion, RN, PhD
Chair and Associate Professor, Acute and Chronic Care Department
Robert Wood Johnson Executive Nurse Fellow
Director, Center for Health Evaluation and Lifestyle Promotion
University of Tennessee Health Science Center
Memphis, Tennessee
Chapter 11

Patricia Caudle, DNSc, CNM, FNP
Faculty
Frontier School of Midwifery and Family Nursing
Heber Springs, Arizona
Chapters 48 and 50

Donna York Clark, RN, MS, CFRN, CMTE
Senior Account Manager
Golden Hour Data Systems
Carmel, Indiana
Chapter 1

Jan Clark, BSN, RN, CWOCN
Wound, Ostomy, Continence Consultant
Wilford Hall Medical Center
Lackland Air Force Base
San Antonio, Texas
Chapter 67

Karen Cooper, RN, MSN, CCRN, CNS, WOCN
Assistant Manager ICU
Kaiser Permanente
Sacramento, California
Chapters 33 and 57

Ellen DeLuca, RN, PhD
Professor of Nursing
Lynchburg College
Lynchburg, Virginia
Chapter 35

Jeromy D. Dyer, PA-C, MPAS
Orthopedic Surgery Specialist
Sutter General Hospital
Sutter Medical Group
Sacramento, California
Chapter 55

Lucie Elfervig, DNS, MSN, BSN, APRN-CS, CRNO, FAAN
Ophthalmic Consultant, Clinician, Researcher, Educator,
and Electrophysiologist
Eye Specialty Group
Memphis, Tennessee
Chapter 71

Peggy Ellis, PhD, RN, ANP, FNP, BC
Associate Professor
Associate Dean, School of Nursing,
Director, DNP Program
Doisy College of Health Sciences
St. Louis University
St. Louis, Missouri
Chapters 20, 65, and 66

Harold Engle, RN, BSN, BS
Program Director
Memorial Hermann Northeast Wound Care Center (R)
Humble, Texas
Chapter 67

Gina Flaharty, RN, BSN, FNP
President & Owner
Passport Health of Northern California
Sacramento, California
Chapter 40

Darlene M. Gilcreast, PhD, RN, MSN, BSN, CLNC
Partner, Diabetes Educator
Gilcreast & Associates, LLC
San Antonio, Texas
Chapter 18

J. Carolyn Graff, PhD, RN, FAAIDD
Associate Professor, College of Nursing
Director, College of Graduate Health Sciences
Chief of Nursing, Boling Center for Developmental Disabilities
University of Tennessee Health Science Center
Memphis, Tennessee
Chapter 11

Michele Grigaitis, MS, FNP-BC, CNRN
Nurse Practitioner, Adult Neurosurgical Services
Barrow Neurological Institute
Phoenix, AZ
Chapter 28

Ginny Wacker Guido, JD, MSN, RN
Associate Dean and Director of Graduate Studies
College of Nursing
University of North Dakota
Grand Forks, North Dakota
Chapter 4

Kori Harder, RN, MS
Clinical Nurse Specialist, Cardiology
Nurse Manager, Cardiovascular
University of California Davis Heart Center
Sacramento, CA
Chapter 40

Ann Harley, EdD, RN
Former Dean/Chair
Nursing Behavioral Health
Carson-Newman College
Jefferson City, Tennessee
Chapter 21

Corinne Harmon, RN, MS, EdD, AOCN
Assistant Professor
Clemson University
Clemson, South Carolina
Chapter 51

Helene Harris, RN, MSN
Instructor
Temple College
Temple, Texas
Chapters 54 and 55

Abby M. Heydman, PhD, RN
Interim President
Samuel Merritt College
Oakland, California
Chapter 52

Reneé Semonin Holleran, RN, PhD, CEN, CCRN, CFRN, CTRN, FAEN
Staff Nurse
Emergency Department
Intermountain Medical Center
Salt Lake City, Utah
Chapters 61 and 73

Rich Keegan, RN, MSN
Lecturer
Division of Nursing
Sacramento State University
Sacramento, California
Chapter 9

Katherine Kelly, RN, MSN, FNP-C, CEN
Lecturer
Sacramento School of Nursing
California State University
Sacramento, California
Chapter 17

Gale Kittle, RN, MPH
Research Nurse Coordinator
Barrow Neurological Institute
Arizona Alzheimer's Center
Phoenix, Arizona
Chapter 30

Dawn Lambie, RN, MSN, CHPN
Clinical Nurse Educator
Clinical Education
Kaiser Permanente
Roseville, California
Chapter 64

Kristine L'ecuyer, MSN, RN
Continuing Nursing Education Director Associate Professor
School of Nursing
Saint Louis University
St. Louis, Missouri
Chapter 37

Joseph Lindsay Jr, MD, FACC
Professor of Medicine
The George Washington University School of Medicine
Director, Emeritus, Division of Cardiology
Washington Hospital Center
Washington, D.C.
Chapter 39

Dawna Martich, RN, BSN, MSN
Director, Education
MCN Healthcare, Inc.
Denver, Colorado
Chapter 70

Bonnie McCracken, RN, NP
UC Davis Medical Center
Sacramento, CA
Chapter 44

Brenda McCulloch, RN, MSN, CNS
Sutter Heart and Vascular Institute
Sutter Medical Center
Sacramento, California
Chapter 43

Arlene McGory, DNSc, RN
Research Nurse
Massachusetts Eye and Ear Infirmary
Boston, Massachusetts
Chapter 69

Joyce Mikal-Flynn, RN, FNP, EdD
California State University, Sacramento
Sacramento, California
Chapter 7

Barbara Moyer, BSN, MS, EdD
DeSales University
Center Valley, Pennsylvania
Chapter 70

Teri A. Murray, PhD, RN
Doisy College of Health Sciences
St. Louis University
St. Louis, Missouri
Chapters 20, 65, and 66

Krisna Ogerio, RN, BScN, CPN(C)
McGill University Health Centre
Royal Victoria Hospital
Montreal, QC
Chapter 26

John Osborn, MD, FACS
Senior Surgeon, The Plastic Surgery Center
Clinical Professor, Department of Surgery
University of California Davis School of Medicine
Sacramento, California
Chapter 49

M. Miki Patterson, PhD, RN, PNP, ONP-C
Past President-National Association of Orthopedic Nurses
UMass Memorial Orthopedics
North Worcester, Massachusetts
Chapter 56

Laurie Quinn, BSN, MSN, PhD
Clinical Associate Professor
College of Nursing
University of Illinois
Chicago, Illinois
Chapter 53

Kismet Rasmusson, FNP-BC, FAHA
Heart Failure Prevention and Treatment Program, NP-Program Development
Intermountain Healthcare
College of Nursing
University of Utah
Salt Lake City, Utah
Chapter 42

Kathleen Richerson
Chief Nursing Officer
North Bay Healthcare
VacaValley Hospital
Vacaville, California
Chapter 3

Katherine Ricossa, MS, RN
Director of Education
Kaiser Permanente San Jose Medical Center
San Jose, California
Chapter 58

Leslie Rittenmeyer, RN, CNS, PsyD
Associate Professor of Nursing
Purdue University Calumet School of Nursing
Hammond, Indiana
Chapter 13

Carol Robinson, RN, MPA, CNAA, FAAN
Director of Nursing/Chief Patient Care Services Officer
University of California Davis Health System
Sacramento, California
Chapter 5

Denita Ryan, MN, RN, ANP-C, CNRN
Nurse Practitioner, Adult Neurosurgical Service
Barrow Neurological Institute
St. Joseph's Hospital and Medical Center
Phoenix, Arizona
Chapters 29 and 30

Ann Sievers, RN, MA, CORLN
Clinical Nurse Specialist
University California Davis Medical Center
University of California Davis
Sacramento, California
Chapter 34

Karen Silady, RN, MN, CNS, CEN
Staff Nurse
East Jefferson General Hospital
Metairie, Louisiana
Chapter 72

Donna Stanbridge, BScN, MA, CPN(C)
Clinical Nurse Specialist
Minimally Invasive Surgery and Surgical Innovation
McGill University Health Centre
Montreal General Hospital
Montreal, QC
Chapter 26

James Stotts, RN, MS
Director
PCS, Practice and Education
Stanford University Medical Center
Stanford, California
Chapter 40

Douglas Sutton, APRN, EdD
Assistant Professor,
Christine E. Lynn College of Nursing
Florida Atlantic University
Boca Raton, Florida
Chapters 45 and 46

Debera Thomas, DNS, RN, CS, ARNP
Assistant Dean and Associate Professor,
Christine E. Lynn College of Nursing
Florida Atlantic University
Boca Raton, Florida
Chapters 45 and 46

Gail Thurkauf, RN, MS
Director of the Department of Nursing Quality
Georgetown University Hospital
Washington, D.C.
Chapter 19

Eileen Trigoboff, RN, APRN/PMH-BC, DNS, DABFN
Clinical Nurse Specialist
Buffalo Psychiatric Center
Buffalo, New York
Chapter 16

Sheila Tucker, MA, RD
Nutritionist, Dining Services
Part Time Faculty, School of Nursing and Lynch School of Education
Boston College
Boston, Massachusetts
Chapter 14

Danielle Vigeant, MScN, CPN(C)
Nurse Manager
Peri-operative Services
McGill University Health Centre
Royal Victoria Hospital
Montreal, QC
Chapter 26

Laurie Walsh, NP
Kaiser Permanente
Sacramento, CA
Chapter 10

Suzanne Watt, RN, MSc(A), CON(C)
McGill University Health Centre
Royal Victoria Hospital
Montreal, QC
Chapter 26
Kathy Yeates, BSN, RN, CCRN
Mercy General Hospital
Sacramento, California
Chapter 60

Supplement Contributors

Sandra N, Berryman, RN, MSN, APN-BC
Assistant Professor
University of Arkansas, College of Nursing
Little Rock, Arkansas
Instructor's Resource Manual
Tracy Blanc, RN, BSN
Nursing Instructor
Ivy Tech Community College
Terre Haute, Indiana
Instructor's Resource Manual
Monica G. Cashiotta-Munn, RN, MFT
Instructor
National University
La Jolla, CA
Instructor's Resource Manual
Kim Cooper, RN, MSN
Nursing Department Chair
Ivy Tech Community College
Terre Haute, Indiana
Instructor's Resource Manual
Test Item File
Karlynne Galczyk, RN, MSN, MPH
Lecturer
Widener University School of Nursing
Chester, Pennsylvania
Instructor's Resource Manual
Test Item File
Rhonda Hutton Gann, RN, MSN
Nursing Informatics Lab Manager
State Fair Community College
Sedalia, Missouri
Test Item File
Margaret Gingrich, RN, MSN
Professor
Harrisburg Area Community College
Harrisburg, Pennsylvania
Instructor's Resource Manual
Test Item File
R. Sue Lasiter PhD (c), RN
Assistant Professor
University of Central Missouri
Warrensburg, Missouri
Instructor's Resource Manual
Wanda K. Lawrence, PhD, RNC, MSN
Assistant Professor of Nursing
Winston-Salem State University
Winston-Salem, North Carolina
Instructor's Resource Manual
Denice Kirchoff, MSN, APRN, BC
Assistant Professor of Nursing
Fairmont State University
Fairmont, West Virginia
Test Item File
Andrea R. Mann, MSN, RN
Instructor and Third Level Chair
Frankford Hospital School of Nursing
Philadelphia, Pennsylvania
Test Item File

Dawna Martich, RN, BSN, MSN
Director, Education
MCN Healthcare, Inc.
Denver, Colorado
Test Item File
Joyce Mikal-Flynn
Assistant Professor
Division of Nursing
Sacramento State University
Sacramento, California
Instructor's Resource Manual
Donna Russo, RN, MSN, CCRN, CNE
Nursing Instructor
Frankford Hospital School of Nursing
Philadelphia, Pennsylvania
Test Item File
Barbara Kim Stevens, MSN, RN
Professor of Nursing
University of Rio Grande
Rio Grande, Ohio
Instructor's Resource Manual
Betsy Swinny MSN, RN, CCRN
Critical Care Educator
St. Lukes Baptist Hospital
San Antonio, Texas
Test Item File
Jane Walker BBA, RN MSN
Walters State Community College
Morristown, Tennessee
Test Item File

REVIEWERS. Our heartfelt thanks go out to our colleagues from schools of nursing across the country who have given their time generously to help create this exciting new medical-surgical nursing textbook. These individuals helped us plan and shape our book and resources by reviewing chapters, art, design, and more. *Medical-Surgical Nursing: Preparation for Practice* has reaped the benefit of your collective knowledge and experience as nurses and teachers, and we have improved the materials due to your efforts, suggestions, objections, endorsements, and inspiration. Among those who gave their time generously to help us are the following:

UNIT REVIEWERS. We are so grateful to our Unit Reviewers, who contributed their valuable time, knowledge, and insight to ensure that the Units are written to the highest standard of accuracy and consistency.

Christi DeLemos, RN, MSN, ACNP-c
UC Davis Medical Center, Department of Neurological Surgery, Sacramento, California
Unit 6
Heidi A. Hotz, RN
Cedars-Sinai Medical Center, Los Angeles, California
Unit 16
Dawn Lambie, RN, MSN, CHPN
Kaiser Permanente, Roseville, California
Immunological, Inflammatory and Hematological Disorders
Units 5, 13, and 14
Mary McDermott, MS, RN
Hospital for Special Surgery, New York, New York
Unit 12
Charlotte Miller, RN
Cool, California
Units 1, 2, and 8
Kim Moody, PhD, RN
University of Southern Maine School of Nursing, Portland, ME
Unit 8
Donna York, RN, MS, CFRN, CMTE
Indiana University School of Nursing, Indianapolis, Indiana
Units 3 and 4
Kelly Karr, BA, MA
Sacramento, California

Academic Reviewers

Faisal H. Aboul-Enein, RN, MSN, MPH, NP, BC
Texas Woman's University College of Nursing, Houston, Texas
Joy Ache-Reed, RN, MSN
Indiana Wesleyan University, Marion, Indiana
Betty N. Adams, PhD
Prairie View A & M University, Houston, Texas
Sheila A. Alexander, RN, PhD
University of Pittsburgh, Pittsburgh, Pennsylvania
Cheryl Alt, RN, MSN
Great Falls College of Technology, Great Falls, Montana
Ella R. Anaya, RN, MSN, CNS
Kent State University, Kent, Ohio
Beverly Anderson, MSN, RN
Salt Lake Community College, Salt Lake City, Utah
Cheryl Anema, RN, MSN
Trinity Christian College, Palos Heights, Illinois
Gail Armstrong, RN, ND
University of Colorado–Denver, Denver, Colorado
Karen Sue Bailey, RN, MSN, APRN-BC-FNP
Marshall University, Huntington, West Virginia
L. Antoinette Bargagliotti, DNSc, RN, ANEF
University of Memphis, Memphis, Tennessee
Shirley Sperinde Baxter, RN, BSN, MSN
University of California Davis Medical Center, Sacramento, California
Randal D. Beaton, PhD, EMT
University of Washington, Seattle, Washington
Julie A. Beck, RN, DEd, CNE
York College of Pennsylvania, York, Pennsylvania
Deborah Becker, PhD, RN, ACNP-BC
University of Pennsylvania, Philadelphia, Pennsylvania
William T. Bester, MSN, RN
The University of Texas at Austin, Austin, Texas
Cynthia Ann Blum, PhD, RN, CNE
Florida Atlantic University, Boca Raton, Florida
Donna W. Bohmfalk, MSN, RN
The University of Texas Medical Branch, Galveston, Texas
Joanne Bonesteel, MS, RN
Excelsior College, Albany, New York
Portia A. Botchway, MSN, RN
Clemson University, Clemson, South Carolina
Sharon McFadden Bradley, MSN, RN, CNL
University of Florida College of Nursing, Gainesville, Florida
Janet Witucki Brown, RN, PhD
University of Tennessee, Knoxville, Knoxville, Tennessee
Cindy L. Brubaker, EdD, RN
Bradley University, Peoria, Illinois
Tammy Bryant, RN, BSN
Southwest Georgia Technical College, Thomasville, Georgia
Kathleen Burke, PhD, RN
Ramapo College, Mahwah, New Jersey
Dorothy Burns, RN, PhD, MS
Hampton University, Hampton, Virginia
Dorothy Stano Carlson, DEd, RN
Edinboro University of Pennsylvania, Edinboro, Pennsylvania
Tracy Carlson, MSN, RN
Kent State University, Kent, Ohio
Monica G. Cashiotta-Munn, RN, MFT, MSN
National University, La Jolla, California
Olivia Catolico, PhD, RN, BC
Dominican University of California, San Rafael, California
Donna York Clark, RN, MS, CFRN, CMTE
Golden Hour Data Systems, San Diego, California
Patricia Clark, RN, PhD
Abraham Baldwin College, Tifton, Georgia
Pamela S. Combs, MSN, RN
University of Louisville, Louisville, Kentucky
Cathy Cormier, PhD, RN
Southeastern Louisiana University, Hammond, Louisiana
Nancy Dentlinger, RN, AS, BS, MS, EdD
Redlands Community College, El Reno, Oklahoma
Susan DeSanto-Madeya, DNSc, RN
University of Massachusetts, Boston, Massachusetts

Patricia Brown Dominguez, RN, MSN
Houston Baptist University, Houston, Texas
Nancy Duffy, RN, CEN, MSN
Medical University of South Carolina, Charleston, North Carolina
Jaibun Earp, FNP, PhD, MA, BSN
Florida Agricultural and Mechanical University, Quincy, Florida
Sandra Eggenberger, PhD
Minnesota State University Mankato, Mankato, Minnesota
Jeanette Embry, RN, MS, PhD
West Texas A&M University, College Station, Texas
Deborah Erickson, PhD, RN
Bradley University, Peoria, Illinois
Geralyn M. Frandsen, EdD, RN
Maryville University, St. Louis, Missouri
Kathy Frum, RN, MSN
West Virginia University at Parkersburg, Parkersburg, West Virginia
Kay E. Gaehle, RN, PhD
Southern Illinois University, Edwardsville, Illinois
Karlynne Galczyk, RN, MSN, MPH
Widener University, Chester, Pennsylvania
Donna Gauthier, PhD, RN, CNE
University of Louisiana, Lafayette, Louisiana
Rebecca Gesler, MSN, RN
Spalding University, Louisville, Kentucky
Margaret M. Gingrich, RN, MSN
Harrisburg Area Community College, Harrisburg, Pennsylvania
Donna Glankler, MSN, RN
College of Mount St. Joseph, Cincinnati, Ohio
Sharron Guillett, PhD, RN
Marymount University, Arlington, Virginia
Susan Sweat Gunby, RN, PhD
Mercer University, Atlanta, Georgia
Polly C. Haigler, PhD, RN
University of South Carolina, Columbia, South Carolina
Lori Rae Hamilton, RN, MSN
Otero Junior College, La Junta, Colorado
Jenny Hamner, DSN
Auburn University, Auburn, Alabama
Chris Hawkins, PhD, RN
Texas Woman's University, Denton, Texas
Connie S. Heflin, MSN, RN, CNE
West Kentucky Community and Technical College, Paducah, Kentucky
Carol Heim, MA, RN
Mount Mercy College, Cedar Rapids, Iowa
Jan Herren, MSN, RNC
Southern Arkansas University, Magnolia, Arkansas
Susan Holmes, RN, MSN, CRNP
Auburn University, Auburn, Alabama
Gail M. Holtzman, MSN, CCRN, CNE
University of Alaska, Anchorage, Alaska
Linda Howe, PhD, CNS, CNE
Clemson University, Clemson, South Carolina
Trinity Ingram, MSN, APRN, CPNP, PCNS
South University and Savannah Technical College, Savannah, Georgia
Pamela B. James, RN, BSN, MSN
Fayetteville Technical Community College, Fayetteville, North Carolina
Cindy K. Jenness, BSN, MAE, MSN
Allen College, Waterloo, Iowa
Michelle Johnson, MSN, RN
Northern Michigan University, Marquette, Michigan
Pam Johnson, MSN, RN, APRN, BC
Viterbo University, LaCrosse, Wisconsin
Karin Jones, RN, PhD
Grambling State University, Grambling, Louisiana
Peggy Kalowes, RN, MSN, CNRN, CNS
California State University, Los Angeles, California
Tamara Kear, MSN, RN, CNN
Gwynedd-Mercy College, Gwynedd Valley, Pennsylvania
Frances Keen, DNSc, RN
Villanova University, Villanova, Pennsylvania
Deborah Kern, MSN, RNCS, FNP
Montana State University, Bozeman, Montana
Joan E. King, PhD, ACNP-BC, ANP-BC
Vanderbilt University, Nashville, Tennessee

Kenn M. Kirksey, RN, PhD, APRN, BC
California State University, Fresno, California
Ina Koerner, RN, MS, PhD
University of Louisiana, Lafayette, Louisiana
Cheryl Lacasse, PhDc, RN, OCN
University of Arizona, Tucson, Arizona
Dawn Lambie, RN, MSN, CHPN
Kaiser Permanente, Roseville, California
R. Shelly Lancaster, MSN, RN
University of Wisconsin, Oshkosh, Wisconsin
Karen M. Lavallee, RNC, CS, ARNP
New Hampshire Technical Institute, Concord, New Hampshire
Wanda K. Lawrence, PhD, RN, MSN
Winston-Salem State University, Winston-Salem, North Carolina
Theresa Gunter Lawson, MS, APRN, FNP-BC
Lander University, Greenwood, South Carolina
Patricia Price Lea, PhD, RNC, MSN, MSEd, BSN
North Carolina Agricultural & Technical State University, Greensboro, North Carolina
Barbara Lee, MSN, RN, BC, MEd, CWOCN
Bellarmine University, Louisville, Kentucky
Elizabeth Lee, MSN, APRN, BC
Harding University, Searcy, Arkansas
Manon Lemonde, RN, PhD, BScN, MScN
University of Ontario Institute of Technology, Ontario, Canada
Linda Lichty, RN
Cosumnes Community Fire Service District, Elks Grove, California
Cynthia A. Logan, PhD, RN
Southeastern Louisiana University, Hammond, Louisiana
Gayla Love, RN, MS, BSN, CCM
Griffin Technical College, Griffin, Georgia
Naomi Lungstrom, MN, FNP
Washington State University, Pullman, Washington
Susan Luparell, PhD, CNS-BC, CNE
Montana State University, Bozeman, Montana
Amy Ma, DNP, APRN, FNP-BC
Long Island University, Brooklyn, New York
Bernadette Madara, BC, EdD, APRN
Southern Connecticut State University, New Haven, Connecticut
Cecilia Jane Maier, MS, RN
Mount Carmel College of Nursing, Columbus, Ohio
Andrea R. Mann, MSN, RN
Frankford Hospital School of Nursing, Philadelphia, Pennsylvania
Bradley J. Manuel, RN, MSN, CNOR(E)
Texas Woman's University, Houston, Texas
Karen S. March, PhD, RN, CCRN, ACNS-BC
York College of Pennsylvania, York, Pennsylvania
Suzanne Marnocha, RN, MSN, PhD, CCRN
University of Wisconsin, Oshkosh, Wisconsin
Janet G. Marshall, PhD, RN
Florida A&M University School of Nursing, Tallahassee, Florida
Brenda Mason, MSN, BSN, RN-FNP
Alderson-Broaddus College, Philippi, West Virginia
Dotti Mathers, MSN, RN
Pennsylvania College of Technology, Williamsport, Pennsylvania
Amy McClune, PhD, RN, BC
Edinboro University of Pennsylvania, Edinboro, Pennsylvania
Emily McClung, RN, MSN
Kent State University College of Nursing, Kent, Ohio
Mary McDermott, MS, RN, APN, NE-C
Hospital for Special Surgery, New York, New York
Barbara McGraw, MSN, RN, CNE
Central Community College, Grand Island, Nebraska
Phyllis McKiernan, MSN, APN-C, RN
Hackensack University Medical Center, Hackensack, New Jersey
Melody McKinney, DNS, RN
Indiana State University, Terre Haute, Indiana
Tara McMillan-Queen, RN, MN, APRN, BC
Mercy School of Nursing, Charlotte, North Carolina
Debbie Metzler, MSN, APNP, GNP-BC
Bellin College of Nursing, Green Bay, Wisconsin
Rita Miller, MSN, RN
Idaho State University–Pocatello, Boise, Idaho

Connie Miller, MSN, FNP-C
University of Northern Colorado, Greeley, Colorado
Donna Molyneaux, PhD
Gwynedd-Mercy College, Gwynedd Valley, Pennsylvania
Kimberly Moody, PhD, RN-CS, ANP
University of Southern Maine, Portland, Maine
Judy K. Moren, BM, RN
California State University, Sacramento, California
Martha C. Morris, PhD, RN
The University of Southern Mississippi, Hattiesburg, Mississippi
Deborah R. Murphy, RN, MSN
West Virginia University at Parkersburg, Parkersburg, West Virginia
Janice A. Neil, RN, PhD
East Carolina University, Greenville, North Carolina
Nancy Noble, RN, MSN, ACNS-BC
Marian University, Fond du Lac, Wisconsin
Catherine M. Nosek, RN, PhD
Winona State University, Winona, Minnesota
Elizabeth Palmer, PhD, RN, CNE
Indiana University of Pennsylvania, Indiana, Pennsylvania
Laurie J. Palmer, RN, MS, AOCN
Monroe Community College, Rochester, New York
Denise Panosky, MSN, RN, CCHP
University of Connecticut, Storrs, Connecticut
Barbara Patterson, RN, PhD
Widener University, Chester, Pennsylvania
Jo Ann Pelaez-Fisher, MSHA, BSN, RN
The College of Southern Nevada, Las Vegas, Nevada
Linda Honan Pellico, MSN, PhD, RN
Yale University, New Haven, Connecticut
Sheila Perrault, MSN
Salem State College, Salem, Massachusetts
Kathleen Perrin, PhD, RN, CCRN
Saint Anselm College, Manchester, New Hampshire
Rebecca Phillip, PhD, RN
The University of Oklahoma Health Sciences Center, Oklahoma City, Oklahoma
Jennifer Ponto, RN, BSN
South Plains College, Levelland, Texas
Christopher B. Powe, PhD(c), ACNP
University of Mississippi Medical Center, Jackson, Mississippi
Rorey D. Pritchard, RN, MSN, CNOR
Chippewa Valley Technical College, Eau Claire, Wisconsin
Anne Purvis, RN, MSN
Gordon College, Barnesville, Georgia
Colleen M. Quinn, RN, MSN
Broward College, Pembroke Pines, Florida
Valeria Ramdin, MS, APRN-BC
Northeastern University, Boston, Massachusetts
Carol Delia Ratta, RN, MS, CCRN
Stony Brook University, Stony Brook, New York
Kathleen M. Rayman, PhD, RN
East Tennessee State University, Johnson City, Tennessee
Anita K. Reed, MSN, RN
Saint Joseph's College, Lafayette, Indiana
Joy Reed, MS, BSS, ADN
Indiana Wesleyan University, Marion, Indiana
Mattie L. Rhodes, RN, PhD, CNS
State University of New York at Buffalo, Buffalo, New York
Gwendolyn E. Richardson, APRN, MN
Midlands Technical College, Columbia, South Carolina
Margaret Richbourg, MSN, BSN, ASN, AA
Florida State University, Tallahassee, Florida
Michelle Robnett, BA, BSN, MA, MBA, PhD
University of Iowa, Iowa City, Iowa
Cheryl Ross, MS, RN
Oklahoma City University, Oklahoma City, Oklahoma
Donna Russo, RN, MSN, CCRN, CNE
Frankford Hospital School of Nursing, Philadelphia, Pennsylvania
Arlene Saliba, MS, RNCS
Andrews University, Berrien Springs, Michigan
Buckie Sasser, RN, MSN
South Georgia College, Douglas, Georgia
Jacalyn M. Schaefer, MSN, RN, CNOR
The Ohio State University, Columbus, Ohio

Gisela Schmidt, RN, MA, MS
Andrews University, Berrien Springs, Michigan
Nancy Schoofs, RN, PhD
Grand Valley State University, Grand Rapids, Michigan
Connie J. Schroeder, MS, RN
Danville Area Community College, Danville, Virginia
Jenny Schuessler, RN, DSN
Auburn University School of Nursing, Auburn, Alabama
Lisa A. Seldomridge, PhD, RN
Salisbury University, Salisbury, Maryland
Joanne Farley Serembus, EdD, RN, CCRN, CNE
Drexel University, Philadelphia, Pennsylvania
Laurie J. Singel, MSN, RN, BC
The University of Texas Health Science Center at San Antonio
San Antonio, Texas
Patricia Slesinski, BS, MS
State University of New York, Middletown, New York
Rose Marie Smith, MSN, RN
Platt College North, Oklahoma City, Oklahoma
Soledad M. Smith, RN, PhD
The University of Louisiana at Lafayette, Lafayette, Louisiana
Marilyn Smith-Stoner, RN, PhD, CHPN
California State University, San Bernardino, California
Cheryl Bruick Sorge, RN, MA
Indiana University, Fort Wayne, Indiana
Sharon Souter, RN, PhD, CNE
University of Mary Hardin-Baylor, Belton, Texas
Martha Spies, PhD
Chamberlain College of Nursing, St. Louis, Missouri
Russlyn A. St. John, RN, MSN
St. Charles Community College, Cottleville, Missouri
Annette Smith Stacy, MSN, RN, AOCN
Arkansas State University, Jonesboro, Arkansas
Barbara Kim Stevens, MSN, RN
University of Rio Grande, Rio Grande, Ohio
James Stotts, RN, MS, CNS
Stanford Hospital and Clinics, Stanford, California
Kathleen Stroh, MA, MSN, RN
Edinboro University of Pennsylvania, Edinboro, Pennsylvania
Ardith L. Sudduth, PhD, GNP, FNP-BC
University of Louisiana at Lafayette, Lafayette, Louisiana
Katherine Elizabeth Sullivan, BSN, MA
Rockland Community College, Suffern, New York
Sheila Cox Sullivan, PhD, RN, CNE
Central Arkansas Veterans Healthcare System, Little Rock, Arkansas
Beth Swart, RN, MES
Ryerson University, Toronto, Canada
Marianne F. Swihart, RN, BSN, MEd, MSN, CRNI, CWON, PCCN
Pasco Hernando Community College–West Campus, New Port Richey, Florida
Judith Tanner, RN, MSN
Sacramento City College, Sacramento, California
Marilyn M. Teeter, RN, MSN
Harrisburg Area Community College, Gettysburg, Pennsylvania
Kathleen Thiede, MA, RN
The College of St. Scholastica, Duluth, Minnesota
Scott Thigpen, RN, BSN, MSN, CCRN, CEN
South Georgia College, Douglas, Georgia
Cindy Thomas, PhD, RN
Mesa State College, Grand Junction, Colorado
Loris A.Thomas, PhD, ARNP, ACNP-BC/ANP-BC
University of Florida College of Nursing, Gainesville, Florida
Shirley Thompson, MSN, CNS, RN
Bethune-Cookman College, Daytona Beach, Florida
Janet P. Tracy, RN, PhD
William Paterson University, Wayne, New Jersey
Lise Turner, RNC, MSN
Mercy School of Nursing, Charlotte, North Carolina
Karla Uhde, RN, MSN, CNE
Ivy Tech Community College of Indiana-Southwest, Evansville, Indiana
Carolyn VanCouwenberghe, RN, PhD
California State University, Sacramento, California
Shellye A. Vardaman, RN, BC, MSN
Troy University, Troy, Alabama

Delayne Vogel, MSN, RN
Viterbo University School of Nursing, La Crosse, Wisconsin
Gerry Walker, MSN, RN
Park University, Parkville, Missouri
Susan Walker, PhD, RN, FNP
University of Texas at Arlington, Arlington, Texas
Patricia Walters, RN, ACNP, CCRN, ACLS, BCLS
Hackensack University Medical Center, Hackensack, New Jersey
Carol L. Warner, MSN, RN, CPN, FNP-BC
St. Luke's School of Nursing, Bethlehem, Pennsylvania
Diane Graham Webb, MSN, RN, CNE
Northwestern State University of Louisiana, Natchitoches, Louisiana
Bonnie K. Webster, MSN, RN, BC
University of Texas Medical Branch, Galveston, Texas
Linda B. Wheeler, RN, MSN
University of North Carolina at Greensboro, Greensboro, North Carolina
Ann White, RN, PhD, MBA, CNA, BC
University of Southern Indiana, Evansville, Indiana
Loretta White, DNS
Indiana State University, Terre Haute, Indiana
Barbara Wilder, DNS, CRNP
Auburn University, Auburn, Alabama
Anna Wilson, RN, BS
California State University, San Bernardino, California
Marion E. Winfrey, EdD, RN
University of Massachusetts, Boston, Massachusetts
Karen M. Wood, RN, DNSc, CCRN, CNL
Saint Xavier University, Chicago, Illinois
Lisa Woodley, MSN, RN
University of North Carolina, Chapel Hill, North Carolina
Kathy Woodruff, MSN, CRNP
University of Maryland, Baltimore, Maryland
Wendy Woodward, PhD, RN
Humboldt State University, Arcata, California
Linda Wray, RN, PhD
Eastern Kentucky University, Richmond, Kentucky
Malou Blanco Yarosh, MSN, RN, CNS
University of California, Los Angeles, California

Clinical Reviewers

Carmalita F. Andrus, CNRN, MN, FNP-C
Lafayette General Medical Center, Lafayette, Louisiana
Susan D. Anthony, MN, RN, APRN
South Plains Health Provider Organization, Plainview, Texas
Elizabeth Archer-Nanda, MSN, ARNP, CNS
Louisville Oncology, Louisville, Kentucky
Traci Ashcraft, BSN, RNBC
West Virginia University School of Nursing, West Milford, West Virginia
Kathleen J. Bailey, BSN, MA, MS, RN, CNM
US Army Landstuhl Regional Medical Center, Landstuhl, Germany
Dian Baker, RN, MA, MSN, CPNP
California State University Hospital, Sacramento, California
Brenda J. Baranowski, RN, CMSRN, CHPN
Froedtert Hospital, Milwaukee, Wisconsin
Shirley Sperinde Baxter, RN, BSN, MSN
University of California, Davis Medical Center, Sacramento, California
Megan Brunson, BSN, RN
St. Joseph's Hospital of Atlanta, Atlanta, Georgia
Christine Greiser Chadwell, MSN, APRN, BC, NP-C
Albright Health Center, Highland Heights, Kentucky
Karen Cheng, RN
Stanford University Medical Center, Stanford, California
Patricia G. Christy, MSN, APRN, BC, CFNP
Prien Lake Medical Clinic, Lake Charles, Louisiana
Regina Ciambrone, RN, BSN
Overlook Hospital, Summit, New Jersey
Donna York Clark, RN, MS, CFRN, CMTE
Golden Hour Data Systems, San Diego, California
John A. Collins, RN, CCRN
Lehigh Valley Hospital, Allentown, Pennsylvania
Damon Cottrell, MS, RN, CCNS, CCRN, APRN-BC, CEN
Providence St. Vincent Medical Center, Portland, Oregon
Janice Ann Cousino, RN, MSN, CNS
Hartford Hospital, Hartford, Connecticut

Diane K. Daddario, MSNc, RN, BC, CMSRN
Pennsylvania College of Technology, Williamsport, Pennsylvania
Yvonne D'Arcy, MS, CRNP, CNS
Suburban Hospital, Bethesda, Maryland
Sherri Davidson, RN, MSN, CS, ACNP
Central Texas Neurological Association, Waco, Texas
Christi DeLemos, RN, MSN, ACNP-c
UC Davis Medical Center, Department of Neurological Surgery,
Sacramento, California
Lisa Duquette, BSN, CCRN, CEN, CFRN, EMT-P
Hartford Hospital, Hartford, Connecticut
Tracey C. Gaslin, RN, MSN, CRNI, CPNP
University of Louisville, Louisville, Kentucky
Barbara Gercke, MSN, FNP
San Diego State Student Health Services, San Diego, California
Denice E. Gibson, MSN
Banner Good Samaritan Medical Center, Phoenix, Arizona
Jean G. Gisler, RN, MSN, FNP-c, CDE
University of Texas Health Science Center at San Antonio, San Antonio, Texas
Theresa M. Glessner, RN, MSN, NP, BC, CCRN
Rochester General Hospital, Rochester, New York
Karen Diane Groller, MSN, RN, BC, CMSRN
Lehigh Valley Hospital, Allentown, Pennsylvania
Melody H. Hale, MSN, APRN-BC
New River Family Health, Scarbro, West Virginia
Lori Harris, RN, BSN, CNOR, CLNC
Mercy Health Center, Oklahoma City, Oklahoma
Amy Herrington, RN, MSN, CEN, NR-EMT-B
Bluegrass Community and Technical College, Lexington, Kentucky
Ellen S. Kane, MSN, RN, CDE
Banner Good Samaritan Medical Center, Phoenix, Arizona
Mary Knudtson, DNSc, NP
University of California Irvine, Irvine, California
Dawn Lambie, RN, MSN, CHPN
Kaiser Permanente, Roseville, California
Marilyn Leshko, RN
Lehigh Valley Hospital, Allentown, Pennsylvania
Patricia Lewis, MSN, FNP, CVN
Bassett Healthcare, Cooperstown, New York
Lori Kennedy Madden, MS, RN, ACNP, CCRN, CNRN
University of California, Davis, Sacramento, California
Kathleen-McCaffrey, RN, MSN
New York University Medical Center, New York, New York

Mary McDermott, MS, RN, NE-BC, APRN
Hospital for Special Surgery, New York, New York
Phyllis McKiernan, MSN, APN-C, RN
Hackensack University Medical Center, Hackensack, New Jersey
Ann McSwain, RN, MSN, CCRN, APRN, BC
St. Mary's Health Center, Jefferson City, Missouri
Peggy Tidikis Menck, PhD, RN
Independent Consultant
Barry M. Mitchneck, RN, MSN, CEN
Lehigh Valley Hospital, Allentown, Pennsylvania
Judy K. Moren, BM, RN
Nursing Education and Collections Training Manager, BloodSource,
Sacramento, California
Maxine L. Morris, BSN
New York Medical Center, New York, New York
Agnes Oblas, ANP-C
Ray Road Medical Center, Phoenix, Arizona
Jaime L. Peters, ADN
Lehigh Valley Hospital, Bethlehem, Pennsylvania
Sherri Reese, RN, BSN, CIC
University of California Davis Medical Center, Sacramento, California
Lory Anne F. Robles, BSN, MSN, RN
Stanford University Hospital, Palo Alto, California
Bonnie Smith Rosario, RN
Assumption Rural Health Clinic, Napoleonville, Louisiana
Sande Rowlee, MS, RN, CNS, ACNP-BC
Sacramento Bariatric Medical Associates, Carmichael, California
Jeremy Sabatino, BSN
Trinitas Hospital, Elizabeth, New Jersey
Debby Skroch, BSN, RN
John C. Lincoln North Mountain Hospital, Phoenix, Arizona
Leonard Sterling, RN, BSN
University of California Davis Medical Center, Sacramento, California
Ann D. Stoltz, PhD, RN
California State University, Sacramento, California
Belinda J. Swearingen, RN, MSN, FNP-C
Corrigan Medical Center, Corrigan, Texas
William E. Trumbore, III, RN, CEN, PHRN, AAS, BSPA
Lehigh Valley Hospital, Allentown, Pennsylvania
Deborah Tuggle, RN, MN, CCNS
Jewish Hospital-St. Mary's Healthcare, Louisville, Kentucky
Patricia Walters, RN, ACNP, CCRN, ACLS, BCLS
Hackensack University Medical Center, Hackensack, New Jersey

Authors Kathleen Osborn, Cheryl Wraa, and Annita Watson and their contributors have written an integrative and comprehensive textbook for preparing basic nursing students for evidence-based practice in medical–surgical nursing. This text places caring practices as conceptualized by the nurse theorist Sr. Simone Roach (1984) at the center of excellent nursing practice. Caring includes six essential components: compassion, competence, confidence, conscience, commitment, and comportment. The authors also place clinical judgment and critical thinking within the context of best evidence-based practice, recognizing that nursing and medicine are subject to ever-changing modes of scientific discovery and validation and that a particular patient may not easily fit into statistical norms. Therefore, the nurse must exercise good clinical reasoning, evaluation of evidence, and critical thinking.

This text invites the student to begin a lifelong journey of learning and clinical knowledge development while providing a clear road map beginning with the general and moving to more complex medical–surgical nursing care. The ability to recognize the nature of an ambiguous, under-determined clinical situation is at the heart of good clinical reasoning and care. The Critical Alert boxes throughout the text help the student focus on essential nursing interventions for attending to a particular patient with specific clinical conditions. Mastering this text will facilitate students' learning so they begin to think like a nurse in a broad range of clinical situations.

The authors are to be commended for fostering a comprehensive and holistic view of nursing practice, as caregiver, patient advocate, educator, researcher, and leader. Clinical vignettes and nurse interviews are included so that the student can develop a clinical imagination for the care of patients with specific clinical conditions and sociocultural characteristics. I highly recommend this book for all nursing students! Studying this text is a great way to gain visions and examples of excellent nursing practice, research, patient advocacy, leadership, and education.

PATRICIA BENNER, RN, PhD, FAAN
Thelma Shobe Endowed Chair in Ethics and Spirituality
University of California, San Francisco,
Department of Social and Behavioral Sciences

As the 21st century evolves, nursing and its place in health care are also evolving. This era is characterized by rapid change, including a growing multicultural population, longer life spans, arrival of new illnesses, and poor health conditions. Explosive advances in technology, ever-changing work settings, and a complex health care environment that is costly and competitive contribute to nursing's evolving environment. The burgeoning level of information affects decision making, and newer, faster modes of communication add to the environment's complexity. The definitions of roles and responsibilities for health care providers are changing; new boundaries are defined in which accountabilities are different, quality indicators are vital, and evidence-based practice is the standard. Ethical considerations must be balanced as nurses are called on to think quickly in establishing short- and long-term goals with the patient and family, in collaboration with the health care team and the community.

Never before in the history of nursing has the profession faced greater challenges to produce enough qualified nurses to practice in such a rapidly changing environment. And at a time when the need for professional nurses is overwhelming, we face a deficit in qualified nurses. Thus, it is time for professional scrutiny, self-determination, and innovation; nursing education is challenged to be innovative in preparing nurses for practice now and in the future. The challenge is to prepare nurses who can provide cognitively skilled care, in a caring manner, with a diverse patient population, and in innovative health care settings.

The authors' vision for this textbook is to meet that challenge. This textbook prepares the learner to be a knowledgeable, caring health care professional. It is a foundation on which to build the nursing practice of today and tomorrow, incorporating the cognitive, affective, and psychomotor skills necessary to practice. This book is not a destination to be achieved, but the beginning of lifelong learning.

Goals

The goal of this book is to expose the learner to concepts basic to the practice of professional nursing, including caring, critical thinking, research, nursing process, and health promotion. Caring is the foundation of nursing practice because of its impact on patients and their families. The authors have adopted Roach's (1984) theory of caring, which includes six components: compassion, competence, confidence, conscience, commitment, and comportment. Within the chapter features the authors have applied these six components when describing the nursing care needed for each of the physical disorders. This helps learners develop their understanding of how to be a caring nurse and makes them aware of these qualities in fellow health care professionals' practice and when advocating for the patient.

The nursing process is used to develop critical thinking and clinical reasoning skills, providing the framework for applying evidenced-based practice. Research is discussed throughout the text, providing opportunities for the reader to examine current research topics and their application to nursing practice.

Health promotion, one of the primary roles of the nurse, is woven throughout the book, so learners will understand the importance of educating the patient/family about healthy habits and lifestyles that prevent illnesses and injuries.

Readers will become active participants in learning about nursing as they progress through the book contents. Learners should be able to demonstrate understanding of the concepts of medical–surgical nursing in a variety of settings by collaborating with the authors in defining requisite content for patient care, arriving at patient diagnoses, and developing plans of care.

The concepts of experiential learning shape the book contents. The intention is that learners will engage in reflective thought and analysis of their practice as they apply the principles and concepts incorporated in the book to clinical practice, using the book as a resource for validating perceptions, expanding their knowledge base, and evaluating their approaches to patient care. The book is organized to introduce learners to the basic concepts of health care in general, and to nursing specifically, before moving on to the concepts underlying health promotion and disease management and the common physiological disorders that are encountered in medical–surgical nursing practice.

The units and chapters are grouped to lead the learner from general concepts to the more complex concepts and challenges of disease management. The information is sequenced to enhance critical thinking skills, thereby promoting the development of clinical judgment.

Knowledge acquisition is enhanced by application, analysis, and evaluation. Thus, this text provides numerous opportunities for learners to participate in activities designed to develop critical thinking and problem-solving skills in collaboration with the nursing experts who have contributed to the book. These learning activities include preparing clinical preparation plans, establishing priorities for care, developing patient care plans, and evaluating knowledge in the affective, cognitive, and psychomotor domains of practice. As learners complete these experiential and interactive activities, they will achieve a holistic, scientific, and caring approach to professional nursing practice for now and the future.

Organization

The book consists of 16 units sequenced from simple, basic concepts to complex, medical–surgical disorders. Units 1 and 2 introduce the reader to general concepts related to health care delivery, followed by basic concepts related to nursing practice. The next two units cover physiological concepts and the theoretical basis of skills that are germane to all areas of nursing practice. Units 5 through 16 focus on physiological disorders common to medical–surgical nursing. Each disorder unit opens with an assessment chapter that provides a template to assess the presenting patient within the specific body system.

THE TEXT FEATURES were designed to highlight the concepts that form the framework for this textbook and that are basic to professional nursing: **caring, research, critical thinking, the nursing process,** and **health promotion.** The capstone feature in each disorders chapter, **Clinical Preparation,** offers learners the opportunity to bring all of the concepts into one summary exercise and thus prepares learners for safe and knowledgeable clinical practice in their future work as professional nurses.

Profiles in Nursing

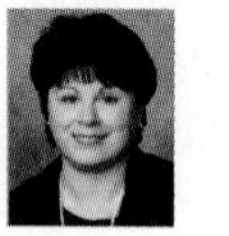

KATHY My name is Kathy and I am the senior management leader for nursing services with the title of Vice President, Chief Nursing Officer (CNO), for NorthBay Healthcare in Northern California. My organization is a nonprofit, independent community health system consisting of two acute care hospitals (190+ beds) offering a full range of services, a variety of outpatient services, and specialty/primary care practices. My position has responsibility for nursing practice throughout the system and operating responsibility for all inpatient nursing units and services for emergency/trauma, perioperative, women's/children's, cardiopulmonary, wound care/HBO, and physician hospitalist programs.

In my role I oversee all aspects of nursing services including staffing/scheduling functions, strategic direction, environment of practice, quality/patient safety, standards of care, and collaborative relationships with other disciplines providing care to patients. I also oversee the financial planning for operating and capital budgets that support the provision of care and the resources needed to meet the demands of our services. This role allows me to interface at many levels within our organization from attending governing board meetings to unit-based staff meetings, medical staff committees and various State and community forums that are focused on health policy and providing care to patients. I feel privileged to represent the nurses and their professional practice in our organization and take every opportunity to highlight the contributions of nursing to our mission. The role of the senior nurse leader is critical in speaking to the balance of the provision of quality, safe patient care and the financial needs of the business of health care.

As the (CNO) I have a very busy schedule that moves me from meeting to meeting with often very diverse agendas. I generally start my day catching up on e-mail and voice mail communications because I know it is important for people to get timely responses to their questions and requests. I also try to keep my door open when I am in my office for "drop-in" conversations and "face time" with my team. Visibility is a key component of my job because staff, physicians, and the nursing management team need to know that I understand what is going on in the environment and that I am listening to their concerns and suggestions. A technique I use to increase my visibility is that when I need information I go to the person or department to communicate with them directly in their environment rather than asking them to come to my office. This way I can check in with people as I travel the hallways and I can observe the environment along the way. My **commitment** to being available to staff and my leadership team is important to ensure I understand their needs in order to represent them well.

The meetings I attend fall into to two categories, group and individual. The majority of my work is done in groups and teams to discuss, debate, and make decisions on policy and direction for all aspects of the organization's business. My **comportment** in meetings is important for me to adequately represent nursing as a credible business and clinical entity. I must also be knowledgeable about issues such as quality and patient safety standards so I can contribute to discussions on improving care and the hospital environment. In many meetings I attend, I may be the only clinical representative participating, so I need to know about how nonnursing departments function also.

Most of the individual meetings I schedule are with the people who report directly to me. These meetings are to discuss their work and mentor them in their roles and in their development. For example, I have some new managers and advanced practice nurses who are working to understand their roles and how best to handle difficult situations. An example of mentoring would be the work I have done with a clinical nurse specialist who was new to her role. Her concerns were about acceptance by the staff as a resource and consultant and for them to ask for her help. We developed a plan to coordinate her schedule so she had time to just be on the nursing units, talk with staff, interact with physicians, and observe the care being given. This enabled her to be present during critical situations in which she could help the staff figure out what was going on with the patients and how to best communicate that with the physicians.

3

Caring

Profiles in Nursing. Each unit opens with a portrait of a nurse who describes "a day in the life" of working in a given specialty area. This profile includes a snapshot of a typical day and highlights the nurse's application of the six components of caring into his or her specialty. The information helps nursing students learn about the possibilities open to them when they are deciding where to spend concentrated clinical rotations or contemplating a job change.

Research

RESEARCH OPPORTUNITIES AND CLINICAL IMPACT RELATED TO CORONARY ARTERY DISEASE

Research Area	Clinical Impact
Stem cell injection after acute myocardial infarction.	Stimulate new growth of myocardial cells and increase myocardial viability.
Gene therapy for chronic CAD patients who have no other alternatives.	Stimulate angiogenesis, thereby decreasing symptoms and increasing quality of life.
Facilitated percutaneous intervention for acute myocardial infarction.	Conjoined mechanical and pharmacologic interventions for AMI will decrease mortality and increase myocardial salvage.
Establish heart-healthy food supplements.	Decrease hyperlipidemia, thereby providing risk factor modification for some predisposed risk factors.
Identify predictors of vulnerable plaque and their impact.	Provide ability to manage plaque and prevent plaque rupture, thus future coronary events.
Establish standard of providing fibrinolytic therapy in the field.	Increase survival for acute myocardial infarction patient.
Effect of community awareness programs on patients with ACS emphasizing early symptom recognition and treatment.	Decrease adverse cardiovascular events and increase survival from out-of-hospital events.
Effect of immediately triaging women with ACS-like symptoms to chest pain unit.	Increase survival in the female population and bring awareness because their symptoms are often missed.
Behavior modification techniques and their effect on CAD and its events.	Lower all modifiable risk factors, thereby decreasing cardiovascular events in a high-risk population.
Effect on established grammar and high school education program teaching about CAD; i.e., signs and symptoms, treatments, outcomes.	Establish an aware and healthier population early on, thereby decreasing total cardiovascular events.

Research Opportunities and Clinical Impact. Current research topics and their clinical impact introduces the learner to prospective research needs that are designed to potentially improve patient care. The purpose is to help the learner focus on future research needs and potential projects to improve patient care.

EVIDENCE-BASED PRACTICE

Heart Failure

Clinical Problem

Heart failure (HF) remains the most common discharge diagnosis in elderly patients, accounting for almost a quarter of all cardiovascular hospitalizations (Stewart et al., 2002). Heart failure patients commonly experience readmissions due to noncompliance, lack of understanding of self-management principles, inadequate treatment, and/or progressive disease. Although a number of pharmacologic treatments have been shown to improve outcomes in patients with HF (Jessup & Brozena, 2003), the prognosis of these patients remains poor (MacIntyre et al., 2000), resulting in frequent readmission to the hospital. Thus, there is a need for other approaches to management.

Research Findings

McAlister, Stewart, Ferrua, & McMurray (2004) conducted a study to determine whether multidisciplinary strategies improve outcomes for HF patients. The researchers searched electronic databases, bibliographies, and contacted experts to find multidisciplinary management programs in HF. Twenty-nine trials (5,039 patients) were identified. The researchers independently reviewed the results of the search strategy and selected all studies reporting the impact of outpatient-based multidisciplinary management strategies on mortality or hospitalization rates in patients with HF. Each type of intervention was then independently assigned to one of four groups: (1) multidisciplinary HF clinic; (2) multidisciplinary team providing specialized follow-up but not in a hospital or practice-based clinic; (3) telephone follow-up or telemonitoring and enhanced communication with primary care physician (including advice to deteriorating patients to see their regular physician); or (4) educational programs designed to enhance patient self-care activities.

The study results reveal that these programs are associated with a 27% reduction in HF hospitalization rates and a 43% reduction in total number of HF hospitalizations. Those strategies that incorporate specialized follow-up by a multidisciplinary team or in a multidisciplinary HF clinic also reduce all-cause mortality by approximately one-quarter and all-cause hospitalizations by one-fifth.

Implications for Nursing Practice

In order to assist the patient in getting ready for discharge from the hospital, it is essential that the nurse have an understanding of the symptoms, diagnosis, and management (medical, device, and self-management). The nurse must stress the importance of compliance with every aspect of care. If the patient has been cared for using a multidisciplinary approach, the nurse typically coordinates each member of the team. The nurse must reinforce teaching and determine the patient/family's understanding of the disease and its management.

When doing discharge planning, the nurse must ask the patient about her resources and support system. A plan needs to be developed that is realistic and manageable for the patient and family. Assistance for patients who may have difficulties taking or obtaining their medications must be provided. Ensure patients have access to urgent care, outside emergency department settings. It could be beneficial if a system for postdischarge telephone follow-up were instituted for these patients.

Critical Thinking Questions

1. Your patient was discharged from the hospital 3 days ago after a heart failure hospitalization. You are the nurse calling him to see how he is feeling since discharge. He states that his daughter was supposed to pick up his medications, but had a family emergency and forgot. He still does not have his medications, and he was discharged 5 days ago. What do you do?
2. You are the nurse in a clinic, and a patient with heart failure says she is taking her medications appropriately and following a low-salt, fluid-restricted diet. Your patient's weight continues to rise, and symptoms are worsening. What do you do to help this patient?
3. Your patient is readmitted for heart failure 2 weeks after his last heart failure hospitalization. What can you do to understand what went wrong at home, and how you can prevent a third admission?

References

Jessup, M., & Brozena, S. (2003). Medical progress heart failure. *The New England Journal of Medicine, 348,* 2007–2018.

MacIntyre, K., Capewell, S., Stewart, S., et al. (2000). Evidence of improving prognosis in heart failure trends in case fatality in 66,547 patients hospitalized between 1986 and 1995. *Circulation, 102,* 1126–1131.

McAlister, F. A., Stewart, S., Ferrua, S., & McMurray, J. J. (2004). Multidisciplinary strategies for the management of heart failure patients at high risk for admission: A systematic review of randomized trials. *Journal of the American College of Cardiology, 44*(4), 810–819.

Stewart, S., Jenkins, A., Buchan, S., McGuire, A., Capewell, S., & McMurray, J. J. V. (2002). The current cost of heart failure to the National Health Service in the UK. *European Journal of Heart Failure, 4,* 361–371.

Evidence-Based Practice. This feature presents examples of evidence and how the studies impact nursing interventions, patient teaching, skills, and professional guidelines. Learners have an opportunity to test their understanding by responding to the critical thinking questions provided for each Evidence-Based Practice feature.

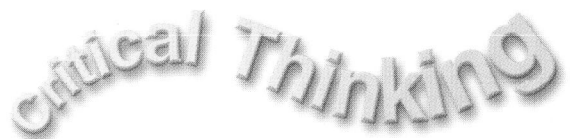

 **ETHICAL ISSUES for Pain Management
at End of Life**

Management of pain at the end of life is the right of the patient and the duty of the caregiver. Many families state that their loved ones suffered from untreated pain at the end of their life (Jackson & Abrahm, 2005). Failure to treat the pain adequately can arise from the caregiver's fear of violating ethical and moral tenets in the administration of pain medication to the dying patient.

At the end of life, the use of opioids, benzodiazepines, and other medications in doses high enough to control the patient's symptoms may unintentionally hasten death. This is referred to as double effect, where an action may have two possible effects, one good and one bad. The action is not considered immoral if it is undertaken with the intention of achieving the good effect without intending the bad effect, even though it may be foreseen. At the end of life not administering a drug to relieve symptoms because it may hasten death would be viewed as causing the patient harm and increased suffering.

Ethical Issues. This feature highlights the diverse ethical dilemmas that nurses face in clinical practice daily.

 **GERONTOLOGICAL CONSIDERATIONS
Weight Management**

Adults over age 65 years can benefit from weight management with improved day-to-day functioning and reduced cardiovascular risk. Before weight loss is recommended or attempted, however, a thorough nutrition assessment should be considered because of the high prevalence of malnutrition among older adults. Improper dieting attempts could unwittingly contribute to increased risk of malnutrition. Patients should be evaluated for their individual risks and benefits associated with potential weight loss. Specific attention should be given to preservation of muscle mass with physical activity. Appropriate referrals should be made for monitoring nutrition and exercise in the elderly.

Gerontological Considerations. The special needs of the fastest growing population are considered in order to help prevent complications and improve the prognoses for elderly patients.

 **CULTURAL CONSIDERATIONS for Therapeutic
Communications**

Munoz and Luckmann (2005) provide a rationale for the growing need for transcultural communication. They cite the increasing ethnic, racial, and cultural diversity of the United States; the increase in the number of patients who represent different culturally influenced patterns of health behavior; the different cultural meanings of health care; the different ways in which patients and families respond to health care; the multicultural nature of health care settings; and the nursing profession's commitment to culturally competent humanistic care. They further contend that talking to strangers about deeply personal issues is often difficult and may be particularly so for patients who are from different cultural backgrounds. They identify several behaviors on the part of nurses that are necessary to encourage patents to talk about themselves. Nurses must convey empathy, show respect, build trust, establish rapport, listen actively, provide appropriate feedback, and demonstrate genuine interest (p. 148). They also identify barriers to effective transcultural communication as follows: nurses' lack of knowledge, bias, ethnocentrism, prejudice, and stereotyping. Further, language differences, differences in the understanding of terminology, and differences in perceptions and expectations also create barriers (p. 162).

Cultural Considerations. These topics teach the learner to be sensitive to the needs of patients with different ethnic/cultural backgrounds, religious practices, and beliefs about health care and end of life, thereby enabling the learner to develop a multicultural approach to care.

 **GENETIC CONSIDERATIONS Implications
for Weight Management**

Speculation about the genetic implications in weight management has existed for some time. The specific roles of genetics as related to risk of obesity and eating disorders are being investigated. Risk factors for the development of eating disorders have been linked to genetic phenotypes for other disorders, such as the traits for obsessive-compulsive disorder and disturbances of dopamine systems (Kaye et al., 2004; Shinohara et al., 2004).

The role of genetics and the possibility of genetic manipulation have been heavily researched in the hope of identifying obesity risk factors and treatment options. Substances involved in appetite regulation, such as neuropeptide Y and ghrelin, proteins involved in thermogenesis, and leptin, and their relation to obesity are among the areas of research (Campion, Milagro, & Martinez, 2004; Marti, Moreno-Aliaga, Hebebrand, & Martinez, 2004). Although the topic of genetic influence on the development of both eating disorders and obesity is intriguing, it is difficult to draw firm conclusions without further research into these areas (Bulik, Sullivan, Wade, & Kendler, 2000; Kaye et al., 2004).

Genetic Considerations. This box contributes vital information about risk factors, therapies, research, legal implications, and counseling/screening, as appropriate.

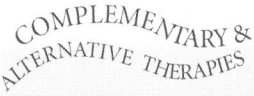 **Music Therapy**

BEHAVIORAL MEDICINE, psychologists, and nurses have focused on prevention and psychosocial influences of cardiovascular diseases for the past 30 years. Music therapy is a viable collaborative, complementary method in the psychosocial arena for alleviating risks and motivating rehabilitation from cardiac events. For the most part, music is listened to via headphones during hospitalization. Cardiac units should stock headphones, CD or other varieties of players, and a wide selection of musical CDs, ranging from country-western to rock and roll to classical scores. Patients can be encouraged to use their music of choice on an outpatient basis prior to discharge.

Research Support:
Research supports the use of music to modulate heart health measurements such as heart rate and blood pressure, to enhance exercise programs, and to relieve stress symptoms. One study (Metzger, 2004) involved administering a music therapy survey to determine current use and preference for music in a cardiac rehabilitation program. Patients attending sessions in a large city hospital completed a survey on which they rated their level of use of music for exercise, relaxation, and enjoyment. Information was also gathered about musical preferences, musical experiences, and pertinent demographics. Patients, mostly white males over the age of 60, showed positive responses to the aesthetically pleasurable aspects of music. The results suggest that education and development of music therapy in a cardiac rehabilitation program are warranted.

A German study with coronary patients (Vollert et al., 2003) concluded that music is able to lower stress and fear, contributing to relaxation in spite of physical exercise. Fifteen patients in a coronary sports unit listened to relaxation music while doing their heart-frequency-adapted exercises. Before the exercises and after listening to music, blood pressures were measured and blood was collected for determination of beta-endorphin. Simultaneous to blood collection, the participants had to perform two psychometric tests: the Perceived Stress Questionnaire (PSQ) of Levenstein, to measure the graduation of subjective perceived stress, and the State-Trait Anxiety

Inquiry (STAI) of Spielberger, as an indicator of coping. The whole protocol was performed one week prior to the mean trial, but without listening to music and without blood collections and blood pressure measurements. In the test trial without music, there were no significant changes in PSQ data. In the mean trial, under the influence of music, values in the section "worries" decreased as a sign of lower worries. STAI values were significantly lower as a sign of reduced fear after listening to music. Beta-endorphin concentration and systolic blood pressure decreased significantly after listening to music. These researchers conclude that worries and fear, patients benefit by the intervention of music (Vollert et al., 2003).

The use of music therapy has been shown to reduce pain, anxiety, and physiological parameters in patients having surgical procedures. One study (Sendelbach et al., 2006) used an experimental design to compare the effects of music therapy versus a quiet, uninterrupted rest period on pain intensity, anxiety, physiological parameters, and opioid consumption after cardiac surgery. A sample of 86 patients was randomized to 1 of 2 groups receiving either 20 minutes of music (intervention) or 20 minutes of rest in bed (control). A significant reduction in anxiety and pain was demonstrated in the group that received music compared with the control group, but no difference was observed in systolic blood pressure, diastolic blood pressure, or heart rate. No reduction in opioid usage occurred in the 2 groups.

References
Metzger, L. K. (2004). Assessment of use of music by patients participating in cardiac rehabilitation. *Journal of Music Therapy, 41*(1), 55–69.
Sendelbach, S. E., Halm, M. A., Doran, K. A., Miller, E. H., & Gaillard, P. (2006). Effects of music therapy on physiological and psychological outcomes for patients undergoing cardiac surgery. *Journal of Cardiovascular Nursing, 21*(3), 194–200.
Vollert, J. O., Stork, T., Rose, M., & Mockel, M. (2003). Music as adjuvant therapy for coronary heart disease. Therapeutic music lowers anxiety, stress and beta-endorphin concentrations in patients from a coronary sport group. *Dtsch Med Wochenschr, 128*(51–52), 2712–2716.

Complementary and Alternative Therapies. The content of this feature introduces the learner to a variety of therapies used by patients that augment mainstream medicine. An understanding of the interactions of these therapies with more traditional therapies is essential for patient safety.

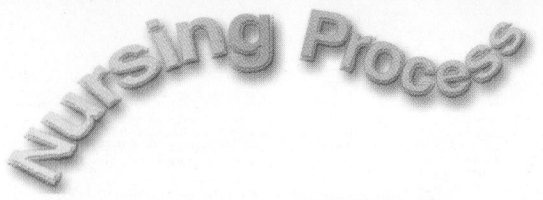

Critical Alerts. This feature alerts the learner to the immediate need for a nursing intervention that will prevent complications and promote learning. The learner will differentiate the critical nature of various clinical situations and determine the need to prioritize interventions.

PHARMACOLOGY Summary of Medications to Treat Inflammatory Heart Disease

Medication Category	Action	Application/Indication	Nursing Responsibility
Inflammatory Heart Disease			
Antibiotics — Erythromycin, Penicillin, Specific type depends on the organism	Inhibits protein synthesis of microorganisms by binding reversibly to a ribosome, thus interfering with transmission of genetic information.	*Rheumatic fever:* treats Lancefield group A beta-hemolytic streptococcus. *Pericarditis and myocarditis:* indicated if it is a bacterial infection. *Endocarditis:* indicated if infecting organism is bacterial and prophylactic for invasive procedures and dental work.	Assessment of history of drug allergies prior to administration. Assessment of clinical manifestations of allergic reaction. Assessment of relief of clinical manifestations to determine drug effectiveness. Patient education regarding need to complete the entire regimen and report any clinical manifestations of drug allergy.
Nonsteroidal Anti-Inflammatory Agents (NSAIDs) — Indomethacin (Indocin), Ibuprofen, Aspirin	Inhibits cyclooxygenase, an enzyme responsible for the formation of prostaglandins. When cyclooxygenase is inhibited, inflammation and pain are reduced.	*Rheumatic fever:* joint pain and fever. *Pericarditis:* chest pain and swelling. *Myocarditis:* pain. *Endocarditis:* fever.	Assess pain before and after administration to determine effectiveness. Medications should not be taken on an empty stomach. Monitor renal and liver function tests for abnormalities related to drug side effects. Assessment of bleeding and gastric ulcer development.
Steroids — Solu-Cortef, Cortisone, Solu-Medrol	Stabilizes leukocyte lysosomal membrane; inhibits phagocytosis and release of allergic substances; reduces capillary dilation and permeability. Modifies immune response to various stimuli.	*Myocarditis:* to prevent cardiac damage when the cause is autoimmune.	Careful assessment of relief of clinical manifestations. Assessment of side effects: Infection due to depressed immune response. Blood glucose monitoring. Gastric bleeding. Emotional lability. Lack of wound healing. Patient education regarding need to eventually reduce dosage.
Cardiac Medications — ACE inhibitors: Lisinopril, Enalapril, Ramipril, Captopril	ACE inhibitor: Lowers peripheral resistance and reduces blood volume by enhancing the excretion of sodium by inhibition of angiotensin-converting enzyme.	*Myocarditis:* heart failure. *Rheumatic fever, pericarditis, and myocarditis:* to control atrial and ventricular dysrhythmias caused by inflammation and stretching of myocardium.	Monitor blood pressure carefully after first dose for hypotension. Educate patient that it takes 2 weeks for therapeutic effect. May experience dizziness.
Antiarrhythmic Agents — Adenosine, Amiodarone, Atropine sulfate, Sotalol	Alters the electrophysiological properties of the heart by either blocking flow through the channels or altering autonomic activity.	To control dysrhythmias.	There is a narrow margin between therapeutic effect and toxicity; careful and ongoing cardiac monitoring is essential. Patient teaching includes avoiding the use of alcohol, drugs, and tobacco.
Diuretics — Furosemide, Torsemide	Blocks reabsorption of sodium and chloride in the loop of Henle. Reduces edema associated with heart failure.	*Myocarditis:* heart failure.	Potassium levels also need monitoring because low levels are a side effect of certain diuretics, especially furosemide. May need potassium replacement. Measure urine output prior to administration to gauge the response to the medication.

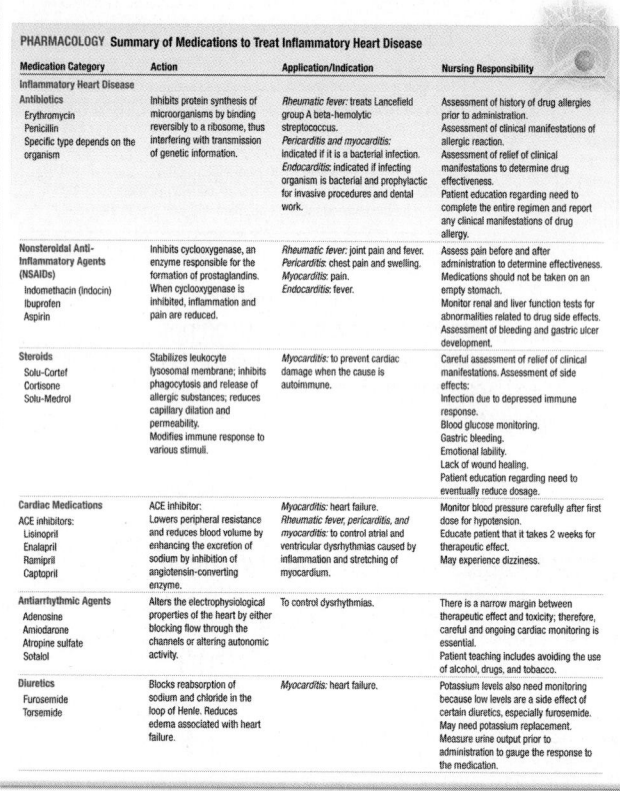

Pharmacology Summary Tables. These four-column tables offer a comprehensive overview of the pharmacology for the chapter disorders, organized by drug categories, and include medications, actions, applications and indications, and the nursing responsibilities.

NURSING PROCESS: Patient Care Plan for Obesity

Assessment of Current Nutritional Status

Subjective Data:
Have you recently gained or lost weight?
Do you prepare your own meals?
How often do you eat in restaurants?
Do you live/eat alone?
Do you have a regular meal schedule? What is it?
Do you eat during the night?

Objective Data:
Current measured weight in pounds/height with minimal clothing and after urination
Serial weights from medical records
Presence of abdominal adiposity

Nursing Assessment and Diagnoses	Outcomes and Evaluation Parameters	Planning and Interventions with *Rationales*
Nursing Diagnosis: *Imbalanced Nutrition: More than Body Requirements* related to imbalance in dietary requirements and energy requirements	**Outcome:** Balanced nutrition. **Evaluation Parameters:** Maintaining BMI within normal range.	**Interventions and *Rationales*:** Perform a complete physical assessment and nutritional history on admission *to assess current nutritional status and to provide a nutritional baseline of data.* Calculate BMI to determine overweight/obesity status. Current weight is compared to BMI charts, height weight charts, and waist measurement *to determine degree of overweight status, overweight, obese, or morbidly obese.* Measure waist circumference *to determine cardiovascular disease risk.* Differentiate weight gain of obesity from weight gain of edema, and other nonadiposity causes *to determine cause of weight gain.*

Assessment of Current Nutritional and Dietary Intake

Subjective Data:
24-hour and possibly 3-day recall of all meals, snacks, liquids
Location of meals
Method of food preparation
Portion size
Meals missed
Other factors that may influence intake, such as recent acute illness or cultural or religious influences on food intake patterns.
Alcohol intake

Objective Data:
Ask spouse or significant other to validate data if patient agrees

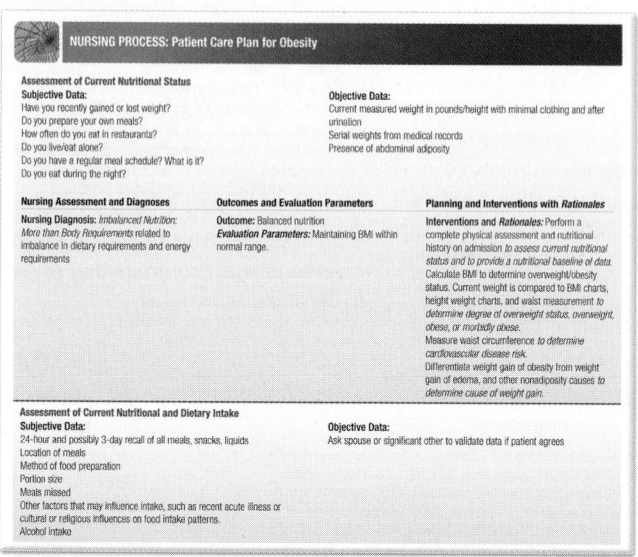

Nursing Process: Patient Care Plan. The nursing process care plan provides the learner with an easy-to-follow, easy-to-apply, succinct way of organizing nursing care, guided by nursing diagnosis, assessment, intervention, and outcome evaluation. It is designed to assist the learner in developing a plan of care specific to the patient with desired patient outcomes and specific nursing interventions for a given diagnosis.

DIAGNOSTIC TESTS for Cardiac Valve Disease

Test and *Normal Values*	Expected Abnormality	Rationale for Abnormality
Echocardiogram and transesophageal echocardiography (TEE) Echocardiogram (ultrasound): *Normal chamber size and normal cardiac structures*	Abnormal structure and function of heart valves, able to identify thickened valve leaflets, vegetative growths, myocardial function, and chamber size. TEE is particularly useful not only for diagnosing but also for tracking the progression of the disease.	Vegetative growths and infection cause a thinning of valve leaflets leading to abnormal function.
Chest x-ray: *Clear lungs and normal heart size*	Pulmonary congestion, cardiac hypertrophy, chamber and great vessel enlargement, and calcification of the valves.	Abnormal valve function causes a change in blood flow leading to changes in chamber size and valve structure.
Cardiac catheterization: *Normal coronary artery blood flow, chamber size, and valve function*	The size of the valve opening and pressure gradients across valve surfaces is abnormal. Pressure in the heart chambers and pulmonary system is increased. Cardiac output typically is decreased.	Abnormal valve structure causes changes in openings leading to increased pressures in the cardiac chambers and decreased cardiac output.
Electrocardiogram (ECG): *Normal conduction time intervals*	Conduction delays, atrial and ventricular dysrhythmias, and the presence of cardiac ischemia. Is useful in detecting increased ischemia and the presence of life-threatening dysrhythmias.	Changes occur due to diminished blood flow to the myocardium due to decreased cardiac output caused by abnormal valvular function.
Cardiac MRI (CMR): *Normal heart valve function*	Valve size and competence.	Abnormal valve structure causes changes in openings, leading to increased pressures in the cardiac chambers and decreased cardiac output.

Diagnostic Tests. These tables inform the learner about the relevant diagnostic tests for the disorder under discussion. Normal result ranges are included, as well as expected abnormalities with rationales.

PATIENT TEACHING & DISCHARGE PRIORITIES for Coronary Artery Disease/Acute Coronary Syndrome

Need	Teaching
Knowledge of disease process and prognosis	Written and verbal instructions for: • Specific diagnosis/treatment; i.e., angioplasty, stent, heart attack, congestive heart failure, CAD • Follow-up labs, test, health care provider appointment • Medications • Diet • Activity. These instructions will reinforce the need to comply with therapy.
Understanding of medications	The patient and family are taught what the purposes of the medications are, their side effects, and their timing. These instructions will reinforce medication compliance and prevent over- or underdosing.
Safety	Stress the importance of wearing an identification bracelet to identify a heart problem to health care workers. Carry stent identification card in wallet to identify implant information to health care workers.
Disease prevention	Teach about dietary consumption. Stress the importance of a low-fat, low-cholesterol, low-salt diet. Teach about an exercise program. Stress the importance of exercise to prevent further CAD and keep current CAD from progressing. Offer cardiac rehabilitation program resources. Teach about behavior modification; decrease stress environment. Stress importance of smoking cessation and offer resources for community programs.
Reportable clinical manifestations	Teach to report chest pain or anginal equivalent. Stress how to take sublingual nitroglycerin should patient experience angina. Stress importance of using 911 emergency response system instead of driving self to emergency department (ED). Teach about fatigue and shortness of breath, as they too may be indicators of an unstable plaque or valve problem exacerbating. Teach about dental prophylaxis if patient was diagnosed with valve problem or had invasive coronary procedure.
Family/support system	Assess availability, knowledge, and compliance with treatment regimen. Assess discharge needs; i.e., home placement, medications, driving. Involve discharge planning if specific needs are not met to offer community resources.
Emotional adjustment of patient/family	Answer questions honestly. Encourage verbalization of frustrations and anger. Encourage positive reinforcement from the family. Provide active listening. Provide additional hospital and community resources, as necessary.

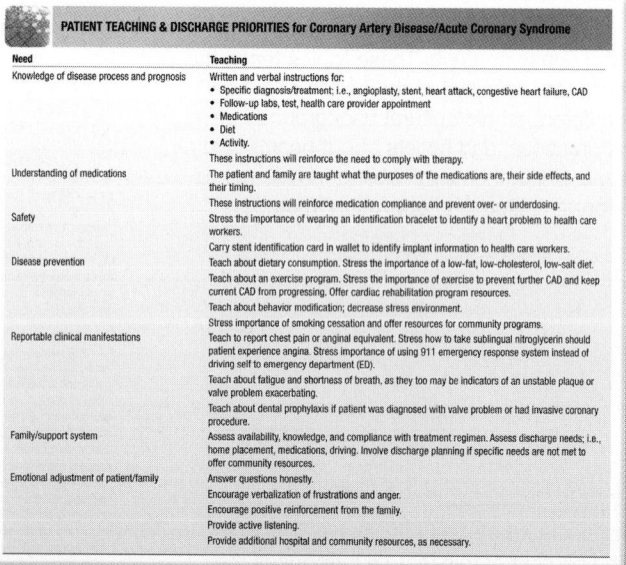

Patient Teaching & Discharge Priorities. This table helps identify priorities for discharge planning while integrating patient teaching with home and community care.

Health Promotion

Risk Factors. These boxes highlight particular items in the patient history and interview that should alert the nurse to possible problems.

Health Promotion. Found as appropriate in many chapters, Health Promotion sections call the learner's attention to one of the primary roles of the nurse, that of educating the patient and family about healthy habits and lifestyles, thereby preventing or ameliorating unhealthy conditions.

RISK FACTORS for Stress

Younger adults	Stress may go unnoticed in the very young and old.
Women in general	Women may be at higher risk than men for stress-related chest pain, but men's hearts may be more vulnerable to adverse effects from long-term stress.
Working mothers	Working mothers face higher stress levels and possibly adverse health effects, most likely because they bear a greater and more diffuse workload than men or other women.
Caregivers of family members	Caregivers of family members with physical or mental disabilities are at risk for chronic stress. They are particularly vulnerable to stress-related health threats such as influenza, depression, and heart disease.
Less educated individuals	Less educated individuals may be at higher risk because they may not be able to differentiate the causes of stress.
Divorced or widowed individuals	Unmarried people generally do not live as long as their married contemporaries.
The unemployed	Being unemployed is an environmental stressor that threatens security.
Isolated individuals	Such individuals usually lack support systems.
People who are targets of racial or sexual discrimination	Discrimination is an environmental stressor that is beyond individual control.
Those without health insurance	This is a threat to one's health that can lead to stress.
People who live in cities	City dwellers may be more stressed as a result of external stressors beyond their control.

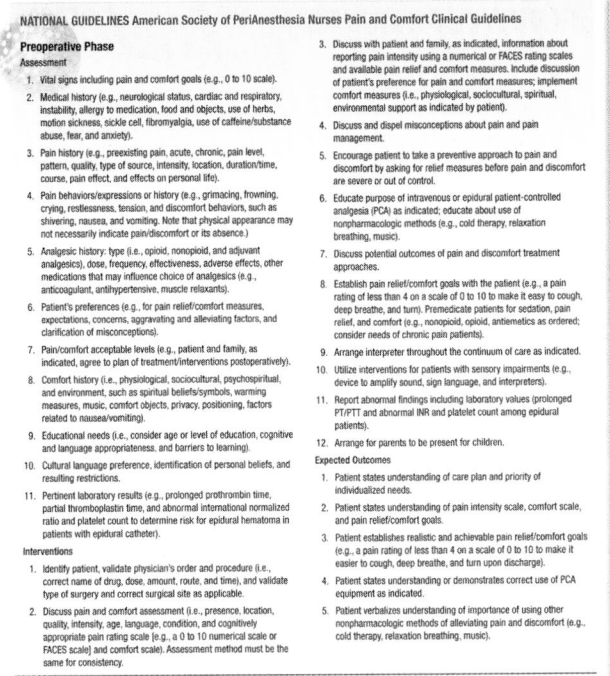

NATIONAL GUIDELINES American Society of PeriAnesthesia Nurses Pain and Comfort Clinical Guidelines

Preoperative Phase

Assessment

1. Vital signs including pain and comfort goals (e.g., 0 to 10 scale).
2. Medical history (e.g., neurological status, cardiac and respiratory, instability, allergy to medication, food and objects, use of herbs, motion sickness, sickle cell, fibromyalgia, use of caffeine/substance abuse, fear, and anxiety).
3. Pain history (e.g., preexisting pain, acute, chronic, pain level, pattern, quality, type of source, intensity, location, duration/time, course, pain effect, and effects on personal life).
4. Pain behaviors/expressions or history (e.g., grimacing, frowning, crying, restlessness, tension, and discomfort behaviors, such as shivering, nausea, and vomiting. Note that physical appearance may not necessarily indicate pain/discomfort or its absence.)
5. Analgesic history: type (i.e., opioid, nonopioid, and adjuvant analgesics), dose, frequency, effectiveness, adverse effects, other medications that may influence choice of analgesics (e.g., anticoagulant, antihypertensive, muscle relaxants).
6. Patient's preferences (e.g., for pain relief/comfort measures, expectations, concerns, aggravating and alleviating factors, and clarification of misconceptions).
7. Pain/comfort acceptable levels (e.g., patient and family, as indicated, agree to plan of treatment/interventions postoperatively).
8. Comfort history (i.e., physiological, sociocultural, psychospiritual, and environment, such as spiritual beliefs/symbols, warming measures, music, comfort objects, privacy, positioning, factors related to nausea/vomiting).
9. Educational needs (i.e., consider age or level of education, cognitive and language appropriateness, and barriers to learning).
10. Cultural language preference, identification of personal beliefs, and resulting restrictions.
11. Pertinent laboratory results (e.g., prolonged prothrombin time, partial thromboplastin time, and abnormal international normalized ratio and platelet count to determine risk for epidural hematoma in patients with epidural catheter).

Interventions

1. Identify patient, validate physician's order and procedure (i.e., correct name of drug, dose, amount, route, and time), and validate type of surgery and correct surgical site as applicable.
2. Discuss pain and comfort assessment (i.e., presence, location, quality, intensity, age, language, condition, and cognitively appropriate pain rating scale [e.g., a 0 to 10 numerical scale or FACES scale] and comfort scale). Assessment method must be the same for consistency.
3. Discuss with patient and family, as indicated, information about reporting pain intensity using a numerical or FACES rating scales and available pain relief and comfort measures. Include discussion of patient's preference for pain and comfort measures; implement comfort measures (i.e., physiological, sociocultural, spiritual, environmental support as indicated by patient).
4. Discuss and dispel misconceptions about pain and pain management.
5. Encourage patient to take a preventive approach to pain and discomfort by asking for relief measures before pain and discomfort are severe or out of control.
6. Educate purpose of intravenous or epidural patient-controlled analgesia (PCA) as indicated; educate about use of nonpharmacologic methods (e.g., cold therapy, relaxation breathing, music).
7. Discuss potential outcomes of pain and discomfort treatment approaches.
8. Establish pain relief/comfort goals with the patient (e.g., a pain rating of less than 4 on a scale of 0 to 10 to make it easy to cough, deep breathe, and turn). Premedicate patients for sedation, pain relief, and comfort (e.g., nonopioid, opioid, antiemetics as ordered; consider needs of chronic pain patients).
9. Arrange interpreter throughout the continuum of care as indicated.
10. Utilize interventions for patients with sensory impairments (e.g., device to amplify sound, sign language, and interpreters).
11. Report abnormal findings including laboratory values (prolonged PT/PTT and abnormal INR and platelet count among epidural patients).
12. Arrange for parents to be present for children.

Expected Outcomes

1. Patient states understanding of care plan and priority of individualized needs.
2. Patient states understanding of pain intensity scale, comfort scale, and pain relief/comfort goals.
3. Patient establishes realistic and achievable pain relief/comfort goals (e.g., a pain rating of less than 4 on a scale of 0 to 10 to make it easier to cough, deep breathe, and turn upon discharge).
4. Patient states understanding or demonstrates correct use of PCA equipment as indicated.
5. Patient verbalizes understanding of importance of using other nonpharmacologic methods of alleviating pain and discomfort (e.g., cold therapy, relaxation breathing, music).

Source: American Society of PeriAnesthesia Nurses. (2003). ASPAN pain and comfort guideline. *Journal of PeriAnesthesia Nursing, 18*(4), 232–236.

National Guidelines. These guidelines are integrated throughout the chapters where appropriate to provide pertinent, specific objectives to increase the awareness of the learner of the need for uniformity of care on national and international levels (i.e., *Healthy People 2010,* HIPAA, and AHA).

Preparation for Practice

Clinical Preparation

CRITICAL THINKING

Read

- History of Current Illness
- Past Medical History
- Physical Exam
- Admitting Medical Orders
- Laboratory Study Results

Document

- Summary of Hospitalization
- Pathophysiology Form
- Laboratory Values
- Laboratory Results Explanation

Apply

- List of Potential Nursing Diagnoses
- Concept Map
- Critical Thinking Questions

**Log on to MyNursingKit.com to download forms you will need and to complete further steps in the Clinical Preparation assignment.*

PEARSON mynursingkit

HISTORY OF PRESENT ILLNESS

As the on-coming nurse on a telemetry cardiovascular care unit, you receive report about Mr. X, who was admitted with a diagnosis of heart failure 48 hours ago. He is a 56-year-old male who presented to his primary care provider with a 2-month history of worsening symptoms of dyspnea on exertion, a nonproductive cough, general fatigue, and decreased activity tolerance. Initially, the patient thought he had the flu, but when the symptoms persisted longer than expected, he sought medical attention. At the office Mr. X was found to have profound jugular venous distention, rales in his lungs, and lower extremity swelling. After admission, he had an echocardiogram and a serum BNP that was 1,560 pg/mL. Coronary angiography was performed to provide a definitive diagnosis that revealed no evidence of coronary artery disease. Echocardiogram shows moderate concentric hypertrophy of the ventricles, moderate left ventricular dysfunction, ejection fraction 33%, mild to moderate mitral regurgitation. Angiogram: normal coronary arteries, ejection fraction 33%, confirmed reduction in ventricular function with a ventriculogram.

Medical Surgical History

Hyperlipidemia: diagnosed 3 years ago
Hypertension: diagnosed this past year
Type 2 diabetes: diagnosed this past year
Obesity: over 20 years
Hypothyroidism: diagnosed 12 years ago
Tonsillectomy: 40 years ago
Cholecystectomy: 4 years ago

Current Medications

Simvastatin 20 mg po qhs
Levothyroxine 0.125 mg po daily
Glipizide 500 mg po bid
Hydrochlorothiazide 25 mg po daily

Physical Exam

Vital signs: HR: 84 beats per minute; BP: 146/84 mmHg; temperature: 36.8°C; oxygen sat: 94% on 2 liters of oxygen.
He is a well-nourished male with appropriate affect and no apparent distress
All extremities have palpable pulses, are warm to touch, and have a capillary refill of less than 3 seconds.
3+ pitting edema is present in his lower ankles bilaterally, which extends to his midcalf; his lungs have bibasilar crackles without wheezing or retractions; he also has a nonproductive cough.
Normal S_1 and S_2 are present. S_3, and the point of maximal impulse is displaced laterally, into the anterior axillary line of his chest.
Positive hepatojugular reflux.
Bowel sounds present and palpation is nontender.

Admitting Medical Orders

Cardiology Service
Diagnosis: acute heart failure
Telemetry floor
Condition guarded
No known allergies
Full code
Bed rest with bathroom privileges
Call house officer: pulse < 60 and > 100/minute; BP < 90 and > 160 systolic; temperature > 38.5; urine output < 30 mL/hr for 2 hours; respiratory rate > 30/minute; oxygen saturation < 92%; Blood sugar < 60 or >120
Continuous cardiac monitor
Oxygen per nasal cannula to maintain oxygen sat > 92%
Vital signs and oxygen saturation q4hours
Daily a.m. weights
IV: saline lock-flush with NS q8h
Blood sugars ac and hs
Cardiac rehab evaluation and management
Low-sodium (< 2,000 mg/day), fluid-restricted (< 2 L/day) diet
Strict I&O
Sequential compression devices (SCD) to lower extremities when in bed
Incentive spirometry 2 hours while awake and q4 at night

Clinical Preparation. This exercise is presented at the end of each disorder chapter to present the learner with a reality-oriented approach to patient assessment and diagnosis. The learner will complete the assignment on the Web in MyNursingKit.

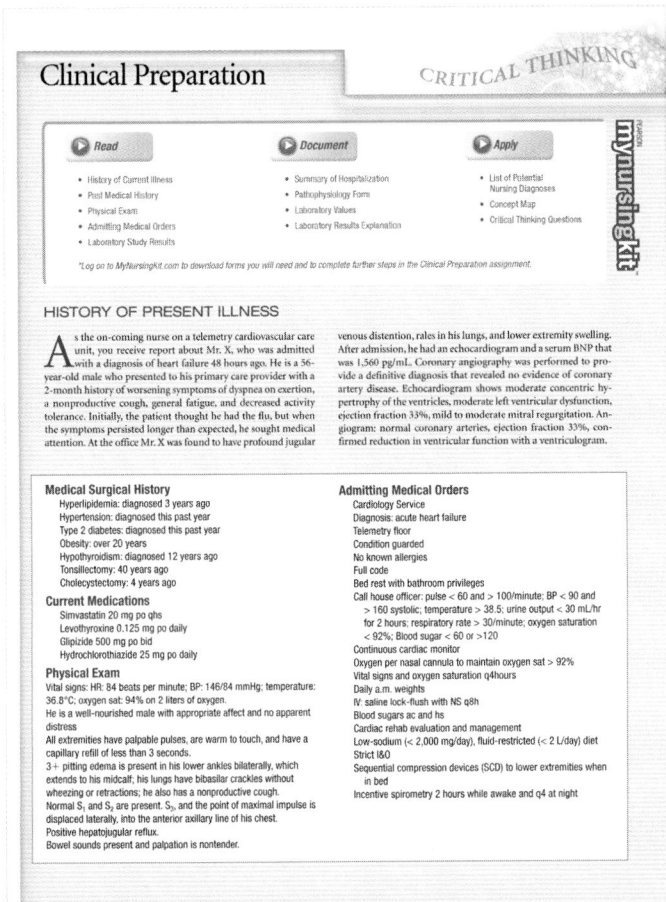

CRITICAL THINKING QUESTIONS

1. When reviewing Mr. X's orders when coming on shift, list them in order of priority.
2. Why would the patient receive daily a.m. weights?
3. Which laboratory values may require notification to the ordering provider?
4. What should you monitor for after giving lisinopril 2.5 mg PO daily?
5. Why is a beta-adrenergic blocker not listed on the ordered medications?

Clinical Preparation Assignments. The assignment helps the learner develop a problem-solving approach to nursing care. By completing the assignments presented at the end of the chapters, the learner will gain experience in critical thinking skills and develop a systematic method for determining a patient's health problem, devising a plan of care, developing evaluation criteria, and determining expected outcomes. The Clinical Preparation assignments also help the learner articulate the patient's needs and learn how to write effective evaluation statements. This, in turn, significantly improves documentation skills and the ability to communicate with other health care team members to provide the safest, most effective, and holistic care for the patient.

ACKNOWLEDGMENTS

In addition to the individuals mentioned in our dedications, we would also like to thank people who were instrumental in the development of the book. The following people assisted us in bringing this project to fruition:

- Marion Waldman, the development editor, for being the glue that kept the project moving in a positive direction. For listening and being patient with our never ending list of questions. We could not have done it without her.

- Kelly Karr for her editing expertise and for the long hours she dedicated to making sure each chapter was error free.

- Susan Poirier for her exacting work in developing, formatting, and editing the pharmacology tables.

- Charlotte Miller for precise review of units to ensure consistency of content, developing the Kardex format, and placing URLs in the chapters.

- Linda Cooke for developing the clinical preparation framework, hand printing the Kardexs, and patiently guiding the authors to ensure consistency.

- Judy Tanner for her endless support, diligence, and patience in the detailed editing of chapters in the first page proofs.

- Mary Ann Shahdi, Jennifer FitzGerald, Andrea Perry, Sonia Garcia, Kathleen Budesa, and Jolie Tietz, nursing students, who generously shared their thoughts and feelings about caring behavior observed in nurses, presented in Chapter 1.

- Mike Osborn, Maddison Thivierge, and Adam Jonathan Davis for very short notice assistance with finalizing content for the book; it was greatly appreciated.

CONTENTS

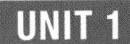

UNIT 4

Complex Skills Related to Nursing Practice 510

UNIT 9

Nursing Management of Patients with Gastrointestinal, Renal, and Urinary Disorders   1364

CHAPTER 44

Nursing Assessment of Patients with Gastrointestinal, Renal, and Urinary Disorders   1366

CHAPTER 45

Caring for the Patient with Gastrointestinal Disorders   1381

CHAPTER 46

Caring for the Patient with Hepatic and Biliary Disorders   1427

CHAPTER 47

Caring for the Patient with Renal and Urinary Disorders   1463

UNIT 10

Nursing Management of Patients with Reproductive Disorders 1502

UNIT 11

Nursing Management of Patients with Endocrine Disorders 1594

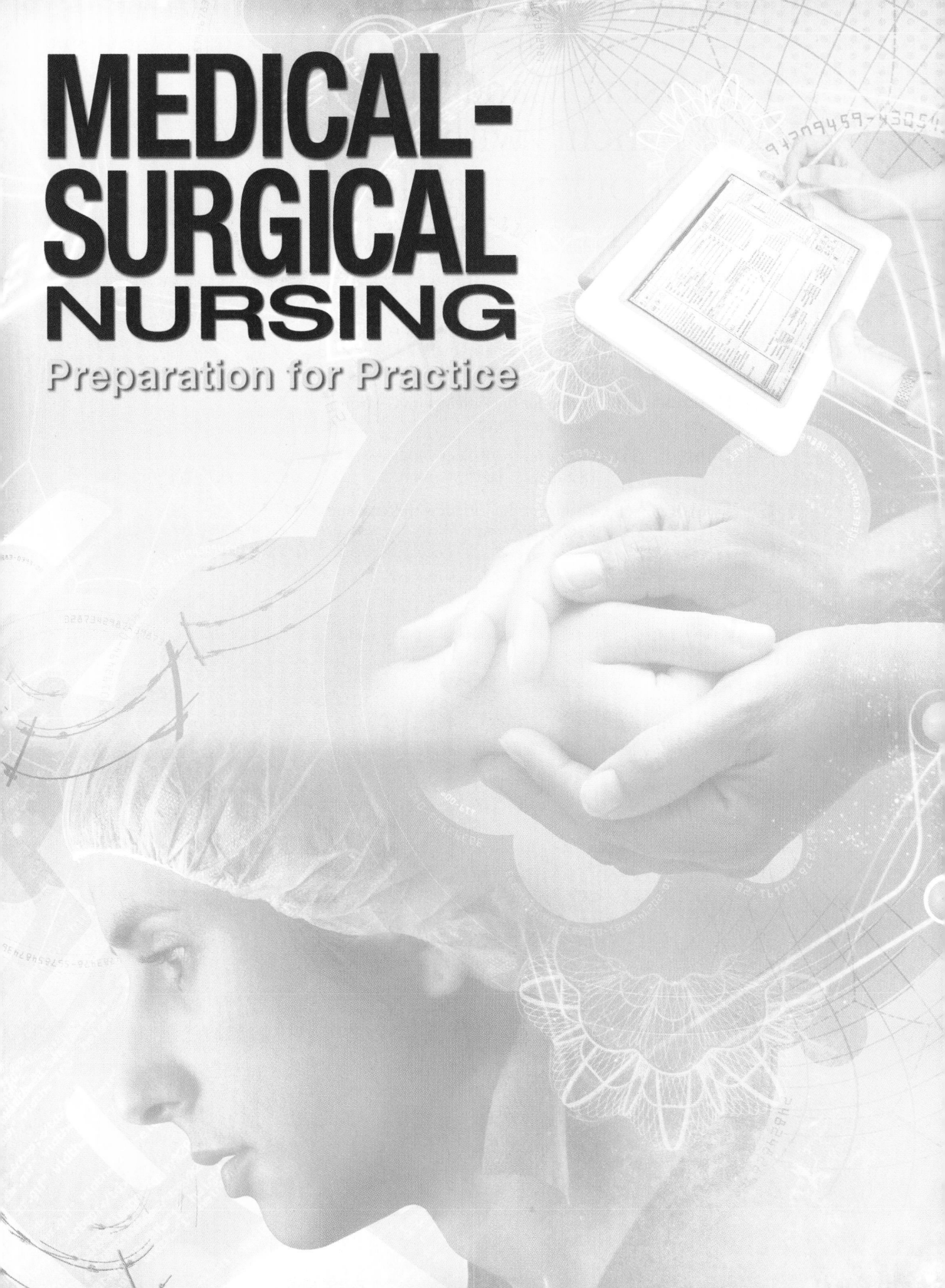

MEDICAL-SURGICAL NURSING
Preparation for Practice

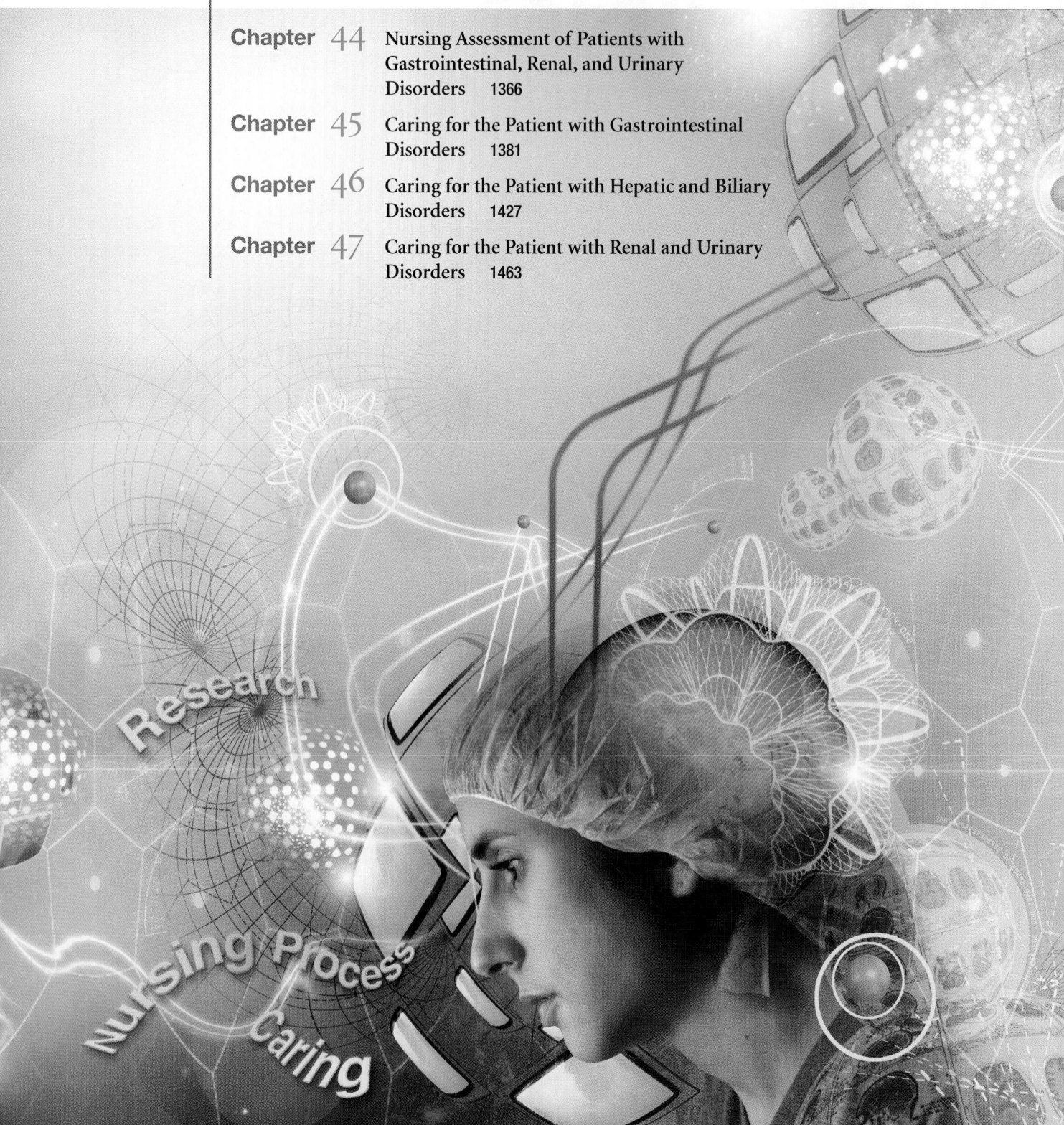

UNIT 9

Nursing Management of Patients with Gastrointestinal, Renal, and Urinary Disorders

Research

Nursing Process

Caring

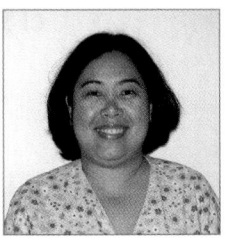

CELESTE   I am Celeste May Padilla, clinical nurse III in the Renal Services Program at the University of California, Davis Medical Center. I am a member of the American Nephrology Nurses' Association and a certified nephrology nurse acknowledged by the Nephrology Nursing Certification Board. I have been working as a nephrology nurse since 1999, and give direct patient care to patients of different ages and varying diagnoses.

The nurses in the Renal Services Program are mobile—we go from different floors and units to provide dialysis. Most of our patients are adults with acute and chronic renal diseases, but we also care for pediatric and geriatric patients. Our average number of patients is 15 a day, but that number can rise to more than 20 patients on busy days. We also provide in-patient dialysis at Shriners Children's Hospital, which is adjacent to our facility.

We use the nursing process to direct the treatment of patients who are experiencing, or at risk for, renal disease. Our program provides different modalities such as *continuous renal replacement therapy* for patients in the intensive care unit (ICU) who are critically ill and diagnosed with acute renal failure. Patients who are at risk for renal impairment benefit from early dialytic management of fluid and solute imbalance. *Slow extended daily dialysis* (SLEDD) is another modality. SLEDD is used when ICU patients need gentle and slow dialysis so they can tolerate fluid removal and have electrolyte imbalances corrected. Intermittent hemodialysis, or regular dialysis, is a modality for patients in the medical–surgical units who can tolerate dialysis and maintain stable vital signs throughout the procedure. We provide interventions to improve patient outcomes based on the nurse's individual clinical judgment and knowledge.

As a nephrology nurse, it is part of my profession and daily life to follow the six components of caring. **Compassion** is being aware of my patient's needs, that is, willing to share and discover another person's meaning and purpose in life, sickness, and health. Providing care to patients who are in the denial stage of their diagnosis is one of my priorities. I show my **commitment** to my profession, department, and colleagues by my attendance on scheduled days to work and by my willingness to be called in to give prompt care to patients who need emergent dialysis.

On occasion, I have been called in the middle of the night to come to the emergency department (ED) to do emergent dialysis for a chronic patient who came in with hyperkalemia, severe chest pain, fluid overload, and very short of breath. The patient may be a noncompliant end-stage renal disease patient who didn't go to dialysis for several treatments and now is in the ED seeking emergent treatment. My **conscience** dictates that I suspend judgment; there is no choice based on whether the patient is compliant or not—we are always ready to render service.

I had one very young pediatric patient who required dialysis. The parents were always at the bedside 24/7, and they had never experienced dialysis before so they had many questions. I understood completely because they wanted to make sure that treatment was appropriate and the patient would be in good hands. As a **competent** nurse I answered them in a way they could easily understand. I showed them each step and demonstrated to them with **confidence** that I practice my profession without hesitation or doubt. My **comportment** helped them to accept the fact that their child needed dialysis.

Being a nephrology nurse involves giving direct care, educating, and coordinating. We complete a thorough assessment, and if a patient is stable enough to start dialysis, then we proceed. But if a certain modality is ordered for this particular patient and we know it's not safe, then we use our own judgment and inform our nephrologists of the patient's change in condition. Our nephrologists value our expertise and listen to our suggestions—after all, we are a team with one purpose: to deliver safe, excellent care.

"As a nephrology nurse, it is part of my profession and daily life to follow the six components of caring. **Compassion** is being aware of my patient's needs, that is, willing to share and discover another person's meaning and purpose in life, sickness, and health."

44 | Nursing Assessment of Patients with Gastrointestinal, Renal, and Urinary Disorders

Bonnie McCracken

Outcome-Based Learning Objectives

After studying this chapter, the learner will be able to:

1. Compare and contrast the significant subjective and objective data that pertain to the gastrointestinal and urinary systems obtained during history taking.
2. Identify the four components of the physical exam.
3. Describe techniques used during the physical assessment of the gastrointestinal and urinary systems.
4. Differentiate abnormal from normal findings of the physical assessment of the gastrointestinal and urinary systems.
5. Describe key aspects that should be included when documenting the physical examination.

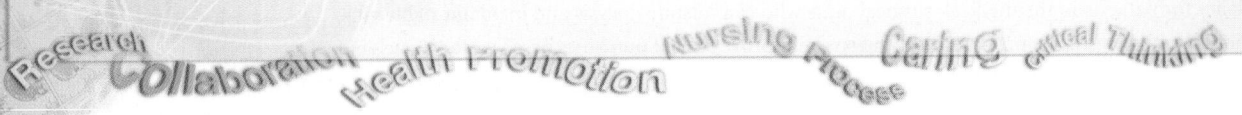

Research   Collaboration   Health Promotion   Nursing Process   Caring   Critical Thinking

THE SYMPTOMS of abdominal pain are frequent presenting medical complaints. The symptoms may represent something very benign or something extremely serious and even life threatening. For example, the complaint of abdominal pain can be either gastroenteritis or an aortic aneurysm. The difference between the two diagnoses can be differentiated by a thorough history and physical examination. In order to perform a proper history and physical examination, the nurse must have a thorough understanding of the anatomy and physiology of the gastrointestinal system (Figure 44–1 ■). The nurse will then be able to determine what is occurring with the patient.

■ Anatomy and Physiology

For the nurse to complete a thorough assessment of the gastrointestinal and urinary systems, it is imperative to understand the anatomy and physiology of each system. This knowledge will assist the nurse in thinking critically and assimilating all data gathered during the assessment.

Gastrointestinal System

The primary purposes of the gastrointestinal (GI) system are to transport and deliver nutrition and water, and to support the function of cells throughout the body. The oral cavity or mouth is at the beginning of the GI tract. This is where food is taken in

and the process of digestion starts. The act of chewing and the mixture with saliva starts the breakdown of the food and makes it a size acceptable for passage through the esophagus. The salivary glands have several roles in this process. First, they add an aqueous component to the food bolus, making it easier to swallow, and second, they lubricate the mouth, facilitating the movement of the lips and tongue during swallowing. This aqueous environment assists in the distribution of the food across the taste buds dispersed across the tongue, making the food palatable and therefore more pleasing to eat. Without these taste buds, food would have no taste and be difficult to eat. An additional property of saliva is the reduction in bacteria in the oral cavity. Saliva contains large amounts of ions, such as chloride, bicarbonate, potassium, thiocyanate, hydrogen, and **immunoglobulin A**, a vital component for destroying oral bacteria (Urdan, Stacy, & Lough, 2006). There are three pairs of major salivary glands: the parotid, sublingual, and submandibular glands. The parotid gland secretes enzymes, which begins the chemical breakdown of large polysaccharides into dextrins and sugars.

The act of chewing is a complex process of using the teeth to masticate and the tongue to move the food bolus backward. Simultaneously, the soft palate lifts and covers the nasal passage while the epiglottis closes the opening, preventing aspiration of food. A change in any of these intricate movements can cause problems with the first step of digestion.

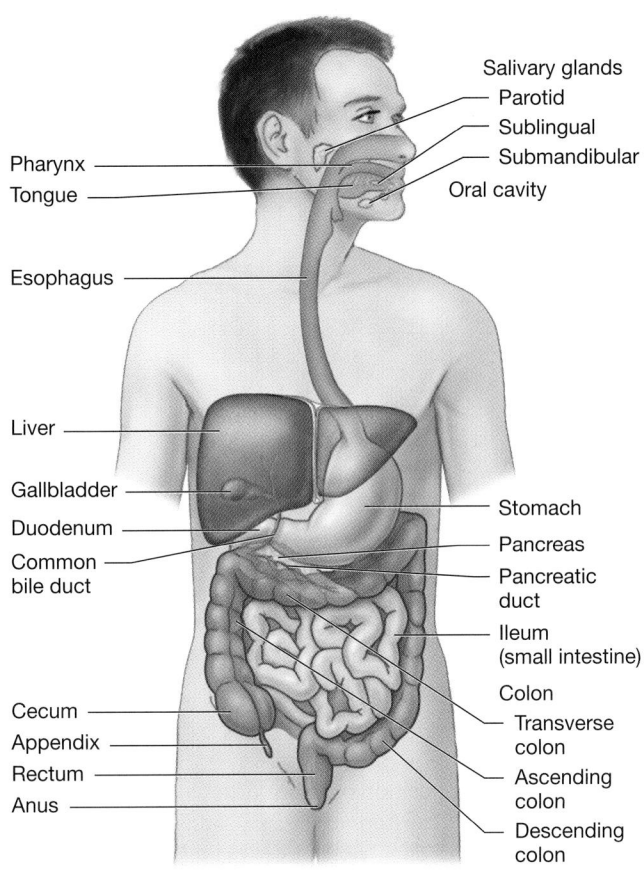

Salivary glands
Parotid
Sublingual
Submandibular
Oral cavity

Pharynx
Tongue

Esophagus

Liver

Gallbladder
Duodenum
Common
bile duct

Stomach
Pancreas
Pancreatic
duct
Ileum
(small intestine)
Colon
Transverse
colon
Ascending
colon
Descending
colon

Cecum
Appendix
Rectum
Anus

FIGURE 44–1 ■ Organs of the gastrointestinal (GI) system.

The food bolus then passes through the **esophagus**. This tubular structure connects the oral cavity to the stomach. There is a segment of the esophagus in the cervical area, the thoracic area, and then it passes through the diaphragmatic hiatus into the abdominal cavity. There are two esophageal sphincters; the upper esophageal or **pharyngoesophageal**, which is created by the cricopharyngeus muscle, and the lower esophageal or **cardioesophageal**. The upper esophageal sphincter inhibits air from entering the esophagus during respiration, and the lower esophageal sphincter controls the food entering the stomach and prevents reflux of gastric contents. After swallowing, the esophageal sphincter in the upper portion closes, which increases the normal pressure within the esophagus. This phenomenon, along with peristalsis, moves the food bolus down to the stomach. **Peristalsis** is caused by the coordinated contraction of the circular and longitudinal muscle fibers making up the musculature of the esophagus. The pressure changes in the esophagus prevent reflux of the food bolus into the pharynx as well as gastric content from entering the lower portion of the esophagus. When reflux from the stomach into the esophagus occurs, it is known as **GERD, gastroesophageal reflux disease**. Commonly called "heartburn," it is a frequent patient complaint. Once the bolus has passed through the esophagus, the pressures return to normal.

The vagus nerve provides the parasympathetic innervation of the pharynx and the esophagus. Pharyngeal branches of the vagus nerve innervate the constrictor muscles of the pharynx with

a small contribution by cranial nerves IX and XI. The upper esophageal sphincter and the upper portion of the esophagus are innervated by branches of the recurrent laryngeal nerves, which originate from the vagus nerve. Patients with injury to these nerves will have functional problems with their vocal cords as well as problems with the upper esophageal sphincter and motility of the esophagus, one of the causes of dysphasia, speech impairment resulting from a brain lesion or neurodevelopmental disorder. A problem with the upper esophageal sphincter also causes an increased risk of aspiration and further respiratory complications resulting from this condition.

The food bolus passes from the esophagus into the stomach. The stomach can be described as a muscular container where food is released into the intestine at a controlled rate. The stomach starts with the lower esophageal sphincter and ends with the pylorus. In between these two structures, the stomach can be divided into three portions: the cardia, the fundus, and the antrum (Figure 44–2 ■, 1368).

The **cardia** is where mucus and bicarbonate are secreted to protect the surface of the stomach from the acidic gastric juices. The lining of the stomach has multiple folds called rugae. Within this lining are deep gastric glands, which further differentiate the areas of the stomach. These glands are shallow in the cardia, medium depth in the antrum, and the deepest are found in the fundus. These deeper glands in the fundus contain secretory cells producing acid and pepsin, important components of the gastric juice. This capability establishes the primary purpose of the fundus as the secretory region of the stomach. The **antrum** is the place of the greatest motility with the purpose of mixing the gastric juices with the food particles and grinding them into smaller particles. The antrum then empties into the small intestine through the pylorus.

An understanding of the vasculature of the stomach is important in order to understand the significance of any bleeding in this area. This is the most vascularized portion of the gastrointestinal tract, which explains why a perforated ulcer can be life threatening due to rapid exsanguination. The largest artery supplying the stomach is the left gastric artery. This arises from the celiac trunk and is divided into the ascending and descending branches along the lesser curvature of the stomach. The second largest artery is the right gastroepiploic artery originating from the gastroduodenal artery. The left gastroepiploic artery arises from the splenic artery. These two arteries supply the greater curvature of the stomach. The fourth artery is the right gastric artery arising from the hepatic artery and runs along the distal stomach.

The venous system draining the stomach parallels the arteries. The left and right gastric veins drain into the portal vein, the right gastroepiploic veins drain into the superior mesenteric vein, while the left gastroepiploic vein drains into the splenic vein.

The nerve innervation of the stomach is with the anterior and posterior trunk of the vagal nerve. Approximately 90% of the nerve fibers are afferent, with the remaining 10% efferent.

The stomach empties through the pylorus into a portion of the small intestine called the duodenum. The duodenum has 12 sections and is responsible for the regulation of digestion and absorption. It is found almost entirely in the **retroperitoneal space**, the anatomic space behind the abdominal cavity. The

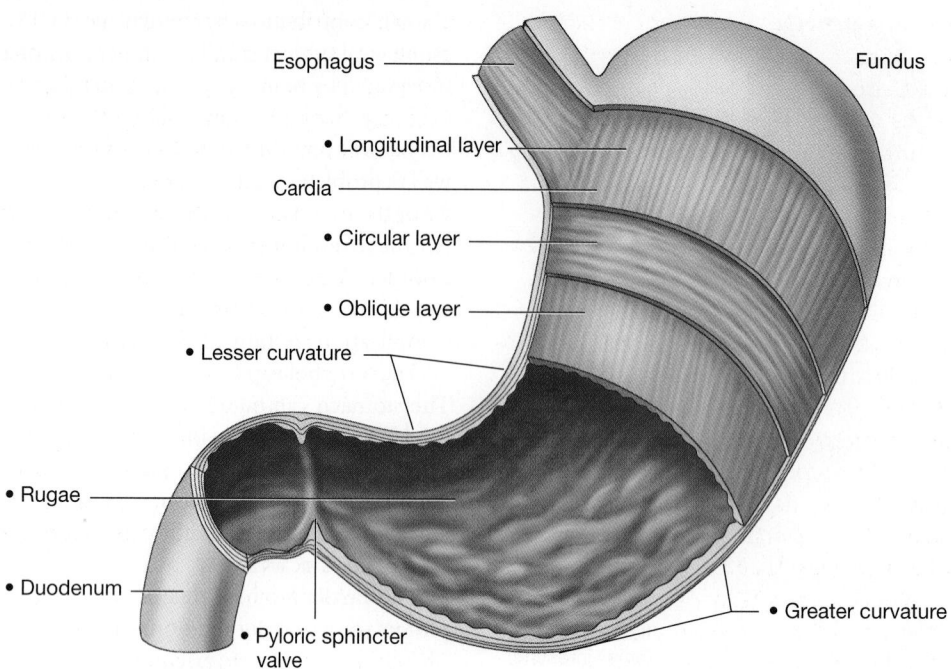

FIGURE 44–2 ■ The stomach.

primary purpose of this portion of the gastrointestinal tract is for the regulation of digestion and the absorption of the luminal contents. The duodenum is divided into four sections. The first, superior, part is approximately 5 centimeters from the pylorus to the second portion. It is in this area that a duodenal ulcer is found, usually along the anterior wall.

The second portion of the duodenum, known as the descending portion, is the area where the pancreatic and common bile ducts enter through the major duodenal papilla, or ampula of Vater. The pressure in the pancreatic duct is greater than in the bile duct to prevent reflux. To assist digestion, the pancreas secretes approximately 500 milliliters of fluid per day (Fisher, Andersen, Bell, Saluja, & Bruinicardi, 2005). The pancreatic juice is secreted from acinic and duct cells. The acinic cells secrete amylase, proteases, and lipases. These enzymes are responsible for the breakdown of carbohydrates, fats, and proteins. The duct cells secrete the water and electrolytes in the pancreatic juice. These cells keep a constant balance between the amount of bicarbonate/chloride and sodium/potassium that is secreted. The secretion of the pancreatic juice is the exocrine function of the pancreas. The endocrine function, although vital, is not discussed in this chapter.

The pancreatic duct carries the pancreatic juice, joins with the bile duct, and enters the duodenum where the contents assist the digestive process. The bile duct originates from the gallbladder, a muscular sac lying beneath and adjacent to the liver (Figure 44–3 ■). A simplistic way of thinking of it is as a conduit and storage receptacle for bile produced by the liver. The bile enters from the liver via the cystic duct and exits via the common bile duct, which then empties into the duodenum. Bile makes the fat molecules water soluble so the body may better utilize them.

The third and fourth portions of the duodenum are called the inferior/horizontal and are the ascending portions. This also describes the anatomic position of these portions of the duodenum. The second and third portions of the small bowel are called the jejunum and the ileum. These portions of the small bowel lie in the peritoneum but are tethered to the retroperitoneum. The surface of the small intestine is covered with small finger-like projections called villi. These in turn are covered with more projections called microvilli. This creates a larger surface area and a greater ability for absorption of nutrients before passing into the large intestine.

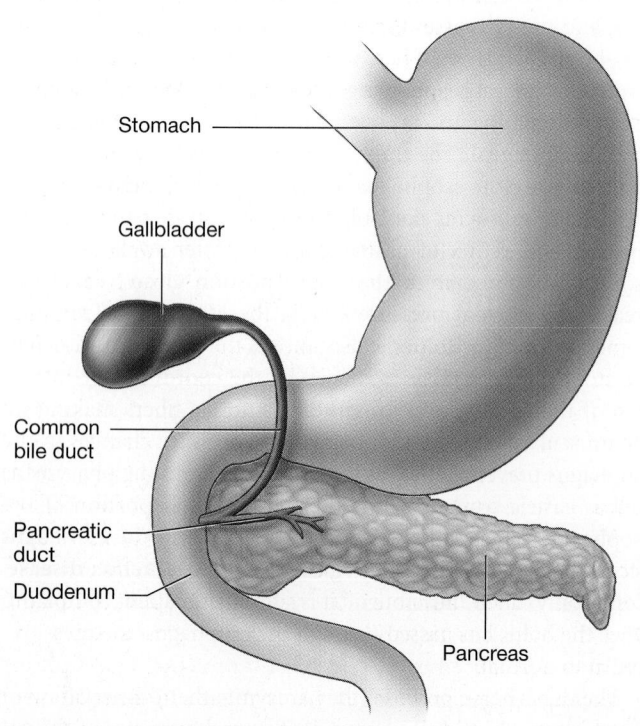

FIGURE 44–3 ■ The pancreas and gallbladder.

The large intestine starts at the ileocecal valve and ends at the anus. There are three anatomic and functional sections: the **colon** (the large intestine from the end of the ileum to the anal canal that surrounds the anus), the **rectum** (lower part of the large intestine between the sigmoid colon and the anal canal), and the **anal canal** (the last part of the large intestine situated between the rectum and the anus). The colon and rectum have five layers: the mucosa, submucosa, inner circular muscle, outer longitudinal muscle, and serosa. The serosa ends at the midrectum, and therefore there is no serosa in the mid and lower third of the rectum. The distal rectum also has inner smooth muscles, which join together to form the internal anal sphincter. The colon is also divided into sections. The cecum is the portion with the widest diameter and the thinnest muscle wall. It is the severe stretching of this thin wall that may lead to perforations. Paradoxically, the wide diameter makes it a rare location of obstruction.

The other terms commonly associated with the colon are *hepatic flexure, transverse colon, splenic flexure*, and *descending colon*. The ascending colon, on the right side of the abdomen, is fixed to the retroperitoneum. The transitional colon is more free and transverses the abdomen after the hepatic flexure. The greater omentum is attached to the superior and anterior portion of this part of the colon. The splenic flexure is the transition point to the descending colon, the portion on the left of the abdomen. The sigmoid colon is the narrowest and most mobile portion of the colon. It is because of this mobility that diseases of this portion of the colon may yield pain in the right lower abdomen, although the sigmoid is generally located in the left lower quadrant. Because of the lack of fixation, this part of the colon is subject to volvulus, when the colon turns into itself and the narrowness leads to common areas of obstruction.

The rectum is approximately 12 to 14 centimeters in length. It ends in the anal canal, which is 2 to 4 centimeters in length and is generally longer in men than in women. The differentiation between the anal canal and the rectum is at the dentate line. It is at this junction that the mucosa changes from the columnar rectal mucosa to the squamous anoderm. There are two sphincters: the internal sphincter and external sphincter at the distal rectum.

The function of the colon is primarily water absorption and electrolyte balance. This is why patients with diarrhea can have such imbalances in electrolytes. As the stool passes quickly through the colon when diarrhea is present, the normal function of absorption is gone. A large amount of water can be absorbed through the colon, up to 5,000 milliliters per day. Along with this is the transport of sodium, potassium, and chloride. Ammonia is produced when there is bacterial degradation of protein and urea. This ammonia is absorbed and transported to the liver, where it is metabolized. The absorption of ammonia is dependent on the intraluminal pH, which can be altered by a change in the bacteria levels leading to poor absorption of ammonia.

Stool is comprised of approximately 30% bacteria with the most prominent being *Escherichia coli,* known to cause grave illness when it contaminates food sources (Bullard & Rothenberger, 2005). Intestinal gas is primarily from swallowed air, but also is produced by intraluminal production and diffusion of blood. Nitrogen and oxygen are derived from the swallowing of air; carbon dioxide is from the breakdown of triglycerides and from the bicarbonate and hydrogen ions; and methane and hy-

drogen originate from the bacteria in the colon. The culmination of these gases is called flatus. The amount is dependent on the food intake, but 400 to 1,200 milliliters is released as flatus each day (Bullard & Rothenberger, 2005).

The motility of the bowel is what produces bowel sounds. Bowel sounds can be present without having a functioning bowel. For instance, with an ileus, there can be bowel sounds present, but as they are discoordinate; there is not resultant bowel movement or passing of gas. The movement of the intestine is called peristalsis. In the small intestine peristalsis occurs with the contraction of the longitudinal muscles causing the bowel to shorten and the contraction of the inner circular muscles resulting in luminal narrowing. This process moves the content along. In the colon the movement is slightly different. The movement of the colon is more in bursts with low and high amplitude contractions. The low amplitude movement moves the intraluminal content both antegrade and retrograde. It is thought this slows the process time through the colon, allowing for greater absorption. The high amplitude contraction is more coordinated, and the purpose is to move the stool mass along the colon to eventual elimination.

Defecation is the elimination of stool. This occurs with the stretching of the rectum, causing the relaxation of the internal sphincter with stool entering the rectal canal. Defecation can then occur as the rectum shortens and peristaltic waves force the stool out of the rectum. A problem with any of these steps can lead to constipation or incontinence.

Other organs involved in the process of digestion are the liver, pancreas, and gallbladder. Both the liver and the pancreas are multifunctional. The liver has functions that contribute to both metabolism and excretory functions. It is one of the largest organs and the largest gland. The pancreas has both endocrine and exocrine functions. The exocrine functions were discussed earlier. Although it is not within the scope of this chapter to discuss all the functions of the pancreas, an understanding of them is important and will be discussed in Chapter 46.

Related Structures

When examining the abdomen, it is important to have knowledge of all structures within the abdomen, even those that are not related to the gastrointestinal system. The abdomen is the only major cavity of the body not encased in bony structures. Although the lower ribs lend some support to the posterior cavity, the anterior cavity receives its structure from the muscle wall. The abdominal wall muscles consist of the rectus abdominus, the internal and external obliques, and the transverse abdominis (Figure 44–4, p. 1370). These muscles support the abdomen, allow for movement, and when contracted increase the intra-abdominal pressure.

The vascular support of the gastrointestinal system was touched on earlier in this chapter. Another major artery to be aware of and examine when doing an abdominal assessment is the aorta. This is the major artery descending from the heart through the diaphragm, through the abdominal cavity, and bifurcating at the lower abdomen into the right and left iliac arteries. The aorta is discussed more thoroughly in Chapter 37.

The spleen can be found in the left upper quadrant and is protected by the lower left ribs. It is directly inferior to the diaphragm.

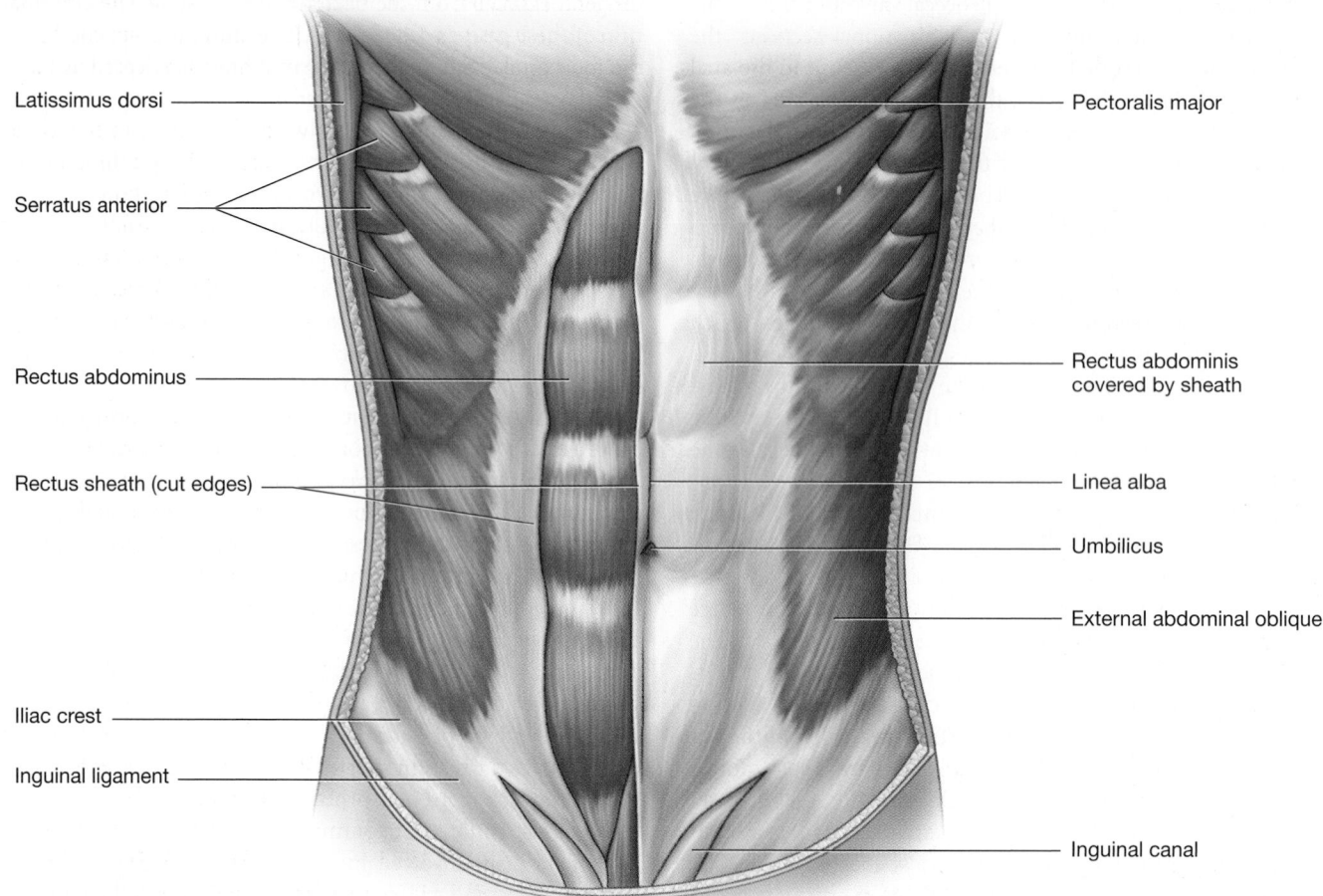

Latissimus dorsi

Serratus anterior

Rectus abdominus

Rectus sheath (cut edges)

Iliac crest

Inguinal ligament

Pectoralis major

Rectus abdominis covered by sheath

Linea alba

Umbilicus

External abdominal oblique

Inguinal canal

FIGURE 44–4 ■ Abdominal muscles.

The primary purpose of the spleen is to filter blood, destroy aged red blood cells, and return their by-products to the liver. Because of its vascular nature, this is an organ that when injured in a trauma to the abdomen, can be life threatening.

Urinary System

The organs of the urinary system lie within the abdomen. The kidneys and bladder lie within the space called the retroperitoneum. This is a space defined the by posterior peritoneum and the posterior body wall. Chart 44–1 lists the organs found in the peritoneal and retroperitoneal spaces.

The kidney is a complex organ and its function is discussed in detail in Chapter 47 ☉. The kidneys are a pair of organs located in the retroperitoneum on each side of the vertebral column. The right kidney is slightly lower than the left due to the presence of the liver. The kidneys are protected by the rib cage both anteriorly and posteriorly. They are also protected by a tough fibrous capsule, cushioned by perirenal fat and supported by the renal fascia. Put simply, the primary roles of the kidneys are to maintain fluid and electrolyte balance, help to achieve acid–base balance, and remove metabolic wastes. The renal system also has an important role in control of blood pressure, bone metabolism, and red blood cell synthesis (Figure 44–5 ■).

The urinary system also includes a drainage system: the ureters, bladder, and urethra. As urine is formed in the kidneys, it flows through the ureters, fibromuscular tubes, by peristalsis

CHART 44–1 **Organs Found in the Peritoneal and Retroperitoneal Spaces**

Peritoneal Cavity	Anterior Retroperitoneal Space	Posterior Retroperitoneal Space
Omentum	Pancreas	Kidneys
Liver	Duodenum	Ureters
Stomach	Ascending colon	Adrenal glands
Gallbladder	Descending colon	
Spleen		
Jejunum		
Ileum		
Transverse and sigmoid colon		
Cecum		
Appendix		

into the bladder. The peristaltic action helps prevent reflux of the urine back into the kidneys. The bladder, which is also muscular, holds the urine and has a capacity of 280 to 500 milliliters. When the bladder is stretched the parasympathetic nervous system signals the smooth muscle of the bladder to contract and expel the urine through the urethra. When urine is expelled, the

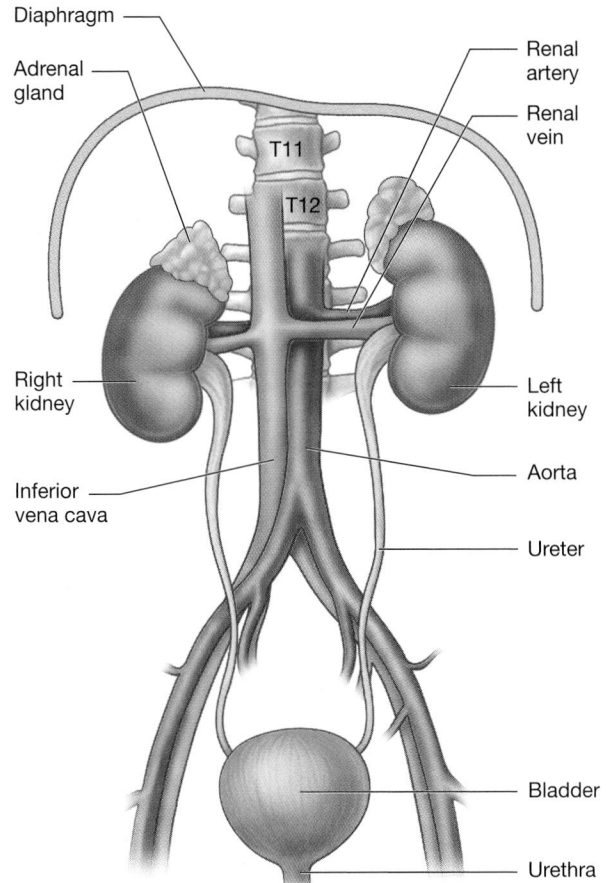

Diaphragm

Adrenal gland

T11

T12

Renal artery

Renal vein

Right kidney

Left kidney

Inferior vena cava

Aorta

Ureter

Bladder

Urethra

FIGURE 44–5 ■ The renal system.

voluntarily controlled external sphincter and the autonomically controlled internal sphincter must open. The length of the urethra is 3 to 5 centimeters in women and approximately 20 centimeters in men.

The reproductive organs are also found in the abdomen. These structures are found in the pelvic region in both males and females. Examination of this system will be addressed in Chapter 48 ☺.

■ History

A thorough history will help the nurse identify gastrointestinal and urinary symptoms as well as current or potential problems that may affect system function. Information learned from a thorough history and physical exam could help prevent undesirable responses to current therapies and treatment plans. The essential assessment data included in the gastrointestinal and urinary history are outlined next.

Biographic and Demographic Data

Biographic and demographic data can lead to a myriad of information to assist the nurse in narrowing the questions, thinking of potential causes of the problem, and formulating how to pose questions and educational plans to meet the patient's needs.

Biographical data should include age, gender, culture, and educational background. Age and gender are important in narrowing the potential causes of the patient's initial complaint. For

instance, **intussusception** is a common cause of intestinal obstruction in children 2 years of age and younger, but is not seen in adults. It is also three times more commonly seen in male children than females (Hackman, Newman, & Ford, 2005). The same is true of **pyloric stenosis**, as this is a cause of regurgitation and poor feeding in infants, generally within the first month, but would not be the cause of similar complaints in adults. Pyloric stenosis is not more gender prominent. Alternately, if an infant were having left lower quadrant abdominal pain, the nurse would not be thinking about diverticulitis in children or adolescents, which would be a common cause in adults and more common in people older than age 40 (Bullard & Rothenberger, 2005).

Demographic data may also glean important information. If a patient lives in an agricultural area or has well water as a source of drinking water, *Giardia* and *Cryptosporidium* infections need to be considered in the case of ongoing diarrhea and abdominal cramping. This might not be the common differential diagnosis for a person who lives in a high-rise apartment in the city.

Cultural Considerations

Cultural background is important in understanding many aspects of communication and care, because it may greatly influence the patient's perception of the complaint, who to speak with in the family, and what interventions the patient may have sought on her own. Additionally, if the patient has recently traveled to her country of origin, it may provide a clue as to other causes not commonly seen. For example, certain types of parasites may be more prevalent in other countries than in the United States.

It is important to consider the patient's cultural background and be sensitive to other therapies the patient might have relied on to decrease his symptoms. In Japanese, Chinese, and East Indian cultures, ginger might have been used for complaints of abdominal pain or digestive issues (Erickson D'Avanzo & Geissler, 2003). If ginger has been used for a period of time, there is a concern regarding bleeding times, because this herb may inhibit platelet aggregation and decrease platelet thromboxane production. This could be catastrophic if the cause of the initial complaint were an ulcer and now the patient is at greater risk from internal bleeding.

Chief Complaint

It is important to allow the patient to express his concerns and explain his problem in his own words. Interruptions should be kept to a minimum, but clarifying questions should be asked. Keep an open mind, because sometimes information that is initially thought of as trivial can be the answer to the problem. A patient with chest pain has a thorough cardiac work-up without any indication of the source of the chest pain. The condition still remains troublesome and the patient mentions an intake of a half gallon of ice cream on a daily basis. Although the symptoms are not common to lactose intolerance, it turns out the chest pain symptoms are resolved after a trial of stopping the ice cream for 2 weeks. This would not have been recognized if the interviewer had not listened to what the patient was saying and kept an open mind.

Taking a history is a very important encounter with a patient. This is a time when a relationship with a patient is started. Therefore, it is vital to develop these skills early in nursing practice.

Because there are core questions when taking a history, it is best to develop a systematic approach that fits one's personal style and comfort level. As a beginner, the nurse should try different methods she has observed used by others. As the nurse becomes an expert, an individual style will emerge, allowing all important information to be gathered and a relationship with the patient established. Characteristics, duration, exacerbation or diminishment of symptoms, and what is wrong or feared by the patient define the chief complaint.

Present Symptoms

Asking the question, Tell me how your symptoms started, is an appropriate way to start an interview. This open-ended question allows the patient to tell the nurse the history of her complaint. Allow the patient the time to answer such questions while giving her nonverbal feedback such as nodding. This can be followed by more clarifying questions, such as, Are there any exacerbating events? Is it reproducible? What has changed since the onset of your symptoms? Does the pain get worse after you eat? Has the character or intensity of the pain changed over time? Can you do something that makes the diarrhea start or go away? These are a few examples of clarifying questions to assist in homing in on the problem. This further clarifies the complaint. If there is pain present, ask the patient to describe it. This is sometimes difficult, especially with children who do not have the verbal skills or the vocabulary to describe what they are feeling.

When interviewing adults, the nurse should have a number of adjectives in his repertoire in order to assist the patient. Typical terms are described in Chart 44–2. *Stabbing, crushing, dull, sharp, radiating, knifelike*, and *burning* are a few of the adjectives that will assist the patient in giving a better description of symptoms. Listen to the words the person uses in characterizing her symptoms, as this can lead to further clues. A complaint of burning or gnawing pain can be associated with ulcers emanating from the duodenum or the stomach. However, these ulcers can be differentiated by the timing and the cause of the symptoms. For example, duodenal ulcers are generally postprandial and awake the subject at night, whereas the pain of the gastric ulcer is precipitated by food. A complaint of burning with urination can be associated with a urinary tract infection.

Duration of Symptoms

How long the problem has been present is very revealing. Has the person waited 4 months to have something evaluated? Possibly there was a change in the characteristic that prompted the sudden attention. Are the symptoms short in duration, but continue to return? Is there something happening in common with the return of the symptoms? A female patient may have had mild symptoms of stress incontinence such as leaking when coughing or sneezing for some time but would just wear a panty liner. Now she is experiencing incontinence when she has the urge to void so the problem has worsened and she is now seeking care.

Exacerbation or Diminishment of Symptoms

Many times a patient will try "home remedies" before presenting for evaluation of a problem. Be open to asking about alternative therapies such as acupuncture, herbal remedies, or moxibustion (an Asian medicine therapy). Did anything the patient tried make the symptoms better or worse? Why did the patient think a certain action would work? The answer to this question can lead into what the patient thinks in wrong. For instance, if the patient thinks his obstructive symptoms were caused by constipation alone, the use of laxatives not only could be ineffective but also could make the symptoms worse by causing increased peristalsis.

What Is Wrong? What Is Feared?

This leads to a very important and sometimes missed area of exploration. What does the patient *think* is wrong with her? Many times, the patient will have a very good idea of what might be the cause of the problem, without really knowing it. Other times, the possibility of exploring the patient's fears of what might be the cause allows the nurse the opportunity to allay her anxieties. Does the patient's culture lead her to believe certain things? For example, in the Hmong culture, illness is believed to be caused by either evil spirits or the loss of a spirit; therefore, it might be difficult for a person of this culture to believe that the cause of diarrhea is from poorly prepared foods (Erickson D'Avanzo & Geissler, 2003).

Is the weight loss due to a fear of eating, or is the person eating frequently in order to make the symptoms subside? Weight loss can be associated with gastric ulcers because of the avoidance of the pain. On the other hand, patients suffering from duodenal ulcers might gain weight as they are eating more frequently to avoid the symptoms. Does the patient notice a change in his skin color or the color of his urine? This could be very important, as hepatitis A can lead to dark-colored urine.

By the end of this part of the interview, the nurse needs to have information regarding the following characteristics: location, quality of the discomfort or pain, severity of the symptoms, onset and duration of the complaint, any changes to the symptoms, and what makes it better or worse. If any of these questions are not answered, the nurse needs to use more focused questions. Examples of sample questions are listed in Chart 44–3.

Past Medical History

Past medical history should always include certain elements; childhood diseases, immunizations, major illnesses, hospitalizations, diagnostic procedures, surgeries, sexual history, medications, and allergies are all considered imperative when gathering data. If the patient is vague regarding the information or does not remember the name of a procedure, assist the patient by giving the best description. For instance, a childhood illness may have required hospitalization or surgery, but the patient might not know whether she had pyloric stenosis or a bowel obstruction. A surgery for a repair of pyloric stenosis is more common in the first 6 months of life, whereas a bowel obstruction from intussusception can be seen up to 2 years of age. Having knowledge regarding surgical procedures and age-

CHART 44–2	**Descriptive Terms**	
Gnawing	Burning	Ripping
Colicky	Stabbing	Dull
Sharp	Crushing	Aching
Localized	Diffuse	

CHART 44–3	**Examples of History Questions**
Location	Where does it hurt the most?
Severity	At the time it is the most painful, how would you rate the pain on a scale of 1–10, with 10 being the worst?
	Does the pain change as it becomes more severe?
Duration	How long does the pain last?
Quality	What does the pain feel like?
Onset	When did the pain start?
	What were the circumstances of the pain starting?
Aggravating factors	What makes the pain worse?
Alleviating factors	What do you do to make the pain better?
Changes	Have your symptoms changed over a period of time?
	Does your pain change from one episode to another?

related diseases can assist in helping the patient clarify possible childhood history.

It is important also to consider where the patient was raised. Practices and availability of medical care and hospitalization will differ between industrialized nations and third world countries. In some circumstances the availability of medical history might be difficult if not impossible to obtain.

Childhood Illnesses and Immunizations

Childhood illnesses should include a history of any significant illnesses. Patients with a history of celiac disease and cystic fibrosis commonly will have an association with stooling problems and obstruction due to the bulking of the stool. A history of streptococcal infection, hypoplastic kidneys, or obstructive uropathy can lead to urinary tract or renal dysfunction as an adult.

Specifically ask about immunizations commonly given for hepatitis, hepatitis B, and hepatitis A. There is also a hepatitis D vaccine, although it is less common. A history of a cholera vaccine may be less common, unless there has been recent travel or if the patient has been residing in another country.

Previous Illnesses and Hospitalizations

A history of major illnesses is important and may impact the chief complaint. For instance, a person whose diabetes is poorly controlled who presents with symptoms of a partial bowel obstruction may be having **gastroparesis**, a slowing in emptying of the stomach due to the diabetes. A patient with hypertension and diabetes may develop renal failure due to the vascular changes with decreased circulation to the kidneys. A history of

Crohn's disease not only can be related to multiple surgeries but also heightens the awareness of the potential for anal fissures and fistulas.

The nurse should ask the patient about medical problems for which the patient is currently being treated. Ask whether there is any diagnosis the patient has been given in the past. A patient may be treated for recurrent hemorrhoids due to intermittent bright-red blood from the rectum. However, if the patient has never had a colonoscopy, the atrioventricular (AV) malformation in the lower colon might be missed as the diagnosis. Chart 44–4 lists common major illnesses.

Diagnostic Procedures and Surgeries

A history of procedures is important in the history of gastrointestinal and urinary diseases. Frequent procedures may include endoscopic evaluations. Common endoscopic evaluations include the following: **endoscopic retrograde cholangiopancreatography (ERCP)**, radiography following injection of a radiopaque material into the papilla of Vater; **flexible sigmoidoscopy**, a sigmoidoscope that uses fiber optics to inspect the sigmoid colon; and **colonoscopy**, visualization of the lower gastrointestinal tract through a flexible endoscope inserted through the anus. Patients might not remember what the name of the test is but would recall what symptoms led to the test. A person would not get an ERCP, which looks for gallbladder and pancreatic causes, if the chief complaint were blood in the stool.

As well as invasive testing, radiologic testing might be utilized in a work-up of GI symptomatology. Upper GI studies as well as a barium enema are common radiologic tests. An upper GI study might be the test of choice in a patient complaining of reflux. On the other hand, a **barium enema** is going to assist in evaluation of diverticular disease or possibly a tumor. For the renal system, a kidney-ureter-bladder (KUB) radiograph, intravenous pyelogram (IVP), renal ultrasound, computed tomography (CT), or magnetic resonance imaging, and renal angiography may help with a diagnosis.

When obtaining medical history from patients with gastrointestinal symptoms, past surgeries also play a major role. It is also important to correlate this information with the physical exam. At times patients will forget a surgery, especially if it was many years ago. Therefore, correlating the history with the scars on their abdomen is a helpful tool. When doing the abdominal examination, confirm what operation relates to which scar. This can also trigger more information from the patient. Pay particular attention to the area around the umbilicus, as laparoscopic scars are small and can be very faint. Chart 44–5 (p. 1374) lists common gastrointestinal surgeries.

Sexual History

A person's sexual practices can have an effect on certain gastrointestinal and urinary complaints. It is important to become comfortable with asking patients not only about their sexual

CHART 44–4	**Major Illnesses with GI-Related Complaints**			
Celiac sprue	Diabetes	Hirschsprung's disease	Crohn's disease	HIV
Alcoholism	Hyperlipidemia	Cystic fibrosis	Cancer	Hepatitis (A, B, C)
Inflammatory bowel disease	Thyroid problems	Hypertension	Hypercholesteremia	Depressive disorders

CHART 44–5	Common Gastrointestinal Surgeries

Appendectomy—removal of the appendix

Cholecystectomy—removal of the gallbladder

Choledochojejunostomy—opening between the common bile duct and the jejunum

Colostomy—opening of the colon through the abdominal wall

Gastrectomy—removal of part or all of the stomach

Ileostomy—opening of the ileum through the abdominal wall

Pyloroplasty—repair of the pylorus or to increase the opening

Vagotomy—resection of the branch of the vagus nerve

activity but also about their individual practices. The more self-conscious and uncomfortable the nurse is with asking these questions, the more the patient is going to be reluctant to self-disclose.

Anal intercourse can be related to disease of the anus and the rectum. Rectal cancer from human *papillomavirus* is important to catch and treat early. It is also possible to get other sexually transmitted diseases such as gonorrhea in the rectum. If the question is never asked, the problem will be overlooked with potential detrimental results for the patient. If a woman has frequent cystitis, it is important to ask and teach her that urinating shortly after intercourse is important to flush any bacteria that might have entered the urethra.

Medications

Medication history should include what is prescribed, what is taken over the counter, and also medications given to the patient by friends or family. Over-the-counter antacid is a commonly overused medication. What type and how often the medication is taken may also be important. Remember to include questions about laxatives and enemas. Inquire as to how frequently patients are using these agents. A frequent use of either can cause a decrease in bowel tone and thus increase the constipation and therefore the use of the laxative.

A history of frequent aspirin or nonsteroidal anti-inflammatory drug (NSAID) use is also significant. Make sure to ask about both. Are patients taking either of these frequently and then following it with an antacid in order to make the stomach pains subside so they can treat the discomfort from arthritis? NSAIDs, antihypertensive drugs that block angiotensin, and aminoglycoside antibiotics can cause an acute or chronic decline in kidney function.

Remember to ask about the use of herbal remedies or supplements. Some of the medications can be hepatotoxic or have other adverse effects not known to the patient. If the medication is a combination of medicines, it is sometimes difficult to verify exactly what the patient is taking, especially if the supplement is a combination of different types of herbs. At times further research is warranted to find all the different ingredients in a powder or tincture.

Allergies

A history of allergies should include not only the offending agent but also the allergic symptom it produces. Many patients mistake nausea as an allergic reaction when it is only a side effect. Also include any food or environmental allergies. Food allergies are especially important when examining a patient for gastrointestinal symptoms. Ask whether there is a certain food that is avoided due to undesirable effects.

Family History

A thorough family history is important and should include a relevant health history of the patient's siblings, parents, and grandparents. Some patients will include a medical history of a relative not related by blood. In other words, a patient may provide a medical history of an uncle, and the nurse may find out the uncle is married to the mother's sister. The nurse must make sure to clarify that she wants only direct relatives included in the history. Some diseases of the gastrointestinal system with hereditary components are Crohn's, familial polyposis, colon cancer, and malabsorption of nutrients such as fructose and folate. Adult onset diseases of the renal system with hereditary components include polycystic disease of the kidney, renal amyloidosis, and some renal cancers.

Social History

Social history includes any alcohol, tobacco, or recreational drug usage, including how often and how much of the substance is used or taken. For example, if a patient has a positive history of smoking, ask how many cigarettes he smokes per day. The same is true for alcohol use to determine whether he is at risk for hepatic disease due to the years of alcohol consumption. Some patients may be reluctant to discuss these habits. Ask these questions in a matter of fact way so the patient does not feel stigmatized or judged. Patients also need to know that this information is confidential and used only to assist in their care.

Habits

Changes in a patient's normal routine can provide clues to the nurse regarding the symptomology of the complaint. This information will also help to guide the nurse's line of questioning.

The nurse should ask the patient about her diet. Have there been any changes related to her current complaint? A recent change in diet can affect gastrointestinal illnesses. An example is the patient who completes a liquid fast and then starts eating again. This sudden stimulation may cause a first attack of cholecystitis, an inflammation of the gallbladder.

Stool patterns also should be included in this section. What is the patient's normal stool pattern? For some patients, stooling 1 to 2 times per week is very normal, whereas others need to have daily movement. Are there changes in consistency or color? Pencil-thin stools can be a concern for colon cancer but also can indicate large hemorrhoids. Is the act of defecation painful? Rectal fissures can be excruciating and lead to constipation due to the fear of defecation.

Patients who are developing renal failure may experience a metallic taste in their mouth from the uremia, which may cause a decrease in appetite. Also, rapid weight gain accompanied by orthopnea may be a sign of fluid overload from renal failure.

Recent Travel

Any recent history of travel is significant information to obtain. Certain gastrointestinal illnesses such as diarrhea are commonly linked to travel. Traveler's diarrhea is a common illness of many travelers both abroad and locally. This is a name commonly used when a person has diarrhea either while traveling or after; but it can be caused by many different agents including viral, bacterial, and parasitic organisms, and is generally contracted through contaminated food or water. It can be self-limiting or cause problems for an extended period of time. Certain organisms such as *Vibrio cholerae* may be common only in certain areas, but *Giardia* can be found in most countries, including the United States. Therefore, it is important to get a complete history of travel, both recent and as far back as several years, if necessary.

Physical Examination

When performing the physical examination of the patient with abdominal complaints, it is imperative that the nurse take a systematic approach to the examination. If it is done out of order, important findings may be obscured due to pain and the patient's subsequent inability to cooperate with the examination. The order is different than when assessing other systems. Inspection should come first, followed by auscultation, percussion, and finally palpation to avoid eliciting or increasing pain. It is important for the nurse to assess the patient's general state of health. Examining a patient experiencing pain from appendicitis is very different from examining a patient with complaints of mild diarrhea. Positioning the patient for the optimal examination does not always mean it is optimal for the examiner. For instance, a patient may not be able to lie flat in a supine position. A more comfortable position may be to have the knees bent. The nurse should work with the patient in establishing a comfortable position for the patient; this will make the examination more productive for both of them.

Inspection

The first element of the physical examination of the abdomen is inspection. This is done initially by just watching the patient. Is the patient able to walk with a normal posture, or is the person walking hunched over, protecting her abdomen? When the patient is sitting, is her posture normal? Is the patient able to sit or is she curled into a fetal position on the examination table or bed? Is the patient able to be still or must she move about due to the colicky pain of **renal calculi** (kidney stones)? These observations are the first part of the data collection and contribute to the ongoing collection of data.

Inspection should include the mouth. Inspect the mucosa for redness, any lesions, and moistness. The tongue should be inspected for any redness, inflammation, fissure, ulcerations, or lesions. The pharynx is evaluated by using a tongue blade to hold the tongue out of the way. Having the patient tilt his head back slightly assists in visualization of the soft palate, uvula, and movement of this structure. Inspect the uvula, tonsils, soft palate, and anterior and posterior pillars. Have the patient say "aah," and the soft palate and uvula should rise symmetrically. Inspection continues after the patient is lying flat and the abdomen is exposed. This might be difficult if the patient is unable to lie flat due to pain. However, inspection can be done with the patient in different positions, although this may not be as optimal.

Before the patient is touched, important data can be collected. Look at the contour of the patient's abdomen both obliquely and straight on. Sometimes masses, fluid waves, or change in contour can be seen. A **ventral hernia**, a hernia through the abdominal wall, is very distinct in an oblique view, particularly when the patient contracts the abdominal muscles. Look at the umbilicus, which is normally midline and inverted. The umbilicus will become everted with pregnancy, ascites, or an underlying mass. It can become enlarged and everted with an umbilical hernia. Observe the skin for any changes such as scars, color changes, hair patterns, or presence of striae. Note that hair patterns will vary between male and female patients. There can also be differences between different races. Female patients with hirsutism, excessive growth of hair in unusual places, may have increased hair growth along the pubic mons extending to the umbilicus. Asian women will demonstrate finer and scarcer patterns than Caucasian or African American women. The nurse should also be cognizant of coloration changes between skin tones. For example, what appears red on a light skin tone will have a different appearance on a darker skin tone. Observe the skin for redness with localized inflammation, jaundice with hepatitis, rashes, or cutaneous angiomas (spider nevi) that occur with portal hypertension or liver disease.

The inspection is the time to ask about the scars and the surgery related to them. Sometimes readdressing questions during this time will assist the patient in recalling further information. It also allows the nurse to ask a question in a slightly different manner, causing further recollection for the patient.

Auscultation

Auscultation is the second step in the physical examination process. This is an important step, and the nurse should become comfortable with auscultation and the sound of the abdomen. However, contrary to previous teaching, in the realm of an abdominal examination, bowel sounds may mean very little. A person can have acute peritonitis but still have bowel sounds. A patient with a postoperative ileus may have very loud bowel sounds, but the patient is distended and the bowels are not functioning in a coordinated pattern. Complete absence of bowel sounds would be significant, but keep in mind that the nurse would have to listen for a minimum of 5 minutes in all four quadrants. That being said, bowel sounds should be auscultated prior to palpation, as the deep palpation can affect the frequency of bowel sounds. The nurse should listen over all four quadrants for a period of 2 to 5 minutes. Note the frequency, pitch, and character of the bowel sounds. Ask the patient about passing flatus. Like all parts of the examination, it should be correlated with the history.

When placing a nasogastric tube, auscultation of the abdomen is imperative. The nurse should always listen over the epigastrium while pushing air in the tube after placement. A gurgling sound over this area should be heard if the nasogastric tube is in the correct position.

The epigastrium and bilateral upper quadrants should be auscultated with both the diaphragm and the bell of the stethoscope. This is the area to listen for the aorta and renal arteries. The nurse is listening for a bruit or schussing sound, which is an indication of an abnormality. Both groins should also be auscultated for bruits of the iliac arteries. Figure 44–6 ■ (p. 1376) indicates sites to listen for vascular sounds.

A ticklish patient may not tolerate the touch of the stethoscope. Having the patient place the stethoscope where the nurse

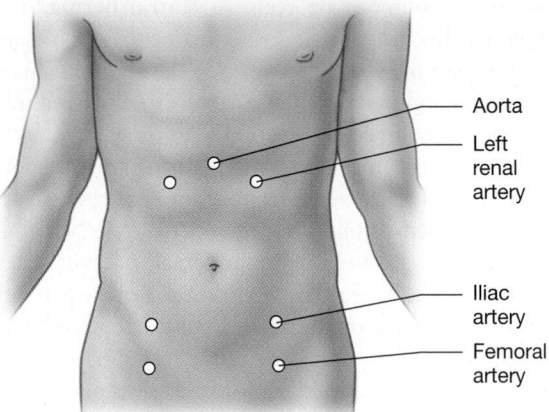

Sites to listen for vascular sounds

FIGURE 44–6 ■ Sites for vascular sounds.

directs will enhance the examination of this type of patient. This not only distracts the patient, but avoids tickling.

Percussion

Percussion, the third step in the physical examination process, is done by placing the nondominant hand flat on the surface of the abdomen. The first joint of the index or third finger is then struck gently with the index or third finger of the dominant hand (Figure 44–7 ■). The nurse should practice this on different types of surfaces and listen to the difference in the sound. A good example is on a melon or even a thigh. The nurse should be able to hear the difference. It is also important to have nails clipped short so as not to cause injury to self or the patient.

Percussing the abdomen will elicit different sounds. There should be the hollow sound, similar to that of tapping on a watermelon, over the epigastric area and sometimes over the bowels. If this hollow sound is throughout the entire abdomen, it is called **tympany** and is indicative of an obstruction or distention of the abdomen. This sound is produced by air in the intestine.

The liver and a full bladder give off a dull sound, similar to that when percussing a piece of meat. The liver edges can be determined by percussing from the lower right abdomen to the edge of the rib. At the transition of the hollow sound to the dull sound, the nurse will find the liver edge. Measure this area by determining how many finger breadths it is from the costal margin.

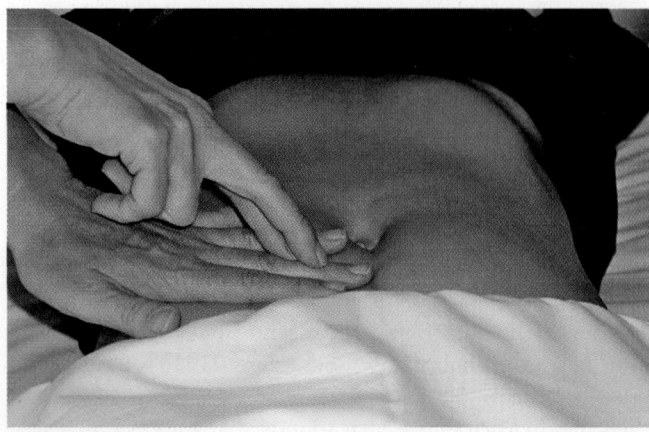

FIGURE 44–7 ■ Percussion of abdomen.
Source: Cheryl Wraa

Similarly, the spleen can be measured in the same fashion. However, the edge of the spleen should not be below the costal margin. It is more likely found near the 10th left rib. If it is below the rib, this is an indication of an abnormal enlargement. Palpation of the area should be done with great care. Percussion can also elicit pain particularly in patients with acute peritonitis, inflammation of the peritoneum.

The size of the bladder can be percussed especially if the patient has a full or distended bladder. In order to percuss the kidney, the patient must be lying on one side or be in a sitting position. The nurse should make a fist and gently strike the patient with the ulnar surface of the fist in the costal vertebral angle. This should be jarring to the patient, but should not elicit any pain. If this action causes pain, it is a sign of kidney infection or injury.

Case Study

A female patient presents with a history of nausea, vomiting, and abdominal pain. On further questioning she reveals she has been tired recently and thinks she has the flu because of generalized body aches. She usually smokes a pack a day but has had only 2 to 3 cigarettes in the past 2 days. She attributes this to not feeling well. She thinks she caught a flu virus because she recently spent over 10 hours on a plane while returning from a trip overseas.

On inspection the nurse notes that the patient has a yellowish tinge to her skin. She has diffused abdominal pain greater in the right upper quadrant. When the nurse percusses the right upper quadrant, there is a dull sound extending 3 finger breadths below the right costal margin. This indicates the patient has hepatomegaly. The most likely cause of this patient's complaints is hepatitis A.

The clinician reaches this conclusion by reviewing the information gathered from both the history and the physical examination.

Palpation

Palpation, the final step in the physical examination process, should start with the mouth and throat area. Any lesions or abnormalities of the oral pharynx should be palpated using a gloved finger. Lesions of the cheek are better felt by placing one finger inside the mouth and one on the cheek. By isolating the lesion between the fingers, the size and shape of the lesion is better defined.

Palpation of the abdomen should be done in a systematic pattern. Start with light palpation. This assists in the identification of muscle resistance and more superficial findings. In patients who are sensitive, even light palpation will cause muscle resistance. Maneuvers to relax the patient are having her bend her legs, using a stethoscope to palpate, or having the patient place her hand under the nurse's, using her hand to press down. After the patient becomes relaxed, the nurse can slide the nurse's hand under the patient's hand. When using the stethoscope to palpate, place the stethoscope on the abdomen, and while listening, the nurse can press harder on the abdomen, eliciting any pain the patient might sense.

The next step is deeper palpation. The nurse should use the palmar surface of the hand and palpate in all four quadrants. If the patient has a complaint of abdominal pain, palpate the area the patient identified as painful last.

The liver edge should be palpable. The nurse should recall where he first percussed the edges of the liver border and place his fingertips below this area. The hand should be placed lateral to the rectus muscle on the right hand side. Press gently down and up toward the ribs (Figure 44–8 ■). The nurse should have the patient take a deep breath. As the patient is inhaling, the liver edge will come down under the nurse's fingertips. A normal liver feels firm, sharp, and has a clear edge. A cirrhotic liver will feel stiffer and the edge will be irregular. The edge will also be palpable farther down on the abdomen.

To palpate the spleen, the nurse should be standing on the patient's right. Reach across with the left hand and place it on the lateral chest wall at the 10th rib. The hand should be placed below the costal margin. While supporting the rib with the left hand, gently palpate up toward and under the costal margin. As the patient takes a deep breath, the tip of the spleen might be palpated as it descends. The spleen is not always palpable, especially in adults. If it is easily palpated below the costal margin, the spleen is considered enlarged and medical staff should be notified.

Both the kidneys should be palpated, but the right kidney is easily palpated and the left kidney is rarely felt. When palpating the right kidney, place the left hand on the right flank area with gentle pressure toward the abdomen. Place the right hand on the abdomen parallel to the costal margin. Press the hands firmly together. The lower pole of the kidney should be felt as the patient takes a deep breath. At times the patient will have a sharp sensation as the kidney pole passes through the nurse's hands. This is not considered a painful sensation.

The left kidney is rarely palpable. However, this area should be examined for any abnormalities. The maneuver is the same. Place the left hand along the flank area. In some patients this can be accomplished from the right side of the table. However, if the patient is large or the left side cannot be reached in this fashion, perform this examination from the left side of the table (Figure 44–9 ■). The kidneys should feel firm and smooth. It is considered abnormal if an irregular surface is palpated, the kidney extends significantly lower than the rib cage, or obvious trauma is noted.

The aorta is palpated in the area above the umbilicus and slightly left. This may be difficult to palpate in the obese abdomen and can sometimes be seen as pulsating in the scaphoid

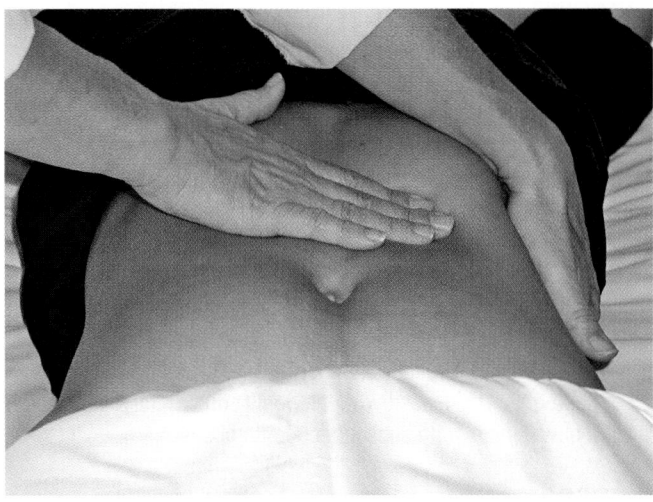

FIGURE 44–9 ■ Palpation of kidneys.
Source: Cheryl Wraa

abdomen. If the pulsation of the aorta is easily palpated, attempt to isolate it between the thumb and finger.

■ Adjunctive Physical Examinations

Certain physical examinations are specific to conditions of the abdomen in particular. These adjunctive exams will assist in narrowing or confirming the nurse's differential diagnosis.

Rebound Tenderness

Rebound tenderness describes tenderness greater when the pressure is released than when it is applied and is a reliable sign of peritoneal inflammation. To perform this test the nurse gently presses into the abdomen and then releases the pressure. Start light and then with greater firmness as the examination warrants. Start away from the area of pain and work toward the area identified by the patient as hurting the most. If a great deal of discomfort is found away from the identified source, stop. There is no further benefit of causing more pain to the patient.

Case Study

A 16-year-old male presents after a motor vehicle crash. On inspection an ecchymotic stripe is seen across the lower abdomen about 4 to 5 centimeters below the umbilicus. There are no other masses visualized. When palpating, the upper quadrants are palpated first, as the ecchymotic area will be the most tender. The initial examination reveals mild tenderness to palpation in the left lower quadrant. There is no rebound at the initial examination.

The continued work-up would include lab tests, primarily a complete blood count (CBC), to examine hemorrhagic anemia or leukocytosis to indicate an inflammatory process.

After several hours, this male patient complains of increased abdominal pain. The CT scan showed some free fluid in the pelvis, but no injury to the spleen or the liver. The concern would be a progressing injury. By reviewing all the information, the most likely cause for the increased pain is a possible bowel injury.

The method in which this patient is examined will be changed to meet his changing complaints. Palpation should always be farthest away from the point of identified pain. At this

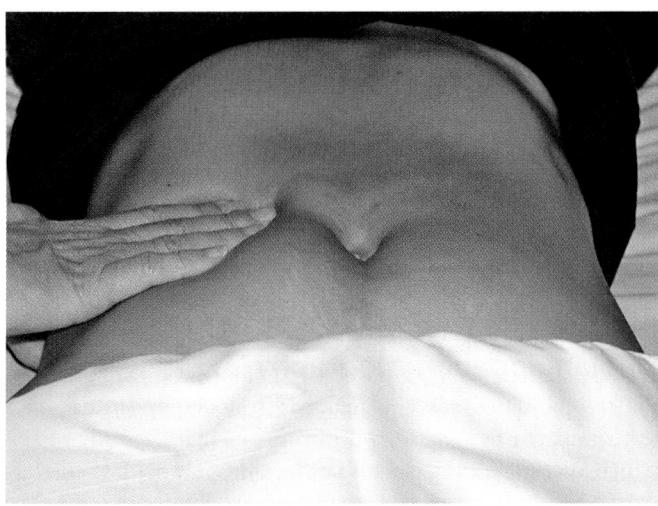

FIGURE 44–8 ■ Palpation of abdomen.
Source: Cheryl Wraa

juncture, palpation should not be done with the fingertips, but rather by placing the middle finger gently on the surface of the abdomen and tapping over the second joint with the finger of the other hand. Pain elicited with this maneuver is common in patients with peritonitis. If the patient has involuntary contraction of the abdominal muscles and pain with this examination, it may not be necessary to proceed further. However, if this does not indicate increased pain, examination for rebound tenderness may be required. This is done by pressing in gently with the fingertips of one hand and releasing rapidly. If the pain is worse at the time the fingertips are released, the examination is positive for rebound tenderness, yet another indication of peritonitis. These positive signs would support the diagnosis of a bowel injury with subsequent peritonitis.

Iliopsoas Sign

When this test is positive, it indicates an inflammation of the psoas muscle, which lies lateral to the lumbar vertebrae and passes deep into the inguinal ligament to the lesser trochanter of the femur. The lumbar plexus of nerves is embedded in the psoas. The iliacus muscle lies along the lateral side of the psoas muscle and extends across the sacroiliac joint to attach to the iliac fossa. Together these muscles form the iliopsoas, the chief flexor of the thigh. Clinically, the **iliopsoas** has relations to the kidneys, ureters, cecum, appendix, sigmoid colon, pancreas, lumbar lymph nodes, and nerves of the posterior abdominal wall. When there is intra-abdominal inflammation or disease of any of theses structures, movement of the iliopsoas causes pain. With the patient lying flat, have the patient flex the leg closest to the examiner. With the nurse's hand flat against the lateral surface of the thigh, have the patient push against the palm with some resistance applied. The test is positive if this causes the patient pain. Repeat on the other side.

Obturator Sign

This test is positive in patients with inflammation along the obturator internus muscle. Positive tests can be related to appendicitis, diverticulitis, and pelvic inflammatory disease, to name a few. The nurse should stand along the side of the bed while performing this test. Have the patient bend her knee and flex at the hip. While supporting the leg, flex the thigh to a right angle and externally and internally rotate the leg. Perform this on both sides.

Murphy's Sign

This test is positive when a person has inflammation of the gallbladder, as seen in cholecystitis. The nurse should stand on the right side of the bed. Place the hand flat on the abdomen with the fingertips just below the right costal margin. Have the patient gently inhale. As the liver and gallbladder descend into the fingertips, pain will be present when there is inflammation.

■ Radiologic Testing

The use of radiologic testing is important in establishing the diagnosis of many abdominal complaints. Although it is not the goal of this chapter to provide education on all radiologic tests, a few will be listed.

Computed Tomography Scan of the Abdomen and Pelvis

The CT scan is very versatile in the information it provides to the clinician caring for the patient. Abscesses, fluid collections, vascular disorders, obstructions, and trauma can be seen. For trauma, however, this test is better for injury to solid organs such as the liver and spleen, rather than to hollow organs such of the bowel or bladder. This test can utilize intravenous, rectal, or oral contrast to enhance the images.

Ultrasound

Ultrasound is used for evaluation of the gallbladder, kidneys, and urinary tract, and at times the appendix. It can also be used for identification of free fluid in trauma patients with suspected intrabdominal injury.

Kidney-Ureter-Bladder (KUB) Versus Three-Way Abdominal Films

A **KUB** stands for kidney, ureters, and bladder and is also known as a "plain film of the abdomen." This is obtained with the patient lying flat and the x-ray plate placed beneath. It helps to determine position, size, and structure of the kidneys and urinary tract. It is useful in evaluating for the presence of calculi and masses. Also, this is an excellent test for obstruction, because it shows the air in the colon nicely. The three-way abdominal series not only incorporates the KUB view but also includes a picture of the abdomen with the patient on his side as well as one upright. This test helps differentiate air fluid levels in the intestinal tract.

Barium Enema

In this radiologic test, barium contrast is inserted in the rectum. The barium fills the colon and shows the contour of the intralumen. This test would enhance intraluminal processes such as colon cancer or diverticular disease.

■ Invasive Procedures

Invasive procedures are uncomfortable and at times painful. For that reason, most of these procedures are done with conscious sedation.

Colonoscopy and Endoscopy

Colonoscopy and endoscopy allow the clinician to visualize the intraluminal space directly. The colonoscopy is a flexible tube with a small camera at the end that is inserted through the rectum and visualizes the intraluminal surface of the colon. This instrument also allows for biopsies to be taken. The same is true for the endoscopy; however, this similar flexible tube visualizes the upper GI tract and is inserted through the mouth.

Endoscopic Retrograde Cholangiopancreatography

Endoscopic retrograde cholangiopancreatography (ERCP) is a test similar to the endoscopy, but this includes a study of the pancreatic and bile ducts. This test is commonly used when evaluating for cholecystitis or pancreatitis. When the scope reaches the duodenum, the endoscopist locates the opening into the ducts or the ampulla. A small tube is placed in the ampulla, and contrast dye is injected that allows for visualization of the ducts. Removal of stones, biopsy, and sphincterotomy may be performed during this procedure.

Common Laboratory Studies

The significance of these laboratory tests (Chart 44–6) will be discussed in more detail in the disorder chapters. Chart 44–6 lists common studies used in the assessment of gastrointestinal, liver, pancreatic, renal, and urinary functions and their clinical significance.

Gerontological Considerations

The aging adult may have increased deposits of subcutaneous fat on the abdomen and hips as it redistributes away from the ex-

tremities. The musculature of the abdomen is thinner and has less tone. If the patient is thin, the nurse may be able to visualize peristalsis when the patient is lying supine. Also, the softer abdominal wall may make palpation of the organs easier. Because the lungs may be distended and the diaphragm depressed, the liver is palpated lower, appearing 1 to 2 centimeters below the costal margin with inhalation.

Summary

All nurses need to have the skills to understand and assess patients with abdominal and urinary complaints. Although these are common complaints of patients, the causes can be very complicated, with a large number of differential diagnoses. Therefore, it is important for the nurse to understand the underlying anatomy and physiology. With practice and further experience, the skills of the interview and examination will improve.

CHART 44–6 **Common Laboratory Studies**

Study	Clinical Significance
Studies of GI function	
• Stool culture	Detection of bacteria, ameba, or worms Large amounts of pus associated with ulcerative colitis, abscesses, and anorectal fistula
Studies of liver function	
• Alkaline phosphatase	↑ with biliary obstruction and hepatitis
• Aspartate aminotransferase (AST)	↑ with hepatocellular injury
• Alanine aminotransferase (ALT)	↑ with hepatocellular injury
• Lactate dehydrogenase (LDH)	↑ with hypoxic and primary liver injury
• Serum bilirubin	
• Indirect	↑ with hemolysis
• Direct	↑ with hepatocellular injury or obstruction
• Total	↑ with biliary obstruction
• Urine bilirubin	↓ with biliary obstruction
• Urine urobilinogen	↑ with hemolysis or shunting
• Albumin	↓ with hepatocellular injury
• Globulin	↑ with hepatitis
• Prothrombin time	↑ with chronic liver disease or vitamin K deficiency
• Partial thromboplastin time	↑ with severe liver disease or heparin therapy
Studies of pancreatic function	
• Serum amylase	↑ with pancreatic inflammation
• Serum lipase	↑ with pancreatic inflammation
• Urine amylase	↑ with pancreatic inflammation
• Stool fat	Decreased pancreatic lipase increases stool fat
Studies of renal function	
• Blood urea nitrogen (BUN)	↑ with poor renal function
• Serum creatinine	↑ with damage to nephrons
• Urine osmolality	↑ fluid volume deficit ↓ fluid volume excess
• Serum osmolality	↑ fluid volume deficit ↓ fluid volume excess

NCLEX® REVIEW

1. An adult patient is experiencing left lower quadrant pain. The nurse realizes this patient might be demonstrating:
   1. Acute appendicitis.
   2. Intussusception.
   3. Pyloric stenosis.
   4. Diverticulitis.

2. The nurse is preparing to conduct a physical examination on a patient. Which of the following should the nurse do first?
   1. Inspection
   2. Percussion
   3. Auscultation
   4. Palpation

3. When percussing a patient's bladder, the nurse hears a dull sound. Which of the following would this sound indicate?
   1. An empty bladder
   2. A bladder obstruction
   3. Kidney stones
   4. A full bladder

4. While assessing a patient, the nurse discovers rebound tenderness. This finding would be indicative of:
   1. Enlarged gallbladder.
   2. A negative obturator sign.
   3. Inflammatory process in the abdomen.
   4. A positive Murphy's sign.

5. A patient states she has had no abdominal surgeries but the nurse sees a large abdominal scar. Which should the nurse do?
   1. Document what the patient stated.
   2. Ask the patient what caused the abdominal scar.
   3. Assume the patient doesn't want to talk about the scar and change the subject.
   4. Palpate the scar.

Answers for review questions appear in Appendix D

KEY TERMS

anal canal *p.1369*
antrum *p.1367*
barium enema *p.1373*
cardia *p.1367*
cardioesophageal *p.1367*
colon *p.1369*
colonoscopy *p.1373*
endoscopic retrograde
   cholangiopancreatography
   (ERCP) *p.1373*

esophagus *p.1367*
flexible sigmoidoscopy *p.1373*
gastroparesis *p.1373*
GERD, gastroesophageal reflux
   disease *p.1367*
iliopsoas *p.1378*
immunoglobulin A *p.1366*
intussusception *p.1371*
KUB *p.1378*

peristalsis *p.1367*
pharyngoesophageal *p.1367*
pyloric stenosis *p.1371*
rectum *p.1369*
renal calculi *p.1375*
retroperitoneal space *p.1367*
tympany *p.1376*
ventral hernia *p.1375*

PEARSON
EXPLORE **mynursingkit™**

MyNursingKit is your one stop for online chapter review materials and resources. Prepare for success with additional NCLEX®-style practice questions, interactive assignments and activities, web links, animations and videos, and more!

Register your access code from the front of your book at
www.mynursingkit.com

REFERENCES

Bullard, K.M., & Rothenberger, D. A. (2005). Colon, rectum and anus. *Schwartz's principles of surgery.* Retrieved February 26, 2006, from http://www. accessmedicine.com/content.aspx?aID=810060&searchStr=colon

Erickson D'Avanzo, C., & Geissler, E. (2003). *Mosby's pocket guide: Cultural health assessment.* St. Louis: Elsevier.

Fisher, W. E., Andersen, D. K., Bell, R. H., Saluja, A. K., & Bruinicardi, F. C. (2005). Pancreas. *Schwartz's principles of surgery.* Retrieved February 24, 2006, from http://www.accessmedicine.com/content.aspx?aID=812451&searchStr=pancreatic+juice#812451

Hackman, D. J., Newman, K., & Ford, H. R. (2005). Gastrointestinal tract. *Schwartz's principles of surgery.* Retrieved February 25, 2007,

from http://www.accessmedicine.com/content.aspx?aID=818606&searchStr=intussusception#818606

Urdan, L. D., Stacy, K. M., & Lough, M. E. (2006). *Thelan's critical care nursing* (5th ed.). St. Louis: Mosby.

Caring for the Patient with Gastrointestinal Disorders

Debera Thomas
Douglas Sutton

Outcome-Based Learning Objectives

After studying this chapter, the learner will be able to:

1. Describe the different causes of stomatitis and related nursing care.

2. Compare and contrast pathophysiology, clinical manifestations, and treatment with related nursing care of patients with peptic ulcer disease (PUD) and gastroesophageal reflux disease (GERD).

3. Develop a teaching plan for patients with celiac disease.

4. Analyze the similarities and differences between different types of inflammatory bowel disease.

5. List the risk factors for developing GERD.

6. Delineate nursing care for a patient with colon cancer.

7. Describe the different intestinal tubes and related nursing care for patients with intestinal obstruction.

8. Discuss the clinical manifestations of the complications of gastric surgery.

9. Outline the nursing care of a patient with an ileostomy, colostomy, and continent ileostomy.

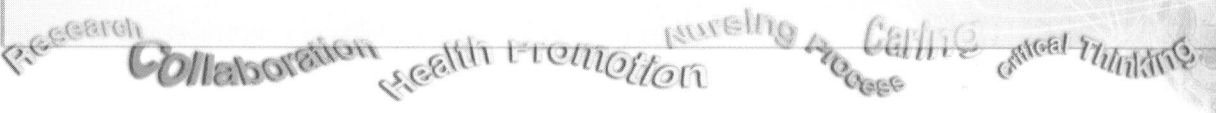

THE GASTROINTESTINAL (GI) tract consists of a hollow tube extending from the mouth to the anus and includes the esophagus, stomach, small intestine, large intestine, and rectum, as well as the accessory organs involved in digestion such as the pancreas, liver, and gallbladder. Anatomy of the gastrointestinal tract is presented in Chapter 44 , and disorders of the liver, gallbladder, and pancreas are discussed in Chapter 46 . Because the major functions of the GI tract are to prepare ingested food for absorption, absorb nutrients, and eliminate wastes, disorders of this system can have devastating effects on nutritional status, lifestyle, body image, and health in general. Most disorders of the GI tract can be classified as inflammatory, ulcerative, structural, or neural in nature.

DISORDERS OF THE MOUTH AND ESOPHAGUS

Disorders of the mouth and esophagus are the result of a variety of causes ranging from viral to nutritional. Likewise, diseases may be as common as a gastroesophageal reflux disease or as serious as esophageal cancer.

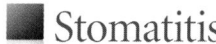 Stomatitis

Stomatitis, the generalized inflammation of the oral mucosa, is classified according to the etiology. Similar to stomatitis is glos-

sitis, or inflammation of the tongue, which is caused by many of the same factors that cause stomatitis, so they may often coexist. These problems may be caused by a virus, bacteria, fungus, trauma, chemical agents, or nutritional deficiencies.

Pathophysiology

The oral mucosa consists of a thin, fragile layer of squamous epithelial cells with a rich blood supply. Cellular turnover is rapid, thus promoting quick healing but also providing an opportunity for cellular mutation and damage to these rapidly dividing cells. Because of the abundant blood supply and the fragility of the epithelial cells, the risks for infection, inflammation, and trauma are increased. Diagnosis is made by noting the history of current symptoms, including the presence of systemic illness or evidence of trauma (e.g., broken teeth, ill-fitting dentures), physical examination, culture, and/or biopsy.

Etiology

Etiology of disorders of the mouth and esophagus include the following: viral, bacterial, fungal, traumatic, chemical, and even nutritional deficiencies.

Viral Causes

Herpetic stomatitis is very common because herpes simplex viral (HSV) infection is widespread in the United States. It is estimated that between 30% and 100% of the U.S. population has HSV-specific antibodies, which indicate a past or dormant infection, and that up to 20% of the adult population is shedding the virus at any given time. Any previous infection of HSV (anywhere on the body) is the primary risk factor for all secondary manifestations of herpes simplex infection (McCaffrey, Thrush, Dunphy, & Porter, 2007).

Initial exposure to HSV results in consistently sized vesicles that are most commonly found on the tongue, on buccal and labial mucosae, and occasionally on the palate. The vesicles rupture and progress to painful ulcerations that are similar to aphthous ulcers and resolve in 10 to 14 days. Any condition that decreases the immune response, such as diabetes mellitus, HIV infection, cancer, chemotherapy, immunosuppressive medications, or aging, can increase the likelihood of viral reactivation causing recurrent stomatitis.

Bacterial Causes

Aphthous stomatitis (or **contact stomatitis**), commonly known as canker sores, is an ulcerative condition limited to the oral cavity. In fact, an estimated 20% of the population is affected at some time and 33% develops recurrent lesions that can continue for 40 years. Although the pathogenesis is unclear, an immunologic response to antigens in the buccal cavity is believed to be responsible for this type of stomatitis. Other possible causes and contributing factors are psychological stress, vitamin deficiencies, genetic predisposition, trauma, allergies, and viruses. The prevalence is higher in people with some autoimmune diseases, such as inflammatory bowel disease (Jackler & Kaplan, 2004), and some women report premenstrual recurrences.

There are four phases in the development of aphthous stomatitis. The premonitory phase is characterized by a tingling, burning, or hyperesthetic sensation that can last up to 24 hours. The preulcerative phase lasts from 18 hours to 3 days and is characterized by painful red macules or papules with erythematous halos. Next, the ulcerative phase, lasting from 1 to 16 days, is characterized by painful ulcers 2 to 10 millimeters in diameter and covered by a grayish yellow membrane. As this phase progresses, the pain ceases. The healing phase can last from 4 to 5 weeks, but the lesions are usually healed in 2 weeks.

Vincent's stomatitis, also known as acute necrotizing stomatitis or "trench mouth," is an acute bacterial infection of the gingiva oral mucous membranes caused most often by the bacteria *Borrelia vincentii*. It occurs in people with conditions that decrease the tissue's resistance, such as poor nutrition, extreme emotional stress, leukemia, severe systemic infections, and other conditions that decrease immunocompetence.

The clinical manifestations of Vincent's stomatitis include erythematous ulceration and necrosis of the gingival margins and oral mucosa. The interdental gingival papillae are red, reduced in size, and appear raw and painful. There is a characteristic purulent gray exudate, and the person complains of pain, increased salivation, gums that bleed easily, and bad breath. There may also be systemic manifestations such as malaise, anorexia, and enlarged lymph nodes in the neck (cervical).

Fungal Causes

Oral candidiasis is extremely common and occurs largely as a result of a compromised immune system or a disruption of the normal oral flora. This type of stomatitis results from an overgrowth of the yeast-like fungus *Candida albicans*. The overgrowth can result from antibiotic therapy, which destroys the normal flora in the oral cavity, as well as from the chronic use of inhaled steroids. When the immune system is compromised by such things as cancer chemotherapy treatments, radiation treatments to the head, immunosuppressive medications (glucocorticoids, antirejection drugs), aging, diabetes, emotional stress, malnourishment, or HIV/AIDS, *Candida* infection often occurs. The manifestations of oral candidiasis include white curd-like patches on the tongue, palate, and oral mucosa. Under the white patches, the surface of the tissue is red and sore, although the person usually complains that the lesions are dry or hot, rather than actually painful (Jackler & Kaplan, 2004).

Traumatic Causes

Traumatic oral ulcers are very common and occur most often at the tongue margins and buccal mucosa. It is often difficult to differentiate traumatic ulcers from aphthous stomatitis other than by history and the report of pain; traumatic ulcers are usually not as painful as aphthous ulcers. Common traumatic causes include thermal injury (hot beverage, hot pizza) and physical injury. Mechanical injury can result from ill-fitting dentures, malocclusion, broken teeth, and habitual cheek biting.

Chemical Causes

Chemical irritation can cause stomatitis. Common chemical irritants include spicy, acidic, or salty foods such as potato chips, pickles, and hot pepper sauce. Dental care products such as mouthwash containing alcohol and peroxide, and toothpaste can also act as chemical irritants. Cancer chemotherapy frequently causes stomatitis because, in addition to attacking cancer cells that are rapidly dividing, chemotherapy agents also attack other rapidly dividing cells, such as the mucous epithelial cells in the oral cavity. The chemical irritation from tobacco, whether smoking, dipping, or chewing, results in nicotinic stomatitis (McCaffrey et al., 2007). Bulimia can be a risk factor for stomatitis because of the repeated exposure of the oral mucosa to stomach acid from vomiting.

Nutritional Deficiencies

Several vitamin deficiencies can cause stomatitis, particularly angular stomatitis, glossitis, cheilosis, or, in other words, a sore mouth. The vitamin deficiencies, although rare in the United States, can be caused by malnutrition, malabsorption, alcoholism, restrictive dieting, and fad dieting. Stomatitis and glossitis are caused from deficiencies in many of the B vitamins. Both vitamin B_2 (riboflavin) and vitamin B_6 (pyridoxine) deficiency cause cheilosis and glossitis, whereas a deficiency in folate or B_{12} (cobalamin) can cause glossitis (Jackler & Kaplan, 2004).

No Known Cause

Benign migratory glossitis, also known as geographic tongue, erythema migrans, and stomatitis areata migrans, as the name implies, is a benign condition occurring in up to 3% of the population and is more frequently reported in people with psoriasis. It is characterized by the loss of papillae in some areas of the tongue. These areas are smooth and erythematous, giving the tongue a "maplike" appearance, hence the name *geographic tongue*. In addition, the areas can change in size, location, and appearance daily. Often the person with this condition complains of soreness or burning of the tongue exacerbated by hot, spicy, or acidic foods (Kelsch, 2007).

Medical Management

Medical management includes treatment of the causative factor if known and relief of symptoms.

Drug Therapy

The health care provider may order topical oral anesthetics such as 2% viscous lidocaine. The nurse should ensure that the patient rinse his mouth with the viscous lidocaine, then spit it out, because swallowing the solution may impair the ability to swallow. However, for patients who have lesions in the upper esophagus, the solution may be swallowed to relieve the pain of these lesions. The nurse should inform the patient that the lidocaine may be used every 3 hours as needed. Using lidocaine before meals may help improve oral intake. Agents that coat the oral mucosa may also be helpful in relieving the discomfort of stomatitis. Agents such as magnesium hydroxide (Milk of Magnesia) and kaolin (Kaopectate) may relieve the pain, particularly of aphthous ulcers, while providing protection of the lesions from further irritation. A mixed solution of 1 part diphenhydramine (Benadryl) for inflammation, 1 part aluminum-magnesium hydroxide (Maalox) for irritation and acidity, and 1 part viscous Xylocaine for pain is frequently ordered to relieve a combination of symptoms and improve appetite/nutritional status.

Anti-infectives will be ordered for the patient with stomatitis caused by viruses, bacteria, or fungus and are dispensed in topical, oral, or intravenous (IV) formulations. Antibiotics such as oral penicillin V potassium (Pen-Vee K) are usually effective for Vincent's stomatitis, but for severe gangrenous cases, IV antibiotics may be required. Antifungal agents such as nystatin suspension are prescribed for *Candida* infection. The nurse instructs the patient to swish the suspension around in the mouth for about 2 minutes and then swallow it. The antifungal agent may also be prescribed in a lozenge, which is held in the mouth until it is dissolved and swallowed. The nurse should instruct the patient to abstain from eating or drinking for 30 minutes after taking the medication.

Antiviral agents are prescribed for herpes simplex stomatitis. For patients with intact immune systems, oral acyclovir (Zovirax) is used. Continued use decreases the frequency and severity of the acute episodes. In patients with compromised immune systems, such as those with HIV/AIDS or those taking immunosuppressive medications, IV acyclovir may be needed. Nursing responsibilities include teaching the patient and the family that the medication does not cure the disease and that the virus remains latent in the body and may recur during times of physical or emotional stress. The Pharmacology Summary (p. 1384) feature outlines medications used to treat stomatitis.

Nursing Management

Assessment

Nursing care focuses on assessing the condition of the oral mucosa and determining how these inflammatory conditions are impacting the patient's well-being, specifically nutritional status.

Planning

The treatment of stomatitis and similar conditions is focused on treating the underlying cause, such as correcting vitamin deficiencies, removing the source of traumatic or chemical irritation, or medicating for the infecting organism.

Interventions and Rationales

For all causes of stomatitis, nursing care focuses on good oral hygiene. Frequent mouth care helps debride oral lesions and can decrease the chance of the patient's developing a superinfection. Mouth care using a soft toothbrush, toothette, or water pick should be done every 2 hours for stomatitis that is not controlled. It is essential to teach patients to avoid harsh mouthwashes, particularly those that contain alcohol, because these can irritate the ulcerated mucosa. The mouth can be rinsed with diluted hydrogen peroxide, warm saline, or sodium bicarbonate solution (1 teaspoon of baking soda per 8-ounce glass of water).

Another important nursing intervention for patients with stomatitis is nutritional assessment. It is often painful for patients to eat or drink when they have stomatitis, so the nurse should encourage a high-calorie, high-protein diet. Often, soft, bland foods are better tolerated and cool or cold foods may be soothing. Acidic foods such as citrus juices and tomatoes should be avoided, as well as spicy or hot foods. Weighing the patient daily can help establish the adequacy of the patient's caloric intake.

Contact stomatitis, or aphthous stomatitis, is an inflammatory reaction of the oral mucosa that occurs as a result of contact with irritants or allergens. Patients who report an allergy to latex may be susceptible to developing contact stomatitis if the nurse uses latex gloves when examining the oral mucosa. The incidence of latex allergy, in both patient and nurse populations, has been steadily increasing during recent years, thus requiring the nurse to determine the presence of latex allergy prior to implementing care (Lopes & Lopes, 2000).

Oral Cancer

Oral cancer can occur on any surface of the mouth, including the lips, tongue, and pharynx. According to the Oral Cancer Foundation (2007), approximately 34,000 people in the United States would be newly diagnosed with oral cancer in 2007. Worldwide, the problem would be far greater, with more than 481,000 new cases expected. Of those diagnosed in 2007, only half will be alive in 5 years, and this number has not been improved in decades. The death rate for oral cancer is higher than that of the brain, liver, testes, kidney, or skin cancer (malignant melanoma). This is in part due to the fact that most oral cancers are found at a late stage. Only 5% of all cancers are oral cancer. The most prevalent risk factor for oral cancer is the use of tobacco, both smoking and smokeless (chewing tobacco). The use of tobacco is associated with 75% of all cases of oral cancer (Lynch, 2007). Other risk factors include drinking alcohol, Betel quid chewing, Areca nut use, human papillomavirus (HPV), abuse of narcotics, cannabis use, and human immunodeficiency virus (HIV) seropositivity. Predisposing risk factors include increasing age, male gender, and genetics (Lynch, 2007). Almost all oral cancers are attributed to lifestyle choices.

PHARMACOLOGY Summary of Medications Used to Treat Stomatitis

Medication Category	Action	Application/Indication	Nursing Responsibility
Anti-Infective Agents			
Antibiotics: Penicillin V potassium (Pen-Vee K)	Exerts bacteriocidal activity by destroying and inhibiting synthesis of bacterial cell wall.	Fusospirochetosis (Vincent's pharyngitis); pneumococcal, streptococcal, and nonpenicillinase-producing staphylococcal infections; endocarditis risk prophylaxis.	Monitor for adverse effects: nausea, vomiting, and diarrhea. Monitor for hypersensitivity reaction: pruititis, urticaria, fever, edema, arthralgia, and anaphylaxis. Give after a meal. Warn female patients that oral contraceptives may be rendered ineffective.
Metronidazole (Flagyl)	Exerts antibacterial and antiprotozoan activity by inhibiting DNA synthesis of infecting organism.	Intestinal amebiasis, colorectal surgery prophylaxis, *H. pylori* eradication, Crohn's disease, diverticulitis, pseudomembranous colitis, anaerobic bacterial infections.	Monitor for adverse effects: nausea, vomiting, anorexia, abdominal pain, dizziness, headache, peripheral neuropathy, seizures, and *Candida* overgrowth. Monitor liver function tests if hepatic dysfunction present. Be aware of multiple drug interactions; monitor for drug toxicities (theophylline, warfarin, disulfiram, and others). Instruct patient not to consume alcohol while taking drug and for at least 24 hours after last dose.
Ciprofloxacin (Cipro)	Exerts bacteriocidal activity on gram-negative and gram-positive bacteria by disrupting DNA replication.	Diverticulitis, infectious diarrhea, intra-abdominal infections.	Monitor for adverse effects: nausea, vomiting, diarrhea, rash, headache, peripheral neuropathy, seizures, and signs of *Candida* overgrowth. Monitor for acute onset of joint pain: notify health care provider. Monitor kidney and liver function if renal or hepatic impairment present. Be aware of multiple drug interactions; monitor for drug toxicities (theophylline, warfarin, procainamide, and others). Give medication 6 hours after or 2 hours before antacid or vitamin administration. Warn patient about possible photosensitivity and need for sunblock. Be aware of extensive IV drug incompatibilities.
Antifungal: Nystatin (Mycostatin, Nilstat)	Exerts fungistatic and fungicidal activity by disrupting permeability of fungal cell wall.	Local *Candida* infections, e.g., oropharyngeal, intestinal candidiasis.	Monitor for signs of contact dermatitis. Instruct patient not to eat or drink for 30 minutes after treatment for oral candidiasis.
Antiviral: Acyclovir (Zovirax)	Decreases viral shedding, formation of new lesions, and healing time by interfering with viral DNA synthesis.	Mucosal and cutaneous herpes simplex virus.	Monitor for adverse effects: headache, nausea, vomiting, and diarrhea. Monitor renal function, especially with IV administration.

Pathophysiology

Most oral cancers are squamous cell carcinoma, arising from the flat cells that line the oral cavity. This form of cancer is slow growing and may not produce symptoms until the tumor is well advanced, usually after invasion of the adjacent tissues and metastasis to other areas has occurred. The tumor ulcerates, produces pain, and may also present other symptoms such as irritation of the tongue, sore throat, and difficulty wearing dentures because of painful irritation. Oftentimes the patient with oral cancer will complain of otalgia (ear pain), which is referred from the oropharynx.

The second most common oral cancer is basal cell carcinoma, which occurs almost exclusively on the lips beyond the vermilion border. The characteristic lesion of this type of cancer is a nodule with an ulcerated center and raised pearly border. Although basal cell carcinoma does not metastasize, it can be locally invasive.

Etiology

The most widely recognized risk factor for the development of oral cancer is tobacco use. Tobacco contains chemicals that are known carcinogens, causing mutations in cellular DNA. Smokeless tobacco is particularly hazardous because the chemicals are absorbed directly through the oral mucosa. Heavy alcohol consumption is also a risk factor for oral cancer and has a synergistic effect with tobacco (Burgess, 2006). Other risk factors include marijuana use, infection with certain types of human papillomavirus, and repeated exposure to chemicals or irritation, such as poorly fitting dentures or broken teeth. Basal cell carcinoma is almost exclusively caused by prolonged sun exposure, placing people who work outdoors in sunny climates at greater risk for this type of cancer.

Medical Management

Elimination of causative factors or sources of irritation, such as all forms of tobacco or alcohol, is the initial treatment for oral cancer. Analgesics, coating agents, and oral anesthetic agents may be prescribed to relieve discomfort. (See the Stomatitis section earlier in this chapter (p. 1381) for a discussion of these agents.) Biopsy of the lesion is needed to diagnose the type of cancer. Tumor staging usually requires additional studies such as a magnetic resonance imaging (MRI) or computed tomography (CT) scan. Treatment is based on the extent of the cancer and presence of metastasis. Radiation may be prescribed before surgery in order to shrink the tumor. Radiation and chemotherapy may be appropriate postoperatively depending on the stage of the tumor and the patient's general health.

Excision of the tumor is usually the treatment of choice unless the tumor is very far advanced and considered unresectable. The goal of surgery is to remove the cancerous tissue, but the surrounding tissue and lymph nodes may also be removed to assure there is no local infiltration of cancerous cells. A radical neck dissection may be performed if the tumor is advanced. This procedure involves the removal of lymph nodes and muscles in the neck and is disfiguring. A tracheostomy will be performed during surgery to maintain adequate respiratory support and may become permanent depending on the extent of the neck dissection and subsequent respiratory function.

■ Nursing Management

Nursing management of the patient with oral cancer centers on elimination of causative factors, care of the oral mucosa, and the nutritional status of the patient before and after surgery. The Nursing Process: Patient Care Plan feature (p. 1386) outlines care for oral cancer.

Health Promotion

Eliminating tobacco use is the single most important factor in risk reduction of oral cancer. Because smokeless tobacco use is highest in males ages 15 to 22, the nurse should target this group for education. Smoking cessation, as well as limiting alcohol consumption, should be encouraged for everyone. Use of sunscreen on the face and lips can reduce the risk of basal cell carcinoma. Routine dental visits are also important in the early detection of oral cancers, as well as for keeping dentition in good repair.

Early detection is key to improving the prognosis of patients with oral cancer. In addition to identifying patients with risk factors, oral inspection may prove invaluable, as seen in the Evidence-Based Practice feature (p. 1387).

■ Hiatal Hernia

A **hiatal hernia** involves the herniation of the upper portion of the stomach into the thorax through the esophageal hiatus. There are two types of hiatal hernia. The most common, the **sliding (direct) hiatal hernia**, occurs 90% of the time (Huether, 2006). The second type is the **rolling (paraesophageal) hernia**. Hiatal hernia is believed to be a very common problem, but the majority of individuals have no symptoms. The incidence of hiatal hernia increases with age.

Gerontological Considerations

Hiatal hernias are more prevalent in Western countries, and the frequency increases with age. Up to 70% of patients who are 70 years of age will develop a hiatal hernia. It is thought that muscle weakening and a loss of elasticity are the primary factors that predispose the elderly patient to have an increased risk of developing a hiatal hernia. Physiologically, as the tissue elasticity is decreased due to aging, the gastric cardia may not return to its original position below the diaphragmatic hiatus. Hiatal hernias are more common in women, and it is thought that this may be due to the increased intra-abdominal pressures associated with pregnancy (Qureshi, 2006).

Pathophysiology/Etiology

The point at which the esophagus and vagus nerve pass through the diaphragm is an inherent area of weakness. In a sliding hiatal hernia, a portion of the fundus of the stomach moves upward through the esophageal hiatus into the thoracic cavity (Figure 45–1A ■, p. 1388). Several factors contribute to this condition, including a congenitally short esophagus, trauma, or weakening of the diaphragm at the gastroesophageal junction (Huether, 2006). The movement of the stomach upward occurs most often when the individual is lying down. Obesity and pregnancy exacerbate this type of hernia, as does anything that increases the intra-abdominal pressure, such as eating a large meal. When the individual assumes a standing position, the hernia slides back into the abdominal cavity. With this type of hernia, there is a **lower esophageal sphincter (LES)** pressure resulting in **gastroesophageal reflux** and esophagitis.

In a paraesophageal hernia (rolling hernia), there is herniation of the greater curvature of the stomach through the esophageal hiatus. The gastroesophageal junction remains in the normal position below the diaphragm (Figure 45–1B ■, p. 1388), and reflux is unusual. However, there can be congestion of the mucosal blood flow in the portion of the stomach in the thorax that can lead to gastritis and ulceration. In rare instances, there can be strangulation of the hernia, causing ischemia and hemorrhage, and this requires surgical intervention.

Both types of hiatal hernia produce similar symptoms, if symptoms are present at all. The primary symptom is reflux and heartburn. Patients often complain of feeling full, belching, and indigestion. Because the stomach herniates into the thoracic cavity near the midline, patients may complain of substernal chest pain and think they may be having a heart attack.

Medical Management

For patients with mild symptoms, the lifestyle changes mentioned earlier may provide symptom relief. The primary care provider may prescribe a **histamine$_2$ (H$_2$)-receptor blocker** (ranitidine, famotidine) or a **proton pump inhibitor (PPI)** (lansoprazole, omeprazole) to reduce gastroesophageal reflux.

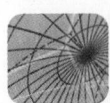

NURSING PROCESS: Patient Care Plan for Oral Cancer

Assessment of Oral Mucosa

Subjective Data:

How long have you had this mouth sore?
Do you smoke or use smokeless tobacco?
Do you drink alcohol? If so, how much?

Objective Data:

Visual inspection of oral cavity including the tongue and under the tongue:
- Lesions may appear as white patches or velvety red.
- Inspect for poorly fitting dentures or teeth in disrepair.

Nursing Assessment and Diagnoses	Outcomes and Evaluation Parameters	Planning and Interventions with *Rationales*
Nursing Diagnosis: *Tissue Integrity, Impaired* related to oral lesion	**Outcome:** Reduced oral cancer risk. **Evaluation Parameters:** No behaviors harmful to oral mucosa: • Smoking cessation. • Limited alcohol consumption. • Dentures/dentition in good repair.	**Interventions and *Rationales*:** Assess for and educate about contributing factors for oral cancer. *To decrease future risk, cause less irritation of lesions present, and improve overall health.* Provide and teach about good oral hygiene.

Assessment of Nutritional Status

Subjective Data:

Do you have difficulty swallowing?
Are there any foods that cause discomfort?
Are you having trouble eating?
Is your appetite good?

Objective Data:

Body weight and appearance.
Skin turgor.
Skin and hair condition.

Nursing Assessment and Diagnoses	Outcomes and Evaluation Parameters	Planning and Interventions with *Rationales*
Nursing Diagnosis: *Nutrition, Readiness for Enhanced* in regard to oral pain or anorexia	**Outcome:** Adequate nutrition. **Evaluation Parameter:** No weight loss.	**Interventions and *Rationales*:** Provide cool, soft foods or liquids that are high in calories. *Cool or cold foods that are soft or liquid are soothing to the oral mucosa.* Daily weight. *Indicator of fluid and nutrition status.* Assess need for dietary consult.

Assessment of Pain

Subjective Data:

Do you have mouth pain?
On a scale of 1–10, with 10 being the worst pain, how would you rate your pain?
Do you take anything for the pain?
What makes the pain better or worse?
Do you have any cultural or religious ways to control your pain?

Objective Data:

Grimacing when swallowing.
Drooling (too painful to swallow secretions).

Nursing Assessment and Diagnoses	Outcomes and Evaluation Parameters	Planning and Interventions with *Rationales*
Nursing Diagnosis: *Pain, Acute* related to oral lesion	**Outcome:** Comfort level maintained. **Evaluation Parameters:** Reports adequate pain control. Consumes meals and snacks without pain.	**Interventions and *Rationales*:** Assess pain using pain scale (1–10) *to increase consistency in quantifying pain.* Assess cultural and religious beliefs about pain and pain relief. *Different cultures and religions may view pain as punishment or may have nontraditional ways of treating pain.* Administer prescribed pain medications or oral anesthetics as ordered. *Adequate pain relief before meals will increase the ability to eat pain free.*

The Pharmacology summary feature (p. 1390) outlines medications used to reduce gastroesophageal reflux. If these medications fail to resolve symptoms, diagnostic evaluation is indicated. A barium swallow or upper endoscopy may be performed to establish the diagnosis. Surgery may be done if the hernia becomes incarcerated or if severe symptoms persist even with medication. The most common surgical procedure for hiatal hernia is the Nissen fundoplication (Figure 45–2 ■, 1388).

Gastroesophageal Reflux Disease

Gastroesophageal reflux is the backward flow of stomach contents (chyme) into the esophagus without associated vomiting. Gastroesophageal reflux is considered a disease when the symptoms are severe, mucosal damage has occurred, or symptoms occur frequently. Ten percent of the adult population in the United States complains of having heartburn daily, while another 45% of these individuals have symptoms at least once a

Oral Cancer

Clinical Problem

The death rate for oral cancer is higher than that of the brain, liver, testes, kidney, or skin cancer (malignant melanoma). This is due in part to the fact that most oral cancers are currently found at a late stage. However, the key to improving survival is identification of risk factors in combination with careful assessment in order to detect early changes in the oral mucosa. Risk factors commonly associated with the development of oral cancer include tobacco use, including pipes, cigars, cigarettes, and chewing tobacco, and alcohol use. Alcohol consumption interacts synergistically with the use of tobacco products to increase the likelihood of developing oral cancer. Nurses must understand how to use evidenced-based findings when caring for patients who are considered to be at risk for developing oral cancer.

Research Findings

Sankaranarayanan and colleagues (2005) reported that periodic examination of the oral cavity can reduce mortality from oral cancer in high-risk individuals. These researchers believed that screening techniques and oral mucosal assessment would improve the identification of those patients who have precancerous lesions or those with early stage oral cancer. The sample consisted of 114,601 adult subjects age 35 or older who were considered to be otherwise healthy. The subjects were randomized to either an intervention group or a control group. Subjects in the intervention group received three rounds of screenings, which consisted of an oral–visual inspection by health workers. The researchers report that, 9 years after the start of the screening, there was a significant 32% reduction in mortality in high-risk individuals in the intervention group. A 42% reduction was found in patients who reported use of tobacco and alcohol products. Overall, these findings suggest that oral cancer screening by health workers could prevent approximately 40,000 deaths worldwide.

Implications for Nursing Practice

This study (Sankaranarayanan et al., 2005) clearly indicates a need for nurses to identify patients who are considered to be high risk for the development of oral cancer. It appears from this study that the

early identification of risk factors, combined with a visual inspection of the oral mucosa for abnormal findings, can improve outcomes for patients who develop oral cancer. Because both the identification of risk factors and simple visual assessment are within the scope of nursing practice, the potential exists for nurses to make a significant contribution to the prevention and reduction of the incidence of and mortality associated with oral cancer. Nurses should include not only the patient but also other family members and significant persons in the teaching of high-risk behaviors associated with the development of oral cancer, and should reinforce the importance of undergoing a simple, noninvasive oral mucosal assessment.

Critical Thinking Questions

1. Which of the following are considered to be significant risk factors for the development of oral cancer? (Select all that apply.)
   A. Smoking a pipe
   B. Eating fresh fruits and vegetables
   C. Using chewing tobacco
   D. Meticulous oral hygiene
   E. Cigarette smoking
   F. Alcohol consumption

2. In addition to the identification of risk factors, what other nursing intervention can significantly improve patient outcomes associated with oral cancer?

3. Describe atypical findings associated with an oral examination that should be reported to the health care provider for further evaluation.

Answers to Critical Thinking Questions appear in Appendix D.

References

Oral Cancer Foundation. (2007). *Descriptive epidemiology*. Retrieved April 17, 2008, from http://www.oralcancerfoundation.org/cdc/cdc_chapter1.htm.

Sankaranarayanan, R., Ranadas, K., Thomas, G., Nuwonge, R., Thara, S., Mathew, B., et al. (2005). Effect of screening on oral cancer mortality in Kerala, India: A cluster-randomized controlled trial. *The Lancet, 365*(9475), 1927–1933.

EVIDENCE-BASED PRACTICE

---

month (Thomas, 2007). It is believed that the number of people experiencing reflux may actually be much higher, but because many H_2-receptor blockers are available without a prescription, a large number of cases go unreported. The incidence of gastroesophageal reflux disease (GERD) increases after age 50, but it can occur at any age and the prevalence is equal across gender, ethnic, and cultural groups.

Pathophysiology/Etiology

Gastroesophageal reflux disease is caused by relaxation of the lower esophageal sphincter (LES). Normal LES pressure is 10 to 30 mmHg and is under muscular, hormonal, and neural control. In patients with GERD, the pressure is less than 10 mmHg. The decreased pressure allows for reflux of stomach contents into the esophagus, particularly during activity that increases intra-abdominal pressure, such as lifting, bending, straining, or recumbency. The esophageal mucosa does not contain the same protective mechanism against the acidic (pH less than 3.9)

stomach contents as does the stomach, and mucosal damage and erosion result.

When the esophagus is exposed to gastric contents, an inflammatory response is initiated. Over time, with repeated exposure, this inflammation becomes chronic. The normal squamous epithelial cells are replaced with columnar epithelium, which is more resistant to damage by acidic stomach contents and supports healing of the erosions. However, this new epithelium, called **Barrett's epithelium**, is a premalignant tissue and increases the risk for esophageal cancer. This is commonly called Barrett's esophagus. Another result of long-term exposure of the esophagus to stomach acid is the development of esophageal strictures.

Many factors increase the risk for developing GERD, such as obesity, pregnancy, and hiatal hernia. In addition, a number of foods and medications decrease the LES pressure and therefore increase the risk of GERD. These include alcohol, caffeine, chocolate, fatty foods, citrus fruit, onions, tomatoes, peppermint,

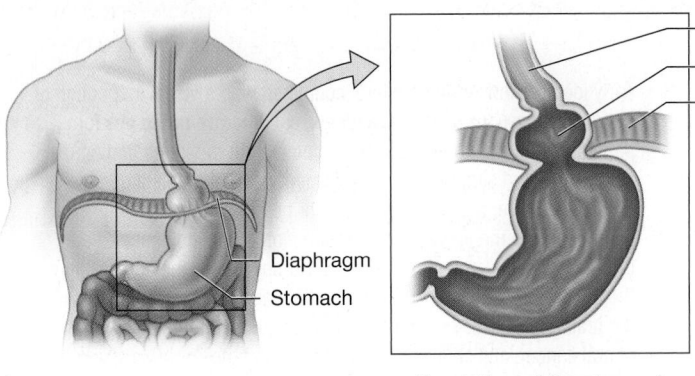

(a)

Herniation of the stomach through the hiatal opening

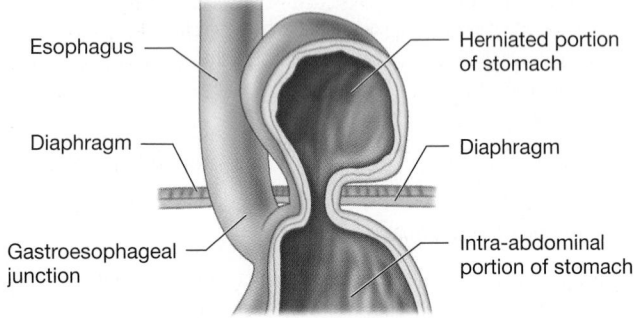

(b)

FIGURE 45–1 ■ (A) Hiatal hernia and (B) Paraesophageal hernia.

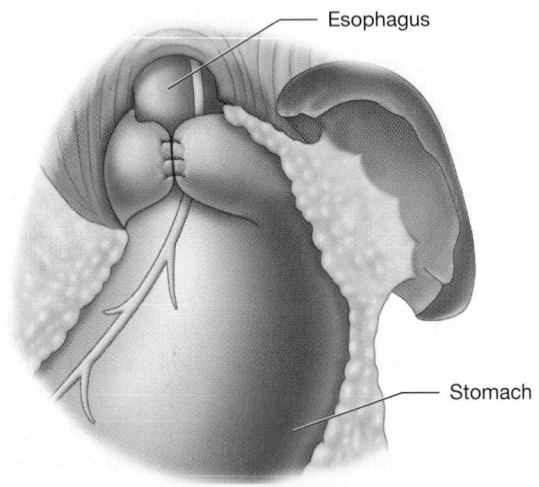

FIGURE 45–2 ■ Nissen fundoplication.

beta-adrenergic blockers (Inderal), calcium channel blockers (verapamil), estrogen, progesterone, diazepam (Valium), and theophylline. Nicotine also lowers LES, including the levels obtained via secondhand smoke (Thomas, 2007).

Clinical Manifestations

The most common symptom of GERD is heartburn, which can be mild to severe in nature. Additional symptoms that commonly occur are a sour taste in the morning on arising, regurgitation, dysphagia, coughing, belching, and chest pain. Atypical symptoms include asthma or a sore throat. There are usually no outward physical signs that the patient has GERD, although the stool may test positive for occult blood due to possible microhemorrhages in the irritated esophageal mucosa.

Medical Management

The medical management of GERD is to educate patients regarding causative factors and assist them to make lifestyle changes. If the symptoms persist, then additional tests will be done to try to identify a cause.

Diagnostic Procedures

The diagnosis of GERD is most often made by symptomatology and predisposing risk factors. Unfortunately, the severity of the disease does not always correlate with the severity of the symptoms. In fact, severe disease may exist with few symptoms. If symptoms persist after 4 weeks of conservative treatment and lifestyle changes, an upper endoscopy may be done to visualize the esophagus directly and obtain tissue samples (Sherman, 2007). The tissue is examined for signs of Barrett's epithelium and malignancy. (Chart 45–1 details nursing care of the patient undergoing endoscopy.) Ambulatory esophageal pH monitoring is the most accurate way to diagnose GERD. In this test, a pH probe is placed 5 centimeters above the LES, and the pH is measured for 24 hours. If the pH is less than 4 above the LES, then GERD is diagnosed, especially if there are corresponding symptoms. Esophageal manometry measures the pressures of the LES and is used to determine its location before 24-hour ambulatory pH monitoring is done. Occasionally a barium swallow may be done to evaluate the esophagus and stomach and visualize a hiatal hernia.

Diet and Lifestyle Modifications

Lifestyle modifications including diet are key in the treatment of GERD. Many patients may have total symptom relief through these efforts alone. Foods that lower LES pressure (mentioned earlier) should be eliminated from the diet or ingested on an infrequent basis following use of medication to prevent symptoms. Because spicy foods may irritate the esophageal mucosa, they should be avoided as well. It is often helpful to eat small frequent meals with the largest meal at midday. The patient should avoid eating anything within 4 hours of bedtime, and the head of the bed should be elevated. Depending on the amount of caffeine an individual drinks, complete withdrawal may cause headaches so gradual elimination is preferred. Weight loss is important in patients who are overweight or obese. A regular exercise program such as daily walking can promote digestion as well as weight loss, thus diminishing symptoms. Tight garments or belts may increase symptoms by increasing intra-abdominal pressure and should be avoided. Smoking cessation should be considered a priority.

Medications

Medications for GERD can be purchased over the counter and prescribed. It is important to know whether the patient has been self-medicating, what the patient has used, and whether it has helped to relieve the symptoms.

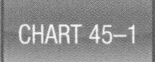

CHART 45–1   Nursing Care of a Patient Undergoing Endoscopy

PREPROCEDURE

- Explain the procedure again (should have been explained by the health care provider), and assure signed consent is in the chart.
- Assure NPO 8 to 12 hours prior to test.
- Record name of person driving the patient home after the test (patient CANNOT drive after the test).
- Place name band on wrist and have the patient change into a hospital gown.
- Have the patient remove any jewelry, dentures, or eyeglasses.
- Ensure the patient empties his bladder before the procedure.
- Take vital signs and start an IV for sedation.
- Answer any questions the patient has about the procedure, and explain that there may be a sensation of pressure as the endoscope is inserted and fullness in the stomach as air is injected to expand the stomach and allow for better visualization.

POSTPROCEDURE

- Frequent vital signs.
- Check gag reflex.
- NPO until gag reflex returns.
- Monitor for signs of complications: pain, dyspnea, tachycardia, or subcutaneous emphysema in the neck.
- Tell the patient to expect flatus or eructation resulting from the instillation of air during the procedure.
- Ensure that the patient does not drive himself home.

Antacids

Antacids are part of the initial treatment of GERD and often provide relief for mild to moderate symptoms. Antacids buffer (increase pH) the gastric contents and help to prevent further mucosal damage. Antacids are available without a prescription and are frequently used by individuals with heartburn even before they seek medical attention. Examples of antacids are Mylanta, Maalox, Tums, Rolaids, and Riopan. Gaviscon, an alginate-antacid, forms a floating barrier and prevents upright reflux.

Histamine₂-Receptor Blockers

Most H$_2$-receptor blockers, such as cimetidine (Tagamet), ranitidine (Zantac), nizatidine (Axid), and famotidine (Pepcid), are available without a prescription and are approved for the treatment of GERD. They are effective in reducing the secretion of gastric acid. They are usually taken twice a day for extended periods of time. The prescription strength of these drugs may be more beneficial if the patient has self-medicated with the lower doses before diagnosis.

Proton Pump Inhibitors

Gastric secretions can also be reduced by proton pump inhibitors such as omeprazole (Prilosec), lansoprazole (Previcid), rabeprazole (Aciphex), esomeprazole (Nexium), or pantoprazole (Protonix). These medications are very effective in treating GERD and have now been approved for long-term use. They may be needed for 6 months or longer. Proton pump inhibitors have been shown to heal the erosive lesions in addition to decreasing acid production.

Other Medications

Drugs such as metoclopramide (Reglan) promote gastric motility and speed gastric emptying, but do not affect acid secretion. By enhancing gastric motility, metoclopramide reduces the amount of time gastric contents have to potentially contact esophageal mucosa. Long-term use is not recommended, and use is associated with side effects such as fatigue, anxiety, ataxia, and even hallucinations. The Pharmacology summary feature (p. 1390) outlines medications used to treat gastroesophageal reflux.

Surgery

Most patients respond favorably to lifestyle modification and drug treatment, but there are some who require surgery to have resolution of GERD. Surgery involves increasing the pressure in the lower esophagus in order to prevent reflux of gastric contents. Several laparoscopic procedures are used either to tighten the LES with sutures or to cause scar tissue to form in the muscles surrounding the sphincter. The most common antireflux surgical procedure is the Nissen fundoplication (see Figure 45–2).

Nursing Management

Nursing care for the patient with GERD focuses primarily on assessment, prevention of complications, and patient/ family teaching. The Nursing Process: Patient Care Plan feature (p. 1391) shows a protocol for the patient with GERD.

Health Promotion

Teach patients and community members that frequent heartburn may be a sign of GERD and that they should seek treatment. The long-term consequences of untreated GERD can be serious and include esophageal strictures, Barrett's esophagus, and the possibility of esophageal cancer.

Achalasia

Achalasia is a motor disorder of the esophagus that is characterized by failure of the LES to relax properly and impaired peristalsis. This is caused by defective innervation of the smooth muscle of the esophagus and LES. Normally, the LES has tonic contractions with intermittent relaxation.

Pathophysiology

In the patient with achalasia, the LES fails to relax in response to swallowing as well as a loss of normal peristalsis. The etiology of this disorder is unknown, but it is believed to be a result of defective inhibitory pathways of the esophageal enteric nervous system. It results in a functional obstruction because the esophagus is unable to empty properly. The clinical manifestations include chronic and progressive dysphagia, regurgitation, and chest pain. Over time, the esophagus may be able to hold as much as 1 liter of material containing old, putrefying food, pus, and fluid. Aspiration pneumonia, esophageal ulceration, and rupture can result.

PHARMACOLOGY Summary of Medications Used to Treat Gastroesophageal Reflux

Medication Category	Action	Application/Indication	Nursing Responsibility
Histamine₂-Receptor Antagonists (H₂ Blockers)			
Ranitidine (Zantac) Famotidine (Pepcid) Cimetidine (Tagamet) Nizatidine (Axid)	Inhibits all phases of gastric acid secretion by blocking histamine receptors in gastric parietal cells; decreases volume and hydrogen ion concentration in gastric secretions.	GERD, duodenal ulcers, gastric ulcers, erosive esophagitis, symptomatic hiatal hernia, chronic hypersecretory conditions.	Monitor for adverse effects: rash, nausea, vomiting, constipation, diarrhea, abdominal pain, dizziness, and headache. Monitor blood count. Monitor elderly and patients with hepatic or renal disease for CNS effects. Administer 2 hours before or after administration of antacids. Consider need for B_{12} replacement if given long term.
Proton Pump Inhibitors (PPIs)			
Lansoprazole (Prevacid), Omeprazole (Prilosec) Rabeprazole (Aciphex) Esomeprazole (Nexium) Pantoprazole (Protonix)	Decreases gastric acid by binding with H+/K+ ATPase in the gastric parietal cells, blocking final phase of acid production.	Short-term treatment of GERD (4–8 weeks), peptic ulcers, duodenal ulcers, erosive esophagitis, and symptomatic hiatal hernia; long-term treatment of chronic hypersecretory conditions.	Monitor for adverse effects: diarrhea, constipation, nausea, vomiting, stomach pain, headache, and dizziness. Monitor for altered absorption of medications, vitamins, and minerals requiring an acid environment. Be aware of multiple drug interactions (warfarin, diazepam, phenytoin, digoxin, theophylline, and others); monitor for signs of elevated serum levels. Evaluate need in elderly for calcium replacement, and evaluate for increased incidence of pneumonia. Instruct patient to take medication 30 minutes prior to meal.
Antacids			
Aluminum hydroxide (Amphojel) Calcium carbonate (Tums) Calcium Carbonate/magnesium hydroxide (Rolaids) Magnesium hydroxide (Milk of Magnesia) Magnesium Hydroxide/aluminum hydroxide (Maalox, Mylanta) Magaldrate (Riopan) Sodium bicarbonate (Alka-Seltzer)	Neutralizes gastric acid by increasing gastric pH.	GERD, esophagitis, gastritis, peptic ulcer disease, hyperacidity.	Monitor for constipation if taking calcium- or aluminum-based product, diarrhea if taking magnesium-based product. Monitor patients with renal or cardiac insufficiency for signs of accumulation of sodium, magnesium, or calcium from selected antacid. Monitor for hypophosphatemia if taking antacid containing aluminum. Be aware of multiple drug interactions; administer 2 hours before or after other oral medications if medication absorption may be affected.
Prokinetic Agent			
Metoclopramide (Reglan)	Increases gastric emptying and intestinal transit, apparently by sensitizing GI smooth muscle to acetylcholine; lowers esophageal sphincter tone; relaxes pyloric sphincter; blocks stimulation of medullary chemoreceptor trigger zone (CTZ) receptors for direct antiemetic effect.	Diabetic gastroparesis, GERD unresponsive to standard treatment, as an antiemetic postoperatively, and in chemotherapy and radiation therapy.	Monitor for adverse effects: restlessness, fatigue, drowsiness, insomnia, headache, dizziness, confusion, depression, hallucinations, involuntary movements, and diarrhea. Monitor for drug interaction (levodopa, digoxin, narcotics, tetracycline, and others). Monitor electrolytes for hypernatremia and hypokalemia, especially in patients with cardiac insufficiency or hepatic disease. Administer oral dose 30 minutes prior to meals. Warn patient to avoid alcohol, sedatives, and other CNS depressants. Be aware of multiple IV drug incompatibilities and light sensitivity.

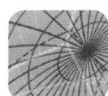

NURSING PROCESS: Patient Care Plan for GERD

Assessment of Discomfort/Pain

Subjective Data:

How often do you experience heartburn?

On a scale of 0–10, with 10 being severe, how would you rate your heartburn?

Do you have a sour taste in the morning when you get up?

Do you ever get a sour or burning sensation in your throat when you bend over or lie down after a meal?

Is your heartburn worse if you wear something tight around your waist?

Are there any foods that cause you discomfort? What are they?

Are you allergic to anything?

Does the pain improve when you eat?

Is your discomfort sharp, dull, gnawing, or burning?

What have you tried to relieve the pain?

Objective Data:

Epigastric tenderness.

Nursing Assessment and Diagnoses	Outcomes and Evaluation Parameters	Planning and Interventions with *Rationales*
Nursing Diagnosis: *Comfort, Readiness for Enhanced* related to esophageal mucosal injury from contact with gastric secretions	**Outcome:** No heartburn. **Evaluation Parameter:** Reports satisfactory control of discomfort.	**Intervention and** *Rationale:* Use pain scale (0–10) to quantify pain and discomfort. *To increase consistency in quantifying pain.*

Assessment of Knowledge of GERD and Treatment

Subjective Data:

What did you have for breakfast, lunch, and so forth?

Do you wear a tight belt or waistband?

Do you wear a girdle or panty hose with a tight waistband?

Do you eat within 2 hours of going to bed?

Do you lie down after eating?

Did you know that GERD is considered a chronic disease? And requires treatment?

Are you aware of the complications associated with GERD if left untreated?

Do you drink coffee, tea, alcohol, citrus juice, or cola?

What medications, OTC, prescription, or herbal, are you taking, and when do you take them?

How often do you eat foods containing mint or drink mint tea?

What are your plans for losing weight?

Nursing Assessment and Diagnoses	Outcomes and Evaluation Parameters	Planning and Interventions with *Rationales*
Nursing Diagnosis: *Knowledge, Readiness for Enhanced* related to treatment and long-term consequences of GERD	**Outcome:** Symptoms reduced. **Evaluation Parameters:** Able to verbalize lifestyle modifications to reduce reflux. Communicates a plan to lose weight. Understands the chronic nature of the disease and long-term consequences as evidenced by ability to articulate the nature of esophageal erosion and Barrett's epithelium.	**Interventions and** *Rationales:* Teach the importance of eating 4–6 small meals a day and to eliminate foods known to decrease lower esophageal sphincter (LES) pressure or cause irritation. *To decrease reflux.* Assess cultural and religious dietary practices. *To explore foods that are culturally based that may decrease LES pressure or cause irritation.* Explain the conversion of squamous epithelial cells to columnar epithelial cells and the possibility of developing cancer if reflux goes untreated over time. *To help the patient understand the consequences of GERD.* Instruct the patient to avoid lying down after eating. *To minimize reflux.* Educate the patient about medication regimen and possible side effects. *To improve adherence to medication regimen.*

Medical Management

The traditional treatment of achalasia has been the use of esophageal dilation or myotomy. Esophageal dilation is done using a balloon catheter (Figure 45–3 ■, p. 1392). The pneumatic dilator (balloon) is placed across the LES, usually under fluoroscopy with local anesthesia. The balloon is inflated to a predetermined level for about 30 to 60 seconds. This causes small tears in the esophageal sphincter muscle fibers, thereby reducing the pressure. The health care provider performs a myotomy using a laparoscope to incise the circular muscle layer of the LES. A less invasive procedure is performed with the injection of botulinum toxin (**Botox**) into the LES through an endoscopic procedure. The disadvantage of this procedure is that it usually requires repeated treatment every 6 to 9 months.

■ Nursing Management

The nursing management for achalasia includes a detailed assessment of the patient's symptoms and nutrition. The focus

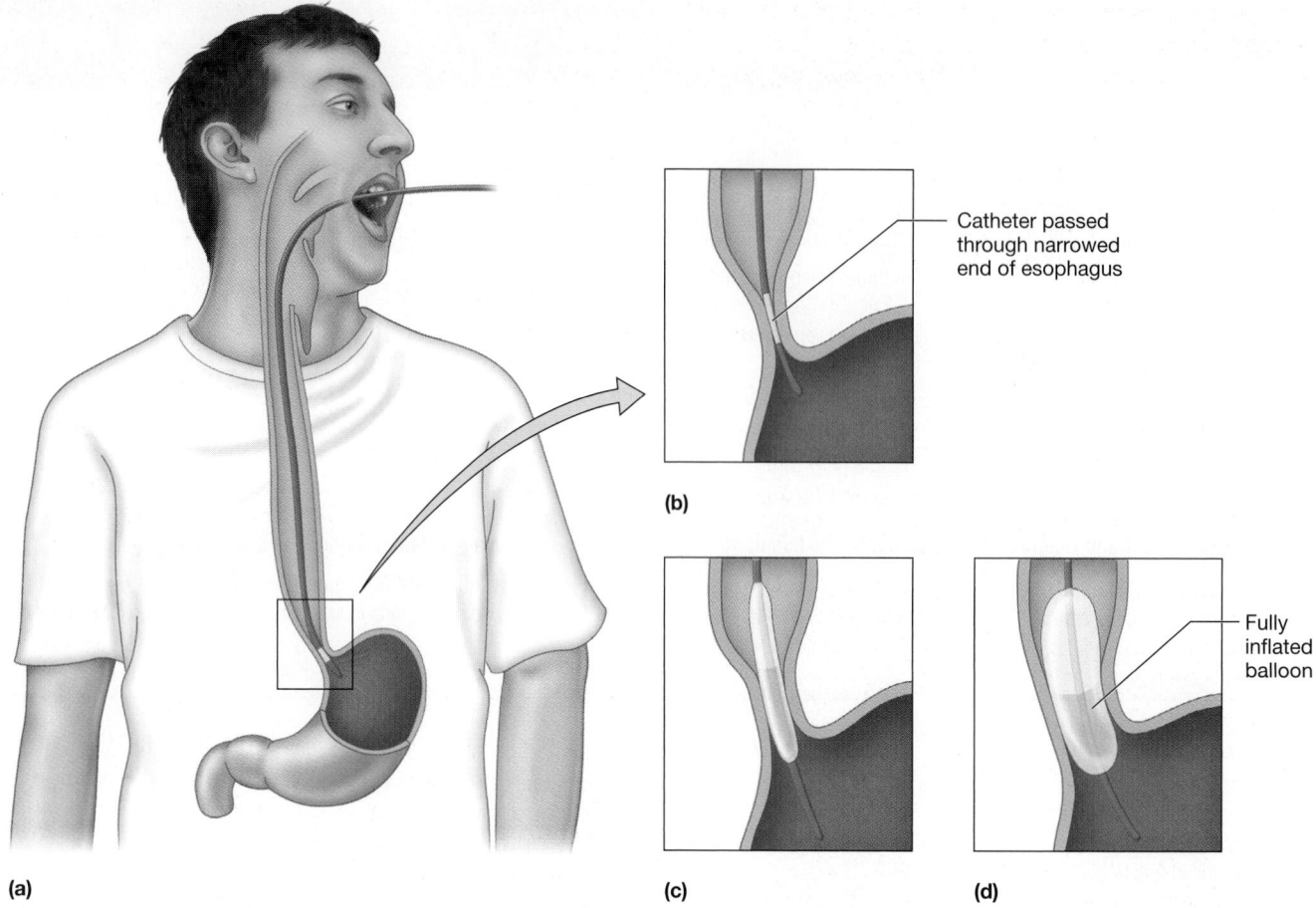

Catheter passed
through narrowed
end of esophagus

(b)

Fully
inflated
balloon

(a)

(c)

(d)

FIGURE 45–3 ■ Esophageal dilation.

then becomes teaching the patient regarding the disease process and helpful dietary changes.

Assessment

Nursing assessment is the first step in caring for a patient with achalasia. The nurse should determine the presence of primary symptoms, their duration, the factors that increase their frequency or intensity, and what the patient has tried to relieve them. A respiratory history is essential because of the potential for aspiration pneumonia. A complete nutritional assessment, including food tolerances and weight loss, will give the nurse an idea of the impact of the esophageal symptoms. The patient with achalasia may have halitosis (foul breath) because of the putrefying food retained in the esophagus.

Interventions

Nursing interventions include advising the patient to try different foods because some foods may be better tolerated than others. Warm, soft foods or liquids are often better tolerated than a standard diet, and small, frequent meals may aid in esophageal emptying. Sleeping either with the head of the bed elevated or in a semisitting position can help prevent nocturnal reflux.

The nurse may assist with endoscopic procedures that are used to ease the pressure in the LES. The nurse should educate the patient and family about what to expect regarding the procedure and symptoms that should be reported after the patient

has left the ambulatory center. The major nursing responsibility is to monitor for respiratory distress and the return of swallowing after the procedure.

■ Esophageal Cancer

Although **esophageal cancer** is uncommon in the United States, it is almost always fatal. The 5-year survival rate is less than 5%. Survival increases if a diagnosis occurs in the early stages. Because the symptoms of esophageal cancer go unrecognized or are associated with other more benign, conditions, it is usually not diagnosed until late in the course of the disease.

Pathophysiology/Etiology

Cancer can occur anywhere along the esophagus, but it is more common in the middle and distal portions. The most common type of esophageal cancer is squamous cell and is more common in African Americans than in whites, peaking at around age 60. Adenocarcinoma is less common but is more common in whites and is associated with the presence of Barrett's epithelium (columnar rather than squamous epithelium) resulting from chronic GERD.

The major risk factor for the development of esophageal cancer is long-term alcohol use. The risk increases as the amount of alcohol consumed increases. Tobacco use increases the risk of esophageal cancer, but pipe and cigar smokers have a higher risk than cigarette smokers. Carcinogenesis is associated with deficiencies of trace elements and vitamins, particularly zinc and vitamin A, which may occur with malnutrition from poor economic conditions, special diets, or alcoholism.

The development of esophageal cancer is facilitated by any process that allows food and drink to remain in the esophagus for prolonged periods, by ulceration and metaplasia usually caused from esophageal reflux, and by long-term exposure of the esophagus to irritants. Malnutrition causes mucosal changes that promote neoplastic changes.

Clinical Manifestations

The clinical manifestations of esophageal cancer are similar to those of GERD, hiatal hernia, and achalasia, and include dysphagia, heartburn, chest pain, and regurgitation. Dysphagia, as the most common and most diagnostic symptom, is usually progressive, beginning with difficulty swallowing solid food, especially meat, and then progressing to difficulty swallowing soft foods and liquids. The dysphagia usually progresses rapidly over the course of weeks or months. Late in the disease, drooling may be noted because the patient can no longer swallow her saliva. Painful swallowing (odynophagia) is common and is described as a steady, dull, substernal pain.

Diagnostic Tests

Diagnosis of esophageal cancer is made with endoscopic visualization and biopsy. A barium swallow may be done initially to identify narrowing of the esophageal lumen or abnormal mucosa. After diagnosis is made, a CT scan or MRI is usually done to assess for metastasis to other organs. Other laboratory tests are done to assess for anemia (complete blood count, or CBC), nutritional status (serum albumin), liver function, and to detect liver metastasis (aspartate aminotransferase, or AST; alanine aminotransferase, or ALT; bilirubin; alkaline phosphatase).

Medical Management

The goal of therapy for the patient with esophageal cancer is to control dysphagia and maintain or improve nutritional status. Surgery is the only definitive treatment and is preferred in patients who are otherwise healthy. Radiation and chemotherapy, in addition to surgery, may enhance results.

Surgery for esophageal cancer involves removal of the affected area of the esophagus and reanastomosis of the remaining esophagus to the stomach. It is usually done in conjunction with radiation and chemotherapy. Radiation and chemotherapy done preoperatively can shrink the size of the tumor, making removal easier. If the cancer is extensive and has invaded the local tissue and metastasized to distant organs, surgery is done for palliation to relieve pain and dysphagia. Laser treatment and stents may be done to keep the esophagus patent in patients who have had surgery, or they may be used as palliation. Tumors in the upper esophagus usually require a tracheostomy and possibly a radical neck dissection with laryngectomy.

Complications following this radical surgery may include hemorrhage, shock, infection, and pneumonia. Additionally, there is the risk of leakage at the anastomosis sites or through the mediastinal space, and depending on the extent of the surgery, peritonitis may occur, leading to serious infection.

Nursing Management

Nursing care for the patient with esophageal cancer will focus on assessing the severity of the symptoms, providing support once diagnosis is made, and educating the patient and family on lifestyle changes needed to facilitate palliative care. Because the disease has a poor prognosis, produces symptoms that are frightening (feelings of choking), and requires a change in eating habits, the nurse assesses the patient's ability to cope, the patient's personal support systems, and acceptance of the diagnosis in order to make appropriate referrals. The nurse should encourage the patient to verbalize fears and feelings. Including the family members in the preoperative teaching and discussions can help the patient deal with the fear associated with the unknown.

Esophageal resection may be recommended, and if so, the nurse should prepare the patient for surgery. General preoperative care is discussed in Chapter 25 🔗. Because the patient with esophageal cancer may be in a nutritionally poor state, nutritional support may be necessary before surgery is done. Patients usually require parenteral or tube feedings either before or after the procedure, and nursing responsibilities should include monitoring the patient's weight, intake and output, fluid and electrolyte balance, as well as assuring that the patient's questions are answered regarding the surgical procedure and postoperative changes. The Nursing Process: Patient Care Plan (p. 1394) presents the plan of care for postoperative patients with esophageal cancer.

DISORDERS OF THE STOMACH AND INTESTINES

The stomach is well suited for storing and mixing food with acid and enzymes. Alterations of the stomach lining or malignancies can cause painful and serious disease. The small intestine is the area of most of the digestion and absorption that occurs in the digestive tract, with the large intestine absorbing the remaining water and concentrating feces. Diseases of the intestines may manifest themselves as diarrhea, constipation, changes in the character of the stool, or in secondary diseases that arise as a result of poor nutrition.

Peptic Ulcer Disease

The word *peptic* comes from the Greek word meaning to digest. **Peptic ulcer** is a generic term used for any ulceration in the digestive surfaces of the upper GI tract. This includes gastric and duodenal ulcers. The word *ulcer* itself denotes disruption in the protective mucosal lining, thereby exposing the submucosal tissue to gastric secretions and digestion of the submucosa (autodigestion).

Gastric Ulcers

Gastric ulcers are more often seen in older patients between the ages of 55 and 70, occurring with equal frequency in men and women. Gastric ulcers occur less frequently than duodenal ulcers but tend to heal more slowly. A family history of ulcers is not usually associated with gastric ulcer disease.

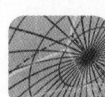

NURSING PROCESS: Patient Care Plan for Postoperative Esophageal Cancer

Assessment of Airway and Gas Exchange

Subjective Data:

Assessing level of consciousness: | What is your name?
Do you know where you are? | Do you know what happened to
What day is it? | you?

Objective Data:

Lung sounds. | Respiratory rate and character.
Oxygen saturation. | Color of skin and nail beds.

Nursing Assessment and Diagnoses	Outcomes and Evaluation Parameters	Planning and Interventions with *Rationales*
Nursing Diagnoses: *Airway Clearance, Ineffective* related to proximity of surgery to the trachea and thoracic incision *Gas Exchange, Impaired* related to possibility of aspiration and general anesthesia	**Outcome:** Adequate oxygenation. **Evaluation Parameters:** Alert and oriented. Normal pulse oximetry and arterial blood gases. Clear lung sounds. Ability to cough to clear secretions. Unlabored respiration.	**Interventions and *Rationales:*** Assess level of consciousness. *Indicates possible decrease in oxygenation and brain hypoxia.* Monitor ABGs and oxygen saturation. *To evaluate gas exchange.* Assess mucous membranes and nail beds for signs of cyanosis. *Indicators of inadequate gas exchange.* Assess for diminished or adventitious breath sounds. *Indicates possible aspiration or decreased inspiratory ability related to surgical pain.* Encourage deep breathing and coughing and use of incentive spirometer at least every hour. *To promote lung expansion, mobilize secretions, and prevent atelectasis.* Assess the need for suctioning. *To maintain a patent airway.* Monitor respiratory rate and character. *To assess for respiratory distress.* Report respiratory distress to the health care provider. *Early intervention can prevent respiratory failure.*

Assessment of Pain

Subjective Data:

What is your level of pain on a scale of 0–10, with 10 being the worst pain?
Are you allergic to anything?
Do you have any cultural or religious practices for dealing with pain?

Objective Data:

Restlessness. | Moaning or groaning.
Grimacing. | Shallow respirations.

Nursing Assessment and Diagnoses	Outcomes and Evaluation Parameters	Planning and Interventions with *Rationales*
Nursing Diagnosis: *Pain, Acute* related to surgery	**Outcome:** Comfort level maintained. **Evaluation Parameters:** Able to communicate level of pain and relief from medications. Able to take deep breaths without pain. Appears restful without restlessness or moaning.	**Interventions and *Rationales:*** Assess pain using pain scale (0–10) to quantify pain level. *To increase consistency in monitoring pain.* Assess level of pain 30 minutes and 1 hour after giving pain medication. *To assess effectiveness of medications.* Explore cultural and religious practices and beliefs about pain and illness. *Different cultures and religions have varying beliefs about pain, suffering, and disease.* Teach nonpharmacologic methods of pain control, such as guided imagery, meditation, and breathing exercises. *This may augment pain relief.*

Assessment of Nutrition

Subjective Data:

How much weight have you lost?
How long did you have difficulty swallowing?
What had you been able to eat?

Objective Data:

Body weight. | Wound healing.
Body mass index. | Physical appearance.
Skin condition. | Serum albumin.

Nursing Assessment and Diagnoses	Outcomes and Evaluation Parameters	Planning and Interventions with *Rationales*
Nursing Diagnosis: *Imbalanced Nutrition: Less than Body Requirements*	**Outcome:** Optimal nutrition. **Evaluation Parameters:** Maintains body weight or gains weight if underweight. Normal serum albumin. Skin is soft without evidence of dryness. Surgical incision healing. No evidence of skin breakdown.	**Interventions and *Rationales:*** Monitor body weight at same time every day. *Indicates a degree of adequate calorie intake and fluid balance.* Assess skin condition and healing. *Adequate dietary protein and calories are needed for wound healing and general skin condition.* Monitor laboratory values particularly serum albumin. Prepare and give parenteral or enteral nutrition as ordered. Assess for edema. *The presence of edema is one indicator of low serum proteins.* Check placement of feeding tube to prevent aspiration.

Pathophysiology/Etiology

Most gastric ulcers develop in the antrum, adjacent to the body of the stomach where acid is produced. Interestingly though, gastric ulcers are not associated with increased acid secretion, but rather with a defect in the mucosal barrier to hydrogen ions, allowing the ions to permeate the mucosa. Chronic gastritis may precipitate gastric ulcers by preventing the mucosa's ability to produce a protective layer of mucus. ***Helicobacter pylori (H. pylori)***, a bacterium causing gastritis, is thought to be responsible for 60% of gastric ulcers (Wollner, 2004).

Another factor contributing to the formation of gastric ulcers is decreased prostaglandin secretion by the mucosa, therefore diminishing its protective ability. Medications such as aspirin and nonsteroidal anti-inflammatory drugs (NSAIDs) inhibit prostaglandin formation (O'Malley, 2003). Therefore, a strong association between the habitual use of these drugs and the development of gastric ulcers has been made.

Duodenal reflux of bile is another contributing factor in the development of gastric ulcers. Bile salts decrease the electrical potential across the gastric mucosal membrane, allowing hydrogen ions to diffuse into the mucosa where they disrupt permeability and cellular structure (Huether, 2006). An inflammatory response is established and histamine is released, stimulating an increase in acid, pepsinogen, blood flow, and capillary permeability leading to edema and minute hemorrhages.

Duodenal Ulcers

Duodenal ulcers are the most common type of peptic ulcer in the United States and are found more often in younger people. There is an association between people with type O blood and the development of duodenal ulcers, although the relationship is not yet clear. As with gastric ulcers, duodenal ulcers occur equally in men and women.

Pathophysiology/Etiology

Almost 80% of duodenal ulcers are caused by *H. pylori* gastritis (Wollner, 2004) and occur in the proximal duodenum. *H. pylori* thrives in the acid environment of the stomach once thought to be inhospitable to any bacteria. *H. pylori* produces urease, the enzyme that catalyzes the hydrolysis of urea to ammonia. Ammonia is toxic to the gastric epithelial cells and causes an inflammatory response that induces cytokine production leading to chronic gastritis.

Other factors contributing to duodenal ulcer formation include hypersecretion of acid and pepsin. The increased acid secretion may be in part related to a greater parietal cell mass, or to vagal activity stimulating the release of gastrin, which in turn stimulates the production of acid and pepsin. There may also be an inadequate secretion of bicarbonate by the duodenal mucosa, which in turn would result in increased secretion of acid (Huether, 2006). Cigarette smoke stimulates acid production, and NSAIDs inhibit prostaglandins, contributing to increased acid and decreased mucosal defenses.

Clinical Manifestations

The common characteristic of both gastric and duodenal ulcers is pain that is located in the upper abdomen. The pain is intermittent and described as gnawing, burning, aching, or hunger-like. Traditionally, the pain of gastric ulcers was considered to be related to food consumption and relieved by antacids and that of duodenal ulcers was relieved by food and commonly occurred before a meal or at night. However, there is wide variability in individual experiences of ulcer pain, and the pattern of pain is not diagnostic. Both duodenal and gastric ulcers produce pain when the stomach is empty that is most often relieved by food or antacids.

Other manifestations, particularly in the elderly, are not as easily associated with peptic ulcer disease (PUD). The patient may present with chest pain, dysphagia, or anemia. Anemia may be the presenting symptom in older adults, especially for those taking NSAIDs. Typically, gastric ulcers are more chronic in nature, whereas duodenal ulcers show periods of remission and exacerbation. Anorexia, weight loss, and vomiting are more common in patients with gastric ulcers, chiefly in older adults.

Complications

Complications of PUD include hemorrhage, perforation, and pyloric or gastric outlet obstruction. All of these complications can prove to be life threatening, but can be avoided with early diagnosis and treatment.

Bleeding is the most common complication of PUD, especially in the elderly, and may occur from an erosion of a small vessel producing a slow and insidious blood loss, or from an erosion of a larger vessel leading to severe hemorrhage and shock. Erosion occurs in smaller vessels; anemia and occult blood in the stool may be the only clinical manifestations. In the erosion of larger vessels, the patient may have bright-red emesis or emesis of partially digested blood, which has a "coffee-grounds" appearance. In addition, these patients usually have melena (dark, tarry stools).

Gastric outlet obstruction (or **pyloric obstruction**) is the result of edema, inflammation, scarring of the pylorus, or a combination of these conditions. As a slowly evolving process, it often begins with a feeling of epigastric fullness progressing to vomiting. If complete obstruction occurs, gastric acid, sodium, and potassium are lost in the vomitus, which can result in metabolic alkalosis and electrolyte imbalance.

The most serious complication of PUD is perforation. Perforation of the ulcer causes severe, sudden upper abdominal pain that radiates throughout the abdomen. Gastroduodenal contents containing acid, pepsin, bile, and pancreatic juice enter the abdominal cavity, causing peritoneal irritation and peritonitis, which triggers a massive inflammatory response. The classic manifestations of peritonitis, rigid boardlike abdomen and absence of bowel sounds, happen almost immediately following the perforation. However, the older adult may not exhibit these classic signs, but may have other nonspecific symptoms, thus delaying diagnosis and treatment.

Diagnostic Tests

The majority of peptic ulcers (80% to 90%) can be detected with a barium swallow (upper GI series), although small or superficial ulcers may be missed. Definitive diagnosis is made by direct visualization of the mucosa in the esophagus, stomach, and duodenum using an endoscope. See Chart 45–1 (p. 1389) for the nursing care of a patient undergoing endoscopy. Tissue specimens can be taken during the endoscopic procedure to detect *H. pylori* and malignancy. Because the majority of peptic ulcers are caused by *H. pylori* infection, testing for the organism is often done. The Diagnostic Tests box outlines the different tests that can be used to detect *H. pylori*.

Medical Management

Treatment for PUD is aimed primarily at relieving symptoms, eradicating *H. pylori* infection, and preventing complications such as hemorrhage, obstruction, or perforation. The health care provider makes the diagnosis of PUD by history and physical examination. With a high suspicion of the disorder, an initial course of drug therapy will be ordered and its effectiveness assessed in 1 month. In the event that there is no relief gained from treatment, or there is evidence of a complication, further diagnostic testing is done.

Medications

Most peptic ulcers can be successfully treated with medications. The goal of pharmacologic intervention is to eradicate *H. pylori* and has a success rate of 75% to 90% (Wollner, 2004). The standard therapeutic regimen at this time includes treatment with two antibiotics and a proton pump inhibitor for 10 to 14 days, but it may also include the use of a bismuth preparation. One regimen uses amoxicillin 1,000 milligrams bid with clarithromycin 500 milligrams bid; another uses metronidazole 500 milligrams bid and clarithromycin 500 milligrams bid; and the third option uses metronidazole 500 milligrams qid combined with tetracycline 500 milligrams qid. Usually after a course of treatment with antibiotics and proton pump inhibitors, the patient is maintained on a once daily dose of a proton pump inhibitor or H_2-receptor blocker (Wollner, 2004). Other medications that are used to treat PUD are antacids, prostaglandin analogs, and mucosal barrier fortifiers. See the Pharmacology Summary feature for drug therapy for *Helicobater pylori* eradication.

Lifestyle Modifications

There are no specific dietary modifications that individuals with PUD should follow because no food is considered ulcerogenic. It is generally believed that any food that does not cause the individual any discomfort can be consumed, and likewise, foods that cause discomfort should be avoided. The patient should be advised not to take NSAIDs or aspirin (or products containing aspirin; i.e., Excedrin, Alka-Seltzer). If the patient requires the anti-inflammatory action of NSAIDs, the health care provider may switch the patient to a COX-2 selective inhibitor, which is less likely to induce an ulcer. However, many of the newer studies show a significant portion of the normal population has similar symptoms when taking the COX-2 inhibitors, so monitoring the patient is paramount. Small amounts of alcohol do not cause harm, but large amounts should be avoided. The rate of healing is slowed and the recurrence rate increased in patients who smoke, so smoking should be discouraged. Because *H. pylori* is found in saliva and feces, increasing the possibility of person-to-person transmission through oral to oral and fecal to oral routes, good hand hygiene should be encouraged. Higher rates of *H. pylori* infection have been found in people living in close contact and where sanitation is not good.

Surgery

Fortunately, with the discovery of *H. pylori* infection as the major cause of peptic ulcers, and the development of medications to eradicate this organism, surgery is rarely necessary. Surgery may be required to treat the complications of PUD if medical treatment fails. (For the nursing care of the patient having gastric surgery, see the Nursing Process: Patient Care Plan for Gastric Cancer and Gastric Resection, p. 1401.)

◼ Nursing Management

Most patients with PUD are treated with medications at home unless complications occur; then hospital admission is necessary. Nursing assessment should include a general health history with a focused assessment on complaints of epigastric pain and heart-

DIAGNOSTIC TESTS for *Helicobacter Pylori*

Test	Method	Results	Nursing Implications
Biopsy urease test	A tissue specimen is obtained during endoscopy and placed in a gel-containing urea.	*H. pylori* produces urease, which changes the color of the gel if the organism is present.	Endoscopy is an invasive procedure. See Chart 45–1 (p. 1389) for care of the patient undergoing endoscopy.
Biopsy examination	A tissue specimen is sent to the laboratory and examined under the microscope for evidence *of H. pylori*.	Presence of *H. pylori* indicates infection.	See Chart 45-1 (p. 1389) for care of the patient undergoing endoscopy
Enzyme-linked immunosorbent assay (ELISA)	A blood sample is tested for antibodies (IgG) against *H. pylori*.	Indicates current or past infection.	There are no food or fluid restrictions. Specimen is collected in a red-top tube.
Urea breath test	Radioactive carbon (C-13 or C-14) labeled urea is given in an oral preparation.	*H. pylori* metabolizes urea and produces carbon that then travels to the lungs and is exhaled. The amount of radioactive carbon in the breath is measured.	The nurse assures the patient that he will not be radioactive after this test and that the 13 C or 14 C is not harmful.
Fecal antigen immunoassay	Stool specimen is examined for *H. pylori*.	Determines active infection.	Confirms presence of *H. pylori*.

PHARMACOLOGY Summary of Drug Therapy for *Helicobacter Pylori* Eradication

Medication Category	Action	Application/Indication	Nursing Responsibility
Anti-Infective Agents Amoxicillin (Amoxil) Clarithromycin (Biaxin) Metronidazole (Flagyl)	Treatment protocols: Triple therapy (2 antibiotics + 1 PPI) Quadruple therapy (2 antibiotics + 1 PPI + bismuth) Sequential therapy (1 antibiotic + PPI followed by 2 antibiotics + 1 PPI) Causes bacterial cell death by inhibition of DNA or bacterial protein synthesis.	Active or inactive peptic ulcer with positive *H. pylori* test.	Monitor for adverse effects: rash, diarrhea, and nausea. Instruct patient to complete medications as ordered; contact health care provider if adverse reaction. Instruct patient not to crush extended-release forms of drug. Multiple drug interactions; monitor for signs of increased drug levels (theophylline, digoxin, warfarin, and others).

burn, including the nature of the pain and relationship to eating, the presence of any symptom associated with a complication (dysphagia, vomiting, and presence of blood in the vomitus), what relieves the pain, and what medications are in use, including NSAIDs or aspirin. The care plan for patients with peptic ulcer disease is presented in the Nursing Process: Patient Care Plan feature (p. 1398).

 Peptic ulcer disease (PUD) is a common disorder that has a major impact on health care costs in the United States; it accounts for approximately 10% of all medical costs associated with digestive diseases. Currently it is thought that PUD is caused by Helicobacter pylori *infection or the chronic use of nonsteroidal anti-inflammatory drugs (NSAIDs). The American Gastroenterological Association (2005) reported that approximately 30 million people take over-the-counter (OTC) and prescription NSAIDs daily for pain relief, headaches, and arthritis. Therefore, it is important for the nurse to determine whether the patient is taking an NSAID and to provide appropriate teaching related to dosage and side effects (Wilcox, Cryer, & Triadafilopoulos, 2005).*

Health Promotion

The thrust of health promotion to prevent PUD is to advise people to avoid known risk factors. As with chronic gastritis and GERD, these include cigarette smoking, excessive and prolonged alcohol ingestion, the use of oral corticosteroids, and the excessive use of NSAIDs and aspirin. Chronic gastritis and GERD do contribute to ulcer formation, and patients should be encouraged to seek treatment for these disorders. Nurses should use every opportunity to clarify misconceptions that ulcers are caused from eating spicy food; however, certain foods may precipitate symptoms in individuals with PUD.

■ Cancer of the Stomach

Gastric carcinoma is the second most common cancer in the world, but it is less common in the United States. It is twice as prevalent in men, with the highest incidences in Hispanics, African Americans, and Japanese Americans (who have retained the traditional diet). There seems to be a genetic predisposition to the development of gastric cancer. The majority of gastric cancer develops in the distal portions of the stomach and can be attributed to *H. pylori* infection. Chronic gastritis, gastric polyps, pernicious anemia, chronic gastric ulcer, and dietary fac-

tors, such as the use of nitrates (used to preserve meats) and smoked meats, may also contribute to the development of gastric cancer. Lack of hydrochloric acid (**achlorhydria**), atrophic gastritis, and history of gastric resection are also known to be risk factors for gastric cancer.

Pathophysiology

The most common type of cancer developing in the stomach is adenocarcinoma; and although it can develop on any mucosal surface, it is most common in the antrum and distal portions of the stomach. Early gastric cancer may involve the mucosa and submucosa and is usually asymptomatic. As the lesion progresses, it spreads to the gastric wall and regional lymph nodes. It may then advance to adjacent organs such as the liver, pancreas, and transverse colon. Because the stomach has a rich blood and lymphatic supply, the cancer spreads via the portal vein to the liver and through the systemic circulation to the lungs. Metastasis has also been found in bone, ovarian, and peritoneal tissue.

Clinical Manifestations

Regrettably, there are rarely any symptoms associated with gastric cancer. The patient may complain of anorexia, indigestion, heartburn, or early satiety, but these are vague and often the patient does not consider them serious. The patient may self-diagnose and self-treat with over-the-counter medications such as antacids, H_2-receptor antagonists, or proton pump inhibitors. Weight loss occurs as the disease progresses and the patient eventually becomes cachectic. When the patient's health fails, he usually seeks medical attention and diagnosis is made. By this time, the disease is far advanced and prognosis is poor.

Diagnostic Procedures

Definitive diagnosis is done through upper endoscopy and biopsy. See Chart 45–1 (p. 1389) for the nursing care of a patient undergoing endoscopy. Because the patient is usually ill at the time of diagnosis, other tests are done first. These include a CBC whereby a decreased hemoglobin and hematocrit may be the first indication of gastric cancer. Abdominal ultrasound may be done, particularly if a mass is felt on physical examination.

Medical Management

The medical management of gastric cancer involves identification of the cancer and in most cases is followed by surgical removal.

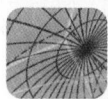

NURSING PROCESS: Patient Care Plan for Peptic Ulcer Disease

Assessment of Pain

Subjective Data:

On a scale of 0–10, with 10 being the worst pain, how would you rate your pain?

What does your pain feel like—burning, gnawing, aching, or stabbing?

When does your pain occur?

Does anything make it worse?

Does anything make it better?

Does eating make it better?

Does eating make it worse?

Does your pain occur before meals?

Does it wake you at night?

What have you used at home to relieve the pain?

Are you allergic to anything?

Do you take any medications such as aspirin, Excedrin, Motrin, or Advil? If so, how much and for how long?

Do you smoke?

Have you felt nauseated?

Did you vomit?

Did the vomit contain blood or brown fluid?

Objective Data:

Vital signs.

Abdominal examination:
- Distention?
- Pain or tenderness on palpation?
- Bowel sounds?
- Soft or rigid?

Stool for occult blood.

Facial grimacing.

Restless, holding abdomen.

Nursing Assessment and Diagnoses	Outcomes and Evaluation Parameters	Planning and Interventions with *Rationales*
Nursing Diagnosis: *Pain, Acute* related to peptic ulceration and irritation of nerve endings	**Outcome:** Pain relieved. *Evaluation Parameters:* Able to communicate level of pain and therapies that relieve it. Able to verbalize need to quit smoking. No restlessness or facial grimacing.	**Interventions and *Rationales:*** Assess pain using scale (0–10) to quantify pain. *To increase consistency in pain measurement.* Assess pain, character and location, and its relationship to food intake, empty stomach, or other factors and what relieves the pain. *To establish a pattern to the pain and make a plan to control contributing factors.* Administer medications ordered *to reduce acid secretion and monitor effectiveness* (see the earlier Pharmacology Summary for details, p. 1390). Teach the importance of following through with medication regimen as ordered. *To increase the effectiveness of H. pylori eradication and decrease the risk of complications.* Provide information about the symptoms of complications of PUD and to have the patient call the health care provider immediately if any should occur. *To decrease the chances of a complication becoming life threatening.*

Surgery

Surgical resection of the stomach is considered the treatment of choice if gastric cancer is diagnosed early, or it may be performed for palliation if the cancer is more advanced. A partial gastrectomy, or removal of a portion of the stomach, can be done in several ways. The two most common partial gastrectomy procedures are the **gastroduodenostomy (Billroth I)**, whereby the lower portion of the stomach is removed and the remainder is anastomosed to the duodenum (Figure 45–4A ▪); and the **gastrojejunostomy (Billroth II)**, which involves removal of a larger distal portion of the stomach with the remainder anastomosed to the jejunum (Figure 45–4B ▪). In total gastrectomy, or the removal of the entire stomach, the esophagus is anastomosed to either the duodenum or the jejunum (Figure 45–4C ▪).

Long-term complications of surgery are not uncommon. The most common problem is dumping syndrome, whereby the pylorus is bypassed and a food bolus enters the duodenum or jejunum rapidly. Because chyme (partially digested food in the stomach containing gastric acid and digestive enzymes) is hyperosmolar, water is pulled into the intestinal lumen to dilute it, causing a rapid decrease in blood volume. When the blood volume is decreased, there is a reflex sympathetic nervous system response manifested by tachycardia, orthostatic hypotension, dizziness, flushing, and di-

aphoresis. Additional symptoms such as nausea, epigastric pain, cramping, and loud, hyperactive bowel sounds (borborygmi) can occur within 5 to 30 minutes of eating. Diarrhea follows shortly.

In response to the hyperosmolar chyme being delivered to the jejunum, there is a rapid rise in blood sugar with a resultant release of excessive amounts of insulin. The insulin causes a secondary hypoglycemia to occur about 2 to 3 hours after eating. In most cases, dumping syndrome lasts from 6 to 12 months after surgery. The symptoms can be managed by eating small, more frequent meals. Carbohydrates should be reduced while increasing the amount of protein and fat in order to help slow the transit time. The patient should be instructed to lie down for 30 to 60 minutes after eating to slow transit time further.

Removal of any portion of the stomach can impact vitamin and mineral absorption. For example, iron is primarily absorbed from the duodenum and proximal jejunum. With the extensive surgery, coupled with the rapid gastric emptying, interference with iron absorption can manifest in anemia. Gastric resection may also decrease the amount of intrinsic factor produced by the parietal cells. Intrinsic factor is needed for the absorption of vitamin B_{12}. Only minute amounts of vitamin B_{12} are needed, and the liver stores enough for up to 2 years, so it may take that long for pernicious anemia to develop.

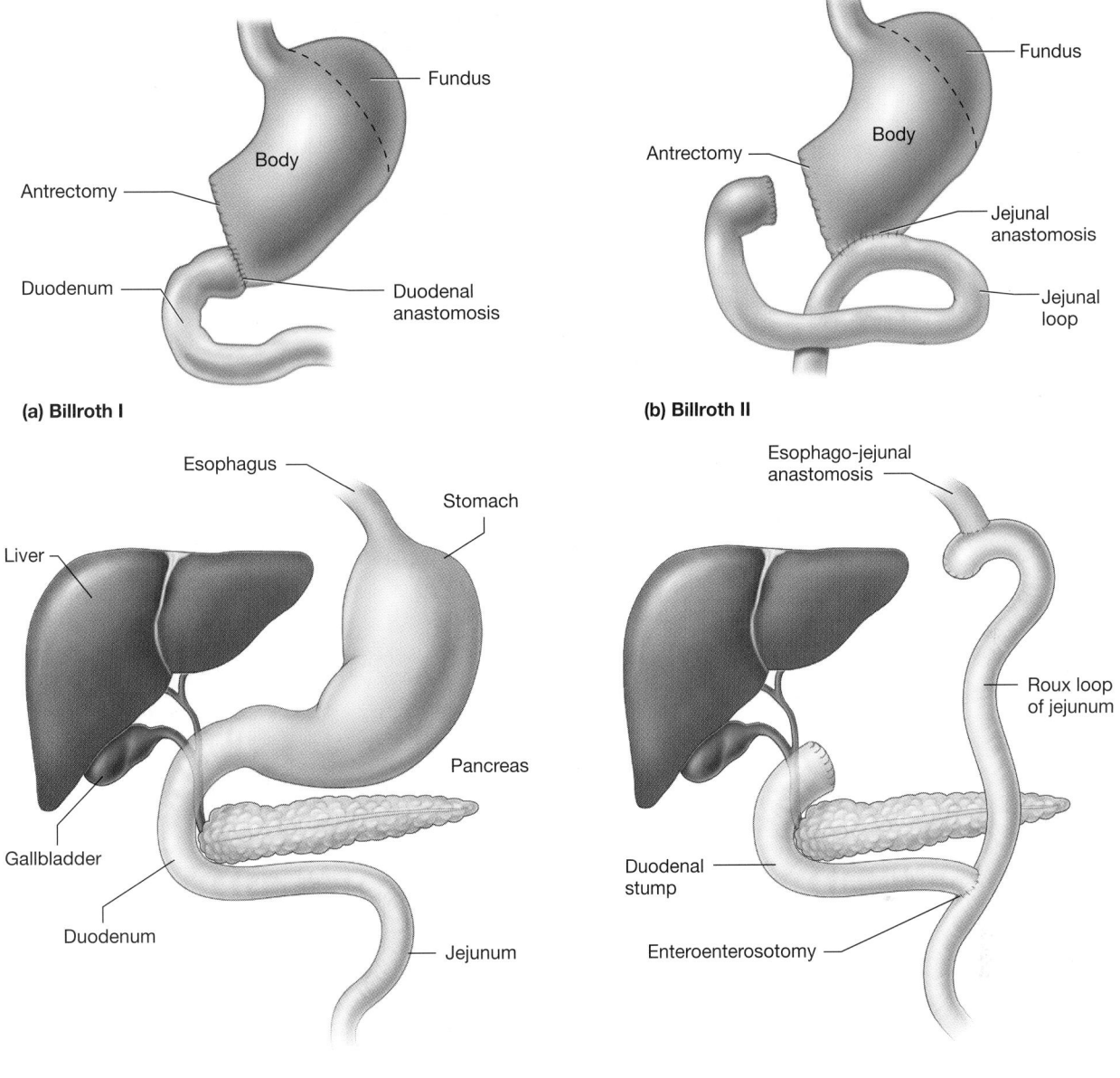

FIGURE 45–4 ■ (A) Billroth I, (B) Billroth II, and (C) total gastrectomy.

Radiation/Chemotherapy

Radiation or chemotherapy may be used to arrest metastatic or lymphatic spread of gastric carcinoma. It is considered palliative in patients with advanced disease to help shrink the tumor and provide some pain relief. However, because of the location of the cancer, these patients will require a feeding tube, in the form of either a gastrostomy tube, if the total stomach has been affected, or, if there is a sufficient portion of the stomach remaining, a jejunostomy tube (Figure 45–5 ■, p. 1400). Chart 45–2 (p. 1400) indicates nursing care of the patient with a feeding tube.

■ Nursing Management

Nursing care of the patient with gastric cancer is mostly supportive. If there is no metastasis, surgical resection of the stomach is performed. For a detailed discussion on care of the patient with cancer, refer to Chapter 64 ⊙. Application of the nursing process can facilitate a comprehensive approach to patient care. The Nursing Process: Patient Care Plan feature (p. 1401) covers the nursing management plan for patients with gastric cancer or having gastric resection.

Health Promotion

The nurse can educate the public about the contributing factors to the development of gastric cancer, such as avoiding or limiting foods containing nitrates, which include smoked meats, bacon, lunch meats, hot dogs, and any other meat product that does not require refrigeration. If a patient is known to have *H. pylori*, the nurse should encourage completion of the prescribed course of medications and return for follow-up to evaluate *H. pylori* eradication.

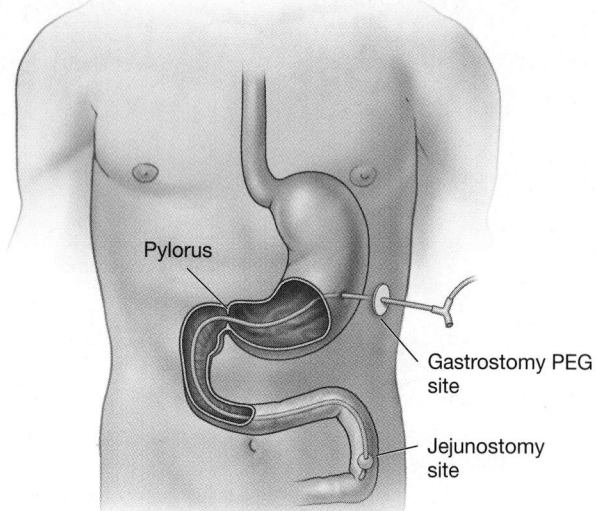

(a) Gastrostomy

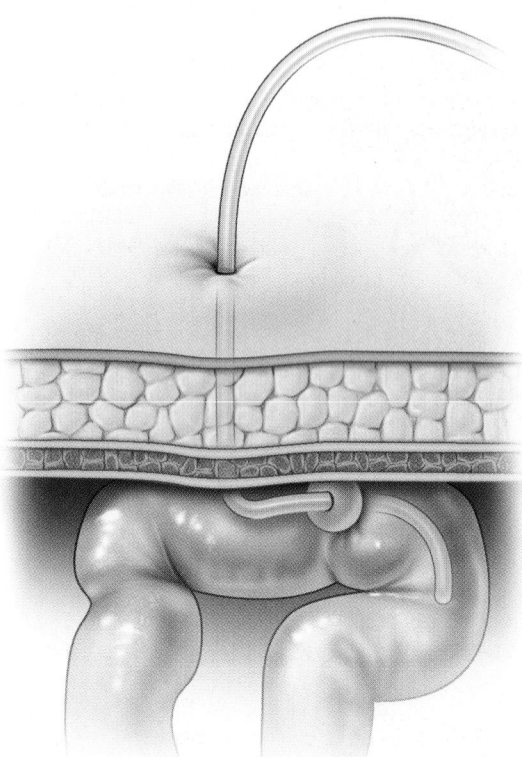

(b) Jejunostomy

FIGURE 45–5 ■ Gastrostomy and jejunostomy tube.

Malabsorption/Maldigestion Syndromes

Malabsorption is considered to be the failure of the small intestine to absorb nutrients from digested food, whereas **maldigestion** is the failure of chemical processes such as inadequate pancreatic enzymes or bile salts to break down food products. Maldigestive disorders result in the malabsorption of nutrients and thus are considered a form of malabsorption. In

---

CHART 45–2 Nursing Care of the Patient with a Feeding Tube

The purpose of a gastrostomy tube or a jejunostomy tube is to provide complete nutrition through the alimentary system. It is safer and has fewer side effects than total parenteral nutrition (TPN), particularly when the patient is to have feedings at home.

CHECK TUBE PLACEMENT
- Aspirate and check pH or aspirate.
- A pH of 5 or less indicates gastric placement.
- A pH of 7 or higher usually indicates intestinal placement.

IRRIGATE TUBE
- *Gently* instill 30 to 50 milliliters of water before and after each feeding or as ordered.
- The lumen of some soft, small-diameter tubes may be cleaned with a special brush to maintain patency.

CLEANSE INSERTION SITE
- Remove old dressing (using clean gloves).
- Inspect site for healing or signs of infection (drainage, redness, or swelling).
- Clean site using saline or what is ordered, using sterile technique if the stoma is not yet healed or clean technique if the site is healed.
- Apply dressing using drain sponge (do not cut gauze dressing; it will fray and threads may enter the wound).

MONITOR FOR INTOLERANCE TO FEEDINGS
- Assess abdomen for distention.
- Auscultate bowel sounds.
- Palpate to assess for tenderness.

CONDUCT PATIENT AND FAMILY TEACHING
- Tube care (patient may clean site in the shower after stoma has healed).
- Feeding schedule.
- Monitoring for side effect of feeding.

---

addition to absorptive failure, malabsorption can be caused by surgical resection of the stomach and intestines, or by vascular disorders or intestinal diseases.

Celiac Disease (Sprue)

Celiac disease, also known as gluten-sensitive enteropathy and celiac sprue, is an autoimmune disorder in which there is a histologic change in the mucosal lining of the small intestine when food containing the gliadin component of gluten (wheat, rye, barley) is ingested (Landzberg, 2006; Young & Thomas, 2004). It was once considered to be a childhood illness and relatively rare. Health care providers now know that celiac disease occurs in individuals at any age and may affect as many as 1 in 200 people (Landzberg, 2006).

Pathophysiology

The development of celiac disease involves a genetic predisposition for the disease, gluten ingestion, and immune mediated

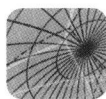

NURSING PROCESS: Patient Care Plan for Gastric Cancer and Gastric Resection

MyNursingKit | Celiac Disease Foundation

Nursing Assessment of Nutrition

Subjective Data:
What are your favorite foods?
How much did you weigh before you found out about your cancer?
Had you noticed any weight loss before that? How much?
Do you feel full after eating a small amount?
Are you nauseated?

Objective Data:
Daily weights.
Intake and output (I&O).
General appearance.
Laboratory studies:
  • Serum albumin
  • H & H

• Transferrin
• Ferritin
• TIBC
• Electrolytes.

Nursing Assessment and Diagnoses	Outcomes and Evaluation Parameters	Planning and Interventions with *Rationales*
Nursing Diagnosis: *Nutrition Imbalanced: Less than Body Requirements* related to removal of part of stomach	**Outcome:** Adequate nutrition. *Evaluation Parameters:* Body weight maintained or increased. Healing incision. Normal serum albumin. Normal serum electrolytes. Normal iron studies. Normal hemoglobin and hematocrit.	**Interventions and *Rationales:*** See Chart 45–2 for nursing interventions for patients with feeding tubes. Weigh daily at the same time and on the same scale. *To provide an accurate assessment of fluid balance and nutritional adequacy.* Measure and record accurate intake and output. *To estimate fluid balance.* Monitor laboratory indicators of nutritional status. *These are better indicators of nutritional status than body weight alone.* Assess skin for breakdown. *Can be an indicator of nutritional status, particularly protein.* Assess wound healing. *Decreased protein and vitamin C can hinder wound healing.* Medicate for nausea and pain as needed before meals. *Pain and nausea often produce anorexia and relief can increase the appetite.* Provide the patient with favorite foods or have family members bring home-prepared food when she is able to eat. *To increase the patient's nutritional intake.* Invite family or friends to visit at mealtime. Gathering for meals is a social function for many families and may improve the patient's intake.

Assessment of Emotional Status

Subjective Data:
What have the doctors told you about your cancer?
Who do you count on for support?
Do you have any religious, cultural, or spiritual beliefs that help you deal with your cancer?

Objective Data:
Family or friends visiting.
Clergy visiting.
Initiates conversations with the nursing staff.

Nursing Assessment and Diagnoses	Outcomes and Evaluation Parameters	Planning and Interventions with *Rationales*
Nursing Diagnosis: *Grieving, Complicated* related to diagnosis of cancer with poor prognosis	**Outcome:** Anxiety and fear controlled. *Evaluation Parameters:* Verbalizes fears about cancer and death. Communicates feelings with significant others.	**Interventions and *Rationales:*** Encourage family and significant others to spend as much time as possible with the patient, especially during difficult times such as visits from the health care provider, during chemo and radiation treatments. *To give purpose to the family and significant others and help them feel a part of the process.* Allow the patient to express any feelings without negating any of these feelings. *Allowing the patient to have hope may aid in coping behavior.* Inquire about the patient's cultural, religious, and spiritual beliefs about illness and death, and facilitate discussion with family and clergy where appropriate. *Spiritual and cultural beliefs can comfort the patient and family during this time.*

(continued)

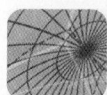

Assessment of Pain

Subjective Data:

On a scale of 0–10, with 10 being the worst pain, how would you rate your pain?

What does your pain feel like—burning, gnawing, aching, or stabbing?

Have you felt nauseated?

Did you vomit?

Did the vomit contain blood or brown fluid?

Objective Data:

Vital signs.

Abdominal examination:

- Distention?
- Pain or tenderness on palpation?

- Bowel sounds?
- Soft or rigid?

Stool for occult blood.

Facial grimacing.

Restless, holding abdomen.

Nursing Assessment and Diagnoses	Outcomes and Evaluation Parameters	Planning and Interventions with *Rationales*
Nursing Diagnosis: *Pain, Acute* related to surgical incision and metastatic cancer	**Outcome:** Pain relieved. *Evaluation Parameters:* Able to communicate level of pain and therapies that relieve it. Abdomen soft, nontender, and bowel sounds present. No restlessness or facial grimacing.	**Interventions and *Rationales:*** Assess pain using scale (0–10) to quantify pain. *To increase consistency in pain measurement.* Assess pain, character and location, and any related symptoms. *To give the nurse clues to the cause of the pain; i.e., incisional pain vs. infection, vs. peritonitis, vs. metastatic cancer.* Administer pain medications as ordered and assess pain level 30 minutes and 1 hour after administration. *To evaluate the effectiveness of the pain medication.*

responses. When a genetically susceptible individual ingests a gluten-containing product, there is a T-cell mediated immune response and chronic inflammation develops if ingestion is continued. Antibodies are produced in response to glutamic acid, which is a product of the digestion of gluten. The antibodies activate leukocytes and the cytokines that release interferon-γ, interlukin-4, and tumor necrosis factor (Young & Thomas, 2004). The microvilli and the brush border of the small intestine are destroyed by the release of cytokines. Continued ingestion of gluten will cause the eventual disappearance of the microvilli and the loss of brush border digestive enzymes, which results in malabsorption.

Clinical Manifestations

Although diarrhea is the most common symptom in children with celiac disease, up to 38% of adult patients are asymptomatic because the small intestine can compensate if the degree of involvement is limited (Presutti, Cangemi, Cassidy, & Hill, 2007). In fact, most adults have signs and symptoms that are unrelated to the GI tract, such as symptoms of rheumatoid arthritis, chronic hepatitis, dental enamel hypoplasia, iron deficiency anemia, neurological dysfunction, osteoporosis, short stature, and reproductive problems. It has been known since the 1970s that diarrhea may not be the primary symptom of celiac disease; however, the patient is usually diagnosed only if diarrhea is present.

Diagnostic Procedures

A biopsy of the small intestine is considered the gold standard for diagnosing celiac disease. When the tissue is examined, the mucosa appears flattened, with an absence of villi, indicating a degree of atrophy. Several new blood tests for celiac disease are proving to be sensitive and specific. They include antigliadin antibody (AGA), antiendomysium antibody (AEA), and tissue transglutaminase (tTG); however, tissue biopsy remains the definitive test (Young & Thomas, 2004).

Medical Management

At the present time, the only treatment for celiac disease is a total gluten-free diet. Gluten is found in wheat, barley, and rye grains (Chart 45–3). Some sources report that oats should also be avoided because they are contaminated by being processed in machines that also process wheat, rye, and barley without interim cleanings and decontamination. Additives, preservatives, and stabilizers may contain gluten, so many food and medicine sources may also cause symptoms.

Nursing Management

Support and education are the major nursing responsibilities in the care of individuals with celiac disease. Because the treatment is total elimination of gluten from the diet, the nurse needs to be well informed about foods that contain gluten in order to teach

CHART 45–3	Celiac Disease: Common Foods Containing Gluten That Should Be Avoided

Barley malt	Gluten	Seitan
Beer	Kamut	Semolina
Bleached flour	Malt	Shoyu (soy sauce)
Bran	Malt extract	Soba noodles
Bread flour	Malt flavoring	Spelt
Brewer's yeast	Malt syrup	Sprouted wheat or
Bulgur wheat	Malt vinegar	barley
Coloring	Matzo	Udon (wheat noodles)
Couscous	Miso	Vegetable starch
Durum wheat	Pasta	Wheat
Edible starch	Pearl barley	Wheat germ
Farina	Rye	Wheat germ extract
Fillers	Seasoned French fries	Wheat germ oil
Food starch	(coated with flour)	Wheat grass

the patient diet modification. Potential hidden sources of gluten should be identified, such as canned or homemade cream soup, cream sauces, gravy, and some candies. Chart 45–3 lists the most common foods that contain gluten. Some items that contain gluten and are often overlooked include stamps, envelopes, and gummed labels; some toothpaste; vitamins; and laxatives. The nurse should be familiar with resources for support, such as the numerous organizations and websites that provide support, information, and gluten-free products.

Lactose Intolerance

Lactose intolerance is caused by a deficiency of lactase at the brush border of the small intestine, resulting in malabsorption. **Lactase** is an enzyme that aids in the breakdown of lactose, a disaccharide found in milk. The enzyme is needed to convert lactose into a monosaccharide, which can be absorbed in the small intestine. The deficiency is usually the result of a congenital defect, but intolerance does not usually develop until adulthood. Lactose intolerance can also be caused by several diseases of the intestine, including celiac disease and Crohn's disease.

Lactase deficiency is very common. In fact, it may affect as many as 90% of Asians and Native Americans and 70% of African Americans (McQuaid, 2004). Because of the lactase deficiency, there is undigested lactose in the intestines, which has two effects. First, intestinal bacteria cause fermentation of the undigested lactose, which produces gas. Second, because lactose is a large molecule, it increases the osmotic gradient in the intestines. These two processes produce the symptoms of lactose intolerance, which include bloating, abdominal distention, flatulence, crampy pain, and diarrhea. However, many individuals may remain symptom free unless large amounts of milk and milk-containing foods are ingested at one time.

Diagnostic Procedures

Lactase deficiency is diagnosed using the lactose breath test. This noninvasive test measures the amount of hydrogen gas exhaled after a 50-gram dose of lactose is given to a fasting patient. Hydrogen gas is a product of the fermentation of lactose in a lactase-deficient individual.

A lactose tolerance test can also be done to determine the degree of lactase deficiency. In this test, a dose of 100 grams of lactose is given orally, and the blood sugar is measured at 30, 60, and 120 minutes postadministration. In normal individuals, there should be an increase in the blood glucose, but in those with lactase deficiency, there is no increase.

Medical Management

Elimination of lactose from the diet will relieve the symptoms of this disorder. Some individuals may tolerate small amounts of lactose and may include in their diet foods that are lower in lactose, such as aged cheese and yogurt. They are cautioned to eliminate these foods if symptoms occur. There are lactase enzymes (Lactaid) available without a prescription to improve lactose tolerance, as well as milk containing lactase available commercially. Individuals, particularly women, may require calcium supplementation in order to get the minimum daily requirement of this mineral, if they must avoid all dairy products. The diet of most Americans is more than adequate in protein, so eliminating dairy products should not cause protein deficiency.

■ Nursing Management

Nursing care for the patient with a lactase deficiency centers on educating the patient and family about sources of lactose and appropriate nutritional alternatives. Lactose is most concentrated in milk, ice cream, and cottage cheese, but is also found in other cheeses, milk chocolate, sherbet, custard, and cream soups. The nurse should teach the patient and family how to read labels in order to detect lactose in food.

Pancreatic Insufficiency

A deficiency of pancreatic enzymes can also cause malabsorption. Lipase, trypsin, chymotrypsin, and amylase are needed to digest fat, protein, and carbohydrates. If these pancreatic enzymes are insufficient, maldigestion occurs. A deficiency in pancreatic enzymes can be caused by pancreatitis, pancreatic cancer, cystic fibrosis, and pancreatic abscess. However, there must be significant pancreatic damage before insufficiency results.

Pancreatic insufficiency results in maldigestion of all nutrients, but because enzymes secreted by the intestinal brush border and salivary amylase help to digest carbohydrates and proteins, maldigestion of these nutrients is not profound. However, these enzymes do not aid in the digestion of fat, so there is a profound inability to digest fats. The consequence is **steatorrhea** (fat in the stools) and weight loss. There could also be problems with the absorption of fat soluble vitamins.

■ Nursing Management

Pancreatic insufficiency is treated with supplemental pancreatic enzymes. The nurse should administer the enzymes (Viokase) before meals. The Pharmacology Summary feature (p. 1404) outlines the use of supplemental enzymes. The nurse should teach the patient and family about the administration of the medication, to monitor for signs of vitamin deficiency, and to notify the health care provider if weight loss or steatorrhea occurs.

Short Bowel Syndrome

Short bowel syndrome results when there is a reduction in the surface of the small intestine from surgical resection of the small bowel, typically because of tumors, Crohn's disease, infarction, trauma, and radiation enteropathy. The degree of the resulting malabsorption depends on the location and extent of the resection. For example, if the duodenum, jejunum, or proximal ileum is removed, severe malabsorption usually occurs.

The absorption of water, nutrients, vitamins, and minerals is hindered in the early postoperative period after small bowel resection. If a large portion of the small intestine is removed, the transit time is significantly reduced. With time, the bowel adapts by enlarging and lengthening the villi that remain, thereby increasing the surface area available for absorption. Some patients may achieve digestion and absorption that is about the same as

PHARMACOLOGY Summary of Medications Used to Treat Pancreatic Insufficiency

Medication Category	Action	Application/Indication	Nursing Responsibility
Digestive Enzymes			
Pancrelipase (Viokase)	Breaks down fats, proteins, and starches in the final stage of digestion for easier absorption.	Steatorrhea from malabsorption syndrome, post pancreatectomy, gastrectomy, or GI surgery (e.g., Billroth II).	Monitor for adverse effects: nausea, abdominal cramps, and diarrhea. Assess for improved nutritional status and decreased steatorrhea. Be aware of religious considerations; drug is pork based.

it was before the resection. However, a significant number of patients have considerable malabsorption that leads to diarrhea, weight loss, dehydration, and nutrient deficiencies.

Medical Management

Treatment for short bowel syndrome focuses on relief of symptoms and methods to maintain nutrition. To maintain nutrition, small, frequent feedings of high-calorie, high-protein foods are usually prescribed if the patient can tolerate oral feedings. If oral feedings are not tolerated, then enteral tube feedings or total parenteral nutrition (TPN) will be ordered. Supplementation with vitamins and minerals is frequently necessary.

If diarrhea is a continued problem, antidiarrheal medications, such as Lomotil, which slows intestinal motility, will be ordered. Proton pump inhibitors such as omeprazole (Prilosec) may be ordered for patients who have gastric reflux or hypersecretion of gastric acid postoperatively. See the Pharmacology Summary feature (p. 1390) which outlines the use of proton pump inhibitors. See the Pharmacology Summary feature of medications used to treat diarrhea.

◼ Nursing Management

Because the patient with short bowel syndrome is at risk for diarrhea, particularly in the early postoperative period, fluid and electrolyte imbalances are possible. Vital signs should be taken frequently and the nurse should monitor the condition of the patient's mucous membranes, daily weight, and record an accurate intake and output including measuring the volume of diarrhea.

The patient is also at risk for nutritional deficits. The health care provider may order total parenteral nutrition (TPN) to maintain the patient's nutritional status until the GI tract has recovered from surgical resection. The nurse monitors the patient's weight, laboratory values, central IV catheter, and insertion site. Once the patient's bowel sounds have returned, oral or enteral feedings may be started. It is important to monitor the patient's tolerance of the feeding once it is begun.

Educating the patient and family members is a major nursing responsibility. The patient will most likely have some problems with digestion and/or absorption for the rest of her life and will need guidance about the recommended diet and ways to maintain nutritional status. If the patient is able to tolerate oral feeding, small, frequent meals may be helpful. Resting in a reclining position after meals may help slow the GI transit time. The patient should be taught to monitor her body weight and to notify the health care provider if there is a consistent weight loss, which could signify either a fluid loss or inadequate calories.

Intestinal Obstruction

Intestinal obstruction can occur anywhere from the pylorus to the rectum and can be either partial or complete. There is impairment of forward movement of intestinal contents because of a mechanical cause (tumors [Figure 45–6C ◼], adhesions [Figure 45–6A ◼], Crohn's disease, diverticular disease, foreign bodies) or a functional cause (surgery, anesthesia, medications). Functional bowel obstructions are also called ileus, paralytic ileus, or adynamic ileus. Most bowel obstructions occur in the

PHARMACOLOGY Summary of Mediations Used to Treat Diarrhea

Medication Category	Action	Application/Indication	Nursing Responsibility
Antidiarrheal Agents **Opioids:** Codeine Camphorated opium tincture (Paregoric) Diphenoxylate/atropine (Lomotil) Loperamide (Imodium) **Other:** Bismuth subsalicylate (Pepto-Bismol)	Increases fluid and electrolyte absorption from the colon by slowing peristalsis. Reduces GI hypermotility by direct antibacterial effect and decreased prostoglandin synthesis.	Moderate to severe diarrhea. Traveler's diarrhea.	Monitor for signs and symptoms of dehydration and altered electrolyte levels. Observe for potential drowsiness. Instruct patient not to drive or perform other potentially hazardous activities until response to drug is known.

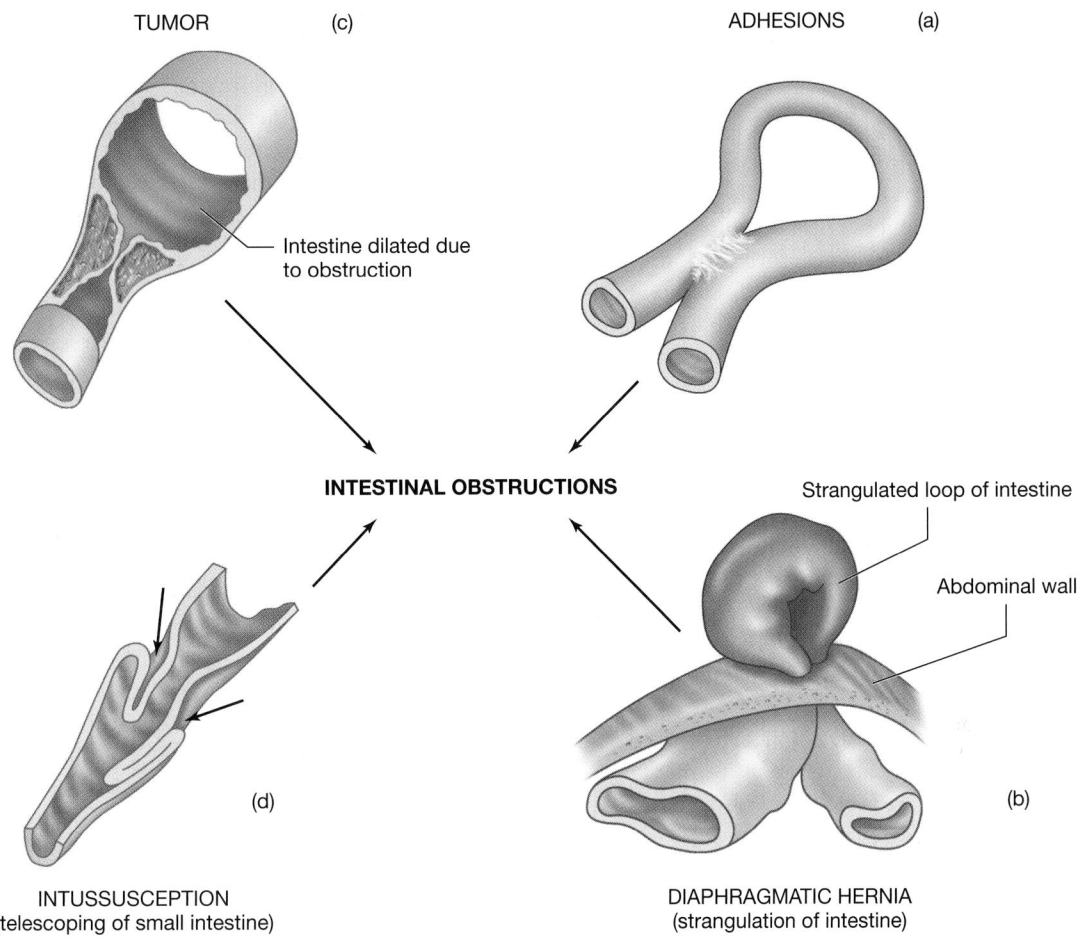

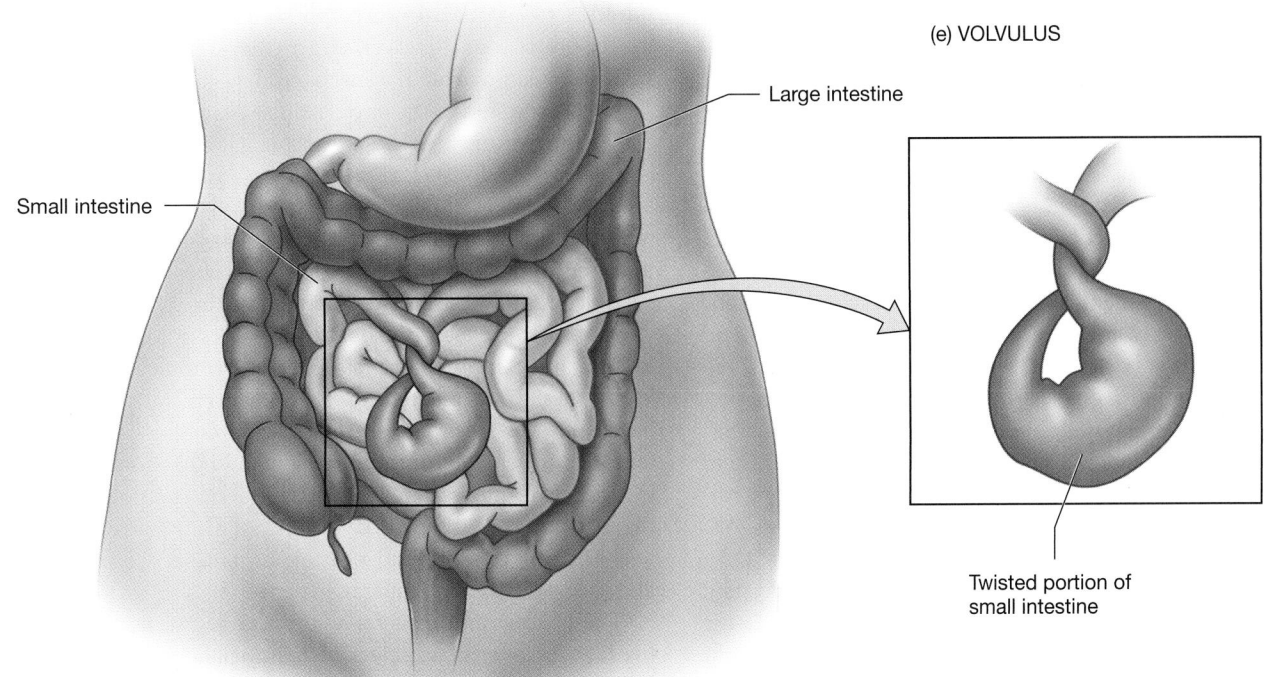

FIGURE 45–6 ■ Causes of intestinal obstruction (A) Adhesions, (B) Hernias, (C) Tumors, (D) Intussusception, (E) Volvulus.

small intestines, with only about 15% occurring in the large bowel.

Pathophysiology

The resultant physiology is the same regardless of the cause of the bowel obstruction. In mechanical obstructions, there is an increase in motility and secretions of the bowel, both proximal and distal to the obstruction. The amount of the secretions may exceed the intestine's ability to reabsorb this fluid, and it results in distention of the bowel. Both the distention and increased motility produce the characteristic cramping abdominal pain (Thomas, 2007). The bowel sounds become high pitched and tinkling, particularly distal to the obstruction. However, as the bowel obstruction progresses, there are diminished or absent bowel sounds.

Bowel obstructions can be classified as simple or strangulated. In a simple bowel obstruction there is no impairment of the vascular or neurological innervation to the intestine. Gas and intestinal secretions accumulate proximal to the obstruction and the distal bowel collapses. An inflammatory response is initiated and the bowel wall becomes edematous and congested. As the process continues there is the possibility of ischemia, necrosis, perforation, and death.

In a strangulated bowel obstruction there is an interruption of blood flow, both venous and arterial, by mechanical means (Thomas, 2007). A strangulated bowel obstruction is extremely serious. Impairment of arterial blood flow leads to ischemia, infarction progressing to gangrene, and perforation and death. This type of bowel obstruction is most often caused by hernias (Figure 45–6B ■), intussusception (telescoping of the bowel; Figure 45–6D ■), volvulus (twisting of the bowel; Figure 45–6E ■), or vascular occlusion, but can also result from surgical adhesions and tumor involvement.

Clinical Manifestations

The manifestations of a bowel obstruction vary depending on the location, type of obstruction, and rapidity of development. The most common symptom is pain. It is usually a cramping or colicky pain that increases as the obstruction progresses. Initially, it may be intermittent but becomes constant with the progression of the obstruction. If the obstruction is in the proximal small bowel, vomiting is common and metabolic alkalosis can result from the loss of gastric acid. If the obstruction is in the distal small bowel, the pain is usually intense and the patient may vomit fecal material.

Abdominal assessment reveals distention resulting from the accumulation of gas, intestinal secretions, and distended and edematous loops of bowel. Early in the obstructive process, visible peristaltic waves may be seen on inspection and hyperactive, high-pitched tinkling bowel sounds may be heard on auscultation of the abdomen. Bowel sounds cease later in the course of the obstruction. However, with a paralytic ileus, there may be diminished or absent bowel sounds throughout the process. Abdominal tenderness may be evident on palpation.

If the obstruction is located in the large intestine, colicky pain and constipation are the most common manifestations. If the pain is severe and continuous, it may indicate bowel ischemia or perforation. There can be massive dilation of the colon, causing pressure and impairing circulation leading to gangrene and perforation. If vomiting develops with a large bowel obstruction, it is usually late in the process.

Diagnostic Procedures

Bowel obstruction is determined with a careful history and physical exam. Confirmation of the diagnosis is made by x-rays and CT scan. Other laboratory tests, although not diagnostic, will be done to determine the presence of infection, fluid and electrolyte imbalances, and acid–base balance.

These laboratory studies usually include a CBC with a differential white blood cell (WBC) count. There will be varying degrees of leukocytosis, but a very elevated WBC count can indicate ischemia or impending strangulation. The serum amylase not only will be elevated in bowel obstruction but also will be elevated with pancreatitis, which has many of the same symptoms. Serum osmolality is elevated if dehydration is present from vomiting and sequestering of fluid in the bowel lumen. If vomiting is severe, hypokalemia and hypochloremia may also be present.

Abdominal x-rays will show distended loops of bowel. If it is a large-bowel obstruction, the entire intestine will be distended all the way to the level of the obstruction. In a small-bowel obstruction there is evidence of gas and fluid in the small bowel. In the upright abdominal x-ray, there are characteristic air–fluid levels within the bowel. Free air under the diaphragm on abdominal x-ray is indicative of bowel perforation.

CT scan with contrast media will be done to determine a mechanical obstruction. A barium swallow is contraindicated because of the possibility of intestinal perforation or a worsening of the obstruction. The contrast media used is diatrizoate meglumine (Gastrografin) and contains iodine. It cannot be used in patients who are allergic to iodine or seafood. A barium enema may be used to diagnose a large-bowel obstruction if there is no threat of perforation.

Medical Management

Treatment for bowel obstruction is centered on relieving the obstruction and resulting pressure in order to avoid perforation. An intestinal tube is placed to decompress the bowel, possibly relieving the obstruction; however, surgery may be necessary if the obstruction is strangulated or mechanical.

Decompression of the bowel using a nasogastric or intestinal tube is the treatment of choice for small bowel obstructions and is very effective for partial obstructions. An intestinal tube is a long tube that is usually inserted through the nose and has a weighted tip that works with gravity to move the tube into the intestine to the point of obstruction. The tube is attached to low suction and the accumulated gas and fluid are removed.

Surgery is needed if the obstruction does not respond to the intestinal decompression or if there is a complete mechanical obstruction or strangulation. Preoperatively, all patients will have a nasogastric (NG) tube inserted to remove stomach contents and to remove continuously any fluid that accumulates in the stomach (unless there is a mechanical obstruction involving the stomach; then insertion of the NG tube is not possible). This will prevent vomiting and possible aspiration during surgery and the immediate postoperative period.

The health care provider will order intravenous fluids to hydrate and correct any electrolyte imbalances before surgery. Isotonic IV fluids (NS, lactated Ringer's) will be given at a rate that will correct fluid balance rapidly but without risk of causing cardiac problems. Because potassium is lost in nasogastric suctioning, as well as through vomiting, potassium is usually added to the IV solution. Blood or blood products may be needed if the obstruction is strangulated or perforated because bleeding may occur. Intravenous antibiotics will be given preoperatively and during surgery to prevent the possibility of infection.

Surgery may involve several procedures including the lysing of adhesions, removal of infarcted or gangrenous bowel, removal of foreign bodies, or tumor resection. A bowel resection is done for most cases of obstruction, except when the cause of obstruction is adhesions. In that case, the adhesions are surgically released. A bowel resection involves removing the section of intestine that is involved and usually an end-to-end anastomosis is performed to reattach the sections of bowel. If a large section of small bowel is removed, the patient may have malabsorption postoperatively. Depending on the cause of the obstruction and the area of bowel affected, ileostomy or colostomy may be necessary.

Nursing Management

Nursing care for the patient with a bowel obstruction focuses on assessment of present condition, instituting fluid and electrolyte replacement, and bowel decompression, by placing either a nasogastric tube or an intestinal tube, and recording the forward progression of the latter. Chart 45–4 outlines care of the patient with a nasogastric tube or nasointestinal tube. If the bowel obstruction cannot be relieved, then surgery will be necessary. The nurse prepares the patient for possible surgery, both physically and emotionally. For complete nursing care for the patient with a bowel obstruction, see the Nursing Process: Patient Care Plan feature (p. 1408).

Diverticular Disease

Diverticular disease results from the occurrence of abnormal saclike outpouchings of the intestinal wall called diverticula. Diverticula can occur anywhere in the gastrointestinal tract except the rectum, but usually occur in the distal large intestine. Diverticular disease includes **diverticulosis**, which is the presence of one or more diverticula, and **diverticulitis**, which is inflammation of the diverticula with possible rupture into the colonic lumen.

Pathophysiology/Etiology

Where arteries penetrate the tunica muscularis are inherent weak points in the intestinal wall. It is at these points, particularly where pressures are normally high in order to push fecal material toward the rectum, that diverticula form. The mucosa herniates through the smooth muscle layers forming the diverticular sac. Diverticula themselves cause few problems; however, if undigested food or bacteria becomes trapped in the diverticula, they form a hard mass called a fecalith and intraluminal pressure increases, resulting in compromise of the blood supply. This results in ischemia of the diverticula and may lead to perforation.

Diverticular disease is common in developed countries, such as the United States, England, Australia, and France, where the diet consists mostly of refined foods. Diverticular disease was virtually unknown until about 1900 when modern grain milling practices began. This process removes two-thirds of the grain's fiber. Socially, only economically disadvantaged people ate brown (whole wheat) bread or brown rice. White, highly refined bread became a status symbol. The incidence of diverticular disease increases as people age and is quite common after age 60, but is rarely found in individuals younger than age 40.

CHART 45–4 Care of the Patient with a Nasogastric (NG) or Nasointestinal (NI) Tube	
NG Tubes (Salem Sump)	**NI Tubes (Cantor, Miller-Abbott, Harris Tubes)**

• Maintain low intermittent suction.
• Check placement every 4 hours.
  1. Aspirate stomach contents and check pH.
  2. Insert 10 milliliters of air rapidly while listening with stethoscope over the stomach to hear the rush of air.
• Monitor skin integrity of nostril of insertion and provide skin care.
• Monitor bowel sounds (suction off).
• Irrigate tube with 30 milliliters NS every 4 hours or as needed to maintain patency.
• Measure NG drainage at least every 8 hours.
• Be sure that the "blue port" is patent, and never irrigate through the port. If the port leaks, do not let the tube hang down, but place it at the patient's shoulder. Do not plug the port unless ordered by the health care provider.
	• Before insertion of Cantor or Harris tube, fill the balloon reservoir with mercury. The balloon on the Miller-Abbott tube is filled with mercury once the distal end has reached the stomach.
	• Once inserted into the stomach, position the patient on his right side.
	• The health care provider may order the tube to be advanced 2–4 inches at a time or to let gravity move the tube into the small intestine.
	• Movement of the patient, either ambulation or changing positions in bed, will assist the forward movement of the tube.
	• The tube is not secured until it reaches the desired position.
	• The tube is not irrigated unless ordered by the health care provider.
	• Placement is checked by x-ray.
	• Low intermittent suction may be ordered once placement is confirmed.
	• Maintain NPO.
	• Mouth care at least every 2 hours.
	• Removal of the tube requires the mercury to be removed from the tube; then withdraw the tube 6 inches every hour until it is removed. The distal end of the tube may have a fecal taste and odor, so mouth care is essential.

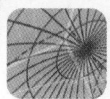

Assessment of Fluid, Electrolyte, and Acid–Base Balance

Subjective Data:

Have you been vomiting? How much? And for how long?

Has your belly become more distended?

Have you been urinating as much as usual?

Do you get dizzy when you stand up quickly?

Objective Data:

Vital signs.

Intake and Output (I&O):

- IV fluids
- Urine output
- NG or NI output
- Fecal output.

Skin color, temperature, turgor.

Abdominal assessment:

- Bowel sounds
- Distention
- Tenderness.

Nursing Assessment and Diagnoses	Outcomes and Evaluation Parameters	Planning and Interventions with *Rationales*
Nursing Diagnosis: *Fluid Volume, Deficient, Risk for* related to bowel obstruction and sequestration of fluid and nasogastric/intestinal suction	**Outcome:** Fluid balance maintained. ***Evaluation Parameters:*** Vital signs normal. Orthostatic blood pressure normal. Intake = output. Skin warm, moist, and pink. Abdomen soft; no increase in girth. Bowel sounds present.	**Interventions and *Rationales:*** Assess frequency and amount of vomiting. *To assess accurately fluid loss prior to hospitalization.* Assess urine frequency prior to hospitalization. *A decrease in urination is a sign of fluid sequestering in the gut.* Monitor orthostatic blood pressure and dizziness. *To assess hypotension and fluid volume deficit.* Monitor and record I&O from all sources every 2–4 hours. *Urine output less than 30 milliliters per hour indicates inadequate glomerular filtration rate, is an indicator of inadequate fluid volume, and is usually the first sign of fluid volume deficit. NG or NI tube drainage is figured into the fluid replacement needs.* Administer IV fluids as ordered to replace lost fluids. *Adequate fluid replacement is necessary to sustain tissue perfusion particularly to the heart and kidneys.* Assess skin color, temperature, and character at least every 4 hours. *When deficient fluid volume exists, cardiac output may decline, triggering a sympathetic nervous system response causing cool, clammy, and pale skin.* Measure abdominal girth at least every 8 hours. *To determine increasing distention and possible fluid sequestering in abdomen.* Assess abdomen for bowel sounds and tenderness. *Hyperactive, high-pitched bowel sounds are present early in a small bowel obstruction. In paralytic ileus there are diminished or absent bowel sounds.*

Assessment of Gastrointestinal Perfusion

Subjective Data:

On a scale of 0–10, with 10 being the worst pain, how would you rate your pain?

Has the character or intensity of your pain changed?

When was your last bowel movement? Was it normal for you?

Objective Data:

Vital signs.

I&O:

- NG or NI drainage
- Urine output
- Feces.

Abdominal assessment:

- Bowel sounds
- Distention
- Tenderness.

Nursing Assessment and Diagnoses	Outcomes and Evaluation Parameters	Planning and Interventions with *Rationales*
Nursing Diagnosis: *Tissue Perfusion, Ineffective Gastrointestinal* related to possible strangulation, volvulus, tumor, foreign body, or vascular congestion resulting from obstruction	**Outcomes:** Adequate GI tissue perfusion. Return of peristalsis. ***Evaluation Parameters:*** Normal bowel sounds. Normal bowel movements. Abdomen soft, nontender, and not distended. Pain free.	**Interventions and *Rationales:*** Assess level of pain every 1–2 hours using a scale of 0–10, with 10 being the worst pain. *A change in the intensity or character of the pain can indicate ischemia, infarction, gangrene, or perforation of the bowel.* Monitor vital signs every 1–2 hours. *Tachycardia can result from pain or a sympathetic response to tissue ischemia. Increased temperature may indicate impending sepsis from bowel perforation or gangrene. Falling blood pressure could signal shock and this. With a low blood pressure, it is difficult to perfuse the intestines, increasing the risk for infarction and possible perforation.* Monitor I&O with particular attention to urine output. *Urine output of less than 30 mL/hr indicates poor perfusion to the kidneys and inadequate glomerular filtration. Urine output declines before changes in the vital signs.* Monitor bowel sounds, abdominal distention, and tenderness. *Increasing abdominal girth and pain could signal perforation or sequestering of fluids in the intestines, causing congestion and impairing perfusion.*

Clinical Manifestations

Most people with diverticular disease are asymptomatic. When diverticulitis develops or the diverticulum hemorrhages, the clinical manifestations typically include left lower quadrant pain, fever with corresponding tachycardia, and possibly nausea, vomiting, and bowel changes, causing either diarrhea or constipation. The pain is usually located in the left lower quadrant because most diverticula form in this portion of the colon. It is initially intermittent, but becomes steady as the inflammatory process progresses and can be mild to severe in quality. The fever is low grade, usually less than 38.2°C (101°F), and can be accompanied by chills. Abdominal distention and flatulence may also occur. On palpation, the abdomen may be tender over the left lower quadrant. The complications of diverticular disease are relatively rare but can include hemorrhage, peritonitis, bowel obstruction, and fistula formation. Clinical manifestations in the elderly may be vague and nonspecific. They may have generalized abdominal pain as well as symptoms of a large bowel obstruction.

Diagnostic Procedures

Diverticular disease may be detected incidentally during diagnostic procedures for other problems or on routine colonoscopy. In the case of asymptomatic and uncomplicated diverticulosis, no other testing is usually indicated.

If symptoms develop, the health care provider will order a CBC with a differential to assess for bleeding and infection. The WBC count will increase and more immature cells will be evident (shift to the left) if the patient has diverticulitis because of inflammation and possible infection. The stool may also be tested for occult blood.

Neither a barium enema nor a sigmoidoscopy will usually be done during the acute phase of the process because of the risk of perforating an inflamed diverticulum. Ultrasonography is a noninvasive test that can detect an abscess or bowel thickening. CT scan not only can be used to detect an abscess but also can assess inflammation. If a perforation is suspected, abdominal x-rays can show free abdominal air, which is characteristic of perforation.

Medical Management

The treatment for diverticular disease can range from dietary modifications to surgical resection of the colon. Patients are usually managed as outpatients when symptoms are mild and fever is less than 38.2°C (101°F). Treatment includes rest, drug therapy, and dietary modifications. Hospital admission is required for higher fevers, persistent (more than 3 days) abdominal pain, dehydration, or the presence of lower GI bleeding. Treatment for more severe diverticulitis includes IV fluids, antibiotics, and possible nasogastric suction. Surgery may be necessary if the patient develops peritonitis from a ruptured diverticulum, abscess, bowel obstruction, fistula, or uncontrolled bleeding.

Dietary Modifications

While the patient is in the acute phase of diverticulitis, a clear liquid diet is recommended. If hospitalized, the patient is usually kept NPO initially and a nasogastric tube may be inserted. Once the acute phase has passed, dietary recommendations include eating a diet high in both soluble and insoluble fiber. The recommended fiber consumption for the general public of the United States is 25 to 30 grams and should be stressed for the person with diverticular disease. Chart 45–5 lists foods high in fiber. For patients with diverticular disease, foods containing small seeds, nuts, and foods with skins such as raisins, grapes, and corn are restricted, because they may become lodged in a diverticulum and cause inflammation and an exacerbation of diverticulitis. These foods are listed in Chart 45–6.

Drug Therapy

Acute diverticulitis is treated with broad-spectrum antibiotics. For mild attacks of diverticulitis, oral metronidazole (Flagyl) and ciprofloxacin (Cipro) may be used. When cost is an issue, trimethoprim-sulfamethoxazole (Bactrim) may be used in the place of the ciprofloxacin. If the diverticulitis is severe and the patient is hospitalized, IV antibiotics effective against gram-negative bacteria and anaerobes will be used. Refer to the Pharmacology Summary feature (p. 1397) for an outline of anti-infective agents.

CHART 45–5 **High-Fiber Foods Recommended for Patients with Diverticular Disease**

Grains and Cereals	Fruits and Vegetables*
Wheat bran	Cooked
Oat bran	• Asparagus
Rice bran	• Fresh beans (lima, green)
Oatmeal	• Broccoli
All-Bran Cereal	• Peas
Raisin bran	• Squash
Shredded wheat	• Greens (kale, spinach)
Whole wheat bread	• Potatoes
Multigrain bread	• Dried beans (pinto, kidney, navy, black-eyed peas)
Whole wheat crackers	
Bulgar (cracked wheat)	Raw
Kasha (buckwheat groats)	• Carrots
Brown rice	• Broccoli
	• Celery
	• Tomatoes
	Peaches
	Apples
	Nectarines
	Oranges
	Pears

* All fruits and vegetables should be eaten unpeeled when possible.

CHART 45–6 **Foods to Be Avoided by Persons with Diverticular Disease**

Popcorn	Berries
Corn	• Strawberries
Sesame seeds	• Raspberries
Poppy seeds	• Blueberries
Sunflower seeds	
Nuts	Figs
Cucumbers	Rye bread with caraway seeds
Okra	

For the patient with diverticulitis experiencing pain, analgesics will be ordered. If the pain is less severe, a mild analgesic is ordered. However, opioid analgesics may be necessary to relieve more severe pain. Meperidine hydrochloride (Demerol) or morphine is used. Pentazocine (Talwin) may cause less colonic pressure and is often used to relieve pain.

Bulk-forming agents, such as psyllium seed (Metamucil) or methylcellulose, are usually prescribed. Laxatives are avoided because they increase motility and intracolonic pressure, although stool softeners (Colace) may be used. See the Pharmacology Summary feature for stool softeners and bulk-forming agents. Enemas are also contraindicated because they increase the intraluminal pressure of the colon and risk diverticular perforation.

Rest

Rest is advocated during acute diverticulitis. The patient should avoid any activity that increases the intra-abdominal pressure, thereby risking perforation. Some of these activities include lifting, straining, coughing, sneezing, and bending.

Bowel rest may be necessary during the acute phase of the illness. Depending on the severity of the inflammation, the patient may be kept NPO. As feeding is resumed slowly, a low-roughage diet may be prescribed. This diet eliminates foods that are high in insoluble fiber, such as whole wheat foods, fruit, nuts, raw vegetables, and dried peas and beans. Fruit juices without pulp are usually permitted. On recovery, high-fiber foods are resumed.

Surgery

If the patient does not improve within 3 days of treatment, or there is deterioration in his condition, surgical intervention may be needed. About 20% to 30% of patients with diverticulitis require surgical treatment (Thomas, 2007). Surgery usually consists of a bowel resection with anastomosis. If surgery is required during the acute phase, a temporary colostomy may be necessary until the inflammation has subsided. The temporary colostomy is closed in 2 to 3 months.

Nursing Management

Because most patients with diverticular disease are symptom free, nursing care focuses on assessing for clinical symptoms of diverticulitis and secondary complications, as well as assessing the diet for fiber content. The Nursing Process: Patient Care Plan feature presents complete nursing care of the patient with acute diverticular disease.

Health Promotion

Health promotion is the number-one responsibility of the nurse. Primary prevention of diverticular disease can be accomplished the majority of the time through a high-fiber diet. Nurses can teach people in the community as well as patients in the hospital of the importance of a high-fiber diet. Nurses can work with local agencies to promote healthy eating, which includes a diet with 25 to 30 grams of fiber.

Inflammatory Bowel Disease

Inflammatory bowel disease (IBD) is an immunologic disease that results in idiopathic intestinal inflammation. It includes two distinct, yet similar conditions: **ulcerative colitis (UC)** and **Crohn's disease**. Both ulcerative colitis and Crohn's disease have common clinical manifestations as well as similar pathophysiology involving an inflammatory process. The cause of IBD remains under investigation, and it is now known that a constellation of factors contribute to the development of the disease. A combination of a genetic susceptibility, an abnormal immune response, an imbalance in beneficial and pathogenic bacteria in the intestines, and intestinal epithelial defects must be present for IBD to develop (Hampton, 2004).

Epidemiology

Approximately 2 million people in the United States are believed to have IBD (Biddle, 2003). The incidence of both ulcerative colitis (UC) and Crohn's disease is similar. The age of onset is usually between ages 15 and 25, although it can occur at any time. IBD is found worldwide, but is more prevalent in the United States, Canada, Europe, and Australia, yet rates are increasing in developing countries. Men and women are affected by IBD equally, although more men have UC and more women have Crohn's disease. The prevalence of IBD is reported for UC and Crohn's disease separately and is 229 per 100,000 for UC and 133 per 100,000 for Crohn's disease (Biddle, 2003).

PHARMACOLOGY Summary for Stool Softeners and Bulk-Forming Agents

Medication Category	Action	Application/Indication	Nursing Responsibility
Bulk-Forming Agents			
psyllium seed (Metamucil) methylcellulose	Improves bowel elimination by increasing stool bulk which promotes peristalsis	Constipation	Monitor for adverse effects: nausea, abdominal cramps, diarrhea. Be aware of drug interactions; monitor warfarin and digoxin levels. Instruct patient to follow each dose with an additional glass of water.
Stool Softeners			
docusate sodium (Colace)	Softens stool by allowing water and fat to penetrate	Constipation, prevention of straining	Monitor for adverse effects: abdominal cramps diarrhea. Instruct patient to increase fluid intake.

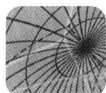

NURSING PROCESS: Patient Care Plan for Acute Diverticulitis

Assessment of Gastrointestinal Integrity

Subjective Data:
Are you having any bleeding?
Are you having any pain?
Have you noticed any abdominal bloating?

Objective Data:
Vital signs.
Abdominal assessment:
- Bowel sounds
- Abdominal girth
- Tenderness
- Guarding.

Stool assessment:
- Color
- Blood
- Consistency.

Nursing Assessment and Diagnoses	Outcomes and Evaluation Parameters	Planning and Interventions with *Rationales*
Nursing Diagnosis: *Tissue Integrity, Impaired* related to acute inflammatory process of diverticulitis	**Outcome:** Normal intestinal tissue. **Evaluation Parameters:** Normal vital signs. Normal bowel sounds in all quadrants. No abdominal distention. No abdominal tenderness. No abdominal guarding. Formed, soft stool. Stool negative for blood.	**Interventions and *Rationales:*** Assess vital signs every 4 hours for tachycardia and tachypnea, *which may indicate increased inflammation resulting in increased vascular leak syndrome and a fluid shift. Increasing fever may indicate perforation and peritonitis as well as increasing inflammation.* Assess abdomen every 4 hours for bowel sounds. *Decreasing bowel sounds may indicate peritonitis or bowel obstruction.* Measure abdominal girth and palpate abdomen for tenderness and guarding. *Increasing girth and/or tenderness and guarding can indicate a ruptured diverticulum, infection, peritonitis, or bleeding in the intra-abdominal cavity.* Examine stools for consistency and character as well as for evidence of blood, occult, or visual. *Diverticulitis can cause lower gastrointestinal bleeding.*

Assessment of Pain

Subjective Data:
On a scale of 0–10, with 10 being the worst pain, how would you rate your pain?
What does your pain feel like—dull, sharp, aching, or stabbing?
Have you felt nauseated?
Did you vomit?

Objective Data:
Vital signs.
Abdominal examination:
- Distention?
- Pain or tenderness on palpation?

- Bowel sounds?
- Soft or rigid?

Facial grimacing.
Restless, holding abdomen.

Nursing Assessment and Diagnoses	Outcomes and Evaluation Parameters	Planning and Interventions with *Rationales*
Nursing Diagnosis: *Pain, Acute* related to diverticulitis and possible ruptured diverticulum	**Outcome:** Comfort level maintained. **Evaluation Parameters:** Communicates reduced or absent pain. No pain behaviors evident: no facial grimacing, not holding abdomen. Abdomen soft with no distention, pain, or tenderness on palpation.	**Interventions and *Rationales:*** Assess pain using pain scale from 0–10, with 10 being the worst pain. *To increase consistency in quantifying pain.* Instruct the patient to inform the nurse if pain gets worse or is not relieved. *Can indicate complications or may need a change in pain medication.* Assess for associated symptoms that could indicate a complication. *Nausea and vomiting can indicate peritonitis.* Notify health care provider if pain increases or there are associated manifestations such as nausea, vomiting, or abdominal distention.

Pathophysiology

The causes of IBD may have a genetic link for some patients. For all, there develops an overly aggressive inflammatory response within the mucosa of the intestine.

Genetic Links

It is clear that some individuals are genetically predisposed to IBD even though only 10% to 15% of cases are familial (Hampton, 2004). The gene that encodes for a protein that possibly mediates epithelial cell-to-cell interactions is found on chromosome 10 and has been linked to Crohn's disease. Additionally, there is a gene on chromosome 7 that has been linked to Crohn's disease. Researchers are trying to identify other IBD-associated genes that mediate the immune response and epithelial integrity (Hampton, 2004).

Immune Response

In the normal intestine, the mucosal immune system works to protect against potentially harmful pathogens and distinguishes self-protein from non–self-protein structures. Antigens are presented to T lymphocytes and B lymphocytes by macrophages, or natural killer cells, and lymphokine-activated cells. The activated lymphocytes initiate the immune response, causing the release of cytokines, specific interleukins, and tissue necrosis factors. The antigen is transported through the lymphatics to the Peyer's patches, causing a release of lymphocytes into the lymph nodes and systemic circulation bound for the lamina propria of the intestines. Once in the intestines, there is an interaction between the lymphocytes and the endothelial cells resulting in the release of substances that support the inflammatory response. In people with IBD, there is a defect in this intestinal immune response (Smith & Bryant, 2002).

Immune Response to Bacteria

There is growing evidence to support that one aspect of IBD is the body's overly aggressive cell-mediated response to bacteria in the gut and/or a persistent infection. A few studies have identified *Mycobacterium paratuberculosis* as a possible pathogen associated with IBD, but further investigation is needed to confirm these studies (Hampton, 2004).

The Epithelium and Immune Response

The epithelial cells lining the intestines form a barrier for protection of the individual against a systemic bacterial infection. However, researchers now understand that the intestinal epithelium also has a role in the immune response. The epithelium communicates with the immune cells, and when the epithelial receptors recognize a bacterial product, they trigger the release of immunoregulatory proteins such as cytokines (Hampton, 2004).

Ulcerative Colitis

Ulcerative colitis (UC) is a disorder that involves chronic inflammation of the mucosal and submucosal layers of the colon and the rectum. It usually begins in the rectum and advances proximally, involving only the large intestine and usually only the sigmoid colon and rectum.

In UC, the inflammation begins at the base of the crypts of Lieberkühn and forms tiny mucosal hemorrhages with the development of abscesses that spread through the submucosa, causing necrosis. This, in turn, causes an increase in the release of inflammatory mediators, which results in congestion and edema leading to tissue friability and ulcer formation. The ulcers bleed easily causing bloody stools, a characteristic manifestation of UC. Atrophy and narrowing of the colon result from chronic inflammation.

Crohn's Disease

Crohn's disease differs from UC in that it can occur in any portion of the gastrointestinal tract from the mouth to the anus; however, it is usually limited to the ileum or ileocecal valve. Crohn's disease involves all layers (transmural) of the intestinal wall, but usually begins in the submucosa, spreading to the mucosa and serosa, while affecting some haustral segments and not others, producing what are called *skip lesions*. The lesions are granulomatous with areas of inflamed tissue circumscribed by scar tissue, giving the intestinal lumen a cobblestone appearance. As the disease progresses, the chronic inflammation causes fibrosis and loss of intestinal flexibility, resulting in obstruction, abscess, and fistula formation.

Malabsorption or malnutrition may develop in Crohn's disease for several reasons. First, Crohn's disease usually affects the jejunum and ileum where many nutrients are absorbed, and the presence of inflamed tissues and ulcers impairs absorption. Second, there may be a loss of exudate from the ulcerated area leading to not only protein loss but also occult or frank blood loss.

Clinical Manifestations

Ulcerative colitis and Crohn's disease have similar clinical manifestations that result from the inflammatory process in the intestines, and it can be difficult to distinguish between the two. Symptoms may be nonspecific and persist for years before diagnosis is made.

- Abdominal pain is usually present in both diseases and is characteristically a cramping type of sensation. The pain can be continuous or intermittent. The pain can be localized to either the right or left lower quadrant or be more diffuse, occurring over the entire lower abdomen.
- Diarrhea is usually present in both UC and Crohn's disease. There may be as many as 10 to 20 bowel movements per day. They can be loose and/or watery and may contain blood, although blood is more common in UC.
- Rectal urgency, incontinence, and tenesmus can be present in either UC or Crohn's disease.
- Systemic manifestations include fever, fatigue, joint pain, mouth sores, fatty liver, uveitis, autoimmune hepatitis, and primary sclerosing cholangitis. It is believed that these extraintestinal manifestations are of an immunologic nature similar to the IBD.

Diagnostic Procedures

Diagnosis of IBD can be difficult, especially when symptoms are nonspecific. The goal of treatment is to eliminate the intestinal inflammation and control the intestinal inflammatory response in the future.

Endoscopy

The gold standard for diagnosing IBD is colonoscopy. During colonoscopy, mucosal biopsy samples are taken at intervals and then examined microscopically for acute and chronic inflammation. UC and Crohn's disease can be differentiated on visualization. The inflammation in UC is continuous, whereas the pattern of inflammation in Crohn's disease is intermittent showing the characteristic skip lesions. An inflamed ileum can most always be attributed to Crohn's disease.

Radiography

A barium swallow with small-bowel follow-through and a barium enema are useful in detecting abnormalities such as ulcerations, strictures, colonic distention, obstruction, and fistulas. Radiography is used cautiously in patients with moderate to severe disease because there is a risk of colon perforation. Fistulas and abscesses, typical in patients with Crohn's disease, can be detected using MRI.

Blood Tests

No blood tests are available to diagnose IBD. A CBC is done to detect anemia resulting from blood loss, chronic inflammation, and malnutrition. An elevated WBC count results from the inflammatory process and abscess formation. The erythrocyte sedimentation rate (ESR) will be elevated but is not specific because it is elevated with any inflammation. Serum electrolytes, glucose, albumin, BUN, creatinine, and serum levels of vitamins are useful in monitoring the degree of malabsorption that may occur in Crohn's disease.

Genetic tests are now available but are not used widely. They are not diagnostic in themselves but are used in conjunction with other tests. Two genetic markers have been developed for clinical use. Anti–*Saccharomyces cerevisiae* antibodies (ASCA) are positive in about 60% of people with Crohn's disease. Perinuclear antineutrophil cytoplasmic antibodies (pANCA) are present in 60% to 80% of patients with UC or UC-like Crohn's disease (Biddle, 2003).

Medical Management

Medical management with medications and dietary changes is the first course of treatment. Only if medical management fails is surgery considered.

Drug Therapy

Medications are used in the treatment of IBD to halt acute exacerbations and minimize or eliminate recurrences. The most common medications act locally to control inflammation and systemically to suppress the immune response.

Sulfasalazine (Azulfidine) has been used to treat UC for more than 60 years. The active ingredient in this sulfonamide antibiotic is 5-aminosalicylic acid (5-ASA). It is safe and effective even when used long term. Patients with allergies to sulfa medications may be sensitive to sulfasalazine as well. This medication cannot be taken during pregnancy. There are now preparations that contain the 5-ASA without the sulfapyridine portion, which have fewer adverse effects, and include mesalamine (Asacol) and olsalazine (Dipentum). The 5-ASA inhibits prostaglandin production in the gut, thereby reducing the inflammatory process.

Corticosteroids, because of their potent anti-inflammatory effects, may be given to terminate an acute exacerbation of IBD. However, their use is avoided whenever possible because of the long-term side effects such as osteoporosis, diabetes mellitus, peptic ulcer disease, and cataracts. If the patient does not respond to 5-ASA treatment, prednisone is added at as low a dose as possible for the shortest time possible.

Immunomodulators such as azathioprine (AZA) and 6-mercaptopurine (6-MP) may be used for immunosuppression in place of corticosteroids. They are being used earlier in the course of IBD than in the past and may be used as a first line treatment. These medications need to be taken for at least 4 months before the full effect can be seen and can result in serious side effects such as bone marrow suppression, which may necessitate discontinuation of the drug if leucopenia or thrombocytopenia develops.

The most promising class of medications currently being developed is that of biologic modifiers. One drug, infliximab, a tumor necrosis factor-α (TNF-α) inhibitor, is approved for use in Crohn's disease. TNF-α is a cytokine that mediates components of the inflammatory process in Crohn's disease, thus, inhibiting TNF-α has proven beneficial in some patients (Rose, Armstrong, Klickstein, & Madsen, 2005). See the Pharmacology Summary feature (p. 1414) on the treatment of Inflammatory Bowel Disease.

Diet Therapy

There is no specific diet to follow for patients with IBD, other than one that is well balanced. Some patients with IBD report that certain foods exacerbate their condition. For example, milk and milk products may increase abdominal pain and diarrhea in some and should therefore be avoided if they cause problems. Conversely, a diet high in fiber may lessen diarrhea and improve tenesmus and rectal urgency. If the patient is known to have strictures or very severe acute symptoms, dietary fiber is contraindicated.

During an acute exacerbation of IBD, particularly Crohn's disease, the patient is allowed no food at all. This "bowel rest" helps relieve symptoms, which supports the theory that some foods and bacteria may be antigenic, causing inflammation in the gut. Total parenteral nutrition (TPN) is usually prescribed during the period of bowel rest. The Complementary and Alternative Therapies box (p. 1415) presents the use of hypnotherapy in treating irritable bowel syndrome.

Surgery

Patients who do not respond to the maximum doses of medication and/or who have complications such as malnutrition, anemia, bowel obstruction, and severe weight loss, are candidates for surgical intervention. The type of surgery will depend on the type of IBD and the location and extent of the lesions. As many as 66% of patients with Crohn's disease will undergo surgery for intractable disease with the average length of time from diagnosis to surgery of 3 years (Biddle, 2003). Only about 20% of people with UC require surgery, which is usually a total colectomy if the disease is extensive.

For patients with severe UC and for some patients with Crohn's disease, the surgical option is usually a total colectomy with an **ileal pouch anal anastomosis (IPAA)**. The entire colon, including the rectum, is removed, and a pouch is fashioned from the terminal ileum. The pouch is then anastomosed to the anus (Figure 45–7 ■, p. 1416). When healed, the pouch can hold enough fecal material to reduce bowel movements to 6 to 8 times a day. In order to allow time for the anastomosis to heal and the pouch to mature, a temporary loop **ileostomy** is done. A loop ileostomy involves bringing a loop of the ileum to the abdominal surface and creating a stoma to allow for the drainage of stool into a collection devise. After about 2 to 3 months, a second surgery is done to close the stoma and repair the bowel.

In patients with extensive Crohn's disease, an ileostomy, either permanent or continent, may be necessary. For these patients, an ileostomy is performed after removal of the entire colon, rectum, and anus. In a permanent ileostomy, fecal material is collected in an external collection bag. Fecal drainage is characteristically continuous and watery, because the large intestine is removed and this is where the majority of water is reabsorbed from feces. Another option is a **continent ileostomy**, also known as **Kock ileostomy or Kock pouch** (Figure 45–8 ■, p. 1417). During ileostomy surgery, the terminal ileum is folded back on itself and the inner wall removed, thereby forming a reservoir and a nipple valve. The end is then brought through the abdominal wall to form a stoma. The nipple valve prevents leaking of fecal contents through the stoma. The reservoir is emptied by a catheter inserted through the stoma. Nursing care of the patient with an ileostomy is outlined in the Nursing Process: Patient Care Plan feature (p. 1418) for patients with IBD.

PHARMACOLOGY Summary of Medications Used to Treat Inflammatory Bowel Disease (IBD)

Medication Category	Action	Application/Indication	Nursing Responsibility
5-Aminosalicylic Acid Agents Sulfasalazine (Azulfidine) Mesalamine (Asacol, Pentasa) Olsalazine (Dipentum)	Reduces inflammation by inhibiting prostaglandin production in the gut.	Mild to moderate inflammatory bowel disease (Crohn's disease, ulcerative colitis), proctosigmoiditis, remission maintenance in ulcerative colitis.	Monitor for adverse effects: headache, abdominal pain, cramps, and diarrhea. Evaluate for aspirin hypersensitivity, contraindicated in these patients. Sulfasalazine contraindicated in patients allergic to sulfa. Monitor BUN and creatinine, especially in presence of renal disease.
Corticosteroids Prednisone (Meticorten) Methylprednisolone (Medrol) Hydrocortisone (Cortef)	Decreases inflammation and immune response through inhibition of phagocytes, lymphocytes, histamine, and prostaglandin synthesis.	Moderate to severe IBD.	Monitor for adverse effects: mood swings, insomnia, nausea, hypertension, oral candidiasis, impaired wound healing, and symptoms of gastric ulcer. Monitor electrolytes and blood sugar. Warn patient not to stop drug abruptly.
Immunosuppressants Azathioprine (Imuran) Methotrexate (MTX)	Suppresses immune response by depressing T cell function.	Severe IBD.	Monitor for adverse effects: nausea, vomiting, and anorexia. Monitor CBC and platelet count. Observe for signs and symptoms of infection.
Biologic Response Modifier Infliximab (Remicade)	Monoclonal antibody that decreases inflammation by reducing production of proinflammatory cytokines.	Moderate to severe IBD.	Monitor for adverse reaction: fever, chills, pruritus, urticaria, chest pain, hypotension, hypertension, or dyspnea. Stop infusion and notify health care provider.
Coating Agents Sucralfate (Carafate) Bismuth subsalicylate (Pepto-Bismol)	Protects ulcer from gastric acid by forming a paste that adheres to ulcer; reduces pepsin.	Active duodenal ulcer, reflux esophagitis, acute erosive gastritis.	Monitor for adverse effects: constipation. Give sucralfate on an empty stomach, 1 hour before meals and at bedtime. Antacids should be given 30 minutes before or after administration. Warn patient about harmless darkening of stools when taking bismuth. Evaluate for aspirin hypersensitivity; bismuth subsalicylate contraindicated in these patients.
Bulk-Forming Agents Psyllium seed (Metamucil) Methylcellulose	Improves bowel elimination by increasing stool bulk, which promotes peristalsis.	Constipation	Monitor for adverse effects: nausea, abdominal cramps, and diarrhea. Be aware of drug interactions; monitor warfarin and digoxin levels. Instruct patient to follow each dose with an additional glass of water.
Stool Softeners Docusate sodium (Colace)	Softens stool by allowing water and fat to penetrate.	Constipation, prevention of straining.	Monitor for adverse effects: abdominal cramps and diarrhea. Instruct patient to increase fluid intake.

■ Nursing Management

Most patients with IBD are managed with medications, dietary changes, and stress reduction. Surgery is done usually as a last resort. Nursing care involves preparing the patient for diagnostic tests, managing the medication regimen, educating the patient about drug treatments and stress reduction, assessing the effectiveness of the interventions, and caring for the patient during the surgical experience, should surgery be necessary. Support networks are vitally important for this very life-disrupting disease. A number of resource groups are available, but the one recommended by most patients with IBD is the Crohn's & Col-

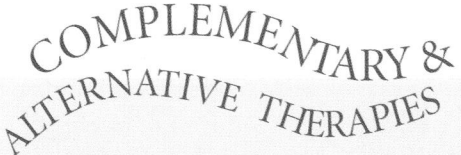

COMPLEMENTARY & ALTERNATIVE THERAPIES   Hypnotherapy

Description:

Irritable bowel syndrome (IBS) is a prevalent gastrointestinal disorder for which no clear cause has been found. Symptoms of IBS include abdominal pain, bloating, and altered bowel habits. Despite the great number of people afflicted with this disorder, there are few effective medical treatments (Tan, Hammond, & Joseph, 2005).

One theory as to the cause of IBS is stress. Hypnotherapy, which is also known as hypnosis, is a form of psychotherapy that uses the power of suggestion to help the patient achieve a deep state of relaxation. Hypnotherapy has been proven effective in many situations such as smoking cessation, headaches, pain, and insomnia.

Research Support:

In a clinical paper, a team of U.S. researchers reviewed 14 published studies to evaluate the effectiveness of hypnotherapy in treating IBS. Eight of the studies had no control group and six had a control group. The researchers found that hypnotherapy produced consistently significant results: Hypnotherapy improved IBS symptoms for the majority of patients. Researchers then evaluated the study results using the efficacy guidelines published by the Clinical Psychology Division of the American Psychological Association (APA). They found that the use of hypnotherapy for IBS qualifies for the APA's highest level of acceptance for both effectiveness and specificity. Researchers then sought to determine how hypnotherapy exerts its action on IBS. They found some evidence that supported both physiological and psychological mechanisms of action (Tan et al., 2005).

In another clinical paper, a team of researchers in Iran reviewed 15 studies on the use of hypnosis for IBS. The researchers based their criteria on the Rome Working Team recommendations for IBS trial design. The team's results showed that hypnosis improved IBS symptoms as well as quality of life, anxiety, and depression, and the improvements lasted from 2 to 5 years (Gholamrezaei, Ardestani, & Emami, 2006).

In a randomized controlled trial conducted in Britain, researchers studied the effect of gut-directed hypnotherapy on primary care IBS patients aged 18 to 65 years. Patients were diagnosed with IBS more than 6 weeks prior to the study and had no success with conventional management treatments. The intervention group received five sessions of hypnotherapy in addition to their usual IBS management. The control group received usual management only. Researchers collected symptom and quality of life data at baseline and again 3, 6, and 12 months posttest. At the 3-month mark, the intervention group showed significantly greater improvements in pain, diarrhea, and overall symptom scores. There were no significant differ-

ences in quality of life between the two groups. Patients in the intervention group, however, were significantly less likely to require medication. The majority of patients in the intervention group described an improvement in their condition. However, there was a lack of significant difference between groups beyond the 3-month mark. The researchers conclusions were that, although gut-directed hypnotherapy showed symptom reduction and reduced medication usage benefits, additional evidence is needed before clinicians can recommend the general introduction of hypnotherapy for IBS patients (Roberts, Wilson, Singh, Roalfe, & Greenfield, 2006).

The final study examined here involved 75 IBS patients in a nurse-led gut-directed hypnotherapy treatment program. Patients recorded their physical symptoms of IBS using 7-day diary cards. The patients' predominant symptoms included abdominal pain (61%), altered bowel habits (32.5%), and abdominal distension/bloating (6.5%). In addition, researchers administered an IBS-specific quality of life questionnaire as well as the Hospital Anxiety and Depression Scale. Statistics showed that patients' reported physical symptoms improved after hypnotherapy. Female patients who reported abdominal pain as their predominant physical symptom showed the most marked improvement. Six of the eight health-related quality of life domains that were measured (emotional, mental health, sleep, physical function, energy, and social role) also showed significant statistical improvement. Anxiety and depression also improved following treatment. Researchers concluded that hypnotherapy, when integrated into conventional care, provides a viable solution for the nursing management of irritable bowel syndrome (Smith, 2006).

References

Gholamrezaei, A., Ardestani, S. K., & Emami, M. H. (2006). Where does hypnotherapy stand in the management of irritable bowel syndrome? A systematic review. *Journal of Alternative and Complementary Medicine, 12*(6), 517–527.

Roberts, L., Wilson, S., Singh, S., Roalfe, A., & Greenfield, S. (2006). Gut-directed hypnotherapy for irritable bowel syndrome: Piloting a primary care-based randomised controlled trial. *British Journal of General Practice, 56*(523), 115–121.

Smith, G. D. (2006). Effect of nurse-led gut-directed hypnotherapy upon health-related quality of life in patients with irritable bowel syndrome. *Journal of Clinical Nursing, 15*(6), 678–684.

Tan, G., Hammond, D. C., & Joseph, G. (2005). Hypnosis and irritable bowel syndrome: A review of efficacy and mechanism of action. *American Journal of Clinical Hypnosis, 47*(3), 161–178.

itis Foundation of America. See the Nursing Process: Patient Care Plan feature (p. 1418) for the complete nursing care of the patient with inflammatory bowel disease.

Colon Cancer

Colon cancer is responsible for more than 56,000 deaths a year, second only to lung cancer with respect to cancer deaths. Men and women are affected equally, and the incidence increases after age 50. If the lesions are confined to the colon and rectum, the 5-year survival rate is as high as 90%. If there is spread to the adjacent tissues, the survival rate drops to 65%; and if there is involvement of distant sites, the survival rate is as low as 8% (Jemal et al., 2007). Early detection is therefore vital. Although the American Cancer Society (ACS) recommends sigmoidoscopy or colonoscopy after age 50, screening rates continue to be low, possibly because of the

personal and embarrassing nature of the test and the financial cost. The Cultural Considerations box (p. 1416) outlines the disparity in the rates of cancer, including colon cancer, among different racial and ethnic groups.

Pathophysiology/Etiology

There is a strong association between the development of colon cancer and genetic events. Researchers have linked an alteration in the p53 gene to 86% of colorectal cancers. Also, when there is an allelic deletion on chromosome 5, 17, or 18, the transformation from normal to malignant colon tissue is promoted (Huether, 2006).

Adenomatous polyps, which result from a mutation on chromosome 5, are considered premalignant tissue, and most colorectal cancers develop from this type of polyp (Huether, 2006). Three different types of polyps develop from mucosal epithelium: tubular, villous, and tubulovillous. Tubular polyps, the most common,

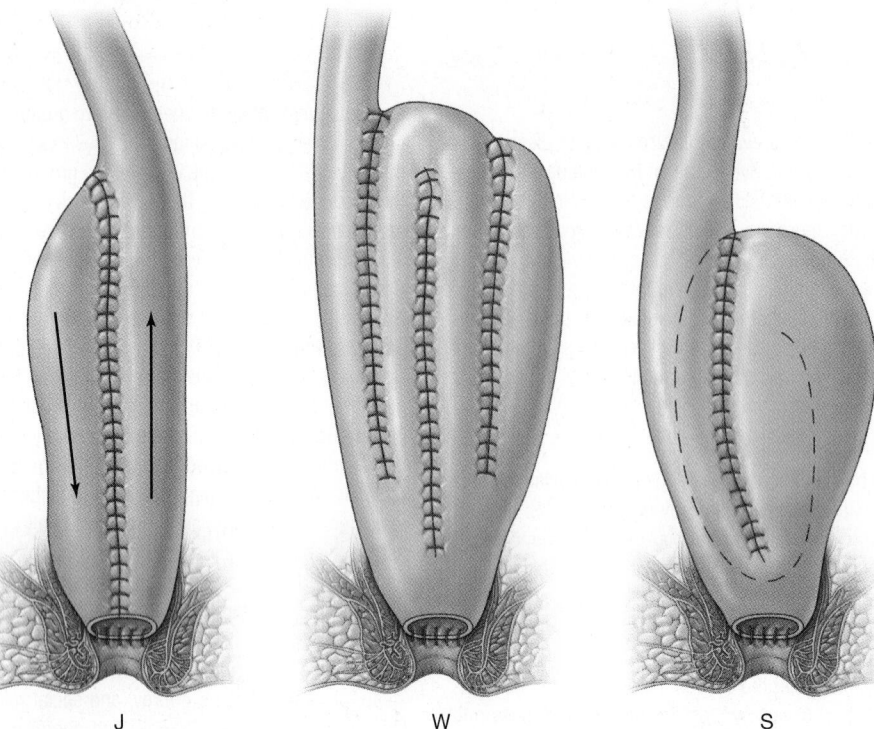

J   W   S

FIGURE 45–7 ■ Ileal pouch anal anastomosis.

CULTURAL CONSIDERATIONS Related to Colon Cancer

According to the American Cancer Society (2007), African Americans are more likely to develop and die from cancer than any other racial or ethnic population. Currently the death rate from cancer among African American males is 38% higher than among white males; for African American females, it is about 17% higher. Overall, racial and ethnic minorities face more obstacles in receiving health care services, including cancer prevention, early detection, and quality treatment. Statistics released from the American Cancer Society Surveillance Research reveal that African American males have the highest incidence and mortality associated with colorectal cancers (Jemal et al., 2007).

consist of a stalk and a spherical structure at the end. The stalk is attached to the intestinal wall. They are also called pedunculated polyps, and their numbers increase with aging. These polyps vary in size from less than 1 centimeter to as large as 5 centimeters. The larger the polyp, the more likely it will transform into malignant tissue. Villous adenomas are less common, are larger than 5 centimeters, and have a high malignant potential. In an autosomal dominant genetic disorder called familial polyposis, there are hundreds of adenomatous polyps present in the large intestine. The polyps in this disorder will transform to malignant tissue 100% of the time, usually by age 40.

There appears to be a link between dietary factors and the development of colorectal cancer. The disease is virtually unknown in poor countries where the diet consists mainly of unrefined grains, fruits, and vegetables. In countries like the United States, where the typical diet is high in animal protein, fat, and calories, the prevalence of colorectal cancer is higher. The largely animal source diet is believed to increase anaerobic bacteria in the colon, where they convert bile acids to carcinogens. The excess dietary animal fat also causes increased deposition of fatty acids within the cell membranes, and an increase in intestinal prostaglandins stimulates cell proliferation. Other nutrients that are associated with a lower risk for colon cancer are folic acid, selenium, vitamin D, and calcium. There is some research to indicate that the use of nonsteroidal anti-inflammatory drugs (NSAIDs), such as aspirin and ibuprofen, and hormone replacement therapy also decreases colon cancer risk. The role of physical inactivity remains controversial.

Recent research indicates that daily alcohol consumption increases the risk for colon cancer and is dose related. In fact, in one study the research found a 70% greater risk of colon cancer in people who drank alcohol daily when compared to their nondrinking counterparts (Su & Arab, 2004). There is also evidence to indicate a link between **C-reactive protein (CRP)** and colon cancer. CRP is a protein released from the liver in response to local inflammation or tissue injury. It has been known for a long time that CRP is a marker for inflammation but only recently discovered that there is a link between inflammation and colon cancer (Erlinger, Platz, Rifai, & Helzlsouer, 2004). This may help explain the association between anti-inflammatory agents and a reduced risk for colon cancer. The chronic inflammation of irritable bowel syndrome (IBS) is also known to increase the risk for developing colon cancer.

Adenocarcinoma is the most common type of colon cancer and accounts for 95% of colon tumors (Thomas, 2007). Adenocarcinomas grow irregularly and form hard, nodular areas. Colon cancer is classified by the tissue type, lymph node involvement, and stage of metastasis (TNM). The National Guidelines box (p. 1420) outlines two tumor classification systems. Colon cancer cells range from well differentiated to poorly differentiated. The cancer is spread first by local invasion and direct ex-

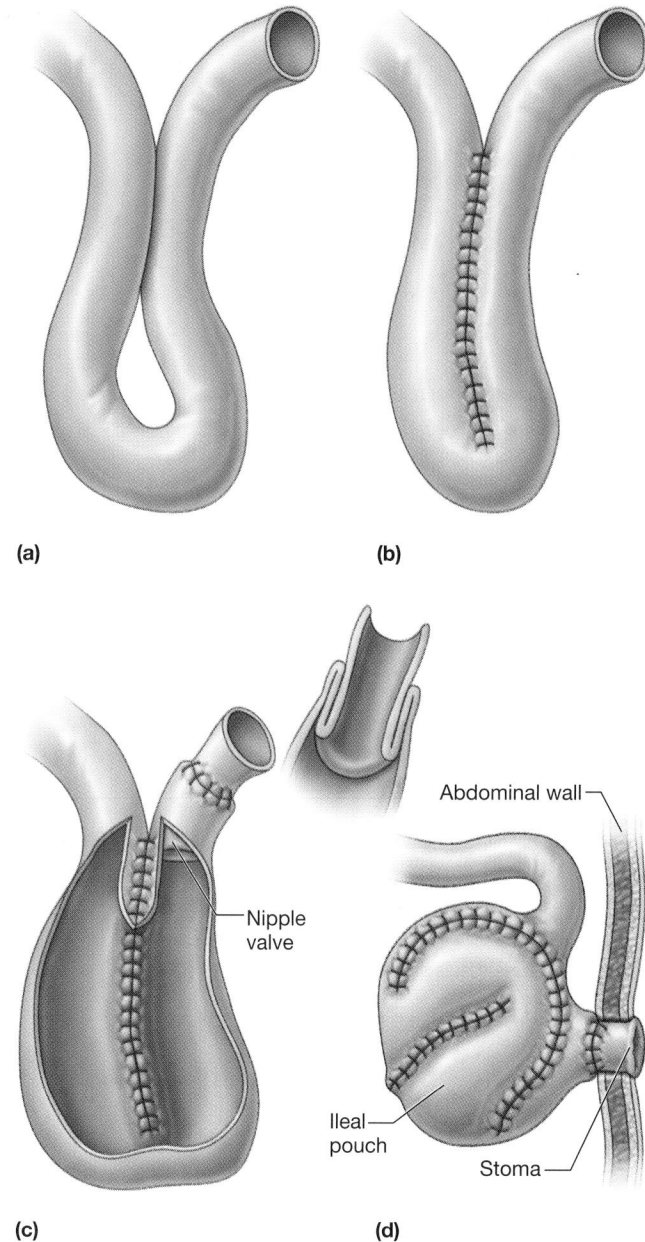

(a)   (b)

Nipple
valve

Abdominal wall

Ileal
pouch

Stoma

(c)   (d)

FIGURE 45–8 ■ Kock ileostomy.

tension. Any tissue or organ in the neighboring area can be affected, such as the liver, duodenum, small intestine, pancreas, and the abdominal wall. Because the lymph system is closely associated with the intestines, cancer is also easily spread to distant sites via this way. It can also reach distant sites by way of the circulation. The most common sites for metastasis of colon cancer are the liver, lungs, brain, and bones.

Clinical Manifestations

Colon cancer is usually asymptomatic until it is well advanced. Most types of colon cancer grow very slowly, taking 5 to 15 years of growth before symptoms are present, and even those symptoms are vague and often misdiagnosed. The symptoms will depend mostly on the location of the tumor and its stage of growth. The most common symptoms are a change in bowel habits, such as constipation or diarrhea, or a change in the caliber of the stools. The symptom that causes the most alarm, and usually prompts

the patient to see her health care provider, is bleeding in the stool. As the disease progresses, there may be weight loss, fatigue, abdominal pain, and anorexia. Anemia may also be a manifestation that presses the patient to seek attention. Some of the complications of colon cancer, such as bowel obstruction and bowel perforation, may be the first manifestations the patient notices.

Tumors in the ascending colon are usually polypoid and extend along one wall of the ascending colon. Because they are bulky tumors, a palpable mass can usually be felt. They tend to develop necrotic areas and ulcerate contributing to the slow blood loss and anemia. Pain is usually a late sign.

Descending colon tumors are usually small and button like. Rather than growing along one wall of the colon as tumors in the ascending colon do, these tumors grow around the circumference of the colon and spread along the entire bowel wall. Because of the circumferential nature of this type of colon cancer, obstruction is common. Constipation is the predominant symptom as the bowel lumen becomes smaller as the tumor grows.

Diagnostic Procedures

The American Cancer Society currently recommends that African American men be screened beginning at age 45 and that all others at age 50 have either an annual fecal occult blood test or a sigmoidoscopy every 5 years or a colonoscopy every 5 to 10 years (Irani & Krevsky, 2007). However, because sigmoidoscopy will detect cancer in only the sigmoid colon and the rectum, most health care providers recommend the colonoscopy, because it can establish the diagnosis of colon cancer with 100% accuracy (Thomas, 2007).

There are no laboratory tests that can establish the diagnosis of colon cancer; however, many tests are used to detect manifestations of colon cancer, such as chronic blood loss. A CBC will detect the anemia that results from blood loss and tumor growth, as well as the leukocyte response to inflammation. As mentioned previously, a C-reactive protein is also ordered to detect inflammation. **Carcinoembryonic antigen (CEA)** is found in 70% of people with cancer of the large intestine, but the test is too insensitive and nonspecific to be useful in screening or diagnosing colon cancer. CEA is useful in monitoring a patient's response to treatment.

The only definitive way to diagnose colon cancer is with a tissue biopsy. This is usually done using colonoscopy and is almost 100% accurate in diagnosing this type of cancer. As mentioned earlier, the TNM system for staging colon cancer is most often used to indicate the extent of the cancer and to judge prognosis. A CT scan is then done to detect possible metastasis in distant locations such as the liver or lungs.

Medical Management

Prevention of colon cancer is the primary goal of collaborative care, followed next by early detection and treatment. Prevention and early detection of colon cancer is done through educating the public about ways to decrease the risk, such as eliminating alcoholic beverages on a daily basis; increasing the amount of fruits, vegetables, and fiber; daily exercise and weight control; and possibly a daily low dose of aspirin.

Surgery

Surgery is the treatment of choice for individuals with colon cancer because it offers the only known cure. Even when metastasis

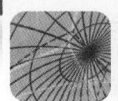

Assessment of Bowel Elimination

Subjective Data:

How many stools do you have a day?
What is the consistency and color?
Is there any blood?
Do you have any abdominal pain or cramping?
How long have you been having this problem?
When did it start?

Does stress in your life make it worse?
Does any food make the diarrhea worse?
Do you have any joint pain or fatigue?
Have you been treated before?
Do you take any home remedies, herbs, or over-the-counter medications?

Objective Data:

Vital signs.
Examination of abdomen:
- Bowel sounds
- Palpation
- Visual exam for contour, scars.

Visual inspection of stools.
Test stool for occult blood.

Nursing Assessment and Diagnoses	Outcomes and Evaluation Parameters	Planning and Interventions with *Rationales*
Nursing Diagnoses: *Diarrhea* related to irritable bowel syndrome (IBS). *Fluid Balance, Readiness for Enhanced* related to the diarrhea.	**Outcome:** Decreased diarrhea. ***Evaluation Parameters:*** Number of stools decreased by at least half. Consistency of stool: formed. Absence of blood in the stool. No abdominal cramping.	**Interventions and *Rationales:*** Take vital signs every 4 hours *to assess for signs of dehydration such as tachycardia, tachypnea, or fever.* Weigh daily *to assess for fluid losses.* Examine skin and mucous membranes *for evidence of dehydration, such as poor turgor, dry mucous membranes, or dry, cracked tongue.* Maintain NPO if ordered *to rest the bowel, which promotes healing and improves diarrhea.* Provide good perianal care with gentle cleansing agents, and apply protective cream or ointment to the area *to prevent skin breakdown.* Administer ordered medications, assess their effectiveness, and monitor adverse effects:

- 5-ASA compounds (sufasalazine, mesalamine, olsalazine) are anti-inflammatory drugs that decrease inflammation of the intestinal mucosa.
  1. Monitor for adverse effects, which include skin rashes, urticaria, pruritus, bleeding or easy bruising, fever, low WBC and platelet counts, low hemoglobin and hematocrit (bone marrow suppression), and decreased urine output (renal failure).
  2. Give and teach patient to take these medications after eating to avoid gastric distress.
  3. Encourage increased fluid intake (2 L/day) to prevent kidney damage.
  4. Teach patient to notify the health care provider if any of the adverse effects occur.
- Corticosteroids—adrenal hormones (prednisolone) that suppress the immune response and have anti-inflammatory properties:
  1. Monitor for side effects such as elevated blood glucose, fluid retention (edema, weight gain, hypertension, heart failure), gastric ulcers, hypokalemia (muscle weakness, nausea, dysrhythmias), and mood swings.
  2. Should be given only with meals to decrease the risk of ulcers and gastric distress.
  3. Teach the patient to increase foods high in potassium (citrus fruit, bananas, potatoes) and reduce intake of sodium (canned soup, bottled salad dressing, processed meats, cheese).
  4. Teach patient NOT TO STOP THE MEDICATION ABRUPTLY (the dose must be tapered).
- Immunomodulators (azathioprine) suppress the immune system.
  1. Be sure to tell the patient that these drugs must be taken for 4–5 months before the full effect is seen.
  2. Monitor for adverse effects such as pancreatitis (usually within the first 2 months), and low WBC or platelet count.
- Infliximab (tumor necrosis factor blocker) used for refractory Crohn's disease.
  1. Given every 2–3 months and must be given intravenously.
  2. Monitor for adverse effects such as infection serum sickness–like reaction and lupus-like syndrome (Biddle, 2003).

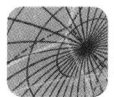

Assessment of Body Image

Subjective Data:
How has this disease/surgery affected your life?
Are you able to continue working? Socializing with friends? Shopping?
Has this affected how you feel about your personal relationships? Sexual activity?

Objective Data:
Facial expressions.
Body language.
Attitude toward stoma.

Nursing Assessment and Diagnoses	Outcomes and Evaluation Parameters	Planning and Interventions with *Rationales*
Nursing Diagnosis: *Disturbed Body Image* related to disease process and/or surgery	**Outcome:** Normal body image. ***Evaluation Parameter:*** Verbalizes acceptance of body image,	**Interventions and *Rationales*:** Assess the patient's current perception of self and demonstrate acceptance of where the patient is now. *Acceptance of the patient's feelings can help establish a caring and trusting nurse–patient relationship.* Provide an environment in which the patient feels comfortable talking about the disease and how it has impacted his life. To build caring nurse–patient relationship. Encourage the patient to talk about ways this disease has affected personal, work, social, and sexual relationships. *To provide understanding and demonstrate acceptance of the patient as a person.* Delineate possible treatment options, including graphic description of surgery and postop possibilities *to give the patient a sense of control.* Provide names and phone numbers of IBS support groups. If possible, arrange for the patient to meet with someone who has the disease. *This shows the patient that she is not the only person facing this problem.*

Assessment of Fecal Diversion (Ileostomy)

Subjective Data:
Are you having any cramping?
Are you passing any gas through the stoma?

Objective Data:
Vital signs.
Abdominal assessment:
- Stoma color
- Stoma drainage/bleeding
- Condition of skin surrounding stoma.

Condition of ostomy appliance.

Nursing Assessment and Diagnoses	Outcomes and Evaluation Parameters	Planning and Interventions with *Rationales*
Nursing Diagnoses: *Bowel Incontinence* related to fecal diversion. *Skin Integrity, Impaired, Risk for* related to ostomy drainage. *Knowledge, Deficient* related to fecal diversion.	**Outcome:** Normal functioning ileostomy. ***Evaluation Parameters:*** Stoma color pink and moist. No bloody effluent. Effluent dark green and viscous initially, gradually turning yellow-brown. Skin around stoma free of irritation and inflammation. Ileoanal skin without irritation or inflammation. Able to communicate necessary stoma care, dietary modification, and stress reduction techniques.	**Interventions and *Rationales*:** Monitor stoma color. *The stoma should be pink, beefy red, and moist with no obvious cyanosis or bleeding. It should extend about 2–3 centimeters from the abdominal wall. Impaired circulation will cause the stoma to be dark, blue, or very pale.* Assess stoma function. *Immediately postop there may be small amounts of blood.* Within 1 or 2 days the drainage will be dark green and viscous, gradually turning yellow-brown and developing an odor. Empty and measure ileostomy drainage when the pouch is one-third to one-half full and explain the procedure to the patient each time. *Emptying the pouch when it is not too full eliminates the possibility of the seal in the pouch breaking and causing leaking. Explaining the procedure to the patient each time gets the patient more comfortable with self-care.* Assess the skin surrounding the stoma and around the perianal area. The skin should be pink and remain free of irritation, excoriation, or inflammation. *Ileostomy drainage is irritating to the skin because it contains bile salts and digestive enzymes that normally get reabsorbed in the large intestine.* Apply a protecting skin barrier under the pouch *to prevent contact of drainage with skin.* Report abnormal assessment findings such as poor stoma color, bulging or retracted stoma, or rash around the stoma. Poor stoma color indicates poor circulation to the section of bowel that forms the stoma; bulging can indicate herniation or prolapse. Teach patient and family members to assess the stoma and to treat it gently. *Because there are no pain receptors in the stoma, it can become injured without feeling pain.* Teach patient to notify health care provider if there is a change in the stoma or if a rash develops in the skin surrounding the stoma. Assess the patient's ability to manage the ileostomy including knowledge of ostomy care, what medications to avoid (laxatives, enteric coated, or capsules), and signs and symptoms to report.

NATIONAL GUIDELINES for Tumor Classification

TNM Classification	American Joint Committee Classification
T (Tumor)	Stage 0:
Tx: tumor cannot be assessed.	Carcinoma in situ.
T0: no tumor.	Stage I:
Tis: carcinoma in situ.	Invasion of submucosa (80–100% 5-year survival).
T1: increasing tumor size.	Invasion of muscularis propria.
T2: invades muscularis.	Stage II (node negative disease) (50–75% 5-year survival):
T3: penetrates through bowel wall.	Invasion into the subserosa or into nonperitonealized pericolic or perirectal tissue.
T4: invades adjacent organs.	Tumor perforates the visceral peritoneum or invades other organs by direct extension.
N (Nodes)	Stage III (node positive disease) (30–50% 5-year survival):
Nx: cannot assess regional lymph nodes.	Bowel wall perforation with lymph node metastasis.
N0: no regional lymph nodes.	
N1: 1–3 pericolic or perirectal lymph nodes.	
N2: 4 or more pericolic or perirectal nodes.	
N3: lymph node metastasis along vascular trunk.	
M (Metastasis)	Stage IV (metastatic disease) (5% 5-year survival):
Mx: not assessed.	Presence of distant metastasis.
M0: no metastasis.	
M1: metastasis present at distant sites.	

Source: Adapted from Tierney, L. M., McPhee, S. J., & Papadakis, M. A. (2004). *Current medical diagnosis and treatment* (43rd ed.). New York: Lange Medical Books/McGraw-Hill.

has occurred, surgical resection can improve the chance of survival. There are several different surgical procedures for the patient with colon cancer depending on the stage, tumor size, and general health of the patient. Surgery can range from abdominoperineal resection with a colostomy to laser photocoagulation. With advances in surgical technique and equipment, thankfully, most patients do not require a colostomy, as was once the case. Tumors of the rectum, however, do usually require removal of the rectum, sigmoid colon, and anus, necessitating a sigmoid colostomy for fecal elimination.

Two procedures can be performed using an endoscope: laser photocoagulation and local excision and fulguration. During laser photocoagulation, an intense beam of laser light is aimed at the tumor where the heat generated destroys the cancerous tissue. This procedure is also helpful as palliative treatment for advanced tumors when the patient is not a good surgical candidate or to remove an obstruction. Local excision can be done by endoscopy or by laparoscopy. This surgical method is used if the tumor is small and well defined. Electrocoagulation or fulguration can reduce the size of a tumor in a patient who is not a good candidate for extensive colon resection.

Occasionally, an end-to-end anastomosis is not possible during colon resection, and the patient requires a colostomy for the diversion of fecal material. The type and permanence of the colostomy depends on the location of the tumor (Figure 45–9 ■). If there is a large bout of inflammation or tissue trauma, a temporary colostomy is created to give the bowel time to heal, and then the bowel is reanastomosed and the colostomy closed at a later date, usually in 3 to 6 months. A sigmoid colostomy, performed for cancer of the rectum, is most usually permanent.

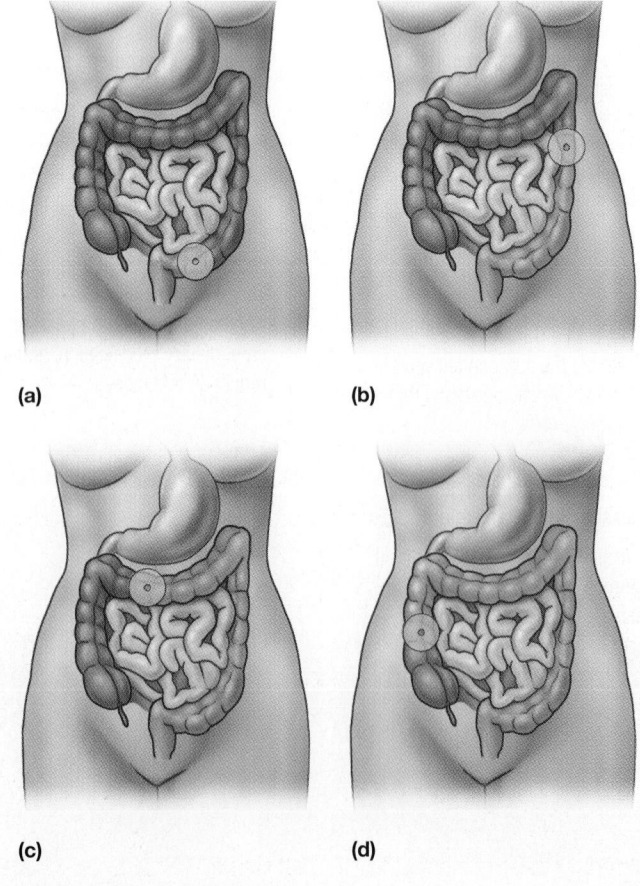

(a)　　　　(b)

(c)　　　　(d)

FIGURE 45–9 ■ Colostomy sites.

A double-barrel colostomy is created in the case of trauma to the colon or severe inflammation. The distal colon is bypassed but not removed, and may be reanastomosed. There are two stomas on the abdominal surface. The distal stoma, also called a mucous fistula because it drains mucus from the distal colon, usually requires only a gauze dressing. The proximal stoma will have fecal discharge and will require the application of an ostomy appliance (bag) to collect feces.

There are several other types of colostomies that are usually temporary in placement. In an emergency, a transverse loop colostomy may be performed. As the name implies, a loop of bowel is brought through the abdominal wall and suspended over a glass or plastic rod, preventing the bowel from slipping back into the abdomen. An ostomy is made in the loop of colon. The rod is removed usually in about 2 weeks. The Hartmann procedure is another technique for creating a temporary colostomy. In this procedure the distal colon is oversewn to close the lumen, and the proximal colon forms the colostomy. It is similar to the double-barrel colostomy, except that the lower portion does not have a stoma on the abdominal wall. Patients require the same care whether the colostomy is permanent or temporary. Nursing care of the patient with a colostomy is discussed in the Nursing Process: Patient Care Plan feature.

Chemotherapy and Radiation Therapy

Chemotherapeutic agents are used as an adjunctive therapy for colon cancer after colon resection. The patient is usually given a period of time to heal postoperatively before chemotherapy is started. Chemotherapy can be combined with radiation therapy to reduce the rate of recurrence. Radiation appears to prolong survival in patients with more advanced cancer, particularly rectal tumors. Radiation can also be used before surgery to shrink large tumors and make them easier to resect surgically.

■ Nursing Management

Because there is a link between lifestyle choices and the development of colon cancer, nursing can impact primary prevention of the disease by teaching and advising patients about lifestyle choices that may decrease the risk. Dietary modifications, including increasing the amount of dietary fiber and reducing the amount of fat, sugar, and meat, can help reduce colon cancer risk. However, it is not enough simply to tell a patient to increase fiber and decrease fat, sugar, and meat. The nurse must give specific information about what foods are high in fiber and those that are high in fat and sugar and should be eaten in limited quantities, and consider cultural, economic, and religious factors when making the suggestions.

Other important aspects of nursing care include teaching patients about the warning signs of colon cancer and when to seek treatment. A frank discussion with patients over age 40 about recommended screening and what each test involves can help dispel their fears and misconceptions.

Because the treatment of choice for patients with colon cancer is surgery, the focus of nursing care is on pre- and postoperative care, and support in dealing with a possible colostomy, chemotherapy, and radiation treatment, and possibly death. Emotional support throughout the course of the illness is paramount. See the Nursing Process: Patient Care Plan feature for complete nursing care of the patient with colon cancer.

■ Research

Research being done regarding gastrointestinal disorders is focused on less invasive approaches to surgical treatments; education regarding screening exams, particularly those with cultural barriers; and multiple alternative therapies. The Research Opportunities and Clinical Impact box (p. 1423) describes current research opportunities for gastrointestinal disorders.

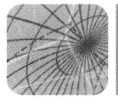
NURSING PROCESS: Patient Care Plan for the Patient with Colon Cancer Having Surgery

Assessment of Preoperative Readiness
Subjective Data:
What did the surgeon tell you about your surgery?
Do you have any questions that you would like to ask?

Objective Data:
Vital signs.
Signed consent.
Character of stool postbowel prep.

Has the enterostomal therapy nurse seen the patient?
Are all preop laboratory reports in the chart?

Nursing Assessment and Diagnoses	Outcomes and Evaluation Parameters	Planning and Interventions with *Rationales*
Nursing Diagnosis: *Fear* related to surgical procedure and diagnosis of cancer	**Outcome:** Ready for surgery. **Evaluation Parameters:** Signed consent. Lab reports in chart. Communicates fears and anxiety. Able to verbalize the nature and extent of the surgery.	**Interventions and *Rationales*:** Ask the patient to tell the nurse what will happen postoperatively. *This helps the nurse assess the patient's understanding of the procedure and what to expect in the postoperative period. It also assesses whether the patient understands what she signed for on the informed consent.* Administer the bowel prep as ordered and examine the stool to assess the effectiveness of the prep. Stool should be liquid and clear by the end of the prep. *The prep cleans the bowel and reduces the risk of infection postoperatively.* Contact the enterostomal therapist to arrange a preop visit with the patient *to help ease fear and anxiety about the possible colostomy.*

(continued)

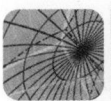

NURSING PROCESS: Patient Care Plan for the Patient with Colon Cancer Having Surgery—*Continued*

Assessment of Postoperative Pain

Subjective Data:
On a scale of 1–10, with 10 being the worst pain ever, how would you rate your pain?
Are you allergic to any pain medications?
Do you have any cultural or religious beliefs that might impact your pain control?

Objective Data:
Vital signs.
Restless and irritable.
Facial grimacing when moving.

Nursing Assessment and Diagnoses	Outcomes and Evaluation Parameters	Planning and Interventions with *Rationales*
Nursing Diagnosis: *Pain, Acute* related to surgical incision	**Outcome:** Comfort level maintained. ***Evaluation Parameters:*** Communicates pain level and effectiveness of analgesia. Reports adequate pain control. No facial grimacing.	**Interventions and *Rationales:*** Use pain scale (1–10) to quantify level of pain *in order to be consistent from nurse to nurse, and time to time, when assessing pain.* Teach the patient to inform the nurse if the pain is not relieved. *Indicates the need to change pain management plan.* Assess cultural and religious beliefs about pain and pain relief. *Different cultures and religions may view pain as punishment or may have nontraditional ways of treating pain.* Medicate the patient prior to ambulation. *Decreased pain increases exercise tolerance, and ambulation increases intestinal motility, preventing ileus, and enhances the respiratory effort, decreasing the chance of pneumonia.*

Assessment of Skin Integrity (Postoperative)

Subjective Data:
Ask the patient whether he has feeling around the stoma.

Objective Data:
Assess stoma and skin around stoma for:
- Redness
- Color of stoma
- Swelling
- Drainage.

Nursing Assessment and Diagnoses	Outcomes and Evaluation Parameters	Planning and Interventions with *Rationales*
Nursing Diagnosis: *Skin Integrity, Impaired* related to colostomy and surgical incision	**Outcome:** Good skin and stomal integrity. ***Evaluation Parameters:*** Stoma pink and moist. Skin surrounding stoma pink, no excoriation.	**Interventions and *Rationales:*** Inspect stoma and surrounding skin for color and edema. A healthy stoma is pink or beefy red and moist due to mucous production. The peristomal skin should be pink and show no signs of irritation, inflammation, excoriation, or rashes. *A bluish purple or dusky stoma indicates impaired blood flow to the stoma. Skin around the stoma can be irritated by the appliance, by a yeast infection, or from a leaking appliance.* Apply caulking agents (Stomahesive or Karaya paste) to maintain a leak-free secure ostomy appliance *to prevent leakage onto skin. Ostomy drainage is very irritating to the skin and can cause skin breakdown.* Assess surgical incision for bleeding, redness, and draining at least every 4 hours. Change dressing as ordered by surgeon to keep the incision clean and dry, *which helps prevent an infected incision.*

Assessment of Bowel Function

Subjective Data:
Are you passing any gas through the stoma?
Do you feel any rumbling in your abdomen?
Have you been nauseated?

Objective Data:
Examination of abdomen:
- Bowel sounds
- Palpation
- Visual exam for contour, condition of stoma, and any drainage.
Color, consistency, and frequency of colostomy drainage.
Test stool for occult blood.

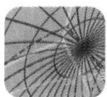

NURSING PROCESS: Patient Care Plan for the Patient with Colon Cancer Having Surgery—*Continued*

Nursing Assessment and Diagnoses	Outcomes and Evaluation Parameters	Planning and Interventions with *Rationales*
Nursing Diagnosis: *Bowel Incontinence* related to surgery and fecal diversion.	**Outcome:** Functioning colostomy. ***Evaluation Parameters:*** Stool from colostomy semiformed. Active bowel sounds.	**Interventions and *Rationales:*** Assess abdomen for bowel sounds, which indicate peristalsis has returned. *Manipulation and anesthesia have the potential for causing an ileus.* Assess for nausea and vomiting, which can also *indicate an ileus.* Assess the characteristics of the colostomy drainage. *Fecal-like drainage and flatulence from the stoma indicate the return of bowel function.*

RESEARCH OPPORTUNITIES AND CLINICAL IMPACT RELATED TO DISORDERS OF THE GASTROINTESTINAL TRACT

Area	Clinical Impact
Physiological Research	
Use of traditional Chinese medicine for gastrointestinal disorders.	Use of non-Western medicine for treatment of GI disorders may improve patient compliance due to fewer side effects and less cost.
Use of complementary and alternative medicine in patients with inflammatory bowel disease.	
Laparoscopic surgery for colon cancer.	Less invasive surgical techniques would decrease complications and patient length of stay.
Relationship between serum antibodies to bacterial antigens and clinical remission in Crohn's disease.	
Drugs for maintenance therapy in inflammatory bowel disease.	Medications or other treatments would decrease the long-term consequences of inflammatory bowel disease, thereby improving the quality of life and longevity.
More sensitive tests for assessing disease activity in inflammatory bowel disease.	
Surgical treatments for gastroesophageal reflux disease.	Because long-term GERD can lead to esophageal cancer, effective treatment can reduce mortality.
Emotional and Psychological Research	
Communicating about screening for colon cancer in culturally diverse groups.	Improved communication between health care providers and culturally diverse groups can increase screening in these groups and hopefully decrease mortality.
Patient satisfaction with photodynamic therapy for Barrett's esophagus.	
Quality of life after bariatric surgery.	
Quality of life after surgery for gastroesophageal cancer.	Understanding issues about quality of life can assist nurses to help patients cope better with life changes.
Music therapy to reduce anxiety before gastrointestinal procedures.	Improve psychological interventions to improve coping.

Clinical Preparation

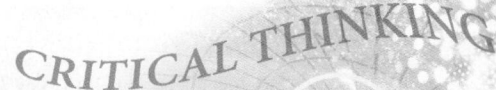
CRITICAL THINKING

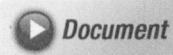 **Read**

- History of Current Illness
- Past Medical History
- Physical Exam
- Admitting Medical Orders
- Laboratory Study Results

Document

- Summary of Hospitalization
- Pathophysiology Form
- Laboratory Values
- Laboratory Results Explanation

 **Apply**

- List of Potential Nursing Diagnoses
- Concept Map
- Critical Thinking Questions

Log on to MyNursingKit.com to download forms you will need and to complete further steps in the Clinical Preparation assignment.

HISTORY OF PRESENT ILLNESS

As a nurse working on a GI floor in a large teaching hospital, you are receiving report about Ms. T, a 35-year-old woman who was admitted 2 days ago with hematemesis and abdominal pain. She reported symptoms of increasing epigastric pain for approximately 3 weeks, and the use of Tums, which had been working most of the time. She also reported taking aspirin daily for prevention of heart disease. The bleeding has stopped now, and she has just returned from an EGD (esophagogastroduodenoscopy), which confirmed a gastric ulcer.

Medical–Surgical History

Her past medical history includes gastroesophageal reflux disease for which she was prescribed Prilosec, but she could not afford to purchase the medication, so she has been taking Tums instead.

Social History

She has a 10 pack-year history of smoking, having quit 3 months prior to this admission. She reports being a "social" drinker. She reports an intentional weight loss of 50 pounds during the last year.

Physical Exam

Her vital signs are temperature 37°C; heart rate 90 and regular; respirations 16 and unlabored; and blood pressure 100/60 sitting. Her skin is pale and dry. Her lungs are clear to auscultation, and her heart is regular with no murmurs or extra heart sounds noted at this time. Her bowel sounds are present in all four quadrants, and her abdomen is soft with tenderness noted in the epigastrium. She has a nasogastric tube set to low intermittent suction that is draining green fluid.

Ms. T's current nursing care, medication schedule, and laboratory study results follow.

Admitting Medical Orders

Service: Medicine
Diagnosis: gastric ulcer
Allergies: none
Vital signs q15min × 4 then q1h × 2 then q4h with oxygen saturation
Activity: up to chair 4 times per day, may ambulate to bathroom
Diet: NPO, may have ice chips
Nasogastric tube to low wall suction; flush NG with 30 mL saline q8h
Call house officer: temp > 38.5°C, HR > 130 or < 60, RR > 30 or < 12, BP sys > 160 or < 90, O_2 sat < 92%, urine output < 120 mL in 4 hours, change in neurological or abdominal exam, any Hct result that is 5 less than the baseline ED Hct
IV: D5NS IV at 125 mL/hr
I&O: q8h
Test each stool for occult blood
Test NG drainage for occult blood q8h

Medications

Omeprazole 40 mg per NG daily (note: clamp NG tube for 2 hours)
Sucralfate 1 g susp daily (note: give through NG at least 3 hours after omeprazole and clamp for 1 hour)

PRN Medications

Hydromorphone 0.2 mg/mL concentration IV per PCA, incremental 0.2 mg, lock-out 6 minutes

Ordered Laboratory Studies

Type and cross match for 2 units packed RBCs (PRBCs)
CBC, electrolytes, retic count daily

LABORATORY STUDY RESULTS

Test	Admission	Day 1	Day 2
CBC	10.5 g/dL	9.5 g/dL	10 g/dL
• Hemoglobin (Hgb)	31%	27%	30%
• Hematocrit (Hct)	3.2 mm³	2.7 mm³	3 mm³
• RBC	2.0%	2.4%	2.4%
• Reticulocytes	72 µm³	68 µm³	70 µm³
• MCV	27 pg	25 pg	26 pg
• MCH	150 mm³	146 mm³	148 mm³
• Platelets	135 mEq/L	135 mEq/L	140 mEq/L
Electrolytes	3.6 mEq/L	3.5 mEq/L	3.9 mEq/L
• Sodium	9 mg/dL	9 mg/dL	9 mg/dL
• Potassium			
• Calcium			

CRITICAL THINKING QUESTIONS

1. What is the physiology mechanism behind the reason that aspirin causes peptic ulcers?

2. Why is omeprazole being given to Ms. T?

3. What is the impact of acute hemorrhage on the results of the CBC?

Answers to Critical Thinking Questions appear in Appendix D.

NCLEX® REVIEW

1. The nurse suspects a patient has Vincent's stomatitis when which clinical manifestation is assessed?
1. Increased salivation and bad breath
2. Painful red maculas with erythematous halos
3. White curd like patches on tongue
4. Oral ulcers covered with a grayish yellow membrane

2. A diagnosis of Barrett's esophagus is made following endoscopic examination of a patient experiencing symptoms of gastroesophageal reflux disease, GERD. The nurse understands this diagnosis is indicative of:
1. Premalignant tissue in the esophagus.
2. Presence of esophageal strictures.
3. Fine tears in the distal esophagus.
4. Ulcerated and inflamed esophageal tissue.

3. A patient is being evaluated for presence of celiac disease. The nurse explains the most definitive test will be a:
1. Gram staining of the stool.
2. Gastric pH analysis.
3. Antigliadin antibody.
4. Biopsy of the small intestine.

4. A patient with a history of irritable bowel disease, IBD, has been recently diagnosed with Crohn's disease. When planning care the nurse understands a manifestation of Crohn's that differs from ulcerative colitis includes:
1. Diarrhea can occur 10–20 times a day.
2. Abdominal pain is cramping in nature.
3. Malabsorption of nutrients often occurs.
4. Incontinence of stool may be a problem.

5. A patient complains of having frequent episodes of belching and heartburn secondary to GERD. The nurse determines the following could be contributing factors. The patient:
1. Has a BMI of 21.
2. Is lactose intolerant.
3. Drinks citrus juice with meals.
4. Eats a lot of high fiber foods.

6. The nurse is preparing education materials on colon cancer to present at a health fair. The following should be included as being risk factors. (Select all that apply.)
1. Daily alcohol intake
2. A low fat diet
3. A history of irritable bowel disease (IBD)
4. Use of daily calcium supplements
5. Daily use of NSAIDs

7. The blue port on a patient's Salem sump tube is leaking clear solution. The nurse should take which action?
1. Place the patient in a high Fowler's position.
2. Plug the port to prevent further leakage.
3. Irrigate the port with 30 mL of saline solution.
4. Place the tube at the shoulder level of patient.

8. A patient has been experiencing symptoms of dumping syndrome following a Billroth II. The nurse should include which interventions in the plan of care?
1. Check for signs of hypoglycemia two hours after a meal.
2. Encourage ambulation in hall after meals.
3. Instruct patient to drink only cold liquids with meals.
4. Remove high fat food from the patient's tray.

9. The nurse is assessing the stoma on a patient with an ileostomy created three days ago. The nurse anticipates the stoma will appear:
1. Beefy red and moist.
2. Pale pink and extending 2–3 cm from abdominal wall.
3. Slightly purple and moist.
4. Pink and flat against the abdominal wall.

Answers for review questions appear in Appendix D

KEY TERMS

achalasia *p.1389*
achlorhydria *p.1397*
adenomatous polyps *p.1415*
anti-infectives *p.1383*
aphthous stomatitis (contact
     stomatitis) *p.1382*
Barrett's epithelium *p.1387*
Botox *p.1391*
carcinoembryonic antigen (CEA) *p.1417*
celiac disease *p.1400*
colon cancer *p.1415*
continent ileostomy (Kock ileostomy or
     Kock pouch) *p.1413*
C-reactive protein (CRP) *p.1416*
Crohn's disease *p.1410*
diverticular disease *p.1407*
diverticulitis *p.1407*
diverticulosis *p.1407*

duodenal ulcer *p.1395*
esophageal cancer *p.1392*
gastric carcinoma *p.1397*
gastric outlet obstruction (pyloric
     obstruction) *p.1395*
gastric ulcer *p.1393*
gastroduodenostomy (Billroth I) *p.1398*
gastroesophageal reflux *p.1385*
gastrojejunostomy (Billroth II) *p.1398*
Helicobacter pylori (*H. pylori*) *p.1395*
herpetic stomatitis *p.1381*
hiatal hernia *p.1385*
histamine$_2$ (H$_2$)-receptor blockers *p.1385*
ileal pouch anal anastomosis (IPAA) *p.1413*
ileostomy *p.1413*
inflammatory bowel disease (IBD) *p.1410*
intestinal obstruction *p.1404*

lactase *p.1403*
lactose intolerance *p.1403*
lower esophageal sphincter (LES) *p.1385*
malabsorption *p.1400*
maldigestion *p.1400*
oral cancer *p.1383*
oral candidiasis *p.1382*
pancreatic insufficiency *p.1403*
peptic ulcer *p.1393*
proton pump inhibitor (PPI) *p.1385*
rolling (paraesophageal) hernia *p.1385*
short bowel syndrome *p.1403*
sliding (direct) hiatal hernia *p.1385*
steatorrhea *p.1403*
stomatitis *p.1381*
ulcerative colitis (UC) *p.1410*
Vincent's stomatitis *p.1382*

EXPLORE PEARSON **mynursingkit**™

MyNursingKit is your one stop for online chapter review materials and resources. Prepare for success with additional NCLEX®-style practice questions, interactive assignments and activities, web links, animations and videos, and more!

Register your access code from the front of your book at
www.mynursingkit.com

REFERENCES

American Cancer Society. (2007). *Cancer facts & figures for African Americans 2007–2008.* Retrieved July 26, 2008, from http://www.cancer.org/docroot/STT/content/STT_1x_Cancer_ Facts_Figures_for_African_Americans_2207-2008_08.asp

American Gastroenterological Association. (2005, January 16). Study shows long-term use of NSAIDs causes severe intestinal damage. *ScienceDaily.* Retrieved July 26, 2008, from http://www. sciencedaily.com/releases/2005/01/050111123706.htm.

Biddle, W. (2003). Gastroesophageal reflux disease: Current treatment approaches. *Gastroenterology Nursing, 26*(6), 228–236.

Burgess, J. A. (2006). Painful oral lesions: What to look for, how to treat: Part 1. *Consultant, 46*(13), 1497–1504.

Erlinger, T. P., Platz, E. A., Rifai, N., & Helzlsouer, K. J. (2004). C-reactive protein and the risk of incident colorectal cancer. *JAMA, 291*(5), 585–590.

Hampton, T. (2004). Scientists explore pathogenesis of IBD. *JAMA, 292*(22), 2708–2713.

Huether, S. E. (2006). Alterations of digestive function. In K. L. McCance & S. E. Huether, *Pathophysiology: The biologic basis for disease in adults and children* (5th ed., pp. 1385–1445). St. Louis: Mosby.

Irani, S., & Krevsky, B. (2007). Colorectal cancer screening: Which test, how often? *Consultant, 47*(2), 138–145.

Jackler, R. K., & Kaplan, M. J. (2004). Ear, nose, & throat. In L. M. Tierney, S. J. McPhee, & M. A. Papadakis (Eds.), *Current medical diagnosis and treatment* (pp. 175–211). New York: Lange Medical Books/McGraw-Hill.

Jemal, A., Siegel, R., Ward, E., Murray, T., Xu, J., & Thun, M. J. (2007). Cancer statistics, 2007. *CA: A Cancer Journal for Clinicians, 57,* 43–66.

Kelsch, R. (2007). *Geographic tongue.* Retrieved April 17, 2008, from http://www.emedicine.com/derm/topic664.htm

Landzberg, B. R. (2006). Celiac disease: Could you be missing the diagnosis? *Consultant, 46*(13), 1458–1465.

Lopes, M. H. B., & Lopes, R. A. M. (2000). Latex allergy in health care personnel. *AORN Journal, 72*(1), 42–3, 45–6, 55–6.

Lynch, D. P. (2007). Oral cancer risk and detection: The importance of screening technology. *RDH, 27*(9), 102–112.

McCaffrey, R., Thrush, S., Dunphy, L. M., & Porter, B. O. (2007). Eyes, ears, nose, and throat problems. In L. M. Dunphy, J. E. Winland-Brown, B. O. Porter, & D. J. Thomas, *Primary care: The art and science of advanced practice nursing* (2nd ed., pp. 229–303). Philadelphia: F. A. Davis.

McQuaid, K. R. (2004). Alimentary tract. In L. M. Tierney, S. J. McPhee, & M. A. Papadakis, *Current medical diagnosis and treatment* (pp. 515–622). New York: Lange Medical Books/McGraw-Hill.

O'Malley, P. (2003). Gastric ulcers and GERD: The new "plagues" of the 21st century update for the clinical nurse specialist. *Clinical Nurse Specialist, 17*(6), 286–289.

Oral Cancer Foundation. (2007). *Descriptive epidemiology.* Retrieved April 17, 2008, from http://www.oralcancerfoundation.org/cdc/ cdc_chapter1.htm

Presutti, R. J., Cangemi, J. R., Cassidy, H. D., & Hill, D. A. (2007). Celiac disease. *American Family Physician, 76*(12), 1795–1802.

Qureshi, W. A. (2006). *Hiatal hernia.* Retrieved April 17, 2008, from http:// www.emedicine.com/med/topic1012.htm

Rose, H. S., Armstrong, L. B., Klickstein, L. B., & Madsen, J. C. (2005). Pharmacology of immunosuppression. In D. E. Golan (Ed.), *Principles of pharmacology: The pathophysiologic basis of drug therapy* (pp. 667–681). Philadelphia: Lippincott Williams & Wilkins.

Sherman, C. (2007). Dyspepsia guidelines emphasize *H. pylori. The Clinical Advisor, 10*(2), 69–74.

Smith, M. M., & Bryant, J. L. (2002). Mind–body and mind–gut connection in inflammatory bowel disease. *Gastroenterology Nursing, 25*(5), 213–217.

Su, L. J., & Arab, L. (2004). Report: Alcohol consumption and risk of colon cancer: Evidence from the national health and nutrition examination survey I epidemiologic follow-up study. *Nutrition and Cancer, 50*(2), 111–119.

Thomas, D. J. (2007). Abdominal problems. In L. M. Dunphy, J. E. Winland-Brown, B. O. Porter, & D. J. Thomas, *Primary care: The art and science of advanced practice nursing* (2nd ed., pp. 473–561). Philadelphia: F. A. Davis.

Wilcox, C. M., Cryer, B., & Triadafilopoulos, G. (2005). Patterns of use and public perception of over-the-counter pain relievers: Focus on nonsteroidal antiinflammatory drugs. *Journal of Rheumatology, 32,* 2218–2224.

Wollner, T. (2004). Eradicate *H. pylori* with effective treatment regimens. *The Nurse Practitioner, 29*(6), 40–44.

Young, L. S., & Thomas, D. J. (2004). Celiac sprue treatment in primary care. *The Nurse Practitioner, 29*(7), 42–45.

Caring for the Patient with Hepatic and Biliary Disorders

Debera Jane Thomas
Douglas Sutton

Outcome-Based Learning Objectives

After studying this chapter, the learner will be able to:

1. Describe the different types of hepatitis virus and the mode of transmission for each one.
2. Discuss the clinical manifestations of hepatitis.
3. Compare and contrast pathophysiology, clinical manifestations, and treatment with related nursing care of patients with cirrhosis.
4. Outline the nursing care of a patient with hepatic encephalopathy.
5. Delineate nursing care for a patient with liver cancer.
6. List the risk factors for gallbladder disease.
7. Compare and contrast the nursing care for patients with an open cholecystectomy and laparoscopic cholecystectomy.
8. Analyze the similarities and differences between acute and chronic pancreatitis.
9. Discuss the causes, clinical manifestations, and treatment for pancreatic cancer.
10. Develop a teaching plan for patients with pancreatitis.

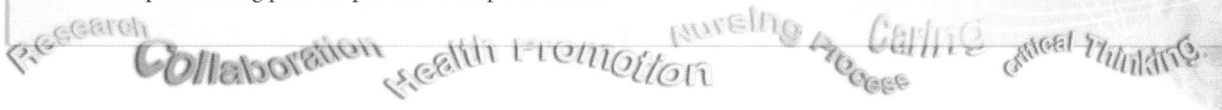

THE LIVER, gallbladder, and **exocrine pancreas** facilitate digestion by secreting hormones, enzymes, and other substances that are necessary for the breakdown of food (Figure 46–1 ■, p. 1428). For example, the liver secretes **bile** that contains salts needed for the breakdown and absorption of fats. Bile is stored and concentrated by the gallbladder for release in response to **cholecystokinin**, which is a hormone secreted from the mucosa of the small intestines. Cholecystokinin, in turn, stimulates the gallbladder to contract and eject bile, as well as stimulating the pancreas to secrete alkaline fluid. In addition to alkaline secretions that help neutralize the acidity of the chyme, the pancreas secretes enzymes that hydrolyze proteins, carbohydrates, and fats. **Trypsin**, **chymotrypsin**, and **carboxypeptidase** are enzymes secreted in inactive form from the pancreas that digest proteins. Pancreatic **alpha-amylase** and **lipase** digest carbohydrates and fats, respectively. This chapter discusses disorders of the liver, gallbladder, and pancreas.

DISORDERS OF THE LIVER

The liver is a complex organ with over 500 identified functions, including metabolic and regulatory functions. Because of its complexity, the clinical manifestations of liver problems can be varied and may include both physiological and psychological symptoms. One of the most amazing features of the liver is its ability to regenerate itself so some level of healing can occur. Liver disorders can result from infectious organisms, toxic substances, and/or tumors that produce either localized or diffuse **hepatocellular** inflammation or destruction.

Hepatitis

Hepatitis is simply defined as inflammation of the liver and is found to be a common problem throughout the world. It can be an acute or chronic infection that may be mild or life threatening, depending on the infectious agent. Inflammation of the liver may also be the result of lifestyle choices such as alcohol or drug abuse.

Etiology

Some of the many causes of liver inflammation include viruses, bacteria, metabolic and vascular disorders, drugs, alcohol, and other toxic substances such as cleaning fluids, industrial toxins, and plant poisons. Chart 46–1 (p. 1428) lists the many causes of hepatic inflammation.

Viral Causes

When most people hear the word *hepatitis,* they think of **viral hepatitis**. At least seven types of viruses are known to cause

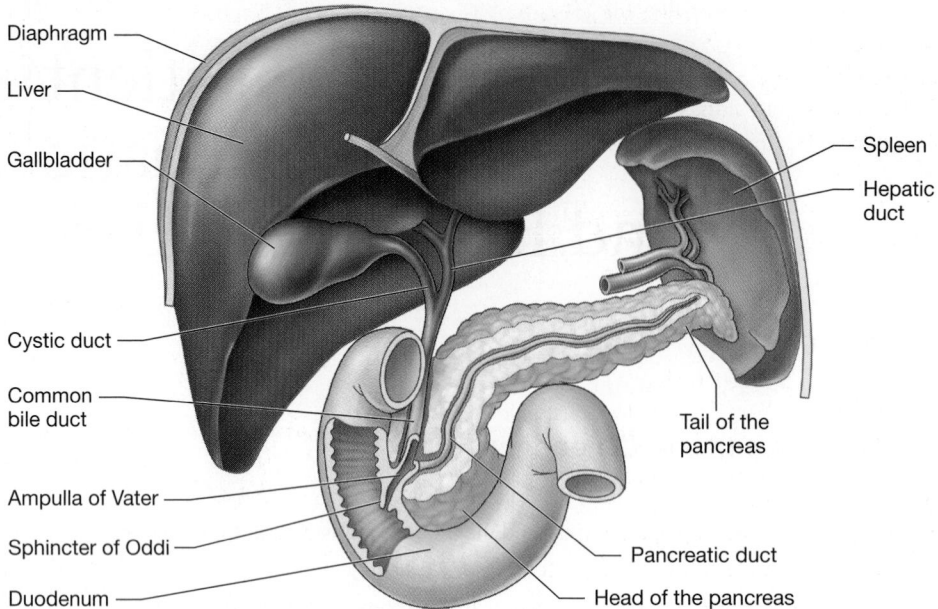

FIGURE 46–1 ■ Liver and biliary system.

CHART 46–1 — Common Causes of Hepatic Inflammation

VIRAL

Hepatitis A, B, C, D, E
(HAV, HBV, HCV, HDV, HEV)

Cytomegalovirus

Epstein-Barr virus

Herpes and varicella-zoster viruses

Yellow fever virus

NONVIRAL

Amebic infiltration (amebic abscess)

Lyme disease

Syphilis

Bacteria

TOXINS

Ethanol (alcohol)

Carbon tetrachloride

Yellow phosphorus

Mushrooms (*Amanita phalloides*)

Herbs (comfrey)

METABOLIC DISORDERS

Alpha$_1$-antitrypsin deficiency

Wilson disease (copper metabolism)

VASCULAR DISORDERS

Budd-Chiari syndrome

Congestive heart failure

Severe hypotension

Shock

DRUGS

Acetaminophen

Allopurinol

Androgens and anabolic steroids

Aspirin (high doses)

Captopril

Carbamazepine

Chlorpromazine

Chlorpropamide

Cholecystographic dyes

Clindamycin

Erythromycin

Estrogen

Halothane

Imipramine

Isoniazid (INH)

Ketoconazole

L-asparaginase

Methotrexate

Methyldopa

Mithramycin

Monoamine oxidase inhibitors (MAOI)

Oral contraceptives

Para-aminosalicylic acid (PAS)

Phenytoin

Procainamide

Sulfonamides

Tetracycline

inflammation of the liver. Because of the diversity of liver function, the effects of hepatitis can be locally diffuse throughout the liver or can manifest as systemic disease. The Cultural Considerations box shows which groups are affected most by which viruses.

Hepatitis A

Hepatitis A virus (HAV), a member of the picornavirus family, is a small RNA virus (Thomas, 2007). It was once known as infectious hepatitis and is endemic throughout the world. Many cases go undiagnosed because symptoms are often nonspecific, mild, and flulike. In the United States, there were an estimated 3,579 cases in 2006, which indicates a steady decline since 2000, when there were 13,397 cases reported (CDC, 2008).

Transmission of HAV is usually through the fecal–oral route, meaning persons contract the virus by drinking water contaminated with sewage, eating uncooked food washed in this water, eating shellfish harvested from contaminated water, or eating food contaminated by a person who is infected and did not wash his hands after using the toilet. It is also considered a sexually transmitted disease, mainly through oral sex. Besides being found in the feces, the virus has been isolated from bile and sera of infected persons, meaning it is possible to transmit the disease through transfusion of infected blood (Huether, 2006). The incubation period (time between exposure and onset of symptoms) for HAV is anywhere from 2 to 6 weeks. The virus is found in the feces up to 2 weeks before symptoms occur and the week following the onset of symptoms, but may be as long as

CULTURAL CONSIDERATIONS Related to Hepatitis in the United States

Cultural groups with the highest reported infections of:

Hepatitis A: American Indians/Alaska Natives

Hepatitis B: non-Hispanic Blacks

Hepatitis C: similar across all racial/ethnic groups.

3 months and is most contagious during this time (Huether, 2006). It takes about 4 weeks for the body to develop antibodies to HAV (anti-HAV). **Serum immunoglobulin M (IgM)** is seen in the acute phase of the illness and begins to decline about 3 months after exposure. **Serum immunoglobulin G (IgG)** levels are slower to peak, but remain elevated years after exposure, conferring immunity against further infection by HAV. Hepatitis A usually causes no long-term damage and a chronic state is unknown for HAV.

Hepatitis B

Hepatitis B virus (HBV) is a DNA virus that replicates in the liver. It was once known as serum hepatitis. Hepatitis B occurs in most places in the world, but the rate of infection varies depending on location. HBV is a complex organism involving three basic components. The intact virus is sometimes called a Dane particle. It has a double-layered outer coat that carries the hepatitis B surface antigen (HBsAg), thereby allowing it to be detected by radioimmunoassay (Huether, 2006). Because of the protective coating, the core antigen (HBcAg) is not detectable in serum; however, a derivative of the core antigen, HBeAg, is detectable, and this serves as a marker of viral replication and infectivity.

HBV may be found in blood, semen, cervical secretions, saliva, and wound drainage with the highest concentration occurring in blood and blood products (Thomas, 2007). The virus is robust, living up to a week in an open environment (Thomas, 2007). Viral transmission is through direct contact with blood and blood products, sexual contact, and contact with contaminated inanimate objects. High-risk groups include health care workers, particularly those working in a laboratory, blood bank, or hemodialysis setting where there is frequent contact with blood and blood products. IV drug users, homosexual men, and people with multiple sex partners are also at risk. Transmission can also occur during pregnancy from mother to fetus, if the mother is infected in the 3rd trimester or at birth.

The incubation period for HBV is longer than that of other hepatic viruses, lasting anywhere from 2 to 6 months, during which time transmission is possible even when symptoms are absent. HBV can exist as a carrier state, and/or it can create a chronic active state of infection, which can progress to cirrhosis and liver failure, thus requiring liver transplantation. HBV infection can lead to an increased risk for developing liver cancer as well.

Hepatitis C

Hepatitis C virus (HCV), once known as non-A, non-B virus, is a large RNA virus with an incubation period of 60 to 150 days (Holloway & D'Acunto, 2006). It replicates at a very high rate, mutating readily, which causes the host immune system to have difficulty building a response. This in turn leads to a high rate of chronic infections.

There are six different genotypes of HCV with three of them occurring most often in the United States. The most common genotype found in the United States is genotype 1, with genotypes 2 and 3 occurring as well. The lack of viral replication is considered a sustained viral response (SVR), which is measured by HCV-RNA or viral load. Genotype 1 has the poorest response to treatment, about a 50% SVR, whereas genotypes 2 and 3 both respond to treatment with a 70% to 80% SVR (Deutsch, 2003).

Antibodies to HCV (anti-HCV) can be detected in acute, recovered, or chronic infection.

The rate of HCV infection has dropped drastically since 2000. The Centers for Disease Control reported that there were 3,197 new cases of HCV infection in 2000 but only 802 in 2006 (CDC, 2008). HCV is found predominantly in blood, blood products, and transplanted tissue. However, there is evidence that HCV can be transmitted sexually, particularly in those having multiple sex partners. In fact, for persons with hepatitis C, the risk appears to be similar for those that report drug use or multiple sex partners (Wasley et al., 2007). The most common cause of HCV transmission in the United States is attributed to injection drug use (CDC, 2008). It is also possible to transmit HCV through other percutaneous exposures, such as tattooing, body piercing, folk medicine practices, and barbering, although records of this transmission are not available.

 Of the reported cases of acute hepatitis C in 2005 (Wasley et al., 2007), the most common risk factor identified was injection drug use (50%). Other risk factors included multiple sexual partners (23%), surgical procedures (14%), and occupational exposure to blood (8%).

Hepatitis D

Hepatitis D virus (HDV), also known as delta virus, is an RNA virus that is defective and must have HBsAg present for its replication; therefore, simultaneous infection with HBV is necessary for HDV. The incubation period lasts from 1 to 6 months and transmission occurs in the same manner as for HBV. IV drug users have a high rate of HDV with a mortality rate of about 3% (Thomas, 2007).

Hepatitis E

Hepatitis E virus (HEV) is an RNA virus with an incubation period of 15 to 60 days (Huether, 2006). It is transmitted via the fecal–oral route and is similar to hepatitis A in clinical manifestations. Unlike HAV, however, the mortality rate for pregnant women who contract HEV is higher at 10% to 20% (Friedman, 2004). HEV is endemic in Southeast Asia, India, North Africa, and Mexico, but is uncommon in the United States.

Hepatitis G

Hepatitis G virus (HGV) is an RNA virus about which little is known. Transmission may occur percutaneously or through sexual contact. The virus has been detected in at least 50% of IV drug users, 30% of patients undergoing hemodialysis, and 15% of patients with chronic HBV or HCV. Infection of HGV is associated with a chronic viremia. Interestingly, it should be noted that if patients with HIV are also infected with HGV, their survival rate is improved (Friedman, 2004).

Pathophysiology

Once the liver is infected with any of these hepatitis viruses, an inflammatory response is initiated when the acini cells develop mononuclear inflammatory infiltrates. The inflammatory response causes edema within the liver and can obstruct the **bile canaliculi,** small channels adjacent to the hepatocytes that move bile toward the common bile duct. It is this intrahepatic obstruction of bile that causes obstructive jaundice. There may also be liver cell necrosis; **Kupffer cells,** cells that line the liver sinusoids and are phagocytic cells; hyperplasia; and scarring.

The cell-mediated immune response (cytokines, toxic T cells, natural killer cells) is responsible for the tissue injury that occurs. If the case of hepatitis is mild, there is little parenchymal damage, but hepatitis B and C usually cause the most severe liver inflammation and damage. Hepatitis C invades the liver cells, causing injury directly; therefore, the inflammation in the hepatocytes is directly related to the viral load. Although rare, acute fulminating hepatitis may be caused by hepatitis B (also coinfection with HDV), resulting in massive hepatocellular necrosis leading to liver failure. Even in severe cases of hepatitis, liver regeneration begins within 48 hours of the tissue injury.

For both HBV and HCV, asymptomatic carrier states may exist. Although these individuals may never develop an active disease process, they carry an increased risk for developing hepatocellular carcinoma (Thomas, 2007). Hepatitis B and C can produce chronic, active infections where the immune system is unable to clear the virus completely. About 10% of individuals infected with HBV will go on to develop chronic infection. In the case of HCV infection, 75% to 85% of those infected will go on to develop chronic HCV.

Additional agents can also cause liver inflammation (hepatitis). Bacteria and circulating bacterial endotoxins can invade the parenchyma during sepsis and cause liver injury. Some medications can also cause hepatitis. For example, toxic metabolites of acetaminophen can damage the cellular structure in the liver, leading to inflammation. Many chemotherapy drugs, such as methotrexate, vincristine, and the combination of 5-fluorouracil and levamisole, have a high potential for causing chemical hepatitis (Baldwin, 2003). But the most common toxic substance that causes chemical hepatitis is alcohol. Liver inflammation can occur after drinking large quantities in a relatively short time or from chronic consumption (alcohol abuse).

Clinical Manifestations

Regardless of the cause, the clinical manifestations of hepatitis are frequently very similar. The severity of the symptoms can range from almost none or asymptomatic, to fulminating hepatitis, progressing to liver failure and death. The patient is usually asymptomatic during the incubation period of viral hepatitis. With HBV infection, there is evidence of HBeAg in the blood, indicating a high degree of infectivity. Later in the incubation period, HBsAg (hepatitis B surface antigen) appears. Following the incubation period, there are three phases in the clinical course of viral hepatitis: the prodromal phase, the icteric phase, and (convalescent) recovery.

Prodromal Phase

It is often difficult to determine the beginning of the **prodromal phase**, the phase of acute hepatitis that occurs between exposure to the virus and the appearance of jaundice, because it starts about 2 weeks after exposure to the virus. Because the time of exposure is often unknown, the prodromal phase will vary depending on the incubation period. The prodromal phase can have either an insidious or a rapid onset. Symptoms may be vague, often flu-like, with anorexia, nausea, vomiting, and malaise, as well as frequent occurrences of myalgia, arthralgia, and easy fatigue (Thomas, 2007). Anorexia usually occurs early in this phase and is frequently accompanied by a distaste of smoking in those patients who are smokers. Additional manifes-

tations may include mild, but constant, abdominal pain in the right upper quadrant (RUQ) or epigastrium, as well as a fever less than 103°F (39.4°C).

Icteric Phase

The **icteric phase** begins with the onset of jaundice, which usually occurs 5 to 10 days after the initial symptoms, although some patients may never develop jaundice. The prodromal symptoms become worse with the onset of jaundice, but then a progressive clinical improvement follows. Due to the increased levels of conjugated **bilirubin**, a product in the breakdown of hemoglobin that is conjugated by the hepatocytes and is excreted in bile, the urine may be dark during this phase.

In 2005, the CDC reported (Wasley et al., 2007) that overall 76% of persons infected with acute hepatitis A developed jaundice, 33% were hospitalized, and 0.6% died. Persons age 5 to 39 were more likely to report the development of jaundice (83%), whereas persons younger than 5 years and persons age 60 or older were less likely (58%).

Convalescent Phase

The **convalescent phase** is characterized by an increased sense of well-being, which usually begins after 2 to 3 weeks of acute illness. The phase is marked by additional signs of improvement such as increased appetite and energy level. The jaundice of the icteric phase and abdominal pain disappear. Complete clinical recovery varies depending on the type of hepatitis, but HAV is usually resolved in 9 to 10 weeks, while recovery may take up to 16 weeks.

Diagnostic Procedures

Tests that assess the degree of liver injury include:

- **Alanine aminotransferase (ALT)** is an enzyme released from hepatocytes when the liver is injured. The ALT is more specific for liver injury than the other enzymes mentioned next. In acute hepatitis, the serum ALT may exceed 1,000 IU/L.

- **Aspartate aminotransferase (AST)** is an enzyme found in hepatocytes and cardiac cells primarily, but it is also found in skeletal muscle cells, the kidneys, and the pancreas. It is released when there is cellular injury in these areas. When the liver is injured, the serum AST level can increase more than 10 times normal and will remain elevated for a longer period of time than in other injuries (Kee, 2002).

- **Alkaline phosphatase (ALP)** is an enzyme found mostly in liver cells and bone. Mild hepatocyte damage will cause a slight increase in the blood level of ALP. Acute hepatitis can cause marked elevations in the ALP, but the level rapidly returns to normal after the acute phase.

- **Gamma-glutamyltransferase (GGT)**, an enzyme found mostly in the liver and the kidneys, is a good way to detect liver parenchymal disease. The GGT will increase 12 to 24 hours after heavy alcohol consumption and remain elevated for weeks after alcohol cessation; in fact, some alcohol rehabilitation programs are using this in planning care for these persons (Kee, 2002).

- **Lactic dehydrogenase (LDH),** an intracellular enzyme, is found in most cells, especially those in active metabolism such as the heart, skeletal muscle, liver, brain, and red blood cells. The subunit, LDH_5, is most specific for liver injury, with levels rising before jaundice develops.

- Serum bilirubin levels become elevated when there is hepatitis. Bilirubin is formed from the breakdown of hemoglobin and processed in the liver to form conjugated bilirubin. If there is intrahepatic edema or another obstruction (cirrhosis), conjugated bilirubin cannot enter the duodenum; therefore, levels of direct (conjugated) bilirubin will be elevated. If function is severely affected, the liver cannot conjugate bilirubin and the indirect (unconjugated) level will rise.

- Specific serological tests for viral antigens, antibodies, or the virus itself are available (Chart 46–2).

- Liver biopsy is done to evaluate chronic hepatitis due to HBV or HCV.

Medical Management

The goals of medical treatment for hepatitis are to identify the cause of the inflammation, either infectious or chemical, provide symptomatic treatment, monitor the damage to the liver, and support the liver's ability to regenerate and heal itself. Laboratory and diagnostic tests give clues to the cause of hepatitis, assess the degree of liver injury, and indicate the degree of healing.

Preventive Drug Treatment

Vaccines are available for HAV and HBV. The vaccine for HBV became available in 1982 and the vaccine for HAV in the early 1990s. In 2001 the Food and Drug Administration (FDA) approved a combination HAV and HBV vaccine that consists of a three-dose series (Wasley et al., 2007).

Anyone in a high-risk group should be vaccinated against HAV and HBV. High-risk groups include health care workers, day care workers, employees at correctional facilities, injection drug users, male homosexuals, and anyone traveling to an endemic area of HAV. Patients on hemodialysis and household and sexual contacts of persons with HBV should be vaccinated as well. Vaccine for HAV is given in 2 intramuscular (IM) doses 6 to 12 months apart. The most common side effect is pain at the injection site. HBV vaccine is given in a series of 3 IM doses, with the first dose followed in 1 month by the second one, and the third one given 5 months later. Side effects of HBV vaccine include pain at the injection site, fatigue, and headache.

Immune globulin (IG) is available for HAV and HBV postexposure prophylaxis. Postexposure prophylaxis is recommended for household and sexual contacts of people with HAV or HBV, health care workers after a needlestick injury, and others exposed to infected blood or body fluids. Postexposure prophylaxis for HAV is a single dose of IG, and it must be given within 2 weeks of exposure. For HBV, IG should be given as soon as possible, but may be given only up to 1 week after exposure, with a second dose given 1 month after exposure. It is recommended that the HBV vaccine be given at the same time as IG in the case of exposure.

Although there is no vaccine for hepatitis C, treatment is initiated to prevent chronic HCV once the diagnosis is made. The goal of treatment is to get a sustained viral response, which

---

CHART 46–2 **Specific Tests for Viral Hepatitis**

Hepatitis A	Hepatitis B	Hepatitis C	Hepatitis D	Hepatitis E
HAV-RNA	**HBV-DNA**	**HCV-RNA**	**HDV-RNA**	**Anti-HEV**
Is viral RNA and is found in stool; peaks 1–2 months after exposure and disappears before month 4.	Is viral DNA and is found in serum just before the second month and disappears by month 5.	Is viral RNA and indicates replicating virus.	Is viral RNA and indicates acute infection.	Is antibody and indicates infection.
Anti-HAV IgM	**HBeAg**	**Anti-HCV**	**HDAg**	
Is found in serum during acute illness, peaking about 2–3 months after exposure and slowly decreasing. It is usually gone by 1 year after exposure.	Is a marker for viral replication and appears about 2 months after exposure.	Is antibody to the virus but does not indicate immunity.	Is hepatitis D antigen and indicates acute infection.	
Anti-HAV IgG	**HBsAg**			
Is found in serum during recovery and indicates immunity to the virus. It remains elevated for years.	Is the surface antigen on the virus and is usually detected 1 week before HBeAg and disappears by month 5. Persistent levels indicate either a chronic or a carrier state.			
	Anti-HBc IgM			
	Is antibody to HBcAg and is found during acute illness and convalescence but may persist for years.			
	Anti-HBs IgM			
	Indicates acute illness and infectivity.			
	Anti-HBs IgG and **Anti-HBc IgG**			
	Both indicate recovery from acute illness.			

means that HCV-RNA is undetectable 6 months after treatment is finished. Standard treatment is with PEG-Intron (pegylated interferon alfa-2b) subcutaneously and oral ribavirin 800 milligrams per day in divided doses for 6 to 11 months (Deutsch, 2003). The side effects of this treatment regimen may include fatigue, muscle aches, headache, fever, and chills. Drinking a lot of water and getting adequate rest can minimize these effects. Patients taking interferon preparations have also reported depression.

Supportive Treatment

Treatment for hepatitis is primarily supportive, regardless of the cause. The keystone of therapy is rest, adequate nutrition, proper diet, and avoidance of alcohol. Few patients require hospitalization, which may be necessary for patients with fulminant liver failure.

The diet recommended for patients with hepatitis is a low-fat, high-calorie diet, with a large portion of the calories coming from complex carbohydrates, such as whole grains, fruits, and vegetables. Depending on the level of functional liver impairment, increased protein intake may also be recommended. Good sources of protein with lower fat concentrations are foods such as egg whites, tofu, beans, and fat-free dairy products. Alcohol and other agents toxic to the liver must be avoided.

Because fatigue can be a common complaint for patients with hepatitis, planned rest periods throughout the day are essential. Although activity is usually restricted during the acute phase of hepatitis, bed rest is rarely indicated. Strenuous activity is discouraged, but may be gradually resumed as the healing process progresses.

Complementary Therapies

Several herbal preparations that have been used for centuries have been shown to be beneficial to the liver. Milk thistle (Silybum marianum) is one of the oldest therapies for liver disease. Its active ingredient, silymarin, has demonstrated its ability to promote hepatocyte growth and reduce liver inflammation, as well as protecting the liver cells from toxic damage (Pelc, 2003). Another herbal preparation for hepatitis uses licorice root, which has both anti-inflammatory and antiviral properties. However, long-term use may cause hypertension and edema because of its chemical resemblance to aldosterone. For patients with HCV receiving the standard treatment, ginger root may help relieve the nausea associated with interferon.

◼ Nursing Management

Nursing care for the patients with hepatitis involves supportive measures and education. Most patients with hepatitis are not hospitalized, but are managed in their own homes. Those requiring hospitalization would be those with fulminant hepatitis, or chronic hepatitis that has progressed to cirrhosis, liver cancer, or liver failure.

Health Promotion

One of the primary responsibilities of nursing with regard to viral hepatitis focuses on prevention and reducing the spread of infection through education. For all types of viral hepatitis, but especially for HAV and HEV, good hand hygiene practices after using the bathroom and before handling food are crucial to prevent transmission. Because many types of hepatitis can be spread through sexual activity, education should include encouraging patients to use safer sexual practices, including barrier protection (condoms), abstinence, and monogamy. There is a high risk of transmitting viral hepatitis through shared needles and other equipment. Some communities therefore participate in a needle exchange program, in which used needles can be traded for sterile ones, thereby reducing the risk of viral hepatitis and HIV.

Nurses are influential in educating the public about vaccinations for HAV and HBV. All people in moderate- and high-risk groups should be encouraged to be vaccinated. Many public health departments offer these vaccines at a reduced cost or no cost for individuals at risk. Postexposure prophylaxis is available for people who have known or probable exposure to HAV or HBV.

Assessment

The focus of the nursing assessment is to identify the patient's responses to hepatitis, both physically and emotionally, and to try to determine the sources of transmission that are controllable if the patient has viral hepatitis. Assessment should include a history of manifestations related to hepatitis, such as complaints of anorexia, nausea, vomiting, abdominal pain, and fatigue. Complaints may also include muscle or joint pain, and patients with hepatitis may notice that their stools become pale or almost white. This results from intrahepatic obstruction of the flow of bile into the duodenum. Conversely, their urine may be dark for the same reason. It is important to assess the onset and duration of symptoms in order to attempt to help patients identify their exposure to hepatitis. The history should include asking questions about sexual practices, injection drug use, chemical exposure, travel history, alcohol use, and dietary practices. Because many drugs and herbal preparations can have adverse effects on the liver, it is important to inquire about these substances, including over-the-counter (OTC) medications and other nonprescription preparations.

Physical assessment should include vital signs, color of the skin, sclera and mucous membranes, color of the stool and urine, and examination of the abdomen for tenderness and contour. Because an elevated bilirubin causes pruritus, there may be evidence of lesions from scratching or a report of generalized urticaria. If liver function is compromised, there may be problems affecting blood clotting factors, and the patient should be observed for signs of bleeding, such as bruising or petechiae.

Interventions

As mentioned earlier, the nursing interventions for patients with hepatitis are mainly supportive. Patients with hepatitis need education about the importance of rest and scheduling rest periods into their daily routines. Diet teaching should include information about specific foods high in complex carbohydrates and protein, low in fat, and abstinence from alcohol, often referred to as a "liver friendly" diet. These diet instructions should consider individual dietary preferences as well as cultural traditions. Specific information about disease transmission should also be included. Because pruritus may be a problem for some patients with hepatitis, specific ways they can relieve the itching and preserve their skin integrity is essential. The Nursing Process: Patient Care Plan

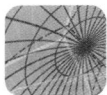

NURSING PROCESS: Patient Care Plan for Hepatitis

Assessment of Fatigue

Subjective Data:
How long have you felt tired or fatigued?
Are you able to maintain your activities of daily living?
How much activity can you tolerate before you feel fatigued?
What makes you feel better?

Objective Data:
Musculoskeletal examination:
- Muscle strength
- Activity tolerance
- Vital signs

Nursing Assessment and Diagnoses	Outcomes and Evaluation Parameters	Planning and Interventions with *Rationales*
Nursing Diagnoses: *Fatigue. Activity Intolerance* related to inadequate liver function	**Outcome:** Reduced fatigue. ***Evaluation Parameters:*** Ability to perform activities of daily living. Increased activity tolerance.	**Interventions and *Rationales:*** Encourage frequent rest periods during the day. *Energy conservation is necessary for tissue rebuilding and regaining well-being.* Facilitate the identification of essential activities and delegate tasks to others. *Energy conservation is necessary for tissue rebuilding and regaining well-being.* Encourage increased activity as fatigue improves. *A feeling of improvement can enhance well-being, self-concept, and a sense of control.*

Assessment of Nutritional Status

Subjective Data:
Are you having trouble eating?
Have you lost any weight?
How is your appetite?
Have you lost a taste for any foods?
Are there foods that you have a taste for?
Has your food consumption changed?
Do you drink alcohol?

Objective Data:
Body weight and appearance
Skin turgor
Skin and hair condition

Nursing Assessment and Diagnoses	Outcomes and Evaluation Parameters	Planning and Interventions with *Rationales*
Nursing Diagnosis: *Nutrition, Readiness for Enhanced* related to anorexia and reduced liver function	**Outcome:** Adequate nutrition. ***Evaluation Parameter:*** No weight loss.	**Interventions and *Rationales:*** Instruct the patient to eat foods that appeal to her, but stress the importance of high-calorie carbohydrates and proteins. *Carbohydrates are necessary for sufficient energy, and proteins are needed for healing.* Explain the importance of avoiding substances that can be toxic to the liver, such as alcohol and acetaminophen *in order to prevent further liver damage or inflammation.* Teach the patient to read food labels and choose foods that are low in fat and have adequate levels of vitamins and minerals, such as Instant Breakfast drink mix, *to improve nutritional status and promote healing.*

Assessment of Skin

Subjective Data:
Does your skin itch?
Have you been scratching your skin?
Have you noticed a change in the color of your skin?

Objective Data:
Examine skin for:
- Jaundice
- Lesions from scratching
- Dryness
- Bruises
- Petechiae

Nursing Assessment and Diagnoses	Outcomes and Evaluation Parameters	Planning and Interventions with *Rationales*
Nursing Diagnosis: *Skin Integrity, Risk for Impaired* related to jaundice and resultant pruritus	**Outcome:** Skin integrity maintained. ***Evaluation Parameters:*** Reports diminished itching. No bruising or petechiae. No lesions from scratching.	**Interventions and *Rationales:*** Instruct the patient to use cool, lightweight, nonrestrictive clothing and avoid woolens. *Clothing made from lightweight fabrics causes less itching.* Explain that a cool environmental temperature and cool water for bathing may increase comfort related to pruritus. Instruct the patient to keep her fingernails trimmed and well cared for *to decrease the likelihood of excoriating when scratching.* Instruct the patient to take antihistamine medication as ordered *to reduce pruritus.*

(continued)

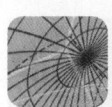

NURSING PROCESS: Patient Care Plan for Hepatitis—*Continued*

Assessment of Infection Transmission

Subjective Data:

Have you ever had a blood transfusion?

Do you have any tattoos or body piercings?

Do you use injectable drugs?

Where have you traveled recently?

Have you eaten any raw fish or seafood?

Where do you work? Child care facility? Correctional facility? Hemodialysis unit?

Do you handle blood or body fluids for your job?

Has anyone you know been sick or had yellow skin?

Do you have multiple sex partners?

When did your symptoms begin?

Objective Data:

Enlarged lymph nodes

Tender liver

Nursing Assessment and Diagnoses	Outcomes and Evaluation Parameters	Planning and Interventions with *Rationales*
Nursing Diagnosis: *Infection, Risk for* related to the transmission of viral hepatitis.	**Outcome:** No spread of the infection. **Evaluation Parameter:** Verbalizes modes of transmission and ways to prevent spread.	**Interventions and *Rationales:*** Use standard or universal precautions when handling blood or body fluids. *Viral hepatitis is transmitted by direct contact with infected feces, body fluids, and blood.* Explain that the time of highest infectivity is before symptoms appear, and that *good hand hygiene can prevent the spread of the disease.* Teach about safe and safer sex practices *to prevent the spread of the virus.* Encourage prophylactic treatment for close contacts and/or vaccination against HAV and HBV. *These measures decrease the risk of contracting the disease or decrease the severity of the illness.*

feature includes specific interventions and application of the nursing process to a patient with hepatitis.

Cirrhosis

Cirrhosis, the 12th leading cause of death in the United States (Askey, 2006), is an irreversible, progressive deterioration of the liver that results from chronic liver disease. Cirrhosis is the result of hepatocellular injury and inflammation usually occurring over time. If the injury or inflammation is short lived, the liver is usually able to regenerate itself. However, severe acute injury, as that seen in hepatitis, can result in cirrhosis. Cirrhosis may be brought about by a variety of causes including chronic hepatitis; alcoholism; prolonged, severe right heart failure; and long-term obstruction to biliary flow. Chart 46–3 lists the causes of cirrhosis. The most common cause of cirrhosis in the United States is alcoholic cirrhosis.

Pathophysiology

Prolonged liver injury from toxins, inflammation, and metabolic derangements causes liver cell damage and cell death. The damaged or dead liver cells are repaired or replaced with tissue that is more fibrous than the original tissue. Fibrotic scarring is the result. Liver cells continue to regenerate but do so in an abnormal pattern. This abnormal liver regeneration creates regenerative nodules. The fibrotic scarring and nodular development

alter the normal lobular architecture. Diffuse, disorganized fibrous bands result, and then as the surviving hepatocytes regenerate, more nodules are formed. The development of cirrhosis depends on several factors, including the length of time the liver is subjected to the injury, the severity of the injury, and the liver's reaction to the assault (Thomas, 2007). As the liver repairs itself, there is distortion in the microcirculation. Collateral vessels develop in the newly regenerated nodule connecting the portal vein to the hepatic artery (Figure 46–2 ■). This results in increased resistance to the flow of blood throughout the liver, causing portal venous hypertension because these vessels are inefficient.

As mentioned earlier, cirrhosis can result from a variety of causes, one of which is alcohol abuse. The ingestion of alcohol causes metabolic changes in the liver in which there is a decrease in the utilization of fatty acids by the liver, increased fatty acid synthesis, increased esterification of fatty acids into triglycerides, and a decreased secretion of fat from the liver (Friedman, 2004). This condition, called fatty liver, can possibly be reversed if no further alcohol is consumed. Continued alcohol use causes liver inflammation leading to necrosis, fibrosis, regenerative nodules, and structural changes.

Prolonged obstruction to the flow of bile within the liver or biliary system can also cause cirrhosis. When the bile ducts within the liver are obstructed, the proximal hepatocytes are injured. There is an inflammatory response to the injury with inflammatory cells infiltrating the liver, leading to fibrosis and

CHART 46–3	**Causes of Cirrhosis**

INFECTIOUS AND DISEASE-RELATED CAUSES

Autoimmune chronic active hepatitis

Biliary cirrhosis

Chronic pancreatitis

Cholelithiasis

Cystic fibrosis

Diabetes mellitus

Hepatitis B and C

Hypertriglyceridemia

Obesity

Sclerosing cholangitis

Syndrome "X" (insulin resistance syndrome)

HEPATOTOXINS

Direct:
- Alcohol
- Carbon tetrachloride
- Phosphorus

Indirect:
- Acetaminophen
- Alkylated anabolic steroids
- Mushroom toxin *(Amanita phalloides)*
- Methotrexate
- Tetracycline

Genetic diseases:
- Galactosemia
- Hemochromatosis
- Wilson disease

Vascular disorders of the liver:
- Budd-Chiari syndrome
- Ischemic hepatitis
- Right heart failure (chronic)

regenerative nodules. This is essentially the same pathway that chronic hepatitis B and C cause cirrhosis; that is, chronic inflammation leading to fibrosis and regenerative nodules.

Clinical Manifestations

Cirrhosis can be asymptomatic until liver function is severely affected and, even then, the onset of symptoms is gradual. Cirrhosis may be found incidentally on the annual physical exam. The manifestations of cirrhosis can be nonspecific and are the result of the hepatocellular damage and portal hypertension. Initially the patient might complain of fatigue, weakness, anorexia, and weight loss, which is caused from the decreased metabolic functions of the liver. Because the liver produces bile, which is needed for the digestion of fat and the formation of fat soluble vitamins, impaired liver function may result in fat soluble vitamin deficiency, particularly of vitamin K. Deficiency of vitamin K

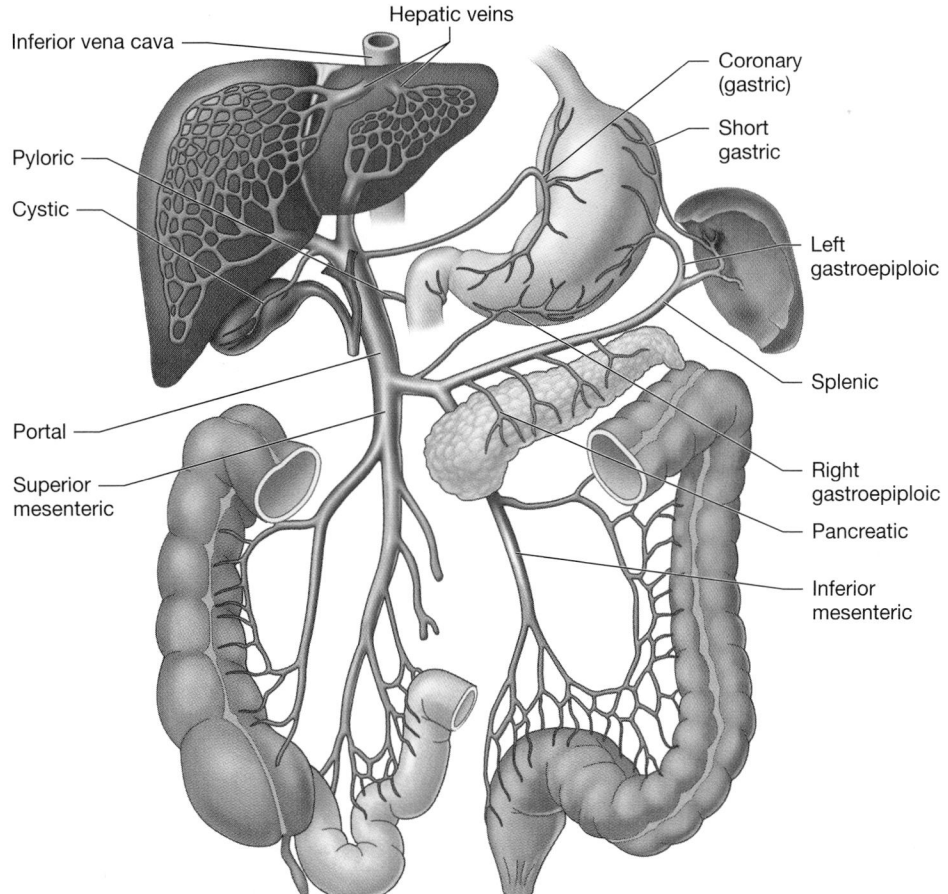

FIGURE 46–2 ■ Portal circulation.

causes problems with blood clotting and fat malabsorption. Other metabolic functions of the liver include **gluconeogenesis** (the making of glucose from noncarbohydrate sources), glycogen storage, synthesis of albumin, clotting factors, and other blood proteins. When liver function is severely compromised and the liver is unable to make albumin, **hypoalbuminemia** leads to edema. Both ascites and peripheral edema develop in part because of the decrease in colloidal osmotic pressure. Because of the architectural changes in the cirrhotic liver structure, there is obstruction to the flow of bile out of the liver, causing jaundice of the skin and sclera. Chart 46–4 contains a list of clinical manifestations of cirrhosis and the physiological basis for each.

Complications

As cirrhosis progresses, severe systemic complications occur, the most significant of which are **portal hypertension**, **hepatic encephalopathy**, and **hepatorenal syndrome**. Each of these conditions has further clinical manifestations and complications.

Portal Hypertension

As the internal architecture of the liver is distorted as a result of scarring, venous blood flow through the portal venous system is impeded. This increases the portal venous blood pressure, from a normal of about 3 mmHg to at least 10 mmHg. Because the portal veins carry blood from the GI tract, spleen, and pancreas to the liver, the obstruction of this blood flow from cirrhosis causes increased pressure in the vessels in the aforementioned organs. The increased pressure causes increased blood flow in collateral vessels, which normally have lower pressure. This causes varices (distended, tortuous, collateral veins) to develop particularly in the esophagus and rectum.

Esophageal varices are thin-walled veins that are prone to rupture, causing massive, life-threatening hemorrhage. Rupture of esophageal varices can result from anything that increases the pressure in the vessel, such as coughing, or from trauma caused by something as simple as eating high-roughage food. However, bleeding from esophageal varices can be slow and chronic leading to anemia and **melena**, the black or maroon, sticky, foul-smelling feces resulting from the digestion of blood. When the varices rupture, there is hemorrhage and vomiting of large volumes of dark-red blood. Contributing to the risk of hemorrhage is erosion by gastric acid, elevated venous pressure, and decreased clotting factors. Individuals who have recurrent esophageal bleeding from portal hypertension usually die within a year (Huether, 2006).

Another consequence of portal hypertension is splenomegaly, or enlargement of the spleen. The splenic vein branches from the portal vein, so when blood flow is obstructed through the portal vein, the subsequent increasing pressure in the splenic vein causes an enlarged spleen as well as the increased rate of blood cell destruction by the spleen. This contributes to the occurrence of anemia. More platelets are removed from circulation and sequestered in the spleen, leading to impaired clot formation, all of which contribute to esophageal bleeding.

Ascites is simply the accumulation of protein-rich fluid in the abdominal cavity. Portal hypertension is the primary cause of ascites, but hypoalbuminemia and accumulation of aldosterone aid in the fluid accumulation. The low serum albumin decreases the colloidal osmotic pressure in the blood vessels causing fluid to escape into the interstitial space, which decreases the circulating blood volume. This, in turn, causes the kidneys to retain sodium and water to increase the blood volume, leading to an increase in hydrostatic pressure and accelerating portal hypertension and ascites formation.

Hepatic Encephalopathy

Hepatic encephalophathy, also known as portosystemic encephalopathy, is the result of an increased level of circulating neurotoxins. The most abundant neurotoxin is ammonia, which forms as the end product of protein digestion. Normally, the hepatocytes convert ammonia to urea, which is then excreted by the kidneys. However, when liver function is impaired, ammonia builds up in the blood causing altered cerebral energy metabolism, interfering with neurotransmitters, and causing cerebral edema. The accumulation of other substances, such as short-chain amino acids, serotonin, and tryptophan, is thought to cause additional symptoms of encephalophathy including **asterixis**, a flapping tremor of the hands when the arms are outstretched, believed to be caused by the accumulation of substances normally detoxified by the liver, agitation, restlessness, and changes in mentation (Huether, 2006).

Hepatorenal Syndrome

Hepatorenal syndrome is characterized by the occurrence of azotemia in a patient with liver failure when other causes of renal failure have been excluded. The cause of this syndrome is unknown, but intense renal vasoconstriction and decreased renal blood flow are present while renal tissue is normal. Type I hepatorenal syndrome is acute and occurs when there is increased serum creatinine to more than 2.5 mg/dL in less than 2 weeks. Type II hepatorenal syndrome is chronic and progresses more slowly. The presence of oliguria, sodium and water retention, hypotension, and peripheral vasodilation indicates a poor prognosis.

Laboratory and Diagnostic Procedures

Because cirrhosis has systemic consequences, nonspecific abnormalities may be found in many laboratory tests. For example, liver function tests (LFTs)—including ALT, AST, alkaline phosphatase (ALP), and GGT, which are indications of liver injury not liver function—not only are all usually elevated in patients with cirrhosis but also are elevated in hepatitis, sclerosing cholangitis, gallbladder disease, and because of some medications. Conversely, these lab results may be normal in the early stages of cirrhosis. The laboratory tests that actually measure liver function include the serum albumin, prothrombin time, partial thromboplastin time, clotting time, bilirubin, and serum ammonia level. The definitive diagnosis of cirrhosis is made through liver biopsy. Other tests give indications of severity and associated complications. The Diagnostic Tests box (p. 1438) outlines the tests and anticipated results for patients with cirrhosis.

Medical Management

The first priority in medical management for the patient with cirrhosis is to prevent or minimize complications such as portal hypertension, esophageal varices, hepatic encephalopathy, and hepatorenal syndrome. This is accomplished through holistic care that addresses physical, spiritual, and psychosocial aspects

CHART46–4   Clinical Manifestations of Cirrhosis and Physiological Causes

Clinical Manifestation	Physiological Cause
Integumentary	
• Jaundice	Blocked outflow of bile from liver due to structural change.
• Palmar erythema	Altered sex hormone metabolism (high estrogen).
• Spider angioma	High capillary pressure.
• Decreased body hair	Altered sex hormone metabolism.
• Pruritus	High levels of bilirubin cause itching.
• Ecchymosis	↓ clotting factors, ↑ platelet destruction by spleen, ↓ vitamin K.
• Caput medusae	Intrahepatic obstruction to portal blood flow.
• Edema	Low serum albumin, high hydrostatic pressure, sodium and water retention.
Gastrointestinal	
• Esophageal varices	Intrahepatic obstruction to portal blood flow.
• Abdominal pain	Stretching of Glisson's capsule or ascites.
• Anorexia	Increased venous pressure in GI tract.
• Ascites	Hypoalbuminemia, ↑ lymph production, ↑ capillary filtration pressure, ↑ renal absorption of sodium and water.
• Light-colored stools	Intrahepatic obstruction of bile flowing into duodenum.
• GI bleeding	Esophageal varices bleed.
• Hemorrhoids	Portal hypertension causes venous congestion.
Neurological	
• Hepatic encephalopathy	Hepatocytes unable to convert ammonia (by-product of protein metabolism) to urea to be excreted by the kidney (↑ ammonia).
• Sensory disturbances	High serum ammonia levels are neurotoxic.
• Asterixis (liver flap)	Caused by high serum ammonia levels.
Cardiovascular	
• Portal hypertension	Intrahepatic obstruction to portal blood flow.
• Bounding pulse	Increased fluid volume from sodium and water retention and ↑ aldosterone.
• Dysrhythmias	Fluid and electrolyte imbalance.
Hematologic	
• Decreased clotting factors	Liver unable to synthesize clotting factors and vitamin K.
• Thrombocytopenia	Enlarged spleen causes ↑ destruction of platelets.
• Anemia	↑ RBC destruction in spleen, bleeding.
Hepatic	
• Atrophic, nodular liver	Scarring.
• Splenomegaly	Intrahepatic obstruction to portal blood flow causes engorgement of spleen.
Respiratory	
• Dyspnea	Ascites cause pressure on diaphragm.
Reproductive	
• Oligomenorrhea (female)	Altered sex hormone metabolism.
• Testicular atrophy	Altered sex hormone metabolism (high estrogen).
• Gynecomastia (male)	Altered sex hormone metabolism (high estrogen).
• Loss of libido	Altered sex hormone metabolism.
Metabolic	
• Hypoalbuminemia	Liver unable to synthesize albumin.
• Hypokalemia	Altered renal excretion.
• Hypocalcemia	Related to low serum protein levels.
• Malnutrition	Impaired metabolism of nutrients.
• Muscle wasting	Muscles are used as protein source.

DIAGNOSTIC TESTS for Cirrhosis

Test	Description	Anticipated Results in Cirrhosis
LIVER FUNCTION TESTS		
ALT (alanine aminotransferase) AST (aspartate aminotransferase)	Enzymes released during liver injury. Primarily found in liver cells. Mainly found in liver and heart muscle.	May be 200–4,000 units/L. The higher elevations result from drug- or chemical-induced liver damage. 10 times or more above the normal (8–38 units/L) and stays elevated for longer period.
ALT/AST	Normally the ALT is more elevated than the AST in liver disease.	In alcoholic cirrhosis, the AST is more elevated.
ALP (alkaline phosphatase)	Primarily found in liver and bone. ALP[1] isoenzyme found in liver. ALP[2] isoenzyme found in bone.	Markedly elevated in severe liver disease—normal is 42–136 units/L; ALP[1] 20–130 units/L.
TESTS THAT INDICATE LIVER FUNCTION		
Bilirubin	Bilirubin is formed from the breakdown of red blood cells (RBCs) and is not water soluble (unconjugated). It is transported to the liver where it is conjugated by the hepatocytes and is then water soluble.	Normal values: 0.1–1.2 mg/dL (total bilirubin); 0.1–0.3 mg/dL direct bilirubin (conjugated). Obstruction to bile flow either within the liver or extrahepatic (gallbladder disease) will cause an increase in direct bilirubin. Indirect bilirubin may be elevated from hemolysis or hepatocyte damage where the liver is unable to conjugate the bilirubin.
Serum ammonia	Ammonia is nitrogenous waste from the breakdown of protein. Liver cells convert ammonia to urea for excretion by the kidneys. Compromised liver function causes ammonia levels to increase.	Normal values: 15–45 mcg/dL; elevated in hepatic failure, hepatic encephalopathy, portacaval shunt, and high-protein diet with liver failure.
Prothrombin time (PT)	PT measures clotting ability that is influenced by factors I (fibrinogen), V, VII, and X.	Prothrombin time: normal is 10–13 seconds or 70–100%. Because the liver makes clotting factors, including prothrombin, compromised liver function will decrease clotting.
Serum albumin	Albumin is synthesized by the liver and makes up more than half of the plasma proteins.	Normal values: 3.5–5.0 g/dL; 52–68% to total protein. Diminished liver function will decrease albumin levels.
Serum glucose	Stored in the liver as glycogen. Decreased liver function may impair glycogen storage.	Normal values: 70–110 mg/dL. Serum glucose may be low due to inadequate glycogen storage.
Serum cholesterol	The liver synthesizes cholesterol.	Normal values: <200 mg/dL. May be decreased in liver failure. May be increased in biliary cirrhosis and cholangitis.
TESTS FOR OTHER SYSTEMIC EFFECTS		
CBC and platelets	Nutritional status may be compromised in patients with liver disease. Folic acid and B_{12} deficiencies are common in alcoholic cirrhosis. Esophageal varices cause bleeding. Splenomegaly, caused by portal hypertension, causes increased destruction of platelets.	Normal values: Hb—male = 13.5–18 g/dL, female = 12–16 mg/dL. Hct—male = 40–54%, female = 36–46%. RBCs—male = 4.5–6 mcg/L, female = 4–5 mcg/L. Platelets—150,000–400,000 mcg/L. These values may all be decreased due to bleeding, folate and B_{12} deficiency, and increased platelet and RBC destruction.
Serum electrolytes	Serum electrolytes include sodium, potassium, magnesium, and phosphate; are affected by malnutrition, fluid retention, and altered renal excretion all due to cirrhosis.	Normal values: Sodium—135–145 mEq/L Potassium—3.5–5.3 mEq/L Magnesium—1.5–2.5 mEq/L Phosphate—1.7–2.6 mEq/L Chloride—95–105 mEq/L Decreased values indicate malnutrition, hemodilution, and altered renal excretion caused from cirrhosis.
OTHER TESTS TO ASSESS THE LIVER		
Abdominal ultrasound	Sound waves are reflected back from tissues and converted to electrical signs by a computer. It is used to determine the size of organs.	The liver may be enlarged earlier in cirrhosis, but is usually small and nodular in advanced disease.
Esophagastroscopy	Endoscopic examination of the esophagus.	This test is used to visualize esophageal varices and may be used to sclerose bleeding varices.
Liver biopsy	A tissue sample is taken via a needle puncture of the liver. It is used to determine the type of liver disease.	In early cirrhosis the histologic changes seen are micronodular. Histologically, there are hepatocellular necrosis and mallory bodies (hyaline endoplasmic reticulum), which indicate the onset of fibrosis. Fatty infiltration and fibrosis are also seen.

of the patient. The Complementary and Alternative Therapies box presents the importance of spiritual care of the patient.

Because alcoholism is a major cause of cirrhosis in the United States, efforts at alcohol abstinence are encouraged. This requires the involvement of the family as well as other forms of support. Comprehensive treatment of cirrhosis includes medications, surgical intervention, diet, and counseling.

Treatment for Ascites

Most medications given to a patient with cirrhosis target the complications of cirrhosis. For example, most patients with cirrhosis have portal hypertension with or without ascites, low serum albumin, and increased renin-angiotensin-aldosterone secretion, complicated by the liver's inability to inactivate aldosterone; and therefore they require diuretic therapy. Spironolactone (Aldactone) is usually given because this diuretic inhibits aldosterone action and increases reabsorption of potassium,

making it a potassium-sparing diuretic. The dose is usually 100 milligrams per day. Furosemide (Lasix), 40 to 60 milligrams per day, may also be given to augment diuresis (Friedman, 2004). Some patients with massive ascites, who also have respiratory compromise, may be given intravenous albumin to increase their oncotic pressure (pressure generated by plasma proteins to maintain vascular fluid volume), but this treatment is very expensive, and the benefits may be minimal. The Pharmacology Summary feature later in the chapter (p. 1446) outlines the medications used to treat hepatic disorders.

Medical Treatment

Many medical therapies for patients with ascites involve a reduction in dietary sodium, which is usually accomplished by restrictions on the patient's fluid and sodium intake. Initially, the sodium restriction is quite severe, with sodium limits of no more than 400 to 800 milligrams per day. Once diuresis occurs,

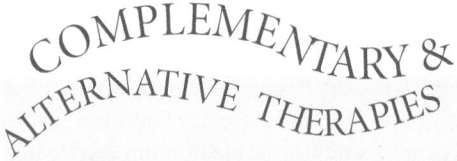

COMPLEMENTARY & ALTERNATIVE THERAPIES   **Spiritual Care**

Description:
Although the concept of "sense of belonging as connectedness" is abstract, there is great potential to positively impact the mental health of many populations when the nurse can gain an understanding of this concept within a cultural worldview. A sense of belonging as connectedness is part of the dynamic nature of human life. Most cultures emphasize the social significance of a sense of belonging to interpersonal relationships and the well-being of individuals, family, and community (Hill, 2006). Some conditions have few allopathic or alternative therapies that are effective. In these cases, the best approach is through spiritual guidance and support, and in some cases, prayer.

Research Support:
An exploratory study identified four nursing competencies for spiritual care: (1) the nurse's role as both a professional and an individual person; (2) delivery of spiritual care using the nursing process; (3) communication with patients, interdisciplinary team members, and clinical/educational organizations; and (4) ensuring ethics in nursing care. Results of this study showed that spiritual care is complex, and requires that nurses be aware of patients' individual uniqueness, including each patient's unique connection between mind, body, and spirit. The study also concluded that nurses must assess each patient's spiritual status during illness and implement holistic care as recommended by the Nursing Code of Ethics (Baldacchino, 2006).

The treatment of Hepatitis C presents many physical and emotional challenges for patients. One study explored patients' experiences during hepatitis C treatment. In order for the nurse to ensure the patient's well-being, it is important for the nurse to understand the patient's experience from a holistic nursing perspective. In this study, patients undergoing treatments for hepatitis C engaged in a dialogue with investigators. The investigators then analyzed the dialogue content, reflection, and pre-understanding. Investigators found that patients' treatment experiences shared four common emotions: sadness, anger, fear, and frustration. This analysis uncovered two themes: (1) "That is not who I am," from patients who rejected the notion of being a "typical" patient, saw treatment as tolerable, felt "different" during treatment, and felt abandoned due to treatment; and (2) "looking beyond the experience" from patients who sought faith and understanding beyond conventional health care (Sheppard & Hubbert, 2006).

The HeartTouch technique is an internal method of changing thoughts and feelings. One study tested the effects of nurses who practice this technique on patients' perceived stress, hardiness, and spiritual well-being. The study used experimental and control groups. The control group participated in an educational session that discussed the effects of thoughts and feelings on stress and health. The experimental group also learned the HeartTouch technique and practiced it for 1 month. Study results showed that nurses who practiced HeartTouch experienced a greater improvement in outcome variables than those who did not practice HeartTouch. Researchers concluded that patients can reduce stress, increase hardiness, and increase spiritual well-being by learning about the power of thoughts and feelings, then using HeartTouch to change them (Walker, 2006).

Eastern spiritual practices emphasize the interconnectedness of body, mind, and spirit. A review paper by Chan and colleagues (2006) proposed that this spirituality does not need to be restricted to any specific religious practice, nor does it need to be pursued in a highly abstract way. Researchers found that nurses can use the body-mind-spirit framework in a flexible way to engage more clients and facilitate the important process of individual exploration and change. Researchers identified key components that include exploring the inner self, utilizing all senses, connecting the body with the mind, and rebalancing one's relationship with the natural and social environment. Researchers concluded that the ultimate goal is to help patients create meaning in their lives and "reach a state of mature spirituality of tranquility and transcendence" (Chan, Ng, Ho, & Chow, 2006).

References
Baldacchino, D. R. (2006). Nursing competencies for spiritual care. *Journal of Clinical Nursing, 15*(7), 885–896.
Chan, C. L., Ng, S. M., Ho, R. T., & Chow, A. Y. (2006). East meets West: Applying Eastern spirituality in clinical practice. *Journal of Clinical Nursing, 15*(7), 822–832.
Hill, D. L. (2006). Sense of belonging as connectedness, American Indian worldview, and mental health. *Archives of Psychiatric Nursing, 20*(5), 210–216.
Sheppard, K., & Hubbert, A. (2006). The patient experience of treatment for hepatitis C. *Gastroenterology Nursing, 29*(4):309–315.
Walker, M. J. (2006). The effects of nurses' practicing of the HeartTouch technique on perceived stress, spiritual well-being, and hardiness. *Journal of Holistic Nursing, 24*(3), 164–175.

sodium intake may be increased slightly. Fluid restrictions are usually set to between 800 and 1,000 milliliters per day.

Some patients with extensive ascites may have difficulty breathing because diuretic therapy was ineffective and the amount of fluid remaining limits movement of the diaphragm. In these patients, a paracentesis may be performed. **Paracentesis** involves removing fluid from the abdominal cavity. After cleansing the lower abdomen, the health care provider will apply local anesthesia and insert a small bore trocar into the peritoneal cavity. Vacuum tubing is connected to the trocar and fluid is drained into a collection bottle. Daily removal of 500 to 1,000 milliliters through paracentesis may be effective without increasing the risk of fluid and electrolyte imbalance. However, large-volume paracentesis, or the removal of 4 to 6 liters of fluid, may be needed and is usually effective in relieving the respiratory symptoms. This can be performed daily as well but increases the risk of fluid and electrolyte imbalance. Intravenous albumin is usually given with a large-volume paracentesis to replace the proteins contained in ascitic fluid. If these are not replaced, a reduction in blood volume because of a shift in oncotic pressure could occur. Chart 46–5 covers nursing care of the patient undergoing paracentesis.

Although it is not a true surgical procedure, a transjugular intrahepatic portosystemic shunt (TIPS) may be used to relieve refractory ascites. This procedure relieves portal hypertension and involves insertion of a catheter into the jugular vein, through which an expandable stent is placed between the hepatic vein and the portal vein. The stent allows blood to flow from the portal vein into the hepatic vein, therefore bypassing the liver and effectively reducing portal pressure. The TIPS procedure has replaced the previous procedure that used peritoneovenous shunts (Friedman, 2004).

Treatment for Hepatic Encephalopathy

Hepatic encephalopathy is a complication of cirrhosis that results from increased levels of ammonia causing a disturbance in mental status. Lactulose, a nonabsorbable synthetic disaccharide that causes the contents of the colon to become more acid, is the most commonly used medication to reduce ammonia levels in the blood. When the colon contents are more acidic, a nonabsorbable form of ammonia (NH_4^+) is created and it is excreted in feces. Lactulose also decreases the presence of those bacteria in the colon that form ammonia when they digest protein in the stool. The standard dose of this medication is 30 milliliters of liquid 3 to 4 times a day. The dose is titrated to a level that results in the patient having two or three loose stools per day. If the patient cannot take oral medication, then 300 milliliters of lactulose is mixed with about 700 milliliters of saline and given as a retention enema, with repetition every 4 to 6 hours (Friedman, 2004). Some patients may also receive neomycin sulfate, which destroys the ammonia-forming bacteria in the intestines, but this practice is used less now than it once was.

Patients with hepatic encephalopathy are often agitated and combative because of the increased level of ammonia and other toxic substances. Oxazepam (Serax), a benzodiazepine that is not metabolized by the liver, is used cautiously to treat marked agitation. The standard dose is usually 10 to 30 milligrams by mouth or through a nasogastric tube. The Pharmacology Summary feature later in the chapter (p. 1446) outlines the medications used to treat hepatic disorders.

Helicobacter pylori generates ammonia in the stomach. There is some evidence that eradicating the *H. pylori* may improve hepatic encephalopathy. The medication regimen for *H. pylori* eradication is discussed in Chapter 45 ⊙.

Patients with hepatic encephalopathy will have dietary protein withheld during acute episodes. Once oral intake is resumed, protein is reintroduced slowly into the diet. Vegetable protein is tolerated better than animal protein. Initially, about 20 grams per day is introduced, increasing the amount 10 grams a day to a maximum of 60 to 80 grams per day (Friedman, 2004).

Treatment for Esophageal Varices

Because many cirrhotic patients with esophageal varices are prone to developing bacterial infections, prophylactic antibiotic medication is often given. Quinolone antibiotics, such as norfloxacin, are preferred. The drug is given orally, via nasogastric tube, or intravenously, twice a day for 7 days.

Medications to reduce portal pressure may be given. The only medication approved in the United States is octreotide, and it is given intravenously as a bolus and then followed by an infusion. It is unclear how the drug works, but it seems to reduce blood flow to the spleen and liver, therefore reducing portal pressure in patients with cirrhosis. Use of this drug in combination with endoscopic therapy has been shown to improve survival (Friedman, 2004).

Vitamin K is often given to patients with cirrhosis and esophageal varices because intrahepatic obstruction to bile flow (from the change in hepatic architecture) causes a vitamin K deficiency (because bile is needed to emulsify fats and vitamin K is fat soluble). Because the healthy liver produces clotting factors, many of which are vitamin K dependent, the person with a cirrhotic liver demonstrates an abnormal prothrombin. The recommended dose of vitamin K is 10 milligrams given subcutaneously. Folic acid and ferrous sulfate are given to treat any underlying anemia.

CHART 46–5   **Nursing Care of the Patient Undergoing Paracentesis**

PREPROCEDURE
- Weigh patient.
- Take vital signs and measure abdominal girth.
- Have the patient empty his bladder.
- Place sitting in an upright position, seated in a chair if possible.
- Assemble needed equipment.

DURING PROCEDURE
- Monitor blood pressure, pulse, and respiratory rate and effort.
- Reassure the patient and family.

POSTPROCEDURE
- Monitor vital signs, especially blood pressure and respiratory effort.
- Monitor for bleeding or excessive drainage from the puncture site.
- Administer albumin if ordered.
- Send specimens to the laboratory for analysis if ordered.
- Change dressing as needed.
- Monitor for infection.

In the case of severe bleeding from esophageal varices, a transfusion of red blood cells, fresh frozen plasma, or platelets may be given. The Pharmacology Summary feature later in the chapter (p. 1446) outlines the medications used to treat hepatic disorders.

The bleeding from esophageal varices must be stopped as quickly as possible. The preferred method is banding. Banding, or variceal ligation, is done during endoscopy and involves the placement of tiny rubber bands on the varices to occlude blood flow. Another treatment done during endoscopy is **sclerotherapy**. This is done by injecting the varices with an agent that causes the vessel to become sclerotic, most commonly ethanolamine or tetradecyl sulfate (Friedman, 2004). Banding has fewer complications than sclerotherapy, but the latter is preferred during active bleeding because of the inability to visualize the varices for banding.

Balloon tamponade of bleeding varices may be used only as a short-term measure in cases in which endoscopy is not immediately available or when bleeding cannot be controlled with pharmacologic or endoscopic techniques. A special three-lumen nasogastric tube (Sengstaken-Blakemore and Minnesota tubes) that has an esophageal balloon, a gastric balloon, and a lumen that opens into the stomach is inserted through the nose. Once in the stomach, the gastric balloon is inflated, applying pressure to the cardiac sphincter at the distal esophagus. Then the esophageal balloon is inflated and tension is applied to the tube. This effectively applies direct pressure to any bleeding vessels. Complications of this treatment, such as aspiration, ulceration and perforation of the esophagus, and airway obstruction, are not uncommon, so this method is rarely used.

Treatment for Hepatorenal Syndrome

Drug therapy for hepatorenal syndrome is generally ineffective. An intravenous infusion of a long-acting vasoconstrictor (ornipressin) and albumin may improve the condition temporarily, but there are numerous ischemic side effects of this therapy. Other combinations of albumin and vasopressors may be used, but they do not improve survival. The Pharmacology Summary feature later in the chapter (p. 1446) outlines the medications used to treat hepatic disorders.

Very few interventions are effective in treating hepatorenal syndrome. A type of modified dialysis, the molecular absorbent recirculating system (MARS), selectively removes substances that are bound to albumin and may prolong survival. Patients with hepatorenal syndrome may also benefit from the TIPS procedure.

Surgical Treatment for End-Stage Liver Disease

Liver transplantation is indicated for patients with end-stage liver disease resulting from cirrhosis; chronic hepatitis B and C; **sclerosing cholangitis**, an inflammatory disorder of the biliary tract that leads to fibrosis and strictures in the biliary system; **primary biliary cirrhosis**, an autoimmune disease where there is inflammation and destruction of the intrahepatic biliary system that results in fibrosis; small hepatocellular carcinoma; and some metabolic diseases where the defect is in the liver. Absolute contraindications for liver transplant include active alcoholism or drug abuse, malignancy, and advanced cardiopulmonary disease. In some cases, transplant is considered for patients over age 70, those with alcohol abstinence of less than 6 months, and patients who are HIV positive. Transplant is not usually considered until the patient demonstrates a deteriorating functional status,

increasing bilirubin, decreasing serum albumin, refractory ascites, recurrent variceal bleeding, or worsening encephalopathy.

Survival rates for liver transplantation have steadily improved in the past 2 decades and currently the 5-year survival is about 80%. The increased survival is due to advances in surgical technique and improved immunosuppression. Immunosuppression is accomplished with a combination of cyclosporine or tacrolimus, prednisone, azathioprine, and mycophenolate mofetil (Friedman, 2004). Side effects of the medications are numerous and include infection, hypertension, hyperlipidemia, neuropsychiatric effects, and weight gain.

◼ Nursing Management

Nursing management of the patient with cirrhosis involves a thorough assessment of risk factors, education regarding lifestyle changes, and developing a plan of care to minimize complications.

Assessment

The focus of the nursing assessment is to evaluate the patient's risk factors and underlying cause of cirrhosis as well as to assess the clinical manifestations of cirrhosis in order to plan care. A thorough health history should consist of an accurate social history (alcohol and substance abuse), sexual history (risk behaviors, lack of libido, impotence), previous exposure to blood products during surgery, and employment history. A review of symptoms by system will help the nurse establish nursing diagnoses. The physical assessment should include vital signs, level of consciousness, skin color and condition, as well as generalized urticaria. The nurse should pay close attention to areas of bruising or **caput medusae**, a term used to describe the engorged, tortuous, and visible blood vessels radiating from the umbilicus in patients with severe liver disorders, which indicate severe liver disease. A methodical abdominal assessment will include general appearance, shape, contour, and girth as well as percussion for the liver margins, noting the size of the liver and palpating for tenderness and a fluid wave.

Interventions

Nursing interventions for the patient with cirrhosis may be directed at many body systems because most body systems are affected when liver function is compromised. The Nursing Process: Patient Care Plan feature (p. 1442) applies the nursing process to a patient with cirrhosis. The Discharge Priorities box (p. 1444) describes the discharge priorities for patients with cirrhosis.

Health Promotion

Because most cases of cirrhosis are preventable, educating the patient and community, especially children and young adults, about high-risk behaviors is essential. The most common cause of cirrhosis in the United States is alcohol abuse, so limiting alcohol intake, especially for women, is the number-one topic for health education. Hepatitis B and especially hepatitis C are risk factors for the development of cirrhosis. Prevention of blood-borne hepatitis is accomplished by sexual abstinence or safe sex practices, and avoidance of injection drug use, as well as unnecessary exposure to blood and bodily fluids.

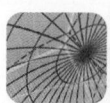

NURSING PROCESS: Patient Care Plan for Cirrhosis

Assessment of Fluid Volume

Subjective Data:

Have you noticed your ankles or feet swelling? For how long?

Have you noticed that your belly has gotten bigger? When did you notice this?

Have you vomited any blood?

Do you have hemorrhoids?

Objective Data:

Vital signs

Abdominal assessment:
- Bowel sounds
- Contour
- Girth
- Liver size
- Tenderness
- Fluid wave

Stool assessment.

Laboratory values:
- Serum albumin
- Serum electrolytes
- Hematocrit
- Creatinine
- BUN

Peripheral edema

Body weight

Jugular venous distention

Intake and output (I&O)

Urine specific gravity

Nursing Assessment and Diagnoses	Outcomes and Evaluation Parameters	Planning and Interventions with *Rationales*
Nursing Diagnosis: *Fluid Volume, Excess* related to portal hypertension and possible hepatorenal syndrome	**Outcome:** Fluid status normal. **Evaluation Parameters:** Decreasing abdominal girth. No peripheral edema. Normal laboratory results. No evidence of active bleeding. No jugular venous distention. Urine specific gravity normal. Urine output at least 30 mL/hr.	**Interventions and *Rationales:*** Weigh daily at the same time of day on the same scale, and monitor I&O. *This gives an accurate assessment of fluid status because a daily change in body weight can be attributed to water retention (or loss).* Measure abdominal girth at the same location on the abdomen at least once a day, but preferably every 8 hours *to monitor progression of ascites.* Restrict dietary sodium to less than 2 grams per day and fluid as ordered. *Sodium promotes water retention, aggravating ascites and portal hypertension.* Monitor lab values and report abnormalities. *Low serum albumin can contribute to ascites and edema. Hyponatremia and hematocrit may indicate hemodilution. Rising BUN and creatinine can indicate impending hepatorenal syndrome.* Examine neck veins for distention and extremities for edema. *Distended jugular veins indicate fluid overload, and edema can result from excess fluid and low serum albumin.* Give prescribed diuretics *to reduce body water.*

Assessment of Nutrition

Subjective Data:

Are you having trouble eating?

Have you lost any weight?

How is your appetite?

Do you drink alcohol? How much?

Objective Data:

Body weight and appearance

Skin and hair condition

Nursing Assessment and Diagnoses	Outcomes and Evaluation Parameters	Planning and Interventions with *Rationales*
Nursing Diagnosis: *Nutrition, Imbalanced: Less than Body Requirements* related to anorexia, impaired protein metabolism, and reduced absorption of fat soluble vitamins because of reduced liver function	**Outcome:** Adequate nutrition. **Evaluation Parameter:** No weight loss.	**Interventions and *Rationales:*** Provide a high-calorie, low-protein, low-sodium diet with 6 small meals per day as ordered. *Protein may be restricted if there is evidence of GI bleeding or encephalopathy in an effort to reduce nitrogenous waste products from protein metabolism.* Weekly weights after discharge. *Short-term fluctuations are usually associated with fluid balance, whereas long-term changes are a better indicator of nutritional status.* Explain the importance of avoiding substances that can be toxic to the liver, such as alcohol and acetaminophen, *in order to prevent further liver damage.* If there is no protein restriction, teach the patient to read food labels and choose foods that are high in protein and have adequate levels of vitamins and minerals, such as Instant Breakfast drink mix, *to improve nutritional status and prevent breakdown of skeletal muscle.*

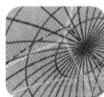

NURSING PROCESS: Patient Care Plan for Cirrhosis—*Continued*

Assessment of Skin

Subjective Data:
Does your skin itch?
Have you been scratching your skin?
Have you noticed a change in the color of your skin?

Objective Data:
Examine skin for:
- Jaundice
- Lesions from scratching
- Dryness
- Bruises
- Petechiae

Nursing Assessment and Diagnoses	Outcomes and Evaluation Parameters	Planning and Interventions with *Rationales*
Nursing Diagnosis: *Skin Integrity, Risk for Impaired* related to jaundice and resultant pruritus	**Outcome:** Skin integrity maintained. **Evaluation Parameters:** Reports diminished itching. No bruising or petechiae. No lesions from scratching.	**Interventions and *Rationales:*** Instruct the patient to use cool, lightweight, nonrestrictive clothing and avoid woolens. *Clothing made from lightweight fabrics causes less itching.* Explain that a cool environmental temperature and cool water for bathing may increase comfort related to pruritus. Hot water causes more pruritus. Instruct the patient to keep his fingernails trimmed and well cared for *to decrease the likelihood of excoriating when scratching.* Instruct the patient to take antihistamine medication as ordered *to reduce pruritus.*

Assessment of Bleeding Potential

Subjective Data:
Have you vomited blood?
Have your stools been dark and tarry looking?
Have you noticed that you bruise easily?

Objective Data:
Vital signs
Test stool for occult blood.
Laboratory values:
- Coagulation studies
- Platelet count
- Hemoglobin and hematocrit

Nursing Assessment and Diagnoses	Outcomes and Evaluation Parameters	Planning and Interventions with *Rationales*
Nursing Diagnosis: Fluid Volume, Deficit: Risk for related to the liver's ability to synthesize clotting factors, portal hypertension with resultant esophageal varices, and hemorrhoids	**Outcome:** No hemorrhage. **Evaluation Parameters:** Stool negative for occult blood. No vomiting blood. Coagulation studies normal. Hemoglobin and hematocrit normal. Vital signs normal.	**Interventions and *Rationales:*** Give vitamin K as ordered. *Vitamin K is synthesized in the liver and may be decreased in cirrhosis.* Teach patient to use a soft toothbrush and avoid using dental floss *because decreased clotting factors make the patient more prone to bleeding.* Monitor for bleeding (stool, skin, urine, and mucous membranes) *because decreased clotting factors make the patient more prone to bleeding.* Instruct patient to refrain from eating rough foods that can cause *trauma to the esophagus and cause varices to bleed.*

Assessment of Mental Status

Subjective Data:
Can you tell me your name, what day it is, and where you are?

Objective Data:
Assess cognitive function
Reflexes

Nursing Assessment and Diagnoses	Outcomes and Evaluation Parameters	Planning and Interventions with *Rationales*
Nursing Diagnosis: Confusion: Risk for related to hepatic encephalopathy	**Outcome:** No disruption in mental status. **Evaluation Parameters:** Alert and oriented to person, place, and time. Able to perform simple computations. Behavior appropriate. Normal reflexes. MMSE score of 25 or better.	**Interventions and *Rationales:*** Administer Mini-Mental Status Exam (MMSE). *Hepatic encephalopathy can cause changes in mentation even in the prodromal phase.* Provide a low-protein diet as ordered *to reduce the nitrogen metabolites of protein digestion.* Administer medications to reduce ammonia level as ordered. *Lactulose, oral or enema, promotes diarrhea and the elimination of ammonia in the feces.* Monitor deep tendon reflexes. *As hepatic encephalopathy progresses, reflexes become exaggerated.*

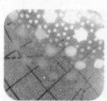

PATIENT TEACHING & DISCHARGE PRIORITIES for Cirrhosis of the Liver

Need	Teaching
Knowledge of disease process and prognosis	Home care needs include verbal and written instructions for: The treatment plan Follow-up care Nutritional and fluid needs.
Diet therapy	Many patients with cirrhosis have special dietary needs and restrictions, particularly related to protein, sodium, and fluid intake. Teaching should focus on each patient's specific dietary plan developed by the health care provider or dietician (Lutz & Przytulski, 2006). Frequently, these patients develop abdominal ascites and fluid retention; the nurse should reinforce the importance of adhering to a sodium-restricted diet (Afdhal, 2007). For the most part, patients with chronic liver disease are protein depleted, which tends to worsen as the disease progresses. The nurse should reinforce the importance of consuming small, frequent meals that are well balanced in order for the body to have sufficient kilocalories and nutrients to prevent catabolism of tissue protein for energy (Afdhal, 2007).
Drug therapy	The nurse should recognize that drug therapy is focused on the alleviation of symptoms and the prevention of complications, but it cannot reverse cirrhosis (Chisholm-Burns et al., 2008). Current drug therapy is available to treat the complications of ascites, varices, spontaneous bacterial peritonitis, hepatic encephalopathy, and coagulation abnormalities (Chisholm-Burns et al., 2008). Patients with liver disease may have several types of medications prescribed; however, commonly prescribed medications include beta-blockers, diuretics and lactulose syrup. It is important for the nurse to provide teaching related to expected effects, prescribed dosage, as well as any side effects in order to improve compliance and promote optimal patient outcomes. Emphasis should be placed on the importance of reporting side effects to the health care provider immediately for further evaluation.
Alcohol abstinence	Abstinence from alcohol is critical and should be reinforced during discharge teaching. The nurse should provide information regarding local support groups and counseling services to facilitate adherence to this critical component of the treatment plan.

Sources: Afdhal, N. H. (2007). *Epidemiology of and risk factors for gallstones.* Retrieved April 24, 2008, from http://www.uptodate.com/patients/content/topic.do?topicKey=~5rphinkcGz/zys; Chisholm-Burns, M. A., Wells, B. G., Schwinghammer, T. L., Malone, P. M., Kolesar, J. M., Rotschafer, J. C., et al. (2008). *Pharmacotherapy principles & practice.* New York: McGraw-Hill; and Lutz, C., & Przytulski, K. (2006). *Nutrition and diet therapy: Evidence-based applications.* Philadelphia: F. A. Davis.

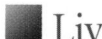 ## Liver Cancer

Cancer of the liver accounts for less than 2% of all deaths from cancer in the United States. Primary liver cancer is rare in the United States but is common in densely populated areas in southern Africa, Asia, and Greece (Huether, 2006). However, the liver is a common site of metastatic spread from cancer in other parts of the body. People with chronic hepatitis B or C are at a high risk for developing primary liver cancer.

Pathophysiology

Cancer of the liver develops from the liver's parenchymal cells (hepatocellular carcinoma) or from the cells in the bile ducts (**cholangiocarcinoma**). Up to 90% of all primary liver tumors are hepatocellular carcinoma. This type of cancer can be nodular, massive, or diffuse, and is most closely related to cirrhosis or hepatitis B and C. Hepatocellular carcinoma metastasizes to the heart, lungs, brain, kidneys, and spleen. Cholangiocarcinoma is more common in southeast China, where liver fluke infestation is common, and has a similar metastatic profile to hepatocellular carcinoma.

Primary liver cancer arises when there is damage to the hepatocellular DNA. Both hepatitis B and C viruses can act as carcinogens especially in the presence of cirrhosis. Exposure to mycotoxins, such as those produced by *Aspergillus flavus* (mold on corn, peanuts, and grain), causes the mutation of the p53 suppressor gene (Huether, 2006). Other risk factors for the development of liver cancer include heavy smoking and drinking, prolonged use of anabolic steroids, and arsenic-contaminated water.

Clinical Manifestations

The clinical manifestations of liver cancer are often general and nonspecific. Symptoms may include weakness, anorexia with weight loss, fatigue, and malaise. These usually occur early, but as the tumor enlarges or more of the liver becomes involved, manifestations include abdominal pain, ascites, jaundice, and a palpable mass in the right upper quadrant. There may also be signs of liver failure such as portal hypertension.

Laboratory and Diagnostic Procedures

There are no specific tests for liver cancer, although most tumors can be identified by magnetic resonance imaging (MRI) and computed tomography (CT) scans. Once a suspicious area is found, a liver biopsy is done to determine the tumor type. Liver enzymes, AST and ALT, are measured and are usually elevated in people with liver cancer. Patients with advanced hepatocellular cancer will have an elevated alpha-fetoprotein (AFP). An elevated AFP is strongly correlated with chronic hepatitis B infection, rapid tumor growth, and poorly differentiated tumors (Huether, 2006).

Medical Management

Surgical resection of the liver is possible only if the tumor is localized and in a lobe of the liver that can be removed. For example, if the tumor is in the posterior section of the right lobe, it

Medications Used in Palliative Care

Clinical Problem

When a patient develops acute or chronic liver failure, the metabolism of medications commonly used for palliation becomes abnormal, requiring a careful and frequently changing dosing regimen. Decreased hepatic blood flow and the shunting of blood cause the medications to be metabolized more slowly and to have an increased bioavailability. For instance, benzodiazepines such as midazolam that are used for sedation may have an increased effect due to the presence of unmetabolized toxins, increased sensitivity to the drug, stimulation of the gamma-aminobutyric acid (GABA) receptors, and reduced cerebral blood flow (Rhee & Broadbent, 2007).

Research Findings

To facilitate care of the patient with liver failure, Rhee and Broadbent (2007) conducted an extensive literature search, as well as a review of major textbooks in pharmacology, palliative care, hepatology, and gastroenterology. From these data they developed a table of functional groups of medications commonly used in palliative care: the pharmacologic half-life with normal liver function and with cirrhosis. When data were available, the medications affected by cirrhosis were further broken down following the Child-Pugh criteria of liver disease. This information may assist in the decision-making process of which medications to use, reduce potential complications, and improve palliation of symptoms for patients with liver failure. As an example, here are the findings for opioid analgesics and nonopioid analgesics. Within the article, the complete table includes comments and

recommendations for changes in dose and frequency with the references used for each drug.

Implications for Nursing Practice

It is important for the nurse to understand the degree of decreased function of the liver and to understand the affect on the metabolism of medications. Patients with end-stage liver disease require palliation. Knowing the expected increase in the half-life of analgesics will allow the nurse to administer medications safely.

Critical Thinking Questions

1. Discuss the effect of liver failure on the metabolism of palliative medication.

2. The health care team prescribes morphine IV for a patient with acute liver failure. Before initiating the prescription, what is most important for the nurse to do?

Answers to Critical Thinking Questions appear in Appendix D.

Reference

Rhee, C., & Broadbent, A. M. (2007). Palliation and liver failure: Palliative medications dosages guidelines. *Journal of Palliative Medicine, 10*(3), 677–687.

Source: Adapted from Rhee, C. & Broadbent, A. M. (2007). Palliation and liver failure: Palliative medications dosages guidelines. *Journal of Palliative Medicine, 10(3),* 677–687.

Medication	Half-Life Normal Liver	Half-Life Cirrhosis	Half-Life Child-Pugh A	Half-Life Child-Pugh B	Half-Life Child-Pugh C
Opioid Analgesics					
Fentanyl	4.4 minutes	5.1 minutes			
Hydromorphone	2.5 hours	No data			
Methadone	18.8 hours	No data	11.3 hours	13 hours	35.5 hours
Morphine (IV)	1.7 hours	4.2 hours	3.4 hours	4.35 hours	4.47 hours
Morphine (oral)	3.3 hours	5.5 hours	6.4 hours	6.85 hours	4.4 hours
Morphine (SR)	4.01 hours	No data	7.36 hours		
Oxycodone	3.4 hours	13.9 hours			
Nonopioid Analgesics					
Aspirin	7.9 hours	7.3 hours			
Ibuprofen	2.2 hours	No data	1.9 hours		2.6 hours
Naproxen	14.14 hours	20.36 hours			

cannot be removed because the right hepatic vein is located in this area. Chemotherapy agents may be given directly into the liver or systemically. Liver transplant is an option for small tumors without evidence of spread. Overall, the survival prospects for patients with liver cancer are less than 6 months.

■ Nursing Management

A goal of nursing care for patients with liver cancer is prevention whenever possible. Nurses can encourage alcohol abstinence

and prevention of HBV and HCV. In those patients who have a risk factor for liver cancer, such as chronic infection with HBV or HCV, the risk for developing liver cancer can be reduced if they abstain from alcohol. Most of the nursing interventions for a patient with liver cancer are similar to those for patients with cirrhosis and liver failure. Nursing care includes helping patients with liver cancer prepare for death, supporting the family, and providing comfort. Refer to Chapter 17 🖙 for nursing management at end of life. See Evidence-Based Practice box for specific medications for palliative care.

PHARMACOLOGY Summary of Medications Used to Treat Hepatic Disorders

Medication Category	Action	Application/Indication	Nursing Responsibility
Antiviral Agents			
Interferons: Peginterferon alfa-2b (PEG-Intron) Interferon alpha-2a (Pegasys)	Inhibits viral replication in infected cells, activates cellular immunity.	Management of chronic hepatitis C.	Monitor for adverse effects: fatigue, muscle aches, headache, fever, and chills. Monitor complete blood count (CBC) with differential, platelets, and renal function. Monitor for severe reactions: depression, psychoses, suicidal ideation, and pancreatitis. Be aware theophylline level may increase. Monitor drug level.
Noninterferons: Adefovir (Hespera)	Exerts antiviral effects by interfering with viral DNA.	Treatment of chronic hepatitis B.	Monitor for adverse effects: muscle weakness, abdominal pain, diarrhea, dyspepsia, nausea, hematuria, headache, and rash. Monitor electrolytes, renal and hepatic function, especially in presence of liver or kidney dysfunction.
Lamivudine (Epivir)	Exerts antiviral effects by interfering with viral DNA replication.	Treatment of chronic hepatitis B.	Monitor for adverse effects: neuropathy, insomnia, dizziness, fever, nausea, and diarrhea. Monitor liver and renal function, CBC with differential. Observe for lactic acidosis.
Oral ribavirin (Rebetol)	Antiviral effect thought to be due to interference with viral RNA synthesis.	Management of hepatitis C in combination with interferon alpha-2b.	Monitor for adverse effects: fatigue, myalgia, nausea, insomnia, headache, irritability, and depression. Monitor hemoglobin, neutrophil count. Observe for development or worsening of cardiac or pulmonary dysfunction.
Diuretics			
Potassium sparing: Spironolactone (Aldactone)	Promotes diuresis through sodium and chloride excretion in distal tubule without loss of potassium.	Hepatic cirrhosis, ascites.	Monitor for adverse effects: hyperkalemia, menstrual irregularities, gynecomastia, and impotence. Monitor electrolytes and I&O. Be aware of multiple drug interactions (digoxin, ACE inhibitors, corticosteroids, NSAIDs, and others). Monitor for altered drug efficacy or toxicity. Monitor digoxin level if given concurrently.
Loop diuretic: Furosemide (Lasix)	Diuretic effect due to reduced reabsorption of sodium and chloride in loop of Henle, proximal tube, and distal tubule.	Edema associated with hepatic cirrhosis.	Monitor for adverse effects: hypotension, hypokalemia, hyponatremia, hypochloremia, hypocalcemia, and metabolic alkalosis. Be aware of multiple drug interactions (digoxin, insulin, NSAIDs, and others). Monitor for altered drug efficacy or toxicity. Be aware of ototoxicity potential with patients on aminoglycoside or if rapid IV administration, especially in presence of decreased renal function or high drug dose. Monitor electrolytes and I&O. Be aware of multiple drug incompatibilities when given IV.
Hyperosmotic Laxative Lactulose	Increases ammonia excretion by acidifying colon contents, reducing diffusion of ammonia from colon to blood.	Prevention and treatment of hepatic encephalopathy.	Monitor for adverse effects: nausea, vomiting, and hypernatremia. Monitor electrolytes. Monitor fluid status.
Aminoglycoside Antibiotic Neomycin sulfate	Reduces blood ammonia by destroying ammonia-forming bacteria.	Cirrhosis, hepatic coma.	Monitor for adverse effects: diarrhea, nausea, and vomiting. Observe for severe adverse reactions: respiratory paralysis, ototoxicity, and nephrotoxicity. Monitor renal function and serum drug levels.

PHARMACOLOGY Summary of Medications Used to Treat Hepatic Disorders—*Continued*

Medication Category	Action	Application/Indication	Nursing Responsibility
Synthetic Hormone			
Octreotide (Sandostatin)	Reduces portal blood flow by inhibiting release of vasodilatory hormone.	Variceal bleeding.	Monitor for adverse effects: nausea and diarrhea. Monitor electrolytes, blood glucose.
Sedative-Hypnotic			
Oxazepam (Serax)	Causes sedative effect by potentiating inhibitory neurotransmitter GABA.	Anxiety, acute withdrawal symptoms in chronic alcoholism, agitation.	Monitor for adverse effects: drowsiness, ataxia, paradoxical stimulant response, and sleep disturbances, especially in elderly. Monitor for drug interactions (other CNS depressants, cimetidine, phenytoin, smoking, and others). Monitor for altered drug efficacy or toxicity. Be aware prolonged use requires slow withdrawal of medication. Caution patient sedative effect is increased with alcohol.
Immunosuppressants			
Cyclosporine[a] (Sandimmune, Neoral) Tacrolimus[a] (Prograf, Protopic) Mycophenolate[a] (CellCept) Azathioprine (Azasan, Imuran)	Suppresses immune response by inhibiting lymphocyte replication or disrupting helper T cells or inhibiting antibody formation.	Adjunct therapy with corticosteroids for transplant rejection, oral form—biliary cirrhosis, Crohn's disease, ulcerative colitis.	Monitor for adverse effects: hypertension, nausea, vomiting, and infection. Observe for signs of toxicity: tremors, seizures, altered mental status, visual disturbances, nephrotoxicity, and neurotoxicity. Monitor CBC, liver, and renal function tests, electrolytes, and blood sugar. Be aware of multiple drug specific interactions (digoxin, NSAIDs, erythromycin, verapamil, cimetidine, allopurinal, ACE inhibitors, warfarin, and others). Monitor for altered drug levels, nephrotoxicity, or leukopenia.

[a]*Monitor blood sugar.*

DISORDERS OF THE GALLBLADDER

The gallbladder is a saclike structure that concentrates and stores bile. Bile is produced by the liver and is necessary for the absorption of dietary fat and fat soluble vitamins. Most gallbladder disorders result in obstructed bile flow from the liver to the gallbladder or from the gallbladder to the duodenum. The most common cause of obstructed flow is gallstones, or **cholelithiasis**. When a gallstone either forms in or migrates to the common bile duct, the resultant condition is called **choledocholithiasis**. Cirrhosis can obstruct the flow of bile from the liver to the gallbladder (Figure 46–3 ■, p. 1448). Other causes of obstructed flow include tumors (rare) and abscesses.

■ Cholelithiasis

Gallstones may form from a combination of factors. If the stone is large, it may obstruct flow from the gallbladder to the duodenum, causing pain.

Etiology and Epidemiology

Gallstones result from a combination of factors including biliary stasis, inflammation of the gallbladder, and abnormal bile composition and reabsorption. There are two types of gallstones: those predominantly composed of cholesterol and those composed of calcium bilirubinate. Cholesterol gallstones are the more commonly occurring, with 80% of gallstones in the United States and Europe being this type. In Japan, however, 30% to 40% of gallstones are the calcium bilirubinate type (Friedman, 2004).

Cholelithiasis is more common in women, but the incidence in both men and women increases as people age. In fact, 20% of women and 10% of men have gallstones by the age of 65. Certain ethnic groups are at a higher risk for gallstones. For example, 75% of Native American Indian women over the age of 25 have gallstones (Chart 46–6, p. 1448). Other risk factors for the development of cholelithiasis are obesity, especially in women; high estrogen states; diabetes; hyperlipidemia; cirrhosis; and Crohn's disease. Rapid weight loss is also associated with gallstone formation, and there is an increased incidence after bariatric surgery. Many drugs can increase the risk for gallstone formation, such as clofibrate, ceftriaxone, oral contraceptives, and hormone replacement therapy.

Pathophysiology

Cholesterol is a normal component of bile, but when the bile is supersaturated with cholesterol, the chances increase for cholesterol crystal formation. The cholesterol crystals aggregate to

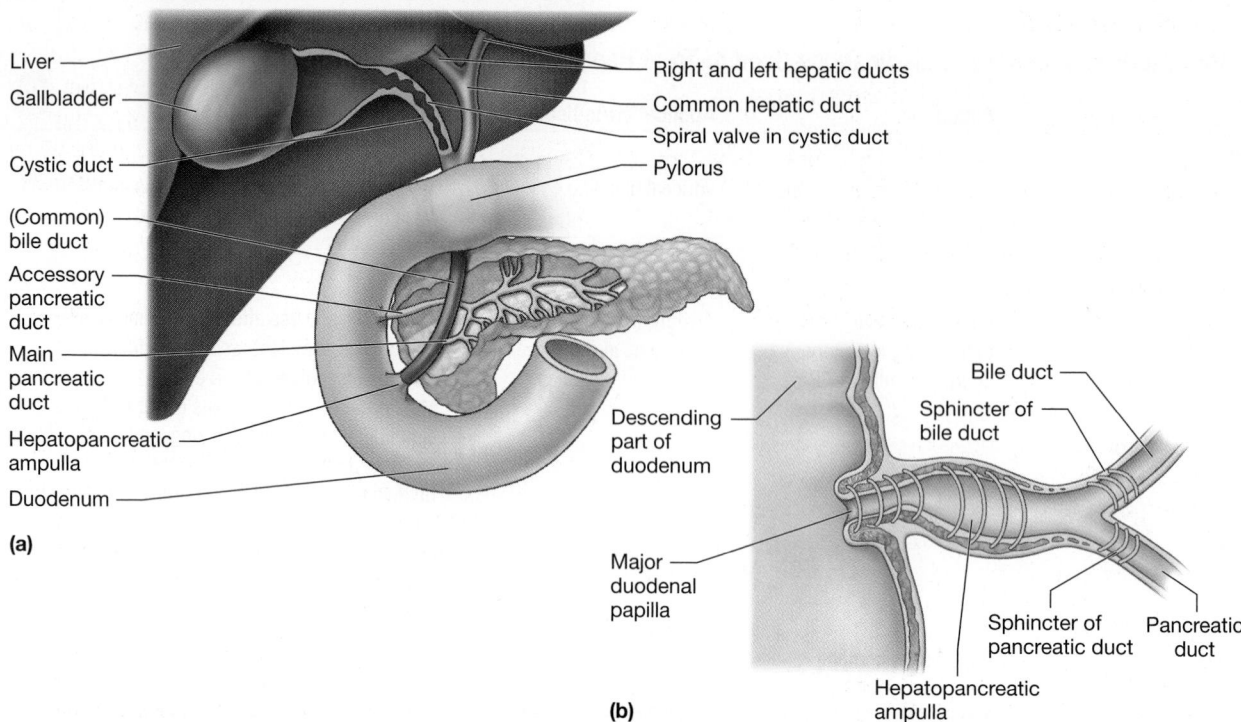

FIGURE 46–3 ■ (A) Extrahepatic bile passages, gallbladder, and pancreatic ducts. (B) Entry of the pancreatic and bile ducts into the hepatopancreatic ampula, then into the duodenum.

CHART 46–6 | **Ethnic/Gender Considerations in Patients with Cholelithiasis**

Many factors influence the prevalence of cholelithiasis, including comorbidities, ethnicity, genetics, and gender. In general, there appear to be higher rates of cholelithiasis in Western Caucasian, Hispanic, and Native American populations and lower rates in eastern European, African American, and Japanese populations (Afdhal, 2007).

Prevalence for the formation of gallstones is also reported to be higher among women. For example, in non-Hispanic white women the prevalence was reported to be 16.6%, compared to 8.6% in non-Hispanic white men. Among Mexican American populations, the disparity is even greater, with 26.7% of Mexican American women developing symptomatic cholelithiasis, whereas only 8.9% of Mexican American men develop gallstones (Afdhal, 2007). This disparity is attributed to the fact that estrogens cause increased cholesterol secretion, and progesterone promotes biliary stasis.

form larger stones. When these "macrostones" obstruct the cystic or common bile duct, the gallbladder becomes inflamed and **cholecystitis** results. It is unclear why the hepatocytes form bile with a high concentration of cholesterol, but it is most likely a combination of factors, including the presence of a defective enzyme that influences the liver cells' synthesis of cholesterol, a decreased secretion of bile acids, and a decreased reabsorption of bile salts from the ileum.

Clinical Manifestations

The most common manifestation of cholelithiasis is epigastric and/or right upper quadrant pain. Most patients also complain of intolerance to fatty foods and nausea. Other symptoms include flatulence, bloating, abdominal distention, diarrhea, and chest pain. Often the pain associated with gallstones is steady and severe with radiation to the mid-upper back, right scapula, and shoulder. Pain usually occurs within 1 hour after eating, may be accompanied by nausea and vomiting, and may last for 4 to 5 hours. If a stone becomes lodged in the common bile duct, the patient may also develop jaundice as a result of hepatocyte damage from bile refluxing into the liver.

■ Cholecystitis

Cholecystitis is simply inflammation of the gallbladder and can be an acute or chronic problem. The most common cause of both acute and chronic cholecystitis is a gallstone lodged in the cystic duct. When the flow of bile out of the gallbladder is obstructed, the gallbladder becomes distended and an inflammatory response is initiated.

Pathophysiology

In at least 90% of the patients with cholecystitis, cholelithiasis is the cause. If the gallstones are in the cystic duct, pressure in the gallbladder increases, causing ischemia of the mucosal wall and inflammation. Prolonged ischemia leads to necrosis and in severe cases gangrene can result. In a severely inflamed gallbladder, or in the case of gangrene, perforation with resultant peritonitis is possible. In patients who are immunosuppressed, infectious organisms such as cytomegalovirus and cryptosporidiosis can cause acute cholecystitis. Chronic cholecystitis can result from persistent irritation of the gallbladder by either repeated bouts of acute cholecystitis or constant presence of many small gallstones in the gallbladder.

Clinical Manifestations

The clinical manifestations of cholecystitis are similar to those of cholelithiasis. Pain is the predominant symptom and is usually severe and steady, lasting up to 12 to 18 hours. As with gallstones, the pain is usually in the right upper quadrant and may radiate to the mid-upper back, right scapula, and shoulder. Unlike cholelithiasis, the patient with cholecystitis can have a fever and chills. The gallbladder may be palpable on abdominal exam if it is extremely inflamed, and there may be tenderness with possible guarding on palpation of the RUQ. Jaundice may be present as well.

◼ Biliary Dyskinesia

Biliary dyskinesia is a term applied to motility disorders of the gallbladder. Although they are uncommon disorders, the clinical manifestations are almost indistinguishable from other problems of the gallbladder. The most common clinical manifestation is episodic abdominal pain. The pain is usually epigastric or in the right upper quadrant and may radiate to the back and right scapula. As with the pain in cholelithiasis, the pain from biliary dyskinesia occurs following a fatty meal and may be accompanied by nausea and vomiting.

Laboratory and Diagnostic Procedures

The diagnostic test of choice for cholelithiasis is an *ultrasound of the gallbladder*. This test is noninvasive and can detect gallstones, dilated ducts, wall inflammation, and abnormal fluid presence. It can also be used to assess the emptying of the gallbladder for patients that may have biliary dyskinesia. Other tests may be performed to identify possible complications or to rule out other possible causes of the symptoms.

- *Serum bilirubin,* both direct (conjugated) and indirect (unconjugated), is measured. If the direct bilirubin is elevated (normal = 0.3 to 1.2 mg/dL), this is most indicative of an obstructive process within the liver or biliary system. Gallstones, cirrhosis, or hepatitis can cause this type of obstruction. On the other hand, indirect bilirubin is elevated when there is RBC hemolysis or when the hepatocytes are unable to conjugate bilirubin, usually due to cellular damage.
- *Serum amylase and lipase* are measured to determine whether the pancreas is involved, possibly due to common bile duct obstruction, or whether pancreatitis is present.
- *AST and ALT* will usually be measured to determine whether any liver injury has occurred as a result of a stone in the common bile duct.
- A *CBC* may indicate an infectious process in the gallbladder if the WBC count is elevated.
- An oral cholecystogram is rarely done any longer. For this test, the patient is given an oral dye that concentrates in the gallbladder, making any stones visible.

Medical Management

Patients with asymptomatic cholelithiasis are usually treated conservatively with dietary modifications and lifestyle changes. However, if the patient has frequent symptoms, very severe symptoms, or cholecystitis, surgery to remove the gallstone and the gallbladder is indicated.

Dietary and Lifestyle Management

For mild cases of cholelithiasis, diet (low fat) and lifestyle changes may be effective in managing the condition. For more severe cases, diet and lifestyle changes are only a part of treatment that will include surgery. For either case, dietary fat intake is limited. Chart 46–7 lists foods with a high fat content. Patients with obstructed bile flow may require supplementation with the fat soluble vitamins A, D, E, and K. For patients who are obese, a weight loss program that includes exercise is recommended. Other contributing factors such as hyperlipidemia and diabetes are treated to minimize recurrence of gallstones.

Surgery

Surgery is the treatment of choice for most patients with cholelithiasis, cholecystitis, and biliary dyskinesia. Removal of the gallbladder, or **cholecystectomy**, is done most often using the laparoscopic surgical method, which is minimally invasive, has fewer complications, and requires a much shorter length of hospital stay than the traditional open cholecystectomy. Patients with a very large or infected gallbladder may not be candidates for laparoscopic cholecystectomy and may require an open cholecystectomy. During the laparoscopic procedure, the surgeon may find it necessary to convert the procedure to an open cholecystectomy. If stones are located in the common bile duct, an exploration of this duct is done, and a T-tube is placed in the common bile duct to maintain patency, allowing bile to pass from the liver into the duodenum until the edema from surgery diminishes. Chart 46–8 (p. 1450) outlines the nursing care of a patient with a T-tube.

Medications

Some patients may not be good surgical candidates or they may refuse surgery. Drugs are available to dissolve the gallstones by reducing the cholesterol content of the stone. Ursodiol (Actigall) or chenodiol (Chenix) may be used but are effective only if the gallstones contain a high concentration of cholesterol and are less than 1.5 to 2 centimeters in diameter. Treatment with these agents is expensive and usually lasts for 1 to 3 years, with recurrent stone formation occurring in 50% of patients after

---

CHART 46–7   Foods High in Fat Content

Full fat dairy products:
- Whole milk
- Cheese
- Cream
- Ice cream
- Cottage cheese
- Sour cream

Cooking and salad oil:
- Olive oil
- Canola oil
- Corn oil
- Sunflower oil

Salad dressing (regular, not lite)

Snack foods:
- Potato chips
- Corn chips
- Pork rinds

Fried food:
- Doughnuts
- French fries
- Hamburgers
- Bacon
- Fried fish, chicken

Nuts

Peanut butter

Chocolate

Gravy

Some cuts of meat:
- Ham
- Pork shoulder
- Lunch meat
- Ground meat

CHART 46–8 Care of the Patient with a T-Tube

- Attach tube to sterile gravity drainage.
  - Place patient in Fowler's position to maximize gravity drainage.
- Monitor drainage and record the amount every 8 hours.
  - The amount may be between 500 and 1,000 milliliters on the first day, decreasing to about 200 milliliters by the 3rd day.
  - Drainage may be blood tinged at first but becomes green-brown.
  - Drainage in excess of 500 milliliters by the 3rd day is excessive, and the surgeon must be notified.
- Monitor color of the stools.
  - Pale stools indicate obstruction of flow of bile to duodenum.
- Clamp the T-tube as ordered, and monitor the patient's response to clamping.
- Keep skin clean and free from bile drainage.
  - Bile is irritating to the skin. Skin can be protected with zinc oxide, karaya, or other barrier.
- Teach the patient how to care for the tube during activities of daily living.
  - The patient may be discharged with the tube in place and should be informed of the signs of infection, such as fever, redness, swelling, or drainage from the site, as well as care for the tube, avoiding any direct pulling or traction on the tube.
  - A daily shower is usually permitted, but a tub bath is not.

treatment is stopped. The Pharmacology Summary feature later in the chapter (p. 1457) outlines medications used to treat biliary disorders.

Other drug treatment for cholelithiasis and cholecystitis includes antibiotics if an infection is suspected. Bile salts accumulate on the skin when the patient is jaundiced and this causes pruritus. Cholestyramine (Questran) binds these bile salts, which are then excreted in the stool. For acute cholecystitis a narcotic analgesic may be needed to relieve the pain.

Ultrasound Therapy
Extracorporeal shock wave lithotripsy (ESWL) is a method to break up large gallstones by using ultrasound waves. After the procedure, the patient may have biliary colic pain when the gallbladder attempts to expel the stone fragments. Patients undergoing ESWL also require oral dissolution therapy to help dissolve the stone fragments. This method of treating cholelithiasis is more than 5 times more expensive than surgery.

Complementary Therapy
The use of the herb goldenseal to treat cholecystitis has had limited research. The active ingredient berberine has been shown to decrease the symptoms of cholecystitis. It appears to stimulate the secretion of bile. Use in pregnancy is contraindicated because of the stimulatory effects on the uterus and should not be used during breast-feeding.

Nursing Management
Nursing care for patients with cholelithiasis or cholecystitis includes assessment, assuring pain relief, preparing the patient for possible surgery, preventing infection, and education regarding future prevention, postoperative care, and dietary modifications.

Assessment
Nursing assessment includes a complete history and physical examination. The history should focus on risk factors for cholelithiasis and cholecystitis; previous history of symptoms; character, duration, and relationship of pain with meals; presence of associated symptoms such as nausea and vomiting; and current medications, activity, and diet. If the patient reports dark-colored urine and light-colored stools, there is a strong suspicion of a gallstone obstructing the common bile duct, the cystic duct, or the hepatic duct.

The physical exam should include a head-to-toe assessment, including body weight and BMI (body mass index). Scleral color, skin color and condition, abdominal palpation for tenderness or guarding, and a visual examination of stool and urine should also be included. The physical exam should include a thorough heart and lung assessment as well, because the patient will most likely be scheduled for surgery.

Interventions
Most patients who have acute cholelithiasis will eventually require surgery, either laparoscopic cholecystectomy or open cholecystectomy. Nursing care centers on comfort measures and preventing complications such as pneumonia, infection, and nausea. The Nursing Process: Patient Care Plan feature presents the complete care for the patient with cholelithiasis and surgery.

Health Promotion
Several risk factors for cholelithiasis can be controlled, such as obesity, hyperlipidemia, and diabetes. Increasing exercise and maintaining a well-balanced low-fat, low-calorie diet can modify obesity. However, rapid weight loss should be discouraged because it could contribute to gallstone formation. Hyperlipidemia can be controlled through medication, by a low-fat, low-cholesterol diet, and with at least 30 minutes per day of regular exercise. Good control of blood sugar in patients with diabetes may also decrease the recurrence of gallstones.

DISORDERS OF THE EXOCRINE PANCREAS
Disorders of the pancreas that will be discussed are pancreatitis, acute and chronic, and cancer of the pancreas.

Pancreatitis
Pancreatitis, or inflammation of the pancreas, can be acute or chronic and is a potentially serious disease. Most cases of pancreatitis occur between age 50 and 60 with incidence the same for men and women. Risk factors for the development of pancreatitis include alcoholism, biliary obstruction, peptic ulcers, trauma, extreme hyperlipidemia, hypertriglyceridemia, and the use of some medications (Huether, 2006). Mortality is high if the patient develops cardiac, pulmonary, or renal complications.

Acute Pancreatitis
Many cases of acute pancreatitis are mild, are self-limiting, and do not require hospitalization. However, about 20% of patients

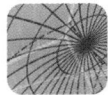

NURSING PROCESS: Patient Care Plan for Cholelithiasis and Surgery

Assessment of Pain:
Acute Cholelithiasis/Cholecystitis; Preoperatively

Subjective Data:
What is your level of pain on a scale of 0–10, with 10 being the worst pain?
Are you allergic to anything?
Do you have any special cultural or religious practices for dealing with pain?
Do you have pain when you eat certain foods, particularly high-fat foods?
Have you ever had this type of pain before? If yes, how long did it last? What relieved the pain in the past?
Do you take oral contraceptives? Or hormone replacement therapy?
Could you possibly be pregnant?

Objective Data:
Vital signs q4h:
- Temperature
- BP
- Pulse
- Respirations

Abdominal examination:
- Bowel sounds
- Tenderness
- Guarding
Restlessness
Grimacing
Moaning or groaning
Shallow respirations

Nursing Assessment and Diagnoses	Outcomes and Evaluation Parameters	Planning and Interventions with *Rationales*
Nursing Diagnosis: *Pain, Acute* related to cholelithiasis/cholecystitis	**Outcome:** Comfort level maintained. *Evaluation Parameters:* Able to communicate level of pain and relief from medications. Able to take deep breaths without pain. Appears restful without restlessness or moaning.	**Interventions and *Rationales:*** Assess pain using pain scale (0–10) to quantify pain level. *To increase consistency in monitoring pain.* Administer pain medication, usually meperidine or morphine (research indicates that morphine does not cause sphincter of Oddi spasms), and assess level of pain 30 minutes and 1 hour after giving medication. *To assess effectiveness of medications.* Explore cultural and religious practices and beliefs about pain and illness. *Different religions have varying beliefs about pain, suffering, and disease.* Teach nonpharmacologic methods of pain control, such as guided imagery, meditation, and breathing exercises. *This may augment pain relief.* Discuss foods that are high in fat and may cause nausea and GI distress even after surgery. *Foods high in fat stimulate contractions of the gallbladder and may cause pain if stones are present.* (See Chart 46–7 (p. 1449) for a list of high-fat foods.)

Assessment of Nutrition

Subjective Data:
How is your appetite?
Are you nauseated?
Are there any foods that make you nauseated?
Have you lost a lot of weight lately?

Objective Data:
Height and weight measurements
BMI

Laboratory results:
- Bilirubin
- Serum albumin
- Glucose
- Cholesterol
- Urinalysis

Nursing Assessment and Diagnoses	Outcomes and Evaluation Parameters	Planning and Interventions with *Rationales*
Nursing Diagnosis: *Nutrition: Readiness for Enhanced* related to anorexia, pain, and nausea from impaired bile flow	**Outcome:** Adequate nutrition. *Evaluation Parameters:* No weight loss. Serum albumin normal. Fasting glucose normal. No reported nausea. No evidence of bleeding.	**Interventions and *Rationales:*** Obtain diet history, history of large rapid weight loss, and height and weight measurements *to help establish current status and possible imbalanced diet with fat soluble vitamin deficiency.* Assess laboratory results and report any abnormal values to the patient's health care provider. *Bilirubin in the urine indicates an obstruction to bile flow and will be reflected in an elevated serum bilirubin. Patients with diabetes mellitus and high serum cholesterol are at risk for gallstones. Protein malnutrition is reflected in a low serum albumin.* Give supplemental vitamins as ordered. *Bile is necessary for the absorption of fat soluble vitamins, so supplements may be necessary.* Educate the patient about avoiding foods that contain a large amount of fat. *Even after removal of the gallbladder, high-fat foods may cause nausea.* Refer to a dietitian for a low-fat diet plan that promotes slow weight loss. *Many patients with gallbladder disease are overweight or obese and will benefit from a sensible weight loss plan.*

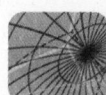

NURSING PROCESS: Patient Care Plan for Cholelithiasis and Surgery—*Continued*

Assessment of Postoperative Status

Subjective Data:

What is your level of pain on a scale of 0–10, with 10 being the worst pain?
Are you nauseated?
How active were you before surgery?

Objective Data:

Vital signs:
- Temperature
- BP
- Pulse
- Respirations

Abdominal examination:
- Bowel sounds
- Tenderness

- Guarding
- Wound inspection

Laboratory values:
- CBC
- Coagulation studies
- Bilirubin

Nursing Assessment and Diagnoses	Outcomes and Evaluation Parameters	Planning and Interventions with *Rationales*
Nursing Diagnoses: *Comfort: Readiness for Enhanced* related to surgical incision. *Nutrition: Readiness for Enhanced* related to postoperative nausea. *Airway Clearance, Ineffective* related to decreased lung expansion, immobility, and anesthesia. *Infection: Risk for* related to surgical incision and ineffective airway clearance.	**Outcome:** Discharge 1–2 days postoperatively. **Evaluation Parameters:** Hemoglobin and hematocrit normal. Vital signs normal. No complaints of nausea. Bowel sounds and bowel movement. Eating soft food without nausea.	**Interventions and *Rationales*:** Assess pain using pain scale (0–10) to quantify pain level, and administer pain medication as ordered or monitor the PCA (patient controlled analgesia) if the patient has an IV pump. *To increase consistency in monitoring pain.* Give antiemetic as ordered *to prevent vomiting that may result from anesthesia.* Discuss previous activity level, and instruct to resume normal activity slowly over 2–3 days after discharge. *An otherwise sedentary patient cannot be expected to be more active after surgery than before.* Give vitamin K as ordered. *Vitamin K is a fat soluble vitamin and may be ordered postoperatively to prevent bleeding.* Position in semi-Fowler's and ambulate as ordered when the patient is alert. *Early ambulation promotes lung expansion and helps prevent postoperative pneumonia, as well as promoting intestinal motility. The upright position allows for fuller lung expansion.* Monitor vital signs every 2–4 hours × 4, then every 4–8 hours as ordered *to detect any complications. Tachycardia, increased respiratory rate, or elevated temperature can indicate pain, bleeding, or infection.* Examine abdomen for return of bowel sounds, signs of peritonitis, and assess wound for drainage and infection. *Increasing abdominal tenderness, guarding, and rigid abdomen may be signs of an intra-abdominal leak of bile or blood.* Assess laboratory results for signs of over-/underhydration, bleeding, biliary obstruction, and infection, and notify the health care provider. *Early detection of complications of surgery, such as hemorrhage, infection, edema of the common bile duct, and fluid overload/dehydration, makes treatment more efficient.*

develop severe pancreatitis, which can lead to necrosis of the pancreas, and must be hospitalized.

Pathophysiology

The precise cause of pancreatitis is unknown, but most cases are associated with either biliary tract obstruction or heavy alcohol use. It is believed that activated pancreatic enzymes, particularly trypsin, leak into the pancreatic tissue and begin the process of autodigestion; the pancreas begins to digest itself. If bile refluxes into the pancreas as a result of biliary obstruction, this activates the pancreatic enzymes and the process of autodigestion. Activated trypsin and lipase begin to break down the cell membranes, which results in edema, vascular leakage, hemorrhage, and necro-

sis. In response to this autodigestion, tissue necrosis factor-alpha (TNF-α), substance P, and many interleukins and kinins enter the systemic circulation causing damage to tissue in the lungs, blood vessels, and kidneys, which results in increased mortality.

Clinical Manifestations

The most prominent manifestation of acute pancreatitis is sudden, severe, steady epigastric pain. The pain is worse when the patient is lying supine or when walking. It may radiate to the right or left side of the back and is made better by sitting, leaning forward with the knees bent. The patient usually complains of nausea and vomits. During a severe attack the patient may appear anxious and sweaty. The patient may also have abdominal distention, decreased bowel sounds, and rigidity. In 3 to 6 days Turner's sign (ecchymosis in the flanks) and Cullen's sign (bruising around the umbilicus) may appear as a result of retroperitoneal bleeding.

Circulating pancreatic enzymes can cause pleural effusions, atelectasis, or pulmonary edema in a small number of patients. Manifestations of these complications include tachypnea, tachycardia, and hypoxia. In addition, transient hyperglycemia may result from glucagon secretion from damaged cells in the pancreatic islets.

Chronic Pancreatitis

Chronic pancreatitis is an irreversible process of gradual destruction of pancreatic tissue with 50% to 80% of the cases attributed to chronic alcohol use (Fox, 2006). However, less than 10% of alcoholics develop chronic pancreatitis. Additional causes of chronic pancreatitis include cystic fibrosis, a genetic mutation in the cystic fibrosis transmembrane conductance regulator gene, and an autosomal dominant trait with high penetrance (Fox, 2006). Obesity, type II diabetes mellitus, and insulin resistance are also associated with chronic pancreatitis (Fox, 2006). Approximately 10% of cases of chronic pancreatitis have no identifiable cause.

Pathophysiology

The pathogenesis of chronic pancreatitis from alcohol ingestion is believed to cause the secretion of insoluble pancreatic proteins that go on to calcify and obstruct the pancreatic duct. As the pancreatic ducts become blocked, inflammation and fibrosis occur, destroying the function of the pancreatic tissue. The resulting pancreatic insufficiency leads to malabsorption and diabetes mellitus may also develop. Other theories as to the pathogenesis of chronic pancreatitis include embryonic defects, resulting in a relative obstruction of pancreatic flow, or trauma causing inflammation in the ductal epithelium, triggering the characteristic inflammatory changes (Fox, 2006).

Clinical Manifestations

The predominant manifestation of chronic pancreatitis is recurrent epigastric and left upper quadrant pain that may be referred to the left lumbar region. Other common symptoms may include anorexia, nausea, vomiting, weight loss, flatulence, and constipation. The pain in chronic pancreatitis is less severe than in the acute disease. The abdomen is usually tender with mild muscle guarding over the pancreas. The attacks initially last from several hours to 2 weeks, but generally become almost continuous as the disease progresses. A late manifestation is **steatorrhea**, which is bulky, fatty, and foul stools from the lack of pancreatic lipase.

Diagnostic Tests for Acute Pancreatitis

The diagnosis of acute pancreatitis is based on a complete history and physical exam, and elevated levels of serum amylase and lipase, and urine amylase. Other tests, such as serum bilirubin and serum alkaline phosphatase, indicate obstruction of the common bile duct, which can result from stones or edema, resulting in acute pancreatitis. An elevated ALT (>80 units/L) in patients with symptoms of acute pancreatitis indicates a biliary pancreatitis.

- Serum amylase increases just hours after the onset of the disease to levels two to three times normal. It will return to normal (25 to 125 units/L) within 3 to 4 days, or sooner in mild cases.
- Serum lipase levels rise rapidly, remain elevated up to 14 days, and then return to normal (<200 units/L).
- Serum alkaline phosphatase will be elevated if there is compression or obstruction of the common bile duct causing the acute pancreatitis. Normal values are 30 to 90 units/L.
- Serum bilirubin will also be elevated in cases of compression or obstruction of the common duct.
- Serum calcium levels may be decreased because of saponification, and this correlates with the severity of the disease. Levels below 7 mg/dL are associated with a poor prognosis (Friedman, 2004).
- C-reactive protein (CRP) elevations after 48 hours indicate the possibility of pancreatic necrosis (Friedman, 2004).
- White blood cell elevation (leukocytosis) is usually present in acute pancreatitis and indicates inflammation.

Imaging tests are ordered for the patient with acute pancreatitis. An abdominal x-ray may show signs of acute pancreatitis such as gallstones, a segment of small intestine in the left upper quadrant that is filled with air, or a gas-filled segment of transverse colon that ends at the area of pancreatic inflammation (Friedman, 2004). A CT scan is ordered after 3 days in order to identify necrotizing pancreatitis. A fluid collection in the pancreas seen on CT scan is an ominous sign and is associated with an increased mortality rate.

Laboratory and Diagnostic Procedures for Chronic Pancreatitis

Laboratory values for patients with chronic pancreatitis are usually similar to those of acute pancreatitis; however, the amylase and lipase may be normal. Most patients with chronic pancreatitis (80%) will develop diabetes after having the disease for 25 years and have elevated blood sugar levels and glycosuria. Stool samples usually show an elevation in fecal fat content as a result of pancreatic insufficiency.

The most sensitive test for chronic pancreatitis is the endoscopic retrograde cholangiopancreatography (ERCP), an imaging test to locate the cause of a biliary obstruction. Contrast media is injected into the duodenal papilla, and the biliary and pancreatic ducts are viewed. It will show dilated ducts, intraductal stones, strictures, or pseudocysts. Newer tests such as **magnetic resonance cholangiopancreatography (MRCP)**, a noninvasive imaging test, and endoscopic ultrasonography with tissue sampling are becoming more common and may replace the ERCP (Swaroop, Chari, & Clain, 2004).

Medical Management of Acute Pancreatitis

Treatment of acute pancreatitis involves resting the pancreas. This includes keeping the patient NPO (nothing by mouth), so a nasogastric tube frequently is inserted and connected to low intermittent suction. This keeps normal secretions from stimulating the pancreas to release digestive enzymes, therefore causing pain. Bed rest may be ordered until the acute phase has subsided. When the patient is free from pain and bowel sounds have returned, a diet of clear liquids is usually ordered. The diet is then advanced slowly to low fat. In severe cases, particularly necrotizing pancreatitis, large amounts of intravenous fluids may be required to maintain the patient's fluid volume. This may require the patient to be transferred to the intensive care unit.

Medications

Pain relief is of primary importance and is usually achieved with narcotic analgesics. Meperidine or morphine sulfate may be ordered every 3 to 4 hours. Antibiotics such as Imipenem or cefuroxime may be prescribed if there is evidence of infection, or in the case of pancreatic necrosis, to prevent infection. In the patient with severe pancreatitis who has been NPO for 7 to 10 days, total parenteral nutrition may be needed to maintain adequate nutritional status. Patients that are hypocalcemic will be given calcium gluconate intravenously to prevent tetany. The Pharmacology Summary feature later in the chapter (p. 1457) outlines medications used to treat biliary disorders.

Surgery

Surgery to debride the pancreas and surrounding tissue is indicated for patients that have infected necrotizing pancreatitis. This process may improve survival for those with multiorgan failure if the pancreatitis does not respond to other treatment within 4 to 6 weeks. If pancreatic abscesses develop, then the patient may require a percutaneous or open surgical drainage. Occasionally, patients with acute pancreatitis develop pseudocysts, which require drainage if persistent pain develops or if there is ductal obstruction.

Medical Management of Chronic Pancreatitis

Patients with chronic pancreatitis require lifelong changes in their lifestyle. Abstinence from alcohol is mandatory because it often will precipitate an acute attack. A low-fat diet should be maintained because of the lack of the pancreatic enzyme lipase, which is responsible for fat synthesis. During an acute exacerbation of chronic pancreatitis, the patient will be treated in much the same way as a patient with acute pancreatitis.

Medications

Although pain is a major manifestation of chronic pancreatitis, narcotic analgesia is avoided when possible because opioid addiction is common in these patients. These patients will require nutritional supplementation with pancreatic enzymes (Chart 46–9). If steatorrhea becomes a major problem, a dietary supplement with a high concentration of lipase will be prescribed. The supplements should be taken with meals. If the medication is not enteric coated, then an H_2-receptor antagonist such as ranitidine or a proton pump inhibitor such as omeprazole is given once or twice a day.

Surgery

Surgical intervention may be needed in patients with chronic pancreatitis to eradicate biliary tract disease, make sure that bile can freely flow into the duodenum, or eliminate obstruction of the pancreatic duct (Friedman, 2004). Pancreatic pseudocysts may need to be drained if they are over 6 centimeters in diameter. Surgery may also be attempted to try and relieve pain.

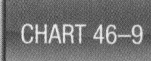

CHART 46–9 **Pancreatic Enzyme Supplement Preparations**

Pancreatic enzymes are purified from pig pancreases.
- Actions:
  - Contains protease, lipase, and amylase
  - Digests proteins, fats, and carbohydrates
- Contraindications:
  - Allergy to pork protein
  - Jews keeping kosher
  - Vegetarians

CONVENTIONAL PREPARATIONS

Viokase

Ilozyme

Cotazym

ENTERIC-COATED PREPARATIONS

Creon

Pancrease

Cotazym-S

Ultrase

 # Nursing Management

The major focus of nursing care for the patient with pancreatitis is pain control, nutrition, and health teaching about alcohol abstinence.

Assessment

Subjective data for both acute and chronic pancreatitis should include a history of the present condition including a comprehensive assessment of the pain and associated symptoms. A social history can give clues to alcohol intake, amount, and duration. For a complete assessment, see the Nursing Process: Patient Care Plan feature for pancreatitis.

Nursing Diagnoses and Interventions

The Nursing Process: Patient Care Plan feature also outlines the nursing diagnoses and interventions for the patient with pancreatitis. The National Guidelines box (p. 1457) presents the practice guidelines for acute pancreatitis.

Health Promotion

Because most cases of pancreatitis are related to alcohol abuse, the focus of prevention is on abstinence from alcohol. After diagnosis, it is essential that patients with pancreatitis abstain from alcohol to prevent future painful episodes. Referral to Alcoholics Anonymous or other treatment programs is recommended.

 # Cancer of the Pancreas

Cancer of the pancreas is the fourth leading cause of cancer death overall. It is estimated that in 2008, 37,680 patients in the United States will be diagnosed with pancreatic cancer and

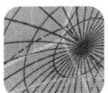

NURSING PROCESS: Patient Care Plan for Pancreatitis

Assessment of Pain

Subjective Data:
What is your level of pain on a scale of 0–10, with 10 being the worst pain?
Are you allergic to anything?
Do you have any special cultural or religious practices for dealing with pain?
Describe the character of your pain? Burning? Steady? Radiate?
Is your pain worse when you are lying down?
Do you have pain when you eat?
Does vomiting relieve the pain?
Have you ever had this type of pain before? If yes, how long did it last? What relieved the pain in the past?
Do you have a history of gallbladder disease?
Do you drink alcohol? How much? How often?

Objective Data:
General appearance:
- Looks distressed
- Sits with knees pulled toward chest
- Restlessness
- Grimacing
- Moaning or groaning
- Clenched fists

Pulse—tachycardia
Shallow rapid respirations
Abdominal tenderness or guarding
Flank or periumbilical ecchymosis
Diaphoresis

Nursing Assessment and Diagnoses	Outcomes and Evaluation Parameters	Planning and Interventions with *Rationales*
Nursing Diagnosis: *Pain: Acute* related to pancreatitis	**Outcome:** Comfort level maintained. **Evaluation Parameters:** Able to communicate level of pain and relief from medications. Appears restful without restlessness or moaning.	**Interventions and *Rationales*:** Assess pain using pain scale (0–10) to quantify pain level. *To increase consistency in monitoring pain.* Administer pain medication, usually meperidine or morphine, and assess level of pain 30 minutes and 1 hour after giving medication. Notify health care provider if pain is unrelieved. *To assess effectiveness of medications.* Explore cultural and religious practices and beliefs about pain and illness. *Different religions have varying beliefs about pain, suffering, and disease.* Teach nonpharmacologic methods of pain control, such as guided imagery, meditation, and breathing exercises. *This may augment pain relief.* Maintain a quiet, darkened, comfortable environment. *This can help decrease physical and mental stimulation, which can lead to decreased pancreatic secretions and less pain.* Maintain bed rest and position the patient in a sitting position *to decrease the pain caused by stretched abdominal muscles that are irritated by inflammation.* Close the patient's door during mealtime *because the smell of food can stimulate pancreatic secretions.* Place a nasogastric tube if ordered, and/or monitor drainage and relief of pain. *This helps to "rest" the pancreas and removes secretions that can stimulate the pancreas to produce enzymes.*

Assessment of Nutrition

Subjective Data:
Are you nauseated?
Have you vomited?
Have you noticed any weight loss?

Objective Data:
Height and weight measurements
BMI
Abdominal examination:
- Diminished or absent bowel sounds

Laboratory results:
- Serum albumin
- Glucose
- Transferrin
- Hemoglobin and hematocrit (H & H)

(continued)

MyNursingKit | National Pancreas Foundation

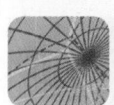

NURSING PROCESS: Patient Care Plan for Pancreatitis—*Continued*

Nursing Assessment and Diagnoses	Outcomes and Evaluation Parameters	Planning and Interventions with *Rationales*
Nursing Diagnosis: *Nutrition, Imbalanced: Less than Body Requirements* related to nausea, vomiting, pain, and possible lack of pancreatic enzymes for digestion	**Outcome:** Adequate nutrition. ***Evaluation Parameters:*** No weight loss. Serum albumin normal. Fasting glucose normal. Hemoglobin and hematocrit normal. No reported nausea.	**Interventions and *Rationales:*** Weigh daily on same scale at the same time. *Fluctuations in weight from day to day are an indicator of fluid balance, but changes over a week reflect nutritional status.* Assess laboratory results and report any abnormal values to the patient's health care provider. *The pancreas produces enzymes that aid in the digestion of protein, fat, and carbohydrates. Protein malnutrition is reflected in a low serum albumin. Transferrin is a protein that transports iron, so this level may be low. The H & H may be decreased in cases of malnutrition. Serum glucose may be elevated if the pancreatitis affects the endocrine function of the gland.* Monitor the frequency, color, consistency, and odor of stools. *Lack of lipase from the pancreas results in poor fat digestion and steatorrhea results. The presence of steatorrhea indicates severe pancreatitis with impaired pancreatic function.* Provide oral hygiene at least every 2 hours while the nasogastric tube is in place *to decrease discomfort and maintain the integrity of the oral and nasal mucosa.* Offer small, frequent meals, beginning with clear liquids once bowel sounds return and pain is relieved. *Smaller meals reduce the secretion of pancreatic enzymes.*

Assessment of Fluid and Electrolyte Status

Subjective Data:

Do you feel dizzy or light-headed?

Objective Data:

Cardiac status:
- Rhythm
- Pulmonary artery pressure
- Peripheral pulses
- Capillary refill

Vital signs:
- BP
- Pulse
- Respirations

Renal function:
- Hourly urine output
- Daily body weight

Neurological function:
- Mental status
- Level of consciousness
- Behavior

Laboratory values:
- Electrolytes
- Hematocrit
- BUN and creatinine

Nursing Assessment and Diagnoses	Outcomes and Evaluation Parameters	Planning and Interventions with *Rationales*
Nursing Diagnoses: *Fluid Volume Deficit* related to vascular leak syndrome resulting from inflammation, and fluid accumulation in the abdominal cavity. Potential for electrolyte imbalance related to nasogastric suction	**Outcomes:** Adequate fluid volume and electrolyte balance. ***Evaluation Parameters:*** Normal blood pressure with no orthostatic changes. Normal sinus rhythm. Stable daily weight with moist mucous membranes. Pulmonary artery pressure 8–12 mmHg. Cardiac output at least 5 L/min. Brisk capillary refill. Good peripheral pulses. Urine output 30 mL/hr. Alert and oriented.	**Interventions and *Rationales:*** Evaluate cardiac status: heart rate and rhythm at least every 4 hours; orthostatic blood pressure, pulmonary artery pressure usually every 4 hours as indicated; peripheral pulses; capillary refill; skin color. *These assessments help establish fluid volume. The body compensates for diminished volume by increasing the heart rate to maintain cardiac output. Capillaries constrict to force more fluid into the general circulation and the signs are weak peripheral pulses and pale skin color. A decreased cardiac output means a decrease in the renal perfusion and decreased urine output and possibly early prerenal renal failure.* Monitor renal function by measuring urine output every hour and notifying the health care provider if the level is less than 30 mL/hr. Daily body weight *is an indicator of fluid status.* Monitor neurological function by assessing level of consciousness and behavior. *Cerebral perfusion may be diminished if there is a fluid volume deficit and the cardiac output is low. Electrolytes, particularly sodium, can cause confusion when the levels are low.* Monitor laboratory values for electrolyte status and renal function. *Electrolytes are lost in nasogastric suction or vomiting. The BUN and creatinine will rise if renal function is compromised.*

NATIONAL GUIDELINES for Acute Pancreatitis

Priorities of Care	Guideline
Supportive care	The nurse should anticipate the need for supportive care with particular attention to the assessment and prevention of hypoxemia and the need to ensure adequate fluid balance. Nursing interventions would include: • Frequent assessment of vital signs. • Frequent assessment of bedside oxygen saturation. • Accurate assessment of fluid status (strict I&O). • Administration of supplemental oxygen therapy, particularly when narcotic agents are being used for pain control. • Aggressive IV fluid therapy is critical to counteract hypovolemia caused by third space losses, vomiting, diaphoresis, and an increased vascular permeability secondary to the presence of inflammatory mediators. • The nurse should also monitor serum laboratory values for signs of inadequate fluid balance and hemoconcentration.
Level of nursing care	A patient with acute pancreatitis who develops organ failure or severe pancreatitis should be transferred to an intensive care or step-down unit to accommodate the evolving high acuity needs. Common indicators of organ failure or increased severity include: • Sustained hypoxemia • Hypotension refractory to IV therapy • Signs of renal insufficiency (such as a serum creatinine > 2 mg/dL) • Hemoconcentration in an elderly client with a history of cardiovascular disease who requires aggressive fluid resuscitation. Additional danger signals that warrant increased evaluation, but may not necessitate transfer to a high acuity bed, include: • Obesity (BMI > 30) • Oliguria (urine output < 50 mL/hr) • Tachycardia with pulse $\geq$ 120 beats/min • Encephalopathy • Increased need for narcotic analgesics.
Nutritional support	When pancreatitis is mild, oral intake is typically restored in 3 to 7 days, thus negating the need for nutritional support. However, during more prolonged periods of inadequate nutritional intake, enteral feedings are preferred over total parenteral nutrition (TPN). Enteral nutrition, administered into the distal jejunum, avoids the stimulation of pancreatic secretions and does not exacerbate the disease. In general, enteral feedings have been found to be safer and less expensive than TPN.

Source: Banks, P. A., & Freeman, M. L. (2006). Practice guidelines in acute pancreatitis. *American Journal of Gastroenterology, 101*(10), 2379–2400.

PHARMACOLOGY Summary of Medications Used to Treat Biliary Disorders

Medication Category	Action	Application/Indication	Nursing Responsiblity
Gallstone-Solubilizing Agents			
Ursodiol (Actigall) Chenodiol (Chenix)	Dissolves gallstones by reducing the cholesterol content of the stone or blocking cholesterol production.	Prevention, dissolution of noncalcified cholesterol gallstones, primary biliary cirrhosis.	Monitor for adverse effects: nausea, vomiting, and dyspepsia. Be aware of drugs that reduce efficacy: bile acid sequestrants, aluminum antacids, estrogens, some lipid lowering agents.
Bile Acid Sequestrants			
Cholestyramine (Questran, LoCholest) Colestipol (Colestid)	Decreases pruritus by decreasing circulation bile acids and decreasing bile acid deposits in skin tissue.	Relief of pruritus secondary to partial biliary stasis.	Monitor for adverse effects: constipation, abdominal pain, nausea, vomiting, indigestion, and headache. Be aware long-term use may require supplementation of fat soluble vitamins. Give 1 hour after or 4–6 hours before other drugs.

34,290 will die from the disease (American Cancer Society, 2008). Risk factors include obesity, chronic pancreatitis, family history of pancreatic cancer, history of abdominal radiation, and cigarette smoking. In fact, smokers have twice the incidence of pancreatic cancer as nonsmokers. There is some evidence that a high-fat diet and diabetes mellitus increase the risk as well, particularly in women. The risk of developing pancreatic cancer increases with age.

Pathophysiology

Most pancreatic cancer is ductal adenocarcinoma that develops from the exocrine cells in the ducts. Rarely, cancer develops in the endocrine cells, and these types of tumors, which are always fatal, are called **apudomas**. Ductal adenocarcinoma begins in the ducts, slowly invades the glandular tissue, and then extends into the surrounding tissue. Roughly 75% of these cancers arise in the head of the pancreas, although they can occur anywhere in the pancreas. When the tumor arises in the head of the pancreas, it usually causes obstruction of the common bile duct early in the course of the disease with resultant jaundice. Survival is longer in these patients, probably because they seek treatment earlier than those with cancer in the body or tail of the pancreas. Because of the vascular structure of the area, cancer cells infiltrate the portal vein, mesenteric artery, vena cava, and aorta, with metastasis to the liver (Huether, 2006).

Clinical Manifestations

Most cases of pancreatic cancer are asymptomatic until the tumor invades surrounding tissue or obstructs the common bile duct. Jaundice may be the first sign. In about 70% of cases, patients recall vague, diffuse epigastric pain that did not cause them alarm. Once jaundice occurs, stools become light in color and the urine becomes dark. Pruritus results from the bilirubin in the skin. The blockage of pancreatic enzymes into the duodenum results in problems of fat and protein digestion and absorption, so the patient may exhibit weight loss, steatorrhea, and malnutrition.

Laboratory and Diagnostic Procedures

Diagnosis of pancreatic cancer is done by history and physical examination. When there is a suspicion of pancreatic cancer, a dual-phase spiral CT or an MRI is done to detect the tumor. The dual-phase method detects 80% of tumors. The next step is to perform a percutaneous needle aspiration to get samples of the tissue for cytologic study (Friedman, 2004). If the CT or MRI is inconclusive, an ERCP may be done to identify any neoplasm. In

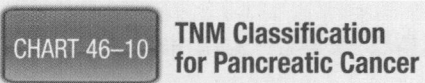

CHART 46–10 **TNM Classification for Pancreatic Cancer**

Tis: Carcinoma in situ.

T1: Tumor is limited to the pancreas and is less than 2 centimeters in size.

T2: Tumor is larger than 2 centimeters but limited to the pancreas.

T3: Tumor spread beyond the pancreas but no involvement of the celiac axis or superior mesenteric artery.

T4: Tumor invasion of the celiac axis or superior mesenteric artery.

about 30% of patients, a laparotomy is performed to establish a definitive diagnosis and determine the extent of the disease. Tumor staging is done based on the TNM system of classification. Chart 46–10 outlines the TNM staging for pancreatic cancer.

Medical Management

Treatment of pancreatic cancer is varied, ranging from surgical intervention to palliation. If the tumor is limited to the head of the pancreas and there is no lymph node involvement or metastasis, then radical **pancreaticoduodenal (Whipple) resection** is done. This procedure has a 5-year survival rate of 20% to 25%. The Whipple procedure involves removal of the head of the pancreas, the duodenum, a distal portion of the stomach, a part of the jejunum, and the lower half of the common bile duct. Unfortunately, most pancreatic cancer is too advanced when first diagnosed for the Whipple procedure to be effective. Radiation and chemotherapy may be used after surgery to enhance recovery efforts or for palliation in patients with unresectable cancer.

Patients with pancreatic cancer require nursing care that focuses on palliation, comfort, and support. Chapter 64 ☻ presents the care of patients with cancer, and Chapter 45 ☻ discusses the care of patients with gastrointestinal surgery.

▮ Research

Research is necessary for improvement in the care of patients with liver, gallbladder, and pancreatic disorders. The goal of research is to identify areas in practice where innovations can impact the patient's health and well-being, and then to develop and test interventions that address the identified problems. The Research Topics Related to Patients with Liver, Gallbladder, or Pancreatic Disorders feature presents a list of research opportunities related to these disorders.

RESEARCH TOPICS RELATED TO PATIENTS WITH LIVER, GALLBLADDER, OR PANCREATIC DISORDERS

Research	Clinical Impact
Physiological Research	
Vaccine for hepatitis C.	Development of a vaccine would decrease the number of people with chronic hepatitis C and possible liver failure.
Drugs to treat hepatitis C genotype most common in the United States.	Effective drug treatment can help decrease the spread of hepatitis C and improve morbidity and mortality.
Drugs to reverse hepatic encephalopathy.	
Effective treatments for hepatorenal syndrome.	Medications or other treatments would decrease the complications of cirrhosis, thereby improving the quality of life and longevity of patients with cirrhosis.
Drugs to prevent esophageal varices.	
Herbal preparations to boost liver function in patients with a compromised liver.	
The management of pain in patients with pancreatitis.	Patient comfort is enhanced with less dependence on narcotics.
Use of acupuncture as an adjunct to pain management in pancreatitis.	

Emotional and Psychological Research	Clinical Impact
Living With the Uncertainty of Chronic Hepatitis C	
Music therapy to reduce anxiety before, during, and after painful procedures such as paracentesis, ERCP, and surgical intervention.	Nurses can help patients cope with an uncertain future and increase patient well-being.
Quality of life after liver transplant.	The goal is to improve psychological interventions to improve coping.
	Understanding the issues after liver transplant can help nurses plan interventions for patients to maximize their recovery.

Clinical Preparation

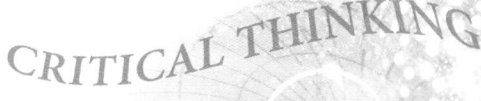
CRITICAL THINKING

PEARSON **mynursingkit**™

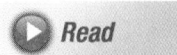 **Read**

- History of Current Illness
- Past Medical History
- Physical Exam
- Admitting Medical Orders
- Laboratory Study Results

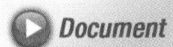 **Document**

- Summary of Hospitalization
- Pathophysiology Form
- Laboratory Values
- Laboratory Results Explanation

 **Apply**

- List of Potential Nursing Diagnoses
- Concept Map
- Critical Thinking Questions

Log on to MyNursingKit.com to download forms you will need and to complete further steps in the Clinical Preparation assignment.

HISTORY OF PRESENT ILLNESS

As the nurse on a medical–surgical floor in a community hospital, you receive report about Mr. M., a 60-year-old construction worker who was admitted 2 days ago with a diagnosis of cirrhosis of the liver.

Medical–Surgical History

According to his wife, Mr. M.'s past medical history includes hepatitis A infection as a young man. He has no history of any other diseases. He has had a "beer belly" for at least 20 years, but his wife notices that it has been getting larger during the last week.

Social History

Mr. M. drinks 6 to 10 beers each night after work and greater amounts on the weekends. He has smoked three packs of cigarettes a day for the last 30 years. He does not take any prescription medications, but uses Tylenol occasionally for headache.

Physical Exam

In report the nurse leaving states that Mr. M. is confused and restless in bed. His vital signs are temperature of 37°C; pulse of 120 beats per minute; respirations 26 and labored; blood pressure of

140/76. She states that he is slightly jaundiced and diaphoretic. His lungs are clear to auscultation, and gynecomastia is noted on the chest exam. His heart sounds indicate a regular rhythm, tachycardia, with no murmurs or gallops.

Mr. M.'s abdomen is large and distended with hypoactive bowel sounds. It is tender to palpation with a positive fluid wave. His spleen is enlarged. His abdominal girth is 56 inches and his stool tests positive for blood. He is confused and oriented to person only. The nurse reports that he has asterixis and hyperactive reflexes.

Admitting Medical Orders

Service: medicine
Diagnosis: cirrhosis of the liver
Allergies: none known
Vital signs q4h including oxygen saturation
Neurological checks q4h
Abdominal girth q shift
I&O q shift
Daily weight
Activity: bed rest
DVT prophylaxis: sequential compression device to lower extremities

Incentive spirometer: q1h while awake
Diet: sodium restriction: 2 g/day; fluid restriction: 1,500 mL/day; high-calorie, low-protein, 20 g/day diet
Call house officer: temp > 38.5°C, HR > 110 or < 60, RR > 30 or < 12, BP sys > 160 or < 90, O_2 sat < 92%, urine output < 120 mL in 4 hours, change in neurological or abdominal exam, any Hct result that is 5 less than the baseline ED Hct
IV: D5NS IV at 10 mL/hr

Scheduled Medications

Multivitamin 1 po daily
Lactulose 30 mL po qid × 3 days then bid
Spironolactone (Aldactone) 100 mg po daily
Lasix 40 mg po daily
Oxazepam (Serax) 10 mg po tid

Ordered Laboratory Studies

Hgb and Hct
Electrolyte panel
Liver function tests
Serum ammonia qam
Chart and test stool for occult blood

LABORATORY STUDY RESULTS

Test	Admission	Day 1	Day 2
Hemoglobin (Hgb)	12.5 g/dL	12.0 g/dL	11.8 g/dL
Hematocrit (Hct)	38%	36%	34%
Bilirubin—total	1.5 mg/dL	1.5 mg/dL	1.5 mg/dL
• Direct	0.6 mg/dL	0.6 mg/dL	0.6 mg/dL
• Indirect	0.9 mg/dL	0.9 mg/dL	0.9 mg/dL
AST	400 unit/L	386 unit/L	352 unit/L
ALT	150 unit/L	149 unit/L	147 unit/L
Alkaline phosphatase	150 unit/L	144 unit/L	144 unit/L
Electrolytes:			
• Sodium	138 mEq/L	140 mEq/L	141 mEq/L
• Potassium	3.5 mEq/L	3.4 mEq/L	3.5 mEq/L
• Calcium	8.6 mg/dL	8.8 mg/dL	8.8 mg/dL
Serum ammonia	50 µ/dL	58 µ/dL	46 µ/dL
Serum albumin	3.0 g/dL	3.2 g/dL	3.0 g/dL

CRITICAL THINKING QUESTIONS

1. What signs and symptoms of hepatic encephalopathy is Mr. M. manifesting?

2. Describe the pathophysiology of cirrhosis and how it relates to each of his clinical manifestations.

3. Why is Mr. M. on a low-protein diet?

4. Why is lactulose given to Mr. M.?

Answers to Critical Thinking Questions appear in Appendix D.

NCLEX® REVIEW

1. A patient is being evaluated for hepatitis C infection. Which question will best assist the nurse in identifying if exposure has occurred?
   1. "Have you traveled outside the country recently?"
   2. "Do you eat a lot of uncooked shellfish?"
   3. "Have you ever had a tattoo?"
   4. "Do you share eating utensils with anyone infected with hepatitis A?"

2. During the prodromal phase of hepatitis the nurse expects to assess which of the following symptoms in the patient:
   1. Hypothermia.
   2. Increased appetite.
   3. Dark colored urine.
   4. Constant epigastric pain.

3. The nurse identifies a patient with cirrhosis of the liver with an albumin level of 2.5 gm/dL is at risk for the development of:
   1. Peripheral edema.
   2. Prolonged blood coagulation.
   3. Jaundice of the skin.
   4. Vitamin A malabsorption.

4. A patient with cirrhosis develops hepatic encephalopathy and is extremely confused and agitated. The nurse places priorty on administering which ordered medication?
   1. Lactulose, Chronulac
   2. Oxazepam, Serax
   3. Propanolzole, Protonix
   4. Phytonadione, Vitamin K

5. A patient diagnosed with liver cancer three months ago has elevated alpha-fetoprotein levels, AFP. The nurse should incorporate which of the following interventions into the plan of care.
   1. Provide supportive and comfort measures to the patient and family.
   2. Explain how the transhepatic portosystemic shunt, TIPS will relieve symptoms.
   3. Prepare the patient and family for the likelihood of a liver transplant.
   4. Restrict dietary proteins and foods high in sodium.

6. The nurse identifies the following factor would have increased the risk to develop stones in a patient diagnosed with cholelithiasis.
   1. The patient consumes a high fiber diet.
   2. The patient recently was treated with aminoglycosides for a urinary tract infection.
   3. The patient has had rapid weight loss secondary to crash dieting.
   4. The patient is of northern European descent.

7. A patient who had a cholecystectomy 2 days ago complains of abdominal pain which is unrelieved by the opioid analgesic given one hour ago. Which action should be taken initially by the nurse?
   1. Administer a second dose of analgesia.
   2. Encourage the patient to ambulate in order to expel flatus.
   3. Examine abdomen for rigidity and tenderness.
   4. Position patient in a side lying fetal position.

8. A patient admitted with complaints of mid epigastric and abdominal pain is being evaluated for pancreatitis. The nurse recognizes which finding would support a diagnosis of chronic pancreatitis rather than acute pancreatitis?
   1. Stools are clay colored.
   2. Amylase level is normal.
   3. Blood sugar is within normal limits.
   4. Abdomen is tender to palpation.

9. A patient who is experiencing jaundice has just been diagnosed with pancreatic cancer. The nurse anticipates the patient will display which other symptoms?
   1. Pale dilute urine
   2. Clay colored stools
   3. Weight gain
   4. Easy bruising

10. When providing discharge instructions for a patient recovering from chronic pancreatitis, the nurse should plan to include which instructions?
    1. Avoid using all over-the-counter analgesics.
    2. Eat a diet low in fat.
    3. Limit alcohol drinks to one a day.
    4. Avoid sharing any eating utensils.

Answers for review questions appear in Appendix D.

KEY TERMS

alanine aminotransferase (ALT) *p.1430*
alkaline phosphatase (ALP) *p.1430*
alpha-amylase *p.1427*
apudomas *p.1458*
aspartate aminotransferase (AST) *p.1430*
asterixis *p.1436*
bile *p.1427*
bile canaliculi *p.1429*
biliary dyskinesia *p.1449*
bilirubin *p.1430*
caput medusae *p.1441*
carboxypeptidase *p.1427*
cholangiocarcinoma *p.1444*
cholecystectomy *p.1449*
cholecystitis *p.1448*
cholecystokinin *p.1427*
choledocholithiasis *p.1447*
cholelithiasis *p.1447*
chymotrypsin *p.1427*

cirrhosis *p.1434*
convalescent phase *p.1430*
esophageal varices *p.1436*
exocrine pancreas *p.1427*
gamma-glutamyltransferase (GGT) *p.1430*
gluconeogenesis *p.1436*
hepatic encephalopathy *p.1436*
hepatitis A virus (HAV) *p.1428*
hepatitis B virus (HBV) *p.1429*
hepatitis C virus (HCV) *p.1429*
hepatitis D virus (HDV) *p.1429*
hepatitis E virus (HEV) *p.1429*
hepatocellular *p.1427*
hepatorenal syndrome *p.1436*
hypoalbuminemia *p.1436*
icteric phase *p.1430*
Kupffer cells *p.1429*
lactic dehydrogenase (LDH) *p.1430*
lipase *p.1427*

magnetic resonance
    cholangiopancreatography
    (MRCP) *p.1453*
melena *p.1436*
pancreaticoduodenal (Whipple)
    resection *p.1458*
pancreatitis *p.1450*
paracentesis *p.1440*
portal hypertension *p.1436*
primary biliary cirrhosis *p.1441*
prodromal phase *p.1430*
sclerosing cholangitis *p.1441*
sclerotherapy *p.1441*
serum immunoglobulin G (IgG) *p.1429*
serum immunoglobulin M (IgM) *p.1429*
steatorrhea *p.1453*
trypsin *p.1427*
viral hepatitis *p.1427*

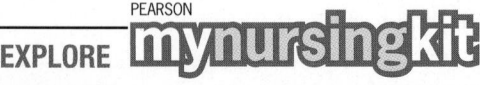

EXPLORE PEARSON mynursingkit™

MyNursingKit is your one stop for online chapter review materials and resources. Prepare for success with additional NCLEX®-style practice questions, interactive assignments and activities, web links, animations and videos, and more!

Register your access code from the front of your book at
www.mynursingkit.com

REFERENCES

Afdhal, N. H. (2007). *Epidemiology of and risk factors for gallstones.* Retrieved April 24, 2008, from http://www.uptodate.com/patients/content/topic.do?topicKey=~5rphinkcGz/zys

American Cancer Society. (2008). *Pancreatic cancer.* Retrieved August 9, 2008, from http://www.cancer.org/docroot/CRI/content/CRI_2_4_1X_What_are_the_key_statistics_for_pancreatic_cancer_34.asp?rnav=cri

Askey, B. D. (2006). Managing cirrhosis in a primary-care setting. *The Clinical Advisor, 9*(12), 22–28.

Baldwin, P. D. (2003). Chemical hepatitis. *Clinical Journal of Oncology Nursing, 7*(1), 99–103.

Centers for Disease Control and Prevention (CDC). (2008). *Viral hepatitis.* Retrieved August 9, 2008, from http://www.cdc.gov/hepatitis/

Chisholm-Burns, M. A., Wells, B. G., Schwinghammer, T. L., Malone, P. M., Kolesar, J. M., Rotschafer, J. C., et al. (2008). *Pharmacotherapy principles & practice.* New York: McGraw-Hill.

Deutsch, K. F. (2003, May). Hepatitis C: The silent epidemic. *The Clinical Advisor,* 10–18.

Fox, K. M. (2006). Chronic pancreatitis. *Clinician Reviews, 16*(6), 46–52.

Friedman, L. S. (2004). Liver, biliary tract, and pancreas. In L. M. Tierney, S. J. McPhee, & M. A. Papadakis, *Current medical diagnosis & treatment* (pp. 623–668). New York: Lange Medical Books/McGraw-Hill.

Holloway, M., & D'Acunto, K. (2006). An update on the ABCs of viral hepatitis. *The Clinical Advisor, 9*(6), 26–37.

Huether, S. E. (2006). Alterations of digestive function. In K. L. McCance & S. E. Huether, *Pathophysiology: The biologic basis for disease in adults and children* (5th ed., pp. 1385–1445). Philadelphia: Mosby.

Kee, J. L. (2002). *Laboratory and diagnostic tests with nursing implications* (6th ed.). Upper Saddle River, NJ: Prentice Hall.

Lutz, C., & Przytulski, K. (2006). *Nutrition and diet therapy: Evidence-based applications.* Philadelphia: F. A. Davis.

Pelc, C. E. (2003). Milking it! *Hepatitis, 5*(3), 15–17.

Rhee, C., & Broadbent, A. M. (2007). Palliation and liver failure: Palliative medications dosages guidelines. *Journal of Palliative Medicine, 10*(3), 677–687.

Swaroop, V. S., Chari, S. T., & Clain, J. E. (2004). Severe acute pancreatitis. *JAMA, 291*(23), 2865–2868.

Thomas, D. J. (2007). Abdominal problems. In L. M. Dunphy, J. E. Winland-Brown, B. O. Porter, & D. J. Thomas, *Primary care: The Art and Science of Advanced Practice Nursing* (2nd ed., pp. 473–561). Philadelphia: F. A. Davis.

Wasley, A., Miller, J. T., & Finelli, L. (2007). Surveillance for acute viral hepatitis—United States, 2005. *Morbidity and Mortality Weekly Report, 56*(SS-3), 1–24. Retrieved, April 24, 2008, from http://www.cdc.gov/mmwr/preview/mmwrhtml/ss5603a1.htm

Caring for the Patient with Renal and Urinary Disorders

Cheryl Wraa

Outcome-Based Learning Objectives

After studying this chapter, the learner will be able to:

1. Discuss the function of the kidney in relation to regulating fluid, electrolyte, and acid–base balance.

2. List common diagnostic tests used to determine kidney function and related diseases.

3. Identify the major diseases of the kidney.

4. Discuss complications of kidney-related diseases.

5. Recognize the signs and symptoms associated with urinary tract disorders.

6. Compare and contrast the underlying principles of hemodialysis and peritoneal dialysis.

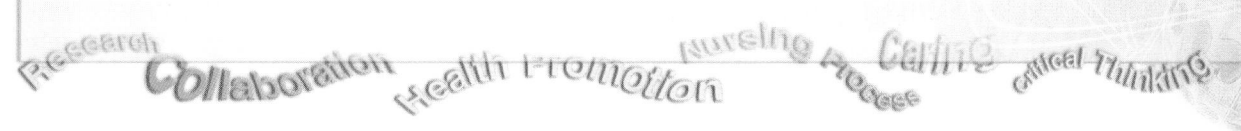

Research Collaboration Health Promotion Nursing Process Caring Critical Thinking

THE KIDNEYS play an important role in maintaining constancy of the internal environment of the body through multiple functions, including:

- Maintaining electrolyte balance, which is a major factor for normal nerve and muscle physiology.

- Helping to regulate acid–base balance through the reabsorption and elimination or conservation of sodium, potassium, hydrogen, chloride, and bicarbonate ions.

- Production of **erythropoietin**, a hormone that stimulates the production of red blood cells in the bone marrow.

- Secretion of **renin** that converts angiotensinogen to angiotensin, which stimulates the release of aldosterone by the adrenal cortex. Aldosterone plays a part in the regulation of sodium and water reabsorption to help elevate blood pressure.

- Activating vitamin D, and regulating calcium and phosphate conservation and elimination, which contribute to the metabolic functions of the skeletal system.

- Regulating the osmolality of the extracellular fluid through action of the antidiuretic hormone (ADH).

- Elimination of metabolic wastes: urea, uric acid, creatinine, and drugs and their metabolites.

Throughout the day the two kidneys process approximately 1,700 liters of blood and combine the waste products to produce approximately 1.5 liters of urine. To put it another way, the kidneys filter a person's entire blood volume 60 to 70 times a day (Porth, 2005; Urden, Stacy, & Lough, 2006).

Physiology

To better understand the disease processes, it is important to be familiar with the physiology of the renal system. The **nephron** is the functional unit of the kidney, and each kidney encompasses approximately 1 million nephrons (Urden et al., 2006). Each nephron consists of a **glomerulus**, a compact tuft of capillaries where blood is filtered (Figure 47–1 ■, p. 1464). The glomerulus is encased in a thin double-walled capsule called **Bowman's capsule**. The capillary walls of the glomerulus are very thin, and the blood pressure within them is higher than the pressure in Bowman's capsule; therefore, fluid from the plasma is filtered into the capsule. This fluid is initial urine, and in the healthy nephron, neither red blood cells nor protein should pass through the filter. Nutrients and water are then reabsorbed by the proximal convoluted tubule and taken back into the capillaries that surround the tubules. Two important electrolytes, sodium and chloride, are reabsorbed during this time according to the body's needs. The waste products of protein metabolism, urea, and creatinine, along with substances that are in excess in body fluids, such as hydrogen ions, are secreted into the distal tubules to be excreted. Finally, urine empties into the renal pelvis, moves down the ureters, is stored in the bladder, and then leaves the body through the urethra.

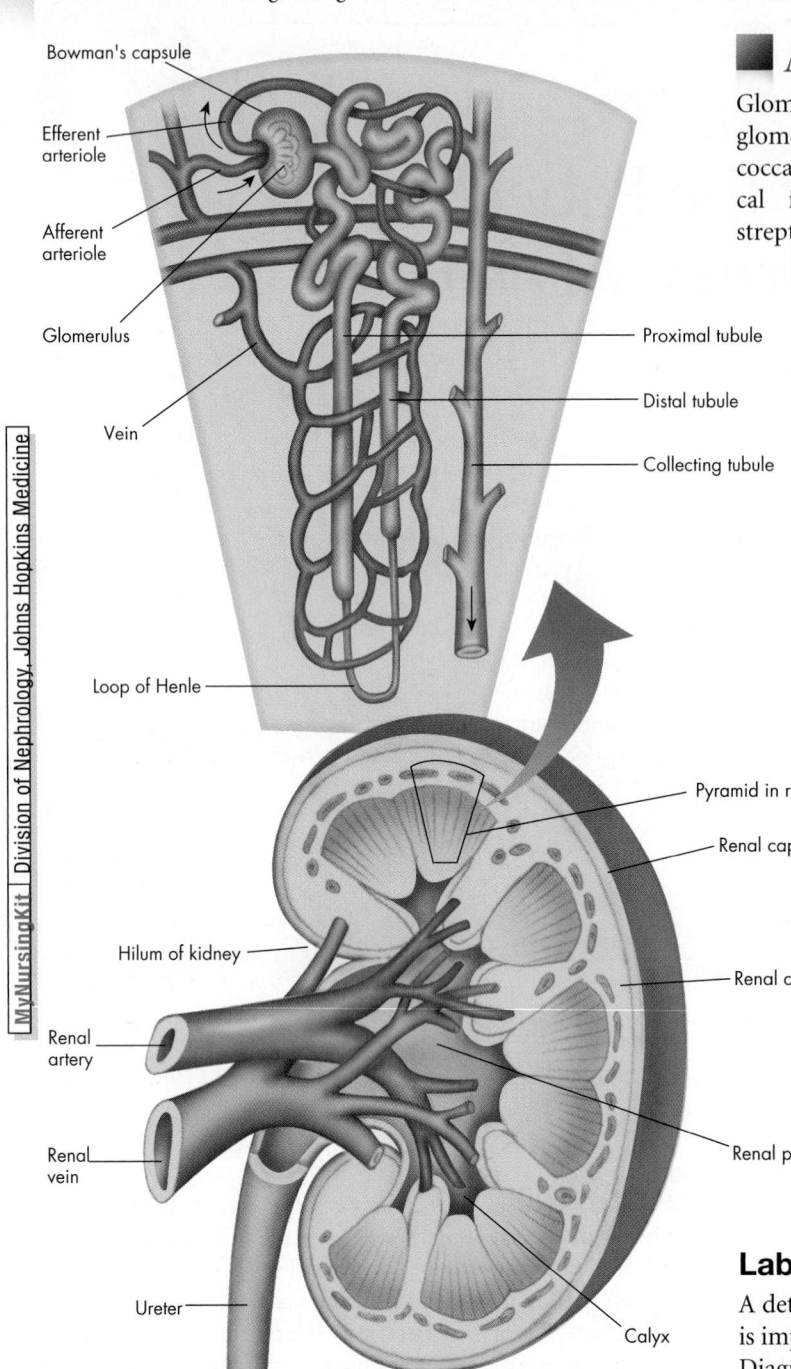

FIGURE 47–1 ■ The kidney and nephron.

DISORDERS OF THE KIDNEY

There are multiple diseases of the kidney, all of which cause loss of filtration capacity. Some are rapidly reversible and others cause permanent damage to the kidneys. When approximately two-thirds of filtration capacity is lost, symptoms of renal failure appear, with end-stage renal disease being the loss of approximately seven-eighths of filtration capacity. The goal of care for all the disease processes is to stop the source of damage to the kidneys and preserve what filtration capacity remains (Walser, 2004).

■ Acute Glomerulonephritis

Glomerulonephritis is a degenerative inflammation of the glomeruli and most commonly results from a previous streptococcal infection, usually of the respiratory tract. The streptococcal infection triggers antibody production against the streptococcal antigen. The antigen–antibody complexes become trapped in the glomeruli, causing an inflammatory response. Other causes can be immunoglobulin A (IgA) nephropathy, thin basement membrane disease, hereditary nephritis (Alport syndrome), lupus, and mesangial proliferative glomerulonephritis (Follin & Lenker, 2004; Post & Rose, 2008c). There is no pus formation associated with glomerulonephritis, nor are any bacteria found. As neutrophils collect in the inflamed loops of the glomeruli, the blood flow to the nephrons is reduced, and less filtration into Bowman's capsule occurs with less urine being formed. The glomeruli begin to degenerate along with the nephron, and the kidney tissue shrinks. The remaining functioning glomeruli become permeable, allowing red blood cells and albumin to appear in the urine. The disease is most common in young males, but can occur at any age (Follin & Lenker, 2004).

Acute glomerulonephritis usually occurs within 1 to 3 weeks after an untreated pharyngitis. Symptoms include mild edema; **oliguria**, decreased urine output of less than 400 milliliters in a 24-hour period; **proteinuria**, the presence of protein in the urine; **azotemia**, an increase in the blood urea nitrogen (BUN) caused when the kidneys are unable to excrete normally; **hematuria**, blood present in the urine; and fatigue.

Laboratory and Diagnostic Procedures

A detailed patient history and assessment of clinical symptoms is important for the diagnosis of acute glomerulonephritis. The Diagnostic Tests box presents tests that are helpful in supporting the diagnosis of acute glomerulonephritis.

Goodpasture's Syndrome

Another cause for acute or rapidly progressive glomerulonephritis is Goodpasture's (anti-GBM antibody) syndrome. In this disorder, circulating antibodies are directed against an antigen intrinsic to the glomerular basement membrane (GBM), resulting in acute glomerulonephritis. It is unknown what stimulus triggers the production of the circulating autoantibodies, and the disease is rare, with an estimated less than one case per million population (Pusey & Kalluri, 2008).

The syndrome presents similarly to other forms of rapidly progressive glomerulonephritis with relatively acute renal failure, urinalysis showing proteinuria, and a nephritic sediment characterized by white cells, dysmorphic red cells, and granular casts. What is different is that 60% to 70% of patients will also pre-

DIAGNOSTIC TESTS for Acute Glomerulonephritis

Test	Expected Abnormality	Rationale for Abnormality
Urinalysis	Presence of protein, red blood cells, white blood cells, and mixed cell casts	Increased permeability of the functioning glomeruli
Serum creatinine	Elevated serum creatinine	Impaired glomerular filtration
Urine creatinine clearance	Decreased	Impaired glomerular filtration
Serum antistreptolysin-O titer	Elevated	Recent streptococcal infection
Throat culture	May show group A beta-hemolytic streptococci	Recent streptococcal infection

sent with pulmonary involvement, usually consisting of alveolar hemorrhage (Pusey & Kalluri, 2008). The patients will complain of shortness of breath, cough, and some will have hemoptysis. Chest radiograph will exhibit pulmonary infiltrates. Goodpasture's syndrome is usually idiopathic, but it can occasionally follow pulmonary infections or be associated with pulmonary injury.

Goodpasture's syndrome should be suspected in any patient with acute glomerulonephritis, especially if the patient also exhibits rapid progression and pulmonary hemorrhage. To diagnose the syndrome, there must be demonstration of anti-GBM antibodies in either the serum or the kidney. Normally a renal biopsy is performed, as it provides information regarding the activity and chronicity of renal involvement.

The medical management of Goodpasture's syndrome is plasmapheresis combined with prednisone and cyclophosphamide (Kaplan, Appel, & Pusey, 2007). The plasmapheresis removes the circulating anti-GBM antibodies and other mediators of inflammation. The immunosuppressive medications minimize new antibody formation. This disorder is typically associated with severe renal injury and, if untreated, progresses quickly to end-stage renal failure.

Alport Syndrome

Alport syndrome, or hereditary nephritis, is a progressive glomerular disease that is genetically heterogeneous with X-linked, autosomal recessive and autosomal dominant variants (see Chapter 11 🔗). The prevalence of the disease is approximately 1 in 50,000 live births (Kashtan, 2007). The disorder occurs from mutations in genes encoding several members of the type IV collagen protein family, the predominant collagenous constituent of basement membranes. The secondary changes in glomerular basement membrane composition that occur due to the mutations predispose to the development of glomerulosclerosis. The histologic changes increase in severity with age.

Patients with Alport syndrome will initially present with asymptomatic microhematuria and episodes of gross hematuria. The plasma creatinine level and blood pressure are normal early in the disease, but hypertension, increasing proteinuria, and renal insufficiency occur with time. End-stage renal disease usually appears in males between age 16 and 35. In females, renal failure may be delayed until age 45 to 60. Patients may also exhibit several extrarenal manifestations including sensorineural hearing loss beginning in the high tones and progressing over time to frequencies in the range of conversational speech; and eye changes such as white or yellow flecking of the perimacular region of the

retina, corneal lesions such as posterior polymorphous dystrophy, and recurrent corneal erosions (Kashtan, 2007).

Diagnosis is usually suspected with a family history of renal failure and deafness. Up to 15% of cases have no family history of renal disease, and the diagnosis is made by renal biopsy with analysis of type IV collagen expression (Kashtan, 2007). There is no specific treatment for Alport syndrome. For patients who develop end-stage renal failure, dialysis or transplantation can be performed, although 3% to 4% of patients develop de novo anti-GBM antibody disease after transplantation (Kashtan, 2007).

Medical Management

The goals of treatment for acute glomerulonephritis are relief of symptoms and prevention of complications. Supportive care includes fluid restrictions, bed rest, dietary sodium restrictions, and correction of electrolyte imbalances. Medical treatment includes diuretics to reduce extracellular fluid and antihypertensives if needed. The Pharmacology Summary feature on page 1490 presents medications used to treat renal disorders.

◼ Nursing Management

Although patient care is primarily supportive, it is important to monitor the patient and watch for signs of acute renal failure. Critical assessments include strict monitoring of intake and output, daily weight, assessment of renal function through serum creatinine, blood urea nitrogen (BUN) levels, and urine creatinine clearance. Consult the dietary department to provide a high-caloric, low-protein, low-sodium, and low-potassium diet. Instruct the patient that follow-up examinations are necessary to detect renal failure. The patient should have his blood pressure, urine protein, and renal function assessed for at least 1 year following to detect recurrence. More detail will be given in the Nursing Management section for the patient with chronic glomerulonephritis later in this chapter.

Although the prognosis for acute glomerulonephritis is generally good, with normal kidney function returning after a period of time, repeated occurrences can lead to chronic glomerulonephritis.

◼ Chronic Glomerulonephritis

Chronic glomerulonephritis is a slow, progressive disease caused by inflammation of the glomeruli that results in sclerosis and scarring. This leaves the remaining glomeruli to do all of the filtration. An elevation of blood pressure is necessary for this to be accomplished; therefore, hypertension often accompanies this disease (Follin & Lenker, 2004).

Common causes of chronic glomerulonephritis include membranoproliferative glomerulonephritis, membranous glomerulopathy, focal segmental glomerulosclerosis, and rapidly progressive glomerulonephritis. Systemic disorders include lupus erythematosus, Goodpasture's syndrome, and diabetes mellitus.

Laboratory and Diagnostic Procedures

Chronic glomerulonephritis usually remains subclinical until the progressive phase begins, which may take years. At any time the disease may become progressive, and the patient will exhibit hypertension, proteinuria, and hematuria. As the disease continues to progress, the patient may exhibit azotemia, nausea, vomiting, pruritus, dyspnea, and fatigue. During the late stages of the disease, mild to severe edema and anemia may develop. The ensuing severe hypertension may cause the heart to hypertrophy and will lead to heart failure, which will accelerate the development of renal failure necessitating dialysis or potential for kidney transplantation. Tests that are helpful in the diagnosis of chronic glomerulonephritis are outlined in the Diagnostic Tests box.

Medical Management

The goals of treatment are control of hypertension with antihypertensives and a sodium restrictive diet; correction of electrolyte imbalances through dietary restrictions and supplements; and reduction of edema and the prevention of heart failure with diuretics. For end-stage glomerulonephritis, treatment may include antibiotics for urinary tract infections, dialysis for renal failure, and potential for transplantation. The Pharmacology Summary feature on page 1490 presents medications used to treat renal disorders.

Nursing Management

Because treatment is primarily supportive, close observation and monitoring of the patient's blood pressure, strict intake and output, and daily weight are necessary to evaluate fluid retention and possible fluid overload. Monitor blood work for signs of electrolyte and acid–base imbalances. Consult the dietary department to plan a low-sodium, high-caloric diet with adequate protein.

Assessment

The nurse should inquire as to the following during the nursing history:

- Amount and frequency of urination
- Headaches, swelling of the lower extremities
- Recent high-risk episodes such as an infection; cardiac, vascular, or biliary surgery; significant trauma; ingestion of aspirin, antibiotics, or other drugs; and allergic response to food, drugs, or a blood transfusion
- Pain in the flank area
- Fatigue or longer than usual sleep periods
- Muscle cramps or difficulty breathing during exercise.

The nurse should assess the patient for the following physical findings:

- Oliguria (less than 400 mL/day)
- Abnormal urine color, clarity, or smell
- Lethargy
- Normal or high blood pressure
- Dyspnea
- Fine crackles with auscultation of the lung fields.

Nursing Diagnoses

Nursing diagnoses for the patient with glomerulonephritis include:

- *Fluid Volume, Excess* related to sodium and water retention
- *Infection, Risk for*
- *Nutrition, Imbalanced: Less than Body Requirements* related to anorexia, nausea, and restricted dietary intake.

Planning

The overall goals for the patient with glomerulonephritis are to prevent further damage to the kidney and prevent renal failure.

Outcomes and Evaluation Parameters

Outcomes and evaluation parameters for the patient with glomerulonephritis include:

- The patient will maintain serum electrolyte levels within acceptable limits.
- The patient will be normovolemic, as exhibited by vital signs and hemodynamic readings within acceptable parameters,

DIAGNOSTIC TESTS for Chronic Glomerulonephritis

Test	Expected Abnormality	Rationale for Abnormality
Urinalysis	Presence of protein, red blood cells, and red blood cell casts	Impaired filtration
Serum creatinine	Rising serum creatinine	Indicates advanced renal insufficiency
Blood urea nitrogen (BUN)	Rising serum BUN	Indicates advanced renal insufficiency
X-ray or ultrasonography	Shows smaller kidneys	Atrophy of the kidney
Biopsy of the kidney	Identifies the underlying disease	Needed to guide therapy

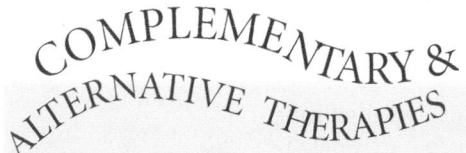

COMPLEMENTARY & ALTERNATIVE THERAPIES   Cranberries

Description:

Urinary-tract infections (UTIs) are very common, and recurrent UTIs have significant implications. Antibiotics are the most prevalent conventional treatment, but antimicrobial resistance and side effects result from frequent use. UTIs result from the colonization and adherence of uropathogens in the urinary tract. It has been shown that cranberries (*Vaccinium macrocarpon*) interfere with uropathogen adherence. Therefore, cranberries provide a promising alternative in the treatment and prevention of UTIs (Beerepoot et al., 2006).

Research Support:

Two randomized controlled trials involved 300 young women with recurrent UTIs who consumed cranberry juice or tablets daily. Results showed that daily use of cranberry reduced the relapse rate for UTI. Of 100 women who consumed cranberry juice or tablets daily for 1 year, 15 to 33 women prevented at least one urinary tract infection. Daily doses of cranberry ranged from 7.5 g of concentrate in 50 mL of water, to 750 mL of juice, to two tablets of concentrate. This same research paper examined two trials that involved elderly patients in hospitals or nursing homes who used cranberry-based products. Results from these studies showed a small reduction in UTI relapse frequency. However, it is important to note that cranberry juice or tablets may interact with warfarin, and may cause bleeding problems for patients taking warfarin concurrently ("Cranberry and Urinary Tract Infections," 2006).

Anthocyanins are components in cranberry that are believed to exert a therapeutic effect on UTIs. In order to determine the amount of absorption and excretion of anthocynanins, another study conducted by a Japanese research team analyzed urine samples from 11 healthy volunteers after they ingested cranberry juice. Volunteers consumed 200 mL of cranberry juice that contained 650.8 mcg of anthocyanins. Researchers collected urine samples within 24 h before and after consumption. Results showed that cranberry anthocyanins are well absorbed and excreted in human urine (Ohnishi et al., 2006).

Sweetened dried cranberries are popular food items available in most grocery stores. Another study determined whether consumption of this type of cranberry product elicited the same urinary antiadherence effect against uropathogens as previously demonstrated with cranberry juice. *Escherichia coli* is one of the most common uropathogens that causes UTI. Levels of *E. coli* were analyzed from urine samples of five women with culture-confirmed UTIs. Of the urine samples collected after the women consumed approximately 42.5 g of dried cranberries, one demonstrated 50% antiadherence activity, two demonstrated 25% activity, and two showed no increased activity. Although this was a very small study, results suggest that sweetened dried cranberries may offer similar therapeutic effects as cranberry juice (Greenberg, Newmann, & Howell, 2005).

References

Beerepoot, M. A., ter Riet, G., Verbon, A., Nys, S., de Reijke, T. M., Geerlings, S. E. (2006). Non-antibiotic prophylaxis for recurrent urinary-tract infections. *Nederlands Tijdschrift voor Geneeskunde, 150*(10), 541–544.

Cranberry and urinary tract infections: Slightly fewer episodes in young women, but watch out for interactions. (2006). *Prescrire International, 15*(84), 145–146.

Greenberg, J. A, Newmann, S. J., & Howell, A. B. (2005). Consumption of sweetened dried cranberries versus unsweetened raisins for inhibition of uropathogenic Escherichia coli adhesion in human urine: A pilot study. *Journal of Alternative and Complementary Medicine, 11*(5), 875–878.

Ohnishi, R., Ito, H., Kasajima, N., Kaneda, M., Kariyama, R., Kumon, H., et al. (2006). Urinary excretion of anthocyanins in humans after cranberry juice ingestion. *Bioscience, Biotechnology, and Biochemistry, 70*(7), 1681–1687.

---

clear lung sounds, minimal peripheral edema, normal skin turgor, and maintenance of weight gain and loss.

- The patient will not show signs of infection, as exhibited by a normal temperature, clean, dry access sites for lines and catheters, negative cultures, and completion of the antibiotic regime.

- The patient will be able to understand and agree to comply with dietary modifications and activity restrictions.

Interventions and Rationales

Nursing interventions and rationales for the patient with glomerulonephritis include:

- Continually assess for signs of infection. Document and report any signs to the health care team. *Uremic syndrome (which may occur) suppresses normal cell metabolism and immune response, placing the patient at greater risk for infection.*

- Provide skin care and use preventive measures to protect against shearing or decubitus formation. Turn the patient every 2 hours, maintain wrinkle-free linens, and use protective pads to bony areas. Provide site care and dressing changes for intravenous lines according to hospital policy. *Skin integrity is compromised due to the edema and accumulation of waste products in the tissues because of the altered metabolism.*

Site care will assist to prevent accumulation of moisture, which serves as growth media for infective organisms.

- Collaborate with the health care team to implement a high-carbohydrate diet that provides small amounts of high-quality proteins; limits fluids, sodium, and potassium; and includes vitamin supplements. *A high-carbohydrate diet supplies calories for energy needs; limiting proteins prevents protein catabolism, as the kidneys are unable to excrete the waste products at this time; fluids and sodium are limited to prevent volume overload, while potassium is limited because the kidneys are unable to excrete it.*

- Administer diuretics as needed and ordered. Document administration and results. *Diuretics may be given to reduce fluid overload and increase fluid volume through the kidneys in an attempt to prevent acute renal failure.*

Evaluation

The patient will remain free of infection, maintain fluid and electrolyte balance, and maintain her weight while following the diet regimen. Topics that should be addressed with patients who have glomerulonephritis and/or their families before discharge are described in the Patient Teaching & Discharge Priorities box (p. 1468).

Pyelonephritis

Pyelonephritis, one of the most common renal diseases, is a sudden inflammation of the kidney and renal pelvis caused by bacteria (Follin & Lenker, 2004). The inflammation is **suppurative** (associated with the formation of pus). The bacteria that usually cause pyelonephritis are normal intestinal and fecal floras that grow readily in urine. Pyelonephritis is more common in women because they have a shorter urethra, and the proximity of the meatus to the vagina and rectum allows the bacteria to reach the urethra and bladder more easily. The most common causative bacteria are *Escherichia coli*, followed by *Proteus, Pseudomonas, Staphylococcus aureus*, and *Streptococcus faecalis* (Hager & Mills, 2008).

The infection usually starts in the bladder and then spreads to the kidney through the ureters. The bacteria can also be introduced by instrumentation such as catheterization, cystoscopy, or urologic surgery; by bacteria translocated by the blood, as in septicemia or endocarditis; and from lymphatic infections. Risk factors for increased incidence of pyelonephritis are included in the Risk Factors box.

Laboratory and Diagnostic Procedures

The signs and symptoms of pyelonephritis include urinary urgency, frequency, and burning; dysuria; nocturia; and hematuria. The urine may appear cloudy and have the odor of ammonia or fish. Due to the inflammatory response to the bacteria, the patient usually experiences high fever, chills, flank pain, and fatigue. If the bacterial infection is not severe, the symptoms may subside within a few days, but a residual bacterial infection is common and may cause recurrence of symptoms if untreated. Tests that are helpful in the diagnosis of pyelonephritis are listed in the Diagnostic Tests box.

Medical Management

Treatment consists of identification of the infecting organism and treatment with the appropriate antibiotics. Intravenous antibiotics are often used initially to control the growth of bacteria. Commonly used antibiotics include sulfa drugs, cephalosporins, amoxicillin, levofloxacin, and ciprofloxacin. If the patient is experiencing urinary urgency and frequency, urinary analgesics such as phenazopyridine are appropriate. The Pharmacology Summary feature on page 1490 presents medications used to treat renal disorders. See

RISK FACTORS for Pyelonephritis

- Inability to empty the bladder. Examples include neurogenic bladder, urinary obstruction due to tumor, kidney stone, prostatic hyperplasia, or urinary stasis.
- Being female due to the proximity of the urinary meatus to the vagina and rectum. Females also lack the antibacterial prostatic secretions produced in males.
- Sexually active women due to the increased risk of bacterial contamination from intercourse.
- Pregnant women. Approximately 5% develop asymptomatic bacteriuria and, if untreated, approximately 40% develop pyelonephritis (Follin & Lenker, 2004).
- Diabetes due to the development of neurogenic bladder, which causes incomplete emptying and urinary stasis. Also, glucose in the urine may support bacterial growth.
- Compromised renal function from other renal diseases increases the susceptibility.

The bacteria that reach the kidney create colonies of infection within 24 to 48 hours. Abscesses frequently form and when they rupture, pus enters the renal pelvis and appears in the urine. Untreated, the abscesses can continue to form and fuse until the entire kidney is filled with pus. If this continues, renal failure occurs and uremia develops. If the infection is less severe, the kidney can heal but will form scar tissue that tends to contract and cause the kidney to shrink and become granular, making it less efficient.

Complementary & Alternative Therapies feature (p. 1467) for nonpharmaceutical adjuncts for prevention of infection.

 If the patient is pregnant, be sure that the prescribed antibiotic is safe to use during pregnancy.

If the infection was caused by an obstruction, surgery may be necessary to relieve the obstruction.

Nursing Management

If the patient has a high fever, administer antipyretics. Encourage the patient to drink enough fluids to maintain a urine output of more than 2,000 mL/day to empty the bladder of contaminated

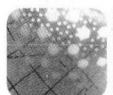

PATIENT TEACHING & DISCHARGE PRIORITIES for Glomerulonephritis

Need	Teaching
Nutrition	Have patient/family work with dietitian to plan a low-sodium, high-caloric diet with adequate protein.
Medications	Stress to the patient the importance of taking prescribed antihypertensives as scheduled, even if patient is feeling better.
	Suggest that diuretics be taken in the morning to decrease disruption of sleep due to need to void.
Skin care	Stress to the patient the importance of good skin care, as the pruritus and edema may cause skin breakdown.
	Teach the patient how to assess ankle edema.
Avoidance of continued infections and scarring	Stress to patient/family the importance of reporting signs of infection, particularly urinary tract infection, and to avoid contact with people who have infections.
	Stress importance of follow-up appointments to assess renal function.

DIAGNOSTIC TESTS for Pyelonephritis

Test	Expected Abnormality	Rationale for Abnormality
Urinalysis	Pyuria: pus in urine; leukocytes appear singly, in clumps, and in casts.	Rupture of abscesses, allowing pus to empty into the urine.
	Low specific gravity and osmolality.	Decreased ability to concentrate urine.
Urine culture	Bacteriuria: more than 100,000 organisms/mcL of urine.	Bacterial growth in urine.
X-ray films of the kidneys, ureters, and bladder (KUB)	May reveal cause of obstruction: renal calculi, tumor, or cysts.	Obstruction causes urinary retention and stasis, increasing risk for infection.

urine but not to drink more than 3 liters of fluid, as that may decrease the effectiveness of the antibiotics. When collecting urine for urinalysis and culture, teach the proper technique for a clean-catch urine specimen, and send the culture within 30 minutes of collection to prevent overgrowth of the bacteria.

Assessment

When taking a patient history, the nurse should consider the following: age; sex; whether a female patient is sexually active; whether the patient has had a recent procedure such as catheterization, cystoscopy, or urologic surgery; and whether the patient has a history of neurogenic bladder. Physical assessment findings may include fever (usually 38.9°C or higher), burning with urination, general fatigue, hematuria, flank pain, and urinary frequency and urgency.

Nursing Diagnoses

Nursing diagnoses that apply to pyelonephritis include:

- *Infection, Risk for* related to insufficient knowledge to avoid exposure to pathogens, neurogenic bladder, or urinary obstruction
- *Urinary Incontinence, Urge* due to infection
- *Fatigue* due to inflammation.

Planning

The goals for the patient with pyelonephritis are to treat the infection and prevent further infections.

Outcomes and Evaluation Parameters

Outcomes and evaluation parameters include:

- The patient is free from infection, as exhibited by follow-up urine culture that is free of growth.
- The patient does not experience urgency or urinary urge incontinence.

- The patient does not suffer fatigue, as exhibited by the ability to do normal activities without tiring.

Interventions and Rationales

Nursing interventions and rationales for the patient with pyelonephritis include:

- The nurse should teach the patient the importance of completing the patient's prescribed antibiotic therapy and the need to drink enough fluids to produce more than 2,000 milliliters of urine per day. *Stopping antibiotics early, even when symptoms subside, may allow the infectious agent to remain. Drinking plenty of fluid helps to empty the bladder of contaminated urine.*
- The nurse should teach the patient to plan activities in short increments to allow for rest time. *Planning activities to allow for rest periods in between will prevent further fatigue.*
- If the patient is having urinary urgency and burning with urination, administer urinary analgesics. *Urinary analgesics relieve the pain of burning, frequency, and urgency arising from irritation of urinary tract mucosa.*

Evaluation

The patient should have a normal temperature, have no burning or frequency with urination, and have no growth on culture of the urine.

Topics that should be addressed with patients who have pyelonephritis and/or their families before discharge are outlined in the Patient Teaching & Discharge Priorities box.

 Hydronephrosis

If an obstruction occurs in the ureter, bladder, or urethra, the kidney can become extremely dilated with urine. The most common

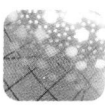

PATIENT TEACHING & DISCHARGE PRIORITIES for Pyelonephritis

Need	Teaching
Prevention	Instruct female patients to wipe the perineum from front to back after defecation.
	Instruct female patients to void after sexual intercourse to flush the bladder and urethra.
Antibiotic therapy	Instruct the patient to complete the prescribed antibiotics even after symptoms subside.
Follow-up treatment	Encourage follow-up care for high-risk patients.
	Teach patients the signs and symptoms of infection: cloudy urine, burning with urination, urgency, frequency, and fever.

causes of obstruction are an enlarged prostate gland, urethral strictures, and renal calculi. Other causes may include stricture or stenosis of the bladder outlet or ureter, abdominal tumors, tumors of the ureter and bladder, blood clots, neurogenic bladder, and congenital abnormalities. If the site of the obstruction is the urethra or bladder, then both kidneys are usually affected. If the obstruction occurs in one ureter, then the hydronephrosis will be unilateral. When the obstruction is in the urethra, distal to the bladder, first the bladder dilates with urine acting as a buffer, which delays the hydronephrosis.

Hydronephrosis is most commonly a chronic condition with slow changes in the kidney that occur with pain or other symptoms. If the obstruction is severe and prolonged, fibrotic changes occur in the kidney, and there is a loss of function of the nephrons that are involved. The finding of hydronephrosis is often accidental, occurring when a radiograph or ultrasound of the abdomen is ordered for another reason.

Laboratory and Diagnostic Procedures

Signs and symptoms of hydronephrosis vary depending on the cause of the obstruction and the extent of the blockage. Symptoms may be as mild as slight discomfort and slightly decreased urine flow. Other patients may experience severe, colicky renal pain or flank pain that radiates to the groin. If the hydronephrosis is unilateral, the pain is only on the affected side. If infection occurs due to stagnation of urine, then the patient will develop fever, nausea, and pain on urination. Tests that are helpful in the diagnosis of hydronephrosis are presented in the Diagnostic Tests box.

Medical Management

Treatment consists of identifying and treating the cause of the obstruction in order to preserve renal function and prevent infection. Removal of the obstruction may include dilation for stricture of the urethra, prostatectomy for prostatic hypertrophy, or surgical removal of calculi or tumor. Inoperable obstructions may require drainage of the kidney using a nephrostomy tube.

Nephrostomy Tube

Nephrostomy tubes are placed percutaneously under fluoroscopy or surgically. The tube is placed through the flank area into the renal pelvis and secured to a closed drainage system to allow drainage via gravity flow. Preprocedure, several precau-

tions are taken: A broad-spectrum antibiotic is given to prevent infection; coagulopathy should be corrected; and uncontrolled hypertension should be corrected. It is important to assess the tube for kinks or clots that may impede drainage. If the tube becomes dislodged, the fistula that was created closes quickly, and it may be impossible to insert another catheter in as little as 30 minutes. Nursing management of the patient that has had a nephrostomy tube placed includes:

- Assess for complications such as bleeding at the site, hematuria, fistula formation, and infection.
- Assess skin at nephrostomy site for signs of inflammation, infection, bleeding, leakage of urine, and skin irritation.
- Assess tube patency. If obstructed, the patient will complain of pain and pressure.
- Use aseptic technique when replacing dressings.
- Encourage oral intake of fluids to promote flushing of the kidney and nephrostomy tube.
- Never clamp a nephrostomy tube.
- Never irrigate a nephrostomy tube without specific orders.

▇ Nursing Management

If the hydronephrosis has already affected renal function, a diet low in protein, sodium, and potassium is indicated to prevent progression of renal failure prior to surgery. Refer to the earlier Nursing Management section for the patient with glomerulonephritis. Prior to the patient's diagnostic tests, inquire regarding allergies to dye or foods that contain iodine such as shellfish. Hydronephrosis can be very painful; administer pain medication as needed. Topics that should be addressed with patients who have hydronephrosis and/or their families before discharge are presented in the Patient Teaching & Discharge Priorities box.

▇ Polycystic Kidney Disease

Polycystic kidney disease is a congenital anomaly that is characterized by multiple clusters of fluid-filled cysts that grossly enlarge the kidneys. The cysts are dilated kidney tubules that do not open into the renal pelvis. As the cysts enlarge and fuse, they usually be-

DIAGNOSTIC TESTS for Hydronephrosis

Test	Expected Abnormality	Rationale for Abnormality
Intravenous pyelogram (IVP)	Identification of stricture or obstruction.	Decrease in or cessation of flow.
	Dilation of the renal pelvis.	Inability to drain renal pelvis.
Renal ultrasonography	Identification of fluid accumulation.	Inability of urine to drain from renal pelvis.
	Identification of area of obstruction.	Stricture, tumor, or calculi will be visible.
Renal function studies:		
Blood urea nitrogen (BUN)	Increased.	Decreased filtration.
Serum creatinine	May rise slightly.	Nephron function loss.
Creatinine clearance	Decreased.	Decreased glomerular function.

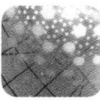

PATIENT TEACHING & DISCHARGE PRIORITIES for Hydronephrosis

Need	Teaching
Prevention	Teach older men, especially those with prostatic hypertrophy, to have routine checkups to monitor progression. Also instruct them to recognize and report symptoms of hydronephrosis, such as colicky pain, blood in the urine, or urinary tract infections.
Nephrostomy tube care	Instruct patient/family in the care of the nephrostomy tube. Teach the importance of checking for bleeding and patency. Stress importance of immediate notification of the health care provider if the tube becomes dislodged.
Signs and symptoms of postoperative complications	Instruct patient/family during hospitalization and at home after discharge.
	Instruct patient/family to report any sign of impending hemorrhage and shock: tachycardia; cold, clammy skin; and a feeling of anxiousness or decreased level of consciousness.
Antibiotic therapy	If there was concurrent infection, instruct the patient to complete the prescribed antibiotics even after symptoms subside.

come infected. The cysts compress and gradually replace the functioning renal tissue, leading to fatal uremia. The disease appears in two forms, infantile or adult, with both types affecting males and females equally (Follin & Lenker, 2004; Hager & Mills, 2008).

Infantile polycystic kidney disease is inherited as an autosomal recessive trait and may cause stillbirth or early neonatal death. If the infant survives, he usually develops fatal renal, respiratory, or heart failure by the age of 2.

Adult polycystic kidney disease is inherited as an autosomal dominant trait and affects 1 of 500 to 1,000 individuals (see Chapter 11 ⊙). The disease usually becomes symptomatic between ages 30 and 50 (Hager & Mills, 2008). This is because, in the adult form, renal deterioration not only is more gradual but also progresses to fatal uremia. Unless the patient receives treatment with dialysis, a kidney transplant, or both, once uremic symptoms develop the disease is usually fatal within 4 years.

Laboratory and Diagnostic Procedures

Adult polycystic kidney disease may go undiagnosed for some time because the symptoms are nonspecific, such as hypertension, polyuria, and urinary tract infections. As the disease progresses, the patient will develop signs and symptoms related to the enlarging kidneys. These include lumbar pain, swollen or tender abdomen, and abdominal pain that is exacerbated by exertion and relieved by lying down. Signs and symptoms that

manifest in the advanced stages are recurrent hematuria, retroperitoneal bleeding from a ruptured cyst, proteinuria, and abdominal pain caused by ureteral passage of clots or calculi.

The diagnosis of polycystic kidney disease is made from both family history and examination revealing grossly enlarged and palpable kidneys. Tests that are helpful in the diagnosis of polycystic kidney disease are outlined in the Diagnostic Tests box.

Medical Management

The goal of treatment is to preserve renal function and prevent infectious complications. Adequate control of hypertension is necessary to help prevent rapid deterioration in function. As the disease progresses, the patient will require dialysis. The Pharmacology Summary feature on page 1490 presents medications used to treat renal disorders.

■ Nursing Management

Young adult patients should be encouraged to seek genetic counseling. Approximately half of the children born to a patient with polycystic kidney disease will have the disease (Walser, 2004). Because the disease is progressive, comprehensive patient teaching and emotional support are extremely important. For more detail, refer to the Nursing Management section for the patient with acute renal failure later in this chapter. Topics that

DIAGNOSTIC TESTS for Polycystic Kidney Disease

Test	Expected Abnormality	Rationale for Abnormality
Ultrasonography, tomography, and radioisotope scans	Enlargement of the kidneys and cysts.	Enlargement is caused by the fluid-filled cysts that displace the renal tissue.
Retrograde ureteropyelography	Enlarged kidneys with elongation of the renal pelvis, flattening of the calyces, and indentations.	Enlargement is caused by the fluid-filled cysts that displace the renal tissue.
Urinalysis	Presence of protein, red blood cells, and red blood cell casts.	Impaired filtration.
Serum creatinine	Rising serum creatinine.	Indicates advanced renal insufficiency.
Blood urea nitrogen (BUN)	Rising serum BUN.	Indicates advanced renal insufficiency.

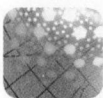

PATIENT TEACHING & DISCHARGE PRIORITIES for Polycystic Kidney Disease

Need	Teaching
Asymptomatic stage	Monitor kidney function carefully: • Obtain a creatinine clearance test every 6 months. • Obtain a urine culture every 6 months.
Follow-up care	Patient/family at home: • Monitor filtration capacity and progression of the disease. • If infection detected, patient should receive antibiotic treatment even if she is asymptomatic.

should be addressed with patients who have polycystic kidney disease and/or their families before discharge are presented in the Patient Teaching & Discharge Priorities box.

Renal Infarction

An occlusion of a renal blood vessel results in renal infarction and an area of necrosis in one or both kidneys. The location of the infarction depends on the site of the occlusion. In approximately 75% of infarctions, the vessel that becomes occluded is the renal artery. The embolic event is secondary to a predisposing cardiovascular disease such as mitral stenosis, atrial fibrillation, microthrombi in the left ventricle, rheumatic valvular disease, endocarditis, or a recent myocardial infarction. Less common causes include atherosclerosis of the renal vasculature, thrombus from flank trauma, sickle cell anemia, and scleroderma (Follin & Lenker, 2004).

The degree of occlusion and rate of decreased blood flow to the kidney determine whether the event will be acute or become chronic as the narrowing progresses. Signs and symptoms include severe upper abdominal pain or constant flank pain with tenderness, fever, nausea, and vomiting. Renovascular hypertension may occur several days after infarction due to the reduced blood flow, which stimulates the renin-angiotensin mechanism.

Renal infarction may also arise from renal vein thrombosis (RVT). A spontaneous renal vein thrombosis is rare in patients who are ambulatory but has been reported in patients with trauma, women taking oral contraceptives, patients with hypovolemia or dehydration, and those with inherited procoagulant defects (Radhakrishnan, 2008). RVT can be unilateral or bilateral, is usually chronic, and may extend into the inferior vena cava. Pulmonary embolus may be the first clue that the patient

has chronic RVT. Acute RVT typically presents with flank pain, microscopic or gross hematuria, a marked elevation in serum lactate dehydrogenase, and an increase in the size of the affected kidney on radiographic study. If the acute RVT is bilateral, the patient may present with acute renal failure.

Laboratory and Diagnostic Procedures

Any patient with predisposing cardiovascular disease, flank trauma, sickle cell anemia, or scleroderma who develops typical signs and symptoms should be further evaluated for renal infarction. Renal vascular angiography or venogram will show the exact location and extent of obstruction, but it is a high-risk procedure due to the adverse effects of the dye load on renal function. Tests that are helpful in the diagnosis of renal infarction are listed in the Diagnostic Tests box.

Medical Management

Therapies to remove the occlusion include administration of intra-arterial streptokinase, lysis of blood clots, catheter embolectomy, and heparin therapy. If the infarcted area becomes infected or is very large, causing hypertension, surgical repair of the occlusion or removal of the kidney may be necessary.

Nursing Management

It is important to monitor the patient's intake and output, daily weight, and electrolyte levels to assess renal function. Encourage the patient to schedule follow-up appointments to monitor return of renal function. Refer to the Nursing Management section for the patient with acute renal failure later in this chapter.

DIAGNOSTIC TESTS for Renal Infarction

Test	Expected Abnormality	Rationale for Abnormality
Urinalysis	Presence of protein, red blood cells, and red blood cell casts	Impaired filtration
Serum enzyme levels	Elevated lactate dehydrogenase (LD), alkaline phosphatase, and aspartate aminotransferase	Result of tissue destruction
Excretory urography	Reveals diminished or absent excretion of contrast	Indicates diminished or nonfunctioning kidney
Isotopic renal scan	Reveals absent or reduced blood flow to kidneys	Indicates the area and extent of occlusion

Renal Carcinoma

Carcinoma of the kidney causes enlargement of the organ and eventually destroys it. Approximately 80% to 85% of all primary renal cell carcinomas originate within the renal cortex. Transitional cell carcinomas of the renal pelvis account for 8%, with other parenchymal epithelial tumors, collecting duct tumors, and renal sarcomas occurring infrequently (Atkins, 2006b). Renal carcinoma represents approximately 2% of total cancer incidence and mortality (Atkins, 2006b). The Risk Factors box presents the risk factors that have been associated with renal carcinoma. The influence of genetic disorders on the risk of developing renal carcinoma is outlined in the Genetic Considerations box.

Laboratory and Diagnostic Procedures

Many patients are asymptomatic until the disease is advanced, and when diagnosed, 25% have either metastases or advanced disease (Atkins, 2006a). The most common presenting symptoms are hematuria, pain, abdominal mass, and weight loss. There is an increasing amount of patients who are diagnosed as an incidental finding of a radiologic procedure performed for another indication. Metastasis to other organs often occurs, with common metastatic sites being the lungs, lymph nodes, liver, bones, and the brain.

Medical Management

Treatment consists of surgical removal. Renal carcinoma is radiation resistant, so this form of treatment is used only if the cancer has spread to the perinephric region or lymph nodes. Chemotherapy has not been shown to be effective against renal cancer. Biotherapy using lymphokine-activated killer cells with recombinant interleukin-2 has shown promise but also causes adverse reactions (Hager & Mills, 2008). Refer to Chapter 64 for the care of the patient with cancer.

Nursing Management

This nursing management section pertains to the immediate preoperative and postoperative care for the patient undergoing a nephrectomy.

Assessment

During the health history, the nurse should focus on:

- Any history of comorbidities such as diabetes, hypertension, or vascular disease
- Any concerns or fears the patient may have regarding normal kidney function after the surgery
- Concerns regarding activity and diet restrictions after the surgery
- Patient's level of weight loss, nausea or vomiting, and fatigue.

During the physical assessment, the nurse should focus on:

- Signs of fluid overload: peripheral edema and distended neck veins
- Hypertension
- Signs of hypovolemia: decreased blood pressure; pale, cool skin; agitation
- Adventitious breath sounds
- Dysuria, hematuria, oliguria, or polyuria
- Skin color, temperature, and turgor.

Nursing Diagnoses

The primary nursing diagnoses for the patient undergoing nephrectomy are:

- *Knowledge, Deficient* related to the procedure
- *Pain, Acute*
- *Fluid Volume, Imbalanced, Risk for*
- *Gas Exchange, Impaired*

Planning

The overall goals for the patient undergoing nephrectomy include understanding of the procedure and postoperative plan

---

RISK FACTORS for Renal Carcinoma

- Cigarette smoking. Smoking increases the risk of renal carcinoma by twofold.
- Occupational exposure to toxic compounds. Exposure to compounds such as cadmium, asbestos, and petroleum by-products has been suggested to increase the risk of renal carcinoma. The exposure may be associated with mutations in genes associated with the pathogenesis of renal carcinoma.
- Obesity. There appears to be a direct correlation between obesity and an increased risk of developing renal carcinoma.
- Acquired cystic disease of the kidney. Patients on dialysis who develop polycystic kidney disease have been estimated to have a risk of developing renal carcinoma that is 30 times greater than that of the general population. The cancer typically develops after 8 to 10 years of dialysis.

Source: Atkins, M. (2006b). *Epidemiology, pathology, and pathogenesis of renal cell carcinoma.* Retrieved April 16, 2007, from http://www.uptodate.com

---

GENETIC CONSIDERATIONS for Renal Carcinoma

Patients with certain inherited disorders show an increased risk of developing renal carcinoma (see Chapter 11). Included are hereditary papillary renal cancer, characterized by a predisposition to development of multiple, bilateral, papillary renal tumors. The inherited papillary cancers usually occur late in life with most patients being in their 70s. Hereditary leiomyoma, or Reed syndrome, is characterized by cutaneous leiomyomas (benign soft tissue neoplasms that arise from smooth muscle), uterine fibroids, and renal carcinomas that may be single, multiple, and bilateral. The renal tumors are aggressive and may metastasize. Von Hippel-Lindau syndrome is an autosomal dominant disorder that has a predisposition to neoplasm. Approximately one-third of patients with this disease develop renal cell carcinoma. Birt-Hogg-Dube syndrome is characterized by skin lesions that develop on the skin of the head and neck, lung cysts with spontaneous pneumothoraces, and a predisposition to kidney neoplasms.

Source: Atkins, M. (2006b). *Epidemiology, pathology, and pathogenesis of renal cell carcinoma.* Retrieved April 16, 2007, from http://www.uptodate.com

(cough and deep breathe, use of incentive spirometer, etc.), control of postoperative pain, and prevention of postoperative complications.

Outcomes and Evaluation Parameters

The major outcomes and evaluation parameters for the patient undergoing nephrectomy are:

- Patient is able to verbalize understanding of operative procedure.
- Patient is able to demonstrate ability to cough and deep breathe, splint the incision site, use the incentive spirometer, and perform leg exercises.
- Postoperative pain is controlled as evidenced by patient rating pain low on a 0–10 scale. Patient maintains vital signs within normal limits.
- The patient's fluid and electrolytes will be balanced as exhibited by a urine output greater than 30 mL/hr initially and 60 mL/hr or greater by time of discharge. Electrolytes will be within normal limits.
- The patient will maintain adequate oxygenation as evidenced by unlabored respirations, clear breath sounds in all lobes, and arterial blood gases within normal limits.
- The patient will have normal bowel function as evidenced by normal, active bowel sounds, ability to eat a regular diet, and ability to have a regular bowel movement.

Interventions and Rationales

Nursing interventions and rationales for the patient undergoing nephrectomy include:

- Discuss with the patient where the incision will be made, if the patient will have a chest tube or any drains, and the effects of positioning after surgery. *Knowledge of what to expect postoperatively will decrease the patient's fear and anxiety, and increase her ability to participate in her postoperative care.*
- Teach the patient regarding postoperative pain management. Let the patient know whether he will have patient-controlled analgesia or epidural infusion. Discuss potential adverse effects and the importance of requesting pain medication before the pain becomes severe. *The patient will be able to better control his pain with an understanding of the plan.*
- Protect the remaining kidney by maintaining adequate hydration. Monitor urine output and specific gravity. Minimize the use of nephrotoxic medications. *Preservation of the remaining kidney is paramount. Appropriate hydration preserves renal function and the removal of waste products. Use of nephrotoxic drugs may damage the remaining kidney.*
- Assist the patient to perform incentive spirometry, encourage the patient to cough and deep breathe, splint the incision site, promote early ambulation, and check pulmonary status frequently. *Atelectasis is an inherent risk of general anesthesia. Also, the patient with a flank incision is at risk because the intercostal muscles were spread and the 12th rib may be removed. Pain involved with this incision limits deep breathing. If atelectasis develops and is not treated, it can lead to pneumonia.*
- Encourage early and frequent ambulation. Encourage fluids and progression of diet as tolerated. Assess the abdomen for distention and bowel sounds. Monitor nasogastric tube drainage. *Manipulation of the bowel during surgery increases the risk of paralytic ileus.*

Evaluation

The patient's pain will be controlled postoperatively, respiratory effort will be unlabored, and breath sounds will be clear in all lobes. The patient will be able to advance her diet and have return of normal bowel function. The patient will be able to take adequate food and fluid orally and will maintain normal fluid and electrolyte imbalance.

Acute Tubular Necrosis

Acute tubular necrosis (ATN) results from damage to the renal tubular epithelium from a nephrotoxic or ischemic injury. ATN is the most common form of intrinsic renal failure and accounts for the majority of acute renal failure admissions to the hospital (Urden et al., 2006). The damage to the epithelium prevents normal concentration of urine, filtration of waste products, regulation of acid–base balance, electrolyte hemostatsis, and fluid balance.

The common causes of ATN can be divided into two categories:

1. Toxic injury is the result of damage from nephrotoxins that cause uniform, widespread damage. Nephrotoxins are usually drugs, chemical agents, or bacterial endotoxins. Sources of nephrotoxins include:
   - Rhabdomyolysis
   - Nephrotoxic medications: cephalosporins, analgesics containing phenacetin, antineoplastic agents, aminoglycosides
   - Contrast media
   - Insecticides, fungicides
   - Methanol
   - Heavy metals: arsenic, mercury, lead, uranium
   - Phencyclidine (PCP).

2. Ischemic injury occurs when perfusion to the kidneys is severely reduced. The damage to the tubular membrane is irregular and causes cast formation. Causes of ischemic injury include:
   - Hemorrhage
   - Severe dehydration
   - Shock: hypovolemic, septic, cardiogenic
   - Crush injuries
   - Transfusion reaction
   - Obstetric complications: severe toxemia, placenta previa, abruptio placentae, uterine rupture.

Laboratory and Diagnostic Procedures

ATN commonly occurs in patients that are debilitated or critically ill. Therefore, it can be difficult to diagnose in the early stages because effects of the primary disease or injury may mask the symptoms. The first sign may be decreased urine output, although only 50% of patients become oliguric (Urden et al., 2006). Oliguria is more common in ischemic damage and carries a higher mortality rate when present.

Accurate diagnosis tends to occur in the advanced stage, as the glomerular filtration is greatly reduced leading to increased uremia, electrolyte abnormalities, and metabolic acidosis. Tests that are helpful in the diagnosis of acute tubular necrosis are outlined in the Diagnostic Tests box.

Medical Management

The acute phase of ATN often requires total support of renal function with hemodialysis. Initially treatment may be the infusion of large volumes of fluid in conjunction with administration of a diuretic to flush the tubules of cellular casts and debris, but the patient must be carefully monitored for fluid overload. Infection is the leading cause of death in patients with ATN (Follin & Lenker, 2004), so the patient must be assessed frequently for any signs of fever and the infection treated with the appropriate antibiotics. The Pharmacology Summary feature on page 1490 presents medications used to treat renal disorders.

With appropriate treatment, renal function will slowly return with the glomerular filtration rate at 70% to 80% of normal within 1 to 2 years. Although most patients recover normal renal function, 33% will have residual renal insufficiency, and approximately 5% will require ongoing hemodialysis (Urden et al., 2006).

Nursing Management

Maintenance of fluid balance is important in the patient with ATN, with fluid overload a common complication of therapy. Therefore it is important to accurately document daily weight, intake and output, including loss from wound drainage, and dialysis balances. Maintain electrolyte balance by monitoring laboratory results, enforcing dietary restriction of foods containing sodium and potassium, and assessing for potassium content in prescribed medications such as penicillin.

The debilitated patient is vulnerable to infection, and because infection is the leading cause of death in patients with ATN, use of aseptic technique is paramount. Monitor for fever, chills, delayed wound healing, and flank pain. Encourage the patient to cough and deep breathe to prevent pulmonary complications. For a more detailed review of additional interventions,

refer to the Nursing Management section for the patient with acute renal failure later in this chapter.

Renal Failure

Renal failure is the inability of the kidneys to clear the blood of the waste products of protein metabolism: urea and creatinine. Urea, an end product of protein catabolism resulting from the breakdown of ammonia in the liver, is the primary method of nitrogen excretion from the body. If the body is unable to excrete the urea, it accumulates and toxicity develops.

Acute Renal Failure

Acute renal failure (ARF) develops suddenly and can usually be reversed with treatment, but if the condition causing the failure is not treated, the patient will progress to end-stage renal disease, uremic syndrome, and death. The causes of acute renal failure can be classified into three categories: (1) prerenal, (2) intrinsic, and (3) postrenal. Chart 47–1 (p. 1476) lists causes within the three categories. The mortality rate remains high for acute renal failure, with rates ranging from 25% to 90%. Influencing factors include the increasing age of patients and the comorbid conditions that accompany aging, such as vascular disease and diabetes (Dirkes & Hodge, 2007).

Laboratory and Diagnostic Procedures

Acute renal failure is a sudden and critical event with early signs being oliguria, azotemia, or **anuria**, a total loss of urine production. As the patient becomes more uremic, he will develop systemic signs and symptoms including headache, irritability, confusion, nausea, vomiting, diarrhea, pruritus, pallor, purpura; hypotension early in the process and then hypertension; **anasarca** (total body edema); altered clotting mechanisms; and bleeding. Reduced tubular hydrogen excretion produces hyperchloremia of low anion gap acidosis. If the glomerular filtration rate becomes severely impaired, the retention of acidic wastes may produce a high anion gap acidosis (see Chapter 19 ☺). As a result of the acidosis, the patient's breath will have the odor of ammonia, and the patient may exhibit **Kussmaul's respirations**,

DIAGNOSTIC TESTS for Acute Tubular Necrosis

Test	Expected Abnormality	Rationale for Abnormality
Urinalysis	Presence of red blood cells and red blood cell casts	Impaired filtration
	Low specific gravity (1.010)	Decreased ability to concentrate urine
	Low osmolality (less than 400 mOsm/kg)	
Serum creatinine	Rising serum creatinine	Indicates advanced renal insufficiency
Blood urea nitrogen (BUN)	Rising serum BUN	Indicates advanced renal insufficiency
Arterial blood gases (ABG)	Metabolic acidosis	Impaired filtration
	pH < 7.35	
	$HCO_3 < 24$ mEq/L	
Electrolytes	Hyperkalemia	Impaired filtration
	Hyperphosphatemia	
	Hypocalcemia	

CHART 47–1 **Types of Acute Renal Failure**

Category	Causes
Prerenal failure	Diminished blood flow to the kidneys causes prerenal failure. The decreased flow may result from: • Hypovolemia • Sepsis • Embolism • Heart failure • Idiopathic thrombocytopenic purpura • Transfusion reactions • Malignant hypertension • Scleroderma.
Intrinsic failure	Intrinsic (parenchymatous) failure results from damage to the kidney. The damage may be a result of: • Acute tubular necrosis • Acute poststreptococcal glomerulonephritis • Systemic lupus erythematosus • Polyarteritis nodosa • Vasculitis • Sickle cell disease • Bilateral renal vein thrombosis • Nephrotoxins • Ischemia • Renal myeloma • Acute pyelonephritis.
Postrenal failure	Postrenal failure is the result of bilateral obstruction of urine outflow. Obstruction may be caused by: • Renal calculi • Clots • Papillae from necrosis • Tumors • Benign prostatic hyperplasia • Strictures • Urethral edema from catheterization.

which are deep, sighing respirations. The most immediately life-threatening electrolyte imbalance that occurs with acute renal failure is severe **hyperkalemia**, an excess of potassium in the blood. The accompanying muscle weakness will cause heart failure and possible cardiac arrest. Sources of potassium should be identified and regulated if possible. Endogenous sources include cell lysis, hematoma reabsorption, and tissue breakdown. Exogenous sources include medications that interfere with potassium regulation, intravenous fluid, and diet. Water and sodium imbalances are common, because the patient can neither conserve nor excrete sodium or water optimally. Hyponatremia and fluid overload are common. The ability of the kidney to excrete phosphorus is impaired when the glomerular filtration rate

drops below one-third of normal. The resulting phosphorus retention leads to the formation of insoluble calcium phosphorus salts that can precipitate in soft tissue.

The progress and severity of the failure can be assessed by measurement of the glomerular filtration rate (GFR). The GFR is evaluated through clearance tests of the waste product creatinine. When the GFR is impaired, the serum creatinine level rises, and the creatinine clearance rate falls.

$$Creatinine\ clearance =$$
$$\frac{Urine\ creatinine\ concentration\,(mg\,\%)\times Urine\ volume\,(mL/min)}{Plasma\ creatinine\ concentration\,(mg\,\%)}$$

The test consists of a 12- or 24-hour urine collection and a blood sample. Normal levels are 88 to 128 mL/min in women and 97 to 137 mL/min in men. Values are slightly decreased in the elderly due to reduced renal plasma flow with aging. A creatinine clearance less than 40 mL/min is suggestive of moderate to severe renal impairment (Kee, 2005). Tests that are helpful in the diagnosis of acute renal failure are outlined in the Diagnostic Tests box.

Medical Management

The goal of treatment is to identify and treat reversible causes. Supportive measures include:

- Restrict protein intake to 0.25 to 0.5 g/kg per day to prevent increased urea synthesis.
- Provide nutrition to ensure a caloric intake of > 400 kilocalories per day to reduce tissue catabolism.
- Monitor potassium. If hyperkalemia occurs, therapy can include hypertonic glucose and insulin infusions, administration of intravenous calcium, and oral or rectal administration of potassium exchange resin. If the patient continues to be hyperkalemic, dialysis may be necessary.
- Restrict free water intake to avoid water overload and hyponatremia.
- Avoid exposure to or administration of nephrotoxic agents (Chart 47–2).
- Adjust doses of all medications that are excreted by the kidneys.
- Avoid nonsteroidal anti-inflammatory drugs (NSAIDs), and angiotensin-converting enzyme inhibitors (ACE inhibitors), as they interfere with potassium regulation.
- Avoid magnesium-containing drugs (antacids).
- Reduce the risk of hospital-acquired infection by using strict aseptic technique and removing indwelling urinary and vascular catheters when feasible.
- Use intermittent hemodialysis or continuous renal replacement therapy.

Continuous Renal Replacement Therapy

Continuous renal replacement therapy (CRRT) is a mode of dialysis that may be used in the hospital to treat acute renal failure. CRRT is a way to remove solute and fluids slowly and continuously in a patient that may be hemodynamically unstable. Described simply, CRRT includes blood flowing from a vascular access point; the blood is then purified in some manner outside the body by use of filters, creating an effluent and returning the purified blood to the body through another vascular access.

DIAGNOSTIC TESTS for Acute Renal Failure

Test	Expected Abnormality	Rationale for Abnormality
Blood urea nitrogen (BUN)	Increased	Impaired glomerular filtration
	Not as reliable an indicator of renal damage as serum creatinine levels, because the BUN is easily changed by protein intake, blood in the gastrointestinal tract, and cell catabolism	
Serum creatinine	Increased	Impaired glomerular filtration
Serum electrolyte levels:		
Potassium	Increased	Impaired filtration
Sodium	Decreased	Dilutional
Phosphorus	Increased	Impaired filtration
Calcium	Decreased	Response to increased phosphorus
Urinalysis	Presence of red blood cell casts, proteinuria	Impaired filtration
	Low specific gravity (1.010)	Decreased ability to concentrate urine
	Low osmolality (less than 400 mOsm/kg)	
Radiography:		
Renal ultrasound	Identification of size of the kidneys	Changes may signify damage to the kidney
Computed tomography *should be done without contrast*	Characterization of the parenchyma and collecting systems	May identify cause of kidney dysfunction
Retrograde pyelography	Identifies urinary tract obstruction	Will identify damage to kidney
Isotopic renal scan	Assesses renal perfusion and function	

CHART 47–2   Nephrotoxic Agents

Antibiotics
- Amphotericin B
- Colistin
- Gentamicin
- Kanamycin
- Neomycin
- Phenazopyridine
- Polymyxin B

Antineoplastic agents

Heavy metals
- Arsenic
- Lead
- Mercury

Iodinated radiographic contrast

Miscellaneous
- Acetaminophen
- Amphetamines
- Cyclosporine
- Heroin
- Silicon

Nonsteroidal anti-inflammatory drugs

Pesticides

Poisonous mushrooms

Solvents
- Carbon tetrachloride
- Ethylene glycol
- Methanol

High-efficiency membranes are used for maximum water and waste removal. The membranes are synthetic and biocompatible. In all forms of CRRT, as blood flows through the hemofilter, water is filtered through the pores in the membrane and produces the ultrafiltrate. The ultrafiltrate is composed primarily of water, electrolytes, wastes, and some dialyzable medications. Indications for use include hypervolemic or edematous patients unresponsive to diuretic therapy, multiple organ dysfunction syndrome (MODS), and large fluid volume removal in hemodynamically unstable patients. Terms that are commonly used with CRRT are:

- **Ultrafiltration**— Process of removing excess water by creating a pressure differential between the blood and fluid compartments. Positive pressure in the blood path and negative pressure in the dialysate path cause the excess water to move from the patient to the dialysate. The negative pressure is a suctioning force applied to the membrane.
- **Diffusion**—Spontaneous movement of solute from an area of higher concentration to an area of lower concentration.
- **Convection**—Movement of solutes through a membrane via an action called a solvent drag.
- **Osmosis**—Spontaneous movement of water from an area of lower concentration to an area of higher concentration.
- **Hemofiltration**—Movement of large amounts of fluid via ultrafiltration, and some movement of solutes via convection.
- **Replacement fluid**—Approximates normal plasma to meet the patient's needs. Fluids given may include lactated Ringer's solution, normal saline, albumin, bicarbonate, and electrolytes.

- **Dialysate**—Solution that surrounds the patient's blood, separated by a filter, and allows solute to cross from one side to the other.

There are several forms of CRRT. The four most frequently used are:

- **Continuous arteriovenous hemofiltration (CAVH)**—The blood is circulated by the patient's own arterial pressure, so a pump is not necessary. There is no concentration gradient, so only filtration of fluid occurs. Electrolytes are eliminated only as they are pulled along with the fluid. Replacement fluid is infused into the venous port to approximate fluid removal or to maintain weight balance.

- **Continuous arteriovenous hemodialysis (CAVHD)**—As with CAVH, the blood is circulated by the patient's own arterial pressure, so a pump is not necessary. CAVHD uses dialysate, which adds the advantages of the filtering properties of dialysis, providing a better clearance of urea. The dialysate solution is infused along with the hemofiltered blood.

- **Continuous venovenous hemodialysis (CVVHD)**—Diffusion and ultrafiltration are used to remove waste products. Dialysate is infused countercurrent to the blood flow in the outside compartment of the hemofilter to provide diffusion of wastes from the blood. CVVHD requires the use of a blood pump to control the flow at specific rates to optimize diffusion.

- **Slow continuous ultrafiltration (SCUF)**—This form of CRRT is used primarily for fluid removal. No dialysate or replacement fluids are used as wastes; electrolyte balance and acid–base balance are not as critical an issue. SCUF is the hemofiltration therapy of choice when the only goal is fluid removal and the patient is not azotemic, as in patients who are refractory to diuretics.

Nursing implications for CRRT include monitoring of fluid and electrolyte balance. Vital signs, hemodynamic status, and intake and output should be monitored hourly. The amount of hourly ultrafiltrate removed depends on an hourly fluid-balance calculation and assessment of the patient's volume status. Excess fluid volume to be removed is ordered by the health care provider and is usually termed as net loss. It may be ordered as 50 to 200 mL/hr more than hourly intake. This would be calculated as the patient's non-CRRT intake, such an intravenous infusions, medications, and feedings, plus fluid loss ordered by the health care provider minus non-CRRT system output, such as chest tube drainage, blood loss, and urine. The CRRT system infuses and removes fluid after the fluid balance is calculated and the desired volumes are input into the system. The system then monitors the amount of replacement fluids and/or dialysate to be infused and the volume of fluid removed. The patient's weight should be checked daily. Assessment and care of the vascular access sites is very important, because patency of the catheter can affect the effectiveness of the therapy.

■ Nursing Management

Fluid balance is critical for the patient with acute renal failure. Intake, output, and daily weight should be closely monitored and documented. Intake of fluids should match the amount of urine output plus 500 to 750 milliliters a day for insensible losses and 400 milliliters a day for metabolic processes (Hogan, 2007). Strict measurement of output should include all body fluids, such as wound drainage. The patient should be instructed to follow the National Renal Diet that contains food exchanges for protein, sodium, potassium, and phosphorus. Monitoring of intake includes the patient's nutritional status. A high-calorie, low-protein, low-sodium, low-potassium diet is key in preventing further progression of the disease. Restrictions should be as follows:

- Sodium intake should only be what is needed to replenish losses, which is approximately 20 to 40 mEq/day (2 to 3 g/day).
- Limit protein to 0.25 to 0.5 g/kg body weight per day to minimize azotemia or nitrogen retention if not being dialyzed. If on dialysis, may increase protein to 1.2 g/kg daily.
- Limit diet potassium to 25 to 40 mEq/day to prevent hyperkalemia until urine volume increases during recovery.
- Parenteral iron may be needed to enhance erythropoiesis.
- Dietary phosphate may need to be restricted, although low-phosphate diets may be poorly accepted. Phosphate-binding antacids may be used to decrease the amount.
- If the patient is anorexic, give her small, frequent meals. (Hogan, 2007)

The patient with acute renal failure is susceptible to infectious complications. The use of aseptic technique is of significant importance in preventing hospital-acquired infections. Prevent complications of immobility with frequent position changes, coughing and deep breathing, and passive range-of-motion exercises. Provide frequent mouth care to prevent stomatitis.

If the patient is uremic, he may be confused and unsteady. Provide safety measures, such as having the bed in low position, three side rails up and one down to prevent falls, and soft restraints, if necessary.

Assessment

Focused nursing assessment during history taking should include:

- Amount and frequency of urination
- Change in urine color and smell
- History of headaches, dependent edema, or palpitations
- Pain around the flank or costal margin areas
- Nausea, loss of appetite, odd taste in mouth
- Weight gain or loss
- Weakness and fatigue
- Inability to concentrate or confusion
- Any job-related exposure to nephrotoxic agents
- Cessation of menstruation or impotence
- Increased irritability.

Focused nursing assessment during physical exam should include:

- Abnormal urine color, clarity, or smell
- Oliguria (<400 mL/day) or anuria (<50 mL/day) or nonoliguric ARF (1 to 2 L/day)
- Lethargy, apathy
- Tremors
- Bounding, rapid pulse with normal or high blood pressure, distended neck veins

- Orthostatic hypotension
- Tachypnea, dyspnea, or adventitious breath sounds
- Kussmaul's respirations (found when patient is acidotic)
- Dependent edema (with hypervolemia), poor skin turgor (with hypovolemia)
- Thin, brittle hair and nails.

Nursing Diagnoses

Key nursing diagnoses for the patient with acute renal failure include:

- *Fluid Volume, Excess*
- *Infection, Risk for*
- *Nutrition, Imbalanced: Less than Body Requirements*
- *Injury, Risk for*
- *Knowledge, Deficient* related to ARF and possible dialysis.

Planning

The overall goals for the patient with ARF are to identify and treat reversible causes, prevent further damage to the kidneys, and maintain fluid and electrolyte balance.

Outcomes and Evaluation Parameters

Patient outcomes and evaluation parameters for the patient with acute renal failure include:

- Maintenance of serum electrolyte levels as evidenced by results of lab work being within normal limits.
- Maintenance of fluid volume as evidenced by vital signs and hemodynamic readings being within acceptable limits.
- The patient will maintain balanced nutrition as exhibited by limited weight loss, muscle wasting, or edema.
- The patient will remain free of infection as exhibited by white blood count (WBC) being within normal range, no increase in temperature, and clean, dry access sites for lines and catheters.
- The patient will not be at risk for injury as exhibited by no signs or symptoms of uremia, such as confusion and tremors.
- The patient will have a clear understanding of the disease process and the plan of care by expressing knowledge of and commitment to comply with treatments.

Interventions and Rationales

Nursing interventions and rationales for the patient with ARF include:

- Monitor and document electrolyte levels as ordered. *The kidneys have lost the ability to regulate electrolyte excretion and reabsorption. This is especially true of potassium, phosphate, calcium, and magnesium. The levels can change quickly and result in complications.*
- Monitor the ECG continuously. Notify the health care team and document any changes. *Electrolyte imbalances can cause dysrhythmias and cardiac arrest.*
- If hyperkalemia is present, notify the health care team and be prepared to administer the following, as ordered: *The kidneys' inability to excrete potassium released by normal cellular metabolism can cause very high potassium levels.*

1. 50% Glucose intravenously and insulin solution. *In an emergent situation, glucose and insulin may transport potassium into the cells, temporarily lowering the serum potassium level.*

2. Calcium chloride or calcium gluconate intravenously. *To protect the heart from the effect of hyperkalemia on the cardiac rhythm, calcium competes with potassium for entry into cardiac cells.*

3. Administration of cation-exchange resins such as sodium polystyrene sulfonate (Kayexalate with sorbitol) orally or rectally as ordered. *Sodium polystyrene sulfonate removes potassium at a rate of 1 mEq/g of medication by exchanging it for sodium in the bowel. The sorbitol helps to remove the bound potassium from the bowel by acting as an osmotic diarrhetic.*

- Limit dietary and drug intake of potassium (penicillin VK or potassium-containing antacids). Limit intake of magnesium-containing antacids. *The kidneys are unable to excrete the potassium or magnesium.*
- Assess for signs of fluid overload, such as weight gain, hypertension, tachypnea, adventitious breath sounds, peripheral edema, and low hematocrit. Maintain a strict record of intake and output. *During ARF the kidneys are unable to maintain normal fluid balance resulting in fluid overload during the oliguric stage and a potential for dehydration during the diuretic stage.*
- Restrict fluid intake to measure output plus 400 mL/day. Compare intake and output records with daily weights. If fluid losses have increased or the patient is losing weight, consult the health care team. *The kidneys are unable to eliminate excess fluids; therefore, intake must be restricted to replacement of lost fluids plus 400 mL/day to cover insensible losses (through lungs and skin).*
- Provide hard candies and frequent mouth care. *Restricting fluids may cause dry mouth and thirst. Hard candy will stimulate salivation, and mouth care will remove debris and add comfort.*
- Administer diuretics as ordered. Document administration and results. Administer vasodilators as ordered, such as low-dose dopamine. *During prerenal conditions, diuretics may be administered in an attempt to prevent ARF by increasing fluid volume through the kidneys. If the kidneys are marginally functioning, diuretics may cause ARF. Vasodilators expand the vascular bed, lessening the congestion and the risk of pulmonary edema. Low-dose dopamine increases renal perfusion by dopaminergic stimulation of the renal blood vessels.*
- Assess for signs of infection (increased temperature, increased WBC, signs of infection at IV and catheter sites). Practice strict asepsis and provide site care and dressing changes according to policy. *The uremic syndrome that develops with ARF suppresses normal cell metabolism and immune response, placing the patient at increased risk for infection. Careful hand hygiene and the use of aseptic technique during procedures help to prevent infection. Site care prevents the accumulation of secretions that serve as growth media for infective organisms. Regular assessment of all site areas and general assessment of the skin will allow for early identification and treatment of infection.*
- Provide skin care and use preventive measures to protect against shearing or decubitus formation. Turn the patient every 2 hours, maintain wrinkle-free linens, and use protective pads to bony areas. Provide site care and dressing changes

for intravenous lines according to hospital policy. *Skin integrity is compromised due to the edema and accumulation of waste products in the tissues due to the altered metabolism. Site care will assist to prevent accumulation of moisture, which serves as a growth medium for infective organisms.*

- Collaborate with the health care team to implement a high-carbohydrate diet that provides small amounts of high-quality proteins; limits fluids, sodium, and potassium; and includes vitamin supplements. *A high-carbohydrate diet supplies calories for energy needs; limiting proteins prevents protein catabolism, as the kidneys are unable to excrete the waste products at this time; fluids and sodium are limited to prevent volume overload, while potassium is limited because the kidneys are unable to excrete it.*

- Monitor BUN, creatinine, uric acid, and pH levels as ordered. Assess for signs and symptoms or uremia (headache, confusion, change in mentation, pruritus, nausea and vomiting, weight loss with muscle wasting, Kussmaul's respirations, seizures). *The accumulation of metabolic waste products and increasing acidosis reflect worsening kidney function. Uremia affects all systems in the body, but the changes may initially be subtle.*

- Assess for signs and symptoms of hemorrhage. *Uremic syndrome places the patient at high risk for stress ulcers and coagulopathy.*

- Monitor the patient for anemia (hematocrit and hemoglobin levels). Administer folic acid and iron supplements, or administer blood as ordered. *In ARF the kidneys' ability to produce erythropoietin, a hormone that stimulates the production of red blood cells (RBCs), diminishes, resulting in anemia. Folic acid and iron supplements stimulate RBC production. Administration of packed red blood cells provides RBCs without causing fluid overload.*

- Provide information and teaching for the patient and significant others as needed regarding the process and stages of ARF, signs and symptoms that should be reported immediately, dietary modifications, activity restriction, and an explanation of any procedures, including dialysis. *Knowledge and understanding of the disease process and the treatment plan help to decrease anxiety and may enhance recovery. If the patient is acutely ill, teaching may need to be done in small time frames.*

Evaluation

The patient should be able to verbalize her understanding of the disease process and the plan of care. The patient will maintain serum electrolyte levels and vital signs within acceptable limits. The patient will not display signs of uremia. The patient will remain free of infection with clean, dry access sites for lines and catheters. The patient will have only limited weight loss with no signs of muscle wasting or edema.

Chronic Renal Failure

Chronic renal failure is generally not reversible and often gets progressively worse. The symptoms of renal failure usually appear when approximately two-thirds of filtration capacity is lost. When the loss of filtration ability reaches approximately seven-eighths, the survival of the patient depends on maintenance dialysis or kidney transplantation. When a patient reaches this stage of failure, the patient is said to have **end-stage renal disease (ESRD)** (Follin & Lenker, 2004; Walser, 2004). If the patient continues

without treatment, uremic toxins accumulate and cause potentially fatal physiological changes in all of the major organ systems.

In the United States, over 300,000 patients have ESRD and are currently on dialysis. Outside of the United States there are another 300,000 to 400,000 patients on dialysis, with many hundreds of thousands of patients in third world countries who suffer from ESRD but do not have dialysis available for economic reasons. In the United States, the number of patients on dialysis increases each year, and it is estimated that by 2010 there will be approximately 650,000 patients with ESRD (Walser, 2004).

Many patients who are developing kidney disease and early renal failure are unaware due to the lack of symptoms in the early stages. There are those who are at risk for renal failure due to inherited susceptibilities or dangerous behaviors. At-risk groups include:

- **Being African American**—This population has almost twice the frequency of ESRD than the population at large and comprises 30% of patients with ERSD (Walser, 2004).

- **Genetics**—Many first-degree relatives, such as siblings or children, of patients with ESRD have signs of renal disease. The explanation is not yet clear, but statistics reveal a strong familial factor (Walser, 2004).

- **Polycystic kidney disease**—As stated earlier in this chapter, polycystic kidney disease is an inherited condition, with half of the children of patients with the disease developing the disorder.

Diseases that lead to an increased risk of renal failure include:

- **Diabetes**—In the United States today, patients with diabetes comprise the largest group of patients starting dialysis (Walser, 2004). The cardiovascular changes that develop with diabetes gradually decrease the circulation to the kidneys and eventually cause irreversible damage. Recent studies have revealed that close control of blood glucose levels in those patients with insulin-dependent diabetes reduces the incidence of renal failure (Follin & Lenker, 2004; Walser, 2004).

- **Hypertension**—Hypertension is one of the most common disorders in the United States (Walser, 2004). Vascular changes with this disease cause a decrease in circulation to the kidneys, gradually damaging the nephrons.

- **Potassium deficiency**—Chronic diarrhea or an overuse of laxatives can cause chronic potassium deficiency. The kidney's ability to produce concentrated urine, and to decrease output in response to dehydration, is impaired by potassium deficiency. Patients with potassium deficiency tend to excrete large amounts of urine even though they have reduced kidney function. If the potassium deficiency is severe, the kidney may never recover and renal failure will occur (Walser, 2004).

- **Urinary tract obstruction**—Diseases that obstruct outflow of urine, such as enlarged prostate in men, will cause back pressure and hydronephrosis. If not treated, the hydronephrosis will distort the shape of the kidney and diminish the function.

- **Chronic glomerular disease**—Chronic glomerulonephritis scars and eventually destroys the ability of the glomeruli to function.

- **Chronic infection**—Chronic infections such as pyelonephritis or tuberculosis will also cause scarring and eventually destroy the ability of the kidney to function.

Laboratory and Diagnostic Procedures

The presence of any type of chronic kidney disease should be established as early as possible and be based on the presence of kidney damage and level of renal function through measurement of the glomerular filtration rate (GFR). Chronic kidney disease in adults is defined as evidence of structural or functional kidney abnormalities as revealed by abnormal urinalysis, imaging studies, or histology; or GFR < 60 mL · min^{-1} · (1.73 m^2)$^{-1}$ that persists for at least 3 months (Post & Rose, 2008c; Michigan Quality Improvement Consortium, 2006). The extent of the disease is classified based on the level of renal function. The National Kidney Foundation defines the stages as:

Stage 1: Kidney damage with normal or increased GFR, GFR ≥ 90 mL · min^{-1} · (1.73 m^2)$^{-1}$

Stage 2: Kidney damage with mild decrease in GFR, GFR = 60 to 89 mL · min^{-1} · (1.73 m^2)$^{-1}$

Stage 3: Moderate decrease in GFR, GFR = 30 to 59 mL · min^{-1} · (1.73 m^2)$^{-1}$

Stage 4: Severe decrease in GFR, GFR = 15 to 29 mL · min^{-1} · (1.73 m^2)$^{-1}$

Stage 5: Kidney failure, GFR < 15 mL · min^{-1} · (1.73 m^2)$^{-1}$ or dialysis.

(Michigan Quality Improvement Consortium, 2006)

Diagnosis of chronic renal failure is made through clinical assessment and a history of progressive debilitation with gradual deterioration of renal function. One of the earliest symptoms of chronic renal failure, and also the most common, is fatigue. The patient may describe feeling tired all of the time or tiring quickly with mild activity. The patient may also describe a loss of the sense of well-being. The cause of fatigue is unclear and is disproportionate to the anemia that develops with chronic renal disease. Fatigue is one of the most prevalent causes of disability in patients with chronic renal failure (Walser, 2004).

Muscle cramps, typically involving the calf muscles, are the second most common complaint of patients with chronic renal failure (Walser, 2004). The cramps can be very painful and are often experienced at night. The exact cause is unknown, but a decreased potassium or sodium level can make the cramps worse.

As the blood urea concentration increases, the patient may have a loss of appetite with accompanying nausea and vomiting. Intensive nutritional counseling and calculation of dietary needs to prevent weight loss are very important for the well-being of the patient with chronic renal failure and will be discussed later in this chapter.

Chronic renal failure eventually produces changes throughout all body systems.

- Cardiovascular changes
  - Hypertension
  - Cardiomyopathy
  - Uremic pericarditis
  - Pericardial effusion
  - Heart failure
  - Peripheral edema
  - Arrhythmias
- Respiratory changes
  - Increased susceptibility to infection due to pulmonary macrophage activity
  - Pulmonary edema
  - Pleural effusions
  - Uremic pleuritis
  - Uremic pneumonitis
  - Dyspnea due to heart failure
  - Kussmaul's respirations due to acidosis
- Gastrointestinal changes
  - Inflammation and ulceration of gastrointestinal mucosa
  - Ulceration and bleeding gums
  - Esophagitis
  - Gastritis
  - Duodenal ulcers
  - Uremic colitis
  - Pancreatitis
  - Proctitis
  - Uremic fetor: ammonia smell to breath
  - Anorexia
  - Nausea and vomiting
- Neurological changes
  - Peripheral neuropathy causing pain, burning, and itching in the legs and feet; eventually progresses to paresthesia and footdrop from motor nerve dysfunction
  - Shortened memory and attention span
  - Drowsiness
  - Irritability
  - Confusion
  - Coma
  - Seizures
- Endocrine changes
  - Stunted growth in children
  - Infertility and decreased libido in both sexes
  - Amenorrhea
  - Impotence and decreased sperm production in men
  - Increased aldosterone secretion due to increased renin production
  - Increased blood glucose levels due to impaired carbohydrate metabolism
- Hematopoietic changes
  - Anemia
  - Decreased red blood cell survival time
  - Blood loss from dialysis and gastrointestinal bleeding
  - Mild thrombocytopenia
  - Platelet defects
  - Increase in bleeding and clotting disorders
- Skeletal changes
  - Calcium–phosphorus imbalance and parathyroid imbalance cause:
    - Skeletal pain
    - Skeletal demineralization
    - Pathologic fractures
    - Calcifications in the brain, eyes, gums, joints, myocardium, and blood vessels

- Cutaneous changes
  - Skin appears yellowish bronze, dry, and scaly
  - Itching
  - Purpura
  - Ecchymosis
  - Petechiae
  - Thin, brittle fingernails with lines
  - Dry, brittle hair that may fall out easily

Tests that are helpful in the diagnosis of chronic renal failure are presented in the Diagnostic Tests box.

Medical Management

Treatment is aimed at slowing the progression of the disease by treating any underlying condition that may be contributing to or causing the failure; treating specific symptoms; and minimizing complications. As the disease progresses, identification of potential patients for dialysis is necessary to prepare them adequately.

Reversible causes of decreased renal function in the patient with chronic renal failure include hypovolemia from vomiting, diarrhea, diuretic use, or bleeding, and hypotension due to myocardial dysfunction, sepsis, or pericardial disease. In the case of hypovolemia, fluid replacement may result in the return of renal function to the previous baseline.

For patients with chronic renal failure, the administration of drugs or diagnostic contrast will adversely affect renal function. The use of drugs that lower the glomerular filtration rate (such as NSAIDs and ACE inhibitors), aminoglycoside antibiotics, and radiographic contrast should be avoided.

Medical Management to Slow Progression

To slow the progression of the failure, protective mechanisms are employed. Studies have suggested that progression may be due in part to secondary factors such as intraglomerular hypertension and hypertrophy; glomerular scarring; hyperlipidemia;

metabolic acidosis; and tubulointerstitial disease (Post & Rose, 2008c). Therefore, antihypertensive therapy is given for both renal protection and cardiovascular protection, because there is a marked increase in cardiovascular risk with chronic renal failure. Patients are usually administered angiotensin-converting enzyme (ACE) inhibitors or angiotensin II receptor blockers (ARBs). The goal is a reduction in blood pressure to less than 130/80 mmHg (Post & Rose, 2008c). If the goal is not reached with an ACE inhibitor or an ARB, then a diuretic is added and, if necessary, diltiazem, verapamil, or a beta-blocker.

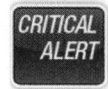 *ACE inhibitors and angiotension II receptor blockers (ARBs) can cause a decrease in renal function and an increase in plasma potassium soon after the onset of therapy. Repeat plasma creatinine and potassium within 3 to 5 days.*

Patients with chronic renal failure without dialysis should have dietary interviews every 3 months with measurement of serum albumin and body weight. The deterioration of the patient's nutritional status often begins early in the course of the disease. Malnutrition in patients that are about to begin maintenance dialysis is a strong predictor of poor clinical outcome (Hogan, 2007). For patients who are not undergoing dialysis, a low-protein diet consisting of 0.60 g/kg per day should be considered. When well monitored, a low-protein, high-energy diet maintains nutritional support while limiting the potentially toxic nitrogenous metabolites, development of uremic symptoms, and occurrence of other metabolic complications. Low-protein diets can decrease the effects of hyperphosphatemia, metabolic acidosis, hyperkalemia, and other electrolyte disorders.

The energy expenditure and requirements of a nondialyzed patient with chronic renal failure is similar to that of healthy adults. A diet providing approximately 35 kcal/kg per day has been shown to maintain neutral nitrogen balance, to promote higher serum albumin concentrations, and to reduce the urea nitrogen appearance (Hogan, 2007). Patients who are age 60 or older tend to be

DIAGNOSTIC TESTS for Chronic Renal Failure

Test	Expected Abnormality	Rationale for Abnormality
Serum electrolytes:		
Urea nitrogen	Increased	Impaired glomerular filtration
Creatinine	Increased	
Potassium	Increased	
Sodium	Increased	
Hemoglobin and hematocrit	Decreased	Insufficient production of erythropoietin
Arterial pH and bicarbonate levels	Decreased	Impaired glomerular filtration
Urinalysis	Presence of red blood cell casts, proteinuria	Impaired filtration
	Low specific gravity (1.010)	Decreased ability to concentrate urine
	Low osmolality (less than 400 mOsm/kg)	
Radiography:		
Renal ultrasound	Reduced kidney size	Permanent damage to the kidney
Computed tomography *should be done without contrast*	Characterization of the parenchyma and collecting systems	
	Reveals decreased function	
Isotopic renal scan	May show decreased perfusion	
Kidney biopsy	Histologic identification of underlying pathology	Identifies pathology

less physically active, so an intake of 30 to 35 kcal/kg per day may be sufficient. It may be difficult for patients to achieve this level of energy intake, and nutritional supplements with high energy density may be necessary.

The patient who is on maintenance dialysis, either hemodialysis or peritoneal dialysis, is recommended to have a dietary protein intake of 1.2 g/kg per day with at least 50% of the protein being of high biologic value. Protein that is considered of high biologic value has an amino acid composition similar to human protein, is usually an animal protein, and tends to be utilized more efficiently by humans to conserve body proteins. Daily energy intake for the patient requiring dialysis is the same as for the patient without dialysis.

Medical Management of Complications of Renal Failure

As stated, renal failure affects many body systems. Multiple complications may arise due to the loss of renal function. The patient should be monitored closely and have any complication treated.

The kidneys are able to maintain sodium and intravascular volume balance until the GFR falls below 10 to 15 mL/min. Even though the patient with mild to moderate failure is able to maintain fluid balance, he is less able to respond to a rapid infusion of sodium and is prone to fluid overload. Most patients with renal failure who experience fluid overload respond to a combination of dietary sodium restriction and diuretic therapy with a loop diuretic given daily.

Hyperkalemia usually develops in the patient who is oliguric and has a high intake of potassium in her diet, increased tissue breakdown, or hypoaldosteronism due in part to the administration of an ACE inhibitor. Hyperkalemia in conjunction with administration of an ACE inhibitor usually occurs when the serum potassium is elevated prior to therapy. If this is the case, institution of a low-potassium diet or use of a loop diuretic in conjunction often decreases the degree of hyperkalemia. For some patients, a low dose of Kayexalate (5 grams with each meal), can lower the serum potassium concentration.

Patients with chronic renal failure tend to retain hydrogen ions and progressively develop metabolic acidosis with serum bicarbonate concentrations between 12 and 20 mEq/L. Treatment of even mild acidemia is desirable, because bone buffering of some of the excess hydrogen ions is linked with the release of calcium and phosphate from the bone, worsening the bone disease. Also, uremic acidosis can increase skeletal muscle breakdown and diminish albumin synthesis, eventually causing loss of lean body mass and weakness. Treatment consists of administration of sodium bicarbonate 0.5 to 1 mEq/kg per day. Sodium citrate may also be used but is avoided in a patient taking aluminum-containing antacids, as it enhances intestinal aluminum absorption.

Phosphate retention starts early in renal disease due to decreased filtration. The condition remains mild with hyperphosphatemia occurring late, but the retention is related to the development of secondary hyperparathyroidism. The parathyroid gland hypersecretes parathyroid hormone (PTH) to correct both hyperphosphatemia and hypocalcemia, and in the early stages of renal disease maintains a phosphate balance in the patient with a GFR greater than 30 mL/min. Dietary phosphate restriction may delay the development of secondary hyperparathyroidism, but this can be accomplished only by limiting protein intake, which is

not acceptable to many. Once the GFR falls below 25 to 30 mL/min, oral phosphate binders are usually required. Guidelines recommend keeping serum phosphorus levels between 2.7 and 4.6 mg/dL in patients with chronic renal failure and between 3.5 and 5.5 mg/dL in patients with end-stage renal disease. The most widely used phosphate binder is calcium carbonate. The dose ranges from 2.5 to 20 g/day and is increased gradually until the serum phosphate falls or hypercalcemia ensues. Close monitoring of the serum calcium concentration is needed, as hypercalcemia is a common complication of this therapy.

 **CRITICAL ALERT** *Phosphate binders are most effective when taken with meals to bind dietary phosphate.*

There is also a nonabsorbable agent, sevelamer, that does not contain calcium or aluminum. Sevelamer is a cationic polymer that binds with phosphate through ion exchange. It is used in patients who cannot tolerate calcium carbonate or who exhibit a persistent hyperphosphatemia. Other phosphate binders such as aluminum hydroxide, magnesium hydroxide, and calcium citrate should be avoided due to their side effects of aluminum toxicity and hypermagnesemia with the magnesium hydroxide. All phosphate binders have limited binding capacity and should be used in conjunction with a carefully planned diet that restricts phosphorus when possible.

Hypertension is present in 80% to 85% of chronic renal failure patients (Post & Rose, 2008c). Fluid retention contributes to the elevation of blood pressure; therefore, control is usually achieved with a combined therapy of ACE inhibitor or ARB and a diuretic. As stated previously, the recommended blood pressure goal is less than 130/80 mmHg.

The anemia associated with chronic renal failure is due primarily to reduced production of erythropoietin and shortened red cell survival. Although anemia is present in most patients with chronic renal failure, the patient should be evaluated for all other causes prior to instituting a therapy. In patients with end-stage renal disease, epoetin alfa (EPO) or darbepoetin alfa therapy helps to correct the anemia. Erythropoietic agents are given to patients who are predialysis with a hemoglobin concentration less than 11 g/dL. Guidelines suggest that the initial erythropoietin dose should be approximately 80 to 120 units/kg per week (Post & Rose, 2008c). The hemoglobin level should be tested weekly, and the dose or frequency adjusted. Darbepoetin alfa, another erythropoietic agent, has a longer half-life and greater biologic activity than recombinant erythropoietin and can be scheduled weekly, every 2 weeks, or monthly. The recommended starting dose for patients with chronic renal failure is 0.45 mcg/kg per week. The drug can be given intravenously or subcutaneously.

For an adequate response to erythropoietin or darbepoetin, the patient must have sufficient iron stores. This usually requires the administration of oral or intravenous iron to maintain a serum ferritin level of greater than 100 ng/mL. Patients are most commonly given 325 milligrams of ferrous sulfate three times daily. Severe anemia may require the infusion of fresh frozen packed cells or washed packed cells.

A tendency to bleed is present in both acute and chronic renal failure due to platelet dysfunction. If the patient is asymptomatic, no therapy is indicated. If the patient is actively bleeding or is scheduled for an invasive procedure, then therapy may consist of the administration of desmopressin acetate (DDAVP), which improves platelet function by increasing levels of factor VIII; cryoprecipitate; and the initiation of dialysis.

Patients with advanced renal failure may present with uremic pericarditis. They will complain of fever, pleuritic chest pain, and have a pericardial friction rub. Because it is a metabolic pericarditis and epicardial injury is uncommon, the electrocardiogram will usually not show the typical diffuse ST and T wave elevation seen with other forms of pericarditis. This development is an indication to institute dialysis. With dialysis, most patients will have a resolution of chest pain and a decrease in the size of the effusion.

If end-stage renal disease goes untreated, the patient will develop uremic neuropathy with dysfunction of the central and peripheral nervous systems, including encephalopathy leading to seizures and coma. Signs of sensory dysfunction, such as restless leg or burning feet syndrome, are frequent presentations of uremic neuropathy. These signs and symptoms are usually absolute indications for the initiation of dialysis.

Nursing Management

With chronic renal failure, management is aimed at slowing the progression of the disease to end-stage renal disease and avoiding complications. Patient education regarding control of underlying causes such as diabetes and hypertension is key. Infection, volume depletion, and the taking of nephrotoxic medications must be avoided to prevent further deterioration of renal function. As the patient reaches end-stage renal disease, management moves to dialysis or renal transplantation. The Nursing Process: Patient Care Plan outlines nursing care for chronic renal failure.

 **CRITICAL ALERT** *Medications that are excreted primarily by the kidneys require modification of dosage and/or frequency. Elderly patients with chronic renal failure that are taking digitalis must have careful dosage titration, as 85% of the drug is excreted by the kidneys.*

Collaborative Management

Working with a renal dietician is very beneficial. To slow progression of the disease, protein and phosphorus are restricted. Carbohydrates are increased to ensure that the patient has adequate caloric intake to prevent tissue catabolism. As the disease progresses, sodium intake is limited and fluids may be restricted. The kidneys' ability to excrete potassium is decreased; therefore, potassium intake is also limited. Providing a fact sheet listing foods that are restricted or limited is helpful. Provide sample menus to help the patient plan daily menus that incorporate these restrictions.

Patients may also benefit from psychological counseling to help them cope with a chronic illness and the uncertain future it entails.

Initiation of Maintenance Dialysis

For patients with chronic renal failure, the decision to initiate maintenance dialysis or renal transplantation involves discussion between the patient and the health care provider with consideration of subjective and objective data. It is important to explore with the patient his perception of his quality of life and the changes that will occur, in the case of dialysis, with a therapy that is technologically complex. With hemodialysis, the treatment regimen is based on two factors: the restriction of certain nutrients and the removal of waste metabolites from the blood by regular dialysis. The management is effective only if the patient adheres closely with the therapeutic regimen. Although hemodialysis can effectively contribute to long-term survival of patients with ESRD, morbidity and mortality of patients on dialysis remain high, especially due to cardiovascular disease. Approximately 33% of patients on hemodialysis survive past 5 years of treatment, whereas 70% of recipients of kidney transplant are alive after 5 years (Denhaerynck et al., 2007).

The absolute clinical indications to initiate renal replacement therapy include:

- Pericarditis
- Volume overload or pulmonary edema that is refractory to diuretics
- Increasing hypertension that is minimally responsive to antihypertensive medications
- Progressive uremic encephalopathy or neuropathy
- Persistent nausea and vomiting
- Plasma creatinine concentration above 12 mg/dL or blood urea nitrogen greater than 100 mg/dL (Ismail, 2008).

Early recognition of chronic renal failure allows for renoprotective therapy such as rigorous blood pressure control and protective dietary changes, as discussed earlier. Early recognition enables dialysis to be initiated at an optimal time and may also permit the recruitment and evaluation of family members for the placement of a renal allograft before the need for dialysis arises (Post & Rose, 2008c).

Relative indications to initiate renal replacement therapy include:

- Anorexia progressing to nausea and vomiting
- Decreased attentiveness
- Decreased cognitive tasking
- Depression
- Severe anemia that is unresponsive to erythropoietin
- Persistent pruritus or restless leg syndrome (Ismail, 2008).

The advantage of starting dialysis when relative indications are present is to enhance the quality of life and to prolong survival. Dialysis has also been shown to improve multiple nutritional indexes including serum albumin, iron, transferrin saturation, creatinine, and the nPNA (protein nitrogen appearance) over the first 6 months of therapy (Ismail, 2008).

When the decision has been made to begin renal replacement therapy, discussion should commence with the patient regarding the advantages and disadvantages of hemodialysis, peritoneal dialysis (continuous or intermittent), and renal transplantation (living or deceased donor).

Hemodialysis

To perform hemodialysis, the patient must have vascular access. For acute access a dual-lumen venous catheter may be used. The outflow openings are proximal to the inflow openings on the opposite side to avoid dialyzing the same blood that was just returned to the vessel. The subclavian, internal jugular, and femoral veins are usually used for this short-term access, and the catheters can be inserted at the bedside. Percutaneous catheters

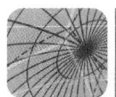

Assessment of Fluid Status

Subjective Data:
How much fluid have you been taking in?
Have you felt short of breath?
Have you gained weight?

Objective Data:
Assess:
Patient weight
Skin turgor

Presence of edema
Blood pressure
Respiratory effort and lung sounds

Nursing Assessment and Diagnoses	Outcomes and Evaluation Parameters	Planning and Interventions with *Rationales*
Nursing Diagnosis: *Fluid Volume, Excess* related to compromised regulatory mechanisms secondary to renal failure	**Outcome:** Neither fluid volume excess nor deficient volume will occur. ***Evaluation Parameters:*** Demonstrates no rapid weight changes. Absence of edema. Normal skin turgor. Reports no difficulty breathing.	**Interventions and *Rationales:*** Assess dietary intake and habits that may contribute to excess fluid volume. *To identify potential sources of fluid such as foods high in sodium, medications that contain fluid, or amount of fluid taken with medications.* Teach patient/family rationale for restrictions. *Understanding promotes cooperation.* Teach and encourage need for frequent oral hygiene. *To minimize dry mouth associated with fluid restriction.*

Assessment of Nutritional Intake

Subjective Data:
Describe your usual intake pattern.
Is this intake sufficient?
Do you have religious dietary restrictions or practices?

How often do you exercise?
Who prepares your meals?
Do you feel you have enough energy?

Objective Data:
Assess:
General appearance
Weight

Hair, nails, and skin
Muscle mass
Edema

Nursing Assessment and Diagnoses	Outcomes and Evaluation Parameters	Planning and Interventions with *Rationales*
Nursing Diagnosis: *Nutrition, Imbalanced: Less than Body Requirements*	**Outcome:** The patient will maintain adequate nutrition. ***Evaluation Parameter:*** Maintenance of weight without loss of muscle mass.	**Interventions and *Rationales:*** Facilitate education with a renal dietary consultant. *Consultation can ensure a diet that provides optimal caloric and nutrient intake.* Encourage frequent oral hygiene. *Poor oral hygiene leads to bad breath and taste in the mouth, which decreases the appetite.* Provide the patient with printed material outlining the dietary needs and restrictions. *To aid the patient in selecting the proper foods.* Promote the intake of protein foods with high biologic value: eggs, meats, and dairy products. *Complete proteins provide positive nitrogen balance needed for growth and healing.*

Assessment of Activity Tolerance

Subjective Data:
Are you able to perform activities of daily living?
Do you experience pain that interferes with activity?
Are there activities you feel you are unable to do?

Objective Data:
Assess strength and balance.
Assess response to activity by taking vital signs at rest and then after performing an activity.
Assess coping strategies.

Nursing Assessment and Diagnoses	Outcomes and Evaluation Parameters	Planning and Interventions with *Rationales*
Nursing Diagnosis: *Activity Intolerance* related to fatigue, anemia, and altered metabolic state	**Outcome:** Patient will have a balance of rest and activity to aid participation without fatigue. ***Evaluation Parameters:*** Alternates rest and activity. Reports a decrease in fatigue and an increased sense of well-being. Participates in self-care activities.	**Interventions and *Rationales:*** Promote independence in self-care as tolerated. *To promote self-esteem.* Encourage naps between activities. *To promote activity within patient's limits.* Assess factors that may be contributing to fatigue: Fluid and electrolyte imbalances Anemia Depression. *To identify factors contributing to fatigue.*

(continued)

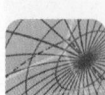

NURSING PROCESS: Patient Care Plan for Chronic Renal Failure—*Continued*

Assessment of Knowledge of Disease Process

Subjective Data:
What causes renal failure?
What is the relationship of fluid and dietary restrictions to renal disease?
What is your understanding of renal failure?

Objective Data:
Patient follows treatment regimen and is able to articulate understanding of disease process.

Nursing Assessment and Diagnoses	Outcomes and Evaluation Parameters	Planning and Interventions with *Rationales*
Nursing Diagnosis: *Therapeutic Regimen Management, Ineffective* related to lack of knowledge of disease process and treatment	**Outcome:** Understands cause of renal failure and need for treatment. *Evaluation Parameters:* Patient can explain fluid and dietary restrictions and their relationship to kidney failure. Uses written information to clarify questions.	**Interventions and *Rationales:*** Assess understanding of disease process. *To provide baseline for teaching needs.* Assist patient to identify ways to incorporate treatment into his lifestyle. *To help build self-esteem.* Assist patient to obtain written information about renal disease. *To give the patient information that can be reviewed at home.*

in the subclavian or jugular vein may be left in place for 1 to 3 weeks. Catheters placed in the femoral vein can remain for up to 1 week.

For patients who require long-term or maintenance dialysis, vascular access is imperative and often a major problem. There are various forms of access, including arteriovenous fistula, arteriovenous graft, and arteriovenous shunt (Figure 47–2 ■). All of these allow access to the arterial circulation and return to the venous circulation.

Arteriovenous (AV) graft is the most common form of access for treating chronic renal failure. The graft consists of a Gortex tube that is surgically implanted into the forearm. A surgical in-

cision is made; an artery and vein are identified; then a tunnel, either straight or U-shaped, is created; and the graft is anastomosed to the artery and vein. After the surgical site is closed, the graft creates a raised area that looks like a large peripheral vein. During dialysis two large-bore needles are placed for outflow from and inflow to the graft. When the needles are removed, firm pressure is required until bleeding subsides.

An AV fistula is formed by creating a surgical incision, identifying a peripheral artery and vein, then creating an opening in both the artery and vein, and anastomosing the two openings. The anastomosis may be side to side, end to end, or end to side. The high pressure from the arterial flow creates a pseudo-

Double lumen catheter

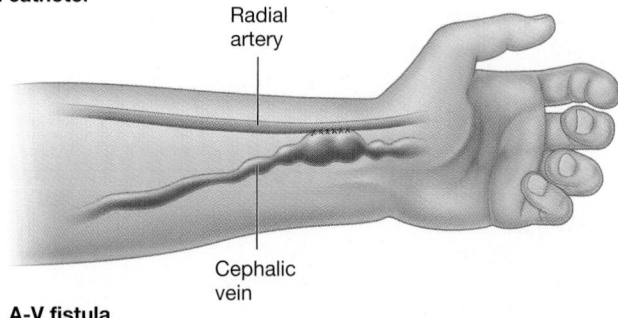

(a)

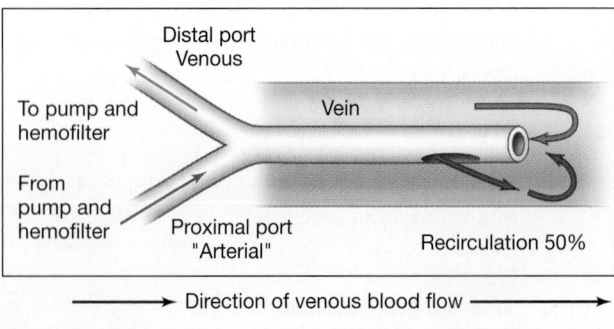

(b)

FIGURE 47–2 ■ Types of vascular access.

aneurysm of the vein that, when healed, a large-bore needle can be inserted into for dialysis. The fistula must mature and may require weeks to months before developing sufficient flow. If the fistula is accessed before it is developed, painful vascular spasm may occur. AV fistulas also have the potential of creating arterial insufficiency due to the high arterial blood flow diverted for dialysis. The symptoms that occur are known as vascular steal syndrome. The extremity becomes pale, cool, and painful. The nurse may assess patency of the fistula by palpation or auscultation. A patent fistula has a thrill when palpated and a bruit when auscultated with a stethoscope. The extremity should also be assessed and should be warm to the touch with good color.

AV external shunts are created by performing a cutdown over a peripheral artery and then a vein; a Teflon silicone cannula is implanted in both the artery and vein and is connected to silicone rubber tubing that exits from the skin. The two ends are then connected by an external U-shaped shunt that has a connector at the midpoint. The connection can be opened after both sides of the shunt are clamped, and then both sides are attached to the dialysis machine. External shunts are associated with complications such as infection and bleeding. Because of these, external shunts are rarely used for chronic maintenance dialysis.

The nursing implications for access devices are to protect the patency of the device and prevent infection. Complications involving access devices are one of the leading causes for hospitalization of patients on renal dialysis. Nursing management of complications of AV fistulas and grafts is described in Chart 47–3.

 **CRITICAL ALERT** *Blood pressure measurements, blood draws, and intravenous lines should never be performed on the arm that has the access device.*

To initiate dialysis, two large-bore needles are placed in the fistula or graft. Arterial blood is sent from the patient to the dialyzer with the assistance of a pump. Prior to dialysis, the machine is primed with saline so no air is in the system. At the beginning of dialysis, the saline is discarded as the blood fills the dialyzer circuit. Heparin is added to the blood as it enters the dialyzer, because blood has a tendency to clot when it encounters a foreign substance. The blood then enters the extracorporeal circuit, a long plastic cartridge that contains thousands of parallel hollow fibers, which are a semipermeable membrane made of a synthetic material. Dialysis fluid, called dialysate, is pumped into the cartridge, bathing the fibers; and through osmosis and diffusion, exchanges of fluid, electrolytes, and toxins from the blood enter the dialysate. The dialysate and blood are pumped in opposite directions through the dialyzer to maintain a high osmotic and chemical gradient. After the blood leaves the dialyzer, it is returned to the patient via the venous line through the second needle. At the end of the procedure, the dialysis machine is filled with saline to return all of the patient's blood to her. Each dialysis treatment takes between 3 and 4 hours, and most patients require treatment three times a week. Although dialysis is very efficient, it does not remove all metabolites. In between each dialysis treatment, electrolytes, toxins, and fluids increase. Contraindications to hemodialysis include hemodynamic instability, lack of access, and inability to anticoagulate. Chart 47–4 lists the complications of hemodialysis. The research topics related to dialysis are outlined in the Research Opportunities and Clinical Impact box (p. 1488). The Evidence-Based Practice box (p. 1488) discusses the success of hemodialysis.

Peritoneal Dialysis

Peritoneal dialysis is the infusion of sterile dialyzing fluid through an implanted catheter in the abdominal cavity. The dialysate fluid bathes the peritoneal membrane that covers the abdominal organs and overlies the capillary beds. As occurs with hemodialysis, excess fluid and solutes travel via osmosis, diffusion, and active transport from the peritoneal capillary fluid through the capillary walls, through the peritoneal membrane, into the dialyzing fluid. After a prescribed amount of time, the fluid is drained from the abdomen by gravity.

Peritoneal dialysis may be performed as continuous or intermittent. Continuous ambulatory peritoneal dialysis, or CAPD, requires multiple exchanges during the day and a continuous

CHART 47–3   Nursing Management of Complications of AV Fistulas and Grafts

Complication	Nursing Management
Grafts and Fistulas	
Infection	Use aseptic technique when cannulating access.
Bleeding	Do not cannulate new access too early.
Thrombosis	Teach patients not to wear anything constrictive on the accessed arm.
Pseudoaneurysm	Avoid multiple cannulations in the same area.
Pain from vascular steal syndrome	Apply warm compresses and administer analgesia.
Fistulas	
Inadequate blood flow	Teach patients to develop blood flow through daily exercises such as squeezing a ball while applying slight impedance to the flow distal to the access point.

CHART 47–4   Complications of Hemodialysis

Complication	Cause
Hypotension	Rapid removal of vascular volume Decreased systemic vascular resistance Decreased cardiac output
Loss of blood	Residual blood not rinsed from the dialyzer Accidental separation of vascular tubing Dialysis membrane rupture Bleeding from access site after removal of needles
Muscle cramps	Rapid removal of sodium and water
Hepatitis	Blood transfusions IV drug abuse
Sepsis	Infection of the vascular access site Introduction of bacteria during dialysis due to poor technique or interruption of tubing
Disequilibrium syndrome (development of cerebral edema)	Rapid changes in the composition of the extracellular fluid due to removal of solutes from the blood more rapidly than from the cerebrospinal fluid and the brain

EVIDENCE-BASED PRACTICE

Hemodialysis

Clinical Problem

Registries within the United States and Europe show an increase in the prevalence and incidence of end-stage renal disease. Only 32% to 33% of patients on hemodialysis survive beyond their fifth year of treatment. In comparison, 70% of patients who have kidney transplants survive beyond their fifth-year post transplant (Denhaerynck et al., 2007). The success of hemodialysis depends on following a regimen of fluid restriction, dietary guidelines, medication prescriptions, and attendance at hemodialysis sessions.

Research Findings

Denhaerynck et al. (2007) reviewed the literature looking at the four aspects of success with hemodialysis. Results of nonadherence regarding fluid restriction, dietary guidelines, medication prescriptions, and attendance at hemodialysis sessions varied greatly depending on how the study was conducted and which country the subjects were from. Most of the studies concentrated on adherence to fluid restriction, but adherence to the entire prescribed medical regimen is crucial for achieving good therapeutic results and reducing morbidity and mortality. Fluid nonadherence can result in fluid overload and provoke shortness of breath, dizziness, anxiety, panic, lung edema, and hypertension. Nonadherence to medication and dietary regimens can result in elevated serum levels of phosphate, which plays a role in the development of secondary hyperparathyroidism and renal osteodystrophy. Elevated levels of phosphate also contribute to coronary artery disease, which significantly increases the risk for mortality. Skipping or shortening dialysis is associated with increased mortality. Denhaerynck and colleagues found in their review of the literature that "In studies in which the delivered dialysis dose was determined by assessing appointment nonadherence, the relationship between the dose and higher mortality or higher blood pressure was significant. Skipping at least one dialysis session per month has been associated with a 25% to 30% higher risk of death."

Implications for Nursing Practice

After reviewing the literature, Denhaerynck et al. (2007) believed that "The prevalence of nonadherence with the different aspects of the dialysis regimen seems considerable. However, assessment of nonadherence has two major obstacles: inconsistencies in definitions and invalid measurement methods." Despite these issues, the evidence suggests that the behavioral dimension of hemodialysis should be considered to guarantee adherence to the treatment regimen and adequate treatment results. Nurses are in an excellent position to affect the behavioral dimension by assessing adherence and by implementing adherence-enhancing interventions and patient teaching that have the ultimate goal of improving clinical outcomes.

Critical Thinking Questions

1. Discuss the consequences of nonadherence to fluid, dietary, and medication regimens.

2. How can the nurse help the patient to be adherent with his hemodialysis regimen?

Answers to Critical Thinking Questions appear in Appendix D.

Reference

Denhaerynck, K., Manhaeve, D., Dobbels, F., Garzoni, D., Nolte, C., & De Geest, S. (2007). Prevalence and consequences of nonadherence to hemodialysis regimens. *American Journal of Critical Care, 16*(3), 222–235.

Source: Adapted from: Denhaerynck, K., Manhaeve, D., Dobbels, F., Garzoni, D., Nolte, C., & De Geest, S. (2007). Prevalence and consequences of nonadherence to hemodialysis regimens. American Journal of Critical Care, 16(3), 222–235.

RESEARCH OPPORTUNITIES AND CLINICAL IMPACT RELATED TO DIALYSIS

Research Area	Clinical Impact
What are the optimum serum bicarbonate and blood pH levels for patients on maintenance dialysis?	Data available for patients without renal insufficiency indicate that a mid-normal or high-normal blood pH range maintains better nutritional status than the low-normal range.
What are the long-term effects of correcting acidemia on clinical and nutrition-related outcomes?	Tight control of acidemia may improve nutritional status, but in the long term how will it affect morbidity and mortality?
Development of a simple and inexpensive method for determining the energy expenditure in individual acutely ill patients.	A simple method would enhance the monitoring of patients with renal failure. It would assist in defining how energy needs may vary with different protein and amino acid intakes.
The effects of different levels of protein intake on outcome and nutritional markers of patients on dialysis.	Increasing protein intake can alter dialysis requirements. It would be valuable to define the effect of higher levels of protein intake on the optimal dose of dialysis.
Which energy sources (protein, amino acids, carbohydrates, and fat) are associated with optimal clinical outcomes for patients with renal failure?	Maintaining optimal nutritional status and energy is crucial to the patient's progression and quality of life.

dwell overnight. The nighttime dwell can be accomplished with an exchange device, which would then perform two exchanges overnight. Continuous cyclic peritoneal dialysis, or CCPD, has a continuous daytime dwell with an exchange device exchanging several cycles overnight.

Intermittent peritoneal dialysis, or IPD, has periods in which dialysate is in the abdomen (wet abdomen) and periods in which the peritoneal cavity has been drained (dry abdomen). Patients who are unable to tolerate the full volume of dialysate or who leak at the catheter site may use a technique called tidal peritoneal dialysis, or TPD. TPD uses exchanges whereby the peritoneal cavity always contains some dialysate, usually up to half the regular amount. TPD is used infrequently, because it requires larger amounts of dialysate, which becomes very expensive.

■ Nursing Management

The amount of, concentration of, and dwell time for the dialysate are determined by the health care provider. When performing IPD, it is important to obtain baseline vital signs and weight for comparison at the end of the drainage. Measurement of abdominal girth and respiratory status is helpful as an indication of fluid retention. Assess for the presence of edema and obtain lab work for status of electrolytes, hematology, and blood glucose levels. When connecting or disconnecting the solution to the catheter, it is imperative to use good aseptic technique to prevent entry of bacteria into the peritoneal cavity. Dialysate fluid should be at least body temperature to provide comfort and enhance exchange. When the fluid is removed, it is important to assess its appearance. The outflow fluid should be straw colored and not be cloudy or blood tinged, which might indicate peritonitis. Compare the amount of dialysate infused to the outflow amount to determine whether less fluid drained out, and the patient is fluid balance positive; or whether there was more outflow volume than was infused, and the patient is fluid balance negative.

If it is anticipated that the patient will be doing CAPD or CCPD, the nursing focus is on teaching the patient/family how to perform the dialysis. Use of aseptic technique and signs and symptoms of infection are particularly important aspects to be taught.

Kidney Transplantation

Kidney transplantation is the treatment of choice for end-stage renal disease because it improves the quality of life and reduces the mortality risk for most patients (Post & Rose, 2008a). Restoring kidney function reverses many of the pathophysiological changes that occur with renal failure. Transplantation eliminates the dependence on and restrictions associated with dialysis. Maintenance of a successful kidney transplant costs much less than the continued need for dialysis.

A kidney for transplantation may be from a living donor, such as a relative with compatible tissue type, or a human cadaver. The success of the transplant is increased if it is received before dialysis is initiated. The success of the transplant is dependent on careful tissue typing before the transplant and immunosuppression after the transplant. Rejection is the major complication related to transplant surgery. These rejections are potentially reversible and are treated with increased immunosuppression. Signs of rejection are oliguria, sudden weight gain, fever, a rise in BUN and serum creatinine, hypertension, and pain over the graft site. The long-term complications, which occur secondary to the use of immunosuppressive drugs, include infection, hypertension, chronic liver disease, bone demineralization, cardiovascular disease, cancer, cataracts, and gastrointestinal hemorrhage.

■ Nursing Management

The greatest risk to patients who have undergone transplantation is infection. Risk for infection occurs from invasive procedures, immunosuppression, and exposure to infected individuals. When caring for transplant patients, use of aseptic technique is paramount. It is important to teach the patient/family that due to the immunosuppressive medications the patient's response to infection will be muted. Teach them the importance of being sensitive to low-grade temperature elevation, any fever, and unexplained tachycardia. Also stress the importance of avoiding exposure to individuals known to have infections. See Chapter 27 ☻ for care of the postoperative patient. A listing of resources about renal failure is included in the National Guidelines box.

NATIONAL GUIDELINES for Renal Failure Resources

- **KDOQI clinical practice guidelines and clinical practice recommendations for anemia in chronic kidney disease. (2) 2007 update of hemoglobin target.**—National Kidney Foundation—Disease Specific Society. 1997 (updated 2006 May; addendum released 2007 Sep). Original guideline: 145 pages; addendum: 60 pages. (NGC:006019)

- **Diagnosis and management of adults with chronic kidney disease.**—Michigan Quality Improvement Consortium - Professional Association. 2006 Nov. 1 page. (NGC:005685)

- **NKF-K/DOQI clinical practice guidelines for peritoneal dialysis adequacy: Update 2006.**—National Kidney Foundation—Disease Specific Society. 1997 (updated 2006). 32 pages. (NGC:005330)

- **NKF-K/DOQI clinical practice guidelines for vascular access: Update 2006.**—National Kidney Foundation—Disease Specific Society. 1997 (updated 2006). 26 pages. (NGC:005331)

- **NKF-K/DOQI clinical practice guidelines and clinical practice recommendations for anemia in chronic kidney disease: 2007 update of hemoglobin target.**—National Kidney Foundation—Disease Specific Society. 1997 (updated 2007). 145 pages; addendum 60 pages. (NGC:006019)

- **NKF-K/DOQI clinical practice guidelines for hemodialysis adequacy: Update 2006.**—National Kidney Foundation—Disease Specific Society. 1997 (updated 2006). 85 pages. (NGC:005329)

Source: National Guideline Clearinghouse. Retrieved August 10, 2008, from http://www.guideline.gov

PHARMACOLOGY Summary of Drugs Used in Renal Disorders

Medication Category	Action	Application/Indication	Nursing Responsibility
Anti-infectives Quinolone Ciprofloxacin (Cipro) Norfloxacin (Noroxcin)	Inhibits DNA gyrase, an enzyme necessary for bacterial replication.	Urinary tract infections, acute pyelonephritis.	Obtain culture and sensitivity prior to administration. Assess for skin rash or other signs of hypersensitivity reaction. Patient teaching: Increase fluid intake while taking mediation. Do not take the following within 2 hours of taking the medication: aluminum or magnesium antacids, iron supplements, multivitamins with zinc, or sucralfate. Avoid exposure to excess sunlight or artificial UV light. Avoid NSAIDs. Do not breast-feed.
Antineoplastic alkylating agent Chemotherapy	Thought to be the result of cross-linkage of DNA strands blocking synthesis of DNA, RNA, and protein.	Cancer.	Monitor leucopenia. Assess for signs of infection. Monitor and report hematuria or dysuria. Protect patient from potential sources of infection. Patient teaching: Adhere to dosage regimen; and do not omit, increase, decrease, or delay doses. Hair loss occurs in some patients and will be noted 3 weeks after therapy begins. Amenorrhea may last up to 1 year after medication is stopped. Do not breast-feed.
Loop diuretic Furosemide (Lasix) Bumetanide Torsamide	Decreases renal vascular resistance. May increase renal blood flow.	Treatment of edema associated with kidney disease, including nephrotic syndrome.	Monitor for signs of hypokalemia: malaise, depressed reflexes, muscle weakness, rapid irregular pulse, hypotension, vomiting, and mental confusion. Monitor blood pressure. Monitor serum and urine electrolytes. Monitor input and output (I&O) ratio and pattern. Patient teaching: Consult health care team regarding allowable salt and fluid intake. Eat potassium-rich foods daily; bananas, oranges, peaches, and dried dates. Signs and symptoms of hypokalemia. Make position changes slowly to prevent dizziness or imbalance. Avoid prolonged exposure to direct sun. Do not breast-feed.
Corticosteroid: Dexamethasone Decadron Prednisolone (Prelone) Delta-Cortef	Immediate-acting synthetic analog of hydrocortisone. Effect depends on biotransformation to prednisolone.	May be used in cancer therapy, in inflammatory conditions, and as an immunosuppressant.	Monitor blood pressure; Report an ascending pattern. Monitor serum electrolytes. Monitor for signs of infection: Use of steroids may mask infection and delay healing. Assess for oral Candida infection. Long-term use: Monitor bone density. Patient teaching: Do not alter dosing regimen or stop medication suddenly. Appetite will improve and a slight weight gain is expected. Avoid alcohol and caffeine, as they may contribute to steroid ulcer development. Report any symptoms of GI distress to the health care team. Do not breast-feed.
Antihypertensives	Refer to Chapter 21 ⊚.	Refer to Chapter 21 ⊚.	Refer to Chapter 21 ⊚.

DISORDERS OF THE BLADDER AND URINARY TRACT

The bladder stores urine and controls the elimination. Disorders affecting storage and elimination can result in incontinence or obstruction of urinary flow, which ultimately will affect renal function.

Nephrolithiasis

Renal and ureteral calculi are formed when substances in the urine come out of solution and form a precipitate that accumulates and grows in size. The calculi may form anywhere in the urinary tract but most commonly develop in the renal pelvis or calyces of the kidneys and are generally referred to as *kidney stones*. In the United States, 1 in 1,000 people require hospitalization for renal calculi, with its being more prevalent in males than in females (Hager & Mills, 2008).

The calculi vary in size and may be single or multiple. They can remain in the renal pelvis or pass through the ureter to the bladder. Small calculi are often passed spontaneously in the urine, whereas larger calculi, when entering the ureter, may damage the renal parenchyma or become lodged and cause pressure necrosis. If the calculi cannot pass through the ureter, they will cause obstruction leading to hydronephrosis, as the kidney is unable excrete urine. A **staghorn calculus** is a calculus or stone that remains in the renal pelvis and becomes so large that it fills the pelvis completely, blocking the flow of urine.

As stated earlier, the calculi are formed from precipitation of substances normally dissolved in the urine. Eighty percent of patients form calcium stones, the most common being calcium oxalate and less commonly calcium phosphate (Curhan, Aronson, & Preminger, 2008). Other types include magnesium ammonium phosphate or, occasionally, urate or cystine. The exact cause is unknown, but predisposing factors include:

- **Infection**—The pH changes provide a favorable medium for formation of calculi, especially magnesium ammonium phosphate or calcium phosphate. Infected tissue also provides a site for the development. Bacteria may serve as the nucleus in calculus formation, which is common in magnesium ammonium phosphate or staghorn calculi.
- **Dehydration**—The decrease in urine production leads calculus-forming substances to become concentrated and to form calculi more easily.
- **Metabolic factors**—Predispositions to the formation of calculi from metabolic abnormalities are hyperparathyroidism; renal tubular acidosis; gout, due to the elevated uric acid levels; defective metabolism of oxalate; genetic defect in the metabolism of cystine; and excessive intake of vitamin D or dietary calcium.
- **Obstruction**—Any condition that results in urinary stasis, such as spinal cord injury, allows the calculus-forming substances to remain and adhere. Stasis also promotes infection, which compounds the problem.

There are also several hereditary diseases by which the patient may develop renal calculi. In patients who have a rare disease called renal tubular acidosis, 70% develop renal calculi. Cystinuria and hyperoxaluria are two other rare, inherited metabolic disorders that also tend to develop calculi. Hypercalciuria is an inherited disease that causes calcium from food to be absorbed in excess and lost into the urine. This high level of calcium in the urine causes calcium oxalate or calcium phosphate crystals and the formation of calculi.

Laboratory and Diagnostic Procedures

Pain is the primary symptom and is usually the result of obstruction. As the calculi attempt to pass, they may occlude the opening to the ureter, increasing the number and force of peristaltic contractions. Typically the pain is severe and colicky, and it travels from the costovertebral angle to the flank, and then to the suprapubic area and external genitalia. If the calculi remain in the renal pelvis and calyces, the pain will be more constant and dull in nature. Because the pain is severe, nausea and vomiting usually occur. The patient may also have hematuria from damage by the calculi. Tests that are helpful in the diagnosis of calculi are outlined in the Diagnostic Tests box (p. 1492).

Medical Management

The majority of renal calculi are smaller than 5 millimeters in diameter and are able to pass without invasive intervention. Treatment focuses on promoting the passage with vigorous hydration and pain control. Diuretics may be given to prevent urinary stasis and continuing calculus formation. The Pharmacology Summary feature on page 1496 presents medications used to treat bladder and urinary tract disorders.

If calculi are too large to pass, surgical intervention or lithotripsy may be required. A cystoscope may be inserted through the urethra to retrieve calculi from the ureter. A ureteroscope may be inserted through the ureter to remove calculi from the kidney. If the attempt to capture the stone is unsuccessful, electrohydraulic lithotripsy or laser lithotripsy may be used to break the stone apart into smaller particles that can pass naturally. Extracorporeal shock-wave lithotripsy is the use of acoustic shock waves that travel through soft tissues to shatter the calculi into fragments, which can then pass normally. The procedure may be performed with the patient immersed in a tank of water and is then called hydrolithotripsy.

Nursing Management

It is important to try to determine the composition of the calculi to prevent further formation. Have the patient strain all urine through a urine strainer and send all solid material obtained to the lab for analysis. Encourage intake of fluids to facilitate passage and encourage the patient to walk. Renal calculi are very painful and frequent monitoring of pain level and administration of analgesics will assist with passage. In the past, patients who form calcium calculi were told to avoid dairy products and foods with high calcium content. Recent studies have shown that foods high in calcium may help prevent calcium calculi, but taking calcium in pill form may increase the risk of developing calculi (National Institute of Diabetes and Digestive and Kidney Diseases [NIDDK], 2007). Also, antacids that have a calcium

DIAGNOSTIC TESTS for Calculi

Test	Expected Abnormality	Rationale for Abnormality
Kidneys/ureters/bladder (KUB) radiograph	Most will show renal calculi.	Calculi are the precipitation of substances and will appear on x-ray.
Excretory urography, Abdominal CAT scan Renal MRI scan	Any of these imaging tests will reveal the obstruction and help determine the size and location of the calculi.	Calculi are the precipitation of substances and will appear on imaging.
Renal ultrasonography	May detect obstructive changes such as hydronephrosis.	If the obstruction is total, urine will be unable to drain, causing hydronephrosis.
Calculus analysis	Reveals mineral content.	Assists in diagnosing cause of calculi.
Urinalysis	Increased specific gravity and acid or alkaline pH. Hematuria. Crystals: calcium, urate, or cystine.	Suitable environment for different types of calculi formation. Damage from the calculi. Precipitate from the calculi.
Blood uric acid levels	May be increased.	Indicates gout as the cause of the calculi formation.

base may need to be avoided. Patients prone to calcium oxalate calculi should limit their intake of the following foods:

- Beets
- Chocolate
- Coffee
- Cola
- Nuts
- Rhubarb
- Spinach
- Strawberries
- Tea
- Wheat bran.

Assessment

Assessment for the patient with renal or ureteral calculi includes:

- Any past history or family history of calculi, gout, or other renal problems
- Blood in the urine
- Painful, urgent, and frequent urination
- Decreasing urine output
- Severe pain in the pelvis; can be dull, constant pain or intermittent, excruciating pain radiating anteriorly down to the vulva in women or testes in men.

Nursing Diagnoses

Major nursing diagnoses for the patient with calculi include:

- *Pain, Acute*
- *Urinary Elimination, Impaired*
- *Knowledge, Deficient* related to disease process

Planning

Overall goals include pain control, passage and identification of the calculi, and understanding of potential causes of calculus formation and the possible need for dietary restrictions and increased fluid intake.

Outcomes and Evaluation Parameters

Outcomes and evaluation parameters for the patient with calculi include:

- Pain is decreased to a tolerable level as evidenced by the patient rating the pain as less than 3 on a 0–10 scale.
- The patient will not exhibit impaired urinary elimination as evidenced by voiding more than 200 milliliters of clear amber urine each void.
- The patient will understand the disease process and plan of care as evidenced by his ability to articulate how calculi are formed and the need for dietary restrictions.

Interventions and Rationales

Nursing interventions and rationales for the patient with calculi include:

- Administer analgesics and antispasmodics as ordered. *Narcotic analgesia is warranted due to the severity of the pain. Antispasmodics relax tense muscles and reduce reflex spasms.*
- Monitor the volume and character of each void. Strain all urine for calculi. Encourage intake of fluid (12–17 eight-ounce glasses of fluid daily). *Adequate urine output indicates proper kidney function. Increased fluid intake is necessary to flush the calculi through the kidney and ureters. The characteristics of the urine can indicate the presence of infection (odorous, cloudy) and hemorrhage.*
- Provide information to the patient and significant others regarding dietary limitations for specific calculi, the need for regular activity, adequate fluid intake, and signs and symptoms of recurrence, such as pain and hematuria. *The patient needs an understanding of preventative strategies in order to comply with the regimen.*

Evaluation

The patient will have a tolerable level of pain as evidenced by a low pain rating on a 0–10 scale. The patient will void more than 200 milliliters of urine each void. The urine will be clear and without foul odor. The patient will be able to articulate an understanding of preventative measures and will agree to comply.

Topics that should be addressed with patients who have renal calculi and/or their families before discharge are presented in the Patient Teaching & Discharge Priorities box.

Cystitis and Urethritis

Cystitis is an inflammation of the urinary bladder and is more common in women than in men due to their urethra being shorter. The most common cause is the introduction of *Escherichia coli* from fecal material into the urethra. The bacteria then travel up to the bladder. Cystitis may also develop following sexual intercourse when organisms around the vaginal opening enter the urethra.

Urethritis is an inflammation of the urethra. As with cystitis, the most common causative microorganism is *Escherichia coli*, followed by *Klebsiella*, *Enterobacter*, *Proteus*, and *Pseudomonas*. Sexually transmitted infections, such as gonorrhea, can also cause cystitis and urethritis (Frazier & Drzymkowski, 2007).

Acute nongonococcal urethritis (NGU) is one of the most common sexually transmitted infections affecting men (Bradshaw et al., 2005). In a study conducted by Bradshaw and colleagues (2005), they found that the cause of the urethritis differed with different clinical and behavioral association. Adenoviruses and herpes simplex virus were associated with sex with men and insertive oral sex. *Chlamydia trachomatis* and *Mycoplasma genitalium* infections were associated with sex with women and unprotected vaginal sex. Insertive oral sex was highly associated with NGU, in which no pathogen was detected.

Laboratory and Diagnostic Procedures

The signs and symptoms of cystitis include increased urinary frequency with a sense of urgency, burning with urination, and at times hematuria. Urinalysis reveals bacteria, pus, and casts in the urine.

Nursing Management

Nursing management for the patient experiencing bladder infections includes treatment of the source and education regarding ways to prevent recurrent infections.

Interventions and Rationales

The nursing interventions and rationales for cystitis include the following. The nurse should encourage the patient to increase fluids. *Fluids assist in flushing bacteria out of the urethra.* Treatment usually consists of an appropriate antibiotic and, if urination is very painful, phenazopyridine, which is taken orally and when excreted by the kidney produces a topical analgesia. Inform the patient that the phenazopyridine will turn urine a bright-orange color that will stain clothing. If the patient is female, discuss the importance of cleansing the genital area from front to back to avoid contamination by fecal material. Also, encourage the female patient to void as soon as possible after having sexual intercourse. *This will flush contaminates that may have entered the urethra.* Encourage male patients to have protected sex. The Pharmacology Summary feature on page 1496 presents medications used to treat bladder and urinary tract disorders.

Neurogenic Bladder

As the renal system creates urine, it is stored in the bladder to be released. For the system to function properly, muscles and nerves work together to hold urine in the bladder and then release it when desired. When the bladder becomes full, nerves carry messages to the brain to let it know. The nerves then carry messages from the brain to tell the muscles either to tighten to block the release of urine or to release to allow the urine to flow out. Problems that affect the ability of the nerves to relay these messages may cause difficulty with bladder control. The most common causes of damage to nerves and nerve pathways are:

- Diabetes: autonomic neuropathies
- Cerebral disorders: stroke, brain tumor, dementia
- Vaginal childbirth
- Infections of the brain or spinal cord
- Traumatic injury to the brain or spinal cord
- Multiple sclerosis, Parkinson's disease
- Heavy metal poisoning
- Collagen diseases: systemic lupus erythematosus
- Herpes zoster. (Follin & Lenker, 2004; NIDDK, 2008)

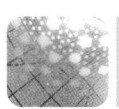

PATIENT TEACHING & DISCHARGE PRIORITIES for Renal Calculi

Need	Teaching
Prevention of further stones	Encourage patient intake of fluids to maintain a urine output of 3 to 4 liters a day. Patient's urine should be diluted and appear colorless.
Acidify urine	If the patient's urine is consistently alkaline (7.2 to 7.7), calcium phosphate or magnesium ammonium phosphate calculi may develop.
	Encourage the patient to drink fruit juices, especially cranberry juice.
Dietary restrictions with gout	Uric acid calculi may develop.
	Instruct patient/family to avoid alcohol and purine-rich foods, such as anchovies, liver, sardine, kidneys, sweetbreads, and lentils.

Bladder Control Problems

Three different kinds of bladder control problems arise from nerve damage:

1. **Urinary retention**—The nerves and pathways are damaged, and the bladder muscles do not receive the message that the bladder is full and it is time to release urine. The bladder then becomes too full, and urine may back up resulting in hydronephrosis, stagnant urine leading to infection, and overflow incontinence.

2. **Poor control of sphincter muscles**—There are sphincter muscles that surround the urethra keeping it closed to hold urine in the bladder. If the nerves or pathways to the sphincter muscles are damaged, the muscles will either become loose, allowing leakage, or remain tight, preventing the release of urine.

3. **Overactive bladder**—The damaged nerves and pathways may send signals to the bladder at inappropriate times causing the muscles to contract without warning. Symptoms of an overactive bladder include urinary frequency, urinating eight or more times a day or two or more times a night; urinary urgency, a strong and sudden need to urinate immediately; and urge incontinence, the leaking of urine that follows a strong, sudden urge.

Laboratory and Diagnostic Procedures

If the history and physical examination lead health care providers to suspect nerve damage, the tests outlined for neurogenic bladder in the Diagnostic Tests box are helpful in supporting the diagnosis.

Treatment for Overactive Bladder

The goal of treatment is to protect the kidney and upper urinary tract, prevent infection, and prevent urinary incontinence by evacuating the bladder. If the patient has an overactive bladder, bladder training may be the first course of treatment.

For bladder training, the patient keeps a diary to include fluid intake, times the patient voids, and any episodes of urine leakage. The diary helps to identify any patterns and helps in planning to avoid incontinence. The patient plans to void at certain times of the day and, as he gains more control, may increase the interval of time between voiding. For women, Kegel exercises are also part of bladder training and are used to strengthen the muscles that hold urine in. The following explains how to do Kegel exercises:

- Have the patient identify the correct muscles by imagining that she is sitting on a marble and wants to pick it up with her vagina. Have her picture sucking the marble into the vagina. Instruct the patient not to tighten her stomach, buttocks, or thigh muscles. Tightening the wrong muscles can put increased pressure on the muscles that control the bladder. Instruct the patient to squeeze the pelvic muscles and not to hold her breath.

- Instruct the patient to tighten the pelvic muscles and hold for a count of 3. Then relax the muscles for a count of 3. Initially tell the patient to do a few sets and gradually work up to 3 sets of 10 repeats. If it is difficult to do in a sitting position, have the patient try the exercise lying down.

- Inform the patient that bladder control may not improve for 3 to 6 weeks. Some patients have noticed an improvement after the first few weeks.

Bladder control treatment may include electrical stimulation of the nerves that control the bladder and sphincter muscles. Depending on which nerves are being treated, the electrical stimulus can be given through the vagina or through patches placed on the skin. Also, a wire can be surgically placed near the coccyx and connected to a stimulator that can be placed under the skin. This device, marketed as the InterStim system, has been approved by the Food and Drug Administration (FDA) to treat urge incontinence, urgency-frequency syndrome, and urinary retention in patients for whom other treatments have failed (NIDDK, 2008).

Medications that help to relax the bladder muscles and prevent bladder spasms include anticholinergics such as oxybutynin chloride (Ditropan), hyoscyamine (Levsin), propantheline bromide (Pro-Banthine), and tolterodine (Detrol). The most common side effect is dry mouth, but larger doses can cause blurred vision, tachycardia, flushing, and constipation. Administering time-release formulations helps to decrease the side effects. The Pharmacology Summary feature on page 1496 presents medications used to treat bladder and urinary tract disorders.

If urinary incontinence is severe and other treatments have failed, a surgery known as augmentation cystoplasty may be considered. The surgery enlarges the bladder by replacing diseased bladder with a section taken from the bowel. This improves the ability to store urine but may make it more difficult to empty, requiring regular catheterization.

Treatment for Urinary Retention

Urinary retention can occur due to the inability of the bladder wall muscle to contract or the inability of the sphincter muscle to relax. Patients can be taught techniques of bladder evacuation including Credé's method, Valsalva's maneuver, and intermittent catheterization.

DIAGNOSTIC TESTS for Neurogenic Bladder

Test	Expected Abnormality	Rationale for Abnormality
Voiding cystourethrography	Vesicoureteral reflux and continence	Poor nerve innervation to the muscles of the neck of the bladder
Uroflow	Diminished urine flow	Lack of muscle contraction
Cystometry	Poor bladder muscle tone with decreased pressures during filling and contraction	Poor nerve innervation with diminished tone
Sphincter electromyography	Decreased sphincter and bladder tone	Poor nerve innervation causing decreased bladder tone or involuntary spasms

Credé's method is the application of manual pressure over the lower abdomen; Valsalva's maneuver is performing a forced exhalation against a closed glottis. Both are used to promote complete emptying of the bladder. Although most patients can learn these methods, they are not always successful, and the patient may still need to perform catheterization.

 Patients with spinal cord injuries who perform Credé's method may develop autonomic dysreflexia, a rise in blood pressure to potentially fatal levels due to the stimulation of the sympathetic nervous system.

Patients and/or their family members can be taught to perform intermittent catheterization at regular intervals to empty the bladder. If patients are unable to catheterize themselves and there is no other family member or caregiver to assist them, then they may need to have an indwelling catheter that can be changed less often. There are several risks associated with indwelling catheters, including infection, bladder stones, and bladder tumors.

When nerve signals to the sphincter muscles that squeeze the urethra shut and the bladder are not coordinated, the bladder and urethral sphincter may contract at the same time, making it difficult to pass urine easily. Medications may be used to reduce muscle spasms and help relax the sphincter. Baclofen (Lioresal) is used to prevent muscle spasms or cramping in patients with multiple sclerosis and spinal injuries. Diazepam (Valium) can also be used as a muscle relaxant. Alpha-adrenergic blockers such as terazosin (Hytrin) and doxazosin (Cardura) can be used to relax the sphincter. Side effects can include low blood pressure, dizziness, and nasal congestion.

Urethral stents, which are small tubelike devices, can be inserted into the urethra and expanded, like a spring, widening the opening for urine to flow out. Risks associated with stents include movement of the stent and infection.

Male patients may consider surgery to prevent urinary retention. The surgeon passes a thin instrument through the urethra to deliver electrical or laser energy to burn away sphincter tissue. The patient may have a sphincter resection, or removal of a section of the sphincter, or a sphincterotomy, which is complete removal of the external sphincter. The surgery causes loss of urine control, and the patient will need to wear an external catheter that fits over the penis like a condom and drains the urine to a leg bag for collection. Complications of the surgery can include bleeding, infection, and problems obtaining an erection.

If conservative treatment has failed and the patient is experiencing frequent urinary retention with damage to the kidney, urinary diversion may be needed. Urinary diversion via an ileal conduit is described in the next section, Cancer of the Bladder. Another form of urinary diversion is the replacement of the bladder with a urinary reservoir, an internal pouch made from sections of bowel or other tissue. The urine is stored inside the body, and a catheter is passed through a stoma to empty the pouch. A third option is an orthotopic neobladder, which consists of a detubularized segment of intestine used to construct a reservoir for urine storage. The ureters are implanted into the reservoir, and the reservoir is anatomosed to the native urethra. The patient is able to control continence via the external sphincter of the urethra.

Nursing Management

Nursing care for patients with neurogenic bladder varies depending on the underlying cause and the method of treatment. It is very important to explain and review the treatment plan frequently. Topics that should be addressed with patients who have neurogenic bladder and/or their families before discharge are outlined in the Patient Teaching & Discharge Priorities box.

Cancer of the Bladder

Bladder cancer is the fourth most common cancer in men and the ninth leading cancer in women in the United States (McGrath, Michaud, & DeVivo, 2006). Tumors may develop on the surface of the bladder wall or grow within the bladder wall. Those that grow within the wall are invasive and usually infiltrate the bladder wall, invading the underlying muscles. Approximately 90% of bladder tumors are transitional cell carcinomas that arise from the transitional epithelium of mucous membranes (Davis, 2006; Follin & Lenker, 2004). Bladder tumors are most common in males over the age of 50 and are more common in populated industrial areas.

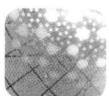

PATIENT TEACHING & DISCHARGE PRIORITIES for Neurogenic Bladder

Need	Teaching
Prevention of calculi formation and infection from urinary stasis	Encourage the patient to increase fluid intake to prevent formation of calculi and infection.
Bladder evacuation	Teach and have patient/family perform evacuation techniques, such as Credé's method, Valsalva's maneuver, and intermittent catheterization. To assist the female patient in learning self-catheterization, use a mirror.
Prevent infection	Teach patient/family the importance of strict aseptic technique during catheterization.
	If the patient has an indwelling catheter, teach the need for cleaning the catheter insertion site with soap and water at least twice a day.
	Teach patient/family to watch for signs of infection including: • Fever • Cloudy or foul-smelling urine.
Enterostomal care	If a urinary diversion procedure has been done, arrange for consultation with an enterostomal therapist.

PHARMACOLOGY Summary of Drugs Used in Bladder and Urinary Tract Disorders

Medication Category	Action	Application/Indication	Nursing Responsibility
Opioid Analgesics			
Morphine sulfate	Binds with and activates opioid receptors in brain and spinal cord to produce analgesia and euphoria.	Treatment of pain.	Regular, frequent assessment of pain and nonpain symptoms: i.e., shortness of breath, anxiety, etc. Safe and timely reduction of pain and symptom levels. Barriers to effective pain management should be addressed, including inappropriate fears of risk of side effects, addiction, and respiratory depression.
Urinary Analgesic			
Phenazopyridine (Pyridium)	Azo dye: exact mechanism of action not known. Therapeutic effect: local anesthetic action on urinary tract mucosa.	Symptomatic relief of pain, burning, frequency, and urgency caused by irritation of the urinary tract mucosa.	Instruct patient: The drug will turn urine a bright-orange color and will stain clothing. Stop use immediately, and contact health care team if skin or sclerae appear to have a yellowish color. Do not breast-feed while taking medication.
Anti-infectives			
Cephalosporins Cefazolin Ancef Kefzol Cefuroxime Kefurox Zinacef Ceftriaxone Rocephin	Binds to one or more of the penicillin-binding proteins located on cell walls of susceptible organisms. This inhibits the final stage of bacterial wall synthesis, killing the bacteria.	Infections of genitourinary tracts.	Determine prior hypersensitivity to cephalosporins and penicillins. Perform culture and sensitivity tests prior to therapy. Monitor input and output (I&O) pattern, especially with patients with impaired renal function and patients older than age 50. Monitor patients for antibiotic-associated pseudo-membranous enterocolitis caused by *Clostridia difficile*. Avoid use of alcohol during and for 48 to 72 hours after taking drug. Yogurt or buttermilk may help protect against intestinal superinfection by maintaining normal intestinal flora. Do not breast-feed while taking medication. For third-generation cephalosporins: Do not give within 2 hours of aluminum- or magnesium-containing antacids or iron supplements.
Sulfonamide Sulfamethoxazole Bactrim Sulfasoxazole Gantrisin	Believed to interfere with folic acid biosynthesis (required for bacterial growth) by competitive inhibition of aminobenzoic acid.	Acute, recurrent, and chronic urinary tract infections.	Obtain culture and sensitivity prior to administration. Monitor I&O. Fluid intake should be enough to create urinary output of at least 1,500 milliliters a day to prevent crystalluria and stone formation. Monitor urine pH daily. Acidic urine increases risk of crystalluria. Monitor temperature. Increased temperature may signify sensitization or hemolytic anemia. Assess for skin lesions, popular or vesicular, especially on sun-exposed areas. Observe patients with diabetes taking oral hypoglycemic medication for hypoglycemic reactions. Patient teaching: may make hormonal contraceptives unreliable. Avoid exposure to ultraviolet light and excessive sunlight. Do not breast-feed while taking medication.
Quinolone Ciprofloxacin (Cipro) Norfloxacin (Noroxcin)	Inhibits DNA gyrase, an enzyme necessary for bacterial replication.	Urinary tract infections, acute pyelonephritis.	Obtain culture and sensitivity prior to administration. Assess for skin rash or other signs of hypersensitivity reaction. Patient teaching: Increase fluid intake while taking mediation. Do not take the following within 2 hours of taking the medication: aluminum or magnesium antacids, iron supplements, multivitamins with zinc, or sucralfate. Avoid exposure to excess sunlight or artificial UV light. Avoid NSAIDs. Do not breast-feed.

PHARMACOLOGY Summary of Drugs Used in Bladder and Urinary Tract Disorders—*Continued*

Medication Category	Action	Application/Indication	Nursing Responsibility
Aminopenicillin Ampicillin Amoxicillin	Inhibits mucoprotein synthesis in cell wall of rapidly multiplying bacteria.	Urinary tract infections.	Obtain culture and sensitivity prior to administration. Determine previous hypersensitivity to penicillins and cephalosporins. Assess for urticarial rash: sign of hypersensitivity. Assess for diarrhea to rule out pseudomembranous colitis. Patient teaching: Take medication as prescribed; do not miss a dose and continue until all medication is taken. Do not breast-feed.
Anticholinergic (parasympatholytic) Oxybutynin (Ditropan)	Exerts direct antispasmodic action, and inhibits muscarinic effects of acetylcholine on smooth muscle.	Relieve symptoms associated with voiding in patients with neurogenic bladder.	Monitor patients for expected responses to therapy. Assess patients with colostomy or ileostomy for abdominal distention and onset of diarrhea—may be early signs of obstruction or toxic megacolon. Patient teaching: Do not drive or engage in potentially hazardous activities until the patient is aware of how the medication affects her. Do not overexert in hot environments; medication suppresses sweating and may cause heatstroke. Do not breast-feed.

Environmental carcinogens such as 2-naphthylamine, benzidine, tobacco, and nitrates have been found to predispose a person to transitional cell tumors. Therefore, those who work in industries where they are exposed to these carcinogens are at high risk for development of this type of tumor. These industries include rubber workers, weavers, leather finishers, hairdressers, aniline dye workers, petroleum workers, and spray painters. The time period between exposure and development of symptoms is approximately 18 years (Follin & Lenker, 2004).

Women also develop bladder cancer but tend to be diagnosed at more advanced stages. Bladder cancers that occur in women include a higher portion of rare cell types such as adenocarcinoma, small cell carcinoma, and squamous cell carcinoma (see Chapter 64 ☺). Also, older women have a thin bladder wall, which may permit a more rapid spread of the tumor. Risk factors for women are for those who smoke, use hair dye, and ingest tap water containing nitrates (Follin & Lenker, 2004).

Laboratory and Diagnostic Procedures

The first sign is most commonly gross, painless, intermittent hematuria. Patients with invasive tumors may have suprapubic pain after voiding.

Diagnostic tests include cystoscopy with anesthesia, so a bimanual examination can be done to determine whether the bladder is fixed to the pelvic wall. Biopsy of the tumor will confirm the type of cancer. Tests that are helpful in the diagnosis of bladder cancer are listed in the Diagnostic Tests box (p. 1498).

Staging and Grading the Tumor

Bladder cancer is categorized according to stage, the tumor's anatomic progression or depth, and to grade, the cell differentiation and aggressiveness. The American Joint Committee on Cancer (AJCC) developed the tumor, nodes, metastasis system, which includes the following stages:

- Stage 0: Cancer cells are found only on the inner surface of the bladder wall.
- Stage I: Cancer cells have invaded the layer of connective tissue under the bladder wall but have not penetrated muscle or spread to lymph nodes or distant sites.
- Stage II: Cancer cells have invaded the muscle layer but have not passed through the muscle to reach the tissue layer surrounding the bladder, nor have cancer cells spread to lymph nodes or distant sites.
- Stage III: Cancer cells have spread into the outer layer of tissue surrounding the bladder and may also invade surrounding structures, but lymph nodes and distant sites are not involved.
- Stage IV: Cancer cells have spread to the pelvic or abdominal wall or metastasized to a distant location such as the lungs, liver, or bones.

Grading compares how abnormal the cancer cells appear in relation to normal tissue of the same type and how aggressive the cells seem to be. Well-differentiated cells resemble normal cells more closely, tend to be less aggressive, grow slowly, and are termed low-grade tumors. Poorly differentiated cells are termed higher grade and are more aggressive (Davis, 2006).

Medical Management

If the tumor has not invaded the muscle, the tumor can be removed by transurethral resection and electrical destruction. If there are superficial tumors in multiple sites, intravesicular chemotherapy is used. The bladder is directly washed with an antineoplastic drug. Tumors may reoccur, and as long as they do

DIAGNOSTIC TESTS for Bladder Cancer

Test	Expected Abnormality	Rationale for Abnormality
Urinalysis	Red blood cells	Invasion of the bladder wall
	Malignant cells	
Excretory urography	Identifies tumor infiltration	Damage by the tumor to the bladder and surrounding structures
	Delineates problems in the upper urinary tract	
	Displays hydronephrosis	
	Detects deformity of the bladder wall	
CAT scan	Displays the thickness of the involved bladder wall	Progression of the cancer
	Detects enlarged retroperitoneal lymph nodes	
Ultrasonography	May detect metastasis outside of the bladder	Progression of the cancer

not invade the muscle layer, treatments may be repeated as needed. Intravesical immunotherapy is a treatment similar to intravesicular chemotherapy except the agent that is instilled to treat the cancer is bacillus Calmette-Guérin (BCG), a form of inactivated tuberculosis bacterium. BCG immunotherapy works by triggering the body's own immune system to destroy the cancer cells. This treatment is indicated for lower stage tumors that have not invaded the muscle wall.

Tumors that are too large to remove transurethrally and are away from the bladder neck and ureteral orifice, require a segmental bladder resection. Tumors that have infiltrated the muscle require a radical cystectomy, removal of the entire bladder. Due to the incidence of metastasis, the surgery involves removal of the bladder, lymph nodes, urethra, the prostate and seminal vesicles in males, and the uterus, ovaries, and adnexa in females. A urinary diversion is created using the intestinal tract and is usually an ileal conduit (Figure 47–3 ■). A segment of ileum is separated from the small intestine and formed into a tubular pouch with the open end being brought to the skin surface, forming a stoma. The ureters are then connected to the pouch and the patient will need to wear an external pouch to collect the urine.

Following a radical cystectomy, another option is the creation of a neobladder, or internal urine collection reservoir formed from the small intestine and connected to the urethra. The patient learns to void normally through the urethra by tightening the abdominal muscles in a Valsalva-type maneuver. The advantage of the neobladder is that the patient can maintain a relatively normal lifestyle. Because the neobladder does not fully empty, the patient will need to learn to perform self-catheterization twice a day to remove residual urine and prevent infection. The patient may also need to irrigate the bladder through the catheter to remove mucus that can accumulate from the neobladder wall.

Following the cystectomy, bladder cancers that are advanced will also require radiation therapy and chemotherapy. Refer to Chapter 64 ☺ for nursing care of the patient undergoing radiation therapy and chemotherapy.

Nursing Management

For general nursing management of the postoperative patient, refer to Chapter 27 ☺. Following radical cystectomy, one of the most important postoperative nursing responsibilities is to monitor urine output. Urine output that drops below 30 mL/hr may indicate shock, hemorrhage, obstructed ureters, or renal dysfunction. Encourage the patient to look at the stoma, and involve the patient in the care of the stoma as soon as possible. Advise the patient that as soon as she can she may participate in most activities except heavy lifting and contact sports. Prior to discharge, referral for home health care or an enterostomal therapist should be made to help coordinate the patient's care. Males will be impotent because the surgery damages the sympathetic and parasympathetic nerves that control erection and ejaculation. The patient may, at a later date, have a penile implant placed that will allow for sexual intercourse without ejaculation. Refer patients with an ostomy to resources such as the United Ostomy Association and the American Cancer Society.

Summary

The key to most renal and urinary disorders is the recognition and treatment of the cause and the preservation of renal function. The nurse is a critical member of the health care team in monitoring changes in the patient's condition and reporting and acting on these changes. Many renal and urinary disorders require lifestyle changes by the patient. The nurse's role in teaching, discussing, and evaluating the patient's understanding is critical to the success of long-term treatment and preservation of renal function.

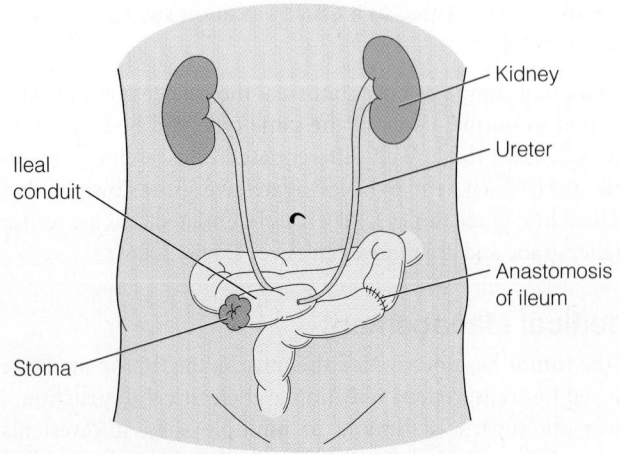

Kidney

Ureter

Ileal conduit

Anastomosis of ileum

Stoma

FIGURE 47–3 ■ Ileal conduit.

Clinical Preparation

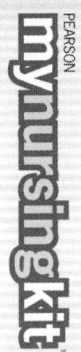

 **Read**

- History of Current Illness
- Past Medical History
- Physical Exam
- Admitting Medical Orders
- Laboratory Study Results

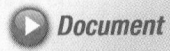 **Document**

- Summary of Hospitalization
- Pathophysiology Form
- Laboratory Values
- Laboratory Results Explanation

 **Apply**

- List of Potential Nursing Diagnoses
- Concept Map
- Critical Thinking Questions

Log on to MyNursingKit.com to download forms you will need and to complete further steps in the Clinical Preparation assignment.

HISTORY OF PRESENT ILLNESS

A 72-year-old male came to the emergency department (ED) complaining of right lower abdominal/groin pain. He stated that the pain was 8/10 and started suddenly after returning from the airport where he had lifted heavy luggage. He was found to have an incarcerated right inguinal hernia with bowel necrosis. He was taken to the operating room for bowel resection and repair of his hernia. Of note, in the ED he received 100 mL of normal saline IV and 300 mL of blood product. His output was 110 mL of urine via Foley catheter and 200 mL gastric content via nasogastric tube.

After the surgery he was admitted to the medical–surgical ward. On postoperative day 1, the patient's total urine output for the day was 230 mL. Despite receiving multiple fluid boluses, his urine output remained low and he had a rise in his serum creatinine and BUN. On the morning of postoperative day 2 he was transferred to the ICU for fluid management and strict monitoring of his intake and output.

Medical–Surgical History

He has no significant medical history and takes aspirin, multivitamins, fish oil, folic acid, and calcium daily. Family history is significant for adult-onset diabetes.

Social History

The patient has never smoked and occasionally drinks alcohol. He is married and lives with his wife.

Physical Exam

You receive the patient in bed with the head of the bed up 30 degrees. He opens his eyes to voice and follows commands. He complains of lethargy and a mild headache. Breath sounds are clear bilaterally. His abdomen is soft and slightly tender at the surgical site. The surgical site is clean, dry, and intact. His bowel sounds are decreased. The extremities are warm with 3+ pulses to all. You note 2+ dependent edema to the lower extremities.

Admitting Medical Orders

  Service: surgical ICU service
  Diagnosis: incarcerated right inguinal hernia, acute renal failure
  Allergies: penicillin
  Diet: renal diet; restrict protein intake to 0.25 to 0.5 g/kg per day; caloric intake of > 400 kcal/day; low sodium and potassium; restrict free water intake
  Vital signs every 1–2 hours and prn with O_2 saturations
  Accu-Cheks: before meals and at bedtime
  Activity: bed rest; up to chair bid

  Call house officer; temp > 38.5°C; SBP > 180 or < 90; pulse > 110 or < 50; resp rate > 30 or < 8; O_2 sat < 92%, urinary output < 30 mL/hr × 2 hours; blood sugar < 70 or > 150
  IVs: D5.45NS; titrate fluids to equal output plus 400 mL/day
  Foley to gravity drainage
  Strict I&O
  Weight daily
  Respiratory care: incentive spirometer every hour when awake
  DVT prophylaxis: sequential compression device to lower extremities

Scheduled Medications

  Metoprolol 5 mg IV q6h
  Famotidine 20 mg IV bid
  Regular insulin SC sliding scale
  Hydromorphone 0.2 mg/mL concentration IV per PCA, incremental 0.2 mg, lock-out 6 min

PRN Medications

  Diphenhydramine 12.5 mg IV q6h prn itching

Ordered Laboratory Studies

  Electrolyte panel qam
  Complete blood count qam

LABORATORY STUDY RESULTS

Test	Day 1	Day 2	Day 3
WBC	$17.8/mm^3$	$21.7/mm^3$	$12.3/mm^3$
RBC	$5.97/mm^3$	$5.80/mm^3$	$5.25/mm^3$
Hgb	17.1 g/dL	16.8 g/dL	15.4 g/dL
Hct	51.1%	49.6%	46.2%
Platelets	$867/mm^3$	$815/mm^3$	$658/mm^3$
Na	138 mEq/L	139 mEq/L	140 mEq/L
K	4.0 mEq/L	4.2 mEq/L	4.9 mEq/L
Cl	104 mEq/L	106 mEq/L	109 mEq/L
Total CO_2	26 mEq/L	25 mEq/L	26 mEq/L
BUN	14 mg/dL	25 mg/dL	33 mg/dL
Creatinine	1.0 mg/dL	1.9 mg/dL	2.1 mg/dL
Glucose	175 mg/dL	151 mg/dL	173 mg/dL

CRITICAL THINKING QUESTIONS

1. What contributed to the patient's acute renal failure?

2. What serum electrolyte changes would you expect to see?

Answers to Critical Thinking Questions appear in Appendix D.

NCLEX® REVIEW

1. The urine output of a patient in cardiogenic shock has been 200 mL for the last 24 hours and serum creatinine level is 1.5 mg/dL. The nurse suspects the patient is in acute renal failure when laboratory values indicate:
   1. BUN is 16 mg/dL.
   2. Calcium is 8.7 mg/dL.
   3. Sodium level is 152 mg/dL.
   4. Potassium is 4.8 mEq/L.

2. A patient with suspected pyelonephritis has urine sent for analysis and culture. The nurse checks for which result to substantiate the diagnosis?
   1. High specific gravity
   2. Low leukocyte count
   3. Casts in the urine
   4. Presence of protein

3. A patient has been diagnosed with the onset of acute renal failure. The nurse recognizes a prerenal precipitating cause in the patient is:
   1. Urinary calculi.
   2. Recent intravenous pylogram with contrast dye.
   3. Congestive heart failure.
   4. Crushing injury.

4. In order to prevent the cardiovascular complications associated with chronic renal failure, the nurse should include which interventions in the plan of care?
   1. Apply a non-drying lotion to the skin.
   2. Maintain a low fat, low carbohydrate diet.
   3. Evaluate ankles for edema daily.
   4. Restrict fluid and salt intake.

5. A patient has a neobladder created following a radical cystectomy. The nurse plans to teach the patient which technique?
   1. Manual Credé
   2. Kegel exercises
   3. Self-catheterization
   4. Stoma wafer change

6. A patient receiving hemodialysis tells the nurse that the worst part of the treatment is the severe leg cramps that he gets a few hours after the procedure. Which of the following should the nurse instruct this patient?
   1. The leg cramps are because of the blood transfusions that you receive.
   2. The leg cramps are because of an infection that will need to be treated.
   3. The leg cramps are because of the extra water and salt that is being removed.
   4. The leg cramps are because you aren't eating enough protein.

Answers for review questions appear in Appendix D

KEY TERMS

anasarca *p.1475*
anuria *p.1475*
azotemia *p.1464*
Bowman's capsule *p.1463*
end-stage renal disease (ESRD) *p.1480*
erythropoietin *p.1463*

glomerulus *p.1463*
hematuria *p.1464*
hyperkalemia *p.1476*
Kussmaul's respirations *p.1475*
nephron *p.1463*

oliguria *p.1464*
proteinuria *p.1464*
renin *p.1463*
staghorn calculus *p.1491*
suppurative *p.1468*

EXPLORE PEARSON **mynursingkit**™

MyNursingKit is your one stop for online chapter review materials and resources. Prepare for success with additional NCLEX®-style practice questions, interactive assignments and activities, web links, animations and videos, and more!

Register your access code from the front of your book at
www.mynursingkit.com

REFERENCES

Atkins, M. (2006a). *Clinical manifestations, evaluation, and staging of renal cell carcinoma.* Retrieved April 16, 2007, from http://www.uptodate.com

Atkins, M. (2006b). *Epidemiology, pathology, and pathogenesis of renal cell carcinoma.* Retrieved April 16, 2007, from http://www.uptodate.com

Bradshaw, C. S., Tabrizi, S. N., Read, T. R., Garland, S. M., Hopkins, C. A., Moss, L. M., et al. (2005). Etiologies of nongonococcal urethritis: Bacteria, viruses, and the association with orogenital exposure. *The Journal of Infectious Diseases, 193,* 336–345.

Curhan, G., Aronson, M., & Preminger, G. (2008). *Diagnosis and acute management of suspected nephrolithiasis in adults.* Retrieved August 4, 2008, from http://www.uptodate.com/patients/content/topic.do?topicKey=~PEEs8wkDGf.awB&selectedTitle=1~150&source=search_result

Davis, C. B. (2006). Bladder cancer: Revealing news about a hidden threat. *Nursing 2006 36*(4), 54–57.

Denhaerynck, K., Manhaeve, D., Dobbels, F., Garzoni, D., Nolte, C., & De Geest, S. (2007). Prevalence and consequences of nonadherence to hemodialysis regimens. *American Journal of Critical Care, 16*(3), 222–235.

Dirkes, S., & Hodge, K. (2007). Continuous renal replacement therapy in the adult intensive care unit. *Critical Care Nurse, 27*(2), 61–81.

Follin, S., & Lenker, E. (Eds.). (2004). *Handbook of diseases* (3rd ed.). Philadelphia: Lippincott Williams & Wilkins.

Frazier, M. S., & Drzymkowski, J. W. (2007). *Essentials of human diseases and conditions* (4th ed.). St. Louis: Elsevier.

Hager, L., & Mills, E. J. (Eds.). (2008). *Nursing: Understanding diseases.* Philadelphia: Lippincott Williams & Wilkins.

Hogan, M. A. (2007). *Nutrition & diet therapy* (2nd ed.). Upper Saddle River, NJ: Prentice Hall Health.

Ismail, N. (2008). *Indications for initiation of dialysis in chronic renal failure.* Retrieved August 9, 2008, from http://www.utdol.com/online/content/topic.do?topicKey=dialysis/18787&selectedTitle=23~150&source=search_result

Kaplan, A., Appel, G., & Pusey, C. (2007). *Treatment of anti-GBM antibody (Goodpasture's) disease.* Retrieved August 3, 2008, from http://www.uptodate.com/patients/content/topic.do?topicKey=~OaJEblyepxfF.0&selectedTitle=1~150&source=search_result

Kashtan, C. E. (2007). The wages of thin. *Journal of the American Society of Nephrology, 18,* 2800–2802.

Kee, J. L. (2005). *Handbook of laboratory and diagnostic tests with nursing implications.* Upper Saddle River, NJ: Prentice Hall Health.

McGrath, M., Michaud, D. S., & DeVivo, I. (2006). Hormonal and reproductive factors and the risk of bladder cancer in women. *American Journal of Epidemiology, 163*(3), 236–244.

Michigan Quality Improvement Consortium (2006). *Diagnosis and management of adults with chronic kidney disease.* Retrieved August 10, 2008, from http://www.guideline.gov

National Institute of Diabetes and Digestive and Kidney Diseases (NIDDK). (2007). *Kidney stones in adults.* Retrieved January 26, 2007, from http://kidney.niddk.nih.gov/kudiseases/pubs/stonesadults/

National Institute of Diabetes and Digestive and Kidney Diseases (NIDDK). (2008). *Nerve disease and bladder control.* Retrieved August 2, 2008, from http://kidney.niddk.nih.gov/kudiseases/pubs/nervedisease/

Porth, C. (2005). *Pathophysiology: Concepts of altered health states* (7th ed.). Philadelphia: Lippincott Williams & Wilkins.

Post, T. W., & Rose, B. D. (2008a). *Diagnostic approach to the patient with acute or chronic kidney disease or renal failure.* Retrieved August 10, 2008, from http://www.uptodate.com

Post, T. W., & Rose, B. D. (2008b). *Diagnostic approach to the patient with acute or chronic kidney disease.* Retrieved August 10, 2008, from http://www.uptodate.com

Post, T. W., & Rose, B. D. (2008c). *Overview of the management of chronic kidney disease in adults.* Retrieved August 10, 2008, from http://www.uptodate.com

Pusey, D. C., & Kalluri, R. (2008). *Pathogenesis and diagnosis of anti-GBM antibody (Goodpasture's) disease.* Retrieved August 3, 2008, from http://www.uptodate.com/patients/content/topic.do?topicKey=~3F_i7b5xj4DwvF&selectedTitle=2~52&source=search_result

Radhakrishnan, J. (2008). *Diagnosis and treatment of renal infarction.* Retrieved August 10, 2008, from http://www.utdol.com/online/content/topic.do?topicKey=renldis/17093&selectedTitle=1~32&source=search_result

Stevens, L., & Perrone, R. (2008) *Assessment of kidney function: Serum creatinine; BUN; and GFR.* Retrieved August 10, 2008, from http://www.uptodate.com

Urden, L. D., Stacy, K. M., & Lough, M. E. (Eds.). (2006). *Critical care nursing* (5th ed.). St. Louis: Mosby.

Walser, M. (2004). *Coping with kidney disease.* Hoboken, NJ: John Wiley.

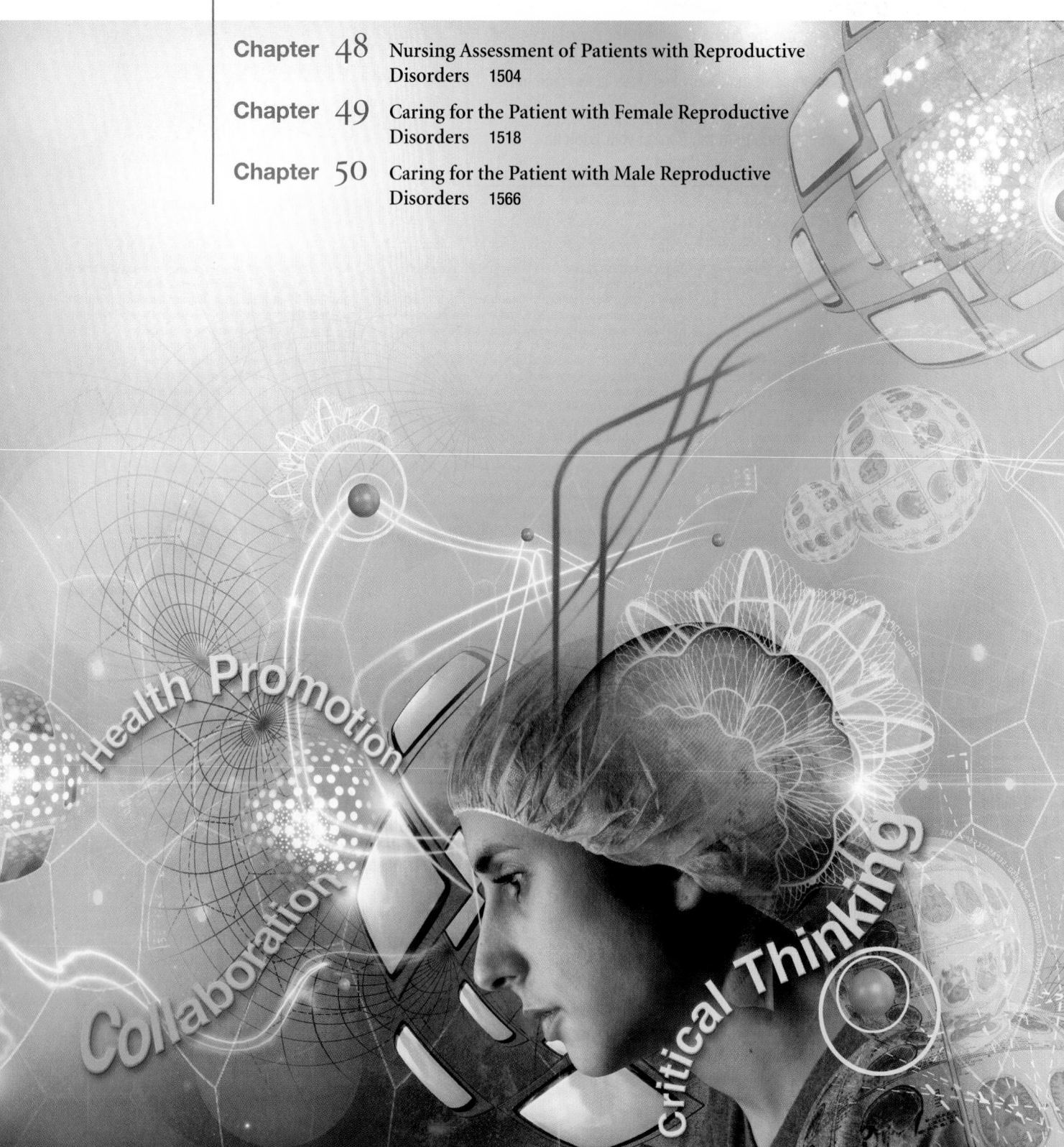

Nursing Management of Patients with Reproductive Disorders

Health Promotion

Collaboration

Critical Thinking

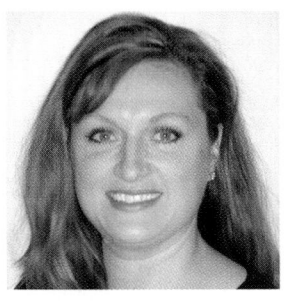

LESLIE My name is Leslie Theilen and I work on the High Risk Maternity Antepartum unit of a large medical center in a metropolitan area. The unit's population spans the spectrum of pregnancy disorders including preterm labor, gestational diabetes, preeclampsia, and premature rupture of membranes. Women stay on the unit from hours to months before they deliver, often experiencing a sense of loss and independence due to separation from their homes and families.

I have worked in this hospital for 17 years. I am a member of the American Association of Women's Health, Obstetrics, and Neonatal Nurses, and hold several national certifications. My practice roles include providing direct patient care, precepting new nurses and nursing students, conducting unit-based audits for performance improvement, participating on the Joint Commission preparation team and staff nurse council, teaching classes as a service excellence adviser, and serving as a mentor coordinator for my unit.

I have wanted to be a nurse since the first time I saw a baby born. I made a **commitment,** to myself and my patients, to be the best nurse I could be. As a nurse caring for pregnant women, I am not only responsible for the well-being of the patient but also that of her unborn child(ren). I have cared for women of childbearing ages from 12 to 50, the poor and wealthy, married and single, addicted and sober, and treated each one as I would want to be cared for. I regularly attend classes and seminars in order to stay up to date with research findings and changes in clinical practice. Recently, I completed my bachelor's degree in nursing from California State University, Sacramento.

A typical day is anything but. I may be the charge nurse for the day, assigned to precept a nursing student or orient a new hire. Or I may be assigned to care for three patients with different needs and acuities. Recently, I cared for a patient who was 22 weeks pregnant with bulging membranes. She arrived on the unit via wheelchair, coming from the doctor's office after a routine ultrasound found her cervix dilated 5 centimeters with the bag of water bulging through into her vagina. She was crying and obviously upset. Offering reassurance, I placed her in the Trendelenburg position in the hopes that gravity would assist with the recession of the bag of water. I explained to her that the first goal was to stop the continued dilation of the cervix, then to get the pregnancy to the 24-week mark that constitutes viability. The patient was alone and had no one to call. I spent most of my time talking with her and listening to her fears. Although I tried for several hours to stop her contractions, her bag of water ruptured. Worried that she had advanced in dilation and the baby would easily pass through the cervix, I notified the doctor and then explained what was happening to the patient, emphasizing that our goal was to keep her pregnant as long as possible. Upon examination, the doctor explained to the patient there was nothing we could do to prevent the birth from happening. The patient began sobbing. I held her hand and promised not to leave her.

The doctor wanted to transfer the patient to labor and delivery to give birth since delivery was not normally done on our unit. I could not in all good **conscience** let this women be moved from her surroundings where she felt safe. This was a time for **compassion** not routine. There was no question; she would stay and I would help her give birth. I knew I had the **competence** to assist the doctor in her delivery and the **confidence** to provide her with the best care I could give. Her labor was short and after a few pushes, she gave birth to a son. He was given a name, pictures of the two of them were taken, and his mother held him until he died. I stayed with her as she counted his fingers and toes, kissing him while she told him how perfect he was. I found myself crying with my patient over the loss of her son. Later, I thanked her for letting me care for her and sharing that very sacred moment in her life. She thanked me for letting her stay on the unit and deliver with the only nurse she had come to know and trust. I was proud that my **comportment** had made an impression and that in thinking outside the box I had made a good decision for my patient.

At the end of each of my workdays, I look back at the people who invited me into their lives. It is with great gratitude that I am allowed to be the hand that calms the anxious, the comforting voice that soothes the ache, the attentive ear that listens to the worries. I am a counselor, care provider, safe haven, and friend. I am a nurse.

"I made a **commitment,** to myself and my patients, to be the best nurse I could be. As a nurse caring for pregnant women, I am not only responsible for the well-being of the patient but also that of her unborn child(ren)."

Nursing Assessment of Patients with Reproductive Disorders

Patricia Caudle
With contribution by:
Laurie Kaudewitz

Outcome-Based Learning Objectives

After studying this chapter, the learner will be able to:

1. Describe the structures and function of the male and female reproductive systems.
2. Identify pertinent subjective and objective data related to the reproductive systems and information about the sexual function that should be obtained.
3. Identify risk factors for reproductive system disorders.
4. Differentiate normal from abnormal findings obtained from the physical assessment for males and females.
5. Describe age-related changes in the male and female reproductive systems.
6. Discuss the implications for health promotion related to the reproductive systems of females and males.

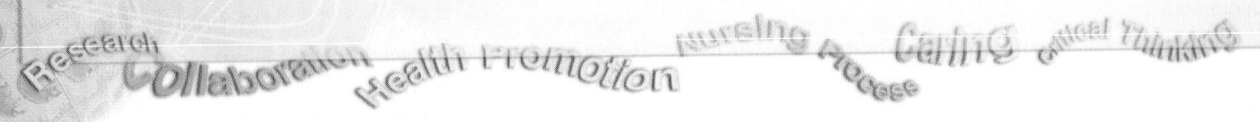

ASSESSMENT OF the female and male reproductive systems requires an understanding of the anatomy, open communications, a nonjudgmental attitude, gentleness, and a high degree of empathy and compassion. Most women and men consider the genital area very private, and many may be reluctant to talk about concerns or to allow examination by the nurse. The nurse should not be offended if the patient asks for an examiner of the same gender. Privacy and confidentiality are very important and should be maintained at all times.

The reproductive systems of the female and male include sexual organs, the lower urinary system, and the anorectal area. This means that assessment of the reproductive system is complex and must include history and physical examination that is inclusive of the three systems. This chapter outlines the important components of the female and male reproductive system assessment. Concepts discussed here introduce the learner to assessment skills needed to care for patients with disorders of the female and male reproductive systems discussed in Chapters 49 and 50 ⊚ .

Female Reproductive System

The female breast tissue extends from the second to the sixth rib on either side of the sternum and covers the pectoralis major muscle (Figure 48–1 ■). The skin over the breasts is the same color as other skin and may have striae (stretch marks). The nipples are on the anterior surface of each breast, surrounded by the areola (pigmented skin around the nipple). The areola has sebaceous glands that may be raised and more active during pregnancy (Montgomery's tubercles). Sebaceous glands help to moisturize the nipple to make it more pliable (Stables & Rankin, 2005). Occasionally, supernumerary nipples are seen along a line (the "milk line") from the axilla to the upper thigh on either side (Figure 48–2 ■). These small nipples may be mistaken for moles. They are considered normal variants and are benign (Bickley & Szilagyi, 2007).

Each breast is made up of glandular, connective, and adipose (fatty) tissue. The glandular tissue includes 15 to 20 lobes suspended from ducts that drain into sinuses. The sinuses are near the nipple and are drained by smaller ducts on the nipple surface. The lobes are further divided into lobules where the milk is produced during lactation. The connective tissue provides support via ligaments within the breast (also called Cooper's ligaments). Adipose tissue completes the structure of the breasts and determines the size of the breast (see Figure 48–1 ■) (Bickley & Szilagyi, 2007).

Physiologically, breast tissue responds to estrogen (steroid female hormone produced by the ovary and placenta),

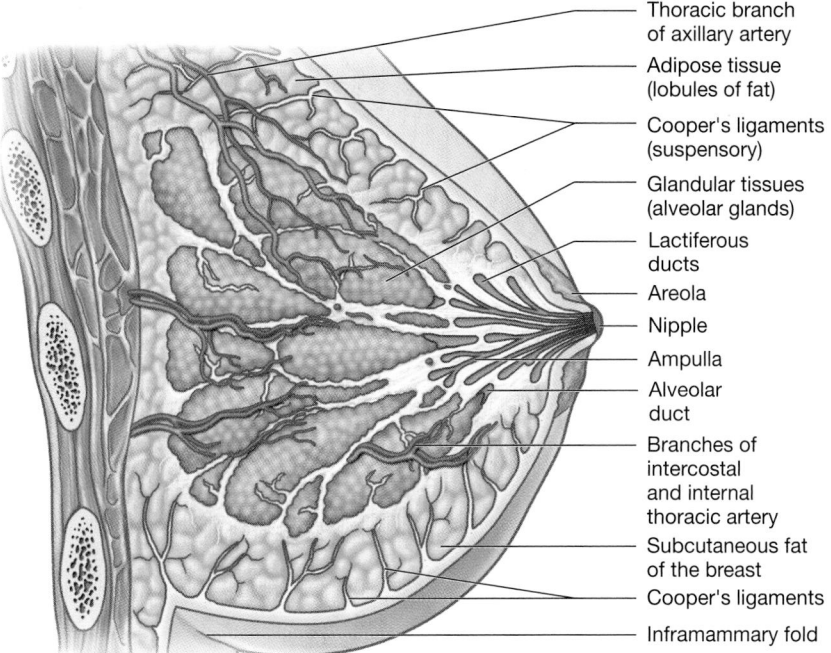

Thoracic branch
of axillary artery

Adipose tissue
(lobules of fat)

Cooper's ligaments
(suspensory)

Glandular tissues
(alveolar glands)

Lactiferous
ducts

Areola

Nipple

Ampulla

Alveolar
duct

Branches of
intercostal
and internal
thoracic artery

Subcutaneous fat
of the breast

Cooper's ligaments

Inframammary fold

FIGURE 48–1 ■ The female breast.

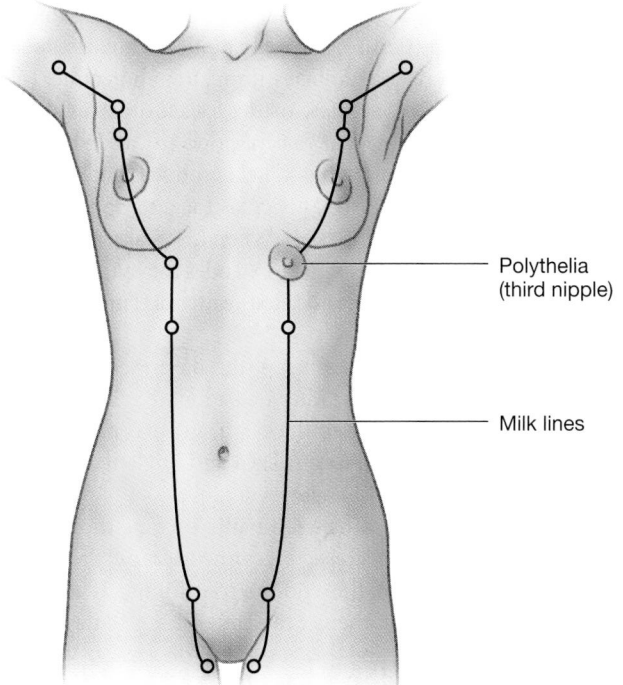

Polythelia
(third nipple)

Milk lines

FIGURE 48–2 ■ Supernumerary nipples.

progesterone (steroid female hormone produced by the ovary and placenta), **prolactin** (hormone produced in the anterior pituitary), and **oxytocin** (hormone produced in the hypothalamus and released by the posterior pituitary) in the processes of **galactogenesis** (the manufacture of milk from available nutrients) and **lactation** (breast-feeding). The cyclic changes in estrogen and progesterone levels each month cause changes in the breasts as they prepare for lactation, even though a pregnancy does not always occur. This cyclic exposure to hormonal change is thought to be a factor in the development of breast cancer (American Cancer Society, 2006b).

Lymph nodes drain the breasts to the axilla, clavicular area, mediastinum, the opposite breast, and into glands in the liver (Stables & Rankin, 2005). The lymph nodes of the axilla and clavicular area are accessible to physical examination.

The female external genitalia depicted in Figure 48–3 ■ (p. 1506) have several components that are important to recognize during examination. These include the mons, the vulva (labia majora and labia minora), the clitoris (erectile tissue at apex of labia minora), the urinary meatus (urinary opening above the vaginal opening), and the introitus (opening to the vagina). The introitus is surrounded by an elastic line of connective tissue called the hymenal ring (Stables & Rankin, 2005).

Internally, the female reproductive organs include the uterus (muscular, hollow organ where the embryo matures before birth), the fallopian tubes (hollow tube from the uterus to the ovaries, where fertilization occurs), and the ovaries (female gonad). The uterus sits between the rectum and the bladder. The opening to the uterus is the cervix, found at the internal end of the vagina (Stables & Rankin, 2005) (Figure 48–4 ■, p. 1506).

The lymph nodes of the female external and internal reproductive organs that are accessible to examination are the superficial inguinal nodes, including the horizontal grouping and the vertical grouping. These nodes are found in the groin on each side. The horizontal group is below the inguinal ligament, and the vertical group lines up along the great saphenous vein. The horizontal group drains the lower abdomen, the superficial external genitalia, the anal canal, the perineum, and the lower vagina. The vertical group drains the upper leg (Bickley & Szilagyi, 2007).

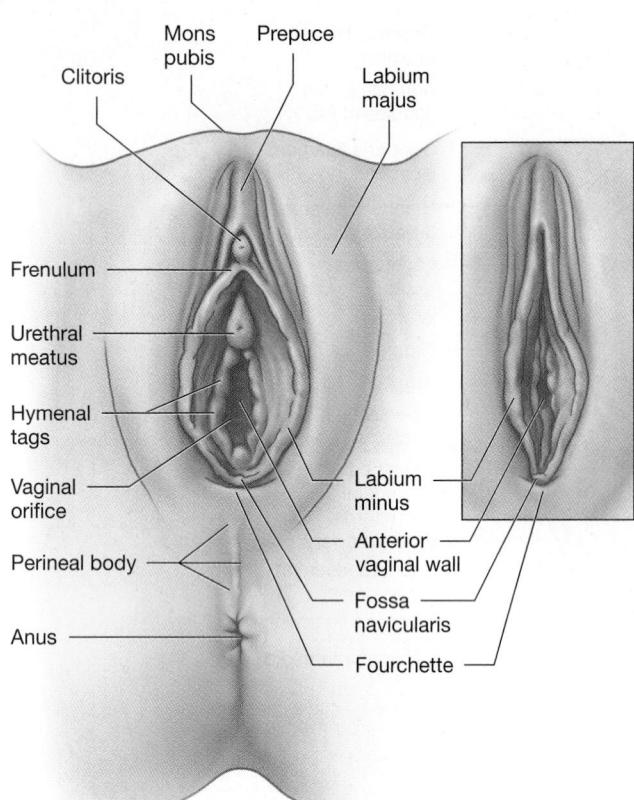

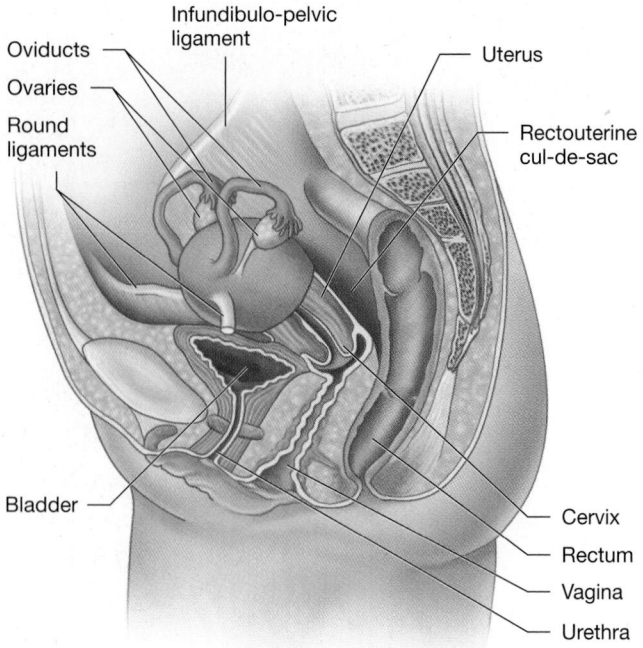

FIGURE 48–4 ■ Female internal genitalia.

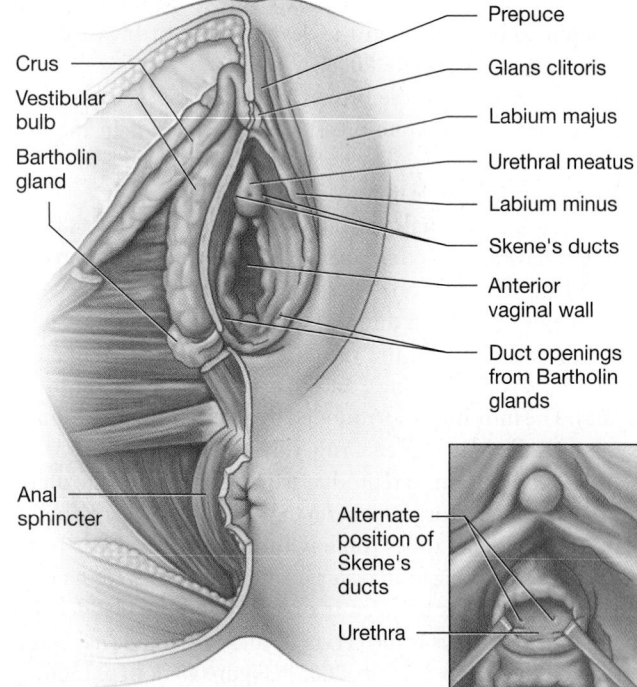

FIGURE 48–3 ■ Female vulva including anus.

Physiology of the Menstrual Cycle

The menstrual cycle is a complex physiological process that involves the hypothalamus, pituitary gland, ovaries, and endometrium. The cycle begins with the first day of menses. Menses, or vaginal bleeding, is the result of the thickened endometrial lining that was constructed during the previous cycle that is being sloughed or shed. As this occurs, the hypothalamus (through

complex signals) recognizes a need to secrete gonadotropin-releasing hormone (GnRH). This hormone stimulates the anterior pituitary to release follicle-stimulating hormone (FSH), which in turn stimulates a few of the follicles that exist on the ovary. From the follicles that first respond to the FSH, one becomes dominant. This growing follicle produces and secretes estrogen. When estrogen peaks, it signals the anterior pituitary to release luteinizing hormone (LH). When LH peaks, ovulation occurs. That is, the dominant follicle extrudes the ovum. The ovum travels to the fallopian tube and into the uterus (Hughes, Steele, & Leclaire, 2006).

Under the influence of estrogen, the uterine lining has been thickening before ovulation. After ovulation, the lining begins to proliferate; that is, it gets even thicker. It now has more nutrients available should the ovum be fertilized and implantation into the endometrial lining occur (Hughes et al., 2006).

After ovulation, the follicle remnants become the corpus luteum (yellow body), which secretes progesterone. Progesterone causes the "fluffing" of the endometrial lining. If a fertilized ovum does not implant, then at the end of 12 to 14 days the corpus luteum regresses and progesterone decreases. When this happens, the endometrial lining sloughs and menses begins (Hughes et al., 2006). Figure 48–5 ■ is a graph that shows when in the cycle each event occurs.

■ Male Reproductive System

The male breast is a small nipple and areola. There is a small amount of undeveloped breast tissue that may enlarge (gynecomastia) in response to certain drugs or illicit drug use. Breast cancer rarely occurs in male breast tissue (Slovik, 2006).

The male external genitalia are pictured in Figure 48–6 ■. External genitalia include the penis and scrotum (skin pouch that contain the testes). The penis is made up of erectile tissue

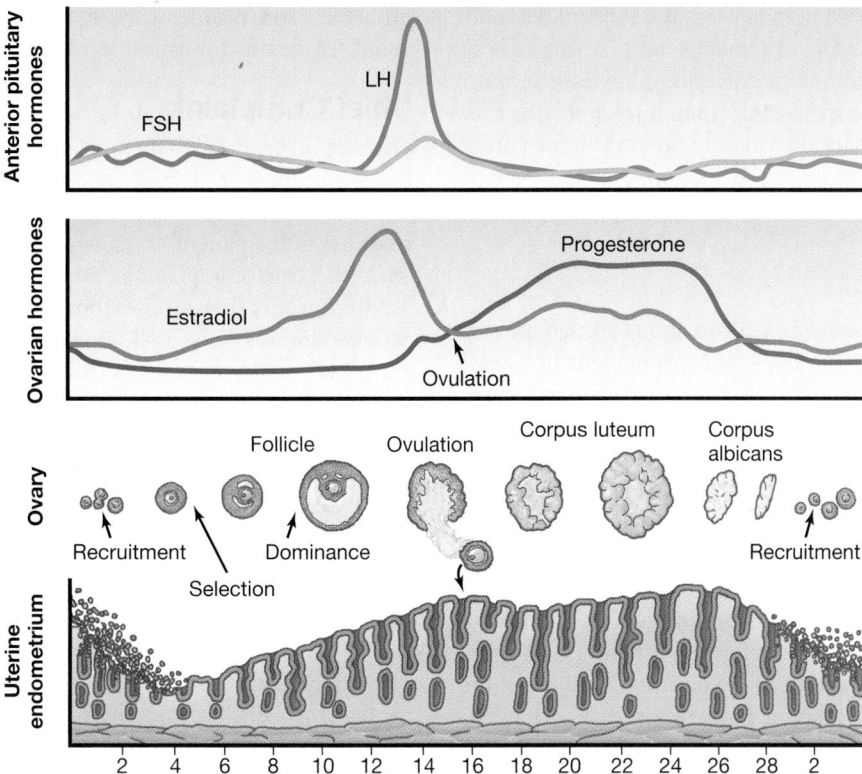

FIGURE 48–5 ■ The menstrual cycle.

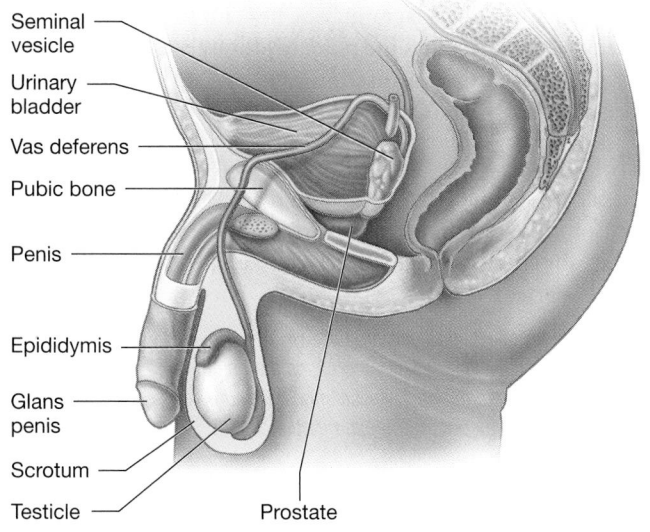

FIGURE 48–6 ■ Male genitalia.

and contains the urethra. At the tip of the penis is the urinary meatus (opening of the urethra to the outside). Within the scrotum are the testis, the epididymis (anatomic structure on the posterior of the testicle), and the spermatic duct. The spermatic duct is surrounded by blood vessels and together they form the spermatic cord (Bickley & Szilagyi, 2007). As the spermatic cord ascends into the abdomen via the inguinal canal, it becomes the vas deferens (duct that carries sperm and semen to the seminal vesicles and prostate). Sperm pass through the vas deferens to the seminal vesicles (finger-like structures behind the prostate), which produce 60% of semen

(Stables & Rankin, 2005), and into the prostate (a gland at the bladder neck; the urethra passes through it) to be mixed with prostate fluid before ejaculation during intercourse. The prostate is about 2.5 centimeters long with a median sulcus (groove) between two lateral lobes. A third, anterior, lobe is not palpable. The prostate is fibrous and firm to touch (Bickley & Szilagyi, 2007).

The inguinal canal (tunnel for vas deferens) is medial to the inguinal ligament and has two openings: the external and internal inguinal rings. The external inguinal ring is accessible to examination. The inguinal canal is the site for direct and indirect inguinal hernias, which are common in men (Bickley & Szilagyi, 2007). Chapter 50 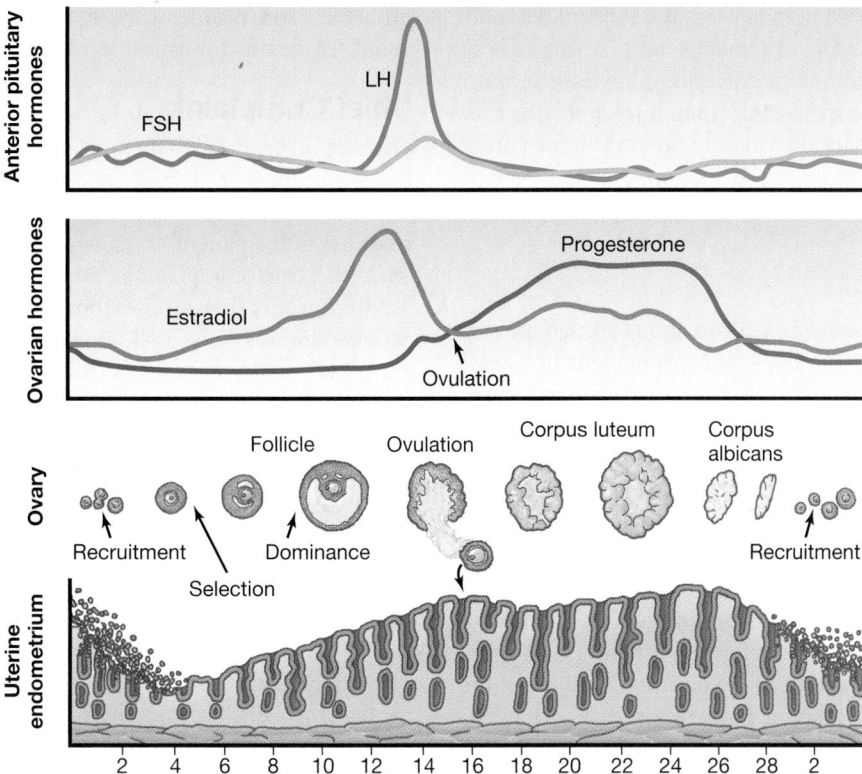 includes an in-depth discussion of hernias.

Inguinal lymph nodes are located below the inguinal ligament in a horizontal configuration at the groin and along the femoral and great saphenous veins vertically on the upper thigh. The horizontal group drains the lower abdomen, buttock, external genitalia, anal canal, and perianal area. The vertical group drains the upper thigh. The testicles drain into lymph nodes in the abdomen. The abdominal lymph nodes are not accessible to palpation (Bickley & Szilagyi, 2007).

Physiology of Male Reproduction

Male reproductive physiology begins with an interaction between the hypothalamus, the pituitary gland, and the testis. The hypothalamus secretes gonadotropin-releasing hormone (GnRH) based on signals from the central nervous system and blood levels of testosterone. The GnRH travels to the anterior pituitary gland and causes the release of luteinizing hormone (LH) and follicle-stimulating hormone (FSH). LH stimulates testosterone and other hormone synthesis in the Leydig cells of the testicle. The role of FSH in the male is not fully understood. It appears to be necessary for spermatogenesis. Leydig cells of the testis produce testosterone. Sertoli cells of the testis support and provide nutrients for spermatids (immature sperm) as they grow to become spermatozoa (mature sperm). Information about sex chromosome disorders is presented in the Genetic Considerations box.

History

History, or what the patient can tell you about himself and his health concerns, is the most important component of assessment. Much of what nurses do is based on what the patient is able to convey about how he or she feels and the symptoms he or she is having. In this section, the health history related to the reproductive system is discussed.

Biographical and Demographic Data

After introductions are completed, the patient is asked about age, marital status, occupation, address, and other data that will identify this history as specifically for this patient. It is important to date and time the history and to note the reliability of the person providing the information. From this interview clues begin to emerge related to reproductive system problems. For instance, the older the female patient, the higher the risks are for breast, endometrial, and uterine cancer. See Chapter 49 for more about risks for cancer in women. The older the male patient, the higher the risks are for sexual dysfunction, prostate

problems, and bladder cancer. See Chapter 50 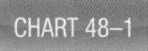 for more about risk factors for cancer in men.

Chief Complaint

This section begins with the chief complaint. The patient is asked to describe the reproductive concern that has brought her or him into the health care system. The chief complaint is usually recorded in the patient's own words (Bickley & Szilagyi, 2007). Once the chief complaint is established, a description of the health concern follows. It is important to ask about the onset, location, duration, associated symptoms, any treatments tried, aggravating factors, and factors (other than treatments) that may alleviate the problem. For example, a male may complain of urinary frequency, urgency, difficulty beginning the urinary stream, and nocturia with gradual onset when he is describing symptoms of benign prostatic hyperplasia (BPH). See Chapter 50 for a complete description of BPH. Chart 48–1 lists specific questions that can be used to elicit history of present illness from a man with benign prostatic hyperplasia.

Current Medications

This section of the history should include a list of prescribed medications, illicit drugs, herbal remedies, over-the-counter drugs, home remedies, or vitamins that the patient is taking. It is important to record the name of the drug or herb, the dosage, and how often it is being taken. Some women who are taking birth control pills may forget to mention this, so it is a good habit to ask women of childbearing age about birth control pills. Ask men with prostate problems whether they are taking saw palmetto. Men who are taking Viagra may be hesitant to discuss this with the nurse. This drug has the potential for interacting with other drugs, such as cardiac medications, and causing harm, so it is important to ask about it.

Allergies

All patients should be asked about allergies to drugs, latex, foods, and environmental substances. For those patients with allergies, the chart should be clearly marked so that the health care team is alerted.

> **CRITICAL ALERT** *Examination of a patient using latex gloves when that patient has a latex allergy increases the risk for an adverse reaction, including anaphylactic shock. Be sure to ask about possible allergy before the examination begins.*

> **GENETIC CONSIDERATIONS for Sex Chromosome Disorders**
>
> Normal sperm occur in two types. One type has 22 autosomes and an X chromosome, and the other has 22 autosomes and a Y chromosome. Only one type of ovum is ready for fertilization, and it has 22 autosomes and an X chromosome. Therefore, it is the sperm contribution to the coupling that will determine the sex of the child. In the assessment of the female and the male, the examiner may examine individuals who have a sex chromosome disorder. The two most common examples are Klinefelter's syndrome and Turner's syndrome.
>
> Klinefelter's syndrome occurs in about 1 in 1,000 births and is usually an extra one or two X chromosomes (XXY or XXXY). This is generally not identified until puberty when the secondary sexual characteristics do not occur. These individuals will have decreased testosterone, testicular atrophy, long legs and arms, feminine hair distribution, gynecomastia, a feminine voice, infertility, and mental retardation (Banasik, 2005).
>
> Turner's syndrome is a monosomy disorder in which the sex chromosome has only one X chromosome and no corresponding X or Y. The phenotype (how the person will look or will display the abnormality) is female, but the ovaries do not develop and secondary sex characteristics such as breast development and pubic hair do not appear. This abnormality is rare, occurring in about 1 in 3,000 live births (Banasik, 2005). Other physical characteristics include short stature, webbing of the neck, amenorrhea (no menses), a wide chest, and heart defects.
>
> *Sources:* Banasik, J. (2005). Genetic and developmental disorders. In L. Copstead & J. Banasik, *Pathophysiology* (3rd ed., pp. 123–148). Philadelphia: W. B. Saunders; and Moore, K., & Persaud, T. (2003). *Before we are born: Essentials of embryology and birth defects* (6th ed.). Philadelphia: W. B. Saunders.

> **CHART 48–1 Interview Questions for History of Present Illness**
>
> After introductions, Mr. Davis tells you he has come to the hospital for surgery on his prostate. Here are some questions that would be asked to find out about his symptoms:
>
> Have you been troubled with frequency of urination?
>
> How often do you have to urinate?
>
> Is this keeping you up at night?
>
> Do you have difficulty starting the urinary stream?
>
> Have you had to be catheterized because you could not void?
>
> Does dribbling of urine occur after you void?
>
> Are you ever incontinent?

Past Medical History

This section of the history includes childhood and adult illnesses; comorbid conditions; immunizations; hospitalizations; surgeries; and menstrual, obstetric, sexual, and social histories. Here the discussion is about some parts of the patient's past history that may affect reproductive health.

Childhood Illnesses and Immunizations

For women, childhood diseases that would have affected her health, fertility, or the health of her children would need to be considered. For instance, any communicable disease that affected her health severely would affect her ability to have children. This could mean that she would need to prevent pregnancy or to have special care if she were to become pregnant. Another example is the woman of childbearing age who has not had rubella or immunization for rubella. If she develops rubella while she is pregnant, this could cause birth defects in her child.

The childhood disease of concern for men is mumps. This viral illness has the potential for affecting the testicles, causing sterility. See Chapter 50 🌐 for further discussion of mumps orchitis.

Previous Illnesses and Hospitalizations

Medical comorbidities that may impact the reproductive system would include diabetes, hypertension, hepatitis, and HIV. The male with diabetes or hypertension treated with certain antihypertensive drugs may experience impotence. Hepatitis and human immunodeficiency virus (HIV) are sexually transmitted infections (STIs) that may be life threatening. Patients (female or male) who have hepatitis or HIV may pass these diseases to their sexual partners. The nurse should determine whether the patient has been diagnosed and treated for a sexually transmitted infection such as chlamydia, gonorrhea, syphilis, or herpes. For women, it is also important to ask whether they have ever had pelvic inflammatory disease (Narrigan, 2006). Ask about hospitalizations for any reproductive health concerns or chronic health problems. Find out when the hospitalization occurred, what the problem was, and how it was treated.

Diagnostic Procedures and Surgeries

Past surgeries that may affect the woman with a reproductive system problem may include breast surgeries, hysterectomy, bilateral tubal ligation, cervical laser or cryosurgery, or any surgery for **endometriosis** (presence of uterine lining in sites other than within the uterus). See Chapter 49 🌐 for further discussion of surgeries of the reproductive system.

Procedures of particular interest in this section of the history for women include screenings or tests for breast cancer and cervical cancer. Mammograms, lump biopsies, or any other procedures for breasts would need to be dated and recorded in the history. It is also important to note the date of the last cervical cancer screening and the results of the Papanicolaou (Pap) smear. If the patient has ever been diagnosed with cervical dysplasia or treated for an abnormal Pap smear, it should be documented.

Men who have had prostate surgery may have increased incontinence or impotence. Other surgeries that may impact the reproductive system or lower urinary system include orchidectomy, vasectomy, or penile reconstruction due to epispadias (the urinary meatus is at the top or dorsal surface of the penis, between the penis and bladder) or **hypospadias** (the urinary

opening is on the ventral or bottom of the penis, between the scrotum and the distal end of the penis). See Chapter 50 🌐 for further discussion of surgeries of the reproductive system.

Menstrual History

For women, the menstrual and obstetric history should be included in the health history. The menstrual history should include age at **menarche** (first menstruation), length of time from first day of menstrual flow to first day of next menstrual flow (one cycle), number of days and characteristics of menses, regularity of cycles, **molimenal** symptoms (symptoms accompanying menstruation), and the first day of her last menstrual period. For older women, ask about menopause including age at onset and symptoms such as hot flashes, vaginal dryness, night sweats, and insomnia (Narrigan, 2006).

Obstetric History

Obstetric history includes the number of pregnancies, premature and term births, and spontaneous and therapeutic abortions. It is also important to determine whether the deliveries were spontaneous vaginal births or cesarean sections and whether there were any complications (Narrigan, 2006).

Sexual History and Risks for Sexually Transmitted Infection

Healthy People 2010 set 10 high-priority public health issues for this decade. Responsible sexual behavior is number 5 on this list of the most important changes people can make to help everyone in the United States be healthier (U.S. Department of Health and Human Services [DHHS], 2007). The steps toward achieving this goal include identifying people who are engaging in risky sexual behavior and helping them to choose safer practices. In working toward this goal, the examiner can ask the patient about the last time the patient had intimate physical contact or sex with someone; whether the patient is happy with her or his sex life; whether the patient has sex with men, women, or both; and any concerns the patient may have about sexual health. If the patient is in a mutually monogamous relationship, then the risks are decreased for sexually transmitted infection (Narrigan, 2006).

In settings where the patients may be at risk for sexually transmitted infection or HIV, more in-depth exploration of sexual practices may be indicated. The Centers for Disease Control and Prevention (CDC) has published a list of five areas to be explored along with counseling about the prevention of sexually transmitted infection and HIV. Chart 48–2 (p. 1510) lists specific questions that the CDC suggests be used to elicit this history.

Family History

Explore the family history of women for mother, sister, maternal grandmother, or aunts with breast cancer. The occurrence of breast cancer in any of these relatives increases the risks for the patient (Lashley, 2005). This is also true of about 10% of cases of ovarian cancer.

There is the possibility that there may be women who are daughters of women who took diethylstilbestrol (DES) to prevent a miscarriage during that pregnancy. These daughters are at 40 times the risk of developing cancer of the vagina and cervix (Wallace & Sanford, 2006). Therefore, it is important to ask women born between 1940 and 1971 whether they were exposed to DES while *in utero*.

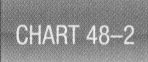

CHART 48–2 Exploring the Five Areas of Concern in the Prevention of Sexually Transmitted Infection (STI)

PARTNERS

"Do you have sex with men, women, or both?"

"In the past 12 months, how many partners have you had sex with?"

PREVENTION OF PREGNANCY

"Are you or your partner trying to get pregnant?" If "no":

"What are you doing to prevent pregnancy?"

PROTECTION FROM STIS

"What do you do to protect yourself from STIs?"

PRACTICES

"To understand your risks for STIs, I need to understand the kind of sex you have had recently."

"Have you had vaginal sex, meaning 'penis in vagina sex'"? If "yes":

"Do you use condoms: never, sometimes, or always?"

"Have you had anal sex, meaning 'penis in anus sex'"? If "yes":

"Do you use condoms: never, sometimes, or always?"

"Have you had oral sex, meaning 'mouth on penis/vagina sex'"?

For Condom Answers

If "never": "Why do you not use condoms?"

If "sometimes": "In what situations or with whom, do you not use condoms?"

PAST HISTORY OF STIS

"Have you ever had an STI?"

"Have any of your partners had an STI?"

Additional Questions to Identify Human Immunodeficiency Virus (HIV) and Hepatitis Risk

"Have you or any of your partners ever injected drugs?"

"Have any of your partners exchanged money or drugs for sex?"

"Is there anything else about your sexual practices that I need to know about?"

Source: Workowski, K., & Berman, S. (2006). Sexually transmitted disease treatment guidelines. *Morbidity and Mortality Weekly Report, 55*(RR-11), 2–3.

Men should be asked whether their father or brother has prostate cancer. Early onset prostate cancer seems to occur in some families. African American men are particularly susceptible. See further discussion of inheritance of susceptibility to prostate cancer in Chapter 50 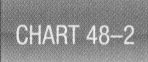.

Social History

Occupations or hobbies by which patients have been exposed to hazardous materials increase their risks for infertility (female and male) and prostate cancer. Ask the patient whether he works around hazardous materials such as excessive heat, radiation, heavy metals, or organic solvents and how he protects himself (Quallich, 2006).

Cigarette Smoking and Substance Abuse

Habits such as cigarette smoking, alcohol use, or illicit drug use should be explored. There is evidence from cohort and case-control research that cigarette smoking and secondhand smoke

increase the risks for cervical cancer (National Cancer Institute, 2007). Alcohol and illicit drug use have been shown to increase the incidence of sexually transmitted infection and HIV (Fogel, 2006b).

It is best to ask directly, "Tell me about your use of alcohol," or "When was your last drink of alcohol?" If the patient answers in such a way that the examiner is suspicious of problem drinking, then screening questions such as the CAGE questionnaire (Chart 48–3) can be used to help identify alcohol abuse. CAGE stands for "cutting down, annoyance if criticized, guilty feelings, eye-openers" (Bickley & Szilagyi, 2007).

The same direct approach should be used in questioning about illicit drug use. Direct questions, such as "Have you ever used any drugs other than those required for medical reasons?" and "Have you ever injected a drug?" work best to elicit this information from the patient (Bickley & Szilagyi, 2007).

Domestic Violence

Violence affects people of all ages, both genders, and of all religions, races, and socioeconomic groups. Domestic violence, whereby intimate partners inflict physical, sexual, or emotional injury, is very prevalent (Harley, 2006; Mick, 2006). In fact, *Healthy People 2010* lists injury and violence as number 7 of the top 10 high-priority health issues in the United States (DHHS, 2007). People who suffer intimate partner violence are more likely to abuse alcohol and drugs, and to have HIV or a sexually transmitted infection (Fogel, 2006b; Wingood, 2006).

Domestic violence is difficult to discuss, but questions about abuse should be asked of all patients, both women and men. The only way to begin to change behavior is to uncover the abuse. Make it a habit to ask patients questions, such as "Are there times in your relationship that you feel unsafe or afraid?" or "Within the last year, have you been hit, kicked, punched, or otherwise hurt by someone you know?" (Bickley & Szilagyi, 2007). Try to conduct the interview in private, away from family or the abusive partner (Harley, 2006).

■ Physical Examination

After the history is completed, the examiner should ask the patient to disrobe and put on a gown for the physical examination. The gown should open in front for better access to the breasts and genitals of both the female and male patient. Assemble the equipment needed for the pelvic examination. The examiner should step out of the room while the patient changes. Hand hygiene and donning of gloves by the examiner needs to occur in the room, in front of the patient.

CHART 48–3 The CAGE Questionnaire

1. Have you ever felt the need to **C**ut down on drinking?

2. Have you ever felt **A**nnoyed by criticism of your drinking?

3. Have you ever felt **G**uilty about drinking?

4. Have you ever taken a drink first thing in the morning (**E**ye-opener) to steady your nerves or get rid of a hangover?

Source: From Mayfield, D., McLeod, G., Hall, P.: The CAGE questionnaire: Validation of a new alcoholism screening instrument. *American Journal of Psychiatry, 131,* 1121–1123, 1974.

Female Examination

Chart 48–4 lists the equipment needed for the female examination. The nurse examiner should be accompanied by an assistant because of the sexual nature of this examination. This is true regardless of the gender of the nurse. During the physical assessment, the nurse should teach the patient about healthy lifestyles and choices.

Breasts

The breast examination is best done with the woman sitting at the end of the examination table. For inspection of the breast, she should be asked to open the gown so that her breasts are fully visible to the examiner. The examiner should inspect the breasts for size, shape, contour, dimpling, and inverted nipples; areas of increased vascularity; and erosion or inflammation of the nipple or areola. The inspection should be carried out while the patient's arms are at her side, then again when she raises her arms above her head or presses her hands to her hips to contract the pectoralis muscle. These maneuvers will move the breast and pull the suspensory ligaments in such a way that a tumor would cause dimpling or a bulge. If the woman has large, pendulous breasts, a bimanual (palpating breast tissue between the two hands of the examiner) examination of the breasts as she leans forward will help to palpate any masses (Narrigan, 2006).

The next portion of the breast examination is palpation. Ask the patient to lie down and raise one arm over her head. Place a small pillow or folded towel beneath the shoulder on the side of the breast to be examined, and palpate all the breast tissue. Palpate in a circular pattern, in smaller circles as you near the center of the breast. Be sure to include all four quadrants of the breast, including the upper outer quadrant and the tail of Spence (a section of breast tissue that extends toward the axilla). End the palpation with a gentle pressure on the nipple between the thumb and forefinger to determine whether there is discharge from the nipple. Repeat the procedure for the other breast. Palpate for masses or tenderness. If there is nipple drainage, collect a specimen on a slide and send it to the laboratory for evaluation (Narrigan, 2006).

Inspect the axilla for lesions, masses, or inflammation. Hold the patient's arm in a relaxed position and palpate for the axillary nodes by grasping the axillary fold and feeling for pectoral nodes along the pectoral muscle. Reach high in the axilla and feel along the humerus for the lateral lymph nodes. Then, change hands so that the arm is supported and the opposite hand can examine for subscapular nodes by feeling inside the posterior axillary fold. Examine along the top and below the clavicle for supra- and infraclavicular nodes. Repeat the entire procedure for the opposite adnexa (Bickley & Szilagyi, 2007).

External Genitalia

While the patient is still lying down, examine the groin for swollen inguinal lymph nodes. When this is completed on both sides, help her move down on the table and to put her feet into the stirrups for the external genitalia and internal genitalia examinations. Her buttocks should be right at the edge of the end of the examination table with her knees flexed and legs spread so that the external genitalia are accessible to examination. This is the **lithotomy** position (Figure 48–7 ■). Raise the head of the examination table to help her be more comfortable and drape her lower body and legs.

The nurse examiner should sit on a stool for the examination and lower the drape so that the nurse can see the patient's face during the examination. Inspect the external genitalia. The nurse tells the patient the nurse is going to touch her before the nurse moves a gloved hand to the vulva to spread the tissues for inspection of the entire vulva and perineum. Look for lesions, warts, vesicles, changes in pigmentation, signs of abuse such as bruises or lacerations, swollen Bartholin glands, or vaginal discharge or blood at the introitus. Figure 48–8 ■ (p. 1512) illustrates the technique for examining the Bartholin glands. Ask the patient to bear down as if to move her bowels, and observe for any bulges of cystocele (relaxation of the anterior vagina wall under the urinary bladder) or rectocele (relaxation of the posterior vaginal wall over the rectum) or prolapsed uterus at the introitus. Cystocele and rectocele are discussed in Chapter 49 . Palpate bulges to differentiate the cystocele from the rectocele. Palpate the Bartholin glands at 7 and 5 o'clock to the introitus. Palpate with one finger for the location of the cervix within the vagina (Bickley & Szilagyi, 2007).

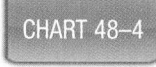 *Discovery of very painful swelling of the Bartholin gland should be referred immediately to a gynecologist for treatment (Birnbaum, 2006).*

Vagina and Cervix

The nurse places a small amount of water soluble lubricant on the speculum and tells the patient that the nurse is about to insert the speculum to visualize the cervix. Grasp the speculum in the dominant hand, spread the labia with the opposite hand, and

---

CHART 48–4 **Equipment Needed for the Female Genitalia Examination**

1. Examination gloves (latex or nonlatex, depending on patient allergy)

2. A good light source (gooseneck lamp or light that attaches to the speculum)

3. Speculum (choose size most appropriate for the patient)

4. Water soluble lubricant

5. Pap smear equipment

6. Culture tubes for STIs or other bacterial infection

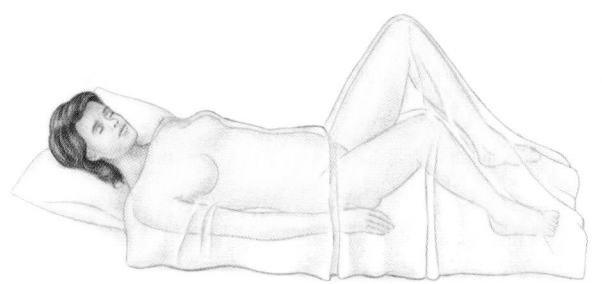

FIGURE 48–7 ■ Female lithotomy position.

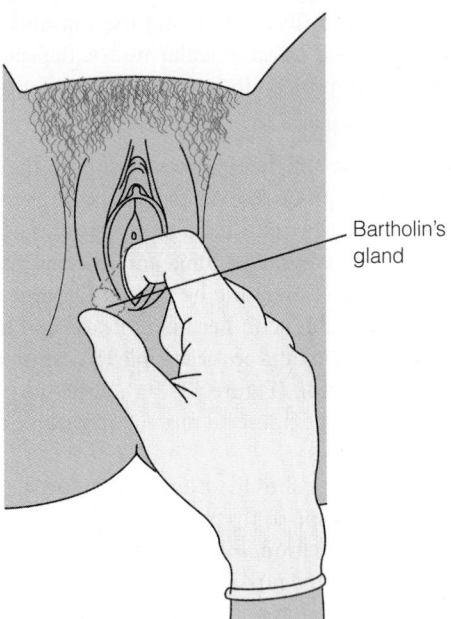

FIGURE 48-8 ■ Palpation of the Bartholin glands.

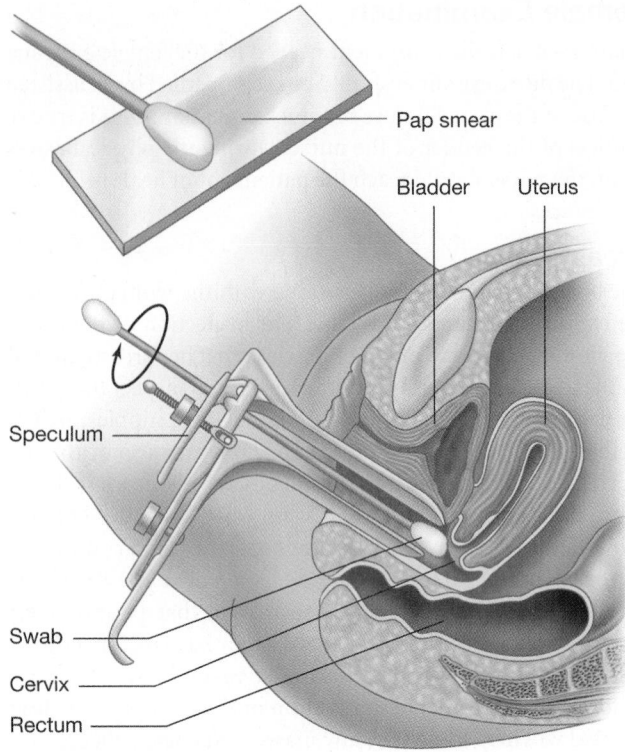

FIGURE 48-10 ■ Obtaining Pap smear.

insert the speculum, pointing it down and back toward the cervix (Figure 48–9 ■). Open the speculum to visualize the cervix. Look for any lesions, warts, or increased vascularization on the cervix or the vaginal walls. Look at the cervical os (opening) for drainage. Obtain specimens for Pap smear or STI cultures as appropriate (Figure 48–10 ■). Note whether the cervix bleeds slightly on contact with the specimen collector. If blood is present, this means that the cervix is **friable** (easily damaged). Rotate the speculum to visualize the remainder of the vagina before removing it. Discard the speculum appropriately (Bickley & Szilagyi, 2007).

Uterus and Adnexa

Lubricate the forefinger and long finger of the dominant hand for the bimanual examination. Explain to the patient that the examination of the uterus and ovaries is next. Insert the lubricated fingers into the vagina and palpate the cervix for motion tenderness by moving it side to side. Perform a bimanual examination with one hand on the lower abdomen just above the symphysis

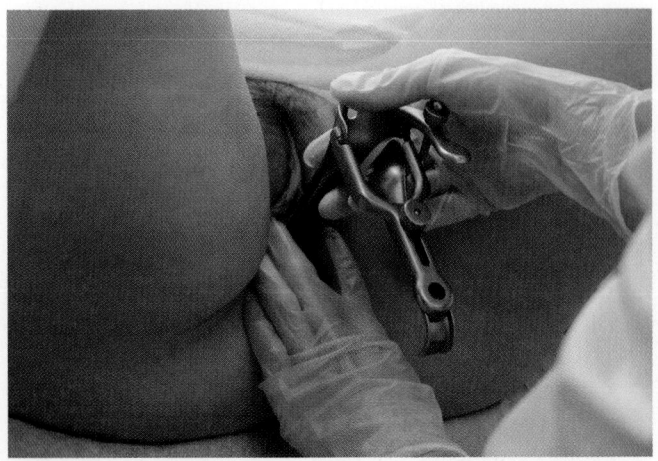

FIGURE 48-9 ■ Speculum insertion.

(pubic bone) and the fingers in the vagina pressing the cervix and uterus upward toward the abdominal hand to determine uterine tenderness, position, size, and shape. Figure 48–11 ■ shows the bimanual exam of the female. Move the hands to the right adnexa and examine bimanually for masses or tenderness. Move the hands to the left adnexa and repeat the examination for masses or tenderness. Figure 48–12 ■ depicts the palpation of the adnexa (Bickley & Szilagyi, 2007).

Rectum

If the woman's history or examination indicates a reason, then a rectal examination should be done. Put on clean examination gloves. Inspect the anal area for hemorrhoids, fissures, lesions, or warts. Lubicate the index and long fingers of the dominant hand, and then place the long finger over the anus and ask the patient to bear down as if for a bowel movement. Insert the finger as the anus opens. Place the forefinger into the vagina. Palpate for lesions, a retroverted uterus, or a fistula between the vagina and rectum. Remove the forefinger from the vagina and palpate the entire rectal wall with the long finger for rectal lesions. After removal of the long finger, place any stool obtained on a hemoculture card and test for occult blood (Bickley & Szilagyi, 2007).

Help the patient to move back on the table before sitting up, so that she is supported by the examination table. Help her down from the examination table, give her some tissue to remove the excess lubricant from the genitalia, and leave the room to give her privacy to dress.

Male Examination

The male breast should be inspected for lesions, piercing, or gynecomastia. If the history or inspection has revealed a problem with the male breast, palpation for masses and tenderness is indicated.

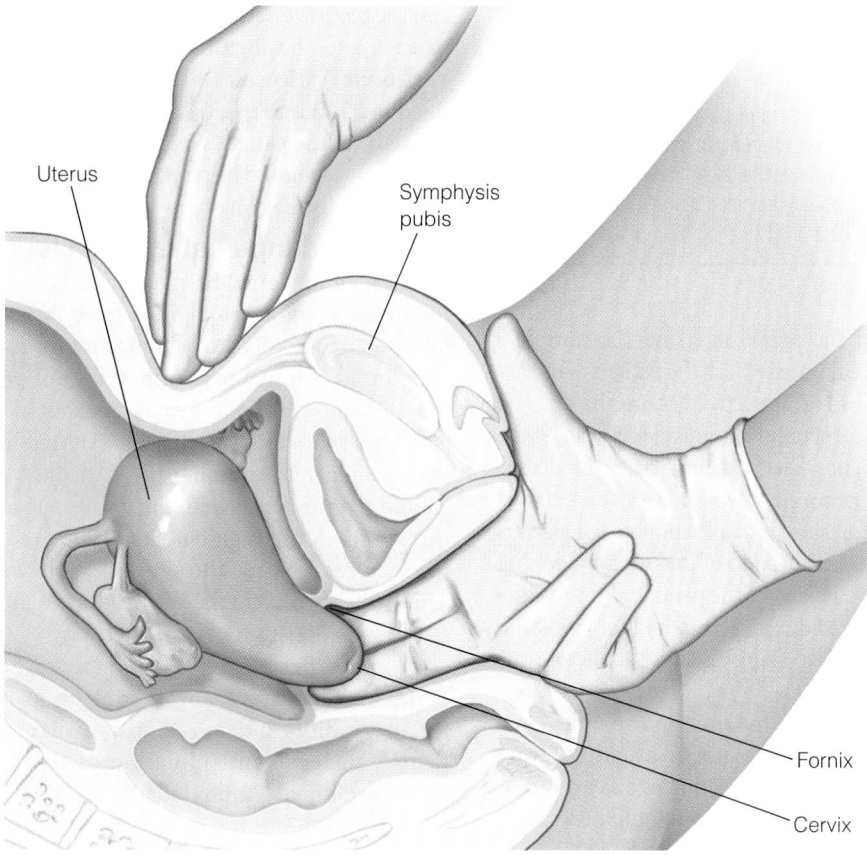

FIGURE 48–11 ■ Bimanual exam female.

The male external genital examination should occur in a warm, private room after the examiner has washed and warmed the examining hands. The patient should be asked whether the room is warm enough. A cold room or cold examining hands will activate the **cremasteric reflex** (testicles rise in the scrotum to the abdominal cavity when the thigh is stroked or the room is cold). The nurse should introduce herself or himself and ask permission before proceeding. This will give the patient an opportunity to ask for a same-sex examiner, if he wishes. During the examination, the patient may be standing or lying down. Drape and gown the patient so that the genitalia can be visualized by having the patient hold up the gown if he is standing or to have a cover over his chest and legs if he is lying down. The examiner should be accompanied by an assistant or the patient's wife because of the sexual nature of the examination (Ceo, 2006). The Cultural Considerations box (p. 1514) notes the importance of respecting cultural attitudes about privacy.

External Genitalia

The examination of the male external genitalia is completed by inspection followed by palpation. Chart 48–5 (p. 1514) lists the equipment that may be needed. With the male standing, the examiner can sit on a stool in front of him and inspect the genitalia for lesions in the pubic hair, on the penis, or on the front or back of the

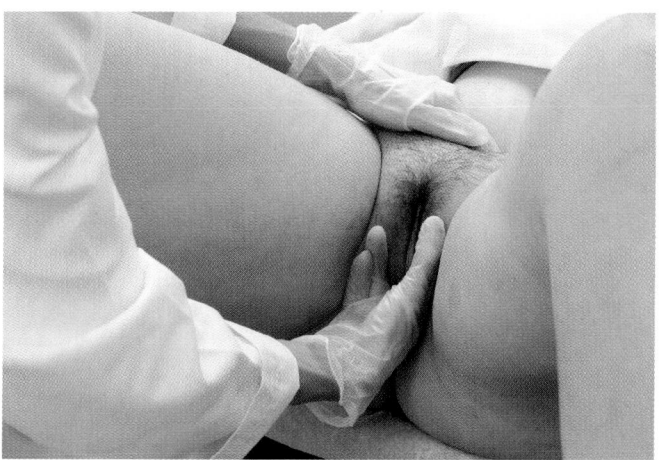
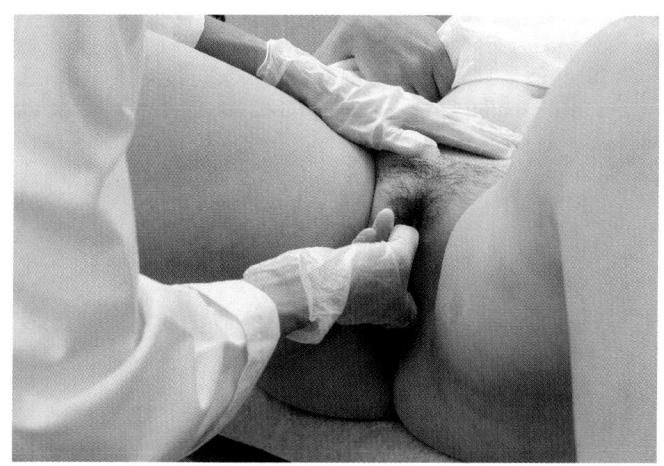

FIGURE 48–12 ■ Palpation of adnexa.

CULTURAL CONSIDERATIONS for Genital Examinations

Before proceeding with a male genital examination with the wife present, ask the wife whether she would prefer to leave. In certain cultures, the wife's presence during a genital examination of her husband would be considered taboo or against cultural mores (Ceo, 2006).

scrotum. The dorsal vein of the penile shaft may be normally prominent. If the male is not circumcised, ask the patient to retract the foreskin so that the glans can be inspected. Lesions that may be seen include **chancres** (ulcers of syphilis), abnormal contour of the scrotum, cancer, warts, herpetic vesicles, or infestation by lice or other insects in the pubic hair. Smegma (white, cheesy material) is a normal finding under the foreskin. Inflammation of the glans is called balanitis. Inspection for the location of the urinary opening follows. Normally, it will be at the end of the penis and free of discharge. If the patient has reported discharge, but it is not visible, he should be asked to strip the penis to bring discharge to the meatus for culture (Bickley & Szilagyi, 2007).

Palpation of the penis is reserved for any abnormalities such as tenderness or plaque formation. The nurse should be aware that the male patient may have an erection during the examination. This is often beyond his control, and he should be assured that this is a normal occurrence (Bickley & Szilagyi, 2007).

If the contour of the scrotum is suspicious, palpation for **cryptorchidism** (an undescended testicle), scrotal **hydrocele** (swelling due to fluid accumulation in the scrotum), or hernia should be done. A hernia with a loop of bowel in the scrotum can be differentiated from hydrocele by translumination (with a light source behind the swelling, look for a glow of clear fluid or no light penetrance). One can also auscultate the scrotal mass with the aid of the stethoscope for bowel sounds (Ceo, 2006).

 CRITICAL ALERT *Discovery of an undescended testicle in a teenager would warrant immediate referral to an urologist. The incidence of testicular cancer is increased when the testicle is undescended (Goroll & Mulley, 2006).*

Palpation of the testis is accomplished by grasping it between the thumb and forefinger and feeling for nodules or masses. The examiner should be aware that too much pressure on the testis can cause deep pain. The epididymis is found on the posterior surface and is palpated in the same way. Cysts or tumors may be identified on the testicle or epididymis. Cysts or tumors in this area may be malignant or benign. From the epididymis, a cord will ascend upward toward the abdomen. This is the vas deferens

CHART 48–5 | **Equipment Needed for the Male Genitalia Examination**

1. Examination gloves (latex or nonlatex, depending on patient allergy)
2. Water soluble lubricant
3. Flashlight or other light source for translumination
4. Stethoscope

and the blood vessels of the spermatic cord. This structure is palpated up to the inguinal ring where it enters the abdomen. **Varicocele** (varicosities of the veins of the scrotum) may be identified here. These "bag of worms" abnormalities are more likely to occur on the patient's left side. Both sides of the scrotum and both testicles should be palpated (Ceo, 2006). See Chapter 50 for more information about varicoceles.

Hernia and Inguinal Lymph Nodes

Femoral and inguinal hernias may be detected by inspection of the inguinal and femoral areas for bulges. These bulges can be intensified by asking the patient to strain down or cough. To palpate for an inguinal hernia that has not presented as a loop of bowel in the scrotum, the examiner should use the right forefinger to examine the patient's left external inguinal ring and the left forefinger to examine the patient's right. This maneuver should start low enough in the scrotum to assure that the fingertip will reach the inguinal ring. While the examining finger is held against the ring, the patient should cough or strain down. This will bring a mass against the examining finger. Figure 48–13 ■ demonstrates this maneuver.

The superficial inguinal lymph nodes are palpated, and if the nodes in the horizontal or vertical group are swollen or tender, this may indicate inflammation or malignancy of the scrotum or penis. Cancer or inflammation of the testicles would affect intra-abdominal lymph nodes that cannot be palpated (Bickley & Szilagyi, 2007).

Prostate

To palpate the prostate, a rectal examination is required. The patient will need to lean over the examining table or lie on his left side with his right knee drawn up (Figure 48–14 ■). The anal area is inspected by spreading the buttocks. The examiner should look for lesions, external hemorrhoids, or warts in this area. The examiner should lubricate the forefinger of the dominant hand generously. To decrease discomfort, the nurse should tell the patient what is about to be done, have the patient bear down as if moving his bowels, and move the examining finger into the anal canal as it opens. The posterior surface of two lobes of the prostate is palpated through the anterior rectal wall. The examiner should identify the median sulcus and note the size and firmness of the prostate, and the presence of any masses or tenderness. When the examination is complete, the examiner removes the

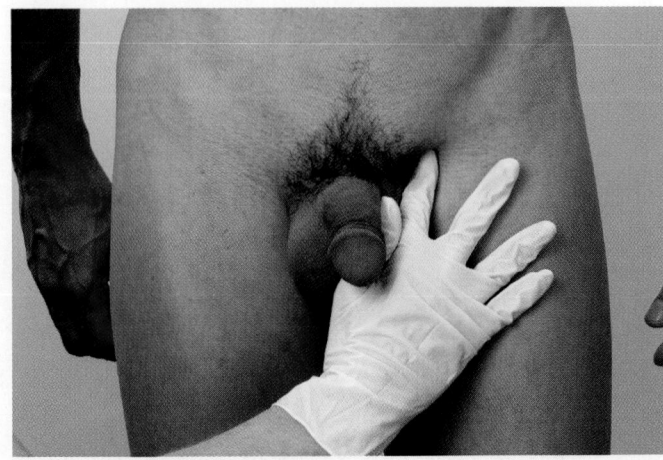

FIGURE 48–13 ■ Palpation for inguinal hernia.

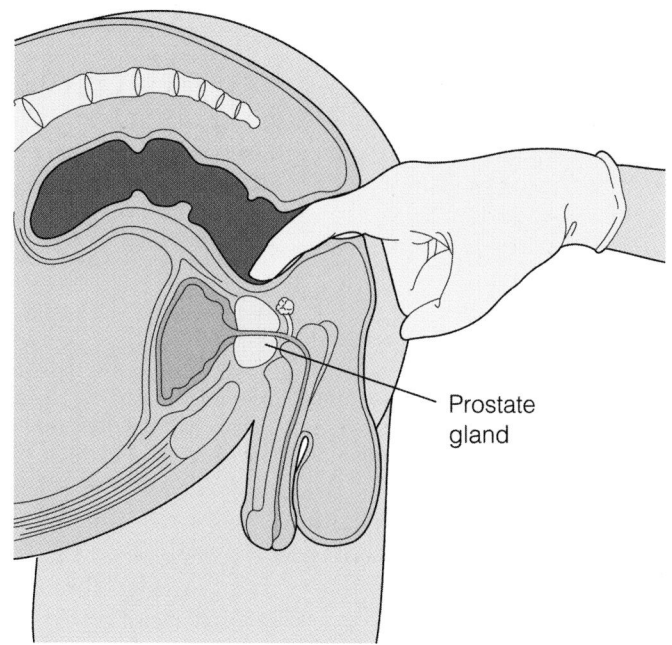

FIGURE 48–14 ■ Digital rectal exam prostate.

finger and wipes the excess lubricant from the anus (Bickley & Szilagyi, 2007; Ceo, 2006).

Gerontological Considerations

As with all systems of the body, the reproductive system undergoes changes with aging. Psychologically, there is reduced libido and decreased sexual satisfaction. This does not mean that men and women over age 65 are not sexual or that they do not enjoy sexual activity. It just means that sex is not as intense or frequent (Fogel, 2006a). On the other hand, libido and sexual feelings may decrease due to loss of a significant other, social isolation related to loss of mobility, or other factors. Some elders experience incontinence of urine, which decreases their willingness to exercise or to socialize with others (Stanley, Blair, & Beare, 2005).

Women experience menopause and the loss of estrogen usually in the early part of the fifth decade. The decrease in estrogen may cause symptoms such as hot flashes (which usually come and go during the first 5 years of menopause) and drying of the vaginal mucosa. Drying of the vaginal mucosa will make sexual intercourse and vaginal examinations uncomfortable. Less frequently, the woman may experience sleep disturbances, decreased ability to concentrate, and depression. Over time, decreased estrogen will contribute to loss of muscle mass and bone, and increased fat of the abdomen. The breast will atrophy as the glandular tissue is replaced by fat. The vulva will lose fat and the mons and vulva will lose hair. There may also be graying of the pubic hair (Ebersole, Hess, Touhy, & Jett, 2005).

Changes in mobility brought on by aging may necessitate a change in the positioning for vaginal examinations. For those women who cannot open their legs at the hips for the lithotomy position, alternate positioning may be needed. A side-lying position with the top leg drawn up will allow for small speculum examination of the vagina and cervix. Another option is to have two assistants support the patient's legs during the examination (Bickley & Szilagyi, 2007).

Men experience **andropause** (decrease in testosterone) beginning gradually in about the third decade. This causes decreased spermatogenesis and a shortening of the penis; the penis is slower to erection, and the scrotum hangs lower. Chronic disease may affect the testicles, causing them to shrink. Depression and a decrease in cognition may occur, just as with women in menopause. Men may have loss of muscle mass and bone mass, but not as much as seen in women (Stanley et al., 2005).

Loss of mobility or inability to stand for long periods may necessitate that the patient lie down for the prostate examination. Lying on the left side, bending at the hips, and drawing the right leg up so that the anal area is accessible to the examiner, is the recommended position (Bickley & Szilagyi, 2007).

Health Promotion

Health promotion means following a lifestyle that is conducive to health. Sexual health requires a healthy mind and body, open communications with the partner, and capacity to enjoy and control sexual impulses according to social norms (Fogel, 2006a). To be sexually healthy is to have a good body image and sexual identity. Sexual health is promoted by mutually monogamous relationships with uninfected partners. It also entails the avoidance of substances such as alcohol or illicit drugs that would decrease inhibitions and cause the female or male to engage in risky sexual behaviors.

National Guidelines for Disease Screening and Self-Examination

Early detection of disease through screening examinations is a tactic for health promotion. For women, cervical and breast cancer screening are recommended. The United States Preventive Services Task Force (USPSTF) recommends that sexually active women have annual Pap smears until age 65. At this point, the benefit of screening seems to diminish (USPSTF, 2003a). For breast screening, the USPSTF recommends screening mammography every 1 to 2 years for women age 40 and older (USPSTF, 2003b). According to the USPSTF, the research to date (worldwide) has not demonstrated that breast self-examination reduces mortality from breast cancer. The USPSTF does not recommend routine screening for ovarian cancer with serum CA-125 levels or transvaginal ultrasound, because research has not established that the benefits outweigh the potential harm (USPSTF, 2003d). The American Cancer Society, however, recommends that women with a strong family history of ovarian cancer be screened with both transvaginal ultrasound and serum CA-125 levels (American Cancer Society, 2006b).

For adolescents and young men, the USPSTF recommends against testicular self-examination and routine screening by clinicians (USPSTF, 2003c). Studies demonstrate that routine examination of the testicles has caused more harm than benefit.

For older men, the USPSTF has found that there is insufficient evidence to recommend for or against routine screening for prostate cancer with serum levels of prostate-specific antigen (PSA) and digital rectal examination (DRE) of the prostate (USPSTF, 2003e). Routine screening has been shown to cause unnecessary anxiety, biopsies, and treatments with severe side effects for a cancer that may never have affected the patient. In addition, there continue to be many false-positive PSAs.

Summary

Assessment of the reproductive systems of women and men has been described. Readers are encouraged to use what has been presented in this chapter in management plans for women and men with reproductive health care concerns, as presented in Chapters 49 and 50 ☺ .

NCLEX® REVIEW

1. The nurse is instructing a teenage patient about menstruation and hormone regulation. Which of the following should the nurse include in this instruction?
    1. The next menstrual cycle begins on the last day of the current menses.
    2. The uterine lining becomes thicker because of estrogen.
    3. Estrogen causes ovulation.
    4. After ovulation, the lining of the uterus becomes thinner.

2. A male patient seeks medical care for a new onset of impotence. Which of the following should the nurse assess in this patient?
    1. Any other chronic illnesses such as diabetes
    2. Past medical history including mumps
    3. History of sexually transmitted infections
    4. Date of first sexual experience

3. A 35-year-old female is having difficulty conceiving. Which of the following can the nurse assess in this patient to aid in determining the cause of the infertility?
    1. Smoking history
    2. Occupations and hobbies
    3. Amount of daily exercise
    4. Amount of daily sleep and rest

4. While assessing the penis of an uncircumcised male, the nurse notes a white cheesy substance under the foreskin. The nurse realizes this finding indicates:
    1. Smegma, a normal finding.
    2. Syphilis.
    3. Inflammation.
    4. Discharge.

5. A 50-year-old female patient believes something is "drastically wrong" because she is "losing hair down there." Which of the following should the nurse respond to this patient?
    1. There could be something wrong.
    2. Hair loss over the mons and vulva is a normal part of the aging process.
    3. I suggest you schedule a complete physical immediately.
    4. Hair doesn't really serve a purpose there anyway.

6. A 70-year-old male patient tells the nurse that he "hates his annual physical" because every year he worries what his PSA level is going to be. Which of the following does this anxiety suggest?
    1. The patient does not like his primary physician.
    2. Routine screening for prostate cancer can lead to unnecessary anxiety.
    3. The patient thinks he has prostate cancer.
    4. The patient is hiding a health concern.

Answers for review questions appear in Appendix D

KEY TERMS

andropause *p.1515*
chancres *p.1514*
cremasteric reflex *p.1513*
cryptorchidism *p.1514*
endometriosis *p.1509*
friable *p.1512*

galactogenesis *p.1505*
hydrocele *p.1514*
hypospadias *p.1509*
lactation *p.1505*
lithotomy *p.1511*
menarche *p.1509*

molimenal *p.1509*
oxytocin *p.1505*
progesterone *p.1505*
prolactin *p.1505*
varicocele *p.1514*

REFERENCES

American Cancer Society. (2006a). *Can ovarian cancer be found early?* Retrieved February 27, 2008, from http://www.cancer.org/docroot/CRI/content/CRI_2_4_3X_Can_ovarian_cancer_be_found_early_33.asp?sitearea=CRI

American Cancer Society. (2006b). *What are the risk factors for breast cancer?* Retrieved April 27, 2007, from http://www.cancer.org/docroot/CRI/content/CRI_2_4_2X_What_are_the_risk_factors_for_breast_cancer_5.asp?sitearea

Bickley, L., & Szilagyi, P. (2007). *Bates' guide to physical examination and history taking* (9th ed.). Philadelphia: Lippincott Williams & Wilkins.

Birnbaum, S. (2006). Medical evaluation of female sexual dysfunction. In A. Goroll & A. Mulley. (2006), *Primary care medicine: Office evaluation and management of the adult patient* (5th ed., pp. 792–795). Philadelphia: Lippincott Williams & Wilkins.

Ceo, P. (2006). Assessment of the male reproductive system. *Urologic Nursing, 26*(4), 290–296.

Ebersole, P., Hess, P., Touhy, T., & Jett, K. (2005). *Gerontological nursing and healthy aging* (2nd ed.). St. Louis: Mosby.

Fogel, C. (2006a). Sexuality. In K. Schuiling & F. Likis (Eds.). *Women's gynecologic health* (pp. 149–167). Boston: Jones & Bartlett.

Fogel, C. (2006b). Sexually transmitted infections. In K. Schuiling & F. Likis (Eds.), *Women's gynecologic health* (pp. 421–468). Boston: Jones & Bartlett.

Goroll, A., & Mulley, A. (2006). *Primary care medicine: Office evaluation and management of the adult patient* (5th ed.). Philadelphia: Lippincott Williams & Wilkins.

Harley, A. (2006). Domestic violence screening: Implications for surgical nurses. *Plastic Surgical Nursing, 26*(1), 24–28.

Hughes, N., Steele, N., & Leclaire, S. (2006). Gynecologic anatomy and physiology. In K. Schuiling & F. Likis (Eds.), *Women's gynecologic health*. Boston: Jones & Bartlett.

Lashley, F. (2005). *Clinical genetics in nursing practice* (3rd ed.). New York: Springer.

Mick, J. (2006). Identifying signs and symptoms of intimate partner violence in an oncology setting. *Clinical Journal of Oncology Nursing, 10*(4), 509–513.

Narrigan, D. (2006). Gynecologic history and physical examination. In K. Schuiling & F. Likis (Eds.), *Women's gynecologic health* (pp. 101–126). Boston: Jones & Bartlett.

National Cancer Institute (NCI). (2007). *Cervical cancer (PDQ): Prevention, health professional version.* Retrieved February 27, 2008, from http://www.cancer.gov/cancertopics/pdq/prevention/cervical/HealthProfessional

Quallich, S. (2006). Examining male infertility. *Urologic Nursing, 26*(4), 277–288.

Slovik, D. (2006). Evaluation of gynecomastia. In A. Goroll & A. Mulley, *Primary care medicine: Office evaluation and management of the adult patient* (5th ed., pp. 707–710). Philadelphia: Lippincott Williams & Wilkins.

Stables, D., & Rankin, J. (Eds.). (2005). *Physiology in childbearing* (2nd ed.). Edinburgh, UK: Elsevier.

Stanley, M., Blair, K., & Beare, P. (2005). *Gerontological nursing: Promoting successful aging with older adults* (3rd ed.). Philadelphia: F. A. Davis.

U.S. Department of Health and Human Services. (2007). *Healthy People 2010 leading health indicators: Priorities for action.* Retrieved February 27, 2008, from http://www.healthypeople.gov/LHI/Priorities.htm

U.S. Preventive Services Task Force (USPSTF). (2003a). Recommendations and rationale: Screening for cervical cancer. In *Guide to Preventive Services* (2nd ed.). (Publication No. 00-P046). Rockville, MD: Agency for Healthcare Research and Quality. Retrieved February 27, 2008, from http://www.ahcpr.gov/clinic/3rduspstf/cervcan/cervcan.htm#clinical

U.S. Preventive Services Task Force (USPSTF). (2003b). Recommendations and rationale: Screening for breast cancer. In *Guide to Preventive Services* (2nd ed.). (Publication No. 00-P046). Rockville, MD: Agency for Healthcare Research and Quality. Retrieved February 27, 2008, from http://www.ahcpr.gov/clinic/3rduspstf/breastcancer/brcanrr.htm

U.S. Preventive Services Task Force (USPSTF). (2003c). Recommendations and rationale: Screening for testicular cancer. In *Guide to Preventive Services* (2nd ed.). (Publication No. 00-P046). Rockville, MD: Agency for Healthcare Research and Quality. Retrieved February 27, 2008, from http://www.ahcpr.gov/clinic/3rduspstf/testicular/testiculrs.htm

U.S. Preventive Services Task Force (USPSTF). (2003d). Recommendations and rationale: Screening for ovarian cancer. In *Guide to Preventive Services* (2nd ed.). (Publication No. 00-P046). Rockville, MD: Agency for Healthcare Research and Quality. Retrieved February 27, 2008, from http://www.ahcpr.gov/clinic/3rduspstf/ovariancan/ovcanrs.htm

U.S. Preventive Services Task Force (USPSTF). (2003e). Recommendations and rationale: Screening for prostate cancer. In *Guide to Preventive Services* (2nd ed.). (Publication No. 00-P046). Rockville, MD: Agency for Healthcare Research and Quality. Retrieved February 27, 2008, from http://www.ahcpr.gov/clinic/3rduspstf/prostatescr/prostaterr.htm

Wallace, M., & Sanford, A. (2006). Gynecologic cancers. In K. Schuiling & F. Likis (Eds.), *Women's gynecologic health*. Boston: Jones & Bartlett.

Wingood, G. (2006). Efficacy of an HIV prevention program among female adolescents experiencing gender-based violence. *American Journal of Public Health, 96*(6), 1085–1090.

49

Caring for the Patient with Female Reproductive Disorders

Katherine Kelly
Kathleen Osborn

With Contributions by:
John M. Osborn
Laurie Kaudewitz

Outcome-Based Learning Objectives

After studying this chapter, the learner will be able to:

1. Differentiate the cause, mode of transmission, prevention, and treatment of sexually transmitted infections.
2. Discuss risk factors, diagnosis, and treatment of breast cancer.
3. Describe the procedure for a breast self-examination.
4. Differentiate the pathophysiology of the most common female reproductive disorders.
5. Discuss the medical treatment and nursing care for the most common female reproductive disorders.
6. Discuss the common causes and treatment of infertility and the related nursing care.
7. Discuss common diagnostic surgical procedures related to female reproductive disorders.
8. Describe key components of the interview of a patient who has been victimized by intimate partner violence.

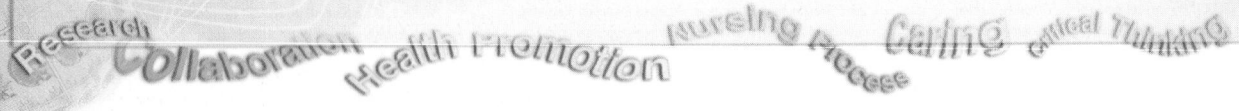

MANY HEALTH concerns of women relate to normal changes that occur in the reproductive cycle, but others involve alterations in normal reproductive functioning. Still others are cancer-related or sexually transmitted problems. This chapter will address specific diseases and disorders that affect the reproductive system and its functioning. It includes the expected signs, symptoms, and treatments as well as the psychosocial impact of each disease or disorder. *Healthy People 2010* guidelines are incorporated throughout the chapter with an emphasis on improving the health of women.

Sexually Transmitted Infections

Sexually transmitted infections (STIs) are also referred to as sexually transmitted diseases (STDs). They are more accurately identified as infections rather than diseases. STIs include more than 25 infections that are passed from person to person during sexual contact (CDC, 2008f).

One of the 28 focus areas in *Healthy People 2010* includes reducing or preventing sexually transmitted infections. Specifically, the goal of this focus area is promoting responsible sexual behavior, strengthening community capacity, and increasing access to quality services in an attempt to prevent sexually transmitted in-

fections (STIs) and their complications. The government recognizes that social, cultural, and behavioral factors play a role in the spread of these infections, and that access to health care is critical to preventing the spread of disease. The Centers for Disease Control and Prevention estimates that 19 million new sexually transmitted infections occur each year, almost half of them among young people ages 15 to 24 (CDC, 2005b). Women comprise two-thirds of these diagnoses (Johnson-Mallard, 2007).

Sexually Transmitted Infections Characterized by Cervicitis

Infectious disease of the cervix is primarily a result of sexual transmission. These infections, although easily transmitted through sexual contact, are often asymptomatic; therefore, women of childbearing age are routinely screened for them. Women are diagnosed with about two-thirds of these diseases, and it is women who suffer the morbidity of these infections in the form of loss of fertility (Johnson-Mallard, 2007).

Chlamydia Infections

The Centers for Disease Control and Prevention (CDC) reports that **chlamydia** is the most frequently reported infectious disease in the United States with 2.8 million new cases each year (CDC, 2008c). Chlamydia is known as a "silent™" disease because about three-quarters of infected women have no symptoms (CDC, 2008c). It is caused by *Chlamydia trachomatis* and transmitted during sexual intercourse. The bacteria initially infect the cervix and the urethra. Women who do notice symptoms often complain of burning urination, vaginal discharge, and mild lower abdominal cramps. Like gonorrhea, it is important to perform routine screening to prevent chlamydia from spreading. Also like gonorrhea, chlamydia that is left untreated can develop into pelvic inflammatory disease up to 40% of the time. Chlamydial infections cannot be distinguished from other urogenital infections by symptoms alone. Laboratory testing is needed to differentiate chlamydial infection from other lower genital tract infections such as urinary tract infection, bacterial vaginosis, and trichomoniasis. Figure 49–1 ■ shows typical objective signs of a chlamydia infection. To test for chlamydia, a small amount of vaginal fluid is needed to culture for the presence of the causative organism. A new urine test also is available that provides a noninvasive, quick mechanism for diagnosis (Quest Diagnostics, 2005). Chlamydia is treatable with antibiotics, typically azithromycin orally in a single dose or doxycycline orally for 7 days. In all diagnosed cases, partner treatment is necessary, and use of condoms is recommended until the infection is gone. Due to the prevalence of the disease, the CDC recommends routine screening for the following groups:

- Women with multiple sexual partners
- Sexually active women under 20 years of age
- Women over 24 years of age who are inconsistent with the use of barrier contraception, or have had new or more than one sex partner during the last 3 months.

The Pharmacology Summary of Medications to Treat Female Reproductive Disorders feature (p. 1552) includes the medications used to treat chlamydia infections.

Lymphogranuloma Venereum

Lymphogranuloma venereum (LGV) is an invasive, systemic infection that is caused by *Chlamydia trachomatis*. The most common clinical manifestation of LGV among heterosexuals is tender inguinal and/or femoral lymphadenopathy that is typi-

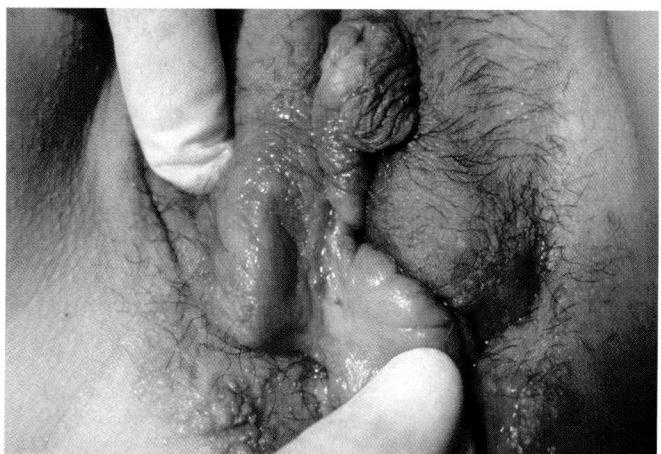

FIGURE 49–1 ■ Chlamydia.
Source: Courtesy, Director-General and Programme Manager Prevention of Blindness, World Health Organization

cally unilateral. Rectal exposure in women can result in proctocolitis, which causes anal pain, constipation, fever, and/or tenesmus. If not treated, LGV proctocolitis might lead to chronic colorectal fistulas and strictures. Treatment with doxycycline or erythromycin cures the infection and prevents further tissue damage. Sexual partners with whom the patient has had sexual contact in the preceding 60 days should also be treated.

Gonorrhea

Gonorrhea is the second most commonly reported sexually transmitted infection in the United States, with 339,593 cases reported in 2005 (CDC, 2005b). It is estimated that only one-half of the actual number of infections are reported. There has been a steady decline in the rate of reported cases of gonorrhea over the past 30 years (since 1975); however, the decline has leveled off in the past 5 to 6 years. Women ages 15 to 19 have the highest rate of infection. Increased prevalence is also noted in those living in the southern United States and African Americans. The incidence of gonorrhea is most prevalent in high-density urban areas among persons who have multiple sex partners and engage in unprotected sexual intercourse.

Gonorrhea is caused by the bacterium *Neisseria gonorrhoeae*, which infects the warm moist environment of the reproductive tract, along with any other mucous membranes in the body, such as the oral mucosa and the mucosa of the eye in a newborn. It is spread by sexual contact with another infected individual. Ejaculation does not have to occur for the infection to be transmitted. Gonorrhea can also be spread from mother to baby during delivery. Gonorrhea in women is often an incidental diagnosis, as it can very often be asymptomatic. For that reason, routine screening is important for all women of childbearing age. Symptoms in women include burning with urination, a vaginal discharge, or vaginal bleeding between periods. Occasionally, patients will have some pelvic pain and fever indicating a more serious pelvic inflammatory disease that has resulted from gonorrhea. Untreated gonorrhea can develop into pelvic inflammatory disease causing damage to the fallopian tubes in the form of scar tissue, which in turn causes infertility or increased risk of ectopic pregnancy.

Gonorrhea is easy to diagnose if the patient presents for care. Cervical discharge can be cultured to confirm the presence of infectious bacteria, when present; then antibiotic therapy is initiated. Some resistance has been detected to the commonly used antibiotics, so the Centers for Disease Control and Prevention (CDC) has updated the recommended regimens. Currently CDC recommendations include ceftriaxone or cefixime. These medications can be given as a single dose. This one-treatment dose is so successful that a follow-up culture is not necessary, but if desired, the most cost-effective approach is to culture 1 to 2 months after treatment. Gonorrhea is highly communicable, and partner treatment is essential. The CDC recommends concomitant treatment for chlamydia, because it frequently coexists most with gonorrhea. Condoms are recommended to prevent reinfection during sexual relations.

Etiology, Epidemiology, and Pathophysiology of Pelvic Inflammatory Disease

Pelvic inflammatory disease (PID) is an infection of the uterus, fallopian tubes, and ovaries. It is a common and a serious complication of many sexually transmitted infections, with up to 80% of cases being related to chlamydia and gonorrhea infections. The

MyNursingKit | Video: Infectious Diseases: Sexually Transmitted—Gonorrhea highest risk for the development of PID is seen in women of child-bearing age who are sexually active. This population tends to have a higher incidence of STIs and bacterial infections that cause PID (CDC, 2008e). It is estimated that more than 1 million women experience an episode of acute PID each year, with more than 100,000 becoming infertile and 300,000 requiring hospitalization as a result. Annually, more than 150 women die from PID or its complications (CDC, 2008e). The Risk Factors box outlines the risk factors for the development of pelvic inflammatory disease. PID is more likely to occur during the first days of the menstrual cycle, so sexual intercourse during menstrual bleeding is also a risk.

Clinical Manifestations of Pelvic Inflammatory Disease

Symptoms vary from none to severe, including lower abdominal pain, fever, foul-smelling vaginal discharge, painful intercourse, painful urination, and irregular menstrual bleeding. Objective findings include fever (38.3°C), abnormal cervical or vaginal discharge, elevated white blood count (WBC) and erythrocyte sedimentation rate (ESR), and pain with palpation of the adenexal areas and/or the cervix. Patients with suspected PID need to have cultures of vaginal secretions to confirm diagnosis and a pelvic ultrasound to rule out a tubo-ovarian abscess and ectopic pregnancy.

Medical Management of Pelvic Inflammatory Disease

PID is curable with antibiotics. Because the causative organism is often unclear, it is important to treat with at least two different broad-spectrum antibiotics that cover a wide range of organisms. Bed rest helps with pain control, but the patient needs to placed in a high Fowler's position to help control spread of infection to the upper abdominal area. Universal precautions need strict adherence if the patient has purulent vaginal drainage and shares a bathroom. Patient teaching should include restriction of sexual relations if vaginal drainage is present. Use of a condom to prevent reinfection is important if an individual is not in a long-term, monogamous relationship with an uninfected partner. A patient's partner should be referred for evaluation and treatment of any sexually transmitted infection. Nurses should provide emotional support and stress the importance of follow-up care and evaluation. Patients should return for a follow-up evaluation 48 to 72 hours after the medication is started and again in 7 to 10 days.

Health Promotion for Diseases Characterized by Cervicitis

Patient and partner education is essential to the prevention and spread of the diseases characterized by cervicitis. The following facts are necessary components of the teaching plan:

- Cervicitis is most often transmitted during vaginal, anal, or oral sex.

RISK FACTORS for the Development of Pelvic Inflammatory Disease

Age (adolescent and young women)
Nonwhite women
Multiple sex partners
History of sexually transmitted infection
Intercourse with a partner who has untreated urethritis
Recent intrauterine device insertion
Nulliparity

- Ejaculation does not have to occur in order for infection to occur.
- These infections can be passed from infected mother to baby during vaginal birth.
- The greater number of sex partners, the greater risk of infection.
- Teenagers and young women are most at risk for cervicitis infections if sexually active.
- Sex partners must be treated in order to prevent recurrence and spread.
- Complications from cervicitis infections include pelvic inflammatory disease, ectopic pregnancy, and infertility.
- Routine screening for cervicitis should occur during yearly exams.
- A single dose of the appropriate antibiotic can cure cervicitis infections.
- Prevention of cervicitis infections is accomplished by being in long-term, mutually monogamous relationship with a partner who has been tested and is known to be uninfected.
- Latex condoms when used consistently and correctly can reduce the risk of transmission of cervicitis.

Sexually Transmitted Infections Characterized by Ulcers

Ulcers found in the genital area can be suspicious for three conditions primarily. Multiple painful vesicles are often herpes simplex virus (HSV). HSV is the most frequently occurring ulcerative disease of the genitals. However, a group of flesh-colored cauliflower-like lesions can be human papillomavirus (HPV), and a single chancroid-type lesion may be indicative of primary syphilis.

Etiology and Epidemiology of Syphilis

Syphilis is a complex sexually transmitted infection that can lead to serious systemic illness and even death if untreated. **Syphilis**, caused by the *Treponema pallidum* bacterium, is a systemic infection and is referred to as the "great imitator" because its symptoms often mimic those of other STIs (CDC, 2008f). Between 2003 and 2004, the cases of syphilis increased in the United States by 8% (CDC, 2004). In 2005 there were 8,724 cases, representing an increase of 9.3% (CDC, 2005b). Most cases occurred in persons 20 to 39 years of age; the incidence of infectious syphilis was highest in women 20 to 24 years of age, with the rate of 3 cases per 100,000 (CDC, 2005b). Rates are very high among young adult African Americans in urban areas and in the southern United States. Experts have attributed current syphilis infections to crack cocaine use, which is accompanied by the practice of exchanging sex for money and drugs (Nakashima, Rolfs, Flock, Kilmarx, & Greenspan, 1996). The CDC also reports that in 2005, 50% of the total number of primary and secondary syphilis cases was reported from 19 counties and 2 cities.

Pathophysiology and Clinical Manifestations of Syphilis

There are three primary stages of syphilis. In the first stage, a painless chancre (Figure 49–2 ■) develops soon after being infected, but will disappear on its own. If identified at this stage, a single dose of penicillin G can cure the infection (CDC, 2008f). If the in-

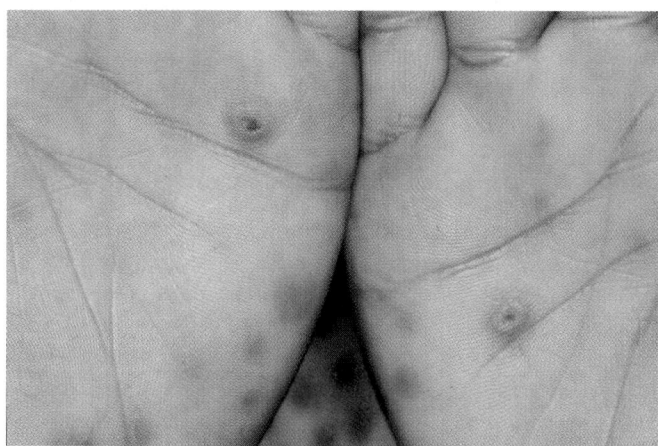

FIGURE 49–2 ■ Syphilis chancre.
Source: Zeva Oelbaum/Peter Arnold, Inc.

fection progresses to the secondary stage, a rough rash will appear on various parts of the body, but in particular on the soles of the feet and the palms of the hands. Other symptoms of the second stage may include fever, weight loss, swollen lymph glands, and muscle aches. A cure is still possible at this stage, but will require larger doses of antibiotics. Without treatment, the infection progresses to the latent and final state of the disease. Latent syphilis is defined as syphilis characterized by seroreactivity without other evidence of disease. The final stage begins after secondary symptoms disappear. The infection remains in the body for years and slowly damages the brain, nerves, eyes, heart, blood vessels, liver, bones, and joints. Symptoms, which typically progress to what is termed *neurosyphilis*, include muscle weakness, difficulty coordinating muscle movements, paralysis, numbness, blindness, dementia, and eventual death. Genital sores (chancres) caused by syphilis make it easier to transmit and acquire HIV infection. There is an estimated two- to fivefold increased risk of acquiring HIV infection when syphilis is present (CDC, 2008f).

Transplacental transmission of an infected mother to her fetus is very possible. If pregnancy occurs while a woman has syphilis, the fetus could develop deformities or could be stillborn. Routine screening of pregnant women is widely performed in the United States (CDC, 2008g). Providers can diagnose syphilis by examining material from a chancre (infectious sore) or using a blood test. Shortly after being infected, the body produces syphilis antibodies that can be detected. Every pregnant woman should have a blood test for syphilis.

Medical Management of Syphilis
A single intramuscular injection of penicillin will cure a person who has had syphilis for less than 1 year. Treatment with penicillin during pregnancy is necessary. If the woman is allergic to penicillin, she may require skin testing with desensitization treatment in order to receive penicillin, because alternate drug choices, such as doxycycline, tetracycline, and erythromycin, are contraindicated in pregnancy (CDC, 2008f). See the Pharmacology Summary feature (p. 1552).

Etiology, Epidemiology, and Pathophysiology of Genital Herpes
Genital herpes is caused primarily by the herpes simplex virus (HSV). It presents as painful multiple vesicular or ulcerative lesions found on the labia, perineum, and vaginal areas. Once one

is infected, HSV becomes a chronic, lifelong viral infection. There are two types of herpes simplex virus. Type 1 has historically been the source of cold sores or fever blisters on the mouth and lips. Type 2 HSV usually refers to herpes infection of the genitals. This distinction, however, has become blurred in recent years. It is no longer uncommon to find HSV types 1 and 2 in both areas of the body.

Genital herpes is considered a sexually transmitted infection; most infections are caused by HSV-2. At least 50 million persons in the United States have genital HSV infection. Many persons have mild or unrecognized infections but shed virus intermittently in the genital tract (CDC, 2008d). Generally, a person can get HSV type 2 only by sexual contact with someone who has a genital HSV type 2 infection. Unfortunately, the infected person does not have to have open lesions to transmit the virus to a partner. This makes it very difficult to prevent transmission between partners. Many people infected with HSV-2 are not aware of their infection.

Clinical Manifestations of Genital Herpes
The signs and symptoms may be transient and very mild. The first outbreak usually occurs within 2 weeks after the virus has been transmitted, and the sores heal within 2 to 4 weeks. During a first outbreak, the patient may have some mild flu-like symptoms including low-grade fever, inguinal lymphadenopathy, and fatigue in addition to the ulcerative lesions in the genital area (Figure 49–3 ■). More women than men are infected with HSV-2, probably because transmission is more likely from man to woman than it is from woman to man (CDC, 2008d). Most people diagnosed with a first episode of genital herpes can expect to have several outbreaks within a year. Over time these recurrences usually decrease in frequency.

Medical Management of Genital Herpes
Diagnosis of HSV-2 can often be made by visual exam; however, cultures from an open lesion can provide confirmation. If there

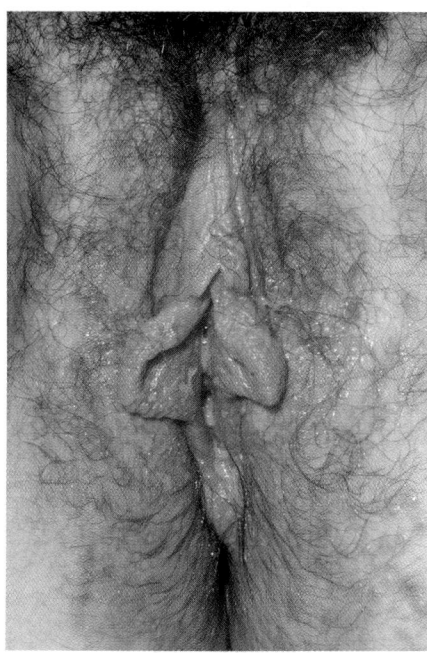

FIGURE 49–3 ■ Herpes simplex virus type 2.
Source: Mediscan/Visuals Unlimited

are no open sores at the time of exam, certain blood tests detect HSV-1 or HSV-2 infection. Although genital herpes causes recurrent outbreaks that are painful and worrisome, the condition is not life threatening unless the patient is immunosuppressed. Potentially lethal infections can occur in patients with HIV. HSV infections can make people more susceptible to HIV. Additionally, HSV-2 can also make HIV-infected individuals more infectious. Pregnant women with HSV-2 risk transmission of HSV to the infant during delivery; therefore, women with HSV-2 frequently deliver by cesarean.

Treatment of HSV-2 can be accomplished with antiviral medications (acyclovir or valcyclovir). These medications cannot cure HSV-2, but they can shorten and prevent outbreaks. Daily suppressive therapy is used for some patients who continue to have repeated outbreaks and to reduce transmission to uninfected partners. Treatment recommendations also include cleaning of lesions daily to prevent secondary infections, sitz baths to increase comfort, loose cotton underwear, and analgesics for discomfort. Abstinence from the first sign of recurrence through complete healing of the lesions is the recommendation, along with condoms between episodes.

Etiology, Epidemiology, Pathophysiology, and Medical Management of Chancroid

A **chancroid** is a bacterial sexually transmitted infection that occurs rarely outside of tropical climates. Although this infection may occur with any sexually active person, it is more common in men, especially those that are uncircumcised. The first symptom is typically a sore or raised bump on the genital organs. Within 5 to 10 days of the initial lesion, the glands on one or both sides of the groin become enlarged, hard, and painful. This infection is transmitted through intercourse as long as there is an open sore. There is no evidence of any natural resistance, and reinfection can occur immediately after treatment with antibiotics, with the lesions healing within about 2 weeks of treatment. Because there is no natural immunity to a chancroid, the individual is considered cured after treatment, but can be reinfected if exposed to the bacterium. Prevention techniques that include limiting the number of sex partners, using a condom, and thorough hygiene after sexual contact will help decrease the spread of this infection.

Etiology and Epidemiology of Human Papillomavirus

Human papillomavirus (HPV), also referred to as genital warts, infection is the most common sexually transmitted viral infection in the United States. The best estimate is that there are over 20 million people infected with HPV in the United States. It is anticipated that there will be 6.2 million new infections yearly. The highest rate of infection occurs in sexually active adolescents, but by age 50, at least 80% of women will have acquired a genital HPV infection (Allred, Cox, & Mahoney, 2006). Approximately 100 types of HPV have been identified. About 30 high-risk forms of HPV are known to cause genital tract cancers including cervical cancer. Many other types are known to cause genital warts, but not cancer.

Pathophysiology and Clinical Manifestations of Human Papillomavirus

Most people who have HPV do not know they are infected. The virus causes **genital warts** that appear as cauliflower-like growths in the genital, anal, and vaginal areas. They can be raised or flat, single or multiple; some are small and some are large. Genital warts are transmitted via sexual contact with an infected person. The warts may appear within weeks or months, or not at all (Figure 49–4 ■). Itching, increased vaginal discharge, and abnormal vaginal bleeding after intercourse are typical symptoms.

Medical Management of Human Papillomavirus

Most women are diagnosed with HPV based on abnormal Papanicolaou smear (Pap smear). A Pap smear, the primary method of screening for cervical cancer, detects precancerous changes in the cervix that may occur as a result of HPV infection. The warts can be treated with topical medications, such as Podofilox solution or Imiquimod cream. Genital warts can also be removed with minor surgery, known as cryotherapy, with liquid nitrogen, or with a shave excision.

On June 8, 2006, the Food and Drug Administration approved the use of a vaccine developed to prevent cervical cancer caused by HPV. The vaccine, known as Gardasil, protects against the four HPV types that are responsible for 70% of cervical cancers and 90% of genital warts. The vaccine is recommended for females aged 9 to 26. Ideally, the vaccine should be administered before the onset of sexual activity. However, females who are sexually active also may benefit from vaccination. The vaccine is recommended at a younger age because research studies demonstrated that titers were higher for young girls than for older females participating in the efficacy trials. The duration of vaccine protection is unclear. Current studies indicate that the vaccine is effective for at least five years (CDC, 2008f). The advent of the HPV vaccine does not change any of the recommendations for cancer screening outlined in the National Guidelines box. The American Cancer Society recommends beginning of screening for cervical cancer within 3 years of initiation of sexual activity or by age 21. Repeat exams should be done every 2 years for women until age 70. Women that have 3 consecutive normal exams and are in a monogamous relationship may extend testing to every 3 years. Likewise, women who are over 70 years of age and have had 3 or more normal cervical screenings in the previous 10 years may opt to discontinue the screenings. Women who have had a total abdominal hysterectomy may be able to discontinue testing if their surgeon agrees. For women who have had a subtotal hysterectomy, cervical cancer screenings should continue (American Cancer Society, 2008).

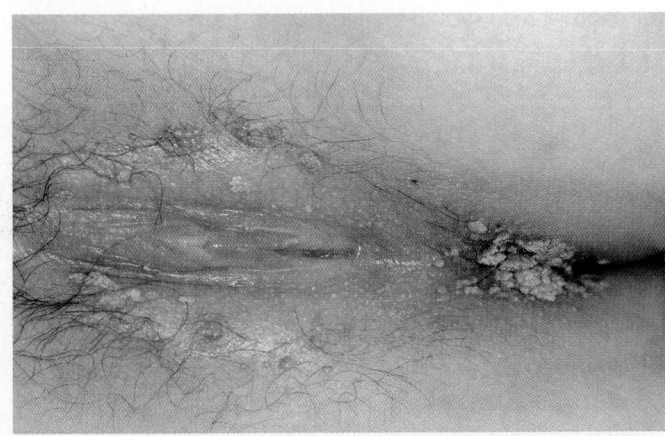

FIGURE 49–4 ■ Human papillomavirus (HPV) genital warts.
Source: ISM/Phototake NYC

NATIONAL GUIDELINES for Cervical Cancer Screening from the American Cancer Society

Criteria	ACS Guidelines
Age to initiate screening	3 years after the onset of sexual activity, no later than age 21
Screening frequency	Screening should be done every year with the regular Pap test or every 2 years using the newer liquid-based Pap test. After age 30, women with 3 consecutive normal tests and in a monogamous relationship may be screened every 2 to 3 years.
	Another option for women over 30 is to get screened every 3 years (but not more frequently) with either the conventional or liquid-based Pap test, plus the HPV DNA test.
	Women who have certain risk factors such as diethylstilbestrol (DES) exposure before birth, HIV infection, or a weakened immune system due to organ transplant, chemotherapy, or chronic steroid use should continue to be screened annually.
Screening after hysterectomy	Women who have had a total hysterectomy (removal of the uterus and cervix) may also choose to stop having cervical cancer screening, unless the surgery was done as a treatment for cervical cancer or pre-cancer.
	Women who have had a hysterectomy without removal of the cervix should continue to follow the guidelines.
Discontinuation of screening	After age 70 and 3 normal cytology exams in previous 10 years, screening can be discontinued.
	Women with a history of cervical cancer, DES exposure before birth, HIV infection, or a weakened immune system should continue to have screening as long as they are in good health.
Routine screening HPV infection	Test for HPV DNA is FDA approved as an adjunct to cervical screening among women age 30 and over.

Source: "American Cancer Society Guidelines for the Early Detection of Cancer: Cervical Cancer" adapted and reprinted by the permission of the American Cancer Society, Inc. from www.cancer.org. All rights reserved.

Health Promotion for Diseases Characterized by Ulcers

Patient and partner education is essential to the prevention and spread of the diseases characterized by genital ulcers. The following facts are necessary components of the teaching plan:

- Any unusual discharge, sore, or rash, particularly in the groin area, should be a signal to refrain from having sex and to seek the care of a health care provider.
- Prevention of sexually transmitted infections is best accomplished by abstaining from sexual contact or being in a long-term, mutually monogamous relationship with a partner who has been tested and is known to be uninfected.
- Condoms are not fully effective in preventing the spread of genital ulcer diseases. Persons with HSV and HPV should abstain from sexual activity with uninfected partners when lesions or other symptoms are present.
- An HSV-infected person who does not have any symptoms can still infect sex partners by shedding virus between outbreaks.
- HPV infection can lead to cervical cancer.
- Avoidance of alcohol and drug use may also help prevent transmission of STIs, as these activities may lead to risky sexual behavior.
- It is important that sex partners talk to each other about their HIV status and history of other STIs so that preventive action can be taken.
- Transmission of an STI cannot be prevented by washing the genitals, urinating, and/or douching after sex.
- Ulcerative STIs that cause sores, ulcers, or breaks in the skin or mucous membranes, disrupt barriers that provide protection against infections such as HIV.

Sexually Transmitted Infections Characterized by Vaginitis

Vaginitis is usually characterized by a vaginal discharge and/vulvar itching and irritation. A vaginal odor might be present. Three infections are associated with vaginitis conditions: trichomoniasis, bacterial vaginosis, and candidiasis.

Etiology, Epidemiology, Pathophysiology, Clinical Manifestations, Diagnosis, and Medical Management of Trichomoniasis

Trichomoniasis is a very common protozoan infection caused by *Trichomonas vaginalis.* Trichomoniasis affects both men and women, but symptoms are more common in women. Symptoms often include burning and itching in the vaginal area. Objective findings include a malodorous, yellow-green vaginal discharge with vulvar irritation, although some women experience minimal symptoms.

Microscopic examination of vaginal secretions can reveal flagellated protozoa, but this method has a sensitivity of only 60% to 70% (Figure 49–5 ■, p. 1524). A nucleic acid probe test is also available and has a higher sensitivity. Vaginal culture is the most sensitive and specific method of diagnosis. This infection is considered the most common curable STI in young people (CDC, 2008f). It is treated with a single dose of metronidazole and abstinence until both partners are asymptomatic. See the Pharmacology Summary feature (p. 1552).

Etiology, Epidemiology, Pathophysiology, Clinical Manifestations, Diagnosis, and Medical Management of Bacterial Vaginosis

Bacterial vaginosis (BV) is the most common bacterial infection in women of childbearing age, and it is seen in 16% of pregnant

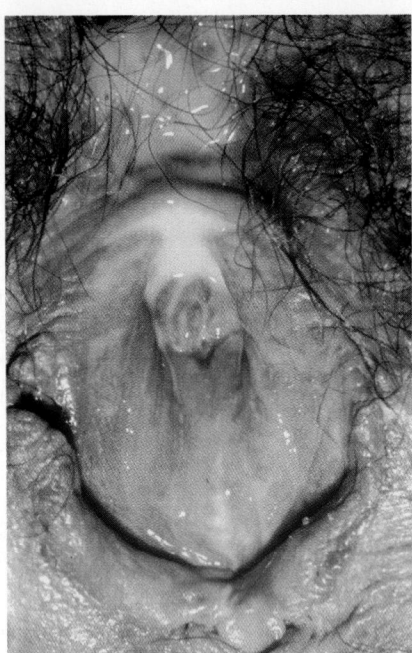

FIGURE 49–5 ■ Trichomoniasis.
Source: NMSB/Custom Medical Stock Photo, Inc.

women (CDC, 2008f). It is not the typical STI, that is, transmitted from one person to the other, although the CDC does list it under the sexually transmitted infection area. The cause of BV is not clearly understood, but it is known that an imbalance in the normal bacteria growth found in the vagina can cause an overgrowth of anaerobic bacteria known as *Gardnerella vaginalis*.

BV is associated with having multiple sex partners, a new sex partner, douching, use of an intrauterine device to prevent contraception, and a lack of vaginal lactobacilli. Women who have never been sexually active are rarely affected. Women with BV have an increased white/gray, typically thin vaginal discharge, with an unpleasant odor. These women may also experience burning on urination or vaginal itching. Objective findings include a thin, white discharge, the presence of clue cells on microscopy, and a fishy odor of vaginal discharge.

There are no complications associated with BV except in pregnancy. Babies are often born prematurely or are of low birth weight. BV can migrate upward and infect the uterus and fallopian tubes, increasing the risk of ectopic pregnancy or infertility and pelvic inflammatory disease (PID). The reason is unclear, but BV increases the woman's susceptibility to HIV, chlamydia, and gonorrhea.

Treatment is necessary to avoid PID because it can lead to infertility and damage to the fallopian tubes, which increases the risk of ectopic pregnancy. Two different medications are prescribed, metronidazole and clindamycin, both being safe if needed during pregnancy. The medications can be either oral or a topical vaginal route. See the Pharmacology Summary feature (p. 1552). BV can recur after treatment. Treatment of male sex partners has not been beneficial in preventing the recurrence of BV.

Etiology, Epidemiology, Pathophysiology, Clinical Manifestations, Diagnosis, and Medical Management of Candidiasis

Candidiasis is a fungal infection, more commonly referred to as a yeast infection. *Candida* organisms are typically found in the genital tract, the gastrointestinal tract, and the mouth. Symptoms develop when there is an overgrowth of *Candida* caused by multiple factors such as pregnancy, diabetes mellitus, and the use of antibiotics and/or corticosteroids that disturbs the pH or hormone balance in these areas (CDC, 2008b). Other causes can include tight-fitting undergarments that maintain a moist environment for fungal growth and frequent douching that may alter the pH balance that is needed to prevent it.

The normal *Candida* flora is rarely passed from person to person (CDC, 2008b), but can be transmitted through oral or genital sexual contact, when a disturbance in pH or hormone balance occurs. Symptoms include a white, cheesy discharge, often with intense itching, a burning sensation, and painful urination. A culture of the genital area is usually sent for testing to confirm the presence of candidiasis.

The treatment of choice is a 3- or 7-day course of antifungal drugs taken orally, topically, or vaginally (CDC, 2008b). Self-treatment is becoming common as more over-the-counter drugs become available. The CDC (2008b) indicates that as many as two-thirds of women who self-treat do not have the disease, leading to an increasing number of resistant infections. Women who have recurrences of what they believe to be candidiasis should seek medical diagnosis to rule out another cause of their symptoms. Recurrent or unresponsive episodes of candidiasis may be due to diabetes mellitus or HIV. Untreated infections may lead to persistent symptoms and an increased chance of passing the infection between partners. Wearing cotton undergarments that allow for better absorption of moisture and limiting douching may decrease the incidence of *Candida* growth in prone individuals.

Health Promotion for Diseases Characterized by Vaginitis

Patient and partner education is essential to the prevention and spread of the diseases characterized by vaginitis. The following facts are necessary components of the teaching plan:

- Observe for changes in color, odor, and amount of vaginal discharge.
- Wear light cotton underwear.
- If a presumed yeast infection does not improve with over-the-counter (OTC) treatment, seek medical care.
- Changes in the environment of the vagina may occur with changes in diet, medications, and new sex partner.
- Recurrent vaginitis or vaginitis that is nonresponsive to treatment requires further consultation with a health care provider.
- Avoid douching.

Acquired Immunodeficiency Syndrome

Acquired immunodeficiency syndrome (AIDS) is a result of an infection with the human immunodeficiency virus (HIV). HIV/AIDS is primarily transmitted by sexual contact, but it also can be acquired through a transfusion with infected blood, by an infant through the childbirth process, via contaminated needles, or through breast-feeding from an infected mother. The HIV virus attacks the immune system, which then places the individual at high risk for opportunistic infections. Due to altered immunity, these individuals are often unable to fight infections and eventually succumb to this disease. Certain medications have been successful at slowing the disease process, but, as of yet, there is no cure (CDC, 2008f).

The CDC (2008f) estimates there are 40,000 new cases in the United States each year and the fastest growing population are heterosexuals under the age of 25. HIV/AIDS is a deadly combination, and to decrease the incidence, a concerted effort must be made on the part of all people. The CDC has initiated an HIV prevention program that details the implemented activities for 2008, evaluation, communication, and plans for 2009. Chapter 60 🌐 includes an in-depth discussion of HIV/AIDS.

Nursing Management

Care of patients with sexually transmitted infections is primarily aimed at health education that prevents infections. Patients should receive results of testing as soon as possible and be encouraged to follow up for treatment. Nurses, who are responsible for revealing results of testing for STIs to patients, should be extremely careful to protect the confidentiality of their patients. Leaving messages on phones or with domestic partners or other family members is strictly prohibited. The Nursing Process: Patient Care Plan feature outlines nursing care specific to sexually transmitted infections (p. 1526).

Collaborative Management

Sexually transmitted infections are a sensitive topic for many patients. Patients are reluctant to seek treatment for these issues and instead hope they will resolve on their own. Nurses and health care providers must work together to help patients feel comfortable discussing possible STIs and the source of infections. Patients should be encouraged to disclose their infection to sexual partners, and for some infections, the disease may be reportable to the public health department (i.e., syphilis, gonorrhea, and chlamydia). On occasion, patients will realize that an STI is the result of an unfaithful partner. At that time it may be reasonable to offer psychological counseling to the patient.

Health Promotion
for Sexually Transmitted Infections

The specific information for patient/partner teaching is included under each STI section when described earlier. In general, health promotion for sexually transmitted infections should be directed at prevention. Once the disorder occurs, the care is directed toward symptom management, decreasing progression when possible, prevention of recurrence, and prevention of infection of others. The care and education need to be individualized to both the type of STI and the patient's needs.

The CDC (2008f) maintains that the primary preventative measure of sexually transmitted infections is to abstain from sexual intercourse and contact (including vaginal, anal, and oral sex) or in being in a long-term, monogamous relationship with an uninfected partner. Because neither of these measures is always followed, safer sex practices are the most common preventative measure. Once the infection is present, early treatment can assist in decreasing its progression. Some STIs are curable,

such as gonorrhea, syphilis, and trichomoniasis, and others are only treatable. To assist with prevention of both transfer to another partner and recurrence, safer sex practices are encouraged.

Breast Disorders

Breast disorders are most often manifested by pain, lumps, or nipple discharge. Sixteen percent of women between the ages of 40 and 69 will have one of these breast complaints (Klein, 2005). Most lumps are benign and are a result of fibrocystic changes, mastitis, or intraductal disorders. Breast malignancies are the most commonly occurring cancer in women and the second leading cause of death in women in the United States (Klein, 2005). The following section will discuss specific common breast disorders.

Pathophysiology of Fibrocystic Breast Abnormalities

Most breast masses are benign and are caused by fibrocystic changes. Fibrocystic breast changes most often occur as a result of hormone shifts around the time of the menses. However, the condition can also be exacerbated by stress or anxiety, nutritional factors, and physical or environmental stimuli.

Fibrocystic breast changes are characterized by an increase in glandular and fibrous tissues in the breast. This increase in fibrous tissue is palpable on examination and also may be seen on mammography. Fibrocystic changes are thought to be caused by estrogen dominance, which is why the changes wax and wane with menses and usually disappear after menopause, but the exact cause is unknown. When the fibrous tissue blocks milk ducts, fluid-filled cysts form. Typically, this condition affects women between the ages of 30 and 50.

Clinical Manifestations of Fibrocystic Breast Abnormalities

The manifestations of fibrocystic breast changes include a smooth, mobile, well-defined, tender lump usually found in the upper outer quadrant of the breast. The mass exhibits no redness, warmth, or overlying skin changes. Patients may sometimes note that coffee, tea, cola soft drinks, and chocolate aggravate the masses and cause increased tenderness. Breast pain (**mastalgia**) may be experienced in women with fibrocystic disease premenstrually but usually disappears after the menses when the influence of hormones diminishes.

Medical Management of Fibrocystic Breast Abnormalities

Fibrocystic changes are not precancerous and do not increase the woman's risk of developing breast cancer, but they can cause pain and anxiety (ACOG, 2000). Medical treatment for pain and tenderness associated with fibrocystic breasts may involve decreasing the estrogen level. Danazol (Danocrine), an antiestrogenic, can be given in severe cases. See the Pharmacology Summary feature (p. 1552).

Nursing Management

Nursing care should include obtaining a focused history of the patient with a breast mass to determine the risk of breast cancer. The Risk Factors box (p. 1527) outlines hormonal and nonhormonal

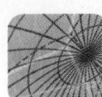

NURSING PROCESS: Patient Care Plan for Sexually Transmitted Infections

Assessment of Impaired Tissue Integrity

Subjective Data:
When did your symptoms begin?
Have you ever had this before?
Describe your symptoms.
Tell about the habits of your sex partner or partners.

Objective Data:
Skin appearance (color, texture, temperature, discharge, etc.)
Describe lesions (type, location, distribution, size, etc.)
Assess for edema and pain

Nursing Assessment and Diagnoses	Outcomes and Evaluation Parameters	Planning and Interventions with *Rationales*
Nursing Diagnosis: *Impaired Tissue Integrity* related to effects of disease process of STIs	**Outcome:** Tissue integrity will be restored. ***Evaluation Parameters:*** Skin tissue will be without breaks or lesions. Skin tissue will be pink without redness, excoriation, pain, or damage.	**Interventions and *Rationales:*** Assess damaged skin. *Gives baseline data to determine healing process.* Instruct patient on healthy hygiene. *Keeping clean and dry will decrease organism growth.* Instruct patient on use of sitz bath or warm soaks. *To cleanse area, increase circulation, and increase healing.* Administer and do home teaching on prescribed medications. *To decrease organism growth and increase healing.*

Assessment of Anxiety

Subjective Data:
Describe for me how you feel about this diagnosis.
What is your greatest concern?

Objective Data:
Verbal statements that indicate concern and anxiety
Nonverbal clues such as facial expressions showing concern or worry, wringing of hands, nervousness, etc.
Is the patient withdrawn/quiet/apathetic?

Nursing Assessment and Diagnoses	Outcomes and Evaluation Parameters	Planning and Interventions with *Rationales*
Nursing Diagnosis: *Anxiety* related to diagnosis of sexually transmitted infection (STI)	**Outcome:** Patient's anxiety level will be reduced. ***Evaluation Parameters:*** Patient will verbalize feeling less anxious. Patient affect will appear less stressed.	**Interventions and *Rationales:*** Assess patient concerns. *Gives baseline for intervention needs.* Provide open atmosphere and nonjudgmental attitude for communication/discussion. *To maintain relaxed atmosphere and nonjudgmental attitude to encourage patient verbalization.* Identify support systems for patient. *To identify whom patient can rely on for encouragement.* Answer questions honestly and openly. *To provide therapeutic environment.*

Assessment of Knowledge

Subjective Data:
What do you know about the prevention/transmission of STIs?
Are you sexually active?
If so, do you have more than one partner?
Do you want to get pregnant?
Do you use birth control?
Do you use any protection from diseases such as condoms?

Objective Data:
Patient's level of knowledge related to STIs
Patient's willingness to learn more about the importance of and the types of protection

Nursing Assessment and Diagnoses	Outcomes and Evaluation Parameters	Planning and Interventions with *Rationales*
Nursing Diagnosis: *Deficient Knowledge* related to disease prevention/transmission	**Outcome:** Disease transmission will be reduced or prevented. ***Evaluation Parameters:*** Patient will verbalize understanding of ways to prevent/reduce transmission. Patient will verbalize understanding of need for partner treatment to reduce reinfection. Patient verbalizes commitment to safer sex practices.	**Interventions and *Rationales:*** Assess knowledge level. *Must have baseline for teaching.* Teach ways to prevent/reduce disease transmission such as abstinence or condoms. *Both ways will decrease direct contact.* Encourage questions. *Giving information increases chance of compliance.* Provide information regarding treatment of partners to reduce reinfection. *Important to reduce transmission.*

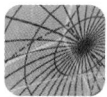

NURSING PROCESS: Patient Care Plan for Sexually Transmitted Infections—*Continued*

Assessment of High-Risk Behaviors

Subjective Data:
Are you aware of the dangers of unprotected sexual contact?
Are you concerned about either contracting or transmitting an STI?

Objective Data:
Evidence of STI based on culture results and/or clinical examination.

Nursing Assessment and Diagnoses	Outcomes and Evaluation Parameters	Planning and Interventions with *Rationales*
Nursing Diagnoses: Self Neglect Related to Ineffective Health Maintenance due to sexual behaviors	**Outcome:** Patient will verbalize understanding of safer sex practices. *Evaluation Parameters:* Patient will verbalize understanding of use of condoms. Patient will advise partner of need for treatment. Patient will avoid further exposure to sexually transmitted infection.	**Interventions and *Rationales:*** Assess understanding of how STIs are transmitted. *Must have baseline for teaching.* Assess understanding of use of condoms. *Must have baseline for teaching.* Supply condoms as needed. *To supply condoms for use with subsequent sexual contacts.* Encourage questions and frank discussion of risks of unprotected sexual contact. *Information provided in a nonjudgmental manner will increase potential for compliance.* Provide resources for pregnancy planning. *To encourage patient to prevent unplanned pregnancy.* Provide resources for treatment of sexual partners. *To emphasize the importance of partner treatment to prevent reinfection.*

risk factors for breast cancer. Relevant history includes family history, age of menarche and menopause, history of breast-feeding, and number of pregnancies and live births. Documentation of oral or transcutaneous contraceptives or hormone replacement therapy is also pertinent.

During the physical assessment, lump characteristics should be documented, including changes in size over time, changes relative to the menstrual cycle, duration, pain, swelling, redness, fever, or discharge from the nipples. A clinical breast exam should be performed to evaluate the mass. Clinical breast exam is described in Chapter 48 👁. Often masses can be preliminarily determined to be benign or malignant based on clinical exam, but mammogram and/or ultrasound, followed by fine needle aspiration, is used to gain definitive diagnosis. Chart 49–1 outlines the differences between benign versus malignant breast masses.

Nursing management includes suggesting a well-fitting support bra, decreasing salt and caffeine, which can increase the size of the cysts, taking ibuprofen (Motrin) (see Pharmacology Summary feature on p. 1552) as an anti-inflammatory agent for the pain, and applying local heat to the area of the mass. More importantly, the nurse needs to allow the patient to express concerns and ask questions regarding the source and implications

RISK FACTORS for Breast Cancer

Hormonal Risks	Nonhormonal Risks
Long menstrual histories	Women with a family history of breast cancer
Use of birth control pills	
Hormone replacement therapy	Lack of regular exercise
Early menarche (<12 years)	Post menopausal obesity
Late menopause (> 55 years)	Increased use of alcohol
Age at first full term pregnancy (after 30 years)	Night shift workers
	Age (65 years +)
	Caucasian women after age 40
	High breast tissue density
	No full term pregnancies
	Never breast-fed
	Higher socioeconomic status
	Tall
	Jewish heritage
	Two or more first-degree relatives with breast cancer at an early age

Source: "American Cancer Society. Breast Cancer Facts and Figures 2007–2008. Atlanta: American Cancer Society, Inc." "Breast Cancer: What are the Risk Factors for Breast Cancer" adapted and reprinted by the permission of the American Cancer Society, Inc. from www.cancer.org. All rights reserved.

CHART 49–1   Differentiation of Breast Masses by Clinical Exam

Benign Mass	Malignant Mass
No skin changes are noted. Breasts are symmetrical.	The mass is fixed to surrounding skin and soft tissue, causing skin dimpling and asymmetry of the breasts.
When palpated, the lump is smooth.	The mass is irregularly shaped.
The consistency of the lump is soft to firm.	The consistency is hard.
The lump is mobile beneath the skin.	The mass is immobile beneath the skin.
The margins are well defined and easily delineated.	The margins are poorly defined and irregular.
The mass is tender to palpation.	The mass is usually nontender.

of the mass. Ensure that the patient understands the terms *benign* and *malignant* and the types of diagnostic evaluations that will be used to make a definitive diagnosis. Impress on the patient the importance of reporting any change in the mass immediately to the treating health care provider.

Etiology, Pathophysiology, Clinical Manifestations, and Treatment of Mastitis

Mastitis, which is an inflammation of the breast tissue, occurs most frequently in women who are breast-feeding. Microorganisms invade the tissue through a portal of entry such as a crack or a fissure in the nipple, or through a duct. Symptoms include breast tenderness, redness typically at the site of inflammation, and edema. The woman may also experience fatigue, malaise, fever, or chills.

Treatment includes rest, fluids, alternating warm and cold compresses, and continued breast-feeding. Alternating warm and cold compresses aids in pain relief and increases circulation to the area.

Continuation of breast-feeding was controversial many years ago because it was thought the infection could cause harm to the nursing infant. Mastitis is inflamed breast tissue, not the milk ducts, and it is often caused from clogged milk ducts in breast-feeding women. Therefore, emptying the breasts frequently and completely is a successful intervention. Antibiotics are prescribed when the infection does not clear with nonpharmacologic methods, or when the health care provider feels the infection may cause additional problems. The woman is instructed to wear a support bra. Nursing care is aimed at prevention of breast tissue damage from engorgement by encouraging breast-feeding, relieving discomfort, treating the infection causing the inflammation, and prevention of recurrence. Women who are nursing infants should use lanolin creams to the nipples regularly to avoid cracking of the nipples and thus preventing invasion of bacteria into the breast tissue. Mastitis occurs primarily in breast-feeding mothers, so instruction on feeding technique and symptoms may prevent progression of this problem.

Etiology and Epidemiology of Breast Cancer

Breast cancer is defined as the formation of a malignant glandular tumor as a result of an uncontrolled growth of abnormal cells in the breast tissue. The malignant cells over time destroy normal breast tissue. Other than skin cancer, breast cancer is the most common cancer in women, with more than 212,000 new cases occurring in 2006 and 41,000 deaths (American Cancer Society [ACS], 2007). Breast cancer accounts for nearly 1 in 3 cancers diagnosed in U.S. women (ACS, 2005). The overall incidence of breast cancer appears to have increased since 1975 when there was both a shift in delaying childbearing and the advent of breast mammography, which detected cancers earlier (ACS, 2005; CDC, 2008a). Therefore, a goal of *Healthy People 2010* is to "reduce the numbers of new cancers as well as the illness, disability, and death caused by cancer" (DHHS, 2000).

Risk Factors for Breast Cancer

The etiology of breast cancer is based on a number of risk factors (Chart 49–2). Several factors are associated with increased risk of breast cancer including age, family history, age at first pregnancy, age of menarche, and age of menopause. These are

nonmodifiable risk factors. Modifiable risk factors include obesity, hormone replacement therapy, alcohol consumption, and sedentary lifestyle.

Besides being female, age is the most important risk factor for breast cancer (Osteen, 2001). The risk increases with age from 1 in 1,984 at age 20 to 1 in 24 at age 70. Currently, a woman living in the United States has a 1 in 8 lifetime risk of developing breast cancer. This has gradually increased over the past three decades in part due to longer life expectancy and more complete diagnosis through the use of mammography screening (ACS, 2005).

Family history is also a significant etiologic factor. Women with a family history of breast cancer, especially in a first-degree relative (mother, sister, or daughter), have an increased risk of developing breast cancer (Loman et al., 2001). Families with extensive history of breast and ovarian cancers are often screened for mutation of the BRCA1 gene. The BRCA1 is a tumor suppression gene when it functions normally. However, the BRCA1 gene can undergo mutation or alteration that causes increased susceptibility of the patient to not only breast cancer but ovarian cancer as well. The BRCA1 gene is located on chromosome 17; a similar gene, the BRCA2 gene, is located on chromosome 11. Five percent to ten percent of breast cancers are related to BRCA1 and BRCA2 gene mutations. Women with BRCA1 and BRCA2 gene mutations have a 40% to 80% lifetime risk of developing breast cancer. BRCA1 and BRCA2 gene mutations are also associated with early onset of breast cancer (Ford et al., 1998).

Reproductive hormones, specifically estrogen and progestin, are thought to influence breast cancer risk through effects on cell proliferation and DNA damage. Early menarche (<12 years of age) and menopause at > 55 years of age increase the exposure to estrogen. Being over age 30 at the time of a first full-term pregnancy and a low number of pregnancies may increase a woman's risk of breast cancer by affecting the endogenous reproductive hormones her body produces (Hulka & Moorman, 2001). The prolonged use of combination hormone replacement (estrogen and progestin) has also been shown to increase the risk of breast cancer (Rossow et al., 2002). The use of oral contraceptives may increase the risk of breast cancer slightly; however, once the woman stops using oral contraceptives for 10 years or more, she has the same risk as the woman who never used oral contraceptives. (Li et al., 2003).

Other modifiable risk factors can be considered in the prevention of breast cancer. There is, of course, no guaranteed way to prevent breast cancer, but decreasing risk factors is an effective strategy in reducing the risk of breast cancer. Obesity increases the risk of postmenopausal, but not premenopausal, breast cancer (Boyles, 2006). In postmenopausal women, circulating estrogen is primarily produced in fat tissue; therefore, having more adipose tissue increases estrogen levels and supports potential tumor formation. A recent American Cancer Society (2005) study showed that women with a body mass index (BMI) of > 25 are 1.3 to 2.1 times more likely to die from breast cancer compared to women with normal weight (BMI of 18.5 to 24.9). Recent studies also indicate that physical activity appears to have a protective effect on women with regard to breast cancer. The protective effect is most apparent in lean women, women who have carried children to term, and premenopausal women (Bianchini, Kaaks, & Vaino, 2002; McTiernan et al.,

CHART 49-2   Overview of Risk Factors for Developing Breast Cancer

Nonmodifiable Risk Factors	Modifiable Risk Factors	Uncertain, Controversial, or Unproven Risk Factors
Gender: • 100 times more common in women.	Childbirth: • Having children later than age 30. • Not having any children.	High-fat diets: • Most studies found that breast cancer is less common in countries where the typical diet is low in total fat, low in polyunsaturated fat, and low in saturated fat. • Many studies of women in the United States have not found breast cancer risk to be related to dietary fat intake.
Age: • About 1 out of 8 invasive breast cancer diagnoses are younger than 45. • Two out of 3 women are age 55 or older.	Oral contraceptive use: • Women now using oral contraceptives have a slightly greater risk. • Risk seems to decline once their use is stopped.	Antiperspirants: • One small study recently found trace levels of parabens (used as preservatives in antiperspirants and other products), which have weak estrogen-like properties, in a small sample of breast cancer tumors. The study did not look at whether parabens had caused the tumors. • A large study of breast cancer causes found no increase in breast cancer in women who used underarm antiperspirants or who shaved their underarms.
Genetics: • Women with mutated breast cancer genes BRCA1 and BRCA2 have an 80% chance of developing breast cancer during their lifetime. Ethnicity: • Caucasian women are slightly more likely to develop breast cancer than are African American women. • African American women are more likely to die from this cancer. • Asian, Hispanic, and Native American women have a lower risk of developing and dying from breast cancer. BRCA mutations are found most often in: • Jewish women of Ashkenazi (Eastern European) population • African American women • Hispanic women	Postmenopausal hormone therapy (PHT): • Combined postmenopausal hormone therapy increases the risk of developing and may also increase the chances of dying from breast cancer. Breast-feeding: • Some studies suggest that breast-feeding may slightly lower risk, especially if continued for 1.5 to 2 years.	
Family history of breast cancer: • Having one first-degree relative (mother, sister, or daughter) with breast cancer approximately doubles a woman's risk. • Having two first-degree relatives increases her risk about fivefold. • A family history of breast cancer in a father or brother increases a woman's risk. • 20–30% of women with breast cancer have a family member with this disease. • 70–80% of women who get breast cancer do not have a family history.	Alcohol: • One alcoholic drink a day has a very small increase in risk. • Two to 5 drinks daily have about 1½ times the risk. • Also known to increase the risk of developing cancers of the mouth, throat, esophagus, and liver.	Night work: • Several studies have suggested that women who work at night may have an increased risk. This is a fairly recent finding, and more studies are in progress to look at this issue. According to some researchers, the effect may be due to disruption in melatonin, a hormone that is affected by light, but other hormones are also being studied.

(continued)

CHART 49–2	Overview of Risk Factors for Developing Breast Cancer—*Continued*

Nonmodifiable Risk Factors	Modifiable Risk Factors	Uncertain, Controversial, or Unproven Risk Factors
History of breast cancer: • Cancer in one breast has a three- to fourfold increased risk of developing a new primary cancer in the other breast or in another part of the same breast. This is different from a *recurrence* of the first cancer.	Overweight or obese: • Increased breast cancer risk, especially for women after menopause due to once the ovaries stop making estrogen, most of a woman's estrogen comes from fat tissue. Having more fat tissue after menopause can increase estrogen levels and thereby increase the risk.	

Abnormal breast biopsy results:
• The *proliferative lesions with atypia* (those with excessive growth of cells in the ducts or lobules of the breast tissue, and in which the cells no longer appear normal) increase risk 4 to 5 times. They include:
  • Atypical ductal hyperplasia (ADH)
  • Atypical lobular hyperplasia (ALH).
	Physical activity:
	• Evidence is growing that physical activity in the form of exercise reduces breast cancer risk. The only question is how much exercise is needed. The Women's Health Initiative (WHI) found that as little as 1.25 to 2.5 hours per week of brisk walking reduced a woman's risk by 18%.
	• Walking 10 hours a week reduced the risk a little more.	

Menstrual periods: • Menstruating at an early age (before age 12). • Menopause after age 55 has a slightly higher risk. Previous chest radiation: • Radiation therapy to the chest area as treatment for another cancer (such as Hodgkin's disease or non-Hodgkin's lymphoma) significantly increases risk. Diethylstilbestrol (DES) exposure: • Slightly increased risk.		

Source: "American Cancer Society. Breast Cancer Facts and Figures 2007–2008. Atlanta: American Cancer Society, Inc."

2003). The underlying mechanism is not well understood at this time. Alcohol consumption is consistently associated with increased breast cancer risk (Li et al., 2003). Alcohol appears to increase estrogen and androgen levels; therefore, the equivalent of two drinks a day may increase breast cancer risk by 21% (Singletary & Gapstur, 2001).

Pathophysiology of Breast Cancer

Breast tissue is made up of glands for milk production, called lobules, and ducts that connect the lobules to the nipple. Cancer arises from the epithelial cells that line the ducts and the lobules. Breast cancers can be *in situ*, which is the term that describes a cancer confined to the ducts or lobules. In 2005, there were 58,490 cases of *in situ* breast cancer (American Cancer Society, 2005). This type of breast cancer is not usually palpable on exam, so it is most often discovered by mammogram. The rates of *in situ* breast cancer have increased markedly since 1980, largely due to the increased diagnostic ability of mammography. Most cases of ductal carcinoma *in situ* (DCIS) are detectable only through mammography (National Cancer Institute, 2000). Approximately 22% of breast cancers are *in situ* (ACS, 2005). Lobular cancer *in situ* (LCIS) is not considered a true cancer by many

oncologists, but more of an indicator of increased risk of invasive cancer. Nearly all cancers at the *in situ* stage can be cured (ACS, 2005).

Invasive or infiltrative cancer starts in the lobules or ducts, but breaks through the walls to invade the surrounding fatty tissue of the breast. The most common type of breast cancer is invasive ductal carcinoma. In 2005 there were 211,240 cases of invasive ductal cancer (ACS, 2005). Once cancer is identified as invasive, it is staged according to the American Joint Committee on Cancer. The National Guidelines box outlines the staging of breast cancer.

Paget's disease is a rare form of breast cancer that is characterized by infiltration of the nipple epithelium. The patient may have itching, burning, and bloody nipple discharge. Some ulceration may be present as well. Treatment delays can be caused by misdiagnosis as infection or dermatitis. Prognosis is good for Paget's disease when the cancer is localized in the nipple.

Another form of breast cancer that is very rare is inflammatory breast cancer. This is a very malignant form of cancer because of its aggressive nature and fast growing character. This type of cancer is described by a finding of *peau d'orange* on the skin of the breast. The skin of the breast, which looks red, feels warm and has a thickened appearance resembling an orange peel.

NATIONAL GUIDELINES for the Staging of Breast Cancer

Stage	Tumor Size	Lymph Node	Metastasis
I	<2 centimeters	No involvement	None
IIA	No evidence of primary tumor	0–3 Axillary or internal mammary nodes	None
IIB	2–5 centimeters	0–3 Axillary or internal mammary nodes	None
IIIA	No evidence of tumor ranging to > 5 centimeters	Yes; 4–9 axillary or internal mammary nodes	None
IIIB	Any size with extension to chest wall or skin	Yes; 4–9 axillary or internal mammary nodes	None
IIIC	Any size	Yes; 10 or more axillary, internal mammary, or infraclavicular nodes	None
IV	Any size	Any type of nodal involvement	Yes

Source: American Joint Committee on Cancers. (2005). *AJCC cancer staging manual.* Retrieved February 27, 2008, from http://www.cancerstaging.org/products/ajccproducts.html

Clinical Manifestations of Breast Cancer

Early stage breast cancer or *in situ* cancer typically produces no symptoms when the tumor is small and most treatable. The most significant finding in breast cancer is a painless mass. The lump is most often in the upper outer quadrant of the breast where the majority of glandular tissue is found. The mass may be noted as a thickening in the breast tissue found during self-breast exam or showering. Other symptoms are an unusual lump in the axilla or above the clavicle. A persistent skin rash near the nipple area can signal Paget's disease, along with flaking or eruption near the nipple. Some tumors can cause dimpling, pulling, or retraction in one breast, creating an asymmetrical appearance. Some patients will complain of a burning, stinging, or prickling sensation in the breast. Nipple abnormalities such as spontaneous discharge, erosion, inversion, or tenderness can occur less commonly (American Cancer Society, 2005).

Diagnosis of Breast Cancer

The key to survival from breast cancer is early detection and intervention, with a 5-year survival rate of 97% for women diagnosed in Stage I (ACS, 2005). Mammography and breast self-exam are the two primary keys to early diagnosis. Breast self-exams, described in Chart 49–3, should be performed monthly beginning in the early 20s. Breast self-examination, along with mammography, can detect breast cancer early, with the cure rate being nearly 100% with early detection (CDC, 2008a). Once an abnormality has been detected, more invasive diagnostic techniques such as breast biopsy are used to make a definitive diagnosis. Diagnostic techniques are discussed next.

Mammography

The CDC (2008a) maintains that mammography is the most effective way to detect breast cancer when it is at a treatable stage. **Mammography** is a low-dose x-ray procedure that allows visualization of the internal structure of the breast. Mammography can identify cancer several years before physical symptoms develop. Modern screen-film units used today result in higher quality images with a considerably lower x-ray dose than the general-purpose x-ray equipment used in the past. The National Cancer Institute (NCI) (2007) and the CDC (2008a) recommend that all women over age 40 have a mammogram every 1 to 2 years. This alone could reduce breast cancer mortality by 20% to 25% over 10 years (CDC, 2008a). Mammography can

CHART 49–3   Breast Self-Exam (Self-Breast Exam)

Beginning in their 20s, women should be told about the benefits and limitations of breast self-exam (BSE). Women with breast implants can do BSE. It may be helpful to have the surgeon help identify the edges of the implant so that you know what you are feeling. Women who are pregnant or breast-feeding can also choose to examine their breasts regularly.

ESTABLISH A REGULAR SCHEDULE

- Perform on day 4–7 of menstrual cycle.
- If no periods, choose a regular day (i.e., the first of each month).
- Know how breasts normally look and feel and report any new breast changes to a health professional as soon as they are found.
- Best time to examine breasts is when the breasts are not tender or swollen.

INSPECT BREASTS

- Lie down and place your right arm behind your head. The exam is done while lying down, not standing up. This is because when lying down the breast tissue spreads evenly over the chest wall and is as thin as possible, making it much easier to feel all the breast tissue.
- Use the finger pads of the 3 middle fingers on left hand to feel for lumps in the right breast.
- Use overlapping dime-sized circular motions of the finger pads to feel the breast tissue.
- Use 3 different levels of pressure to feel all the breast tissue. Use each pressure level to feel the breast tissue before moving on to the next spot.
  - Light pressure is needed to feel the tissue closest to the skin.
  - Medium pressure to feel a little deeper.
  - Firm pressure to feel the tissue closest to the chest and ribs. A firm ridge in the lower curve of each breast is normal.

IMPORTANT POINTS TO REMEMBER

- Many lumps are benign.
- Early detection through breast self-exam and mammography increases the survival rate.

Source: "How to Perform a Breast Self-Exam adapted and reprinted by the permission of the American Cancer Society, Inc. from www.cancer.org. All rights reserved."

detect about 80% to 90% of breast cancers in women without symptoms; testing is somewhat more accurate in postmenopausal than in premenopausal women (Kerlikowski & Barclay, 1997). Approximately 60% of women over the age of

40 have had a mammogram within the previous year; however, a woman who has no health insurance, who has not graduated from high school, or who has recently immigrated to the United States is much less likely to have access to mammogram or clinical breast exam.

Terms associated with mammography include *screening* versus *diagnostic* and *film* versus *digital*. A screening mammogram simply indicates that the breast is being evaluated for any lumps or signs of potential cancer. A diagnostic mammogram is utilized when the screening mammogram or a clinical breast exam finds a suspicious area of the breast requiring closer evaluation. The diagnostic mammogram is often specific to the area in question and may utilize an enhancement mechanism to better view this area. Film mammography uses a film to both capture and display the breast tissue being evaluated. Film mammography is limited with dense breast tissue, seen in a population at higher risk for breast cancer (NCI, 2007). Digital mammography stores the electronic image in a way that allows for it to be enhanced, magnified, or manipulated to evaluate areas in question more fully.

Breast Ultrasound

Breast ultrasound is not as effective a screening tool as is mammography. It is used more often in the office setting for further characterization and guided biopsy of breast masses and suspicious axillary nodes. Ultrasound is very useful in differentiating solid masses and cystic lesions. Sound waves bounced off of the cystic lesion reveal lobulated and nonechogenic lesions with well-defined borders. The surgeon can use ultrasound to aid in locating and excising nonpalpable breast lesions and achieving clean lumpectomy margins. The future may find ultrasound being used to ablate tumors.

Breast Biopsy

A breast biopsy is performed to evaluate a lump or cyst that is found to be of a suspicious nature on mammography. There are four primary types of biopsies: fine needle aspiration biopsy, incisional biopsy, excisional biopsy, and stereotactic needle biopsy. Each is unique in its own way and used for specific reasons.

A fine needle aspiration (FNA) biopsy uses a fine gauge (typically 22 or 25 gauge) needle to pierce the skin and remove fluid from a cyst or remove cells from a solid mass. The tissue is removed by inserting the needle in the mass and aspirating fluid or cells, which are then sent to a pathology lab for analysis. The procedure is done under mammography or ultrasound guidance to pinpoint the exact location of the mass. This is usually an outpatient procedure, not requiring any stitches, and many patients resume normal activities that same day. Prior to discharge from the outpatient facility, assessment of the puncture site, vital signs, and pain evaluation are done. Discharge instructions include signs and symptoms of infection, pain-relief measures, and health care provider follow-up appointment. An FNA is considered the easiest form of breast biopsy, with rapid results (Imaginis, 2006). It is limited in that it samples only a small portion of tissue or cells.

Impalpable lesions are often evaluated using an image guided core needle biopsy. The patient needs to understand that the lesion will only be sampled, not excised. The core needle biopsy is less expensive than open biopsy, takes less time, and leaves only a tiny scar. Limitations of the procedure include the possibility

of a sampling error that will cause the examiner to miss the lesion, causing equivocal findings that will require follow-up.

An open surgical incisional biopsy is considered the gold standard against which other methods are compared (Imaginis, 2006). Surgical incisional biopsies involve a less than 2-inch incision in the breast done under local anesthetic or intravenous (IV) sedation, and, like FNA, are usually considered an outpatient procedure. Prior to the procedure the surgeon will use mammography to locate and mark the specific area. Marking is done by several methods. If the abnormality can be felt by examination, the surgeon will mark the area using a marker or skin dye. If it cannot be felt by examination, the surgeon will use ultrasound to insert a small hollow needle into the mass, followed by insertion of a thin wire into the hollow bore of the needle. The needle is removed once the wire is placed. The patient is taken to the operating room for removal of all or part of the abnormality.

An excisional biopsy is done when complete removal of the abnormality and some surrounding tissue is planned. In this case, the pathologist will evaluate whether the margins of the lesion are free of abnormal cells, indicating that the entire lesion was removed. An incisional biopsy is performed when the lesion is large enough that removal through the small incision is not possible. A part of the lesion is removed in this case and sent for pathology evaluation, with follow-up surgery or treatment based on the pathology report. Pain control, vital signs, incisional assessment, and emotional needs are evaluated by the nurse. A follow-up appointment is made with the health care provider.

A stereotactic needle biopsy refers to the method in which the needle is guided into the abnormality. Stereotactic mammography is a three-dimensional mammography whereby the woman lies on her stomach on a mammography table with her breast protruding through a hole in the table. The breast is compressed as with a mammogram and an image taken. A biopsy is taken under a local anesthetic using a fine gauge needle. This procedure does not require surgery and is only mildly uncomfortable, but will produce a biopsy sample similar to the surgical route. The disadvantage is that the size of the abnormality is not clearly understood with this method. There are no special discharge instructions for the patient, and follow-up is scheduled with the health care provider.

Treatment of Breast Cancer

Breast cancer treatment is usually multileveled. Most women will require some form of surgery, and this may be followed by radiation, chemotherapy, hormone therapy, or monoclonal antibody therapy. A **lumpectomy**, removal of the cancerous growth and a small amount of surrounding normal tissue, is the least invasive form of surgery and is usually followed by 6 to 7 weeks of radiation. This is coupled with axillary node dissection and radiation therapy to improve long-term survival. A woman who chooses lumpectomy and radiation therapy will have the same expected long-term survival as if she had chosen a more invasive surgery such as mastectomy (American Cancer Society, 2005; Fisher et al., 2002).

Other surgical techniques include a simple (also called a total) **mastectomy**, which is removal of the entire breast, or a modified radical mastectomy, which is removal of the entire breast along with the surrounding lymph nodes. This surgery does not include removal of the chest wall muscles, as is done in radical mastectomy. Radical mastectomy is very rarely used today because of the disfiguring nature of the surgery. Radical mastectomy is not any more effective than other procedures. A complication of axillary node dissection is the problem of lymphedema, a serious swelling of the arm caused by retention of lymph fluid (Bumpers, Best, Norman, & Weaver, 2002).

Radiation is used to destroy cancer cells remaining in the breast tissue, chest wall, or underarm lymph nodes. Currently technology increases the ability to target radiation therapy accurately and decrease the side effects from radiation therapy. Radiation therapy can be used in conjunction with surgery and chemotherapy to improve long-term survival in women with lymph node positive disease.

Chemotherapy is a systemic method of destroying cancer cells that may have migrated to other parts of the body. Chemotherapy also is used to reduce the size of a tumor to allow a more conservative, rather than radical, approach to surgery. Hormone therapy is used to block the effects of estrogen on the growth of breast cancer cells. Tamoxifen, the most common medication used in breast cancer, blocks the tumor's ability to utilize estrogen in both pre- and postmenopausal women. Tamoxifen has been shown to reduce the rate of recurrence by 26%, and has reduced the death rate by 14% (American Cancer Society, 2005). Another group of antiestrogen agents known as aromatase inhibitors (anastrozole, letrozole) has been successfully used to block estrogen production by tissues other than the ovaries in postmenopausal women (ACS, 2005). Trastuzumab, a monoclonal antibody, targets a protein of breast tumors called HER2. Trastuzumab has been shown to improve survival for women with metastatic disease as well as late stage and recurrent disease (ACS, 2005; National Cancer Institute, 2000). See the Pharmacology Summary feature (p. 1552). A complete discussion of monoclonal antibodies is found in Chapter 59. Additional information on aspects of diagnosis and treatment of breast cancer may be found in Chapter 64 .

Breast Reconstruction

Reconstructive breast surgery occurs after mastectomy for breast cancer. Advances in techniques have made breast reconstruction a more desirable procedure for women requiring mastectomy. Reconstructive surgery can be done at the time of the mastectomy or it can be delayed, based on the woman's preference. Immediate breast reconstructive surgery does not delay administration of chemotherapy or radiation, nor does it prevent detection of recurrent disease. It is now thought to be beneficial to perform the breast reconstruction immediately after the mastectomy. An immediate breast reconstruction is more cost-effective, allows for a quicker recovery, and makes for reduced inconvenience, as well as greater satisfaction, for the patient (Harcourt & Rumsey, 2001). (Breast reconstruction is discussed in detail in the Diagnostic and Surgical Procedures section later in the chapter.)

Predicting Breast Cancer Survival

Breast cancer survival is dependent on multiple factors. The time since diagnosis is a factor; eighty-eight percent of women survive 5 years after diagnosis, 80% survive 10 years after diagnosis, 71% survive 15 years after diagnosis, and 63% survive 20 years after diagnosis (Smigal, et al, 2006). The 5-year survival

rate is slightly lower among women diagnosed with breast cancer before age 40. This may be due to tumors in this age group being more aggressive and less responsive to hormonal therapy (Kroman et al., 2000).

The stage of cancer at diagnosis also determines survival rate. Naturally, the survival rate is lower among women with more advanced state of disease; the 5-year survival rate is 98% for localized disease and 81% for regional disease with only a 26% survival rate for women diagnosed with distant-stage disease (Smigal, et al., 2006). In addition, larger tumor size at diagnosis is associated with decreased survival. A tumor is considered to be large when it is greater than 5.0 centimeters. Survivability can also depend on race or ethnicity and socioeconomic factors. African American women with breast cancer are less likely than Caucasian women to survive 5 years (Smigal, et al., 2006). Aggressive tumor characteristics associated with poorer prognosis appear to be more common in African American women (Chlebowski, Prentice, & Adams-Campbell, 2005). The presence of additional illnesses, lower socioeconomic status, unequal access to medical care, and disparities in treatment may contribute to the observed differences in survival between lower and higher income breast cancer patients. Chapter 64 provides an in-depth discussion of cancer staging and treatment.

Nursing Management

The patient with breast cancer requires a comprehensive interdisciplinary care plan to address the complex nature of the disease. The Nursing Process: Patient Care Plan feature (p. 1534) provides a complete care plan for the patient with breast cancer. The Patient Teaching & Discharge Priorities box (p. 1536) outlines the discharge teaching for the patient with breast cancer.

Health Promotion for Breast Cancer

Patient and family education is essential for the prevention of breast cancer. The following facts are necessary components of the teaching plan:

- Self-breast exam
- Weight management
- Avoidance of excessive alcohol use
- Mammograms every 2 years after age 40
- Caution with use of hormone replacement therapy during menopause.

The United States (U.S.) Preventive Services Task Force recommends screening mammography, with or without clinical breast examination, every 1 to 2 years for women aged 40 or older. This task force found evidence that mammography screening every 12 to 33 months significantly reduces mortality from breast cancer. Evidence is strongest for women aged 50 to 69, the age group generally included in screening trials. For women aged 40 to 49, the evidence is weaker that screening mammography reduces mortality from breast cancer, and the absolute benefit of mammography is smaller, than it is for older women (U.S. Preventive Services Task Force, 2002).

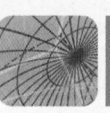

NURSING PROCESS: Patient Care Plan for Breast Cancer

Assessment of Patient History

Past medical history, relative risk factors, menstrual history, pregnancy history, reproductive cancers, such as ovarian or endometrial, benign breast disease, previous breast cancer.

Subjective Data:

Do you have pain in your back or other bone?

How is your appetite?

Have you had any change in breast size or symmetry, or skin changes over the breast?

Objective Data:

Signs of anxiety or stress, axillary or supraclavicular lymphadenopathy, changes in lung sounds (indicative of lung metastasis); hepatomegaly, jaundice, or ascites; obesity; or cachexia.

Nursing Assessment and Diagnoses	Outcomes and Evaluation Parameters	Planning and Interventions with *Rationales*
Nursing Diagnosis: *Deficient Knowledge* related to disease process, medications, treatment options, and complications	**Outcome:** Increased understanding of diagnosis, disease process, and treatment. *Evaluation Parameter:* Patient asks pertinent questions related to disease process, treatment, and symptoms.	**Interventions and *Rationale:*** Provide information to patient regarding disease process, medications, and treatment options. Encourage patient to ask questions regarding disease process, medications, and treatment options. Explain assessment findings to patient and encourage her to relate changes in signs and symptoms. *To increase knowledge about the disease.*

Assessment of Signs and Symptoms of Pain

Subjective Data:

Tell me your level of pain on a scale of 0–10, with 10 being the worst pain you have ever had.

Describe the location, intensity, and quality of your pain.

Objective Data:

Assess vital signs

Signs of stress and tension due to pain

Nursing Assessment and Diagnoses	Outcomes and Evaluation Parameters	Planning and Interventions with *Rationales*
Nursing Diagnosis: *Acute Pain* related to breast cancer and surgical intervention	**Outcomes:** Comprehensive pain management. Patient reports tolerable pain. Patient uses analgesic and nonanalgesic measures appropriately. *Evaluation Parameters:* Reduction in pain to patient acceptance. Patient reports pain is under control.	**Interventions and *Rationales:*** Perform a comprehensive pain assessment. Provide for quiet and restful environment. Reposition for comfort as needed. Provide for diversion with music, television, or relaxation techniques. Provide patient teaching regarding use of analgesics or PCA as appropriate. Advocate for patient when needed to change or increase pain medications. Encourage patient to use pain control measures before pain becomes severe and out of control. *To ensure the patient is as comfortable as possible.*

Assessment of Coping Abilities

Subjective Data:

Do you have a history of reproductive cancers?

Do you have any questions about your treatment plan?

Do you feel less anxious with more or less information?

Tell me what you are feeling regarding your illness?

Who are your support systems?

Objective Data:

Signs of anxiety and stress

Reduced communicative efforts

Withdrawal from social support

Insomnia

Crying

Nursing Assessment and Diagnoses	Outcomes and Evaluation Parameters	Planning and Interventions with *Rationales*
Nursing Diagnosis: *Disturbed Body Image* related to anticipated physical effects of treatment modalities	**Outcomes:** Development of effective coping behaviors. Development of attitude of realistic hope. *Evaluation Parameters:* Patient verbalizes feelings and fears about illness. Patient accepts social support. Patient reports decrease in symptoms of stress and anxiety. Patient reports increase in psychological well-being.	**Interventions and *Rationales:*** Encourage verbalization of feelings, perceptions, and fears *to reduce stress and anxiety.* Encourage patient to seek social support in the form of outreach groups *to feel less alone.* Encourage interaction with other women with breast cancer *to feel less alone.* Encourage patient to verbalize feelings of helplessness, and provide information regarding progress with treatments *to decrease stress level.* Encourage family members to verbalize concerns regarding the diagnosis, treatment, and potential complications *to decrease stress level.*

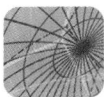

NURSING PROCESS: Patient Care Plan for Breast Cancer—*Continued*

Assessment of Signs and Symptoms of Infection

Subjective Data:
Do you have any increased pain, redness, or drainage from surgical site?

Objective Data:
Fever and chills
Changes in white blood count (WBC)
Drainage from the wound
Positive wound cultures
Decreased healing

Nursing Assessment and Diagnoses	Outcomes and Evaluation Parameters	Planning and Interventions with *Rationales*
Nursing Diagnosis: *Risk for Infection* related to neutropenia	**Outcome:** Avoidance of infection. *Evaluation Parameters:* Healed wound. No fever. Diminishing or absent pain.	**Interventions and *Rationales:*** Instruct patient and family members in hand hygiene *to prevent wound contamination.* Monitor surgical site for signs of infection for redness, odor, drainage, and lack of healing *that would indicate an infection.* Provide patient education about infection signs and symptoms and what to report to the surgeon. *To institute medical intervention as soon as possible.*

Assessment of Acceptance of Body Image

Subjective Data:
How do you feel about the changes in your body since surgery?
Do you plan to have reconstruction done?
Do you have any questions?

Objective Data:
Ability to participate in care
Willingness to interact with social support persons
Willingness to touch affected breast

Nursing Assessment and Diagnoses	Outcomes and Evaluation Parameters	Planning and Interventions with *Rationales*
Nursing Diagnosis: *Disturbed Body Image* related to anticipated physical effects of treatment modalities	**Outcome:** Acceptance of body image. *Evaluation Parameters:* Patient exhibits willingness to touch affected breast. Patient shows acceptance of social support. There is an interaction with individuals with similar change in body image. Patient discusses changes in body image. Patient demonstrates willingness to use strategies to enhance appearance.	**Interventions and *Rationales:*** Encourage patient to interact with Reach to Recovery volunteer *to develop hope for the future.* Encourage patient to attend breast cancer support group where she can draw on experiences of other women with breast cancer. Provide information on support groups available to patient. Facilitate contact with individuals with similar change in body image.

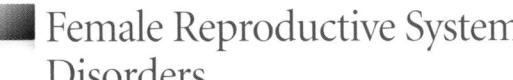

Female Reproductive System Disorders

Reproductive system disorders are varied and do not have age barriers. This section will discuss the more common disorders, their clinical manifestations, and treatment modalities, along with some prevention methods where applicable. Further information on general reproductive assessment can be found in Chapter 48 🔗.

Etiology, Epidemiology, Pathophysiology, and Clinical Manifestations of Uterine Fibroid Tumors

Fibroid tumors of the uterus, also known as leiomyomas and myomas, occur in more than 30% of women 40 to 60 years of age but are almost always benign (Evans & Brunsell, 2007). They occur with higher prevalence in African American women, and some studies indicate that African American women are more likely than Caucasian women to have more symptomatic tumors (Kjerulff, Langenberg, Seidman, Stolley, & Guzinski, 1996). Leiomyomas are the most common female reproductive tract tumors (Evans & Brunsell, 2007). The lesions are growths aris-

ing from the tissue of the uterine muscle for unknown reasons (Figure 49–6 ■, p. 1536). They develop slowly in women ages 25 through 40, and tend to enlarge during pregnancy and after menopause; fibroids often decrease on their own, due to decreased estrogen production. Fibroids often cause no symptoms, so many are undiscovered unless the patient has dysfunctional uterine bleeding, pelvic pain, and infertility or pregnancy loss. Uterine tumors can add pressure to surrounding organs, causing pain, constipation, urinary problems, menorrhagia (heavy bleeding), and metrorrhagia (irregular bleeding). Risk factors for uterine fibroid tumors include 40 years of age or older, nulliparity, obesity, family history, African American, and hypertension.

Diagnosis and Medical Management of Uterine Fibroid Tumors

Diagnosis is accomplished based on an internal examination using transvaginal ultrasonography and hysteroscopy to help visualize the tumor and determine its exact location and size. The surgeon can then determine the best approach for treatment. The options for treatment of uterine fibroid tumors have increased substantially in the last 20 years. There are currently multiple treatment options that depend on the size of the tumor,

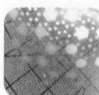

PATIENT TEACHING & DISCHARGE PRIORITIES for Breast Cancer

Need	Teaching
Analgesics	Take analgesics as prescribed.
Patient	Encourage patient to take analgesics as prescribed.
Family/support system	Advise patient to report to health care provider if analgesics are inadequate.
Activity	Range of motion exercises to maintain muscle tone and improve lymph and blood circulation.
Patient	Assist patient with items that are heavy and discourage strenuous activity.
Family/support system	
Diet	Regular, well-balanced diet as soon as desired.
Patient	Adequate amount of protein to ensure healing and immunity.
Family/support system	Encourage a healthy diet.
Postoperative	The value of a well-fitting prosthesis.
Patient	Provide resources for prosthetic bra.
Family/support system	Assist patient as needed with resources and provide emotional support.
Coping needs	Explain implications of a loss of a breast as it relates to self-image. Provide resources for counseling.
Patient	Spouse may need assistance in dealing with emotional needs of patient. Provide resources for counseling.
Family/support system	
Complications	Signs and symptoms of complications to include surgical site changes that indicate infection.
Patient	New or worsening pain, especially back pain (bone metastasis), shortness of breath, or change in sensorium.
Family/support system	Advise family members of important findings for which they should notify the patient's health care provider or seek emergency care.

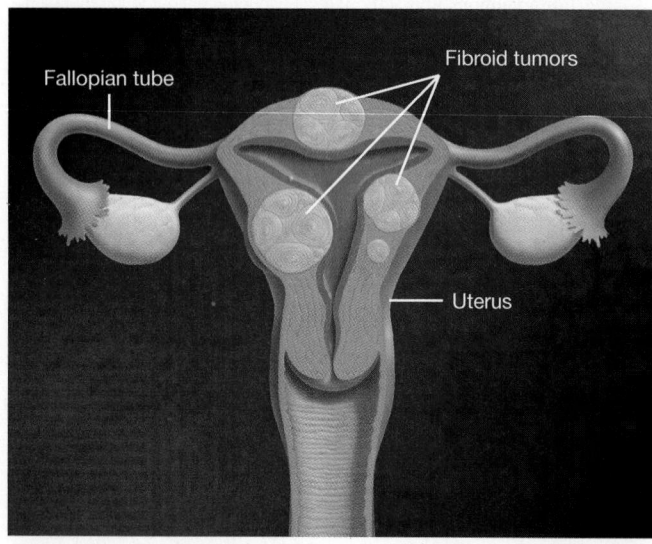

FIGURE 49–6 ■ Uterine fibroid tumor.
Source: Jane Hurd/Phototake NYC

the age of the patient, and the severity of symptoms. Choice of options also depends on whether fertility needs to be preserved. Observational management is increasingly recognized as a reasonable course for women with asymptomatic tumors. Conservative treatment involves drug therapy such as nonsteroidal anti-inflammatory drugs (NSAIDs) to control pain, birth control pills, and hormone therapy to decrease the size of the fibroids and the associated discomfort.

Uterine fibroid embolization, a nonsurgical treatment done under intravenous sedation that shrinks the fibroid, may also be used. This procedure is minimally invasive and avoids surgery. It is an interventional radiologic procedure that occludes the uter-

ine arteries that feed the fibroid. Intravenous (IV) conscious sedation is needed to assure patient comfort during the embolization procedure and is usually adequate, although some operators may prefer epidural or spinal analgesia. Patients usually experience pelvic pain immediately after the procedure. Nursing personnel are responsible for monitoring sedated patients and should be prepared to manage sedation and the analgesia required immediately after the procedure. This procedure will not preserve fertility.

In women whose symptoms are severe, or if the fibroid is very large, treatment can range from simple fibroid removal (myomectomy) to hysterectomy. Laser surgery is often used for myomectomy. A new technique that may prevent the need for a hysterectomy consists of destroying the uterine lining with heated water that is circulated into the uterus (MedlinePlus Medical Encyclopedia, 2007). This procedure is advantageous in that it can preserve fertility. Hysterectomy is the procedure that is used the most often for fibroid tumors. Justification for this recommendation includes the risk that tumors that are large could potentially mask other adnexal pathology and increase operative complication rates.

Etiology and Epidemiology of Endometriosis

Endometriosis affects approximately 10% of women in the United States (Mounsey, Wilgus, & Slawson, 2006). That makes it one of the most common health problems for women. Generally, women who have endometriosis are in the age range of 20 to 30 with the average age being 27. Women have symptoms for an average of 2 years before a definitive diagnosis is made.

Pathophysiology of Endometriosis

Endometriosis is a condition in which endometrial-like cells that are normally found only in the uterus are found outside of the uterus. These cells attach to ovaries, fallopian tubes, the bowels, or abdominal organs. During the menstrual cycle, these cells respond to hormone production and may swell and bleed. In response, the body will surround these lesions with scar tissue, which can form adhesions on the area of attachment. These adhesions respond to the hormones that stimulate the monthly period with the proliferation of blood and tissue. Tissue and blood that are shed into the body cause inflammation, scar tissue, and subsequently pain. As the misplaced tissue grows, it can cover and grow into the ovaries and block the fallopian tubes, causing problems of infertility (U.S. Department of Health and Human Services, Office on Women's Health, 2006).

Clinical Manifestations of Endometriosis

Endometriosis can produce mild symptoms of discomfort, to severe symptoms of pain, and infertility. The symptoms include pain in the lower abdomen and pelvis radiating down the thighs and to the lower back. There is often a feeling of rectal pressure and discomfort when defecating. Patients with endometriosis have dysmenorrhea and pain with sexual intercourse (dyspareunia) along with abnormal uterine bleeding. These women also have difficulty conceiving a child. Endometriosis is associated with infertility because of adhesions that distort the pelvic anatomy and cause impaired ovum release and implantation. A meta-analysis of 22 studies evaluating *in vitro* fertilization (IVF) outcomes found that patients with endometriosis had a pregnancy rate of nearly one-half that of patients without endometriosis (Barnhart, Dunsmoor-Su, & Coutifaris, 2002).

Risk Factors for Endometriosis

Risk factors for endometriosis include a family history, menstrual flow of greater than 6 days, and menstrual cycle of less than 28 days. Women at risk for endometriosis experienced menarche at an early age and have very heavy menses; they also have periods that last more than 7 days. Some studies suggest that women may lower their chances of developing endometriosis if they exercise regularly and avoid alcohol and caffeine.

Diagnosis and Medical Management of Endometriosis

Endometriosis is diagnosed using pelvic ultrasound and laparoscopy. Treatment ranges from palliative over-the-counter pain medications to prescription medications and surgery. The most commonly prescribed medication is oral contraceptives. Other medications prescribed include high-dose progesterone, gonadotropin-releasing hormone (Gn-RH), and danazol, all of which alter the production of hormones causing the symptoms associated with endometriosis, or shrink the sites of adhesions that will reduce symptoms. See the Pharmacology Summary feature (p. 1552). Laparoscopic surgery to examine reproductive organs and remove or obliterate endometrial tissue is an alternative treatment. A hysterectomy may be indicated in extreme cases.

▆ Nursing Management and Health Promotion

Nursing management for the patient with endometriosis is primarily about patient education. The patient needs to understand the disease process and the accompanying signs and symptoms. Patients need to understand the treatment options and the use of medications that are used to treat endometriosis. NSAIDs and heat are often helpful. Hormone medications may stop periods but can cause side effects similar to menopause (hot flashes and vaginal dryness). Sometimes these side effects will subside if patients take an estrogen pill every day. Patients should not get pregnant while taking medications for endometriosis. Women who want to get pregnant may need surgery to treat their endometriosis. Even with surgery, women with endometriosis may still need fertility treatments. Endometriosis will probably go away with the onset of menopause.

Nursing Diagnoses

Nursing diagnoses associated with endometriosis include:

1. Potential for *Tissue Perfusion, ineffective* from prolonged and heavy periods
2. *Fatigue* related to anemia
3. *Chronic Pain* and *Acute Pain* related to pelvic lesions
4. *Deficient Knowledge* related to management of symptoms and treatment options
5. *Ineffective Sexuality Pattern* related to dyspareunia
6. *Anxiety* and *Grieving* related to decreased fertility.

Outcomes

Expected outcomes associated with endometriosis include:

- A normal menstrual pattern with periods lasting up to 5 days and menstrual cycles extending to 28 days.
- Menstrual bleeding that does not require more than 1 pad in 2 hours.
- Menstrual discomfort that is controlled and does not interfere with patient's normal activities.
- Patient verbalizes understanding of management of the symptoms and treatment options.
- Patient reports less discomfort with sexual intercourse.
- Patient seeks specialized care for infertility as indicated.

Interventions

Nursing interventions associated with endometriosis include:

- Monitoring of complete blood count (CBC) to determine changes in hemoglobin and hematocrit. Report a drop of 1 gram or more in the hemoglobin or a drop of 3% or more in the hematocrit.
- Encourage the patient to pace activities to avoid fatigue.
- Instruct patient in pain management techniques, including use of NSAIDs and heat, along with relaxation techniques and diversion.
- Provide a nonjudgmental environment in which to discuss problems with dyspareunia and sexual dysfunction. Provide resources for further counseling.
- Provide resources for infertility counseling as indicated.

Etiology, Epidemiology, Pathophysiology, Clinical Manifestations, and Medical Management of Cystocele and Rectocele

A **cystocele** occurs when the wall between the bladder and the anterior vagina weakens and the bladder protrudes into the vaginal vault (Figure 49–7 ■). This frequently occurs following multiple vaginal deliveries. Symptoms include urine leakage when the woman sneezes, coughs, or laughs, or incomplete emptying of the bladder. The woman will often describe a feeling of pelvic pressure. When cystoceles are large, the bladder may not empty completely, and the patient will be susceptible to urinary tract infections.

A **rectocele** occurs when the posterior vaginal wall is weakened and the rectum bulges into the vagina (Figure 49–8 ■). The most frequent symptom is difficulty initiating a bowel movement, with resultant constipation, and rectal pressure. This can occur in women who have had conditions that involve repetitive bearing down, such as chronic constipation, chronic coughing,

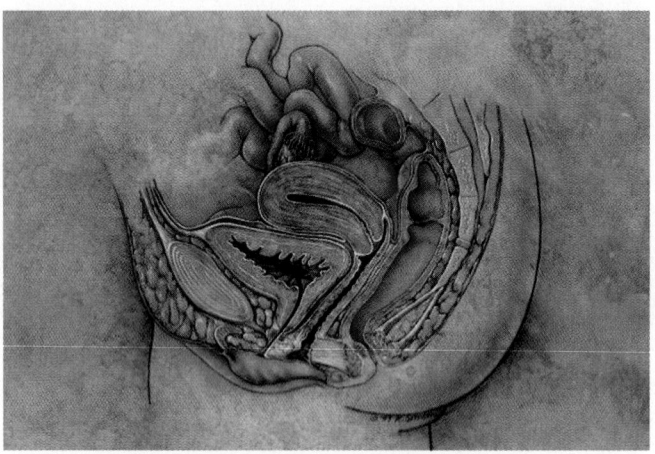

FIGURE 49–7 ■ Cystocele with uterine prolapse.
Source: Kevin A. Somerville/Phototake NYC

Cystocele   Rectocele

Urethrocele   Enterocele

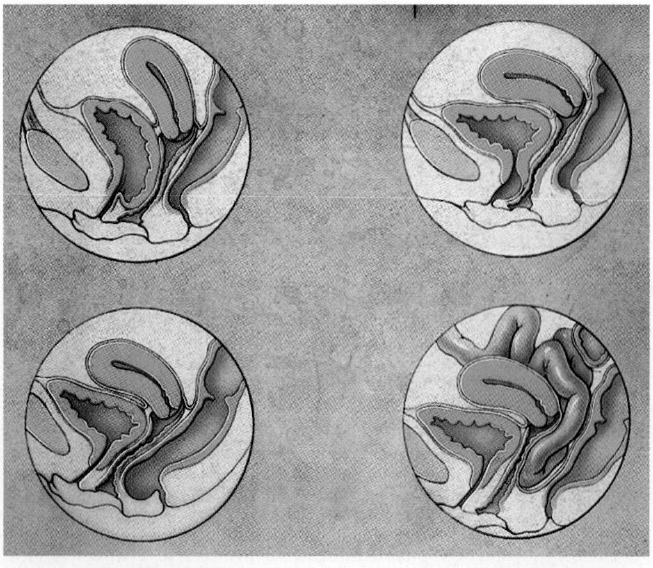

FIGURE 49–8 ■ Rectocele.
Source: Kevin A. Somerville/Phototake NYC

or repetitive heavy lifting. Simple Kegel exercises (intermittent tightening of the perineal and vaginal muscles) will help to prevent the development of these problems.

For women with mild to moderate symptoms, a pessary may be an option. A **pessary** is a device that, when inserted into the vagina, will help support the vaginal walls, reducing the bulging into the vagina; therefore, it is used for management of pelvic support defects such as cystocele, rectocele, and uterine prolapse. The pessary is also used before and after pelvic surgery such as hysterectomy to support the pelvic floor muscles. For those patients who are not good candidates for extensive surgery to repair defects of the pelvic floor, the pessary is an important management option. The pessary is one of the oldest medical devices available. Currently, there are a number of different types of pessaries and health care providers are becoming reacquainted with their use. Pessaries should not be used if there is evidence of active pelvic infection such as vaginitis or pelvic inflammatory disease. Patients should be compliant with follow-up visits.

Complications of pessaries include vaginal irritation, infection, discharge, pressure sores, or allergy to the components of the pessary. Patients should know that although the pessary can be worn during sexual intercourse, it does not provide any method of birth control or protection against sexually transmitted infections. Last, the patient must be taught effective placement and removal of the pessary and how to care for and clean it.

Surgery can correct the issues of cystocele and rectocele when the symptoms are moderate to severe. Cystoceles and rectoceles are repaired using a procedure called a colporrhaphy, also referred to as an anterior/posterior (A&P) repair, depending on whether one or both procedures are done. The anterior wall repair, done for a cystocele, involves repair and resultant strengthening of the weakened area by either shortening the pelvic muscles providing greater support for the bladder or suspending the urinary bladder in the proper position. The posterior repair is used for the rectocele and tightens the pelvic floor muscles to provide greater support for the rectum. Risks are minimal but can include bleeding and infection. Postoperative assessment includes monitoring vital signs, observing vaginal bleeding greater than simple spotting, signs of infection, and adequate hydration. The woman will have a Foley catheter for 1 or 2 days, and intake and output should be monitored accordingly. Stool softeners may be needed to avoid straining with bowel movements, and encouraging a well-balanced, high-fiber diet will assist in maintaining normal bowel function. Discharge instruction should include avoiding activities that might stress the incision, including intercourse or placing anything in the vagina until released by the health care provider. Avoiding long periods of standing, coughing, and sneezing will also decrease strain on the surgical site. Adequate fluids and continuing a well-balanced, high-fiber, high-protein diet will aid in healing and regaining normal bowel function.

Etiology, Epidemiology, Pathophysiology, Clinical Manifestations, and Treatment of Uterine Prolapse

Uterine **prolapse** is another common structural disorder that occurs as a result of weakening of the pelvic floor musculature. The structures supporting the uterus are sometimes weakened during pregnancy and childbirth. There is an increased risk for uterine prolapse with obesity, chronic coughing, and straining during bowel movements. In addition, multiple pregnancies, congenital weakness, and loss of elasticity and muscle tone due to the aging process can contribute to the problem. The result is the uterus is displaced downwardly into the vaginal canal. The uterus can prolapse enough to be seen outside the vagina. The prolapse pulls on surrounding structures and puts pressure on the bladder and rectum. This pressure can cause symptoms of incontinence or retention, and may be aggravated by coughing or lifting heavy objects. Generally, the treatment of choice is surgery to suture the uterus into place and tighten the musculature supporting it. Occasionally, a hysterectomy is done, although a pessary to support the uterus can be inserted into the vagina to support the uterus.

Etiology, Epidemiology, Pathophysiology, Clinical Manifestations, and Medical Management of Ectopic Pregnancy

An **ectopic** pregnancy is implantation of the products of conception outside the uterine endometrium (Figure 49–9 ■). Approximately 2% of all pregnancies are ectopic (Sepilian, 2007). The most common location for an ectopic pregnancy is the fallopian tube (95%). The other 5% may occur in such places as the cervix, ovary, or abdomen. Causes of ectopic pregnancy are varied but often include problems that may leave scar tissue or prevent movement of the fertilized ovum appropriately down the fallopian tube and into the uterine cavity. These problems include pelvic inflammatory disease (PID), previous ectopic pregnancy, endometriosis, tubal surgery, and use of an intrauterine device (IUD) for birth control. Also contributing to the risk of ectopic pregnancy are procedures used in infertility treatments, including *in vitro* fertilization and embryo transfer.

Any condition that leaves residual scar tissue can cause partial or complete blockage of the fallopian tubes. The scar tissue impedes the passing of the fertilized egg into the uterus. As the

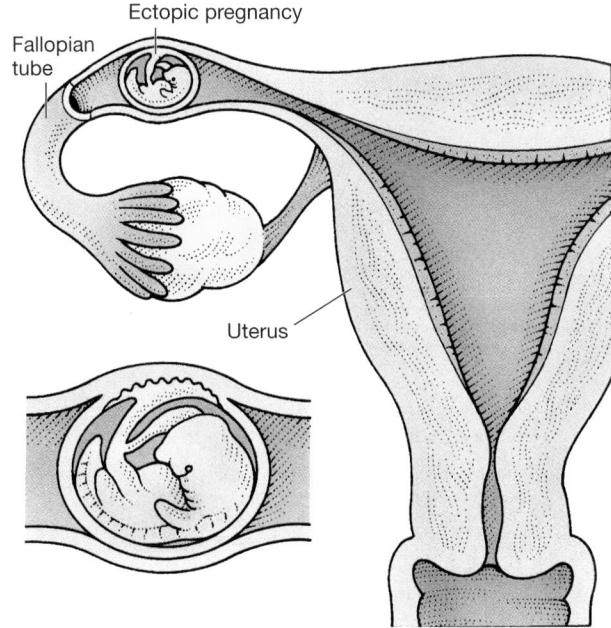

FIGURE 49–9 ■ Ectopic pregnancy.
Source: © Dorling Kindersley

cells divide, the gestational sac expands against the tubal wall. If allowed to continue, the tube expands until it ruptures, causing acute lower abdominal pain and internal bleeding.

Often the patient will present with typical symptoms of pregnancy, including an elevated quantitative human chorionic gonadotropin (HCG), amenorrhea, and nausea, but with pelvic pain and in some cases light vaginal bleeding. The prime time for the manifestations of ectopic pregnancy is at approximately 7 weeks after a missed period. These findings are very nonspecific and are certainly common to patients who may be having a spontaneous abortion, acute appendicitis, ovarian torsion, pelvic inflammatory disease, and renal calculi. Therefore, the positive HCG is very important to making the diagnosis of ectopic pregnancy. Because the implantation is not inside the uterus where space for the growth of the embryo is adequate, the growth puts pressure on the surrounding tissues and structures causing discomfort and pain. If the fallopian tube ruptures, the patient experiences intense, sharp, unilateral pain with pain referred to the shoulder as a result of irritation of the diaphragm by blood in the abdominal cavity. When this happens, there is risk of hemorrhage and hypovolemic shock. This is treated as a medical emergency.

Due to the life-threatening potential of ectopic pregnancy, all women of childbearing age who present with lower abdominal or pelvic pain should be tested for pregnancy. If the test is positive, then the patient will need a transvaginal ultrasound to examine the ovaries, uterus, and fallopian tubes. Quantitative HCG is a serum test used to determine the duration of the pregnancy. Under normal circumstances, this value doubles every 48 hours in early pregnancy. If the HCG level fails to double, the pregnancy is not viable, and an ectopic pregnancy is assumed until proven otherwise. The transvaginal ultrasound will be accurate in determining the presence of an intrauterine pregnancy when the quantitative HCG has reached 1,500 to 2,000 mLU/m. (Lozeau & Potter, 2005).

Medical treatment of ectopic pregnancy is preferred over surgical treatment. Methotrexate, a drug often used in cancer treatment, is the current drug of choice and will act on the ectopic cells as it does in cancer treatment: to destroy the cells. It is given if the ectopic is unruptured and the patient is in stable condition. It is given intramuscularly and often as an outpatient procedure. Successful treatment may require more than one dose of methotrexate.

Failure of beta HCG levels to decrease by at least 15% from day 4 to day 7 after methotrexate administration indicates the need for an additional dose of methotrexate or surgery (ACOG, 1998).

If surgery is indicated with a ruptured ectopic pregnancy, it consists of repair of the tube if future pregnancies are desired. Removal of the tube may be necessary if repair is not possible or may be desired if future pregnancies are not planned. Approximately 30% of women treated for ectopic pregnancy later have difficulty conceiving. Rates of recurrent ectopic pregnancy are between 5% and 20% (Lozeau & Potter, 2005).

Reproductive System Cancers

Reproductive system cancers include cervical, vulvar, endometrial, ovarian, and vaginal cancers. See Chart 49–4 (p. 1540) for a comparison of these cancers. Chapter 64 💿 has an in-depth discussion of the pathophysiology of cancer development and progress.

CHART 49–4 Comparison of Female Reproductive Cancers

Etiology	Assessment	Interventions
Cervical Cancer		
Third most common reproductive cancer. 90% Squamous cell. 10% Adenocarcinoma. Average age 40–50. Increased risk with human papillomavirus (HPV) and herpes 2, multiple partners, and decreased socioeconomic status. Increased in African American and Hispanic women.	Preinvasion is often asymptomatic. Invasive shows postcoital bleeding and abnormal bleeding. Late symptoms include rectal bleeding, hematuria, back and leg pain, and anemia. Pap smear is the single most reliable diagnostic test (it will show 90% of early cervical cancers). Other diagnostic tests include colposcopy, biopsy, and conization.	Preinvasive lesions often entail cryosurgery, laser surgery, or loop electrosurgical excision procedure (LEEP: an electrically charged thin wire is used to remove a thin layer of cells from the cervix). Typically done as an outpatient procedure. Invasive treatment is hysterectomy with internal or external radiation.
Vulvar Cancer		
Fourth most common gynecologic cancer. Average age 60–70. Those under 35 are linked to condolymata. 90% Squamous cell. Slow growing. 90% Survival even with late diagnosis if nodes are negative. Less than 50% survival with node involvement.	Lesion usually asymptomatic until 1–2 centimeters. Symptoms include vulvar pruritus and burning pain. Diagnosed by biopsy with histologic evaluation using toluidine blue.	Local, wide excision, or vulvectomy. External radiation.
Endometrial Cancer		
Most common gynecologic malignancy. Average age 50–65. Risk factors include obesity, nullipara, infertility, diabetes mellitus, hypertension, family history, Caucasian, and hormone imbalance, which is the most significant risk factor.	Symptoms include abnormal uterine bleeding, lower back pain, lower pelvic pain, uterine enlargement, and positive Pap smear. Diagnosis by fractional curettage or endometrial biopsy.	Total abdominal hysterectomy with bilateral salpingectomy and oophorectomy. Radiation (internal or external) before or after surgery. Chemotherapy with advanced stage or recurrent.
Ovarian Cancer		
Second most frequent gynecologic cancer. Causes more deaths than any other reproductive cancer. Risks include nullipara, infertility, and family history. Affects all ages but increased in the 50s.	No definitive tests. Often diagnosed in late stage. Symptoms include lower abdominal discomfort and digestive complaints. Increased pain, weakness, and malnutrition are late signs.	Treatment varies from removal of the ovary to total hysterectomy. Chemotherapy. Antineoplastic drugs. Radiation is controversial.
Vaginal Cancer		
Rare. Two types: squamous cell (increased in ages 60–80) and adenocarcinoma (increased in ages 12–30). Risks include young women of mothers who received diethylstilbestrol (DES) in 1945–1970 as a treatment for miscarriage.	Bleeding or discharge not related to menstruation. Pain during intercourse (dyspareunia). Pelvic pain.	Treatment depends on the stage of the cancer and may include: • Surgery (to remove the cancer) • Radiation (to kill cancer cells and/or shrink tumors) • Chemotherapy (to kill the cancer cells).

Source: "Detailed Guides for Cervical, Vulva, Endometrial, Ovarian and Vaginal Cancer" adapted and reprinted by the permission of the American Cancer Society, Inc. from www.cancer.org. All rights reserved.

Etiology, Epidemiology, Pathophysiology, Clinical Manifestations, and Treatment of Orgasmic Dysfunction

One phase of the sexual response cycle is the orgasmic phase. When there is difficulty reaching orgasm, it is called orgasmic dysfunction, or **anorgasmia**. Anorgasmia is considered to be one of the most common sexual problems among women; however, less than 20% of cases are related to physiological issues. Anorgasmia is frequently found to be psychological in nature and results from unresolved conflicts about sexual activity or marital conflict (Phillips, 2000). Primary dysfunction is when the woman has never had an orgasm following any means of sexual stimulation. Secondary dysfunction occurs when the woman has had orgasms in the past, but is unable to achieve them now. Causes of anorgasmia can be disease that results in general debility such as multiple sclerosis, diabetes, spinal cord injuries, and hormonal conditions that affect sexual response. Drugs such as antidepressants, alcohol, and other central nervous system (CNS) depressants can also inhibit sexual response. Chart 49–5 outlines medications that interfere with sexual function.

Menopause and oophorectomy (surgical removal of the ovaries) create a hypoestrogenic state, which may increase the likelihood of orgasmic dysfunction. Testosterone decreases with menopause and oophorectomy, and is considered an essential female hormone for sexual desire as well as in males. Testosterone appears to have a direct role in sexual desire. However, studies are limited at this point, so there are no guidelines for testosterone replacement therapy for women with disorders of desire (Phillips, 2000). Use of testosterone supplementation in conjunction with estrogen replacement therapy has shown success in increasing sexual desire and orgasm (Phillips, 2000). Orgasmic disorders can be treated with Kegel exercises and masturbation. The purpose is to maximize stimulation and minimize inhibition.

Treatment of both physical and psychological circumstances may benefit from counseling therapy. When medical conditions prevent the ability to reach orgasm, therapy may be directed at alternative ways of satisfaction, such as simple holding each other close, touching, or exploring individual ways that make each other feel satisfied. When secondary dysfunction is the cause, counseling is directed at the couple and the root of their discord.

CHART 49–5	**Medications That Interfere with Sexual Function**

PSYCHOACTIVE MEDICATIONS

Antipsychotics

Barbiturates

Benzodiazepines

Selective serotonin reuptake inhibitors

Lithium

Tricyclic antidepressants

CARDIOVASCULAR AND ANTIHYPERTENSIVE MEDICATIONS

Antilipid medications

Beta-blockers

Clonidine

Digoxin

Spironolactone

CENTRAL NERVOUS SYSTEM AGENTS

Anticholinergics

Antihistamines

H_2 blockers

Methyldopa

Amphetamines

Anorexic drugs

Narcotics

Phenytoin

Etiology, Epidemiology, Pathophysiology, Clinical Manifestations, and Treatment of Dyspareunia

Dyspareunia, painful intercourse, can be a result of several factors including both physiological and psychological ones. Endometriosis is an example of a physiological cause, which is due to displaced endometrial tissue in the peritoneal cavity. Menopause is another physiological cause, resulting from a decrease in hormone production, which in turn decreases the normal lubricating mechanism of the vagina. In addition, the vagina may become somewhat smaller during menopause, causing a more difficult penetration. Other physiological causes may include an imperforate hymen or vaginal scarring.

Psychological causes may be related to early traumatic events such as sexual abuse or rape, triggering an involuntary reflex known as vaginismus. **Vaginismus** is a condition in which the vaginal muscles at the introitus contract very tightly, making vaginal penetration painful.

Hormonal treatment of endometriosis, often with danazol (Danocrine), an androgenic steroid, has been successful in regression of the displaced endometrial tissue. Hormone replacement therapy and lubricating gel can assist in the treatment of dyspareunia related to menopause. Psychological causes require counseling.

■ Nursing Management

Use of the nursing process provides an effective framework to guide the nursing management for patients experiencing the various disorders of the reproductive system. During the nursing assessment it is important to obtain a history from the woman about the type of reproductive disorder that is occurring. The nurse should be careful not to ask questions in a manner so as to allude to bias toward heterosexuality or homosexuality. Establishment of the patient's sexual orientation is necessary for appropriate evaluation and management. Nonjudgmental, direct questions best achieve this goal (Phillips, 2000). The interviewer must be careful to ensure privacy and confidentiality. During the interview the nurse gains a complete history of the patient symptoms include timing, situation, and duration. Questioning the patient about her insight into the cause may be very helpful. It is important to collect history regarding chronic illness, injuries, and a psychiatric history. Prescription and over-the-counter medications as well as the use of recreational drugs and alcohol must be listed accurately. Surgical interventions and malignancies such as breast cancer can alter self-image and cause decreased sexuality. Questions regarding relationships should be asked to determine level of partner support and previous problematic or violent relationships.

A complete physical needs to be done with a pelvic exam to determine the existence of vaginismus, vulvar dystrophy, dermatitis, vaginal atrophy, infectious disease, scar tissue, postoperative changes, fibroids, masses, endometriosis, tenderness, or structural defects. The goal of the examination is detection of disease; however, the examination also provides an opportunity to educate the patient about normal anatomy and sexual function, and to reproduce and localize pain encountered during sexual activity (Phillips, 2000).

Nursing Diagnoses

Nursing diagnoses associated with female reproductive dysfunction include:

- *Disturbed Body Image*
- *Ineffective Sexuality Pattern*
- *Risk for Situational Low Self-Esteem* related to sexual difficulties
- *Chronic Pain*
- *Compromised Family Coping*
- *Decisional Conflict* related to treatment options
- *Deficient Knowledge* related to disease process
- *Disturbed Thought Process* related to sense of inadequacy
- *Fear*

Outcomes

Expected outcomes of care for patients experiencing reproductive dysfunction include:

- Enhanced knowledge related to sexual functioning
- Decreased anxiety and fear
- Acceptance of body image
- Adequate decision making regarding treatment options
- Improved family coping
- Adequate health seeking behaviors
- Adequate sexual functioning and identity
- Enhanced self-esteem related to sexual difficulties
- Adequate pain relief and ability to cope with pain.

Planning and Intervention

Care of the patient with sexual dysfunction requires education, support, and therapeutic interventions. Information regarding normal anatomy, sexual function, and the normal changes of aging, pregnancy, and menopause are important. Encourage discussion of sexual issues in the context of a medical condition or a new medication agent prescribed. Depression is frequently associated with reproductive disorders; therefore, psychological counseling may be necessary. Women with long-standing dysfunction, multiple dysfunctions, or history of sexual abuse need to be referred to a gynecologist and/or psychological counseling.

Health Promotion
for Female Reproductive Disorders

Patients frequently have difficulty discussing sexual problems with their health care provider. But up to 70% of couples have a problem with sex at some time during their relationship. Promoting good sexual health is dependent on providing an accepting environment in which patients can discuss problems with sexual response. Encouraging patients to explain their problems openly and honestly with their health care provider can result in possible treatments. It is also important for couples to communicate regarding concerns. A mutually satisfying relationship that includes respectful and caring behaviors on the part of both partners provides the best hope for a gratifying sex life.

■ Menstrual Disorders

Menstrual disorders involve not only physical symptoms but emotional symptoms as well. Because the menstrual cycle is related to the reproductive ability of a woman, any problems may be a cause of great concern. Almost all women will experience some form of menstrual disorder in their lifetime, such as missing a period, heavy periods, or painful periods. The most common ones are discussed next.

Etiology, Epidemiology, Pathophysiology, Clinical Manifestations, and Medical Management of Amenorrhea

Amenorrhea is defined as the absence of menstruation. It is considered primary when the girl/woman has not started her menstrual cycles by the age of 16. It is secondary when menstruation has been present but ceases for more than 3 months and is not related to pregnancy. Secondary amenorrhea is more common than primary amenorrhea. Causes of amenorrhea are varied and may be related to stress, athleticism, weight changes, and disease/hormonal processes. Chart 49–6 outlines the various causes of amenorrhea.

Primary amenorrhea can be caused by a congenital absence of a part of the reproductive tract such as ovaries, uterus, or vagina. Another cause could be the presence of the imperforate hymen. Imperforate hymen is a congenital defect in which the opening to the vagina does not form, and as a result there is no exit from the vagina. Imperforate hymen occurs in 1 in 1,000 women. A procedure using local anesthetic can correct the defect.

In adolescence, stress, eating disorders, exercise, and ovulation abnormalities can cause irregular periods. This is especially pertinent in the patient in which fat comprises less than 10% of the body. Bulimia, anorexia, obesity, and malnutrition may alter the hormone balance in the body, as some are produced by fat cells. This change in hormone production or utilization may cause amenorrhea. Excessive exercise, usually more than 20 hours a week for a prolonged number of weeks, triggers a reduction in reproductive hormones, in particular, leptin. Decreased leptin can interfere with the production of luteinizing hormone, which is necessary for ovulation.

There is a triad of symptoms that has been identified in the female athlete that reflects the health issues of females who exercise more than 20 hours week. The components include amenorrhea or oligomenorrhea, eating disorder (anorexia or bulimia), and decreased bone mineral density (Sherman & Thompson, 2004). Alternatively, women who are obese also have a higher incidence of amenorrhea.

Elevated prolactin levels may inhibit ovulation and consequently cause amenorrhea. The elevated levels may be related to pituitary tumors and can cause breast milk production not related to pregnancy (galactorrhea). Elevated prolactin levels need to be evaluated by an endocrinologist. Treatment of amenorrhea depends on the cause. Frequently, correcting pituitary disorders, thyroid disorders, or inducing appropriate nutrition and exercise levels can result in normal menstruation.

CHART 49–6   Causes of Amenorrhea

Hormone Alteration

Thyroid disease: hypothyroidism
Pituitary dysfunction
Menopause
Pregnancy
Cushing's syndrome
Polycystic ovary syndrome

Chronic Disease

Liver failure
Renal failure
Cancer (bronchogenic, renal cell CA)
Autoimmune diseases
Chemotherapy
Pelvic radiation
Central nervous system tumor
Diabetes
Immunodeficiency
Inflammatory bowel disease
Thyroid disease
Severe chronic depression

Structural Defects

Imperforate hymen
Congenital defect causing absence of ovaries, fallopian tubes, or uterus
Cervical stenosis
Transverse vaginal septum

Medications

Oral contraceptives
Antipsychotics
Antidepressants
Antihypertensives
Histamine H_2-receptor blockers
Opiates, cocaine

Exercise and Nutrition

Anorexia or bulimia nervosa
Excessive exercise
Excessive weight loss
Malnutrition

Alterations in Growth and Development

Constitutional delay of growth and puberty
Acromegaly
Congenital adrenal hyperplasia
Mumps
Genetic defects

Etiology, Epidemiology, Pathophysiology, Clinical Manifestations, and Treatment of Polycystic Ovary Syndrome

Polycystic ovary syndrome (PCO or PCOS) is an endocrine disorder that results from high levels of androgens (male hormones), especially testosterone. The incidence of PCOS is relatively common at 5% to 10% (U.S. Department of Health and Human Services, Office on Women's Health, 2007). It is the most commonly occurring endocrine disorder in women of childbearing age and the most common cause of infertility (U.S. Department of Health and Human Services, Office on Women's Health, 2007). The causes of PCOS are unknown at this time, but scientists are studying genetic mutations that may be at the root. It is known that there is a familial tendency for PCOS. It is also known that poor utilization of insulin increases production of the male hormones (androgens) that cause many of the manifestations of PCOS.

The high level of male hormones often causes an associated low follicle-stimulating hormone (FSH) production, which prevents mature egg production. Egg production is required for the stimulation of progesterone. Without progesterone a woman's menstrual cycle is irregular or absent. When there is no mature egg produced, the follicles fill with fluid and form cysts. The cysts that form make male hormones, which also prevent ovulation. As cysts continue to form, some may become the size of grapefruit.

The associated low or absent progesterone production, increased estrogen levels, and increased androgen production may produce the following manifestations: increased facial hair and acne, oligomenorrhea (few periods), infertility due to anovulation, pelvic pain due to ovarian cyst formation, anxiety or depression due to appearance and infertility, obesity, and elevated lipids and blood glucose. On rare occasions PCOS may produce the male characteristics of deepening voice and clitoral enlargement.

It is important that the woman maintain a regular schedule of medical visits so the growth of the cysts can be monitored. Treatment is directed at the symptoms causing the most concern and may involve pharmacologic interventions or surgery. Oral contraceptives are used to suppress ovulation by inhibiting the release of luteinizing hormone (LH) and decreasing testosterone levels. In addition, this often improves hirsuitism. Gonadotropin-releasing hormone (Gn-RH) may be used if the oral contraceptives do not reduce the size of the cysts. If a pregnancy is desired, the use of oral contraceptives is replaced by ovulation-inducing medications.

Cysts that are greater than 8 centimeters are typically surgically removed. Analgesics may be used for pain management associated with pressure from the enlarging cysts. Additionally, the patient should be treated with oral hypoglycemics such as metformin to control blood glucose and lower testosterone production. This will aid in slowing abnormal hair growth and ovulation may return after a few months. Metformin will also decrease body mass and improve cholesterol levels. See the Pharmacology Summary feature (p. 1552).

Nursing interventions are directed toward pain management and education in the areas of treatment options. Women who adopt a healthy lifestyle by maintaining normal weight and getting regular exercise can help manage PCOS. Even 10% loss in body weight can restore a normal period and make a woman's cycle more regular (Master-Hunter & Heiman, 2006).

Women with PCOS have a 4 to 7 times' higher risk of coronary artery disease and myocardial infarction than do women of the same age without PCOS. Additionally, PCOS patients are at greater risk of having high blood pressure. The increased risk for the development of endometrial cancer is another concern for women with PCOS. Irregular menstrual periods and the absence of ovulation cause women to produce the hormone estrogen, but not the hormone progesterone. Progesterone causes the endometrium to shed its lining each month as a menstrual period. Without progesterone, the endometrium becomes thick, which can cause heavy bleeding or irregular bleeding. Over time, this can lead to endometrial hyperplasia and the potential for cancer cells to develop (U.S. Department of Health and Human Services, Office of Women's Health, 2007). Resources for women looking for more information about PCOS include the Polycystic Ovarian Syndrome Association, Inc. and the American Association of Clinical Endocrinologists.

Etiology, Epidemiology, Pathophysiology, Clinical Manifestations, and Treatment of Dysmenorrhea

Dysmenorrhea is defined as painful menstruation. It is generally described as cramping-type pelvic pain that begins shortly before or at the onset of the monthly menses. Most women experience the discomfort for approximately 3 days. Adolescents report the highest incidence of dysmenorrhea. A recent study in Sweden found a prevalence of dysmenorrhea of 90% in women 19 years of age and 67% in women 24 years of age (French, 2005). Dysmenorrhea is classified as primary, which is associated with increased uterine contractility, or secondary, which is caused by some form of pelvic pathology, such as endometriosis or fibroid tumors.

With primary dysmenorrhea, there is an increase in uterine muscle contractions due to an increase in the prostaglandin level in the second half of the menstrual cycle. Systemic response to increased prostaglandin levels is manifested in pain in the lower back and lower abdomen, nausea, diarrhea, headache, and weakness. It is seen only with ovulatory cycles because both estrogen and progesterone are necessary for it to occur. It is also seen primarily in adolescents and women in their early 20s, with the incidence and severity often declining with age. Risk factors for dysmenorrhea include adolescent age, nulliparity, heavy menstrual flow, attempts to lose weight, depression and anxiety, and smoking.

Evaluation of the patient with dysmenorrhea should include a history of symptoms and menstrual cycles, including age of menarche and level of flow. An abdominal exam alone is performed on the adolescent who is not yet sexually active. A pelvic examination should be performed in females who have been sexually active to screen for sexually transmitted infections. A transvaginal ultrasound can be used to rule out anatomic abnormalities such as masses, ovarian cysts, and endometriosis. Laparoscopic surgery may be needed to further identify and define causes of dysmenorrhea.

Management varies depending on the severity of symptoms. Chart 49–7 shows the nonpharmacologic therapies most often prescribed. The pharmacologic therapies are listed in the Pharmacology Summary feature (p. 1552). Being cognizant of the increased incidence of bleeding that occurs with certain pain relievers is essential.

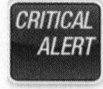 **CRITICAL ALERT** *Do not use nonsteroidal anti-inflammatory drugs (NSAIDs) for patients with hemophilia, those with bleeding ulcers, those allergic to aspirin or other NSAIDs, or those taking anticoagulant medications. Be sure to take NSAIDs with milk or food to help prevent gastric irritation and possible bleeding.*

Secondary dysmenorrhea is pain associated with a specific condition, such as endometriosis, pelvic inflammatory disease, or

CHART 49–7 Nonpharmacologic Therapies for Dysmenorrhea

Therapy	Rationale
Heating pad/hot bath and fetal position	Increases vasodilation Relaxes uterine muscle Decreases uterine ischemia
Lower back massage	Relaxes paravertebral muscles Increases pelvic blood supply
Effluerage (rhythmic rubbing)	Distraction and focal point
Exercise	Increases vasodilation Decreases ischemia Releases natural endorphins Decreases prostaglandins Decreases stress
Dietary changes: Decreased salt Increased water intake	Reduces fluid retention Natural diuretic

Source: Lowdermilk, D. L., & Perry, S. E. (2004). *Maternity & women's health care* (8th ed.). St. Louis: Mosby.

uterine fibroids. In contrast to primary dysmenorrhea, this discomfort is often characterized by dull, lower abdominal aching that radiates to the back and thighs, bloating, and pelvic fullness.

Management is directed at removing the underlying cause, often necessitating surgery to excise the displaced tissue or remove the fibroids. Pharmacologic pain-relief measures are the same as with primary dysmenorrhea. Nursing care is directed at education of the woman regarding the cause or treatment modalities. Patients should be advised to maintain a healthy diet and exercise level, take in plenty of fluids, and use heat and NSAIDs in moderation to help with symptoms. Patients who do not respond to simple measures should seek care to determine the possibility of secondary causes. Also patients should seek care for dysmenorrhea that occurs later in life, pain that occurs at other times besides the first couple of days of a period, any vaginal discharge, or abnormal bleeding between periods.

Etiology, Epidemiology, Pathophysiology, Clinical Manifestations, and Treatment of Menorrhagia

Menorrhagia is defined as excessive or prolonged menstruation. The menses of young women may vary from month to month, and a single heavy period is not necessarily cause for concern. However, high-volume periods that last more than 7 days are cause for concern. A woman who requires pad or tampon changes every 1 to 2 hours is considered to have menorrhagia. Menorrhagia can be caused by endometriosis, pelvic inflammatory disease, intrauterine devices for birth control, uterine fibroids, or functional ovarian cysts. Also women with hypothyroid conditions can have very heavy periods. Health care providers will also check for clotting disorders.

Treatment is dependent on the cause. Alternative contraceptive methods may be utilized if that is the cause. Fibroids may be surgically removed or shrunk through use of medications. Infections may indicate the need for antibiotic drug therapy. Assessment of the amount of bleeding is done through saturated pads or tampon counts. Hemoglobin analysis can be used to determine the extent of blood loss. Other pertinent laboratory values include a thyroid-stimulating hormone to determine the presence of a hypothyroid condition, and serum or urine HCG to test for pregnancy.

Etiology, Epidemiology, Pathophysiology, Clinical Manifestations, and Treatment of Metrorrhagia

Bleeding between menstrual periods is called **metrorrhagia**. A small amount of spotting may be seen around the time of ovulation and is considered normal. Use of low-dose oral contraceptives reduces the amount of hormones available in the body and is also associated with breakthrough bleeding. Pathologic causes of metrorrhagia include endometritis, STIs, pregnancy-related problems, ovarian cysts, or uterine fibroid tumors. Postmenopausal bleeding may be caused by uterine polyps, inappropriately prescribed hormone therapy, or uterine cancer. Early evaluation of this concern is extremely important. The hormone frequently in deficient status and causing metrorrhagia is progesterone, which is accompanied by a relative excess of estrogen. This results in hyperplasia of the endometrial lining of the uterus. Without adequate progesterone, sloughing of the lining occurs, resulting in vaginal bleeding that is not in accordance with the woman's monthly cycle. Hormone imbalances can be caused by anovulation, stress, and emotional upheavals. However, of utmost concern is that abnormal bleeding from the vagina, whether menorrhagia or metrorrhagia, can be an indicator of neoplasm and should be evaluated urgently.

Treatment is directed at the cause, such as drug therapy for endometritis and STIs; removal or shrinkage of cysts and fibroids; and surgery, drug, or chemotherapy/radiation for cancers. Pregnancy-related problems must be dealt with on an individual basis. Nursing care involves education regarding the causes of and treatments for metrorrhagia and addressing the fatigue associated with anemia and the relative dehydration.

Etiology, Epidemiology, Pathophysiology, Clinical Manifestations, and Treatment of Premenstrual Syndrome

Premenstrual syndrome (PMS) is a common, but complex, often misunderstood condition, involving physical, psychological, and behavioral symptoms. The Committee on Gynecologic Practice of the American College of Obstetricians and Gynecologists (ACOG) indicates that up to 80% of women of childbearing age have physical symptoms during menstruation: Twenty percent to forty percent have symptoms consistent with PMS; 2% to 4% indicate that their symptoms cause severe disruption of their daily activities (ACOG, 2005). These symptoms vary widely among women, so much so that it is difficult to define PMS. When present, the symptoms occur in the luteal phase, the time from ovulation until the start of the menstrual period of the cycle. Chart 49–8 shows the more common symptoms related to PMS, but symptoms can number 100 (Cronje & Studd, 2002). The diagnosis of PMS should meet specific criteria: symptoms occur in the luteal phase and resolve with menses; no symptoms occur during the follicular phase; and symptoms recur with repeated cycles (Lowdermilk & Perry, 2004).

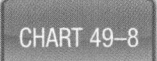

CHART 49–8 Symptoms Commonly Associated with Premenstrual Syndrome

Abdominal bloating

Lower extremity edema

Breast tenderness

Weight gain

Depression

Irritability

Loss of concentration

Food cravings/binges

Headache

Fatigue

Backache

Mood swings

Source: Cronje, W., & Studd, J. (2002). Premenstrual syndrome and premenstrual dysphoric disorder. *Primary Care, 29*(1), 1–12.

The etiology and pathophysiology of PMS is poorly understood. There is a biologic trigger that is exacerbated by psychosocial factors. Serotonin neurotransmitter is also considered to be a factor. It does appear there is a genetic or familial tendency associated with PMS. Additionally, estrogen and progesterone imbalances may play a role as well as nutritional deficiencies such as of vitamin B_6 and magnesium.

Management of PMS symptoms is difficult because of the diversity of symptoms in different women. Diet and exercise provide some relief for some women, along with the reduction of salt, sugar, and caffeinated beverages. The diet needs to be high in carbohydrates, limited in simple sugar, and limited in alcohol use to minimize hypoglycemia. Caffeine intake should be limited to decrease irritability. Women who exercise regularly appear to have fewer symptoms of anxiety and depression due to the increase in endorphin levels. Education is by far the most important part of management. The nurse can assist the woman in symptom evaluation, in cyclic relationships, and in counseling and support. Alternative and complimentary therapies have been found to help manage symptoms for some women. For example, the use of black cohosh root helps relieve anxiety and depression by suppressing estrogen, as presented in the Complementary and Alternative Therapies box (p. 1546). Bugleweed decreases prolactin levels and decreases breast discomfort (Lowdermilk & Perry, 2004). Medications may be used when other treatments fail to improve the PMS symptoms. Diuretics, prostaglandin inhibitors, which are the nonsteroidal anti-inflammatory drugs (NSAIDs), progesterone, and oral contraceptives have been shown to relieve symptoms. Fluoxetine (Prozac), 20 milligrams a day, is the only FDA-approved drug for PMS (Jones, 2001). See the Pharmacology Summary feature on p. 1552.

Etiology, Epidemiology, Pathophysiology, Clinical Manifestations, and Treatment of Premenstrual Dysphoric Disorder

Premenstrual dysphoric disorder (PMDD) is recognized as a separate syndrome, with similar, but more severe symptoms, often overwhelming the woman (Elliot, 2002). PMDD is a severe form of PMS that includes five or more symptoms of depression for most of the time during the last week of the luteal phase that begin to remit within a few days after onset of the follicular phase of the menstrual cycle (Bhatia & Bhatia, 2002). Symptoms include those of atypical severe depressive disorders (depressed mood, interpersonal rejection, hypersensitivity, carbohydrate craving, and hypersomnia). Women have depressed mood with feelings of hopelessness, anxiety, tension, and feelings of being "on edge." Many women describe marked anger or irritability and increased interpersonal conflicts. Friends and family notice decreased interest in usual activities and hypersomnia. Patients also complain of lethargy, easy fatigability, and marked lack of energy with changes in appetite and food cravings. Women with PMDD state they feel overwhelmed and out of control. Physical symptoms include breast tenderness and swelling, headaches, joint and muscle pain, and bloating.

There is a significant correlation between depression and PMDD; however, not all patients have depressive symptoms, so PMDD is not considered just a variant of depression. The etiology of PMDD is a combination of biologic, psychological, environmental, genetic, and social factors. Seventy percent of women whose mothers have been affected by PMS and PMDD have the disorders as well. Additionally, there is a 93% correlation rate in monozygotic twins compared with a rate of 44% in dizygotic twins (Bhatia & Bhatia, 2002). It is also reasonable to believe that PMDD has a hormonal basis because PMDD affects only women of childbearing age.

Treatment of PMDD must incorporate lifestyle changes, nutritional supplements, stress management, and pharmacologic interventions. Lifestyle changes include aerobic exercise and dietary changes that include small frequent balanced meals rich in complex carbohydrates, decreasing caffeine and sodium, restricting alcohol, and smoking. Nutritional supplements that are recommended include vitamin B_6, calcium carbonate, magnesium, and tryptophan. Nonpharmacologic treatments are also pertinent recommendations and include stress management, anger management, individual and couple's therapy, and patient education regarding the cause of, diagnosis of, and treatment for PMS and PMDD. Psychologists also recommend light therapy with 10,000 lux cool-white fluorescent light. Pharmacologic treatments include antidepressant and anxiolytic medications. Selective serotonin reuptake inhibitor (SSRI) antidepressants are considered first line. Fluoxetine 20 milligrams per day may be used during the luteal phase or throughout the full menstrual cycle (Bhatia & Bhatia, 2002). Alprazolam or another anxiolytic has also been shown to be effective in patients with PMS and PMDD. There is an issue with dependency on benzodiazepine-type medications, so this should be used for a short term only and only as a second line therapy if SSRIs fail. Hormonal therapies that are used are the gonadotropin-releasing hormone agonists; these suppress ovulation and cause amenorrhea, thereby providing significant relief of symptoms in those who do not also have significant depressive symptoms. These medications can cause symptoms of menopause such as hot flashes, vaginal dryness, and fatigue and irritability, so use is limited. Danazol is a weak androgen that is sometimes prescribed for women with endometriosis and fibrocystic breast disease. It is sometimes used to treat PMDD. Danazol can reduce symptoms, but has side effects of anovulation and masculinization. Gonadotropin-releasing hormone agonists and danazol have limited use due to the side effects and cost. See the Pharmacology Summary feature (p. 1552).

COMPLEMENTARY & ALTERNATIVE THERAPIES

Black Cohosh for Menopausal Symptoms

Description:
Many women seek complementary and alternative treatments as well as lifestyle modifications for their menopausal symptoms instead of using prescription HRT (Nachtigall et al., 2006). Black cohosh, in particular, is very commonly used as an herbal medicine for menopausal symptoms in both America and Europe over the past several decades. However, its bioactive components are still unknown (Jiang, Kronenberg, Balick, & Kennelly, 2006).

Research Support:
A review of randomized controlled trial evidence showed that black cohosh had a high level of support for treatment of menopausal symptoms (Dennehy, 2006). Another review of clinical trials showed that black cohosh significantly reduced menopause-related depression and anxiety in all studies reviewed (Geller & Studee, 2006).

A research team in the Czech Republic investigated a black cohosh extract to assess its effect on endometrial tissue of 400 postmenopausal women. Over the course of 52 weeks, participants received a daily dose of 40 mg of black cohosh extract. Results showed a lack of endometrial proliferation as well as improvement of menopausal complaints after the 1-year treatment period (Raus, Brucker, Gorkow, & Wuttke, 2006).

References
Dennehy, C.E. (2006, November–December). The use of herbs and dietary supplements in gynecology: An evidence-based review. *Journal of Midwifery and Womens Health,* 51(6), 402-409.

Geller, S. E., & Studee, L. (2006, December 28). Botanical and dietary supplements for mood and anxiety in menopausal women. *Menopause.* [Epub ahead of print]

Jiang, B., Kronenberg, F., Balick, M. J., & Kennelly, E. J. (2006). Analysis of formononetin from black cohosh (Actaea racemosa). *Phytomedicine,* 13(7), 477–486.

Nachtigall L., E., Baber, R. J., Barentsen, R., Durand, N., Panay, N., Pitkin, J., et al. (2006). Complementary and hormonal therapy for vasomotor symptom relief: A conservative clinical approach. *Journal of Obstetrics and Gynaecology Canada,* 28(4), 279–289.

Raus, K., Brucker, C., Gorkow, C., & Wuttke, W. (2006, July-August). First-time proof of endometrial safety of the special black cohosh extract (Actaea or Cimicifuga racemosa extract) CR BNO 1055. *Menopause,* 13(4), 678–691.

■ Nursing Management

Ideally all women should be screened for PMS and PMDD on a routine basis. Incorporate screening questions into a self-assessment that is routinely collected during intake. Much of the basic subjective data can be collected via a structured questionnaire. The following screening questions are effective:

- Do you ever have pelvic pain or cramps during or around the time of your period?
- Are you able to treat this pain so it does not bother you?
- Do you ever have other physical or mood discomforts during or around the time of your period?
- Are you able to treat these discomforts so they do not bother you?

Assessment of PMS and PMDD

Conduct a focused nursing assessment for women with PMS and PMDD for whom current treatments or self-care therapies are ineffective. An interview by a nurse can confirm self-report data as well as collect additional data. Start with a focused health history whenever possible to identify the individual woman's pattern of PMS or PMDD. The menstrual cycle may be divided into three phases: premenstrual, early menstrual (days 1 to 3 or days of heavy flow), and late menstrual (day 4 and onward or days of lighter flow).

The following areas should be assessed:

- Pattern of severity of PMS or PMDD across premenstrual and early menstrual phases
- Rating of overall distress caused by PMS or PMDD
- Pattern of severity of other cyclic discomforts across premenstrual and early menstrual phases
- Rating of overall distress caused by cyclic discomforts
- Influences on the cyclic pain symptoms; for example, work stress, diet, or exercise.

Identify the individual woman's pattern of symptom management by gathering the following information:

- Interventions, including self-care strategies
- Pattern of use across premenstrual and early menstrual phases
- Rating of relief obtained from intervention
- Rating of satisfaction with pain and symptom control
- Rating of adherence (i.e., consistent use of treatment).

Conduct a focused history and physical assessment using data from the history as a basis. The assessment data need to be organized into symptom patterns. Chart 49–9 provides a template for this organization.

Planning Expected Outcomes and Care for PMS and PMDD

Review assessment data together with the woman, and identify the outcomes important to the woman and amenable to nursing intervention. Expected outcomes for PMS and PMDD management may include the following:

CHART 49–9 Organization of Assessment Data for Premenstrual Syndrome and Premenstrual Dysphoric Disorder

Pelvic pain	Abdominal cramps Nausea, vomiting Backache Change in bowel frequency
Perimenstrual physical discomforts	Fatigue Headaches Fluid retention Joint aches and pain Breast tenderness Leg and thigh discomfort Change in energy and appetite
Perimenstrual mood discomforts	Depression, irritability Tension, impatience Anxiety, anger Mood swings, hostility Guilt, tearfulness Feeling out of control Change in sexual desire

- Improvements in PMS and PMDD symptoms' frequency, severity, distress, and pattern
- Improvements in discomfort symptoms' frequency, severity, distress, and pattern
- Increased comfort level (physical and psychosocial well-being)
- Successful use of treatments to manage symptoms
- Relief of pain and discomfort
- Enhanced role performance (work, family, friends, school, leisure)
- Patient understanding of the cost of various forms of treatment.

Review symptom patterns and establish expected outcomes through mutual goal setting with the woman. Use the assessment as an opportunity to educate women about managing pain and discomfort. Develop an individualized treatment plan, incorporating the multimodal treatment strategies and participant involvement through personal choice whenever possible.

Interventions for PMS and PMDD

Because PMS and PMDD are a complex mixture of physiological and psychological clinical manifestations, is it essential to implement a comprehensive plan that focuses on symptom management interventions. This plan will provide the patient with the knowledge and interventions to manage the disorder. The nurse along with the patient must identify goals of care and explore ways to best achieve the goals. To enhance coping, the nurse must provide an atmosphere of acceptance and give factual information concerning diagnosis, treatment, and prognosis. Mutual goal setting is essential for the plan to be successful.

Keeping a log of when and what stressors increase the clinical manifestations will assist in identifying appropriate interventions. The patient needs to be instructed to self-monitor stressors and habits that impact the disorders and then identify effective interventions. Chart 49–10 outlines the pharmacologic and nonpharmacologic interventions for PMS and PMDD.

Evaluation of PMS and PMDD

Following the interventions outlined in Chart 49–10, the nurse needs to assess the effectiveness of the plan. Ideally, the same assessment tools should be used for both the initial assessment and the follow-up evaluation. The evaluation assesses the achievement of expected outcomes initially identified by the woman in collaboration with her health care provider. When a woman is referred to another health care provider for additional evaluation or treatment, follow up on the woman's progress whenever possible and indicated.

Etiology, Epidemiology, Pathophysiology, Clinical Manifestations, and Treatment of Toxic Shock Syndrome

Toxic shock syndrome (TSS) affects 1 to 2 women in every 100,000 in the United States, from 15 to 44 years of age (CDC,

2005a). It is caused by the *Staphylococcus aureus* (*S. aureus*) bacterium, which is thought to be found in tampons and intravaginal contraceptive devices. Although *S. aureus* is colonized commonly on skin surfaces, it can cause multisystem problems when it invades the body through a break in the skin. Symptoms of TSS include sudden onset of fever, chills, vomiting, diarrhea, intense muscle pain, and a diffuse red rash. Chart 49–11 outlines the signs and symptoms associated with TSS.

Toxic shock is an urgent condition that can rapidly progress to severe and intractable hypotension and multisystem dysfunction. Desquamation of the palms of the hands and the soles of the feet are later signs. This infection can lead to shock and kidney and liver failure (McKinley Health Center, 2002). Hospitalization is often recommended if there is a rapid progression of severe symptoms requiring intravenous fluids and antibiotics. Mortality rate will vary, depending on the organism involved. Although *S. aureus* is the primary organism involved, TSS has been associated with *Streptococcus pyogenes exotoxin*. The mortality rate with *S. aureus* is less than 3%, but with *S. pyogenes exotoxin* it is as high as 70% (Salandy & Brenner, 2002). Primary prevention techniques include avoiding the super plus tampons and/or changing them every 2 to 4 hours, and using the smallest size tampon that will ab-

---

CHART 49–10 **Interventions for Premenstrual Syndrome and Premenstrual Dysphoric Disorder**

Self-Monitoring Interventions

Tracking symptoms.
Tracking stressors, function, and health status.

Pharmacologic Symptom Management

Over-the-counter (OTC) pain medication:
- Nonsteroidal anti-inflammatory drugs (NSAIDs).
- Timing and strength of the medication are critical to pain relief.
- Take an adequate dose of medication at the first sign of pain or before bleeding occurs.
- Manufacturers' recommendations for OTC medications should not be exceeded.
- Read labels of other OTC medications taken concomitantly, particularly cold and sleep remedies.
- Be advised regarding appropriate duration of use because of the potential for gastrointestinal distress or other side effects.

Hormones:
- Combination estrogen–progestin oral contraceptives.
- Progesterone intrauterine device.

Nutritional supplements:
- Calcium: 1,200 mg/day (do not exceed 2,500 mg/day).
- Magnesium: 250 mg/day (do not exceed 500 mg/day).
- Essential fatty acids.
- Vitamin B complex: B_6 50–200 mg/day, B_1 100 mg/day.

Antidepressant medication:
- Refer to a mental health professional as indicated for symptoms of depression.

Topical/cutaneous symptom management:
- Heat application: heating pad, hot baths, disposable heat wraps.
- Therapeutic massage.
- Acupressure and acupuncture.
- Transcutaneous electrical nerve stimulation (TENS).

Behavioral/Cognitive Symptom Management

Behavioral relaxation:
- Breathing exercises.
- Stretching exercises.
- Progressive muscle relaxation.
- Autogenic training.

Cognitive relaxation:
- Thought-stopping strategies.
- Thought substitution.
- Decreased negative self-talk.
- Meditation.
- Mindfulness meditation.
- Guided imagery.
- Prayer.
- Affirmations.
- Biofeedback.
- Distraction.

Lifestyle Modifications as Indicated

General dietary modification:
- Decreasing intake of caffeine, simple sugars, and salt.
- Eating frequent, small meals.
- Increasing water and fluid intake to 6–8 glasses per day.
- Reducing alcohol intake.
- Increasing intake of foods that can decrease symptoms such as:
  Those that are rich in essential fatty acids
  Those that are rich in B complex vitamins
  Those that are rich in calcium and magnesium.
- Use a daily multivitamin and mineral supplement.
- Use a premenstrual syndrome formula vitamin and mineral supplement during premenses.
- Smoking cessation.
- Exercise. Encourage one or more of the following types of exercise as indicated and as can be tolerated:
  Regular aerobic exercise
  Nonaerobic exercise (e.g., yoga, t'ai chi, stretching/relaxation
  Exercise modification across the menstrual cycle.

Environmental modification interventions:
- Environmental stress management.
- Time management.
- Social support.

CHART 49-11   Signs and Symptoms of Toxic Shock Syndrome

Sudden high fever
Low blood pressure
Vomiting and/or diarrhea
A rash similar to a sunburn, found mostly on the palms of hands and soles of feet; may also see peeling of the skin on hands and feet
Confusion/delirium
Muscle aches
Redness of eyes, mouth, and throat
Seizures
Headache

sorb the menstrual flow without leakage for 2 to 4 hours. Once toxic shock has been diagnosed or suspected, the woman should avoid tampons altogether and use sanitary pads exclusively.

Diagnosis of TSS is based on fever, low blood pressure, rash that peels after 1 to 2 weeks, and at least 3 organs with signs of dysfunction. In some cases, blood cultures may be positive for growth of *S. aureus* (MedlinePlus Medical Encyclopedia, 2006b). Treatment includes intravenous fluids, vasopressors to control hypotension, antibiotics, and dialysis as needed for acute renal failure.

Patient education regarding toxic shock syndrome should include information regarding signs and symptoms and when the patient should seek care. Women should be advised that superabsorbent tampons that are left in place for too long become a breeding ground for bacteria and put young women at risk for toxic shock syndrome. Women should also be advised that using a diaphragm or contraceptive sponge can cause toxic shock syndrome. One can reduce chances of developing toxic shock syndrome by changing a tampon every 4 to 8 hours and using the lower absorbency tampon. It can also help to alternate using tampons and sanitary napkins whenever possible.

Etiology, Epidemiology, Pathophysiology, and Medical Management of Menopause

Menopause is the process by which the ovaries cease to function. The process can take 10 to 15 years as the regression of follicles within each ovary starts to accelerate after age 35. Symptoms begin as early as age 42 and end usually by age 58. More than 90% of women have ceased having periods by their early 50s. This process is accelerated by smoking. Once a woman has experienced 1 year of amenorrhea, she is considered postmenopausal. The average age of natural menopause is 51. A hysterectomy is referred to as surgical menopause. **Perimenopause** is the time during which periods may increase, decrease, and become irregular as the function of the ovaries waxes and wanes. As the ovaries become nonfunctional, the follicles cease to respond by producing estrogen. As the estrogen levels are depleted, a number of signs and symptoms appear. Irregular vaginal bleeding is common, and vasomotor symptoms manifest as hot flashes. Patients may experience vaginal drying and thinning of the mucosa, which causes atrophic vaginitis causing dyspareunia. The same mucosal changes occur in the bladder as well, causing a de-

crease in bladder capacity and loss of tone. These changes can cause dysuria and frequency even when no infection is present. This is often a somewhat difficult time for many women psychologically, as they experience emotional lability and changes in sleep patterns.

Health problems can become an issue at this time of life because the cardiovascular, musculoskeletal, and endocrine systems are affected. Cholesterol levels may begin to change, increasing the cardiovascular risks. The high density lipoproteins (good cholesterol) decrease and the low density lipoproteins (bad cholesterol) increase. The loss of estrogen, which begins a steady decline in bone density, puts the woman at risk for osteopenia, osteoporosis, and the potential for fractures.

The symptoms that the perimenopausal or menopausal woman may present should be considered carefully before determination of menopause. The possibility of thyroid dysfunction, anemia, and depression can present with many of the same symptoms. Laboratory tests that are valuable include an estrogen level and FSH level. The FSH (>35 international units per liter) is elevated and the estrogen level is decreased with menopause.

The most significant concern for the woman presenting with menopausal symptoms is how to manage her symptoms. Women have received volumes of conflicting information regarding hormone therapy during menopause. Most women know that hormone therapy provides relief from symptoms, but they also know that there are increased risks of breast cancer, stroke, heart disease, deep venous thrombosis, and pulmonary emboli. Thus, women are very conflicted about using hormone therapy to help with symptoms. If women want to consider taking hormone therapy for short-term treatment of menopausal symptoms, the risks and benefits should be explained fully. All options should be considered. Estrogen alone may be prescribed for the woman that has had her uterus removed. Estrogen and progesterone must be prescribed for the woman who still has a uterus. Unopposed estrogen causes hyperplasia of the endometrial lining and places the patient at risk for endometrial cancer. Progesterone has side effects that are problematic including increased appetite, weight gain, irritability, depression, headache, and breast tenderness. There are numerous preparations of hormone therapy, combination preparations with estrogen and progesterone, separate preparations and topical creams, gels, rings, and dermal patches. Vaginal creams are usually specific for atrophic vaginitis, but do not provide relief from vasomotor symptoms. One very important aspect of patient teaching for the woman considering hormone therapy is the high risk of fatal pulmonary emboli in the women who smoke and take hormone therapy.

Other therapies are available; for example, antidepressants can be used to help with situational depression that can accompany menopause. Fluoxetine, paroxetine, and venlafaxine are sometimes effective alternatives to hormone therapy in managing symptoms. Vasomotor symptoms can be relieved even if the patient is not depressed. Selective estrogen receptor modulators (SERMs) such as raloxifene can be used to prevent bone loss in patients at risk for osteoporosis. See the Pharmacology Summary feature (p. 1552).

Nonpharmacologic therapies can often be a better alternative for the woman with family history of endometrial, ovarian, or breast cancer. Managing the environment and reducing caffeine and alcohol can reduce the effects of vasomotor symptoms. Vitamin E (800 international units) may also help reduce vasomotor symptoms. Kegel exercises and lubricants can aid in vaginal dryness and associated dyspareunia. Well-balanced nutrition, exercise, and good sleep habits can decrease anxiety and depression and maintain a sense of well-being. Weight-bearing exercise also reduces the loss of bone density and prevents weight gain. Aerobic exercise helps the patient manage her weight and improves cardiovascular health. The patient who takes calcium supplements and maintains a diet high in complex carbohydrates and vitamin B complex will maintain optimal weight and minimize symptoms. The American Cancer Society recommends yearly exams after 40 to detect cancers. Health teaching should address alcohol and tobacco abuse, diet, and exercise.

Etiology, Epidemiology, Pathophysiology, and Medical Management of Infertility

Infertility is generally considered a viable diagnosis when a couple has been unable to achieve a pregnancy after 12 months of unprotected intercourse, and it affects about 10% of the reproductive population (American Society for Reproductive Medicine [ASRM], 2002). Primary infertility refers to a couple who has never been pregnant, whereas secondary infertility refers to a couple who has been pregnant in the past but has been unable to achieve another pregnancy. There are many religious and cultural considerations necessary when discussing infertility with couples. For instance, the Roman Catholic Church deems technical procedures such as *in vitro* fertilization, donor insemination, and the freezing of embryos as unacceptable. Protestant and Muslim groups support *in vitro* fertilization with the husband's sperm, and Christian Scientists support both husband and donor insemination (Lowdermilk & Perry, 2004). Many cultures blame the woman for fertility difficulties and sometimes believe her infertility is caused by her sins or due to evil spirits (D'Avanzo & Geissler, 2003).

Both male and female factors are involved with infertility. The American Society for Reproductive Medicine (2002) simplifies the statistics and states that one-third is male related, one-third is female related, and one-third is a combination or unexplained. In male infertility, the cause is most commonly related to a decreased sperm count, but could be related to retrograde ejaculation, impotence, hormone deficiency, a varicocele (distended testicular veins), or scarring from a sexually transmitted infection. Female-related causes are most commonly related to ovulatory dysfunction. Other causes may include hormone imbalance, ovarian cysts, or pelvic infections. Age has also been associated with fertility difficulties. The woman reaches peak fertility in her early 20s, and the likelihood of conceiving after age 35 or 40 is less than 10% per month (MedlinePlus Medical Encyclopedia, 2008). In addition to age-related factors, couples at risk for infertility involve those with multiple sexual partners, those with a sexually transmitted infection, endometriosis, men with a history of orchitis or a history of undescended testicles, past history of diethylstilbestrol (DES) exposure for both men and women, and those with chronic diseases such as diabetes or thyroid disorders.

Diagnosis is determined through a complete history and physical examination of both partners, and the reported inability of a couple to conceive after 1 year of unprotected intercourse. The year time frame is often decreased in older couples due to the premium time frame for conception. The Diagnostic Tests box presents the typical diagnostic tests for reproductive disorders.

Treatment for infertility must be directed at the cause. Sometimes all that is necessary is counseling regarding timing of intercourse. As much as 85% to 90% of couples can be treated with conventional methods that involve medications or surgical repair of reproductive organs (ASRM, 2002). Assisted reproductive therapies (ARTs), for example, *in vitro* fertilization, have brought hope and success to many infertile couples. These procedures are used less than 5% in the treatment of infertility (ASRM, 2002), in part because of the cost, which can run into the thousands of dollars. Chart 49–12 (p. 1553) outlines the assisted reproductive therapies available to infertile couples.

Etiology, Epidemiology, Pathophysiology, and Medical Management of Abortion

Abortion is defined as the ending of a pregnancy before what is thought to be the age of fetal viability. This age of viability is decreasing due to an increase in medical technology; it ranges from 22 to 24 weeks' gestation (Lowdermilk & Perry, 2004). Some literature even supports the age of viability as low as 20 weeks' gestation (MedlinePlus Medical Encyclopedia, 2006a). There are two types of abortions: spontaneous, the naturally occurring loss of the pregnancy, and elective or induced, the intentional termination of the pregnancy. A miscarriage is considered a "lay term" for spontaneous abortion.

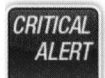 **CRITICAL ALERT** *Because of the negative connotation associated with the term abortion, when asking the patient about her pregnancy history, it might be beneficial to ask whether she has ever had a spontaneous loss or an elective loss of a pregnancy, rather than use the single term abortion or miscarriage. A patient may say yes to a miscarriage, but may not include the fact that she has also had an elective abortion, because the lay public often confuses the terms.*

Spontaneous abortion has four classifications: incomplete, complete, threatened, and inevitable (Chart 49–13, p. 1553). Not all symptoms will end in a spontaneous loss of the pregnancy. For example, only 30% of women with vaginal bleeding during the first trimester, with or without abdominal cramping, will have their pregnancy end in abortion (MedlinePlus Medical Encyclopedia, 2006a). When spontaneous abortion does occur, it is usually because the fetus has died, often due to chromosomal or developmental abnormalities (MedlinePlus Medical Encyclopedia, 2006a). Other causes of spontaneous abortion include maternal endocrine disease, such as thyroid or diabetes, or infection. It is thought that up to 50% of pregnancies may be spontaneously lost, most before the woman even realizes she is pregnant, and a 10% loss for known pregnancies (MedlinePlus Medical Encyclopedia, 2006a).

Symptoms of all types of spontaneous abortion include cramping and vaginal bleeding associated with a pregnancy, and they occur between what would be considered normal menstrual periods. Low back or abdominal pain, described as dull,

DIAGNOSTIC TESTS for Reproductive Disorders

Test	Expected Abnormality	Rationale for Abnormality
Herpes simplex virus (HSV)	Positive viral culture. Positive serologic test.	Indicates presence of HSV-1 or HSV-2.
Chlamydia	Positive culture.	Indicates presence of bacteria.
Syphilis	Venereal Disease Research Laboratories (VDRL): positive. Rapid plasma reagin (RPR): positive.	Indicates presence of serologic markers indicative of *Treponema*.
Gonorrhea	Positive culture.	Growth of *N. gonorrhoeae* bacteria from specimen.
Bacterial vaginosis	Positive vaginal culture.	Presence of *G. vaginalsis* from specimen.
Trichomoniasis	Microscopy positive for flagellates.	Indicative of presence of *Trichomonas* in specimen.
Vulvovaginal candidiasis	Microscopy positive for pseudohyphae. Positive culture of vaginal discharge.	Presence of *Candida* in specimen.
Human papillomavirus (HPV)	Nucleic acid probe positive for specific type of HPV. Liquid-based cytology with positive HPV finding. Carcinoma *in situ* noted from Pap smear.	Presence of genital warts, also known as HPV.
Mammogram	Positive for breast mass.	Suspicious for breast cancer. Mammography can detect 80–90% of breast cancers in women without symptoms. Requires biopsy for confirmation.
Breast cancer genes BRCA1 BRCA2	Positive for gene mutation.	Increases lifetime risk of developing breast cancer by 40–80%.
Transvaginal ultrasound Pelvic ultrasound	Positive for uterine mass, ectopic pregnancy, or ovarian cyst. Positive for fetal demise.	Determines size and location of masses and helps with the decision for or against surgery. Determines presence of ectopic pregnancy.
Urine human chorionic gonadotropin (HCG) Serum HCG Quantitative HCG	Positive: indicative of pregnancy. A quantitative HCG that doubles in 48 hours is indicative of pregnancy that is continuing. A quantitative HCG that fails to double in 48 hours is indicative of fetal demise.	Serum HCG is most accurate. Quantitative HCG is helpful in determining the length of pregnancy, and serial quantitative HCG tests are performed to determine the possibility of spontaneous abortion.
Blood culture	Positive for *S. aureus*.	Possible toxic shock syndrome.
Follicle-stimulating hormone	Greater than 35 international units per liter.	Indicative for menopause.
Semen analysis	2–3 days after complete abstinence.	Determines adequacy of volume, viscosity, sperm count, and motility.
Basal body temperature	Daily temperature of the woman before rising.	Determines ovulation if temperature rise of 0.5–1 degree is noted during the cycle.
Cervical mucus	Daily or every other day.	Notes cyclic changes in mucus to determine whether sperm can pass. Ideally needs thin, stretchy mucus for optimal sperm movement.
Serum progesterone	Late cycle (day 20–25).	Determines corpus luteum production of progesterone necessary for maintenance of a pregnancy.
Postcoital test	1–2 days before ovulation and 2–8 hours after intercourse.	Evaluates sperm motility in cervical mucus.
Commercial urine test for ovulation	Around the time of ovulation.	Determines luteinizing hormone, which is necessary for ovulation.
Hysterosalpingogram	Day 7–10 of cycle.	Assesses patency of uterine cavity and fallopian tubes.
Laparoscopy	Anytime.	Direct visualization of the pelvic cavity.

Sources: Adapted from Lowdermilk, D. L., & Perry, S. E. (2004). *Maternity & women's health care* (8th ed.). St. Louis: Mosby; MedlinePlus Medical Encyclopedia. (2008). *Infertility.* Retrieved February 28, 2008, from http://www.nlm.nih.gov/medlineplus/ency/article/001191.htm; and Mount Sinai Medical Center. (2008). *Reproductive endocrinology.* Accessed August 8, 2008, from http://www.mountsinai.org/Patient%20Care/Service%20Areas/Women/Procedures%20and%20Health%20Care%20Services/Reproductive%20Endocrinology

PHARMACOLOGY Summary of Medications to Treat Female Reproductive Disorders

Medication Category	Action	Application/Indication	Nursing Responsibility
Antibiotics: Azithromycin or erythromycin (Zithromax or ERY-C)	Disrupts cell wall synthesis of susceptible bacteria.	Chlamydia infection.	Large single dose given. Consider prevention for nausea. Take with food.
Doxycycline (Doryx)	Disrupts cell wall synthesis of susceptible bacteria.	Chlamydia infection.	Take with large glass of water. Not for patients under 18 years of age.
Penicillin G	Disrupts cell wall synthesis of susceptible bacteria.	Syphilis.	Intramuscular (IM) injection.
Metronidazole (Flagyl)	Disrupts cell wall synthesis of susceptible bacteria.	Trichomoniasis.	Caution patient not to drink alcohol while taking.
Clindamycin (Cleocin)	Disrupts cell wall synthesis of susceptible bacteria.	Bacterial vaginosis.	Can be given po or as vaginal ovules.
Nonsteroidal anti-inflammatory drug (NSAID): Ibuprofen (Motrin)	Cyclooxygenase-1 (COX-1) inhibitor with anti-inflammatory, analgesic, and antipyretic effects.	Premenstrual syndrome (PMS), premenstrual dysphoric disorder (PMDD), fibrocystic breast disease.	Caution patient to take with food to avoid stomach irritation.
Antineoplastic hormone antagonist: Tamoxifen (Nolvadex)	Nonsteroidal gonad-stimulating drug with potent antiestrogenic activity.	Palliative or adjunctive treatment for advanced breast cancer. Can reduce the recurrence or incidence of breast cancer in women at high risk.	Monitor white blood count for neutropenia.
Antiestrogen agents: Aromatase inhibitors Anastrozole (Arimidex) Letrozole (Femara)	Nonsteroidal competitive inhibitor of the enzyme system that converts androgens to estrogens.	Blocks estrogen production by other tissues in women who are postmenopausal.	Menopausal symptoms may increase.
Monoclonal antibody antineoplastic agent: Trastuzumab (Herceptin)	Recombinant DNA monoclonal antibody that selectively binds to the human epidermal growth factor to inhibit tumor growth.	Treatment of patients with metastatic breast cancer whose tumors express a protein known as HER2/neu.	Monitor for congestive heart failure. Not for use in patients with preexisting cardiac disease or dysfunction.
Antineoplastic antimetabolite: Methotrexate (Rheumatrex)	Antimetabolic and folic acid antagonist, thereby interfering with mitotic processes.	Nonsurgical treatment of ectopic pregnancy.	Generally one or two doses given. Most adverse effects are seen in long-term use such as with rheumatoid arthritis. Methotrexate will be excreted in breast milk.
Androgen: Danazol (Danocrine)	Mild androgenic effects that suppress follicle-stimulating hormone (FSH) and luteinizing hormone (LH).	Treatment of endometriosis and fibrocystic breast disease.	Monitor for masculinity effects, virilization, menstrual irregularities, and gastrointestinal (GI) distress.
Female hormones: Estrogen	Natural or synthetic steroid hormone secreted by the ovaries.	Treatment of menopausal symptoms from natural occurrence or surgical occurrence. Low doses can be used to control metrorrhagia.	Monitor for irregular vaginal bleeding and breast tenderness. Increased potential for deep venous thrombosis, especially if patient is a smoker.
Progesterone	Steroid hormone that opposes estrogen.	Prevents endometrial hyperplasia. Treatment for anovulation.	Monitor for dysfunctional or irregular vaginal bleeding.
Oral hypoglycemic: Metformin (Fortamet)	Increases binding to insulin receptor sites.	Lowers testosterone production in the patient with polycystic ovary syndrome.	Monitor for hypoglycemia and GI distress.
Antidepressants: Fluoxetine (Prozac) Paroxetine (Paxil) Venlafaxine (Effexor)	Selective serotonin reuptake inhibitor.	Approved for PMS and PMDD.	Avoid abrupt withdrawal of the medication. Avoid alcohol. Take in the morning to avoid insomnia.

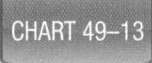

CHART 49–12 Assisted Reproductive Therapies

Reproductive Therapy	Indications	Procedure
In vitro fertilization (IVF) *In vitro* fertilization and embryo transfer (IVF-ET)	Blocked fallopian tubes; severe male infertility/sterility; cervix has an unfavorable environment due to acidic secretions. Shortens life span of sperm.	Ova retrieved from female and sperm from male; fertilization takes place in laboratory; fertilized eggs transferred a few days later to uterus in hopes of implantation (50% success rate for women under age 40).
Intrauterine insemination (IUI)	Severe male infertility/sterility; cervical hostile environment.	Husband or donor sperm are passed through a catheter into the uterus at the time of ovulation.
Intracytoplasmic sperm injection (ICSI)	Severe male infertility or failure to inseminate via IVF.	Harvest a single sperm and inject into ova and then inseminated via IVF.
Gamete intrafallopian transfer (GIFT)	Same as IVF but must have at least one tube patent.	Ova retrieved from ovary and fertilized in catheter with washed motile sperm; immediate transfer to fimbriated ends of fallopian tube.
Zygote intrafallopian transfer (ZIFT)	Same as GIFT.	Same as IVF but fertilized ova transferred to fallopian tube during zygote stage.

Sources: Adapted from Lowdermilk, D. L., & Perry, S. E. (2004). *Maternity & women's health care* (8th ed.). St. Louis: Mosby; and Mount Sinai Medical Center. (2008). *Reproductive endocrinology.* Accessed August 8, 2008, from http://www.mountsinai.org/Patient%20Care/Service%20Areas/Women/Procedures%20and%20Health%20Care%20Services/Reproductive%20Endocrinology

CHART 49–13 Classification of Spontaneous Abortions

Incomplete. Not all products of conception are expelled.

Complete. All productions of conception are expelled.

Threatened. Signs/symptoms of abortion are present and indicate the loss could happen.

Inevitable. Signs/symptoms of abortion cannot be stopped and the loss will eventually happen.

Symptoms of all types of abortion include vaginal bleeding with or without abdominal cramping.

Source: Lowdermilk, D. L., & Perry, S. E. (2004). *Maternity & women's health care* (8th ed.). St. Louis: Mosby.

sharp, or cramping, may be constant or intermittent. If tissue is passed, the abortion is usually considered inevitable. It is worth noting that up to 20% of all women experience some vaginal bleeding in the first trimester, but less than half of them experience an abortion (MedlinePlus Medical Encyclopedia, 2006a).

On examination, the cervix is often thin and dilated, and there may be evidence of rupture of the amniotic membranes. Human chorionic gonadotropin (HCG) levels will drop after a fetal death. Other laboratory tests that may be beneficial with a pregnancy loss include a complete blood count (CBC) to determine blood loss and a white blood count (WBC) to identify any infection. An ultrasound, transvaginal or abdominal, will assist with the diagnosis of fetal death and/or the presence of placental fragments that may have been retained in the uterus after a pregnancy loss.

Nothing can be done to treat an abortion that is inevitable, although there are palliative interventions that may help maintain the integrity of a pregnancy by providing a quiet uterine environment. These interventions include bed rest and abstaining from intercourse.

When an abortion occurs, it must be determined that all placental fragments and products of conception were fully expelled.

If not, a procedure called a dilation and curettage (D&C) may be performed to scrape the uterine lining clean of fragments. The amount of postprocedure uterine bleeding must be monitored. It is expected after a complete abortion or a D&C that the amount of bleeding is about the same as a normal menstrual period. Bleeding that continues longer, is heavier, or contains tissue fragments or any signs of infection, such as fever or foul-smelling vaginal discharge, should be reported to the health care provider. It is recommended to prevent another pregnancy for approximately the length of gestation of the current loss (i.e., if 8 weeks' gestation, then wait 8 weeks before attempting another pregnancy).

The second type of abortion is elective or induced. This may be done because of the desire of the woman to terminate the pregnancy due to not desiring a child or because of the results of fetal medical tests; for example, the potential for Down syndrome or a congenital illness such as hemophilia. The woman herself may have an illness that would put the fetus or herself at risk for harm, such as a serious heart condition, cancer, or advanced diabetes. When done for medical necessity, the term *therapeutic abortion* is often used. *Roe v. Wade* is the hallmark case in 1973 that legalized abortion in the United States for any reason before the 24th week of gestation. Third-trimester abortions may be performed only when the life or health of the mother is endangered by the pregnancy.

Induced abortions may be completed through the use of drugs or surgery. Surgical abortion methods include uterine evacuation, vacuum aspiration, dilation and curettage (D&C), and induced procedures. With uterine evacuation, a small cannula is inserted through the cervix. The products of conception are suctioned out of the uterus using a syringe during the 4th through 8th weeks of gestation. A vacuum aspiration is normally used from the 6th through the 14th week of gestation. The cervix is dilated and a cannula is inserted into the uterus. This canula is attached to a vacuum device that will remove the products of conception. Uterine evacuation and vacuum aspiration are procedures often done in an office setting. A D&C can be performed between the 6th and 16th weeks of gestation. The procedure involves dilating the cervix and scraping the lining of the uterus with a curette to remove the contents. A variation of this procedure is a D&E, dilation and evacuation, which is more difficult but can be done up to the 24th week of gestation. An induced abortion is the usual procedure between the 16th and 24th weeks of gestation. To perform an induced abortion, a small amount of amniotic fluid is replaced with a prostaglandin or pitocin solution. Approximately 24 to 48 hours later, the uterus will begin to contract and expel the fetus. The D&C, D&E, and induced abortion are done under general anesthesia.

Complications of any abortion procedure include bleeding, infection, cervical or uterine tear, retained products of conception, or even missed abortion whereby the pregnancy continues. Along with these physical complications, the woman may experience emotional upset surrounding the circumstances, which may require counseling to come to terms with the decision or necessity of the abortion. Nursing care involves education on complications, referral as needed, and emotional support.

Diagnostic and Surgical Procedures

There are several surgical procedures specific to women's health. These include exploratory laparoscopy, colposcopy, bladder suspension, and hysterectomy. An exploratory laparoscopy is a minimally invasive procedure that involves a small incision through which a laparoscope is inserted that allows visualization of the internal organs and structures to assess for disease processes. Carbon dioxide is instilled into the abdomen to elevate the abdominal wall and create a larger work area. After the procedure, the incision is sutured to secure the edges for healing. The patient may experience shoulder pain as the carbon dioxide dissipates from the abdomen. Instruct the patient to sit up and walk to promote gas diffusion and reduce pain. The nurse should be careful to assess the following:

- Incisions and any drainage
- Vital signs, bowel sounds
- Nutrition.

A **colposcopy** is a test to evaluate the cells of the cervix. The cervix is visualized with the use of a bright light and magnification, in order to see abnormal cells. Biopsies of unusual cells can be taken at precise spots. The procedure can be done in an office setting. The patient is encouraged to take ibuprofen or extra strength Tylenol shortly before the procedure to help control the pain of the procedure. It is important to remind the patient not to insert anything into the vagina, including not having intercourse, for 24 to 48 hours before the procedure. Spermicides, tampons, and semen can interfere with test results. Risks and complications are rare but can include slight spotting to heavy bleeding after the procedure. The patient should be taught signs and symptoms of infection and that she should report any pelvic or abdominal pain.

A **bladder suspension**, or Burch procedure, is done to suspend the bladder and correct urinary incontinence. During childbirth, the bladder ligaments are sometimes weakened and cause the bladder to sink in the pelvic cavity, causing leakage of urine, or incontinence. This is a common complaint of women typically over 40 years of age that have given birth to one or more children. The bladder suspension can be done using an abdominal incision, or it can be done utilizing a laparoscope, which lessens the length of hospitalization. As with any surgery, bleeding is a complication that needs assessing, and the patient is instructed that normal bladder function often does not return for up to 2 months. Specific discharge instructions for a bladder suspension that the nurse should carefully review with the patient are outlined in the Patient Teaching & Discharge Priorities box.

Hysterectomy

Hysterectomy is a surgical procedure to remove the uterus. Approximately 600,000 hysterectomies are performed each year in the United States (CDC, 2008h). The surgery can be done as a total abdominal hysterectomy removing the uterus, ovaries, and fallopian tubes, or as a vaginal hysterectomy in which the uterus is removed through the vagina. Hysterectomies are performed for four conditions primarily: uterine fibroids (leiomyoma, myoma), endometriosis, cancer, and uterine prolapse. Other reasons necessitating a hysterectomy include severe, chronic pelvic pain; long-term, chronic vaginal bleeding; or cancers involving the cervix, ovaries, or uterus.

A hysterectomy involves removal of the uterus, which can be done in one of three ways: through an abdominal incision, through the vagina, or through laparoscopic incisions in the abdomen. The reason for the removal will determine which procedure to use and whether other organs besides the uterus are to be removed. A partial hysterectomy is the removal of the upper portion of the uterus, leaving the cervix intact. A total hysterectomy involves removal of the entire uterus and the cervix. A radical hysterectomy is the removal of the uterus, the cervix, and the upper part of the vagina. The procedure chosen will depend on the extent of the pathology necessitating the surgery. For example, uterine fibroids may require only a partial hysterectomy, whereas extensive cancer could require a total or radical hysterectomy.

Nursing care for the woman having a hysterectomy includes addressing the following nursing diagnoses:

Anxiety related to fear of surgery and related diagnosis

Risk for Infection related to surgical procedure

Readiness for Enhanced Fluid Balance from electrolyte imbalance related to urinary retention

Potential for *Altered Tissue Perfusion* related to hemorrhage

Potential for *Altered Tissue Perfusion* related to deep venous thrombosis

Deficient Knowledge related to surgical procedure and risks and benefits

Acute Pain related to incision

Fatigue related to blood loss

Disturbed Body Image related to perceived loss of femininity.

Risks associated with hysterectomy are the same as those related to any major abdominal surgical procedure including reactions to medications, bleeding, infection, and bladder and bowel injury. Recovery is fastest with the vaginal or laparoscopic procedure, and the patient may experience less pain. The patient usually has a urinary catheter for 1 to 2 days while hospitalized,

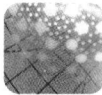

PATIENT TEACHING & DISCHARGE PRIORITIES for a Bladder Suspension

Need	Teaching
Analgesics	Take analgesics as prescribed.
Patient	Encourage patient to take analgesics as prescribed.
Family/support system	Advise patient to report to health care provider if analgesics are inadequate.
Activity	Avoid lifting, straining, driving, or other strenuous activity for 2–4 weeks.
Patient	Assist patient as needed to allow adequate rest and avoidance of strenuous activity.
Family/support system	
Diet	Regular, well-balanced diet as soon as desired.
Patient	Avoid spicy foods, caffeine, and alcohol, as they may irritate the bladder during healing.
Family/support system	Encourage a healthy diet.
Bladder/catheter care	Urinate regularly and use self-catheterization as taught (as often as after each void until residual amount is less than 100 milliliters).
Patient	
Family/support system	Assist patient as needed.

Sources: University of Maryland Medical Center. (2004). *Anterior vaginal wall repair.* Retrieved February 27, 2008, from http://www.umm.edu/ency/article/003982.htm

and some health care providers order injectable heparin for those at higher risk for blood clots. Ambulation is essential as soon as feasible, and a regular diet is encouraged after bowel function returns. Discharge instructions should include no heavy lifting, regular diet, rest, and nothing in the vagina, including intercourse, until released by the health care provider in 6 to 8 weeks. Menopause is immediate for women who also have their ovaries removed during the hysterectomy, and estrogen replacement therapy should be discussed with the patient.

The Maryland Women's Health Study and the Maine Women's Health Study were large, prospective studies designed to measure outcomes of hysterectomy for benign conditions. These studies demonstrated that hysterectomy substantially improves symptoms and quality of life in women with multiple and severe symptoms associated with gynecologic disorders. Medical therapy for abnormal bleeding and chronic pelvic pain produced significant improvements, but one-quarter of the nonsurgical group subsequently underwent hysterectomy (Kjerulff et al., 2000).

Salpingo-oophorectomy is the procedure whereby the fallopian tubes and ovaries are removed. Removal of just the fallopian tube is a salpingectomy. Oophorectomy is the removal of just the ovary. These can be unilateral or bilateral depending on the pathology that requires the procedure. These surgeries are done for ectopic pregnancy, ovarian cysts, or cancers of the ovary. In the case of cancer of the endometrium or ovaries that is spreading, the salpingo-oophorectomy may be done in conjunction with a total abdominal hysterectomy and the procedure may be abbreviated as TAH-BSO (total abdominal hysterectomy and bilateral salpingo-oophorectomy). A procedure such as this creates surgical menopause. The symptoms can be more intense than the gradual menopause that occurs naturally. The patient may be treated for these symptoms with a variety of estrogen replacements if the surgery is not done for cancer. Remember that estrogen is generally not given to women with reproductive cancer because many of these types of cancer are estrogen dependent. The care of these patients is very similar to that of the patient with a hysterectomy.

Mammoplasty

Cosmetic and reconstructive surgery on the breast is performed to increase or decrease its size, to lift the breast tissue, or for replacement after mastectomy. Augmentation or enlargement of the breast is generally done for cosmetic purposes. Breast reduction is often done for functional reasons because large breasts can cause back and shoulder pain and contribute to poor posture, possibly allowing this surgery to be covered financially by insurance. A mastopexy is a surgical procedure performed to improve drooping (ptotic) breasts. Breast reconstruction following mastectomy also is possible and is usually covered by insurance.

Breast Augmentation

Augmentation of the breast involves the implantation of a manufactured silicone shell implant filled with either silicone gel or saline, or, in some cases, a double lumen implant consisting of each of these substances. The implants are placed in a surgically created pocket either subglandular (beneath the breast tissue but in front of the muscle fascia) or submuscular (under the pectoralis muscle and sometimes the serratus anterior and upper part of the rectus abdominus muscles). The surgery is typically done on an outpatient basis either under local anesthesia and conscious sedation or under general anesthesia. Surgical incisions are made in one of four areas: around the periareolar margin; in or just above the inframammary fold; in the axilla; or in and around the umbilicus. Figure 49–10 ■ (p. 1556) shows a patient both before and after an augmentation mammoplasty.

Complications are rare and include hypertrophic scars, hematoma formation, infection, deflation or rupture of the implant, asymmetry of the breasts, temporary or permanent loss of sensation, and contracture of scar tissue. Formation of scar tissue around the implant is normal to "wall it off" as a foreign body. However, the scar tissue can sometimes thicken and contract, making a smaller pocket, which can then lead to breast firmness referred to as capsule contracture. The cause of this condition is usually unknown, but the incidence is thought to be increased by hematoma and seroma formation,

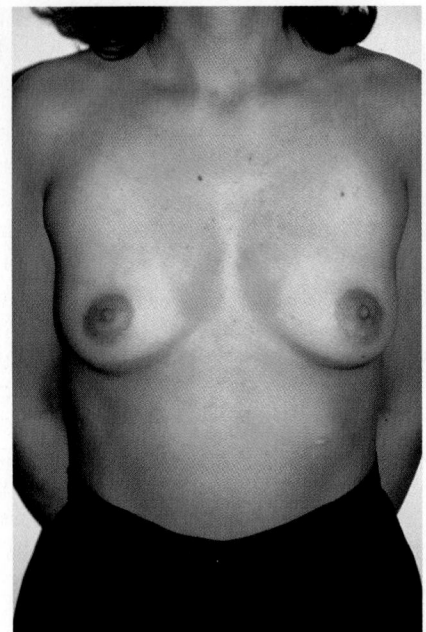

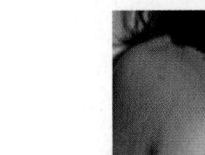

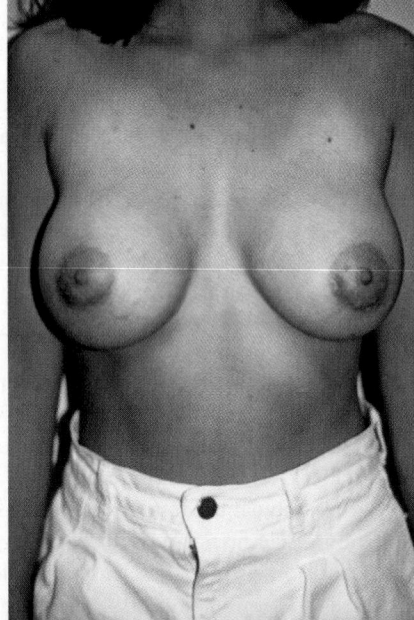

FIGURE 49–10 ■ Breast augment (A) before and (B) after.
Source: Custom Medical Stock Photo, Inc.

or subclinical infections. Treatment is usually surgical, incising the scar to allow the surrounding tissues to expand and create a larger pocket, thus, allowing the implants to feel softer and drape more naturally. Recently the Erchonia laser is being used to soften the capsules, resulting in a more natural feel and appearance of the breasts. The long-term effects of laser use are yet to be determined, and the results are variable among patients. Women with breast augmentation have the same incidence of developing a malignancy as those without implants and therefore should continue to do regular breast self-examination and mammograms (American Cancer Society, 2007).

Silicone is used to make breast implants because it is the least reactive substance placed in the body and is not rejected, as most

foreign bodies are. For this reason, it is also used for facial, testicular, penile, and joint implants. It is used for shunts, pacemakers, and as a coating to lubricate needles and syringes. However, in 1990, concerns were raised about the safety of the breast implants and the possibility that they might be contributing to many of the immunologic diseases that usually occur in women, such as chronic fatigue syndrome, fibromyalgia, lupus, scleroderma, and so forth. In 1992, the FDA restricted the use of the gel-filled implants only to women undergoing breast reconstruction following mastectomy for cancer, to those having replacement of previously placed gel implants, or to those undergoing augmentation with a mastopexy at the same time. Women undergoing augmentation only were restricted to using saline-filled implants. This restriction was lifted in 2006, 14 years later, after the FDA became reassured that there did not seem to be confirmation of these concerns either scientifically or statistically.

Breast Reduction

Breast reduction is usually done for complaints of pain and discomfort related to large breasts but can be done for cosmetic reasons as well. Breast reduction relieves pain in the back, neck, and shoulder; increases the patient's feelings of self-worth; and potentially decreases anxiety and depression (Iwuagwu et al., 2006). Breast reduction is a surgical procedure in which breast tissue and skin are removed from the center and lower parts of the breast. Usually the nipple and areolar complex are relocated superiorly, keeping the complex attached to the subcuticular breast tissues to retain circulation and sensation. In women with very large breasts, it may be necessary to remove the nipple and areolar complex completely during the procedure and relocate the complex as a full thickness skin graft after the breast tissue and skin have been removed and the remaining breast tissue and skin sculpted to give a natural-looking breast appearance.

Breast reduction also can be performed using liposuction if much of the breast is made up of fat cells. Liposuction may or may not use ultrasonic energy to emulsify fat cells. This technique removes a significant volume of breast fat, and in younger patients with good elasticity, it lifts the breast while leaving minimal scarring. Liposuction for breast reduction is not indicated for older women or for women with very large breasts.

Breast reduction is usually done under general anesthesia and, depending on the patient's age and condition, can be done as either an outpatient or an inpatient. Complications include blood loss, infection, hematoma, asymmetry of breasts, loss of sensation, and hypertrophic scarring. In childbearing women, this surgical procedure may result in the inability to breast-feed. The scar from this procedure extends around the areola and straight down from the center of the inferior portion of the areola to the inframammary fold. Sometimes there is also a scar across the inframammary fold. Women tend to be extremely satisfied with the results because of the increased comfort and appearance.

Mastopexy

Mastopexy is a surgical procedure performed in women who have nursed, have lost weight, or have breasts that have settled due to the aging process. This procedure lifts the nipple and areolar complex superiorly, excises excess skin, and reshapes the remaining skin without removing breast tissue. An implant may be inserted during a mastopexy to improve breast fullness and give a more natural shape. This procedure does have some degree of visible scarring.

Breast Reconstruction

There are several approaches for reconstructing the breast following a mastectomy. The goal of breast reconstruction is to create a mound that creates a normal appearance in a bra or a bathing suit and improves the woman's self-image. It also is possible to re-create a pigmented circle with a mound in the center that looks like a normal nipple and areola in thin clothing. It is not possible to restore the normal breast function of lactation or nipple sensation or erectility. The process of reconstructing the breast can begin immediately when the mastectomy is being performed, or it can be delayed and begun in a separate surgery later. The timing is based on patient and surgeon preference, along with the possible need for chemotherapy and/or radiation.

Symmetry of the breasts is usually easier to achieve when doing bilateral reconstruction. No matter which technique is used, it is sometimes difficult to match a normal side that is too large, ptotic, or has had other changes associated with the aging process. Sometimes a mastopexy, augmentation, or reduction is done on the normal side for symmetry. In some states the law mandates that both breasts' procedures be covered by the patient's insurance carrier.

Tissue Expanders and Implant Reconstruction

Breast reconstruction using an implant is usually a multistep process. It begins after the mastectomy with the placement of a tissue expander under the skin and pectoral, serratus anterior, and rectus abdominus muscles in order to stretch the muscle and skin and create a pocket for subsequent placement of an implant. The tissue expander is minimally inflated on insertion and gradually filled with weekly injections of saline inserted into a self-sealing valve in the expander. This facilitates a gradual expansion of skin and muscle tissue until the desired breast size is reached (Figure 49–11 ■). Once the size is reached, the expander is surgically removed and a permanent implant is inserted. Although not commonly used, some expanders are designed also to be the permanent implant, thereby eliminating the need for a second surgery.

Tissue Transfer Reconstruction

It is possible to use the patient's own tissue to reconstruct the breast by using tissue transferred from other areas of the body. The three types of tissue transfers include the latissimus dorsi muscle of the back, the transverse rectus abdommis muscle (TRAM) of the lower abdomen, and the microvascular free flaps from the lower abdomen or buttocks. The placement of this tissue will replace skin and breast tissue removed during the mastectomy.

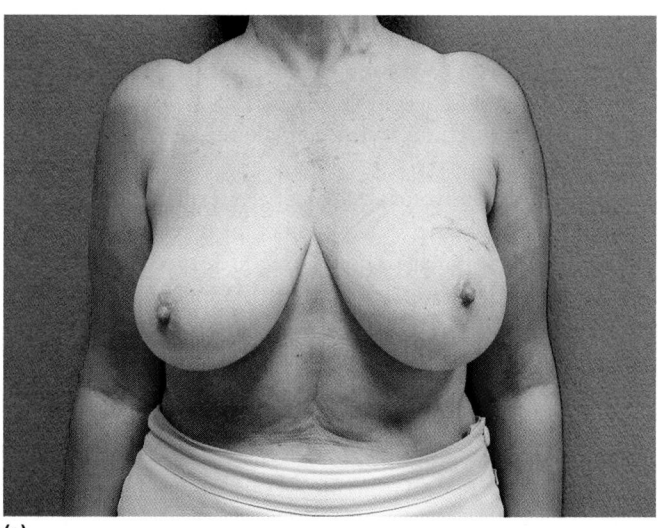

(a)

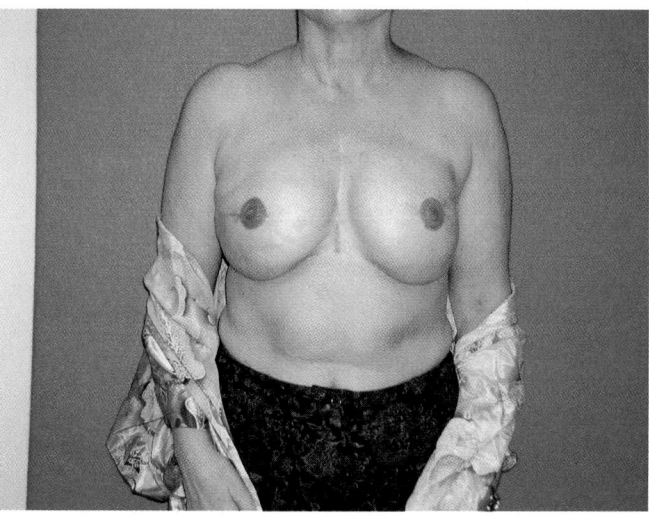

(b)

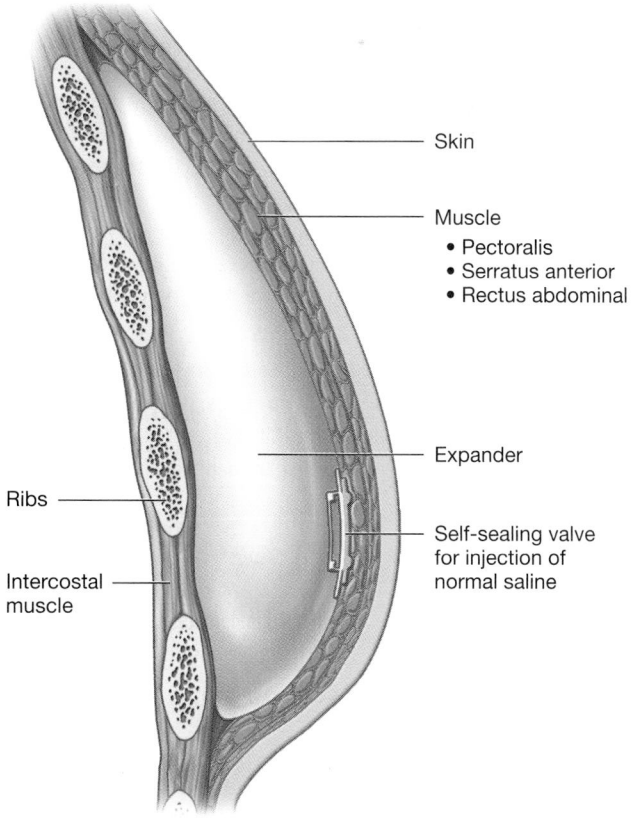

(c)

FIGURE 49–11 ■ Tissue expander (C) and breast reconstruction photos (A) before, (B) after.
Source: (a) and (b): Kathleen Osborn

A latissimus dorsi flap consists of a skin island attached to the latissimus dorsi muscle, which gets its blood supply from axillary vessels to which it is attached. Usually an implant is inserted beneath muscle to augment the volume when a latissimus dorsi flap is used.

A TRAM flap consists of skin from the lower abdomen left attached to the rectus abdominus muscle for its blood supply that is then tunneled up under the remaining abdominal skin and carefully inserted and sculpted into the deficient breast area to create a mound that resembles a breast. If there is sufficient abdominal tissue, this technique can be used to reconstruct both breasts at the same time, splitting the skin in the center and leaving each half attached to its respective rectus muscle. The main trade-off for this procedure is that it does weaken the abdominal musculature. Implants may or may not be used with a TRAM flap, depending on the amount of fatty tissue available, the patient's preference for size, and the amount of volume required for symmetry.

Some patients may be better candidates for a microvascular free flap reconstruction in which skin and fat are taken from either the abdomen or the buttock, along with their vascular supply, which are then sutured using microvascular techniques to the surrounding recipient vessels for circulation. Patients who smoke, patients with diabetes, and patients with some previous abdominal scars may not be good candidates for this procedure, because of the already compromised vascular supply to the skin and muscle.

Nipple-Areolar Reconstruction

Once the mound is reconstructed, there are several methods for reconstructing the nipple and areolar complex. The techniques used involve various combinations of local flaps, skin grafts, and sometimes tissue from the nipple on the normal side, if it is of adequate size. After the nipple and areola have been reconstructed, the final step is to use micropigmentation (tattooing) to darken the area to match the contralateral breast for unilateral reconstruction. This completes the reconstruction and helps to make women feel "whole" again.

Complications of breast reconstruction include wound infection, hematoma, dehiscence, asymmetry, rupture of the expander or implant, and capsule contracture. Wound infection may occur especially if the woman is immunosuppressed due the cancer itself and/or is under treatment with chemotherapy. Capsule contracture was discussed earlier in this chapter. Previous radiation may result in various degrees of fibrosis of the skin and muscle and may make expansion more difficult.

Papanicolaou (Pap) Smears

Annual Papanicolaou (Pap) smears are highly successful in diagnosing early cancer of the cervix (NCI, 2007). The National Cervical Cancer Coalition (2005) recommends women begin Pap smears 3 years after becoming sexually active or by age 21. There are two primary classification systems in use, the cervical intraepithelial neoplasia (CIN) and the Bethesda systems. A comparison of these systems will help with understanding of Pap smear results (Chart 49–14).

■ Interpersonal Violence

Sexual assault is an act of violence. It is defined as the forcible perpetration of a sexual act on a person without his or her consent. According to the National Violence Against Women Survey (2005), 1 in 6 women will be the victim of rape or attempted rape. The immediate reactions to rape include shock, fear, confusion, and disbelief. Some who have been raped may deny the incident occurred or withdraw from rescuers. Those who have been raped may sustain physical injuries as well, which include bruising and lacerations to the genital area, head and neck injuries, and abdominal trauma.

Initial care of the woman who has been sexually assaulted centers on the person's safety. Treatment of the urgent and emergent injuries and emotional responses requires specifically trained professionals who have experience in dealing with those who have been sexually assaulted and can provide not only the crisis intervention that makes a difference at the time of the incident but also the continuing care over the course of her recovery. Readily available rape advocates, specially trained law enforcement personnel, and sexual assault nurse examiners (SANEs) should be involved with the patient from the very beginning of the patient's presentation. The importance of careful and meticulous evidence collection is the second priority after assuring the patient's safety

CHART 49–14	Classification of PAP SMEARS (CIN Versus Bethesda System)	
Description	**Cervical Intraepithelial Neoplasia (CIN Grading)**	**Bethesda System (2001)**
Normal	Normal	Normal
Atypia	Atypia	Atypical squamous cells of undetermined significance (ASCUS)
Human papillomavirus (HPV)	HPV	Low-grade squamous intraepithelial lesion (SIL)
Atypia with HPV	Atypia (condylomatous atypia)	Low-grade SIL
Mild dysplasia	CIN I	Low-grade SIL
Moderate dysplasia	CIN II	High-grade SIL
Severe dysplasia	CIN III	High-grade SIL
Carcinoma *in situ*	CIS	High-grade SIL
Invasive cancer	Invasive cancer	Invasive cancer

Source: National Cervical Cancer Coalition. (2005). *Cervical cancer.* Retrieved February 28, 2008, from http://www.nccc-online.org/patient_info/cervical_cancer.html

and treatment of injuries. Sexual assault nurse examiners are specially trained to collect this evidence according to the protocol of the local jurisdiction. Sexual assault exams are for the express purpose of collecting evidence and have no bearing on the patient's medical care. The victim of a sexual assault must consent to the collection of evidence in total or in part. The process is laborious and time consuming, and many who have been victimized become exhausted and frustrated with the process without the appropriate support from the rape advocate and the sexual assault examiner. The evidence that should be collected and usually included in local protocols includes a history of the assault, collection of seminal fluid and possible sperm, combing pubic hair for foreign hair and matter, fingernail scrapings, collecting the patient's blood for typing and DNA screening, collecting torn or stained clothing, taking photographs of the injuries, and creating an accurate body map of the injuries. The handling of evidence is critical, and therefore, the sexual assault nurse examiner carefully labels all evidence and seals it for transfer to law enforcement. This is referred to as "creating a chain of evidence," which is critical to maintaining the integrity of the evidence. No unnecessary personnel should be involved in handling evidence.

Assessment findings of the victim of rape may be unpredictable. Emotionally, some victims of rape may be extraordinarily calm and controlled. Others may be hysterical and difficult to calm. Many cry uncontrollably and express anger and fear; others may be silent and withdrawn. Physical findings include oral, vaginal, and rectal injuries, bruises to the neck and arms, head injuries, and multiple scrapes and cuts. One of the most important findings in a woman who has been raped is a slight tear to the posterior fourchette of the vaginal opening. This small physical indication is frequently an indication of forced penetration. Many victims of rape show very few or no injuries because they cooperate with their attacker out of fear for their life. All these women should be monitored carefully during evidence collection for delayed response to the assault. Decreasing level of consciousness or changes in vital signs will require that evidence collection be halted and the patient be assessed for occult injuries. Most evidence collection protocols include toxicology and blood alcohol levels to determine whether the person who was raped was under the influence of drugs or alcohol, which may have impacted her ability to fight off her attacker. Screening for sexually transmitted infections is also part of the exam, and prophylactic treatment with antibiotics is offered to the patient. Additionally, the patient is offered emergency contraception. Victims of sexual assault should never be allowed to leave the hospital alone after treatment. Rape advocates should be available to ensure the patient's safety once released from the hospital. A safe house, family member's home, or women's shelter may be possible options for the patient.

Nurses can help prevent sexual assaults by educating young women about self-defense and avoiding risky situations. Encour-

agement of patients to participate in self-defense classes can improve situational awareness and confidence. Female patients should also be encouraged to practice safe habits in lighting entrances to home, locking doors, and avoiding opening doors to strangers. Women patients should protect their identification as a single occupant in phone books, in mailbox listings, and on answering machines. Remind patients of the dangers of walking in deserted areas especially after dark. Encourage patients to pay attention to suspicious behaviors and avoid being alone in offices or elevators with unknown persons. In social situations, patients should avoid becoming intoxicated or accepting mixed drinks from casual acquaintances. All women should proceed very cautiously with online correspondence. Providing resources to female patients for obtaining whistles or pepper spray and encouraging them to keep it accessible will add to the general safety of women.

Many communities have rape crisis centers or phone lines that are staffed 24 hours a day. The programs provide counseling and advocacy and ensure appropriate treatment during medical and legal procedures. Victim financial assistance can be arranged to offset lost time from work and added expenses for medical care, psychological counseling, transportation, and housing. In 2002 the Association for Genitourinary Medicine established national guidelines for the treatment of adult victims of sexual assault, which are outlined in the National Guidelines box (p. 1560). Recent research that improves practice is discussed in the Evidence-Based Practice feature (p. 1561).

■ Gerontological Considerations

As women age, they are more prone to some conditions and less prone to others. In general, the geriatric population is rapidly growing, and health issues need to be addressed by the health care providers. Information on the effects of aging on the female population is widely available. For example, much information exists on menopause and the effects it has on sexual desire and sexual response. There is a plethora of information on breast cancer and the need for screening mammography, even in the aging population. The National Institute on Aging provides information on many topics, including women's health issues.

■ Research

Research on women's health issues has been in the forefront for many years. Both the Office of Research on Women's Health and the National Institute on Aging are involved in research on menopause, fibroids, and cancer, to name only a few topics. The Research Opportunities and Clinical Impact box (p. 1561) outlines potential research topics related to female reproductive disorders and trends in the care of women.

NATIONAL GUIDELINES for the Management of Adult Victims of Sexual Assault

Ensure local law enforcement is aware of patient.

Forensic exam is useful up to 7 days postassault.

The orifices used in the assault, the timing of the assault, prior and subsequent consenting sexual intercourse, use of condoms by the assailant, and whether or not ejaculation had occurred should be documented.

Signed consent is essential if any information is subsequently disclosed to the police. This should be with the understanding that the court may order disclosure of all information divulged during the legal proceedings.

Injuries requiring immediate attention will take precedence over any other examination.

If the assault is recent, accurately document injuries found on the genital inspection. Petechial hemorrhages on the palate should be sought with a history of forced oral penetration. Anal examination including proctoscopy should be performed if there is a recent history of forced anal penetration, noting any trauma.

A full screening for sexually transmitted infections at presentation is recommended.

Exam should include cultures for *Neisseria gonorrhoeae* and tests for *Chlamydia trachomatis* from any sites of penetration or attempted penetration.

Vaginal slides for microscopy and yeasts, bacterial vaginosis, and *Trichomonas vaginalis*.

Blood should be drawn for syphilis serology.

Hepatitis B, HIV, and hepatitis C testing should be offered.

Sexually transmitted infection (STI) prophylaxis:
    Ciprofloxacin 500 milligrams immediately, doxycycline 100 milligrams twice daily bid for 7 days, or
    ciprofloxacin 500 milligrams immediately and azithromycin 1 gram immediately.
    Hepatitis B vaccination should be offered if the patient has not received it previously.
    A discussion about HIV infection should be part of the interview with the patient and follow-up testing and counseling. The patient can be offered postexposure prophylaxis in line with the postexposure prophylaxis guidelines for occupational exposure. This should be started within 72 hours after a high-risk exposure.

Pregnancy prevention:
    Postcoital oral contraception can be issued if within 72 hours of the assault and no risk of preexisting pregnancy.
    Levonorgestrel 0.75 milligram for 2 doses 12 hours apart.

Counseling:
    Post-traumatic stress disorder is common following sexual assault; however, there is no evidence that brief psychological debriefing reduces this.
    Links with local victim support organization, rape crisis groups, and local psychologist should be present to facilitate referral if needed.
    As psychological sequelae may develop months or years later, communication with the general health care provider to ensure continuity of care should be encouraged.

Source: Andrews, R. T., Spies, J. B., Sacks, D., Worthington-Kirsch, R. L., Niedzwiecki, G. A., Marx, M. V., et al. (2002). *National guidelines on the management of adult victims of sexual assault.* London: Association for Genitourinary Medicine (AGUM), Medical Society for the Study of Venereal Disease.

Sexual Assault Nurse Examiners (SANE)

Clinical Problem

Care of individuals who have been a victim of sexual assault is complex and multifaceted. There are obvious emotional needs along with physical as well as legal issues. Research is need to evaluate the most effective approach to ensure a comprehensive plan is in place. These researchers evaluated the use of sexual assault nurse examiners (SANEs) as opposed to staff nurses and health care providers.

Research Findings

Plichta, Clements, and Houseman (2007) conducted a study to assess the impact of SANE programs in the care of victims of sexual assault. The findings of this study include evidence that emergency departments with forensic nurse examiners for victims of sexual assault generally provide better and timelier care to these patients and are also better at conducting the forensic exam. Those emergency departments with full coverage models of SANE programs were significantly more likely to offer a full forensic exam, to have a relationship with a rape crisis center, and to participate in a community-wide sexual assault response team (SART). They are also more likely to offer victims emergency contraception and shower facilities as well as fresh clothing. Additionally, emergency departments with SANE programs were more likely to offer staff training and annual in-services on the care of victims of sexual assault.

Implications for Nursing Practice

Sexual assault nurse examiners and emergency department nurses have been proactive in the development of standards of care for victims of sexual violence. The potential for improving care and determining referrals for those who have been sexually assaulted will create the opportunity for the victim to recover more fully from the event with fewer complications. The SANE model allows for comprehensive services to victims and a coordinated response from law enforcement, district attorney, health care, and advocacy services. The follow-up care includes crisis intervention and witness protection. The forensic exam that is conducted using the guidelines for forensic exams is more effective in aiding in the subsequent prosecution of the sexual offender. Each emergency department needs a written policy regarding the care of survivors of sexual assault and written protocols on the care of the victim and the training of the staff. There should be well-defined working relationships with other agencies and cooperation between agencies to achieve the best outcome for the victim of sexual assault.

Critical Thinking Questions

1. The following priorities should be addressed for the patient entering the emergency department with a chief complaint of sexual assault:
   a. A phone to contact a friend for a ride home
   b. Assessment of injuries
   c. Reassurance of her safety
   d. Report to law enforcement for possible investigation
   e. B, C, D
   f. A and C

2. The chain of evidence in a sexual assault exam:
   a. Must be kept as clear as possible with as few people as possible handling the evidence
   b. Dictates that rape kits must not be opened until the forensic exam begins
   c. Requires the nurse performing the forensic exam to sign the rape kit over to the investigating officer when complete
   d. Allows the rape kit to be left alone in the nurses' station while awaiting collection by the investigating officer
   e. A and D
   f. A, B, C

3. The role of the rape advocate in a sexual assault includes:
   a. Providing emotional support to the patient during and after the forensic exam
   b. Explaining findings from the forensic exam to family members
   c. Ensuring safe shelter for the patient immediately after the forensic exam
   d. Explaining investigative procedures to the victim
   e. A and B
   f. A, C, D

Answers to Critical Thinking Questions appear in Appendix D.

Reference

Plichta, S. B., Clements, P. T., & Houseman, C. (2007). Why SANES matter: Models of care for sexual violence victims in the emergency department. *Journal of Forensic Nursing, 3*(1), 15–23.

EVIDENCE-BASED PRACTICE

RESEARCH OPPORTUNITIES AND CLINICAL IMPACT RELATED TO FEMALE REPRODUCTIVE DISORDERS

Research Area	Clinical Impact
Clinical Trials	
Hormone replacement therapy	Will assist with information on the impact of short- versus long-term therapy on heart disease, breast cancer, Alzheimer's disease, stroke, and dementia
Physiologic Research	
Research on why some fibroids grow to become problems and others do not	May help develop strategies to prevent fibroids and to develop new strategies to decrease the need for hysterectomy
Breast cancer	Cause, treatment, prevention, and survival
Menopause	Treatment options for prevention of symptoms
Pregnancy	Prenatal care and prevention of complications and fetal abnormalities and death
Infertility	Ability to have children

Source: Office of Research on Women's Health. (2008). *Annual NIH research priorities for women's health.* Retrieved August 10, 2008, from http://orwh.od.nih.gov/research/priorities.html

Clinical Preparation

CRITICAL THINKING

PEARSON mynursingkit™

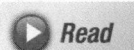 **Read**

- History of Current Illness
- Past Medical History
- Physical Exam
- Admitting Medical Orders
- Laboratory Study Results

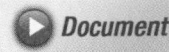 **Document**

- Summary of Hospitalization
- Pathophysiology Form
- Laboratory Values
- Laboratory Results Explanation

 **Apply**

- List of Potential Nursing Diagnoses
- Concept Map
- Critical Thinking Questions

Log on to MyNursingKit.com to download forms you will need and to complete further steps in the Clinical Preparation assignment.

HISTORY OF PRESENT ILLNESS

Mrs. G is a 54-year-old admitted early yesterday morning for a scheduled total abdominal hysterectomy and bilateral salpingo-oophorectomy. The patient has had heavy menstrual periods all her life, but for the last 2 years she has felt confined to the house due to the amount of bleeding she experienced. Her health care provider has put her on various medications in an attempt to control the heavy bleeding without success. Mrs. G also has several uterine fibroid tumors that cause severe discomfort. She and her health care provider decided a total abdominal hysterectomy with bilateral salpingo-oophorectomy was warranted.

During morning report, it was reported that the occlusive dressing on the abdominal incision has been marked for a moderate amount of bleeding, but that it appears to have stopped as the drainage marks have gotten no bigger in the last 6 hours. The patient was scheduled for a hemoglobin and hematocrit this morning. She is currently receiving patient-controlled analgesia with morphine. The day nurse enters the patient's room at 0745 and begins the initial assessment. Temp: 99.4°F P: 96 RR: 22 BP: 108/62. IV D5½ NS with 20 KCL infusing at 125 mL/hr, without signs of redness or swelling at the IV site. Lung sounds: clear to auscultation.

Patient is lying quietly in bed, eyes closing as if she is very tired. Patient reports pain is increasing, is 7 on a 1–10 scale. When the covers are pulled back to examine the dressing, the nurse notes bright-red blood oozing from the edges of the dressing. Further assessment reveals approximately 20 milliliters of bright-red blood staining the top sheet that was covering the patient. The nurse pushes the patient call light and asks the secretary to please page the attending surgeon. The surgeon arrives and requests a suture kit and local anesthetic to put in retention sutures in an attempt to control the bleeding. The equipment arrives, and the surgeon removes the occlusive dressing to reveal an oozing incision, without redness, edema, slight ecchymosis, and edges remain approximated with staples. The surgeon asks for the most recent laboratory work that was drawn earlier in the morning. After placing 6 retention sutures and observing that the oozing has stopped, the surgeon leaves the floor after writing orders for antibiotics every 6 hours.

Medical/Surgical History

Mrs. G had 3 vaginal deliveries of live children. She had an appendectomy at age 15.

Social History

Mrs. G lives with her husband and has 3 grown children who all live in the local area. She has never smoked or used illicit drugs. She has a glass of wine in the evening with her dinner. Mrs. G runs an average of 20 miles per week.

Physical Exam

Temp: 97.4°F P: 82 RR: 16 BP: 108/62

Oxygen sat 98% on RA

HEENT: normal

Heart: regular rate and rhythm, normal S_1, S_2

Lungs: clear to auscultation in all fields

Abdomen: soft, nontender, bowel sounds present

Normal neuro exam

No rash

Chest x-ray: clear

ECG: WNL

Weight: 130 lb

Height: 5.4 ft

Admitting Medical Orders

Surgical service

Admit to surgical floor

Admitting diagnosis was menorrhagia and uterine fibroid tumors. Status post total abdominal hysterectomy with salpingo-oophorectomy.

No known allergies

Call house officer: pulse < 60 and > 130/minute; BP < 90 and > 160 systolic; temperature > 38.5; urine output < 30 mL/hr for 2 hours; respiratory rate > 30/minute

Ambulate qid beginning postoperative day 1

IV D5½ NS with 20 KCL at 125 mL/hr

Vital signs q4hours

Sequential compression device (SCD) to lower extremities until ambulating without assistance

Incentive spirometer q2h while awake

I&O q8hours

Progressive postoperative diet as tolerated post-nausea

Scheduled Medications

PCA: morphine sulfate 1mg/mL, incremental dose 1mg, lock out 6 minutes

Unasyn 2 grams IV q6h.

PRN Medications

Phenergan 25 mg q6h prn nausea

Ativan 0.5–2 mg IV q6–8h prn anxiety (not to exceed 10 mg/24 hours)

Tylenol 650 mg PO/PR q4h for pain

Benadryl 25-50 mg IV q6hours PRN insomnia or itching

Ordered Laboratory Studies

CBC morning after surgery

LABORATORY STUDY RESULTS

Test	1 Day Prior to Surgery	4 Hours After Surgery	0500 Today
HGB	14.3 g/dL	11.9 g/dL	9.5 g/dL
HCT	43%	38%	32%
Platelets	230,000/mm³	165,000/mm³	90,000/mm³
WBC	8,000/mm³	12,000/mm³	14,000/mm³
RBC	4.9/mm³	4.1/mm³	3.92/mm³

CRITICAL THINKING QUESTIONS

1. What action by the nurse would be top priority?

2. What should the nurse do next?

3. Based on this situation and the 3 days of lab values, which of the interventions outlined below should receive the highest nursing priority?

- Assess incision q30min × 2, then q1h × 2, then q2h × 2, then prn for signs of bleeding or infection.
- IV at 200 milliliters q1h for 4 hours, then decrease to 150 milliliters per hour.
- Administer analgesic as prescribed.
- Unasyn 2 grams IV q6h.
- Vital signs and oxygen saturation q4h.
- CBC stat.
- Call laboratory results to the health care provider.
- Educate patient on safety measures for low hemoglobin and platelets.
- Change patient linens to provide comfortable environment.
- Encourage oral fluids and increased protein and iron in diet.

Answers to Critical Thinking Questions appear in Appendix D.

NCLEX® REVIEW

1. A female patient is diagnosed with a chlamydia infection. The nurse realizes that this patient will most likely be treated with:

1. Penicillin G.
2. Flagyl.
3. Doryx.
4. Cleocin.

2. A female patient wants to reduce her risk of developing breast cancer. Which of the following should the nurse instruct this patient?

1. Do not have any children.
2. Do not use underarm antiperspirants.
3. Limit dietary fat intake.
4. Have children before the age of 30.

3. The nurse is reviewing the technique for self-breast examination with a post-menopausal female. Which of the following should be included in this instruction?

1. Do the exam at least one time each month.
2. Use a mirror to examine the shape and size of each breast.
3. Always examine in a lying down position.
4. If you feel a lump, prepare yourself emotionally for the diagnosis of breast cancer.

4. A patient with uterine fibroids was told that the size of the fibroids has decreased. The nurse realizes that the decrease in size could be due to:

1. Constant uterine bleeding.
2. Decreased estrogen production.
3. Pregnancy.
4. Menopause.

5. A patient is diagnosed with an unruptured ectopic pregnancy. The nurse realizes this patient will most likely be treated with:

   1. Surgical removal of the fallopian tube.
   2. Methotrexate.
   3. A pessary.
   4. Colporrhaphy.

6. The nurse is assessing a 24-year-old female's reproductive status. Which of the following assessment findings would increase this patient's risk of infertility?

   1. Type I diabetes mellitus.
   2. Diagnosis of scoliosis.
   3. Menses began at the age of 13.
   4. Parents had 4 children, all live births.

7. A patient is recovering from an exploratory laparoscopy. Which of the following should the nurse instruct this patient to reduce the pain caused by carbon dioxide?

   1. Splint the incision before moving.
   2. Ambulate.
   3. Lay flat in bed for at least 16 hours.
   4. Ingest clear liquids only for at least one day.

8. A female victim of personal violence is brought into the emergency department by the local police. Which of the following should the nurse do first?

   1. Have the patient sign a consent form to collect evidence.
   2. Obtain the patient's name and address.
   3. Find three additional staff members to be with the patient during the assessment.
   4. Locate a SANE immediately.

Answers for review questions appear in Appendix D

KEY TERMS

abortion *p.1550*
anorgasmia *p.1540*
bacterial vaginosis (BV) *p.1523*
bladder suspension *p.1554*
breast cancer *p.1528*
candidiasis *p.1524*
chancroid *p.1522*
chlamydia *p.1518*
colposcopy *p.1554*
cystocele *p.1538*
dysmenorrhea *p.1544*
dyspareunia *p.1541*
ectopic *p.1539*
endometriosis *p.1536*

fibrocystic breast *p.1525*
fibroid tumor *p.1535*
genital herpes *p.1521*
genital warts *p.1522*
gonorrhea *p.1519*
human papillomavirus (HPV) *p.1522*
hysterectomy *p.1554*
lumpectomy *p.1532*
lymphogranuloma venereum (LGV) *p.1519*
mammography *p.1531*
mastalgia *p.1525*
mastectomy *p.1532*
mastitis *p.1528*

menorrhagia *p.1544*
metrorrhagia *p.1545*
pelvic inflammatory disease (PID) *p.1519*
perimenopause *p.1549*
pessary *p.1538*
premenstrual dysphoric disorder (PMDD) *p.1545*
premenstrual syndrome (PMS) *p.1545*
prolapse *p.1538*
rectocele *p.1538*
syphilis *p.1520*
trichomoniasis *p.1523*
vaginismus *p.1541*

REFERENCES

Allred, S., Cox, J. T., & Mahoney, M. (2006). HPV prevention and the promise of the new vaccines. *Journal of the American Academy of Nurse Practitioners, 18*(Suppl. 2), 1–11.

American Cancer Society (ACS). (2003). *Updated breast cancer screening guidelines released.* Retrieved February 27, 2008, from http://www.cancer.org/docroot/NWS/content/NWS_1_1x_Updated_Breast_Cancer_Screening_Guidelines_Released.asp

American Cancer Society (ACS). (2005). *Breast cancer facts and figures 2005–2006.* Retrieved February 27, 2008, from http://www.cancer.org/downloads/STT/CAFF2005BrF.pdf

American Cancer Society (ACS). (2007). *What are the risk factors for breast cancer?* Retrieved February 27, 2008, from

http://www.cancer.org/docroot/CRI/content/CRI_2_4_2X_What_are_the_risk_factors_for_breast_cancer_5.asp?rnav=cri

American Cancer Society (ACS). (2008). *Cervical cancer: Prevention and early detection.* Retrieved August 12, 2008, from http://www.cancer.org/docroot/CRI/content/CRI_2_6x_cervical_cancer_prevention_and_early_detection_8.asp?sitearea=PED

American College of Obstetricians and Gynecologists (ACOG). (1998). Medical management of tubal pregnancy (Number 3, December 1998). Clinical management guidelines for obstetricians-gynecologists. *International Journal of Gynecology & Obstetrics, 165,* 97–103.

American College of Obstetricians and Gynecologists (ACOG). (2000). *Fibrocystic breast changes.* Retrieved February 27, 2008, from

http://www.rgoa.yourmd.com/ypol/user/userMain.asp?siteid=1744043&content=userViewContentInFramework&bcx=My+Doctor^TAB~Web+Site^MNU~ROCHESTER+GYNECOLOGIC+%26+OBSTETRIC+ASSOCIATES%2C+P.C.^PST^1744043~Our+Practice^CAT^1~Article^MAP^ZZZLF2SXODC&cid=ZZZLF2SXODC&secure=2&rndm=0.4799626

American College of Obstetricians and Gynecologists (ACOG). (2005). *Premenstrual syndrome* (ACOG Practice Bulletin No. 15). Washington, DC: Author.

American Joint Committee on Cancers. (2005). *AJCC cancer staging manual.* Retrieved February 27, 2008, from http://www.cancerstaging.org/products/ajccproducts.html

American Society for Reproductive Medicine (ASRM). (2002). *Frequently asked questions about infertility.* Retrieved February 27, 2008, from http://www.asrm.org/Patients/faqs.html

Andrews, R. T., Spies, J. B., Sacks, D., Worthington-Kirsch, R. L., Niedzwiecki, G. A., Marx, M. V., et al. (2002). *National guidelines on the management of adult victims of sexual assault.* London: Association for Genitourinary Medicine (AGUM), Medical Society for the Study of Venereal Disease.

Barnhart, K., Dunsmoor-Su, R., & Coutifaris, C. (2002). Effect of endometriosis on *in vitro* fertilization. *Fertility and Sterility, 77*, 1148–1155.

Bhatia, S. C., & Bhatia, S. K. (2002). Diagnosis and treatment of premenstrual dysphoric disorder. *American Family Physician, 66*(7), 1235–1251.

Bianchini, F., Kaaks, R., & Vainio, H. (2002). Weight control and physical activity in cancer prevention. *Obesity Reviews, 3*(1), 5–8.

Boyles, S. (2006). Age, Obesity, and Breast Cancer Risk: Extra Weight May Lower Risk for Younger Women. *WebMD.* Retrieved August 16, 2008 from http://www.webmd.com/breast-cancer/news/20061127/breast-cancer-risk-age-and-obesity

Bumpers, H. L., Best, I. M., Norman, D., & Weaver, W. L. (2002). Debilitating lymphedema of the upper extremity after treatment of breast cancer. *American Journal of Clinical Oncology, 25*(4), 365–367.

Centers for Disease Control and Prevention (CDC). (2004). *Trends in reportable sexually transmitted diseases in the United States, 2004.* Retrieved February 27, 2008, from http://www.cdc.gov/std/stats04/04pdf/trends2004.pdf

Centers for Disease Control and Prevention (CDC). (2005a). *Toxic shock syndrome.* Retrieved February 28, 2008, from http://www.cdc.gov/ncidod/dbmd/diseaseinfo/toxicshock_t.htm

Centers for Disease Control and Prevention (CDC). (2005b). *Trends in reportable sexually transmitted diseases in the United States, 2005.* Retrieved August 12, 2008, from http://www.cdc.gov/std/stats05/trends2005.htm

Centers for Disease Control and Prevention (CDC). (2008a). *Breast cancer.* Retrieved August 12, 2008, from http://www.cdc.gov/cancer/breast/

Centers for Disease Control and Prevention (CDC). (2008b). *Candidiasis.* Retrieved February 28, 2008, from http://www.cdc.gov/nczved/dfbmd/disease_listing/candidiasis_gi.html#21

Centers for Disease Control and Prevention (CDC). (2008c). *Chlamydia.* Retrieved February 27, 2008, from http://www.cdc.gov/std/chlamydia/the-facts/default.htm

Centers for Disease Control and Prevention (CDC). (2008d). *Genital herpes.* Retrieved February 28, 2008, from http://www.cdc.gov/std/Herpes/default.htm

Centers for Disease Control and Prevention (CDC). (2008e). *Pelvic inflammatory disease—CDC fact sheet.* Retrieved February 28, 2008, from http://www.cdc.gov/std/PID/STDFact-PID.htm#What

Centers for Disease Control and Prevention (CDC). (2008f). *Sexually transmitted diseases.* Retrieved February 27, 2008, from http://www.cdc.gov/nchstp/dstd/disease_info.htm

Centers for Disease Control and Prevention (CDC). (2008g). *STDs and pregnancy—CDC fact sheet.* Retrieved February 28, 2008, from http://www.cdc.gov/std/STDFact-STDs&Pregnancy.htm#test

Centers for Disease Control and Prevention (CDC). (2008h). *Women's reproductive health: Hysterectomy.* Retrieved August 13, 2008, from http://www.cdc.gov/reproductivehealth/WomensRH/Hysterectomy.htm

Chlebowski, R. T., Prentice, R., & Adams-Campbell, A. (2005). Re: Ethnicity and breast cancer: Factors influencing differences in incidence and outcome. *Journal of the National Cancer Institute, 97*(21), 1619–1620.

Cronje, W., & Studd, J. (2002). Premenstrual syndrome and premenstrual dysphoric disorder. *Primary Care, 29*(1), 1–12.

D'Avanzo, D., & Geissler, E. (2003). *Mosby's pocket guide to cultural health assessment* (3rd ed.). St. Louis: Mosby.

Elliot, H. (2002). Premenstrual dysphoric disorder. *North Carolina Medical Journal, 63*(2), 72–75.

Evans, P., & Brunsell, S. (2007). Uterine fibroid tumors: Diagnosis and treatment. *American Family Physician, 75*(10), 1503–1507.

Fisher, B., Anderson, S., Bryant, J., Margolese, R. G., Deutsch, M., Fisher, E. R., et al. (2002). Twenty-year follow-up of a randomized trial comparing total mastectomy, lumpectomy, and lumpectomy plus irradiation for the treatment of invasive breast cancer. *The New England Journal of Medicine, 347*, 1233–1241.

Ford, D., Easton, D. F., Stratton, M., Narod, S., Goldgar, D., Devilee, P., et al. (1998). Genetic heterogeneity and penetrance analysis of the BRCA1 and BRCA2 genes in breast cancer families. *American Journal of Human Genetics, 62*, 676–689.

French, L. (2005). Dysmenorrhea. *American Family Physician, 71*(2), 285–290.

Harcourt, D., & Rumsey, N. (2001). Psychological aspects of breast reconstruction: A review of the literature. *Journal of Advanced Nursing, 35*(4), 477–487.

Hulka, B. S., & Moorman, P. G. (2001). Breast cancer: Hormones and other risk factors. *Maturitas, 28*, 103–113.

Imaginis. (2006). *Breast cancer diagnosis.* Retrieved February 28, 2008, from http://www.imaginis.com/breasthealth/biopsy/core.asp

Institute for Clinical Systems Improvement (ICSI). (2006). *Initial management of abnormal cervical cytology (Pap smear) and HPV testing.* Bloomington, MN: Author.

Iwuagwu, O. C., Walker, L. G., Stanley, P. W., Hart, N. B., Platt, A. J., & Drew, P. J. (2006). Randomized clinical trial examining psychosocial and quality of life benefits of bilateral breast reduction surgery. *British Journal of Surgery, 93*(3), 291–294.

Johnson-Mallard, V. (2007). Increasing knowledge of sexually transmitted infection risk. *Nurse Practitioner, 32*(2), 26–32.

Jones, C. (2001, March). Premenstrual dysphoric disorder. *Advances for Nurse Practitioners*, 87–90.

Kerlikowski, K., & Barclay, J. (1997). Outcomes of modern screening mammography. *Journal of the National Cancer Institute, Monographs, 22*, 105–111.

Kjerulff, K. H., Langenberg, P., Rhodes, J. C., Harvey, L. A., Guzinski, G. M., & Stolley, P. D. (2000). Effectiveness of hysterectomy. *Obstetrics & Gynecology, 95*, 319–325.

Kjerulff, K. H., Langenberg, P., Seidman, J. D., Stolley, P. D., & Guzinski, G. M. (1996). Uterine leiomyomas. Racial differences in severity, symptoms and age of diagnosis. *Journal of Reproductive Medicine, 41*, 483–490.

Klein, S. (2005). Evaluation of Palpable Breast Masses.American Family Physician: A peer reviewed journal of the American academy of family physicians. Retrieved August 15, 2008 from http://www.aafp.org/afp/20050501/1731.html.

Kroman, N., Jensen, M. B., Wohlfahrt, J., Mouridsen, H. T., Andersen, P. K., & Melbye, M. (2000). Factors influencing the effect of age on prognosis in breast cancer: Population based study. *British Medical Journal, 320*, 474–478.

Li, C. et al. (2003). The Relationship between Alcohol Use and Risk of Breast Cancer by Histology and Hormone Receptor Status among Women 65–79 Years of Age. *Cancer Epidemiology Biomarkers & Prevention* Vol. 12, 1061-1066, American Association for Cancer Research. Retrieved on August 14, 2008 from http://cebp.aacrjournals.org/cgi/content/abstract/12/10/1061

Loman, N., Johannsson, O., Kristoffersson, U., et al. (2001). Family history of breast and ovarian cancers and BRCA1 and BRCA2 mutations in a population-based series of early-onset breast cancer. *Journal of the National Cancer Institute, 93*, 1215–1223.

Lowdermilk, D. L., & Perry, S. E. (2004). *Maternity & women's health care* (8th ed.). St. Louis: Mosby.

Lozeau, A. M., & Potter, B. (2005). Diagnosis and management of ectopic pregnancy. *American Family Physician, 72*(9), 1707–1714.

Master-Hunter, T., & Heiman, D. L. (2006). Amenorrhea: Evaluation and treatment. *American Family Physician, 73*(8), 1374–1382.

McKinley Health Center. (2002). *Toxic shock syndrome and tampons.* Retrieved February 28, 2008, from http://www.mckinley.uiuc.edu/Handouts/toxic_shock_syndrome.html

McTiernan, A., Kooperberg, C., White, E., Wilcox, S., Coates, R., Adams-Campbell, L., et al. (2003). Recreational physical activity and the risk of breast cancer in postmenopausal women. *JAMA, 290*(10), 1331–1336.

MedlinePlus Medical Encyclopedia. (2006a). *Abortion—spontaneous.* Retrieved February 28, 2008, from http://www.nlm.nih.gov/medlineplus/ency/article/001488.htm

MedlinePlus Medical Encyclopedia. (2006b). *Toxic shock syndrome.* Retrieved February 28, 2008, from http://www.nlm.nih.gov/medlineplus/ency/article/000653.htm

MedlinePlus Medical Encyclopedia. (2007). *Hysterectomy.* Retrieved February 28, 2008, from http://www.nlm.nih.gov/medlineplus/ency/article/002915.htm

MedlinePlus Medical Encyclopedia. (2008). *Infertility.* Retrieved February 28, 2008, from http://www.nlm.nih.gov/medlineplus/ency/article/001191.htm

Mounsey, A. L., Wilgus, A., & Slawson, D. C. (2006). Diagnosis and management of endometriosis. *American Family Physician, 74*(4), 594–600.

Mount Sinai Medical Center. (2008). *Reproductive endocrinology.* Accessed August 8, 2008, from http://www.mountsinai.org/Patient%20Care/Service%20Areas/Women/Procedures%20and%20Health%20Care%20Services/Reproductive%20Endocrinology

Nakashima, A. K., Rolfs, R. T., Flock, M. L., Kilmarx, P., & Greenspan, J. R. (1996). Epidemiology of syphilis in the United States, 1941–1993. *Sexually Transmitted Diseases, 23*(1):16–23.

National Cancer Institute (NCI). (2000). *SEER summary staging manual—2000.* Retrieved February 28, 2008, from http://seer.cancer.gov/tools/ssm/

National Cancer Institute (NCI). (2007). Screening Mammograms: Questions and Answers. Retrieved on January 1, 2009 from http://www.cancer.gov/cancertopics/factsheet/detection/screening-mammograms

National Cervical Cancer Coalition. (2005). *Cervical cancer.* Retrieved February 28, 2008, from http://www.nccc-online.org/patient_info/cervical_cancer.html

Osteen, R. (2001). Breast cancer. In R. E. Lenhard, R. T. Osteen, & R. Gansler (Eds.), *Clinical oncology* (pp. 251–268). Atlanta, GA: American Cancer Society.

Phillips, N. (2000). Female sexual dysfunction: Evaluation and treatment. *American Family Physician, 62*(1), 127–136, 141–142. Retrieved February 28, 2008, from http://www.aafp.org/afp/20000701/127.html

Plichta, S. B., Clements, P. T., & Houseman, C. (2007). Why SANES matter: Models of care for sexual violence victims in the emergency department. *Journal of Forensic Nursing, 3*(1), 15–23.

Quest Diagnostics. (2005). *Chlamydia tests.* Retrieved February 28, 2008, from http://www.questdiagnostics.com/kbase/topic/medtest/hw4046/howdone.htm

Roussow, J. E., Anderson, G. L., Prentice, R. L., LaCroix, A. Z., Kooperberg, C., Stefanick, M. L., et al. (2002). Risks and benefits of estrogen plus progestin in healthy postmenopausal women: Principal results from the Women's Health Initiative randomized controlled trial. *JAMA, 288*(3), 321–333.

Salandy, D., & Brenner, B. (2002). *Toxic shock syndrome.* Retrieved February 28, 2008, from http://www.emedicine.com/emerg/topic600.htm

Sepilian, V. P. (2007). Ectopic Pregnancy. *eMedicine.* Retrieved August 16, 2008 from http://www.emedicine.com/med/topic3212.htm.

Sherman, R. T., & Thompson, R. A. (2004). The female athlete triad. *The Journal of School Nursing, 20*(4), 197–202.

Singletary, K. W., & Gapstur, S. M. (2001). Review of epidemiologic and experimental evidence and potential mechanisms. *JAMA, 286*(17), 2143–2151.

Smigal, C. et al. (2006). Trends in Breast Cancer by Race and Ethnicity: Update 2006. *Cancer Journal;* 56:168-183 doi: 10.3322/canjclin.56.3.168

University of Maryland Medical Center. (2004). *Anterior vaginal wall repair.* Retrieved February 27, 2008, from http://www.umm.edu/ency/article/003982.htm

U.S. Department of Health and Human Services (DHHS). (2000). *Healthy People 2010 understanding and improving health.* Washington, DC: Author.

U.S. Department of Health and Human Services (DHHS), womenshealth.gov. (2006). *Endometriosis.* Retrieved February 28, 2008, from http://www.4woman.gov/faq/endomet.htm

U.S. Department of Health and Human Services (DHHS), womenshealth.gov. (2007). *Polycystic ovarian syndrome (PCOS).* Retrieved February 28, 2008, from http://www.4woman.gov/faq/pcos.htm

U.S. Preventive Services Task Force. (2002). Screening for breast cancer: Recommendations and rationale. *Annals of Internal Medicine, 137*(5, Pt. 1), 344–346.

Caring for the Patient with Male Reproductive Disorders

Patricia Caudle

With contributions by:
Laurie Kaudewitz

Outcome-Based Learning Objectives

After studying this chapter, the learner will be able to:

1. Identify the most common male reproductive disorders.
2. Discuss the etiology, pathophysiology, clinical manifestations, and treatments of testicular, penile, and prostatic disorders.
3. Interpret diagnostic test results for male reproductive disorders.
4. Identify nursing management goals when caring for males with reproductive disorders.
5. Apply nursing diagnoses and nursing process to the care of the male patient with testicular and prostatic cancer.
6. Discuss health education, health promotion, and disease prevention specific for male health.

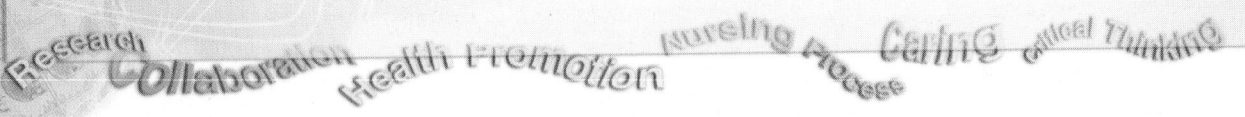

Research Collaboration Health Promotion Nursing Process Caring Critical Thinking

MALE REPRODUCTIVE disorders are often complex as they involve both sexual functioning and the urinary system. Disorders of the male reproductive system may also be a source of embarrassment for the male. Nursing care should include both the physical and emotional aspects associated with these disorders. This chapter will differentiate some of the major male reproductive disorders and will discuss both medical and nursing management. Figure 50–1 ■ portrays the normal anatomy of the male genitourinary system.

■ Testicular Disorders

Testicular disorders may arise from inflammation, infection, trauma, or cancer. The most common disorders are discussed here, along with appropriate treatment modalities and nursing care. Health education and prevention are important aspects of nursing care in this section.

Epididymitis: Etiology

Epididymitis is an infection or inflammation of the ductus epididymidis, a crescent-shaped structure found on the posterior aspect of each testicle (Cole & Vogler, 2004). The epididymis functions in the transport of sperm from the testicle to the vas deferens.

An infection of the epididymis may originate at the prostate, the urethra, or the urinary bladder and migrate via the urinary system to the vas deferens and the epididymis (see Figure 50–1 ■).

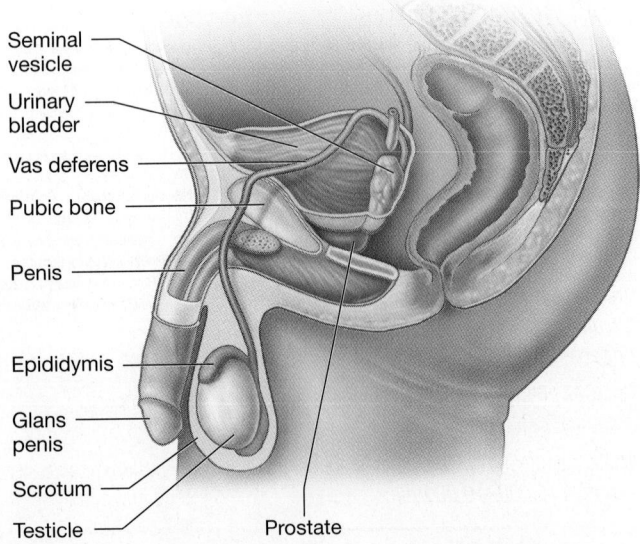

Seminal vesicle
Urinary bladder
Vas deferens
Pubic bone
Penis
Epididymis
Glans penis
Scrotum
Testicle
Prostate

FIGURE 50–1 ■ Normal anatomy of the male genitourinary system.

Infection of the epididymis in men younger than age 35 is more likely to be the result of gonococcal, chlamydial, or ureaplasma organisms. In older men, infection is more likely to be the result of prostatitis, instrumentation of the urinary system, or a structural lesion such as carcinoma of the testis (Goroll & Mulley, 2006). In these cases, the coliform bacteria, especially *Escherichia coli*, are most frequently identified as causative (Cole & Vogler, 2004).

Clinical Manifestations

Symptoms include tenderness and swelling of the epididymis that may spread to the testicle causing a large, tender scrotal mass (Goroll & Mulley, 2006). When a sexually transmitted organism is the cause, dysuria, penile discharge, fever, and pus in the urine or semen may be seen. Inguinal lymph nodes may be enlarged, especially on the side where the location may be situated. The tests outlined in the Diagnostic Tests box can be used to determine a diagnosis of epididymitis.

Medical Management

Medical management of epididymitis includes antibiotics specific to the causative organism identified, analgesics, and nonsteroidal anti-inflammatory agents (NSAIDs). See Chapter 15 ⊚ for a discussion of pain assessment and management. The Pharmacology Summary feature (p. 1585) presents medications used to treat male reproductive disorders.

▪ Nursing Management

Nursing management includes encouraging the patient to maintain bed rest and elevating the scrotum with a towel sling. Elevation and the application of cold to the scrotum will help decrease swelling and pain. Figure 50–2 ▪ (p. 1568) depicts one form of towel sling. Ambulation requires a soft scrotal support that keeps the scrotum close to the body (Karlowicz, 1995). Patients need education about epididymitis, the medications used, and how to avoid a recurrence of the ailment.

Orchitis: Etiology

Orchitis is an inflammation or infection of one or both testes. Infection may be caused by viral or bacterial agents. One viral cause is mumps orchitis which may be seen 7 to 10 days after mumps parotitis or, rarely, it may occur spontaneously (Goroll & Mulley, 2006). Mumps orchitis usually is unilateral and may cause infertility. Men who have never had the mumps and are exposed to the mumps virus require treatment. Like epididymitis, the causative bacterial agents include gonorrhea, chlamydia, and *Escherichia coli*.

 CRITICAL ALERT *Men exposed to the mumps virus who have never had mumps should receive gamma globulin immediately to aid in decreasing the severity of the disease and preserving fertility.*

Clinical Manifestations

Symptoms and diagnostic testing are the same as for epididymitis. It is important to be aware that the symptoms of orchitis closely resemble testicular torsion, a surgical emergency described in the next section of this chapter.

Medical Management

Medical treatment includes the use of antibiotics when appropriate, analgesics, and NSAIDs (see the Pharmacology Summary feature, p. 1585). Viral causes are treated with rest, fluids, and NSAIDs.

▪ Nursing Management

Nursing management includes minimizing activity, elevation of the scrotum using a towel sling or soft support (see Figure 50–2 ▪, p. 1568), and cold compresses to decrease edema and pain. The goal of treatment is to prevent testicular atrophy, infertility, abscess, and impotence. Emotional support is important because of the reproductive concerns. In cases in which antibiotics are needed, teaching should stress the importance of completing the full course of medication prescribed.

Testicular Torsion: Epidemiology and Etiology

Testicular torsion occurs when a mobile testicle causes a twisting of the spermatic cord, essentially closing off the blood supply to the testicle. Loss of blood supply to the testicle will cause ischemia, necrosis, and loss of the testicle if it is not relieved within 6 to 12 hours (Cole & Vogler, 2004).

DIAGNOSTIC TESTS for Epididymitis

Test and Normal Values	Expected Abnormality	Rationale for Abnormality
Urinalysis: *Normally will not have any white blood cells or bacteria*	Elevated white count.	Due to inflammatory/infectious process.
Cultures of any discharge: *Normally will be negative for bacteria*	May be positive for chlamydia, gonorrhea, *Escherichia coli*, etc.	Sexually transmitted infections and coliforms may cause epididymitis.
White blood cells (WBC): *Normal = 5,000–10,000/mm³*	Elevated white count. Shifts indicating acute infection.	Due to inflammatory/infectious process.

Sources: Adapted from Cole, F., & Vogler, R. (2004). The acute, nontraumatic scrotum: Assessment, diagnosis and management. *Journal of the American Academy of Nurse Practitioners, 16*(2), 50–56; and Fischbach, F. (2003). *A manual of laboratory and diagnostic tests* (7th ed.). Philadelphia: Lippincott Williams & Wilkins.

Towel sling scrotal support

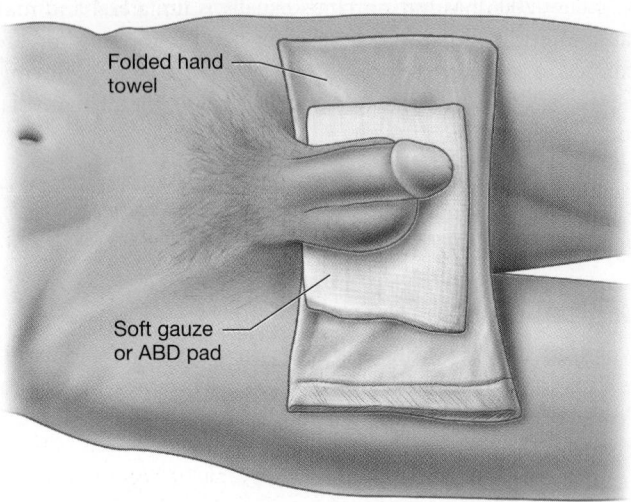

Folded hand towel

Soft gauze or ABD pad

FIGURE 50–2 ■ Scrotal supports.

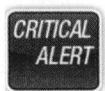
CRITICAL ALERT *Sudden onset of scrotal/testicular pain without injury in an adolescent should be considered testicular torsion until proven otherwise. Surgical intervention to preserve the testicle should occur within 6 to 12 hours of occurrence.*

Annually, 1 in 4,000 males under the age of 25 experience testicular torsion (Ringdahl & Teague, 2006). The process for the development of this problem begins with the congenital absence of attachment of the testicle to the tunica vaginalis. Without this attachment, the testicle hangs freely and can easily twist on the cord (Cole & Vogler, 2004). The left testicle is more at risk because of the longer spermatic cord.

Clinical Manifestations

Clinical manifestations include sudden, severe pain in one testicle, nausea, vomiting, and light-headedness. On examination, the testicle will be high in the scrotum due to the shortening of the spermatic cord. Figure 50–3 ■ depicts the twisting and shortening of the spermatic cord. The affected testicle may also feel larger than normal, and the cremasteric reflex (the testicle will rise in the scrotum when the thigh near the scrotum is stroked) will be absent (Ringdahl & Teague, 2006). Diagnosis is confirmed with Doppler ultrasound.

Medical Management

Medical treatment for testicular torsion is immediate surgery. The testicle and cord are untwisted, and if the testicle is viable, it is anchored to the scrotum (**orchiopexy**) to prevent recurrence. If the testicle is nonviable, then it is removed (**orchiectomy**). Before and after surgery, the patient will require analgesia (Ringdahl & Teague, 2006). See Chapter 15 for a discussion of pain assessment and management.

■ Nursing Management

Nursing care of boys and men experiencing testicular torsion usually begins in the postoperative period and includes bed rest, observation for bleeding or drainage on the dressing, monitor-

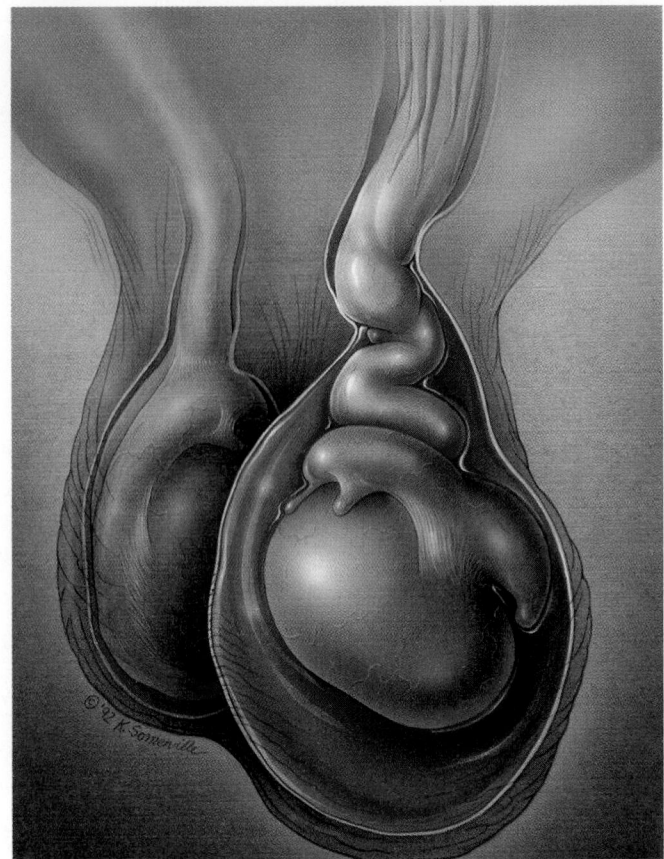

FIGURE 50–3 ■ Testicular torsion.
Source: Kevin A. Somerville/Phototake NYC

ing vital signs, administering analgesics, and providing scrotal support. The towel sling (see Figure 50–2 ■) can be used while the patient is in bed. Ambulation will require a soft scrotal support that keeps the scrotum close to the body (Karlowicz, 1995). Education of the patient and his parents would include information about the analgesic action and side effects and the importance of follow-up visits with the urologist or surgeon. When the adolescent reaches ages 14 to 16, a testicular prosthesis can be implanted if desired (Ringdahl & Teague, 2006).

Hydrocele: Epidemiology and Etiology

The space between the tunica vaginalis and the testicle may fill with fluid causing a hydrocele (Goroll & Mulley, 2006). This is the most common cause of scrotal swelling. In the newborn male, hydrocele develops when fluid that surrounds the testicles does not absorb after the closure of the tunica vaginalis *in utero*. In older males, hydrocele may develop after infection in the scrotum, injury, radiation, or testicular cancer. There are also incidences of idiopathic hydrocele among elderly males (Every, Mikkelsen, & Bailey, 2005).

Clinical Manifestations

Clinical manifestations include scrotal swelling that transluminates (light source behind the swollen scrotum will cause a glow as the light penetrates the fluid). The swelling is not painful unless there is so much fluid that it causes increased pressure on the testes (Goroll & Mulley, 2006).

Medical Management

Medical management is usually conservative, as the fluid will be reabsorbed in time. Should the swelling increase to painful levels, the fluid can be aspirated or surgically drained to prevent damage to the testes (Every, Mikkelsen, & Bailey, 2005).

■ Nursing Management

Nursing care depends on the extent of the hydrocele. For newborns with hydrocele, the care is the same as for all newborns. For adults, elevation of the scrotum may help. If surgery is required, postoperative care is similar to the postoperative care for testicular torsion.

Spermatocele: Etiology, Epidemiology, and Clinical Manifestations

Spermatoceles are painless, sperm-containing cysts that occur on the upper portion of the testis near the epididymis. These cysts are thought to be caused by an occlusion of the efferent (outflow) spermatic ducts of the testis. Usually only one testis is affected and the cyst is 1 centimeter or less in size (Scrotal Masses, 2005).

While most spermatoceles go unnoticed, some become large enough to annoy the male or the cyst may be found coincidentally in males who seek help for infertility (Bazar et al., 2003). On physical examination, the cyst is palpable and transluminates. Translumination helps differentiate this fluid-filled cyst from a solid nodule that is more likely to be testicular cancer. Diagnosis is verified by ultrasound (Goroll & Mulley, 2006).

Medical Management

Medical management for those rare spermatoceles that grow large enough to disfigure or cause pain is inguinoscrotal surgery to remove the mass (Bazar et al., 2003). Patients who require surgery can be reassured that the procedure does not affect fertility or virility (Goroll & Mulley, 2006).

Varicocele: Epidemiology and Etiology

A varicocele is an enlargement of the veins of the pampiniform plexus within the scrotum. It develops because of incompetent venous valves just like varicose veins in the legs. Varicoceles are most likely to occur on the left because the left spermatic vein empties directly into the renal vein causing increased hydrostatic back pressure within the vein when the patient stands (Goroll & Mulley, 2006). About 15% of all males and 40% of males who have infertility have varicocele (Quallich, 2006). The cause is unknown and there are no specific risk factors.

Clinical Manifestations

Signs and symptoms of varicocele include a "bag of worms" appearance to the scrotum that decreases in size when the patient is recumbent. The varicocele is usually not painful, but some men will notice a dull ache and fullness or pulling to the affected side of the scrotum after prolonged standing (Quallich, 2006).

Medical Management

Medical management is not necessary unless there are symptoms or infertility. Surgical treatment may be used to seal the affected

vein and redirect blood flow to a normal vein if the varicocele is painful. Surgery has not improved fertility (Quallich, 2006).

Undescended or Mispositioned Testicles: Epidemiology, Etiology, and Clinical Manifestations

When one or both testes are not in the scrotum at birth, it is called cryptorchidism. During gestation, the testes form inside the abdomen and, normally, move down into the scrotum at term. Occasionally, the testicle may be misdirected as it emerges from the inguinal canal into areas other than the scrotum (Every, Mikkelsen, & Bailey, 2005). Figure 50–4 ■ depicts some of the extrascrotal sites.

Cryptorchidism occurs in 0.7% to 1% of male infants at birth (Every, Mikkelsen, & Bailey, 2005). The cause may be a testicular or hormonal defect. Undescended testicles become fibrotic and spermatogenesis does not occur. In addition, there is an increased risk for testicular cancer in the cryptorchid testes.

Medical Management

Medical treatment is usually postponed until the child is 1 year of age. If the testis is still undescended at this time, the testis is brought down into the scrotum and orchiopexy is performed. This is an outpatient procedure with few side effects and the baby recovers quickly.

Testicular Cancer: Etiology and Epidemiology

Cancer that forms in the tissue of the testis usually occurs in men between the ages of 20 and 39. It is the most common form of cancer in Caucasian men between the ages of 15 and 34 (National Cancer Institute [NCI], 2007c). It is estimated that testicular cancer will occur in 7,920 men in the United States in 2007. Of these, approximately 380 will die of the disease (NCI, 2007c). Men of Scandinavian descent are at greatest

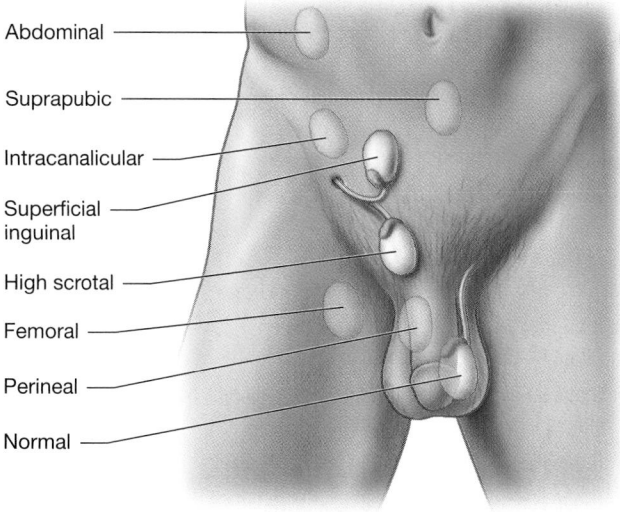

Ectopic testes
Cryptorchism

Abdominal

Suprapubic

Intracanalicular

Superficial inguinal

High scrotal

Femoral

Perineal

Normal

FIGURE 50–4 ■ Extrascrotal testicular sites.

risk, but overall the rate of occurrence has increased by 200% in the last 40 years. Other risk factors include familial history (especially siblings), prior personal history, cryptorchidism, Klinefelter's syndrome, natural exposure to gestational estrogen, and exposure to insecticides (Brown, 2004; Goroll & Mulley, 2006).

Pathophysiology

Testicular cancer may arise from a germ cell, stromal cell, or nongerm cell of the testes. Nongerminal neoplasms originate from Leydig cells or stromal cells and occur less frequently. Germinal tumors account for 95% of testicular tumors and are generally divided into two groups: seminomas that are slow growing and nonseminomas that are more aggressive. Nonseminomas have four subtypes: embryonal, yolk sac, choriocarcinoma, and teratoma (Every, Mikklesen, & Bailey, 2005; Stevenson & McNeill, 2004). Teratoma subtypes are the least likely to metastasize, whereas choriocarcinomas are the most likely to metastasize (NCI, 2007c).

Clinical Manifestations

Usually, a solid, painless, nontransluminating lump is found on the testicle of a young man. Some men will have a dull discomfort or heaviness in the scrotum and lower abdomen. Occasionally, the scrotum will swell. Many testicular cancers are first diagnosed as epididymitis or orchitis and treated with antibiotics. When the lump does not resolve, further studies reveal the malignancy. Testicular tumors have also been found coincident to sports injuries to the groin or genitals. A small number of men may first seek medical advice because of **gynecomastia** (enlargement of the male breast) caused by testicular tumors that secrete beta human chorionic gonadotropin (HCG) (Brown, 2004). Men with metastatic disease may complain of cough, hemoptysis, and weight loss. Chapter 64 @ has an in-depth discussion of the diagnosis and treatment of cancer.

Diagnostic Testing and Staging

The first line of diagnostic testing after a lump is found is ultrasonography of the scrotum. Ultrasound is excellent for differentiating cancer from epididymitis or hydrocele. Once the tumor is identified, chest x-ray, computed tomographic (CT) scan of the abdomen, and serum markers are obtained in order to stage the cancer (Brown, 2004). The commonly used staging system appears in Chart 50–1. Testicular cancer produces a predictable spread to the retroperitoneum, lungs, and mediastinum (Stevenson & McNeill, 2004). Fine needle or open biopsy is never done because of the danger of seeding the scrotum with the cancer cells

and causing a more rapid dissemination of the cancer to the abdomen and lungs (Goroll & Mulley, 2006; NCI, 2007c).

Serum tumor markers include beta human chorionic gonadotropin (secreted by most choriocarcinomas and about 50% of other nonseminomas), alpha-fetoprotein, and lactate dehydrogenase. These serum markers are used to detect disease, to monitor response to treatment, and as a surveillance tool following treatment (NCI, 2007c). A rise in the serum markers during chemotherapy indicates relapse or failure to respond to treatment. An elevation in serum markers a year after treatment indicates recurrence and the need for chemotherapy. The Diagnostic Tests box offers further explanation of tumor markers.

Medical Management

Medical management decisions depend on the type of tumor, the stage of the disease, and tumor markers. Seminomatous testicular tumors, Stages I and II, are treated by orchiectomy via an inguinal route and retroperitoneal node irradiation (NCI, 2007c). This combination will result in 100% cure rates. Side effects of radiation therapy include fatigue, skin changes, loss of appetite, nausea, diarrhea, and reduced sperm production. Sperm production from the remaining testicle does recover, but it will take 1 to 2 years after radiation. Seminomatous tumors at Stage III or above may be treated pre- and postorchiectomy with cisplatin-based chemotherapy that results in cure rates of about 90% (Goroll & Mulley, 2006). See the Pharmacology Summary feature (p. 1585).

Nonseminomatous testicular tumors in Stages I and II require only the surgical removal of the affected testicle. The cure rate for surgery is about 95% (Goroll & Mulley, 2006). Higher stages of the nonseminomatous tumors require chemotherapy. Cisplatin-based multiple-agent chemotherapy is highly effective, even in patients with metastatic disease. This newest chemotherapy for testicular cancers has decreased the need for wide lymphadenectomy.

Follow-up medical surveillance is very important. For the first year, the patient is seen monthly. For years 2 and 3, he is evaluated every other month; every 3 months in the third year; and every 6 months in the fourth and fifth years. The majority of recurrences will occur within the first 2 years, but relapse can occur even beyond that time. Examinations should include physical examination, tumor markers, chest x-ray, and CT scans of the abdomen and pelvis should be done every 3 to 6 months (NCI, 2007c; Segal et al., 2001).

■ Nursing Management

Nursing care for men newly diagnosed with testicular cancer requires a high degree of emotional support. The men experiencing this cancer face altered sexuality, body image, role function, and fertility. They often fear loss of masculinity and must come face to face with their own mortality. Reassurance that orchiectomy does not cause **impotence** (problems associated with ejaculation or orgasm, in addition to erectile dysfunction) or infertility and that masculinity will remain intact is important. Open discussion of sexuality and the genitalia will allow the patient to express his worries without embarrassment. Review of the surgical procedure, the treatment planned, and the cure rates of these treatments will also help alleviate fear. Keep communications with the patient clear, concrete, and open.

CHART 50–1 **Staging of Testicular Cancer**

- Stage I—Cancer is confined to the testicle.
- Stage II—Cancer has spread to retroperitoneal nodes, but disease is limited to below the diaphragm.
- Stage III—Cancer has spread above the diaphragm.
- Stage IV—Tumor has spread to other organs.

Source: Adapted from Goroll, A., & Mulley, A. (2006). *Primary care medicine: Office evaluation and management of the adult patient* (5th ed.). Philadelphia: Lippincott Williams & Wilkins.

DIAGNOSTIC TESTS for Testicular Cancer Using Tumor Markers

Test and *Normal Values*	Expected Abnormality	Rationale for Abnormality
Human chorionic gonadotropin (HCG): *Produced in the syncytiotrophoblasts Normal range < 2 ng/mL or no measurable amount*	Increased in seminoma, embryonal, and choriocarcinoma tumors.	Used to detect tumors too small to be detected by x-ray or computed tomography (CT) scan.
Alpha-fetoprotein (AFP): *Produced in the liver, GI tract, fetal yolk sac Normal range < 15 ng/mL*	Elevated in yolk sac tumors.	Used to detect tumors too small to be detected by x-ray or CT scan. Also elevated when there is liver damage.
Lactate dehydrogenase (LDH): *Normal range 70–250 units/L*	Nonspecific.	Useful in staging of seminomas and nonseminomatous germ cell tumors. Also elevated in hemolysis, liver and muscle disease, and myocardial infarction.

Source: Adapted from National Academy of Clinical Biochemistry (NACB). (2006). *Tumor markers PDF. Practice guidelines and recommendations for use of tumor markers in the clinic: Testicular Cancer (section 3A).* Retrieved March 30, 2007, from http://www.aacc.org/Pages/default.aspx

Nursing Interventions and Health Promotion

Preoperatively, the patient will need information about postoperative incision care, analgesia, and pulmonary toileting. Presurgical laboratory tests will need to be obtained. See Chapter 25 ⊙ for review of preoperative teaching. The possibility for testicle prosthesis may be discussed, should the patient feel that this would improve his body image (Brown, 2004).

There is usually bowel preparation because an abdominal inguinal incision is used, even for simple orchiectomy. This may be done at home before admission for surgery or after admission. The patient needs to know that he should avoid aspirin and other NSAIDs about a week prior to surgery to decrease bleeding risks (Stevenson & McNeill, 2004). This is a very stressful time and education will need to be repeated and reinforced.

Some patients with testicular cancer may be receiving chemotherapy before surgery. If one of the agents used is bleomycin, lung toxicity may have occurred and pulmonary risks are increased. Close monitoring of respiratory function will be needed.

Postoperatively, emotional support is needed as staging the cancer proceeds. Anxiety and fear may require that the nurse continue to repeat information. If the surgery includes extensive retroperitoneal lymph node removal, the patient may be in the hospital for about a week. During the recovery time, pain control, fluids, monitoring the incision for bleeding or infection, pulmonary toileting, and monitoring vital signs for elevated temperature or shortness of breath are all part of routine care. (See Chapter 27 ⊙ for postoperative care and Chapter 15 ⊙ for pain assessment and management.) All postoperative patients are at increased risk for deep venous thrombosis and should begin to ambulate on the first day. Pain management before ambulation will ease the discomfort and help them to be more willing to move.

Patients who have seminomas will begin radiation therapy before discharge. Radiation therapy will involve the retroperitoneal area and will require education for the patient about what to expect. Side effects of irradiation include nausea, vomiting, diarrhea, fatigue, skin changes, and loss of appetite (Brown, 2004; NCI, 2007d). An antidiarrheal and an antiemetic will be needed. Cisplatin-based multiagent chemotherapy will begin for pa-

tients with nonseminomas or cancers that have spread outside the testicle. Chemotherapy offers systemic therapy, reaching cancer cells anywhere in the body. Common side effects are nausea, hair loss, fatigue, diarrhea, vomiting, fever, chills, cough, mouth sores, and skin rash. Other, less common side effects include numbness, loss of reflexes, impaired hearing, and decreased to absent sperm production (NCI, 2007c). Nursing care will include emotional support, assistance with oral hygiene, antidiarrheal and antiemetic medications such as Zofran (ondansetron), and skin care. See the Pharmacology Summary feature (p. 1585).

Discharge priorities for the patient with testicular cancer are delineated in the Patient Teaching & Discharge Priorities box (p. 1572).

Health Promotion

Young men at risk for testicular cancer are not likely to receive education about self-testicular examination. In addition, they are not likely to have a testicular examination on routine physical or during a visit to the health care provider for another reason (Brown, 2004). Nurses are in a key position to encourage and to teach self-testicular examination in their community. The Testicular Cancer Resource Center has patient instruction programs to help nurses reach young men with this important information (Testicular Cancer Resource Center, 2007).

It has been recommended that men over age 50 receive Digital rectal exam (DRE) and PSA tests every year. If the screening tests indicate a need, then transrectal ultrasound guided biopsy should be done and repeated every 3 years (Gray & Sims, 2006).

Health fairs or community programs designed to include the African American man can be especially beneficial. African American men have the highest incidence of prostate cancer in the world (NCI, 2007b). In addition, they are less likely to seek care. A culturally sensitive program within the community is more apt to attract these men and to save lives (Ward-Smith, 2006).

■ Prostate Disorders

The prostate gland is located under the urinary bladder at the bladder neck and in front of the rectum in men (see Figure 50–1 ■, p. 1566). It is primarily made up of smooth muscle and

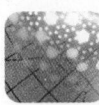

PATIENT TEACHING & DISCHARGE PRIORITIES for Testicular Cancer

Need	Teaching
Knowledge of disease process and prognosis	Home care needs include verbal and written instructions for: 1. The treatment plan, including continued radiation therapy or chemotherapy appointments 2. Follow-up care and appointments with the health care provider 3. Activity restriction.
Understanding of medications	If chemotherapy is to continue, patient/family is taught how to care for the infusion site using aseptic technique. Teach the purpose, dose, timing, and possible side effects of all medications.
Reportable clinical manifestations	Instruct patient/family to report: 1. Bleeding or drainage at the incision site 2. Fever 101°F 3. Signs of deep venous thrombosis 4. Signs of pulmonary embolism or other lung problems.
Patient/family support system	Assess availability of, knowledge of, and compliance with treatment regimen. Assess home environment for need for assistive devices. Assess for need for professional home health services. Offer cancer support resources.
Emotional adjustment of patient/family due to diagnosis of cancer	Answer questions honestly. Encourage verbalization of frustration and anger. Discuss adjustments that will need to be made at home.

collagen enclosed in a fibrous capsule. The urethra passes through the prostate. When semen moves through the prostatic portion of the urethra, the prostate secretes prostatic fluid that increases the pH of semen to help sperm survive in the more acidic female reproductive system (Every, Mikkelsen, & Cagle, 2005). Disorders of the prostate include inflammation, infection, hyperplasia, and cancer. This section discusses each of these disorders.

Prostatitis: Etiology

Inflammation of the prostate gland (**prostatitis**) may be acute, chronic, infectious, or noninfectious. Chronic prostatitis is more common and may persist long after the bacteria are eradicated. In fact, 90% of patients with chronic prostatitis have sterile ejaculate and urine (Goodson, 2006). The National Institutes of Health has developed a consensus classification system for prostatitis, which is outlined in the National Guidelines box.

Acute prostatitis may arise from ascending urinary infection, rectal infection, or bloodborne pathogens. Gram-negative coliforms are the usual causative bacteria, especially *Escherichia coli*, *Proteus*, *Klebsiella*, and enterococci. Less frequently, sexually transmitted *Chlamydia*, ureaplasma (virus), or *Trichomonas* may be the causative agent (Goodson, 2006). Causes of chronic or abacterial prostatitis are not always identifiable. It has been theorized that increased levels of purine, uric acid, or pyrimidine may have gotten into the prostatic ducts causing inflammation. Some health care provider researchers believe it may be an autoimmune disorder (McNaughton Collins, MacDonald, & Wilt, 1999/2008).

Clinical Manifestations

The clinical presentation differs depending on the type of prostatitis the patient has contracted. Chart 50–2 summarizes the symptoms according to prostatitis type.

Laboratory and Diagnostic Procedures

Diagnostic testing for prostatitis would include urinalysis, pre- and postprostatic massage urine, and a digital rectal examination (DRE). For older men, a urine cytology should also be done.

NATIONAL GUIDELINES for the Classification of Prostatitis

I. Acute bacterial prostatitis

II. Chronic bacterial prostatitis

III. Chronic prostatitis/chronic pelvic pain syndrome
   IIIa Inflammatory
   IIIb Noninflammatory

IV. Asymptomatic inflammatory prostatitis (discovered incidentally)

Source: Adapted from NIH Consensus Classification System for Prostatitis in Prostatitis: Prostate disease (2005). *Merck manual professional.* Retrieved March 30, 2007, from http://www.merck.com/mmpe/sec17/ch240/ch240c.html

---

CHART 50–2	Clinical Manifestations of Acute and Chronic Prostatitis
Acute Prostatitis	**Chronic Prostatitis**
Flu-like symptoms: fever, chills, myalgia, malaise Pain in genitalia, pelvis, or low back Dysuria, nocturia, urgency, frequency Hematuria Painful ejaculation	Recurrent episodes of infection Symptoms same but milder Abacterial prostatodynia Pain in pelvis Painful ejaculation

Sources: Adapted from Porche, D. (2006). Prostatitis. *Journal of Nurse Practitioners, 2*(10), 662–663; and Prostatitis: Prostate disease (2005). *Merck manual professional.* Retrieved March 30, 2007, from http://www.merck.com/mmpe/sec17/ch240/ch240c.html

Prostate Cancer

Clinical Problem

Early diagnosis and treatment of prostate cancer has increased the time the patient and his spouse must cope with treatment regimens for the cancer. These treatments cause severe side effects including fatigue, incontinence, sexual dysfunction, threatened body image, and loss of masculinity. These insults to quality of life have a profound effect on the patient and his wife. Sometimes the health care team does not include the spouse in the patient's care. This can also have a pervasive effect on the wife and the patient. Nurses, especially, should be attuned to the needs of the spouse and assist her whenever possible.

Research Findings

Hawes et al. (2006) conducted a descriptive, cross-sectional study of 66 couples in their homes as part of an experimental intervention program in problem-solving therapy. The spouses of patients were asked to report two problems they believed were important to solve during the study. From this descriptive arm of the study, it was learned that the spouse issue of maintaining a balanced life and emotional wellness was most often listed as a concern. Second most listed was the patient's issue of lack of communication, fear, and depression. The third most frequently listed issue was treatment and side-effect issues.

Implications for Nursing Practice

Wives of men with prostate cancer need support and guidance. Nurses should recognize that the problems wives face when their husbands are ill are not solely from the husband's diagnosis and treatment regimen. Wives should be given the opportunity to discuss problems with balancing their lives and maintaining emotional wellness. If there are problems within the relationship, such as lack of communication, these could undermine the couple's ability to cope with treatment-related issues. Nurses can begin a discussion with the wife, explore what she finds stressful, and offer problem-solving guidelines.

Anticipating problems when a new treatment regimen is planned and initiating discussions with the patient and his wife will help them both to cope and problem solve.

Critical Thinking Questions

1. Why should spouses of men with prostate cancer be offered support and be included in care planning for the patient?

2. In this descriptive study, the investigators discovered three leading problems identified by the participants. Using these identified problems as a guide, describe the most important points about guiding and nurturing spouses and patients with prostate cancer.
   a. Help the wife balance multiple demands and maintain emotional balance.
   b. Help the wife by anticipating problems and preparing her for challenges.
   c. Initiate discussions with spouses and patients to help them problem solve.
   d. Involve the spouse in medical decision making along with her husband, the patient.

Answers to Critical Thinking Questions appear in Appendix D.

Reference

Hawes, S., Malcarne, V., Ko, C., Sadler, G., Banthia, R., Sherman, S., et al. (2006). Identifying problems faced by spouses and partners of patients with prostate cancer. *Oncology Nursing Forum, 33*(4), 807–814.

EVIDENCE-BASED PRACTICE

The urinalysis is collected in four different sterile containers. The first 10 milliliters of urine is from the urethra, the midstream urine is from the bladder, and the last few drops are premassage prostatic urine. After massage of the prostate, another urinalysis is obtained. All of the urine samples are cultured, with the infective agent to the prostate recovered from the postmassage specimen (Goodson, 2006; Porche, 2006). A prostate-specific antigen (PSA) test may be done. It is expected to be higher and it is nonspecific, but it does give supporting evidence for a diagnosis of prostatitis.

Medical Management

Medical management decisions depend on the type of prostatitis the patient has and the infective agent identified. Bacterial prostatitis is treated with appropriate antibiotics. The Pharmacology Summary feature (p. 1585) gives more details about antibiotic treatment. Antibiotics are given orally for a period of 30 days in an attempt to prevent chronic prostatitis. If the patient becomes septic, he may be admitted for care and be given IV antibiotic therapy until he is afebrile for 24 to 48 hours (Prostatitis: Prostate Disease, 2005). When the patient is discharged, oral therapy will continue for 4 to 6 weeks.

Some health care providers will use other drugs such as alpha blockers, NSAIDs, muscle relaxants, stool softeners, and in the case of chronic pelvic pain, anxiolytics (Porche, 2006; Prostatitis: Prostate Disease, 2005). Symptomatic treatments may include sitz baths, prostate massage, pelvic floor exercises, and microwave therapy. Microwave therapy is a transurethral heat treatment used more often in benign prostatic hyperplasia, which is discussed later in this chapter.

■ Nursing Management

Nursing care for patients with prostatitis includes education about the disease, the medications used, and the treatments to help decrease pain and swelling of the prostate. If the patient is admitted for sepsis related to prostatitis, IV antibiotic therapy will be given. This will require education of the patient about the medication and its side effects and close monitoring of the patient for signs of worsening condition. The nurse will also help with sitz baths and other comfort measures. When the patient is discharged, he and his family will need education about the disease; the medications; the need to continue the antibiotic for 4 to 6 weeks as prescribed and why; and the importance of follow-up visits with the health care provider. The Patient Teaching & Discharge Priorities box (p. 1574) lists some teaching points important for the patient with prostatitis.

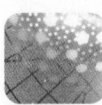

PATIENT TEACHING & DISCHARGE PRIORITIES for Prostatitis

Need	Teaching
Patient/Family/support system	Continue antibiotics as prescribed.
Patient/Family/support system	Report continuation or worsening of symptoms to health care provider.
Patient	Regular voiding and complete emptying of bladder.
Patient	Increase fluids, such as water, to 64 to 128 ounces per day to flush the bladder.
Patient	Avoid beverages and food that are irritating to the bladder: • Alcohol • Caffeine • Citrus juices • Hot/spicy foods.

Benign Prostatic Hyperplasia

Benign prostatic hyperplasia (BPH) is nonmalignant, nodular growth of prostatic tissue that eventually compresses the urethra, causing lower urinary tract symptoms (LUTS) (Beckman & Mynderse, 2005; McVary, 2006). BPH is a common disorder of aging men, occurring in as many as 90% of men ages 85 and older (Kuritzky, Rosenberg, & Sadovsky, 2006; McVary, 2006).

Etiology and Epidemiology

The exact cause of BPH is not known; however, one theory is that BPH may result from a "restart" of the same induction process of the prostate that occurs in the embryo (McVary, 2006). Another theory is that testosterone and estrogens levels change with age (Alper & Crawford, 2005).

Pathophysiology

Nodules form at the transition zone, or innermost aspect of the prostate gland, along the urethra in response to the change in hormones (McVary, 2006). Because the prostate is expandable and elastic, urethral constriction may not occur until the prostate is significantly enlarged. Also, neuronal control over prostatic smooth muscle differs among men, making lower urinary tract symptoms unpredictable.

As the urinary urethra constricts, it causes increased pressure to urinate, thereby causing bladder distention, eventual hypertrophy of the detrusor muscle, bladder diverticula, urinary stasis, infection, and bladder stone formation. If the obstruction is prolonged, **hydronephrosis** (backflow of urine into the renal pelvis) will occur and cause damage to the kidneys (Benign Prostatic Hyperplasia, 2005).

Clinical Manifestations

Clinical manifestations of BPH are varied. Some men who have BPH do not develop lower urinary tract symptoms (LUTS) or acute urinary retention (AUR) (O'Leary, 2006). Others will present with obstructive or irritative symptoms that significantly affect their quality of life. Chart 50–3 lists the signs and symptoms of BPH. The American Urological Association (AUA) has developed a symptom index tool that can be used to quantify the symptoms of BPH for each patient. The AUA Symptom Score is used both in diagnosing and for monitoring therapeutic response. It is a seven-question exploration of symptoms that

CHART 50–3 Clinical Manifestations of Benign Prostatic Hyperplasia

Urinary hesitancy and intermittency

Weak urine stream

Nocturia, frequency, and urgency

Sensation of incomplete bladder emptying

Terminal dribbling of urine

Overflow incontinence

Complete urinary retention

Hematuria if straining at urination is severe

Enlarged, rubbery prostate that has lost the median furrow

Full urinary bladder palpable on abdominal examination

Urinary tract infection

Bladder stones and diverticuli

Renal damage, insufficiency, and failure after prolonged urinary retention

Sources: Adapted from Benign prostatic hyperplasia (BPH). (2005). *Merck manual professional.* Retrieved April 4, 2007, from http://www.merck.com/mmpe/sec17/ch240/ch240b.html; O'Leary, M. (2006). Treatment and pharmacologic management of BPH in the context of common comorbidities. *American Journal of Managed Care, 12*(Suppl. 5), S129–S140; and McVary, K. (2006). BPH: Epidemiology and comorbidities. *American Journal of Managed Care, 12*(Suppl. 5), S122–S128.

the patient can answer while waiting to be seen. The score allows the health care provider to match treatment options with the severity of the symptoms for each patient (Beckman & Mynderse, 2005; Benign Prostatic Hyperplasia, 2005).

Laboratory and Diagnostic Procedures

Diagnostic testing for BPH begins with the AUA Symptom Index. The next step is history and physical examination, including evaluation for neurological deficits and a digital rectal examination (DRE) of the prostate gland. Chapter 48 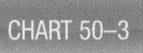 describes the DRE more fully. Other tests that may be used include urinalysis, serum blood urea nitrogen and creatinine, postvoid residual urine measurement, and uroflow rate studies that assess voiding patterns. If hematuria, urinary tract infection, or signs of renal failure are discovered, then renal imaging, urine cytology studies, and cystoscopy may be done (Alper & Crawford, 2005). The prostate-specific antigen (PSA) is sometimes used to differenti-

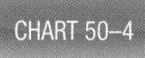

ate BPH from prostate cancer. The PSA is described more fully in the Cancer of the Prostate section later in this chapter.

Medical Management

Patients who have developed LUTS seek medical advice because of the discomfort. Treatment will depend on the impact on the patient's quality of life, the presence of comorbidities such as diabetes or heart disease, and the severity of the urinary problem (O'Leary, 2006). Treatment modalities vary from watchful waiting to radical surgery.

Medication and Treatments

Patients with mild symptoms who are willing to make some lifestyle changes can usually postpone medical or surgical intervention for a time. Lifestyle changes would include such things as decreasing fluid intake at bedtime to decrease nocturia, decreasing caffeine and alcohol intake because of the irritation to the urinary system, and limiting prescription and over-the-counter drugs that may affect urination (Beckman & Mynderse, 2005; O'Leary, 2006). Chart 50–4 lists medications that may affect urination. Patients who choose watchful waiting are evaluated annually or when worsening symptoms occur.

Medication therapy has replaced surgery as the most common treatment of BPH (Beckman & Mynderse, 2005). Two primary drug types are used to reduce LUTS: alpha-adrenergic antagonists and 5-alpha reductase inhibitors. Alpha-adrenergic antagonists work by relaxing the bladder neck and prostatic muscle tone, thereby relieving obstruction. Newer alpha-adrenergic antagonists selectively reduce the prostatic smooth muscle tone and do not affect the blood pressure (Barry, 2006).

The second class of medication for BPH is the 5-alpha reductase inhibitors that work by reducing the conversion of testosterone. This slows prostate growth; however, it takes 6 to 12

CHART 50–4	**Medications That May Affect Urination**

Diuretics cause urinary frequency.

Sympathomimetic agents such as ephedrine cause increased urethral sphincter contractility.

Anticholinergic drugs such as atropine, Spiriva, and Vesicare cause decreased detrusor contractility.

Antihistamines and antidepressants have caused lower urinary tract symptoms (LUTS) in older men.

Over-the-counter drugs, especially cold remedies, cause LUTS by various mechanisms.

Opiates (Oxymorphone, meperidine) may cause urinary retention and urinary tract spasms.

Skeletal muscle relaxants (methocarbamol) may cause renal impairment.

Sources: Adapted from Alper, B., & Crawford, E. (2005). Benign prostatic hyperplasia. *The Clinical Advisor, 8*(10), 119–121; and Beckman, T., & Mynderse, L. (2005). Evaluation and medical management of benign prostatic hyperplasia. *Mayo Clinic Proceedings, 80*(10), 1356–1362.

months of drug therapy to see the full effect (Beckman & Mynderse, 2005). More about the different drugs used for BPH can be found in the Pharmacology Summary feature (p. 1585).

Many men wanting to prevent or decrease symptoms of BPH choose herbal remedies such as *Pygeum africanum* (African star grass), African plum tree bark, rye grass pollens, stinging nettle, and cactus flower (Buck, 2004). The most popular of the herbal remedies is saw palmetto (*Serenoa repens*). The Complementary and Alternative Therapies box presents some types of alternative therapies that are available. Saw palmetto has been studied in

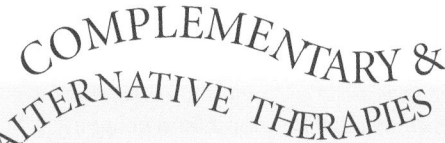

COMPLEMENTARY & ALTERNATIVE THERAPIES   **Types of Therapies**

Type of Therapy	Proposed Clinical Use	Nursing Responsibility
Nutriceuticals Vitamin E Vitamin K (para-aminobenzoate) Lycopene, selenium, Vitamin E, calcium, green tea, phytoestrogens	Varied success in treatment of Peyronie's disease. Decrease risk for prostate cancer, under study.	Fat soluble vitamins in excess are harmful. Investigate the amount the patient is taking. Not associated with adverse affects and good for overall health.
Saw palmetto (*Serenoa repens*)	Antiandrogenic, anti-inflammatory, and antiproliferative actions have been claimed. A recent study seems to show there is no difference in lower urinary tract symptoms (LUTS) among men who take this herbal versus placebo.	Ask the patient with prostate problems whether he has been taking saw palmetto. This will cause changes in the prostate-specific antigen (PSA).
Pygeum Africanum	Antiandrogenic action slows growth of prostate; relieves nocturia.	Ask the patient whether he is using this alternative. No adverse effects but questionable efficacy.

Sources: Adapted from Argyriou, A., Chroni, E., Koutras, A., Iconomou, G., et al. (2006). A randomized controlled trial evaluating the efficacy and safety of vitamin E supplementation for protection against cisplatin-induced peripheral neuropathy: Final results. *Supportive Care in Cancer: Official Journal of the Multinational Association of Supportive Care in Cancer, 14*(11), 1134–1140; Bent, S., et al. (2006). Saw palmetto for benign prostatic hyperplasia. *New England Journal of Medicine, 354*(6), 557–566; Buck, A. (2004). Is there a scientific basis for the therapeutic effects of *Serenoa repens* in benign prostatic hyperplasia? Mechanisms of action. *The Journal of Urology, 172*(5, Pt. 1), 1792–1799; Gray, M., & Sims, T. (2006). Prostate cancer: Prevention and management of localized disease. *The Nurse Practitioner, 31*(9), 15–28; Ishani, A., MacDonald, R., Nelson, D., Rutks, J., & Wilt, T. (2000). *Pygeum africanum* for the treatment of patients with benign prostatic hyperplasia: A systematic review and quantitative meta-analysis. *American Journal of Medicine, 109*(8), 654–664; and Peyronie's disease: Penile and scrotal disorders. (2005). *Merck manual professional.* Retrieved March 31, 2007, from http://www.merck.com/mmpe/print/sec17/ch239/ch239f.html

Europe and the United States and has been proven safe. However, a double-blind, randomized trial that included 225 men over age 49 studied the effects of saw palmetto versus placebo and found that the two groups had similar LUTS at the end of 1 year (Bent et al., 2006).

Surgery

Although many men with BPH respond to medication therapy, there are those who do not want to take the medication for life, who are unable to tolerate the medications, or whose prostate continues to enlarge. These men are candidates for more invasive therapy. The mainstay of surgeries for BPH is transurethral resection of the prostate (TURP), wherein a resectoscope is passed through the urethra, a cystoscope is passed through the resectoscope to visualize the bladder and urethra, and a removable loop of resectoscope cuts prostate tissue and coagulates bleeding vessels. Continuous irrigation is needed to prevent blood clotting. Postoperative side effects may include erectile dysfunction, **retrograde ejaculation** (backflow of semen into the bladder at ejaculation), and, in about 1% of cases, incontinence (Benign Prostatic Hyperplasia, 2005; Nickel, 2006).

Transurethral microwave heat treatment (TUMT) and transurethral needle ablation (TUNA) are forms of thermoablation of the prostate. These are alternative operative therapies wherein microwave heat is used to coagulate prostate tissue. A microwave antenna is placed in the urethra and radiofrequency is passed into the prostate via needles. The device is surrounded by a cooling jacket to protect the urethra. These outpatient procedures are cheaper than TURP and there is less bleeding, but heat ablation usually has to be repeated in 1 to 2 years (Goroll & Mulley, 2006; Nickel, 2006).

Other treatments include transurethral vaporization of the prostate (TUVP) and transurethral incision of the prostate (TUIP). In TUVP, the urologist uses laser or electrical vaporization to destroy or remove prostate tissue. TUIP involves making surgical incisions in the prostate to enlarge the urethral opening. TUIP is less destructive than TURP and TUVP, making it a better choice for younger men. It is less likely to cause retrograde ejaculation or erectile dysfunction (Goroll & Mulley, 2006).

Acute urinary retention of BPH can rapidly become an emergent condition, requiring catheterization. If a standard catheter cannot be passed through the urethra, a stiffer catheter may be used. It the blockage still cannot be penetrated, the patient must undergo cystoscopy and the use of dilators to open the urethra and drain the bladder. Eventually, an overfull bladder will cause hydroureter, hydronephrosis, and renal failure (Benign Prostatic Hyperplasia, 2005).

■ Nursing Management

When a patient with BPH comes to the hospital because of LUTS, bladder infection, urinary retention, or hydronephrosis, he is seeking relief and is anxious about any procedures that may have been planned with his health care provider. The nurse will need to do a careful assessment of the patient's condition, elimination patterns, medications, and the patient's knowledge of his condition and any planned procedure. He and his wife or family will need to receive education about the procedure, medications that will be used, and what to expect from the proce-

dure. Preoperative preparation is similar to that of other surgeries and is discussed more fully in Chapter 25 ☺.

If the patient is admitted with acute urinary retention, catheterization is needed. It is very important to maintain a closed, sterile system while the catheter is in place. As for any patient with a renal or urinary problem, intake and output records should be maintained. Review Chapter 44 ☺ for care of the patient with urinary impairment.

Postsurgical care following a TURP will include maintenance of continuous bladder irrigation to decrease clot formation and bleeding. A three-way catheter is placed after surgery and a steady flow of saline is used to flush the bladder. The nurse should be sure that the catheter is secured to the patient's thigh with a Velcro strap to prevent injury to the urethra and bladder neck. The irrigation and drainage tubing should be checked often for kinks that would block flow. Clot formation will cause obstruction and fluid retention. If a clot should occlude the catheter, the system can be opened and direct irrigation with saline can be done, but this should be a sterile procedure and avoided unless absolutely necessary.

Monitoring for bleeding is very important. If the output becomes redder, the irrigation should be increased. Bright-red heavy bleeding would indicate an arterial bleed requiring that the health care provider be called.

TURP is painful surgery and bladder spasms occur because the catheter irritates the bladder mucosa (Karlowicz, 1995). The patient should be encouraged not to strain against the catheter or try to urinate around the catheter, as this will increase the spasm. Also, straining at stool will be very uncomfortable for the patient. Analgesia and stool softeners are indicated. Review Chapter 15 ☺ on pain assessment and treatment for more information about care of patients with postoperative pain.

Prevent infection by keeping the irrigation system closed and cleaning the urinary meatus with soap and water at least twice a day. Monitor the vital signs and the patient for any indication of infection. Encourage increased fluid intake to keep urine output at about 50 milliliters above the irrigation fluid being used. Encourage ambulation and pulmonary toilet as with all patients who have had surgery.

In 24 to 48 hours, the irrigation will stop if the bleeding has stopped. The catheter may be removed in 1 to 5 days (Benign Prostatic Hyperplasia, 2005). The patient should be monitored for urinary retention and assisted as needed when he attempts to void. Some men prefer to stand to void. Some may be able to void if sitting in a warm bath.

Discharge planning and education should begin early so that the patient and his family have time to ask questions. The Patient Teaching & Discharge Priorities box lists the discharge teaching needed for the patient with BPH who has experienced TURP.

Cancer of the Prostate: Etiology and Epidemiology

A man's lifetime risk for prostate cancer is 1 in 6, making this disease the most common cancer in men in the United States and the second leading cause of death. It is estimated that there will be 218,890 new cases and 27,050 deaths due to prostate cancer in 2007 (NCI, 2007a, 2007b). The incidence is increasing as

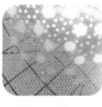

PATIENT TEACHING & DISCHARGE PRIORITIES for Transurethral Resection of the Prostate (TURP) Used to Treat Benign Prostatic Hyperplasia

Need	Teaching
Knowledge of disease process and prognosis	Home care needs including verbal and written instructions for: Urinary incontinence, lower urinary tract symptoms (LUTS), and sexual function will improve. Rest; avoid lifting heavy objects or sitting for long periods. Practice pelvic exercises, stopping urinary stream, and contracting and relaxing pelvic muscles. Follow-up with the health care provider in 1 week.
Understanding of medication	Use of analgesic for bladder pain; how much and how often. Purpose, dose, and possible side effects of alpha-adrenergic blocker if ordered for improvement of voiding.
Safety	Pain medication and alpha-adrenergic blocker may cause hypotension. Rise slowly and move carefully to avoid falls.
Danger signs	Inability to void, shortness of breath, and bleeding from the urinary tract are signs of emergent conditions; and patient needs to come to the emergency department.
Family/support system	Assess availability of, knowledge of, and compliance with the treatment plan. Assess home environment for need of assistive devices. Assess for need for professional home health care.
Emotional adjustment	Answer questions honestly. Encourage verbalization of frustrations with LUTS. Encourage positive reinforcement from the family.

the population ages. In fact, aging is the most powerful risk factor for prostate cancer. African American men have a 60% higher incidence rate of it than do Caucasian men. The Genetic Considerations box outlines the influence of mutated genes on developing prostate cancer. Other risk factors for this cancer are presented in the Risk Factors box.

Pathophysiology

The prostate has three zones: central zone, peripheral zone, and transitional zone. These zones are surrounded by a fibromuscular casing. The peripheral zone, where prostate cancer usually originates, occupies about 70% of the gland. The cause of prostate cancer is unknown (Gray & Sims, 2006).

Prostate cancer occurs in two forms: latent or slow growing and aggressive or fast growing. The aggressive form is more likely to occur in African American and younger men (Gray & Sims, 2006).

Clinical Manifestations

Prostate cancer may be asymptomatic if it is of the slow-growing type. Some men have prostate cancer for many years and die of other causes. Often signs and symptoms are not noticed until

GENETIC CONSIDERATIONS for BRCA2 Mutation

About 10% to 15% of cases of prostate cancer may result from mutated breast cancer genes. BRCA2 mutations are linked with an increased risk for early onset prostate cancer.

Although this association is not as strong as the association between BRCA1 and breast cancer, it is advisable for men with a potential for BRCA2 mutation to begin screening prostate-specific antigen (PSA) and digital rectal examination (DRE) as early as age 40. Men with a brother or father who had prostate cancer are more likely to have the BRCA2 mutation.

Source: Adapted from Lashley, R. (2005). *Clinical genetics in nursing practice* (3rd ed.). New York: Springer.

RISK FACTORS for Prostate Cancer

Age: usually occurs in men over age 65.

Ethnicity: African American men.

Family history: especially father or brother with the disease; 5% to 10% may be due to high-risk inherited gene factors.

Diet: high fat and meat consumption.

Body weight.

Smoking increases risk of fatal prostate cancer.

Sources: Adapted from Gray, M., & Sims, T. (2006). Prostate cancer: Prevention and management of localized disease. *The Nurse Practitioner, 31*(9), 15–28; and National Cancer Institute. (2007d). *Prostate cancer.* Retrieved April 7, 2007, from http://www.cancer.gov/cancertopics/types/prostate

after metastasis has occurred. Chart 50–5 (p. 1578) lists the more common signs and symptoms of prostate cancer.

Diagnostic Testing and Staging

With the advent of prostate-specific antigen (PSA) as a screening tool, many men with asymptomatic, early prostate cancer have been identified. PSA is a serum kinase that originates from the prostate epithelial cells. It is not specific enough to diagnose prostate cancer as a single test and must be used with digital rectal examination (DRE) to increase the likelihood of identifying a cancer. PSA levels less than 4 ng/mL are normal and levels higher than 10 ng/mL have a 67% predictive value for prostate cancer (Mahon, 2005).

An abnormal DRE and an elevated PSA level indicate a need for further testing. A transrectal ultrasound guided biopsy is used to identify and help stage and grade the disease. There is one system for staging and one system for grading: the tumor, node, metastasis (TNM) staging system and the Gleason histologic grading system (Gray & Sims, 2006). Chart 50–6 (p. 1578) outlines the TNM system.

CHART 50–5	Common Signs and Symptoms of Prostate Cancer

Frequent urination

Urinary retention

Trouble starting or holding back urine

Weak or interrupted urine stream

Dysuria

Hematuria

Painful ejaculation

Nocturia

Pain in the lower back, hips, or upper thigh if cancer has metastasized

Source: Adapted from National Cancer Institute. (2007d). *Prostate cancer.* Retrieved April 7, 2007, from http://www.cancer.gov/cancertopics/types/prostate

CHART 50–6	Tumor, Node, Metastasis (TNM) Staging System for Prostate Cancer

T1 = microscopic, not visible by transrectal ultrasound

T2 = palpable, appears confined to the prostate

T3 = protruding beyond the capsule or into the seminal vesicles

T4 = fixed and extends well beyond the prostate

Source: Adapted from Walsh, P., Retik, A., Vaughan, E., & Wein, A. (Eds.). (2007). *Campbell's urology* (9th ed.). Philadelphia: W. B. Saunders. Cited in Gray, M., & Sims, T. (2006). Prostate cancer: Prevention and management of localized disease. *The Nurse Practitioner, 31*(9), 15–28.

The Gleason grading system is based on histologic patterns in the cellular structure of the prostate. The pathologist looks at the two most common patterns within the sample and gives a grade to the first and second most frequently occurring patterns. This gives a score such as 4 + 3 or 3 + 4 with the 4 + 3 being the sample with the poorest prognosis. Gleason scores of less than 7 indicate a lower risk of metastasis, and scores higher than 7 indicate a higher risk (Gray & Sims, 2006).

The PSA and the Gleason score are used in planning further medical diagnostic testing and intervention (Goroll & Mulley, 2006). If the PSA is greater than 20 ng/mL, then bone metastasis is probable and a bone scan is recommended. CT scans are used only for men whose Gleason scores are over 6.

Medical Management

Once the diagnosis is established and the tests for staging and grading are completed, then the next step is medical intervention. Compounding factors include the patient's age and any co-morbidities. If the tumor is slow growing and the patient's life expectancy is affected by other health problems, the decision may be to do nothing or to begin a program of watchful waiting. In this case, a DRE and serum PSA would be done every 3 to 12 months, and the patient would be monitored for LUTS and signs that the cancer may have metastasized. Transrectal ultrasound guided biopsy may be done every 3 years, but these examinations are painful and the patient may choose not to have them done (Gray & Sims, 2006). During this time, lifestyle interventions to improve diet, exercise, and stress management can be instituted. Group support may be helpful, also. The Complementary and Alternative Therapies box discusses the benefits of a healthy lifestyle.

Radiation therapy is used for localized tumors and can be delivered by external beam radiation or implant therapy (brachytherapy). Brachytherapy has fewer side effects than radical surgery or external beam radiation, including less frequent occurrence of erectile dysfunction and urinary incontinence. This therapy will cause swelling of the prostate that will alter urination patterns and can last up to 12 months (Goroll & Mulley, 2006; Zeroski, Abel, Butler, Wallner, & Merrick, 2005). External beam radiation occurs over about 6 weeks, and there are several side effects including cystitis, proctitis, and dermatitis that occur near the end of the treatment period and may last for as much as 6 weeks after the treatments have stopped (Gray & Sims, 2006). External beam radiation is discussed in Chapter 64 🔗. Patients who choose either of the radiation treatments have the potential for needing medication to help them to void and reduce the risk of urinary retention. Conversely, these patients may need medication to alleviate frequency and urgency.

If the tumor is the more aggressive type and the patient is younger, he may choose radical **prostatectomy** or removal of the prostate, seminal vesicles, and adjacent tissues. This can be done as open surgery or by laparoscopic or robot-assisted open surgery. Robot-assisted laparoscopic radical prostatectomy offers smaller incisions, less blood loss, and shorter hospital stays but requires a high degree of skill for the surgeon and it is more expensive (Gray & Sims, 2006; Rigdon, 2006).

Hormone therapy (androgen suppression) or orchiectomy is used to decrease the level of testosterone, thereby slowing disease progression (Goroll & Mulley, 2006). This therapy is being used in localized disease and for advanced, symptomatic metastatic disease. Often, it helps to relieve the pain and other symptoms of advanced disease. Medications used to decrease testosterone include estrogen and the Gn-RH agonist. Chemotherapy is a last resort in prostatic cancer. Its use does not seem to alter survival rates significantly (Goroll & Mulley, 2006).

A new development has just been announced by the American Cancer Society. A vaccine called Provenge is being studied and may soon be approved by the United States Food and Drug Administration (FDA) for use in treating advanced prostate cancer. This vaccine is the first to be designed to treat existing cancer. It is made of the patient's own cells and a protein that stimulates the immune system and causes it to attack the cancer. If approved, this vaccine will offer a treatment option for men who have metastatic disease (ACS, 2007).

Treatment guidelines for prostate cancer and support of the senior oncology patient may be accessed via links in the National Guidelines box (p. 1580).

◼ Nursing Management

The nurse's role in the diagnostic stage of prostate cancer may include assisting with the diagnostic examinations, education of the patient and his partner about the diagnostic tests and what to expect, physical care postbiopsy, and emotional support. If the patient and his partner should choose watchful waiting, the nurse may educate them concerning the timing of follow-up vis-

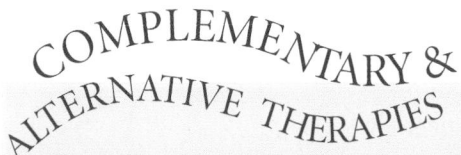

COMPLEMENTARY & ALTERNATIVE THERAPIES — Healthy Lifestyle

Description:

Many herbal products claim to enhance male virility and overall health, such as saw palmetto seed. However, these claims have little validation in the scientific research. Considering this absence of evidence-based data on herbal products, the best approach to ensuring optimal male reproductive health includes the well-validated behaviors of regular exercise, weight management, and a healthy diet.

Research Support:

The lifestyle habits of smoking and obesity cause a large burden of disease, including a negative impact on male reproductive health. However, one study showed that, although eliminating smoking and obesity does increase good health, it may not absolutely reduce morbidity (van Baal, Hoogenveen, de Wit, & Boshuizen, 2006).

Another study evaluated the effects of changes in health behaviors including reduction in dietary fat intake, increase in exercise, and stress management on coronary risks and psychosocial factors. Over the course of 3 months, 869 nonsmoking CHD patients enrolled in the health insurance-based Multisite Cardiac Lifestyle Intervention Program. Results showed that patients experienced a significant overall improvement in coronary risk as well as perceived stress and hostility. These results suggest that multi-component programs that focus on diet, exercise, and stress management may benefit patients (Daubenmier et al., 2007).

The Health Professionals Follow-up Study monitored 42,847 men for a period of 16 years. Participants, who were from 40 to 75 years of age and free of disease, completed questionnaires that assessed five lifestyle factors that were identified as low risk. The five lifestyle factors were (1) the absence of smoking, (2) body mass index less than 25 kg/m², (3) moderate-to-vigorous activity of at least 30 minutes per day, (4) moderate alcohol consumption of 5 to 30 grams per day, and (5) the top 40% of the distribution for a healthy diet score. Over the course of the study, researchers found that men who were at low risk for these five lifestyle factors had a lower risk of coronary heart disease (CHD) as compared to men who were at low risk for no lifestyle factors. Sixty-two percent of coronary events in this cohort may have been prevented with better adherence to these 5 healthy lifestyle practices. Among men taking medication for hypertension or high cholesterol, 57% of all coronary events may have been prevented with a low-risk lifestyle. Compared to men who did not make lifestyle changes, those who adopted at least two additional low-risk lifestyle factors had a 27% lower risk of CHD. Results showed that adherence to lifestyle practices including exercise, weight management, not smoking, moderate alcohol consumption, and a healthy diet may prevent a majority of CHD events among U.S. men. In addition, men that are healthier as a result of these lifestyle behaviors will likely have better reproductive health (Chiuve, McCullough, Sacks, & Rimm, 2006).

References

Chiuve, S. E., McCullough, M. L., Sacks, F. M., & Rimm, E. B. (2006). Healthy lifestyle factors in the primary prevention of coronary heart disease among men: Benefits among users and nonusers of lipid-lowering and antihypertensive medications. *Circulation, 114*(2), 160–167.

Daubenmier, J. J., Weidner, G., Sumner, M. D., Mendell, N., Merritt-Worden, T., Studley, J., et al. (2007). The contribution of changes in diet, exercise, and stress management to changes in coronary risk in women and men in the multisite cardiac lifestyle intervention program. *Annals of Behavioral Medicine, 33*(1), 57–68.

van Baal, P. H., Hoogenveen, R. T., de Wit, G. A., & Boshuizen, H. C. (2006). Estimating health-adjusted life expectancy conditional on risk factors: Results for smoking and obesity. *Population Health Metrics, 4*, 14l.

---

its with the health care provider for DRE, PSA, and transrectal ultrasound (TRUS) guided biopsy. The nurse may also guide the patient in improving his diet, exercise regimen, and stress management. Referrals to groups in the local community for support of patients with newly diagnosed prostate cancer would also be appropriate. See Evidenced-Based Practice box on page 1573.

Patients with prostate cancer may be seen in the emergency department for urinary retention. The nurse's role here is to offer emotional support, to educate about the catheter's being used to relieve the retention, and the need for slowed release of urine from a distended bladder. The patient and his partner will need emotional support and education about the catheter and the use of any incontinence pads or devices.

When the medical plan is for radiation therapy in the form of external beam radiation or brachytherapy, the nurse's role will be teaching about the procedure and the side effects. Chapter 64 discusses the various types of radiation therapy. The patient and his partner should be alert to signs of urinary retention secondary to prostate swelling and should seek care immediately if it occurs. The patient will need education about proctitis, cystitis, and dermatitis and demonstrations on how to use the skin protectant and the medications ordered (see the Pharmacology Summary feature, p. 1585).

Radical prostatectomy may be chosen. In this event, the preoperative preparation is much the same as for other surgeries. Refer to Chapter 25 for preoperative preparation. The patient will need to know about the use of the suprapubic catheter and the pain management plan for him. He will need emotional support as he faces some of the complications such as urinary incontinence, erectile dysfunction (depending on the operative approach), possible rectal injury, and anal damage. Urinary incontinence is most likely right after surgery and will improve over the next 6 months to 2 years by about 50% (Gray & Sims, 2006).

Reinforcement of education and repeated information is needed for the anxious patient and his partner. The diagnosis is a difficult one and will change their lives substantially. His body image is changing and the patient will have many life adjustments to make.

Hormone therapy or orchiectomy may be done if the cancer has spread beyond the prostate. If orchiectomy is chosen, the surgery is quick and usually recovery goes well. The loss of the testicles, however, may have a profound effect on the patient. The loss of masculinity can mean depression due to altered body image and function. Hormone therapy in the form of diethylstilbestrol or luteinizing hormone-releasing hormone agonists will lower the testosterone level, but the side effects may be further debilitating to the patient. The nurse can help find ways of decreasing the side effects and offer support to the couple as they cope with the changes.

NATIONAL GUIDELINES for Treatment and Support of Patients with Prostate Cancer

Principles of Expectant Management

Expectant management means that active monitoring of the course of the disease with the expectation to intervene if the cancer progresses.
Localize cancer monitoring includes:

- Digital rectal exam (DRE) and prostate-specific antigen (PSA) every 6 months, or at least every 12 months.
- Needle biopsy of prostate may be repeated within 6 months of diagnosis if initial biopsy was < 10 cores or palpable tumor contralateral to the side of the positive biopsy.
- Needle biopsy of the prostate may be repeated within 18 months of diagnosis if initial biopsy was > 10 cores.

Cancer progression may have occurred if:

- Primary Gleason grade 4 or 5 is found with repeat prostate biopsy.
- Prostate cancer is found in a greater number of prostate biopsies or occupies a greater extent of prostate biopsies.
- PSA doubling time < 3 or PSA velocity is > 0.75.

A repeat prostate biopsy is indicated for signs of disease progression by exam or PSA.
Advantages of expectant management:

- Avoid unnecessary therapy and its side effects
- Quality of life maintained
- Risk of unnecessary treatment of small, indolent cancers is reduced

Disadvantages of expectant management:

- Chance of missed-opportunity for cure
- Risk of progression and/or metastases
- Subsequent treatment may be more intense with increased side effects
- Nerve sparing may be more difficult, which may reduce chance of potency preservation after surgery
- Increased anxiety
- Requires frequent medical exam and periodic biopsies
- Uncertain long-term history of prostate cancer

Source: National Comprehensive Cancer Network. (2008). *Clinical practice guidelines in oncology: Prostate cancer* [V.1.2008]. Retrieved August 11, 2008, from http://www.nccn.org/professionals/physician_gls/PDF/prostate.pdf

---

Chemotherapy may be needed if the patient's disease has spread to other organs. Nursing care for cancer patients is discussed in Chapter 64 ⊙.

The Nursing Process: Patient Care Plan feature provides further information about treating a patient who has undergone radical prostatectomy. Refer to the Patient Teaching & Discharge Priorities box for information on discharge planning after radical prostatectomy (p. 1584).

■ Collaborative Management

Prostate cancer is a complex disease and requires a team approach for optimal care. The urologist is assisted by nurses, the oncologist, anesthesiologists, nutritionists, counselors, and community resources. Open communication between specialties will facilitate the best care possible for the patient. The health care team should include the spouse or partner and the patient's family in all aspects of the plan of care.

The urologist is a specialist in the care of patients with renal and urinary disorders. The urologist is the team leader and responsible for surgery. Nurses assist in the many roles discussed earlier. The oncologist, a specialist in chemotherapy and radia-

tion treatment for cancer, will be called if the tumor has grown outside the prostate and metastasized to other organs. Anesthesiologists direct the general anesthesia or epidurals needed during surgery or as a palliative measure for severe pain. Nutritionists help the patient and his spouse to choose nutritious foods that help in healing and restoration of the body. Counselors help the couple to cope with this stressful life event. The counselor may help with problem-solving methods, stress relief, or biofeedback and relaxation techniques. Community resources include the different institutions that offer information and support groups, such as the American Cancer Society and the National Cancer Institute. Other community resources may be home health care, physical therapy, massage therapists, and local support groups for the spouse or the couple.

■ Penile Disorders

There are a number of penile disorders, many of which may cause an alteration in sexual functioning. Treatment for the various disorders may range from simple medication to radical surgery. Psychological counseling is an integral part of the treatment and follow-up phases of care for patients with these conditions. The most common penile disorders are discussed in this section.

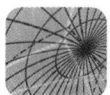

NURSING PROCESS: Patient Care Plan for Prostate Cancer After Radical Prostatectomy

Assessment of Anxiety and Fear

Subjective Data:

Tell me about your concerns.

Are you concerned that treatments may affect your quality of life?

Do you understand your diagnosis?

Do you understand your health care provider's plan for you?

Who are your support people?

Have you ever had cancer before?

How have you coped with stress in the past?

Are you aware that there will be a loss of sexual function that may or may not be permanent?

Objective Data:

Body language: look of concern or anguish

Nursing Assessment and Diagnoses	Outcomes and Evaluation Parameters	Planning and Interventions with *Rationales*
Nursing Diagnoses: *Anxiety* related to diagnosis, treatment plan, and prognosis *Ineffective Sexuality Pattern* related to prostate cancer and treatments *Disturbed Body Image* related to diagnosis, orchiectomy, and side effects of other treatments	**Outcome:** Reduced stress and improved ability to cope. ***Evaluation Parameters:*** Appears more relaxed. States that he feels less anxious. Reiterates information about diagnosis, treatment, and prognosis in calm manner.	**Interventions and *Rationales:*** Clarify information and help patient to cope by helping him to understand. *Often anxious patients are not able to understand as well.* Be there for him. *Quiet presence helps alleviate fear.* Offer support and open communication with him and his partner. *An atmosphere of acceptance and openness will help him to be more willing to talk.* Answer questions honestly and reiterate information often and in concrete terms. *Anxiety reduces cognition.* Encourage him to verbalize his concerns about sex and changes in his physical appearance. *Verbalizing fear is the first step in alleviating fear.*

Assessment of Pain

Subjective Data:

Do you have pain?

Where is the pain?

Is it getting worse?

On a pain scale of 1–10, with 10 being the worst, how would you rate your pain?

Assess gender, cultural, and religious impact on patient response to pain.

Objective Data:

Body language, facial grimace, confusion, and anxiety may be signs of pain

Nursing Assessment and Diagnoses	Outcomes and Evaluation Parameters	Planning and Interventions with *Rationales*
Nursing Diagnosis: *Readiness for Enhanced Comfort* related to postoperative prostatectomy pain	**Outcome:** Comfort level maintained. ***Evaluation Parameters:*** Patient will be able to communicate pain level and therapies that help alleviate it. Pain reduced and/or absent as evidenced by patient report and no pain behaviors. Nonpharmacologic method of pain control is effective, as evidenced by patient report and no pain behaviors. Patient reports satisfaction with pain management.	**Interventions and *Rationales:*** Instruct patient not to strain against the catheter in an attempt to void. *Straining will cause bladder spasms and increased pain.* Instruct patient to inform the nurse if the pain is not relieved. *Indicates need to change pain management plan.* Obtain clear description of location of pain. *To assist in developing a pain management plan.* Provide supportive atmosphere so that patient is comfortable asking for assistance with pain. *Open communications facilitate pain management.* Ask the patient about pain and encourage him to use the pain medication prescribed. *Men are more stoic and less likely to request medication for pain.* Use pain control measures before pain becomes severe. *To increase comfort, decrease anxiety, and decrease need for pain medication.* Record patient response to pain medication. *Record of relief or lack of relief helps health care team plan for better pain relief.*

(continued)

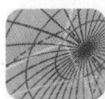

NURSING PROCESS: Patient Care Plan for Prostate Cancer After Radical Prostatectomy—*Continued*

Assessment of Knowledge

Subjective Data:

Tell me what you understand about the surgery planned for you.

Have you had surgery before?

Do you know what to expect after surgery?

What is your understanding about the catheter used after surgery?

Do you know how to use an incentive spirometer?

Do you know how to use support hose?

Objective Data:

Patient unable to answer questions correctly

Patient asks questions that indicate lack of knowledge

Nursing Assessment and Diagnoses	Outcomes and Evaluation Parameters	Planning and Interventions with *Rationales*
Nursing Diagnosis: *Deficient Knowledge* related to the treatment plan and care needs	**Outcome:** Patient will be more cooperative and willing to participate in his care. **Evaluation Parameters:** Patient verbalizes understanding of surgical procedure planned. Patient verbalizes understanding of need for pulmonary toilet, support hose, early ambulation, and need for catheter, and the pain management plan. Patient demonstrates use of incentive spirometer. Patient verbalizes understanding of how to use and why to use support hose.	**Interventions and *Rationales:*** Provide education in simple terms. *Simplicity enhances the anxious patient's ability to learn.* Explain what to expect with surgery and the recovery period. *Knowledge assists the patient to be less fearful.* Explain that the urinary catheter is also a splint to help maintain the surgical reconnection of the urethra. *Knowing the reason for the catheter increases tolerance of the discomfort.* Explain what will be experienced. *Knowing a little about how it will feel will reduce fear.* Allow to ask questions. *Open communication enhances learning.* Allow patient to become familiar with spirometer. *Handling equipment makes it familiar and easier to use after surgery.* Demonstrate how support hose are used. *Support hose are used to help prevent thrombosis and pulmonary embolism.*

Assessment of Urinary Elimination

Subjective Data:

Preoperative:

    What is your usual pattern of urination?

    When was the last time you voided?

    Does your bladder feel full?

    Are you dribbling urine?

Postoperative:

    Is the catheter uncomfortable?

Objective Data:

Preoperative:

    Bladder distention, dribbling urine, or incontinence

Postoperative:

    Yellow, pink-tinged urine

    Catheter and tubing intact and free of kinks

    Catheter secured to inner thigh

Nursing Assessment and Diagnoses	Outcomes and Evaluation Parameters	Planning and Interventions with *Rationales*
Nursing Diagnosis: *Urinary Retention* due to urethral obstruction secondary to prostate enlargement	**Outcome:** Normal urinary output. **Evaluation Parameters:** Preoperative: Urinary retention relieved. Patient is dry and comfortable. Postoperative: Output at 50 milliliters or more per hour. Balance to intake and output. No retention related to kinks in catheter tubing. Patient does not strain against catheter. Catheter is secured to inner thigh at all times.	**Interventions and *Rationales:*** Preoperative: Usual pattern gives baseline. *Return to usual pattern is goal to work toward.* Relieve urinary retention. *Urinary retention will cause damage to the bladder, and, if severe and prolonged, hydroureter, hydronephrosis, and renal failure.* Postoperative: Maintain strict intake and output records. *High output is needed to clear blood from bladder to prevent clots and obstruction. Output less than intake indicates retention.* Monitor color and amount of output. *Increased bleeding must be identified early and corrected.* Keep catheter secured to thigh and prevent dislodging. *Dislodging the catheter can cause damage to the urethra anatomosis or bladder neck.* Keep tubing coiled on the bed and free of kinks. *To facilitate urine flow and prevent obstruction.* Use incontinence pads and other equipment to keep patient dry. *Urine is irritating and can cause skin breakdown.*

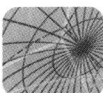

NURSING PROCESS: Patient Care Plan for Prostate Cancer After Radical Prostatectomy—*Continued*

Assessment of Bowel Elimination

Subjective Data:
When was your last BM?
Are you using a stool
softener or laxatives?

Objective Data:
Frequency and consistency of bowel movements
Type and amount of stool softeners and/or laxatives

Nursing Assessment and Diagnoses	Outcomes and Evaluation Parameters	Planning and Interventions with *Rationales*
Nursing Diagnosis: Potential for Pain, Acute, related to Constipation and straining at stool	**Outcome:** Regular bowel movement (BM) without straining. **Evaluation Parameter:** Patient reports regular BM that is soft and passed without straining.	**Intervention and *Rationale:*** Administer stool softener and encourage increased fluids. *Straining at stool can cause bleeding and increased pain.*

Assessment of Skin and Fluid Volume

Subjective Data:
Have you had problems with urine leaking from your catheter?
Are you able to keep you skin dry?
Are you thirsty?
Does your urine appear concentrated?
Have you had a fever or chills?
Does your urine appear cloudy or clear?

Objective Data:
Inspect skin exposed to urine or tape
Inspect incision and catheter site
Vital signs

Nursing Assessment and Diagnoses	Outcomes and Evaluation Parameters	Planning and Interventions with *Rationales*
Nursing Diagnoses: *Risk for Impaired Skin Integrity* related to urinary incontinence *Risk for Infection* related to surgery and urinary retention *Risk for Deficient Fluid Volume* related to blood loss	**Outcomes:** No skin breakdown. No infection at the incision. **Evaluation Parameters:** Skin is intact. Patient has no complaints of skin itching or burning. Vital signs are normal for the patient.	**Interventions and *Rationales:*** Inspect skin. Keep skin clean and dry. *Clean, dry skin does not break down.* Monitor surgical wound and drain sites for infection or signs of healing. *Early identification of infection decreases morbidity.* Monitor vital signs for elevated temperature. *Indication of infection.* Monitor pulse and blood pressure for signs of blood loss. *High pulse and lower blood pressure indicate blood loss.* Assist in early ambulation. *Ambulation improves circulation and enhances healing.*

Phimosis and Paraphimosis

Phimosis occurs when a tight foreskin cannot be retracted over the penile glans (Figure 50–5 ■, p. 1586). Phimosis is usually the result of inflammation or infection secondary to poor hygiene. Treatment includes antibiotics for infection and circumcision if the phimosis interferes with urination (Every, Mikkelsen, & Bailey, 2005).

Paraphimosis occurs when a retracted foreskin becomes trapped over the glans (see Figure 50–5 ■, p. 1586). The retracted foreskin causes a tourniquet effect, decreasing the circulation to the glans. Swelling develops swiftly, further tightening the foreskin band. Compressing the glans and moving the foreskin forward should be attempted as soon as possible. If the foreskin cannot be manually reduced, circumcision is needed and may have to be done as an emergency procedure to prevent ischemia and necrosis of the glans (Every, Mikkelsen, & Bailey, 2005).

Nursing care includes education about hygiene, emotional support, monitoring vital signs for evidence of a worsening condition, and administration of analgesics. Circumcision is usually an outpatient surgery and does not require hospitalization.

Peyronie's Disease

Peyronie's disease is a penile condition where palpable, fibrous plaque forms on the corpora cavernosa. The plaque will cause abnormal curvature of the penis and painful, incomplete erections. Peyronie's disease affects middle-aged and older men (Figure 50–6 ■, p. 1586). The cause is unknown.

There are no completely effective treatments for this condition. Limited success has occurred with vitamin E and aminobenzoate potassium (Potaba). Alternative therapies may be helpful. Surgery is a last resort, but removing the plaque and repairing the corpora cavernosa with a graft has offered relief of pain (Every, Mikkelsen, & Bailey, 2005).

Nursing management would include emotional support, education about the condition and medications used, preoperative care, and postoperative care for those who have surgery. If the surgery is extensive, a suprapubic catheter may be placed so that the penis can heal more quickly.

Urethral Stricture

The urethra is the most distal portion of the urinary tract (see Figure 50–1 ■, p. 1566). It allows urine and semen to pass out of the body. Stricture within the urethra may occur as the result of trauma, an enlarged or nodular prostate, instrumentation, or infection that causes scarring. Strictures will block the flow of urine and ejaculate. Urinary retention may result, and if the stricture is severe enough, hydronephrosis may result. Signs and

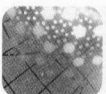

PATIENT TEACHING & DISCHARGE PRIORITIES for Prostate Cancer After Radical Prostatectomy

Need	Teaching
Knowledge of self-care and need for follow-up visit with health care provider	Home care needs including verbal and written instructions for: May go home with catheter in place. Needs education about home including maintaining patency of the tubing and cleansing the urinary meatus. Urinary incontinence may follow removal of catheter but will improve. Rest; avoid lifting heavy objects, sitting for long periods, or straining at stool. Maintain increased oral intake at about 2–3 quarts a day, unless medically contraindicated. Practice pelvic exercises, stopping urinary stream, and contracting and relaxing pelvic muscles. Follow-up with the health care provider in 1 to 3 weeks.
Understanding of medication	Use of analgesic and antimuscarinic for bladder pain; how much and how often and what the side effects may be. Purpose, dose, and possible side effects of alpha-adrenergic blocker if ordered for improvement of voiding.
Safety	Pain medication and alpha-adrenergic blocker may cause hypotension. Rise slowly and move carefully to avoid falls.
Danger signs	If the catheter comes out before it is supposed to, if unable to void after the catheter is removed, if patient experiences any shortness of breath, bleeding from the urinary tract, or high fever, he should be sent to his health care provider.
Family/support system	Assess availability of, knowledge of, and compliance with the treatment plan. Assess home environment for need of assistive devices. Assess for need for professional home health care. Seek support groups for spouse or partner to help her cope. Respite care may be needed.
Emotional adjustment	Answer questions honestly. Encourage verbalization of frustrations and fears. Encourage positive reinforcement from the family.
Institutional and community resources and support groups	Suggest National Cancer Institute, American Cancer Society as resources. Offer community-based programs and support group addresses and phone numbers.

symptoms include decreased urinary stream, spraying of urine, urethral discharge, bladder infection secondary to retrograde urination, and urinary retention. Diagnosis is made by cystoscopy or urethrography (Every, Mikkelsen, & Bailey, 2005).

Medical management includes surgical procedures to dilate or reconstruct the urethra. These procedures may be done under general or epidural anesthesia on an outpatient basis. Chapter 47 includes a discussion of the treatment for urinary disorders.

Nursing care depends on the extent of the stricture and surgical procedures to correct the stricture. Most of the patients will need pre- and postoperative teaching, analgesia, careful monitoring of vital signs, and observation for bleeding or drainage. See Chapter 15 for information about pain assessment and management. Many of these patients need emotional support if the stricture has become severe enough to warrant surgery.

Epispadias

An epispadias is an abnormal urethral opening on the dorsal or top of the penile shaft just under the urinary bladder. It is a congenital condition that usually occurs with exstrophy of the bladder where the abdominal wall fails to form below the umbilicus (Every, Mikkelsen, & Bailey, 2005).

Medical management involves staged surgical procedures to reconstruct the bladder and urethra. Usually these repairs are

completed by school age, but if the congenital disorder was severe, particularly with exstrophy of the bladder, there may be problems with incontinence, impotence, and fertility.

Nursing management includes emotional support of the child and his parents, education, and preoperative and postoperative care. Chapter 47 includes a discussion of the treatment for urinary disorders.

Hypospadias: Etiology

Hypospadias is a congenital disorder wherein the urinary opening occurs on the ventral or lower portion of the penis. Embryonic development of the male urethra begins as a cleft in the genital area during gestation at about 8 to 14 weeks of life. Incomplete closure of the cleft will cause the meatus to occur anywhere along the lower penis, including the scrotum and the perineum (Carmichael et al., 2005).

Medical management includes staged reconstruction of the penis. For those infants in which the meatus occurs on the scrotum or perineum, studies are conducted to determine whether there is insufficient masculinization (Every, Mikklesen, & Bailey, 2005).

Nursing care includes emotional support of the baby and his parents, education about the defect, and preoperative and postoperative care. Chapter 47 includes a discussion of the treatment for urinary disorders.

PHARMACOLOGY Summary of Medications to Treat Male Reproductive Disorders

Medication Category	Action	Application/Indication	Nursing Responsibility
Antibiotics: Macrolides (Biaxin) Penicillin (Pen-Vee K) Fluoroquinolones (Cipro) Trimethoprim-sulfamethoxazole (Bactrim) Doxycycline (Doryx) Specific type depends on causative agent.	Varies with antibiotic; may be bactericidal or bacteristatic.	Used for infections of susceptible organisms including sexually transmitted infection, epididymitis, orchitis, prostatitis, coliforms, and any postoperative infections.	Assess for drug allergies before beginning any antibiotic. Assess for any manifestation of allergic reaction. Assess for improvement of symptoms, especially decreased fever and pain. Educate patient concerning importance of completing full course of antibiotics.
Nonsteroidal anti-inflammatory agents (NSAIDs): Ibuprofen (Advil) Naproxen sodium (Aleve)	Prostaglandin synthetase inhibition.	Used for fever reduction, for pain relief, and for decreasing inflammation.	Assess for drug allergies before beginning any drug. Give with food. Assess for gastrointestinal side effects, including ulcer and gastrointestinal (GI) bleeding. Assess for relief of symptoms.
Chemotherapy: Cisplatin (Platinol-AQ) Bleomycin (Blenoxane), Etoposide (Toposar)	Alkylates DNA, RNA; inhibits enzymes that allow synthesis of amino acids in proteins; activity is not cell cycle phase specific.	Used for testicular cancer.	Assess for drug allergies. Prepare for anaphylactic reaction with first dose. Monitor renal and liver function tests for abnormalities related to chemotherapy side effects. Side effects of cisplatin include nausea, vomiting, alopecia, fatigue, neutropenia, azoospermia, peripheral neuropathy, and ototoxicity. Bleomycin may cause fibrosis, pneumonitis, and lung toxicity. Etoposide may cause hepatotoxicity and nephrotoxicity.
Antiemetics and antidiarrheals (especially for side effects of chemotherapy): Ondansetron (Zofran)	Ondansetron blocks serotonic 5-HT3 receptor, decreasing nausea. Antidiarrheals work directly at intestinal muscle to decrease peristalsis or increase bulk.	Side effects of chemotherapy include vomiting and diarrhea. Ondansetron (Zofran) has been especially efficacious for this type of nausea.	Assess for drug allergies. Assess for untoward effects such as headache and dizziness. Assess for relief of symptoms.
Benign Prostatic Hyperplasia Alpha blockers: Doxazosin (Cardura) Terazosin (Hytrin) Tamsulosin (Flomax) Alfuzosin (Uroxatral) 5-Alpha reductase inhibitors: Finasteride (Proscar) Dutasteride (Avodart)	Alpha blockers work by relaxing the bladder neck and prostatic smooth muscle tone. Blocks conversion of testosterone to androgen, thereby decreasing size of the prostate.	Improves urinary flow; relieves hesitancy, urgency, and frequency. Blocks conversion of testosterone to potent androgen, thereby reducing size and growth of prostate. More efficacious for men with larger prostates.	Assess for drug allergies. Monitor blood pressure and heart rate. Assess for side effects such as dizziness, headache, and nausea. Observe for improvement of symptoms. Warn patients to limit Viagra to 25 milligrams at least 4 hours before or after using alpha blockers. Assess for allergies before administering. Monitor for side effects such as decreased libido, ejaculatory problems, and lower prostate-specific antigen (PSA) levels.
Medications for Side Effects of Radiation Therapy Antimuscarinics: Tolterodine (Detrol LA) Oxybutynin (Ditropan) Phenazopyridine (Baridium) Trypsin, castor oil, and balsam of Peru (Xenaderm)	Relaxes smooth muscle in urinary tract: Exerts analgesic, anesthetic action on the urinary mucosa. Antispasmodic. Skin protectant.	Radiation cystitis: helps relieve frequency and urgency. Relieves discomfort of bladder irritation. For relief of proctitis symptoms. Skin irritation due to radiation. Soothes and promotes healing.	Assess for allergies to any drugs. Monitor for side effects. Assess for relief of symptoms. Encourage diet low in irritants such as coffee, spicy foods, and alcohol. Encourage diet high in fluid intake and roughage to keep stool soft and movements regular.

(continued)

PHARMACOLOGY Summary of Medications to Treat Male Reproductive Disorders—*Continued*

Medication Category	Action	Application/Indication	Nursing Responsibility
Hormone Therapy for Prostate Cancer			
Diethylstilbesterol (DES) Leuprolide Eligard® Lupron® Lupron Depot®	Antiandrogen. Luteinizing hormone-releasing hormone agonist.	Slows or stops prostate cancer growth by lowering androgen levels to those of castration. Lowers androgen levels to those similar to castration.	Monitor for side effects: feminization and loss of libido. Erectile dysfunction. Explain side effects. Help patient find ways to cope. Monitor for side effects such as hot flashes, impotence, and loss of libido.

Sources: Adapted from Barry, M. (2006). Approach to benign prostatic hyperplasia. In A. Goroll & A. Mulley, *Primary care medicine: Office evaluation and management of the adult patient* (5th ed., pp. 909–914). Philadelphia: Lippincott Williams & Wilkins; Gray, M., & Sims, T. (2006). Prostate cancer: Prevention and management of localized disease. *The Nurse Practitioner, 31*(9), 15–28; Kuritzky, L., Rosenberg, M., & Sadovsky, R. (2006). Efficacy and safety of alfuzosin 10 mg once daily in the treatment of symptomatic benign prostatic hyperplasia. *International Journal of Clinical Practice, 60*(3), 351–358; National Cancer Institute (NCI). (2007d). *Treatment choices for men with early-stage prostate cancer.* Retrieved April 9, 2007, from http://www.cancer.gov/cancertopics/prostatecancer-treatment-choices.; RxList the Internet Drug Index. (2007a). *Cisplatin.* Retrieved March 31, 2007, from http://www.rxlist.com/cgi/generic/cisplatin_ids.htm; RxList the Internet Drug Index. (2007b). *Motrin.* Retrieved March 31, 2007, from http://www.rxlist.com/cgi/generic/ibup.htm; RxList the Internet Drug Index. (2007c). *Zofran injection.* Retrieved March 31, 2007, from http://www.rxlist.com/cgi/generic/ondansetron.htm; and Wilt, T., Howe, R., & Rutks, I. (2000). Terazosin for benign prostatic hyperplasia. *Cochrane Database Systematic Reviews 2000.* In *The Cochrane Library,* 2007, Issue 1. Retrieved March 31, 2007, from www.thecochranelibrary.com

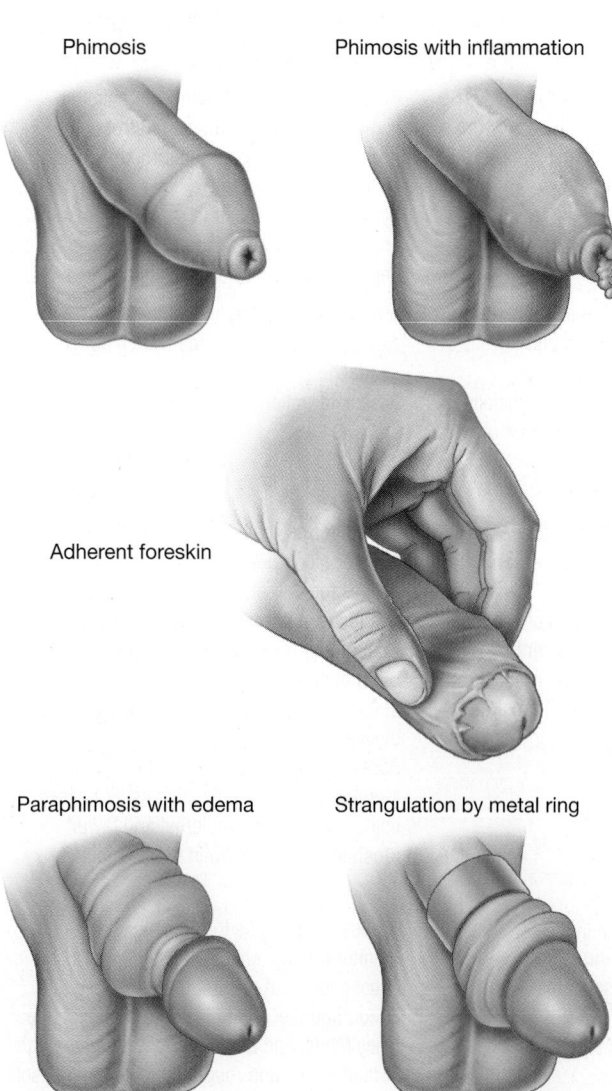

Phimosis

Phimosis with inflammation

Adherent foreskin

Paraphimosis with edema

Strangulation by metal ring

FIGURE 50–5 ■ Phimosis and paraphimosis.

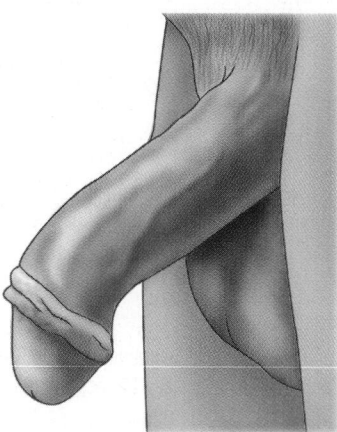

FIGURE 50–6 ■ Peyronie's disease.

Penile and Scrotal Injuries

Men are more likely than women to experience genital trauma. Scrotal injuries may be the result of infections, burns, or gunshot wounds. Testicular injuries are more likely to be blunt trauma that may cause hematoma or even rupture of the testicle. Penile injuries may occur from pant zippers, amputations, animal bites, gunshot wounds, battlefield injuries, or ruptures of the corpus cavernosum caused by severe bending of the penis during an erection (Genital Trauma: Genitourinary Tract Traumas, 2005/2007).

Medical care includes identification of the extent of the injury and surgical repair as needed. Antibiotic therapy and analgesia will be needed. Nursing care depends on the extent of the injury. Preoperative and postoperative education and emotional support are imperative.

Cancer of the Penis

Penile cancer is very rare in North America and Europe, accounting for approximately 0.2% of cancers in men and 0.1% of cancer deaths in men in the United States. Penile cancer is more common in some parts of Africa and South America, where it accounts for up to 10% of cancers in men (American Cancer Society, 2008). More than 95% of penile carcinomas are squamous cell carcinomas (Goodman, Hernandez, & Shvetsov, 2007).

RISK FACTORS for Penile Cancer

Poor local hygiene

Phimosis

Human papillomavirus infection (risk for this infection is increased by sexual intercourse at an early age, many sexual partners, sex with a partner who has had many partners, or unprotected sex)

Smoking

Age (most cases occur in men over age 65)

AIDS

Not being circumcised

Source: Adapted from American Cancer Society. (2008). *Detailed guide: Penile cancer.* Retrieved April 4, 2007, from http://www.cancer.org/docroot/CRI/CRI_2_3x.asp?dt=35

CHART 50–7	**Drugs That May Cause Erectile Dysfunction**

Clonidine	Alcohol
Spironolactone	Cocaine
Beta-blockers	Opioids
Tricyclics	Anticholinergics
Selective serotonin reuptake inhibitors (SSRIs)	

Source: Adapted from Male sexual dysfunction. (2005). *Merck manual professional.* Retrieved April 4, 2007, from http://www.merck.com/mmpe/sec17/ch227/ch227c.html

Causes of the various types of penile cancer are not known. Research has shown that two proteins produced by high-risk human papillomavirus can interfere with tumor suppressor genes, thereby allowing cancer to grow (ACS, 2007). Risk factors for penile cancer are listed in the Risk Factors box.

Medical care for penile cancer is usually surgery. This may be circumcision or laser ablation for smaller lesions or partial or total **penectomy** (removal of part of or the entire penis) for larger lesions. Radiation therapy is used if the cancer has not spread beyond the local lymph nodes. Chemotherapy is used when the cancer is widely spread, with little success (Penile Cancer: Genitourinary Cancer, 2005).

Nursing care depends on the extent of the cancer. Preoperative and postoperative education and emotional support are imperative. Care of the patient undergoing cancer treatment is discussed in detail in Chapter 64 ⊚ .

▪ Sexual Functioning

In order to impregnate a female, a male must have normal **spermatogenesis** (the manufacture of normal sperm in high numbers), and he must have the ability to transmit the sperm into a woman's vagina. This means that he needs to be able to have and sustain an erection and to have a normal ejaculation (Hatcher et al., 2004). If a male does not want to produce children but wishes to continue sexual relations, he can use condoms or undergo sterilizing surgery called vasectomy. This section will explore selected topics related to male sexual function, including erectile dysfunction, male infertility, andropause, and vasectomy.

Erectile Dysfunction

Erectile dysfunction (ED) is the inability to achieve or sustain an erection firm enough for intercourse. In the United States, it is estimated based on imprecise data that 10 to 20 million men over age 18 have had at least a few instances of ED. The prevalence increases to 50% of men aged 40 to 70 (Male Sexual Dysfunction, 2005).

Epidemiology and Etiology

ED may be primary (a man has never achieved erection) or secondary (a man has had erections but is no longer able). It is estimated that about 80% of ED events are physiological and the remaining events have a psychological cause, including but not limited to guilt, depression, performance anxiety, and fear of intimacy (Male Sexual Dysfunction, 2005).

The major organic causes include diabetes, stroke, atherosclerosis, spinal cord injuries, and complications of prostate surgery. Hormones, significant smoking, drugs, and structural problems may also contribute to ED. Chart 50–7 lists some drugs that may cause ED.

Laboratory and Diagnostic Procedures

Diagnostic tests will include a complete history to reveal disease, congenital defects, medication use, and any associated psychological concerns. The physical examination would focus on secondary sexual characteristics, any evidence of circulatory problems, anatomical abnormalities of the penis, and neurological deficits. Laboratory tests may include testosterone serum levels, prolactin levels, tests for diabetes, a lipid profile, and thyroid function tests, depending on the findings of the history and physical examination (Male Sexual Dysfunction, 2005). Chapter 48 ⊚ on reproductive assessment details male reproductive history and physical examination.

Medical Management

Medical management of ED depends on the underlying cause. Contributory drugs can be changed or discontinued, depression can be treated, and patients and their partners can be educated about ED and sexual intimacy alternatives to intercourse (Krebs, 2006).

Devices are available to help achieve and sustain an erection. If mechanical devices are not acceptable to the patient and his partner, drug therapy may be used. The most popular of these drugs is sildenafil (Viagra), which enhances nitric oxide release needed for an erection. Sildenafil will cause coronary vasodilation and hypotension and should not be used with other nitrates such as nitroglycerine. Also, it should be used in lower dosage and with extreme caution if the patient is taking an alpha blocker for BPH (Male Sexual Dysfunction, 2005).

Other drugs may be injected into the urethra or into the penis to produce an erection. These medications have a higher incidence of injury to the penis and are more likely to cause **priapism** (an erection that lasts more than 4 hours). There are also penile prostheses that may be surgically implanted.

▪ Collaborative Management

Collaborative management is indicated for men with ED. First on the team is his sexual partner. Education, counseling, emotional support, acceptance, and open communication are essential.

Health care providers, nurses, counselors, and community support groups may have a role in providing holistic care for this couple on a long-term basis.

Male Infertility

General information about infertility may be found in Chapter 49 ⊘. Achieving a pregnancy requires both male and female contributions. When a couple cannot achieve a pregnancy after 1 year of unprotected intercourse, the male factor alone is the cause in about 20% of cases and will contribute in 30% to 40% of all couples who seek medical help for infertility (Quallich, 2006). There are reversible and irreversible causes of male infertility, many of which are listed in Chart 50–8.

The most common test for evaluating male infertility is semen analysis. This test gives information about male hormone cycle integrity, spermatogenesis, and the patency of the genital tract. Refer to Chart 50–9 for the parameters for semen analysis.

Medical care for infertility depends on the underlying cause and is highly specialized. Most of the medical interventions are completed on an outpatient basis from infertility clinics.

Andropause

Unlike women, men begin to decrease the production of sex hormones at about age 30. The decrease is gradual and the rate of decline varies greatly among individual men. Both cross-sectional and longitudinal studies have demonstrated that about 25% of men over age 70 have a significant testosterone deficiency (Seidman, 2006). Whether or not this age-dependent reduction in testosterone levels requires hormone replacement is under debate.

Physiologically, men aged 40 to 70 experience a decrease in total, free, and bioavailable testosterone and an increase in sex hormone-binding globulin (SHBG). The decrease in testosterone is associated with an increase in follicle-stimulating hormone (FSH) and a modest increase in luteinizing hormone (LH). These changes suggest an age-related impairment in the secretion of hypothalamic gonadotropin-releasing hormone (Tan & Pu, 2004). Unlike women in menopause who stop ovulating, men with lower levels of testosterone remain fertile.

Androgen decline in aging males (ADAM), or andropause, may cause mood changes, decreased libido, decreased muscle mass, increased abdominal fat, thinning of bones, decreased energy, slowed mathematical thinking, and lower blood counts (Organon, 2002a). Often, the symptom severity does not correlate with the level of testosterone in serum (Tan & Pu, 2004).

Diagnostic and Laboratory Procedures

After a thorough history and physical, laboratory measurement of **bioavailable testosterone** (both free testosterone and testosterone that is loosely bound to albumin) is the most appropriate test to diagnose andropause in men over age 65. Testing methods include radioimmunoassay and saliva testing. The Endocrine Society Andropause Consensus Statement has recommended treatment with androgen replacement if the older man has both significant symptoms and a low bioavailable testosterone level. Serum levels of testosterone are highest soon after awakening, so test results should be evaluated based on the timing of the sample (Tan & Pu, 2004).

Medical Management

Testosterone replacement therapy has not proven effective in reversing most andropause symptoms (Seidman, 2006). Haren et al. (2005) assessed the effect of 12 months of oral testosterone on self-reported andropause symptoms in older men with low plasma testosterone levels and found that testosterone undecanoate (Andriol) 80 milligrams twice a day did not improve symptoms. There was some evidence that Andriol may preserve mood and some erectile function, but only in men with the lowest testosterone levels before treatment (Haren et al., 2005).

Andriol should not be used if the older male has ever had breast or prostate cancer, allergies to androgens, or use of anticoagulant medications. It is used with caution if there is preexisting liver disease, heart or blood vessel disease, edema, prostatic hyperplasia, kidney disease, or diabetes mellitus (Organon, 2002b).

Men experiencing andropause seem to benefit from counseling, decreasing stress, losing excess weight, increasing zinc intake, adequate nutrition, and weight training to build muscle mass. Weight training and increased muscle mass have increased endogenous testosterone levels (Tan & Pu, 2004).

■ Nursing Management

Nursing care of older men with andropause symptoms includes education about what andropause is and the lifestyle changes that can improve symptoms. An excellent website for information about andropause and the use of androgen replacement therapy is produced by Organon, the pharmaceutical company that manufactures Andriol.

CHART 50–8	Causes of Male Infertility

Reversible Causes	Irreversible Causes
Varicocele	Klinefelter's syndrome
Heavy smoking	Congenital bilateral absence of vas deferens
Hypercholesterolemia	
Some forms of erectile dysfunction	Spinal cord injuries
	Antisperm antibodies
Hypogonadism	Some forms of erectile dysfunction
Obesity	Impaired spermatogenesis
Recreational drug use	
Alcohol intake	

Source: Adapted from Quallich, S. (2006). Examining male fertility. *Urologic Nursing, 26* (4), 277–288.

CHART 50–9	Semen Analysis Parameters

Volume	2–5 milliliters
pH	7–8
Sperm count	>20 million/mL
Motility	>50%
Morphology	>14% with normal morphology (World Health Organization [WHO] criteria)
White blood count (WBC)	1–3 per high-power field

Source: Adapted from Sperm disorders. (2005). *Merck manual professional.* Retrieved April 4, 2007, from http://www.merck.com/mmpe/sec18/ch256/ch256b.html

Vasectomy

Vasectomy is male sterilization surgery whereby the vas deferens on each side is identified, cut, and the cut ends are ligated or cauterized closed (Sterilization, 2007). Vasectomy is highly effective in preventing pregnancy if at least two semen-free ejaculates have been analyzed and documented. This is needed to assure that the vas deferens was cut and closed and that all sperm have been cleared from the system. The procedure can be done in the health care provider's office under local anesthesia in about 20 minutes.

Inguinal Hernia

Abdominal **hernias**, protrusions of abdominal contents through a weakness in the abdominal wall, are very common. About 700,000 surgeries for abdominal hernia occur in the United States each year (Hernias of the Abdominal Wall, 2005). About half of all abdominal hernias are **indirect inguinal hernias** (present via the inguinal canal and exit at the external inguinal ring) and another 25% are **direct inguinal hernias** (occur above the inguinal ligament, close to the pubic tubercle and the external inguinal ring). See Figure 50–7 ■ for a depiction of direct and indirect inguinal hernias.

Inguinal hernias are usually congenital but may become symptomatic due to trauma or chronic cough (Goroll & Mulley, 2006). Signs and symptoms depend on the severity of the hernia and include a visible bulge, discomfort or pain, tenderness, bowel obstruction, and infarction. Chart 50–10 lists clinical manifestations specific to inguinal hernias.

Medical Management

Medical management includes diagnosis and surgery to repair the hernia with placement of mesh to reinforce the repair. Surgery for hernia repair may be conventional or laparoscopic depending on the skill of the surgeon. Occasionally, when the hernia is small and asymptomatic, a watchful waiting approach will be taken. Hernia repair surgery is considered elective unless incarceration occurs (Goroll & Mulley, 2006; Hernias of the Abdominal Wall, 2005).

Nursing Management

Nursing care depends on the severity of the hernia. Education is of particular importance because the patient who is scheduled for surgery will need to know the signs and symptoms of incarceration and strangulation so that he can seek help immediately. Patients

CHART 50–10	**Clinical Manifestations of Inguinal Hernias**

Reducible; Mass appears on standing, reduces when supine.

Incarcerated: Contents cannot be replaced into the abdomen, even when supine.

Strangulated: Irreducible hernia where blood supply to trapped bowel has been cut off and bowel obstruction has occurred.

Source: Adapted from Goroll, A., & Mulley, A. (2006). *Primary care medicine: Office evaluation and management of the adult patient* (5th ed.). Philadelphia: Lippincott Williams & Wilkins.

CHART 50–11	**Sexually Transmitted Infections by Presenting Sign**

Presenting Sign	Sexually Transmitted Infection
Urethritis	Gonococcal
	Nongonococcal: chlamydia, trichomoniasis
Genital ulcers	Herpes, primary syphilis, chancroid, granuloma inguinale, lymphogranuloma venereum
Genital warts	Human papillomavirus (HPV)
Immune deficiency	Human immunodeficiency virus (HIV); acquired immunodeficiency syndrome (AIDS)

Source: Adapted from Centers for Disease Control and Prevention. (2006). Sexually transmitted disease treatment guidelines, 2006. *Morbidity and Mortality Weekly Report,* 55(RR-11), 1–94. Retrieved April 7, 2007, from http://www.cdc.gov/mmwr/preview/mmwrhtml/rr5511a1.htm

usually want to know that they will be up the same day of surgery, return to light work in 2 to 3 weeks, and return to full activity in 3 to 6 weeks. There should be no effect on sexual function (Goroll & Mulley, 2006). Many hernia surgeries are done in outpatient surgery. See Chapter 25 ⊚ for a review of preoperative nursing.

If the hernia is strangulated, it may require bowel resection as well as hernia repair. Postoperatively, analgesia, pulmonary toilet, and monitoring of vital signs and for bleeding or drainage on the dressing will be needed. Patients who have bowel surgery usually have a nasogastric tube and require IV therapy. See Chapter 45 ⊚ for a description of care of the patient after bowel surgery.

Sexually Transmitted Infections

Surveillance data from the Centers for Disease Control and Prevention (CDC) indicate that the incidence of sexually transmitted infections (STIs) continues to increase each year.

The CDC has categorized STIs by their primary presentation. Chart 50–11 refers to each abnormality and the STIs it may involve.

Treatment of STIs should include both the patient and his partner. Both should receive an examination for any coexisting STI; medication as appropriate; and education and counseling to prevent reinfection, complications, and spreading the infection to others. Male condom use does protect the male from infection, and it prevents the transmission of sperm and infection to his partner. A more complete discussion of STIs can be found in Chapter 49 ⊚ on female reproductive disorders and Chapter 60 ⊚ on immune response disorders.

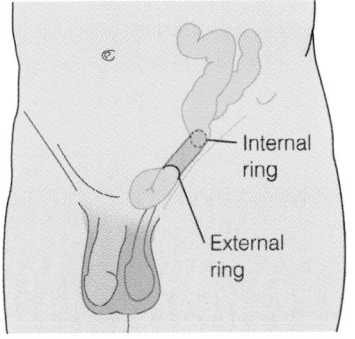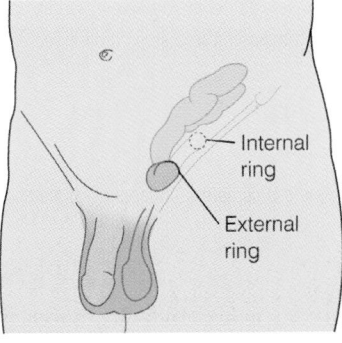

FIGURE 50–7 ■ Direct and indirect inguinal hernia.

Gerontological Considerations

As discussed earlier, diseases of the prostate are most likely to occur in older men. This is also a time that other diseases tend to occur, complicating the prostate condition and treatment. Because of the changes in the body caused by aging, special consideration for skin care and bowel elimination become more important to nursing care for older men presenting with reproductive disorders. Nursing assessment of the older male should also include hearing and vision. If the older male is hard of hearing or unable to see as well as he used to, then education must be

modified to fit his needs. Communication must be clear, simple, and direct.

Research

To improve care of males experiencing abnormalities with their reproductive system, it is imperative that nurses be knowledgeable and that research continue to refine this knowledge. The Research Opportunities and Clinical Impact box outlines potential research topics related to male reproductive disorders.

RESEARCH OPPORTUNITIES AND CLINICAL IMPACT RELATED TO MALE REPRODUCTIVE DISORDERS

Research Area	Clinical Impact
Examination of why prostate cancer risks are higher for African American men.	African American men are much more likely to develop and die from prostate cancer.
Determination of whether selenium and vitamin E may help prevent prostate cancer.	Research currently underway. Prevention of prostate cancer is much preferred to treating it.
Use of complementary and alternative therapies among patients with cancer.	Nurses should know more about complementary and alternative therapies so that they can give information about safety and efficacy to their patients.
Prostate cancer outcomes study (PCOS) is examining the impact of treatments for prostate cancer on quality of life.	Important for the patient to know all about his options and potential outcomes before choosing a treatment.
Identifying problems faced by partners of men with prostate cancer.	Nurses are recognized support persons, and wives or partners will turn to them when they need help dealing with decreased affection from or depression in their partner. Support of the partner helps in support of the patient.
Predicting the use of complementary and alternative therapies among patients with cancer.	Nurses need to be asking patients about the complementary and alternative therapies they may be using such as herbs, vitamins, and homeopathic medications that may impact their medical care.

Clinical Preparation

CRITICAL THINKING

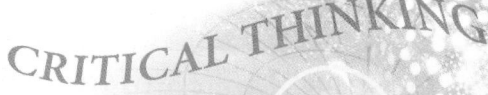

mynursingkit PEARSON

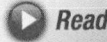 **Read**
- History of Current Illness
- Past Medical History
- Physical Exam
- Admitting Medical Orders
- Laboratory Study Results

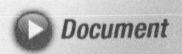 **Document**
- Summary of Hospitalization
- Pathophysiology Form
- Laboratory Values
- Laboratory Results Explanation

 **Apply**
- List of Potential Nursing Diagnoses
- Concept Map
- Critical Thinking Questions

Log on to MyNursingKit.com to download forms you will need and to complete further steps in the Clinical Preparation assignment.

HISTORY OF PRESENT ILLNESS

You are the nurse receiving report on Mr. Hyatt, a 60-year-old male patient who is 3 days postoperative from a suprapubic prostatectomy. The patient was first seen 2 weeks ago

in his health care provider's office with complaints of increasing difficulty voiding during the past 4 months. The physical exam and elevated PSA strongly suggested prostate cancer, and a transrectal ultrasound guided biopsy was done. The results showed a T2, Gleason 2 + 2 tumor. The patient was given the option of radiation therapy or surgery. The patient opted for an immediate prostatectomy. The patient was admitted early yesterday morning for surgery.

You begin your shift rounds and greet the patient as you enter the room. You note an IV in the right forearm, without redness or edema, infusing at 100 mL/hr. A suprapubic catheter is in place and draining well. The outflow bag contains red-tinged fluid. The patient is in a semi-Fowler's position with the overbed table in front of him. The tray on the table contains unopened apple juice, chicken broth, and coffee. When questioned about his untouched food, he states he is just not hungry. You continue the assessment and examine the occlusive suprapubic dressing, which appears moist under the tape. Patient states that his pain on a 1–10 point scale, with 10 being the worst, is 6 mostly around the suprapubic catheter. You give the patient an analgesic and help him to a more comfortable position.

You change the suprapubic dressing around the catheter and note a thick yellow odorous discharge on the dressing with a streak of red on the gauze. A sterile dressing is reapplied to the site, which appears inflamed, with slight edema, minimal bruising, with pale yellow drainage at the catheter insertion site. A suture is visible that is holding the catheter in place. When you return to the nurses' station, the laboratory results for the patient have returned. The health care provider is notified of the CBC values.

Medical–Surgical History

Past medical history was on the chart and is remarkable for hypertension and insulin-dependent diabetes. The patient had all the "usual" childhood illnesses including measles, mumps, and rubella. He had a broken arm requiring casting at age 15 as a result of a baseball injury. There were no major illnesses or medical events until the patient was in his 40s. At age 42, the patient was diagnosed with hypertension requiring 150 milligrams of irbesartan (Avapro) once daily. At age 48, the patient was diagnosed with diabetes, which was controlled with diet therapy until 3 years ago when he started taking a sliding-scale insulin lispro (Humalog) with meals. His blood sugars average in the 120s most days.

Social History

Lives with wife independently. Has three adult children all of whom live out of state. He smoked for 30 years and quit about 10 years ago. He drinks alcohol socially.

Physical Exam

Vital signs: temp 100°F, P 88, R 18, and BP 134/90

Cardiovascular: JVP not elevated; normal S_1 and S_2; regular rate and rhythm, no significant murmur, rub, or gallop; carotids 2+ without bruits

Lung sounds: clear

Bowel sounds: hypoactive in all four quadrants; abdomen is tense

HEENT: scleras anicteric, oropharynx clear

Neck: supple, no lymphadenopathy

Lungs: clear to auscultation bilaterally

Extremities: no edema

Neurological: normal, alert, and oriented $\times$ 3

CXR: normal

ECG: normal sinus rhythm with bundle branch block

Admitting Medical Orders

Diagnosis: cancer of the prostate; prostatectomy

Surgery/urology

Admit to surgical floor

No known allergies

Vital signs and oxygen saturation q4h

Call house officer: pulse < 60 and > 130/minute; BP < 90 and > 160 systolic; temperature > 38.5; urine output < 30 mL/hr for 2 hours; respiratory rate > 30/minute; oxygen saturation < 92%; blood sugar > 120

IV: D51/2NS at 100 mL/hr

Clear liquids postnausea; advance to regular diet as tolerated

Ambulate qid beginning postoperative day 1

Sterile dressing change daily and prn beginning postoperative day 1

Continuous sterile NS bladder irrigation

Fingerstick glucose ac and at bedtime beginning on postoperative day 1

I&O q8h

Incentive spirometer q2h during the day and q4h at night

Sequential compression devices (SCDs) to lower extremities

Scheduled Medications

Humalog S_Q sliding scale per patient home routine

Unasyn (ampicillin sodium) 1.5 g IV daily

Avapro 150 mg po daily beginning postoperative day 1

PRN Medications

Demerol 100 mg IM q4h prn pain

Lortab 7.5 mg po q4h prn pain

Phenergan 25 mg IV or IM q4h prn nausea

Ordered Laboratory Studies

CBC and glucose daily

LABORATORY STUDY RESULTS

Test	Postoperative Day 1	Postoperative Day 2	Postoperative Day 3
White blood cell count (WBC)	12,000/mm³	15,000/mm³	18,000/mm³
Platelets	410,000/mm³	380,000/mm³	378,000/mm³
Hemoglobin (HGB)	14 g/dL	12 g/dL	10 g/dL
Hematocrit (HCT)	48%	42%	39%
Red blood cells (RBC)	4.92/mm³	4.2/mm³	3.5/mm³
Platelets	298,000 mm³	308,000 mm³	310,000 mm³
Hemoglobin A1c	7.2 %	—	—
Serum glucose	114 mg/dL	105 mg/dL	114 mg/dL

CRITICAL THINKING QUESTIONS

1. Which nursing assessment should take priority for this patient?
2. Why should the nurse assess the suprapubic catheter when assessing the patient's pain?
3. What significance is there to the thick yellow drainage at the suprapubic insertion site?
4. What impact do the hemoglobin and diabetes have on the patient's recovery?
5. What significance does the temperature have at this point in the patient's postoperative course?

Answers to Critical Thinking Questions appear in Appendix D.

NCLEX® REVIEW

1. The nurse is caring for a young male patient with an infection of the epididymis. The nurse realizes this infection is most likely the result of:
   1. Inflammation from a sports-related injury.
   2. Exposure to the mumps.
   3. Sexually transmitted infections.
   4. *Escherichia coli* spread from the urinary tract.

2. A 30-year-old male patient is admitted with symptoms of cancer. The nurse realizes that the most common type of reproductive cancer in males under 35 years of age is:
   1. Prostate.
   2. Testicular.
   3. Penile.
   4. Urethral.

3. The nurse working in a urology clinic asks a male client to complete an AUA Symptom Index Tool for the purpose of:
   1. Assisting to diagnose sexual dysfunction disorders.
   2. Determining risk factors for urinary tract malignancy.
   3. Assessing the symptoms associated with incontinence.
   4. Quantifying the symptoms of benign prostatic hypertrophy.

4. The nurse is providing care to a male patient with continuous bladder irrigation after a TURP. The care priority for this patient would be:
   1. Running in one liter per hour of irrigation fluid.
   2. Securing the catheter to the bedrail to promote drainage.
   3. Manually irrigating the catheter several times per shift.
   4. Checking the drainage tubing for kinks on a regular basis.

5. The nurse is providing care to a patient recovering from an orchiectomy for testicular cancer. Which of the following nursing diagnoses should the nurse include when planning this patient's care?
   1. Risk for Infection
   2. Altered Mobility
   3. Disturbed Body Image
   4. Impaired Urinary Elimination

6. The nurse is instructing a 52-year-old male on reproductive health. Which of the following should this instruction include?
   1. Encourage to receive a DRE and PSA test annually.
   2. Teach testicular self-examination.
   3. See a health care provider only if experiencing changes in urinary elimination patterns.
   4. Educate that a lifetime risk for prostate cancer is 1 in 10.

Answers for review questions appear in Appendix D

KEY TERMS

benign prostatic hyperplasia (BPH) *p.1574*
bioavailable testosterone *p.1588*
direct inguinal hernia *p.1589*
epididymitis *p.1566*
erectile dysfunction (ED) *p.1587*
gynecomastia *p.1570*
hernia *p.1589*
hydronephrosis *p.1574*
impotence *p.1570*

indirect inguinal hernia *p.1589*
orchiectomy *p.1568*
orchiopexy *p.1568*
orchitis *p.1567*
paraphimosis *p.1583*
penectomy *p.1587*
Peyronie's disease *p.1583*
phimosis *p.1583*

priapism *p.1587*
prostatectomy *p.1578*
prostatitis *p.1572*
retrograde ejaculation *p.1576*
spermatocele *p.1569*
spermatogenesis *p.1587*
testicular torsion *p.1567*
vasectomy *p.1589*

REFERENCES

Alper, B., & Crawford, E. (2005). Benign prostatic hyperplasia. *The Clinical Advisor, 8*(10), 119–121.

American Cancer Society (ACS). (2007). *ACS News Center. Prostate cancer vaccine one step closer to approval.* Retrieved April 7, 2007, from http://www.cancer.org/docroot/NWS/content/NWS_1_1x_Prostate_Cancer_Vaccine_One_Step_Closer_to_Approval.asp

American Cancer Society (ACS). (2008). *Detailed guide: Penile cancer.* Retrieved April 4, 2007, from http://www.cancer.org/docroot/CRI/CRI_2_3x.asp?dt=35

Argyriou, A., Chroni, E., Koutras, A., Iconomou, G., et al. (2006). A randomized controlled trial evaluating the efficacy and safety of vitamin E supplementation for protection against cisplatin-induced peripheral neuropathy: Final results. *Supportive Care in Cancer: Official Journal of the Multinational Association of Supportive Care in Cancer, 14*(11), 1134–1140.

Barry, M. (2006). Approach to benign prostatic hyperplasia. In A. Goroll & A. Mulley, *Primary care medicine: Office evaluation and management of the adult patient* (5th ed., pp. 909–914). Philadelphia: Lippincott Williams & Wilkins.

Bazar, H., Baydar, S., Boyunaga, H., Batislam, E., Basar, M., & Yilmaz, E. (2003). Primary bilateral spermatocele. *International Journal of Urology, 10*, 59–61.

Beckman, T., & Mynderse, L. (2005). Evaluation and medical management of benign prostatic hyperplasia. *Mayo Clinic Proceedings, 80*(10), 1356–1362.

Benign prostatic hyperplasia (BPH). (2005). *Merck manual professional.* Retrieved April 4, 2007, from http://www.merck.com/mmpe/sec17/ch240/ch240b.html

Bent, S., et al. (2006). Saw palmetto for benign prostatic hyperplasia. *New England Journal of Medicine, 354*(6), 557–566.

Brown, C. (2004). Testicular cancer: an overview. *Urologic Nursing, 24*(2): 83–93.

Buck, A. (2004). Is there a scientific basis for the therapeutic effects of *Serenoa repens* in benign prostatic hyperplasia? Mechanisms of action. *The Journal of Urology, 172*(5, Pt. 1), 1792–1799.

Carmichael, S., Shaw, G., Laurent, C., Lammer, E., Olney, R., & the National Birth Defects Prevention Study. (2005). Hypospadias and maternal exposure to cigarette smoke. *Paediatric and Perinatal Epidemiology, 19*, 406–412.

Cole, F., & Vogler, R. (2004). The acute, nontraumatic scrotum: Assessment, diagnosis and management. *Journal of the American Academy of Nurse Practitioners, 16*(2), 50–56.

Every, M., Mikkelsen, D., & Bailey, D. (2005). Alterations in male genital and reproductive function. In L. Copstead & J. Banasik, *Pathophysiology* (3rd ed., pp. 790–805). St. Louis: Elsevier Saunders.

Every, M., Mikkelsen, D., & Cagle, C. (2005). Male genital and reproductive function. In L. Copstead & J. Banasik, *Pathophysiology* (3rd ed., pp. 772–789). St. Louis: Elsevier Saunders.

Fischbach, F. (2003). *A manual of laboratory and diagnostic tests* (7th ed.). Philadelphia: Lippincott Williams & Wilkins.

Genital trauma: Genitourinary tract traumas. (2005/2007). *Merck manual professional.* Retrieved April 4, 2007, from http://www.merck.com/mmpe/print/sec21/ch314/ch314c.html

Goodman, M.T., Hernandez, B. Y. & Shvetsov, Y. B. (2007). Demographic and Pathologic Differences in the Incidence of Invasive Penile Cancer in the United States, 1995–2003. *Cancer Epidemiology Biomarkers & Prevention* 16, 1833-1839. doi: 10.1158/1055-9965.EPI-07-0221. *American Association for Cancer Research.* Retrieved August 17, 2008 from http://cebp.aacrjournals.org/cgi/content/abstract/16/9/1833?ck=nck

Goodson, J. (2006). Management of acute and chronic prostatitis. In A. Goroll & A. Mulley, *Primary care medicine: Office evaluation and management of the adult patient* (5th ed., pp. 914–919). Philadelphia: Lippincott Williams & Wilkins.

Goroll, A., & Mulley, A. (2006). *Primary care medicine: Office evaluation and management of the adult patient* (5th ed.). Philadelphia: Lippincott Williams & Wilkins.

Gray, M., & Sims, T. (2006). Prostate cancer: Prevention and management of localized disease. *The Nurse Practitioner, 31*(9), 15–28.

Haren, M., Chapman, I., Coates, P., Morley, J., & Wittert, G. (2005). Effect of 12 month oral testosterone on testosterone deficiency symptoms in symptomatic elderly males with low-normal gonadal status. *Age and Aging, 34*(2), 125–130. Retrieved November 5, 2007, from *Cochrane Central Register of Controlled Trials (CENTRAL)*, 2007, Issue 4.

Hatcher, R., et al. (2004). *Contraceptive technology.* New York: Ardent Media.

Hawes, S., Malcarne, V., Ko, C., Sadler, G., Banthia, R., Sherman, S., et al. (2006). Identifying problems faced by spouses and partners of patients with prostate cancer. *Oncology Nursing Forum, 33*(4), 807–814.

Hernias of the abdominal wall. (2005). *Merck manual professional.* Retrieved April 4, 2007, from http://www.merck.com/mmpe/print/sec02/ch011/ch011f.html

Ishani, A., MacDonald, R., Nelson, D., Rutks, J., & Wilt, T. (2000). *Pygeum africanum* for the treatment of patients with benign prostatic hyperplasia: A systematic review and quantitative meta-analysis. *American Journal of Medicine, 109*(8), 654–664.

Karlowicz, K. (Ed.). (1995). *Urologic nursing: Principles and practice.* Philadelphia: W. B. Saunders.

Krebs, L. (2006). What should I say? Talking with patients about sexuality issues. *Clinical Journal of Oncology Nursing, 10*(3), 313–315.

Kuritzky, L., Rosenberg, M., & Sadovsky, R. (2006). Efficacy and safety of alfuzosin 10 mg once daily in the treatment of symptomatic benign prostatic hyperplasia. *International Journal of Clinical Practice, 60*(3), 351–358.

Lashley, R. (2005). *Clinical genetics in nursing practice* (3rd ed.). New York: Springer.

Mahon, S. (2005). Screening for prostate cancer: Informing men about their options. *Clinical Journal of Oncology Nursing, 9*(5), 625–627.

Male sexual dysfunction. (2005). *Merck manual professional.* Retrieved April 4, 2007, from http://www.merck.com/mmpe/sec17/ch227/ch227c.html

McNaughton Collins, M., MacDonald, R., & Wilt, T. (1999). Interventions for chronic abacterial prostatitis (review). *Cochrane Database of Systemic reviews.* In *The Cochrane Library*, 2007, Issue 1. Retrieved August 11, 2008 from http://www.mrw.interscience.wiley.com/cochrane/clsysrev/articles/CD002080/frame.html

McVary, K. (2006). BPH: Epidemiology and comorbidities. *American Journal of Managed Care, 12*(Suppl. 5):, S122–S128.

National Academy of Clinical Biochemistry (NACB). (2006). *Tumor markers PDF. Practice guidelines and recommendations for use of tumor markers in the clinic: Testicular Cancer (section 3A).* Retrieved March 30, 2007, from http://www.aacc.org/members/nacb/lmpg/onlineguide/draftguidelines/tumormarkers/pages/tumormarkerspdf.aspx

National Cancer Institute (NCI). (2007a). *Genetics of prostate cancer (PDQ).* Retrieved April 7, 2007, from http://www.cancer.gov/cancertopics/pdq/genetics/prostate/HealthProfessional/

National Cancer Institute (NCI). (2007b). *Prostate cancer.* Retrieved April 7, 2007, from http://www.cancer.gov/cancertopics/types/prostate

National Cancer Institute (NCI). (2007c). *Prostate cancer treatment (PDQ): Stage information.* Retrieved August 11, 2008, from http://www.cancer.gov/cancertopics/pdq/treatment/prostate/HealthProfessional/page4#Section_88

National Cancer Institute (NCI). (2007d). *Testicular cancer: Questions and answers.* Retrieved March 22, 2007 from http://www.cancer.gov/cancertopics/factsheet/sites-types/testicular#5

National Cancer Institute (NCI). (2007e). *Treatment choices for men with early-stage prostate cancer.* Retrieved April 9, 2007, from http:/www.cancer.gov/cancertopics/prostate-cancer-treatment-choices

National Comprehensive Cancer Network. (2008). *Clinical practice guidelines in oncology: Prostate cancer* [V.1.2008]. Retrieved August 11, 2008, from http://www.nccn.org/professionals/physician_gls/PDF/prostate.pdf

Nickel, J. C. (2006). BPH: Costs and treatment outcomes. *The American Journal of Managed Care, 12*(Suppl. 5), S141–S148.

O'Leary, M. (2006). Treatment and pharmacologic management of BPH in the context of common comorbidities. *American Journal of Managed Care, 12*(Suppl. 5), S129–S140.

Organon. (2002a). *Impact of low testosterone.* Retrieved November 5, 2007, from http://www.andropause.com/about_andropause/impact.asp

Organon. (2002b). *Understanding risks.* Retrieved November 5, 2007, from http://www.andropause.com/treatment_options/understanding.asp

Penile cancer: Genitourinary cancer. (2005). *Merck manual professional.* Retrieved April 4, 2007, from http://www.merck.com/mmpe/print/sec17/ch241/ch241d.html

Peyronie's disease: Penile and scrotal disorders. (2005). *Merck manual professional.* Retrieved March 31, 2007, from http://www.merck.com/mmpe/print/sec17/ch239/ch239f.html

Porche, D. (2006). Prostatitis. *Journal of Nurse Practitioners, 2*(10), 662–663.

Prostatitis: Prostate disease. (2005). *Merck manual professional.* Retrieved March 30, 2007, from http://www.merck.com/mmpe/sec17/ch240/ch240c.html

Quallich, S. (2006). Examining male fertility. *Urologic Nursing, 26*(4), 277–288.

Rigdon, J. (2006). Home study program: Robotic-assisted laparoscopic radical prostatectomy. *AORN Journal, 84*(5), 759–762, 764, 766–774.

Ringdahl, E., & Teague, L. (2006). Testicular torsion. *American Family Physician, 74*, 1739–1743.

RxList the Internet Drug Index. (2007a). *Cisplatin.* Retrieved March 31, 2007, from http://www.rxlist.com/cgi/generic/cisplatin_ids.htm

RxList the Internet Drug Index. (2007b). *Motrin.* Retrieved March 31, 2007, from http://www.rxlist.com/cgi/generic/ibup.htm

RxList the Internet Drug Index. (2007c). *Zofran injection.* Retrieved March 31, 2007, from http://www.rxlist.com/cgi/generic/ondansetron.htm

Scrotal masses. (2005). *Merck manual professional.* Retrieved November 3, 2007, from http://www.merck.com/mmpe/print/sec17/ch239/ch239i.html

Segal, R., Lukka, H., Klotz, L., Eady, A., Bestic, N., & Johnston, M. (2001). Cancer Care Ontario Practice Guidelines Initiative Genitourinary Cancer Disease Site Group. Surveillance programs for early stage nonseminomatous testicular cancer: A practice guideline. *Canadian Journal of Urology, 8*(1), 1184–1192. In *Database of Abstracts of Reviews of Effects*, 2007, Issue 1. Retrieved March 29, 2007, from http://www.mrw.interscience.wiley.com/cochrane/

Seidman, S. (2006). Normative hypogonadism and depression: Does "andropause" exist? *International Journal of Impotence Research, 18*, 415–422.

Sperm disorders. (2005). *Merck manual professional.* Retrieved April 4, 2007, from http://www.merck.com/mmpe/sec18/ch256/ch256b.html

Sterilization. (2007). *Merck manual professional.* Retrieved August 14, 2008, from http://www.merck.com/mmpe/sec18/ch255/ch255c.html

Stevenson, T. D., & McNeill, J. A. (2004). Surgical management of testicular cancer. *Clinical Journal of Oncology Nursing, 8*(4), 355–360.

Tan, R., & Pu, S. (2004). Is it andropause? Recognizing androgen deficiency in aging men. *Postgraduate Medicine, 115*(1), 62–66.

Testicular Cancer Resource Center. (2007). *How to do a testicular self examination.* Retrieved April 1, 2007, from http://tcrc.acor.org/tcexam.html

Walsh, P., Retik, A., Vaughan, E., & Wein, A. (Eds.). (2007). *Campbell's urology* (9th ed.). Philadelphia: W. B. Saunders.

Ward-Smith, P. (2006). Cultural disparities in the diagnosis and treatment of prostate cancer. *Urologic Nursing, 26*(5), 397–405.

Wilt, T., Howe, R., & Rutks, I. (2000). Terazosin for benign prostatic hyperplasia. *Cochrane Database Systematic Reviews 2000.* In *The Cochrane Library*, 2007, Issue 1. Retrieved March 31, 2007, from www.thecochranelibrary.com

Zeroski, D., Abel, L., Butler, W. M., Wallner, K., & Merrick, G. S. (2005). Factors affecting patient selection for prostate brachytherapy: What nurses should know. *Clinical Journal of Oncology Nursing, 9*(5), 553–560.

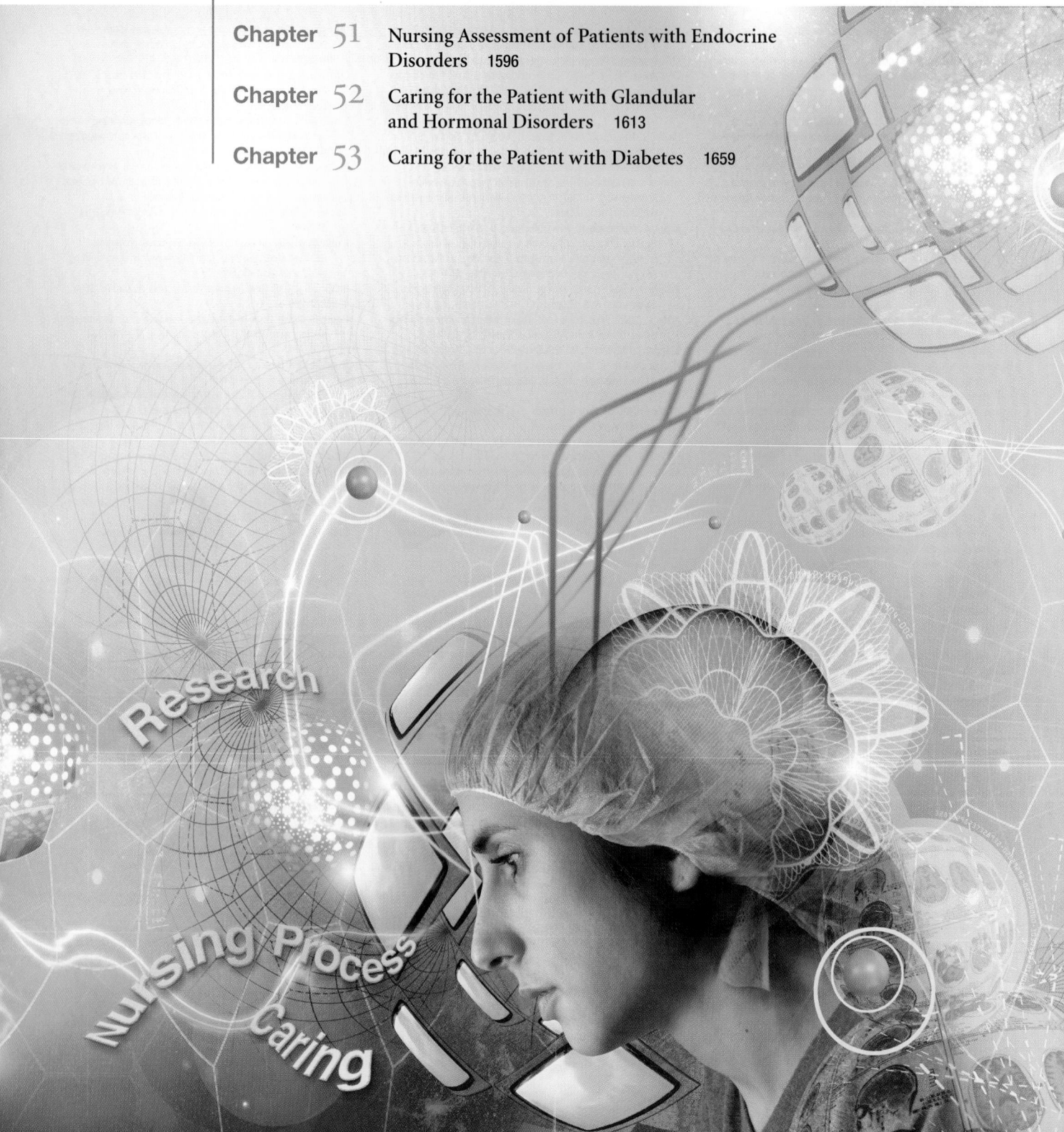

UNIT **11**

Nursing Management of Patients with Endocrine Disorders

Research

Nursing Process

Caring

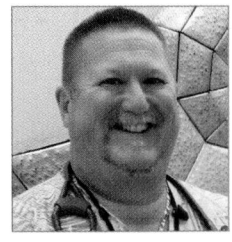

RICH   My name is Rich and I am a clinical resource nurse (CN III) on a medical–surgical unit at a 540-bed teaching hospital. As a tertiary facility, we receive patients from all of Northern California as well as a large population of underserved patients who seek health care when they are at their sickest. As a resource nurse, I do patient care and precept new nurses. I care for patients with diabetes, pancreatitis, acute liver failure, chronic renal failure, antibiotic-resistant serious infections, and for those who require long-term ventilator support.

I chose to work at this hospital because it is a teaching facility where state-of-the-art practices are implemented, and it has a nursing body that encourages personal growth and career movement and doctors who value the input of the nursing staff and truly work as a team to provide the utmost in quality patient care. This hospital uses the primary nursing model, in which the nurse is at center stage when orchestrating the care required by each patient. As their primary nurse, I am able to help patients understand what the plan of treatment is for them.

I also teach in a local nursing program as a clinical instructor. Both as a clinical nurse and as part-time faculty, I have the opportunity to teach new nurses and students the six components of caring. I also value the importance of these six components in the care that I give to my patients. On a typical day, I can be caring for three to four patients with complex problems. My **commitment** to each of the patients is that I will do my utmost to provide them the nursing care that will enable them to heal and ultimately be discharged from the hospital. We care for long-term ventilator patients and our commitment to them as a unit is to provide the highest level of care to afford them the ability to have quality time with their families as we attempt to wean them from the ventilator or, in some cases, as we prepare both the patient and families for a life of being ventilator dependent.

Compassion is an integral part of my daily interactions with my patients. Patients come to our unit with a variety of unhealthy habits, such as alcohol and drug abuse, that over time have put them into various states of organ failure. It can be very easy to become jaded when dealing with this type of patient. My compassion for these individuals allows me to provide them with the nonjudgmental care that is required to bring them back to their prior state of wellness. Often these patients have become so debilitated that they are no longer able to do the simplest of activities of daily living and my **conscience** dictates that I assist them with these tasks in a dignified manner.

Because I have 26 years of experience as a nurse, I am able to perform my nursing care in a **confident** manner. In doing so, I put patients at ease by letting them know that I have performed my nursing skills many times. My confidence in performing procedures serves to decrease patients' anxiety levels. I pride myself in being a very **competent** nurse. I have had physicians tell me that they have been glad that I was caring for their patients because they know my level of competence. This also allows me to feel comfortable precepting a novice nurse. As a preceptor, I am able to guide new nurses in applying what they have learned and can help make their transition to this busy and often demanding unit less stressful. My **comportment**, or how I interact with my patients and their families, is a professional nurse–patient relationship. I let them know that I will be their advocate while they are under my care.

Being able to think critically is essential, because it is the nursing assessments that indicate when a patient is not doing well and what information needs to be communicated to physicians. Critical thinking is essential when caring for the complex ventilator patient because they can decompensate at any given moment during the weaning stages. Clinical reasoning also is paramount in dealing with the patients who have illnesses or comorbidities that may hamper their efforts at a full recovery. It is the task of nurses to use their broad nursing knowledge to prioritize the care required of the particular patient. Nurses must be able to communicate with the health care team in a concise and focused manner about these priorities. I have had the opportunity on many occasions to analyze patients' vital signs and physical appearance and demeanor and been able to summon the medical team to evaluate any patient who in my estimation has taken a turn for the worst. This ability is something that has evolved over time as I have evolved into the professional nurse that I am today.

> "My **commitment** to each of the patients is that I will do my utmost to provide them the nursing care that will enable them to heal and ultimately be discharged from the hospital."

Nursing Assessment of Patients with Endocrine Disorders

Corinne Harmon

Outcome-Based Learning Objectives

After studying this chapter, the learner will be able to:

1. Identify the components of the endocrine system.
2. Explain the general structure and function of hormones.
3. Explain the concept of hormonal regulation as it relates to the hypothalamus, pituitary, thyroid, parathyroid, adrenals, gonads, and pancreas glands.
4. Explain subjective and objective data related to the general assessment of the endocrine system.
5. Discuss the purpose, preparation, and nursing functions related to diagnostic testing of the endocrine system.

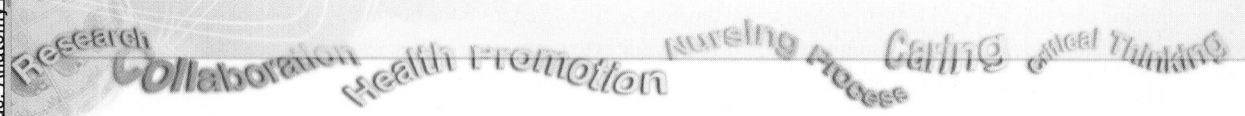

THE ENDOCRINE SYSTEM is truly a marvel. This system of glands and specialized tissue located throughout the body is involved in maintaining the body's overall function and homeostasis. This is accomplished through the release of hormones. Hormones exert their effect only on specific target tissues. This specificity of action and the fact that glands are ductless makes the endocrine system unique.

Anatomy and Physiology Review

The endocrine system is composed of glands, glandular tissue, and target tissue or receptors. The organs of the endocrine system are known as glands. Glands arise from glandular epithelial tissue during embryonic development. These glands include

- Hypothalamus
- Pituitary gland
- Adrenal glands
- Thyroid gland
- Parathyroid glands
- Islet cells of the pancreas
- Gonads.

The term **endocrine** refers to the process of an active biological agent being secreted into the bloodstream. These biological agents are known as hormones. The functions of the glands and their production of hormones may be age contingent as is discussed sequentially under each gland and hormone produced.

General Structure and Function of Hormones

Hormones are chemical substances that have a regulatory action on target tissues. They act as chemical messengers to stimulate certain functions while retarding others. Because glands are ductless, hormones are released directly into the circulation. The hormone then travels thorough the bloodstream where it will exert its action on target cells or receptors. Target tissues (cells) or **receptors** represent those tissues or organs upon which the specific hormone acts. The receptors within the endocrine system are able to distinguish a specific hormone from all other chemicals in circulation and bind to it in a lock-and-key type manner. This binding process then triggers the target tissues or organs to produce the desired response. The organs and target tissue of the endocrine system are located throughout the body.

The endocrine system's functioning is intimately connected to that of the nervous system. Together, these systems provide a mechanism for communication between cells and organs. This connection is referred to as *neuroendocrine regulation*. The systems work synergistically to regulate overall physiological functioning by regulating responses to the internal and external environment. Through the combined efforts of the two systems, growth and development, maintenance of homeostasis, the adaptability to changes in the external environment, and reproduction can occur.

Hormone Classification and Function

Hormones travel through the bloodstream to reach target tissues or receptors. They exist as proteins, peptides, lipids, or amino acid analogues. As they circulate in the bloodstream, they may be free or bound. The majority of hormones are secreted in their active form. Others must undergo metabolic conversion to their active form in peripheral tissue. Hormones also function in other ways. If hormones affect cells within the vicinity of their release, it is known as **paracrine functioning**. Hormones are said to have **autocrine functioning** when the hormones produced act on the cells that created them.

General Hormone Regulation

All hormones are interrelated to some degree, and a number of complex interactions control their secretion. Overall, hormone regulation involves the interplay of individual hormone responses, while counterbalancing the influence of other hormones by integrating mechanisms for terminating or attenuating their response. These mechanisms operate to maintain an intricate balance of the internal environment, ensuring precise control in order to maintain homeostasis. Hormone release may be regulated by one or more mechanisms. Common regulatory mechanisms at work within the endocrine system include basal hormone release, circadian or infradian rhythms, brain-mediated neural stimulation or inhibition of hormone release, and feedback systems.

In basal hormone release, small amounts of hormones are released continuously. **Circadian rhythms** refer to cyclical biological activities. The phenomenon denotes that there is an orderly change or variation in hormonal activity during a 24-hour period. An example of this is the release of cortisol, whose peaks and troughs have been demonstrated by serum analyses. **Infradian rhythms** are those that last for more than 24 hours. This is seen in females in the menstrual cycle. Neural regulation of hormone secretion, suppression, or release also occurs.

A feedback system is a regulatory system that keeps certain body functions within a prescribed range to sustain homeostasis (Figure 51–1 ■). Feedback systems can be positive or negative. In **negative feedback**, an alteration in a hormone level stimulates a series of changes to return the level to normal. **Positive feedback** occurs when the increased secretion of a hormone causes another gland to release a hormone. The best example of this is the release of leuteinizing hormone in response to higher estrogen levels.

Feedback loops can be simple or complex. A simple loop is seen with insulin and glucagon; with hyperglycemia, insulin is released, whereas with hypoglycemia, glucagon is released. In more complex loops, control is accomplished by releasing factors made in the hypothalamus as well as by stimulating factors made in the pituitary.

Hypothalamus Gland

The hypothalamus gland is located in the third ventricle of the brain and is composed of nervous tissue. It shares its circulatory system with the anterior pituitary, and it plays a role in the func-

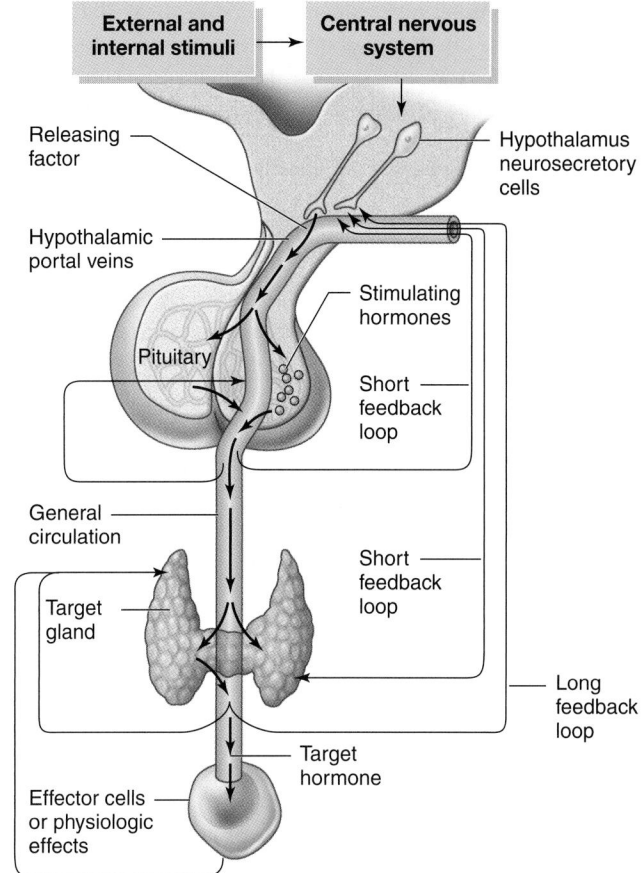

FIGURE 51–1 ■ General feedback loop.

tion of both the anterior and posterior pituitary. The hormones produced in the hypothalamus are secreted directly into the anterior pituitary gland via the hypothalamic-hypophyseal portal system. These hormones, called neurohormones, may be stimulatory or inhibitory. They act directly on the tissues of the pituitary gland to control the secretion of the anterior pituitary hormones. Inhibiting hormones are released by the hypothalamus to stop the formation and secretion of target hormones; the most important of these is prolactin inhibitory factor. Tropic or stimulating hormones, which are made by the pituitary, act on target tissue or glands to release hormones needed for homeostasis, growth maturation, and reproduction of the individual.

The hypothalamus receives signals from almost all possible sources, including the cerebral cortex. These sources send pain and psychological messages, causing release of tropic hormones. Therefore, prolonged stress can alter cortisol, thyroid, and growth hormone levels and cause menstruation to cease. Because of this interrelation and the wide range of functions that these hormones exert in maintaining the body's function, the hypothalamus is considered by some to be the true "master gland."

Pituitary Gland

The pea-sized pituitary gland is located at the base of the brain above the sphenoid bone. It is divided into two parts, the anterior pituitary (adenohypophysis) and the posterior pituitary (neurohypophysis). The anterior pituitary is glandular tissue and the posterior pituitary is actually an extension of the hypothalamus.

The posterior pituitary is made up of nervous tissue and its primary function is the release of antidiuretic hormone, to be discussed later, and oxytocin. Oxytocin in females is responsible for the secretion of milk from the breasts and causes the contraction of the uterus during labor.

The anterior pituitary originates from epithelial tissue and comprises approximately 80% of the gland's mass. Its cells secrete hormones that are regulated by the releasing and inhibiting hormones produced by the hypothalamus. Five specialized cell types within the anterior pituitary are responsible for the secretion of the six major hormones: growth hormone, thyroid-stimulating hormone or thyrotropin, adrenocorticotropin hormone or corticotropin, prolactin, follicle-stimulating hormone, and luteinizing hormone. Most of these hormones are tropic hormones. Releasing and inhibiting hormones produced by the hypothalamus control the secretion of the hormones produced by the anterior pituitary (Chart 51–1). Each of these is discussed under a separate section.

Assessment

Hormones are involved in the use and production of energy, growth and development, sexual development and maturation, and maintaining homeostasis. These vast, encompassing functions make it clear that the assessment of endocrine function is an involved task. Disorders may not produce any associated symptoms or may be so vague as to be attributed to any number of problems other than endocrine dysfunction. Abnormalities are produced by five indistinct mechanisms: difficulty with the appropriate transport of a hormone, production of hormones by hypersecretion (excessive production) or hyposecretion (decreased production), inability of target tissues to respond to a secreted hormone, and inappropriate stimulation of target tissue.

Health History

Assessing for normal and abnormal hormonal variations entails a thorough assessment of the patient's history along with a systematic, complete physical examination. Assessment should include examination of past medical history, family history, current complaints, general and functional health evaluation, and diagnostic testing. General health screening and focused screening of chief complaints will assist in the identification of the origin of suspected endocrine disorders.

Exploration of the patient's history is essential. Questioning should seek to assess the onset, characteristics, and severity of symptoms. The nurse also should seek to identify any alleviating or aggravating factors, associated symptomatology, and timing of symptoms. The patient is asked about previous head injuries, hospitalizations, illnesses, surgeries and treatments, changes in appearance, sleep and rest patterns, elimination problems, sexual dysfunction, changes in diet or appetite, and medication usage. Cognitive function, including sensory and perception, along with affect, also may be altered with endocrine dysfunction.

Along with a review of the entire medical history, family, occupational, and social histories are evaluated. Disorders of the endocrine system tend to occur in a familial pattern. There is a high correlation of diabetes, thyroid disorders, and obesity among families. Knowing this information should assist the interviewer in conducting a more focused assessment. Dietary patterns and involuntary weight losses and gains should be explored. Exposure to chemicals, use of drugs and alcohol, smoking, coping with stress, and behavioral patterns are all areas to be investigated.

Health Assessment Across the Adult Life Span

Generally endocrine disorders should be assessed for all patients across the adult life span. However, certain hormonal disorders are prone to develop in certain age groups. For example, disorders of the pituitary and related hormones tend to affect chil-

CHART 51–1	**Anterior Pituitary Hormone Production and Function**	
Cell Type	**Hormone Produced**	**Hormone Function**
Somatotropic	Growth hormone (GH) or somatotropin	• Stimulates growth and development of skeletal muscle and long bones. • Metabolizes carbohydrates, fats, and protein.
Lactotrophic	Prolactin	• Stimulates the production of breast milk following childbirth. • Increases response of the follicles to luteinizing hormone (LH) and follicle-stimulating hormone (FSH).
Thymotrophic	Thyroid-stimulating hormone (TSH)	• Stimulates the production and synthesis and release of thyroid hormone from the thyroid.
Corticotrophic	Adrenocorticotrophic hormone (ACTH)	• Stimulates the release of hormones from the adrenal cortex.
Gonadotrophic	Follicle-stimulating hormone (FSH) Luteinizing hormone (LH)	• In women, stimulates the development of ovarian follicles and estrogenic female sex hormones. • In men, functions in the development and maturation of sperm. • In women, stimulates ovulation and formation of corpus luteum from an ovarian follicle. • In men, stimulates production of male sex hormones.
Melanocytic	Melanocyte-stimulating hormone (MSH)	• Stimulates the production and release of melanin (melanogenesis) by melanocytes in skin and hair.

dren and young adults. Hyperpituitarism, or oversecretion of the growth hormone is evident in adulthood after puberty. Gigantism begins before the epiphyseal closure of the bones; the disease is progressive. It affects children as evidenced by an increasing growth rate. Acromegaly develops between the ages of 30 and 50; and dwarfism occurs as a result of failure of the pituitary gland and is evident in young adults. Deficiency in hormones produced by the pituitary gland also may affect sexual development of males and females and cause consequences in postpartum lactation.

Age differences also are noted in diabetes mellitus (DM), type 1 and type 2, generated by decreased production of insulin by the pancreas or by decreased ability to use insulin. Type 1 DM typically occurs in people before the age of 30, peaking at ages 5 to 11. Type 2 usually develops after the age of 30, often in middle age. Gestational diabetes starts or is first recognized during pregnancy, usually becoming apparent during the 24th to 28th weeks of pregnancy. It is important to recognize these age variations in assessing patients because they can help guide the assessment process and recognition of presenting symptoms.

Relative to the aging population the most frequent sign of hormonal imbalance is hypothyroidism (Bharaktiya, Orlander, Woodhouse, & Davis, 2007). This is discussed in detail under the discussion of the thyroid gland. Disorders related to each of the hormonal imbalances referenced above are discussed in Chapters 52 and 53 🔵.

Current Health Problems

Because the endocrine system functions in the storage and production of energy, the patient should be asked about energy levels and the ability to carry out activities of daily living (ADLs) independently. The patient may report not being able to "do what I used to" or may complain of generalized weakness and fatigue." Patients are more likely to report a gradual decline than an abrupt change in activity tolerance. Assessment of a patient's energy level also will be important in developing the ongoing plan of care. Thyroid and adrenal dysfunction are common reasons for altered energy levels (see these sections later in this chapter).

Physical Examination

The only endocrine glands that can be palpated are the thyroid, ovaries, and testes. All others are located within the body and examination of function relies on the examination of the end result of hormone function on target tissue and diagnostic testing. The physical exam should be thorough and systematic. This section provides a general overview. More findings are included in the specific endocrine disorder section.

General appearance, skin, hair, nails, facial contours, and body symmetry can provide clues to the endocrine gland experiencing dysfunction. Normal growth and development patterns are compared to physical findings in the client. Alterations of temperature, heart rate, and blood pressure all may be attributed to endocrine dysfunction. Comparisons to normal stature and usual body weight may yield clues to pituitary or thyroid dysfunction.

The physical exam should begin with vital sign measurement, height and weight, and mental status exam. The skin and its appendages also are examined. The skin is assessed for temperature, color, homogeneous pigmentation pattern, turgor,

texture, edema, and presence of masses. The skin also is assessed for the presence of lesions or striae. Nail angle, thickness, and pigmentation are reviewed for abnormalities. Hair distribution pattern and texture are noted. The presence of acne, hirsutism, ecchymosis, striae, thinning skin, and alopecia may be associated with steroid-excess states. Excessive sweating and coarse dry skin also can be associated with endocrine dysfunction.

Assessment of the head and neck involves both internal and external examination. Visually, the examination begins with the inspection of the face and neck for contours, symmetry, and masses. The oral cavity is examined for color, size, intactness, lesions, and condition of teeth, tongue, and gums. The neck also is examined for bulging and masses along with the position of the trachea. The eyes are assessed for bulging. Visual acuity, field of gaze, and lid movement should be evaluated.

The chest is visualized for its overall appearance. Symmetry of chest movement is noted. Heart sounds are auscultated and the patient is examined for the presence of bruits (turbulent blood flow through a vessel or artery). Heart rhythm is assessed for regularity and the presence of abnormality and is compared to peripheral pulses. Lung sounds are assessed. Measurement of oxygen saturation will provide information that may be important in evaluating mental status and cognitive function. The size of the heart can be affected by endocrine disease. The presence of adventitious (abnormal) breath sounds may indicate increased fluid retention that may be seen in patients with endocrine dysfunction.

Peripheral pulses are palpated and pulse volume is noted. The abdomen usually is assessed for skin color, pigmentation pattern, and presence of striae. It also is inspected for distention, masses, pulsations, and dilated veins. Bowel sounds are auscultated, noting frequency and character. Palpation is done to assess for the presence of masses, tenderness, or pain. Unintentional weight loss due to loss of appetite, weight gain, constipation, and bouts of diarrhea can all be seen in patients experiencing endocrine dysfunction. Liver impairment also may be seen in the endocrine disorders of diabetes and myxedema. Abdominal obesity has been associated with metabolic syndrome.

The upper and lower extremities are examined visually for general appearance, pigmentation pattern, skin texture, and hair distribution. Symmetry of muscle mass along with appropriateness of size as dictated by normal parameters of growth and development are assessed. Deep tendon reflexes, motor movement, sensation, and strength are assessed. Proprioception, coordination, and the presence of tremors are noted.

Nervous system complaints are common in endocrine dysfunction because nearly all hormones have a demonstrated influence on the central nervous system. Headache is a common complaint. Patients also may display tremors, lethargy, and convulsions. Electrolyte imbalances produced by endocrine disorders can produce considerable muscle weakness or spastic muscle activity. Neuropathies, myopathy, osteoporosis, osteomalacia, gouty arthritis, and distortion of bone growth all can be seen in endocrine dysfunction.

A number of endocrine disorders are associated with urinary dysfunction. Patients may complain of frequency, urgency, and nocturia with diabetes mellitus or insipidus. Nephrolithiasis (kidney stones) can occur with hyperparathyroidism, Cushing's disease, and acromegaly. Patients with diabetes mellitus are prone to urinary tract infections. Congenital urinary abnormalities are seen in Turner's syndrome. The next section focuses on specific subjective and objective findings for different endocrine disorders.

Specific Hormonal Functions and Assessment of Hormonal Imbalances

Each hormone has a specific function. Hormones act on the target tissue by different mechanisms. They can alter the function of the target tissue by interacting with chemical receptors located either on the cell membrane or in the interior of the cell. Imbalances, either hypersecretion or hyposecretion of the hormone, can lead to specific hormonal disorders.

Growth Hormone

Like the other hormones controlled by the pituitary in a complex feedback loop, growth hormone (GH) is secreted by the pituitary directly into the blood throughout the life cycle in a double feedback loop. GH synthesis and release is controlled by the hypothalamus through growth hormone releasing factor (GHRF) and growth hormone release-inhibiting hormone (GHRIH), which stimulate the pituitary to release GH. Once released into circulation, GH stimulates the production of insulin-like growth factor-1 (IGF-1), also known as somatomedin C (SM-C). Growth hormone stimulates growth of all tissues. When the epiphyses of the bones close at approximately age 21, bone growth will cease.

Assessment

A tumor of the pituitary with GH hypersecretion can cause excess growth or gigantism in children. The nurse should take a careful history of size of other family members to rule out genetic causes for very tall children. The nurse assessing extremes in size should consider a tumor of the pituitary as the source.

In adults, the name for hypersecretion of GH is acromegaly. More than 95% of acromegaly cases are caused by a pituitary adenoma that secretes excess amounts of GH. Ectopic production of GH and GHRH by malignant tumors accounts for other causes (Khandwala, 2005). Hypersecretion causes growth of the cartilage, resulting in enlargement of the ears and jaw, protrusion of the tongue, and disproportionately large hands and feet with thick fingers and toes. There is skeletal thickening, hypertrophy of the skin, and enlargement of the heart and liver. Other findings include weakness, delayed onset of puberty, and irregular menstruation. Because GH is an insulin antagonist, the nurse should assess for hyperglycemia. Because tumors of the pituitary may erode into the oral mucosa, the mouth needs careful inspection.

Insufficient GH causes a child to be a perfectly proportioned midget, in contrast to dwarfism, a genetic defect in which there is failure of the long bones to grow. Children who are not on the growth chart need referral to an endocrinologist.

Laboratory and Diagnostic Procedures

Growth hormone (somatotropin) is increased in gigantism and acromegaly, and decreased in dwarfism. However, random GH measurements are often not diagnostic because of the episodic secretion of GH, its short half-life, and the overlap between GH concentration in patients with acromegaly and healthy subjects. Because IGF-1 has a long half-life, its measurement is useful to gauge integrated GH secretion, to screen for acromegaly, and to monitor the efficacy of therapy (Khandwala, 2005). A computerized tomography (CT) or magnetic resonance imaging (MRI) scan will show pituitary tumor in gigantism. X-rays may show spotting or stippling near the epiphyses of the bones in dwarfism. Chart 51–2 summarizes growth hormone testing.

Antidiuretic Hormone

Antidiuretic hormone (ADH) or vasopressin is synthesized in the cell bodies of neurons located in the hypothalamus and transmitted to the posterior pituitary along axons in response to neural stimulation. ADH is responsible for the reabsorption of water in the renal tubules resulting in an increase in circulatory volume, and is released in response to increased osmolality of the blood. Excessive ADH, secreted by tumors or ectopic sources, causes fluid retention and is known as syndrome of inappropriate ADH (SIADH). Lack of ADH causes fluid loss and is known as diabetes insipidus.

Assessment

The nurse should take a careful history of the cardiac and renal systems when assessing fluid balance to eliminate these as causes for fluid retention. Excessive weight gain without overt edema is

CHART 51–2	Growth Hormone Testing		
Laboratory Test and Normal Values	**Gland Tested Diagnostic Significance**	**Disorders Associated with Abnormal Levels** *(symptoms are italicized)*	
		Increased	**Decreased**
Growth hormone (somatotropin) Adult (fasting and at rest) 2–5 ng/mL	Anterior pituitary (origin) Muscle and bone (target)	*Gigantism in children, acromegaly in adults,* benign pituitary gland tumor, severe malnutrition states, hyperpituitarism, multiple endocrine neoplasia, neurofibromatosis	*Dwarfism in children,* hypopituitarism, Seckel's syndrome, congenital GH deficiency, pituitary fibrosis, or calcification
IGF-1 Concentrations vary with age. An assay in which reference ranges have been stratified in such a manner is required.	Anterior pituitary (origin) Muscle and bone (target)	*Gigantism in children, acromegaly in adults,* benign pituitary gland tumor, severe malnutrition states, hyperpituitarism, multiple endocrine neoplasia, neurofibromatosis	*Dwarfism in children,* hypopituitarism, Seckel's syndrome, congenital GH deficiency, pituitary fibrosis, or calcification

characteristic of SIADH, as are hyponatremia, nausea, vomiting, muscle cramps, confusion, convulsions, inappropriately elevated urine osmolality (>200 mOsm/kg), excessive urine sodium excretion (UNa >30 mEq/L), and decreased serum osmolality. These findings occur in the absence of diuretic therapy; in the presence of normal volume without edema; and in the setting of otherwise normal cardiac, renal, adrenal, hepatic, and thyroid function (Rafailov, 2007). This syndrome may occur as a result of ectopic secretion in association with oat-cell lung cancer, pancreatic cancer, prostate cancer, and Hodgkin's disease as well as a number of other disorders.

 Hyponatremia with serum sodium < 115 mEq/L causes osmotic shifts of fluid from the blood into the brain. This increases the pressure and can cause lethargy, headaches, decreased responsiveness, seizures, and coma.

Excessive urination, decreased urine specific gravity, thirst, and dehydration are found with lack of ADH, known as diabetes insipidus (DI). The term *insipidus* means lacking character, referring to the clear colorless urine. Trauma or autoimmune response can cause a lack of ADH. The most common form is central DI. Central DI results from damage to the pituitary gland, which disrupts the normal storage and release of ADH. Nephrogenic DI results when the kidneys are unable to respond to ADH. Rarer forms occur because of a defect in the thirst mechanism (dipsogenic DI) or during pregnancy (gestational DI) (National Kidney and Urologic Diseases Information Clearinghouse, 2006).

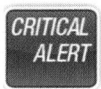 *Trauma to the head may damage the pituitary and result in decreased production of ADH, resulting in extreme diuresis or diabetes insipidus. Trauma patients who produce excessively large amounts of urine are at risk of hypovolemic shock.*

Laboratory and Diagnostic Procedures

Serum osmolarity testing is done to determine ADH balance. Increased serum osmolality indicates lack of ADH and dehydration; decrease in serum osmolality indicates SIADH and fluid overload. Serum sodium is also decreased when fluid is retained; it is increased with diabetes insipidus and dehydration. Urine osmolality testing will be decreased in diabetes insipidus due to large volumes of very dilute urine. Chart 51–3 summarizes antidiuretics hormone tests of the posterior pituitary used to determine disorders of associated abnormal levels.

Gonads

The gonads are the body's primary source of sexual hormones. They are controlled in a triple feedback loop. The hypothalamus makes follicle-stimulating hormone releasing factor (FRF) and luteinizing hormone releasing factor (LRF). FRF from the hypothalamus causes release of follicle-stimulating hormone (FSH) and luteinizing hormone (LH) from the anterior pituitary gland. FSH in women promotes maturation of the ovarian follicle, which produces estrogen. As levels of estrogen rise, there is an increase in LH. Together FSH and LH induce ovulation. In men, FSH produces spermatogenesis, and the LH stimulates secretion of androgens.

Gonads are important for the progression into puberty and they control other physical traits that differentiate men from women. The principal hormone produced by the testes is testosterone. The primary hormones produced by the ovaries are estrogen and progesterone. For males, testosterone maintains reproductive functioning and secondary sexual characteristics. Sexual hormones also promote the production and maturation of sperm and stimulate most cells into protein synthesis.

In women, the ovaries secrete estrogen and progesterone to maintain reproductive functioning and secondary sexual characteristics. Progesterone in females also promotes the growth of the lining of the uterus for the implantation of a fertilized ovum and prepares the mammary glands for lactation. Some sexual hormones, called androgens, also are produced by the adrenal gland.

Assessment

Assessment of reproductive and sexual functioning entails the visualization of age-appropriate sexual development along with questioning concerning changes in libido, fertility, impotence, and menstrual irregularities. Hair distribution and character also are noted, particularly pubic hair, which decreases with decreased sex hormones. The breasts are observed for contours, masses, tenderness, and the presence of inappropriate lactation. Males are assessed for gynecomastia (enlarged breasts), which occurs when the liver does not destroy female hormones made by the adrenal gland. The testes are palpated in males and a pelvic examination conducted in females. Clitoral enlargement in women may indicate an endocrine disorder. Precocious puberty in the young may be caused by premature release of gonadotropin-releasing hormone (GnRH) by the hypothalamus. Lack of secondary sexual characteristics in adults may be seen in pituitary hypofunction.

The patient should be assessed for sexual maturation using Tanner's stages (Estes, 2002); (Chart 51–4, p. 1602). Failure to develop secondary sexual characteristics of pubic hair and genital growth by the age of 16 should be investigated and referred by the nurse.

CHART 51–3 Antidiuretic Hormone Testing

Laboratory Test and Normal Values	Gland Tested Diagnostic Significance	Disorders Associated with Abnormal Levels *(symptoms are italicized)*	
		Increased	Decreased
Antidiuretic hormone If serum osmolarity is >290 mOsm/kg: 2–12 pg/mL or SI: 1.85–11.1 pmol/L If serum osmolarity is <290 mOsm/kg: <2 pg/mL or SI: <1.85 pmol/L	Posterior pituitary (origin) Kidneys (target) Used to diagnose diabetes insipidus and syndrome of inappropriate antidiuretic hormone release (SIADH)	Pituitary hyperplasia, drugs, severe pain, stress, hyperthermia, *SIADH, weight gain, hyponatremia,* ectopic production from cancer, pneumonia, tuberculosis, cerebrovascular disease	Pituitary failure, *diabetes insipidus, psychogenic polydipsia, enuresis, nephrotic syndrome*

CHART 51–4	Tanner's Stages		
Tanner Stage	**Pubic Hair (Both Male and Female)**	**Genitals (Male)**	**Breasts (Female)**
I	No pubic hair at all (prepubertal state) (ages 10 and under)	Prepubertal (testicular volume is less than 1.5 mL; small penis of 3 cm or less).	No glandular tissue; areola follows the skin contours of the chest (prepubertal).
II	Small amount of long, downy hair with slight pigmentation at the base of the penis and scrotum (males) or on the labia majora (females) (ages 10–11)	Testicular volume between 1.6 and 6 mL; skin on scrotum thins, reddens, and enlarges; penis length unchanged.	Breast bud forms, with small area of surrounding glandular tissue; areola begins to widen.
III	Hair becomes more coarse and curly, and begins to extend laterally (ages 12–14)	Testicular volume between 6 and 12 mL; scrotum enlarges further; penis begins to lengthen to about 6 cm.	Breast begins to become more elevated, and extends beyond the borders of the areola, which continues to widen but remains in contour with surrounding breast.
IV	Adult-like hair quality, extending across pubis but sparing medial thighs (ages 13–15)	Testicular volume between 12 and 20 mL; scrotum enlarges further and darkens; penis increases in length to 10 cm and circumference.	Increased breast size and elevation; areola and papilla form a secondary mound projecting from the contour of the surrounding breast.
V	Hair extends to medial surface of the thighs (ages 16+)	Testicular volume greater than 20 mL; adult scrotum and penis of 15 cm in length.	Breast reaches final adult size; areola returns to contour of the surrounding breast, with a projecting central papilla.

Laboratory and Diagnostic Procedures

Testing involves FSH and LH levels. Pituitary malfunction causes a lack of these hormones, which will result in lack of menses in women and lack of secondary sexual characteristics in boys and girls. Testosterone levels are done when there is precocious puberty or delayed male sexual development. Refer to Chart 51–5.

Adrenal Glands

The triangular-shaped adrenal glands sit on the upper poles of the kidneys. Within the adrenal glands there are two distinct layers that have specialized functions. The outer layer is known as the adrenal medulla. The inner layer is the adrenal cortex. These glands are responsible for secretion of catecholamines and steroids, which are released to assist the body in maintaining homeostasis when exposed to stressors.

The adrenal medulla produces the catecholamines epinephrine and norepinephrine, substances that play an important role in the body's physiological response to stress. Epinephrine is a potent vasoconstrictor that, when released, increases heart rate, force of cardiac contraction, and blood pressure. Epinephrine also stimulates release of glucocorticoids in order to increase the serum glucose. Norepinephrine is an even more potent vasoconstrictor, mostly released at the neuromuscular junction, which also increases the heart rate and force of cardiac contractions. It constricts blood vessels throughout the body. Essential hypertension is sometimes caused by benign adrenal medulla tumors, called pheochromocytoma (see Chapter 21 ).

The adrenal cortex secretes corticosteroids of which there are two types, mineralocorticoids and glucocorticoids; both are essential to life. Mineralocorticoids, such as aldosterone, exert control over the retention of sodium and water in maintaining blood pressure and body fluid volume. The glucocorticoids function in carbohydrate metabolism, assist in immune func-

tion, are released in response to stress, and are controlled by a complex feedback loop. A drop in the cortisol level to the hypothalamus stimulates the release of cortisol releasing factor (CRF), a neurohormone that subsequently causes the pituitary to release adrenocorticotropic hormone (ACTH). ACTH then directly stimulates an increase in cortisol by the adrenal cortex. If the cortex is not responsive (primary failure or Addison's disease), the pituitary increases production of ACTH in an effort to raise cortisol levels. Increased ACTH stimulates melanocytes, causing darkening of the skin with Addison's disease. The perception of stress impacts the hypothalamus, and increased stress from illness, surgery, or psychological trauma can increase cortisol levels up to 30 times normal levels. Figure 51–2 ■ illustrates the adrenal gland feedback loop.

CRITICAL ALERT *When patients take cortisone, the increased levels in the blood inhibit production of CRF and ACTH, and the patient's adrenal gland stops functioning. Because ACTH stimulates the release of the mineralocorticoid aldosterone, a sudden cessation of the medication may result in cardiovascular collapse.*

Assessment

The nurse must complete a careful history about the onset of symptoms and medications taken to eliminate other possible etiologies. Two major disorders may be caused by adrenal cortex malfunction. The first adrenal cortex disorder is Cushing's disease, caused by an excess of cortisol. Cortisol causes breakdown of fat and muscle from the extremities for conversion to glucose (gluconeogenesis), which is subsequently deposited as fat in the abdomen and face and back. Symptoms of Cushing's disease include truncal obesity, thin arms and legs, moon face, buffalo hump, severe fatigue and muscle weakness, hyperglycemia, easy bruising, gastrointestinal bleeding, depression, and osteoporosis. Because hyperfunction of the adrenal cortex also can include increased aldosterone and androgens, hypertension may be present.

| CHART 51–5 | **Gonadal Gland Testing** | | |

Laboratory Test and Normal Values	Gland Tested Diagnostic Significance	Disorders Associated with Abnormal Levels *(symptoms are italicized)*	
		Increased	**Decreased**
Follicle-stimulating hormone (FSH) *Males:* 4–15 mU/mL *Females:* 4.6–22.4 mU/mL pre- and postovulation 13–41 mU/mL midcycle peaks	Anterior pituitary (origin) Ovaries and testes (target) Controls the growth and maturation of ovarian follicles in women and the production of sperm in men	Ovarian failure of menopause, hysterectomy, castration, anorchism, hyperthyroidism, hyperpituitarism, hypothalamic tumor, acromegaly, *primary amenorrhea*	*Infertility,* adrenal hyperplasia, *secondary amenorrhea,* anorexia nervosa, neoplasm, hypogonadotropism, hypophysectomy
Luteinizing hormone (LH) *Males:* 3–18 mU/mL *Females:* 2.4–34.5 mU/mL pre- and postovulation 43–187 mU/mL midcycle peaks	Anterior pituitary (origin) Ovaries and testes (target) In women, responsible for the ovulation and stimulation of the ruptured follicle to produce progesterone. In men, stimulates the production of androgens, which support development of secondary sexual characteristics	Menopause, anorchism, hyperpituitarism, Klinefelter, liver disease, pituitary tumors	*Hypogonadism (primary or secondary),* pituitary insufficiency, adrenal hyperplasia or tumor, *amenorrhea* (pituitary failure, *secondary gonadal insufficiency*), malnutrition, hypophysectomy
Testosterone *Males:* 270–1,070 ng/dL *Females:* 8–86 ng/dL	Gonads (origin) Assesses precocious sexual development in young males; assesses the activity of ovaries and testes in adults	*Precocious puberty (in boys), masculinization in women and girls, adrenogenital syndrome,* adrenal hyperplasia, adrenal tumor, testicular tumor	*Failure of the testes to develop,* pituitary insufficiency, *male impotence,* cirrhosis, *hypogonadism,* orchiectomy, *gynecomastia, obesity*

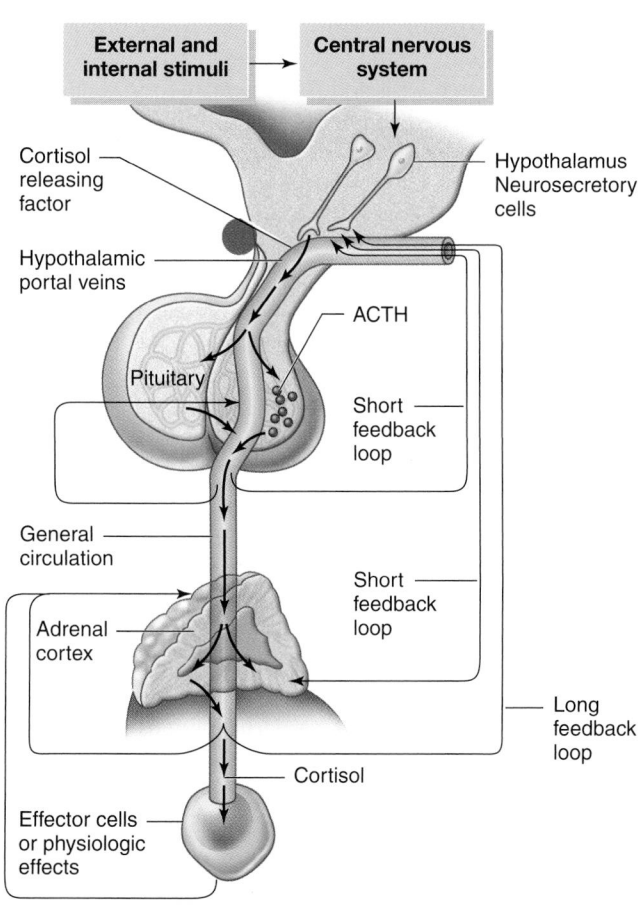

FIGURE 51–2 ■ Adrenal gland feedback loop.

Distribution and location of facial hair should be noted. The presence of hirsutism and deepening of the voice in women can occur with androgen excesses. Cushing's disease is caused by tumor or trauma and is to be differentiated from Cushing's syndrome, an iatrogenic condition caused by exogenous administration of cortisone.

The second cortex disorder is Addison's disease, caused by an autoimmune response that destroys the adrenal cortex. It is characterized by lack of aldosterone, a mineralocorticoid responsible for sodium and water reabsorption from the kidney tubules. Aldosterone, a mineralocorticoid, acts at the level of the distal tubular sodium/potassium exchange system to increase potassium excretion while facilitating sodium reabsorption. Mineralocorticoid deficiency causes increased urinary losses of sodium, chloride, and water, along with decreased excretion of potassium. The results of hyponatremia are loss of extracellular fluid, decreased cardiac output, and hyperkalemia. Hyperkalemia results as the kidney tubules reabsorb other cations because they cannot absorb sodium ions. The nurse should assess for hypotension, muscle weakness, dysrhythmias, and fatigue. The heart may be smaller in Addison's disease due to a reduction in volume of circulating fluid (Odeske & Nagelberg, 2006).

If the disorder is caused by primary adrenal cortex failure, the resulting increase in ACTH causes a dark skin color or tanned appearance that is most prevalent on the areas exposed to sun. Increased pigmentation of the oral mucosa also may indicate Addison's disease. Hypoglycemia and weight loss are symptoms caused by decreased levels of cortisol from primary failure of the entire adrenal gland. Lack of androgen causes decreases in body, axillary, and pubic hair, especially in women who have no other source of androgen hormones. Other symptoms include nausea, vomiting, anorexia, a craving for salty foods, and the inability to tolerate stress.

 *Acute adrenal insufficiency is called Addisonian crisis and is a life-threatening event triggered by a stressful situation such as surgery, trauma, or severe infection. The patient may die from hypotension from volume depletion.*

Hyperaldosteronism (Conn's syndrome) is most commonly caused by adrenal adenoma and is characterized by increased secretion of aldosterone. This mineralocorticoid causes increased sodium retention with potassium and hydrogen ion excretion. The nurse should assess for increased blood pressure, hypernatremia, hypokalemia, and metabolic alkalosis.

If assessment includes severe hypertension and other symptoms including shakiness, anxiety, cold diaphoresis, and headache, the nurse should consider an adrenal medulla disorder. Pheochromocytoma is a benign tumor of the adrenal medulla that produces excess adrenaline and accounts for less than 1% of all hypertensive cases. It can occur at any age, but is most common in people between the ages of 40 and 60. Ninety percent of cases are sporadic. However, 10 percent can be linked to hereditary causes (American Urological Association, 2007).

Laboratory and Diagnostic Procedures

Laboratory tests ordered for adrenal cortex disorders first include checking cortisol levels, which follow a diurnal pattern in the body. If there is an abnormal level, ACTH stimulation tests determine if the disorder is caused by adrenal (primary failure) or pituitary (secondary failure) malfunction. Normally, the ACTH stimulation test will cause an increase in cortisol levels. If the pituitary is not functional (secondary failure), the hypothalamus increases production of CRF, but the ACTH and cortisol levels will still be low. In tertiary failure of the hypothalamus, all three hormone levels will be low. Another test is 17 ketosteroids; it measures the urinary excretion of metabolites from cortisol and is elevated with hypersecretion or Cushing's and low with Addison's. Aldosterone levels will also be depressed with Addison's. X-rays and CT scans may show an adrenal tumor. Tuberculosis testing can eliminate TB of the kidney as a cause of failure.

Testing for adrenal medulla disorders includes urinary catecholamines and metanephrines, measured in a 24-hour urine collection. If these are more than two times the normal level, imaging studies are usually done to look at the adrenal glands. Levels are elevated with pheochromocytoma and decreased with adrenal gland hypofunctioning. Chart 51–6 summarizes adrenal gland tests. See Chapter 59 for additional information 🔗.

Thyroid Gland

The thyroid gland is located in the neck anterior to the upper part of the trachea and just inferior to the larynx. It has two lobes, which are in the shape of a butterfly connected by a structure known as the isthmus. The thyroid has both glandular and follicular tissue, which produces the hormones secreted by the thyroid, triiodothyronine (T_3) and thyroxine (T_4), as well as calcitonin hormones, which are responsible for cellular metabolism, for growth and development in children, and for the regulation of calcium levels.

The thyroid is controlled by a complex feedback loop. A drop in thyroid levels to the hypothalamus stimulates production of thyroid releasing factor (TRF), a neurohormone that subsequently causes the pituitary to release thyroid-stimulating hormone (TSH), which then causes release of thyroid hormone (TH). In primary failure of the thyroid gland, there is low TH with increased TSH, the pituitary's attempt to increase TH levels. In secondary failure of the pituitary, there is low TH and low TSH with increased TRF, the hypothalamus's attempt to increase TH levels. In tertiary failure of the hypothalamus, all three hormones are low: low TRF results in low TSH, which results in low TH. Figure 51–3 ■ (p. 1606) shows the thyroid feedback loop.

Assessment

Thyroid malfunction is one of the most common endocrine disorders. Congenital hypothyroidism, formerly known as cretinism, can be endemic, genetic, or sporadic. If untreated, it results in mild to severe impairment of both physical and mental growth and development. Infants are screened at birth for this condition. Short stature may indicate insufficient thyroid hormone in a child. Lack of secondary sexual characteristics in adults may be caused by lack of thyroid hormone.

Because thyroid hormone controls the metabolic rate, the nurse should assess the patient for fatigue and weight gain. Elevated cholesterol levels are common with hypothyroidism. There may be heavy menstrual periods and constipation from decreased peristalsis. There are decreased deep tendon reflexes. The hair is thinned and dry and loses its shine, and the skin is dry. Patients with hypothyroidism may complain of cold intolerance and have bradycardia. Because hypothyroidism causes slow mentation, cognitive disorders, and decreased orientation, a mental status exam should be completed. Hypothyroidism is sometimes associated with nodular goiters and the swallowing process may be involved and needs to be assessed.

Profound hypothyroidism is associated with myxedema, which refers to a deposit of mucopolysaccharides that causes a nonpitting edema. The cardinal manifestation of myxedema coma is a deterioration of the patient's mental status, which may be subtle, manifesting as apathy, neglect, or a decrease in intellectual function (Wall, 2000). Typically, patients with myxedema have primary hypothyroidism manifested by low T_4 levels and elevated TSH levels.

Graves' disease is the most common cause of hyperthyroidism, accounting for 60% to 80% of all cases. It is an autoimmune disease caused by an antibody, active against the TSH receptor, which stimulates the gland to synthesize and secrete excess thyroid hormone (Reid & Wheeler, 2005). Hyperthyroidism increases the metabolic rate and causes vasodilation in attempts to decrease body temperature. Patients complain of heat intolerance and may have lower blood pressure and compensatory tachycardia, palpitations, and functional heart murmurs. The increased metabolism causes weight loss and fatigue. Diarrhea and shorter or lighter menstrual periods may be seen in clients with hyperthyroidism. The patient may have difficulty sleeping. There may be exaggerated deep tendon reflexes. Hyperthyroid disorders may impair coping ability and are known to cause psychosis (Fenton & Gold, 2006).

Hyperthyroidism is associated with "fullness" in the neck. The swallowing process is observed along with the character and

CHART 51–6   Adrenal Gland Testing

Laboratory Test and Normal Values	Gland Tested Diagnostic Significance	Disorders Associated with Abnormal Levels *(symptoms are italicized)*	
		Increased	Decreased
ACTH stimulation *Rapid test:* cortisol levels increase > 7 mg/dL above baseline *24-hour test:* cortisol level > 40 µg/dL *3-day test:* cortisol level > 40 µg/dL	Adrenals (target) Pituitary (origin) Evaluates the ability of the adrenal gland to respond to ACTH administration	Exaggerated response: Cushing's syndrome Bilateral adrenal hyperplasia: more cortisol is released in response to ACTH dose	Normal or below response: adrenal insufficiency (Addison's) results in less cortisol release in response to stimulation because the gland is not functioning
Serum ACTH *a.m.:* <80 pg/mL or <18 pmol/L (SI units) *p.m.:* <50 pg/mL or <11 pmol/L (SI units)	Anterior pituitary (origin) Adrenals (target) To assess etiology of either overproduction (Cushing's disease) or underproduction of cortisol (Addison's disease)	Ectopic ACTH producing tumors, stress, Addison's disease (primary adrenal insufficiency), surgical removal of the adrenals, adrenal suppression with long-term exogenous steroid therapy. If the adrenal glands are less functional, ACTH production increases via the feedback loop	Pituitary insufficiency; Cushing's syndrome, (exogenous steroid administration) or Cushing's disease caused by bilateral adrenal hyperplasia will cause decreased levels via feedback loop
Serum cortisol *8 a.m.:* 5–23 µg/dL or 138–635 nmol/L (SI units) *4 p.m.:* 3–13 µg/dL or 83–359 nmol/L (SI units)	Adrenals (origin) Measures serum cortisol levels Diurnal functioning with peak levels of 6–8 morning and lowest levels around midnight	*Cushing's disease*, stress including burns, ectopic ACTH producing tumors, *obesity*, hyperpituitarism, hyperthyroidism, pregnancy	*Addison's disease*, hypopituitarism, hypothyroidism; low cortisol levels cause hypoglycemia
Urinary cortisol 20–70 µg/ 24 hr or 25–95 ng/mg of creatinine	Adrenals (origin) Assess for adrenal hyperfunction	Cushing's syndrome, stress, ectopic ACTH-secreting tumors, pregnancy, hyperthyroidism, obesity	Addison's disease, hypopituitarism, hypothyroidism
17-Hydroxycorticosteroids (Porter–Sibler test, 17-OCHS) *Males:* 4–10 mg/24 hr or 8.3–27.6 µmol/day (SI units) urine specimen *Females:* 2–8 mg/24 hr or 5.2–22.1 µmol/day (SI units) urine specimen	Adrenals (origin) Assess for adrenal hyperfunction	Cushing's syndrome, cortisone administration, ACTH-secreting ectopic tumors, obesity, hyperthyroidism, Cushing's disease	Addison's disease, congenital adrenal hyperplasia or lack of cortisol, hepatic disorders, renal disorders, hypopituitarism, hypothyroidism
17–Ketosteroids (17KS) *Males:* 6–20 mg/24 hr or 20–70 µmol/day (SI units) *Females:* 6–17 mg/24 hr or 20–60 µmol/day (SI units)	Adrenals (origin) Measures the metabolites of steroids from both the adrenal cortex and the testes except for the androgen testosterone	Adrenogenital syndrome, tumors of the adrenal cortex and testes, ACTH administration, hyperpituitarism, *Cushing's syndrome*	*Addison's disease*, severe debilitating disease, severe stress and infection, chronic disease, hypogonadism, castration, certain adrenal adenomas, hypopituitarism
Aldosterone *Serum* *Supine:* 3–10 ng/dL or 0.08–0.30 nmol/L (SI units) *Sitting upright for at least 2 hours:* *Males:* 6–22 ng/dL or 0.17–0.61 nmol/L (SI units) *Females:* 5–30 ng/dL or 0.14–0.80 nmol/L (SI units) Urine 2–26 units/24 hr or 6–72 nmol/24 hr (SI units)	Adrenals (origin) Kidney tubules (target) To diagnose hyperaldosteronism Hyponatremia and hyperkalemia stimulate increased aldosterone release Decreased aldosterone results in less reabsorption of sodium from the renal tubules causing hyponatremia	Primary or secondary hyperaldosteronism (Conn's), adrenal tumor or hyperplasia, laxative abuse, poor perfusion states, pregnancy, oral contraceptives, *hypertension*	Addison's disease, primary hypoaldosteronism salt-wasting syndrome, antihypertensive therapy; steroid therapy may interfere with feedback loop, *hypotension*

(continued)

CHART 51–6	Adrenal Gland Testing—*Continued*		

Laboratory Test and Normal Values	Gland Tested Diagnostic Significance	Disorders Associated with Abnormal Levels *(symptoms are italicized)*	
		Increased	**Decreased**
Plasma renin assay *Supine:* 0.3–3.0 ng/mL per hour *Upright:* 1.0–9.0 ng/mL per hour	Adrenals (target) Glomerulus (origin) Evaluation of hypertension To make differential diagnosis of primary versus secondary hyperaldosteronism. In primary, both renin and aldosterone are increased; in secondary, renin is decreased and aldosterone is increased	*Hypertension*, Addison's, secondary hyperaldosteronism, hypokalemia, cirrhosis, salt-losing GI disease, renal disease	Primary hyperaldosteronism, congenital adrenal hyperplasia, steroid therapy
Urinary Catecholamines *Dopamine:* 65–400 mcg/24 hr *Epinephrine:* 1.7–22.4 mcg/24hr *Norepinephrine:* 12.1–85.5 mcg/24 hr *Metanephrines:* 24–96/mcg/24hr *Vanillylmandelic acid (VMA):* 1.4–6.5 mg/24hr *Homovanillic acid (HVA):* 0.0–15.0 mg/d	Adrenal medulla (origin) To assess adrenal medullary function	Pheochromocytoma, neuroblastomas, adrenocortical adenoma, *seizures, stress (severe anger or anxiety)*	Profound hypofunctioning, Addison's disease, chronic disease

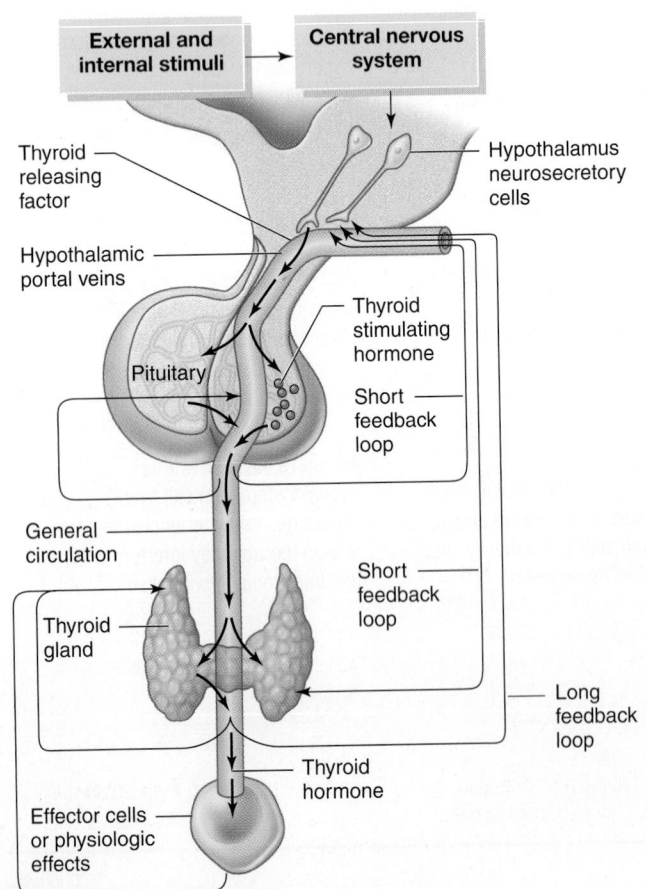

FIGURE 51–3 ■ Thyroid gland feedback loop.

quality of voice. When patients experience thyroid enlargement, they will have palpable or visible enlargement of the thyroid, which can displace the trachea and thus affect breathing and swallowing.

Because of the close association to catecholamines, the patient may experience nervousness and anxiety, shaking, irritability, tremors, and diaphoresis. Prolonged hyperthyroidism causes deposits of fat in the pads behind the eyes, causing bulging of the eyes (exophthalmos) and, occasionally, double vision or loss of vision. Any of these symptoms should motivate the nurse to investigate further.

Laboratory and Diagnostic Procedures

There is no consensus on screening for thyroid disease (see the Health Promotion section on the next page). T_3 and T_4 levels are lower in hypothyroidism and elevated in hyperthyroidism. TSH levels are commonly checked to determine thyroid homeostasis; they are elevated with primary failure of the thyroid gland. TRF (made by the hypothalamus) is elevated with secondary failure (of the pituitary). Because of the connection to the hypothalamus, increased perception of stress can alter TH production. Chart 51–7 summarizes types of glandular failure and related

CHART 51–7	Differentiation of Thyroid Gland Hormone Testing and Glandular Failure		
	T_3 and T_4	TSH	TRH
Primary failure (thyroid gland)	Low	High	High
Secondary failure (pituitary gland)	Low	Low	High
Tertiary failure (hypothalamus gland)	Low	Low	Low

diagnostic test results of thyroid stimulating hormone (TSH) and thyrotropin-releasing hormone (TRH). Chart 51–8 summarizes different thyroid function tests. The Gerontological Considerations box (p. 1608) discusses the effects of hypothyroidism and hyperthyroidism on elderly patients.

 Severe hyperthyroidism (thyrotoxicosis or Graves' disease) can cause tachycardia in excess of 150 beats per minute and is considered a medical emergency; beta-blockers are given to decrease the heart rate until ablation of the thyroid gland is accomplished.

Health Promotion Related to Thyroid Imbalances

Hypothyroidism can be associated with obesity. According to new guidelines issued by the American Thyroid Association (ATA), everyone should be screened at 5-year intervals at a minimum, for thyroid problems beginning at age 35 (Ladenson et al., 2000). Those with symptoms should be checked even more frequently. The American College of Physicians has been recommending thyroid screening for women ages 50 and older for the past few years because it is estimated that thyroid dysfunction affects 5% to 15% of women (Helfand & Redfern, 1998). Although men are less affected by this problem, the ATA is suggesting screening of both sexes, because the blood test used to detect levels of TSH is inexpensive. They state that screening is important because thyroid problems can easily go undetected and can lead to other serious conditions.

Parathyroid Glands

There are four to six parathyroid glands embedded on the posterior surface of the lobes of the thyroid gland. The chief cells secrete parathyroid hormone (PTH) in response to a drop in calcium levels. PTH is responsible for the regulation of the serum calcium level through a simple feedback loop. This balance is maintained by the excretion of phosphorus and reabsorption

CHART 51–8   Thyroid Gland Testing

Laboratory Test and Normal Values	Gland Tested Diagnostic Significance	Disorders Associated with Abnormal Levels *(symptoms are italicized)*	
		Increased	**Decreased**
Antithyroglobin antibodies (thyroid autoantibody) Titer < 1:100	Thyroid (origin) Presence of antibodies to several components, which may cause inflammation and destruction of thyroid gland	Thyroiditis, rheumatoid arthritis, pernicious anemia, *hypothyroidism* or hyperthyroidism, thyroid cancer, Graves' disease, Hashimoto's thyroiditis, systemic lupus erythematosus	Normal is a negative titer or titer of less than 1:100
Thyroxine index, Free (FT$_4$) 0.8–2.4 ng/dL or 10–31 pmol/L (SI units)	Thyroid (origin) Evaluates thyroid function	*Hyperthyroidism, acute psychiatric illness*	*Hypothyroidism, anorexia nervosa,* severe illness
Triiodothyronine uptake (T$_3$ resin uptake) 24–34% or 24–34 AU (arbitrary units, SI units)	Thyroid (origin) Measures amount of T$_3$ bound to protein and the evaluation of thyroid function	Hyperthyroidism, hypoproteinemia	Hypothyroid, hypothyroid states, hepatitis, cirrhosis
Thyrotropin releasing hormone (TRH) Euthyroid < 10	Thyroid function Hypothalamus (origin) Pituitary (target) Evaluation of thyroid function	Primary hypothyroidism (thyroid disease), secondary hypothyroidism (pituitary disease) or TRH secreting tumor in hypothalamus	Hyperthyroid, secondary hyperthyroidism (pituitary disease) or nonfunctional hypothalamus
Thyroid stimulating hormone (TSH) assay 2–10 mU/L (SI units)	Anterior pituitary (origin) Thyroid (target) Differentiate primary and secondary hypothyroidism	Primary hypothyroidism (thyroid dysfunction), Addison's, anti-TSH antibodies, goiter, hyperpituitarism or pituitary adenoma, postop thyroidectomy	Secondary hypothyroidism (pituitary disorder with decreased secretion); high doses of dopamine or corticosteroids, Hashimoto's, primary hyperthyroidism
Thyroxine (T$_4$) *Males:* 51–154 nmol/L (SI units) *Females:* 64–154 nmol/L (SI units) *>60 yr:* 64–124 nmol/L (SI units)	Thyroid (origin) Assess thyroid function, monitor replacement and suppression therapy	Hyperthyroidism, acute thyroiditis, porphyria, cirrhosis, excess dietary intake of iodine, goiter, Graves', thyrotoxicosis	Hypothyroidism, pituitary insufficiency, hypothalamic failure, protein malnutrition, iodine insufficiency, Hashimoto's thyroiditis, nephrotic syndrome, thyroidectomy
Thyroid scan Homogeneous uptake of radioactive tracer and normal size, shape, and position of gland	Thyroid gland (origin) Differentiates between causes of nodules	Increased uptake in hyperfunctioning nodule or "hot nodules"; not usually malignant	Normal uptake; decreased uptake in "cold nodules"; are more likely to be malignant

and excretion of calcium in the urine, gastrointestinal tract, and from bone. Increases in phosphorus, which bind to and lower calcium ions, stimulate PTH release.

A sudden decreased PTH level can result in tetany (carpopedal spasm), a life-threatening condition. This most commonly occurs due to accidental removal of the glands during thyroid surgery, or from autoimmune destruction. A reduced total serum calcium can also result from a decrease in albumin secondary to liver disease, nephrotic syndrome, or malnutrition.

Increased PTH levels can be primary from tumor, resulting in hypercalcemia, or secondary, resulting from hypersecretion. Renal failure causes hyperphosphatemia, leading to hypocalcemia, and subsequent secondary hyperparathyroidism. Calcitonin is released from the thyroid gland in response to hypercalcemia; it shifts calcium from the blood into the bones. Homeostasis of calcium balance is dependent on normal levels of vitamin D.

Assessment

Hypocalcemia causes neuromuscular irritability and tetany. Patients usually complain of numbness and tingling sensations in the perioral area or in the fingers and toes. Muscle cramps are common in the back and lower extremities and may progress to tetany. Neurological symptoms, including irritability, impaired intellectual capacity, depression, and personality changes, may be present. Respiratory disturbances may develop from laryngospasm and bronchospasm.

Hypocalcemia seen in parathyroid disorders can produce spastic contraction of the arm when a blood pressure cuff is applied (Trousseau's sign) or facial muscle contraction when the facial nerve is tapped (Chvostek's sign). Alkalosis induces tetany due to a decrease in ionized calcium. In severe cases, hypocalcemia may lead to arrhythmias, hypotension, and heart failure. Seizures of all types can occur in patients with hypocalcemia.

 **CRITICAL ALERT** *Hyperventilation causes respiratory alkalosis, which drops the ionized calcium in the blood and can result in tetany and respiratory arrest. Carpopedal spasm (Trousseau's sign) and spasm of the facial nerve when tapped (Chvostek's sign) are earlier signs of impending tetany.*

Hypercalcemia is caused by overactive parathyroid glands and also by metabolic cancers to the bone and from some medications. The nurse should assess for symptoms of dehydration, dry skin, confusion, thirst, nausea and vomiting, constipation, fatigue, and decreased deep tendon reflexes.

Laboratory and Diagnostic Procedures

Calcium levels help evaluate calcium metabolism, ionized and nonionized calcium in serum, and parathyroid functioning. PTH levels can also be measured; they will be elevated if calcium levels are decreased, and decreased with hypercalcemia. Because a gradual drop does not create symptoms, a low serum calcium does not always correlate with tetany. The nurse must correlate the clinical picture with the blood levels. Calcitonin and serum phosphorous levels also help evaluate parathyroid functioning. Chart 51–9 outlines the laboratory tests used to evaluate the parathyroid gland (Porth, 2007).

Pancreas

The pancreas lies beneath the peritoneum and behind the stomach, with its head and neck in the curve of the duodenum. Its body extends horizontally across the horizontal posterior abdominal wall and its tail touches the spleen. The pancreas is unique in that it has both endocrine and exocrine functions. The islet cells within the pancreas provide endocrine functioning. These cells are responsible for carbohydrate metabolism and regulation of glucose levels through secretion and inhibition of insulin and glucagons. There are four types of islet cells: alpha, beta, delta, and PP cells.

Alpha cells are responsible for the production of glucagon. This hormone decreases the oxidation of glucose and promotes an increase in the serum glucose level by signaling the liver to release glucose from the glycogen stores. Beta cells are responsible for the production of insulin. Insulin facilitates the uptake and use of glucose by the cells and prevents excessive breakdown of glycogen in the liver and muscle. Together, insulin and glucagon control blood sugar levels by a simple feedback loop. Delta cells produce somatostatin, which inhibits GH, TSH, and gastrointestinal hormones, such as glucagon and insulin, by the alpha and beta cells of the pancreas. PP cells produce pancreatic polypeptide, or digestive enzymes, which are responsible for the exocrine activity of the pancreas.

Assessment

Diabetes mellitus is a disorder characterized by either lack of insulin (type 1) or impaired use of insulin (type 2). Either results in hyperglycemia, which in turn creates an osmotic pull of fluid off the tissues, causing polyuria, polydipsia, dehydration, and confusion leading to stupor or coma. The patient may have severe dehydration with volume depletion and hypotension. Hyperglycemia also causes osmotic fluid shifts in the vitreous fluid resulting in blurred vision. Because insulin normally suppresses breakdown of fat, and there is no insulin in type 1 diabetes, this disorder is also characterized by acidosis from conversion of stored fat to fatty acids. Acidosis causes nausea, vomiting, hunger, low pH, and compensatory Kussmaul's respirations. The nurse should assess for rapid, shallow respirations, as well as a fruity odor to the breath and urine.

The risk factors for type 1 DM include genetic factors plus a viral infection causing autoimmune destruction. Type 2 DM has been linked genetically with, and is strongly correlated to, obesity, age, ethnic minorities, physical inactivity, and gestational diabetes (National Diabetes Information Clearinghouse

CHART 51–9   Parathyroid Gland Testing

Laboratory Test and Normal Values	Gland Tested Diagnostic Significance	Disorders Associated with Abnormal Levels (symptoms are italicized) Increased	Decreased
Parathyroid hormone (PTH) 10–65 pg/mL or 10–65 ng/L (SI units)	Parathyroid (origin) Bone and gut (target) Evaluation of hypocalcemia and hypercalcemia; also monitored in patients with chronic renal failure	Increased as a response to low serum calcium levels: *hypocalcemia, rickets*, malabsorption syndrome, vitamin D deficiency, parathyroid adenoma, ectopic PTH producing tumors, *renal hypercalciuria*, chronic renal failure (secondary hyperparathyroidism)	Decreased as a response to high serum calcium levels: hypercalcemia of malignancy, metastatic bone tumor, sarcoidosis, vitamin D intoxication; hypoparathyroidism due to surgical ablation or immunoablation
Osteocalcin *Males:* 5.8–14 ng/mL *Females:* 3.1–13.4 ng/mL	Parathyroid function Bone (origin) Evaluation of bone turnover in diseases that affect bone density	Hyperparathyroidism, osteoporosis, Paget's disease, acromegaly, hyperthyroidism, low calcium intake, low estrogen production	Hypoparathyroidism, steroid therapy, multiple myeloma, hypercalcemia from malignancy
Total serum calcium 9–10.5 mg/dL or 2.25–2.75 mmol/L	Parathyroid function Bone (origin) Evaluation of calcium metabolism, ionized and nonionized calcium in serum and parathyroid functioning	Hyperparathyroidism, bone metastasis, hypercalcemia, Addison's, acidosis, hypervitaminosis, immobility, renal calculi	Hypoparathyroidism, renal failure, rickets, vitamin D deficiency, osteomalacia, alkalosis, burns, chronic renal disease, parathyroidectomy, hypoproteinemia
Calcitonin *Males:* 3–26 pg/mL or 3–26 ng/L (SI units) *Females:* 2–17 pg/mL or 2–17 ng/L (SI units)	Thyroid (origin) Parathyroid (target) Responsible for lowering the calcium ion levels	Anemia, cancer, chronic renal failure, parathyroid adenoma or hyperplasia; *increased levels result in hypocalcemia*	autoimmune thyroiditis; *decreased levels result in hypercalcemia*
Serum phosphorus/phosphate 3–4.5 mg/dL or 0.97–1.45 mmol/L (SI units)	Parathyroid function Diet (origin) Evaluation of parathyroid and calcium abnormalities	Hypoparathyroidism, renal failure, bone tumors, hyperthyroidism, diabetic acidosis, increased dietary intake of phosphorus; *increased levels result in hypocalcemia*	Hyperparathyroidism, chronic antacid ingestion, chronic alcoholism, burns, malnutrition, vitamin D deficiency and myxedema, Crohn's, dialysis, sprue
Serum alkaline phosphatase (ALP) 30–120 unit/L	Parathyroid function Multiple origins Evaluation of bone and liver diseases	Hyperparathyroidism, primary cirrhosis, biliary obstruction, *healing fractures,* Paget's disease, rheumatoid arthritis, hyperthyroidism	Hypophosphatemia, malnutrition, pernicious anemia, scurvy, celiac disease, malnutrition, hypothyroidism

[NDIC], 2006. Long-term changes associated with DM include retinopathy, nephropathy, vascular and cardiac disease, and hypertension. The nurse needs to take a careful history about the onset of symptoms and complete a thorough examination of the heart, extremities, kidneys, and eyes.

Because of regulatory mechanisms, it is unusual for a nondiabetic patient to have episodes of severe hypoglycemia. When this occurs, the nurse should suspect an islet-secreting tumor of the pancreas. Low blood sugar causes release of epinephrine, which stimulates hunger, tachycardia, diaphoresis, and feelings of nervousness. Hypoglycemia can cause confusion, sudden unconsciousness, seizures, and brain injury.

Laboratory and Diagnostic Procedures

DM is diagnosed in the presence of any random blood sugar higher than 200 mg/dL and/or a fasting blood sugar of >125 mg/dL (NDIC, 2006). Prediabetes is diagnosed with a fasting blood sugar of between 110 and 125 mg/dL. One test done to diagnose borderline diabetes is a glucose tolerance test (GTT). A carbohydrate load is given and then blood sugars are checked prior to and at intervals afterward. Fasting and before meals blood test-

ing is done in the home and hospital setting. The most accurate test of long-term control of blood sugar is the hemoglobin A1c test, which measures the glucose attached to hemoglobin and gives information about the average blood sugar level in the previous 6-week period. A microalbuminuria test is the best indicator of early renal involvement. Chart 51–10 (p. 1610) summarizes pancreatic gland testing.

In type 2 diabetes, there may be insulin resistance at the cellular level, resulting in high blood sugar despite increased insulin levels. Insulin resistance has been linked to metabolic syndrome. In 1999, the World Health Organization criteria for metabolic syndrome required the presence of diabetes mellitus, impaired glucose tolerance, impaired fasting glucose, or insulin resistance, *and* two of the following:

- Blood pressure ≥ 140/90 mmHg
- Dyslipidemia: triglycerides ≥ 1.695 mmol/L and/or high-density lipoprotein cholesterol ≤0.9 mmol/L (male), ≤1.0 mmol/L (female)
- Central obesity: waist-to-hip ratio > 0.90 (male), > 0.85 (female), and/or body mass index > 30 kg/m²

CHART 51–10	Pancreatic Gland Testing		
Laboratory Test and Normal Values	**Gland Tested Diagnostic Significance**	**Disorders Associated with Abnormal Levels *(symptoms are italicized)***	
		Increased	**Decreased**
Fasting glucose <100 mg/dL normal fasting glucose 100–126 mg/dL impaired fasting glucose >126 mg/dL diagnostic for diabetes	Pancreas (target) Diet (origin) Glucose homeostasis	*Impaired fasting glucose, hyperglycemia,* diabetes mellitus, IV fluids, physiological stress	*Hypoglycemia,* insulinomas
Oral glucose tolerance test <140 mg/dL normal glucose tolerance 140–200 mg/dL impaired glucose tolerance >200 mg/dL diagnostic for diabetes	Pancreas (target) Diet (origin) Glucose metabolism	Diabetes mellitus, *impaired glucose tolerance,* Cushing's syndrome, hepatic tumors, pregnancy, pheochromocytoma, hyperthyroidism	Insulinomas, Addison's, celiac disease, hepatic disease, hypothyroidism
Hemoglobin A1c or glycosylated hemoglobin 4–6%; <7% for diabetics	Pancreas (target) Diet (origin) Glucose metabolism	Diabetes mellitus, gestational diabetes	Insulinomas, Addison's, celiac disease, hepatic disease, hypothyroidism

- Microalbuminuria: urinary albumin excretion ratio ≥20 mg/min or albumin-to-creatinine ratio ≥30 mg/g (Harmel & Mathur, 2003).

Critical Thinking Related to Assessment Data

As previously noted, when conducting a focused endocrine assessment, it is critical to begin with a thorough history of the patient's chief complaints. The nurse needs to elicit any experience with signs or symptoms of endocrine disease or disorders. Symptoms usually are manifested according to which endocrine hormone is being overproduced and secreted or underproduced and secreted. Thus, it is incumbent on the nurse to understand the functions on the endocrine system.

When assessing the endocrine system, the nurse likely will perform a problem-focused assessment, following a comprehensive assessment. The focused assessment may need to be repeated periodically when an interval or abbreviated assessment shows a change in status from the last assessment or report received. When a new symptom emerges or the patient experiences some distress, a focused endocrine assessment also should be considered.

Physical exam techniques consist of the same techniques used in a general exam: inspection, auscultation, palpation, and percussion. With inspection, the nurse is looking forward for anything that can be observed with eyes, ears, or nose, for example, skin color, locations of lesions, bruises or rashes, symmetry, size of body parts, and abnormal sounds or odors.

Auscultation is used in the focused endocrine assessment before palpation or percussion. Findings that may be auscultated include murmurs, cardiac irregularities, adventitious breath sounds, and alterations in bowel sounds.

Palpation is another physical exam technique that is used in the focused endocrine assessment. Palpation allows the nurse to assess for texture, tenderness, temperature, moisture, pulsations, masses, and internal organs (Porth, 2007).

Percussion is used to allow the nurse to elicit tenderness or sounds that point to underlying problems. When percussing directly over suspected areas of tenderness, the patient should be monitored for signs of discomfort.

Examples of Data Collection

Data is acquired through the history and physical exam and is enhanced with laboratory testing. With endocrine disorders, the history is the most essential piece of data collection. Many times, patients will have a constellation of symptoms that do not clearly fit into one hormone imbalance. The nurse is in a unique position to analyze the data to determine the relevance of each symptom to the underlying disorder. Abnormal findings need to be reported to the primary care provider and patient education initiated. With proper education, patients can be empowered to manage and improve their personal health.

Diagnostic Evaluation

Providing patient education, allaying patient's fears regarding the testing process, and ensuring that testing is done appropriately are parts of the nurse's role in diagnostic assessment and evaluation of the endocrine system. Proper preparation for diagnostic testing is essential for ensuring accurate evaluation of endocrine system function. Testing may require special diets, fasting, or use of drugs in order to assess proper functioning. It is the nurse's role to assist the patient in preparing for these tests.

Laboratory and Diagnostic Procedures

Laboratory tests for endocrine function involve serum hormone levels, suppression and stimulation, and urine hormone levels. In most cases, elevated hormone levels are associated with increased function of the gland. Suppression and stimulation testing is used to determine glandular function in feedback loops.

Urine hormone levels give information about increased and decreased function of specific glands. Radiological examinations also are used to made diagnostic decisions.

Serum Hormone Levels

Diagnostic testing of the endocrine system begins with examination of serum hormone levels. Some tests may involve a single specimen, whereas others require multiple blood samples. Laboratory testing of a specific endocrine organ involves the measurement of the specific hormone or tropic hormones. If the serum concentration of hormone is deficient, further testing is needed to assess whether the deficiency is related to dysfunction of the associated gland; this is known as primary dysfunction. If the deficiency is due to the dysfunction of another gland or a stimulating hormone, it is known as secondary dysfunction. If the deficiency is due to dysfunction of the neurohormone, as in TRF or CRF, it is known as tertiary dysfunction.

Suppression and Stimulation Testing

Suppression and stimulation testing also may be used to assess endocrine function. This type of testing is accomplished by the administration of a drug that stimulates or suppresses the release of hormones. This type of testing is especially useful in differentiation of primary or secondary dysfunction. Numerous tests may be necessary to definitively confirm an endocrine system disorder.

A record of the medications that the patient is receiving as well as those that should be withheld, foods that should be avoided during testing, and instructions regarding the purpose and procedure for the test are provided by the nurse. Special materials may need to be obtained from the laboratory for the specimen collection. Special handling of the specimens also may be necessary (e.g., adding acid to the specimen or keeping the specimen on ice).

Urine Hormone Levels

Measurements of urinary hormone or hormone metabolite excretion often are done on a 24-hour urine sample which provides a better measure of hormone levels during that period than hormones measured in an isolated blood sample. The advantages of a urine test include the relative ease of obtaining the urine sample and the fact that blood sampling is not required, though it is recognized that reliability timed urine collections often are difficult to obtain. Because many urine tests involve the measure of a hormone metabolite, rather than the hormone itself, drugs or disease states that alter hormone metabolism may interfere with the test results. Some urinary hormone metabolite measurements include hormones from more than one source and are of little value in measuring hormone secretion from a specific source. "For example, urinary 17-ketosteroids are a measure of both adrenal and gonadal androgens" (Porth, 2007, page 671).

Radiologic Examination

Radiologic examination with simple x-rays, CT scanning, or MRI scanning can be used to visualize endocrine glands to assess for size, atrophy, hypertrophy, or neoplasm. The nurse provides explanations of the purpose and procedures for radiologic exams. Allergies to iodine, shellfish, or contrast media also must be determined prior to examination by CT scans requiring contrast. Pregnancy should be ruled out for female patients prior to any type of x-ray examination. If the patient is to have an MRI, nurses should inquire about claustrophobia, previous surgeries, implantable devices, and any previous injuries involving metals such as gunshot wounds or pellet injuries.

In summary, conducting the health history, physical examination, and preparation for and interpretation of laboratory tests and procedures takes experience and practice. It is not enough to simply ask the right questions and perform the physical exam. The nurse must critically analyze all of the data obtained, synthesize the data into a relevant problem focus, and then identify a plan of care for the patient based on this synthesis. Examples of plans of care based on assessment data are found in Chapters 52 and 53 ⊚ .

Health Promotion

Health promotion in general is based on knowing and identifying the risk factors and overt symptoms of hormonal imbalances. These vary with the type of hormonal imbalance experienced, but the public should be made aware of common symptoms, such as headache, sudden weight gain or loss, thinning of hair, lethargy, localized pain, nausea, irritability, nocturia, heat intolerance, insomnia, and others. The public should be made aware of the Internet sources or health promotion pamphlets available through health care providers' offices or localized outlets that provide information related to specific hormonal imbalances. An annual physical examination may alert patients to potential problems. Patients also should be counseled as to when to report aberrant symptoms to the physician or health care provider.

■ Summary

In conclusion, endocrine disorders cause changes in almost every system in the human body. The nurse must carefully assess each system for alterations in function and appearance to discern the system involved. Some physical changes can be caused by more than one endocrine imbalance. Careful examination and laboratory testing are essential to accurate diagnosis and treatment.

NCLEX® REVIEW

1. A patient with diabetes does not understand how an injection of insulin can take the place of insulin secreted from the pancreas. Which of the following should the nurse respond to this patient?

   1. It does not; insulin is for another purpose.

   2. Insulin helps the pancreas work well.

   3. It works by a negative feedback mechanism.

   4. Insulin is a hormone and works through the bloodstream.

2. The nurse is explaining to a patient how the hormones secreted by the ovaries work on the ovaries to cause an egg follicle to mature. This nurse is instructing the patient on which of the following?

   1. Neuroendocrine regulation

   2. Paracine functioning

   3. Autocrine functioning

   4. Basal hormone release

3. A patient has been diagnosed with cancer that has metastasized to the outer layer of his adrenal glands. Which of the following hormones will be affected by this disease?

   1. Mineralcorticoids

   2. Glucocorticoids

   3. Epinephrine

   4. Calcitonin

4. During an assessment a patient says "I eat but am losing weight! And I'm so thirsty and seem to always have to pass water." Which of the following should the nurse say in response to this patient?

   1. Does frequent urination keep you up at night?

   2. Do you use tobacco?

   3. Everyone thinks that they weigh less than they really do.

   4. Does anyone in your family have diabetes?

5. A 50-year-old female patient asks the nurse why a follicle-stimulating hormone test was done. Which of the following should the nurse respond to this patient?

   1. It measures the amount of hormones your adrenal glands are making.

   2. It measures the hormones being made by your thyroid.

   3. It checks for ovarian function and might indicate if you are approaching menopause.

   4. It predicts how well you metabolize carbohydrates, proteins, and fats.

Answers for review questions appear in Appendix D

KEY TERMS

autocrine functioning *p.1597*
circadian rhythm *p.1597*
endocrine *p.1596*

infradian rhythm *p.1597*
negative feedback *p.1597*
paracrine functioning *p.1597*

positive feedback *p.1597*
receptors *p.1596*

REFERENCES

American Thyroid Association. (2008). *NACB thyroid guidelines.* Retrieved June 9, 2008, from http://www.thyroid.org

American Urological Association. (2007). *Pheochromocytoma.* Retrieved September 12, 2007, from http://urologyhealth.org/adult/index.cfm?cat=02&topic=114

Bharaktiya, S., Orlander, P. R., Woodhouse, W. T., & Davis, A. B. (2007). *Hypothyroidism.* Retrieved June 9, 2008, from http://www.emedicine.com/med/topic1145.htm

Estes, M. E. (2002). *Health assessment and physical exam* (2nd ed.). New York: Delmar Publishing.

Fenton, C. L., & Gold, J. G. (2006). *Hyperthyroidism.* Retrieved June 8, 2008, from http://www.emedicine.com/ped/TOPIC1099.HTM

Harmel, A., & Mathur, R. (2003). *Davidson's diabetes mellitus.* St. Louis: Elsevier.

Helfand, M., & Redfern, C. C. (1998). Screening for thyroid disease: An update. *Annals of Internal Medicine, 129*(2), 144–158.

Khandwala, H. M. (2005). *Acromegaly.* Retrieved September 2007 from http://www.emedicine.com/med/topic27.htm

Ladenson, P. W., Singer, P. A., Ain, K. B., et al. (2000). American Thyroid Association guidelines for detection of thyroid dysfunction. *Archives of Internal Medicine, 160*(11), 1573–1575.

National Diabetes Information Clearinghouse. (2006). *Am I at risk for diabetes?* Retrieved September 12, 2007, from http://diabetes.niddk.nih.gov/dm/pubs/riskfortype2/index.htm#6

National Kidney and Urologic Diseases Information Clearinghouse. (2006). *Diabetes insipidus.* Retrieved September 2007 from http://kidney.niddk.nih.gov/kudiseases/pubs/insipidus/index.htm

Odeske, S. & Nagelberg, S. B. (2006). Addison disease. *eMedicine.* Retrieved June 8, 2008, from http://www.emedicine.com/med/TOPIC42.HTM

Porth, C. M. (2007). *Essentials of pathophysiology: Concepts of altered health states.* Philadelphia: Lippincott Williams & Wilkins.

Rafailov, A. (2007). *Syndrome of inappropriate antidiuretic hormone secretion.* Retrieved September 2007 from http://www.emedicine.com/emerg/topic784.htm

Reid, J. R. & Wheeler, S. F. (2005). Hyperthyroidism: Diagnosis and treatment. *American Family Physician, 72*(4). Retrieved June 9, 2008, from http://www.aafp.org/afp/20050815/623.html

Singh, S. (1999). Low levels of thyroid hormone blamed on age. *Geriatrics and Aging, 2*(6). Retrieved June 9, 2008, from http://www.geriatricsandaging.ca/fmi/xsl/article.xsl?-lay=Article&-recid=220&-find=-find

Trivalle, C., Doucet, J., Chassagne, P., et al. (1996). Differences in the signs and symptoms of hyperthyroidism in older and younger patients. *Journal of the American Geriatrics Society, 44*(1), 50–53.

Wall, C. R. (2000). Myxedema coma: Diagnosis and treatment. *American Family Physician, 62*(11). Retrieved September 2007 from http://www.aafp.org/afp/20001201/2485.html

Caring for the Patient with Glandular and Hormonal Disorders

Abby Heydman

With contributions by:
Annita Watson
Kathleen Osborn

Outcome-Based Learning Objectives

After studying this chapter, the learner will be able to:

1. Describe the anatomic location and function of the endocrine glands, including the physiological effects of the hormones that each gland produces.
2. Compare the common pathophysiological syndromes caused by under- and overproduction of hormones for each of the endocrine glands, including the thyroid, parathyroid, hypothalamus and pituitary, and adrenal glands.
3. Identify clinical manifestations, treatment, and nursing interventions for hypo- and hypermetabolic conditions.
4. Describe the complex neurological and immunologic effects of common glandular disorders.
5. Develop a plan of care for patients with each of the common endocrine gland disorders, including the patient teaching and discharge needs.
6. Describe the potential gerontological implications for each glandular disorder.
7. Identify implications for nursing research when caring for persons with glandular disorders.

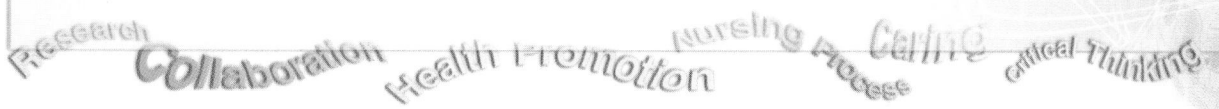

Research   Collaboration   Health Promotion   Nursing Process   Caring   Critical Thinking

THE HUMAN BODY is a complex organism that functions as a result of exquisite control by the glandular system in constant interaction with the neurological and immune systems. All major organ systems and physiological processes such as cell metabolism, bone metabolism, growth, homeostasis, regulation of energy, and reproduction are regulated by the glandular system and its feedback control systems. This chapter focuses on disorders of the major endocrine glands: the thyroid, parathyroid, hypothalamus and pituitary, and the adrenal glands. Disorders of the thyroid gland are emphasized because these are the most common problems seen by nurses in clinical practice.

Endocrinology

Endocrinology is a broad field of science and medicine that involves the study of the glands and tissues that produce hormones that serve as chemical messengers orchestrating a multitude of physiological processes. The endocrine glands specifically include the thyroid, parathyroid, adrenals, pituitary, hypothalamus, thymus, pancreas, pineal, ovaries, and testes. The ovaries and testes are discussed in Chapters 48, 49, and 50 ☺. The thymus gland is involved in regulation of the immune system and is discussed in Chapters 59, 60, and 61 ☺. The pancreas produces insulin and it is discussed in Chapter 53 ☺. The pineal gland is a tiny structure located in the middle of the brain and it secretes melatonin, which is involved with biological rhythms and reproductive functions. Researchers are still learning about the role of the pineal gland and it has not been cited as a major factor in human disease. For this reason, the pineal gland is not discussed in this chapter. The anatomic location of each of the endocrine glands is illustrated in Figure 52–1 ■, (p. 1614).

Hormones

Hormones are substances that circulate like chemical messengers to produce cellular actions and to regulate physiological processes throughout the body. Hormones include amino acid derivatives, small neuropeptides, large proteins, steroid hormones, and vitamin derivatives, which act primarily by stimulating target cells that are uniquely responsive to them. The target tissue for a hormone includes all of the cells that have receptor sites for that hormone. Sometimes target tissue is localized in a single gland and, in some cases, the target tissue is located throughout the body.

Hormone Production

Hormone production is stimulated by the body in three ways. First, several hormones are controlled by a **negative feedback**

The endocrine glands secrete hormones which regulate various functions throughout the body

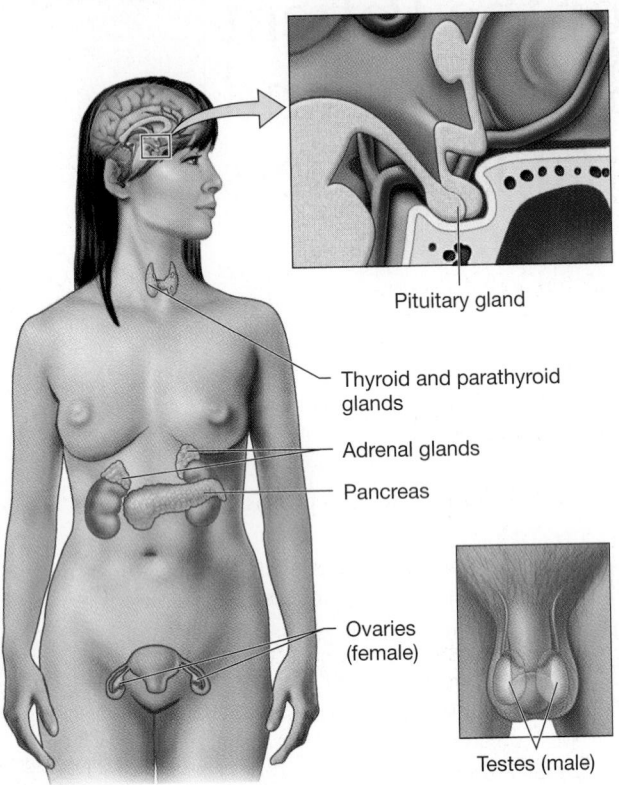

Pituitary gland

Thyroid and parathyroid glands

Adrenal glands

Pancreas

Ovaries (female)

Testes (male)

FIGURE 52–1 ■ Location of the endocrine glands in the male and female bodies.

system in which hormone production is stimulated if body receptors indicate that the concentration of a needed hormone is low. Second, hormone production can be stimulated by a hormone produced by another organ. Hormone-stimulating hormones are called tropic hormones. For example, the pituitary gland produces thyroid-stimulating hormone (TSH), which acts on the thyroid gland to stimulate production of thyroid hormone. Third, hormones can be produced by direct nervous system stimulation.

Hormones are produced by both the endocrine glands and the exocrine glands, which include specialized tissues in the gut and other parts of the body (Braunwald et al., 2001). Hormones produced by the endocrine glands, also known as ductless glands, are secreted internally into the blood, whereas hormones secreted by the exocrine system are secreted through ducts or tubes (Chart 52–1). An example of an endocrine hormone is thyroxine, a hormone that is produced by the thyroid gland. An example of an exocrine hormone is gastrin, which is produced by the gastric mucosa for the purpose of stimulating the production of hydrochloric acid and the enzyme pepsin to aid in the digestion of food. Other exocrine glands include the small intestine, which secretes the hormones secretin and cholecystokinin; the heart, which produces atriopeptin; and the placenta of a pregnant woman, which produces chorionic gonadotropin. In recent years, research has demonstrated that peptide hormones also are produced by brain tissue, leading to a new field of neuroendocrinology. This chapter focuses on common disorders of the major endocrine glands and the clinical situations nurses are most likely to see in practice.

Endocrine Disorders

Endocrine disorders are linked to several factors including aging, illness, stress, environmental substances, congenital birth defects, and genetics. In addition, surgery, trauma, cancerous and benign tumors, infection, and autoimmune disorders may all trigger endocrine dysfunction. The major clinical problems seen in the endocrine glands are those related to underproduction or overproduction of hormone, and those cases in which there is resistance to the action of the hormone. Generally, hormone underproduction can be treated by hormone replacement therapy and overproduction can be treated by reducing hormone levels through surgical intervention or the use of medications to lower hormone levels.

The endocrine system is studied by measuring hormone levels in the blood. Endocrine disorders are classified as primary, secondary, or tertiary based on the particular physiological system involved in causing the disease. Primary endocrine disease occurs when the organ itself is diseased. Secondary disease occurs when the pituitary and its stimulating hormones are affected by some pathology. Tertiary disease occurs when dysfunction occurs within the hypothalamus. Chart 52–2 (p. 1617) shows disorders of the endocrine system.

The Effect of Aging on the Endocrine System

The aging process takes a toll on normal cells and gradually leads to altered hormone production and secretion, changes in hormone metabolism and hormone levels, slowed response of target cells to hormones, and changes in physiological body rhythms such as menstruation. Secretion of some hypothalamic hormones and related pituitary response may be impaired due to aging. As a person ages, the pituitary gland often becomes smaller and may fail to work as effectively, leading to decreased muscle mass, decreased heart function, and osteoporosis. Infections or trauma may quickly destabilize older patients because the aging body is less capable of responding to either internal or external stressors due to a decline in endocrine functioning.

■ Disorders of the Thyroid Gland

The thyroid gland is a small butterfly-shaped and highly vascular organ located in the front of the neck with lobes connected by an isthmus resting on the anterior side of the trachea (Figure 52–2 ■, p. 1618). The primary function of the thyroid gland is to produce thyroid hormone, which regulates body metabolism.

Disorders of the thyroid gland are the most common of the diseases of the endocrine system, and include hypothyroidism, hyperthyroidism, and thyroid nodules. **Hypothyroidism** is a condition in which the thyroid gland produces an inadequate amount of thyroid hormone. **Hyperthyroidism** occurs when an excess of thyroid hormone is secreted. Thyroid nodules are lumps in or on the thyroid gland and they may be small or large. Thyroid nodules are of four general types: overgrowth of normal thyroid tissue, a fluid-filled cyst, or a benign or malignant tumor (American Association of Clinical Endocrinologists [AACE], 2005d). Because the thyroid gland affects the functioning of most of the body processes, signs and symptoms may be diffuse and difficult to diagnose. For this reason, the health care provider will need to rely on discriminating laboratory tests of

CHART 52–1	**Glands and Their Hormones**

Endocrine Gland and Hormone Source	Hormone(s)	Action Site	Physiological Effects
Hypothalamus	Thyrotropin-releasing hormone (TRH)	Anterior pituitary	Stimulates release of TSH and prolactin.
	Gonadotropin-releasing hormone (GnRH)	Anterior pituitary	Responsible for release of FSH and LH.
	Growth hormone-releasing hormone (GHRH)	Anterior pituitary	Promotes growth hormone secretion.
	Corticotropin-releasing hormone (CRH)	Anterior pituitary	Promotes release of ACTH.
	Somatostatin	Pituitary Pancreas GI tract	Inhibits secretion of GH, TSH, gastric hormones. Prolongs gastric emptying. Suppresses pancreatic hormones.
	Dopamine	Anterior pituitary	Inhibits release of prolactin.
Pituitary gland			
Anterior lobe (adenohypophysis)	Human growth hormone (GH)	Systemic	Stimulates growth and cell reproduction.
Posterior lobe (neurohypophysis)	Thyroid-stimulating hormone (thyrotropin) (TSH)	Thyroid	Stimulates release of thyroid hormone.
	Adrenocorticotropin (ACTH)	Adrenal cortex	Stimulates the cortex of the adrenal gland and boosts the synthesis of corticosteroids, mainly glucocorticoids, and also mineralocorticoids and sex steroids (androgens).
	Follicle-stimulating hormone (FSH)	Ovaries	Stimulates growth of immature graafian follicles to maturation.
		Testes	Essential in spermatogenesis.
	Luteinizing hormone (LH)	Ovaries	Stimulates production of the sex hormones. Triggers ovulation and development of the corpus luteum during the menstrual cycle.
	Prolactin	Mammary glands	Stimulates mammary glands to produce milk.
	Melanocyte-stimulating hormone	Skin and hair	Stimulates production and release of melanin by melanocytes in skin and hair.
	Antidiuretic hormone (ADH) (vasopressin)	Kidneys	Causes kidneys to concentrate urine. Stimulates thirst.
	Oxytocin	Breasts Uterus	Causes milk to "let down" into mammary ducts. Aids uterine contraction and cervical dilation during labor and delivery.
		Testes	Facilitates sperm transport in ejaculation.
Thyroid gland	Thyroxine (T_4) Triiodothyronine (T_3)	Systemic	Controls metabolic rate, metabolism, growth, and development.
	Thyrocalcitonin (calcitonin)	Bone	Reduces the level of calcium in the blood. Lowers bone reabsorption.
Parathyroid gland	Parathyroid hormone (parathormone) (PTH)	Bone, kidney, and intestine	Increases calcium absorption, raises calcium levels in blood, promotes bone reabsorption.
Adrenal glands Cortex Medulla	Mineralocorticoids (aldosterone and similar hormones)	Kidneys	Stimulates active reabsorption of sodium, passive reabsorption of water, and the active secretion of potassium in the distal convoluted tubule, thus increasing blood pressure and blood volume.
	Glucocorticoid (cortisol)	Receptors in most tissues and cells	Regulates or supports cardiovascular, metabolic, immunologic, and homeostatic functions.
	Androgens (including testosterone)	Gonads	Stimulates or controls the development and maintenance of masculine characteristics. Is the precursor for estrogen.
	Epinephrine (adrenalin)	Cardiac muscle, smooth muscle, glands	Increases heart rate and stroke volume, dilates the pupils, constricts arterioles in the skin and gut while dilating arterioles in leg muscles. Elevates the blood sugar level by increasing hydrolysis of glycogen to glucose in the liver, and begins the breakdown of lipids in fat cells.
	Norepinephrine (noradrenalin)	Sympathetic nervous system	Activates the sympathetic nervous system to directly increase heart rate, release energy from fat, and increase muscle readiness.

(continued)

CHART 52–1 **Glands and Their Hormones—*Continued***

Endocrine Gland and Hormone Source	Hormone(s)	Action Site	Physiological Effects
Thymus	Thymosin	Immune system	Aids in development of the body's immune system.
Pineal gland	Melatonin	Gonads	Can suppress sexual desire. Influences the circadian rhythm.
Pancreas Islets of Langerhans	Insulin	Muscles and tissues	Lowers blood sugar, controls utilization and storage of carbohydrates. Increases glycogen synthesis.
	Glucagons	Liver	Raises blood glucose, glycogenolysis.
	Somatostatin		Lowers blood glucose by interfering with release of growth hormone and glucagon.
Gonads			
Testes (males)	Androgens (testosterone)	Gonads Muscle tissues	Stimulates male sex characteristics. Promotes enlargement of muscle mass.
Ovarian follicle (females)	Inhibin	Ovaries, pituitary, placenta	Inhibits FSH synthesis and secretion and participates in the regulation of the menstrual cycle.
	Oestrogens (estrogen)	Breasts Uterus	Promote the development of female secondary sex characteristics, such as breasts, and are also involved in the thickening of the endometrium and other aspects of regulating the menstrual cycle.
Corpus luteum	Testosterone	Endometrium	Responsible for the thickening of the endometrium and its development in pregnancy.
	Progesterone	Endometrium	Converts the endometrium to its secretory stage to prepare the uterus for implantation.
Placenta	Human chorionic gonadotropin (HCG)	Endometrium	Prevents disintegration of the corpus luteum of the ovary and thereby maintains progesterone production that is critical for a pregnancy.
	Human placental lactogen (hPL)	Placenta	Ensures nutrient supply to the fetus.
	Progesterone	Placenta	Supports gestation and embryogenesis.
	Corticotropin-releasing hormone (CRH)	Placenta	Helps determine duration of the pregnancy.
Gastrointestinal tract (stomach and intestines)	Gastrin	Stomach	Produces gastric juices.
	Enterogastrone	Stomach	
	Secretin	Liver and pancreas	Inhibits secretion and motility.
	Pancreozymin	Pancreas	Produces pancreatic juices rich in enzymes.
	Ghrelin	Pituitary	Is associated with growth hormone release and appetite stimulation.
	Cholecystokinin (CCK)	Gallbladder	Provides for contraction and emptying of the gallbladder.
Liver	Insulin-like growth factor	Nerve, muscle, and other cells	Has insulin-like effects. Regulates cell growth and development.
	Angiotensinogen	Vascular	Constricts blood vessels and raises blood pressure.
		Brain	Increases thirst.
		Kidneys	Increases glomerular filtration rate.
		Adrenals	Increases production of aldosterone.
	Thrombopoietin	Bone marrow, platelets	Regulates the production of platelets.
Kidney	Calcitriol (1,25-dihydroxyvitamin D)	Intestine	Stimulates calcium absorption from the gut.
	Renin	Kidneys	Stimulates the renin-angiotensin-aldosterone system.
	Erythropoietin (EPO)	Bone marrow	Increases red blood cell production.
Brain	Peptide hormones	Brain and nervous system	May be used as neurotransmitters in the nervous system.
Heart	Atrial-natriuretic peptide (atriopeptin) (ANP)	Heart	Is involved in the homeostatic control of body water and sodium.

CHART 52–1	Glands and Their Hormones—*Continued*

Endocrine Gland and Hormone Source	Hormone(s)	Action Site	Physiological Effects
Adipose tissue	Leptin	Brain and nervous system	Decreases appetite and food intake, reduces insulin secretion and fat storage, increases sympathetic activity and metabolic rate.
	Resistin	Adipose cells	Suppresses insulin's ability to stimulate glucose uptake by adipose cells.
Skin	Calciferol (vitamin D)	Kidneys Intestines Bones	Contributes to the maintenance of normal levels of calcium and phosphorus in the bloodstream. Aids in the absorption of calcium for the formation of bones and teeth.
Bones	Osteocalcin	Pancreas and fat cells	Aids in sugar metabolism.

Sources: Braunwald, E., Hauser, S. L., Fauci, A. S., Longo, D. L., Kasper, D. L., & Jameson, J. L. (2001). *Harrison's principles of internal medicine* (15th ed.). New York: McGraw-Hill; Colorado State University, (2000). *Pathophysiology of the endocrine system.* http://www.colostate.edu; EndocrineWeb. (2002a). *Hyperthyroidism, overactivity of the thyroid gland. Part 2: Causes of hyperthyroidism.* Retrieved September 19, 2005, from http://endocrineweb.com/hyper2.html; EndocrineWeb. (2002b). *Pheochromocytoma.* Retrieved March 10, 2006, from http://endocrineweb.com/pheo.html; Hormone Foundation. (2006). *Endocrine glands.* Retrieved January 24, 2006, from http://www.hormone.org/endo101/index.html.

CHART 52–2	Disorders of the Endocrine System

Gland	Disorders of Hypometabolism	Hormone Involved	Disorders of Hypermetabolism
Thyroid	Hypothyroidism Cretinism Hashimoto's thyroiditis Postpartum thyroiditis	Thyroid hormone	Hyperthyroidism Graves' disease Postpartum thyroiditis Toxic goiter Hot nodules
Parathyroids	Hypoparathyroidism	Parathyroid hormone	**Hyperparathyroidism**
Anterior Pituitary	Hypopituitarism Sheehan's syndrome* Infertility	Growth hormone Prolactin ACTH	**Hyperpituitarism** Gigantism (children and youths) **Acromegaly (adults)** **Prolactin adenoma** Cushing's syndrome
Posterior Pituitary	Diabetes insipidus*	ADH	**SIADH***
Adrenal Cortex	Adrenal insufficiency* Addison's disease Congenital adrenal hyperplasia	Cortisol Aldosterone	**Cushing's syndrome** **Primary aldosteronism/Conn's disease***
Adrenal Medulla		Adrenalin (epinephrine)	**Pheochromocytoma***

*Described in an abbreviated form in the chapter.

thyroid function. Chart 52–3 (p. 1618) shows hypo- and hypermetabolic disorders of the thyroid.

Hypothyroidism

Hypothyroidism is a common endocrine disorder resulting from deficiency of thyroid hormone. It usually is a primary process, but also may be a secondary process. Primary hypothyroidism, caused by thyroid gland malfunction, is a common condition in which the thyroid gland fails to produce sufficient thyroid hormone to sustain normal metabolic function. This type of hypothyroidism may be caused by Hashimoto's disease, an autoimmune disease, surgical removal of the organ, therapeutic radiation as a result of treatment for hyperthyroidism, congenital hypothyroidism (**cretinism**, a condition caused by congenital absence that affects 1 in 4,000 newborns), or atrophy of the thyroid gland (Bharaktiya, Orlander, Woodhouse, & Davis, 2007).

Other causes include aging, iodine deficiency, tumors of the thyroid gland, or discontinuation of thyroid hormone replacement therapy or supplementation in cases where this therapy is being used (Greco, 2001). Secondary hypothyroidism occurs when the cause is related to pituitary tumors and other pituitary disorders and results from alterations in the hypothalamic–pituitary axis (Elliott, 2000; Greco, 2001). Tertiary thyroid disease originates at the level of the hypothalamus (Holcomb, 2002c).

Epidemiology and Etiology

Primary hypothyroidism is much more common than secondary and tertiary hypothyroidism (Porth, 2007). Hypothyroidism is defined as a deficiency in the production of TSH and is found in approximately 4.6% of the population (Kajantie et al., 2006). It is more common in women with small body size at birth and low body mass index during childhood. Generally, thyroid disease is much more common in females than in males,

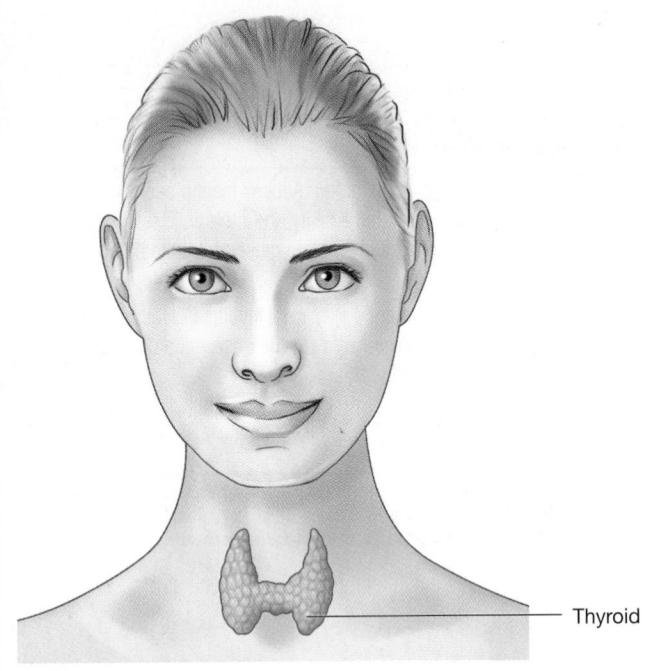

FIGURE 52–2 ■ The thyroid gland.

Thyroid

with reports of prevalence being two to eight times higher in females (Bharaktiya et al., 2007). Note also that the frequency of hypothyroidism, goiters, and thyroid nodules increases with age. Hypothyroidism is most prevalent in elderly populations, with as much as 2% to 20% of older age groups having some form of hypothyroidism (Bharaktiya et al., 2007). From a racial perspective the prevalence of hypothyroidism has been reported to be higher in Caucasians than in people of Hispanic descent or African Americans (Hollowell et al., 2002).

Primary hypothyroidism may result from **thyroidectomy** (removal of the thyroid) or ablation of the gland with radiation. Certain goitrogenic agents such as lithium carbonate and the antithyroid drugs propylthiouracil and methimazole in continuous dosage can produce hypothyroidism and goiter, as can iodine deficiency (which is very uncommon in the United States) (Porth, 2007).

The most common cause of hypothyroidism is a condition known as **Hashimoto's thyroiditis**, also known as **chronic lymphocytic thyroiditis**, a disorder in which the body's own immune system attacks the thyroid gland. The inflammatory response damages thyroid tissue and reduces the thyroid gland's ability to produce thyroid hormone. Studies in China indicate

---

CHART 52–3 **Hypothyroid and Hyperthyroid Metabolic Disorders**

	Hypothyroidism	Hyperthyroidism
Types of Thyroid Disorders and Therapy	A hypometabolic condition in which the thyroid gland fails to produce adequate thyroid hormone, resulting in a slowdown of metabolism and cellular function.	A hypermetabolic condition in which the thyroid gland produces an excess of thyroid hormone and the body increases cellular function in response.
Primary Disease (causative source is the thyroid gland itself)	*Hashimoto's thyroiditis:* an autoimmune disease leading to underproduction of thyroid hormone. May result from surgical removal of the thyroid, therapeutic radiation of the thyroid gland, endemic cretinism, and postpartum thyroiditis.	*Graves' disease:* an autoimmune disease causing overproduction of thyroid hormone. May result from postpartum thyroiditis and a "hot" thyroid nodule. Stress also may be a contributing factor.
Secondary Disease (causative source is largely due to pituitary dysfunction)	The pituitary gland becomes unable to produce adequate TSH, thus thyroxine levels drop, causing hypothyroidism. Causes include adenoma, infarction, infiltrative disease, surgery, and trauma.	The pituitary continues to produce TSH, stimulating the thyroid gland to produce more T_3 and T_4, leading to hyperthyroidism.
Tertiary Disease	Caused by impaired production of TRH from the hypothalamus, which fails to stimulate the pituitary to produce TSH.	
Pharmacologic Intervention	Administer synthetic thyroid hormone. Patient should take drug (usually levothyroxine) daily in the early morning on an empty stomach.	Administer antithyroid drugs: propylthiouracil, methimazole, or potassium iodide to inhibit thyroid hormone secretion. Hydrocortisone may be given to block TSH and for adrenal insufficiency. Calcium channel blockers and beta-blockers may be given to slow the heart rate and reduce atrial fibrillation.
Medical Intervention	*Primary disease:* administer synthetic thyroid hormone. Monitor thyroid levels regularly. *Secondary disease:* assess and treat pituitary disease. *Tertiary disease:* treat problem arising from the hypothalamus.	*Primary disease:* administer antithyroid drugs or radioactive iodine to partially or completely eliminate thyroid hormone production. *Secondary disease:* administer antithyroid drugs and treat pituitary disease.
Surgical Intervention	*Primary disease:* surgical removal of the thyroid if large goiter or nodules present.	*Primary disease:* surgical removal of part or all of the thyroid gland to reduce or eliminate hormone production.

Sources: Adapted from Holcomb, S. (2002). Thyroid diseases: A primer for the critical care nurse. *Dimensions of Critical Care Nursing, 21*(4), 127–133; Porth, C. M., 2007.

that excessive intake of iodine may increase the incidence and prevalence of autoimmune thyroiditis (Teng et al., 2006).

Pathophysiology

The thyroid gland functions with a negative feedback system through the involvement of three organs, the hypothalamus, the anterior pituitary, and the thyroid glands. The hypothalamus secretes thyrotropin-releasing hormone (TRH), the initiating hormone, which stimulates the anterior pituitary to release TSH, causing the thyroid to secrete thyroid hormone (T_3, T_4) (Larson, Anderson, & Koslawy, 2000; Porth, 2007). The dynamic feedback regulatory and compensatory responses of the pituitary and the thyroid gland are known as the hypothalamus–pituitary–thyroid axis (Holcomb, 2002c).

Follicles within the thyroid gland produce thyroxine (T_4), which constitutes approximately 95% of the thyroid hormone initially produced by this gland, as well as triiodothyronine (T_3) and calcitonin. Much of the T_4 is eventually converted into T_3, thus these are referred to collectively as thyroid hormone (Larson et al., 2000; Porth, 2007). Both thyroxine and triiodothyronine require iodine for their synthesis. With iodine deficiency, the thyroid is unable to secrete sufficient thyroid hormone. Calcitonin, also known as thyrocalcitonin, is secreted in response to high levels of calcium, reducing plasma calcium by depositing calcium in the bones. The pathophysiology of thyroid disease can involve autoimmune response disorders, inflammation, infection, atrophy of the gland, hyperplasia of tissues, tumor growth, or genetic mutations or abnormalities. See the Risk Factors for Hypothyroidism box.

Clinical Manifestations

Vague complaints of fatigue, weight gain, cold intolerance, constipation, and mental lethargy may make diagnosis of hypothyroidism difficult until the disease has progressed significantly. Dry skin, hair thinning or loss, and enlargement of the thyroid gland may be observed on physical examination. In cases of primary thyroid disease, laboratory tests will reveal a high level of TSH, because the pituitary will respond to an underproduction of thyroid hormone. In such cases, free T_4 (FT_4) (thyroxine) will be lower than normal. A major problem is that symptoms are very insidious and patients may have chronic **thyroiditis**, an inflammation of the thyroid gland, for years before a diagnosis is made and intervention initiated.

Long-standing or severe hypothyroidism may lead to a serious condition known as **myxedema**, a term used to describe the accumulation of mucopolysaccharides in tissues. This condition is characterized by signs of serious physiological compromise, including profound lethargy, muscle weakness, facial edema, thick tongue, mental decline, and personality change. Infection or trauma may precipitate myxedema as the body becomes increasingly compromised and unable to respond due to inadequate thyroid hormone.

Laboratory and Diagnostic Procedures

Thyroid function is evaluated using laboratory tests, thyroid scanning, fine-needle biopsy, and ultrasonography. Measurement of TSH in the blood and also the thyroxine level is a key diagnostic tool in suspected cases of hypothyroidism. Measurement of the FT_4 serum level reflects the amount of unbound

RISK FACTORS for Hypothyroidism

Risk factors for hypothyroidism include familial history of thyroid disease, a history of autoimmune disease, pernicious anemia, aging, an inadequate supply of dietary iodine, and previous treatment for hyperthyroidism. Hypothyroidism can occur at any age but is particularly common in older adults, affecting 17% of women and 9% of men over age 60 (Thyroid Federation International, 2003). An iodine-deficient diet also is a risk factor in the development of hypothyroidism. Iodine is needed as a raw material for the production of thyroid hormone and an inadequate supply leads to a decrease in thyroid hormone production. This condition results in overstimulation of the thyroid gland through the production of TSH by the pituitary gland, resulting in an enlarged gland or a goiter. A **goiter** is a significant enlargement of the thyroid gland.

Fortunately, goiters caused by iodine deficiency are rarely seen in developed countries due to the addition of iodine to salt and other foods, but may be seen in underdeveloped countries where natural sources of iodine are low and nutrition is poor. Patients who have had previous treatment for hyperthyroidism also are at risk following treatment, because radiation therapy or surgery may significantly reduce the production of thyroid hormone over time. Some drugs and foods inhibit thyroid production and are known as **goitrogens**. For example, lithium, a drug commonly used for the treatment of bipolar disorders, may cause hypothyroidism. Similarly, the drug rifampin, which is used to treat tuberculosis, is known to impair thyroid secretion (Takasu, Takara, & Komiya, 2005). Another drug implicated in thyroid dysfunction is amiodarone. Used for cardiac arrhythmias, amiodarone may cause abnormal results on thyroid tests and either thyrotoxicosis or hypothyroidism (Porsche & Brenner, 2006).

thyroxine in the blood and is considered the best clinical measure of thyroxine levels. Total T_3 and total T_4 are considered to be less reliable indicators of thyroid level because they are affected by drugs and other protein-binding factors.

The pituitary–thyroid negative feedback loop quickly responds when a low level of thyroid hormone is perceived. Small decreases in thyroid hormone level will result in a rapid increase in output of TSH, and increases in thyroid hormone will lead to a decrease in TSH production. Low levels of T_3 and T_4 (or FT_4) in the presence of high levels of TSH indicate that the problem is due to disease of the thyroid gland. Low levels of TSH in combination with low levels of T_3 and T_4 (or FT_4) indicate potential problems with the pituitary gland. Treatment for primary hypothyroidism, in which the thyroid gland itself is functioning poorly, is directed at hormone replacement therapy. When the problem is caused by failure of the pituitary to release TSH, further diagnostic work will be required to determine a course of therapy. Symptoms and physical findings in thyroid disease are shown in Chart 52–4 (p. 1620).

Monitoring of TSH and FT_4 will continue to be important during hormone replacement therapy as a means to evaluate the effectiveness of treatment over time. A test for thyroid antibodies also may reveal Hashimoto's thyroiditis (hypothyroidism) or Graves' disease (hyperthyroidism). In addition, thyroid scanning can be used by the health care provider when evaluating thyroid nodules, which are fairly common, occurring in 1% to 4% of the population over age 50 (AACE, 2005a). A scan involves administration of a small dose of radioactive isotope, which becomes concentrated in the thyroid tissue. Following the

CHART 52–4 Symptoms and Physical Findings for Thyroid Disease

Physiological System	Symptoms of Hypothyroidism	Symptoms of Hyperthyroidism
Cardiopulmonary	Slowed heartbeat/pulse, high blood pressure, high cholesterol levels, cardiac enlargement, congestive heart failure, ascites	Rapid heartbeat/pulse, palpitations, angina, irregular heart rhythm, heat intolerance, and hot flashes
Neuromuscular	Drowsiness, fatigue, mental lethargy, forgetfulness, depression, muscular weakness, emotional lability, and paranoia	Insomnia, jitteriness, shaking, nervousness, irritability, hand tremors, muscle weakness, myalgia, and muscle cramps
Gastrointestinal	Enlarged tongue, constipation, reduced bowel sounds	Difficulty swallowing, more frequent bowel movements, diarrhea
Skin/hair	Dry patchy skin, coarse and thinning hair (alopecia), fluid retention in skin, cold intolerance, decreased perspiration, edema of face and eyelids	Thinning hair or alopecia, warm, moist skin (sweating), heat intolerance
Other	Weight gain, fatigue, heavy and irregular menstrual periods, lowered body temperature	Unexplained weight loss, change in or lighter menstrual cycles, bulging eyes (exophthalmos), goiter (thyroid enlargement), accelerated loss of calcium from bones
Diagnostic lab values	Elevated cholesterol levels Serum TSH (will be low if the pituitary is involved and high if the thyroid gland is the affected tissue) Decreased or absent T_4 and T_3 levels Low basal metabolic rate (BMR) Presence of thyroid antibodies	Low level of TSH Elevated serum free T_4 and free T_3 Elevated BMR

Source: Adapted from American Association of Clinical Endocrinologists. (2005b). *Hyperthyroidism: Information for patients.* Retrieved September 19, 2005, from http://www.aace.com/members/brochures.php; American Association of Clinical Endocrinologists. (2005c). *Hypothyroidism: Information for patients.* Retrieved September 19, 2005, from http://www.aace.com/members/brochures.php; Hadley, M. E. (2000). *Endocrinology* (5th ed.). San Francisco: Benjamin Cummings.

ingestion or injection of the isotope, a picture is taken of the gland to determine the nature of the nodule, a majority of which are benign. The thyroid scan shows whether a nodule is hot or cold (nonfunctioning). Ultrasound also can be useful in evaluating the size and shape of nodules, whether a nodule is a cyst (cysts are normally benign) or solid, but it is less useful in differentiating benign from malignant growths. A fine-needle biopsy is the most accurate method used to determine whether a nodule is malignant or benign. Ultrasonography of the thyroid may be most useful in guiding the placement of a needle for biopsy to obtain a good specimen (AACE, 2005b; Larson et al., 2000). See the Diagnostic Tests for Thyroid Disorders box.

Medical Management

The treatment for hypothyroidism involves the replacement of thyroid hormone as indicated by the physiological functioning of the gland. In hypothyroidism, therapeutic actions are directed at stimulating the production of or replacing thyroid hormone. Hypothyroidism is easily treated with the administration of the synthetic thyroid hormone levothyroxine. The dosage is determined by the amount needed to bring TSH levels into the normal range and to provide abatement of symptoms. Approximately 70 to 100 mcg of levothyroxine is given daily based on age, weight, hormone levels, and symptoms. Initial adult doses vary from 25 to 100 mcg, with smaller doses given to the elderly and patients with diabetes or cardiac disease.

To ensure maximum absorption of the hormone, it is advised that levothyroxine be taken in the early morning on an empty stomach. Synthetic thyroid hormone can be taken safely concurrently with some medications, but patients taking medications such as anticoagulants, beta-blockers, cholesterol-lowering

drugs, or seizure control drugs should check with the pharmacist for potential drug interactions. Although administration of levothyroxine will bring thyroid hormone levels within normal limits, it may suppress TSH, which increases the risk of osteoporosis, a side effect that can be avoided by the ingestion of calcium carbonate. However, if the two preparations are taken together, the calcium can interfere with absorption of thyroid hormone. Thus patients should be advised to take any over-the-counter (OTC) vitamins, minerals (including iron), and antacids at least 4 hours earlier or later than thyroid hormone (Neafsey, 2004). Patients also need to be advised that they will be taking thyroid replacement hormone for life.

- *Because the absorption of the synthetic thyroid hormone levothyroxine is altered by food and selected drugs, herbs, vitamins, and minerals, the nurse should advise the patient to take this drug on an empty stomach, usually as a single dose before breakfast and to hold food intake for at least 1 hour. Patients should ingest this medication at least 4 hours before taking antacids, iron, or vitamin/mineral supplements.*

- *Because the bioavailability of the drug varies with different manufacturers, patients should continue taking the same brand continuously or should have thyroid function studies done 6 to 8 weeks after a change in prescription.*

- *Patients should be advised they will be taking thyroid replacement therapy for the remainder of their lives and not to discontinue this medication without consulting with their health care provider.*

Symptoms of hypothyroidism gradually fade over a period of 3 to 6 weeks as therapy is initiated. Blood levels of TSH and FT_4 should be tested 6 to 8 weeks after therapy is initiated and regularly thereafter until hormone levels stabilize and symptoms disappear.

DIAGNOSTIC TESTS for Thyroid Disorders

Test	Nature of the Test	Normal Ranges*	Use in Diagnosis	Nursing Implications
Thyroid-stimulating hormone (TSH) test	Laboratory test of blood.	*Adults:* 2–12 microinternational unit/mL	Differentiating primary from secondary hypothyroidism. Elevation of TSH occurs in primary hypothyroidism. In secondary hypothyroid states where pituitary pathology exists, TSH may be absent or very low, even with low levels of T_3 and T_4.	Prepare patient for blood test. Does not require fasting. Recent administration of radioisotopes for other diagnostic tests may affect test results.
TSH stimulation test	A laboratory examination of the blood.	Evidence of increased thyroid function with administration of TSH.	Helps differentiate primary and secondary hypothyroidism. Patients with primary disease are unable to increase the production of thyroid hormone when stimulated with TSH.	Prepare patient for blood test. Fasting is not required.
Thyrotropin-releasing hormone (TRH) test	An IV bolus of TRH is given.	A quick rise in TSH levels within 30 minutes after receiving TRH.	Reveals the responsiveness of the anterior pituitary to TRH. Confirms the presence of primary hyperthyroidism because little or no increase in TSH is seen due to the suppression effect of excess circulation of thyroid hormone. A TSH level that rises too high may indicate early hypothyroidism.	Prepare patient for blood test. Does not require fasting. Explain procedure to patient. Check site of drug administration.
Thyroxine (T_4) screen	A laboratory test with blood.	*Adults:* 4–11 mcg/dL	Provides a direct (but not always reliable) measure of T_4 in the blood. Increased levels indicate hyperthyroidism and low levels indicate hypothyroidism.	Results may be affected by iodine contrast scans. Level also may be affected by medications such as estrogen, oral contraceptives, seizure medications, and opiates such as heroin, lithium, steroids, and antithyroid drugs.
Thyroxine index, free (FT$_4$ index)	A laboratory test of blood.		Measures the amount of free T_4, which is not affected by thyroid-binding globulin abnormalities. Reflects the real hormonal status more effectively than does a total T_4 or T_3 blood test. Increased levels indicate hyperthyroidism and decreased levels indicate hypothyroidism.	Explain the procedure to the patient.
Triiodothyronine (T_3) radioimmunoassay	A laboratory test of blood.		Accurately measures thyroid function. When levels are below normal, hypothyroidism generally exists.	May be affected by pregnancy, recently administered radioisotope administration, and selected drugs. Does not require fasting.

(continued)

DIAGNOSTIC TESTS for Thyroid Disorders—*Continued*

Test	Nature of the Test	Normal Ranges*	Use in Diagnosis	Nursing Implications
Triiodothyronine (T₃) uptake test	A laboratory test of blood.	25–35%	Indirectly quantifies thyroid-binding globulin and thyroid-binding prealbumin, which may be elevated due to pregnancy, oral contraceptive use, or genetic factors. Adds information in the diagnosis of hypothyroidism and hyperthyroidism.	May be affected by recent radioisotope scans and selected drugs. Does not require fasting.
Iodine uptake scan	Patient takes an oral dose of radioactive iodine on an empty stomach. The amount of iodine that is taken up by the thyroid gland is measured during the next several hours.	Measures how much iodine is taken up by the thyroid gland.	Hypothyroid patients take up little iodine and hyperthyroid patients take up a lot of iodine.	Patient should be NPO before exam. Usually done in conjunction with thyroid lab studies.
Thyroid scan	A radioactive substance is given to enhance visualization of the gland. An image of the gland is recorded as the scan passes over the gland.	Reveals normal size, shape, position, and function. No areas of decreased or increased uptake are apparent.	Particularly useful in differentiating thyroid nodules, Graves' disease from Plummer's disease, and metastatic tumors.	Contraindicated in pregnancy and with allergies to iodine.
Thyroid ultrasound	Ultrasound.	Reveals normal size, shape, and position of gland.	Useful in differentiating cystic from solid thyroid nodules. Can be used to aid in placement of needle for biopsy. A safe procedure when thyroid scan cannot be done due to pregnancy.	Prepare patient for procedure.

*Normal ranges are best determined by the laboratory administering the tests.

Sources: Adapted from EndocrineWeb.com. (2008). Retrieved August 29, 2008 from http://www.endocrineweb.com/; Larson, J., Anderson, E., & Koslawy, M. (2000). Thyroid disease: A review for primary care. *Journal of the American Academy of Nurse Practitioners, 12*(6), 226–232.

Following stabilization, thyroid hormone levels then should be checked annually to ensure that the appropriate medication level has been reached and to avoid drug-induced hyperthyroidism.

◼ Nursing Management

Nursing care for patients with hypothyroidism is guided by the severity of the disease process and related symptoms. Typically, the nurse is an objective observer and recorder of patient signs and symptoms, both during diagnosis and following treatment, a role that is particularly important given the frequency with which the diagnosis of hormonal disorders is delayed or missed. Patients with hypothyroidism will report weight gain, dry skin and hair, constipation, fatigue, and mental lethargy. In cases of long-standing disease or seriously decreased hormone levels, cardiac problems may be apparent as evidenced by bradycardia, high blood pressure, high cholesterol levels, cardiac enlargement, and congestive heart failure.

Nursing care should be directed at symptom management and improvement of the patient's physiological status with hormone replacement therapy. Patients should be instructed on the nature of the hormone replacement and the importance of taking thyroid hormone on an empty stomach. The primary goal of treatment is to return patients to a **euthyroid**, or normal thyroid, status. Patients are started on small to moderate doses of levothyroxine to begin their hormone replacement therapy. Patients with diabetes should be monitored carefully during this period because their blood sugars may be more labile due to hypothyroidism. See the Nursing Process: Patient Care Plan for Hypothyroidism, which details the nursing process used in caring for patients with hypothyroidism.

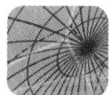

NURSING PROCESS: Patient Care Plan For Hypothyroidism

Assessment of Current Body Characteristics

Subjective Data:

Is your pulse slower than normal?

Has your weight changed, either increased or decreased in recent months?

Do you feel energetic or fatigued much of the time? Are you sleeping a great deal but still feeling tired?

Has there been any change in your activity tolerance?

How would you describe your mental alertness and memory?

Describe your menstrual pattern. Has there been any change in the frequency or flow during your menstrual periods?

Objective Data:

Weight gain

Edema around eyes and facial puffiness

Thick tongue

Bradycardia and dyspnea

Low body temperature

Enlargement of the thyroid gland (goiter)

TSH level high

FT_4 low

Unable to process thoughts rapidly

Nursing Assessment and Diagnoses	Outcomes and Evaluation Parameters	Planning and Interventions with *Rationales*
Nursing Diagnosis: *Fatigue*, and *Activity Intolerance* secondary to hypometabolic state with decreased cardiac output	**Outcome:** Patient is able to manage self-care and explain rationale for therapeutic plan, including medication regime and instructions. **Evaluation Parameters:** Patient is able to repeat instructions for taking medications and can describe symptoms of both hypo- and hyperthyroidism. TSH and FT_4 levels return to normal range. **Outcome:** Patient does not use sedatives or opiates during acute phase of illness. **Evaluation Parameter:** Patient and health care team express awareness of risks associated with use of sedatives, opiates, or alcohol.	**Interventions and *Rationales*:** Instruct patient on administration of hormone replacement medication, signs and symptoms of hypo- and hyperthyroidism, and self-care practices. *To ensure patient takes hormone replacement medication on an empty stomach for optimal absorption. To inform patient to be alert for signs of hypo- or hyperthyroidism.* Patient and health care providers are warned to avoid use of sedatives, opioids, analgesic medications, or alcohol products, which would further depress metabolic functions and increase risk of myxedema crisis. *To prevent further suppression of the patient's metabolic state and possible serious complications such as coma, particularly in the elderly.*

Assessment of Skin and Nail Characteristics and Wound Healing

Subjective Data:

Have you noticed any change in your skin, hair, or nails lately?

Are your nails brittle, thick, and often breaking or splitting?

Is your skin cold, dry, or itchy? Do you bruise easily? Do wounds heal slowly?

Objective Data:

Skin cool and dry

Evidence of itching skin

Brittle nails

Hair dry, sparse, coarse, and brittle

Generalized interstitial edema

Nursing Assessment and Diagnoses	Outcomes and Evaluation Parameters	Planning and Intervention with *Rationales*
Nursing Diagnosis: *Risk for Impaired Skin Integrity* secondary to thyroid hormone deficiency	**Outcome:** Verbalizes satisfaction with improved condition of skin, hair, and nails, with less itching and breaking. **Evaluation Parameters:** Skin intact, soft, and moist with no evidence of patient itching or scratching. Patient's hair is soft and thick.	**Interventions and *Rationales*:** Avoid use of soaps, astringents, or other agents such as alcohol. Liberally apply emollient skin lotion. Consider using an alternating air mattress if needed. *To counteract drying of skin, hair, and nails due to hormone loss and to protect skin from injury.*

Assessment of Gastrointestinal Function and Disturbances

Subjective Data:

Have you observed any changes in your bowel habits?

Have you experienced frequent constipation or abdominal pain?

Is your cholesterol high?

Objective Data:

Abdomen distended

Bowel sounds decreased

Weight gain

Increased TSH level

Decreased T_4

Presence of thyroid antibodies

Nursing Assessment and Diagnoses	Outcomes and Evaluation Parameters	Planning and Interventions with *Rationales*
Nursing Diagnosis: *Constipation* secondary to lethargy, activity intolerance, and hypometabolic state	**Outcome:** Observed bowel function is normal with no reports of constipation or abdominal pain. **Evaluation Parameters:** Abdomen soft, not distended. Active bowel sounds. Patient's normal bowel pattern is resumed.	**Interventions and *Rationales*:** Administer stool softeners as prescribed. Gradually increase fluid intake and fiber in diet. Increase activity level with short, frequent walks and mild exercise. *To maintain or regain normal bowel function and to prevent bowel obstruction or megacolon.*

(continued)

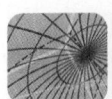

NURSING PROCESS: Patient Care Plan For Hypothyroidism—*Continued*

Assessment for Hypothermia

Subjective Data:
Are you feeling too cold or too hot?
Do you feel anxious or restless?

Objective Data:
Wearing multiple layers of clothing
Skin is cool and dry
Hypothermia (in severe myxedema) with low body temperature

Nursing Assessment and Diagnoses	Outcomes and Evaluation Parameters	Planning and Interventions with *Rationales*
Nursing Diagnosis: *Hypothermia* secondary to metabolic dysfunction	**Outcome:** Patient is able to tolerate typical ambient temperatures without distress. **Evaluation Parameters:** Body temperature within normal range. Patient appears comfortable with no reports of distress related to ambient temperature.	**Interventions and *Rationales*:** Monitor the environment to provide a warm room for patient comfort. *To minimize patient discomfort while patient's body is adapting to stabilization of hormone levels.*

Assessment of Cognition Level and Memory Impairment

Subjective Data:
Do you feel mentally alert?
Are your thought processes slowed?
Is your short- or long-term memory impaired?
Are you irritable or confused?

Objective Data:
Responds appropriately to questions
Able to follow directions
Recalls objects when asked to
Recognizes individuals by name and/or position

Nursing Assessment and Diagnoses	Outcomes and Evaluation Parameters	Planning and Interventions with *Rationales*
Nursing Diagnosis: *Confusion, Acute* secondary to hypothyroidism	**Outcomes:** Patient oriented to time, place, and circumstances. Able to recall instructions regarding medications and activity prescriptions. Mood stable. **Evaluation Parameters:** Alert and oriented. Evidence of effective short- and long-term memory. Family reports stable affect and mood.	**Interventions and *Rationales*:** Reduce stimuli and mental demands while hormone deficiency is replaced. Instruct family about potential mood swings, depression, and irritability. Provide instructions to patient and family in writing as well as orally. *To minimize distress and disorientation while patient's body is adapting to stabilization of hormone levels.*

Discharge Priorities

Discharge priorities include ensuring patient's understanding of the need for lifelong hormone replacement therapy and annual monitoring of hormone levels once a stable, therapeutic level of hormone has been reached. Some authorities advise patients to be wary of changing brands or suppliers of hormone replacement drugs because of the variability in bioavailability of the drug in different products (American Thyroid Association, 2005; Holcomb, 2002c; Thyroid Foundation of America, 2004b). If the brand name drug or generic drug is changed, the patient should be retested about 6 weeks after starting on the new medication. Consultation with an endocrine specialist is advised, particularly if the patient is diabetic or pregnant.

Gerontological Considerations

Hypothyroidism is seen clinically at an increasing rate in women over age 50. Clinical manifestations, unless severe, may be too subtle to easily recognize, thus making diagnosis and intervention more difficult. In rare cases, **myxedema coma**, a rare life-threatening complication in which there is overwhelming cardiopulmonary failure, may be seen in elderly patients, usually precipitated by some untoward event such as infection, trauma, surgery, or neurological disorder (Figure 52–3 ■). Patients

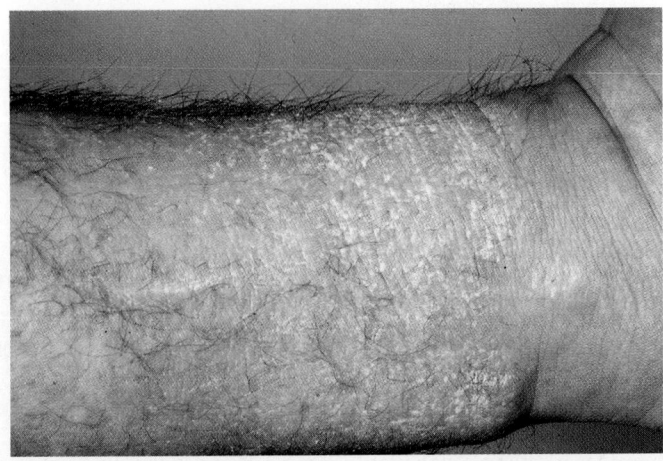

FIGURE 52–3 ■ Patient with myxedema.

present with all the usual, but exacerbated and serious symptoms of hypothyroidism, and they typically have body temperatures below normal as well. Hypothermia, with body temperature lower than 35°C (95°F), is a key sign that myxedema coma may be impending. In addition, patients with myxedema coma may demonstrate serious cardiac symptoms, impaired ventilation, and neuromuscular weakness. Timely diagnosis and intervention is essential in such cases because mortality rates are high.

In addition, it is essential that the underlying problem be identified and treated since patients may have other problems such as myxedema megacolon, an abnormal dilation of the colon that is not caused by mechanical obstruction, due to reduced intestinal motility caused by hypothyroidism. This condition may lead health care providers to consider surgery when the primary need is for hormone replacement therapy.

Fortunately, abdominal symptoms usually subside when synthetic thyroid hormone is administered to the patient (Greco, 2001). In emergency situations, levothyroxine sodium, a more powerful injectable form of triiodothyronine, may be administered intravenously for treatment of myxedema coma. Nurses must be particularly vigilant in assessment and reporting of cardiac symptoms, impaired ventilation, and neuromuscular weakness in these cases. Patients may require ventilator assistance and other support measures to ensure survival.

- *Immediately report signs of myxedema, a severe, life-threatening illness with symptoms including facial edema, thick tongue (macroglossia), mental confusion, irritability, severe mood swings, significant hypothermia (91°F to 95°F), severely slowed pulse and respirations, decreased blood pressure, profound neuromuscular weakness, anemia, and signs of psychosis, because the mortality rate is high.*
- *Avoid use of sedatives, opiates, or alcohol to prevent congestive heart failure and circulatory collapse.*
- *Provide respiratory support with administration of oxygen and ventilation if needed.*
- *Administer intravenous fluids with care, observing for plural effusion and congestive heart failure.*
- *Be prepared to administer fast-acting intravenous thyroid hormone to restore the body's thyroxine level.*
- *Slowly rewarm the patient to avoid causing refractory hypotension and increased oxygen demand.*
- *Observe for signs of infection and treat infections immediately to avoid further compromise of the patient.*

Health Promotion
The thyroid gland requires iodine to manufacture thyroid hormone. Until iodine was added to salt sometime in the 1920s, hypothyroidism was not uncommon in some parts of the United States. Patients should be encouraged to eat a healthy diet, to purchase salt enhanced with iodine, and ensure that iodine is ingested regularly. Another food source high in iodine is seafood. Health promotion for patients with thyroid disease most often revolves around instruction regarding medications for hormone replacement therapy since therapy will be required for the remainder of the patient's lifetime. Some patients will find it difficult to accept the notion that lifetime drug therapy is advised

for treatment of this disorder. For this reason, it is important for the nurse to assess the patient's understanding of the disorder and the need for hormone replacement therapy.

The Genetic Considerations for Hypothyroidism box discusses the nurse's role if a familial predisposition to hypothyroidism is suspected.

Collaborative Management
Patients with thyroid disease will need the support of several members of the health care team. Following diagnosis, the patient with hypothyroidism will benefit from instruction by the pharmacist regarding medication for replacement of thyroid hormone and medications to treat other symptoms such as anemia. The nutritionist or dietitian can provide helpful consultation on diet to address the hypometabolic needs of the patient's body while therapy corrects and stabilizes thyroid hormones.

Hyperthyroidism
Hyperthyroidism, a condition in which there is excess production of thyroid hormone, is caused by an increase in thyroid function for any reason. This condition may lead to **thyrotoxicosis**, a clinical syndrome that results when tissues are exposed to high levels of circulating thyroid hormone (Greenspan, 2004).

Epidemiology and Etiology
Hyperthyroidism may be due to Graves' disease, toxic multinodular goiter, painful subacute thyroiditis caused by a viral infection, other types of thyroiditis, adenomas of the thyroid gland, and excessive iodine or thyroid hormone intake. **Graves' disease**, a disorder named for an Irish physician who described the syndrome, is an autoimmune disorder that is the most common cause of hyperthyroidism, with it being more prevalent in women (Porth, 2007; Yeung & Habra, 2007). In Graves' disease, thyroid stimulating immunoglobulins (TSIs) activate TSH receptors on the thyroid follicular cells, resulting in increased production of thyroid hormones and symptoms of hyperthyroidism such as increased appetite, unexplained weight loss, heat intolerance, exertional dyspnea, increased heart rate, fatigue, nervousness, goiter, and palpitations (Waltman, Brewer, & Lobert, 2004). Generally, thyroiditis involves the entire thyroid gland and is eight times more common in women than men between the ages of 30 and 50 years (Figure 52–4 ■, p. 1626).

Other causes of thyroiditis with resulting temporary hyperthyroidism include subacute thyroiditis (also known as De Quervain's thyroiditis), and silent thyroiditis (lymphocytic and postpartum thyroiditis). These may be caused by a viral infection, and there are indications that trauma and stress, such as

GENETIC CONSIDERATIONS for Hypothyroidism

Patients should be advised of any familial predisposition to thyroid disease based on a family history of thyroid and autoimmune disorders in order to advise other family members of this particular health risk.

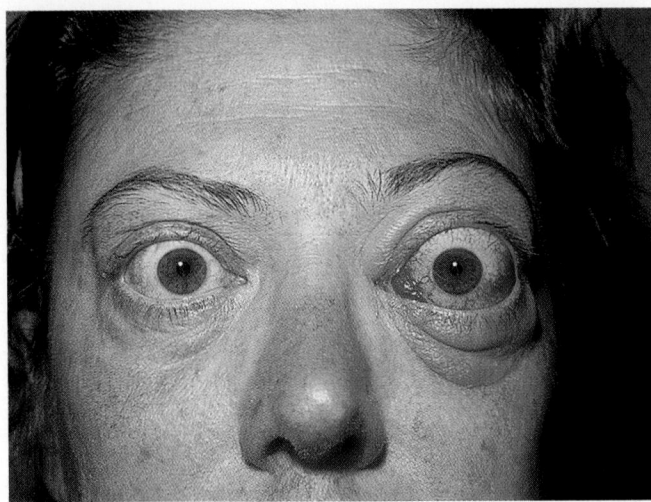

FIGURE 52–4 ■ Patient with Graves' disease.

pregnancy, also may influence the development of the disease. In subacute thyroiditis, patients often experience pain as well as enlargement of the thyroid gland. Many patients with these conditions will resume normal thyroid function over time, but sometimes treatment is required for subsequent hypothyroidism (AACE, 2005d).

Multiple or single "hot" nodules in the thyroid gland may excrete excess thyroid hormone. These conditions are called toxic multinodular goiter or toxic nodule. Thyroid nodules are fairly common and only a small percentage are malignant. Nodules may occur simply due to excess growth of normal thyroid tissue, fluid-filled cysts, inflammation (thyroiditis), or benign or cancerous tumors. A single enlarged nodule may cause hyperthyroidism because it can produce a very large amount of thyroid hormone. For more information, see the Risk Factors for Hyperthyroidism box.

Pathophysiology

Hyperthyroidism is a condition in which excessive levels of thyroid hormone stimulate the body's metabolic processes, resulting in symptoms indicative of the hypermetabolic state, including loss of weight, nervousness, rapid pulse, and warm, moist skin. Thyrotoxicosis is an inclusive term that describes severe hypermetabolic conditions caused by the thyroid hormones. Hyperthyroidism may be due to primary disease

RISK FACTORS for Hyperthyroidism

There appears to be a genetic predisposition to autoimmune disorders that cause hyperthyroidism, or Graves' disease. Situational physiological changes such as the stress of pregnancy or viral illness can stimulate the onset of the disease. Excessive iodine intake and excessive thyroid hormone replacement therapy can also be predisposing factors (Holcomb, 2002c). A history of amiodarone therapy for cardiac arrhythmias is also a risk factor for hyperthyroidism because amiodarone is 37% iodine by weight (Porsche & Brenner, 2006). Hyperthyroidism occurs most often in women in their middle years but can occur in older adults and children as well.

involving the thyroid itself or it may be caused by unchecked pituitary secretion of TSH. In primary hyperthyroidism, inflammation of thyroid cells occurs due to thyroiditis with accumulation of white blood cells and fluid causing thyroid enlargement. In secondary hyperthyroidism, increased growth and proliferation of thyroid cells may also occur due to stimulation by TSH produced by the pituitary. Long-standing or very acute illness states can lead to cardiac complications and **exophthalmus**, bulging of the eyes.

Clinical Manifestations

The clinical signs of hyperthyroidism will vary depending on the severity of thyrotoxicosis, patient age, and individual response to high levels of thyroid hormone. Key indications of hyperthyroidism are unexplained weight loss, fine tremors of the hand and tongue, hyperactivity, heat intolerance, palpitations, tachycardia (with heart rate greater than 100 beats/min), fatigue, and weakness. See Chart 52–3 (p. 1618) for a comparison of signs and symptoms in hypothyroidism and hyperthyroidism. The symptoms of hyperthyroidism may be very subtle initially in elderly patients, presenting with complaints of fatigue and/or weight loss. Elderly patients are easily misdiagnosed and may be thought to have depression, given that they report insomnia, fatigue, and impaired concentration and memory.

Graves' Disease During Pregnancy

Pregnant women normally have some increase in thyroid stimulation during pregnancy and the thyroid gland will enlarge somewhat. However, significant **thyromegaly**, abnormal growth in thyroid tissue, and goiter are unusual physical findings and should cause the clinician to evaluate a pregnant woman for possible hyperthyroidism. Graves' disease is the most common endocrine disorder other than diabetes in pregnancy and may put mother and fetus at risk for preterm delivery, perinatal morbidity, heart failure, and thyroid storm. During pregnancy, Graves' disease is managed best with antithyroid drugs (medications that inhibit the production of thyroxine), because radioactive iodine will affect the fetus's thyroid gland and surgery will increase the risk of miscarriage or preterm delivery (Waltman et al., 2004).

Laboratory and Diagnostic Procedures

The same diagnostic tests described earlier in the section on hypothyroidism are used in the assessment of patients with suspected hypermetabolic thyroid states. Measurements of TSH and FT_4 are commonly used to assess patients with suspected hyperthyroidism. A decrease in TSH in combination with a high level of FT_4 indicates hyperthyroidism. Refer to the earlier Diagnostic Tests for Thyroid Disorders box (p. 1621) for an overview of the thyroid tests used to assess thyroid functioning during diagnosis and treatment of thyroid disorders.

Medical Management

Hypermetabolic thyroid states, including Graves' disease, can be difficult to treat, depending on the responsiveness of thyroid tissue to treatment modalities (Fenton, Gold, & Sadeghi-Nejad, 2006). There are three common ways to treat Graves' disease:

- Antithyroid drugs, which inhibit production or conversion of active thyroid hormone

- Radioactive iodine, which destroys all or part of the thyroid gland and makes it unable to produce excessive thyroid hormone
- Subtotal thyroidectomy, in which most of the thyroid gland is removed, making it unable to produce excessive thyroid hormone.

Medical options usually are tried first since complications, including hemorrhage, damage to the parathyroid glands, and impairment of the vocal cords, can occur with surgical intervention. Antithyroid drug therapy has the benefit of lower cost and is safer for patients such as pregnant women, adolescents, and children. Moreover, antithyroid drugs can be of great value in autoimmune diseases such as Graves' disease because antithyroid drugs improve the autoimmune process (Cooper, 2005). However, selection of treatment for hyperthyroidism will depend on age, physical condition, pregnancy, degree of illness, and personal preferences.

Antithyroid drugs, such as propylthiouracil (PTU) and methimazole (Tapazole, Carbimazole), may be used in both the initial and long-term treatment of hyperthyroidism. Methimazole, taken in just one daily dose, has an advantage over PTU, which must be given in three divided doses. Thus, methimazole, which yields more rapid improvement in serum concentrations of thyroxine and triiodothyronine, also enhances better patient compliance.

Short-term use of antithyroid drugs may be prescribed to reduce thyroid hormone levels over a period of a few weeks since radioactive iodine can initiate acute thyroiditis, causing the release of more stored thyroid hormone. Iodine solutions may also be given orally for up to 2 weeks to reduce thyroxine production prior to surgery but this approach is of short-term benefit. Antithyroid drug therapy is also used in vulnerable, elderly patients at risk for cardiac complications and for pregnant patients for whom other therapies present a special risk (Holcomb, 2002c; Waltman et al., 2004). It is essential that when such patients are hospitalized, careful attention be given to ensuring that they are receiving their antithyroid medications (Harris, 2007).

Antithyroid drugs are associated with a variety of side effects. Skin rashes may be managed with the administration of an antihistamine. Other minor side effects include arthralgias, nausea, and abnormal taste or smell. PTU and methimazole can cause more serious side effects such as liver inflammation, a severe deficiency of white blood cells, and polyarthritis, thus patients should be advised to stop the drug and notify their health care provider if they experience jaundice of the skin, fever, or sore throat. Propylthiouracil is the preferred antithyroid drug in pregnancy because methimazole is known to cause rare congenital anomalies (Cooper, 2005).

Antithyroid drugs may be effective over a period of several months to a few years and the hyperthyroidism may subside. However, patients with severe hyperthyroidism often require more aggressive therapy because antithyroid drugs may not manage symptoms adequately. Patients whose antithyroid drugs have been discontinued should have their thyroid function evaluated regularly since reoccurrence of hyperthyroidism may occur (Cooper, 2005). Medications used to treat hyperthyroidism are shown in the Pharmacology Summary (p. 1628).

Graves' disease also is routinely treated with radioactive iodine therapy (except in pregnancy as noted) and offers the advantage of rapid oblation of the thyroid gland. Radioactive iodine concentrates in thyroid tissues, thus it does not present a risk to the rest of the body. It has the additional advantage that it can be taken on an outpatient basis, thus the patient may avoid hospitalization. Outcomes, including partial or complete elimination of thyroid hormone production, depend on the dosage of the radioactive iodine and sensitivity of tissues. Because of the potential for permanent elimination of all thyroid hormone production over time, patients should be given both oral and written instructions on symptoms of hypothyroidism, and thyroid hormone levels should be taken at regular intervals until the patient has stabilized over a period of several months. In rare cases, treatment may need to be repeated.

Surgical intervention may be selected if antithyroid drugs are ineffective or if the patient is not a candidate for either drug therapy or radioactive iodine therapy for some reason. Surgery is warranted when there is suspicion of malignancy, compression of the trachea or esophagus due to thyroid enlargement, difficult-to-manage hyperthyroidism during pregnancy, or substernal thyroid. Lifetime replacement of thyroid hormone is needed when a major portion or all of the thyroid gland has been removed or oblated through surgery or radioactive iodine. Other drugs such as beta-blockers or calcium channel blockers also will be prescribed during episodes of hyperthyroidism in order to control cardiac arrhythmias such as tachycardia and/or atrial fibrillation.

A rare, but serious complication of hyperthyroidism is **thyroid storm**, a life-threatening condition in which the body decompensates in overwhelming thyrotoxicosis. The most vulnerable patients for thyrotoxicosis are the elderly and those patients who are prone to infection or postsurgical complications, are pregnant or postnatal, and those subject to antithyroid medication withdrawal (Harris, 2007). Thyrotoxicosis is characterized by sinus or supraventricular tachycardia, hyperpyrexia (with temperature above 40°C [104°F]), confusion, delirium, and coma. Immediate treatment is essential to prevent fatalities, which occur in 20% to 30% of cases (Waltman et al., 2004).

■ Nursing Management

The goal in nursing management of the patient with hyperthyroidism is to support the treatment plan, which is directed at reducing or eliminating the output of thyroid hormone and addressing the symptoms attendant to the hypermetabolic state. Instruction on the action, benefits, and side effects of antithyroid drugs is a key role for the nurse. It is essential that patients understand that therapy should not be abruptly halted unless there are signs of serious side effects. Immediate consultation with the health care provider should occur if antithyroid drugs are discontinued. This is a vulnerable time when thyroid storm could occur, thus patients must be advised to observe for worsening signs of hyperthyroidism and report such signs to their health care provider. Should the patient be hospitalized, the nurse must note signs of significant change in a patient's condition and alert the health care provider so that immediate action can be taken to counteract the cascade of thyroid hormone to prevent fatalities, which occur in a significant percentage of those patients who develop thyroid storm.

PHARMACOLOGY Summary of Medications to Treat Thyroid Disorders

Medication	Action	Side Effects	Nursing Care
Propylthiouracil (PTU)	Controls hyperthyroidism by slowing thyroid hormone production. May be given over several months and may cause temporary or long-term remission of hyperthyroidism.	Allergic reaction with rash, hives, fever, joint pain. Decrease in white blood cells, sore throat, fever, joint aches, infection. Impaired liver function, jaundice, fever, loss of appetite, and abdominal pain.	Instruct patient to have regular follow-up of thyroid function since hyperthyroid activity may reoccur. Monitor white blood cell count. Monitor liver function. Report fever or sore throat to health care provider immediately.
Methimazole (Tapazole, Carbimazole)	Inhibits synthesis of thyroid hormone.	Caution in patients with liver disease, bone marrow disorders, and previous allergies to other antithyroid drugs. Congenital anomalies.	Instruct patient to take at same time daily at regular intervals. Monitor liver function. Avoid giving when the following drugs are being taken: anticancer drugs, iodine-containing drugs, lithium, sulfonamides, interferon.
Iodide or iodide products (Lugol's solution, sodium iodide, potassium iodide)	Inhibits synthesis and release of thyroid hormone and decreases size and vascularity of the thyroid. Effective for relatively short-term therapy (7–14 days).	Diarrhea, vomiting, nausea, abdominal pain. Skin rash, GI bleeding may signal adverse reaction.	Advise patient to drink all of solution, to use a straw to avoid discoloration of teeth, and not to withdraw drug abruptly. Discourage use of OTC drugs without health care provider consultation. Have patient report symptoms of iodism: abdominal symptoms.
Propranolol (Inderal)	Beta-adrenergic blocking agents. Decreases the effects and some symptoms of excess thyroid hormone.	Decreases heart rate and myocardial oxygen consumption. Lowers blood pressure.	Contraindicated in patients with asthma, sinus bradycardia, and heart block. Instruct patient not to discontinue abruptly. Discourage use of OTC drugs without health care provider consultation.
Radioactive iodine (sodium iodide [I-131], Iodotope)	Radioactive iodine destroys thyroid tissue with maximum benefit apparent in 3–6 months. Radioactive iodine concentrates in thyroid tissues and is excreted in a few days.	No serious complications reported so this has become the treatment of choice.	Instruct patient to: Have thyroid hormone levels monitored regularly. Take thyroid replacement hormone on an empty stomach. Take hormone replacement for life. Do not change brands of hormones without follow-up monitoring. Follow radiation precautions as directed.

Sources: Adapted from EndocrineWeb.com. (2007). Endocrine disorders & endocrine surgery. Retrieved August 29, 2008 from http://www.endocrineweb.com/; Jordan, S. (2005). Prescription drugs: Uses and effects. Thyroid disorders: Symptom control. *Nursing Standard, 19*(23), 56–58; Medline Plus. (2001). *Cabergoline (systemic).* Retrieved March 7, 2006, from http://www.nlm.nih.gov/medlineplus/druginfo/uspdi/203584.html; *Physician's drug handbook* (11th ed.). (2005). Philadelphia: Lippincott Williams & Wilkins; Sachse, D. (2001). Acromegaly. *American Journal of Nursing, 101*(11), 69, 71, 73–75.

- *Thyroid storm occurs in severe hyperthyroidism and may be triggered by surgery, trauma, infection, postpartum status, or withdrawal of antithyroid drugs, resulting in severe tachycardia, heart failure, hyperthermia, and shock.*
- *Ensure adequate oxygen and ventilation.*
- *Control dysrhythmias if they occur.*
- *Administer IV fluids, monitoring glucose and electrolyte levels.*
- *Administer antithyroid drugs to inhibit the biosynthesis and block the release of thyroid hormone. (Iodide preparations should not be given for at least 1 hour after other antithyroid medications because they may be used to synthesize more T₄.)*

   Patients choosing radioactive iodine therapy as their treatment option need both instruction and reassurance regarding the benefits of this therapy, as well as any information about radiation pre-

cautions that must be taken during the first few days after therapy is initiated. Specific instructions will be provided to patients by the health care provider or the radiology staff but generally patients will be instructed to avoid close contact with other persons for a period of days. Patients with small children will need to arrange alternative care during this period. Patients should use a private toilet and be instructed to flush two times after each use. They should not be involved in handling food preparation for others and should launder towels and linens they use separately from others. Use of disposable eating utensils and plates is suggested (AACE, 2005c).

   Patients will need to know the signs and symptoms of hypothyroidism because radioactive iodine treatment is likely to result in hypothyroidism over a period of several weeks to months. Written instructions regarding signs of hypothyroidism and the need for regular evaluation of thyroid function should be given to the patient at discharge. In addition, it is essential to stress the importance of continuous hormone replacement in the event of hypothyroidism since inadequate thyroid hormone replacement increases the risk of hyperlipidemia and increased heart disease (Franklin, Sheppard, & Maisonneuve, 2005).

If surgical intervention is planned in the case of hyperthyroidism, the nurse prepares the patient for surgery and provides immediate postoperative care. Surgical intervention may include a subtotal thyroidectomy, a partial resection, or removal of the thyroid gland. Postoperatively the nurse should pay particular atten-tion to the patient's airway, because hemorrhage and swelling may compromise respiratory status. It is advisable to have emergency supplies such as a tracheostomy tray available at the bedside or close by on an emergency response cart. Accidental removal of the parathyroids is also a potential risk, thus intravenous calcium also should be available if needed. The critical response team should be alerted as early as possible should there be indications that the patient will need rapid intervention. The patient care plan for patients with hyperthyroidism is shown in the Nursing Process: Patient Care Plan for Hyperthyroidism. Chart 52–5 (p. 1631) shows life-threatening conditions related to thyroid disease.

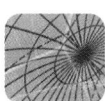 **NURSING PROCESS: Patient Care Plan for Hyperthyroidism**

Assessment of Cognition Level

Subjective Data:
What medications have you been taking?
Does your family have a history of any particular disease(s)?
Has your weight changed during the past year?
Is there unexplained change in body weight?
Do you feel anxious, nervous, or restless?
Have you noticed any insensitivity to changes in room temperature?
Are you "wound up" or "feeling like you are in overdrive"?
How much exercise are you getting?
Are you experiencing any muscle weakness?
Is there anything affecting your ability to be active?

Objective Data:
Skin warm and diaphoretic
Hair loss
Agitation, hand tremors
Enlarged thyroid, exophthalmos of the eyes
Hyperthermia Tachypnea, Tachycardia (heart rate >100 beats/min)
Hyperreflexia
Elevated serum T_3, T_4

Nursing Assessment and Diagnoses	Outcomes and Evaluation Parameters	Planning and Interventions with *Rationales*
Nursing Diagnosis: *Anxiety* and restlessness, fine hand tremors, and insomnia secondary to hypermetabolism	**Outcome:** Patient expresses relief from symptoms of excess thyroid hormone. *Evaluation Parameters:* Patient reports less anxiety and restful sleep through the night. Patient's tremors and blood levels of free T_3 and free T_4 decrease and stabilize. Patient is comfortable in an environment with a normal range in ambient temperature. Patient's vital signs are within normal range.	**Interventions and *Rationales:*** Decrease environmental stimuli and promote a restful environment. Eliminate chemical stimulants such as caffeine from diet. Administer antithyroid drugs as prescribed. *To eliminate stimulants that will exacerbate sleep deprivation and anxiety.*

Assessment of Understanding of Disorder

Subjective Data:
Have you lost or gained weight during the past year?
Did you take any specific steps to cause this change in your weight?
Describe your appetite for me.
How do you feel most of the time: anxious? calm?

Objective Data:
Patient underweight for height
Clothing too large for size/frame

Nursing Assessment and Diagnoses	Outcomes and Evaluation Parameters	Planning and Interventions with *Rationales*
Nursing Diagnosis: *Imbalanced Nutrition* secondary to anxiety, restlessness, and hypermetabolic state	**Outcomes:** Patient regains normal weight and reports resumption of appetite. Patient can describe symptoms of hypo- and hyperthyroidism. *Evaluation Parameters:* Patient's weight is maintained or returned to normal. Nutritional deficiencies eliminated. Patient reports appetite and intake are satisfactory. Patient able to describe symptoms of hypo- and hyperthyroidism.	**Interventions and *Rationales:*** Monitor weight daily. Offer patient a well-balanced diet with nutritional supplements and nutritional consultation as needed. Teach patient about effects of hypo- and hyperthyroidism on weight. *To ensure patient regains health and lost weight if desirable and to enable patient to report early signs of change in metabolic state that might indicate a need for further medical intervention.*

(continued)

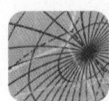

NURSING PROCESS: Patient Care Plan for Hyperthyroidism—*Continued*

Assessment of Ocular Characteristics and Function

Subjective Data:
Have you noticed any facial changes, swelling, redness, or protrusion of the eyes?

Objective Data:
Eyes appear dry and reddened
Eyes protrude (exophthalmos)
Patient unable to close eyelids completely
Visible sclera

Nursing Assessment and Diagnoses	Outcomes and Evaluation Parameters	Planning and Interventions with *Rationales*
Nursing Diagnosis: *Risk for Injury* to eyes secondary to exophthalmos and inability to close eyelids completely	**Outcome:** Eyes are moist and patient reports no eye pain or discomfort. *Evaluation Parameter:* No evidence of eye damage or corneal ulceration or abrasion.	**Interventions and *Rationales:*** Encourage patient to flush eyes with warm water at intervals while awake, to use artificial tears to keep eyes moist, and to cover eyes while sleeping and as needed if patient is unable to close eyes completely. *To keep eyes moist and to prevent corneal ulceration or abrasion.*

Assessment of Cardiac Function

Subjective Data:
Have you noticed any change in your pulse or heart rate?
Have you experienced any chest pain recently?
Have you observed any swelling in your feet?
What is your energy level?

Objective Data:
Tachycardia with heart rate >100 beats/min
Atrial fibrillation
Edema
Cardiac enlargement
Chest pain

Nursing Assessment and Diagnoses	Outcomes and Evaluation Parameters	Planning and Interventions with *Rationales*
Nursing Diagnosis: *Decreased Cardiac Output* related to hypermetabolic state	**Outcomes:** Cardiac function within normal limits. Patient free from symptoms of pulmonary edema and heart failure. *Evaluation Parameters:* Assessment reveals that heart rate has decreased and stroke volume has increased. No dyspnea present. No coughing and wheezing present. Tissues free from edema. Patient verbalizes feeling less tired and free of anxiety. Patient expresses having an appetite. Patient oriented to time, place, and person. No evidence of pink frothy sputum.	**Interventions and *Rationales:*** Evaluate vital signs frequently. Administer antithyroid and cardiac medications as prescribed. Maintain a restful, calm supportive environment. Assess toleration of physical activity and work with patient to gradually increase activity as tolerated. *To reduce risk of congestive heart failure in patients with a hypermetabolic state.*

CRITICAL ALERT

- *Following a thyroidectomy, it is essential that during the immediate postoperative period, the patient be observed closely for signs of hemorrhage or swelling in the operative site, as well as damage to the vocal cords or parathyroid glands. Check behind the neck for signs of pooling blood.*

- *The postop patient should be readily observable by the nurse and have a call bell in order to get immediate attention should symptoms of respiratory distress be noted. The location of the thyroid gland in proximity to the trachea and vocal cords also presents a threat to the airway, should swelling or hemorrhage cause obstruction. A tracheostomy set should be readily available in case of this emergency.*

- *In the event of accidental removal of part or all of the parathyroid glands, intravenous calcium should also be readily available.*

Discharge Priorities

Discharge priorities with thyroid disease include patient education about thyroid functioning, particularly symptoms of both hypothyroid disease and hyperthyroid disease since treatments for either condition may result in the opposite condition. Patients need to understand that they should receive regular follow-up laboratory work to assess thyroid function since treatments for hyperthyroidism, including antithyroid drugs, radioactive iodine, and surgery, may result in a significant decrease or cessation in thyroid hormone production over time. On the other hand, administration of levothyroxine in dosages that are too high may lead to symptoms of hyperthyroidism. Patients need careful instruction about the need for follow-up after treatment for thyroid disorders until there is evidence that hormone levels are normal and have stabilized. Certain vulnerable patients with hyperthyroidism or hypothyroidism should be instructed to avoid additional stress or infections until their disease is under control. Postsurgical patients should receive instruction about wound care and signs and symptoms of infection that should be reported immediately to the health care provider. Hyperthy-

CHART 52–5	Life-Threatening Complications of Thyroid Disorders	
	Hypothyroidism Myxedema Coma	**Hyperthyroidism Thyroid Crisis/Storm**
Life-Threatening Conditions	Myxedema coma occurs when a precipitating event such as trauma, infection, or sedation compromises the *hypothyroid* patient (usually older adults with long-standing primary thyroid disease).	Acute thyrotoxicosis/thyroid crisis/thyroid storm occurs when there is failure of the compensatory metabolic, thermoregulatory, and cardiovascular systems in the *hyperthyroid* patient.
Early Symptoms	Weight gain, extreme fatigue or lack of energy, bradycardia, lethargy, mental dullness, memory impairment, cold intolerance.	Significant unexplained weight loss, warm, moist skin, heat intolerance, cardiac palpitations and tachycardia. Tachypnea and dyspnea on exertion.
Signs or Symptoms of Serious Complications	Very low body temperature (32.8°–35°C [91°–95°F]) Skin very cool and dry Seizures, severe bradycardia, delayed deep tendon reflexes Nonpitting edema (particularly around face and eyes), enlarged tongue, decreased awareness and loss of consciousness Profound mood disturbance and psychosis may occur	Tachycardia (greater than 140 beats/min), atrial fibrillation, arrhythmias, increased stroke volume, symptoms of high output heart failure with pulmonary edema. Very high body temperature (up to 40°C [105°F]) restlessness, agitation, abdominal pain, nausea, vomiting, coma, emotional lability, exophthalmos, goiter, and coma.
Laboratory Values	Low TSH (if the pituitary is involved) and very high TSH (if the thyroid gland is the affected tissue) Low serum FT_4 Hyponatremia, hypoglycemia, hyperlipidemia Respiratory acidosis ECG: prolonged QT intervals Pleural and pericardial effusions Presence of antithyroid antibodies	Low level of TSH High serum FT_4 Elevated liver function tests Elevated alkaline phosphatase
Assessment	Vital signs, level of consciousness, lab work	Body temperature, blood glucose levels
Treatment	Hormone replacement therapy	Antithyroid drugs Surgery

Sources: Adapted from Greco, L. K. (2001). Hypothyroid emergencies. *Topics in Emergency Medicine, 23*(4), 44–50; Dahlen, R. (2002). Managing patients with acute thyrotoxicosis. *Critical Care Nurse, 22*(1), 62–69; Holcomb, S. (2003). Detecting thyroid disease, Part 1. *Nursing, 33*(8), 32cc1–32cc4; Waltman, P. A., Brewer, J. M., & Lobert, S. (2004). Thyroid storm during pregnancy: A medical emergency. *Critical Care Nursing, 24*(2), 74–79.

roidism in the elderly population is addressed in the Gerontological Considerations box.

Health Promotion

Optimal health in terms of endocrine function requires a healthy diet, including a reliable source of iodine for the production of thyroid hormone. Patients should be encouraged to plan a healthy diet that includes fish and foods supplemented with iodine such as iodized salt. Health promotion for patients with thyroid disorders requires careful attention to prescribed medications such as

hormone replacement therapy or antithyroid drugs. Symptoms of the hypo- or hypermetabolic state will reoccur if appropriate hormonal levels are not maintained. Patients may be advised to avoid additional stress when experiencing acute thyroid disease until such time as their condition stabilizes. For more on hyperthyroidism in certain populations, see the Cultural Considerations and Genetic Considerations boxes.

GERONTOLOGICAL CONSIDERATIONS Related to Hyperthyroidism

Hyperthyroidism is more common among the 30- to 50-year-old age group, whereas hypothyroidism is a more common problem in patients over age 50. Elderly patients are most vulnerable to serious complications from either hypothyroidism or hyperthyroidism. Diagnosis may be difficult until metabolic function is significantly altered due to the insidious nature of the disease. Infection, trauma, surgery, and stress may precipitate a serious crisis in elderly patients with hypo- or hypermetabolic diseases of the thyroid. Use of medications such as sedatives or opiates also may put these patients at great risk. The nurse must consider the potential for myxedema coma or thyroid crisis in elderly patients and those made more vulnerable due to coexisting illness or stress.

CULTURAL CONSIDERATIONS for Hyperthyroidism

Patients with thyroid disorders may have to take long-term drug therapy or lifelong hormone replacement therapy. Chronic illness is not well accepted in some cultures and poor understanding of the outcomes of rejecting medical therapy may lead to life-threatening consequences. The nurse will need to assess patient and family acceptance and understanding of the disease in order to tailor patient instruction and support appropriately.

GENETIC CONSIDERATIONS for Hyperthyroidism

Researchers know that there is a genetic predisposition to thyroid disease, although the exact genetic problem has not yet been identified. Parents affected by thyroid disease should be advised to share that information with their children so that they are alerted to potential health problems in the future.

Complementary and Alternative Approaches

Patients with thyroid disease may find complementary care such as meditation, massage therapy, and acupuncture to be beneficial in balancing the immune system and in improving one's sense of well-being. However, herbal therapies should be used with extreme caution at this time and only with consultation with the patient's primary care physician, given the potential for drug interactions. Overall, complementary and alternative therapy should not be seen as a replacement for traditional medical therapy in thyroid disease. For more about one type of complementary therapy, aromatherapy, see the Complementary and Alternative Therapies box.

Collaborative Management

As noted when discussing collaborative management of patients with hypothyroidism, patients with hyperthyroidism also will need the support of several members of the health care team. The pharmacist has a role in instruction of hyperthyroid patients who may have to take antithyroid drugs and beta-blockers or calcium channel blockers if they have cardiac symptoms. A radiologist specializing in radiation therapy may administer radioactive io-

dine, which is the preferred treatment for hyperthyroidism. In some cases, the patient with hyperthyroidism may be referred to a surgeon for surgical removal of the thyroid gland if the patient is not a candidate for radioactive iodine therapy or if surgery is needed to remove a large goiter or malignant nodule. The nutritionist also can provide helpful consultation on diet to address the hypermetabolic needs of the patient's body while therapy corrects and stabilizes thyroid hormones.

Disorders of the Parathyroid Gland

The parathyroid glands are four small, highly vascular glands located behind the thyroid gland (Figure 52–5 ▪). Anatomic variation in the number and location of parathyroid glands occurs with some frequency. Approximately the size of a grain of rice, the parathyroid glands regulate the blood calcium level within a very narrow range (8.5 to 10.5 mg/dL) to maintain the effective functioning of the body's muscles and nerves. Calcium-sensing receptors in the parathyroid glands are stimulated to release parathyroid hormone into the blood when serum calcium levels

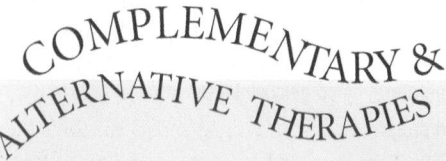

COMPLEMENTARY & ALTERNATIVE THERAPIES Aromatherapy

Description:
Aromatherapy literally means using a scent (aroma) as healing therapy. The products used in aromatherapy are made from herbs and flowers that have been reduced to their aromatic essence. These aromatic essences are then combined with a "carrier oil" such as almond oil, and either applied to small areas of the skin or inhaled. These products are then used as an inhalant. Aromatherapy may be either self-administered, or administered by aromatherapy practitioners (aromatherapists) who are trained in the use of the inhalant, including its indication, quality and dose, and the length of time the patient should use the inhalant. Aromatherapy is often used to treat conditions such as dysmenorrhea, stress, and insomnia—all of which can be related to glandular and hormonal problems.

Research Support:
One randomized placebo-controlled trial explored the effect of aromatherapy with lavender, clary sage, and rose on dysmenorrhea symptoms. The trial involved 67 female college students whose primary dysmenorrhea symptoms were menstrual cramps. Participants rated their menstrual cramps as greater than 6 on a 10-point visual analogue scale. Participants had no systemic or reproductive diseases and were not taking contraceptive drugs. Three groups of participants were randomized: an experimental group who received aromatherapy, a placebo group, and a control group. The aromatherapy procedure involved applying two drops of lavender (*Lavandula officinalis*), one drop of clary sage (*Salvia sclarea*), and one drop of rose (*Rosa centifolia*) in 5 mL of almond oil to the abdomen. In the placebo group, the same treatment was used but only with almond oil. The control group received no treatment. Participants rated their menstrual cramp levels with a visual analogue scale. The aromatherapy group showed significantly improved menstrual cramps than the placebo and control groups at both post-test time points (first and second day of menstruation after treatment). Researchers concluded that the topical application of aromatherapy with lavender, clary sage, and rose is an effective

part of nursing care to women experiencing dysmenorrhea (Han, Hur, Buckle, Choi, & Lee, 2006).

Another study examined the use of aromatherapy with lavender to improve mild insomnia. This small, single-blind, randomized pilot study involved 10 participants (5 males and 5 females). Participants inhaled lavender using an Aromastream® electric diffuser over the course of the 4-week trial. Researchers measured outcomes using the Pittsburgh Sleep Quality Index. Results showed that aromatherapy with lavender created an improvement of insomnia. Women and younger volunteers with a milder insomnia experienced the largest improvement. Researchers concluded that, although a larger trial is needed to draw definitive conclusions, outcomes favor aromatherapy with lavender for mild insomnia (Lewith, Godfrey, & Prescott, 2005).

Cortisol is known as the "stress hormone." A third study examined the use of aromatherapy with lavender and rosemary on cortisol levels. Participants included 22 healthy volunteers who inhaled the lavender and rosemary aromas for 5 minutes. Then, saliva samples were collected from each participant and cortisol levels were tested. Results showed that lavender and rosemary decrease cortisol (Atsumi & Tonosaki, 2007).

References
Atsumi, T., & Tonosaki, K. (2007, February 28). Smelling lavender and rosemary increases free radical scavenging activity and decreases cortisol level in saliva. *Psychiatry Research, 150*(1), 89–96.
Han, S. H., Hur, M. H., Buckle, J., Choi, J., & Lee, M. S. (2006, July-August). Effect of aromatherapy on symptoms of dysmenorrhea in college students: A randomized placebo-controlled clinical trial. *Journal of Alternative and Complementary Medicine, 12*(6), 535–541.
Lewith, G. T., Godfrey, A. D., & Prescott, P. (2005, August). A single-blinded, randomized pilot study evaluating the aroma of Lavandula augustifolia as a treatment for mild insomnia. *Journal of Alternative and Complementary Medicine, 11*(4), 631–637.

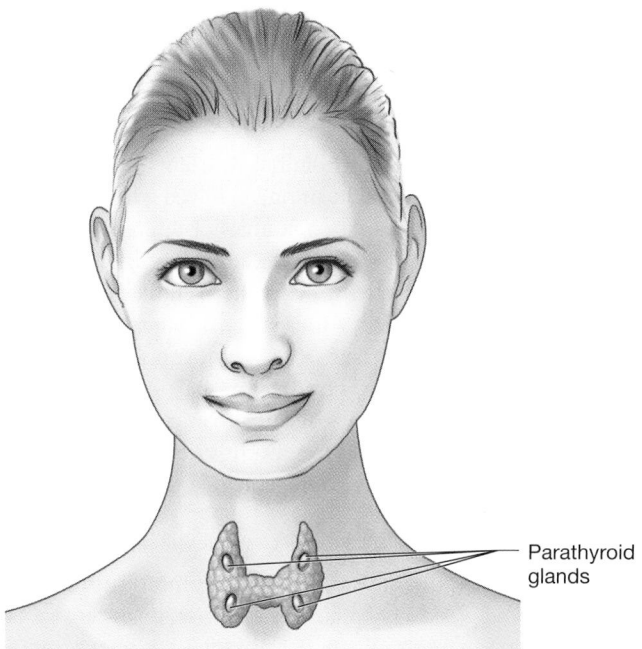

FIGURE 52–5 ■ The parathyroid glands.

drop below a normative level. Parathyroid hormone (PTH) is a small protein that acts directly on both the bone and kidneys where it stimulates release and reabsorption of calcium. It also acts indirectly on the intestines, causing them to reabsorb calcium. Thus PTH contributes to the finely tuned homeostasis of calcium in the body (Braunwald et al., 2001).

As is true with the other endocrine glands, disorders of the parathyroid gland include **hypoparathyroidism**, in which there is inadequate secretion of parathyroid hormone, and **hyperparathyroidism**, in which there is excessive secretion of PTH. Both conditions are rare, frequently missed for long periods because of vague symptoms, and may be identified through routine laboratory testing for other conditions. Genetics may play a role in parathyroid disorders, as discussed in the Genetic Considerations for Parathyroid Disorders box.

■ Hypoparathyroidism

Hypoparathyroidism is a rare condition that occurs when the parathyroid glands do not make enough parathyroid hormone.

Parathyroid hormone helps regulate the levels of calcium and phosphorus in the blood.

Epidemiology and Etiology

When a deficient amount of PTH is produced, hypocalcemia (lower than normal levels of calcium in the blood) results, and there is too little phosphorus in the blood. This syndrome typically results from iatrogenic causes or is one of many rare diseases (Gonzalez-Campoy, 2007). Hypoparathyroidism may be either inherited or acquired (from injury to the glands or, more rarely, from surgery on the thyroid gland).

Pathophysiology

Patients with primary hypoparathyroidism have a low level of serum calcium with a high level of phosphorus in the absence of renal failure or tissue trauma. Pseudohypoparathyroidism (PHP), a hereditary syndrome that becomes apparent in adolescence, involves target tissues that are unresponsive to PTH, causing symptoms like those of hypoparathyroidism (Braunwald et al., 2001). Acquired hypoparathyroidism may occur due to complications from thyroid or neck surgery, but this is seen infrequently because surgical techniques have improved.

When other factors are at play in the cause of hypoparathyroidism, PTH may simply be ineffective (as with renal failure) or overwhelmed (due to severe hyperphosphatemia). Medications, severe trauma, sepsis, and acute pancreatitis are all factors that can cause acute, transient hypocalcemia but may be short term and not require treatment. Chronic hypocalcemia on the other hand, caused by hereditary hypoparathyroid disease, typically becomes symptomatic and does require intervention. See the Risk Factors for Hypoparathyroidism box.

Clinical Manifestations

Typically, hypoparathyroid patients complain about weakness; muscle cramps, particularly of wrists and feet; abnormal paresthesias with tingling, numbness, and burning of hands; excessive nervousness; loss of memory; and headaches. Nerve excitability, triggered by low blood calcium, causes continuous nerve impulses, which stimulate nerve contraction.

Other symptoms may include malformations of the teeth and fingernails, spasms of facial muscles (**Chvostek's sign**), and contraction of carpal muscles with mild compression of the nerves (**Trousseau's sign**)(Urbano, 2000). Chvostek's sign can be induced by tapping on the inferior margin of the zygoma, which

GENETIC CONSIDERATIONS for Parathyroid Disorders

Research is shedding new light on the genetic variations associated with parathyroid disease. At present, this information is useful primarily in diagnosis of new cases of the disease. Genetic counseling is advisable for families with hereditary parathyroid disease but patients may be reluctant to initiate this step if hereditary conditions are considered to be shameful or something to be hidden due to poor cultural acceptance. Families may become more open to genetic counseling with appropriate information about the benefits of this service.

RISK FACTORS for Hypoparathyroidism

Risk factors for hypoparathyroidism include family history and heredity, neck surgery, or the presence of other disease. The precise cause is unknown except in those cases where the parathyroid glands have been removed. The disease may occur singularly or concomitantly with other endocrine disorders. Hypoparathyroidism affects both genders equally, and generally is seen in children under age 16 and adults over age 40. Symptoms of hypocalcemia in older persons should be explored fully because these are more likely due to nutritional deficiencies, renal failure, intestinal disorders, or neck surgery than to primary hypoparathyroidism (Braunwald et al., 2001).

will cause facial spasms, and Trousseau's sign can be elicited by inflating the blood pressure cuff and maintaining the cuff pressure above systolic, which will produce carpal spasms if the serum calcium level is low. Transient cases of hypocalcemia occur due to trauma, burns, medications, and a variety of serious illnesses, and these must be differentiated from true hypoparathyroidism because transient symptoms require little intervention, whereas chronic hypoparathyroidism requires lifetime treatment.

Laboratory and Diagnostic Procedures

Diagnosis begins with a careful history including attention to nutritional history and calcium intake, a history of hereditary disease, the presence of other endocrine disorders, duration of illness, clinical signs and symptoms, renal failure, and an analysis of medications the patient is taking. Diagnostic tests, in addition to serum calcium and phosphatase, include PTH immunoassay and tests for vitamin D metabolites. In primary hypoparathyroidism, the level of PTH is low in spite of low levels of serum calcium.

Medical Management

Treatment of hypoparathyroidism is managed with supplementation of calcium, calcitriol (an active form of an artificial vitamin D), and high doses of oral vitamin D daily. Two or 3 grams of calcium are given daily to patients with primary hypoparathyroidism.

 # Nursing Management

Nursing care for patients with hypoparathyroidism is directed at hormone replacement, symptom management, and support of patient self-care. Because primary disease lasts a lifetime, patients require thorough explanations about their condition and long-term treatment. Instruction on calcium and vitamin D supplements and their role in disease management should begin early after diagnosis. Patients also may find support from patient networks established by others who have the same disease, such as the Hypoparathyroid Association; thus a nursing referral to community groups is suggested. The Gerontological Considerations box gives more information about the effects of hypoparathyroidism on elderly patients.

Discharge Priorities

Discharge priorities for patients with parathyroid disease are focused on compliance with the prescribed medication regime and safety related to falls and fracture prevention. Follow-up home visits are warranted to assess how the patient has modified

---

> ### GERONTOLOGICAL CONSIDERATIONS Related to Hypoparathyroidism
>
> Older patients are particularly vulnerable to bone fractures, so the condition of hypoparathyroidism must be carefully managed as adults age. Careful attention to nutrition, with a high intake of calcium and vitamin D is important. Compliance with the medical regime, which includes high doses of oral calcium, calcitriol, and vitamin D, may be difficult but is essential in the elderly. The nurse will want to initiate a fall prevention program to decrease the risk of fractures. Patients should be encouraged to do a careful analysis of their home environment to remove throw rugs or other items that might put them at risk for a fall.

the environment to enhance safety and to determine whether the patient needs further support in compliance with prescribed calcium and vitamin D supplementation.

Health Promotion

Vitamin D and calcium are essential nutrients in the human diet. Vitamin D is actually a hormone involved with the metabolism of bone and other tissues. Sources of vitamin D include both diet and exposure to sunlight because vitamin D is synthesized by the skin. Patients living in northern climates are susceptible to vitamin D deficiency for several months out the year during which daylight hours are short. Thus supplementation of the diet with vitamin D may be advisable, particularly for those with lower than desirable levels of calcium and those considered to be vulnerable to bone fractures. Daily, brief periods of exposure to sunlight should be encouraged when this is feasible.

Hyperparathyroidism

Primary hyperparathyroidism, the most common problem of the parathyroid glands, is a relatively common disorder that occurs when one or more of the parathyroid glands oversecrete parathyroid hormone.

Epidemiology and Etiology

The incidence of hyperparathyroidism is 1 in 500 to 1,000, and it tends to occur in those over age 50 and in women more than men (Tangiera, 2004). Secondary hyperparathyroidism occurs when another medical condition causes the parathyroid glands to produce too much PTH in response to chronically low levels of circulating calcium. Kidney failure, malabsorption problems, and rickets, a disease caused by severe vitamin D deficiency, are the main causes of this type of hyperparathyroidism.

Physiology and Risk Factors

Hyperparathyroidism results in excessive PTH, leading to hypercalcemia, an excessive level of calcium, and hypophosphatemia, a low level of phosphatase, in the blood. Primary hyperparathyroidism is most commonly caused by a benign tumor, an adenoma, or hyperplasia in one or more of the parathyroid glands. Cancer is the cause of hyperparathyroidism in less than 1% of cases. When one parathyroid gland oversecretes PTH, the other glands will become dormant, responding to the high levels of calcium in the blood (Porth, 2007). Symptoms may be mild or severe depending on the size and impact of the tumor. Hyperparathyroidism may cause **osteitis fibrosa cystica**, a complication in which bone softens and becomes deformed or forms cysts. Secondary hyperparathyroidism may be due to rickets, vitamin D deficiency, or chronic renal failure (Gonzales-Campoy, 2007). Hypercalcemia also may develop secondary to malignancies in the body, in which parathyroid hormone-related peptide is released by tumor cells. This results in a syndrome that mimics hyperparathyroidism (Braunwald et al., 2001).

Primary hyperparathyroidism is rare but more common in middle-aged and older women. Evidence suggests that there is a genetic factor in its development. Neck radiation increases the incidence of the disease.

Clinical Manifestations

Patients with hyperparathyroidism may present with symptoms of bone tenderness, bone cysts, or polyuria due to excretion of high levels of calcium. In severe cases of the disease, the bones may lose significant calcium, seriously affecting bone density, and become brittle, with overt signs of osteopenia (mild loss of bone density) and osteoporosis (moderate to severe loss of bone density resulting in "brittle bones"). This may lead to susceptibility to bone fractures, a particular problem for older patients. High levels of calcium in the blood also may cause inflammation of the gastric lining and the pancreas, leading to a higher risk for ulcers and acute pancreatitis. Kidney stones, caused by high blood levels of calcium and the constant effort of the kidneys to excrete excess calcium, are another potential problem for patients with hyperparathyroidism. Parathyroid pathology often produces vague symptoms over a long period and may simply be discovered in laboratory blood work associated with routine physical examinations.

Laboratory and Diagnostic Procedures

A diagnosis of hyperparathyroidism is most accurately determined with tests of the parathyroid hormone, serum calcium, and alkaline phosphatase levels. In hyperparathyroidism, the blood parathyroid hormone level and the serum calcium level will be elevated and the alkaline phosphatase level will be abnormally low.

Medical Management

At one time invasive surgery under general anesthesia was required to remove a diseased parathyroid tumor. Locating the diseased parathyroid gland could be a problem because of its small size as well as the fact that the gland may have migrated to another location during fetal development. Such surgeries always carried the risk of hemorrhage, as well as damage to the vocal cords. Today, expert surgeons can remove the diseased parathyroid gland under local anesthesia by doing a minimally invasive, radioguided parathyroidectomy. Radioactive tracers facilitate faster and safer surgical intervention. Function of the hyperparathyroid glands can be assessed during surgery using radioactive ratios or PTH assays.

In cases of secondary hyperparathyroidism, the objective is to treat the underlying cause, although chronic kidney failure is the most common etiologic factor (Gonzalez-Campoy, 2007). Damaged kidneys cannot convert vitamin D to the active form, so an active form of vitamin D is used to reduce the production of PTH. After many years, vitamin D treatment can lose its effectiveness in some people, and excessively high levels of both calcium and phosphorus may occur. The drug cinacalcet (Sensipar) can reduce PTH levels, which lowers the chance of this occurring.

A new drug, paricalcitol (Zemplar), has recently been approved for administration orally as well as by injection during hemodialysis therapy. Dosage is determined by serum plasma parathyroid hormone levels, which are tested, along with serum calcium and serum phosphorus, at 2-week intervals for the first 3 months, then monthly for 3 months. Once it has been determined that the patient is stable, testing can be reduced to a quarterly schedule. Patients taking this drug should avoid medications that include large amounts of aluminum such as Maalox, Mylanta, Gaviscon, and Amphojel (Pavlovich-Danis, 2006).

■ Nursing Management

Nursing management for the patient with hyperparathyroidism is focused on patient teaching about the disease, preparation and follow-up for surgical intervention, and instruction about medications and the need for laboratory studies for regular follow-up. Because minimally invasive surgery is the intervention of choice, the patient will be discharged quickly. Thus discharge planning and postoperative instructions should include instruction on dressing changes and follow-up medical visits with regular evaluation of serum calcium levels. If the glands have been completely removed, patient instruction prior to discharge should include information about foods that are good sources of calcium such as milk and other dairy products, tofu, broccoli, kale, mustard greens, oysters, salmon, and sardines.

If the patient and health care provider choose long-term follow-up for milder cases of the disease, the patient should drink lots of water, get plenty of exercise, and avoid diuretics, such as those in the thiazide classification. Immobilization and gastrointestinal illness with vomiting or diarrhea can cause calcium levels to rise. If these conditions develop, patients with hyperparathyroidism should seek medical attention.

Discharge Priorities

Discharge priorities include patient instruction on postsurgical care including observation of the operative site and dressing changes as indicated by the health care provider. The importance of follow-up with laboratory studies to monitor serum calcium levels should be stressed in concert with follow-up visits with the surgeon and endocrinologist.

Surgical removal of the affected gland provides relief of major symptoms and problems related to hypercalcemia. Close follow-up of patients is warranted to ensure that serum levels of calcium are maintained within recommended ranges.

Health Promotion

Following surgery, patients should feel a significant improvement in their health status. With return to normal or near-normal parathyroid functioning, patients should maintain a healthy diet with good sources of calcium and vitamin D essential for a healthy musculoskeletal system. As noted earlier, optimal synthesis of vitamin D in the body warrants at least brief exposure to sunlight daily. Outdoor activity, such as walking, would be beneficial to patients and accomplish both their need for vitamin D synthesis and cardiovascular benefits.

■ Collaborative Management of Parathyroid Disorders

Patients with parathyroid disorders can benefit from care provided by a wide array of health care providers, including the pharmacist, the nutritionist, the endocrinologist, and the genetic counselor, as well as the nurse. Parathyroid problems are rare and typically should be dealt with by an endocrinologist and highly trained surgeons who have experience working with the parathyroid glands. The pharmacist will provide essential information on drug therapies and vitamin and mineral supplementation, not only to the patient but to members of the health care team.

Complementary Care Related to Parathyroid Disorders

Complementary therapies may aid the patient's overall sense of well-being and should be encouraged for this reason. However, such therapies do not substitute for traditional Western medical therapies such as surgery for hyperparathyroidism or calcium and vitamin supplementation for hypoparathyroidism.

Symptom management is very important for patient comfort and well-being. Complementary therapies may be particularly useful in the management of parathyroid disease symptoms, such as fatigue, myalgia, and paresthesias. Acupuncture has been found to ease the symptoms of hyperthyroidism, and may be useful if used alongside traditional medical techniques. Aromatherapy also is considered helpful. Substances such as clove or myrtle are recommended for problems of the thyroid, and they can be made up into oils that are burned. The vapors can then be inhaled or used as bath oils or lotions. In addition, reducing stress and improving the body's immune response are desired outcomes because it may take several months for the body to respond to traditional therapy and for hormone levels to return to normal.

Disorders of the Hypothalamus and Pituitary Glands

Although the pituitary gland is often referred to as the "master" gland because it is responsible for cellular homeostasis and growth, the pituitary gland is so anatomically and physiologically connected with the hypothalamus that it is really the integrated functioning of these glands that affects most of the body's physiological processes. For this reason, this section provides a brief overview of the integrated functioning of these two glands, followed by common disorders that nurses may see in clinical practice.

Diseases of the hypothalamus and pituitary glands may become apparent early or late in life and include conditions caused by insufficient production and overproduction of hormones. As is true for many endocrine disorders, signs and symptoms of hypothalamic or pituitary disease may be subtle and insidious, leading to delayed or missed diagnosis.

Physiological Integration of the Hypothalamus and Pituitary Glands

Located in the middle of the base of the brain, the hypothalamus encapsulates the ventral portion of the third ventricle. The pituitary gland lies immediately beneath the hypothalamus, lying in a depression of the sphenoid bone of the skull called the sella turcica (Figure 52–6 ■). The pituitary is composed of two structures, the anterior pituitary, or adenohypophysis, and the posterior pituitary, called the neurohypophysis. Hormones produced by the hypothalamus control secretions of the anterior pituitary through a rich and direct vascular network that enables the pituitary to respond to miniscule amounts of concentrated hypothalamic hormone. The posterior pituitary, which is more of an extension of the hypothalamus, is composed of neurological cells and tissues (Dorton, 2000; Porth, 2007).

The hypothalamus produces a variety of releasing hormones that stimulate the production of other hormones by the pituitary gland. Secretion of the releasing hormones in the hypothalamus is affected by the perceived level of circulating pituitary hormones. When the level of a circulating pituitary hormone falls, the hypothalamus increases production of a releasing hormone, stimulating hormone production by the pituitary in what is called a

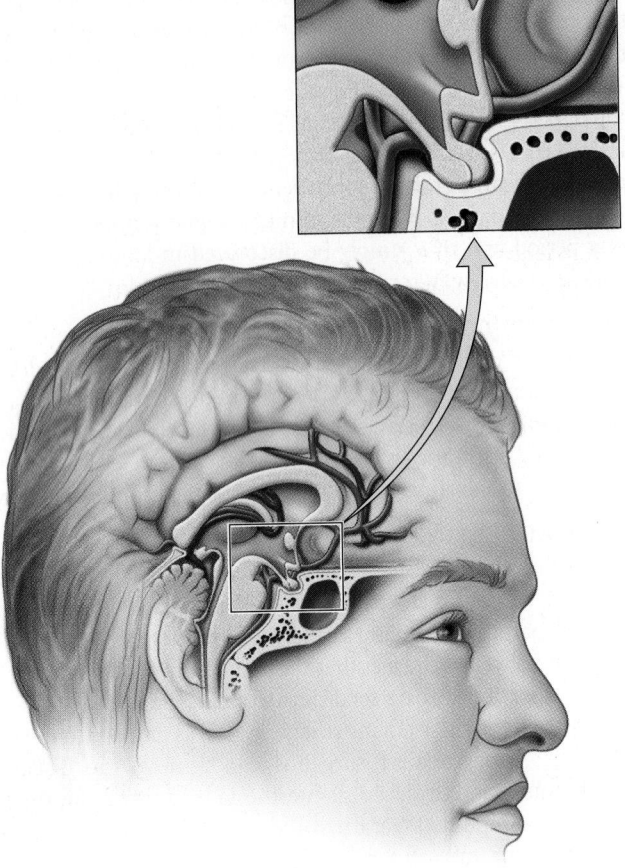

The pituitary secretes hormones that are essential to growth and reproduction

FIGURE 52–6 ■ The pituitary gland.

negative feedback system. Releasing hormones secreted by the hypothalamus include thyrotropin-releasing hormone (TRH), gonadotropin-releasing hormone (GnRH), growth hormone-releasing hormone (GHRH), corticotropin-releasing hormone (CRH), and somatostatin and dopamine. Should the hypothalamus be unable to produce one or more of the releasing hormones or should disease cause overproduction of a releasing hormone, pituitary gland functioning would be altered, leading to symptoms of pituitary dysfunction.

Hypothalamic Disorders

Disorders of the hypothalamus, as well as the pituitary, result from birth defects, genetic abnormalities, trauma (including hemorrhage), neoplasms, vascular disruptions, inflammatory disorders, infiltrative disease (such as tuberculosis), or radiation exposure.

Symptoms usually occur because of failure of the pituitary gland to secrete tropic hormones due to suppression of hypothalamic-releasing hormones. Thus, treatment is generally sought by patients because of metabolic problems related to an underproduction or overproduction of pituitary hormones. A key role for the health care provider is to determine whether the etiology of the endocrine problem is one related to the hypothalamus or the pituitary gland. In some cases, both glands may be affected by the disease process. Although there are a few, very rare genetic disorders and birth defects of the hypothalamus, most nurses will not see these in the clinical setting, thus the focus of this section is on common pituitary disorders that result from an excess or a deficit of the pituitary tropic hormones.

Hypometabolic Disorders of the Anterior Pituitary Gland: Hypopituitarism

Pituitary disorders result in inadequate secretion of one or more pituitary hormones. **Hypopituitarism** is a term used to describe the inadequate secretion of some of the hormones produced by the anterior pituitary gland, whereas **panhypopituitarism** is a term used to describe a disorder in which there is inadequate secretion of all of the anterior pituitary hormones. The pituitary hormones are shown in Chart 52–6.

Epidemiology and Etiology

The most common cause of pituitary disorders is pituitary tumors, which are described as secretory and nonsecretory. Secretory tumors cause problems with excessive secretion of one or more hormones. Nonsecretory, endocrine-inactive, or null tumors, as they are sometimes described, do not produce hormones but may create problems of hyposecretion of hormones if size and mass of the tumor impairs normal pituitary functioning (Pituitary Network Association [PNA], 2006b). A high percentage of hypopituitary disorders are due to pituitary adenomas. Acute pituitary insufficiency may also occur after severe postpartum hemorrhage in a syndrome called Sheehan's syndrome or infarction of a pituitary tumor (Kattah, 2006; Mayo Clinic, 2006). Congenital malformation, exposure to radiation or chemicals, and other unknown factors may also cause pituitary dysfunction.

In the United States, the prevalence of pituitary adenomas is high (10% to 20%); however, the actual presence of clinical disease is quite uncommon. Approximately 2 to 6 in 100,000 persons per year present with symptoms attributed to pituitary tumors (PNA, 2006a). There do not appear to be significant differences between genders in developing adenomas, with the exception of postpartum pituitary necrosis.

Risk Factors

Congenital malformations of the pituitary may develop during fetal growth and are the cause of some hypopituitary problems in infants and children. DNA mutations leading to tumors may also occur due to exposure to radiation or carcinogens, but idiopathic factors also cause pituitary tumors. Some purport that a few types of pituitary tumors appear to run in families, but the precise mechanism is not clear (Ferry & Shim, 2006).

Pathophysiology of the Anterior Pituitary

Each of the two pituitary structures has very distinct functions. The anterior pituitary, or adenohypophysis, produces growth hormone (GH), also known as somatotropin, TSH, adrenocorticotropic hormone (ACTH), prolactin, luteinizing hormone (LH), follicle-stimulating hormone (FSH), and melanocyte-stimulating hormone.

Normally growth hormone is produced episodically in short bursts, followed by periods of inactivity. Growth hormone production is more frequent and of higher volume in youth and gradually declines with age (Sachse, 2001). Protein, lipids, and carbohydrate metabolism are all influenced by growth hormone. TSH acts on target tissue in the thyroid gland, causing the release of thyroid hormones that influence metabolism. Similarly, ACTH acts on target tissue in the adrenal cortex, stimulating steroid biosynthesis and secretion. Prolactin stimulates milk production in the mammary gland and is thought to have some action on testicular function. FSH and LH act on tissue in the ovaries and testes, stimulating production of ovarian follicles in females, and the first steps of sperm production in males.

CHART 52–6 **Pituitary Hormones**

Pituitary Source	Hormone	Location of Target Tissue	Role/Function
Posterior pituitary/ neurohypophysis	Oxytocin	Mammary glands Uterus Ovaries Testes	Milk ejection Uterine contractions
	Antidiuretic hormone (arginine, vasopressin)	Kidney	Water conservation
Anterior pituitary/ adenohypophysis	Adrenocorticotropic hormone (ACTH)	Adrenal cortex	Steroid biosynthesis and secretion
	Growth hormone (somatotropin)	Liver Adipose tissue	Growth promotion
	Thyroid-stimulating hormone (TSH)	Thyroid gland	Triggers thyroid hormone release
	Melanocyte-stimulating hormone	Melanocytes	Production of melanin in the fetus and infant
	Follicle-stimulating hormone (FSH)	Ovaries Testes	Development of ovarian follicles Spermatogenesis
	Prolactin	Mammary glands	Milk production
	Luteinizing hormone (LH)	Ovaries Testes	Reproduction Spermatogenesis

Melanocyte-stimulating hormone acts on melanocytes, enhancing melanin production (Dorton, 2000).

Clinical Manifestations

The clinical picture of hypopituitarism is dependent on disease causation and which hormone(s) is (are) being undersecreted and the degree to which secretion has been affected. For example, deficiency in growth hormone may occur because this seems to be one of the first hormones to be decreased in patients with pituitary tumors. GH continues to be important after childhood and is essential to an individual's optimal sense of physical and emotional well-being. Patients with depressed GH levels will complain of fatigue and lack of energy and vitality and will report the need to sleep during the day. Deficiency in growth hormone is evident in symptoms of central obesity, reduced muscle mass, and increased body fat. Other patient complaints may include reduced capacity for exercise, impaired psychological well-being, poor body image, and social isolation. Deficiency in GH is the most common of the selective hypopituitary problems with gonadotropin deficiency occurring less frequently (Porth, 2007).

When pituitary tumors are present, clinical signs are likely to include headache and visual disturbances, as well as symptoms indicative of hyposecretion of specific pituitary hormones. Nonsecretory tumors, which suppress pituitary function because of their size or mass, may lead to symptoms such as vomiting, decreased mental alertness, loss of libido, infertility, and amenorrhea (PNA, 2006b).

Panhypopituitarism, a complete hypopituitarism that causes metabolic dysfunction, sexual immaturity, and growth retardation, can be caused by failure of either the pituitary or the hypothalamus. In this syndrome, there is inadequate secretion of all of the anterior pituitary hormones. It can occur early in life or in adulthood and may become apparent only during extreme stress when the body is unable to respond effectively to maintain homeostasis (Anderson, 2002; Kattah, 2006).

Laboratory and Diagnostic Procedures

Magnetic resonance imaging (MRI) or computerized tomography (CT) scans are indicated to identify the size and location of a pituitary tumor. Laboratory blood tests also are used to evaluate levels of the pituitary hormones affected by the tumor such as GH, ACTH, FSH, LH, TSH, and antidiuretic hormone (ADH). Because blood levels of GH vary throughout the day, blood testing for GH must be done after a stimulus to GH production is initiated. Stimulation tests include the insulin tolerance test or an arginine stimulation test. Hypoglycemia normally increases GH secretion. Blood levels of GH are tested in 30-minute intervals following administration of insulin. Failure to secrete growth hormone in response to hypoglycemia is an indicator of impaired GH secretion. Arginine stimulation may be used as a diagnostic tool for patients for whom hypoglycemia might be a risk. Failure to produce growth hormone following administration of arginine is indicative of pituitary disease. The effects of some of these tests on the elderly is discussed in the Gerontological Considerations box.

Medical Management

Hormone replacement may be needed for any of the pituitary hormones that are being undersecreted due to tumor growth, trauma, or congenital deformity. Cortisol replacement is partic-

GERONTOLOGICAL CONSIDERATIONS Related to Tests for Hypopituitarism

Older patients and patients with a history of cardiac disease may not endure the insulin tolerance test well, so other diagnostic measures such as the arginine stimulation test should be considered. Given the complexity of endocrine clinical problems, consultation with an endocrine specialist is advised.

ularly important in those cases where this hormone is suppressed because it regulates blood glucose and blood pressure. Treatment of hypopituitary function involving growth hormone insufficiency is by administration of synthetic GH by injection. Patients are taught how to self-administer growth hormone. Initial dosage is based on body weight and size, with long-term dosage determined by laboratory studies and patient response. Surgery for removal of a pituitary tumor may be warranted and this treatment is discussed under the treatment section for hyperpituitarism later in this chapter.

■ Nursing Management

Instruction in self-care, particularly administration of hormone replacement medications, may require that the nurse teach the patient how to give injections safely because some hormones are available only in injectable form. Low hormone production may make the patient more vulnerable to stress, both physical and psychological, so patients should be advised to report signs and symptoms of impending illness promptly to their health care provider.

Discharge Priorities

Understanding of the disease process and related symptoms is important for the patient. Change in symptoms may occur only over a period of several months after treatment is initiated, so patients must continue to update their health care provider on current symptoms and state of well-being. Synthetic growth hormone has been available for treatment of adult growth hormone deficiency for approximately two decades but it is expensive. Patients on limited incomes may need assistance in applying to pharmaceutical firms for free or low-cost supplies of the drug.

Health Promotion

Head trauma is a potential cause of pituitary gland dysfunction. Helmets should be worn by individuals who participate in sports that have the risk of head injury, including bicycling, motorcycling, or skateboarding. Nurses are important role models and teachers with regard to public safety including the use of helmets during high-risk activities.

Hypermetabolic Disorders of the Anterior Pituitary Gland: Prolactinomas and Acromegaly

Prolactinoma is a condition in which a noncancerous tumor (adenoma) of the pituitary gland in the brain overproduces the hormone prolactin. The major effect of increased prolactin is a decrease in normal levels of sex hormones—estrogen in women and testosterone in men. Although prolactinoma isn't life-threatening, it can cause visual impairment, infertility and other effects. Prolactinoma is one of several types of tumors that can develop in the pituitary gland.

Acromegaly is a hormonal disorder that results from too much growth hormone (GH) in the body. In acromegaly, the pituitary produces excessive amounts of GH. Usually the excess GH comes from benign, or noncancerous, tumors on the pituitary. These benign tumors are called adenomas.

Epidemiology and Etiology

Pituitary tumors are the most common cause of hyperpituitary disorders. According to some authorities, the most common type of pituitary adenoma is a prolactin-secreting prolactinoma, leading to problems with fertility and lactation (Braunwald et al., 2001). A second type of hyperpituitary disorder is one that involves the overproduction of growth hormone, resulting in one of two syndromes depending on the age at which the disorder occurs.

Prolactinomas account for 30% to 50% of pituitary tumors. In women, symptoms include absence of menstrual periods, infertility, and **galactorrhea**, the spontaneous flow of milk in a breast unassociated with childbirth or nursing. In men, symptoms include loss of libido, infertility, or signs of central nervous system compression. Goals of treatment are reduction in hyperprolactinemia, reduction in tumor size, resumption of menses and fertility, and improvement of galactorrhea (Braunwald et al., 2001).

Diagnosis of this specific type of pituitary tumor is done by measuring the prolactin level, and in men, measuring the testosterone level (Medline Plus, 2004). Prolactinomas are treated like other types of pituitary tumors as described later in this chapter.

Pituitary tumors also may produce an excess of growth hormone. The overproduction of GH results in two conditions that present with different physical manifestations depending on the timing of the disorder in one's physical development. **Gigantism** occurs in children when overproduction of pituitary hormone occurs before the closure of epiphysial plates in the long bones. Such children may grow as tall as 8 feet in height. On the other hand, **acromegaly** is a disorder that occurs when there is overproduction of pituitary hormone in adults whose epiphysial plates have closed.

Pathophysiology of Hyperpituitary Disorders

Tumors that produce growth hormone account for up to 15% of pituitary adenomas (Ferry & Shim, 2006). Normally, the hypothalamus produces GHRH, which stimulates the anterior pituitary to produce GH. GH stimulates the liver to produce insulin-like growth factor-1 (IGF-1), a hormone that causes bones and other tissues to grow and signals the pituitary to reduce production of GH. Continued production of GH by the pituitary gland leads to unwanted growth of bones and organs, as well as elevation of blood glucose levels, resulting in glucose intolerance (Sachse, 2001).

Hyperpituitarism evolves as two different syndromes depending on the age at which gland dysfunction occurs. As mentioned above, gigantism is the syndrome in which oversecretion of growth hormone begins early in life before there is closure of

the epiphysial plates. Without treatment, growth in height and weight continue throughout adulthood, leading to extremely abnormal height. Over time the physiological demands on the body exceed its capacity to maintain cardiovascular and musculoskeletal homeostasis and the individual typically dies a premature death of cardiovascular failure. Acromegaly, which occurs when there is an excess of growth hormone in adulthood, results in gradual but marked changes in facial characteristics, hands, feet, and ears (Figure 52–7 ■, p. 1640) (Chan, Ziebert, Maas, & Chan, 2005). The most common cause of gigantism and acromegaly is a pituitary adenoma; only in rare instances are these disorders caused by a nonpituitary tumor.

Risk Factors

About 3% of pituitary adenomas run in families and are due to inherited DNA mutations. Acquired mutations can occur due to exposure to radiation or cancer causing chemical agents. Other genetic mutations occur for unknown reasons (American Cancer Society, 2006).

Clinical Manifestations

As is true in pituitary disorders leading to hypopituitarism, the clinical picture in hyperpituitarism depends on the size of the adenoma and the type of hormone secretion, if any, that it produces. As noted previously, the most common pituitary adenoma, accounting for about 30% to 50% of tumors, is a prolactin-secreting prolactinoma. The primary symptom of this tumor is lactation. Growth hormone-secreting tumors, which cause acromegaly, also are seen with some frequency (Braunwald et al., 2001; Pituitary Disorders Education and Support, 2006a). Acromegaly causes excessive bone and soft tissue growth, leading to subtle and gradual coarsening of facial features over a period of years. The periorbital ridge, lips, and nose enlarge, and skin becomes coarse and oily (see Figure 52–7 ■, p. 1640). Patients may experience weakness and fatigue, headaches, loss of peripheral vision, and intermittent sweating as well as separation of teeth and a change in facial appearance (Ferry & Shim, 2006; Song & Weil, 2005). Complaints of osteoarthritis and myalgia are common. The physical changes caused by acromegaly are insidious because they occur gradually and may be attributed to a number of physical findings. Patients may have hyperpituitarism for years before a diagnosis is made.

Laboratory and Diagnostic Procedures

Diagnosis of hyperpituitary disease is based on the clinical picture, patient history, and laboratory results. Tests may be done to evaluate each of the target hormones produced by the pituitary gland in order to determine the extent of pituitary impairment. If a prolactin adenoma is suspected, prolactin hormone levels are tested, and in men, testosterone levels are evaluated because production of testosterone is inhibited in the presence of high levels of prolactin. With suspected growth hormone-secreting tumors, the plasma GH level is measured by radioimmunoassay.

Stimulation tests, such as an insulin tolerance test (ITT), arginine stimulation test, and GHRH test, may be given to assess the pituitary response and the ability to produce hormones. Elevation in GH level following a glucose suppression test will lead to concerns about the possibility of acromegaly. In addition, the IGF-1 level, which is a more stable measure, also is evaluated. Elevated IGF-1 levels are almost always indicative of acromegaly

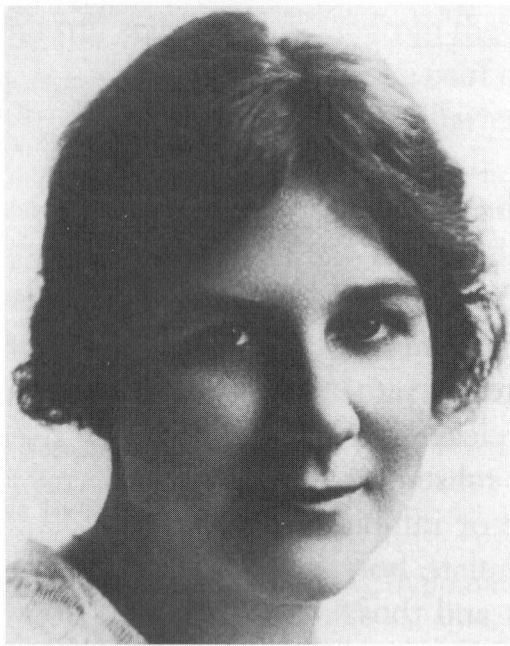

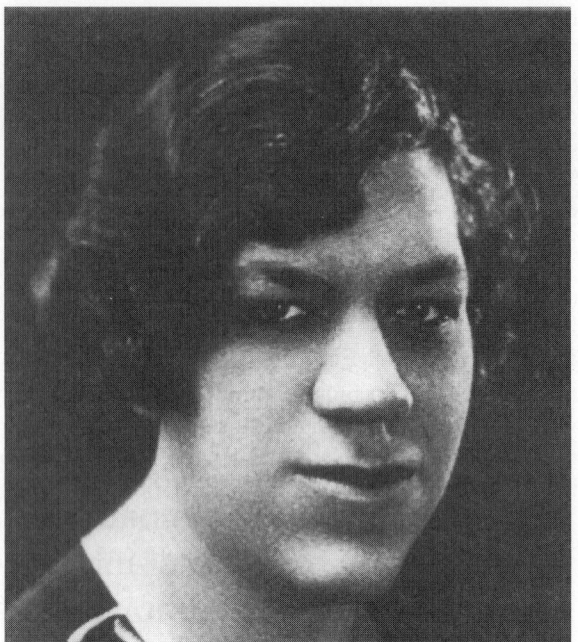

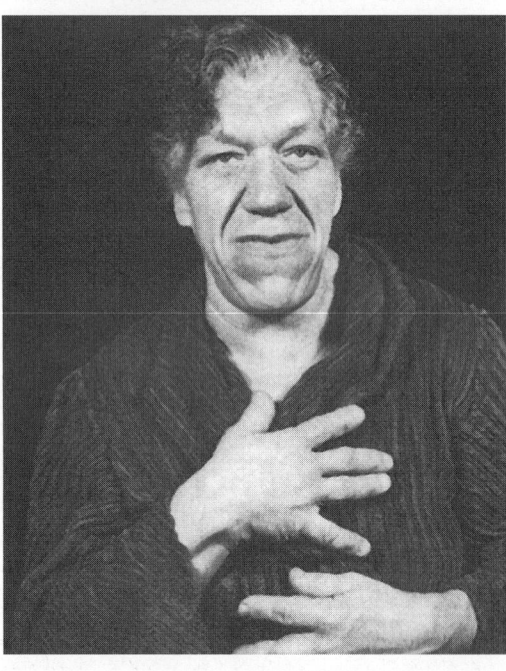

FIGURE 52–7 ■ Patient with development stages of acromegaly.
Source: (a) and (b) © Dr. William H. Daughaday, University of California/Irvine. American Journal of Medicine (20) 1956. With permission of Excerpta Medica Inc.; (c): Reproduced by permission from American Journal of Medicine 20:133, 1956 Copyright © 1956 by Elsevier Science Ltd.

(Sachse, 2001). Examination of the field of vision is another examination that can be done because patients with pituitary tumors sometimes experience a loss of peripheral vision due to the tumor pressing on nerves leading into the eye (Pituitary Disorders Education & Support, 2006a).

Medical Management

Primary treatment of acromegaly and many other hyperpituitary disorders is surgical intervention to remove the adenoma. This surgery is most successful with patients who have a small, localized tumor. Radiation therapy and pharmacologic intervention following surgery will depend on patient response to the initial

surgery. Tumor resection frequently reduces growth hormone production significantly and patients subsequently will experience a reduction in serum GH and alleviation of symptoms. Unfortunately, facial characteristics will remain largely unchanged.

Transsphenoidal microsurgery, with the surgical approach through the nose, along the front of the nasal septum, or under the lip and through the upper gum, into the sphenoid sinus cavity, is the most common treatment for removal of pituitary tumors. This surgical procedure usually eliminates the need for a craniotomy and permits much shorter hospital stays.

Radiation may be selected as a treatment modality if the patient is not a good candidate for surgery. A number of targeted radiosurgery approaches are available, including gamma knife and proton beam therapies. In these approaches, an MRI scan is used to create an image of the brain and the exact location of the tumor. The MRI is used to map locations for application of high-dose radiation beams, which are used to destroy tumor tissue while avoiding surrounding healthy tissue. This approach may take several months for resolution of symptoms and for this reason, radiation therapy is typically used as an adjunct to other treatments.

Radiation therapy may be the primary method of treatment for patients who are poor surgical risks. With this method, however, reduction in growth hormone levels takes much longer, often a period of years. Radiation therapy also is used when the hormone level remains high if surgical intervention is unable to remove all of the adenoma. Medications, including somatostatin analogues or dopamine agonists, which lower serum growth hormone, may also be used in treatment. Medications used to treat hyperpituitary disorders are shown in the Pharmacology Summary.

Octreotide is a somatostatin analogue medication that has proven effective in the treatment of acromegaly. The drug usually causes a marked reduction in symptoms of headache, sweating, and joint pains. Administered by intramuscular or subcutaneous injection, this medication is typically used as adjunctive therapy for patients who have residual tumor following surgery (Katznelson, 2006).

PHARMACOLOGY Summary of Medications to Treat Pituitary Disorders

Medication	Action	Side Effects	Nursing Care
Hyperpituitary Disorders			
Bromocriptine (oral tablet or capsules) Initiate therapy with small doses moving to 20 mg daily.	A dopamine agonist. Decreases sweating and soft tissue edema. Reduces high prolactin levels and restores ovulation and ovarian function in women with amenorrhea.	GI upset: nausea and vomiting, postural hypotension, depression, and nightmares. May cause intolerance to alcohol. Contraindicated in patients with uncontrolled hypertension or toxemia of pregnancy and those with hypersensitivity to ergot derivatives.	Explain that it may take several weeks for menses to resume. Take with meals to avoid GI distress. Rise slowly from supine position to avoid fainting, dizziness. Avoid use of alcohol. Avoid pregnancy (use mechanical barrier methods, not birth control pills).
Pergolide (oral tablet) 0.05 mg given orally daily for 2 days increasing gradually as directed to maximum dose of 5 mg/day. Doses should be divided into 3 doses daily.	Dopamine agonist. Inhibits prolactin secretion and decreases growth hormone levels.	GI distress/pain, constipation, light-headedness, sedation, hypotension, dry mouth.	Increases risk of atrial premature contraction and sinus tachycardia in patients with history of arrhythmia. Administer first dose at night with patient lying down to decrease dizziness. Reduced oral salivation requires good oral hygiene.
Cabergoline (oral tablet) 0.25 mg two times per week. May be increased every 4 weeks up to 1 mg two times per week.	Dopamine agonist. Antihyperprolactinemic. Stops pituitary secretions of prolactin hormone. Will resolve menstrual problems. Reduces lactation.	Abdominal pain, vertigo, changes in vision, difficulty concentrating, dizziness, swelling of hands or feet.	Do not drive until you know how this drug affects you. Get up slowly from supine position to avoid fainting. Avoid pregnancy (see above).
Octreotide 50–500 mg tid (available in forms that can be administered subcutaneously or by IM injection)	Somatostatin analogue. Relieves symptoms such as headache, sweating, and joint pain.	Gallstones, nausea, abdominal pain, diarrhea.	Tell patients to report GI symptoms because drug may cause gallstones.

Sources: Adapted from EndocrineWeb.com. (2007). Endocrine disorders & endocrine surgery. Retrieved August 29, 2008 from http://www.endocrineweb.com/; Jordan, S. (2005). Prescription drugs: Uses and effects. Thyroid disorders: Symptom control. *Nursing Standard, 19*(23), 56–58; Medline Plus. (2001). *Cabergoline (systemic)*. Retrieved March 7, 2006, from http://www.nlm.nih.gov/medlineplus/druginfo/uspdi/203584.html; *Physician's drug handbook* (11th ed.). (2005). Philadelphia: Lippincott Williams & Wilkins; Sachse, D. (2001). Acromegaly. *American Journal of Nursing, 101*(11), 69, 71, 73–75.

Dopamine agonists are a second class of drugs used to treat hyperpituitary disorders. They inhibit prolactin secretion and also cause a decrease in growth hormone. Dopamine agonists such as bromocriptine, pergolide, and cabergoline have varying mechanisms of action but can be useful in the management of symptoms caused by an excess of prolactin and GH in hyperpituitarism. Common side effects include drowsiness, headache, nausea, vertigo, and hypotension, particularly when therapy is initiated and if the client is supine. Gradual dosage titration is necessary with dopamine agonists to minimize side effects. Taking the medication with meals or milk helps patients avoid nausea. Patients should be advised to use care in driving until they know how the drug will affect them. These medications should not be given with estrogen preparations or birth control pills, and women of childbearing age should be advised to use mechanical barrier forms of birth control while taking the drug to avoid pregnancy. Patients taking dopamine agonists should be advised to consult with a pharmacist to ensure that other drugs they are taking do not counteract their action or cause untoward drug interactions (Medline Plus, 2005).

Nursing Management

Nursing assessment of patients with hyperpituitarism is critical to providing effective patient care. This condition often is associated with visual field defects and bony erosion. Thus, the nurse is assessing for mass effects of hormone excess including: headache, double vision, excessive sweating, hoarseness, milk secretion from the breast, sleep apnea, carpal tunnel syndrome, joint pain, limitation of motion, muscle weakness, and numbness or tingling of the skin (Porth, 2007).

Nursing Diagnosis

A diagnosis of hyperpituitarism may be made when evidence of hormonal imbalance surfaces during a time of stress such as hospitalization for other problems. The diagnosis of hyperpituitarism may be missed for years unless patients have severe headaches or marked physical changes in a short period of time. Nurses can offer strong support during the diagnostic period with explanation of and preparation for diagnostic tests. A primary nursing goal is to prepare patients for surgery and postoperative recovery for adenoma tumor resection. The fact that minimally invasive surgery is available may not lessen the patient's and family's fears about surgery.

Interventions and Rationales

Preoperative nursing care includes installation of antibiotic nose drops, discussion about mouth breathing, oral hygiene, early ambulation and activity, pain management, and hormone replacement therapy. A skilled neurosurgeon can remove the tumor with transsphenoidal microsurgery if the tumor is small and localized. Padding may be required for a brief period after surgery but sometimes this is not necessary. Postoperative complications include increased intracranial pressure due to cerebrospinal fluid (CSF) leak, meningitis, transient diabetes insipidus, and hypopituitarism with hormone replacement for life (Pituitary Network Association, 2006c).

Postoperative nursing care includes neurological assessment due to the risk of increased intracranial pressure, observations of temperature, pupils, vital signs, and fluid balance. The head of the patient's bed should always be elevated at a 30-degree angle to reduce headaches and pressure on the entry point in the sella turcica. The patient should be cautioned to avoid coughing, sneezing, straining at stool, or other activities that would initiate the Valsalva maneuver to prevent leakage of cerebrospinal fluid. Leaking of CSF, which is signaled by complaints of persistent generalized or supraorbital headache, increases the risk of meningitis and warrants prophylactic antibiotics, bed rest, and continued elevation of the head of the patient's bed. Nasal drainage, if present, should be tested by the lab for glucose, which indicates leakage of CSF.

Caution should be taken with provision of oral hygiene to avoid trauma to the surgical site. Use of a toothbrush should be discontinued for up to 10 days, and oral hygiene should be provided by the nurse at 4-hour intervals. Seizure precautions should be taken and mild analgesia provided for pain. Because transient diabetes insipidus may occur following surgery due to loss of ADH stored in the pituitary, urine output and serum and urine osmolality should be monitored (Laws, Vance, & Thapar, 2000). Patients generally will have a short hospital stay and should be advised to avoid exercise and unusual activities at home until cleared to do otherwise by the health care provider.

Somatostatin analogues and dopamine agonists are used in pharmacologic therapy to inhibit secretion of pituitary hormones. Patients who are prescribed medications to counteract hormone overload may need repeated explanations of the pharmacologic benefit of these preparations and instructions on potential side effects. Consultation with the pharmacist on dosage, timing, and route of administration, as well as common side effects and contraindications, is advised given that nurses typically are not administering these medications with great frequency in their practice.

Discharge Priorities

Changes in physical appearance and energy levels may have a long-term effect on patient relationships. Patients often report that quality of life is significantly altered by this disorder, even after treatment (Baird, Sullivan, Zafar, & Rock, 2003). Contin-

ued follow-up of patients is required after initial treatment to ensure that hormone levels return to normal and that efforts are made to address patient symptoms and complaints. Nurses may be able to offer vital emotional support for patients during diagnosis, treatment, and follow-up.

Gerontological Considerations

Older patients may be overwhelmed when trying to understand the nature of this rare disease. If the pituitary adenoma is large and cannot be entirely removed, or if the patient is not a candidate for surgery, medications may have to be used to inhibit hormone production. Older patients may need simple but clear instructions on medications and potential side effects. Resolution of symptoms may take some time leading to discouragement, and lack of change in physical appearance may be particularly disheartening and lead to depression. Patients may experience improvement in their field of vision with tumor excision, but failure to remove the tumor, even if other symptoms are controlled, may lead to diminished quality of life for patients who are unable to drive.

Health Promotion

Case studies indicate that patients with pituitary adenoma can have an improved quality of life with appropriate follow-up and case management (Carr, 2001). Patients should be instructed on signs of hypopituitarism, including severe chronic fatigue, central obesity, and reduced muscle mass, because they may experience this syndrome following treatment of the pituitary adenoma. Management of related endocrine disorders also is important. Referrals to support groups and organizations devoted to the needs of patients with pituitary problems may be another health promotion strategy for nursing consideration.

Disorders of the Posterior Pituitary Gland

The posterior pituitary, composed largely of axons of hypothalamic neurons, produces both antidiuretic hormone and oxytocin. Oxytocin stimulates uterine smooth muscle contraction at birth and also stimulates milk ejection and let-down in lactating mothers. Research also has indicated that oxytocin plays some role in the birth process and maternal behavior, but further research is needed on this action. The clinical disorders that the nurse is most likely to see in practice are those that involve an insufficient production of or insensitivity to ADH or an excess of ADH.

Hypometabolic Disorders of the Posterior Pituitary

Diabetes insipidus (DI) is a hypometabolic condition characterized by excretion of large amounts of severely diluted urine, which cannot be reduced when fluid intake is reduced. It signifies inability of the kidney to concentrate urine. There are four types of DI and treatment of the syndrome depends on the particular cause of the disease.

Epidemiology and Etiology

Diabetes insipidus is caused by a deficiency of antidiuretic hormone, also known as vasopressin, due to the destruction of the back or "posterior" part of the pituitary gland where vasopressin is normally released from, or by an insensitivity of the kidneys to that hormone. It can also be induced iatrogenically by various drugs.

This hypometabolic syndrome is not common, with a prevalence of 1 case per 25,000 people (Cooperman, 2008). The etiology of disorders related to the secretion of ADH may be linked to the pituitary gland itself or they may be caused by several other physiological disorders. There are no significant sex differences in DI. Male and female prevalences are equal. Mortality is rare in adults as long as water is available. Severe dehydration, hypernatremia, fever, cardiovascular collapse, and death can ensue in children, elderly people, or in those with complicating illnesses.

Pathophysiology and Risk Factors

Antidiuretic hormone is essential in maintaining fluid and electrolyte balance in the human body. ADH controls the concentration of urine through action on the collection tubules within the kidneys. Diabetes insipidus involves a permanent or transient deficiency in the synthesis or release of ADH or a decreased renal responsiveness to ADH. The four types of diabetes insipidus are discussed next.

Neurogenic Diabetes Insipidus

Neurogenic diabetes insipidus (also known as central, primary, or pituitary DI) is caused by a deficiency of ADH. Risk factors can include damage to the posterior pituitary by tumors, infection, head trauma, infiltrations, and genetic abnormalities. About half of the cases appear to be genetic in origin and half are idiopathic, that is, they occur for unknown reasons. Symptoms of this disorder may be apparent in early childhood or may suddenly appear later in life. Patients typically report constant thirst, along with polyuria, and the patient's urine is almost clear in color. Symptoms can be managed with synthetic hormone replacement using desmopressin (DDAVP), usually administered intranasally or orally. Once treatment is initiated, patients should be monitored for fluid overload and hypernatremia (Holcomb, 2002a).

Nephrogenic Diabetes Insipidus

Nephrogenic diabetes insipidus (NDI) is caused by resistance of the kidneys to ADH, rendering the ADH ineffective. This syndrome may be chronic if caused by a genetic defect or it may be acquired and transient if it occurs as a side effect of drugs such as lithium, colchicine, methoxyflurane, amphotericin B, gentamicin, and more. Eliminating selected medications may resolve acquired NDI. Inherited NDI usually appears early with symptoms of polyuria and polydipsia, but there are genetic patterns that differ, leading to mild or more serious symptoms. Diagnosis may be more difficult in such cases.

Genetically induced NDI is treated by prevention of dehydration through the provision of adequate fluid intake, dietary sodium restriction, and the use of a thiazide diuretic alone or in combination with a prostaglandin inhibitor to reduce urine output. Paradoxically, the thiazides tend to have an antidiuretic effect in DI (Loffing, 2004). Patients may require potassium supplementation to avoid depletion of potassium (Nephrogenic Diabetes Insipidus Foundation, 2005a).

Gestational Diabetes Insipidus

Gestational diabetes insipidus is caused by a deficiency of ADH that occurs only during pregnancy if the pituitary is damaged or if the placenta destroys the hormone too quickly. Treatment involves short-term hormone replacement therapy because the disease disappears 4 to 6 weeks after delivery. It may reoccur with future pregnancies.

Dipsogenic Diabetes Insipidus

Dipsogenic diabetes insipidus is a syndrome that causes primary polydipsia, abnormal thirst, and extreme intake of water and other fluids. It is caused by disease or damage to the part of the brain that regulates thirst. This is the one form of DI in which patients are not dehydrated. Patients ingest a large volume of water leading to water intoxication, decreased plasma osmolality, and a decrease in sodium concentration.

Symptoms include headache, loss of appetite, and nausea. Rarely, this disorder may be caused by **psychogenic polydipsia** in which excessive thirst occurs for psychogenic reasons. Hormone replacement may help manage symptoms but does not address the underlying cause of the disease (Nephrogenic Diabetes Insipidus Foundation, 2005a).

Tumors, trauma, surgery, infection, pregnancy, congenital defects, and genetic disorders are all factors that contribute to the development of diabetes insipidus but there is a significant percentage of cases with idiopathic etiology.

Clinical Manifestations

Each of the different forms of diabetes insipidus is characterized by polyuria (excretion of large amounts of dilute urine) and polydipsia (excessive thirst). Patients with DI present with dry mucous membranes, poor skin turgor, and other signs of dehydration. In untreated cases, symptoms of tachycardia and hypotension signal impending hypovolemic shock, which can be life threatening (Innis, 2002b).

Laboratory and Diagnostic Procedures

Diagnostic tests will help to determine the origin of diabetes insipidus and direct the appropriate therapy since treatment varies depending on the etiology. Blood and urine levels of ADH will be taken before and during a water deprivation or dehydration test, which will determine whether DI is neurogenic or nephrogenic in nature. Serum electrolytes and the osmolality of serum and urine will be determined. Serum will reveal an elevated osmolality and high sodium level (hypernatremia). Urine will be poorly concentrated, with low osmolality and decreased specific gravity (Holcomb, 2002b). An MRI will be used to rule out the presence of a pituitary tumor. A family history and genetic testing will be done to determine whether the disease has been inherited or whether there has been recent stress or trauma to the pituitary (Holcomb, 2002a).

A stimulus test such as fluid deprivation or administration of DDAVP, a synthetic replacement for antidiuretic hormone, to assess the impact of secretion of vasopressin may be done to differentiate neurogenic DI from dipsogenic DI. Unlike pituitary DI, DDAVP eliminates both excessive urination but not the symptoms of increased thirst and fluid intake in dipsogenic DI. In fact, water intoxication is a serious concern with this disorder. Patients will complain of headache, lethargy, and nausea and will have low levels of plasma sodium concentration (hyponatremia).

Medical Management

Treatment is dependent on the type of DI the patient is experiencing. Neurogenic DI may be treated by resolving the pituitary problem causing the disorder. For example, surgery for a pituitary tumor may be indicated. If irreparable damage has been done to pituitary tissues by tumor, infection, head injury, a congenital defect, or some other unexplained factor, then DI is likely to be permanent and must be managed with drugs including desmopressin or DDAVP. These will control the symptoms of constant thirst, drinking, and urination. On the other hand, gestational DI will generally resolve within 4 to 6 weeks following the conclusion of pregnancy but is likely to reoccur with subsequent pregnancies.

Nephrogenic DI, caused by genetic defects, drugs, or kidney disease, can be managed through a combination of hydration strategies, a low-sodium and sometimes low-protein diet, and the use of diuretics to reduce the volume of urine output. A thiazide diuretic, alone or in combination with a prostaglandin inhibitor, or a potassium-sparing diuretic may be ordered as part of the treatment regimen. If diuretics are used, potassium levels should be monitored. Potassium supplements may be needed to prevent hypokalemia. If DI is a side effect of lithium or other drugs, it is important to ensure that the therapeutic drugs selected for treatment do not impair their excretion (Nephrogenic Diabetes Insipidus Foundation, 2005b). It may be necessary to modify drug therapy for patients unable to tolerate lithium due to diabetes insipidus (Innis, 2002a).

Nursing Management

The primary goal in nursing care for patients with neurogenic, gestational, and nephrogenic DI is to prevent serious dehydration by ensuring that patients have an adequate fluid intake. Intravenous fluid replacement and an abundance of oral fluids should be readily available and administered. Vital signs and intake and output should be monitored very closely. Hormone replacement therapy is provided when appropriate, and electrolytes may be supplemented as needed. Diuretics may be used in nephrogenic DI to help kidneys eliminate sodium and decrease the glomerular filtration rate, resulting in conservation of urine. Patients will have a lifetime commitment in the management of hyperpituitarism unless the treatment resolves the underlying problem by pituitary tumor resection, or termination of pregnancy.

Discharge Priorities

Discharge priorities focus on patient instruction regarding the nature of the disease and the importance of hydration and strategies to ensure the availability of fluid at all times. Medic alert jewelry and a medical identification card should always be carried by the patient so that the patient's condition is known and in emergency situations the treatment is efficient. Patients should be made aware of community resources, including organizations that promote education and research on DI.

Hypermetabolic Disorder of the Posterior Pituitary: SIADH

The posterior pituitary secretes the hormones ADH and oxytocin. An excess of oxytocin has not been reported to be problematic, but oversecretion of ADH does occur and is considered potentially life threatening if untreated. This disorder is called **syndrome of inappropriate antidiuretic hormone (SIADH)**.

Epidemiology and Etiology

SIADH results from a failure of the negative feedback system that regulates the release and inhibition of ADH. In persons with this syndrome, ADH secretion continues even when serum osmolality is decreased, causing marked water retention and dilutional hyponatremia (Bayless, 2003; Porth, 2007). It occurs in adults and premature infants, and is caused by a variety of pathophysiological conditions.

Although SIADH is not unusual in adults, it is rare in the pediatric population, and other causes of hyponatremia are more common. It is the most common cause of hypotonic normovolemic hyponatremia in children. Exact incidence figures are not available.

The presence of hyponatremia, its severity, and delay in initiating adequate treatment appear to be the main indicators for both morbidity and mortality. The mortality rate in hyponatremic patients is 50-fold higher than in patients who do not develop hyponatremia. Moreover, the mortality rate in patients with serum sodium concentrations of less than 120 mmol/L is 25%, or twice that, of patients with mild hyponatremia. Acute decreases in serum sodium in adults are associated with a cited mortality rate of 5% to 50%, depending on the severity and rate of development, whereas in children it is only about 8%. Infants probably tolerate cerebral edema with fewer untoward effects because of their expandable cranium. Symptomatic postoperative hyponatremia can result in high morbidity and mortality rates in children of both sexes, which is due, in large part, to inadequate brain adaptation and lack of timely treatment (Ferry & Pascual-y-Baralt, 2007). Controlled studies in adults have shown that women and men are equally likely to develop hyponatremia and hyponatremic encephalopathy after surgery. Menstruating women who develop hyponatremic encephalopathy are 25 times more likely to die or have permanent brain damage than either men or postmenopausal women. The Risk Factors box addresses the risk factors for SIADH.

Although genetic factors may be involved in the etiology of pituitary disorders, not enough is known at present to offer dis-

RISK FACTORS for SIADH

SIADH occurs in patients who have central nervous system disorders, patients who have experienced shock, trauma, stress, or surgery, and patients with malignancies or pulmonary infections such as TB, bacterial pneumonia, or a lung abscess. Selected drugs including narcotics, tranquilizers, barbiturates, general anesthetics, thiazide diuretics, hypoglycemic agents, antidepressants, and some chemotherapeutic agents also are associated with rare cases of SIADH. A high percentage of patients with SIADH have a malignancy, often a small cell or oat cell carcinoma lung cancer, but other forms of cancer also have been found to cause this disorder. Malignant cells can secrete ADH or ADH-like chemicals, which serve as an ectopic source of ADH. Seriously ill ventilated patients and the elderly may experience an increase in the release of ADH (Langfeldt & Cooley, 2003; Terpstra & Terpstra, 2000).

ease prevention strategies. Consultation with the health care provider on the potential benefit of genetic screening should be considered but may offer limited benefit at this time.

Pathophysiology

Several mechanisms regulate sodium and water balance in the human body. The hypothalamus contains strategically located osmoreceptors that maintain a feedback control system for ADH secretion. Changes in the extracellular fluid resulting from a decrease or increase in the sodium ion concentration stimulate the osmoreceptors to increase or decrease the firing rate of the osmoreceptor cells, which stimulates or reduces production of ADH accordingly. Circulating ADH increases the permeability of distal tubules and the collecting duct by attaching to receptor sites in these tissues. Thus when stimulated by increasing plasma osmolality, the osmoreceptors of the hypothalamus secrete ADH and the kidneys respond by reabsorbing more water into the capillary network. As a consequence, a smaller volume of concentrated urine is excreted. When plasma osmolality is low, ADH secretion decreases and little water reabsorption occurs, resulting in the excretion of a large volume of dilute urine.

Decreases in blood pressure and volume, which are communicated by stretch receptors in the heart and large arteries, also stimulate the secretion of ADH. Thus if a patient has experienced extreme blood loss, the body will respond by increasing the output of ADH significantly (Colorado State University, 2003). SIADH occurs when ADH hormone continues to be secreted in spite of hyponatremia (low serum sodium levels).

Clinical Manifestations

Symptoms develop due to gradual water intoxication as evidenced by low serum sodium levels, and patients will exhibit headache, nausea, anorexia, thirst, increase in weight, oliguria, muscle cramps, weakness, and fatigue. As hyponatremia increases, mental confusion, irritability, and disorientation will occur. Seizures and coma can occur along with cerebral edema. When serum sodium drops below 110 to 115 mEq/L, the risk of death is high (Langfelt & Cooley, 2003). Critical care nurses should be alert to symptoms in patients who are known to be at risk for development of SIADH. Culture may play a part in a patient's response to the symptoms of pituitary disorders, as discussed in the Cultural Considerations for Pituitary Disorders box.

Laboratory and Diagnostic Procedures

Laboratory tests of electrolytes, serum and urine osmolality, urine specific gravity, and blood urea nitrogen (BUN) can be useful in the diagnosis of SIADH. Serum sodium is usually moderately or severely low depending on patient condition. Clinical diagnostic measures will be focused on eliminating other potential causes for hyponatremia and fluid retention such as congestive heart failure and cirrhosis. Once the syndrome is identified, the underlying cause should be explored with further diagnostic studies as needed.

Medical Management

Treatment is first directed at the problem of hyponatremia and water intoxication through fluid restriction and gradual correction of the serum sodium level with intravenous electrolytes,

CULTURAL CONSIDERATIONS for Pituitary Disorders

Both hypopituitarism and hyperpituitarism can cause symptoms that will be problematic for patients in terms of cultural acceptance. In patients with long-standing hypersecretion of growth hormone, changes in facial characteristics present a special problem. Body image may be distorted due to coarsening of facial features and may cause the patient particular problems in those cultures where appearance is highly valued. Unexplained lactation is another untoward symptom that may create cultural complications for patients since this typically occurs independent of pregnancy and normal lactation. In addition, the fact that it may take several months for hormone levels, let alone symptoms, to return to normal is often very disturbing for patients.

food, and fluids. The degree of fluid restriction is dependent on the severity of hyponatremia. Lower levels of serum sodium require more aggressive fluid restriction. Too rapid a correction of hyponatremia is ill advised because a complication can occur that will result in cerebral edema, seizures, permanent brain damage, and death a few days after treatment. If a patient is ambulatory, the health care provider may prescribe the use of medications that will block the action of ADH, such as demeclocycline or lithium, in order to avoid strict fluid restriction.

Along with efforts to correct fluid and electrolyte balance, efforts must be made to address the underlying cause of SIADH. Surgical excision of the tumor mass, radiation therapy, or chemotherapy to decrease tumor size may be attempted. Antibiotics should be initiated if the cause is believed to be an infection. Drugs suspected in the etiology of SIADH should be discontinued (Carr, 2001).

■ Nursing Management

Nurses in critical care and oncology settings should be particularly alert in their physical assessment of patients at high risk for SIADH. Assessment of hydration including skin turgor, mucous membranes, intake and output, daily weight, and monitoring for fluid overload is important. Nursing care for patients with suspected SIADH includes meticulous recording of intake and output, urine specific gravity, weight, and vital signs.

During the acute phase of SIADH, the nurse should monitor the patient's neurological status and take seizure precautions. The nurse also should work with the patient and family on a plan for monitored fluid intake and restriction throughout the day. Fluids that are relatively high in sodium such as tomato juice, milk, or broth should be encouraged. Dry mouth may be addressed with sugarless gum or candies, mouth moisturizers, or artificial saliva products (Langfelt & Cooley, 2003).

Patient and family education should include strategies to deal with SIADH as well as the underlying disease and related nursing care. Patients or their caregivers should be instructed on how to record the patient's daily weight and intake and output measurements for ongoing evaluation. Increased weight and decreased output should be reported because further treatment may be required.

Discharge Priorities

Discharge priorities include attention to postoperative instructions and routine follow-up with the health care provider. If patients are taking antipituitary drugs to counteract excess hormone production, instructions should include signs and symptoms of drug side effects. It is not uncommon for further treatment to be required if the tumor is not completely removed and continues to grow over time. Patients should be advised to continue follow-up evaluations with the endocrinologist so that additional treatment such as radiation therapy or medications can be used to reduce symptoms and to improve quality of life (Carr, 2001).

Collaborative Management

Care of patients with pituitary disorders typically will require close teamwork between and among the endocrinologist, neurosurgeon, primary care provider, nurses, and diagnostic imaging staff at the very least. Pharmacists and dietitians also may be involved in planning the care of the patient. The goal of treatment should be to eliminate the pituitary tumor, stabilize hormone production, and improve quality of life for the patient, which often has been severely compromised over time. Research and surgical advances in the field of treatment of neurological and endocrine disorders will require that health professionals work together and update their knowledge of contemporary standards of care when patients present with these rare clinical diagnoses.

Complementary and Alternative Approaches

Complementary approaches to care may offer considerable enhancement of the well-being of patients following treatment for diseases of the pituitary gland. Elimination of symptoms may take several months following initiation of treatment and complementary measures may offer particular benefit during this period. Again, complementary measures do not substitute for medical treatment aimed at eliminating causative factors such as

benign tumors, but they can be important in improving quality of life. Some studies have shown that patients with pituitary tumors report quality of life to be diminished even after hormone levels return to normal following traditional treatment (Baird et al., 2003). This suggests that additional study is needed to determine how these patients can be restored to optimal health, potentially with the use of complementary approaches.

Disorders of the Adrenal Gland

The adrenal glands, like the other endocrine glands, can be affected by a variety of conditions including congenital malformations, genetic disorders, autoimmune disease, infection, hemorrhage, and tumors, all of which can cause either hypofunction or hyperfunction of the glands. The adrenal glands produce hormones that are essential to the body's "fight-or-flight" response and general adaptation to stress (see Chapter 12). Thus hypo- or hypersecretion of hormones of the adrenal glands can have significant and pervasive effects on health.

Although each adrenal gland is described as one unit, in reality, the gland is composed of two very distinct parts, the cortex and the medulla, with cells and tissues that secrete different hormones and have different functions. Chart 52–7 lists hypo- and hyper-metabolic disorders of the adrenal gland. Note that hypometabolic disorders have been identified involving the adrenal cortex but not the adrenal medulla, but hypermetabolic disorders occur in both the adrenal cortex and adrenal medulla.

Hypometabolic Adrenal Disorders: The Adrenal Cortex

Hypofunction of the adrenal glands can occur for many reasons and the degree of dysfunction determines whether the symptoms are mild, moderate, or life threatening. However, any level of impairment puts the individual at risk during times of stress or disease because the body's ability to produce essential hormones to maintain homeostasis has been compromised. Although this condition is fairly rare, adrenal insufficiency may be acute or chronic. The two major hypometabolic disorders of the

CHART 52–7 **Hypometabolic and Hypermetabolic Disorders of the Adrenal Glands**

Adrenals	Disorder	Hormones	Clinical Picture
Adrenal cortex, hypometabolic disorders	Congenital adrenal hyperplasia	Cortisol and aldosterone deficiency with an excess in androgen hormone	Adrenal crisis with dehydration and shock Masculinization of females and early puberty; short stature
	Adrenal insufficiency	Cortisol deficiency	Adrenal crisis
	Addison's disease	Cortisol deficiency	Adrenal crisis
Adrenal cortex, hypermetabolic disorders	Cushing's syndrome Primary aldosteronism/Conn's disease	Cortisol excess Aldosterone excess	Hypertension Abdominal obesity Muscle wasting Hypertension with hypokalemia
Adrenal medulla, hypometabolic disorders	None identified	None identified	None identified
Adrenal medulla, hypermetabolic disorders	Pheochromocytoma	Adrenalin excess	Hypertension

adrenals are primary adrenal hyperplasia and Addison's disease. Congenital adrenal hyperplasia is hereditary and becomes apparent at birth or childhood, whereas Addison's disease usually occurs later in life. Adrenal insufficiency caused by long-term administration of corticosteroid drugs is not a disease per se, but is a disorder with symptoms like those of Addison's disease.

Addison's disease is adrenocortical insufficiency due to the destruction or dysfunction of the entire adrenal cortex. It affects both glucocorticoids and mineralocorticoid function. The onset of disease usually occurs when 90% or more of both adrenal cortices are dysfunctional or destroyed (Odeke & Nagelbereg, 2006).

Epidemiology and Etiology

In the mid-19th century, primary adrenal insufficiency was first described by a physician, Thomas Addison, for whom the condition was later named. At that time, the most common cause of the disease was tuberculosis (TB) infection and this remains the second most common cause today. However, the incidence of Addison's disease secondary to an increase in opportunistic infections related to human immunodeficiency virus (HIV) is rising (Holcomb, 2006). Addison's disease is a rare condition caused by a severe or total deficiency of hormones produced by the adrenal cortex, and results from partial or complete destruction of the adrenal glands. In a normal state, when the body perceives the need for greater energy, the pituitary gland secretes ACTH, which stimulates the release of cortisol by the adrenal glands. In adrenal gland insufficiency, secretion of cortisol is impaired leading to a serious imbalance in homeostasis. The body becomes unable to respond to new and differing demands for adrenal hormones. In most cases of adrenal insufficiency, the adrenal cortex is primarily affected but when the medulla is involved, catecholamine deficiency also may occur. A patient with Addison's disease is shown in Figure 52–8 ■.

The leading cause of Addison's disease is autoimmune disease in which the body's immune system makes antibodies that gradually destroy the cells of the adrenal cortex (Odeke & Nagelbereg, 2006). Autoimmune destruction of the cortex involves a long process, typically occurring over months and years. Chronic infections such as TB, histoplasmosis, or cytomegalovirus may cause Addison's disease, but infection is much less commonly involved today. Cancer (usually caused by metastasis from other tissues such as the breast), hemorrhage into the adrenal gland, tumors, bilateral adrenalectomy, and sudden withdrawal of long-term corticosteroid therapy are other, less frequently noted causes of Addison's disease (Anderson, 2002; National Adrenal Diseases Foundation, 2006a).

Currently the prevalence of Addison's disease in the United States is 40 to 60 cases per 1 million population. Internationally, the condition is rare, and is not associated with a racial predilection. Idiopathic autoimmune Addison's disease tends to be more common in females and children. The most common age at presentation in adults is 30 to 50 years, but the disease could present earlier in patients with any of the polyglandular autoimmune syndromes, congenital adrenal hyperplasia (CAH), or if onset is due to a disorder of long-chain fatty acid metabolism (Odeke & Nagelbereg, 2006).

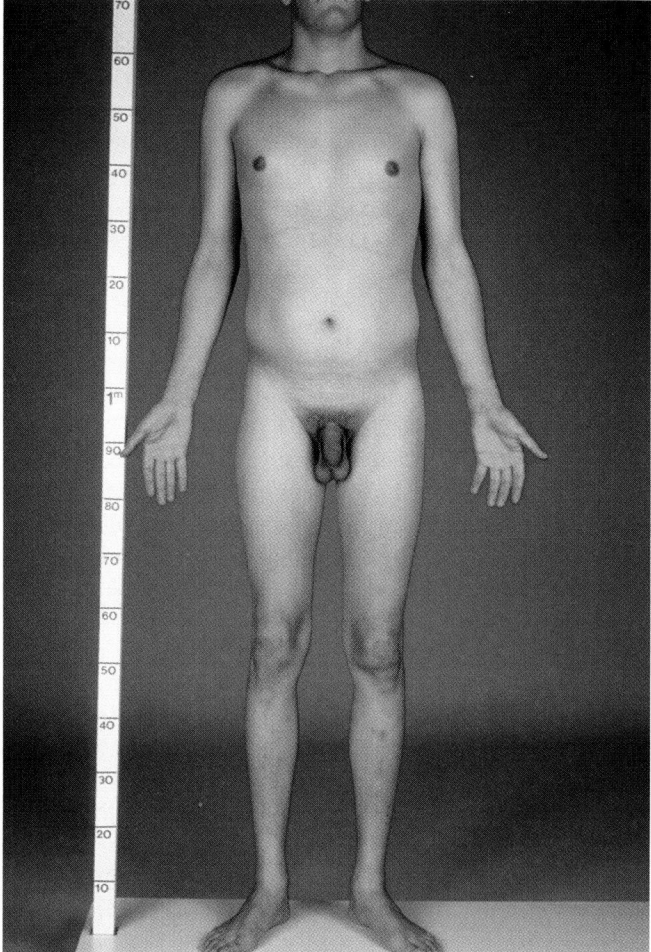

FIGURE 52–8 ■ Patient with Addison's disease.
Source: Bart's Medical Library/Phototake NYC

Pathophysiology

There are two adrenal glands, one located above each kidney in the human body, and they have two distinct parts: the cortex, which is the outer portion, and the medulla, the inner portion. The adrenal cortex produces two essential hormones: cortisol and aldosterone. These hormones are key to the body's general adaptation to stress and illness. The adrenal cortex also produces androgens, which are important in the development of the gonads and male sexual characteristics. Cellular receptors for cortisol exist in cell cytoplasm throughout the entire body. Thus the presence of a normal level of the adrenal hormone cortisol is essential for maintaining cell homeostasis and viability (Coursin & Wood, 2002).

The medulla produces the hormones epinephrine (also known as adrenalin) and norepinephrine. Adrenalin increases heart rate and stroke volume, dilates the pupils, and constricts arterioles in the skin and gut while dilating arterioles in leg muscles. Adrenalin also elevates the blood sugar level by increasing hydrolysis of glycogen to glucose in the liver, and begins the breakdown of lipids in fat cells. Norepinephrine activates the sympathetic nervous system to directly increase heart rate, release energy from fat, and increase muscle readiness.

The hormones of the adrenal glands are produced through the interaction of the negative feedback control of both the hypothalamus and the pituitary glands (Figure 52–9 ■). The hypothalamus produces CRH, which stimulates the pituitary to produce ACTH, to signal the need for production of glucocorticoids in the adrenals. Glucocorticoid levels vary naturally throughout the day, with lower levels typically being produced in the evening hours and production peaking in the early morning hours. Under conditions of stress such as illness, surgery, or trauma, the normal body can dramatically increase the synthesis of cortisol (Coursin & Wood, 2002).

Adrenal insufficiency is a condition in which the body fails to produce adequate amounts of adrenal hormones. **Primary adrenal insufficiency** occurs in conditions when most (up to 90%) of the adrenal gland has been destroyed, resulting in an absence of sufficient glucocorticoids (cortisol), mineralocorticoids (aldosterone), and androgens. The disease process originates within the adrenal gland and may involve autoimmune disease, infection, or hemorrhage. Congenital adrenal hyperplasia is an inherited form of adrenal insufficiency. **Secondary adrenal insufficiency**, caused by impaired pituitary secretion of ACTH, occurs when there is an inadequate secretion of cortisol but an adequate amount of aldosterone. The diseases are similar in that in both conditions there is a loss of cortisol (Coursin & Wood, 2002). Primary adrenal hyperplasia differs from these forms of adrenal insufficiency in that the adrenals are able to respond to signals from the pituitary and attempt to compensate for a decline in cortisol and aldosterone by significantly increasing production of androgen.

Although Addison's disease is rare, a more common problem that may occur in critically ill adults is secondary adrenal insufficiency, which can occur when the patient has received long-term administration of therapeutic glucocorticoids, such as prednisone. These drugs commonly are given for inflammatory conditions and autoimmune disorders such as rheumatoid arthritis, asthma, and ulcerative colitis. Administration of cortisone drugs suppresses the normal stimulation response of the hypothalamus to release CRH and the pituitary to release ACTH, which would trigger the production of increased cortisol in the adrenals. Disruption in the hypothalamic–pituitary–adrenal

(HPA) axis function may last for a long period and is a major reason why abrupt withdrawal of cortisone therapy is ill advised and may put the patient at serious risk (Pfadt & Carlson, 2006). Resumption of normal HPA activity after a long period of hormone therapy may take up to a year (Coursin & Wood, 2002). Thus cortisone drugs should always be discontinued with gradually diminishing doses over an extended period of time. The risk factors for adrenal disorders are discussed in the Risk Factors box.

Clinical Manifestations

Patients with Addison's disease experience severe and chronic fatigue and loss of appetite and weight. Nausea, vomiting, and diarrhea occur in many cases. Patients feel light-headed because their blood pressure is low, and they may experience orthostatic hypotension, that is, low blood pressure upon standing (Løvås & Husebye, 2005). Hyperpigmentation of skin is common, with scars, skinfolds, and pressure points such as elbows, knees, and knuckles becoming characteristically dark. In women, menstruation cycles and patterns may change. Patients may crave salt and may experience low blood sugars. **Addisonian crisis** (or **adrenal crisis**) occurs when symptoms of the disease become exacerbated due to stress, causing severe pain in the lower back, abdomen, or legs; vomiting, or diarrhea with severe dehydration; and low blood pressure and loss of consciousness (Pituitary Network Association, 2006a). Patients with adrenal insufficiency for any reason may experience adrenal crisis if hormone replacement is not initiated, is inadequate, or if other factors increase the physiological demand for adrenal hormones.

Laboratory and Diagnostic Procedures

The physical examination and patient history give the first indications of adrenal insufficiency. The most specific laboratory test is the short ACTH stimulation test, an exam in which a baseline blood sample is drawn and then a synthetic form of ACTH is given by injection, followed by the measurement of blood and, in some cases, urine cortisone levels at 30, 60, and 90 minutes. Patients with adrenal insufficiency are unable to respond to stimulation by producing more cortisol, and do not produce more cortisol (Whiteman, 2006). A prolonged ACTH stimulation test may be given to clarify whether the disease is primary or secondary. A CT scan may be ordered to enhance diagnosis in terms of cause of the disease (Luken, 1999).

Medical Management

Patients with Addison's disease or adrenal insufficiency are treated with hormones designed to replace cortisol (Cortef, prednisone, or cortisone) and aldosterone (fludrocortisone [Florinef]). In addition, the doctor may recommend treating

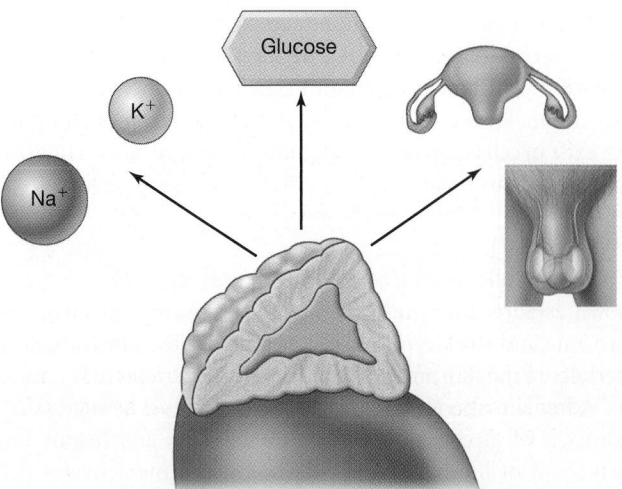

Adrenal glands secrete hormones which help regulate chemical balance, regulate metabolism, and supplement other glands

FIGURE 52–9 ■ Adrenal gland hormone secretion.

RISK FACTORS for Adrenal Disorders

Risk factors for the development of hypoadrenal functioning include a family history of congenital adrenal disorders, autoimmune disease, personal history of TB or other infections such as AIDS, cancer, pituitary disease, or long-term corticosteroid therapy. Nurses are most likely to encounter patients with acquired adrenal insufficiency in older patients over age 55, secondary to corticosteroid therapy, which results in suppression of cortisol production in response to infection, trauma, or stress (Ezell, 2006).

androgen deficiency with an androgen replacement called dehydroepiandrosterone. Some studies indicate that, for women with Addison's disease, androgen replacement therapy may improve their overall sense of well-being, libido, and sexual satisfaction.

Oral doses of hydrocortisone or cortisone acetate, 20 to 30 mg/day, are given in divided doses morning and evening. Typically, two-thirds of the medication is given in the morning and one-third in the evening to mimic the normal output of cortisol throughout the day. Hydrocortisone should be taken with meals, milk, or antacids to avoid increasing gastric acidity and distress. Aldosterone is replaced with a synthetic aldosterone steroid, fludrocortisone tablets (Florinef), taken once daily to prevent loss of sodium, hyperkalemia, and intravascular depletion. If the patient is unable to take replacement therapy by mouth, medications are administered intravenously.

Patients in adrenal crisis are seriously ill and require fluid replacement with intravenous saline and dextrose in saline solution immediately, along with intravenous hydrocortisone for 48 to 72 hours. Patients should be monitored for their electrolyte balance, blood count, and plasma as a means to determine appropriate adjustments to drug dosages. In children with primary adrenal hyperplasia, androgen blocking drugs and growth hormone may be used to block the effects of excess androgen production and to enhance growth in height (National Adrenal Diseases Foundation, 2006b).

■ Nursing Management

Nurses play a key role during adrenal crisis in managing fluid replacement, administering hormone replacements, and measuring vital signs, weight, and fluid intake and output. Once the crisis is resolved, a plan for patient and family education must be developed in cooperation with the medical staff. Patients will require instruction on lifetime drug therapy and risks during periods of stress and illness. Patients should be encouraged to keep a small amount of medications with them at all times in the event of a disaster because interruption of drug therapy can be catastrophic. It is advisable that patients learn how to administer intramuscular injections so that they can self-administer hydrocortisone if unable to take medications by mouth due to nausea or vomiting. Patients should consult with their physician about the advisability of carrying a syringe and a dose of injectable cortisol with them in case of emergency. Cortisol hormone replacements will need to be increased during stress and illness to avoid complications and the mineralocorticoid fludrocortisone acetate should be increased during summer months or periods of intense exercise when sweating increases. The Nursing Process: Patient Care Plan for Acute Adrenal Insufficiency explains the nursing process to be used in caring for patients with this disorder, and the Gerontological Considerations box (p. 1650) addresses additional teaching for the elderly with this disorder.

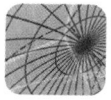

NURSING PROCESS: Patient Care Plan for Acute Adrenal Insufficiency

Assessment of Cognitive Level, Muscle Strength, and Ability to Perform ADLS Independently

Subjective Data:
Have you been taking any steroid medications, such as prednisone, cortisone, or any other steroid drugs?
What other medications, herbs, or dietary supplements have you been taking?
Have you been able to maintain your usual activities of daily living?
What has your appetite been like?
Have you noticed any food cravings lately?
How much salt or sodium do you get in your diet?
Have you experienced any nausea or vomiting?
Do you feel mentally alert?
Are you sleeping well?
Have you experienced any stress, trauma, or illness recently?

Objective Data:
Low blood pressure
Orthostatic hypotension
Poor skin turgor
Tender abdomen
Face appears round, edematous
Muscle weakness noted
Low serum sodium, high potassium noted

Nursing Assessment and Diagnoses	Outcomes and Evaluation Parameters	Planning and Interventions with *Rationales*
Nursing Diagnosis: *Deficient Fluid Volume* and *Hyponatremia* secondary to adrenal insufficiency	**Outcomes:** Free of symptoms of adrenal insufficiency. ***Evaluation Parameters:*** Vital signs within normal limits. Patient able to stand at bedside without vertigo. Abdomen soft, bowel sounds normal. Patient reports appetite has returned with no food cravings. Patient verbalizes feeling less fatigued. Skin turgor appears elastic. Serum sodium and sodium serum levels within normal range. No evidence of nausea, vomiting, or diarrhea.	**Interventions and *Rationales*:** Administer IV therapy, which may include 0.09% saline solution or 5% dextrose in saline to improve fluid and electrolyte balance *to raise blood pressure and improve perfusion of oxygen to tissues.* Administer IV hydrocortisone for first 48–72 hours, followed by oral administration for essential hormone replacement to be taken with meals *to provide hormone needed due to suppression of HPA axis due to long-term corticosteroid therapy and to prevent GI distress.*

(continued)

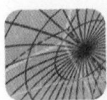

Nursing Process: Patient Care Plan for Acute Adrenal Insufficiency—*Continued*

**Assessment of Emergency Preparedness
in the Event of Adrenal Insufficiency Crisis**

Subjective Data:

Do you carry a medical identification card with a list of your medications on it?

Do you wear a medical ID bracelet or other jewelry?

Have you informed family members or caregivers of your history with corticosteroid drugs?

Tell me what your understanding is about how corticosteroid drugs affect your body.

Are you experiencing any pain?

Please describe the location and intensity.

Objective Data:

Blood pressure: 84/40

Temperature: 101°F

Heart rate: 124

Diaphoretic

Appears confused, disoriented as to time and place

Vomited during interview

No medic alert noted on patient on admission to ICU

Family members report patient has been taking corticosteroids for rheumatoid arthritis

Medications found in patient's purse

Nursing Assessment and Diagnoses	Outcomes and Evaluation Parameters	Planning and Interventions with *Rationales*
Nursing Diagnosis: *Risk of Ineffective Therapeutic Regimen Management*	**Outcomes:** Prepared to care for self and to prevent insufficiency crisis. ***Evaluation Parameters:*** Patient wears a medical alert bracelet on next clinic visit and shows nurse her medical ID in purse. Patient reports notifying other health care providers (podiatrist, ophthalmologist, and dentist) of medication regimen. Patient able to describe rationale for safety precautions related to long-term use of corticosteroid drugs and the need for gradual tapering off of drugs when they are discontinued.	**Interventions and *Rationales:*** Develop teaching plan with patient and family to ensure adequate understanding of benefits and risks of corticosteroid therapy and measures to be taken for patient safety, including use of medical alert jewelry and ID card, notification of other health care providers, and need for gradual tapering off of corticosteroid medications when these are discontinued. *To enable patient to manage self-care with better understanding of medications and side effects, to enhance safety of patient when undergoing medical procedures with other health care providers, and to alert health care providers to patient's history of corticosteroid use in the event of emergency.*

GERONTOLOGICAL CONSIDERATIONS Related to Adrenal Insufficiency

Older patients are more vulnerable to serious problems with adrenal insufficiency and may require more frequent monitoring and observation. The nurse will want to instruct not only the patient, but a spouse or other caregiver about signs and symptoms of impending crisis so that assistance can be obtained if the patient is unable to seek medical assistance in a timely way, for example, when there is infection or nausea and vomiting.

Discharge Priorities

Preparation of patients for discharge must include instruction regarding the need to take hormone replacement therapy for life. Of particular importance is for patients to understand that stress or illness is likely to increase their need for hydrocortisone. In such situations, they should increase the dosage of hormone as advised by their health care provider.

Persistence of vomiting or diarrhea indicates a need for urgent care, which may include intravenous saline and intramuscular hydrocortisone. Flu-like symptoms should never be ignored because they may be the initial indicators of adrenal crisis. The nurse should coordinate care with a home care or community health agency because effective patient and caregiver education may require the patient to be in more optimal health and because sufficient time must be provided to cover key aspects of care.

Health Promotion

Patients with a history of adrenal insufficiency should wear a medical identification bracelet or necklace and keep an identification card with medical instructions in their wallet or purse. A medical alert in the form of medical identification may enable health care personnel to respond to a patient's need for immediate hormone and fluid replacement and could be life saving. Knowledge about the disease is essential for self-management, particularly during illness or added stress. Thus the patient and a reliable family member should have appropriate follow-up with home care to ensure that they have adequate information and skill to manage the demands of the chronic form of the disease. Patient referral to the appropriate support group is suggested.

Collaborative Management

It is important for the pharmacist, rehabilitation professional, and home health nurse to be involved in providing follow-up care with the patient diagnosed with an adrenal crisis. The patient must be advised about permanent hormone injections and the method of self-administration of intramuscular injections. The pharmacist also should be involved in providing instructions on how to take medications, which is particularly important during periods of stress and illness. It is advisable to have a physical therapist or rehabilitation professional collaborate with the patient in establishing an exercise regimen that can be adapted throughout the year to accommodate seasonal changes.

Hypermetabolic Disorders of the Adrenal Cortex: Cushing's Syndrome

Hypermetabolic disorders of the adrenal cortex include **Cushing's syndrome**, which involves an excess of cortisol, and primary aldosteronism, which involves an excess of aldosterone, which is discussed later in the chapter.

Epidemiology and Etiology

Cushing's syndrome occurs with long-term secretion or exposure to excessive adrenocortical hormones, particularly cortisol and related corticosteroids, and to a lesser extent androgens and aldosterone. Factors known to trigger Cushing's syndrome include problems in the HPA axis that cause excess cortisol release from the adrenal glands, iatrogenic sources such as prednisone therapy, and ectopic courses such as tumors outside of the pituitary that produce ACTH (Holcomb, 2005).

The female-to-male incidence ratio is approximately 6:1 for Cushing's syndrome due to an adrenal or pituitary tumor. Ectopic ACTH production is more frequent in men than in woman because of the increased incidence of lung tumors in the population. The peak incidence of Cushing's syndrome due to either an adrenal or pituitary adenoma occurs in persons ages 25 to 49 years. Ectopic ACTH production due to lung cancer occurs later in life (Holcomb, 2005).

Pathophysiology

An excess of cortisol stimulates anti-inflammatory effects and rapid catabolism of protein and peripheral fat to support hepatic glucose production. One of two mechanisms may be at play. Excess cortisol may be produced because of elevated ACTH levels from the pituitary, which stimulate the adrenal cortex to produce more hormones. Or an excess of cortisol may be produced independent of ACTH production, due to the presence of hormone-producing tumor cells or the administration of cortisone and steroid drugs. The presence of excess cortisone causes systemic physiological manifestations including lipidosis, hypertension due to retention of water and sodium, increased gastric secretions and decreased gastric mucus, increased hepatic gluconeogenesis and insulin resistance, increased antibody formation and lymphocyte production, suppressed inflammatory response, and osteoporosis. These physiological alterations in turn lead to heart disease and/or heart failure, peptic ulcer, impaired glucose tolerance, frequent infections and poor wound healing, and pathologic fractures (Kirk, Hash, Katner, & Jones, 2000).

A majority (approximately 70%) of Cushing's syndrome cases are caused by overproduction of ACTH by the pituitary. Other cases are due to the presence of a tumor outside of the pituitary. Such tumors are usually malignant and often involve a small cell carcinoma of the lung or a pancreatic tumor. Another common cause of Cushing's syndrome is administration of synthetic glucocorticoids or steroids, which are commonly used for chronic inflammatory or immune diseases such as rheumatoid arthritis, ulcerative colitis, systemic lupus, and asthma.

Clinical Manifestations

Patients with Cushing's syndrome will present with a particular pattern of fat deposition on their face and bodies. The face will be round and typically referred to as "moon face" and the trunk will appear large and the patient will be obese with slender arms and legs (Figure 52–10 ■). Acne and purple striae will appear on the face. Fat will be concentrated in fat pads above the clavicle and over the upper back in what is sometimes described as a "buffalo hump." Patients may report a history of poor health, frequent infections with poor wound healing, and sudden weight gain (Holcomb, 2005). Vital signs will indicate hypertension and further evaluation may reveal left ventricular hypertrophy.

Androgen production will cause emphasis of secondary sex characteristics in women with hirsutism, virilism, hypertrophy of the clitoris, and amenorrhea or oligomenorrhea. Muscle wasting and pathologic fractures complete the picture in males and females affected with Cushing's disease (National Adrenal Diseases Foundation, 2006b). Family members also may report that the patient has been irritable and emotionally labile, and cases of steroid-induced psychosis may be seen (Shirk, 2003).

Laboratory and Diagnostic Procedures

Specific laboratory tests of blood and urine will be done to test for excess levels of cortisol. Cortisol production is usually low in the evenings, thus high levels will support a diagnosis of Cushing's syndrome. Specialized suppression tests, such as the dexamethasone suppression test, will be used to help differentiate ACTH-dependent Cushing's syndrome (pituitary dependent or ectopic) from non–ACTH-dependent (adrenal tumor) forms. Blood chemistry for sodium, potassium, and glucose will reveal abnormalities such as high serum sodium and glucose levels. A 24-hour urine sample will be collected for determining free cortisol. A CT scan and MRI will help localize tumors if these are

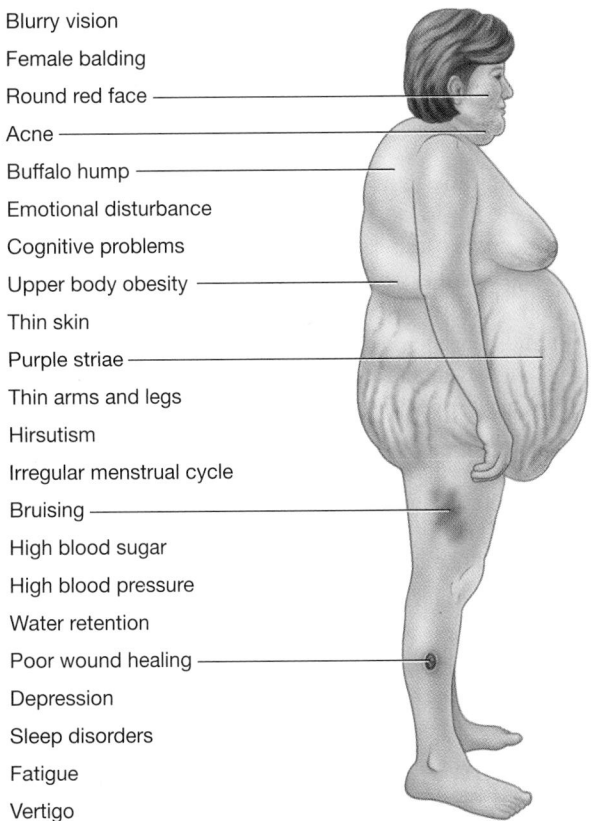

Blurry vision
Female balding
Round red face
Acne
Buffalo hump
Emotional disturbance
Cognitive problems
Upper body obesity
Thin skin
Purple striae
Thin arms and legs
Hirsutism
Irregular menstrual cycle
Bruising
High blood sugar
High blood pressure
Water retention
Poor wound healing
Depression
Sleep disorders
Fatigue
Vertigo

FIGURE 52–10 ■ Patient with Cushing's syndrome.

DIAGNOSTIC TESTS for Cushing's Syndrome

Test	Clinical Value
Urinary free cortisol excretion	Shows excess cortisol excreted in urine, indicating Cushing's syndrome.
Low-dose dexamethasone suppression tests	Helps distinguish pituitary from ectopic corticotrophin-dependent Cushing's syndrome.
Late night serum and salivary cortisol	Demonstrates presence of Cushing's syndrome if late night levels of cortisol are high.
CRH stimulation test	Aids in diagnosing ectopic corticotrophin production.
Inferior petrosal sinus sampling	Localizes the site of ACTH production.
CT scan	Provides evidence of pituitary or other tumor/malignancy.
MRI	Provides evidence of pituitary or other tumor/malignancy.

Sources: Adapted from Boscaro, M., Barzon, L., Fallo, F., & Sonino, N. (2001). Cushing's syndrome. *Lancet, 357,* 783–791; Kirk, L. F., Hash, R. B., Katner, H. P., & Jones, T. (2000). Cushing's disease: Clinical manifestations and diagnostic evaluation. *American Family Physician, 62*(5), 1119– 1127, 1133–1134; Porth, 2007.

causing the disease. Refer to the Diagnostic Tests for Cushing's Syndrome box for a list of the tests that can be used for differential diagnosis in hypermetabolic adrenal states.

Medical Management

Management of Cushing's syndrome is directed at the etiology of the disease. Surgery is the primary intervention for tumors of the adrenal or pituitary glands or other tissue such as the lung. Transsphenoidal microsurgery, as described earlier in this chapter, is used to remove pituitary tumors that are stimulating excessive ACTH production. Radiation therapy also may be used for tumors in the pituitary or other locations. In some cases, surgery may not be indicated and drugs may be used to counter the effect of excess production of adrenal hormones. One such drug is Mitotane (Lysodren), an adrenal cytotoxic preparation, which suppresses adrenal gland function and helps to reduce blood glucose and blood pressure. Mitotane decreases the size of adrenal tumors and reduces symptoms caused by excess hormone secretion. Aminoglutethimide (Cytadren) is another adrenal steroid inhibitor, which can be used to decrease production of adrenal hormones. Side effects of both drugs include gastrointestinal symptoms, lethargy, dizziness, depression, and vertigo. Patients can minimize effects by taking the medication with meals or a snack (Anderson, 2002). Caution should be used in the event a patient experiences trauma, infection, or other physiologically stressful event while taking mitotane or aminoglutethimide since these drugs may seriously impair the patient's ability to increase hormone production in response to the stress.

In patients for whom Cushing's syndrome is caused by long-term administration of corticosteroid drugs, a plan for gradual withdrawal or reduction of medication is indicated. Corticosteroids cannot be abruptly withdrawn because the patient may experience an adrenal crisis with symptoms of hypoadrenal function. Gradual reduction in dosage and administration of medications on alternate days will help minimize the suppression of normal hormone production.

The Gerontological Considerations box discusses elderly patients with Cushing's syndrome.

■ Nursing Management

Nursing care for patients with transsphenoidal surgery, indicated for patients whose Cushing's syndrome is caused by

GERONTOLOGICAL CONSIDERATIONS Related to Cushing's Syndrome

Quality of life for patients with Cushing's syndrome is often compromised by changes associated with the disorder, including distorted body image and the physical and psychological symptoms of excess hormone production. Elderly patients are most vulnerable to stress and other factors that may precipitate a crisis to which their bodies cannot readily respond because of a disorder of the adrenal glands. Observation and careful assessment of elderly patients with Cushing's syndrome will reduce the incidence of complications and death in this population. Elderly patients may be poor surgical risks, thus medical management of Cushing's syndrome is the preferred treatment option.

ACTH stimulation from the pituitary gland, was described earlier in this chapter. Routine nursing care will focus on regular assessment of vital signs, symptoms of hormone or drug toxicity, signs of fever or infection, and complications such as cardiovascular events, diabetes mellitus, depression, and suicide.

Assessment

Specific nursing assessments for suspected Cushing's syndrome will relate to the presence of excess cortisol and ACTH. When taking a patient history for Cushing's syndrome the nurse must be alert for potential precipitating factors such as hypothalamus or pituitary dysfunction or corticosteroid therapy. Face and body distribution of fat must be noted. Acne and purple striae on the face may be present, as well as the development of secondary sex characteristics in women such as hirsutism, virilism, and menstrual dysfunction. Vital sign assessments may indicate the presence of hypertension. Musculoskeletal strength should also be noted. Subjective complaints of weight gain are important, as are family reports of irritability and emotional changes.

Nursing Diagnosis

Primary nursing diagnoses for the patient with Cushing's syndrome will focus on improvement of self-esteem and body image, as well as complications of the disease process. Interpersonal relationships may also have been affected by body changes in patients. Problems related to cardiovascular and musculoskeletal complications may also be present.

Planning

Planning care of the patient with Cushing's syndrome will relate to nursing diagnoses that focus on body image, self-esteem, and relationships. The nurse must prepare the client for multiple diagnostic testing, which will include both serum and urine samples. Some treatment protocols involve surgery, as well as radiation and other pharmacologic interventions. Planning for the management of side effects from treatment must be a priority for the nurse.

Outcomes and Evaluation Parameters

As mentioned in the medical management section, the goals of treatment for Cushing's syndrome focus on the etiology of the disease. Because surgery is often the primary intervention, the nurse should establish goals related to pre- and postoperative patient care and the prevention of complications following surgery. Radiation and or pharmacologic therapy may also be indicated.

The nurse should then establish patient care goals related to adherence to a medical regimen, as well as goals that foster an improvement in the patient's body image, self-esteem, and interpersonal relationships.

Interventions and Rationales

The nurse should monitor the patient for baseline and ongoing measurements related to body characteristics and vital signs. Cardiovascular and musculoskeletal assessments should be monitored. Educational sessions for teaching must be a priority to assist the patient and family members to understand the changes that have occurred in the patients' bodies. Interventions to enhance self-esteem and interpersonal relationships will also be a priority. In the case of surgery, nursing interventions related to both pre- and postoperative care must be implemented.

Evaluation

While undergoing medical care for Cushing's syndrome, the patient should verbalize the rationale for adhering to the treatment regimen. Patients and family members should be able to verbalize what is causing the changes to their bodies, and how these changes have an impact on their physical and emotional well-being. When surgery is indicated, the patient should verbalize an understanding of the procedure, as well as the pre- and postoperative care required.

Discharge Priorities

The goal of care is to return adrenal function to normal and to stabilize hormone levels within a normal range. Prevention and early identification of infection is another goal in light of the body's compromised ability to respond to such stress. Patients who have had a long-standing surplus of corticosteroid hormone are likely to be emotionally labile and subject to serious depression and psychosis. Suicide precautions may be necessary and family members should be alerted to the need to report signs of worsening emotional stability to health care providers.

Hypermetabolic Disorders of the Adrenal Cortex: Hyperaldosteronism

Hyperaldosteronism is a disorder in which the adrenal cortex overproduces the hormone aldosterone, leading to hypertension in affected individuals. Primary hyperaldosteronism occurs when the adrenal gland itself is diseased and secondary hyperaldosteronism occurs when the etiology is outside of the adrenal glands. At one time it was believed that this disorder was responsible for a very small percentage of patients with hypertension, but improvements in screening techniques indicate the incidence is more prevalent (Mayo Clinic, 2005; Mulatero et al., 2004).

Pathophysiology, Risk Factors, and Clinical Picture

Primary aldosteronism, which is responsible for up to 70% of cases, usually is caused by a benign adenoma that produces excess aldosterone or stimulates adjacent cells to secrete excess hormone. Conn's disease, a condition in which the kidneys retain sodium and excrete potassium, is the name given to the disorder when it involves an adrenal adenoma. Other, less common causes of the disease are adrenal cancers and genetic mutations (which are rare) and adrenal hyperplasia (overactivity of both glands).

Patients present with hypertension, which does not respond well to medication or other treatment, as well as headache, orthostatic hypotension, muscle weakness and cramps, fatigue, temporary paralysis, constipation, numbness, pricking, tingling sensations, excessive thirst, and urination (HealthAtoZ, 2002). Hypokalemia and low plasma renin also are noted. Hypertension in combination with hypokalemia should receive further investigation for aldosteronism because the presence of hypokalemia is often indicative of high levels of aldosterone (Shah, 2006). A condition that causes high blood pressure in children and young adults is a rare type of this disease that runs in families and is called glucocorticoid-remediable aldosteronism (GRA) (Mayo Clinic, 2005).

Laboratory and Diagnostic Procedures

Laboratory measurements of aldosterone and renin levels are taken to measure hormone levels. An adrenal vein sample of blood may be drawn by the radiologist from the right and left adrenal veins to determine if aldosterone levels are high in one or both adrenal glands. This will help determine which gland has an adenoma or whether both glands are affected by hyperplasia. An oral salt or saline loading test or fludrocortisone suppression test (FST) may be administered to determine whether the aldosterone level remains high when it would normally decline. A CT scan will help to confirm the presence and location of an adenoma. Screening and detection of aldosteronism is important because studies indicate a high incidence of cardiovascular events such as stroke in patients with the disease.

Medical Management

Surgical removal of the aldosteronoma can bring significant symptom relief and is the treatment of choice. Hypertension may continue to be a problem, but it can often be controlled more effectively with medications. Management of hypertension will reduce the risk of kidney disease, as well as strokes and other cardiovascular problems (HealthAtoZ, 2002). Antihypertensive drugs such as calcium channel blockers may be prescribed for treatment. Potassium-sparing diuretics are another treatment option to reduce blood volume through diuresis. Potassium levels should be monitored for patients on diuretics.

A widely used drug for this condition is spironolactone, however, it is not advised in patients with kidney disease. Long-term spironolactone drug therapy causes impotence and gynecomastia in men, so this medication is generally used only for women. Another drug, amiloride, is the drug of choice for control of symptoms in men (Shah, 2006).

Nursing Management

Patients' vital signs should be monitored frequently and they should be advised to check their blood pressure at home in order to provide regular reports to their health care provider. In addition to monitoring vital signs and dressings postoperatively, the nurse should work with the patient and family to develop an instructional plan to cover monitoring medications, diet, and activity at home. If hypertension continues to be a problem, the nurse will recommend stress reduction strategies, including meditation, biofeedback, yoga, massage therapy, and diet and exercise to assist in reduction of blood pressure.

Hypermetabolic Disorder of the Adrenal Medulla: Pheochromocytoma

Pheochromocytoma is a rare, usually nonmalignant tumor of the adrenal medulla that causes a hypermetabolic condition characterized by excess production of the hormones of the adrenal medulla.

Pathophysiology, Risk Factors, and Clinical Manifestations

The adrenal medulla produces hormones known as catecholamines, including the hormones epinephrine and norepinephrine. Epinephrine stimulates the heart rate and stroke volume and raises blood sugar levels. Norepinephrine stimulates the sympathetic nervous system. Pheochromocytoma, a rare tumor of the adrenal medulla, causes hypertension by producing an excess of epinephrine (adrenalin) and norepinephrine. The disease typically strikes men and women equally between 40 and 60 years of age. About 5% to 10% of cases appear to have a hereditary component, particularly those cases in which there is involvement of both glands (American Urological Association, 2006; Braunwald et al., 2001). Hypertension may be episodic or long standing, and it can become life threatening. Hypertensive paroxysms in which the patient experiences dangerously high blood pressure, profuse sweating, nausea, and other symptoms may be triggered by specific events such as emotional stress, trigger foods, abdominal pressure, tobacco, and selected drugs, including histamine and glucagon. In addition to hypertension, patients with pheochromocytoma may experience headache, tachycardia, and palpitations (American Urological Association [AUA], 2006).

Laboratory and Diagnostic Procedures

Diagnostic tests include 24-hour blood and urine measurements of catecholamine metabolites. Upper limits for catecholamines are 590 to 885 nmol per 24 hours. In patients with pheochromocytoma, values of 1480 nmol and higher are seen. Assays of free or unconjugated catecholamines are also helpful in diagnosis. CT scans and MRI can be used to determine location and size of the tumor (Braunwald et al., 2001).

Medical Management

Treatment involves laparoscopic surgical removal of the tumor, which may involve one or both adrenal glands. A laparoscopic approach minimizes scarring, lowers the risk of hernias at the surgical site, reduces postoperative pain, and provides for shorter hospital stays and recovery time. Surgery is more successful in reducing blood pressure if symptoms have been of short duration. Long-standing hypertension is more difficult to reverse, even with surgery (AUA, 2006). Medical management of hypertension may be required following surgery, and drugs such as alpha-adrenergic blockers may be given to block excess hormone and lower blood pressure.

Nursing Management

Most surgical procedures for adrenal tumor removal today are non-invasive in nature; therefore, making the patient's recovery course and period easier than open surgery. Postoperatively, the nurse will be concerned with observation of the operative site, management of the patient's pain, and management of the patient's blood pressure and vital signs. Postoperative teaching includes informing the patient that she may engage in light activity while at home after surgery and can remove any dressings and shower the day after the operation. Normal routine activities, such as driving, may be resumed within a week. Typical postoperative care is discussed at length in Chapter 27 🔗.

Health Promotion in Hypermetabolic Adrenal Disorders

Adrenal hormone levels will decline and begin to return to normal with treatment whether it is through elimination of a tumor or gradual withdrawal of corticosteroid therapy. Physiological and psychological changes may occur in the patient over several weeks. Patients should be encouraged to maintain a low-sodium, moderate-carbohydrate, low-fat diet to counteract the effects of excess hormone.

An exercise plan should be initiated with gradual resumption of activities. Such a program enhances cardiovascular health and builds muscle and bone tissues that become weakened in cases of Cushing's syndrome. Hypertension should be monitored on a long-term basis because treatment may be required for persistent hypertension in spite of removal of tumor tissue.

Collaborative Management in Adrenal Disorders

Collaborative care will involve the primary care provider, endocrinologist, surgeon, pharmacist, and nutritionist. Management of these rare disorders will require specialized expertise for optimal results. Communication and coordination among members of the health care team will be essential as the patient moves from clinic to hospital to home settings. Patient support and instruction on these complex medical problems will help to allay anxiety and decrease stress. Instruction and involvement of family members is essential given that patients may have to rely on family members for assistance in the event of a medical crisis.

Cultural and Genetic Considerations for Adrenal Disorders

Individuals with congenital or long-term adrenal insufficiency and patients with successful surgical treatment of pituitary tumors may require a lifetime of replacement hormone therapy. In some cultures, a need for continued therapy will stigmatize the individual as "sick" or illness prone, making it more difficult for the individual to maintain a normal life. Patient's and families may not be aware that one of the most famous U.S. presidents, John F. Kennedy, had Addison's disease and in spite of a heavy regimen of medications he was able to stand for election and serve in one of the most demanding jobs in the world. Patients should be encouraged to become as well informed about their disease as possible to enhance effective self-care of adrenal insufficiency.

Autoimmune disorders and congenital adrenal hyperplasia, genetics, and pituitary tumor development cause adrenal insufficiency through either hypo- or hypermetabolic function of the adrenal glands. Early screening of newborns will help to prevent avoidable deaths due to adrenal crisis that may go unrecognized. Parents also may benefit from genetic counseling, which will explain how a disease such as congenital adrenal hyperplasia or other disorders are inherited and options for future pregnancies. Research on genetic causes of adrenal disorders and potential gene therapies offer much potential for the future.

Research

Significant advances have been made in the diagnoses and treatment of endocrine disorders in recent years due to the development of new diagnostic imaging technologies, an immunoassay test of hormones, improved laboratory techniques for genetic studies, and new synthetic hormones and hormone agonists. The development of minimally invasive surgeries for pituitary, parathyroid, and adrenal tumors has been beneficial in the treatment of endocrine disorders. There have also been significant advances in the understanding of genetic factors underlying many endocrine disorders. The role of infection, stress, autoimmune disease, and genetics continues to impact the exploration of endocrine disease etiology and pathology. The field of genetics, genetic counseling, and gene therapy all hold significant promise in endocrinology in the future.

Improvement in clinical management of endocrine diseases is another important frontier in research. Although medical and surgical interventions, as well as hormone replacement therapy, have reaped big rewards in patient management and outcomes, some patients report decreased quality of life despite treatment. This suggests that although hormone levels may appear to be normal after therapy is initiated in endocrine disease, other complex physiological and psychological factors are at play in restoring patients to optimal health. Nurses in ambulatory clinics could play a role in investigating quality-of-life issues for patients with endocrine disease.

Many of the endocrine problems described in this chapter are rare, but they are very debilitating and even life threatening when they occur. Prevention of these diseases offers the most hope for optimal clinical impact because usually when endocrine disorders are established, the treatment is for a lifetime. Increasing the genetic screening of infants at birth for potentially treatable endocrine diseases such as congenital adrenal hyperplasia would certainly save lives. Studies on the genetic etiology of endocrine disease and potential gene therapy also offer significant potential benefits in terms of disease prevention. However, ethical questions abound and funding for this kind of research may not be seen as a top priority.

Other avenues of research that could have a significant clinical impact are those that focus on early identification and treatment of hormonal disorders such as severe hypo- or hyperthyroidism, Cushing's syndrome, gigantism, and acromegaly. Early diagnosis would prevent some of the irreversible physiological changes that occur with such diseases. Studies to determine the etiology of autoimmune disorders of the endocrine glands also hold promise for prevention and treatment. The endocrine system is exquisitely designed to maintain homeostasis in the body in spite of rapidly changing environmental conditions. Disease disrupts and interferes with the exquisite balance and adaptability that exists in an optimally functioning endocrine system. In this situation, regaining optimal health is a bit like putting Humpty Dumpty back together again. Advances in biochemistry, technology, genetics, and pharmacology all offer hope in the search for cures and care of the patient with endocrine problems.

Clinical Preparation

 CRITICAL THINKING

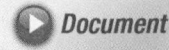

▶ Read	**▶ Document**	**▶ Apply**
• History of Current Illness • Past Medical History • Physical Exam • Admitting Medical Orders • Laboratory Study Results	• Summary of Hospitalization • Pathophysiology Form • Laboratory Values • Laboratory Results Explanation	• List of Potential Nursing Diagnoses • Concept Map • Critical Thinking Questions

Log on to MyNursingKit.com to download forms you will need and to complete further steps in the Clinical Preparation assignment.

HISTORY OF PRESENT ILLNESS

Mrs. B is a 49-year-old female who has been seen in your clinic for her primary health care needs for several years. On a recent visit, you note that she has gained approximately 20 pounds during the past year. She complains of constant fatigue, cold intolerance, and difficulty concentrating. She indicates that her performance at work has declined, that she does not feel as mentally alert as usual, and that she is slower to complete tasks than previously.

Medical–Surgical History

Mrs. B has had an unremarkable medical history with the exception of a short episode of rheumatoid arthritis in her early 30s. The disease responded well to treatment and she has been in remission since that time. Until now she has maintained good physical health. She takes no medications except a daily multivitamin and an occasional aspirin. She has had no surgeries. Regular Pap smears and mammograms have been negative for disease.

Social History

Mrs. B does not smoke, and drinks alcohol only rarely. She works as an administrative assistant in a local engineering firm. She is divorced and a single parent with two healthy adult children.

Physical Examination

Physical examination reveals dry skin and hair that is dry and thinning in spots. The thyroid gland appears enlarged upon palpation. Lungs are clear. The abdomen is slightly distended. Abdominal sounds are diminished and, upon questioning, the patient reports recent bouts of constipation. Vital signs are within normal limits.

Laboratory Studies

Laboratory studies to assess the level of free T_4 and TSH are completed. The TSH level is high and the free T_4 level is low, indicating an underfunctioning thyroid.

Nursing Care

The patient is given a prescription for thyroid hormone replacement therapy and instructed about its use. She is to take levothyroxine each day early in the morning on an empty stomach. Follow-up appointments are scheduled for 8-week intervals during the next 6 months for continued evaluation of hormone levels to determine whether the dosage is adequate, symptoms abate, and the thyroid gland changes in size. The patient is encouraged to increase fluid and dietary fiber intake and exercise to reduce constipation and to aid in weight loss.

CRITICAL THINKING QUESTIONS

1. Identify prevailing symptoms of Mrs. B, with underlying rationale, that led to assessing her for hypothyroidism.
2. Explain the relevance of a low T_4 level and high TSH level in arriving at a diagnosis of hypothyroidism.
3. In developing an outpatient plan of care for the home setting, what key elements with rationale would you consider discussing with Mrs. B?

Answers to Critical Thinking Questions appear in Appendix D.

NCLEX® REVIEW

1. A patient is diagnosed with gastric and duodenal ulcers. The nurse realizes that this patient might experience alterations in which of the following hormones?
   1. Progesterone
   2. Enterogastrone
   3. Angiotensinogen
   4. Calcitriol

2. A 13-year-old patient is diagnosed with an overproduction of a hormone produced by the anterior pituitary gland. The nurse realizes this patient is experiencing:
   1. Gigantism.
   2. Acromegaly.
   3. Sheehan's syndrome.
   4. Infertility.

3. A patient with hypothyroidism is prescribed levothyroxine. Which of the following should the nurse instruct this patient?
   1. Take with an antacid.
   2. Take the medication first thing in the morning on an empty stomach.
   3. Expect the symptoms to subside immediately.
   4. This medication is taken temporarily until the symptoms subside.

4. A patient is admitted with palpitations, hand tremors, muscle weakness, and muscle cramps. Which of the following endocrine disorders should be considered as the cause of this patient's symptoms?
   1. Pheochromocytoma
   2. Hyperthyroidism
   3. Hypothyroidism
   4. Diabetes insipidus

5. The nurse is planning discharge instructions for a patient with diabetes insipidus. Which of the following should be included in these instructions?
   1. The need for frequent rest periods
   2. Strategies to have access to fluids at all times
   3. Availability of high sodium foods
   4. Progressive ambulation activities

6. An elderly patient recovering from back surgery is demonstrating signs of hypothermia. Which of the following should the nurse do to assist this patient?
   1. Increase fluids.
   2. Provide oxygen.
   3. Consider the onset of myxedema coma and contact the health care provider.
   4. Provide warm blankets.

7. A patient recovering from an endocrine disorder tells the nurse that even though the hormone levels are considered "normal," she still feels "terrible." Which of the following should the nurse respond to this patient?
   1. What part of your life is terrible?
   2. That is to be expected.
   3. Everyone goes through this.
   4. I'm sure that you will feel better in time.

Answers for review questions appear in Appendix D

KEY TERMS

acromegaly *p.1639*
Addisonian crisis (adrenal crisis) *p.1648*
Addison's disease *p.1647*
adrenal insufficiency *p.1648*
chronic lymphocytic thyroiditis *p.1618*
Chvostek's sign *p.1633*
cretinism *p.1617*
Cushing's syndrome *p.1651*
diabetes insipidus (DI) *p.1642*
euthyroid *p.1622*
exophthalmus *p.1626*
galactorrhea *p.1639*
gigantism *p.1639*

goiter *p.1619*
goitrogen *p.1619*
Graves' disease *p.1625*
Hashimoto's thyroiditis *p.1618*
hyperparathyroidism *p.1633*
hyperthyroidism *p.1614*
hypoparathyroidism *p.1633*
hypopituitarism *p.1637*
hypothyroidism *p.1614*
myxedema *p.1619*
myxedema coma *p.1624*
negative feedback *p.1613*
osteitis fibrosa cystica *p.1634*

panhypopituitarism *p.1637*
pheochromocytoma *p.1654*
primary adrenal insufficiency *p.1648*
psychogenic polydipsia *p.1643*
secondary adrenal insufficiency *p.1648*
syndrome of inappropriate antidiuretic hormone (SIADH) *p.1644*
thyroid storm *p.1627*
thyroidectomy *p.1618*
thyroiditis *p.1619*
thyromegaly *p.1626*
thyrotoxicosis *p.1625*
Trousseau's sign *p.1633*

REFERENCES

American Association of Clinical Endocrinologists. (2005a). *Hashimoto's thyroiditis: Information for patients.* Retrieved September 19, 2005, from http://www.aace.com/members/brochures.php

American Association of Clinical Endocrinologists. (2005b). *Hyperthyroidism: Information for patients.* Retrieved September 19, 2005, from http://www.aace.com/members/brochures.php

American Association of Clinical Endocrinologists. (2005c). *Hypothyroidism: Information for patients.* Retrieved September 19, 2005, from http://www.aace.com/members/brochures.php

American Association of Clinical Endocrinologists. (2005d). *The thyroid nodule: Information for patients.* Retrieved September 19, 2005, from http://www.aace.com/members/brochures.php

American Cancer Society. (2006). *Do we know what causes pituitary tumors?* Retrieved June 12, 2008, from http://www.cancer.org/docroot/CRI/content/CRI_2_4_2X_Do_we_know_what_causes_pituitary_tumors_61.asp?rnav=cri

American Thyroid Association. (2005). *ATA Alliance for Thyroid Patient Education.* Retrieved September 19, 2005, from http://www.thyroid.org/patients/links.html

American Urological Association. (2006). *Pheochromocytoma.* Accessed March 7, 2006, from http://www.UrologyHealth.org.adult/index

Anderson, T. (2002). *Atlas of pathophysiology.* Springhouse, PA: Springhouse Corporation.

Baird, A., Sullivan, T., Zafar, S., & Rock, J. (2003). Quality of life in patients with pituitary tumors: A preliminary study. *Quality Management in Health Care, 12*(2), 97–105.

Bayless, P. (2003). The syndrome of inappropriate antidiuretic hormone secretion. *International Journal of Biochemistry and Cellular Biology, 35,* 1495–1499.

Bharaktiya, S., Orlander, P. R., Woodhouse, W. R., & Davis, A. B. (2007). Hypothyroidism. *eMedicine.* Retrieved June 19, 2008, from http://www.emedicine.com/med/topic1145.htm

Boscaro, M., Barzon, L., Fallo, F., & Sonino, N. (2001). Cushing's syndrome. *Lancet, 357,* 783–791.

Braunwald, E., Hauser, S. L., Fauci, A. S., Longo, D. L., Kasper, D. L., & Jameson, J. L. (2001). *Harrison's principles of internal medicine* (15th ed.). New York: McGraw-Hill.

Carr, S. (2001). Acromegaly management in the community. *Journal of the American Geriatric Society, 50*(5), 970–972.

Chan, M., Ziebert, M., Maas, D., & Chan, P. (2005). Photo quiz: "My rings won't fit anymore." *American Family Physician, 71*(9), 1766–1767.

Colorado State University. (2000). *Pathophysiology of the endocrine system.* Retrieved on March 6, 2003, from http://www.colostate.edu

Colorado State University. (2003). *Congenital adrenal hyperplasia.* Retrieved March 8, 2006, from http://www.colostate.edu

Cooper, D. S. (2005). Antithyroid drugs. *New England Journal of Medicine, 352*(9), 905–917.

Cooperman, M. (2008). Diabetes insipidus. *eMedicine.* Retrieved June 12, 2008, from http://www.emedicine.com/med/topic543.htm

Coursin, D. B., & Wood, K. E. (2002). Corticosteroid supplementation for adrenal insufficiency. *Journal of the American Medical Association, 287*(2), 236–240.

Dahlen, R. (2002). Managing patients with acute thyrotoxicosis. *Critical Care Nurse, 22*(1), 62–69.

Dorton, A. M. (2000). The pituitary gland: Embryology, physiology, and pathophysiology. *Neonatal Network, 19*(2), 9–17.

Elliott, B. (2000). Diagnosing and treating hypothyroidism. *The Nurse Practitioner, 25*(3), 92–103.

EndocrineWeb. (2002a). *Hyperthyroidism, overactivity of the thyroid gland. Part 2: Causes of hyperthyroidism.* Retrieved September 19, 2005, from http://endocrineweb.com/hyper2.html

EndocrineWeb. (2002b). *Pheochromocytoma.* Retrieved March 10, 2006, from http://endocrineweb.com/pheo.html

Ezell, J. (2006). What is secondary adrenal insufficiency? *Nursing, 36*(5).

Fenton, C. L., Gold, J. G., & Sadeghi-Nejad, A. (2006). Hyperthyroidism. *eMedicine.* Retrieved June 8, 2008, from http://www.emedicine.com/ped/TOPIC1088.HTM

Ferry, R. J., & Pascual-y-Baralt, J. F. (2007). Syndrome of inappropriate antidiuretics hormone secretion. *eMedicine.* Retrieved June 12, 2008, from http://www.emedicine.com/ped/topic2190.htm

Ferry, R. J., & Shim, M. (2006). Hyperpituitarism. *eMedicine.* Retrieved June 12, 2008, from http://www.emedicine.com/PED/topic1092.htm

Franklin, J. A., Sheppard, M. C., & Maisonneuve, P. (2005). Thyroid function and mortality in patients treated for hyperthyroidism. *Journal of the American Medical Association, 294*(1), 71–80.

Gonzalez-Campoy, J. M. (2007). Hypoparathyroidism. *eMedicine.* Retrieved June 12, 2008, from http://www.emedicine.com/MEDS/Topic1131.htm

Greco, L. K. (2001). Hypothyroid emergencies. *Topics in Emergency Medicine, 23*(4), 44–50.

Greenspan, F. S. (2004). The thyroid gland. In F. S. Greenspan & D. G. Gardner (Eds.), *Basic and clinical endocrinology* (7th ed., pp. 215–294). New York: Lang Medical Books/McGraw-Hill.

Harris, C. (2007). Recognizing thyroid storm in the neurologically impaired patient. *Journal of Neuroscience Nursing, 39*(1), 40–42, 57.

HealthAtoZ. (2002). *Hyperaldosteronism.* Retrieved March 8, 2006, from http://www.healthatoz.com

Holcomb, S. (2002a). Diabetes insipidus. *Dimensions of Critical Care Nursing, 21*(3), 94–97.

Holcomb, S. (2002b). Stopping the cascade of diabetes insipidus. *Nursing, 32*(3), 32cc1–32cc2, 32cc4, 32cc6.

Holcomb, S. (2002c). Thyroid diseases: A primer for the critical care nurse. *Dimensions of Critical Care Nursing, 21*(4), 127–133.

Holcomb, S. (2003). Detecting thyroid disease, Part 1. *Nursing, 33*(8), 32cc1–32cc4.

Holcomb, S. (2005). Confronting Cushing's syndrome. *Nursing, 35*(9), 32hn1–32hn6.

Holcomb, S. (2006). Do the clues add up to Addison's disease? *Nursing 2006, 36*(3), 64hn1–64hn4.

Hollowell, J. G., Staehling, N. W., Flanders, W. D., Hannon, H., Gunter, E. W., Spencer C. A., et al. (2002). Serum TSH, T_4, and thyroid antibodies in the United States population (1988 to 1994): National Health and Nutrition Examination Survey (NHANES III). *Journal of Clinical Endocrinology & Metabolism, 87*(2), 489–499.

Hormone Foundation. (2006). *Endocrine glands.* Retrieved January 24, 2006, from http://www.hormone.org/endo101/index.html

Innis, J. (2002a). Recognizing lithium induced diabetes insipidus. *Nursing, 32*(6), 32cc12, 32cc15.

Innis, J. (2002b). Treating nephrogenic diabetes insipidus. *Dimensions of Critical Care Nursing, 21*(3), 98–99.

Jordan, S. (2005). Prescription drugs: Uses and effects. Thyroid disorders: Symptom control. *Nursing Standard, 19*(23), 56–58.

Kattah, J. (2006). Pituitary tumors. *EMedicine.* Retrieved August 28, 2008 from http://www.emedicine.com/NEURO/topic312.htm

Kajantie, E., Phillips, D. I., Osmond, C., Barker, D. J., Forsen, T., & Eriksson, J. G. (2006). Spontaneous hypothyroidism in adult women is predicated by small body size at birth and during childhood. *Journal of Endocrinology Metabolism, 91*(12), 4953–4958.

Katznelson, L. (2006). *Medical management of acromegaly with octreotide.* Retrieved March 7, 2006, from Massachusetts General Hospital website: http://pituitary.mgh.edu/e-f-943.htm

Kirk, L. F., Hash, R. B., Katner, H. P., & Jones, T. (2000). Cushing's disease: Clinical manifestations and diagnostic evaluation. *American Family Physician, 62*(5), 1119–1127, 1133–1134.

Langfeldt, L. A., & Cooley, M. E. (2003). Syndrome of inappropriate antidiuretic hormone secretion in malignancy: Review and implications for nursing management. *Clinical Journal of Oncology Nursing, 7*(4), 425–430.

Larson, J., Anderson, E., & Koslawy, M. (2000). Thyroid disease: A review for primary care. *Journal of the American Academy of Nurse Practitioners, 12*(6), 226–232.

Laws, E. R., Vance, M. L., & Thapar, K. (2000). Pituitary surgery for the management of acromegaly. *Hormone Research, 53*(Suppl. 3), 71–75.

Loffing, J. (2004). Paradoxical antidiuretics effect of thiazides in diabetes insipidus: Another piece in the puzzle. *Journal of the American Society of Nephrology, 15,* 2948–2950.

Løvås, K., & Husebye, E. S. (2005). Addison's disease. *Lancet 365*(9476), 2058–2061.

Luken, K. K. (1999). Pearls for practice: Clinical manifestations and management of Addison's disease. *Journal of the American Academy of Nurse Practitioners, 11*(4), 151–154.

Mayo Clinic. (2005). *Primary aldosteronism.* Retrieved from http://www.mayclinic.com/health/primary-aldosteronism

Mayo Clinic. (2006). *Sheehan's syndrome.* Retrieved February 10, 2006, from http://www.mayoclinic.com/health/sheehans-syndrome/AN01084

Medline Plus. (2001). *Cabergoline (systemic).* Retrieved March 7, 2006, from http://www.nlm.nih.gov/medlineplus/druginfo/uspdi/203584.html

Medline Plus. (2004). *Prolactinoma.* Retrieved March 7, 2006, from http://www.nlm.nih.gov/medlineplus/ency/article/000336.htm

Medline Plus. (2005). *Octreotide (systemic).* Retrieved March 7, 2006, from http://www.nlm.nih.gov/medlineplus/druginfo/uspdi/202421.html

Mulatero, P., Stowasser, M., Loh, K., Fardella, C., Gordon, R., Mosso, L., et al. (2004). Increased diagnosis of primary aldosteronism, including surgically correctable forms, in centers from five continents. *The Journal of Clinical Endocrinology & Metabolism, 89*(3), 1045–1050. Retrieved March 8, 2006, from http://jcen.endojournals.org

National Adrenal Diseases Foundation. (2006a). *Adrenal diseases—Addison's disease.* Retrieved January 24, 2006, from http://www.medhelp.org/nadf/diseases/addisons.htm

National Adrenal Diseases Foundation. (2006b). *Adrenal diseases—Cushing's syndrome.* Retrieved January 24, 2006, from http://www.medhelp.org/nadf/diseases/cushings.htm

Neafsey, P. J. (2004). Levothyroxine and calcium interaction: Timing is everything. *Home Health Nurse, 22*(5), 338–339.

Nephrogenic Diabetes Insipidus Foundation. (2005a). *Facts and statistics: Definition.* Retrieved February 12, 2006, from http://www.ndif.org/facts/html

Nephrogenic Diabetes Insipidus Foundation. (2005b). *Facts and statistics: Description.* Retrieved February 12, 2006, from http://www.ndif.org/facts/html

Odeke, S., & Nagelbereg, S. B. (2006). Addison disease. *eMedicine.* Retrieved June 8, 2008, from http://www.emedicine.com/med/TOPIC42.HTM

Pavlovich-Danis, S. (2006). Zemplar: New treatment option for secondary hyperparathyroidism. *Nursing Spectrum, 16*(6), 23.

Pfadt, E., & Carlson, D. (2006). Action stat: Acute adrenal crisis. *Nursing 2006, 36*(8), 80.

Physician's drug handbook (11th ed.). (2005). Philadelphia: Lippincott Williams & Wilkins.

Pituitary Disorders Education & Support. (2006a). *Pituitary conditions and treatment.* Retrieved February 10, 2006, from www.pituitarydisorder.net/pituitary_conditions_treatments.html

Pituitary Network Association. (2006a). *Adrenal insufficiency: Secondary Addison's or Addison's disease.* Retrieved February 10, 2006, from http://www.pituitary.org/disorders/addisons_disease.aspx

Pituitary Network Association. (2006b). Adult growth hormone (GH). Deficiency. Retrieved February 10, 2006, from http://www.pituitary.org/disorders/gh_deficiency.aspx

Pituitary Network Association. (2006c). *Endocrine—inactive (i.e., non-functional tumors).* Retrieved February 10, 2006, from http://www.pituitary.org/disorders/non-functioning_tumors.aspx

Pituitary Network Association. (2006e). *Hypopituitarism.* Retrieved February 10, 2006, from http://www.pituitary.org/disorders/hypopituitarism.aspx

Porsche, R., & Brenner, Z. (2006). Amiodarone-induced thyroid dysfunction. *Critical Care Nurse, 26*(3), 34–42.

Porth, C. M. (2007). *Essentials of pathophysiology: Concepts of altered health states* (2nd ed.). Philadelphia: Lippincott Williams & Wilkins.

Sachse, D. (2001). Acromegaly. *American Journal of Nursing, 101*(11), 69, 71, 73–75.

Shah, N. (2006).Unexplained weakness in a newly diagnosed hypertensive. *Clinical Advisor for Nurse Practitioners, 9*(10), 106.

Shirk, M. (2003). Hallelujah! A case of steroid psychosis and unorthodox intervention. *American Journal of Nursing, 103*(9), 31.

Song, J. K., & Weil, R. J. (2005). Pathologic quiz case: An unusual cause of acromegaly. *Archives of Pathology and Laboratory Medicine, 129*(3), 415–416.

Takasu, N., Takara, M., & Komiya, I. (2005). Rifampin-induced hypothyroidism in patients with Hashimoto's thyroiditis. *New England Journal of Medicine, 352*(5), 518–519.

Tangiera, E. C. (2004). Hyperparathyroidism. *American Family Physician, 69,* 333–340.

Teng, W., et al. (2006). Effect of iodine intake on thyroid diseases in China. *New England Journal of Medicine, 354*(26), 2783–2793.

Terpstra, T. L., & Terpstra, T. L. (2000). CESieries: Syndrome of inappropriate antidiuretic hormone secretion: Recognition and management. *MEDSURG Nursing, 9*(2), 61–68.

Thyroid Federation International. (2003). *Thyroid videos online.* Retrieved September 19, 2005, from http://www.thyroid-fed.org./intro/thyroidvideos.html

Thyroid Foundation of America (2004a). Thyroid disorders and treatments: Overview. Retrieved August 21, 2005, and September 19, 2005, from http://www.allthyroid.org/disorders/ondex.html

Thyroid Foundation of America (2004b). Thyroid patient organizations. Retrieved September 19, 2005, from http://www.allthyroid.org/resources/patient.html

Urbano, F. L. (2000). Signs of hypocalcemia: Chvostek's and Trousseau's signs. *Hospital Physician,* March 2000, 43–45.

Waltman, P. A., Brewer, J. M., & Lobert, S. (2004). Thyroid storm during pregnancy: A medical emergency. *Critical Care Nursing, 24*(2), 74–79.

Whiteman, K. (2006). ACTH stimulation: Testing the Adrenals. *Nursing, 36*(7), 24–25.

Yeung, S. C. J., & Habra, M. A. (2007). Graves' disease. *eMedicine.* Retrieved June 12, 2008, from http://www.emedicine.com/med/TOPIC929.HTM

Caring for the Patient with Diabetes

Laurie Quinn

With contributions by:
Cynthia Fritschi

Outcome-Based Learning Objectives

After studying this chapter, the learner will be able to:

1. Discuss the epidemiology of diabetes and pre-diabetes (impaired glucose tolerance and impaired fasting glucose).
2. Differentiate between the classifications of pre-diabetes and diabetes as they relate to clinical manifestations and health care management.
3. Compare and contrast the pathophysiology of pre-diabetes and diabetes.
4. Identify the major acute and chronic complications associated with diabetes.
5. Identify risk factors for adults associated with the development of pre-diabetes and diabetes.
6. Discuss the pharmacologic and nutritional management of diabetes as contrasted between diabetes type 1 and type 2.
7. Discuss the role of physical activity and exercise in the prevention and treatment of diabetes.
8. Describe the clinical signs and symptoms, diagnosis, medical therapy, nursing assessment, and management of diabetes.
9. Compare and contrast the clinical signs and symptoms, diagnosis, treatment, nursing assessment, and management of diabetic ketoacidosis, hyperglycemic hyperosmolar syndrome, and hypoglycemia.
10. Describe the prevention, progression, clinical signs and symptoms, nursing assessment, and management of lower extremity disease as it relates to diabetes.

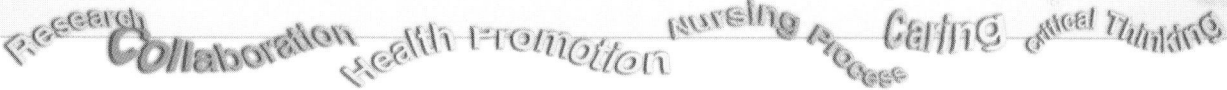

Research   Collaboration   Health Promotion   Nursing Process   Caring   Critical Thinking

MyNursingKit | Video: Endocrine and Metabolic Disorders: Diabetes—Type 1, Type 2, Gestational

DIABETES MELLITUS (DM) is a disorder of carbohydrate, protein, and fat metabolism resulting from an imbalance between insulin availability and insulin need. It is not actually a single disease but a group of metabolic disorders characterized by **hyperglycemia** (high blood glucose) resulting from defects in insulin secretion, insulin action, or both (DeFronzo, 2004). The hormone **insulin,** which is secreted by the beta cells of the islets of Langerhans, is used by the body to break down blood sugars and starches into energy. Diabetes can represent an absolute insulin deficiency, impaired release of insulin by the **pancreatic beta cells,** inadequate or defective insulin receptors, or the production of defective insulin that is destroyed before it can carry out its action (Porth, 2007). The intent of this chapter is to discuss diabetes mellitus and abnormal glucose tolerance generally, and then specifically as the concepts apply to the hospitalized patient with diabetes.

The most recent criteria for the diagnosis and classification of diabetes and abnormal glucose tolerance were published by the American Diabetes Association (ADA) in 1997 with minor updates since that time (American Diabetes Association, 2007). These newer criteria are based on the etiology of diabetes rather than the phenotypical presentation of the disease. In the past when an understanding of the mechanisms underlying the cause of diabetes was less mature, its classification was either related to age or conventional treatment regimens (e.g., diet, insulin, oral medications). These newer classification criteria allow for the diagnosis and classification of five types of diabetes and pre-diabetes: type 1 diabetes, type 2 diabetes, gestational diabetes mellitus, other types of diabetes, and pre-diabetes. Type 1 and type 2 diabetes are the most common forms of diabetes. The development of both type 1 and type 2 diabetes is initiated by interplay between genetics and the environment.

Type 1 diabetes mellitus (DM) is a catabolic, autoimmune disorder in which circulating insulin is very low or absent and plasma glucagon is elevated. The pancreas shows lymphocytic infiltration and destruction of insulin-secreting cells of the islets of Langerhans, causing insulin deficiency. Patients need exogenous insulin to reverse this catabolic condition, prevent ketosis, decrease hyperglucagonemia, and normalize lipid and protein metabolism (Hussain & Vincent, 2007). Type 1 diabetes, previously referred to as juvenile diabetes mellitus, insulin-dependent diabetes mellitus, and type I diabetes mellitus, affects 5% to 10%

of the diabetes population (Centers for Disease Control and Prevention [CDC], 2005). This type of diabetes is associated with destruction of the pancreatic beta cells, the cells that secrete insulin. In the majority of people with type 1 diabetes, the destruction is mediated by an autoimmune process. Because individuals with type 1 diabetes produce no insulin, they require pharmacologic insulin therapy for survival.

Type 1 diabetes can occur at any age, but is frequently diagnosed before 30 years of age; however, there is an adult form of autoimmune type 1 diabetes termed **latent autoimmune diabetes in adults (LADA)** (Pozzilli & Di Mario, 2001). In addition, there are uncommon forms of non–immune-mediated forms of type 1 diabetes. Individuals with type 1 diabetes are usually thin or normal weight at diagnosis and have an abrupt onset of symptoms. In addition, those with type 1 diabetes are more prone to the development of diabetic ketoacidosis, an acute life-threatening complication.

Type 2 diabetes mellitus, previously referred to as adult-onset diabetes or non–insulin-dependent diabetes mellitus (NIDDM) or simply type 2 diabetes, describes a condition of hyperglycemia that occurs despite the availability of insulin (referred to as relative insulin deficiency). Unlike type 1 diabetes mellitus, patients are not absolutely dependent on insulin for life, even though many of these patients are ultimately treated with insulin (Ligaray & Isley, 2007). Type 2 diabetes usually is diagnosed after the age of 30 years, but is beginning to occur more frequently at younger ages. Individuals with type 2 diabetes are not dependent on exogenous insulin to sustain life; however, insulin therapy and/or oral medications may be needed to control hyperglycemia. These individuals are often obese and have a strong family history of type 2 diabetes.

Diabetes also can result from certain specific genetic conditions (e.g., maturity onset-diabetes of the young), surgery (e.g., pancreatectomy), drugs (e.g., corticosteroids), infections (e.g., congenital rubella), and other illness. The initial diagnosis and clinical presentation of the diabetes in this group varies with the underlying disorder. **Maturity onset diabetes of the young (MODY)** is an autosomal dominant subtype of type 2 diabetes that is often diagnosed at younger ages (Tattersall, 1998). An important point is that MODY is not early-onset type 2 diabetes; it is instead a group of monogenetic (single-gene) defects resulting in impaired insulin secretion (Malecki & Klupa, 2005). The clinical presentation of MODY usually is associated with mild hyperglycemia. MODY typically presents in children or during young adulthood and is inherited as an autosomal dominant pattern (Velho & Robert, 2002).

Gestational diabetes mellitus (GDM) refers to a condition in which the onset of diabetes is first diagnosed during pregnancy. This form of abnormal glucose tolerance affects about 4% of pregnancies or 135,000 women in the United States annually (CDC, 2005). Though a specific cause has not been identified, it most commonly affects women with a family history of diabetes, those with glycosuria, and those with a history of stillbirth or spontaneous abortion. Other possible considerations include advanced maternal age and five or more previous pregnancies (Porth, 2007). It also is believed that the hormones produced during pregnancy reduce a woman's sensitivity to insulin, resulting in high blood sugar levels.

Those diagnosed with GDM require dietary treatment and possibly insulin therapy to control hyperglycemia. Uncontrolled hyperglycemia during pregnancy can result in fetal and maternal complications. Gestational diabetes mellitus poses an increased risk for the development of type 2 diabetes with as many as 50% of women with GDM developing type 2 diabetes later in life (CDC, 2005).

Pre-diabetes is a term used to identify people who are at increased risk for developing diabetes. Pre-diabetes can be determined in two different ways. Patients may have fasting plasma glucose levels above normal or they may have abnormal results on an oral glucose tolerance test. In either case the results are abnormal but do not meet the diagnostic criteria for diabetes. The two types of glucose intolerance included in this category include **impaired fasting glucose (IFG)** (a condition that exists when blood sugar levels are higher than normal but not high enough to say that one has diabetes) and **impaired glucose tolerance (IGT)**. IGT is a pre-diabetic state of dysglycemia that is associated with insulin resistance and increased risk of cardiovascular pathology. Individuals with pre-diabetes are at increased risk for developing type 2 diabetes. Approximately 41 million individuals in the United States have pre-diabetes (CDC, 2005).

Epidemiology and Etiology of Diabetes and Other Forms of Glucose Intolerance

The prevalence of diabetes for all age groups worldwide has been estimated to be 6.0% or 246 million in the year 2007 (International Diabetes Federation, 2006). Approximately 23.5 million or 10.7% of the U.S. population over 20 years of age has diabetes (ADA, 2008f). The prevalence of diabetes differs by factors such as race, ethnicity, and geographic location. Some of these factors are explored in the following paragraphs.

Its increasing prevalence has deemed diabetes mellitus a major public health problem in the United States that is affecting millions of individuals, of which an estimated 6.6 million are undiagnosed. From 2002 to 2007, the number of individuals diagnosed with diabetes increased from 12.1 to 17.5 million. In addition, an estimated 54 million individuals have abnormalities in glucose tolerance that place them at high risk for developing diabetes (ADA, 2008f). The global prevalence of diabetes is expected to increase from 171 million in the year 2000 to 366 million in the year 2030 (Wild, Roglic, Green, Sicree, & King, 2004). Among those born in the United States during the year 2000, the lifetime probability of developing diabetes is 32.8% for males and 38.5% for females (Narayan, Boyle, Thompson, Sorensen, & Williamson, 2003). Obesity, population growth, aging, urbanization, and physical inactivity are primary factors accounting for this epidemic.

A variety of serious acute and chronic complications are associated with diabetes. The acute complications are medical emergencies and include diabetic ketoacidosis, hyperosmolar hyperglycemic syndrome, and hypoglycemia. The chronic complications include disorders associated with **microvascular** (small vessel) changes in the eyes, nerves, and kidneys, along with **macrovascular** (large vessel) changes in the heart, veins and arteries. These changes result in retinopathy (eye disease), neuropathy (nerve disease), nephropathy (kidney disease), and accelerated development of coronary heart disease (CHD), cerebrovascular disease, and peripheral vascular disease (PVD). These complications are associated with excessive morbidity and mortality from heart disease, blindness, kidney failure, extremity amputations, and other chronic conditions.

Diabetes and its related complications are associated with significant personal, social, and economic costs. The economic impact of diabetes and diabetic complications on the U.S. economy is substantial. Medical expenditures attributed to diabetes in 2007 were estimated at $174 billion including $116 billion dollars in medical costs and $58 billion dollars in indirect costs (ADA, 2008f). *Direct* medical costs include expenditures related to hospital inpatient care, diabetes medications and supplies, retail prescriptions for diabetes complications, and health care provider office visits. *Indirect* medical costs include costs resulting from increased absenteeism from work, reduced productivity at work and home, unemployment, disability, and loss of productivity due to premature death (ADA, 2008f). Successful treatment of diabetes is essential for reducing the personal, social, and economic costs associated with this disorder. As the prevalence of diabetes increases, the complications of diabetes also will increase, unless aggressive treatment strategies are employed. Because patients with diabetes are so frequently seen in clinical practice, it is essential for nurses to be knowledgeable about the care and treatment of patients with diabetes. The hospitalized patient with diabetes presents a series of unique challenges. The purpose of this chapter is to explore the clinical management of the medical–surgical patient with diabetes.

Type 1 DM accounts for approximately 5% to 15% of all diagnosed diabetes (CDC, 2005; Hussain & Vincent, 2007). Approximately 1 in every 400 to 600 children and adolescents has type 1 diabetes (CDC, 2005) making it one of the most common severe chronic disorders of childhood. Type 1 diabetes affects 0.22% or 176,500 thousand people under the age of 20 years (CDC, 2005). In addition, type 1 diabetes affects approximately 1.4 million in the United States and perhaps 10 million to 20 million individuals globally (Wild et al., 2004).

Type 2 diabetes accounts for approximately 90% to 95% of all diabetes, both nationally and globally (CDC, 2005). There has been a dramatic increase in the prevalence of type 2 diabetes, especially among newly Westernized countries. Only India and China exceed the United States in the number of individuals diagnosed with diabetes (International Diabetes Federation, 2006).

Cultural and Ethnic Considerations of Diabetes Development

The prevalence of diabetes increases with age and varies among different ethnic groups. Approximately 10.6 million, or 20.9%, of the U.S. population ages 60 years or older have diabetes. Age-adjusted rates for diabetes among Mexican Americans and non-Hispanic blacks are 1.7 and 1.8 times, respectively, greater than the rate for non-Hispanic whites (CDC, 2005). In general, the U.S. prevalence of diabetes is highest in Native Americans. The total age-adjusted prevalence of diabetes among Alaska Natives and American Indians in the southern United States is 8.1% and 27%, respectively. Total prevalence data are not available for Asian Americans or Pacific Islanders. In Hawaii, however, Native Hawaiians, Asians, and other Pacific Islanders over 20 years of age have age-adjusted rates of diagnosed diabetes that are more than two times those of non-Hispanic whites (CDC, 2005).

Type 2 diabetes, a disease traditionally associated with adults, has been increasing among children and adolescents. There are no large-scale epidemiologic studies on the prevalence of type 2 diabetes in children and adolescents. A variety of clinic-based reports and small population studies, however, indicate that this increased prevalence of type 2 diabetes among youth is highest among Native American, African American, and Hispanic youth (Bobo et al., 2004; Fagot-Campagna et al., 2000; Rosenbloom, House, & Winter, 1998; Rosenbloom, Joe, Young, & Winter, 1999; Young & Rosenbloom, 1998). In these reports, the percentage of type 2 diabetes among children and adolescents with pediatric diabetes has increased from <5% before 1994 to 30% to 50% in subsequent years (Fagot-Campagna et al., 2000; Kaufman, 2002; Ligaray & Isley, 2007).

Normal Physiology of Fuel Metabolism

The pancreas is located in the posterior portion of the upper abdomen and is divided into the exocrine and endocrine pancreas. Chapters 51 and 52 ⊘ provide more information on endocrine assessment and glandular and hormonal disorders. The exocrine pancreas produces hormones primarily involved in digestion, whereas the endocrine pancreas produces hormones associated with endocrine function.

The exocrine pancreas primarily is composed of small glands called acini, whereas the endocrine pancreas is made up of small cells called islets of Langerhans. These islet cells are distributed throughout the exocrine pancreas and are divided into the alpha cells, beta cells, delta cells, and F cells. Alpha cells secrete the hormone **glucagon**, beta cells secrete the hormone insulin, delta cells secrete the hormone somatostatin, and F cells (or pancreatic polypeptide cells) secrete the hormone **pancreatic polypeptide**. Somatostatin is a hormone that is produced in the delta cells of the pancreas and other locations, including the gastrointestinal tract and the hypothalamus. Somatostatin inhibits the release of insulin from the beta cells and glucagon from the alpha cells of the pancreas. Pancreatic polypeptide is a complex peptide hormone whose role is not entirely understood. In relation to diabetes, the most important of these hormones are insulin and glucagon. These hormones are discussed in greater detail throughout the chapter.

Interrelationships among insulin, glucagon, cortisol, growth hormone, and the catecholamines epinephrine and norepinephrine control fuel metabolism. The effects of insulin are most prominent in liver, adipose tissue, and muscle. The primary functions of insulin in these tissues include the synthesis of **glycogen** (the storage form of glucose) in liver and muscle, the synthesis of protein (a large complex molecule made up of one or more chains of amino acids) in liver and muscle, and the synthesis of triglycerides (molecules consisting of a glycerol backbone with three fatty acids) in adipose tissue and to a smaller extent in muscle.

Insulin is necessary for **glycolysis**, the biochemical pathway that results in the generation of high-energy compounds such as adenosine triphosphate (ATP) and nicotinamide adenine dinucleotide NAD and for glucose transport, the movement of glucose into insulin-sensitive tissues, such as muscle. Most importantly, insulin suppresses **gluconeogenesis** (formation of glucose from noncarbohydrate substrates), **glycogenolysis** (breakdown of glycogen to glucose), and **lipolysis** (breakdown of triglycerides to free fatty acids [FFAs] and glycerol). Insulin promotes glucose uptake and utilization in tissues. Skeletal muscle is the major site of insulin-mediated glucose disposal during the fed state (period following meals) and is critical for preventing hyperglycemia and maintaining glucose homeostasis.

Collectively, glucagon, cortisol, growth hormone, epinephrine, and norepinephrine are referred to as **counterregulatory hormones** because their actions oppose the effects of insulin. The functions of each of these hormones in intermediary metabolism are presented in Chart 53–1. Glucagon is secreted from the alpha cells of the pancreas. The primary functions of glucagon include hepatic gluconeogenesis, glycogenolysis, lipolysis, and **ketogenesis** (formation of ketones [energy substrates] from FFAs). Cortisol, a hormone secreted by the adrenal cortex, causes protein catabolism and lipolysis, therefore, providing precursors for gluconeogenesis and ketogenesis. Growth hormone, secreted by the anterior pituitary, causes lipolysis and provides precursors (glycerol and FFAs) for gluconeogenesis and ketogenesis. Of the catecholamines, epinephrine has the greatest role in fuel metabolism. This hormone is secreted by the adrenal medulla and is associated with glycogenolysis, gluconeogenesis, and lipolysis.

The primary goal following a meal is maintenance of normal blood glucose levels. Following the ingestion of carbohydrates (CHO), mainly sugars and starches, insulin levels rise and stimulate glucose uptake into insulin-sensitive tissues, primarily muscle. Glucagon levels decrease, so there is a higher ratio of insulin to glucagon. Glucose is the primary oxidative fuel for all tissues during the absorptive state. Glucose that is in excess of the oxidative needs of the major tissues is stored as glycogen or lipids.

The primary goal of fuel metabolism during the fasted state is to provide glucose for the brain and nervous tissue. The fasted state is generally considered to be 10 to 12 hours following an overnight fast. The ratio of glucagon to insulin is higher during this time. Hepatic glycogenolysis and gluconeogenesis increase plasma glucose levels. Free fatty acids, released from adipose tissue lipolysis, are oxidized by muscle for energy. As fasting continues, insulin remains suppressed, glucagon levels remain elevated, and the principal source of hepatic glucose production is gluconeogenesis. In addition, ketones can be oxidized by the brain for energy.

In summary, normal fuel metabolism is regulated by a series of complex relationships among insulin, glucagon, and other counterregulatory hormones. Normal plasma glucose levels are tightly regulated by the following three processes: hepatic glucose production, glucose uptake and utilization by peripheral tissues (primarily skeletal muscle), and the actions of insulin and counterregulatory hormones, primarily glucagon. Insulin and glucagon have opposing effects on glucose metabolism. Higher glucagon levels and lower insulin levels facilitate hepatic gluconeogenesis and glycogenolysis during fasted states, thereby preventing hypoglycemia. Fasting plasma glucose levels are determined primarily by hepatic glucose production. Plasma insulin levels increase and glucagon levels decrease as blood glucose levels rise during the fed state.

Pathophysiology and Fuel Metabolism in Diabetes

The hormonal-fuel relationships described above are abnormal in all types of diabetes. In type 1 diabetes, there is a nearly complete loss of insulin production, whereas in type 2 diabetes, there is decreased insulin production and insulin resistance. **Insulin resistance** is generally described as the inability of either endogenous or exogenous insulin to achieve its normal biologic response in its target tissues. The abnormalities of fuel metabolism associated with diabetes result from a deficiency in insulin and an increase in glucagon and other counterregulatory hormones. These hormonal abnormalities most profoundly affect the muscle, liver, and adipose tissue. Hyperglycemia results from decreased glucose transport into insulin-sensitive tissues (e.g., skeletal muscle), hepatic gluconeogenesis, and hepatic and muscle glycogenolysis. In type 1 diabetes, the increased mobilization of free fatty acids from adipose tissue leads to increased hepatic synthesis of ketone bodies and results in the acute complication of diabetic ketoacidosis. In type 2 diabetes, the amount of free fatty acids that are converted to ketone bodies is usually not sufficient for the development of diabetic ketoacidosis.

Physiological Manifestations of Systemic Complications of Diabetes Mellitus

Diabetes complications affect major body systems and organs. These major complications are discussed next.

CHART 53–1	Effects of Insulin and Counterregulatory Hormones on Intermediary Metabolism				
Insulin Resistance	**Insulin**	**Glucagon ↑**	**Cortisol ↑**	**Growth ↑ Hormone**	**Epinephrine/ ↑ Norepinephrine**
Glycogen Synthesis	↑	↓			↓
Glycogenolysis	↓				↑
Gluconeogenesis	↓	↑	↑	↑	↑
Lipolysis	↓		↑	↑	↑
Ketogenesis	↓	↑			
Protein Synthesis	↑		↓	↑	
Proteolysis	↓		↑		

Note: ↓ = inhibits or decreases; ↑ = stimulates or increases.

Diseases of Heart and Vessels

CHD, PVD, and cerebrovascular disease are more common, occur earlier, and are more severe in people with diabetes. Heart disease death rates in adults with diabetes are about 2 to 4 times higher than in adults without diabetes (CDC, 2005). The risk for stroke is 2 to 4 times higher among people with diabetes, and about 65% of deaths among people with diabetes are due to heart disease and stroke (CDC, 2005). CHD is the leading cause of diabetes-related deaths. In the United States, more than 60% of nontraumatic amputations are in patients with diabetes and usually result from the combination of PVD and neuropathy (CDC, 2005). In 2002 about 82,000 nontraumatic lower limb amputations were performed on people with diabetes (CDC, 2005). About 75% of adults with diabetes have blood pressure readings ≥130/80 mmHg or use prescription medications for hypertension (CDC, 2005).

Kidney Disease

Diabetes is the leading cause of chronic kidney disease (CKD) in the United States, accounting for 44% of new cases annually (CDC, 2005). In 2002, in the United States and Puerto Rico, 44,400 people with diabetes began treatment for end-stage renal disease (ESRD) (CDC, 2005). In the same year, a total of 153,730 people in the United States and Puerto Rico with diabetes-related ESRD were living on chronic dialysis or with a transplanted kidney. The Third National Health and Nutrition Examination Survey (NHANES III), conducted from 1988 to 1994, obtained information on the health and nutritional status of the U.S. population through interviews and direct physical examinations. Data from NHANES III demonstrated that approximately 25% to 30% of adults with type 2 diabetes have evidence of early renal disease, as evidenced by **microalbuminuria,** small amounts of protein (30 to 299 mg/24 hours) in the urine, whereas another 5% to 13% have evidence of overt nephropathy, as evidenced by albuminuria ≥300 mg/24 hours (Harris, 2001).

Blindness and Other Visual Disorders

Diabetes remains the leading cause of new cases of blindness among adults 20 to 74 years old (CDC, 2005). Visual impairment among persons older than 50 years of age with and without diabetes has been estimated at 23.5% and 12.4%, respectively (CDC, 2004). The primary causes of visual impairment and blindness among patients with diabetes include diabetic retinopathy, cataracts, macular degeneration, and glaucoma (CDC, 2004). The prevalence of diabetic retinopathy among persons older than 50 years of age is approximately 10.2%. People with diabetes have substantially greater age-adjusted prevalence of cataracts (31.8% vs. 21.2%) and glaucoma (8.0% vs. 4.3%) than the general population (CDC, 2004). Visual disorders are discussed more in Chapter 71 .

Neuropathy

About 60% to 70% of people with diabetes have mild to severe forms of nervous system damage (CDC, 2005). The results of such damage include, but are not limited to, peripheral neuropathy (e.g., impaired sensation or pain in the hands, legs, and feet) and autonomic neuropathy (e.g., delayed gastric emptying, bladder dysfunction, impotence, orthostatic hypotension, and cardiac abnormalities). Approximately 6% of U.S. hospitalizations for diabetes result from some form of neuropathy (CDC, 2005).

Complications of Pregnancy

Elevated glucose levels prior to conception and during the first trimester of pregnancy can cause major birth defects in 5% to 10% of pregnancies and spontaneous abortions in 15% to 20% of pregnancies (CDC, 2005). In addition, chronic hyperglycemia diabetes during the second and third trimesters of pregnancy can result in macrosomia (excessively large babies), resulting in neonatal and obstetrical risks (CDC, 2005).

Diabetic Ketoacidosis

Diabetic ketoacidosis (DKA) is a state of absolute or relative insulin deficiency aggravated by ensuing hyperglycemia, dehydration, and acidosis-producing derangements in intermediary metabolism. The most common causes are underlying infection, disruption of insulin treatment, and new onset of diabetes. DKA is typically characterized by hyperglycemia greater than 300 mg/dL, low bicarbonate level (<15 mEq/L), and acidosis (pH <7.30) with ketonemia and ketonuria (Porth, 2007; Rucker, 2008).

It is one of the most serious complications of diabetes and is most commonly associated with type 1 diabetes. This complication is listed on approximately 3% to 4% of all hospital discharges among people with diabetes (National Center for Chronic Disease Prevention and Health Promotion, 2004). The highest mortality rates from DKA are noted among African American males (36.8%) and elderly men and women older than 75 years of age (ADA, 2001). From 1980 to 2001, the number of deaths with DKA as the underlying cause has remained relatively stable. In 1980 there were 1,772 deaths due to DKA, and in 2001 that number was 1,871 (National Center for Chronic Disease Prevention and Health Promotion, 2004).

Hyperosmolar Hyperglycemic Syndrome

Hyperosmolar hyperglycemic syndrome (HHS) is a hyperglycemic crisis characteristically found in the elderly infirm who are unable to meet their fluid needs; however, this syndrome is beginning to occur at younger ages (ADA, 2001; Nugent, 2005). An estimated 11,000 hospital discharges mention HHS and 70% occur in those older than 64 years of age. Mortality rates for HHS range from 10% to 50% and are largely attributed to underlying illnesses (ADA, 2001).

Hypoglycemia

Hypoglycemia (low blood glucose) in patients with diabetes results from pharmacologic treatment with insulin or oral hypoglycemic medications. Prevalence rates for mild hypoglycemia are difficult to estimate because some degree of hypoglycemia is characteristically associated with intensive diabetes management. In the **Diabetes Control and Complications Trial (DCCT)**, approximately 6% of the intensively treated patients had episodes of moderate to severe hypoglycemia (DCCT Trial Research Group, 1993).

Risk Factors and Pathophysiology of Type 1 Diabetes

Type 1 diabetes appears to result from an interaction between genetics, environment, and autoimmunity. There is a great deal of research involving the etiology of this disorder, but the prevailing theories are detailed next.

Genetics

A familial predisposition to the development of type 1 diabetes does exist; however, the exact mode of genetic inheritance remains unclear. Among U.S. Caucasian populations, the overall risk of developing type 1 diabetes is approximately 0.2% to 0.4% (Hussain & Vincent, 2007; Porth, 2007; Muir, Schatz, & Maclaren, 1992). A sibling of a person with type 1 diabetes has a 6% risk of developing the disorder (Muir et al., 1992). The offspring of a father with type 1 diabetes has a greater chance of developing the disorder (6%) than the offspring of a mother (3%) (Muir et al., 1992). Most significantly, however, is that there is a higher concordance for type 1 diabetes among monozygotic twins (25% to 50%) than dizygotic twins (6%) (Muir et al., 1992). If the development of type 1 diabetes were determined completely by genetic inheritance, the concordance rate would be 100%. This fact that the concordance rate among identical twins is 25% to 50% supports the fact that there is an environmental trigger that initiates the transition from genetic predisposition to type 1 diabetes. The Genetic Considerations box discusses the genes involved in the development of type 1 diabetes.

Environmental

A triggering event in those at risk for developing type 1 diabetes initiates a series of autoimmune events ending in pancreatic beta-cell destruction. A variety of environmental triggers have been proposed as initiating events, but no single factor has been consistently associated with the risk of type 1 diabetes. Among the many possible initiating events, viral infections, dietary factors, and toxins have been identified as possible environmental triggers in the development of type 1 diabetes.

Congenital rubella syndrome is strongly associated with the development of type 1 diabetes, but this syndrome represents a small number of cases (Lammi, Karvonen, & Tuomilehto, 2005). The observation that children frequently develop type l diabetes following a viral illness has provided anecdotal evidence that a virus may be the initiating event in type 1 diabetes. In particular, it has been postulated that enteroviruses may initiate the development of type 1 diabetes in those genetically at risk for the disorder (Akerblom, Vaarala, Hyoty, Ilonen, & Knip, 2002).

Of the possible dietary etiologic factors, cow's milk proteins have received the main attention. Studies indicate an association between early exposure to dietary cow's milk proteins and an increased risk of type 1 diabetes, but the data remain controversial (Akerblom et al., 2002; Dahlquist, 1997; Gerstein, 1994; Knip, 2003). Toxins that have gained attention as possible environmental triggers for type 1 diabetes are the N-nitroso compounds. Nitrate is found in vegetables, and nitrate and nitrite are found in meat products. In the gut, nitrate is reduced to nitrite. Nitrite is transformed in the gut by reaction with amines and amides to nitrosamines and nitrosamines. Evidence such as this suggests that there is a relationship between nitrates and nitrites in type 1 diabetes, but this relationship is under investigation.

Autoimmunity

A number of circulating autoantibodies to pancreatic beta-cell components have been identified in those with type 1 diabetes. These autoantibodies include cytoplasmic islet cell antibodies (ICAs), insulin autoantibodies (IAAs), antibodies directed against the enzyme glutamic acid decarboxylase (GAD), and antibodies against islet tyrosine phosphatase (i.e., IA2 and IA2beta) (Kaufman & ADA, 2008). Unaffected relatives are at risk for the development of type 1 diabetes. The presence of two or more antibodies, together with alterations in insulin secretion, is highly predictive of the development of type 1 diabetes within 5 years (Kaufman & ADA, 2008). These autoantibodies serve as markers of an ongoing autoimmune process.

Sequence in the Development of Type 1 Diabetes

The proposed scheme for the development of type 1 diabetes is detailed in Figure 53–1 ■.

Environmental factors trigger an immune response with the development of ICAs, IAAs, and other islet cell antigens, such as GAD (Kaufman & ADA, 2008). These antibodies are markers of a progressive loss of pancreatic beta-cell mass. These can be helpful in the diagnosis of type 1 diabetes. As noted in Figure 53–1 ■, when the beta-cell mass is reduced by 80% to 90%, marked *impairments in insulin release* and *overt* type 1 diabetes develop. This is followed by a period of endogenous insulin production

> ### GENETIC CONSIDERATIONS for Type 1 Diabetes
>
> Approximately 40% to 50% of the genetic predisposition to the development of type 1 diabetes is conferred by genes on the short arm of chromosome 6, either within or in proximity to the Class II human leukocyte antigen (HLA) region of the major histocompatibility complex (MHC) (Kaufman & ADA, 2008). The inheritance of particular HLA alleles can account for more than half of the genetic risk of developing type 1 diabetes. HLA-DR and HLA-DQ are most strongly linked with type 1 diabetes. In type 1 diabetes at least one allele of DR3 or DR4 is found in 95% of Caucasians, and individuals with both DR3 and DR4 are particularly susceptible to type 1 diabetes. Conversely, the DR2 allele is protective against type 1 diabetes. (Kaufman & ADA, 2008).

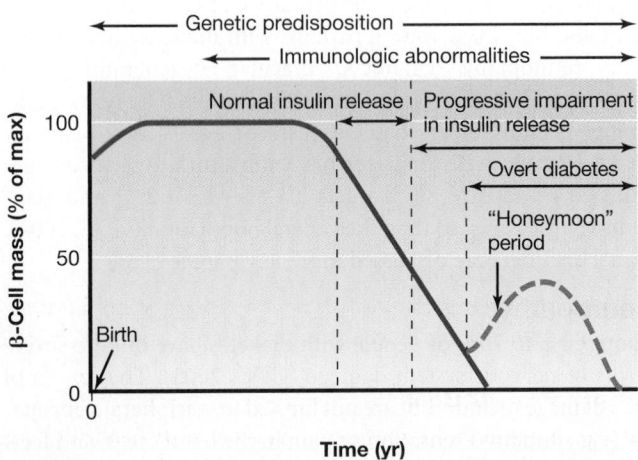

FIGURE 53–1 ■ Proposed scheme of natural history of the beta-cell defect.

called the **honeymoon period**. This "honeymoon period" represents the period of time during which exogenous insulin requirements are reduced. The clinical presentation of the honeymoon period varies from moderate reductions in insulin requirements to normalization of glucose tolerance (Harmel, Mathur, & Davidson, 2004). This period is relatively short lived, usually a few weeks to several months (Harmel et al., 2004) and is followed by loss of insulin production and dependence on exogenous insulin secretion.

Relationship Between Environmental Triggers and Beta-Cell Destruction

The question remains as to how the environmental trigger actually initiates the cascade of events leading to pancreatic beta-cell dysfunction. Currently two theories have been proposed to explain how an environmental trigger can initiate the autoimmune process.

The first theory is that an environmental trigger, such as a virus, directly induces tissue damage and inflammation. This subsequently leads to the release of beta-cell antigens and the recruitment and activation of lymphocytes and additional inflammatory leukocytes to the tissue.

The second theory, known as **molecular mimicry**, postulates that an environmental trigger, such as a virus, produces an immune response against autoantigens. This theory suggests that a susceptible host encounters an environmental trigger, such as a virus, that has antigens that are immunologically similar to the host antigens; however these antigens differ sufficiently enough to induce an immune response when presented to T cells. As a result, the tolerance to autoantigens breaks down, and the immune response cross reacts with host structures to cause tissue damage and disease (Albert & Inman, 1999).

◼ Risk Factors and Pathophysiology of Type 2 Diabetes

A number of risk factors are associated with the development of type 2 diabetes, as discussed next.

Genetics

Though there are genetic determinants of both type 1 and type 2 diabetes, the genetic linkage is stronger in those with type 2 diabetes. A small number of cases of type 2 diabetes are caused by a single-gene defect, such as MODY. The genetic component of the more common form of type 2 diabetes appears to be complex, involving the interactions of several genes and environmental factors (So et al., 2000).

Ethnicity

There is wide variability in the risk of type 2 diabetes among different racial and ethnic groups. Ethnic differences were described earlier in this chapter in the Epidemiology and Etiology of Diabetes and Other Forms of Glucose Intolerance section.

Racial Admixture

Data from populations whose origins are a mixture of different ethnic groups with varying risks for type 2 diabetes have provided *indirect* evidence that there is a genetic predisposition to this disease. Many Hispanics living in the southwestern United States share genes with Native Americans, such as the Pima Indians, and with non-Hispanic Caucasians, who are at much lower risk for developing diabetes. A study of Mexican Americans indicated that the prevalence of type 2 diabetes in this group is associated with the proportion of Native American genes in this population (Gardner et al., 1984). Though dated, the results of this study still are relevant to understanding the etiology of diabetes. The prevalence of type 2 diabetes in the group with the lowest amount of Native American admixture had a prevalence of diabetes at 5%, whereas the group with the highest Native American admixture had a prevalence of 14.5%. The Strong Heart Study, which examined the prevalence of cardiovascular disease (CVD) among three groups of Native Americans, noted that the prevalence of type 2 diabetes in adults ages 45 to 74 years increased with increasing levels of Native American ancestry (Lee et al., 1995).

Family History

Family history is an established risk factor for the development of type 2 diabetes. Twin studies have demonstrated that type 2 diabetes is highly concordant in monozygotic twins, but to a lesser degree in dizygous twins (Newman et al., 1987). The high concordance rate for type 2 diabetes among monozygotic twins supports the evidence that genetic factors play a significant role in the development of type 2 diabetes.

Diet

During times of reduced caloric intake, such as in food shortages during wars, there is a decline in morbidity and mortality from type 2 diabetes (ADA, 2001). Therefore, there appears to be an association between the amount of caloric intake and development of type 2 diabetes. However, the independent effects of caloric restriction on prevention of type 2 diabetes are difficult to discern from the effects of reducing or maintaining normal body weight. The exact dietary composition of diet in the prevention of type 2 diabetes also is not clear. High-CHO and low-fat diets appear to deteriorate insulin sensitivity, but high-fat and low-CHO diets may decrease satiety and lead to higher energy intake.

Obesity

Obesity is strongly associated with the development of type 2 diabetes (Gregg et al., 2004). There has been an increased emphasis on the role of central or visceral obesity (weight centered around the abdomen) in the development of type 2 diabetes. Central body obesity appears as a prognostic marker for glucose intolerance, hyperinsulinemia, and hypertriglyceridemia. Type 2 diabetes and pre-diabetes are manifestations of an underlying disorder termed *metabolic syndrome* (Burant & ADA, 2008).

Metabolic syndrome refers to a group of metabolic abnormalities that predisposes individuals to CVD and type 2 diabetes. The primary abnormalities included in this syndrome include insulin resistance, glucose intolerance, hyperinsulinemia, increased triglycerides and decreased HDL cholesterol, central obesity, and hypertension. The most common criteria used to define metabolic syndrome were developed by the Adult Treatment Panel III (ATP III) National Cholesterol Education Program Expert Panel on Detection, Evaluation, and Treatment of High Blood Cholesterol in Adults (Ford & Giles, 2003). Three or more of the following abnormalities must be present:

- High blood pressure ≥130/85 mmHg
- Hypertriglyceridemia ≥150 mg/dL
- Low high density lipoprotein cholesterol: ≤40 mg/dL in men; ≤50 mg/dL in women
- Abdominal obesity: waist circumference ≥102 cm in men; ≥88 cm in women
- Elevated fasting glucose ≥100 mg/dL.

Physical Inactivity

A number of epidemiologic studies during the last two decades have demonstrated that high levels of physical activity protect against the development of type 2 diabetes (Haffner, 1997; Helmrich, Ragland, Leung, & Paffenbarger, 1991; Hu et al., 2001; Manson et al., 1991, 1992). Two intervention studies have confirmed the value of lifestyle changes in the prevention of type 2 diabetes (Knowler et al., 2002; Tuomilehto et al., 2001). The Finnish Diabetes Prevention Study examined whether type 2 diabetes could be prevented through lifestyle modification in subjects with impaired glucose tolerance (IGT) (Tuomilehto et al., 2001). In this study, subjects were assigned to either an intervention or a control group. Subjects in the intervention group received individualized counseling aimed at weight reduction, dietary fat reduction, saturated fat reduction, increased dietary fiber, and increased physical activity. The risk of diabetes was reduced by 58% in the intervention group.

In the U.S. **Diabetes Prevention Program (DPP),** approximately 3,234 adults with elevated fasting and postload plasma glucose concentrations (i.e., those with pre-diabetes) were randomized into three groups: placebo, medication metformin (an oral hypoglycemic medication), or a lifestyle modification program (Knowler et al., 2002). The lifestyle intervention program reduced the incidence of diabetes by 58% and metformin reduced the incidence by 31% when compared with placebo. The study concluded that to prevent one case of diabetes during a 3-year period, 6.9 persons would have to participate in the lifestyle intervention program, and 13.9 would have to receive metformin. Therefore, the lifestyle intervention was more effective than the metformin.

Urbanization

When certain populations migrate from rural to urban settings, they have an increased prevalence of type 2 diabetes when compared to those whose relatives remain in the original setting. Because urbanization is associated with changes in diet, physical activity, socioeconomic activity, and obesity, the risk of type 2 diabetes increases. This is best exemplified by the Pima Indians of the Southwestern United States, who have a greater than 50% chance of developing type 2 diabetes in their lifetime, but whose relatives in Mexico (who have a traditional lifestyle) have a very low risk of diabetes (Valencia et al., 1999).

Socioeconomic Status and Education

Socioeconomic status (SES) also is associated with the development of type 2 diabetes. Individuals in the lowest SES brackets have the highest risk of type 2 diabetes (ADA, 2001). In addition, lower levels of education also are inversely related to diabetes risk in the United States (ADA, 2001).

Intrauterine Environment

Intrauterine factors may increase the risk of type 2 diabetes. For example, low birth weight has been associated with an increased risk for developing diabetes. It has been hypothesized that this relationship is the result of undernutrition *in utero*, which causes a limited development of pancreatic beta cells, whose number is fixed at birth (Rich-Edwards et al., 1999).

Sequence in the Development of Type 2 Diabetes

Type 2 diabetes is a heterogeneous group of disorders characterized by decreased liver, muscle, and adipose tissue sensitivity to insulin, and a defect in insulin secretion from the pancreatic beta cell. Because both insulin resistance and a reduction in insulin secretion are present at diagnosis of type 2 diabetes, it is difficult to determine which of these metabolic abnormalities the initial defect is. Nonetheless, the development of type 2 diabetes follows a typically evolving course, which can be divided into three distinct stages.

In the first stage, genetic factors probably influence both insulin sensitivity and insulin secretion. As noted previously, environmental factors, such as obesity and physical inactivity, are usually associated with the development of insulin resistance. There is an initial period of hyperinsulinemia in which the pancreatic beta cell is able to overcome insulin resistance and maintain normal glucose tolerance. At this stage, although there is an underlying defect in insulin secretion, the pancreatic cell is able to produce a high level of insulin, and normal glucose homeostasis is maintained by a compensatory hyperinsulinemia (Figure 53–2 ■).

In the second stage, insulin resistance increases and this compensatory hyperinsulinemia becomes insufficient to maintain normal glucose homeostasis. Under conditions of insulin resistance, visceral adipose tissue is very sensitive to the effects of catecholamines and is associated with enhanced lipolysis. This leads to increased free fatty acids (FFA) production and mobilization, exacerbating insulin resistance in liver and muscle. In addition, impairments in insulin-mediated glucose uptake, particularly at the muscle, become evident. Insulin-mediated glucose transport into skeletal muscle, the major target for glucose disposal, becomes impaired. Fasting plasma glucose levels remain normal but postprandial (after a meal) plasma glucose levels rise (Figure 53–3 ■).

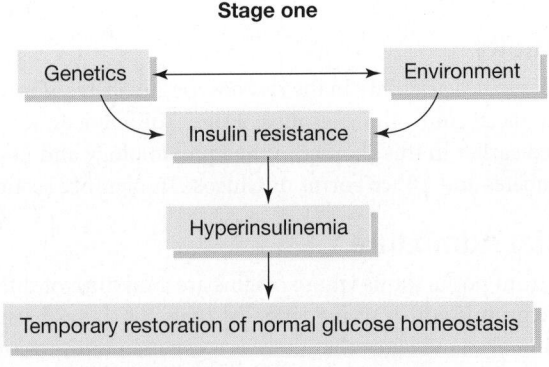

Stage one

Genetics ⟷ Environment

Insulin resistance

Hyperinsulinemia

Temporary restoration of normal glucose homeostasis

FIGURE 53–2 ■ Stage 1 development of type 2 DM.

Stage two

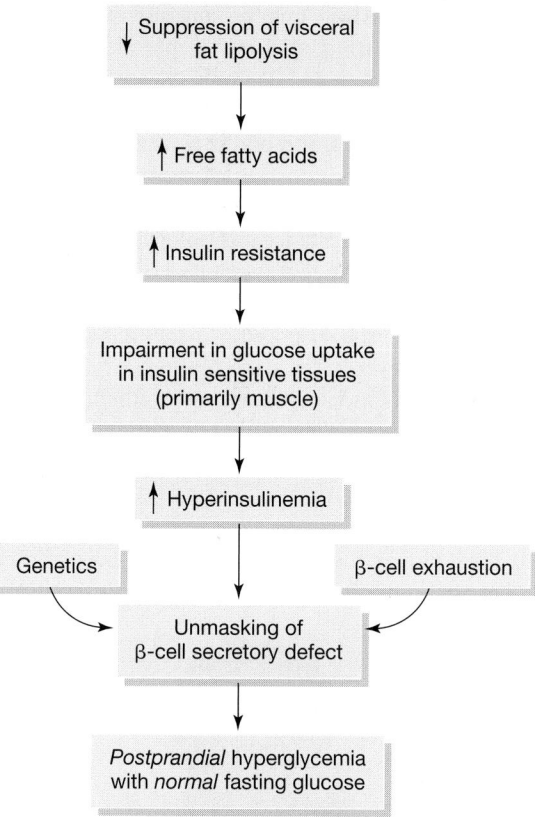

FIGURE 53–3 ■ Stage 2 development of type 2 DM.

Stage three

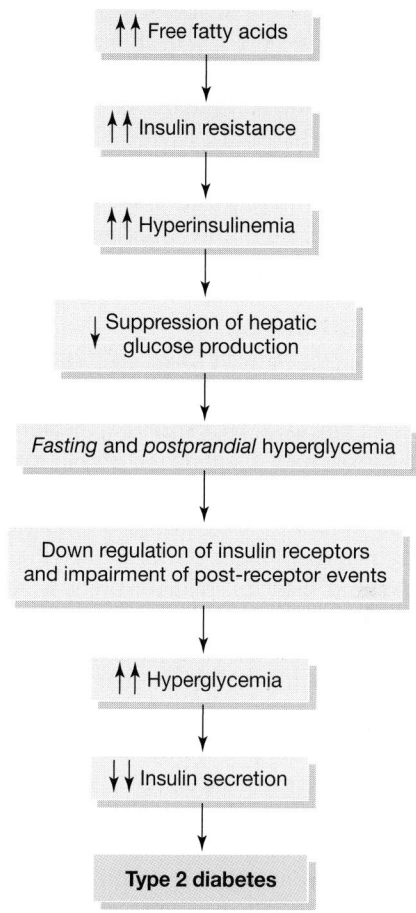

FIGURE 53–4 ■ Stage 3 development of type 2 DM.

In the third stage, there is a further increase in insulin resistance. The restraining effects of insulin on hepatic glucose production become impaired and plasma glucose levels increase. In addition, the worsening hyperglycemia has toxic effects on the pancreatic beta cell, and insulin secretion subsequently declines. With increasing insulin resistance, there is an even greater increase in FFA production and mobilization. The increase in FFAs causes a further increase in insulin resistance. Fasting and postprandial hyperglycemia result from increased insulin resistance, unrestrained hepatic glucose production, and glucose toxicity (Figure 53–4 ■).

Clinical Manifestations

In general, the clinical signs and symptoms of type 1 diabetes originate from hyperglycemia and ketosis, whereas the clinical signs and symptoms of type 2 diabetes originate from hyperglycemia. HHS is a medical emergency primarily associated with type 2 diabetes. The following are signs and symptoms of diabetes *uncomplicated* by DKA or HHS:

- *Glucosuria* (glucose in urine) is associated with an **osmotic diuresis,** an increase in urine volume caused by an osmotic substance (glucose) in the renal tubules.
- *Polyuria* (increased urination) is the primary clinical manifestation of the osmotic diuresis.
- *Nocturia* is frequent urination at night associated with *polyuria.*

- *Osmotic diuresis* is associated with dehydration and volume depletion.
- *Hypotension* (low blood pressure) occurs as a result of dehydration and volume depletion.
- *Tachycardia* (increased heart rate) also occurs as a result of dehydration and volume depletion.
- *Polydipsia* (increased thirst) is a compensatory response to the dehydration and volume depletion.
- *Polyphagia* (increased appetite) results from the significant loss of calories that occurs through the loss of calories in the urine. For example, the amount of glucose in the urine can exceed over 300 kcal/day (Funk, 2003).
- Weight loss occurs through dehydration, volume depletion, and the loss of calories in the urine.
- Fatigue is most likely related to alterations in CHO, protein, and lipid metabolism, especially protein catabolism.

Laboratory and Diagnostic Procedures

Diabetes is a chronic disease requiring frequent monitoring of blood glucose levels so that appropriate diagnoses are made and therapeutic goals can be accomplished through adjustments in diet, physical activity, and pharmacologic therapy. These determinations are performed in a clinical laboratory setting. Following the initial diagnosis of diabetes, patients are taught to measure blood glucose levels several times each day using portable glucose meters. This is called self-monitoring of blood glucose. In the following paragraphs, the laboratory measurement of blood glucose levels, measurement of longer term blood glucose control (e.g., glycosylated proteins), measurement of short-term glucose control, and miscellaneous indices of glycemic status (e.g., urine glucose, blood and urine ketones) are discussed.

Blood Glucose Levels

A fasting blood glucose level is performed using whole blood, plasma, and serum glucokinase, or hexokinase enzymatic methods (McPherson, Pincus, & Henry, 2007). The normal range of fasting blood glucose levels is approximately 60–100 mg/dL. The fasting blood glucose level is measured following an overnight fast (no food or drink with the exception of water) for 10 to 12 hours. Fasting blood glucose levels can be used in the diagnosis of pre-diabetes and diabetes. Additionally it is an important measurement in the daily monitoring of glycemic control.

Oral Glucose Tolerance Tests

As noted previously, **oral glucose tolerance tests (OGTTs)** can be used as diagnostic tools for pre-diabetes and diabetes in nonpregnant adults. Oral glucose tolerance tests normally are not used to diagnose diabetes, but can be useful in confirming the diagnosis of diabetes in atypical clinical presentations of diabetes. Patients are asked to fast for approximately 10 hours prior to the OGTT; they are asked to make certain that their intake of CHO is 150 g/day for the 3 days prior to the test (Joslin & Kahn, 2005). In addition, they are asked to refrain from smoking during the test and participate in their usual activity on the day prior to the test. In the standard OGTT, blood glucose levels are drawn prior to and 1/2, 1, 2, and 3 hours following ingestion of 75 grams of glucose (as in a commercial glucose preparation of glucose dissolved in water). As noted earlier, the diagnosis of pre-diabetes or diabetes is made on the 2-hour value ($\geq$140 to <200 mg/dL; and $\geq$200 mg/dL, respectively). The intermediate glucose levels (1/2, 1, and 3 or more hours) are used primarily for research purposes. Note that different criteria are used for the diagnosis of diabetes in pregnant women (Joslin & Kahn, 2005).

Self-Monitoring of Blood Glucose

One of the most important developments in the management of diabetes is self-monitoring of blood glucose (SMBG). The process of SMBG allows patients to measure blood glucose levels at any time and make changes in diet, physical activity, and pharmacologic therapy. The information can be used to make immediate decisions (e.g., insulin dose prior to meals) or this information can be used to make decisions on therapeutic changes based on blood glucose trends over time. Patients routinely are instructed to perform preprandial blood glucose measurements (i.e., immediately prior to meals and snacks), postprandial blood glucose measurements (i.e., approximately 2 hours after a meal or snack), or in the assessment of clinical symptoms (e.g., hypoglycemia). Patients and health care

providers can review the results of SMBG measurements together and discuss overall changes in management.

The process of SMBG involves measurement of capillary blood glucose levels using a variety of portable blood glucose meters (Figures 53–5A ■ and B). In this process, patients puncture their fingers with a small lancet device, obtaining a small drop of blood. This drop of blood is placed on a strip that has been placed in a small monitoring device. The meter technology falls into two general categories, reflectance and sensor methods. In meters using reflectance technology, the blood is placed directly on a reagent strip that is inserted over a glucose sensor. The blood reacts with an enzyme on the reagent strip; the meter shines a light on the strip and provides a digital readout of the blood glucose level. In sensor technology, a reaction between the glucose in the blood and an enzyme in the test strip generates an electrical charge. The charge is measured by the meter and a digital readout of the blood glucose level is provided (Harmel et al., 2004).

Whether blood glucose levels are measured in a home, hospital, or clinic setting, the meters need to have the highest degree of accuracy. In hospitals and clinics, strict quality control proce-

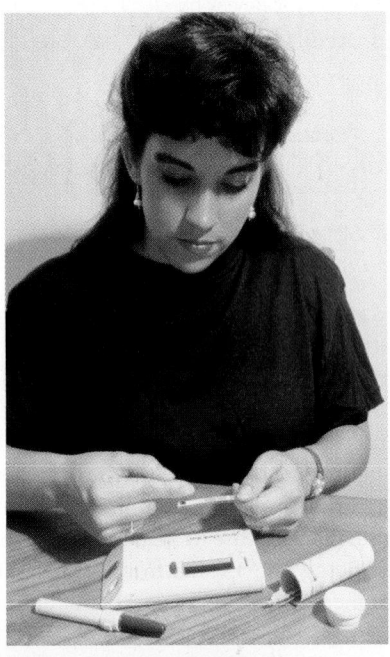

(a)

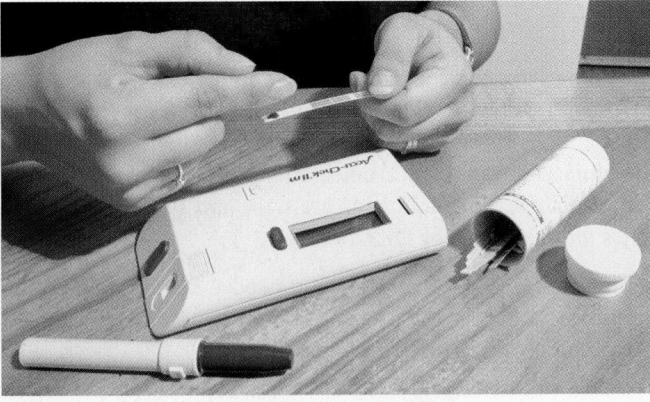

(b)

FIGURE 53–5 ■ Blood glucose monitor.
Source: Tony Freeman/PhotoEdit Inc.

dures are needed to maintain the accuracy of these devices, which are used by multiple operators on several patients. Each hospital or clinic has detailed quality control procedures to ensure that the meters are measuring blood glucose levels accurately and the operators are performing the test correctly. At minimum the procedures will include checking the meters against high, normal, and low standard solutions and periodically assessing operator technique. The standard solutions have specific glucose concentrations in the high, normal, and low ranges. When these solutions are placed on glucose test strips, they should yield a specific concentration. The nursing staff often is responsible for maintaining quality control checks and assessing their own performance. In addition to strict quality control procedures, the following steps are important in obtaining accurate blood glucose levels (Harmel et al., 2004):

- Strips must be current and properly stored at appropriate temperatures.
- The meter must be calibrated to the correct lot number of strips.
- The meter must be clean. This is particularly true of reflectance meters.
- An adequate amount of blood must be placed on the strip.
- The finger must be clean and dry prior to the puncture.

The timing of blood glucose measurements should correlate with the patient's meal status, clinical condition, and insulin regimen.

 CRITICAL ALERT *A hospitalized patient eating four times (three meals and a bedtime snack) per day should have a blood glucose measurement performed prior to each meal or snack. There should not be major gaps between glucose determinations and administration of food. For example, when calculating the prebreakfast dose of rapid-acting insulin, the calculation should be based on a glucose determination made shortly before breakfast, not several hours prior. Patients who are not eating also should have their glucose levels checked four times per day, but it may be more appropriate to check blood glucose levels every 6 hours, depending on their insulin regimen. In addition, patients who are more unstable may need determinations more frequently (e.g., every 2 hours).*

Continuous Blood Glucose Monitoring

During the past few years, blood glucose sensing devices have been developed that provide continuous intermittent measurement of the glucose level in interstitial fluid. The continuous blood glucose monitoring system (Medtronics, Inc.) measures glucose levels in interstitial fluid every 10 seconds and provides an average blood glucose level every 5 minutes (Figure 53–6 ■). The sensor is a small device with tubing and a small cannula; the cannula is inserted into the subcutaneous tissue, usually in the abdomen. The sensor is connected to a small monitor, roughly the size of a pager. At least three times each day the patient takes a fingerstick blood glucose level and programs it into the monitor for calibration purposes. The patient also programs events, such as meals and exercise, into the monitor.

In older versions of the sensor, the patient removes the device after 3 days and returns it to the health care provider who

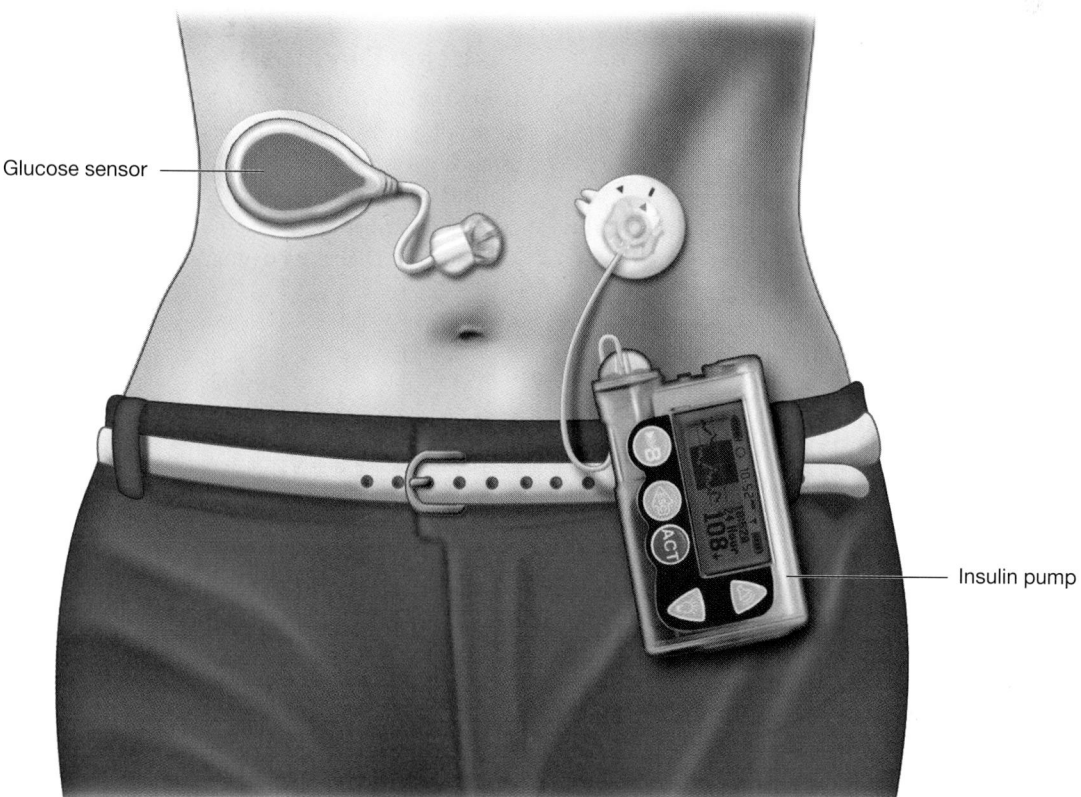

FIGURE 53–6 ■ Continuous blood glucose monitoring system.

downloads the blood glucose data. Together the patient and the health care provider discuss trends in the blood glucose patterns. Mutual decisions between the health care provider and the patient can be made regarding treatment decisions. Newer versions of the sensing device will allow the data to be accessed by the patients.

Hemoglobin A$_{1c}$ Test

The primary laboratory test used for monitoring longer term glucose control is the **hemoglobin A$_{1c}$ (HbA$_{1c}$) test**. A normal HbA$_{1c}$ is <6%. This test also is known as glycated hemoglobin or glycosylated hemoglobin, although it is most often referred to as "A1C." Hemoglobin A$_{1c}$ is formed when glucose in the blood binds irreversibly to hemoglobin to form a stable glycated hemoglobin complex. Protein glycation is the nonenzymatic reaction of sugars with proteins. Because the normal life span of red blood cells is 90 to 120 days, the HbA$_{1c}$ reflects the average blood glucose values of the previous 2 to 3 months and is directly proportional to the ambient concentration of plasma glucose in the blood over the life span of the red blood cells. This test is the most widely used measure for assessment of glucose control (Goldstein et al., 2004).

Glycated Serum Proteins

In addition to hemoglobin, there are a number of additional **glycated serum proteins** (GSPs) in diabetes. In particular, glycated albumin constitutes approximately 80% of the major proteins that undergo glycosylation (Barr, Nathan, Meigs, & Singer, 2002; McFarland, Catalano, Day, Thorpe, & Baynes, 1979). Because the half-life of albumin is 17 to 20 days, measurement of glycated albumin reflects short-term glycemic control (Harmel et al., 2004). Measurements of total GSPs and glycated serum albumin correlate can be useful, particularly in situations where the HbA$_{1c}$ cannot be measured or may not be of use (e.g., in the presence of hemolytic anemias). The fructosamine assay is the most widely used method of quantifying total GSPs or total glycated hemoglobin (Barr et al., 2002), reflecting short-term glycemic control.

Urinary Glucose

SMBG has replaced the measurement of urinary glucose as the measure of glycemic control. The urinary measurement of glucose involves the semiquantitative measurement of glucose, usually in a single urine specimen. Prior to the introduction of blood glucose monitoring devices, patients would make several assessments throughout the day of urinary blood glucose using chemical reagents to assess glycemic control. Urinary glucose is no longer used to routinely monitor glucose control; however, it is part of a routine urinalysis. Ordinarily, glucose should not be detectable in the urine. If glucose is present in a urine specimen, further evaluation is warranted.

Urinary and Blood Ketones

Urinary ketone testing is an essential part of diabetes self-management for patients with type 1 diabetes, pregnancy with preexisting diabetes, and gestational diabetes (Goldstein et al., 2004). Patients use chemical reagents to provide an estimate of urinary ketones, usually ranging from "trace" to "large" amounts. Normally ketones are not detectable in the urine. Urinary ketones may be present in nondiabetic individuals following fasting. In addition, urinary ketones may be present in the first morning urine of pregnant women.

The presence of detectable amounts of urinary ketones in the urine of patients with diabetes is reflective of impending large amounts of serum ketones, which are associated with the development of DKA. It is recommended that patients with type 1 diabetes test their urine for ketones, during times of stress or infection, when blood glucose levels are consistently elevated (>300 mg/dL) and when classic symptoms of DKA (e.g., abdominal pain, nausea, and vomiting) are present (Goldstein et al., 2004). In addition to urinary ketone assessment, bedside and self-testing kits can be used to quantify blood ketone (e.g., beta hydroxybutyrate) levels in a manner similar to those used to test capillary blood glucose levels (Bektas, Eray, Sari, & Akbas, 2004).

Diabetes Diagnosis

Using the laboratory tests just described, diabetes and other forms of glucose intolerance can be diagnosed using the criteria established by the ADA, which serve as a national guideline for diabetes diagnoses (ADA, 2007). Typically, any one of the three criteria described in the National Guidelines for Establishing a Diagnosis of Diabetes box may be used.

NATIONAL GUIDELINES for Establishing a Diagnosis of Diabetes

Diabetes Diagnosis

Any one of the following three criteria may be used to establish a diagnosis of diabetes:

- A random plasma glucose (PG) concentration of ≥200 mg/dL with symptoms of hyperglycemia, for example, polydipsia (excessive thirst), polyuria (excessive urination)
- A fasting plasma glucose (FPG) concentration of ≥126 mg/dL on more than one occasion with or without symptoms of hyperglycemia
- An elevated PG concentration (≥200 mg/dL) at 2 hours following consumption of 75 grams of glucose during an OGTT.

    Important: In the absence of unequivocal hyperglycemia, these criteria should be confirmed by repeat testing on a different day.

Pre-Diabetes Diagnosis

Pre-diabetes includes two categories: impaired fasting glucose (IFG) and impaired glucose tolerance (IGT). The criteria for each are as follows:

- Impaired fasting glucose is a condition in which the FPG is ≥100 and <126 mg/dL on two occasions.
- Impaired glucose tolerance is a 2-hour plasma blood glucose level ≥140 and <200 mg/dL following 75 grams of oral glucose.

Source: American Diabetes Association. (2007). Nutrition recommendations and interventions for diabetes: A position statement of the American Diabetes Association. *Diabetes Care, 30* (Suppl. 1), S48–S65.

Medical Management

The current philosophy of diabetes management is based primarily on the results of two major studies, the Diabetes Control and Complications Trial (DCCT) (DCCT Trial Research Group, 1993) and the **United Kingdom Prospective Diabetes Study (UKPDS)** (U.K. Prospective Diabetes Study Group [UKPDSG], 1998b). The DCCT and the UKPDS demonstrated in type 1 and type 2 diabetes, respectively, that any level of hyperglycemia is associated with the development of diabetes-related complications. In both of these studies, improvements in glycemic control were associated with reductions in microvascular complications (i.e., neuropathy, nephropathy, and retinopathy). The Evidence-Based Practice box (p. 1672) discusses glycemic control and its relationship to diabetes-related complications in more detail.

In the UKPDS, hypertension was associated positively with the development of microvascular complications, and improved blood pressure control was associated with reductions in microvascular disease (UKPDSG, 1998b). Thus the overall goal of diabetes management is the prevention of chronic long-term complications (such as those previously described), with distinctions between short-term and long-term goals. The short-term goals of diabetes management include prevention of severe hypoglycemia, hyperglycemia, and acute complications such as DKA and HHS. Long-term glycemic goals include normalizing blood glucose levels and preventing systemic complications. Laboratory tests for the monitoring short- and long-term glycemic control are detailed in Chart 53–2 (p. 1673).

Although the DCCT (DCCT Trial Research Group, 1993) and the UKPDS (UKPDSG, 1998b) demonstrated that improved glycemic control resulted in reductions in CVD, these reductions did not reach statistical significance. This suggests that the development of diabetes-related CVD is caused by a variety of factors, including glycemic control, dyslipidemias, hypertension, and prothrombotic factors. The target glycemic and metabolic goals for patients with diabetes are as follows (McCarren & ADA, 2007):

- Glycemic goals:
  - HbA_{1c}: <7.0% (These goals are individualized; some patients may establish more stringent glycemic goals, e.g., a normal A1C of <6%.)
  - Preprandial blood glucose: 90 to 130 mg/dL
  - Postprandial blood glucose: <180 mg/dL (The postprandial measurements are generally made 1 to 2 hours following the meal.)
- Blood pressure goals: <130/80 mmHg
- Lipid goals:
  - Low density lipoprotein (LDL) cholesterol: <100 mg/dL
  - Triglycerides: <150 mg/dL
  - High density lipoprotein (HDL) cholesterol: > 40 mg/dL

Current management strategies for the treatment of diabetes include a combination of exercise, nutrition, miscellaneous lifestyle changes (e.g., smoking cessation), and pharmacologic therapy directed toward normalization of blood glucose, blood pressure, and blood lipid levels. An extensive review of antihypertensive and lipid-lowering drugs is beyond the scope of this chapter, however, the role of glucose-lowering drugs is discussed next.

Pharmaceutical Management of Hyperglycemia

The pharmacologic treatment of both types 1 and 2 diabetes has undergone a revolution during the past two decades. The exact relationship between blood glucose levels and the development of chronic diabetes-related complications was debated for several years. Some researchers thought that these complications were the result of poor glycemic control, whereas others believed that there was no relationship. The DCCT (DCCT Trial Research Group, 1993) and the UKPDS (UKPDSG, 1998a) clarified that diabetes-related chronic complications could be prevented or reduced by maintaining **normoglycemia** (normal blood glucose levels). Patients with diabetes now use intricate pharmacologic regimens (along with medical nutrition therapy and exercise) to normalize blood glucose levels. Newer insulin preparations, insulin delivery systems, and oral medications have been developed to assist patients in maintaining normal blood glucose levels.

Because the basic pathophysiological defect in type 1 diabetes is a deficiency of insulin production, the pharmacologic treatment of type 1 diabetes involves the use of exogenous insulin to replace the insulin deficiency. Type 2 diabetes is characterized by insulin resistance and reduced insulin secretion, so the pharmacologic therapy of type 2 diabetes involves oral medications, insulin, or a combination of both. The general mechanisms of insulin and oral diabetes medication are discussed next, followed by discussion as to more specific pharmacologic treatment regimens for both type 1 and type 2 diabetes. This information is presented not to replace a pharmacologic text, but to highlight the important aspects of pharmacologic management.

Insulin Preparations

Until the mid-1980s insulin was produced from beef (bovine) and pork (porcine) sources. Beef and pork insulin preparations are no longer manufactured or marketed in the United States and current insulin products are produced synthetically.

Human insulin is produced by recombinant DNA technology; the structure of recombinant human insulin matches the amino acid sequence of human insulin. Insulin analogs have been developed through amino acid rearrangement, substitution, addition, and deletion in the structure of this synthetically produced human insulin. Insulin **analogs** are altered forms of insulin, different from the insulin secreted by the human pancreas, but still available to the human body for performing the same action as human insulin in terms of glycemic control. These insulin analogs have absorption and biologic activity that mimic the normal physiological pattern of endogenous insulin secretion more precisely than traditional insulin preparations.

Time Profile of Insulin Preparations

Insulin preparations are characterized by *onset, peaks, and duration* of action. Normal physiological insulin secretion involves both basal and meal-stimulated insulin release. Under normal physiological conditions, serum glucose and insulin responses are closely matched; when glucose levels rise, there is a corresponding rise in insulin levels. Under basal conditions (i.e., overnight, between meals, and during fasting) plasma glucose is maintained within a narrow range with a comparable response in insulin secretion. Following a meal, plasma glucose levels rise

Glycemic Control

Clinical Problem

Patients with diabetes often develop severe diabetes-related complications (neuropathy, nephropathy, retinopathy, and an accelerated development of all forms of cardiovascular disease). Nurses and other health care providers must apply evidence-based findings to reduce the development of these complications.

Research Findings

Two major studies have examined the relationship between glycemic control and the development of diabetes complications: the Diabetes Control and Complications Trial (DCCT Trial Research Group,1993) and the United Kingdom Prospective Diabetes Study (UKPDSG,1998a, 1998b). The results of these studies changed diabetes management and are the primary foundation for our current recommendations for glycemic control in diabetes.

The DCCT and UKPDS were prospective, randomized, controlled trials of intensive versus standard glycemic control of patients with type 1 and 2 diabetes, respectively. The DCCT demonstrated definitively that improved glycemic control is associated with sustained, decreased rates of microvascular complications (retinopathy, nephropathy, and neuropathy) in type 1 diabetes. The UKPDS demonstrated that, in patients with newly diagnosed type 2 diabetes, intensive use of medications (metformin, sulfonylureas, insulin) and lifestyle interventions reduced the development of microvascular disease. In the UKPDS there was a trend toward reduction in CVD, as noted by a statistically nonsignificant reduction ($p = 0.052$) in the risk for combined fatal and nonfatal myocardial infarction and sudden death.

In both of these studies, the mean HbA_{1c} of the intensive group was approximately 7%. Thus, the American Diabetes Association recommends that the target HbA_{1c} in patients with diabetes is 7%. Epidemiologic data have demonstrated an incremental benefit (although small in absolute terms) to lowering HbA_{1c} into the normal range (Stratton et al., 2000); however, this reduction must be balanced against the risk of hypoglycemia and other comorbidities.

The recommendations of the ADA (2008e) regarding glycemic control are as follows:

- Lowering HbA_{1c} to an average of ~7% has clearly been shown to reduce microvascular complications of diabetes and, possibly, macrovascular disease. Therefore, the HbA_{1c} goal for nonpregnant adults in general is <7%.

- Epidemiologic studies have suggested an incremental benefit to lowering HbA_{1c} from 7% into the normal range. Therefore, the HbA_{1c} goal for selected individual patients is as close to normal (<6%) as possible without significant hypoglycemia.

- Less stringent HbA_{1c} goals may be appropriate for patients with a history of severe hypoglycemia, patients with limited life expectancies, children, individuals with comorbid conditions, and those with long-standing diabetes with minimal or stable microvascular complications.

Implications for Nursing Practice

Attaining tight glycemic control in patients with diabetes requires a balance of diet, physical activity, and medications. This is not an easy task! Nurses are in a unique position to help patients self-manage their diabetes. Nurses need to develop strong assessment skills that examine the patient from clinical, cultural, behavioral, and psychosocial perspectives. Appropriate plans of care can be structured from this assessment.

Critical Thinking Questions

1. Joe S. is a 16-year-old patient with newly diagnosed type 1 diabetes. He refuses to check his blood glucose levels on a regular basis. When he asks "What is the big deal about checking my blood sugar?" which of the following would be your response?
   a. Keeping your blood glucose levels in the normal range is necessary to prevent diabetes complications!
   b. We know that keeping your blood sugar in the normal range is important in preventing complications and overall making you feel better, but let's talk about how things are going with your diabetes, in general.

2. Mary B. is a 44-year-old patient with type 2 diabetes. When she states "I have the adult form of diabetes; it is not a problem. I don't really need to check my blood sugar," how do you respond?
   a. There is a relationship between blood glucose levels and the development of complications that can occur regardless of the age at which you develop diabetes. Do you have the strips and a meter to check your sugar?
   b. You are correct! Diabetes that is diagnosed as an adult is far less serious than diabetes that is diagnosed as a child.

3. Sally J. is a 90-year-old women who was recently hospitalized for a hip fracture that occurred following a fall. During a home visit, the nurse finds that the patient (with the help of the family) is checking her blood glucose level two times per day and administering multiple daily injections of insulin. When you ask the family about this treatment regimen, they reply that they have a grandson with type 1 diabetes and understand the importance of "tight" glucose control. The patient has a HbA_{1c} of 6.0%. On discussions with her primary health care provider, you find that he has tried to have the patient and family target Sally's insulin therapy to a more reasonable goal of 7% to 7.5% but has had no success. How would you approach this?
   a. Tell the family that the risk of hypoglycemia (and falling again) is greater than the risk of developing complications.
   b. Organize a meeting with the social worker, physician, and other health care providers to discuss the best way to approach the patient and family, knowing (as above) that the risk of falling is greater than that of developing complications. If the patient and family still want "tight" glycemic control, then a monitoring plan should be developed to prevent hypoglycemia (accessible snacks, more frequent monitoring).

Answers to Critical Thinking Questions appear in Appendix D.

References

American Diabetes Association. (2008e). Standards of medical care in diabetes—2008. *Diabetes Care, 31*(Suppl. 1), S12–S54.

DCCT Trial Research Group. (1993). The effect of intensive treatment of diabetes on the development and progression of long-term complications in insulin-dependent diabetes mellitus. *New England Journal of Medicine, 329*(14), 977–986.

Stratton, I. M., Adler, A. I., Neil, H. A., Matthews, D. R., Manley, S. E., Cull, C. A., et al. (2000). Association of glycaemia with macrovascular and microvascular complications of type 2 diabetes (UKPDS 35): Prospective observational study. *British Medical Journal, 321*, 405–412.

U.K. Prospective Diabetes Study Group. (1998a). Effect of intensive blood-glucose control with metformin on complications in overweight patients with type 2 diabetes (UKPDS 34). *Lancet, 352*(9131), 854–865.

U.K. Prospective Diabetes Study Group. (1998b). Tight blood pressure control and risk of macrovascular and microvascular complications in type 2 diabetes (UKPDS 38). *British Medical Journal, 317*(7160), 703–713.

EVIDENCE-BASED PRACTICE

CHART 53–2 **Tests Used to Monitor Glycemia and Ketosis in Diabetes**

Test	Results	Comments
Blood glucose levels	70–110 mg/dL prior to meals <120 mg/dL 2 hours after a meal	
Hemoglobin A_{1c} (HbA_{1c} or A1c)	≤5%	Normal ranges may vary slightly depending on the laboratory used; reflects glucose control over the previous 3 months.
Glycosylated serum proteins (GSPs) Fructosamine Glycated albumin	0–285 µmol/L* 0.6–3%*	Reflects glucose control over the previous 2–3 weeks; higher levels reflect worsening glucose control.
Urine glucose	Negative	
Urine ketones	Negative	Often reported as "trace," "small," "moderate," or "high" with higher levels reflecting a greater degree of ketosis.
Serum ketones	Negative	Often reported in dilutions (e.g., 1:8, 1:16) with higher dilutions reflecting a greater degree of ketosis.

*Values from Associated Regional and University Pathologists, Inc. (ARUP) Laboratories, http://www.aruplab.com/guides.

and there is a rapid increase in insulin secretion. Therefore, insulin secretion often is referred to as basal or meal stimulated. The goal of insulin therapy is to mimic this normal pattern of insulin secretion. Therefore, pharmacologic insulin preparations are often characterized by their ability to mimic basal or meal-stimulated properties. In clinical practice the amount of insulin that is given to match the meal-stimulated insulin response is provided as an insulin "bolus."

Commercial insulin preparations are divided into rapid-, short-, intermediate-, and long-acting preparations based on onset, peak (highest concentration of insulin), and duration of action. The comparative actions of each preparation are detailed in Chart 53–3.

Five insulin analogs are currently available: lispro, aspart, glulisine, detemir, and glargine. Insulins lispro, aspart, and glulisine have rapid absorption profiles, whereas insulins detemir and glargine have delayed insulin absorption. The actions of insulins lispro, aspart, and glulisine most closely resemble meal-stimulated insulin responses, whereas insulins glargine and detemir most closely resembles basal insulin secretion.

CHART 53–3 **Comparative Effects of Common Insulin Preparations**

Type/Generic Name	Brand Name(s)	Onset (hours)	Peak (hours)	Duration (hours)
Rapid Acting				
Insulin lispro (analog) Insulin aspart Insulin glulisine	Humalog NovoLog Apidra	<0.25	1–2	3–4
Short Acting				
Regular	Humulin R Novolin R Humulin R (U-500)*	0.5–1.0	2–3	3–6
Intermediate Acting				
NPH (isophane)	Humulin N Novolin N	2–4	4–10	12–18
Long Acting				
Insulin glargine Insulin detemir	Lantus Levemir	2–4 0.8–2	Peakless Relatively flat	20–24 ~ 24
Combinations				
50% lispro protamine/50% insulin lispro	Humalog Mix 50/50	0.5–1	Dual	~18–24
70% NPH/30% regular	Humulin 70/30 Novolin 70/30	0.5–1	Dual	~18–24
50% NPH/50% regular	Humulin 50/50	0.5–1	Dual	~18–24
75% aspart protamine/25% aspart	NovoLog Mix 75/25	<0.25	Dual	~18–24
75% lispro protamine/25% lispro	Humalog Mix 75/25	<0.25	Dual	~18–24

*The concentration of commercial insulin in the United States is 100 units/mL (U-100); however, regular insulin is also available as 500 units/mL (U-500). This concentration is usually used only in patients who are extremely insulin resistant.

Rapid-Acting Insulin   The time-action profiles of the rapid-acting insulin analogs are detailed in Chart 53–3 (p. 1673). These preparations have an onset of action of approximately 15 minutes after injection, and reach peak biologic action within approximately 1 to 2 hours. They are most effective in reducing postprandial glycemia.

 *Because the onset of action of rapid-acting insulin preparations is so quick, they should be injected as close to the meal or snack as possible to avoid hypoglycemia. A critical role of the nurse is to be alert for signs and symptoms of hypoglycemia and educate patients and family about how to prevent and treat hypoglycemic reactions.*

Rapid-acting insulin preparations are routinely administered before a meal or snack; however, in certain situations these agents may be administered following a meal. For example, often it is difficult to predict the caloric intake of patients who are acutely or chronically ill because they may have changes in taste or appetite. In these situations, the actual amount of food consumed (particularly the CHO content) can be determined and a postmeal dose of rapid-acting insulin administered. This method helps to reduce the potential for hypoglycemia since the food intake and amount of insulin are more accurately matched.

Short-Acting Insulin   The only available short-acting insulin preparation is Regular insulin, which is injected prior to meals. To match the peak action of insulin with the postprandial rise in glucose, Regular insulin should be injected approximately 30 to 45 minutes prior to a meal. The use of Regular insulin has been largely replaced by rapid-acting insulin analogs. Because the rapid-acting preparations have a more rapid onset of action and a greater peak effect, they resemble meal-stimulated endogenous insulin secretion more closely than Regular insulin.

Intermediate-Acting Insulin   The only intermediate-acting insulin preparation currently available is Neutral Protamine Hagedorn (NPH) insulin. With a slow onset of action, prolonged peak effect, and lengthened duration of action, NPH insulin traditionally has been used to provide basal insulin coverage (usually with two injections per day). However, the use of NPH as basal insulin is somewhat limited due the high plasma insulin concentrations during peak action, thus increasing the risk of hypoglycemia.

Long-Acting Insulin   Long-acting insulin was produced to provide basal insulin coverage with relatively small peak biologic action. Glargine is a long-acting acting insulin analog that has no "peak" action, mirroring basal insulin secretion more precisely. Detemir, a newer long-acting insulin analog that has a relatively flat peak, also is used as basal insulin. Slight differences are seen in the onset, peaks, and duration of these preparations. These differences are detailed in Chart 53–3 (p. 1673).

Premixed Insulins

Premixed insulins are combinations of rapid- or short-acting insulin preparations mixed with intermediate-acting insulin in specific proportions. The most common premixed insulin contains 70% NPH and 30% Regular insulin (70/30). Other forms of premixed combinations are listed in Chart 53–3 (p. 1673). These premixed insulins are helpful in patients who have difficulty mixing insulin doses, however, they do not permit easy adjustment of premeal and basal insulin. For example, if a patient using 70/30 insulin needed an increase in pre-meal Regular insulin, it would be impossible to make this adjustment without also increasing the dose of NPH.

Incretin Mimetics

Exenatide injection (Byetta) (Amylin Pharmaceuticals, 2007) is an injectable medication used as adjunctive mealtime therapy to improve glycemic control in patients with type 2 diabetes mellitus who are taking metformin, sulfonylureas, or a combination of metformin and sulfonylureas. This medication belongs to a class of medications called **incretin mimetics**. An incretin mimetic enhances glucose-dependent insulin secretion from the pancreatic beta cell. Therefore, the greatest effect of exenatide is a reduction in postprandial glucose levels. In addition, the incretins suppress elevated glucagon levels, promoting satiety, decreasing food intake, and slowing gastric emptying.

The primary side effect of exenatide is nausea. The nausea may be minimized by increasing the medication dosage slowly. Exenatide should be administered subcutaneously 60 minutes prior to meals. Exenatide may decrease the rate at which orally administered drugs are absorbed. Therefore, oral medications that require rapid absorption that are dependent on threshold concentrations for effective action (e.g., antibiotics and oral contraceptives) should be administered 1 hour prior to administration of the exenatide.

Amylin Analog

Pramlintide acetate injection (Symlin) (Amylin Pharmaceuticals, 2007) is a synthetic analog of human amylin, a hormone secreted by the pancreatic beta cell. Pramlintide can reduce postprandial blood glucose control by slowing gastric emptying, suppressing glucagon secretion, and promoting satiety. Pramlintide is injected subcutaneously immediately before meals (Gutierrez, 2008) and is indicated for improving glycemic control in type 2 diabetes. It also can be used as adjuvant mealtime therapy for the treatment of type 1 diabetes. Pramlintide may decrease the rate at which drugs affecting gastrointestinal motility and alpha-glucosidase inhibitors are absorbed. Such medications should be administered 1 hour before or 2 hours after administration of pramlintide.

Insulin Delivery Devices

A number of insulin delivery devices are available for the administration of insulin. These vary from syringes to pens to cartridges. The ADA publishes a product directory every January in its *Diabetes Forecast* magazine. This is an excellent resource for exploring the ever-changing spectrum of diabetes products (e.g., insulin pumps, sensors, pens, cartridges, and meters).

The traditional method of delivering insulin is a disposable insulin syringe and needle. Recently, however, a variety of pens and insulin cartridges have been developed to add flexibility in insulin dosing and administration. The spectrum of pens and cartridges include disposable and reusable devices and a variety of insulin preparations.

Insulin Pumps

Continuous subcutaneous insulin infusion (CSII) is a method of intensive insulin therapy that is used in the management of diabetes. An insulin pump is made up of a pump reservoir (syringe) filled with insulin, a small battery-operated pump, and a computer chip that allows the patient to program and deliver a specific amount of insulin on a regular basis (Figure 53–7 ■). The reservoir is connected to tubing with a needle or flexible cannula at the end, through which the insulin is delivered. The cannula is inserted subcutaneously, usually on the abdomen. The entire infusion set is changed routinely every 2 days.

The pump delivers insulin 24 hours a day in programmed rates specific to each patient. Insulin pumps are designed to help mimic the basal and meal-stimulated patterns of endogenous insulin secretion. During insulin pump therapy, a small amount of short- or rapid-acting insulin is infused continuously. This rate helps to maintain blood glucose levels within a normal range between meals and during the night.

The pump can be programmed to infuse differing basal rates throughout the 24-hour period. For example, a patient who exercises every day at a particular time may elect to decrease the basal rate during the exercise period. Prior to meals and snacks, the patient injects a specific calculated dose or "bolus" of insulin through the pump. This dose of insulin is calculated based on the premeal/snack blood glucose levels and the CHO content of the meal/snack and reflects meal-stimulated insulin secretion.

Oral Diabetes Medications

Currently six classes of oral medications are approved for the treatment of type 2 diabetes in the United States: *sulfonylureas, meglitinides, α-glucosidase inhibitors, biguanides, thiazolidinediones,* and *dipeptidyl peptidase-4 (DPP-4) inhibitors.* Broadly these medications are grouped into those that enhance insulin secretion (sulfonylureas and rapid-acting secretagogues), reduce hepatic glucose production (biguanides), delay digestion and absorption of intestinal CHO (alpha-glucosidase inhibitors), improve insulin sensitivity (thiazolidinediones and biguanides), and increase postprandial insulin secretion (DPP-4 inhibitors).

The general characteristics of medications within these classes are detailed in the Pharmacology Summary (p. 1678). General information regarding the major classes of drugs used to treat type 2 diabetes is also provided in the Pharmacology Summary (p. 1678). More detailed information regarding drugs within each of these classes is included in the following paragraphs. This information is not meant to replace a pharmacology text, but to highlight important information.

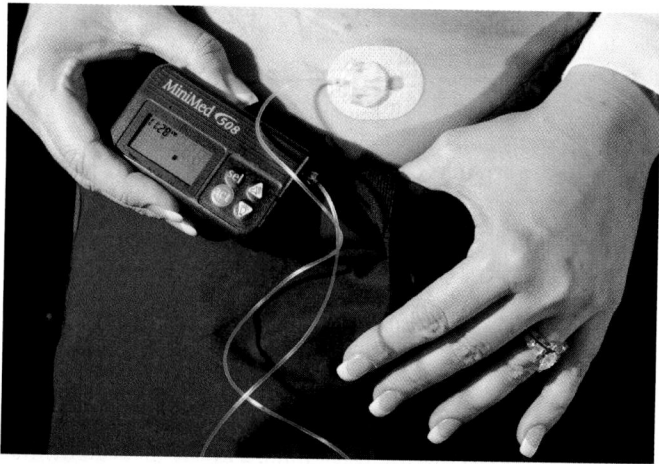

FIGURE 53–7 ■ Insulin pump.
Source: Spencer Grant/Photo Researchers, Inc.

Sulfonylureas

Sulfonylureas are indicated for the treatment of type 2 diabetes and have been an important part of diabetes therapy for several decades. These medications are grouped into first-generation and second-generation compounds. The first-generation products are associated with greater adverse events and interactions. These compounds have been replaced largely by the second-generation compounds.

The primary mechanism through which sulfonylureas exert their effects is by stimulating insulin secretion from the pancreatic beta cell. The secretion of insulin is regulated by ATP-dependent potassium channels, located in the plasma membrane of the pancreatic beta-cell. Sulfonylureas bind to the sulfonylurea receptor and close ATP-dependent potassium channels. As potassium accumulates within the beta cell membrane, the beta cell depolarizes, leading to an influx of calcium. The increased concentration of calcium causes insulin granules to migrate to the cell surface, where the granules rupture and release the insulin by exocytosis (Campbell & White, 2000).

The most common side effect of oral sulfonylureas is hypoglycemia. In addition, there are two specific issues that are important to note. First, there is some cross-sensitivity with sulfa medications, suggesting that some patients who are allergic to sulfa will also be allergic to sulfonylureas. Second, the combination of chlorpropamide and alcohol can result in a disulfiram (medication used in the treatment of alcoholism) reaction characterized by warmth, flushing, headache, nausea, vomiting, sweating, and thirst (Harmel et al., 2004). Although chlorpropamide is seldom used, patients are still advised to avoid alcohol when prescribed second-generation sulfonylureas are used (e.g., glipizide, glyburide, glimepiride).

Meglitinides

Meglitinides are indicated as an adjunct to nutrition and exercise in patients with type 2 diabetes to reduce hyperglycemia. Meglitinides comprise a new class of insulin secretagogues that are structurally and pharmacologically distinct from sulfonylureas (Krentz & Bailey, 2005). This class of medications causes rapid secretion of insulin from the pancreatic beta cells. They are given prior to meals in order to reduce postprandial hyperglycemia.

Meglitinides bind to the sulfonylurea receptor on the plasma membrane of the pancreatic beta cell at a site distinct from the sulfonylurea binding site. This results in the closure of ATP-dependent potassium channels. The closure of these channels inhibits potassium efflux from the cell, and causes membrane depolarization and calcium influx (Campbell & White, 2000). This influx of calcium stimulates the secretion of insulin from the beta cell as described previously with respect to sulfonylureas. There are distinct differences, however, between the onset and duration of action of sulfonylureas and meglitinides. Whereas, sulfonylureas cause insulin to be released in a sustained fashion and are associated with a longer duration of action, meglitinides cause insulin to be released rapidly and are associated with a shorter duration of action (Campbell & White, 2000). The rapid absorption pattern of meglitinides makes them ideal agents to be administered prior to each meal to reduce postprandial hyperglycemia.

Because the meglitinides induce a rapid insulin response, hypoglycemia is a potential risk. Patients need to be counseled to eat within 20 minutes after oral administration to prevent hypoglycemia.

Alpha-Glucosidase Inhibitors

There is increasing emphasis on the contribution of postprandial hyperglycemia to the development of diabetes-related complications. Alpha-glucosidase inhibitors have the ability to reduce the postprandial rise in blood glucose levels and improve glucose control.

Alpha-glucosidase inhibitors are named for their ability to reversibly bind to alpha-glucosidase enzymes (i.e., sucrase, maltase, isomaltase, and glucoamylase) in the brush border of the small intestine. The alpha-glucosidase enzymes break down disaccharides and oligosaccharides into glucose and other monosaccharides that can be absorbed in the small intestine. The competitive reversible binding by the alpha-glucosidase inhibitors to these enzymes delays the absorption of CHOs from the gastrointestinal tract, which leads to a more even absorption of sugars throughout the gut. As a result, there is a blunting of the normally sharp rise in postprandial blood glucose levels that follow a meal.

The gastrointestinal side effects, such as softer stools, diarrhea, flatulence, and bloating, are self-limiting and can be reduced with a lower initial starting dose and a slower dose titration. However, alpha-glucosidase inhibitors are contraindicated in a number of gastrointestinal problems including inflammatory bowel disease, colonic ulceration, and partial intestinal obstruction (Campbell & White, 2000). In addition, alpha-glucosidase inhibitors are contraindicated in the presence of any chronic intestinal disease associated with marked alterations in digestion and absorption and any gastrointestinal conditions that may deteriorate as a result of increased intestinal gas formation (Campbell & White, 2000). Hypoglycemia can occur with alpha-glucosidase inhibitors; hence, patients need to be counseled to use pure glucose, such as fruit juices, glucose tablets, and glucose gels to treat their reactions because the absorption of other CHO may be delayed.

Biguanides

Biguanides are a class of medications that has been used extensively in Europe since the 1950s. One of the earlier compounds, phenformin, was approved for use in the United States in 1959. Federal approval for this medication was withdrawn in 1976 after several cases of fatal lactic acidosis (Krentz & Bailey, 2005). Metformin is another biguanide that has been used extensively in Europe for several decades and has a well-established safety profile. In 1995, this compound was approved for use in the United States.

Metformin has a number of effects on CHO and lipid metabolism. Metformin enhances the sensitivity of peripheral and hepatic tissues to insulin. This compound has multiple effects on the liver, reducing both hepatic glycogenolysis and gluconeogenesis and increasing glycogen synthesis. This reduction in hepatic glycogenolysis and gluconeogenesis results in decreased hepatic glucose production and lowers blood glucose concentrations.

The primary side effects of metformin are gastrointestinal disturbances such as nausea, vomiting, and diarrhea. These side effects can largely be prevented through slow titration of the dosage. A rare but important adverse reaction associated with metformin is lactic acidosis. As noted previously, metformin is excreted primarily by the kidney. Therefore, in the presence of renal insufficiency, the medication accumulates and the risk of lactic acidosis increases. Although lactic acidosis is not a frequent complication of metformin therapy, when it does occur, it can be life threatening. Therefore, careful screening of patients at greatest risk for developing lactic acidosis is the best prevention.

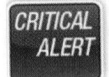
Metformin is contraindicated in patients with acute or chronic metabolic acidosis, who have known hypersensitivity to metformin, heart failure requiring pharmacologic management, renal disease or dysfunction as evidenced by serum creatinine levels ≥ 1.5 mg/dL (males) and ≥ 1.4 mg/dL (females) or abnormal creatinine clearance, and age >80 years with an abnormal creatinine clearance.

Radiological studies often are associated with nephrotoxic contrast dyes. The diabetic kidney is particularly vulnerable to these dyes. In patients treated with metformin, deterioration in renal function can result in accumulation of lactic acid and development of lactic acidosis. Metformin should be withheld for at least 48 hours after procedures in which iodinated radio contrast dyes are used and restarted when serum creatinine levels are normal. In addition, metformin should be discontinued temporarily for any surgical procedure and should be reinstituted only after it has been established that postprocedure renal function is normal.

A number of medical conditions, such as heart failure, acute myocardial infarction, and septic shock, are associated with hypoxia, decreased tissue perfusion, and lactic acidosis. As such, metformin is contraindicated during these situations. Because patients who consume excess alcohol have a greater propensity for lactic acidosis, metformin should be used cautiously in chronic alcohol abusers. Impaired hepatic function also is associated with lactic acidosis and thus metformin should be used cautiously in such patients.

Thiazolidinediones

The thiazolidinediones are a unique class of antihyperglycemic medications that improve insulin sensitivity through multiple actions on gene regulation. These drugs, which are often termed *insulin sensitizers*, require that circulating levels of insulin be present for these drugs to be effective.

The action mechanisms of thiazolidinediones are not completely understood. The effects of thiazolidinediones are mediated through a family of nuclear receptors, called the peroxisome-proliferator-activated (PPAR) receptors. The PPAR family of receptors is responsible for the modulation of lipid homeostasis, adipocyte differentiation, and insulin action. In particular, thiazolidinediones bind and activate the PPAR isoform, improving blood glucose control through enhancement of hepatic and peripheral insulin sensitivity. The thiazolidinediones also show some cross reactivity with other isoforms in the PPAR family, which accounts for their potential roles in a variety of cellular processes, such as regulation of lipid metabolism.

The first thiazolidinedione, troglitazone, was associated with fatal liver toxicity and was withdrawn from the U.S. market in 2000. Because pioglitazone and rosiglitazone are biochemically related to troglitazone, strict guidelines were developed by the U.S. Food and Drug Administration (FDA) regarding how frequently liver function should be monitored. Active liver disease does remain a contraindication to the use of thiazolidinediones, even though pioglitazone and rosiglitazone have not been associated with hepatotoxicity (Krentz & Bailey, 2005). In 2004, the FDA recommendation for monitoring of liver enzymes was relaxed. Liver enzymes must be drawn prior to the initiation of thiazolidinediones and periodically thereafter, based on the clinical judgment of the health care provider.

Fluid retention and weight gain are the main adverse effects in human trials of thiazolidinediones. The fluid retention can result in edema and cases of heart failure have been precipitated. Patients who had significant heart failure, categorized as New York Heart Association (NYHA) class III and IV, were excluded from phase III trials of rosiglitazone and pioglitazone because troglitazone was associated with volume expansion, increased preload, and adverse cardiac effects in animal models of hypoglycemia (Campbell & White, 2000). Therefore, the thiazolidinediones are contraindicated in patients with NYHA class III and IV heart failure.

Dipeptidyl Peptidase-4 Inhibitors

The newest class of oral diabetes medications is the DPP-4 inhibitors. These medications are a part of incretin-related therapies that exert their effects by increasing meal-related insulin secretion and reducing postprandial blood glucose levels.

Incretin hormones, including glucagon-like peptide 1 (GLP-1) and glucose-dependent insulinotropic polypeptide (GIP), are released by the intestine throughout the day, and levels are increased in response to a meal. These hormones are rapidly inactivated by the enzyme dipeptidyl peptidase 4. When blood glucose concentrations are normal or elevated, GLP-1 and GIP increase insulin synthesis and release from pancreatic beta cells. GLP-1 also lowers glucagon secretion from pancreatic cells, leading to reduced hepatic glucose production.

Sitagliptin currently is the only DDP inhibitor approved in the United States; however, a number of newer DDP inhibitors are in clinical trials. One rare complication of sitagliptin is Stevens-Johnson syndrome, a life-threatening hypersensitivity reaction affecting the skin (Burant & ADA, 2008). In general, no dosage adjustment is needed for patients with mild to moderate liver or kidney disease; however, lower dosages are recommended for patients with moderate and severe kidney disease or ESRD requiring hemodialysis.

Approach to Insulin Therapy in Type 1 Diabetes

As previously noted, patients with type 1 diabetes rely on exogenous insulin to sustain life. The goal of insulin therapy in type 1 diabetes is the normalization of blood glucose levels. This is best achieved using combinations of insulin in a manner that most closely resembles basal and meal-stimulated insulin release. See the Pharmacology Summary of Medications to Treat Type 2 Diabetes (p. 1678).

Some of the options for insulin regimens are presented next.

Twice-Daily Injection Regimen

The insulin regimens discussed in this section are examples of a two-injection regimen, combining Regular or rapid-acting insulin (lispro) with an intermediate-acting insulin (NPH) prior to breakfast and prior to supper (Figure 53–8 ■).

The lispro peaks when the blood glucose level rises after breakfast and dinner and the NPH insulin provides basal insulin coverage. The Regular insulin peaks later and the peaks are not

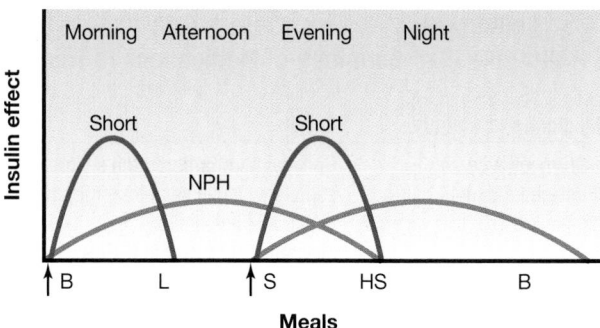

(a)

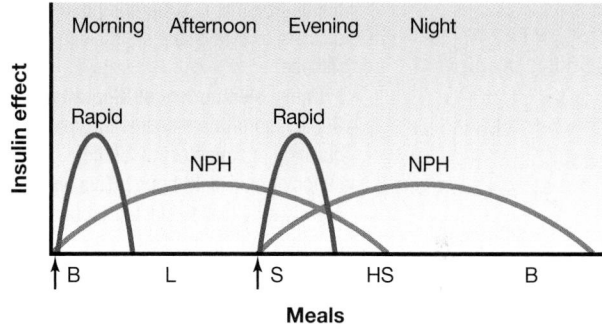

(b)

FIGURE 53–8 ■ Twice-daily split and mixed insulin regimen.

as high. Because no rapid-acting insulin is provided at lunch, the peak of the NPH insulin helps to reduce blood glucose levels following lunch. Using this regimen, patients with type 1 diabetes can attain *adequate* glucose control. The peak effect of NPH predisposes patients to hypoglycemia if meals are skipped. This regimen provides the patient little flexibility in changing mealtimes.

Three-Times-Daily Injection Regimen

The regimen discussed here is an example of a three-times-daily injection regimen (Figure 53–9 ■, p. 1682), combining Regular or rapid-acting insulin with NPH prior to breakfast, Regular or rapid-acting insulin prior to dinner, and NPH prior to bedtime. The major difference in this method with the method described in the previous paragraph is that the NPH is injected prior to bedtime. The movement of the NPH to bedtime means that the NPH will peak in the middle of the night, when the glucose is rising in response to the normal increase in endogenous growth hormone secretion. This method has value in individuals who have high fasting glucose levels on awakening.

There are two major causes of fasting hyperglycemia, the **dawn phenomenon** and the **Somogyi effect**. The dawn phenomenon is defined as fasting hyperglycemia without prior nocturnal hypoglycemia, and the Somogyi effect is defined as fasting hyperglycemia with prior hypoglycemia (Sheehan, 2004). The dawn phenomenon occurs when growth hormone, a counterregulatory hormone, is secreted during the night. Patients awake with elevated fasting blood glucose levels, precipitated, in part, by growth hormone. Moving the timing of the NPH insulin to bedtime means that the NPH insulin will peak as growth hormone rises.

PHARMACOLOGY Summary of Medications to Treat Type 2 Diabetes

Medication/Category	Action	Application/Indication	Nursing Responsibility
Chlorpropamide (First-generation sulfonylurea)	**General Mechanism:** Sulfonylureas stimulate insulin secretion from the pancreatic beta cells. **Mechanism of Action (MOA):** These medications bind with a cell surface protein on the pancreatic beta cell. The binding of the sulfonylurea with the sulfonylurea receptor (SUR) results in the closure of potassium channels and depolarizes the cell membrane, opening calcium channels and stimulating insulin release. **Primary Mechanism of Clearance:** Renal chlorpropamide has the longest duration of action of any of the sulfonylureas (>48 hours). This enhanced activity may place selected groups (e.g., elderly, renal disease) at risk for hypoglycemia.	Used to lower blood glucose in patients with type 2 diabetes.	Assess patient for allergy to other sulfonylureas or sulfa medications. Assess patient for renal or liver disease. Assess patients who are at high risk for injury from hypoglycemia (e.g., elderly). Assess patient for signs and symptoms of hyponatremia (chlorpropamide specific effect). Assess patient for weight gain. Instruct patient on the signs and symptoms of hypoglycemia. Instruct patient on the treatment of hypoglycemia. Instruct patient to avoid ingesting alcohol with medication to prevent a disulfiram reaction.
Tolbutamide (First-generation oral sulfonylurea)	**General Mechanism:** Sulfonylureas stimulate insulin secretion from the pancreatic beta cells. **MOA:** See above **Primary Mechanism of Clearance:** Hepatic	Lowers blood glucose in patients with type 2 diabetes.	As above
Tolazamide (First-generation sulfonylurea)	**General Mechanism:** Sulfonylureas stimulate insulin secretion from the pancreatic beta cells. **MOA:** See above **Primary Mechanism of Clearance:** Hepatic and renal	Lowers blood glucose in patients with type 2 diabetes.	As above
Glyburide (Second-generation sulfonylurea)	**General Mechanism:** Sulfonylureas stimulate insulin secretion from the pancreatic beta cells. **MOA:** See above **Primary Mechanism of Clearance:** Hepatic and renal	Lowers blood glucose in patients with type 2 diabetes.	As above
Glipizide (Second-generation sulfonylurea; available in extended-release formulations)	**General Mechanism:** Sulfonylureas stimulate insulin secretion from the pancreatic beta cells. **MOA:** See above **Primary Mechanism of Clearance:** Hepatic	Lowers blood glucose in patients with type 2 diabetes.	As above *In addition:* Instruct patient to take glipizide with meals.
Glimepiride (Second-generation sulfonylurea)	**General Mechanism:** Sulfonylureas stimulate insulin secretion from the pancreatic beta cells. **MOA:** See above **Primary Mechanism of Clearance:** Hepatic and renal	Lowers blood glucose in patients with type 2 diabetes.	As above

PHARMACOLOGY Summary of Medications to Treat Type 2 Diabetes—*Continued*

Medication/Category	Action	Application/Indication	Nursing Responsibility
Metformin (Biguanide) (available in extended-release formulations)	**General Mechanism:** Metformin reduces hepatic glucose production and improves insulin sensitivity. **MOA:** Metformin reduces hepatic glucose production through decreased hepatic glycogenolysis and decreased hepatic gluconeogenesis. It also improves insulin sensitivity through mechanisms that are not entirely clear. **Primary Method of Clearance:** Metformin is not metabolized but is cleared rapidly from the kidney. Metformin is contraindicated in patients with renal, cardiorespiratory, hepatic dysfunction, and alcohol abuse. These conditions may precipitate lactic acidosis, which is a rare, but life-threatening, complication. Renal dysfunction is defined as: Serum creatinine: $\geq$1.5 mg/dL in males; $\geq$1.4 mg/dL in females; or abnormal creatinine clearance. Elderly patients need a 24-hour urine for creatinine clearance prior to starting on metformin.	Lowers blood glucose in patients with type 2 diabetes.	Assess patient for allergy to metformin. Assess patient for contraindications to metformin (renal, cardiorespiratory, hepatic dysfunction, and alcohol abuse). Assess patient for the development of gastrointestinal symptoms, such as diarrhea, nausea, vomiting, flatulence, abdominal discomfort, and indigestion. Encourage patients to report continued gastrointestinal symptoms to their health care provider, because the symptoms may resolve with slower titration of the metformin dose. Discuss with patient the risk of lactic acidosis. Instruct patient on the signs and symptoms of hypoglycemia. In general, metformin does not cause hypoglycemia as monotherapy. However, hypoglycemia may occur when metformin is combined with other medications. Discuss with patients the need to discontinue metformin prior to any procedure using a radiocontrast dye, and to resume the medication only when normal renal function has been assessed.
Acarbose (Alpha-glucosidase inhibitor)	**General Mechanism:** Alpha-glucosidase inhibitors reduce postprandial hyperglycemia. **MOA:** The actions of the alpha-glucosidase inhibitors occur in the intestinal lumen where they competitively inhibit enzymes that convert polysaccharides into simple sugars. The alpha-glucosidase inhibitors delay the absorption of dietary carbohydrates until they reach the distal bowel. As a result, these inhibitors reduce postprandial hyperglycemia. **Primary Method of Clearance:** Renal and feces	Lowers postprandial hyperglycemia in patients with type 2 diabetes.	Assess patient for allergy to alpha-glucosidase inhibitors. Assess patient for any gastrointestinal conditions (e.g., inflammatory bowel disease, colonic ulceration, partial intestinal obstruction) that may deteriorate as a result of increased intestinal gas formation. Instruct patient to contact her health care provider for continued bloating and flatulence, because the symptoms may resolve with slower titration of the alpha-glucosidase dose. Instruct patient to take the medication with the first bite of each meal. Instruct patient to recognize the signs and symptoms of hypoglycemia. In general, alpha-glucosidase inhibitors do not cause hypoglycemia when used as monotherapy. Hypoglycemia can occur when used in combination with other hypoglycemic medications. Instruct patient on the treatment of hypoglycemia. Patients using alpha-glucosidase inhibitors need to treat their reactions with pure glucose, such as glucose gels, glucose tablets, or fruit juice, because the absorption of other carbohydrates may be delayed.

(continued)

PHARMACOLOGY Summary of Medications to Treat Type 2 Diabetes—*Continued*

Medication/Category	Action	Application/Indication	Nursing Responsibility
Miglitol (Alpha-glucosidase inhibitor)	**General Mechanism:** Alpha-glucosidase inhibitors reduce postprandial hyperglycemia. **MOA:** See above **Primary Method of Clearance:** Renal	Lowers postprandial hyperglycemia in patients with type 2 diabetes.	As above
Repaglinide (Meglitinide)	**General Mechanism:** Meglitinides cause a rapid increase in insulin secretion. **MOA:** Meglitinides are nonsulfonylureas medications that act through the SUR on the pancreatic beta cells. The meglitinides bind with the SUR at a site distinct for the traditional sulfonylureas (see above). The binding of the sulfonylurea with the SUR results in the closure of potassium channels and depolarizes the cell membrane, opening calcium channels and stimulating insulin release. The meglitinides differ from the sulfonylureas in that the insulin response is rapid and exerts it major effect on postprandial hyperglycemia. **Primary Method of Clearance:** Hepatic	Lowers postprandial hyperglycemia in patients with type 2 diabetes.	Assess patient for any allergies to meglitinide. Instruct patient to take the medication at the start of the meal and to withhold the dose if no meal is eaten. Instruct patient on the signs and symptoms of hypoglycemia. Instruct patient on the treatment of hypoglycemia.
Nateglinide (Meglitinide)	**General Mechanism:** Meglitinides cause a rapid increase in insulin secretion. **MOA:** See above **Primary Method of Clearance:** Hepatic and renal	Lowers postprandial hyperglycemia in patients with type 2 diabetes.	As above
Sitagliptin (Dipeptidyl peptidase-4 [DPP-4] inhibitor)	**General Mechanism:** DPP-4 inhibitors lower postprandial hyperglycemia. **MOA:** Glucagon-like peptide 1 (GLP-1) is a hormone that is secreted by the intestinal L-cell, which suppresses elevated glucagon levels, promotes satiety, decreases food intake, and slows gastric emptying. DPP-4 is an enzyme that inactivates the GLP-1 peptide. DPP-4 inhibitors slow the breakdown of GLP-1 and thereby extend the effects of the hormone. **Primary Method of Clearance:** Hepatic and renal	Lowers postprandial hyperglycemia in patients with type 2 diabetes.	Assess patient for allergies to DPP-4 inhibitors. Instruct patient to notify health care provider if a skin rash develops.
Pioglitazone (Thiazolidinedione)	**General Mechanism:** Thiazolidinediones improve insulin sensitivity. **MOA:** The actions of thiazolidinediones occur through the actions of a group of nuclear regulatory proteins, peroxisome-proliferator-activated (PPAR) receptors, which are important in fat and carbohydrate metabolism. Thiazolidinediones bind and activate the PPARγ isoform and improve insulin sensitivity. **Primary Method of Clearance:** Hepatic	Lowers postprandial hyperglycemia in patients with type 2 diabetes.	Assess patient for the presence of liver disease. Monitor patient for weight gain and fluid retention. Instruct patient to contact his health care provider if shortness of breath, edema, and fatigue develop. Instruct patient to contact her health care provider if signs and symptoms develop of liver disease: nausea, vomiting, fatigue, jaundice, and dark urine. Instruct anovulatory premenopausal women (e.g., polycystic ovarian syndrome) that these medications may cause ovulation to resume and pregnancy to occur.

PHARMACOLOGY Summary of Medications to Treat Type 2 Diabetes—*Continued*

Medication/Category	Action	Application/Indication	Nursing Responsibility
Rosiglitazone (Thiazolidinedione)	**General Mechanism:** Thiazolidinediones improve insulin sensitivity. **MOA:** See above **Primary Method of Clearance:** Hepatic	As above	As above
Exenatide (Incretin mimetics)	**General Mechanism:** Exenatide reduces postprandial hyperglycemia. **MOA:** Exenatide is an analog of GLP-1 (see DPP-4 inhibitors) that suppresses elevated glucagon levels, promotes satiety, decreases food intake, and slows gastric emptying. The medication is injected prior to meals to reduce postprandial hyperglycemia. **Primary Method of Clearance**: Renal	Lowers postprandial hyperglycemia in patients with type 2 diabetes.	Assess patient for any allergies to incretin mimetics. Instruct patient on proper injection techniques. Instruct patient to check the injection site for swelling and irritation. Instruct patient to inject medication prior to meals. Instruct patient on the signs and symptoms of hypoglycemia. Instruct patient on the treatment of hypoglycemia. Instruct patient to call his health care provider with continued gastrointestinal symptoms, because slower titration of the dose may alleviate this problem.
Pramlintide (Amylin analog)	**General Mechanism:** Pramlintide reduces postprandial hyperglycemia. **MOA:** Amylin is a neuroendocrine hormone that is secreted with insulin from the pancreatic beta cells. This hormone can reduce postprandial blood glucose control through slowing gastric emptying, suppressing glucagon secretion, and promoting satiety. Pramlintide is an amylin analog that is injected prior to meals to reduce postprandial hyperglycemia. **Primary Method of Clearance:** Renal	Pramlintide is used in patients with type 1 diabetes and insulin-treated type 2 diabetes. Patients with type 1 diabetes are amylin deficient. Patients with type 2 diabetes have a poor amylin response to meal. Treatment with pramlintide can address each of these problems,	Assess patient for any allergies to pramlintide. Assess patient for gastroparesis and hypoglycemic unawareness because these conditions may predispose the patient to severe hypoglycemia. Instruct patient on proper injection techniques. Instruct patient to check the injection site for swelling and irritation. Instruct patient to inject medication prior to meals. Instruct patient on the signs and symptoms of hypoglycemia. Instruct patient on the treatment of hypoglycemia.

Sources: American Diabetes Association. (2008a). *Diabetes forecast resource guide 2008.* Alexandria, VA: Author; Burant, C. F., & American Diabetes Association. (2008). *Medical management of type 2 diabetes* (6th ed.). Alexandria, VA: American Diabetes Association; Campbell, R. K., & White, J. R., Jr. (2000). *Medications for the treatment of diabetes.* Alexandria, VA: American Diabetes Association; Gutierrez, K. (2008). *Pharmacotherapeutics: Clinical reasoning in primary care* (2nd ed.). St. Louis: W. B. Saunders; Kaufman, F., & American Diabetes Association. (2008). *Medical management of type 1 diabetes* (5th ed.). Alexandria, VA: American Diabetes Association; Youngkin, E. Q., Sawin, K. J., Kissinger, J. F., & Isreal, D. S. (Eds.). (2005). *Pharmacotherapeutics* (2nd ed.). Upper Saddle, NJ: Pearson Prentice Hall.

Prior to initiating this regimen, it probably is best to assess whether the patient has dawn phenomenon or the Somogyi effect. In the Somogyi effect, hypoglycemia occurs during the middle of the night. When the hypoglycemia occurs there is a release of glucose from the liver. This release of glucose from the liver is associated with a rise in glucose and an elevated fasting blood glucose level. As a result, patients awake with an elevated fasting blood glucose level. The best way to assess for whether this is the Somogyi effect or the dawn phenomenon is to test the blood glucose levels in the middle of the night. If hypoglycemia is present in the middle of the night, it is likely that the elevated morning blood glucose level is rebound hyperglycemia or the

Somogyi effect. If hypoglycemia is not present during this time, it is more likely that the elevated morning blood glucose level is a result of the dawn phenomenon.

Four-Times-Daily Injection Regimen

The regimen described here requires four injections of insulin per day (Figure 53–10 ■, p. 1682): NPH is given at breakfast and bedtime, while the rapid- or short-acting insulin is give prior to each meal. The premeal insulin helps reduce the postprandial hypoglycemia. The NPH provides "basal" insulin. As noted previously, NPH has a characteristic peak action that predisposes the patient to hypoglycemia.

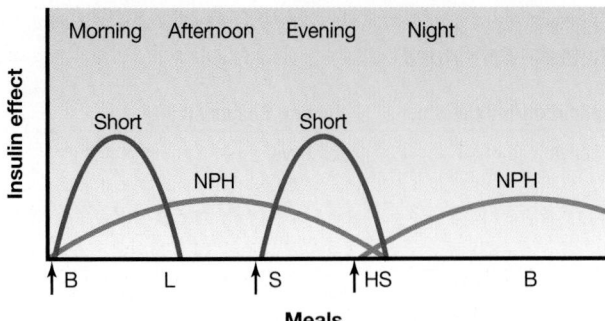

(a)

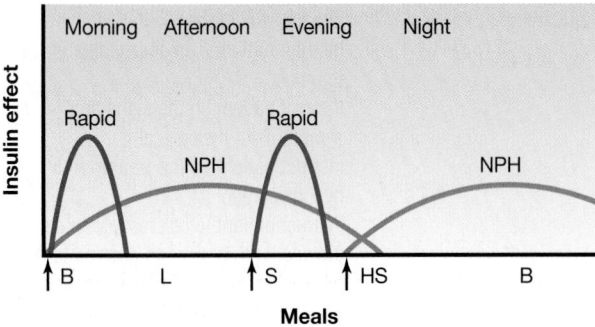

(b)

FIGURE 53–9 ■ Three-times-daily insulin injection regimen.

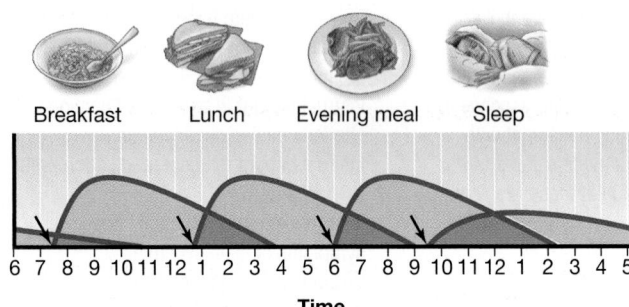

FIGURE 53–10 ■ Four-times-daily insulin injection regimen.

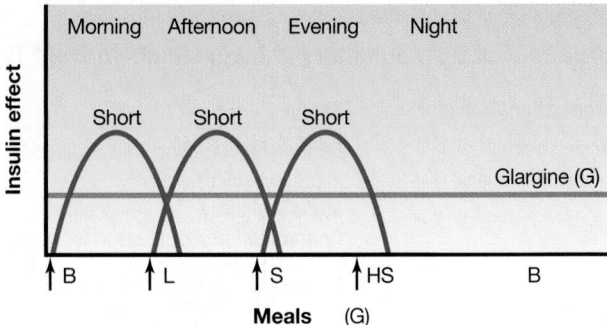

(a)

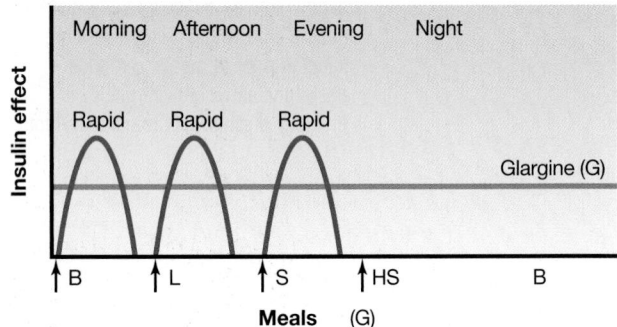

(b)

FIGURE 53–11 ■ Multiple daily dose regimen.

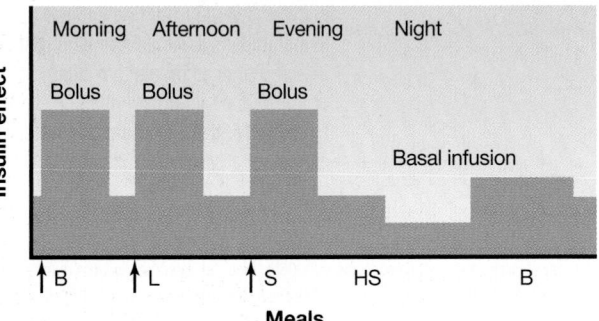

(a)

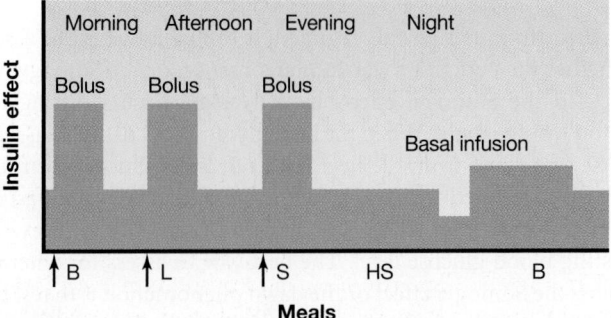

(b)

FIGURE 53–12 ■ Continuous subcutaneous insulin infusion.

"Peakless" insulins, such as glargine, provide better basal insulin coverage. The multiple-dose regimen using glargine is widely used by patients with diabetes and is illustrated in Figure 53–11 ■. In this regimen, long-acting insulin (i.e., glargine) is used in combination with a rapid-acting insulin (lispro) prior to each meal. The glargine insulin has no peak; therefore, it resembles endogenous insulin more precisely.

One of the most effective ways to mimic normal insulin secretion is through the use of an insulin pump, which can provide continuous subcutaneous insulin infusion. The insulin pump, described earlier, is programmed to infuse rapid doses of short-acting insulin continuously at a basal rate, with patients determining bolus insulin injections prior to meals and snacks. The actions of the insulin pump are shown (Figure 53–12 ■). One of the important features of this insulin delivery system is that the basal rate can be changed to match the needs of individual patients. For example, higher rates of insulin can be delivered throughout for those patients who have high fasting glucose levels, presumably due to counterregulatory hormone secretion (e.g., growth hormone) during the night.

Pharmacologic Treatment of Type 2 Diabetes

The traditional approach to the treatment of type 2 diabetes has employed diet and exercise as a "first-line" therapy, introducing pharmacologic therapy when patients cannot meet their glycemic goals with diet and exercise alone. During the past decade, there have been some fundamental differences in the understanding of diabetes that have caused reevaluation of this approach.

Health care providers often are faced with the question as to when to initiate sequential (i.e., diet and exercise, followed by pharmacologic therapy, if indicated) or complementary therapy (i.e., introduction of simultaneous pharmacologic, diet, and exercise therapy) in the treatment of hyperglycemia. The majority of patients with type 2 diabetes are obese, having attempted to lose weight over several years. Increasingly, health care providers are introducing medications at the diagnosis of diabetes to be used in combination with diet and exercise. Some of the newer medications (biguanides and thiazolidinediones) used in the treatment of type 2 diabetes are unlikely to produce hypoglycemia when used as monotherapy; these medications can be safely used at diagnosis in patients with mild to moderate hyperglycemia. Metformin may be used in combination with diet and exercise in patients who have been diagnosed with pre-diabetes.

Although many patients with type 2 diabetes initially are treated successfully with monotherapy, eventually one type of medication is not sufficient to maintain normal blood glucose levels. Because medications have specific mechanisms of action that revolve around several major processes (e.g., augmenting insulin supply, decreasing insulin resistance, decreasing glucose absorption), these medications can be used in combination to maintain normoglycemia. Some of these combinations include sulfonylureas and metformin, sulfonylureas and alpha-glucosidase inhibitors, sulfonylureas and thiazolidinediones, and metformin and meglitinides. Additionally, there are a number of newer medications that combine different medications in one pill. These include metformin and Glyburide (Glucovance), metformin and rosiglitazone (Avandamet), metformin and Glipizide (Metaglip), metformin and pioglitazone (ACTOplus Met), metformin and sitagliptin (Janumet), pioglitazone and glimepiride (Duetact), and rosiglitazone and glimepiride (Avandaryl). The specific properties of each of the classes (e.g., thiazolidinediones, sulfonylureas) are detailed in the Pharmacology Summary (p. 1678) earlier in this chapter.

Oral Medications

Some general principles apply when combining oral medications (Riddle, 1999). First, when a patient fails oral monotherapy, combining drugs of different classes is usually more effective than stopping one and substituting another. Second, when a patient requires near-maximum doses of one medication, adding another drug usually is better than increasing the dosage of the original medication. Third, secondary failure of the two-drug combination in patients with type 2 diabetes is expected eventually. In these patients, a three-drug combination is potentially useful, but one should consider the addition of insulin to the existing regimen or insulin alone should be considered.

Insulin Therapy in Type 2 Diabetes Mellitus

The purpose of insulin therapy in patients with type 2 diabetes is to provide adequate insulin to supplement the reduction in insulin secretion and to overcome insulin resistance. Type 2 diabetes is a progressive disease with patients responding to oral medications early in their disease, but requiring insulin treatment for adequate glucose control over time (UKPDSG, 1998a). Insulin therapy remains a viable and often necessary option for achieving optimal glucose control. When introducing insulin therapy for patients with type 2 diabetes, any of the previously described regimens are useful.

Insulin also may be provided in combination with selected oral medications. For example, sulfonylureas may be provided throughout the day with a dose of NPH or glargine given at bedtime. The goal of this regimen is to suppress hepatic glucose production during the night. Theoretically, the patient awakes with a lower fasting blood glucose level and the sulfonylureas are more effective during the day. In addition, insulin can be added to regimens consisting of metformin and thiazolidinediones. However, edema is a side effect of thiazolidinediones, particularly when combined with insulin. Both patients and health care providers should be cognizant of the risk of heart failure when thiazolidinediones are used in patients with type 2 diabetes.

Nutrition and Diabetes

Nutrition and physical activity also fall within the realm of medical management, as well as nursing management and self-management. Historically, the American Diabetes Association attempted to identify the "ideal diabetes diet" based on estimated caloric needs and percentages of **micronutrients** (nutritional components such as vitamin or minerals that are needed in small quantities for living organisms) and **macronutrients** (nutritional components such as protein, CHO, and fat that are needed in larger quantities for living organisms). Currently, **medical nutrition therapy (MNT)** in diabetes consists of meal planning approaches that are determined by clinical evidence, cultural, social, and ethnic preferences, and patient motivation. There is greater liberalization of macronutrient content, particularly in the amount of CHOs, as long as both glycemic and lipid goals are met. See Chapter 14 ⊘ for more information on nutrition.

The American Diabetes Association has extensively reviewed and revised their dietary guidelines (ADA, 2007). These national guidelines now include recommendations for the role of nutrition in the prevention of diabetes (primary prevention), the prevention of complications (secondary prevention), and the treatment of complications (tertiary prevention). These goals are outlined in the National Guidelines for MNT in Individuals at Risk for Diabetes or Pre-Diabetes box (p. 1684).

Target Micronutrients and Macronutrients in the Diet

The ADA recommendations for treatment of pre-diabetes, diabetes, and diabetes complications are fairly extensive and beyond the scope of this chapter. However, the recommended micronutrients and macronutrients are summarized in Chart 53–4 (p. 1684). It is extremely important to note that the macronutrient (i.e., CHO, fats, and protein) content is highly individualized, and may need to be modified in response to lipid and blood pressure goals.

NATIONAL GUIDELINES for MNT in Individuals at Risk for Diabetes or Pre-Diabetes

The goals for MNT for individuals at risk for diabetes or pre-diabetes are as follows:

- To decrease the risk of diabetes and CVD by promoting healthy food choices and physical activity leading to moderate weight loss.
- To decrease the risk of diabetes and CVD through maintenance of this weight loss.

The goals of MNT for individuals with diabetes are as follows:

- Achieve and maintain blood glucose levels in the normal range or as close to normal as is safely possible.
- Achieve and maintain a lipid and lipoprotein profile that decreases the risk for the development of CVD.
- Achieve and maintain normal blood pressure levels in the normal range or as close to normal as is safely possible.
- Prevent or decrease the rate of the development of chronic diabetes complications by modifying nutrient intake and adapting healthy lifestyle changes.
- Address nutritional needs, taking into account each individual's personal and cultural references and willingness to change.
- Maintain the pleasure of eating by only limiting food choices where there is scientific evidence in support of excluding these choices from the diet.

The goals of MNT that apply to specific situations are as follows:

- Provide adequate calories to ensure normal growth and development in youth with type 1 diabetes, youth with type 2 diabetes, and in pregnant and lactating women.
- Provide self-management training for safe conduct of exercise, including the prevention and treatment of hypoglycemia in individuals treated with medications that cause hypoglycemia.
- Provide self-management training for diabetes treatment during acute illness.

Source: American Diabetes Association. (2007). Nutrition recommendations and interventions for diabetes: A position statement of the American Diabetes Association. *Diabetes Care, 30* (Suppl. 1), S48–S65.

CHART 53–4 **General Macronutrient and Micronutrient Recommendations in Individuals with Diabetes**

CARBOHYDRATES (CHO)

- Dietary patterns including CHO from fruits, vegetables, whole grains, legumes, and low-fat milk are encouraged.
- Low-CHO diets, restricting total carbohydrate to <130 g/day, are not recommended in the management of diabetes.
- Monitoring CHO (e.g., CHO counting, exchanges, experience) is an important strategy in the nutritional treatment of diabetes.
- The use of the glycemic index (i.e., a ranking system that evaluates the effect of CHO on blood glucose levels; higher glycemic index foods are associated with a higher postprandial rise in blood glucose) and load (i.e., a ranking system that takes into consideration the glycemic index and portion size) may provide a modest additional benefit over that observed when total carbohydrate is considered alone.
- Sucrose-containing foods can be substituted for other CHO in the meal plan. If these foods are an addition to the meal plan, they can be covered with insulin or other glucose-lowering medications.
- Many more choices are available today than in the past for including the CHO intake into the diet of individuals with diabetes; however, care should be taken to avoid increased caloric intake.
- Sugar alcohols and nonnutritive sweeteners are considered safe as long as they are consumed within the daily intake levels established by the FDA.

FAT AND CHOLESTEROL

- Limit saturated fat to <7% of total calories.
- Intake of *trans* fat should be minimized.
- Dietary cholesterol should be limited to <200 mg/day.

PROTEIN

- In diabetic patients with normal renal function, there is little evidence to suggest that usual protein intake (15–20% of caloric intake) should be modified.
- Ingested protein can increase the plasma insulin response without increasing blood glucose levels; therefore, protein should not be used to treat acute or prevent nocturnal hypoglycemia in patients with type 2 diabetes.
- High-protein diets are not recommended as a method for weight loss at this time.

ALCOHOL

- If adult patients with diabetes consume alcohol, their daily intake should be limited to a moderate amount (women: ≤1 drink per day; men: ≤2 drinks per day).
- Alcohol should be consumed with food to reduce the risk of nocturnal hypoglycemia in individuals using insulin or oral medications that enhance insulin secretion.
- Moderate alcohol consumption (ingested alone) has no acute effect on blood glucose and insulin concentrations; when CHO is combined with alcohol (i.e., in a mixed drink), the blood glucose level may rise.

MICRONUTRIENTS

- Vitamin or mineral supplementation in patients with diabetes (compared with the general population) does not provide any additional medical benefits.
- Supplementation with antioxidants, such as vitamins E and C and carotene, is not advised; the benefits have not been established and there are concerns about safety.
- Chromium supplementation is not recommended because the benefits have not been established.

Source: American Diabetes Association. (2007). Nutrition recommendations and interventions for diabetes: A position statement of the American Diabetes Association. *Diabetes Care, 30* (Suppl. 1), S48–S65.

Medical Nutrition Therapy

There is no longer a single "diabetes diet"; patients work as partners with their diabetes care team to attain and maintain healthy eating habits that foster the goals of MNT. Meal plans are individualized for each patient, taking into account the patient's lifestyle, culture, food preferences, and ability to make changes. Different educational resources and approaches may be needed during different phases of the educational process. Ideally, every patient with diabetes should be referred to a dietician with training in diabetes MNT. Nurses, physicians, and other members of the health care team are important players in reinforcing healthy eating habits.

Specific considerations need to be addressed when developing meal plans. These primary considerations include glycemic and lipid goals, the type of diabetes, and the pharmacologic treatment regimen being used. In patients with type 1 diabetes using intensive insulin therapy, such as CSII and multiple daily injections (MDIs), meals and physical activity can be coordinated with their insulin doses. Meal planning in the patient using CSII or MDI can be relatively flexible, whereas meal planning in patients with more traditional insulin regimens (e.g., split-mixed insulin) needs to be consistent. For example, patients using CSII or MDI may elect to delay meals for a period of time by maintaining a basal insulin rate and administering the short-acting insulin dose immediately before the meal. In contrast, patients using split-mixed insulin dosing (NPH and short-acting insulin prior to breakfast and prior to dinner) cannot easily change the time of the insulin dose to accommodate meals.

Meal planning for patients with type 2 diabetes also is dependent on the pharmacologic treatment regimen. As noted previously, the patient with type 2 diabetes may use a variety of pharmacologic treatment regimens including oral medications and insulin therapy. In addition, some patients with type 2 diabetes may control their blood glucose levels with a combination of diet and exercise without medications. Many patients with type 2 diabetes are obese and require caloric restriction and weight loss. Diet, weight loss, and pharmacologic therapy need to be finely coordinated. For example, dosages of medications often need to be decreased with caloric restriction or weight loss to prevent hypoglycemia. Otherwise the amount of caloric intake needed to prevent and treat hypoglycemia may interfere with weight loss. With both type 1 and type 2 diabetes, frequent blood glucose testing is necessary to determine the effectiveness of pharmacologic treatment combined with MNT.

Many patients who have been diagnosed with diabetes for a long period of time were taught a system of meal planning using "ADA Exchange Lists." In the ADA Exchange List method all foods were categorized into groups (e.g., bread/starches, meats, fruits, vegetables, fats) and assigned portion sizes representing "1 exchange" or "1 serving" of a particular food. Each exchange had a specific amount of carbohydrates, proteins, and fats. Patients were prescribed a daily meal plan based on a total amount of daily calories (e.g., 1,200 calories per day) equaling a predetermined number of servings from each exchange group.

The ADA Exchange List is not used extensively anymore; however, the principles of the exchange system still may be used for easily determining CHO servings. Because one serving of CHO is 15 grams, patients may be given a meal plan with a specified number of CHO servings at each meal or snack. The patients are free to choose among all CHO foods of equal CHO value. This method is simple, requiring little calculation. Books are available that list portion sizes of commonly eaten CHO-containing foods. (Evert, Hess-Fischl, & ADA, 2006; Fairview Health Services, 2003; McCarren & ADA, 2007).

Individuals using insulin therapy may learn how to adjust their premeal rapid-acting insulin based on the amount of CHO in the meal. Carbohydrate counting is a method of tracking nutritional intake of CHO and relating the CHO quantity to an insulin dosage. Patients use this ratio to calculate the dose of insulin they must take with meals or snacks. Most adults with type 1 diabetes require 1 unit of rapid-acting insulin (such as insulin lispro or aspart) for every 10 to 15 grams of CHO. The ratio may be different with each meal and change with varying levels of physical activity. The following example shows how a patient with type 1 diabetes can calculate her insulin dose:

Prelunch blood glucose level: 104 mg/dL

Insulin-to-CHO ratio: 1:12

Prelunch insulin dose: 4 units

Food	CHO Amount (grams)
1 cup black bean chili	32
1 1/2 cups green salad with tomatoes	10
2 tbsp vinaigrette dressing	6
Total CHO grams:	48

As can be seen from the calculations, the total amount of CHO from a variety of food sources is 48 grams. Because the ratio of insulin to CHO (grams) in the preceding example is 1:12, the premeal dose of rapid-acting insulin is 4 units.

Patients are instructed to read food labels (Figure 53–13 ■, p. 1686) to determine the total amount of CHO in a food item. Serving size must also be monitored because food choices may contain several servings in one item (e.g., 2 servings of CHO in a 12-ounce can of soda pop). This method requires calculations prior to each meal and is an essential skill for those using insulin pump therapy or intensive MDI therapy. As noted in the previous example, the amount of insulin required to cover a specified number of CHO grams is called the insulin-to-CHO, or insulin:CHO, ratio. The ratio is determined through careful monitoring of blood glucose levels before and after meals, frequent communication between all members of the health care team, and trial and error (Bode, 2004).

Nutritional Needs of Hospitalized Patients

As in any catabolic illness, nutritional needs in diabetic patients are compromised. In patients with diabetes, there is an added dilemma of providing adequate calories to maintain nutritional status and promote healing while maintaining glycemic control. The caloric needs of most hospitalized patients can be met through provision of 25 to 35 kcal/kg body weight (McMahon & Rizza, 1996). Protein requirements are variable based on the degree of physiological stress. For example, mildly stressed patients with normal hepatic and renal function require 1.0 g/kg body weight, whereas moderately to severely stressed patients with normal hepatic and renal function may need 1.5 g/kg body weight (McMahon & Rizza, 1996).

Nutrition Facts

Serving Size 1 container (170 grams)

Amount Per Serving

Calories 170

	% Daily Values*
Total Fat 1.5g	**2%**
Saturated Fat 1g	**5%**
Cholesterol 10mg	**3%**
Sodium 130mg	**5%**
Potassium 300mg	**9%**
Total Carbohydrate 33g	**11%**
Fiber 0g	**0%**
Sugars 30g	
Protein 6g	**12%**
Calcium	**20%**
Vitamin B_{12}	**10%**
Riboflavin	**15%**
Phosphorus	**15%**

FIGURE 53–13 ■ Example of food nutrition label.

The preferred route of feeding is the oral route, however, if adequate intake is not possible, then enteral or parenteral feedings will be needed. CHO counting is integrated into the diet of the hospital patient in various ways. For example, in some hospital protocols, a specific amount of CHO is provided with each meal and an estimated insulin:CHO ratio is determined. Therefore the nursing staff can administer the insulin dose immediately prior to the meal. In other hospital protocols, the estimated insulin:CHO ratio is determined and administered based on the variable amount of CHO in the meal. In general, such protocols provide provisions for patients who have poor appetites, nausea, vomiting, and other gastrointestinal disorders. In these cases, the nurse may administer the rapid-acting insulin dose at the end of the meal, when he can observe the amount of CHO eaten. For information about how the diet of patients with diabetes is affected by cultural and aging considerations, see the Cultural Considerations and Gerontological Considerations boxes.

Exercise and Physical Activity

Regular exercise and a physically active lifestyle provide numerous benefits for people with type 1 and type 2 diabetes, as well as those at risk for developing diabetes. Results of a recent multicen-

CULTURAL CONSIDERATIONS Related to Diet for Patients with Diabetes

An important factor in adherence to a dietary plan is to develop diets that best reflect the ethnic practices of each individual. The ADA website provides a number of useful materials about dietary instruction. The materials, which can be downloaded and printed, are available in a variety of languages and provide information on various ethnic and regional dietary habits. These are very important because a patient's adherence to dietary recommendations may increase when traditional foods, practices, and cultural, and dietary customs are included in educational instruction.

GERONTOLOGICAL CONSIDERATIONS Related to Diet for Patients with Diabetes

Many elderly patients are undernourished due to a variety of physiological, psychological, social, and economic considerations. These may include, but are not limited to, changes in smell, taste, and thirst; side effects of medications; inability to shop for food or prepare meals; cognitive impairment, depression, isolation, and loneliness; and inadequate resources to purchase food (Gilden, 1999). For elderly patients it may be necessary to modify their nutritional diet by changing the nutrient composition or density, modifying the food consistency, or using supplements.

ter research trial clearly demonstrated that lifestyle intervention including regular exercise is superior to metformin at preventing the onset of diabetes in high-risk individuals (Knowler et al., 2002). Benefits for those already diagnosed with type 1 or type 2 diabetes include lower blood glucose levels, improved insulin sensitivity, improvements in cardiovascular risks such as blood lipids and blood pressure levels, improved cardiac conditioning, increased strength and flexibility, and improved personal well-being. Exercise also may help in weight loss when used in conjunction with a calorie-restricted diet (Lebovitz & ADA, 2004).

Although the benefits of exercise outweigh the risks of exercise in most instances, many factors must be taken into account prior to initiating an exercise program. In nondiabetic individuals substrate metabolism is tightly balanced by neuroendocrine mechanisms to maintain normoglycemia. Fuel mobilization from muscle and liver stores during exercise may be 20-fold higher than during sedentary activity to maintain normal blood glucose levels. During exercise, glucose transport into working muscles is enhanced, while cellular resistance to insulin is decreased. Plasma insulin levels decrease, while levels of circulating counterregulatory hormones such as glucagon, cortisol, epinephrine, and norepinephrine increase to maintain glucose homeostasis and avoid hypo- or hyperglycemia. However, individuals with diabetes may have impaired neuroendocrine responses to exercise.

In general, patients with diabetes using pharmacologic therapy are at greater risk for hypoglycemia during and following exercise. In fact, the hypoglycemic effect of exercise can persist for several hours; therefore, patient education about preventing and treating exercise-related hypoglycemia is essential.

Individuals with type 1 diabetes can participate in all levels of physical activity, including leisure time activities and professional sports, if they are in good metabolic control and do not have complications (Zinman, Ruderman, Campaigne, Devlin, & Schneider, 2004). For these individuals, the metabolic response to exercise may vary dramatically in relation to plasma glucose levels at the time of exercise, timing of the last food eaten, type of exercise, and level of insulin usage. The use of exogenous insulin plays a key role, potentiating hypoglycemia in those who are overinsulinized and hyperglycemia with possible ketosis in those who are underinsulinized. Exercise-induced hypoglycemia is common, and may occur for many hours after the exercise is completed. Individuals in poor metabolic control are at risk for worsening of hyperglycemia and ketosis. Guidelines for exercise in this population include the following (Zinman et al., 2004):

- Avoid exercise if blood glucose is >250 mg/dL and ketones are present; use caution if blood glucose levels are >300 mg/dL without ketosis.
- Ingest CHO-containing foods if blood glucose levels are <100 mg/dL prior to exercise.
- Monitor blood glucose levels before, after, and more frequently during the postexercise period because the blood glucose-lowering effects of exercise may last many hours after exercise.
- Self-monitor blood glucose responses to different activity levels to determine appropriate changes to diet and insulin.
- Maintain a supply of readily available CHO-containing foods during and after exercise.

The use of intensive insulin therapies, such as MDI therapy or CSII, allows for greater flexibility in making appropriate adjustments to insulin and food, thus decreasing the risk of exercise-induced hypo- or hyperglycemia. The importance of blood glucose monitoring and record keeping cannot be overemphasized because these are the primary means of monitoring glycemic responses to exercise and determining the necessary insulin and dietary changes required to avoid hypo- or hyperglycemia.

For individuals with type 2 diabetes, regular exercise plays a key role in improving long-term metabolic control due to its positive impact on insulin resistance. Exercise, like insulin, decreases blood glucose levels by enhancing glucose uptake into skeletal muscles. Enhanced glucose utilization and insulin sensitivity may last for up to 24 hours after the exercise bout (Devlin, Hirshman, Horton, & Horton, 1987). Although exercise-induced hypoglycemia is less problematic in individuals with type 2 diabetes, those treated with insulin or insulin secretagogues need the same precautions for prevention of hypoglycemia as those with type 1 diabetes.

 *Patients with diabetes can learn to decrease their insulin dose prior to intense exercise to prevent hypoglycemia; however, most exercise is unplanned and patients are often unable to make such adjustments. Because the glucose-lowering effects of exercise can persist for several hours after an exercise bout, patients (especially those using exogenous insulin) are at particular risk for postexercise hypoglycemia. Therefore, nurses should counsel patients to monitor blood glucose levels closely following exercise to prevent hypoglycemia. In particular, patients should monitor their blood glucose prior to sleep to prevent nocturnal hypoglycemia.*

Exercise and Diabetes Complications

The long-term complications associated with diabetes pose special concerns and require extra consideration when planning an exercise program. The ADA recommends that all individuals with diabetes undergo a detailed medical evaluation with appropriate diagnostic studies prior to beginning an exercise program (Zinman et al., 2004). Recommendations include use of a graded exercise test in high-risk individuals. A preexercise assessment for all individuals with diabetes should include an evaluation of PVD, retinal examination, evaluation of renal function, and assessment of autonomic and peripheral neuropathy. The presence of complications does not preclude participation in exercise, but does require attention by members of the health care team.

Exercise Prescriptions

Exercise prescriptions should be individualized to each person, with an emphasis on enjoyment of the activity. Generally, an exercise bout should include 5 to 10 minutes of warm-up, such as low-intensity walking or cycling, 5 to 10 minutes of gentle stretching, a period of aerobic activity, such as swimming, walking, or dancing, and 5 to 10 minutes of cooldown. Moderate to vigorous aerobic activity should be prescribed based on individual preferences, current level of fitness, and risk factors. For example, an individual with decreased or absent lower extremity sensation should be instructed to participate in non–weight-bearing activities such as swimming or bicycling (Zinman et al., 2004). The exercise bouts should be done three to five times per week to achieve cardiovascular conditioning and glycemic control. If weight loss is a goal, the frequency should be increased (Lebovitz & ADA, 2004).

Health Promotion

Exercise offers many benefits for individuals with diabetes and should be encouraged as part of a healthy lifestyle. Although exercise does pose special risks for patients with diabetes, individualized exercise plans can be developed for the majority of patients with diabetes. Through careful clinical assessment and planning, most risks can be minimized or prevented so that most people with diabetes can enjoy the benefits of regular physical activity. Exercise education should include a review of the signs, symptoms, and treatment for hypoglycemia, ketone testing for individuals with type 1 diabetes, proper hydration during exercise, and foot protection measures including proper footwear and self-assessment prior to and immediately after exercise. Positive reinforcement and inclusion of friends and family members in the exercise plan may help to improve motivation.

Complementary and Alternative Medicine and Glycemic Control

An extensive systematic review of published literature on the efficacy and safety of herbal therapies and vitamin/mineral supplements for glycemic control in patients with diabetes was published in 2003 (Yeh, Eisenberg, Kaptchuk, & Phillips, 2003). Results of the review concluded that there is insufficient evidence to actively recommend or discourage the use of any particular supplement; however, most appeared to be generally safe. In addition, the review concluded that the seven most promising supplements included *Coccinia indica*, American ginseng, *Momordica charantia*, nopal, L-carnitine, *Gymnema sylvestre*, aloe vera, and *vanadium*. The Complementary and Alternative Therapies box (p. 1688) discusses the antidiabetic potential of certain spices.

Randomized clinical trials are needed to assess the efficacy of these types of supplements. Most importantly, sound clinical judgment is needed when patients report the use of these plant foods for treatment for diabetes treatment. In particular, nurses and other health care professionals must understand that these medications are supplemental therapy; such supplements claim to enhance insulin secretion, but do not take the place of exogenous insulin. Because patients with type 1 diabetes lack the ability to produce insulin, claims that a supplement will increase insulin secretion in type 1 diabetes are misleading and can be dangerous. In the future, however, as we refine our knowledge of these supplements, there may be a place for them in diabetes treatment.

Management of Hospitalized Patients with Diabetes

For several decades the management of diabetes in the hospitalized patient has focused on the treatment of the acute complications of diabetes, DKA and HHS. The stress of critical illness, however, worsens glycemic control in patients with diabetes and often precipitates hyperglycemia in individuals with no history of diabetes or glucose intolerance. During the last decade, the deleterious effects of hyperglycemia on the clinical outcomes of acutely ill patients with and without diabetes have been estab-

lished. The following paragraphs focus on the treatment of hyperglycemia in patients who are acutely ill along with general treatment strategies for DKA, HHS, and hypoglycemia.

Hyperglycemia in Acute Illness

Physiological stress, such as acute illness, causes an increase in counterregulatory hormones, glucagon, cortisol, growth hormone, and catecholamines. These hormones increase insulin resistance and hepatic glucose production and decrease glucose transport, resulting in hyperglycemia. Investigations into the relationship between hyperglycemia and poor recovery from acute illness have gained momentum during the past few years; however, hyperglycemia has been known to interfere with recovery from infections and wound healing for several decades.

In clinical practice alterations in immune response contribute to the severity of common infections, such as lower extremity ulcers (Lioupis, 2005) along with the development of more severe infections. Recent studies have shown that hyperglycemia also has deleterious effects on recovery from critical illness (Van den Berghe & Bouillon, 2004), myocardial infarction (Malmberg, 2004), stroke (Capes, Hunt, Malmberg, Pathak, &

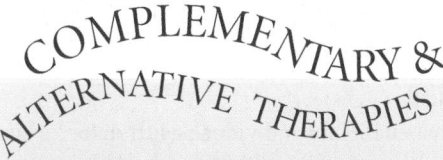

COMPLEMENTARY & ALTERNATIVE THERAPIES **Garlic and Other Spices**

Description:

It is well established that diet plays a large role in the management of diabetes mellitus. Although garlic and spices are well known as a vital part of flavoring foods for increased taste enjoyment, some spices also have therapeutic effects including antidiabetic effects.

In addition to providing flavor and therapeutic physiological properties, spices can partially or wholly replace less health-promoting ingredients such as salt, sugar, and added saturated fat. Current nutritional guidelines for patients with diabetes include increasing intake of vegetables, yet many people do not enjoy eating vegetables. Spices can improve the flavor of vegetables and help patients to adhere to dietary guidelines (Tapsell et al., 2006).

Research Support:

Diabetes mellitus is characterized by increased protein glycation and advanced glycation end product (AGEP) formation. Glycation and AGEP formation have been implicated in diabetic complications, as well as the formation of damaging free radicals through glucose and protein autoxidation. Compounds that have both antiglycation and antioxidant properties may have therapeutic potential in the treatment of diabetes mellitus. Several studies have shown that aged garlic extract (AGE) is a potent antioxidant and can inhibit the formation of AGEPs *in vitro*. AGE may also inhibit the formation of glycation-derived free radicals (Ahmad & Ahmed, 2006).

Another study identified the following spices as having antidiabetic and hypoglycemic properties:

- Fenugreek seeds (*Trigonella foenumgraecum*)
- Garlic (*Allium sativum*)
- Onion (*Allium cepa*)
- Turmeric (*Curcuma longa*)
- Cumin seeds (*Cuminum cyminum*)
- Ginger (*Zingiber officinale*)
- Mustard (*Brassica nigra*)

- Curry leaves (*Murraya koenigii*)
- Coriander (*Coriandrum sativum*) (Srinivasan, 2005).

Onion (*Allium cepa L.*) and garlic (*Allium sativum L.*) have a long history as both spices and medicine. One study found that the therapeutic properties of garlic and onion can be attributed to volatile sulfur compounds called thiosulfinates, which also create the strong odor and flavor of these spices (Lanzotti, 2006).

Another study investigated the effects of garlic oil on glycemic control in rats with streptozotocin-induced diabetes. Diabetic rats were fed garlic oil by gavage (100 mg/kg body weight) every other day for 16 weeks after the induction of diabetes. Although garlic oil did not affect oral glucose tolerance, it significantly improved oral glucose tolerance at 4, 8, 12, and 16 weeks. The researchers concluded that garlic oil can be used in the long-term treatment of diabetes to improve oral glucose tolerance (Wong, Lii, Hse, & Sheen, 2006).

References

Ahmad, M. S., & Ahmed, N. (2006, March). Antiglycation properties of aged garlic extract: Possible role in prevention of diabetic complications. *Journal of Nutrition 136*(3 Suppl), 796S–799S.

Lanzotti, V. (2006). The analysis of onion and garlic. *Journal of Chormatograpy A, 1112*(1–2), 3–22.

Srinivasan, K. (2005). Plant foods in the management of diabetes mellitus: Spices as beneficial antidiabetic food adjuncts. *International Journal of Food Science and Nutrition, 56*(6), 399–414.

Tapsell, L. C., Hemphill, I., Cobiac, L., Patch, C. S., Sullivan, D. R., Fenech, M., et al. (2006, August 21). Health benefits of herbs and spices: The past, the present, the future. *Medical Journal of Australia, 185*(4 Suppl), S4–S24.

Wong, P. L., Lii, C. K., Hse, H., & Sheen, L. Y. (2006). Antidiabetic effect of garlic oil but not diallyl disulfide in rats with streptozotocin-induced diabetes. *Food Chemistry and Toxicology, 44*(8), 1377–1384.

Gerstein, 2001), and cardiac surgery (Furnary, Wu, & Bookin, 2004). Evidence supports the fact that normoglycemia in hospitalized patients results in decreased morbidity and mortality in patients (Umpierrez et al., 2002).

Target Glycemic Goals for Hospitalized Patients

During a consensus conference on inpatient diabetes and metabolic control (Garber, Seidel, & Ambruster, 2004), target glycemic goals for hospitalized patients were established. The upper limits for these goals are as follows:

- Intensive care unit (ICU): 110 mg/dL
- Non–critical care units: preprandial, 110 mg/dL
- Maximum blood glucose: 180 mg/dL.

Insulin Protocols Designed to Meet Treatment Goals in Hospitalized Patients

Evidence supports the use of intravenous insulin infusions in the ICU among hyperglycemic critically ill patients (e.g., during myocardial infarction, following surgeries) regardless of whether or not there is a history of diabetes. In addition, evidence also supports the use of intravenous (IV) insulin in patients who have fluctuating blood glucose levels regardless of whether the patients are treated in the ICU or another unit. However, it is not always practical or standard hospital policy to have IV insulin infusions on non–critical care units.

Various protocols are used to maintain target glucose levels during hospitalization. There is no one standard protocol because each individual's response to insulin depends on a variety of factors. In general, the protocols include infusion of glucose to help prevent hypoglycemia and wide fluctuations in blood glucose levels. Insulin infusion protocols have been found to be of importance in use with patients who are NPO (nothing by mouth), receiving parenteral nutrition, and receiving enteral tube feedings. The use of an IV insulin infusion allows for greater flexibility in changing the insulin dosage and preventing hypoglycemia. An example of an insulin infusion algorithm is described in Chart 53–5.

As can be noted in Chart 53–5, there are three *hypothetical* insulin dosing schemes or algorithms. Patients are started on algorithms based on individual characteristics. For example, "algorithm 1" may be most appropriate for the majority of hospitalized patients. "Algorithm 2" may be most appropriate for patients who have had coronary artery bypass grafting (CABG) or a solid organ transplant or have been treated with glucocorticoids. Ordinarily patients may not be initially treated on "algorithm 3," but this algorithm may be used if blood glucose control is suboptimal on algorithm 2. Each set of algorithms is accompanied by a set of strict criteria as to when to move up or down *within* algorithms or *between* algorithms.

In addition, protocols are currently available for the use of subcutaneous insulin to meet target glucose levels, to transition from IV insulin infusions to subcutaneous insulin (especially when transferring from the ICU to non–critical care units), or to use subcutaneous insulin as a starting point to meet target glycemic control. Standardized insulin protocols have three major components: a premeal insulin dose (e.g., 3 units lispro), a basal insulin dose (e.g., 20 units Glargine qhs), and a "correction factor" (e.g., 5 units lispro). The *correction factor* is an additional amount of insulin that is provided with each meal based on the premeal blood glucose. For example, if a patient routinely uses 3 units of lispro prior to lunch, but her prelunch blood glucose is 250 mg/dL, an additional 5 units of lispro may be administered. In the outpatient setting, patients work with their health care provider to determine their premeal correction factor. In the hospital setting, the determination of the correction factor is based largely on predetermined protocols (Moghissi & Hirsch, 2005).

Diabetic Ketoacidosis

As mentioned earlier, diabetic ketoacidosis is a life-threatening complication precipitated by an acute or relative deficiency in insulin secretion and characterized by profound disturbances in CHO, fat, and protein metabolism. Typically, DKA is treated in the ICU. DKA and HHS have been considered complications of

---

CHART 53–5 **Hypothetical Algorithmic Approach to Diabetes Treatment in the Hospitalized Patient**

Algorithm 1		Algorithm 2		Algorithm 3	
Blood Glucose (mg/dL)	Insulin Infusion Rate (units/hr)	Blood Glucose (mg/dL)	Insulin Infusion Rate (units/hr)	Blood Glucose (mg/dL)	Insulin Infusion Rate (units/hr)
<70	No infusion	<70	No infusion	<70	No infusion
70–110	0.2	70–110	0.4	70–110	0.8
111–120	0.5	111–120	1.0	111–120	2.0
121–150	1.0	121–150	2.0	121–150	4.0
151–180	1.5	151–180	3.0	151–180	6.0
180–210	2.0	180–210	4.0	180–210	8.0
211–240	2.5	211–240	5.0	211–240	9.0
241–270	3.0	241–270	6.0	241–270	10.0
271–300	3.5	271–300	7.0	271–300	11.0
301–330	4.0	301–330	8.0	301–330	12.0
331–360	4.5	331–360	9.0	331–360	14.0
< 360	6.0	< 360	12.0	< 360	16.0

Sources: John, R., & Fogelfeld, L. (2004). Inpatient management of diabetes and hyperglycemia. *Disease-a-Month, 50*(8), 438–479; Moghissi, E. S., & Hirsch, I. B. (2005). Hospital management of diabetes. *Endocrinology Metabolism Clinics of North America, 34*(1), 99–116.

type 1 and 2 diabetes, respectively. Although generally this is true, DKA and HHS can occur in both types of diabetes (Umpierrez & Kitabchi, 2003). The overlap is becoming more apparent as type 2 diabetes occurs with increasing frequency at younger ages (Harmel et al., 2004).

Hyperosmolar Hyperglycemic Syndrome

Hyperosmolar hyperglycemic syndrome is a life-threatening complication characterized by serum hyperosmolarity, dehydration, and hyperglycemia; it is usually restricted to patients who cannot recognize their thirst or express their need for water. Such patients may include the infirm; people who are neglected, very young, very old, or institutionalized; and those who have mental deficiencies. In addition, this syndrome also is seen in patients with excessive unreplaced fluid losses, secondary to massive glycosuric diuresis, and following gastrointestinal fluid losses and limited fluid intake.

Hypoglycemia

Hypoglycemia results from an imbalance between glucose production and glucose utilization that occurs when glucose use exceeds glucose production. Hypoglycemia results in a low blood glucose level (<60 mg/dL) and is associated with a variety of adrenergic and neuroglycopenic symptoms.

Hypoglycemia Unawareness

Hypoglycemia unawareness is defined as the loss of autonomic nervous system responses to hypoglycemia. Symptoms, such as tachycardia, sweating, or palpitations, normally prompt patients to eat in order to prevent progression to severe hypoglycemia. Hypoglycemia unawareness results from altered counterregulation, particularly deficient glucagon and epinephrine responses to hypoglycemia. Subjects with hypoglycemic unawareness are clearly at risk for severe hypoglycemia and injury. The probability of hypoglycemic unawareness and its associated risks should be considered in patients with an increased emphasis on normalization of blood glucose control using intensive insulin regimens and oral hypoglycemic combination therapy.

Etiology and Precipitating Factors of DKA, HHS, and Hypoglycemia

A number of precipitating factors are associated with the development of DKA, HHS, and hypoglycemia, as detailed in Chart 53–6.

Pathophysiology

Short synopses of the pathophysiology of each of the three major complications are given next, starting with DKA.

Diabetic Ketoacidosis

The development of DKA is related to the effects of insulin deficiency on CHO, fat, and lipid metabolism. Although these derangements occur simultaneously, it is helpful to consider them individually in order to correlate the pathophysiology, clinical symptoms, and treatments. The separate effects of insulin lack on CHO, fat, and protein metabolism are described in the following subsections.

Insulin Deficiency and CHO Metabolism

A relative or absolute insulin deficiency results in decreased glucose use by the peripheral tissues, particularly adipose tissue and muscle. Blood glucose levels increase as a result of decreased glucose transport, hepatic and muscle glycogenolysis, and hepatic gluconeogenesis. Glycosuria and osmotic diuresis occur when blood glucose levels exceed the renal threshold. The osmotic diuresis occurs because there is increased urine flow due to an abnormally high concentration of glucose that is reabsorbed incompletely by the proximal tubule. As water reabsorption occurs in the proximal tubule, secondary to Na^+ reabsorption, the concentration of glucose builds up and its osmotic presence impedes the reabsorption of water. In addition, the failure of water to follow Na^+ causes the Na^+ concentration in the proximal tubular lumen to fall below that of the interstitial fluid. The concentration difference between the proximal tubular lumen and the interstitial fluid impedes some Na^+ reabsorption. Thus both Na^+ and water reabsorption are impeded in an osmotic diuresis. This osmotic diuresis results in volume depletion and a reduced glomerular filtration rate (GFR). Reductions in GFR cause decreased renal excretion of glucose, further increasing the hyperglycemia.

CHART 53–6	**Common Precipitating Factors of Diabetic Ketoacidosis, Hyperosmolar Hyperglycemic Nonketotic Syndrome, and Hypoglycemia**[a]		

Diabetic Ketoacidosis	Hyperosmolar Hyperglycemic Syndrome	Hypoglycemia
• Infection	• Undiagnosed diabetes	• Excessive insulin
• Cessation of insulin	• Acute infection	• Wrong type of insulin (e.g., administering rapid-acting instead of long-acting insulin)
• Undiagnosed diabetes	• Cerebrovascular accident	• Missing meals or snacks
• Myocardial infarction	• Myocardial infarction	
• Pancreatitis	• Acute pancreatitis	
• Trauma/shock	• Acute pulmonary embolus	
• Stroke	• Hemodialysis	
	• Peritoneal dialysis	
	• Renal failure	
	• Total parenteral nutrition	
	• Medications (e.g., cimetidine, phenytoin thiazide diuretics)	

*Patients treated with insulin or oral diabetes medications.

Adults with an intact thirst mechanism and normal renal function initially may become only mildly hyperglycemic during DKA since the kidneys are able to excrete some of the filtered glucose load. Adults *without* intact thirst mechanisms (e.g., following a stroke) may not be able to compensate for their fluid loss and become severely hyperglycemic. This loss of water and electrolytes leads to dehydration and hemoconcentration. There is a marked reduction in circulating blood volume leading to peripheral circulatory failure progressing to shock, hypotension, and anuria. In addition, there is generalized tissue anoxia, with a shift to anaerobic metabolism, resulting in increasing concentrations of lactic acid in the blood. Coma and death subsequently result after the development of peripheral circulatory failure. See Chapter 42 ⊘ .

Insulin Deficiency and Fat Metabolism

Insulin deficiency results in mobilization of depot fat in the blood. The liver is flooded with FFAs, which are converted to ketone bodies (acetoacetate and beta-hydroxybutyrate). These ketone bodies are weak acids that are buffered after release from the liver, decreasing the body's buffering capacity. The developing ketonemia leads to progressive metabolic acidosis, which in turn initiates the characteristic deep and rapid respirations accompanied by an acetone odor to the breath (Kussmaul breathing). These Kussmaul respirations are a compensatory response to metabolic acidosis, designed to reduce CO_2. As ketonemia exceeds the renal threshold for ketone body reabsorption, ketones appear in the urine. The ketones are excreted with sodium, which contributes to the net sodium loss. A severe metabolic acidosis results in depression of the respiratory vasomotor center, compromised cardiovascular output, and reduced vascular tone. This may result in cardiovascular collapse with the generation of lactic acid, which adds to the existing acidosis.

Insulin Deficiency and Protein Metabolism

Insulin deficiency results in decreased protein synthesis and promotes net protein catabolism, particularly in muscle. This results in a net loss of nitrogen from the body and increased blood urea nitrogen (BUN) levels. This is accompanied by net loss of K^+, particularly from muscle protein breakdown. Progressive dehydration results in protein catabolism and additional K^+ is subsequently lost in the urine. The final result is that there is a net body loss of K^+.

Counterregulatory Hormones

DKA causes increased plasma glucagon levels, resulting in accelerated rates of hepatic glucose production and ketogenesis. *Catecholamines* stimulate both hepatic and muscle glycogenolysis and adipose tissue lipolysis. The FFAs and glycerol resulting from the lipolysis are converted subsequently to ketones and contribute to glucose production in the liver through ketogenesis and gluconeogenesis, respectively. *Cortisol* increases proteolysis, providing amino acid precursors for gluconeogenesis. *Growth hormone* causes an increase in lipolysis, contributing to ketogenesis and glucose production. *Catecholamines, cortisol,* and *growth hormone* all cause insulin resistance and decreased peripheral glucose uptake.

Hyperosmolar Hyperglycemic Syndrome

The pathogenesis of HHS is similar to that of DKA, but there are specific differences. The pathogenesis of HHS includes hyper-

glycemia and severe dehydration, but does not include metabolic acidosis. Individuals with HHS have a significant reduction in GFR related to dehydration and volume depletion. The reduction in GFR results in an inability to dispose of some of the excess glucose through the kidneys and potentiates hyperglycemia.

The metabolic acidosis does not develop, presumably because the underlying plasma insulin levels are sufficient to inhibit unrestrained lipolysis, but not sufficient to normalize plasma glucose levels. Theoretically, the amount of FFAs that reach the liver is less than in DKA and the production of ketones is restrained. The emergent symptoms associated with metabolic acidosis, are not present to prompt early medical intervention. HHS may evolve over a period of days to weeks, leading to more profound hyperglycemia, dehydration, and hyperosmolality than is seen in DKA.

Hypoglycemia

Glucose is the obligate fuel for the brain and central nervous system. The brain is not able to synthesize or store glucose and must rely on circulating blood glucose levels for survival. Normal blood glucose levels are maintained through the complex interplay between insulin, glucagon, and other counterregulatory hormones. In patients who do not have diabetes, plasma insulin levels decline as blood glucose levels decline; and serum insulin levels increase as plasma glucose increase. However, in patients using exogenous insulin and insulin secretagogues, plasma insulin levels and blood glucose are not appropriately suppressed. Therefore, blood glucose levels may decrease, but the insulin levels remain elevated.

Clinical Manifestations of DKA, HHS, and Hypoglycemia

There are a variety of clinical signs and symptoms of DKA, HHS, and hypoglycemia. In general, these signs and symptoms result predominantly from hyperglycemia, dehydration, hyperosmolality, metabolic acidosis, and electrolyte disturbances. There is overlap between the signs and symptoms of DKA and HHS, with some exceptions. As noted previously, HHS is not associated with a metabolic acidosis. In addition, the degree of hyperglycemia, dehydration, and hyperosmolality is much more severe in HHS than DKA. The general causes of these clinical signs and symptoms are listed in Chart 53–7 (p. 1692).

Laboratory and Diagnostic Procedures

Hyperglycemia is present in both DKA and HHS due to a relative or absolute deficiency of circulating insulin. The hyperglycemia associated with HHS generally is greater than in DKA (Chart 53–8, p. 1692). Because HHS is not associated with emergent symptoms of metabolic acidosis and many of the affected patients are unable to articulate their needs, the course of the disease may evolve over a longer period of time. Additionally, the reduction in GFR during the severe dehydration of HHS decreases urinary loss of glucose, further increasing the blood glucose level.

- **Metabolic acidosis**—Metabolic acidosis is present in DKA as reflected in a *reduced arterial pH, reduced plasma bicarbonate,* and *increased anion gap* and is due primarily to the accumulation of ketone bodies. In addition, some degree of lactic acidosis exists from hypoperfusion, which also contributes to the acidosis.

- **Ketoacids**—The ketoacids beta-hydroxybutyrate and acetoacetate accumulate in the serum causing metabolic acidosis. The

| CHART 53–7 | Signs and Symptoms of Diabetic Ketoacidosis, Hyperosmolar Hyperglycemic Syndrome, and Hypoglycemia |

Diabetes Ketoacidosis

- *Polyuria* is caused by an osmotic diuresis induced by hyperglycemia.
- *Polyphagia* is caused by inability to use energy substrates (CHO, protein, and fats) appropriately.
- As the metabolic acidosis progresses, *polyphagia* is generally replaced by *anorexia*, due to the effects of ketones.
- *Polydipsia* is a compensatory response to dehydration and volume depletion.
- *Weight loss* results from *dehydration* and altered utilization of CHO, protein, and fats.
- *Fatigue* occurs in response to altered CHO, protein, and lipid metabolism, especially protein catabolism, but likely other factors (e.g., dehydration) also contribute to fatigue.
- *Blurred vision* occurs in response to hyperglycemia. Fluid accumulates in the lens of the eye, causing refractory changes.
- *Hypotension, tachycardia,* and *poor skin turgor* result from dehydration and volume depletion.
- As the *metabolic acidosis, dehydration*, and *volume depletion* progress, orthostatic hypotension develops.
- *Cardiac arrhythmias* result primarily from electrolyte disturbances, such as abnormal K^+.
- *Nausea and vomiting* are thought to result from the accumulation of serum ketones. The cause of abdominal pain is not certain but may be related to potassium depletion. Nausea and vomiting also may be related to the precipitating cause of DKA or HHS.
- *Kussmaul's respirations* (deep rapid respirations) are a compensatory mechanism to decrease $PaCO_2$.
- The *red, flushed face*, seen along with Kussmaul's respirations, is due to the increased levels of $PaCO_2$, which have a vasodilating effect.
- *Decreased mental status* and *coma* are primarily due to dehydration and serum hyperosmolality.
- *Hypothermia* results from a variety of causes, the most common being peripheral vasodilation, severe dehydration, and in DKA, metabolic acidosis. In addition, *hypothermia* may be a manifestation of the precipitating event (e.g., sepsis).

Hyperosmolar Hyperglycemic Syndrome

- *Polyuria* (as above).
- *Polyphagia* (as above).
- *Polydipsia* (as above).
- *Weight loss* and *dehydration* (as above).
- *Fatigue* (as above).
- *Blurred vision* (as above).
- *Hypotension, tachycardia,* and *poor skin turgor* (as above).
- *Cardiac arrhythmias* (as above).
- *Decreased mental status* and *coma* are primarily due to dehydration and serum hyperosmolality.
- *Hyperglycemia, dehydration,* and *serum hyperosmolality* are usually much more severe than in DKA. This results in *cerebral dehydration,* which is associated with neurological symptoms such as hemiparesis, seizures, and coma.
- *Hypothermia* results from a variety of causes, the most common being peripheral vasodilation and severe dehydration. In addition, hypothermia may be a manifestation of the precipitating event (e.g., sepsis).
- *Vascular thrombosis* results from severe dehydration. Patients with HHS are at greater risk because of the severity of dehydration and hyperosmolality.

Hypoglycemia

- The clinical symptoms of hypoglycemia are generally divided into autonomic and neuroglycopenic categories.
- The autonomic symptoms are subdivided into adrenergic (e.g., tremors, palpitations, nervousness, anxiety) and cholinergic (e.g., sweating and hunger) categories.
- The neuroglycopenic symptoms (irritability, confusion, drowsiness, weakness, difficulty speaking, unresponsiveness, unconsciousness, seizures, and coma) result from glucose deprivation to the central nervous system.

| CHART 53–8 | Laboratory Values in Diabetic Ketoacidosis, Hyperosmolar Hyperglycemic Nonketotic Syndrome, and Hypoglycemia |

Diabetic Ketoacidosis	Hyperosmolar Hyperglycemic Syndrome	Hypoglycemia
Random plasma glucose (>250 mg/dL)	Random plasma glucose (usually >600 mg/dL)	Random plasma glucose (usually <60 mg/dL)
Arterial pH <7.3	Arterial pH: >7.3	
7.25–7.30: associated with mild DKA	Serum bicarbonate: >15 mEq/L	
7.00–7.24: associated with moderate DKA	Anion gap: <12	
<7.00: associated with severe DKA	Serum ketones: negative or small	
Serum bicarbonate <15 mEq/L (decreases with moderate to severe DKA)	Urine ketones: negative or small	
	Serum osmolality: (>340 mOsm/kg)	
Anion gap: >10 (increases with moderate to severe DKA)		
Serum ketones: positive		
Urinary ketones: positive		
Serum osmolality: variable		

hydrogen ions of the ketoacids are buffered by bicarbonate, which causes reduced serum bicarbonate.

- **Serum Na⁺**—The serum Na⁺ in DKA or HHS may be low, normal, or high. The presence of increased levels of glucose in the extracellular space causes the movement of water from the intracellular to the extracellular space; this dilutes and lowers the serum Na⁺ concentration. As the fluid volume deficit increases, water in the extracellular space is lost in excess of Na⁺ and the serum Na⁺ concentration increases.

The serum K⁺ level may be low, normal, or elevated at the initial clinical presentation of both DKA and HHS. In both DKA and HHS, there is a loss in total body stores of K⁺ from cellular destruction and urinary losses. In an attempt to buffer the metabolic acidosis, however, K⁺ shifts from the intracellular to extracellular space in exchange for hydrogen ions, which move from the extracellular to the intracellular space. With initiation of insulin therapy, K⁺ moves back into the cell and the serum K⁺ drops from the initial serum level. Therefore, insulin infusion and K⁺ are usually begun simultaneously.

- **Serum PO₄⁻**—The serum PO₄⁻ level may also be normal on clinical presentation of DKA or HHS. However, as in DKA, these levels do not reflect actual body deficits that exist when phosphate shifts from intracellular to extracellular during DKA or HHS.
- **Serum creatinine**—The serum creatinine levels are elevated in both DKA and HHS due to severe dehydration and hyperosmolality. The serum creatinine levels in HHS usually are elevated above those in DKA, reflecting possible renal impairment.
- **BUN**—The serum BUN levels are elevated in both DKA and HHS due to dehydration, serum hyperosmolality, and protein catabolism. As with serum creatinine, the BUN levels in HHS usually are elevated above those in DKA, reflecting possible renal impairment.
- **Serum osmolality**—The serum osmolality may be elevated in both DKA and HHS, and is typically higher in HHS than DKA. The rising plasma glucose level increases serum osmolality.
- **White blood count (WBC)**—The WBC may be elevated in DKA. This may reflect a normal leukocytosis that frequently accompanies DKA or the presence of actual infection.

Medical Management of DKA, HHS, and Hypoglycemia

The overall treatment of DKA and HHS revolves around general measures, insulin treatment, fluids, and electrolytes. Overall general measures in the treatment of DKA and HHS include the following:

- Identification of those patients who require hemodynamic monitoring
- Protection of airway in stuporous or comatose patients
- Insertion of a nasogastric tube in patients with a vulnerable airway
- Hourly measurement of serum glucose
- Frequent (every 1 to 4 hours) measurement of arterial blood gases (ABGs), serum ketones, and electrolytes
- ECG monitoring for dysrhythmias (e.g., hypokalemia and hyperkalemia)

- Hourly assessment of urinary output, vital signs, and neurological status
- Chest x-ray and imaging studies as indicated
- Use of a flow sheet to monitor vital signs, urine output, glucose, ABGs, serum ketones, blood chemistries, electrolytes, and IV fluids
- Hourly assessment and documentation of clinical status as treatment progresses.

Insulin Treatment

The preferred method of insulin delivery in DKA and HHS involves Regular insulin as a low-dose IV infusion. The continuous insulin infusion helps to prevent both rapid changes in serum glucose along with hypokalemia and hypoglycemia. In addition, the insulin infusion allows for flexible adjustment of the infusion rate in response to changes in plasma glucose. An IV bolus injection of Regular insulin (0.1 unit/kg body weight) is usually administered prior to beginning the insulin infusion. This bolus should be followed by a continuous infusion of $0.1 \text{ unit} \cdot \text{kg}^{-1} \cdot \text{hr}^{-1}$ (approximately 5 to 10 units/hr) until the plasma glucose concentration is 250 to 300 mg/dL and the arterial pH is ≥7.3 or HCO₃⁻ is ≥18 mEq/L. Important points of this insulin therapy are as follows:

- Blood glucose levels should be monitored hourly during the insulin infusion with a goal of reducing the plasma glucose gradually at a rate of 80 to 100 $\text{mg} \cdot \text{dL}^{-1} \cdot \text{hr}^{-1}$.
- The insulin infusion should be decreased to 2 to 3 units/hr until the blood glucose is 250 to 300 mg/dL and the bicarbonate is HCO₃⁻ is ≥18 mEq/L. The plasma glucose is likely to be corrected prior to the correction of acidosis.
- The insulin infusion should be continued in the presence of acidosis even if the glucose level is continuing to decline toward normal levels. Glucose should be administered at 5 to 10 g/hr intravenously to prevent hypoglycemia.
- Subcutaneous insulin should be given approximately 30 minutes prior to stopping the infusion to make certain that there is no delay that could cause relapse of DKA.

Fluid Therapy

Increased plasma glucose, as seen in DKA and HHS, results in a shift of water from the intracellular to the extracellular space. There is an initial deficit in intracellular fluid, followed by extracellular (intravascular compartment) fluid loss, precipitated by osmotic diuresis. In addition, there may be ongoing losses of fluid (e.g., nausea and vomiting), which further dehydration and volume contraction.

The first goal of fluid therapy in DKA or HHS is the restoration of intravascular fluid volume, thereby, maintaining adequate blood pressure, treating or preventing shock, and reestablishing renal perfusion. The use of isotonic normal saline (0.9 NS) is necessary as a first-line treatment in DKA and HHS. As hyperglycemia is corrected, water is shifted back into the intracellular space. This could potentially lead to circulatory collapse, if 0.9 NS, which remains in the intravascular space, is not administered concurrently with insulin.

After correcting the intravascular fluid losses, the second goal of fluid therapy is to restore the free water deficit by infusing hypotonic solutions such as 0.45 NS. As dehydration is corrected in HHS, normal renal perfusion is established and glucose is lost through urinary glucose disposal. Therefore, patients with HHS may have significant reductions in serum glucose during the process of rehydration alone, requiring less insulin to correct hyperglycemia.

In adult patients (with no underlying comorbidities such as cardiac, renal, and liver disease), 1 to 2 liters of 0.9 NS should be infused for prompt correction of hypotension and hypoperfusion over the first hour. During hours 1 through 4, 750 to 1,000 mL/hr of 0.9 NS or 0.45 NS should be infused for severe volume depletion; or 250 to 500 mL/hr of 0.9 NS or 0.45 NS should be infused for moderate volume depletion. During hours 4 through 24, the infusion rate should be adjusted depending on the patient's intake, urinary output, and hydration status. The composition of the fluid is dependent on serum sodium and plasma osmolality measurements. In addition, the rate of fluid replacement does depend on each patient's overall cardiopulmonary status and the presence of comorbidities.

Electrolyte Management

Phosphate replacement is not recommended routinely in either DKA or HHS, although other electrolytes such as magnesium and calcium may be supplemented as needed. With insulin treatment during DKA and HHS, however, potassium is shifted from the intracellular to the extracellular space, thus placing patients at particular risk for hypokalemia. Some important points regarding potassium replacement are discussed next.

The results of the admission serum K^+ level should be obtained prior to initiating K^+ replacement therapy. If the patient is anuric, the K^+ supplementation should be held. If the patient is anuric and hypokalemic, adults may be given 10 to 30 mEq KCl over 1 to 2 hours, provided close ECG monitoring can be established and serum potassium levels can be assessed frequently. During hours 2 through 8, K^+ supplementation usually is added as 20 to 40 mEq KCl/L is infused depending on the serum K^+ level and estimated K^+ deficit during hours 8 through 48. Bicarbonate therapy is recommended only in the following situations: life-threatening hyperkalemia, severe lactic acidosis, and severe acidosis (pH < 6.9).

Hypoglycemia Management

As noted previously, the blood glucose level in DKA may normalize faster than resolution of the metabolic acidosis. This necessitates the infusion of IV glucose (D10%W or D5%W) for prevention of hypoglycemia. In HHS the glucose level may decline fairly quickly; as renal function improves urinary glucose disposal increases. Patients in this situation need close monitoring to avoid rapid shifts in blood glucose, serum osmolality, and hypoglycemia. This involves slowing the insulin infusion rate as the blood glucose levels decline and providing IV glucose as indicated. When patients with DKA and HHS treated with IV insulin infusions develop hypoglycemia, the lower blood glucose level can be treated with intravenous glucose (D50%W), unless the patient is able to eat and drink appropriately.

 *In hospital settings, insulin drips have been used for DKA and HHS for many years. Currently, insulin drips are being used to maintain normal blood glucose levels in non-DKA or non-HHS patients to maintain normal blood glucose levels. As a result, nurses must assess patients on insulin drips frequently for signs and symptoms of hypoglycemia and assess blood glucose levels on a planned basis (more intense insulin regimens require more frequent monitoring) and anytime hypoglycemia is suspected.*

As just mentioned, in the hospital setting, D50%W is available to treat severe hypoglycemia (or hypoglycemia in patients who cannot eat); at home, however, patients are taught to inject intramuscular or subcutaneous glucagon for severe insulin reactions. Occasionally, glucagon may be administered in the hospital setting. The usual adult dose is 1 mg S_Q or IM; since the major adverse effect of glucagon is nausea and vomiting, patients should rest on their side following administration to prevent aspiration. Adult patients with mild or documented asymptomatic hypoglycemia can be treated with 10 to 20 grams of glucose in the form of juice, soda, liquid glucose, or glucose tablets. If these patients are using alpha-glucosidase inhibitors, they need to be treated with 10 to 20 grams of pure glucose, such as glucose gels and glucose tablets; this is because there will be delayed absorption of other forms of CHO. Following treatment, the patient's blood glucose level should be checked and treatment repeated every 10 to 20 minutes until the blood glucose level returns to normal (Harmel et al., 2004).

Management of Acute Diabetes Complications

A number of complications can occur in patients with DKA and HHS. The most common complications include electrolyte imbalances such as hypokalemia, hypoglycemia, and hypercalcemia. The most emergent and dreaded complication of DKA is cerebral edema (Brown, 2004). The development of cerebral edema typically occurs approximately 6 to 12 hours after therapy has begun when the severe acidosis has been partially corrected, the blood glucose has been reduced, blood pressure restored, and the patient appears to be recovering. This complication most commonly occurs in children (Harmel et al., 2004).

 *The development of cerebral edema is marked by abrupt changes in mental status, abnormal neurological signs, progression to coma, and brain herniation and death.*

There have been a number of proposed causes of cerebral edema. Such causes include a rapid fall in glucose with movement of water from the extracellular to intracellular space, causing brain swelling; a rapid decrease in plasma oncotic pressure resulting from the use of protein-free solutions; and altered cerebral pH with paradoxical cerebrospinal cord acidosis resulting from bicarbonate administration. The failure of serum sodium to rise despite correction of hyperglycemia appears to signify excessive administration of free water and such patients are at risk for cerebral brain swelling (Dunger et al., 2004; Hale et al., 1997).

Despite the fact that no one particular cause of cerebral edema in DKA has been identified, it appears prudent to avoid a rapid fall in plasma osmolality by using 0.9 NS as the initial hydrating solution as in the protocol described previously. In addition, it appears prudent to allow the plasma glucose levels to fall slowly as described previously. If cerebral edema occurs, therapeutic measures include the use of mannitol and dexamethasone.

Medical Management of Chronic Complications of Diabetes

As noted previously, various chronic complications are associated with diabetes. These complications are broadly divided into macrovascular and microvascular complications.

Macrovascular Complications

The leading cause of death among patients with type 2 diabetes mellitus is CVD, with the majority of these deaths attributed to

CHD. The process through which the metabolic derangements of diabetes accelerate the development of CVD in diabetes has yet to be determined and remains an area of intense investigation, focusing on hyperglycemia and insulin resistance (particularly in type 2 diabetes) as major underlying contributors. The topic of CVD is discussed in Chapter 40 ⊘, so it is not discussed extensively in this chapter. As in all complications of diabetes, early detection of CVD is likely to yield better outcomes. Lifestyle interventions including increasing physical activity, weight loss, eating a healthy diet, smoking cessation, and management of prothrombotic factors (through the use of daily aspirin if not contraindicated) are most likely to decrease the risk of macrovascular disease; however, the management of dyslipidemias and hypertension are of the utmost importance.

Microvascular Complications

The microvascular complications of diabetes include retinopathy, neuropathy, and nephropathy. These complications were discussed earlier in the chapter, and also are discussed in other chapters in the text (see Chapters 43, 47, and 71 ⊘).

Retinopathy The national guidelines proposed by the ADA recommend that health care providers work closely with patients and families (Burant & ADA, 2008). For more details, see National Guidelines for Diabetic Retinopathy box.

Nephropathy The development of diabetic nephropathy is often asymptomatic, such that it usually is detected on routine laboratory screening tests. The natural history of diabetic nephropathy is a progression from a period of hyperfiltration, which is characterized by an increased GFR, to ESRD, which is characterized by nephrotic range proteinuria, decreasing GFR, and increasing creatinine. The development of diabetic nephropathy is largely dependent on duration of disease and level of glycemic control. The DCCT clearly demonstrated that there is a relationship between level of glycemia and the development and progression of nephropathy. The first sign of developing nephropathy is the presence of microalbuminuria (>30 mg albumin/24 hours) (Burant & ADA, 2008). Microalbuminuria should prompt the health care provider to aggressively treat even minor elevations in blood pressure in order to preserve renal function. In particular, angiotensin-converting enzyme (ACE) inhibitors and angiotensin receptor blockers (ARBs) are most beneficial in delaying the progression of nephropathy in patients with diabetes and microalbuminuria. In addition to hypertension, other factors such as neurogenic bladder, infections, and nephrotoxic drugs, including selected radiocontrast dyes, are associated with a decline in renal function among those patients with diabetes (see Chapter 45 ⊘).

The ADA guidelines, as listed in the National Guidelines for Diabetic Nephropathy box, highlight the information considered to be the most important in the treatment of nephropathy (Burant & ADA, 2008).

Neuropathy Diabetic neuropathy can affect any area of the body and exists primarily as diabetic polyneuropathy, autonomic neuropathy, or combinations of both. It is beyond the scope of this text to explore this topic in detail; however, attention will focus on some major issues associated with autonomic and peripheral neuropathy.

Autonomic Neuropathy Diminished autonomic nerve function can cause a variety of symptoms. In particular, autonomic polyneuropathy is associated with the development of gastroparesis, neurogenic bladder, diabetic diarrhea, and impaired cardiovascular reflexes (e.g., orthostatic hypotension and tachycardia) and sexual dysfunction (e.g., impotence).

Cardiovascular autonomic neuropathy is associated with a variety of clinical manifestations, most particularly resting tachycardia (>100 beats per minute), orthostasis (a decrease in systolic blood pressure of >20–30 mmHg on standing) (ADA, 2008c). Patients may complain of dizziness or weakness, nausea, vomiting, and syncope when standing up quickly (Harmel et al., 2004). Patients with severe orthostasis may need fludrocortisone and/or compression stockings.

Gastrointestinal disturbances are common in diabetes and may include esophageal disturbances, gastroparesis, diarrhea, and fecal incontinence (ADA, 2008c). *Gastroparesis* is a syndrome

---

NATIONAL GUIDELINES for Diabetic Retinopathy

- Instruct patients to report visual symptoms promptly.
- Instruct patients about the relationship between hyperglycemia, hypertension, and diabetic retinopathy, focusing on risk factor control to preserve eyesight.
- Inform patients about the importance of an annual dilated examination.
- Inform patients that isometric exercise can raise intraocular pressure; as such, these exercises can worsen proliferative retinopathy.
- Inform patients about support programs and community services for patients with visual impairments and visual loss.

Source: Burant, C. F., & American Diabetes Association. (2008). *Medical management of type 2 diabetes* (6th ed.). Alexandria, VA: American Diabetes Association.

NATIONAL GUIDELINES for Diabetic Nephropathy

- Optimizing glycemic control can prevent or delay the progression of diabetic nephropathy.
- Annual tests for microalbuminuria can detect early diabetic nephropathy.
- Regular blood pressure checks can identify hypertension; hypertension can damage the kidney, precipitate the onset of nephropathy, and accelerate the progression.
- Treatment of hypertension with medication, weight loss, and sodium restriction can prevent the development and decrease the progression of diabetic nephropathy.
- The increased risk of infections in patients with chronic hyperglycemia can result in infections, such as pyelonephritis, with decline in renal function. Patients need to report signs and symptoms of infection to their health care provider.
- Patients who have progressive diabetic nephropathy need to explore options such as dialysis and transplantation with their health care provider.

Source: Burant, C. F., & American Diabetes Association. (2008). *Medical management of type 2 diabetes* (6th ed.). Alexandria, VA: American Diabetes Association.

characterized by the impaired transit of food from the stomach to the duodenum in the absence of a mechanical obstruction. This condition is characterized by early satiety, nausea, vomiting, and abdominal discomfort. These symptoms are often accompanied by fluctuations in blood glucose levels due to delayed gastric emptying or retention of food products. These fluctuations are most pronounced in individuals on insulin therapy. Insulin may peak during periods of delayed gastric emptying causing hypoglycemia; the absorption of food while the actions of insulin are waning may cause hyperglycemia. Treatment of gastroparesis largely relies on diet and medications, and nutritional support may be needed in the most severe cases. Improved glycemic control may actually improve gastric emptying. Frequent (six to eight per day) low-fat, low-fiber meals, especially liquids, may be indicated in gastroparesis (Harmel et al., 2004). Metoclopramide, a dopamine agonist, improves gastric emptying time and has a central antiemetic action (Harmel et al., 2004). Erythromycin is a motilin agonist that stimulates gastric motor activity and can provide some symptomatic relief in the treatment of gastroparesis (Harmel et al., 2004).

Diabetic diarrhea is characterized by the frequent passage of loose stools occurring primarily after meals and during the night. Some patients have alternating periods of diarrhea and constipation. The cause of the diarrhea is unknown and diagnosis is made after other causes of diarrhea (e.g., infection) are excluded. The treatment is largely empirical involving the use of antidiarrheal agents, such as loperamide.

Diabetic autonomic neuropathy also is associated with genitourinary track disturbances. These may include bladder and and/or sexual dysfunction. Neurogenic bladder is characterized by a pattern of frequent, small voiding, and incontinence leading to urinary retention. An evaluation of bladder dysfunction should be performed in patients with diabetes who have recurrent urinary tract infections, pyelonephritis, urinary incontinence, or a palpable bladder (ADA, 2008c). In males, diabetic neuropathy may result in the loss of penile erection and/or retrograde ejaculation (ADA, 2008c). Therapy with selective phosphodiesterase-5 inhibitors (e.g., sildenafil, vardenafil) is now the first line of therapy for male erectile dysfunction (Joslin & Kahn, 2005). However, vacuum devices, intrapenile injections of vasodilating substances (e.g., papaverine), and the implantation of an inflatable or semirigid prosthesis may allow the patient to resume sexual activity.

Polyneuropathy Polyneuropathy is most commonly seen in the legs, feet, and hands. This is called **diabetic peripheral neuropathy (DPN)** and is clearly a significant factor in the pathway leading to lower extremity ulceration (Burant & ADA, 2008). Although DPN is predominantly associated with sensory loss, motor and autonomic nerve fibers also can be affected. Distal symmetric sensorimotor polyneuropathy is the most common form of DPN. As the name implies, it usually appears first in the distal portions of the extremities, moving proximally in a "stocking-glove" distribution. It encompasses both sensory and motor nerve damage and affects both limbs.

Clinical symptoms associated with sensory nerve damage may include numbness, pain, burning, tingling, and eventual partial or total loss of sensation. The pain associated with DPN

is first felt distally, in the lower legs, and usually worsens at night. The pain can be persistent or intermittent, occurring over periods of weeks or months. This pain is usually described as aching or burning in nature. Improvement of pain without medication is usually accompanied by the loss of protective sensation and an increase in the risk of foot and lower limb injuries, including ulceration.

Vascular and Neuropathic Complications Leading to Lower Extremity Amputations

Lower extremity amputations in patients with diabetes result from a combination of pathologic events working in tandem. Most diabetic lower extremity amputations originate from diabetic foot ulcers, peripheral arterial disease (PAD), PVD, peripheral neuropathy, minor trauma, deformity, increased plantar pressures, and infection contributing to the development and progression of these ulcers.

Assessment of Sensory Loss Testing for large fiber sensory changes in the diabetic foot can be cost effective and easily performed in any setting with a Semmes-Weinstein monofilament (Mayfield, Reiber, Sanders, Janisse, & Pogach, 2004). The monofilament is a single nylon fiber attached to a handle that buckles under a specified amount of force. A range of monofilaments are available, but the preferred is the 5.07, or 10 grams. The patient is asked to close his eyes and the monofilament then is applied bilaterally to various points on the plantar surface of the toes and metatarsal heads where discriminatory ability is best appreciated. The patient is then asked to give a verbal cue when the monofilament is felt. The inability to perceive the monofilament in any area is considered loss of protective sensation (LOPS). A screening form can be used to document and track where there is loss of protective sensation (Chart 53–9).

Loss of protective sensation also can be established by testing the vibratory perception threshold (VPT), a technique used to measure sensory neuropathy. The simplest and least expensive method uses a 128-Hz tuning fork that is rapped against the clinician's hand and then held to a bony prominence on the foot or the hallux. The patient is asked to indicate when she stops feeling the vibration. If she is unable to feel vibration, she is considered at risk for ulceration.

Treatment for Neuropathic Pain Neuropathic pain is often refractory to traditional analgesic therapy and provides a challenge in pain management. The primary classes of medications used to treat DPN include tricyclic drugs (e.g., amitriptyline, nortriptyline, imipramine), anticonvulsants (e.g., gabapentin, carbamazepine, pregabalin), 5-hydroxytryptamine and norepinephrine uptake inhibitor (e.g., duloxetine), and substance P inhibitor (e.g., capsaicin cream) (ADA, 2008c).

Charcot Deformity Together, distal symmetric polyneuropathy and peripheral autonomic neuropathy can lead to neuropathic osteoarthropathy, or *Charcot deformity*. The underlying assumption is that autonomic neuropathy damages the sympathetic nerves innervating the small blood vessels of the lower extremities. This causes a loss of constrictive tone resulting in vasodilation, increased peripheral perfusion, and expedited

PLANTAR SENSORY TESTING

Fill in the following blanks with an "R", "L", or "B" to indicate positive findings on the right, left, or both feet, respectively:

Has there been a change in the foot since the last evaluation?	Yes___	No___
Is there a foot ulcer now, or history of foot ulcer?	Yes___	No___
Does the foot have an abnormal shape?	Yes___	No___
Are the nails thick, too long, or ingrown?	Yes___	No___
Does the patient currently perform daily foot care?	Yes___	No___

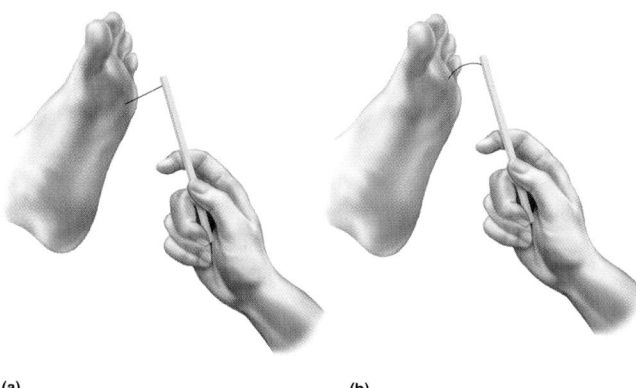

(a)   (b)

Picture of Semmes-Weinstein Monofilament being used

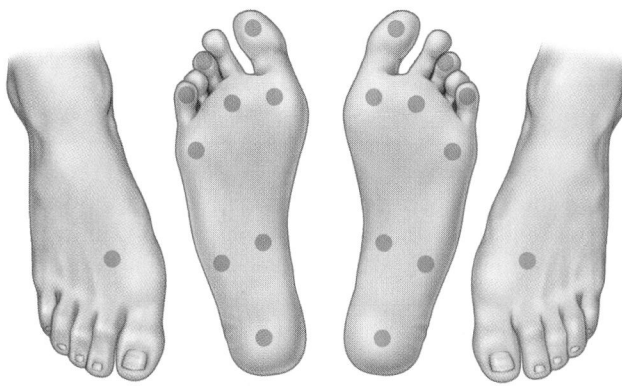

Marked areas indicative of loss of protective sensation as determined by use of monofilament

Risk Category		Action
0	No loss of protective sensation	0 and 1: Teach foot care guidelines.
1	Loss of protection sensation (no deformity, callus, preulcer, or hx of ulceration)	
2	Loss of protective sensation with deformity, preulcer, callus, or corn	2 and 3: Refer immediately to primary care provider/foot care specialist.
3	History of plantar ulceration	

bone resorption and osteopenia. The salient features and therapy for Charcot deformity are detailed in Chart 53–10 (p. 1698).

Peripheral Vascular Disease   Inadequate perfusion to the lower extremities deprives the tissues of oxygen, nutrients, and antibiotics, and impairs waste removal, thus placing the limb at risk for impaired wound healing and gangrene. Clinical findings in PVD include diminished or absent peripheral pulses and intermittent claudication (pain with walking that is relieved by rest). If patients complain of deep, aching pain at night or with rest, severe vascular disease may be present and ulceration or gangrene may follow soon. Additionally, pain may not be present in patients with concurrent neuropathic sensory loss. Unfortunately, gangrene may be the first sign of severe PVD.

Additional signs and symptoms of PVD are shown in Chart 53–11 (p. 1698). Peripheral vascular disease also is discussed in Chapter 43 ⬯.

Assessment of vascular status is important to adequately determine risk in a healthy foot, to define the underlying problem in the presence of an ulcer, and to determine the location of a blockage prior to bypass surgery. After gathering data about the patient's medical history and current self-described pain, the health care provider should proceed with a general inspection of the extremities. The dorsalis pedis and posterior tibial pulses should be assessed and graded as palpable or nonpalpable. In the event the pulse is diminished or absent, a second evaluation should be made by another health care provider. The continued absence of a pulse warrants further work-up. The last step in the assessment is to auscultate for femoral bruits. If bruits are present, an arterial brachial index (ABI) should be performed. The ABI is a test that measures the blood pressures in the arm and ankle both at rest and during treadmill walking; a numerical calculation is performed that is used to predict the severity of PVD.

Literature on the diabetic foot has indicated that, by instituting a regular, organized plan of foot care, most diabetic foot problems can be prevented, but the first step is assessment of risk. Following is a list of the factors that have been associated with increased risk for lower extremity ulcers and amputations (Burant & ADA, 2008):

- Patients who have been diagnosed with DM > 10 years
- Male gender
- Patients with poor glucose control
- Patients with cardiovascular, retinal, or renal complications.

Conditions related to the feet that are associated with higher risk for amputations include:

- Peripheral neuropathy with loss of protective sensation
- Altered biomechanics (in the presence of neuropathy)
- Evidence of increased pressures (erythema, hemorrhage under a callous)
- Bony deformity
- Peripheral vascular disease
- A history of ulcers or amputation
- Severe nail pathology.

The ADA recommends that all patients with diabetes should receive a thorough foot examination annually. The foot examination

CHART 53–10	Stages, Clinical Findings, and Therapy for Charcot Deformity		
Charcot Stage	**Features**	**Clinical Findings**	**Therapy**
1. Acute	• Weakened ligaments are allowed to stretch beyond their normal range of motion, causing spontaneous dislocation of the foot • Joint effusions and bone resorption also occur • Easily confused with osteomyelitis	**Physical Exam** • Visible reddening of foot • Warmth • Edema • Easily palpable pulses • May require advanced imaging technologies because microfractures and joint effusions may be missed by x-ray	• Immediate elimination of weight-bearing on affected limb • If compliance is questioned, hospitalization may be necessary • Continue until redness, edema, and foot temperatures return to normal
2. Progressive	• Dislocation and fragmentation of bone • Further fracture • Osseous tissue and muscle have been weakened from nonuse and will need progressive return to full weight-bearing rather than an abrupt return	Radiography usually shows fractures at the metatarsal joints	• Total non–weight-bearing • Crutches and walkers are not recommended, because they may overstress the contralateral limb. Use of a wheelchair is a better option • Use of total contact or walking casts assure immobilization of joint, but can be walked in, thus undermining non–weight-bearing
3. Advanced	• Collapse of the plantar arch from multiple fractures and joint collapse	"Rocker-bottom" foot	• Prevention of foot ulcer and amputation • Referral for custom orthotic footwear • Surgical intervention may be warranted to reduce or excise bony prominences and/or ulcers if present • Fusion of unstable joints or severely deformed feet may provide a safer base for accepting weight-bearing stress and reducing the risk for further ulceration and collapse

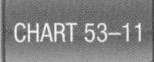

CHART 53–11 Signs and Symptoms of Peripheral Vascular Disease

- Feet cold to touch
- Blanching on elevation
- Dependent rubor
- Loss of hair on foot or toes
- Atrophy of subcutaneous fatty tissue
- Absent or diminished pulses
- Delayed venous filling time after elevation (>25 sec)
- Shiny skin
- Thickened nails, often with fungal infection
- Blue toe syndrome

does not need to be time consuming or require expensive or specialized equipment. All health care providers who treat patients with diabetes should be proficient in conducting simple screening examinations. The findings from this risk assessment should guide the plan for prevention and care of foot problems.

During the initial encounter, and throughout the process, the health care provider should assist the patient to change any modifiable risk factors such as smoking, home foot care practices, activity levels, and glycemic control. A variety of home foot care practices have been devised that help decrease the development of foot ulcers and amputation in patients with diabetes and neuropathy. These practices are detailed in the next section.

It is important to note practices that place the patient at higher risk for injury. These include walking without shoes, walking with ill-fitting shoes, decreased attention to daily inspections, and cutting toenails when vision is too poor to visualize the extremity. Activities such as jogging on concrete sidewalks may be contraindicated in patients with diabetes and neuropathy because they may result in trauma to the extremities. Poor glycemic control is associated with poor wound healing and infection. Care for the high-risk foot should not be delayed while waiting on lifestyle changes or glycemic improvement.

Patient Education for Prevention of Lower Extremity Disease As the foundation for all intervention, patient diabetes self-management education should be a priority in every clinical setting. Patients should be taught the following principles of foot care (Ahroni, 2003):

1. **Inspection**—The feet and interdigital areas should be checked daily for blisters, sores, cuts, and calluses. A magnifying glass or handheld mirror may be helpful in viewing the tops, sides, and bottoms of the feet. If patients have cognitive

or visual impairments, a family member should be instructed in assisting or performing the foot examination. The shoes and socks also should be inspected for foreign objects, holes, or raised seams that could cause skin breakdown.

2. **Daily care**—Feet should be washed with warm, soapy water and dried thoroughly; soaking of the feet in water is not advisable. Water temperature should be checked by forearm or elbow to avoid burns. Minor calluses may be *gently* removed with a pumice stone. Thick calluses should be inspected and reduced by a foot care specialist. Nails should be trimmed straight across and the edges filed. If a patient has any visual difficulty, he should not attempt to trim nails. Lotion should be applied daily or more often if skin is dry, avoiding the area between the toes.

3. **Footwear**—Patients should be taught never to go barefoot to prevent injury to their feet. The decreased sensation associated with neuropathy may cause an injury to go unnoticed. Shoes and slippers should be inspected prior to use to make certain that no objects (e.g., coins) have accidentally dropped into them. In addition, when purchasing shoes, patients should ensure that the size is correct. Patients should be advised to break their shoes in slowly, always wear socks or hose, and replace socks rather than attempt to darn them. Because garters restrict blood flow, they should be avoided.

4. **Special care**—Patients should be taught not to use over-the-counter chemical agents to remove corns and warts.

The irritation caused by such chemicals may result in irritation and subsequent ulceration. In addition, sharp instruments or razor blades should never be used to self-treat foot problems such as ingrown toenails. The health care provider should be notified if any problem arises (cuts, blisters, nonhealing wounds, signs of infection, redness, or swelling).

■ Nursing Management

The nursing care needs of hospitalized patients with type 1 or type 2 diabetes, regardless of their admitting diagnosis, require ongoing attention to subjective and objective changes in diabetes status. The nurse often will be the first to notice improvement or deterioration in blood glucose control, which ultimately can hasten or delay recovery. The assessment data, which include sample questions specific to diabetes, are found in the Nursing Process: Care Plan for the Hospitalized Patient with Diabetes (p. 1700). The care plan applies the nursing process to the relevant nursing diagnoses and provides a comprehensive nursing approach for any hospitalized patient with type 1 or type 2 diabetes. This care plan should be used in conjunction with the care plans for concomitant diagnoses.

The nurse should also be aware of the discharge priorities associated with patients who have diabetes. Some examples are listed in the Patient Teaching & Discharge Priorities box.

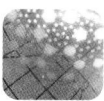

PATIENT TEACHING & DISCHARGE PRIORITIES for Diabetes

Need	Teaching
Physiological teaching needs	Discharge education needs should be evaluated as soon as possible when patients are admitted to the hospital.
	The education needs should be individualized to each patient, but should minimally address those "survival skills" necessary for the patient to be able to self-manage his or her diabetes in the outpatient setting.
	Education should be an ongoing process throughout the hospitalization and nurses should take advantage of every possible "teachable moment" to reinforce learning.
	Survival skill assessment and education should result in the patient or the patient's caregiver being able to: • Describe medication name, dosage, timing, side effects, and refill information. • Demonstrate appropriate technique for preparation and administration of insulin injection (if patient requires insulin). • Demonstrate appropriate technique for monitoring capillary blood glucose levels at home, and verbalize when testing should be done. • Verbalize target blood glucose goals and when to call the health care provider. • Describe the signs, symptoms, and treatment for hypoglycemia. • Describe the signs and symptoms and action to take for hyperglycemia. • Describe how to manage diabetes during illnesses such as the flu. • Verbalize basic understanding of healthy-eating concepts and timing of meals if insulin-requiring. • Verbalize when to call a health care provider.
	If patients are newly diagnosed with diabetes or pre-diabetes during this admission, or they have never received formal diabetes self-management education, or if they have had changes in their health or therapy, they should be referred for further outpatient diabetes education and follow-up.
Psychosocial teaching needs	Patients with diabetes must learn to cope with the daily stress of caring for a chronic disease. The incidence of depression and other psychological disturbances is much higher in people with diabetes than the general population. It is important for the nurse to assess psychosocial needs, family support, and coping skills to foster the patient's ability to self-manage his diabetes, while maintaining optimal quality of life.
	Discharge planning for patients who need further psychosocial support may include: • Referral for social work services • Information about local diabetes support groups • Referral for psychological evaluation.

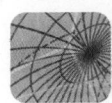

NURSING PROCESS: Patient Care Plan for Hospitalized Patient with Diabetes

Assessment of Blood Glucose Level

Subjective Data:

"I feel shaky."

"I am so thirsty and I am urinating every few hours."

"I can't get any sleep because I am urinating all night long."

Objective Data:

Elevated blood glucose	Palpitations
Polyuria	Mood changes
Polyphagia	Irritability
Weight loss	Unresponsiveness
Fatigue	Unconsciousness
Diaphoresis	Convulsions
Tremors	Coma

Nursing Assessment and Diagnoses	Outcomes and Evaluation Parameters	Planning and Interventions with *Rationales*
Nursing Diagnosis: *Risk for Unstable Blood Glucose*	**Outcome:** Patient will have an acute reduction in hyperglycemia. **Evaluation Parameters:** Evidence of a decrease in blood glucose levels. Common target blood glucose levels are: *Critically ill patients:* 110–180 mg/dL *Non–critically ill patients:* 90–130 mg/dL premeal; <180 mg/dL at 2 hours postmeal. **Outcome:** Patient will have resolution of hypoglycemia. **Evaluation Parameter:** Evidence of normalization of blood glucose levels.	**Interventions and *Rationales:*** In the event of hyperglycemia, administer medications to reduce blood glucose as ordered. These may include insulin, incretin mimetics or oral diabetes medications alone or in combination. In critically ill settings insulin may be administered intravenously (see text). *All of the medications listed above have a glucose-lowering effect.* **Interventions and *Rationales:*** In the event of hypoglycemia, administer medications or food to raise the blood glucose levels. Examples of foods that raise blood glucose levels include: 3–4 glucose tablets 1/2 cup of fruit juice 5–6 pieces of hard candy. Medications to raise blood glucose levels include: Dextrose 50% H_2O Glucagon *All of the medications listed above will increase blood glucose levels.* **Interventions and *Rationales:*** Check the blood glucose level prior to administering glucose-lowering medications. Consult with the medical team if a change in dose may be indicated due to abnormally low (hypoglycemic) or high (hyperglycemic) values. *Because blood glucose levels are affected by factors such as medications (in general), diabetes medications, diet, exercise and physiological stress, fluctuations in blood glucose levels are common in hospitalized patients.* Sustained hyperglycemia in response to treatment may reflect a poor response to therapy, necessitating a change in treatment plan. As the illness resolves, blood glucose levels decline; this may result in hypoglycemia, necessitating a change in the treatment plan. Check blood glucose as ordered. *The frequency and the timing of the blood glucose monitoring will differ depending on the therapy (see text).* Monitor for signs and symptoms of hypoglycemia or worsening hyperglycemia; if either is suspected, test blood glucose levels immediately. *Bedside blood glucose monitoring allows the nurse to verify if the patient has hypoglycemia or hyperglycemia and treat accordingly.*

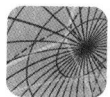

NURSING PROCESS: Patient Care Plan for Hospitalized Patient with Diabetes—*Continued*

Assessment of Fluid Volume Alterations

Subjective Data:
"I feel weak and light-headed."
"My mouth is very dry and I am always thirsty."

Objective Data:
Hypotension
Orthostatic hypotension
Tachycardia

Poor skin turgor
Decreased urine output

Nursing Assessment and Diagnoses	Outcomes and Evaluation Parameters	Planning and Interventions with *Rationales*
Nursing Diagnosis: *Deficient Fluid Volume* with potential for hypoglycemic shock	**Outcome:** The patient will have restoration of fluid volume. **Evaluation Parameters:** Resolution of hypotension. Resolution of orthostatic hypotension. Resolution of tachycardia. Improved skin turgor.	**Interventions and *Rationales:*** General measures include: Encourage fluid intake (in awake and alert patients). Rehydrate with 0.9 NS for intravascular fluid loss. Rehydrate with 0.45 NS for intracellular fluid loss (if indicated). *0.9 NS will reestablish extracellular fluid volume losses; 0.45 NS will restore intracellular volume losses.* Monitor oral fluid intake. Monitor vital signs. Monitor urine output. *To assess hydration status or adequacy of fluid replacement.*

Assessment of Acid–Base Imbalances

Subjective Data:
"I'm breathing fast."
Complaints of headache, altered sleeping pattern, and occasional chest pain

Objective Data:
Decreased arterial pH
Increased anion gap
Decreased serum bicarbonate
Positive serum ketones
Positive urinary ketones

Kussmaul's respirations
Acetone odor to breath
Red, flushed face
Decreased mental status

Nursing Assessment and Diagnoses	Outcomes and Evaluation Parameters	Planning and Interventions with *Rationales*
Nursing Diagnosis: *Risk for acute confusion related to alteration in Acid–Base Balance*	**Outcome:** Patient will have resolution of acid–base imbalance by: **Evaluation Parameters:** Normal arterial pH. Normal anion gap. Normal serum bicarbonate. Negative urinary ketones. Negative serum ketones. Improvements in mental status. Resolution of Kussmaul's breathing, facial flushing, and acid odor to breath.	**Interventions and *Rationales:*** Administer intravenous insulin as ordered. *Insulin will correct the metabolic acidosis.* Obtain the following laboratory tests as ordered and monitor the results closely: ABGs, anion gap, serum ketones, urinary ketones, and serum bicarbonate. The timing of the laboratory tests will change based the acuity of the patient and response to treatment. *The monitoring of these values will help monitor the patient's response to treatment.* Monitor for resolution of the following signs and symptoms: Kussmaul's respirations; fruity odor to breath; red, flushed face; and mental status changes. *Monitoring for resolution in signs and symptoms will help to assess the response to therapy.*

Assessment of Electrolyte Imbalances

Subjective Data:
Experience of muscle spasms.
Describes feelings of weakness, twitching, or confusion.

Objective Data:
Decreased serum potassium level (hypokalemia)

(continued)

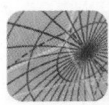

NURSING PROCESS: Patient Care Plan for Hospitalized Patient with Diabetes—*Continued*

Nursing Assessment and Diagnoses	Outcomes and Evaluation Parameters	Planning and Interventions with *Rationales*
Nursing Diagnoses: Decreased cardiac output related to alteration in serum potassium levels (lower than normal) Increased serum potassium level, higher than normal (hyperkalemia) Decreased serum sodium level (hypokalemia)	**Outcome:** Normalization of serum potassium level. ***Evaluation Parameter:*** Serum potassium level is within normal limits.	**Interventions and *Rationales:*** Administer IV potassium (as ordered), usually in the form potassium chloride or potassium phosphate. *Total body potassium stores are often decreased in DKA or HHS. Patients often present with normal or increased potassium levels. Regardless, when exogenous insulin is administered, the serum potassium levels will decrease (see text). Administration of IV potassium is usually indicated to maintain normal potassium levels.* Monitor patients for signs and symptoms of hypokalemia such as: Muscle weakness Anxiety Lethargy Depression Confusion Fatigue Muscle cramps Constipation Abnormal cardiac rhythms such as T-wave flattening, inverted T waves, prominent U wave, ST segment depression, ventricular arrhythmias (e.g., premature ventricular contractions), and atrial arrhythmias. Monitor patients for signs and symptoms of hyperkalemia such as: Muscle twitching Paralysis Gastrointestinal hypermotility Abdominal cramping Diarrhea Muscle cramps Irritability Anxiety Abnormal cardiac rhythms such as tall peaked T waves, widened QRS, and ventricular fibrillation. *Monitoring for signs and symptoms of hypokalemia and hyperkalemia will help assess patient response to treatment.*

Note: This list is not meant to be all inclusive but reflects common issues in the hospitalized patient with diabetes.

Health Promotion, Diabetes Education, and Cultural Implications

Much of the previous portion of this chapter has focused on the clinical presentation and the acute management of patients with diabetes. Diabetes care is a complex balance between the patient and health care providers. The majority of diabetes management decisions are made by the patient, far from the supervision of health care providers. The patients must be provided with the tools necessary to manage their disease.

Diabetes self-management education is an interactive and collaborative process between the patient and the health care team than leads to better diabetes control and health outcomes. Strategies of diabetes self-management education include providing the patient and significant other with the knowledge necessary to the successful management of diabetes. This information may include, but is not limited to (ADA, 2008d):

- Describing the pathophysiology of diabetes and treatment options
- Incorporating nutritional management and physical activity into lifestyle
- Using diabetes medication(s) safely to achieve maximum therapeutic effectiveness
- Monitoring blood glucose and other parameters and interpreting and using the results to make self-management decisions
- Preventing, detecting, and treating acute and chronic complications
- Developing personal strategies to address psychosocial issues and concerns to promote health and behavior changes.

The behavioral context on which the patient learns diabetes self-management skills is based on the complex interplay between culture and perceptions of health and illness. According to

Fleury-Milfort (2004), "the culture and the religious background of a patient and (of the diabetes educator) provide the context in which the patient develops certain values, beliefs, behaviors, attitude, self-care habits and relationships with healthcare providers." When a nurse is engaged in diabetes self-management teaching, she should assess the patient's beliefs about the causes of diabetes and diabetes complications, perceptions of the effect of diabetes and diabetes treatment on one's life, the role of family members on health care decisions and responsibilities, and the importance of customs and observances influencing the treatment plan (Fleury-Milfort, 2004). An understanding of such issues can form the basis of culturally sensitive self-management educational experiences.

Collaborative Management

Optimal care of patients with diabetes requires a multidisciplinary team approach to their care. Physicians, nurses, and dieticians work as a team to monitor blood glucose results, make changes in medication or nutrition therapies, and assess the response to those changes. As the health status of the patient improves or deteriorates, diabetes status also may change rapidly. Healing of infections or increases in mobility (and, thus, ambulation) may cause rapid lowering of blood glucose levels. Addition of some medications, such as corticosteroids may cause elevations in blood glucose levels, requiring alterations in med-

ication dosage by the health care provider. Hyperglycemia, if left untreated, will delay healing and may lead to longer hospitalizations. Careful assessment and monitoring by the nurse is crucial in alerting other members of the health care team to changes in diabetes status that can change the course of patient recovery. The dietitian plays a key role in adjusting diets and nutrients. The physical therapist and occupational therapist also may be involved in the case of mobility and self-care issues.

Summary

Diabetes is a chronic disease and the occurrence and progression of diabetes-related complications can be decreased through intensive glucose, hypertension, and lipid control. In addition, there is mounting evidence that the actual development of diabetes can be decreased through lifestyle modification including increased physical activity and weight maintenance or weight loss (if indicated). Acute complications of diabetes can be avoided through careful monitoring and attention to precipitating factors; yet when these acute complications occur, intensive medical management can decrease mortality and morbidity from these complications. Because the incidence of diabetes is increasing worldwide, health care professionals need to stay current with new treatment measures to address the personal, social, and economic problems associated with diabetes.

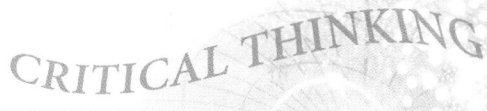

Clinical Preparation

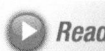 **Read**

- History of Current Illness
- Past Medical History
- Physical Exam
- Admitting Medical Orders
- Laboratory Study Results

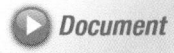 **Document**

- Summary of Hospitalization
- Pathophysiology Form
- Laboratory Values
- Laboratory Results Explanation

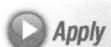 **Apply**

- List of Potential Nursing Diagnoses
- Concept Map
- Critical Thinking Questions

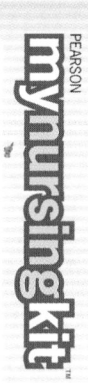

Log on to MyNursingKit.com to download forms you will need and to complete further steps in the Clinical Preparation assignment.

HISTORY OF PRESENT ILLNESS

The patient is a 20-year-old college student who presented to the local emergency department (ED). He reported that he and several other students had a gastrointestinal virus over the past few weeks. The primary symptoms were nausea, vomiting, and diarrhea, which usually resolved within 24 to 48 hours. John reported that he never completely recovered from his illness, feeling tired and listless during the previous week. During the past 2 to 3 days he noted increased thirst and increased urination, along with fatigue during this time period. John has been nauseated and vomiting during the last 2 hours, and has vomited twice in the ED.

The following medications were administered in the ED: an initial bolus of regular intravenous insulin (10 units) followed by an intravenous regular insulin drip of 6 units/hour. In addition, a potassium chloride (KCl) rider (20 mEq/hr) was initiated after it was established that the patient had adequate urinary output (>30 mL/hr).

Nursing care while in the ED revolved around assessing and providing interventions for any emergency needs (i.e., vascular fluid replacement); obtaining the diagnostic laboratory values: arterial blood gases (ABGs), serum ketones, complete blood count

(CBC), serum blood chemistries, serum electrolytes, and urinalysis (UA). In this particular patient, the current nursing care plan calls for initiating fluid replacement therapy (0.9 normal saline at 1 L/hr); obtaining a capillary glucose reading; performing an electrocardiogram (ECG); and sending a stool specimen to the laboratory for culture and sensitivity.

The patient was transferred to the medical intensive care unit (MICU) where you are assigned to care for him.

Medical–Surgical History

The patient's general medical history is noncontributory. There is no history of major medical illnesses, surgeries, or traumas. He does not use any medications, but does report using an "over-the-counter" drug to stop diarrhea during the previous episode of the "flu."

Mother (age 45) has rheumatoid arthritis; father (age 50) has hypertension. Siblings: brother (age 16) has no major illnesses; sister (age 14) has no major illnesses; and brother (age 10) has type 1 diabetes.

Social History

Patient reports social drinking (4 to 6 beers on weekends); has never smoked cigarettes, but smokes approximately 1 to 2 cigars every 2 to 3 months; he indicates that he has never used recreational drugs.

Physical Exam

Patient is a thin acutely ill male; 6'0" and 155 lbs. The following clinical signs are noted: poor skin turgor, dry mucous membranes, facial flushing, and deep rapid breathing with fruity odor to breath. His chest is clear to auscultation; his heart examination reveals tachycardia and is otherwise normal; the abdominal examination reveals a diffusely tender abdomen; the neurological examination reveals increasing lethargy, otherwise his neurological status is normal.

Vital signs: temperature is 99°F. In a supine position, his blood pressure is 100/70, pulse 100 beats per minute, and respirations 32. In a standing position, his blood pressure is 90/60; pulse, 115 beats per minute, and respirations are 32.

Admitting Medical Orders

Admit to Medical ICU
Admitting diagnosis: newly diagnosed type 1 diabetes; diabetic ketoacidosis (mild to moderate)
Allergies: none noted
Vital signs q1h
Neuro checks q1h
Activity: bed rest with bathroom privileges
I&O q8h
Sequential compression stockings (SCDs) to lower extremities
Diet: 1,800-calorie diabetic diet
Call house officer: HR < 60 or > 120, systolic BP < 90 or > 160, temperature > 38.5°C, RR < 10 or > 30, urinary output < 240 mL in 8 hours, O_2 saturation < 92%, glucose level < 70 or > 130, serum sodium level < 135 or > 145, serum potassium level < 3.8 or > 4.5, increased lethargy per neuro checks
IVs: normal saline 0.45 at 100 mL/hr

Scheduled Medications

Insulin drip at 6 units/hour
Potassium chloride (KCl) IV at 20 mEq/hr

PRN Medications

Phenergan for nausea 25 mg IV q4–6h prn
D50%W 25 g IV prn if Accu-Chek less than 70 mg/dL

Ordered Laboratory Studies

Serum K, Na, Cl, HCO_3 q2h
Serum K every hour if unstable
ABGs, CBC, Chem panel, serum acetone, and urine ketones q4h
Accu-Cheks q1h
Stool culture q24h × 3 days

Ordered Diagnostic Studies

ECG on admission and q4h
The patient has a relatively uneventful course during hospitalization with one exception. After approximately 8 hours of treatment, the patient was noted to be increasingly lethargic and confused. The two primary differential diagnoses for this condition include hypoglycemia and cerebral edema. A capillary blood glucose level taken at that time revealed a blood glucose level of 60 mg/dL, which confirms the hypoglycemia. The patient is given 25 g of dextrose 50% in water (D50%W). After administration of the D50%W, the patient is alert and oriented and the subsequent blood glucose reading is 100 mg/dL. The results of other pertinent tests at this time are shown below in the Laboratory Study Results table.
Because the patient's diabetic ketoacidosis has resolved and the patient is able to take fluids and food, the insulin drip is discontinued. Prior to discontinuing the drip, the patient is started on an insulin protocol with an initial starting dose of Glargine 20 units subcutaneously. The premeal lispro dose will be titrated depending on the meal and overall appetite of the patient. In general an insulin:carbohydrate (CHO) ratio of 1:20 (1 unit of lispro insulin to 20 mg of CHO) will be used.
The nursing care at this time is centered on (1) monitoring response to therapy and (2) patient education. In particular, patient education revolves around teaching survival skills (insulin injection, basic nutrition teaching, blood glucose monitoring) and helping to transition to an outpatient education program.

LABORATORY STUDY RESULTS

Test	Result on Admission	4 Hours Post-Admission	8 Hours Post-Admission
Serum glucose	450 mg/dL	250 mg/dL	60 mg/dL
Arterial pH/PO$_2$/PCO$_2$	7.1/105/22	7.2/100/35	7.4/100/38
Serum bicarbonate (HCO$_3$)	9 mEq/L	13 mEq/L	20 mEq/L
Serum Na$^+$	135 mEq/L	138 mEq/L	142 mEq/L
Serum K$^+$	5.3 mEq/L	5.0 mEq/L	4.8 mEq/L
Serum Cl$^-$	98 mEq/L	100 mEq/L	100 mEq/L
Serum acetone	1.16 dilutions	1.8 dilutions	Negative
Serum creatinine	1.4 mg/dL	1.2 mg/dL	—
Serum blood urea nitrogen (BUN)	25 mg/dL	20 mg/dL	—
Hemoglobin	17 g/dL	15 g/dL	14 g/dL
Hematocrit	47%	44%	42%
White blood count	15,000 cells/mm^3	10,000 cells/mm^3	5,000 cells/mm^3
Urine ketones	Large	Moderate	Negative
ECG	Normal sinus tachycardia	Normal sinus rhythm	Normal sinus rhythm
Stool (culture)	Negative		

CRITICAL THINKING QUESTIONS

1. What are the four major biochemical derangements in diabetic ketoacidosis?

2. What are the clinical signs and symptoms (as noted in this scenario) that are derived from these biochemical derangements?

3. How do nursing interventions for diabetic ketoacidosis (DKA) develop from identification of each of these derangements?

4. The patient in this scenario has mild to moderate DKA. How might clinical signs, symptoms, laboratory tests, and treatments differ if the patient had severe DKA?

5. What discharge plans would you anticipate for this patient?

Answers to Critical Thinking Questions appear in Appendix D.

NCLEX® REVIEW

1. The nurse recognizes the following is true regarding the prevalence of diabetes.
   1. The most common form is type 1.
   2. Approximately 20% of Americans over age 60 have diabetes.
   3. The lowest prevalence occurs among Native Americans.
   4. The highest incidence worldwide is in the United States population.

2. The nurse determines a patient has the criteria for pre-diabetes when the following are identified on assessment:
   1. The patient is 20 years old and requires therapy with oral hypoglycemic agents.
   2. The patient was diagnosed with gestational diabetes with her last pregnancy.
   3. Fasting blood sugar (FBS) level is 130 mg/dL.
   4. Glucose tolerance test shows normal blood sugar levels.

3. The nurse identifies the following patient to be most at risk to develop type 1 diabetes:
   1. The adolescent who had chronic bacterial ear infections as a child
   2. A school age child whose mother has type 1 diabetes
   3. A toddler with a monozygotic twin who has type 1 diabetes
   4. A pre-school age child with a dizygotic twin who has type 1 diabetes

4. The nurse recognizes the following assessment findings in a patient with type 2 diabetes are associated with the metabolic syndrome.
   1. Elevated triglycerides and HDL levels
   2. Abdominal obesity and decreased HDL level
   3. Elevated LDL level and hypertension
   4. Elevated blood sugar and decreased triglyceride level

5. A patient with type 1 diabetes is experiencing early signs of proliferative retinopathy. The nurse includes the following instructions for management and prevention of further complications.
   1. "Be sure to have a dilated eye examination every two years."
   2. "Avoid doing any isometric exercises."
   3. "Restrict protein in the diet to 10 grams a day."
   4. "Keep your blood sugar level less than 150 mg/dL."

6. The nurse incorporates the following interventions in the plan of care for a patient receiving a meglitinide oral hypoglycemic agent.
   1. Administer the medication with meals.
   2. Check for signs and symptoms of hyperglycemia one hour after the meal.
   3. Check for allergies to sulfa.
   4. Instruct patient to eat within 20 minutes of taking the medication.

7. The nurse should give the following instructions to a patient with Type 2 diabetes who takes oral hypoglycemic agents and is planning to begin an exercise program.

   1. "You will be at increased risk for hyperglycemia up to two hours after exercising."
   2. "Avoid eating anything before you start exercising."
   3. "Exercise may lower your blood sugar for several hours after completing the activity."
   4. "Eat only simple carbohydrates if you become hypoglycemic after exercising."

8. The nurse determines a patient is experiencing side effects of an alpha-glucosidase inhibitor when these symptoms are manifested sixty minutes after taking the medication.

   1. Abdominal bloating and diarrhea
   2. Elevated temperature
   3. Tremors and palpitations
   4. Fatigue

9. An elderly patient is seen in the emergency department. The family reports the patient has "diabetes" and has not eaten well for the past few days; the patient's blood sugar is 475 mg/dL. Which assessment finding would indicate the patient is experiencing diabetic ketoacidosis (DKA) rather than hyperosmolar hyperglycemic syndrome (HHS)?

   1. Face is flushed and red.
   2. Skin turgor is inelastic.
   3. Patient is lethargic and difficult to arouse.
   4. Blood pressure is 80/40.

10. The nurse recognizes which of the following patients with diabetes is most at risk to develop lower extremity ulcers and/or amputation.

   1. A male who was diagnosed with diabetes two years ago
   2. An elderly female who maintains her blood glucose between 100–140 mg/dL
   3. A male patient with chronic renal failure (CRF)
   4. A female patient who recently had a myocardial infarction (MI)

Answers for review questions appear in Appendix D

KEY TERMS

analog *p.1671*
continuous subcutaneous insulin infusion (CSII) *p.1674*
counterregulatory hormones *p.1662*
dawn phenomenon *p.1677*
Diabetes Control and Complications Trial (DCCT) *p.1663*
Diabetes Prevention Program (DPP) *p.1666*
diabetic ketoacidosis (DKA) *p.1663*
diabetic peripheral neuropathy (DPN) *p.1696*
gestational diabetes mellitus (GDM) *p.1660*
glucagon *p.1661*
gluconeogenesis *p.1662*
glycated serum proteins (GSPs) *p.1670*
glycogen *p.1661*
glycogenolysis *p.1662*
glycolysis *p.1661*

hemoglobin A_{1C} (Hb A_{1C}) test *p.1670*
honeymoon period *p.1665*
hyperglycemia *p.1659*
hyperosmolar hyperglycemic syndrome (HHS) *p.1663*
hypoglycemia *p.1663*
hypoglycemic unawareness *p.1690*
impaired fasting glucose (IFG) *p.1660*
impaired glucose tolerance (IGT) *p.1660*
incretin mimetics *p.1674*
insulin *p.1659*
insulin resistance *p.1662*
ketogenesis *p.1662*
latent autoimmune diabetes in adults (LADA) *p.1660*
lipolysis *p.1662*
macronutrients *p.1683*
macrovascular *p.1660*

maturity onset diabetes of the young (MODY) *p.1660*
medical nutrition therapy (MNT) *p.1683*
microalbuminuria *p.1663*
micronutrients *p.1683*
microvascular *p.1660*
molecular mimicry *p.1665*
normoglycemia *p.1671*
oral glucose tolerance test (OGTT) *p.1668*
osmotic diuresis *p.1667*
pancreatic beta cells *p.1659*
pancreatic polypeptide *p.1661*
pre-diabetes *p.1660*
Somogyi effect *p.1677*
type 1 diabetes mellitus *p.1659*
type 2 diabetes mellitus *p.1660*
United Kingdom Prospective Diabetes Study (UKPDS) *p.1671*

EXPLORE **PEARSON mynursingkit™**

MyNursingKit is your one stop for online chapter review materials and resources. Prepare for success with additional NCLEX®-style practice questions, interactive assignments and activities, web links, animations and videos, and more!

Register your access code from the front of your book at
www.mynursingkit.com

REFERENCES

Ahroni, J. H. (2003). Diabetic foot care and education. In M. J. Franz (Ed.), *Diabetes and complications* (5th ed., pp. 67–83). Chicago: American Association of Diabetes Educators.

Akerblom, H. K., Vaarala, O., Hyoty, H., Ilonen, J., & Knip, M. (2002). Environmental factors in the etiology of type 1 diabetes. *American Journal of Medical Genetics, 115*(1), 18–29.

Albert, L. J., & Inman, R. D. (1999). Molecular mimicry and autoimmunity. *New England Journal of Medicine, 341*(27), 2068–2074.

American Diabetes Association. (2001). *Diabetes: Vital statistics* (p. v). Alexandria, VA: Author.

American Diabetes Association. (2007). Nutrition recommendations and interventions for diabetes: A position statement of the American Diabetes Association. *Diabetes Care, 30*(Suppl. 1), S48–S65.

American Diabetes Association. (2008a). *Diabetes forecast resource guide.* Alexandria, VA: Author.

American Diabetes Association. (2008b). National standards for diabetes self-management education. *Diabetes Care, 31*(Suppl. 1), S97–S104.

American Diabetes Association. (2008c). Standards of medical care in diabetes—2008. *Diabetes Care, 31*(Suppl. 1), S12–S54.

American Diabetes Association. (2008d). *Total prevalence of diabetes and pre-diabetes.* Retrieved June 27, 2008, from http://www.diabetes.org/diabetes-statistics/prevalence.jsp

American Diabetes Association. (2008e). Standards of medical care in diabetes—2008. *Diabetes Care, 31*(Suppl. 1), S12–S54.

American Diabetes Association. (2008f). Total prevalence of diabetes and pre-diabetes. Retrieved June 27, 2008, from http://www.diabetes.org/diabetes-statistics/prevalence.jsp

Amylin Pharmaceuticals. (2007). *Product information.* Retrieved June 9, 2007, from http://www.amylin.com

Barr, R. G., Nathan, D. M., Meigs, J. B., & Singer, D. E. (2002). Tests of glycemia for the diagnosis of type 2 diabetes mellitus. *Annals of Internal Medicine, 137*(4), 263–272.

Bektas, F., Eray, O., Sari, R., & Akbas, H. (2004). Point of care blood ketone testing of diabetic patients in the emergency department. *Endocrine Research, 30*(3), 395–402.

Bobo, N., Evert, A., Gallivan, J., Imperatore, G., Kelly, J., Linder, B., et al. (2004). An update on type 2 diabetes in youth from the national diabetes education program. *Pediatrics, 114*(1), 259–263.

Bode, B. W. (Ed.). (2004). *Medical management of type 1 diabetes.* Alexandria, VA: American Diabetes Association.

Brown, A. F. (2004). Aetiology of cerebral oedema in diabetic ketoacidosis. *Emergency Medicine Journal, 21*(6), 754–755.

Burant, C. F., & American Diabetes Association. (2008). *Medical management of type 2 diabetes* (6th ed.). Alexandria, VA: American Diabetes Association.

Campbell, R. K., & White, J. R., Jr. (2000). *Medications for the treatment of diabetes.* Alexandria, VA: American Diabetes Association.

Capes, S. E., Hunt, D., Malmberg, K., Pathak, P., & Gerstein, H. C. (2001). Stress hyperglycemia and prognosis of stroke in nondiabetic and diabetic patients: A systematic overview. *Stroke, 32*(10), 2426–2432.

Centers for Disease Control and Prevention. (2004). Prevalence of visual impairment and selected eye diseases among persons aged >/=50 years with and without diabetes—United States, 2002 *Morbidity and Mortality Weekly Report, 53*(45), 1069–1071.

Centers for Disease Control and Prevention. (2005). *National diabetes fact sheet: General information and national estimates on diabetes in the United States, 2005.* Retrieved from http://www.cdc.gov/diabetes/pubs/factsheet05.htm

Dahlquist, G. G. (1997). Viruses and other perinatal exposures as initiating events for beta-cell destruction. *Annals of Medicine, 29*(5), 413–417.

DCCT Trial Research Group. (1993). The effect of intensive treatment of diabetes on the development and progression of long-term complications in insulin-dependent diabetes mellitus. *New England Journal of Medicine, 329*(14), 977–986.

DeFronzo, R. A. (2004). Pathogenesis of type 2 diabetes mellitus. *Medical Clinics of North America, 88*(4), 787–835, ix.

Devlin, J. T., Hirshman, M., Horton, E. D., & Horton, E. S. (1987). Enhanced peripheral and splanchnic insulin sensitivity in NIDDM men after single bout of exercise. *Diabetes, 36*(4), 434–439.

Dunger, D. B., Sperling, M. A., Acerini, C. L., Bohn, D. J., Daneman, D., Danne, T. P., et al. (2004). ESPE/LWPES consensus statement on diabetic ketoacidosis in children and adolescents. *Archives of Disease in Childhood, 89*(2), 188–194.

Evert, A. B., Hess-Fischl, A., & American Dietetic Association. (2006). *Pediatric diabetes: Health care reference and client education handouts.* Chicago, IL: American Dietetic Association.

Fagot-Campagna, A., Pettitt, D. J., Engelgau, M. M., Burrows, N. R., Geiss, L. S., Valdez, R., et al. (2000). Type 2 diabetes among North American children and adolescents: An epidemiologic review and a public health perspective. *Journal of Pediatrics, 136*(5), 664–672.

Fairview Health Services. (2003). *Guide to carbohydrate counting: A simple meal-planning method for people with diabetes* (3rd ed.). Minneapolis: Fairview Publications.

Fleury-Milfort, E. (2004). Diabetes self-management education. In A. P. Harmel & R. Matchur (Eds.), *Davidson's diabetes mellitus: Diagnosis and treatment.* Philadelphia: W. B. Saunders.

Ford, E. S., & Giles, W. H. (2003). A comparison of the prevalence of the metabolic syndrome using two proposed definitions. *Diabetes Care, 26*(3), 575–581.

Funk, J. (2003). Pathophysiology of disease: An introduction to clinical medicine. In S. McPhee, V. Lingappa, & W. Ganong (Eds.), *Disorders of the endocrine pancreas.* New York: McGraw-Hill.

Furnary, A. P., Wu, Y., & Bookin, S. O. (2004). Effect of hyperglycemia and continuous intravenous insulin infusions on outcomes of cardiac surgical procedures: The Portland diabetic project. *Endocrinology Practice, 10*(Suppl. 2), 21–33.

Garber, A. J., Seidel, J., & Armbruster, M. (2004). Current standards of care for inpatient glycemic management and metabolic control: Is it time for definite standards and targets? *Endocrinology Practice, 10*(Suppl. 2), 10–12.

Gardner, L. I., Jr., Stern, M. P., Haffner, S. M., Gaskill, S. P., Hazuda, H. P., Relethford, J. H., et al. (1984). Prevalence of diabetes in Mexican Americans. Relationship to percent of gene pool derived from Native American sources. *Diabetes, 33*(1), 86–92.

Gerstein, H. C. (1994). Cow's milk exposure and type I diabetes mellitus. A critical overview of the clinical literature. *Diabetes Care, 17*(1), 13–19.

Gilden, J. L. (1999). Nutrition and the older diabetic. *Clinics in Geriatric Medicine, 15*(2), 371–390.

Goldstein, D. E., Little, R. R., Lorenz, R. A., Malone, J. I., Nathan, D., Peterson, C. M., et al. (2004). Tests of glycemia in diabetes. *Diabetes Care, 27*(7), 1761–1773.

Gregg, E. W., Cadwell, B. L., Cheng, Y. J., Cowie, C. C., Williams, D. E., Geiss, L., et al. (2004). Trends in the prevalence and ratio of diagnosed to undiagnosed diabetes according to obesity levels in the U.S. *Diabetes Care, 27*(12), 2806–2812.

Gutierrez, K. (2008). *Pharmacotherapeutics: Clinical reasoning in primary care* (2nd ed.). St. Louis: W. B. Saunders.

Haffner, S. M. (1997). Impaired glucose tolerance, insulin resistance and cardiovascular disease. *Diabetic Medicine, 14*(Suppl. 3), S12–S18.

Hale, P. M., Rezvani, I., Braunstein, A. W., Lipman, T. H., Martinez, N., & Garibaldi, L. (1997). Factors predicting cerebral edema in young children with diabetic ketoacidosis and new onset type I diabetes. *Acta Paediatrica, 86*(6), 626–631.

Harmel, A. P., Mathur, R., & Davidson, M. B. (2004). *Davidson's diabetes mellitus: Diagnosis and treatment* (5th ed.). Philadelphia: W. B. Saunders.

Harris, M. I. (2001). Racial and ethnic differences in health care access and health outcomes for adults with type 2 diabetes. *Diabetes Care, 24*(3), 454–459.

Helmrich, S. P., Ragland, D. R., Leung, R. W., & Paffenbarger, R. S., Jr. (1991). Physical activity and reduced occurrence of non-insulin-dependent diabetes mellitus. *New England Journal of Medicine, 325*(3), 147–152.

Hu, F. B., Manson, J. E., Stampfer, M. J., Colditz, G., Liu, S., Solomon, C. G., et al. (2001). Diet, lifestyle, and the risk of type 2 diabetes mellitus in women. *New England Journal of Medicine, 345*(11), 790–797.

Hussain, A. N., & Vincent, M. T. (2007). *Diabetes mellitus, type* Retrieved July 1, 2008, from http://www.emedicine.com/MED/topic546.htm

International Diabetes Federation. (2006). *Diabetes atlas* (3rd ed.). Brussels, Belgium: International Diabetes Federation.

Joslin, E. P., & Kahn, C. R. (2005). In C. Ronald Kahn et al. (Eds.), *Joslin's diabetes mellitus* (14th ed.). Philadelphia: Lippincott Williams & Wilkins.

Kaufman, F., & American Diabetes Association. (2008). *Medical management of type 1 diabetes* (5th ed.). Alexandria, VA: American Diabetes Association.

Kaufman, F. R. (2002). Type 2 diabetes mellitus in children and youth: A new epidemic. *Journal of Pediatric Endocrinology and Metabolism 15*(Suppl. 2), 737–744.

Knip, M. (2003). Cow's milk and the new trials for prevention of type 1 diabetes. *Journal of Endocrinological Investigation, 26*(3), 265–267.

Knowler, W. C., Barrett-Connor, E., Fowler, S. E., Hamman, R. F., Lachin, J. M., Walker, E. A., et al. (2002). Reduction in the incidence of type 2 diabetes with lifestyle intervention or metformin. *New England Journal of Medicine, 346*(6), 393–403.

Krentz, A. J., & Bailey, C. J. (2005). Oral antidiabetic agents: Current role in type 2 diabetes mellitus. *Drugs, 65*(3), 385–411.

Lammi, N., Karvonen, M., & Tuomilehto, J. (2005). Do microbes have a causal role in type 1 diabetes? *Medical Science Monitor, 11*(3), RA63–69.

Lebovitz, H. E., & American Diabetes Association. (2004). *Therapy for diabetes mellitus and related disorders* (4th ed.). Alexandria, VA: American Diabetes Association.

Lee, E. T., Howard, B. V., Savage, P. J., Cowan, L. D., Fabsitz, R. R., Oopik, A. J., et al. (1995). Diabetes and impaired glucose tolerance in three American Indian populations aged 45–74 years. The strong heart study. *Diabetes Care, 18*(5), 599–610.

Ligaray, K. P. L., & Isley, W. O. (2007). *Diabetes mellitus, type 2.* Retrieved July 1, 2008, from http://www.emedicine.com/med/topic547.htm

Lioupis, C. (2005). Effects of diabetes mellitus on wound healing: An update. *Journal of Wound Care, 14*(2), 84–86.

Malecki, M. T., & Klupa, T. (2005). Type 2 diabetes mellitus: From genes to disease. *Pharmacologic Reports, 57*(Suppl.), 20–32.

Malmberg, K. (2004). Role of insulin-glucose infusion in outcomes after acute myocardial infarction: The diabetes and insulin-glucose infusion in acute myocardial infarction (DIGAMI) study. *Endocrinology Practice, 10*(Suppl. 2), 13–16.

Manson, J. E., Nathan, D. M., Krolewski, A. S., Stampfer, M. J., Willett, W. C., & Hennekens, C. H. (1992). A prospective study of exercise and incidence of diabetes among U.S. male physicians. *Journal of the American Medical Association, 268*(1), 63–67.

Manson, J. E., Rimm, E. B., Stampfer, M. J., Colditz, G. A., Willett, W. C., Krolewski, A. S., et al. (1991). Physical activity and incidence of non-insulin-dependent diabetes mellitus in women. *Lancet, 338*(8770), 774–778.

Mayfield, J. A., Reiber, G. E., Sanders, L. J., Janisse, D., & Pogach, L. M. (2004). Preventive foot care in diabetes. *Diabetes Care, 27*(Suppl. 1), S63–S64.

McCarren, M., & American Diabetes Association. (2007). *American Diabetes Association guide to insulin and type 2 diabetes.* Alexandria, VA: American Diabetes Association.

McFarland, K. F., Catalano, E. W., Day, J. F., Thorpe, S. R., & Baynes, J. W. (1979). Nonenzymatic glucosylation of serum proteins in diabetes mellitus. *Diabetes, 28*(11), 1011–1014.

McMahon, M. M., & Rizza, R. A. (1996). Nutrition support in hospitalized patients with diabetes mellitus. *Mayo Clinic Proceedings, 71*(6), 587–594.

McPherson, R. A., Pincus, M. R., & Henry, J. B. (2007). *Henry's clinical diagnosis and management by laboratory methods* (21st ed.). Philadelphia: W. B. Saunders.

Moghissi, E. S., & Hirsch, I. B. (2005). Hospital management of diabetes. *Endocrinology Metabolism Clinics of North America, 34*(1), 99–116.

Muir, A., Schatz, D. A., & Maclaren, N. K. (1992). The pathogenesis, prediction, and prevention of insulin-dependent diabetes mellitus. *Endocrinology Metabolism Clinics of North America, 21*(2), 199–219.

Narayan, K. M., Boyle, J. P., Thompson, T. J., Sorensen, S. W., & Williamson, D. F. (2003). Lifetime risk for diabetes mellitus in the United States. *Journal of the American Medical Association, 290*(14), 1884–1890.

National Center for Chronic Disease Prevention and Health Promotion. (2004). *Data and trends: National diabetes surveillance system: Mortality due to diabetic ketoacidosis.* Retrieved June 9, 2007, from http://www.cdc.gov/diabetes/statistics/mortalitydka/source.htm

Newman, B., Selby, J. V., King, M. C., Slemenda, C., Fabsitz, R., & Friedman, G. D. (1987). Concordance for type 2 (non-insulin-dependent) diabetes mellitus in male twins. *Diabetologia, 30*(10), 763–768.

Nugent, B. W. (2005). Hyperosmolar hyperglycemic state. *Emergency Medical Clinics of North America, 23*, 629–648.

Porth, C. M. (2007). *Essentials of pathophysiology: Concepts of altered health states.* Philadelphia: Lippincott Williams & Wilkins.

Pozzilli, P., & Di Mario, U. (2001). Autoimmune diabetes not requiring insulin at diagnosis (latent autoimmune diabetes of the adult): Definition, characterization, and potential prevention. *Diabetes Care, 24*(8), 1460–1467.

Rich-Edwards, J. W., Colditz, G. A., Stampfer, M. J., Willett, W. C., Gillman, M. W., Hennekens, C. H., et al. (1999). Birth weight and the risk for type 2 diabetes mellitus in adult women. *Annals of Internal Medicine, 130*(4, Part 1), 278–284.

Riddle, M. C. (1999). Oral pharmacologic management of type 2 diabetes. *American Family Physician, 60*(9), 2613–2620.

Rosenbloom, A. L., House, D. V., & Winter, W. E. (1998). Non-insulin dependent diabetes mellitus (NIDDM) in minority youth: Research priorities and needs. *Clinical Pediatrics (Philadelphia), 37*(2), 143–152.

Rosenbloom, A. L., Joe, J. R., Young, R. S., & Winter, W. E. (1999). Emerging epidemic of type 2 diabetes in youth. *Diabetes Care, 22*(2), 345–354.

Rucker, D. W. (2008). *Diabetic ketoacidosis.* Retrieved July 1, 2008, from http://www.emedicine.com/emerg/topic135.htm

Sheehan, J. P. (2004). Fasting hyperglycemia: Etiology, diagnosis, and treatment. *Diabetes Technology and Therapeutics, 6*(4), 525–533.

So, W. Y., Ng, M. C., Lee, S. C., Sanke, T., Lee, H. K., & Chan, J. C. (2000). Genetics of type 2 diabetes mellitus. *Hong Kong Medical Journal, 6*(1), 69–76.

Tattersall, R. (1998). Maturity-onset diabetes of the young: A clinical history. *Diabetic Medicine, 15*(1), 11–14.

Tuomilehto, J., Lindstrom, J., Eriksson, J. G., Valle, T. T., Hamalainen, H., Ilanne-Parikka, P., et al. (2001). Prevention of type 2 diabetes mellitus by changes in lifestyle among subjects with impaired glucose tolerance. *New England Journal of Medicine, 344*(18), 1343–1350.

U.K. Prospective Diabetes Study Group. (1998a). Effect of intensive blood-glucose control with metformin on complications in overweight patients with type 2 diabetes (UKPDS 34). *Lancet, 352*(9131), 854–865.

U.K. Prospective Diabetes Study Group. (1998b). Tight blood pressure control and risk of macrovascular and microvascular complications in type 2 diabetes (UKPDS 38). *British Medical Journal, 317*(7160), 703–713.

Umpierrez, G. E., Isaacs, S. D., Bazargan, N., You, X., Thaler, L. M., & Kitabchi, A. E. (2002). Hyperglycemia: An independent marker of in-hospital mortality in patients with undiagnosed diabetes. *Journal of Clinical Endocrinology and Metabolism, 87*(3), 978–982.

Umpierrez, G. E., & Kitabchi, A. E. (2003). Diabetic ketoacidosis: Risk factors and management strategies. *Treatments in Endocrinology, 2*(2), 95–108.

Valencia, M. E., Bennett, P. H., Ravussin, E., Esparza, J., Fox, C., & Schulz, L. O. (1999). The Pima Indians in Sonora, Mexico. *Nutrition Reviews, 57*(5, Part 2), S55–S57; discussion S57–S58.

Van den Berghe, G., & Bouillon, R. (2004). Optimal control of glycemia among critically ill patients. *Journal of the American Medical Association, 291*(10), 1198–1199.

Velho, G., & Robert, J. J. (2002). Maturity-onset diabetes of the young (MODY): Genetic and clinical characteristics. *Hormone Research, 57*(Suppl. 1), 29–33.

Wild, S., Roglic, G., Green, A., Sicree, R., & King, H. (2004). Global prevalence of diabetes: Estimates for the year 2000 and projections for 2030. *Diabetes Care, 27*(5), 1047–1053.

Yeh, G. Y., Eisenberg, D. M., Kaptchuk, T. J., & Phillips, R. S. (2003). Systematic review of herbs and dietary supplements for glycemic control in diabetes. *Diabetes Care, 26*(4), 1277–1294.

Young, R. S., & Rosenbloom, A. L. (1998). type 2 (non-insulin dependent) diabetes in minority youth: Conference report. *Clinical Pediatrics (Philadelphia), 37*(2), 63–65.

Zinman, B., Ruderman, N., Campaigne, B. N., Devlin, J. T., & Schneider, S. H. (2004). Physical activity/exercise and diabetes. *Diabetes Care, 27*(Suppl. 1), S58–S62.

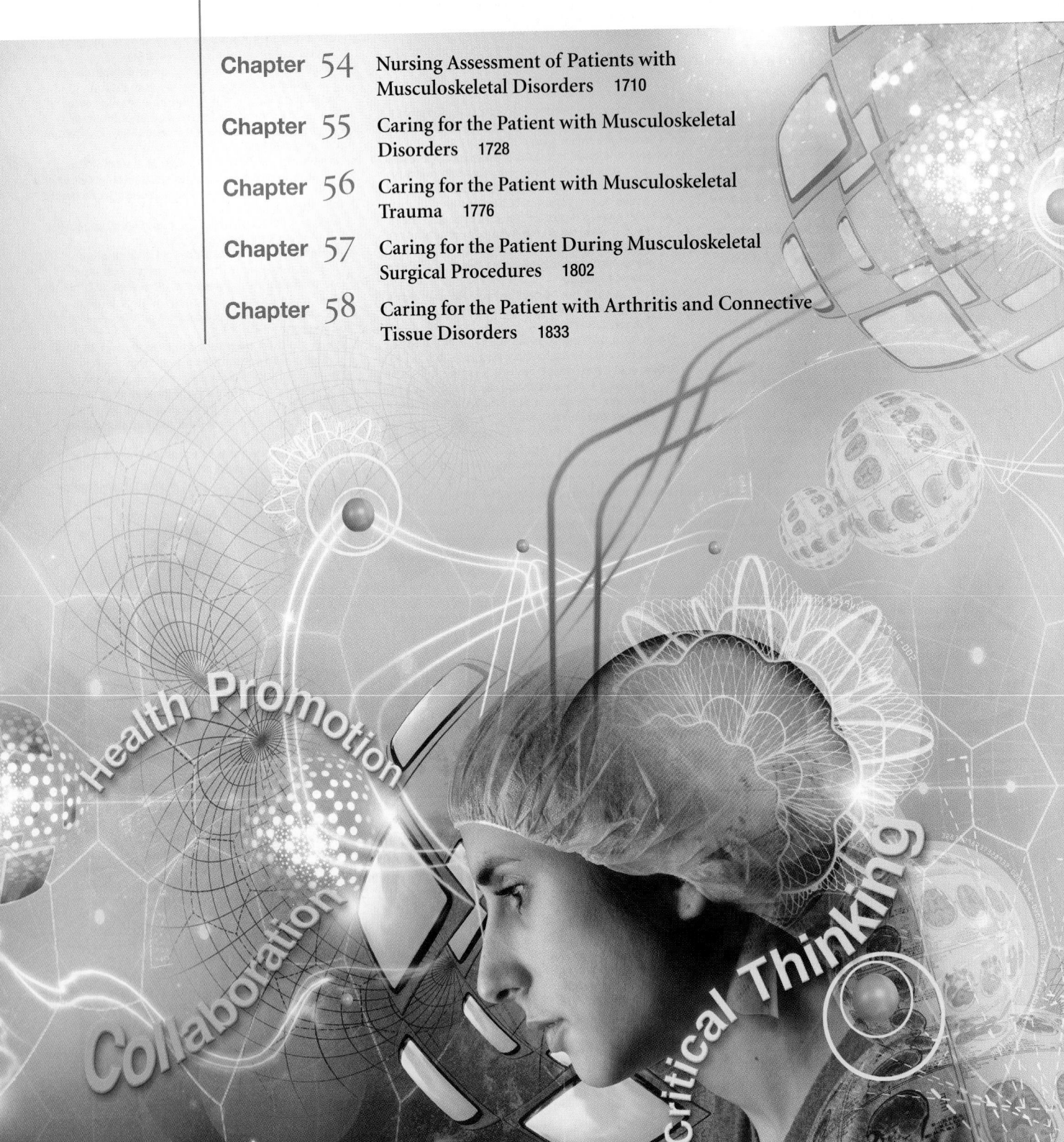

UNIT 12

Nursing Management of Patients with Musculoskeletal Disorders

Health Promotion

Collaboration

Critical Thinking

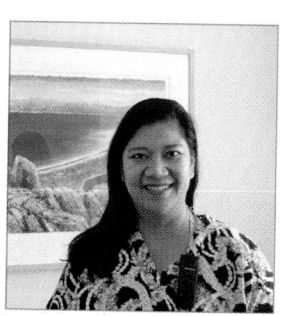

MELISA   My name is Melisa Agustin Jager and I am a clinical resource nurse for a 36-bed orthopedic unit at a Level 1 trauma center that facilitates care to patients in the quickly growing area of Northern California. The orthopedic unit population encompasses the range of orthopedic/trauma practice. The orthopedic nursing staff provides wide-ranging types of care to patients having routine and scheduled orthopedic knee, hip, and spine surgeries to the traumatic injuries, including multiple fractures, sustained from motor vehicle crashes.

As a clinical resource nurse on the unit, I engage in a multitude of key practices including these: assisting with the implementation of quality assurance and problem-solving techniques to help employees meet their professional goals; providing methodology for the technological advances and equipment we use during our daily orthopedic practices, including devices to improve range of motion and the intricacy of fixators and tractions; arranging routine in-service programs for staff that will impart shared knowledge so staff can keep up with the ever-changing dynamics of medicine; and encouraging collaborative care by achieving interpersonal communication with ancillary staff such as the physical/occupational therapist in order to receive guidance regarding safe mobility transfers and developing a plan with the pain pharmacist for the orthopedic patient to achieve comfort during his hospital stay.

A day in the life of an orthopedic nurse has the instrumental characteristics of caring. **Compassion** should be common practice in your nursing care. One example is to speak to patients with soft and empathetic tones—as you would speak to a loved one. Compassionate nursing goes beyond the mere implementation of medical techniques/practices; it involves providing a positive, interactive environment in which rapport and trust develop between nurse and patient. Particularly in orthopedic nursing, the patient who is immobile and not able to care for herself often looks to the nurses for strength and hope.

Resource nurses are leaders who have had significant experience and **competence** in the implementation of orthopedic procedures. Being competent when providing direct care for a patient with posterior hip precautions is distinctly different than anterior precautions to prevent dislodging the hip. Often as a resource nurse, I act as a mentor for less experienced nurses by demonstrating the appropriate techniques involved in caring for patients with specialized needs.

As a resource nurse it is important for me to show **confidence** when speaking with patients and their families. Patients and their families trust a confident/assertive nurse rather than a nurse who cannot articulate a clear plan of care or is not able to explain a procedure effectively.

When caring for a patient, if something is not ethically right, I act with **conscience** and provide tactful advocacy. I facilitate calling a care conference with the health care team, ancillary staff, and family. With long-term patients on the orthopedic unit in particular, a conference facilitates updating the plan of care and provides optimal health services. Our population is culturally diverse so it is important to be culturally sensitive and acknowledge the patient's beliefs.

It is important for me to show pride and **commitment** to my profession. I demonstrate my commitment with a positive attitude when stress is high on the unit. It is important to boost morale and commitment to team building when another person exhibits toxic behavior. On the orthopedic unit critical thinking skills are lifesaving attributes. If a nurse on our unit does not recognize the signs and symptoms of compartment syndrome, the patient is at great risk of loss of circulation to that limb, leading to amputation.

At this hospital, the hallmark is its teaching environment. Clinical resource nurses are motivated to instill proactiveness and commitment and to develop a sense of autonomy in order to achieve a higher standard of proficiencies among the employees and most importantly to incorporate excellence in patient care.

> "Compassionate nursing goes beyond the mere implementation of medical techniques/practices; it involves providing a positive, interactive environment in which rapport and trust develop between nurse and patient."

54

Nursing Assessment of Patients with Musculoskeletal Disorders

Helene Harris

Outcome-Based Learning Objectives

After studying this chapter, the learner will be able to:

1. Identify basic anatomy and physiology of the musculoskeletal system.

2. Analyze the process of obtaining a history on the musculoskeletal system.

3. Identify the general guidelines required for a musculoskeletal examination.

4. Identify the process of assessment of the following structures: temporomandibular joint, shoulders, elbows, wrists, hands, fingers, neck, spine, hips, knees, ankles, and feet, as well as assessment of gait.

5. Compare and contrast normal and abnormal findings associated with the temporomandibular joint, shoulders, elbows, wrists, hands, fingers, neck, spine, hips, knees, ankles, feet, and gait.

6. Compare and contrast the normal and abnormal range of motion for the temporomandibular joint, shoulders, elbows, wrists, hands, fingers, neck, spine, hips, knees, ankles, feet, and gait.

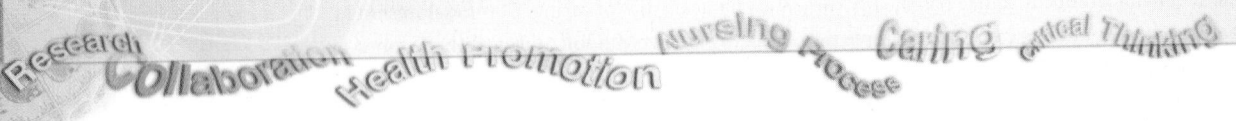

THE MUSCULOSKELETAL system is composed of bones, joints, ligaments, tendons, and cartilage. Each one of these parts plays a key role in the maintenance of a healthy, functioning system. The musculoskeletal system plays a definitive role in determining a person's quality of life because it not only allows movement but also protects inner organs, produces red blood cells, and supports the body.

People in every age group at some time in their lives may be afflicted with either temporary or permanent disabilities related to musculoskeletal problems. Injuries can occur in all stages of life, but children are particularly prone to accidents, and the elderly are inclined to succumb to falls and subsequent fractures. In a study by Lillicrap, Byrne, and Speed (2003), it was noted that out of 100 patients hospitalized for reasons other than orthopedic problems, 63% of them had some degree of musculoskeletal dysfunction.

Anatomy and Physiology of the Musculoskeletal System

Because of the importance of the musculoskeletal system, and the number of patients with primary or secondary orthopedic problems, it is imperative for the nurse to understand how to conduct a musculoskeletal assessment. Each component of the musculoskeletal system must undergo a thorough and systematic evaluation to identify abnormalities so that they can be treated or so further problems can be prevented.

Bones

Bones are composed of collagen fibers, which, in turn, are made up of calcium and phosphate. The human skeleton is constructed of 206 separate bones that have the ability to change structure according to their current function. The skeletal system develops from the middle layer of embryonic tissue. Development begins at approximately the fourth week in the embryo and continues to grow during the first two decades of life. Bones also have the ability to repair themselves after injury through a process of resorption and regeneration. The process involves formation of a hematoma that provides the basis for blood vessel and fibroblast infiltration, proliferation of osteoblasts, callus formation, ossification of the callus, and remodeling of the fracture site. The bone is made up of osteoblasts, which are cells that form the bone itself, and osteoclasts, which are cells that reabsorb bone during repair, for instance, of a fracture (Porth, 2007).

Bones in the human body can be classified into three types: (1) long bones, which have a tubular shaft and articular surfaces, or surfaces that form a joint, at each end; (2) flat bones, which are thin with broad surfaces; and (3) short or irregular bones that vary in size and shape (Bickley, 2003). Chart 54–1 provides examples of the three types of bones.

The functions of bone are many: They provide support for the body; protect internal organs from injury; store calcium, phosphorus, and other minerals; provide for movement in conjunction with muscles; and, in long bones, produce red and white blood cells (Porth, 2007).

Muscles

Muscles are contractile tissues that are attached by tendons to bone and other body parts. They are found in three types throughout the body.

Smooth muscle is stimulated by the autonomic nervous system, meaning it is not under voluntary, or conscious, control. Smooth muscle is found in the skin, internal organs, reproductive system, major blood vessels, and the excretory system. These muscles contract when needed to perform the function of the particular organ system, such as peristalsis. Skeletal, or striated, muscles are called voluntary muscles because they are under conscious control and are supplied with nerves from the central nervous system.

Skeletal muscles are connected to bones via tendons. The skeletal muscles, together with the bones they attach to, allow the body to move, such as in walking or picking objects up with the fingers.

Cardiac muscle, comprising most of the heart, is under autonomic system control and not voluntary control. Like the skeletal muscle, cardiac muscle is striated and contains actin and myosin filaments. The filaments are smaller and more compact than skeletal muscle cells and contain many large mitochondria due to the continuous energy needs. The contractions of the cardiac muscle provide the heartbeat and the pumping of blood through the heart (Porth, 2007).

Cartilage

Cartilage is an elastic, flexible connective tissue. The main function of cartilage is as a "cushioner." It covers the surfaces of joints, protecting them when sliding or moving over one another and thus preventing damage and friction to the joints. For instance, costal cartilages join the ribs to the sternum and vertebrae. The articular cartilages, such as those in the shoulder or hip joint, protect the bone ends and allow easy movement of the joint. Once damaged, cartilage cannot be repaired (Weber & Kelley, 2007).

Ligaments

Ligaments play a crucial role in the function of the skeletal joints in that they bind the ends of different bones together, preventing **dislocations** (displacement of a bone from its normal position). An example is the knee joint connecting the femur with the patella, tibia, and fibula (Bickley, 2003) (Figure 54–1 ■).

Tendons

Tendons connect muscle to bone. The dense tissue is composed largely of intercellular bundles of collagen fibers arranged in the same direction. This provides great tensile strength and can withstand tremendous pull in the direction of fiber alignment. If the musculotendinous unit is stretched to injury, it is called a strain. The most common sites for strains are the lower back and the cervical area of the spine (Porth, 2007).

Joints

A joint is where two or more bones meet or come together. Joints are responsible for a person's **range of motion (ROM)**, or extent and type of movement. In assessing joints it is important to understand and differentiate between three different mechanical configurations of joints: spheroidal joints, hinge joints, and condylar joints. *Spheroidal joints* are located in the shoulders and hip. They have a ball-and-socket contour, which allows for a broad range of motion—not just in a back-and-forth direction, but also swiveling actions. *Hinge* joints are flat and slightly curved. The hinge joint allows movement in only one axis, namely, flexion and extension, as in the elbow. Examples of *condylar joints* include the knee, where the articulating ends of the bones are not connected directly but are linked by a strong fibrous capsule that surrounds the joint and is continuous with the periosteum. There is also additional support from ligaments that extend between the bones of the joint (Bickley, 2003; Weber & Kelley, 2007). Figure 54–2 ■ (p. 1712) illustrates the three

CHART 54–1	Types of Bones	
Long Bones	**Flat Bones**	**Short/Irregular Bones**
Femur	Ribs	Vertebral column
Tibia	Scapula	Carpal
Fibula	Sternum	Tarsal
Humerus	Ilium	
Radius		
Ulna		
Clavicle		
Metacarpals		
Metatarsals		
Phalanges		

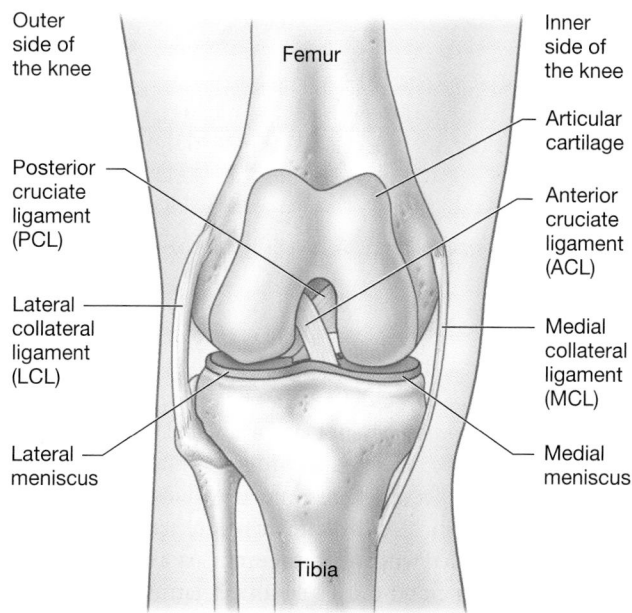

FIGURE 54–1 ■ Ligaments of the knee joint.

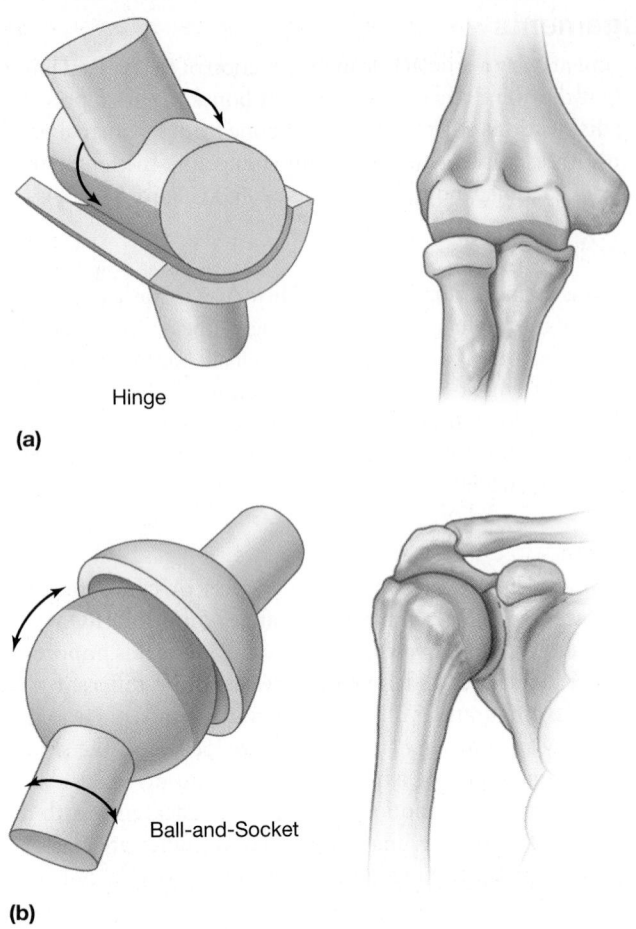

Hinge

(a)

Ball-and-Socket

(b)

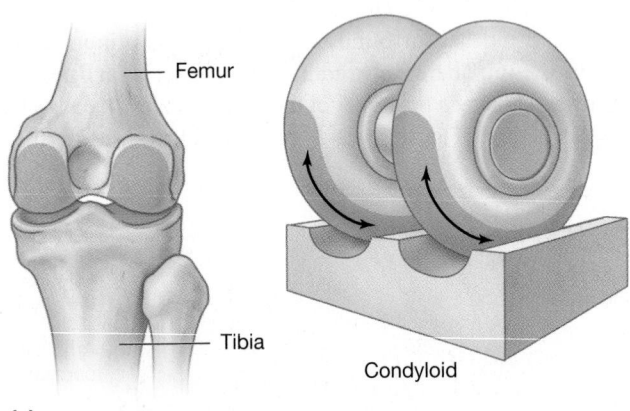

Femur

Tibia

Condyloid

(c)

FIGURE 54–2 ■ Types of joints: (A) hinge; (B) ball-and-socket; (C) condyloid.

CHART 54–2	Vocabulary of Range of Motion
Abduction	Moving an extremity away from the midline of the body
Adduction	Moving an extremity toward the midline of the body
Circumduction	Moving an extremity in a circular motion
Extension	Straightening the extremity of a joint; increasing the angle of the joint
Hyperextension	Moving a joint beyond its normal range
Flexion	Bending an extremity at a joint; decreases the angle of the joint
Eversion	Moving the foot outward
Inversion	Moving the foot inward
Pronation	Facing downward
Supination	Facing upward
Plantar flexion	Placing the foot downward
Dorsal flexion	Placing the foot upward
External rotation	Turning away from the midline of the body
Internal rotation	Turning toward the midline of the body

Sources: Adapted from Kozier, B., Erb, C., Berman, A., & Snyder, S. (2008). *Fundamentals of nursing. Concepts, process and practice* (8th ed.). Upper Saddle River, NJ: Pearson Prentice Hall; Magee, D. (2008). *Orthopedic physical assessment* (5th ed.). Elsevier; Weber, J., & Kelley, J. (2007). *Health assessment in nursing* (3rd ed.). Philadelphia: Lippincott Williams & Wilkins.

slide over one another, such as the knee. The bone surfaces of these joints are covered with cartilage, which allows the two bones to slide over one another and be freely movable. The bones of the joint are separated by a synovial capsule, which surrounds the joint and secretes synovial fluid, a lubricant that also promotes the sliding movement of the bones.

A further aid to movement in the synovial joints is the **bursae** (sacs containing viscous lubricating fluid; singular, *bursa*), which lie between the skin and surface of the bone or joint, contain synovial fluid, and are located in areas where tendons, muscles, and bones have the tendency to rub against one another, such as the acromion process in the shoulder, wrists, knees, hips, and ankles. *Cartilaginous joints* are only slightly movable and are located between the vertebrae and the symphysis pubis. They are separated by a fibrous disk and joined by interosseous ligaments (Bickley, 2003; Weber & Kelley, 2007).

History

The nursing assessment of a patient presenting with a musculoskeletal complaint should start with a thorough history and physical assessment of the musculoskeletal system. A detailed history of the system is vital in determining a patient's ability to function and perform activities of daily living (ADLs). In turn, this determination plays an important role in developing an effective plan of care, because disabilities related to musculoskeletal disorders can affect every aspect of a patient's life.

In gathering subjective data, the nurse should ask the patient a series of open-ended questions regarding past and present mus-

types of joints. Chart 54–2 defines the vocabulary used when describing the type of movement being evaluated.

Joints can also be classified according to material composition. *Fibrous joints* occur where bones are joined together with connective tissue, such as the sutures of the skull. There is no movement associated with a fibrous joint. *Synovial joints* are the most common type and most relevant in terms of injury and loss of range of motion. The synovial joints are the joints between bones that do not come in contact with one another but culoskeletal illnesses, injuries, related diagnostic procedures, surgeries, and treatments. The questioning should start with the chief complaint, or the symptom or condition that has compelled the patient to seek medical care. These questions should be formulated to allow the patient to describe her own impressions of the condition. Next, the past medical history of the patient is important because previous musculoskeletal injuries or disorders can have lingering effects on the neurological system, leading to new conditions. Chronic health conditions can also have a profound effect on the musculoskeletal system, and questions that reveal these disorders will help in the diagnosis of the presenting symptom. Social history and psychosocial history add to the fullness of the patient's medical history by revealing lifestyle habits, such as smoking or level of exercise, and coping mechanisms that can be important both in diagnosis and in treatment of the condition.

History taking is an important part of assessment. During this time the nurse establishes a caring relationship with the patient. It is important to let the patient describe his issues in his own words. Keep an open mind and listen carefully as this information will direct your clarifying questions.

Biographical and Demographic History

Biographical data should include age, gender, culture, and educational background. This information will assist the nurse in narrowing the questions, thinking of potential causes of the problem, and formulating how to pose questions and educational plans to meet the patient's needs. Demographic data may be helpful in determining causes of injury. For instance, if the patient has a job where she is sitting and typing on a computer all day, she may complain of back and neck pain from sitting in a chair that does not support her back, or pain in the joints of the hand, wrist, or arm from the repetitive motion during typing or improper height of the desk placing strain on the joints.

Cultural Considerations

It is important to take into consideration the patient's cultural background and conversational norms. Refer to Chapter 9 ⊙ for a more detailed discussion on cultural norms. Ask the patient if he has used any healing herbs or other alternative treatments such as acupuncture.

Chief Complaint

Characteristics, length of duration, exacerbation or diminishment of symptoms, and what is wrong or feared by the patient helps to define the chief complaint. Ask the patient open-ended questions. Allow her time to answer fully, giving encouragement with nonverbal cues such as nodding your head. Clarifying questions that may be useful include the following:

- What brings you to the facility/office/hospital today?
- How long have you had this symptom?
- When did it start?
- What have you done to alleviate it?
- What makes it better? What makes it worse?
- How has it affected your lifestyle?
- Has the symptom gotten worse since it first started? In what way has it gotten worse? When did it get worse? Did anything precipitate it getting worse? If so, what?

- Is pain associated with the symptom? If the patient answers "yes," ask this follow-up question: Are you experiencing any pain associated with the symptom?
- Where is the pain?
- Does it radiate anywhere?
- How long does it last?
- Have you taken any medication for the pain? What have you taken? How much? How often? Does the medication alleviate the pain? Does it reduce the intensity of the pain?
- How does the pain affect your daily lifestyle?
- What other treatments besides pain medication have you used?
- Do you have any other symptoms? Swelling? Can you describe the type of weakness?

Past Medical History

When obtaining a past medical history, the patient may be asked the following questions:

- Have you had any past surgeries? Where? When? For what reason?
- Do you have any permanent problems associated with past injuries or surgeries?
- Do you know if you have any other health problems that may affect medication therapy, or, due to respiratory problems or fatigue, inhibit ambulation or performance of ADLs ?
- Do you have diabetes? Sickle cell anemia? Systemic lupus erythematosus (SLE)? These are important questions because diabetes can cause neuropathies that can affect ambulation, and sickle cell anemia and SLE can lead to osteoporosis and osteomyelitis (Weber & Kelley, 2007).
- Does anyone in your family have rheumatoid arthritis or osteoporosis? These diseases tend to be hereditary and may predispose a patient to these conditions (Weber & Kelley, 2007).
- Have you had a tetanus or polio vaccine recently? Recent tetanus and polio vaccines may cause joint stiffness. If the patient has never had a polio vaccination, ask if he has traveled to a third world country recently; if so, the patient may have contracted the disease at that time.
- What medications do you take regularly? Include all over-the-counter (OTC) medications.
- Do you have any allergies? If so, to what? (Be specific: medications, environmental.)
- *If the patient is female:* Have you started menopause? Are you on hormone replacement therapy? The lack of estrogen in a menopausal woman can lead to osteoporosis.

A social history provides additional information about the patient's lifestyle that may affect the potential disorder or complaint. The nurse should consider the following questions:

- Do you smoke? If so, how much and how often? Smoking raises the risk of osteoporosis.
- Do you drink alcohol? If so, how much? Excessive alcohol intake raises the risk of osteoporosis.

- Do you have a regular exercise regime? Can you describe it? Do you engage in exercise outside of a routine? How often? What type of exercise?
- Please describe your occupation. Does it involve heavy lifting, pushing, or pulling, or do you sit at a desk all day? Heavy strenuous activities may precipitate back problems, while sitting may lead to posture anomalies, which can lead to other problems such as respiratory disorders.
- Do you use an **assistive device** such as a cane, walker, or brace? If so, which do you use? Why?
- Does your musculoskeletal problem affect your lifestyle or activities of daily living? How?

The nurse should ask the patient how she copes with the injury or illness and whether the illness/injury affects family and personal relationships. Observe the patient's nonverbal cues, note whether the patient appears depressed, angry, or anxious when the history is taken.

Physical Examination

In the physical examination, the nurse uses inspection and palpation to collect objective data. These data are then recorded and made available to the health care team. A full musculoskeletal exam will take time; document findings during the exam for accuracy.

General Guidelines for Musculoskeletal Assessment

General guidelines for conducting a musculoskeletal assessment are as follows:

- Inspect for deformities.
- Inspect and palpate any swelling.
- Feel the area for increased temperature and observe for redness.
- Palpate for tenderness around a joint.
- Assess for range of motion.

 Do not force a body part past its normal range. Discontinue ROM when the patient complains of pain or discomfort.

Inspection

Abnormal appearance of a joint may be due to a musculoskeletal or neuromuscular disease, dislocation, tumor, mass, degenerative change, contracture, or atrophy of the muscle. When inspecting compare corresponding paired joints for symmetry. The nurse observes for skin color, scars, shape of the site, deformities, **muscle atrophy** (shortening of a muscle), masses, or swelling. Also inspect for **fasciculations** (an abnormal contraction or shortening of a bundle of muscle fibers) and **tremors** (an involuntary movement of a body part), which can be related to neuromuscular disorders.

Swelling may be due to an inflammation of the joint (reaction of tissue to irritation, injury, or infection), intra-articular swelling or effusion (escape of fluid into the tissue), a swollen bursa, synovial membrane thickening, or a bony overgrowth. A "boggy" feel-ing over an edematous area may indicate an edematous synovial membrane, which can be indicative of a soft tissue injury (Magee, 2008). If there is swelling, the nurse should note the size and shape of the edematous area, the site, and signs of inflammation such as redness. When inspecting a joint, observe for alignment.

Palpation

The nurse will feel the skin at the site with the back of his fingers to assess the skin's temperature. Note whether the skin is hot, warm, cool, or cold to the touch. Heat and redness over a joint may be indicative of inflammation or a septic joint (infection of a joint). Cold or cool temperatures may indicate a circulation problem (Weber & Kelley, 2007). The nurse will feel for skin texture, dryness, or moisture. Excessive dryness may indicate an acute, **gouty joint** (inflammation of a big toe, heels, elbows, ankles, dorsum), whereas moisture is often associated with a septic joint (Magee, 2008).

Palpate the muscles surrounding the joint and bony articulations. Note any tenderness, swelling, or masses. A normal joint is not tender to palpation. The patient should be asked if the palpation causes any tenderness or pain. Tenderness around a joint may be due to arthritis, a septic joint, inflammation, bursitis, or osteomyelitis (Weber & Kelley, 2007).

Palpate for **nodules** (small raised areas) that may not be visible. While palpating inquire about any numbness, tingling, or weakness in the area.

Range of Motion

Range of motion may be decreased due to pain, muscle spasms, weakness, and atrophy. Decreased ROM occurs in joints where there is inflammation, arthritis, lack of use, dislocation, masses, or pain.

The nurse can test the ROM of all joints by asking the patient to actively move the joints one at a time. Compare each joint for flexibility and mobility, and assess the patient's ability to move the joint through its normal full range of motion. Familiarize yourself with the normal ROM for each type of joint so you will recognize a limitation.

 When assessing joints, muscles, and movements, always assess on both sides of the body for purposes of comparison.

A **goniometer** measures the angle of the joint in degrees, and can assist in the assessment of ROM of a joint (Figure 54–3 ■).

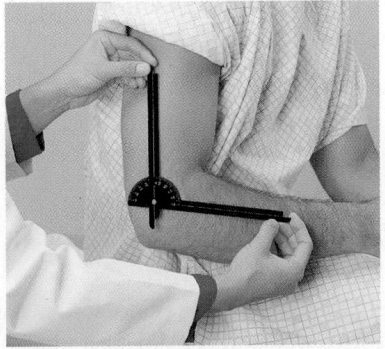

FIGURE 54–3 ■ Goniometer.

To measure the joint angle, place the goniometer exactly at the angle of the joint. The nurse will document, for example, "the right knee flexes from 20–60 degrees." This is important in describing the degree of decreased ROM from normal and also provides a baseline for future measurement (Magee, 2008).

Testing Muscle Strength

Muscle strength is measured by placing your hand firmly against the body part in question and asking the patient to push hard against your hand. Perform the test on both sides and compare your findings, knowing that the dominant side of the body will be stronger. For example, if the nurse is testing the trapezius muscle in the shoulders, she will place her hand against the patient's shoulder and push to allow resistance for the patient and then ask the patient to push against her hand. The nurse will then document the strength of the patient's ability to push by describing the strength as *normal, slightly weak, weak,* or *severely weak* or by recording that the patient was unable to push at all. Chart 54–3 describes a grading system for the documentation of muscle strength.

■ Head-to-Toe Musculoskeletal Assessment

It is important to be methodical when assessing the musculoskeletal system so as not to miss any abnormalities.

Temporomandibular Joint

The temporomandibular joint (TMJ) is the hinge of the jaw. It is located anterior to the external ear and is constantly opening and closing when a patient talks, eats, chews, and yawns (Bickley, 2003). To examine the TMJ, have the patient in a sitting position. Examination includes inspection and palpation. To assess the TMJ, the nurse should place his index and middle fingers anterior to the external ear, just in front of the tragus. The patient is asked to open her mouth as wide as possible. At this time the nurse's fingers should slide into the "groove" or joint space. The nurse moves the patient's jaw back and forth, palpating for masses or nodules. The nurse also inspects the area for redness and swelling indicating inflammation.

CHART 54–3	Muscle Strength Grading	
Functional Level		**Grade**
No evidence of contractibility (inability to contract muscles)—paralysis		0
Slight contractibility—severe weakness		1
ROM without gravity—passive ROM performed by examiner		2
Active ROM with gravity—moderate weakness		3
Complete active ROM against gravity with some resistance—minimal weakness		4
Complete ROM against gravity with resistance—normal		5

Source: Adapted from Bickley, L. (2003). *Bates' guide to physical assessment and history taking* (8th ed.). Philadelphia: Lippincott; Kozier, B., Erb, C., Berman, A., & Snyder, S. (2008). *Fundamentals of nursing. Concepts, process and practice* (7th ed.). Upper Saddle River, NJ: Pearson Prentice Hall; Weber, J., & Kelley, J. (2007). *Health assessment in nursing* (3rd ed.). Philadelphia: Lippincott Williams & Wilkins.

The patient is then asked to open and close the mouth. While the patient does this, the nurse notes the range of motion and questions the patient as to any tenderness. The nurse also listens for any "clicking" sounds. Soft clicking sounds without any complaints of discomfort or ROM difficulty may not be indicative of any problems; however, if the clicking sounds are hard or grating, accompanied by pain or discomfort, and are affecting range of motion, this can be indicative of arthritic changes or a possible dislocation (Magee, 2008).

Normal Findings

- Patient is able to open and close the mouth without difficulty about 2.5 to 5 cm (1 to 2 in.).
- Jaw moves laterally without pain or tenderness.
- Some clicking may be heard and felt during movement.

(Weber & Kelley, 2007).

Abnormal Findings

- Unable to open mouth 2.5 to 5 cm (1 to 2 in.).
- A grating, clicking, or popping sound is noted with a TMJ problem, possibly a dislocation.
- Patient complains of pain, tenderness with opening and closing of the mouth, which may indicate arthritis.
- Masses, nodules felt during palpation.
- Inability to hold mouth open.
- Decreased muscle strength.

Shoulders

The shoulder is composed of the clavicle, acromion process, and the humerus and is able to move in many directions due to various joints, bones, and muscle groups called the shoulder girdle. The clavicle and acromion process are responsible for the stability of the shoulder girdle.

The nurse will need to inspect the shoulders **anteriorly** (the front plane of the body) and **posteriorly** (the back plane of the body). Observe for any swelling, change in skin color, deformity, atrophy, fasciculations, and **asymmetry** (unequal in size and proportion). Patients with scoliosis may have one shoulder higher than the other, causing asymmetry. Inspect for swelling or redness over the joint capsule anteriorly or a bulge under the deltoid, which may be indicative of a problem in the bursa (Bickley, 2003).

Assess range of motion to include **abduction** (away from the midline of the body—in this case, raising the arm away from the body), **adduction** (moving toward the midline of the body—in this case, moving the arm across the front of the body), flexion, extension, hyperextension, internal rotation, and external rotation. Explain to the patient that you will be testing the range of motion of the shoulders and will ask them to perform seven movements (Figure 54–4 ■, p. 1716).

1. Begin by having the patient stand straight with arms at the sides. Observe the area for symmetry.
2. To test for abduction, ask the patient to raise the arms to shoulder level.

3. To test for adduction, ask the patient to raise the arms above the head with the palms facing each other.

4. To test for flexion and extension, ask the patient to bend and straighten out the elbows.

5. To test for external rotation, ask the patient to place both hands behind the neck with elbows out to the side.

6. To test for internal rotation, ask the patient to place the hands behind the lower back.

7. Ask the patient to clasp his hands and bring them around the lower back as far as he can.

Normal Findings

The patient should be able to:

- Raise the arms 90 degrees to the shoulder level.
- Flex arms to 180 degrees and fully extend the arms.
- Hyperextend arms behind the back 50 degrees.
- Place hands behind the neck and lower back at 90 degrees without crepitus, pain, or decreased ROM.
- Shrug shoulders against resistance.

(Weber & Kelley, 2007)

Abnormal Findings

- Pain and decreased ROM are associated with rotator cuff tears, tendonitis, sprains, and bursitis.
- Decreased ability to shrug shoulders or inability to shrug shoulders against resistance may indicate a lesion of cranial nerve XI.
- Weakness in performance of ROM exercises indicates joint disease or muscle disuse.
- Shoulders that are flat or asymmetrical may be dislocated.
- Any redness, heat, or swelling may be associated with sprains, strains, degenerative joint disease, and arthritis.
- Atrophy is associated with nerve damage or disuse.

(Bickley, 2003; Magee, 2008; Weber & Kelley, 2007)

While the patient is performing these tasks, palpate the joints for **crepitus** (grating produced by bone rubbing against bone), and question the patient regarding any associated pain (Jarvis, 2008; Magee, 2008; Weber & Kelley, 2007).

To test the muscle strength of the shoulders, the nurse asks the patient to perform a number of movements and exercises. To assess the deltoid muscle, the patient should hold her arms upward while you try to push them down. To assess the biceps, the patient should flex the arm while you try to extend it. To assess the triceps, the patient should extend the arm while you try to flex it. Finally, to assess the trapezius muscle, the patient should shrug her shoulders while you try to hold the shoulders down (Bickley, 2003; Weber & Kelley, 2007).

Normal Findings with Muscle Grading

- Muscle strength of 3 or greater.
- Muscle strength greater in dominant side.
- Coordinated and painless movements.

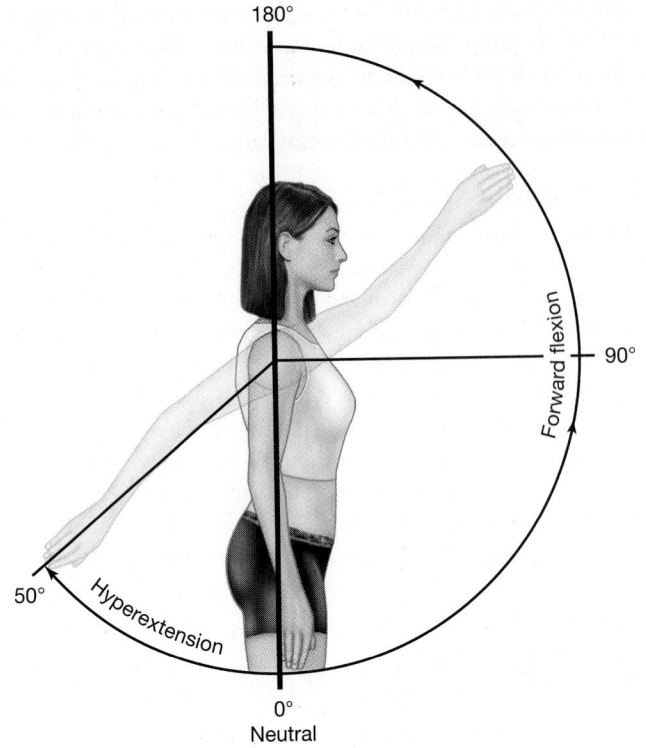

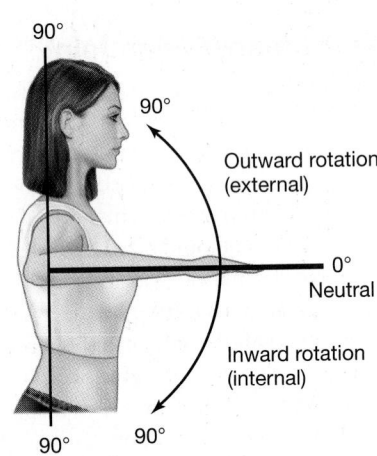

FIGURE 54–4 ■ Shoulder ROM.

Abnormal Findings

- Muscle strength is less than 3.
- Patient is unable to push against resistance.
- Assistance is required to perform exam.

 *Some patients who complain of shoulder pain can be experiencing or possibly already have had a cardiac event. Further assessment is required.*

Elbows

The elbow is a complex joint where the humerus, radius, and ulna come together and are enclosed in a synovial capsule. The elbow can move in extension and flexion, using the joint of the humerus and ulna (humeroulnar joint), and in pronation (palm downward) and supination (palm upward), using the radius. The ulnar nerve passes through the elbow, around the medial epicondyle of the humerus (Bickley, 2003).

During inspection it is best to support the patient's arm with your nonexamining hand. Flex the patient's elbow to approximately 70 degrees. This prevents the patient's muscles from tightening during the examination. Inspect the elbow for shape, deformities, size, redness, swelling, nodules, and bulging. With the tips of your middle fingers and thumb, palpate the olecranon process, epicondyles, and the grooves on either side of the olecranon process. Assess for heat, swelling, tenderness, and nodules (Bickley, 2003; Weber & Kelley, 2007).

To test for range of motion, ask the patient to flex the elbow and bring the hand to the forehead, then extend or straighten the elbow (Figure 54–5 ■). Note any deviations in the angle or deformities. Ask the patient to hold the arm out and supinate (turn the palms up) and pronate (turn the palms down). Have the patient then flex and extend the arm with your resistance. Repeat flexion and extension with the patient supinating and pronating the palms. Assess for deformities, tenderness, swelling, and nodules (Bickley, 2003; Magee, 2008).

 Never force a patient to perform ROM tests if the patient is unable or unwilling.

Normal Findings

- The elbows are symmetrical without nodules, deformities, swelling, or redness.
- Patient is able to perform flexion, extension, supination, and pronation without evidence of swelling, tenderness, or any visible nodules.

Abnormal Findings

- Redness, swelling, deformity over the olecranon process may indicate injury, arthritis, or bursitis.
- Inability to perform range of motion without pain, swelling, deformity, or nodules needs further investigation. Nodules noted during ROM exercises may indicate rheumatoid arthritis (an autoimmune disease that causes inflammation to the joints) or rheumatic fever. Pain and tenderness on movement may indicate tennis elbow, which is due to overuse of the elbow.
- Deformity or displacement of the joint during palpation or range of motion may indicate a fracture (broken bone) or dislocation of the elbow.

Wrists

The wrist joint contains the articulation of the distal radius and double row of carpal bones intertwined to form a malleable hinge. The wrist is a condyloid articulation that allows 3 degrees of freedom. Its movements include flexion, extension, abduction, adduction, and circumduction (Figure 54–6 ■). The joint is surrounded by a capsule and strengthened by multiple ligaments.

The examination should start with the nurse inspecting and palpating the wrist. Inspect the wrist for symmetry, size, shape, deformities, nodules, and swelling. Palpate the wrist for nodules, movement, and tenderness by holding the patient's wrist between your two hands and palpating the lateral and medial surfaces, as well as the groove of each wrist joint with your thumbs.

Normal Findings

- The wrist is symmetrical, without any deformities, swelling, or nodules.

Abnormal Findings

- Swelling, tenderness, and nodules may indicate rheumatoid arthritis.
- Pain, tenderness, and a deformity may indicate an injury or trauma to the wrist.
- A round, painless, swollen, fluid-filled area may indicate a ganglion cyst.

(Jarvis, 2008; Weber & Kelley, 2007)

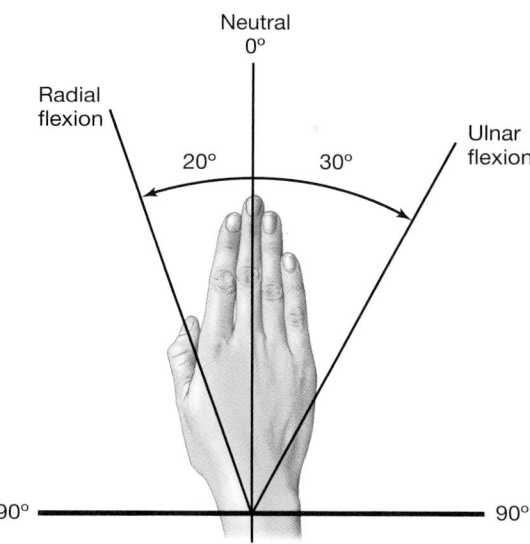

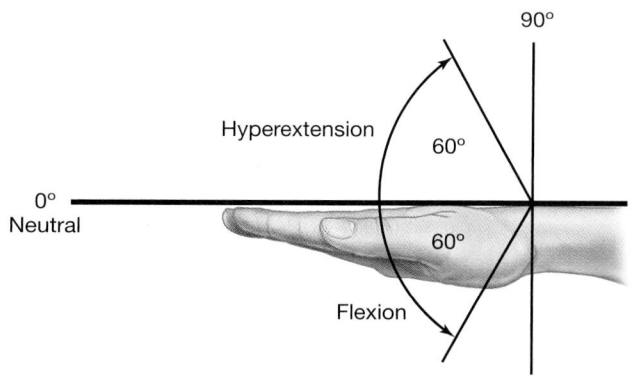

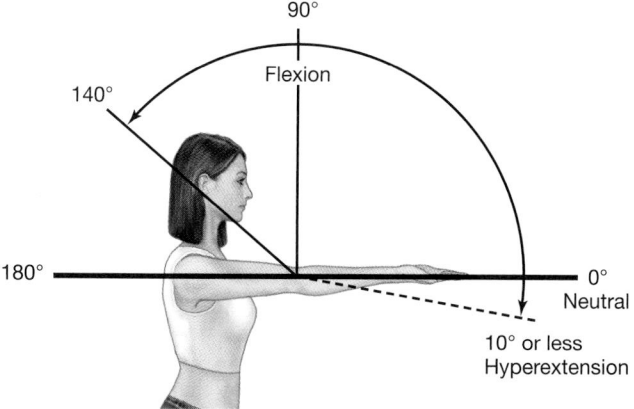

FIGURE 54–5 ■ Elbow ROM.

FIGURE 54–6 ■ Wrist ROM.

Next, the nurse should test the patient's range of motion in the wrist. To test for flexion and extension, ask the patient to bend the wrist back and forth. To test for ulnar or radial deviations, ask the patient to hold the wrist straight out in front of his body, with the palm downward, and move the hand inward toward and outward from the body. Finally, the nurse should palpate the anatomic snuffbox, just lateral to the thumb toward the middle of the hand.

Now repeat the exercises, but with resistance. The nurse should stabilize the patient's forearm on a table or hard surface, place the patient's wrist in extension, and then place her fingertips in the patient's palm. Ask the patient to flex the wrist against gravity. Stabilize the patient's forearm and ask the patient to flex the wrist. The nurse places her hand on the patient's dorsal metacarpals, just below the wrist, and asks the patient to extend the wrist against gravity.

Normal Findings

- Patient should have 90 degrees of flexion and the ability to hyperextend to 70 degrees without pain or swelling.
- Patient should be able to move the wrists laterally and medially.
- Patient should be able to have full range of motion against resistance (Magee, 2008).

Abnormal Findings

- Inability to perform full ROM needs further investigation. An example of a common abnormal condition of the wrist is carpal tunnel syndrome.

Carpal tunnel syndrome occurs when the median nerve is compressed as it travels with the flexor tendons through a canal made by the carpal bones and the transverse carpal ligament (Figure 54–7 ■). Carpal tunnel syndrome is caused by repetitive motion with the wrist flexed, such as with typing. Patients with

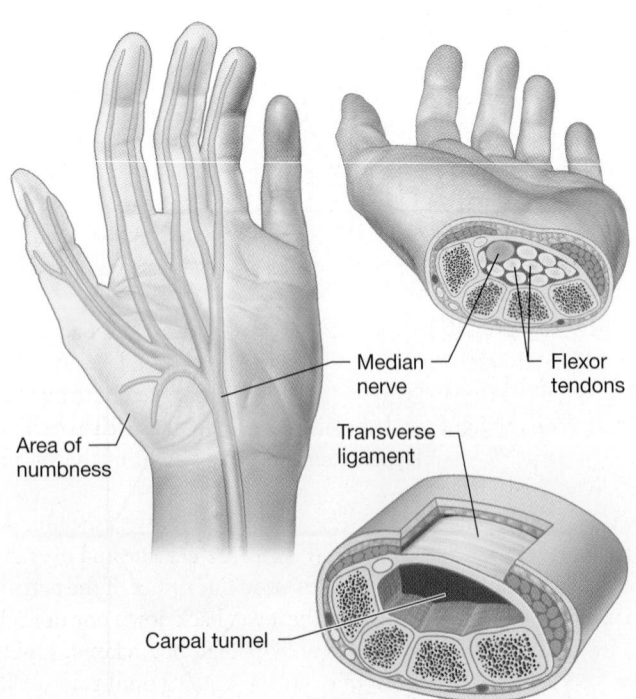

— Median nerve
— Flexor tendons
Area of numbness
Transverse ligament
Carpal tunnel

FIGURE 54–7 ■ Carpal tunnel.

carpal tunnel syndrome complain of numbness, tingling, and pain in the wrists and fingers.

To assess for carpal tunnel syndrome, the patient is asked to perform three tests:

1. **Thumb abduction**—Ask the patient to raise the thumb perpendicular to the palm. The nurse applies pressure to the distal phalanx. If the patient has difficulty performing this maneuver, the median nerve may be compressed.
2. **Tinel's sign**—With your finger, percuss lightly over the course of the medial nerve, located in the medial, inner aspect of the wrist.
3. **Phalen's test**—Ask the patient to place the back of each hand against one another while flexing the wrists 90 degrees for 60 seconds (Bickley, 2003; Magee, 2008; Weber & Kelley, 2007).

Abnormal findings include numbness, tingling, or pain at the wrist or fingers.

Hands and Fingers

The joints of the hands include the **metacarpophalangeal joint** (the joint between the metacarpal bones of the hand and the phalangeal bones of the fingers), the proximal interphalangeal joint and the distal **interphalangeal joint** (the joints between the phalanx bones of the fingers). Because there is very little protection to the bones in the fingers and hands, they are susceptible to trauma and disability. Inspection and palpation are the techniques used in examination of the hands and fingers (Bickley, 2003).

Inspect the palmar and dorsal surfaces of the hands and fingers for size, shape, deformity, color, swelling, nodules, and tenderness. Assess the fingers at rest and while in motion. Palpate the metacarpophalangeal joints at the distal fingers. Then palpate the proximal, middle, and distal interphalangeal joints using your thumb and index finger.

Normal Findings

- The fingers are in a straight line and symmetrical, without deformity, swelling, or nodules.
- Swelling, nodules, and complaints of tenderness are not noted on palpation.

Abnormal Findings

- Swelling of the phalanges, in addition to stiff tender fingers, may indicate acute rheumatoid arthritis.
- Hard, painless nodules at the joints of the fingers may indicate osteoarthritis (progressive loss of cartilage at a joint). **Bouchard's nodes** are found over the proximal interphalangeal joints. **Heberden's nodes** are seen over the distal interphalangeal joints (Figure 54–8 ■).
- "Swan neck" deformity is characterized by a hyperextension of the proximal interphalangeal joint with a fixed flexion of the distal joint.
- Swelling and thickening of the metacarpophalangeal joint.
- **Boutonniére deformity** is flexion of the proximal interphalangeal joint (Figure 54–9 ■).

(Bickley, 2003; Weber & Kelley, 2007)

Test range of motion of the fingers and hands. To test for abduction, ask the patient to extend and spread the fingers apart. To test for adduction, ask the patient to make a fist. To text for

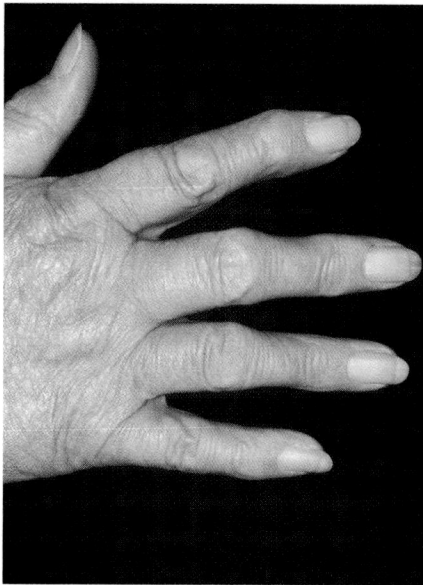

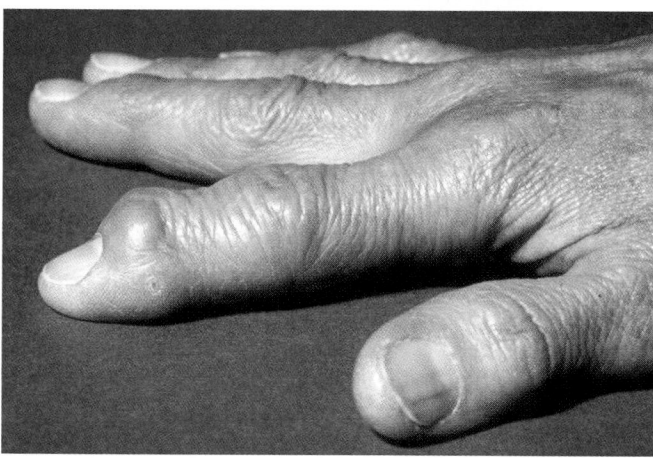

FIGURE 54–8 ■ Bouchard's nodes and Heberden's nodes.
Source: (top): © Pulse Picture Library/CMP Images/Phototake All rights reserved; (bottom): Bart's Medical Library/Phototake All rights reserved.

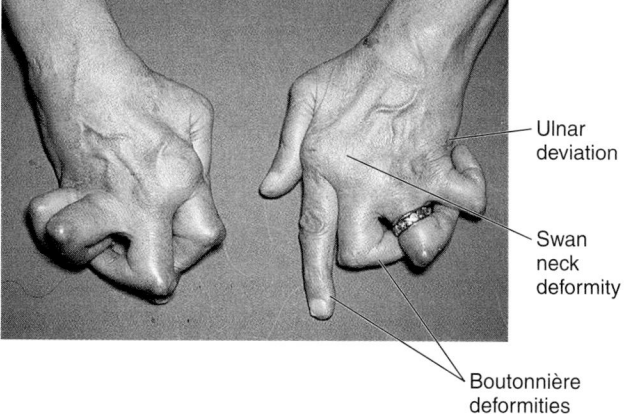

Ulnar deviation

Swan neck deformity

Boutonnière deformities

FIGURE 54–9 ■ Deformities of the hand.

flexion and hyperextension, ask the patient to bend the fingers down and then hold them up.

To test for flexion of the thumb, ask the patient to move the thumb across the palm and touch the fifth finger. To test for extension of the thumb, ask the patient to move the thumb across the palm away from the rest of the fingers. To test for abduction

and adduction of the thumb, ask the patient to move the thumb anteriorly away from the palm, then back. To test for opposition, or movement of the thumb across the palm, ask the patient to touch each of the fingertips with the thumb.

Normal Findings

- Patient is able to perform all ROM exercises without pain or swelling.
- The thumb should move to and away from the other fingers without difficulty.
- All fingers should abduct and adduct without pain and swelling.
- Hyperextension should occur without any difficulty at about 30 degrees.

Abnormal Findings

- Inability to perform any of the ROM tests without discomfort, swelling, and deformity needs further investigation.
- Difficulty or an inability to extend the ring or fifth finger is a sign of **Dupuytren's contracture**.
- Slight flexion of a finger, pain on extension, swelling, and tenderness may be indicative of acute **tenosynovitis**, an infection of the flexor tendon sheaths.

(Bickley, 2003; Weber & Kelley, 2007)

Neck and Spine

The spine or vertebral column is composed of alternating vertebrae and fibrocartilaginous disks that are connected by ligaments and supported by muscles that extend from the skull to the pelvis. This provides axial support to the body. The bony vertebra is composed of an anterior body and a posterior arch made up of two pedicles and two laminae that are united to form the spinous process. On either side of the arch is a transverse process and superior and inferior articular processes. The articular processes articulate with the adjacent vertebrae to form synovial joints. The articular processes account for the degree of flexion, extension, or rotation possible in each segment of the vertebral column. The transverse and spinous processes act as levers for the muscles attached to them.

As the spinal column progresses from the head, the vertebral body size increases. The intervertebral disks connecting the vertebral bodies act like shock absorbers for stresses applied to the vertebral column. There are four distinct curvatures to the vertebral column: (1) the cervical curve, which is concave; (2) the thoracic curve, which is convex; (3) the lumbar curve, which is concave; and (4) the sacral curve, which is convex (Bickley, 2003).

Examination of the spine includes inspection and palpation. Have the patient stand straight with arms at the sides and begin by examining the curvature of the cervical, thoracic, and lumbar areas from the right and left sides of the patient as well as behind the patient. Observe for differences in the height of the shoulders and iliac crests.

Palpate the spinous processes of each vertebra with the thumb, the paravertebral muscles on both sides of the spine and over the sacroiliac joint on the posterior superior iliac spines. If the patient complains of pain moving from the lower back down one or both legs, perform Lasègue's test: Have the patient in a relaxed, supine position. Ask the patient to raise the affected leg until pain is felt, then lower the leg until the pain is relieved; at this point the foot is dorsiflexed to reproduce the pain. Pain that shoots down one or both legs during dorsiflexion may indicate sciatic nerve involvement, a condition that may be caused by a herniated disk or pressure on the spinal cord (Magee, 2008; Weber & Kelley, 2007).

Normal Findings

- The cervical and lumbar curves should be concave; the thoracic and sacral curves should be convex when observed on either side of the patient.
- The spine is straight when observed from behind the patient.
- The shoulders, iliac crests, and gluteal folds should be aligned.

(Weber & Kelley, 2007)

Abnormal Findings

- *Scoliosis:* Lateral deviation or curvature of the thoracic spine, with a downward slant of the thoracic cage on the affected side. The pelvis tilts upward on the opposite side, usually at the chest level. Noticed first in adolescents (Figure 54–10B ■).
- *Kyphosis:* An extreme thoracic curve (hunchback or humpback) often occurs with aging (Figure 54–10D ■).
- *Lordosis:* Excessive inward curve of the spine. Patient appears to be swaybacked.
- Flattening of the lumbar spine may be indicative of a herniated disk at the lumbar area or **ankylosing spondylitis** (inflammation of the spine and the sacroiliac joints).
- Pain between the spinous processes may indicate arthritis, fracture or other trauma, infection, or herniated disks.
- Tenderness on palpation of the posterior superior iliac spine (the dimple just above the buttocks) may indicate ankylosing spondylitis.
- Pain on palpation of the paravertebral muscles may indicate degenerative changes or inflammation to the muscles.
- Pain radiating down one or both legs may indicate sciatic nerve involvement.

(Bickley, 2003; Magee, 2008; Weber & Kelley, 2007)

Range of Motion of the Neck

To test the range of motion of the cervical spine, have the patient touch the chin to the chest (flexion) and then look up at the ceiling (extension). To test rotation of the neck, have the patient turn the head from side to side, looking over the shoulder. To test lateral bending of the neck, have the patient tilt the head and touch the ear to the corresponding shoulder.

Normal Finding

- Full range of motion without pain.

Abnormal Findings

- Decreased range of motion can result from arthritis, muscle spasms, or cervical strain.
- Pain in the neck, shoulders, and arms can be due to spinal cord compression.
- Numbness may indicate spinal cord compression.
- Neck pain with decreased ROM accompanied by fever and chills may be due to an infection, such as strep throat or meningitis.

(Bickley, 2003; Magee, 2008)

Range of Motion of the Spine

To test for flexion, ask the patient to bend forward and touch the toes. To test for hyperextension, stabilize the patient's hips from behind the patient, and ask the patient to bend backward. To test for lateral bending of the spine, ask the patient to bend sideways, and to test for rotation, ask the patient to twist the shoulders to the right and then to the left and vice versa.

Normal Findings

- Patient is able to perform full ROM exercises without pain/deformity.
- When bending down to touch toes, the back flattens.
- No exaggerated curvatures of the spine are noted.
- Muscles display symmetry.

Abnormal Findings

- Pain on movement in the thoracic and lumbar areas can be due to muscle or soft tissue injury, osteoarthritis, ankylosing spondylitis, and any **congenital** (describes a condition that was present at birth) conditions.
- Deformity of the thorax on bending indicates scoliosis.
- Lumbar lordosis indicates ankylosing spondylitis.
- Asymmetrical muscle movements, fasciculations, and decreased or exaggerated angles need further investigation.
- Pain radiating from the lower back to one or both legs may indicate nerve involvement.

(Bickley, 2003; Magee, 2008; Weber & Kelley, 2007)

Hip

The hip is located inside the pelvis. The bones that make up the pelvis include the sacrum, pubis, ileum, and ischium. The hip joint is a ball-and-socket joint formed by the articulation of the rounded head of the femur and the cuplike acetabulum of the pelvis. It forms the primary connection between the bones of the trunk and pelvis with the lower extremity. Both joint surfaces are covered with a strong but lubricated articular hyaline cartilage. The hip is important because it bears the weight of the upper body and it contains the hip joint, which allows the leg to move freely.

To examine the hip, inspect the patient's anterior and posterior pelvis for bruising, asymmetry in height, and muscle atrophy. In addition, inspect the buttocks for symmetry. Observe the patient's **gait**, or way of walking. Ask the patient to remove all clothing except underwear and examine the patient walking to and from you barefooted. If one of the patient's legs is longer than the other, then the nurse should measure them by having the patient lie down with the legs extended. The nurse then measures from the anterior superior iliac spine across the leg medially to the medial malleolus (Weber & Kelley, 2007).

Observe for the hip motion, knee flexion, and a heel-to-heel distance of 5 to 10 cm (2 to 4 in.). Inspect the spine for any abnormal curvatures. Question the patient regarding pain; specifically, where in the gait phase the pain occurs. With the patient standing, palpate the hips and pelvis for tenderness, crepitus (grating sound), and nodules (Bickley, 2003; Weber & Kelley, 2007).

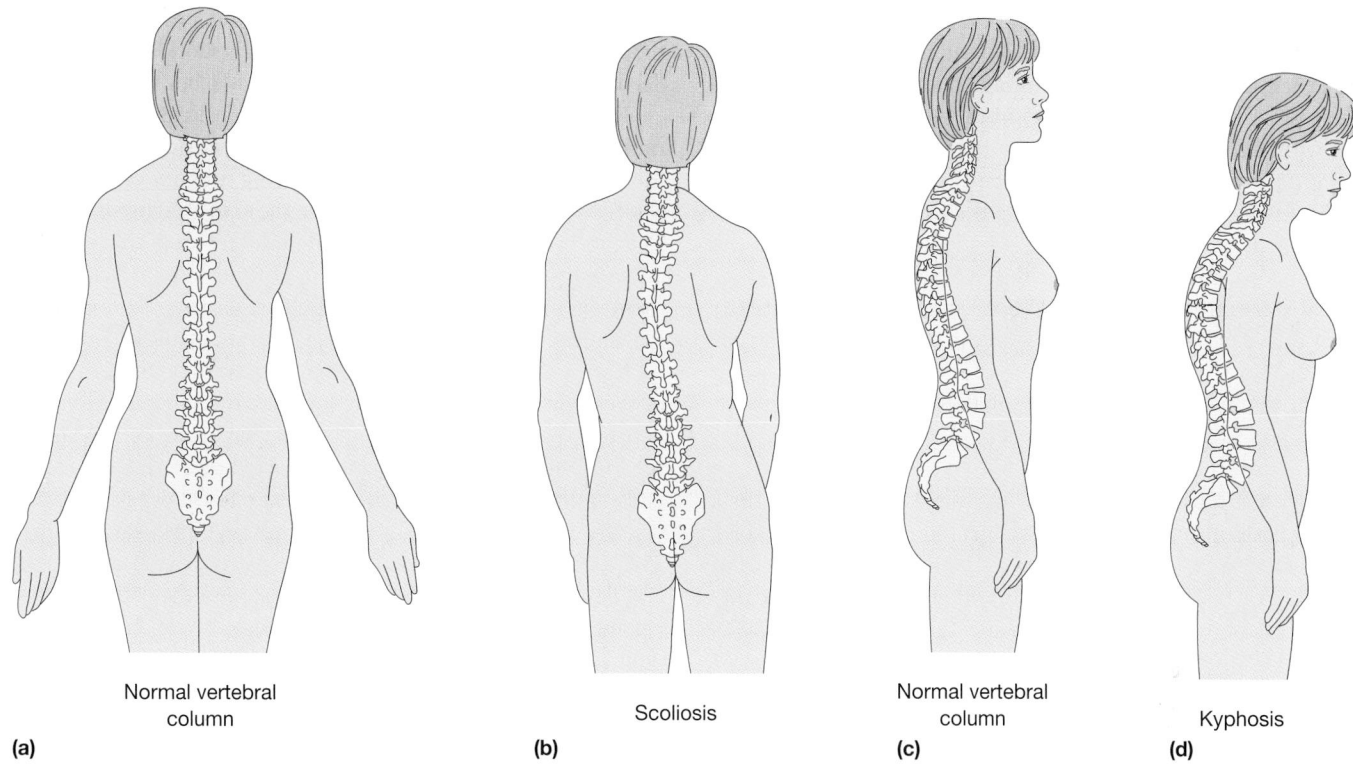

Normal vertebral column
(a)

Scoliosis
(b)

Normal vertebral column
(c)

Kyphosis
(d)

FIGURE 54–10 ■ Normal spine and its deformities: (A) normal vertebral column, posterior view; (B) scoliosis; (C) normal vertebral column, lateral view; (D) kyphosis.

Normal Findings

- The pelvis, on anterior and posterior inspection, is symmetrical in height and shape.
- The buttocks are equal in size.
- Patient is able to bear weight on both legs without pain.
- The gait is rhythmic, nonstaggering, and without a limp.
- The feet are lifted off the ground and are then replanted firmly on the ground.
- Crepitus is not noted by the patient during walking.
- The arm swing is in conjunction with the walking gait.
- During walking the patient's hips are equal and move rhythmically with the gait.
- Patient is able to walk on his toes and on his heels without difficulty or pain.
- Both legs are the same length.
- The knee is flexed while walking, except when the heel touches the ground.
- With the feet forward in a normal standing position, the heel-to-heel distance is 5 to 10 cm (2 to 4 in.).

Abnormal Findings

- An asymmetric pelvis is indicative of hip dislocation, fractured hip, arthritis, **degenerative joint disease** (osteoarthritis), muscle weakness, or atrophy.
- Difficulty in ambulation with an irregular gait may indicate a dislocation or fracture of the hip, degenerative joint disease, or muscle weakness.
- Abnormal curvature of the spine during ambulation may indicate scoliosis or lordosis.
- Leg shortening could mean muscle deformities or hip fracture.
- Unequal leg length may indicate scoliosis.
- Wide heel-to-heel base may indicate a foot or cerebellar problem.

(Weber & Kelley, 2007)

Range of Motion of the Hip

To test ROM of the hip, have the patient lie in the supine position (Figure 54–11 ■). Raise one leg above the body while keeping

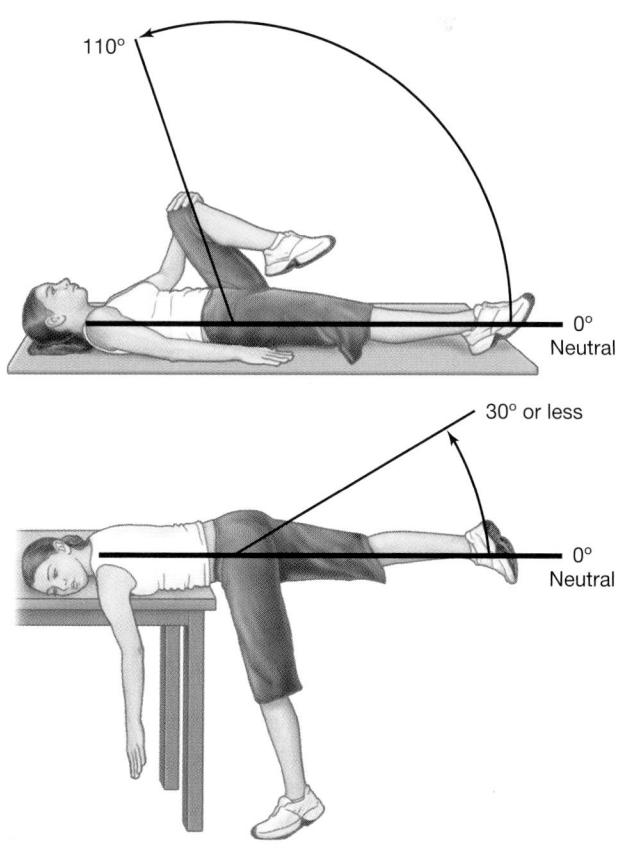

FIGURE 54–11 ■ Hip ROM.

the knee extended and then bring one knee to the chest while keeping the other leg extended. Repeat the exercise with the other leg. To assess for abduction and adduction, have the patient swing one leg laterally away from the body as far as possible while keeping the knee straight and then bring the leg back toward the midline of the body. Repeat with the other leg.

To assess internal rotation, have the patient bend one knee and rotate the knee so that the knee moves inward toward the opposite leg, and then repeat with the other knee. To assess external rotation, have the patient bend one knee and rotate the knee outward, and then repeat with the other knee. To further test ROM, ask the patient to assume a prone position and swing one leg in the air, and then repeat on the other side. Ask the patient to stand and swing one leg behind the body, and then repeat on the other side.

To assess muscle strength, the nurse places the patient in a supine position, and then asks the patient to raise an extended leg while the nurse tries to hold it down. The nurse then asks the patient to push both legs against the nurse's hands while the hands are placed on the outer side of the patient's knees (Bickley, 2003; Magee, 2008; Weber & Kelley, 2007).

Normal Findings

- Patient should be able to raise the legs to at least 90 degrees of flexion with the knee straight and to 120 degrees of flexion with the knee flexed.
- Patient should be able adduct leg to 20 to 30 degrees and abduct it 45 to 50 degrees.
- Patient should be able to internally rotate to 40 degrees and externally rotate to 45 degrees.
- Patient should be able to hyperextend the leg at least 15 degrees.
- Patient should be able to move the extremities against resistance.

(Magee, 2008; Weber & Kelley, 2007).

Abnormal Findings

- Deformity of one or both hips during flexion may indicate a hip deformity.
- Inability to flex knees may indicate a hip deformity.
- Inability to abduct hip is indicative of hip disease, such as arthritis.
- Inability to internally rotate the hip may be indicative of hip disease, such as arthritis.

(Bickley, 2003; Weber & Kelley, 2007)

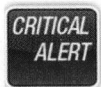 **CRITICAL ALERT** *If the patient has had a hip replacement or hip surgery, do not perform any ROM exercises without the permission of the health care provider.*

Knees

The knee joint is the articulation of the femur, patella, and the tibia. The knee is actually two joints: (1) The *femoropatellar joint* consists of the patella, a bone that sits within the tendon of the anterior quadriceps muscle, and the patellar grove on the femur through which it slides. (2) The *femorotibial joint* articulates the femur with the tibia. The joint is bathed in synovial fluid contained inside the joint capsule. The medial meniscus and the lateral meniscus are two cartilaginous menisci within the joint that protect the ends of the bones from rubbing on each other, act as shock absorbers, and deepen the tibial sockets where the femur attaches.

The knee allows flexion, extension, and slight rotation. The muscles that help move the joint are the quadriceps muscles on the front of the knee and the hamstring muscles on the back. Multiple ligaments help to stabilize the joint (Figure 54–12 ■). The two cruciate ligaments located in the center of the knee, the anterior cruciate ligament (ACL) and the posterior cruciate ligament (PCL), are the major stabilizing ligaments of the joint. The PCL prevents the femur from sliding forward on the tibia, and the ACL prevents the femur from sliding backward on the tibia. Both of these ligaments stabilize the knee in a rotational fashion also and, if damaged, the knee may become unstable when planting the foot and pivoting, causing the knee to buckle and give way.

Examination of the knee includes inspection and palpation. Assess the patient during ambulation for a rhythmic, smooth flow. The knee should be extended when the foot is striking the ground, and flexed during the other phases of gait. Ask the patient to first assume a supine position and then a sitting position. Assess the patient for symmetry of the knees, swelling, redness, size, shape, deformities, and alignment. Assess for atrophy of the quadriceps muscles and the hollows on either side of the knee (Bickley, 2003; Weber & Kelley, 2007).

Palpate the knee while the patient is sitting on the edge of the table with the legs dangling. Palpate for tenderness, heat, swelling, crepitus, and nodules. Begin by palpating 10 cm (about 4 in.) above the patella. Using fingers and thumb, move

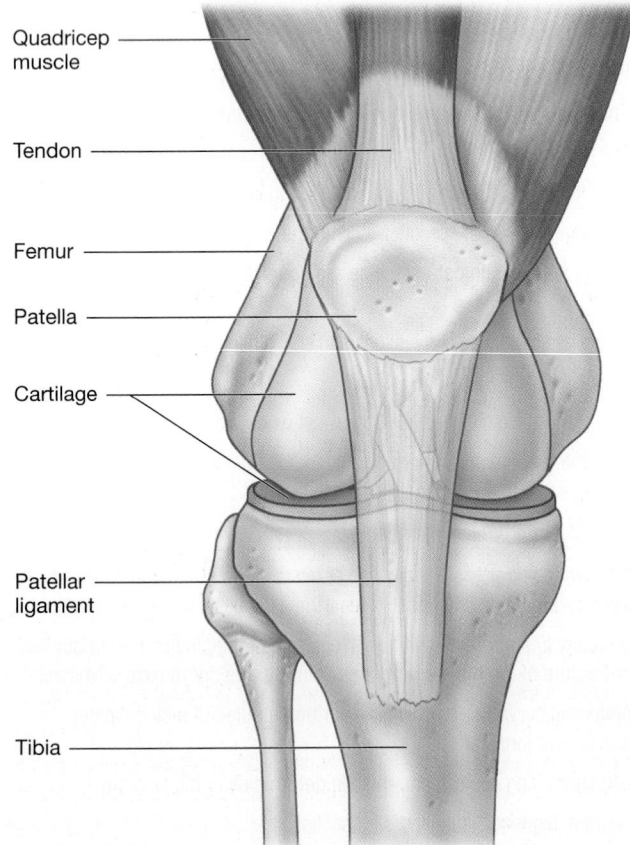

FIGURE 54–12 ■ Knee joint.

downward toward the knee (Bickley, 2003). If swelling is encountered, the following further tests are performed with the patient in the supine position:

1. The *bulge sign* is used to detect fluid in the knee. Place the hand on the medial aspect of the patient's knee and push upward two to four times to displace the fluid. Then place the hand on the lateral side of the knee and look for a bulge of fluid in the hollow area medial to the patella.

2. The *balloon sign* is performed by placing the thumb and index finger of one hand on each side of the patella while the other hand compresses the suprapatellar pouch against the femur. This allows the nurse to feel the fluid entering the spaces next to the patella.

3. The *ballottement test* is used to assess large amounts of fluid, particularly in the suprapatellar pouch. Press against the sides of the patella with the thumb and index finger of one hand, while pushing the patella against the femur with the opposite hand. While pressing on the sides of the patella, fluid is displaced in the suprapatellar pouch. While pushing the patella against the femur, the fluid returns to the pouch and the nurse is able to feel a "wave" as the fluid returns to the pouch (Bickley, 2003; Weber & Kelley, 2007).

Normal Findings

- Both knees are symmetrical.
- Both legs are the same length.
- The hollows are present on both sides of the patella.
- There is no redness, swelling, or tenderness.
- No deformities are noted.
- No nodules are noted.
- The muscles are firm and taut.
- No crepitus is felt or heard.

Abnormal Findings

- Knees turn outward, called bowlegs or genu varum.
- Knees turn inward, called knock-knees or genu valgum.
- Irregular bony ridges may be indicative of osteoarthritis.
- Pain and tenderness may be indicative of bursitis.
- Heat may be indicative of osteoarthritis.
- Pain and crepitus may indicate a rough surface between the femur and the back of the patella.
- Pain on movement by means of quadriceps contraction may indicate a degenerative patella.
- Pain over a tendon or an inability to extend the leg may indicate a tear of a tendon or ligament.
- Thickness, warmth, and bogginess on the sides of the patella may indicate synovitis or osteoarthritis.
- Swelling or bulges of the lateral or medial aspects of the knee or above the knee may indicate an effusion (leaking of fluid into the knee) of the knee or synovial thickening.
- Inability to walk without stumbling or pushing the knee into extension may indicate a weakening of the quadriceps.

Range of Motion of the Knee

To test for ROM of the knee, have the patient in a sitting position and do the following tests. To test for flexion, ask the patient to bend the knee. To test for extension and hyperextension, ask the patient to straighten the knee. To test for internal and external rotation, ask the patient to rotate the foot medially and laterally (Figure 54–13 ■).

To test muscle strength, the nurse asks the patient to extend the leg as the nurse tries to bend it. This tests quadriceps muscle strength. Then the nurse asks the patient to flex the knee while the nurse tries to straighten it. This tests hamstring muscle strength.

Normal Findings

- Patient should be able to flex the knee to 120 to 130 degrees (Weber & Kelley, 2007).
- Patient should be able to extend the knee without difficulty and hyperextend the knee to 15 degrees.
- Patient should have full ROM against resistance.

Abnormal Findings

- Difficulty with ROM may indicate osteoarthritis or a muscle or joint problem.
- Crepitus is noted in osteoarthritis.

Be aware that pain and abnormal or decreased ROM may also indicate a ligament injury or meniscus tear to the anterior or posterior cruciate ligaments and the medial and lateral collateral ligaments. Pain on the lateral sides of the knee, "popping" or "clicking" sounds with movement, patient complaints of the knee "locking," or difficulty in fully extending the knee may indicate damage to the meniscus. To assess for a torn meniscus, perform the McMurray test. With the patient in a supine position, the nurse asks the patient to flex one knee and hip. The nurse then cups one hand over the knee and places her index finger and thumb on opposite sides of the knee. With the other hand, the nurse grasp the patient's heel and rotates the lower leg and foot laterally and medially. Gently and slowly extend the knee, and note any abnormal sounds (Weber & Kelley, 2007).

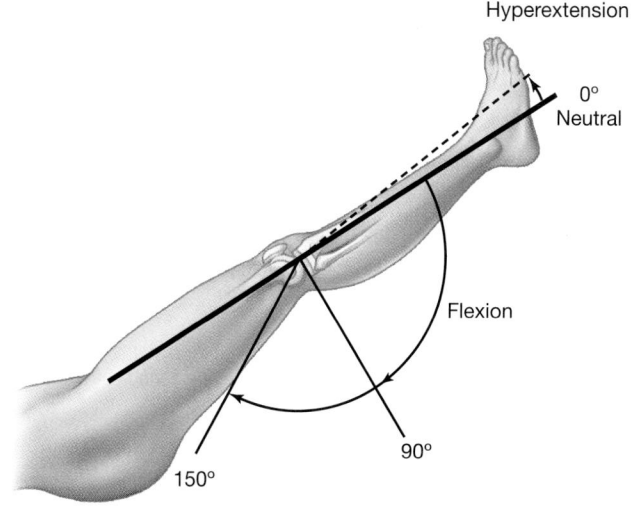

FIGURE 54–13 ■ Knee ROM.

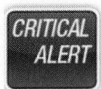

Ankles and Feet

The ankle is the joint between the lower tibia, the fibula, and the talus. The feet are made up of many small bones. Both the ankle and foot have many ligaments and thick padding to cushion the foot against the weight of the body during ambulation (Bickley, 2003).

Ask the patient to stand, walk, and sit. Observe the ankles and feet for shape, deformities, nodules, corns, calluses, bunions, and swelling. Note the position of the toes. Ask the patient to walk barefoot and note the ability to walk normally on the heels and on the toes. Ask the patient to walk placing one foot in front of the other and to walk backwards. Ask the patient to sit with the feet dangling at the sides of the table. Observe the position of the feet and toes. Inspect for roundness and smoothness of the medial malleolus.

Assess ROM by asking the patient to point his toes toward the floor (plantar flexion), point toes toward his nose (dorsiflexion),

Normal Findings

- The toes should point straight ahead and be in alignment with the feet, though some may point slightly inward or slightly outward.

- No nodules, calluses, corns, or bunions are noted.

- The medial malleolus should be round and smooth.

- No pain elicited on palpation.

- The Achilles tendon is without nodules or tenderness.

Abnormal Findings

- A great toe that is deviated medially and abducted to the first metatarsal with an inflamed bursa or bunion on the medial side is indicative of hallux valgus.

- A hot, tender, red, swollen metatarsophalangeal joint is indicative of gouty arthritis.

- A flattened longitudinal arch, so that the sole is very close to the ground or touches the ground may be indicative of flat foot (evident only when patient is ambulating).

- An abnormally high arch may be indicative of cavus foot.

- Hyperextension of the metatarsophalangeal joint of the second toe is referred to as hammer toe.

- Painful thickening over the skin over a bony prominence is a corn.

- An area of thickened skin over a region of pressure points is a callus.

- A wart located over the thick skin of the sole of the foot is referred to as a plantar wart, or verruca vulgaris.

- Painful, inflammation over the great toe may be indicative of gout.

- Tenderness between the ankle joints is indicative of arthritis, infection, or injury to the ankle.

- Painful movement may be indicative of arthritis.

- Pain or nodules around the Achilles tendon may be a result of rheumatoid arthritis, bursitis, or tendonitis.

- Pain at the calcaneus may be due to bone spurs.

- Pain and tenderness of the metatarsals and grooves may indicate arthritis or circulatory compromise.

(Bickley, 2003; Magee, 2008; Weber & Kelley, 2007)

turn the soles of the feet out, then in (eversion, inversion), and then flex and straighten the toes (Figure 54–14 ■).

Palpate with your thumbs at the anterior aspect of each ankle joint, the heel, and the posterior and anterior calcaneus. Palpate the metatarsophalangeal joints, as well as in between them for tenderness, and the Achilles tendon for tenderness, swelling, heat, and nodules (Bickley, 2003; Magee, 2008; Weber & Kelley, 2007).

Gait (Ambulation)

To assess gait, or ambulation, ask the patient to walk away from you using the heel-to-toe gait, swinging her arms. Next have the patient walk toward you. Then ask the patient to walk on tiptoes toward you, and away from you on her heels. Observe the patient during the two phases of walking: The first is the stance phase of gait. This occurs when the foot is on the ground and the patient is weight bearing or walking on the foot. The second phase is the swing phase. This occurs when the patient moves the foot forward and is not bearing weight. Observe for difficulty in weight bearing, gait anomalies, symmetry of legs, rate, rhythm, and arm motion.

Inspect the patient during ambulation for ability to walk heel to toe; arm swing in conjunction with walking; base of support; and posture; limping, or leaning to one side; inability to bear weight on one or both legs.

Normal Findings

- Patient is able to ambulate with smooth, rhythmic movement; arms swing in conjunction with walking.

- No leaning or limping noted; patient is able to keep balance.

- Toes point straight ahead.

- Patients is able to walk heel to toe.

- Back is straight with a wide base of support.

Abnormal Findings

- Leaning or limping may indicate a neurological problem.

- Toes pointing inward or outward may be indicative of bunions or arthritis.

- Arms extended to sides to maintain balance may indicate a neurological problem.

- Shuffling or the inability to take coordinated steps may indicate Parkinson's disease.

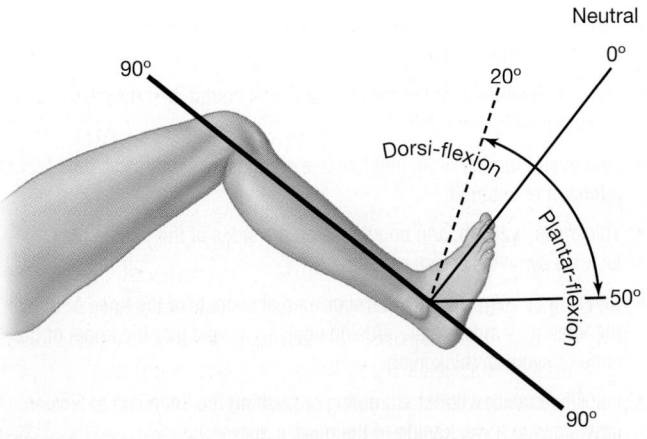

FIGURE 54–14 ■ Ankle ROM.

Gerontological Considerations

As "baby boomers" age, persons 50 years and older will make up the largest population group in the United States, so it is important to understand the numerous changes in the musculoskeletal system that occur with age. When assessing older patients with musculoskeletal ailments, the nurse needs to recognize several important aspects:

1. Flexibility and strength tend to decrease as people age.
2. Because of changes to bone and muscle, older people may find it hard to maintain the various positions required for a proper assessment. Lying supine for a long period of time is difficult for patients with cardiopulmonary problems.
3. Bones become weaker as calcium reabsorption lessens with age.
4. As the bones become weaker, fractures can become more prevalent.
5. Women who are menopausal or postmenopausal are subject to osteoporosis.
6. Articular hyaline cartilage becomes thinner at the joints, restricting ROM.
7. Osteoarthritic changes occur with age, particularly in postmenopausal women. Osteoarthritis causes smooth articular surfaces to become rough and painful.
8. Rheumatoid arthritis causes inflammation and decreased or limited movement of the fingers. The condition is painful and affects a person's ability to perform ADLs.
9. The elderly are prone to **pathologic fractures** (fractures that occur without trauma) due to thinning of the bones.
10. Skeletal muscle mass decreases with age, leading to cramping and severe pain.

Assessing the Elderly Patient

Obtain a current history to include all medications, including OTC drugs. Inquire about pain, discomfort, limitation in movement, and any difficulty performing ADLs. Assess the patient as he ambulates, walks, grasps your hand, and bends over. Note any weakness. Inspect the hands and fingers for rheumatoid nodules or swelling and note any circulatory impairment by blanching the finger/toe nails. Chart 54–4 provides more details for assessing elderly patients.

 Note any signs of depression (crying, monotone voice, lethargy). A limitation in mobility may cause a person to become depressed and possibly suicidal.

Documentation

Documentation of the examination of the musculoskeletal system entails noting subjective data as well as objective data. Include the patient's response to various parts of the examination, including the patient's inability to perform a particular task of an examination or the performance of only part of the task. Note complaints of pain and tenderness, swelling, redness, nodule formation, noticeable deformity, or dizziness.

CHART 54–4	Assessing the Elderly Patient
System	**Difference with the Elderly**
Shoulders	Inability to perform ROM without discomfort
Elbows	Inflammation, swelling, and decreased ROM due to arthritis
Wrist	Decreased ROM, swelling
Hands/fingers	Swelling and thickening of the metacarpophalangeal joint and the proximal interphalangeal joint, decreased ROM, due to rheumatoid arthritis Heberden's nodules over the distal interphalangeal joint and Bouchard's nodes over the proximal interphalangeal joints due to osteoarthritis
Neck	May have difficulty performing ROM
Spine	Kyphosis
Hip	Decreased ROM, crepitus due to arthritis and degenerative joint disease
Knee	Bowleggedness due to loss of muscle control
Ankles	Decreased strength and ROM due to bone thinning and decreased muscle mass
Gait	Wider base of support; slower paced, nonrhythmic walking; use of assistive devices

Sources: Adapted from Magee, D. (2008). *Orthopedic physical assessment* (5th ed.). Elsevier; Weber, J., & Kelley, J. (2007). *Health assessment in nursing* (3rd ed.). Philadelphia: Lippincott Williams & Wilkins.

Nursing Diagnoses

Nursing diagnoses for the musculoskeletal system are based on the subjective and objective data obtained. Nursing diagnoses applicable for the musculoskeletal examination include the following:

- *Activity Intolerance* related to difficulty with ambulation, decreased ROM, pain, swelling, muscle weakness, pain, joint deformity
- *Mobility, Impaired* related to difficulty with ambulation, decreased ROM, pain, swelling, muscle weakness, pain, joint deformity
- *Pain, Acute* related to a specific condition
- *Pain, Chronic* related to a specific condition
- *Disuse Syndrome, Risk for* related to difficulty with mobility, decreased ROM
- *Injury, Risk for* related to difficulty with mobility, decreased ROM, pain
- *Trauma, Risk for* related to difficulty with mobility, decreased ROM
- *Activity Intolerance, Risk for* related to difficulty with ambulation, decreased ROM, pain, swelling, muscle weakness, pain, joint deformity
- *Falls, Risk for* related to decreased mobility, decreased ROM
- *Powerlessness* related to loss of independence.

Health Promotion

Many musculoskeletal disorders are due to individual behaviors as well as social and environmental factors. Many individuals do not participate in regular physical activities, such as jogging, bicycling, or walking. Physical activity is important for many reasons, but as far as the musculoskeletal system is concerned, regularly scheduled physical activity increases muscle and bone mass. Physical activity can prevent thinning of bones as well as muscle atrophy. The increase in muscle mass coincides with a decrease in falling in the elderly, which allows for independence and an ability to perform ADLs.

Obesity also affects the musculoskeletal system in that people who are overweight and obese have a difficult time engaging in physical activity as they become short of breath and fatigued more easily. Cigarette smoking causes lung problems, which again can affect an individual's ability to participate in physical activity.

To maintain one's quality of life, it is important for everyone to engage in some degree of regular physical activity to help maintain a strong musculoskeletal system.

Summary

The musculoskeletal system plays a major role in a patient's mobility and quality of life. As a nurse it is imperative to understand all of the components and how to conduct a thorough assessment of the system. Performing a systematic evaluation to identify abnormalities will assist with timely treatment and the prevention of future complications.

NCLEX® REVIEW

1. A patient sustains a fracture to the ribs. The nurse realizes that the type of bone injured is considered:
   1. Long.
   2. Short.
   3. Flat
   4. Irregular.

2. While assessing a patient with a musculoskeletal injury the nurse asks if the patient uses any assistive devices. This question would be considered as being a part of which of the following areas of the patient's history?
   1. Chief complaint
   2. Social
   3. Demographic data
   4. Biographical data

3. During the musculoskeletal assessment, the nurse notes atrophy of the patient's left thigh muscles. The assessment technique the nurse used to determine this finding would be:
   1. Palpation.
   2. Percussion.
   3. Inspection.
   4. Range of motion.

4. The nurse asks a patient to raise the arms above the head with the palms facing each other. The body area that the nurse is currently assessing would be the:
   1. Elbow.
   2. Shoulders.
   3. Wrist.
   4. Hand.

5. The nurse is assessing a patient's feet. Which of the following would be considered a normal finding during this assessment?
   1. Hallux valgus
   2. Cavus foot
   3. Verruca vulgaris
   4. Toes pointing inward

6. The nurse is assessing a patient's hip range of motion. Which of the following is considered a normal finding?
   1. Leg adduction 10 degrees
   2. Leg abduction 25 degrees
   3. External rotation 45 degrees
   4. Internal rotation 20 degrees

Answers for review questions appear in Appendix D

KEY TERMS

abduction *p.1715*
adduction *p.1715*
ankylosing spondylitis *p.1720*
anteriorly *p.1715*
assistive device *p.1714*
asymmetry *p.1715*
Bouchard's nodes *p.1718*
boutonniére deformity *p.1718*
bursae *p.1712*
carpal tunnel syndrome *p.1718*

congenital *p.1720*
crepitus *p.1716*
degenerative joint disease *p.1721*
dislocation *p.1711*
Dupuytren's contracture *p.1719*
fasciculations *p.1714*
gait *p.1720*
goniometer *p.1714*
gouty joint *p.1714*
Heberden's nodes *p.1718*

interphalangeal joint *p.1718*
metacarpophalangeal joints *p.1718*
muscle atrophy *p.1714*
nodules *p.1714*
pathologic fractures *p.1725*
posteriorly *p.1715*
range of motion (ROM) *p.1711*
tenosynovitis *p.1719*
tremors *p.1714*

EXPLORE PEARSON mynursingkit™

MyNursingKit is your one stop for online chapter review materials and resources. Prepare for success with additional NCLEX®-style practice questions, interactive assignments and activities, web links, animations and videos, and more!

Register your access code from the front of your book at
www.mynursingkit.com

REFERENCES

Bickley, L. (2003). *Bates' guide to physical assessment and history taking* (7th ed.). Philadelphia: Lippincott.

Jarvis, C. (2008). *Pocket companion for physical examination and health assessment* (5th ed.). St. Louis: W. B. Saunders.

Lillicrap, M. S., Byrne, E., & Speed, C. A. (2003). Musculoskeletal assessment of general medical in-patients—joints crying out for attention. *Rheumatology, 42*, 951–954.

Magee, D. (2008). *Orthopedic physical assessment* (5th ed.). St. Louis, MO: Elsevier, Inc.

Porth, C. M. (Ed.). (2007). *Pathophysiology: Concepts of altered health states* (7th ed.). Philadelphia: Lippincott Williams & Wilkins.

Weber, J., & Kelley, J. (2007). *Health assessment in nursing* (3rd ed.). Philadelphia: Lippincott Williams & Wilkins.

Caring for the Patient with Musculoskeletal Disorders

Helene Harris
Karen Bawel-Brinkley
Cheryl Wraa

Outcome-Based Learning Objectives

After studying this chapter, the learner will be able to:

1. Compare and contrast the etiology, pathophysiology, clinical manifestations, and medical and nursing management for bone diseases.
2. Explain the rationale and type of preventive therapy necessary for patients with bone disease.
3. Describe the unique treatment and prevention needs of the gerontological population.
4. Compare and contrast the etiology, pathophysiology, clinical manifestations, and medical and nursing management for muscular diseases.
5. Differentiate between the five types of myopathies, various treatment modalities, and nursing care of a patient diagnosed with a myopathy.
6. Discuss the causative factors, treatment modalities, and nursing care related to a patient diagnosed with fibromyalgia.

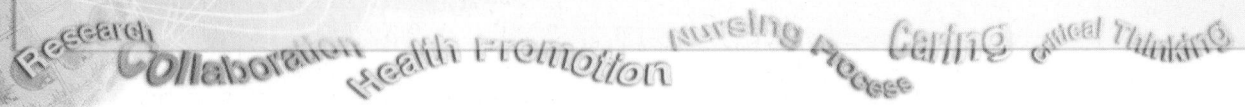

THE MUSCULOSKELETAL system consists of bones, muscles, ligaments, tendons, and other connective tissue. Organic (collagen fibers), inorganic materials (mineral salts), and water combine to form bone tissue that provides protection for crucial internal organs, storage for calcium and other minerals, and sites for formation and development of the cells of the blood (Copstead & Banaski, 2005; Seeman, 2002).

Bone disorders can result from disuse, nutritional deficiencies, chemotherapy, genetic or environmental influences, and traumatic injuries or accidents. Because individuals with bone disease may experience loss of function and independence, the nurse must have a clear understanding of the effects of bone disease and how the disorder or disease will impact the patient's life.

■ Bone Physiology

This section presents a brief overview of bone physiology and bone formation. Because anatomy and physiology provide the foundation for medical and nursing goals and care, the reader is encouraged to review bone physiology and formation.

Characteristics

The study of bones and bone structure of the human body is referred to as **osteology**. The human body consists of the axial and appendicular skeleton comprising 206 bones. These bones have some degree of elasticity and toughness that provide an anchor against which muscles, connected by means of ligaments and tendons, can exert force.

The bone/bone marrow system includes bone cells, fat cells, blood vessels, and nonliving materials including water and minerals. Bones are classified as osseous tissue that is formed from calcium phosphate. This tissue is considered to be a hard **endoskeletal** connective tissue. The body has 80 axial bones (head, facial, hyoid, auditory, trunk, ribs, and sternum) and 126 appendicular bones (arms, shoulders, wrists, hands, legs, hips, ankles, and feet) (Porth, 2005). Bones provide structural support, protect vital organs, act as attachment sites for muscles that permit the mechanics of human motion, and serve as a mineral reservoir and a way to catch unsafe minerals (e.g., lead). Chart 55–1 presents a summary of the classification of bones and their characteristics.

Bone Tissue

Bone tissue has the ability to be strong, lightweight, and adaptable to meet the functional needs of the body (Beers & Porter, 2006; Chan & Duque, 2002). Bone is covered with a fibrous membrane known as the **periosteum**. The blood supply to bone is achieved through blood vessels running through two layers of

CHART 55–1	**Classification of Human Bones and Characteristics**	
Classification of Bone	**Example Bone in Human Body**	**Characteristic of Bone**
Long bones	Femur Tibia	• Tubular • Regions of the bone: diaphysis, epiphysis, and metaphysis • Hollow with bone marrow • Shaft made of compact hard bone and thickest in the middle • Trabecular bone toward the end of the bone • Increases in size in one dimension during growth
Short bones	Wrist Ankle Carpal Tarsal	• Cuboidal in shape • Cancellous bone in the center and compact bone outer shell
Flat bones	Cranium Scapula	• Spongy bone between two layers of compact bone • Generally curved in structure (inner and outer diploe)
Irregular bones	Bones of the face Vertebrae	• Irregular shape • Does not fit into any other category
Sesamoid	Patella	• Occur in tendon leading to exposure to friction

the periosteum: the thick outer layer, which is composed of connective tissue, and the inner layer, which is composed of elastic fibers. In addition, fine nerves and lymphatic vessels run through the thick fibrous tissue covering the bone. The periosteum tightly covers the bone and is connected to both ends of the bone with the epiphyseal cartilage except where tendons and ligaments attach to the bone, and then the periosteum is integrated with them. Two results of the aging process are that the periosteum becomes thinner and vascularity declines (Porth, 2005).

The human body has three types of bone tissue: compact, cancellous, and subchondral tissue (Figure 55–1 ■) **Compact** (or **cortical**) **bone** is resistant to compression, is dense, and is laid down in concentric layers. **Cancellous** (having a hard outer casing with the interior being porous, spongy, and meshwork-like in structure) or **trabecular** (cancellous bone found at the ends of the long bones [e.g., femur], in vertebrae, and in the flat bones of the pelvis) **bone** is laid down in response to stress and shape to accommodate loads placed on the bone (Figure 55–2 ■). The arrangement of plates, rods, arches, and braces in the interior of trabecular bone provides the strength needed for weight bearing. **Subchondral bone** is the smooth tissue at the ends of bones that is covered with cartilage. Cartilage is the specialized, tough connective tissue that is present in adults, and the tissue from which most bones develop in children. Both compact and trabecular bone are **lamellar bone** or mature bone. In the human body, lamellar bone is a slow-forming bone with cellular distribution being orderly and the direction of the collagen fibers standardized (Gupta et al., 2005).

Cortical (outer layer) or compact bone provides about 80% of the skeletal mass and is the major component of tubular bones. Cortical bone has a densely packed, calcified intercellular matrix that makes it more rigid than cancellous bone. **Haversian canals**, which contain one or two capillaries and nerve fibers that serve as the transport systems for nutrients, are located in the cortical bone.

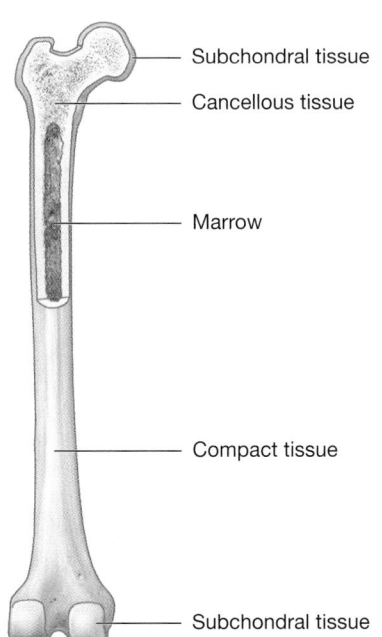

FIGURE 55–1 ■ Bone tissues.

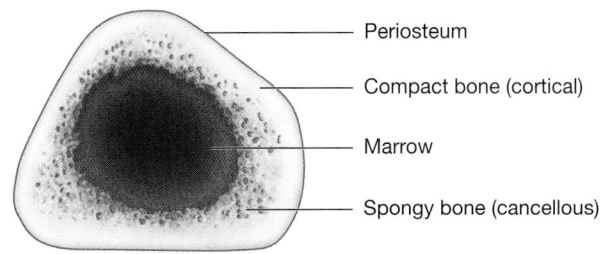

FIGURE 55–2 ■ Cortical and cancellous bone.

Cell communication in cortical bone tissue depends on osteons or the Haversian system (Figure 55–3 ■) (Gupta et al., 2005). Cortical bone is less porous and dense than trabecular bone, resulting in higher resistance to bending and torsion. Consequently, cortical bone provides a protective outer shell around every bone in the body including cancellous bone. In fact, cortical bone is found in the appendicular skeleton and on the outside of the shaft of the long bones of the upper and lower extremities.

Bone marrow is found between and around the plates and braces of the trabecular bone. Age and specific site are two variables that can influence the mechanical properties of cancellous bone. Morphologically, cancellous bone is similar to cortical bone except that it has lower calcium content than cortical bone (McCance & Huether, 2006).

Bone disorders are associated with both types of bones. For example, osteoporosis can affect both cortical and cancellous bone. The underlying etiology of bone disease can be found in the changes within the bone tissue. Because the type of bone is dependent on the genetic composition of the bone tissue, it is important to continue the discussion beyond the structure to the actual composition of bone tissue.

It has been estimated that the composition of bone is 70% mineral, 22% protein, and 8% water by weight. Collagen contributes 89% to 90% of the total organic matrix, with the remaining 10% composed of a variety of classes of other molecules, including noncollagenous proteins, lipids, and carbohydrates. Each of the different categories of bones varies in structure and chemical composition. Therefore, bone tissue is classified on the basis of porosity and the unit microstructure (Beers & Porter, 2006).

The interior of the bone is a mesh-like substance that is a chemical composition of organic and inorganic materials. The percentage of each component depends on the developmental age, gender, and site within the skeletal system. The strength of the bone depends on the matrix-mineral composition. Calcium and phosphate ions are the building blocks of the matrix-mineral composition. Magnesium phosphate, sodium chloride, and sulphate are the other components (Chan & Duque, 2002). The role of calcium and phosphate is presented later along with the influence of hormones on bone structure.

Bone tissue is composed of organic and inorganic materials, yielding a light but functional structure. Three types of bone cells, as discussed next, emerge from the developmental process of the human and are responsible for maintaining the bone tissue.

Bone Cells

Bone tissue is composed of protein fiber bundles arranged in layers with dense accumulation of mineral crystals, resulting in a structure that is strong, functionally adaptable, and light. Bone tissue is composed of three different types of cells: osteoblasts, osteoclasts, and osteocytes (Porth, 2005). Other cells include fat cells and hematopoietic cells found in the bone marrow.

Osteoblasts are any cells that form bone within the body. **Osteocytes** are mature osteoblasts that maintain the bony matrix and participate in the dynamic task of releasing calcium into the bloodstream. Osteoblasts are found in the endosteal bone surfaces, in Haversian systems, and occasionally on periosteal surfaces. A characteristic of osteoblasts is that they produce two type of proteins: type I collagen and noncollagenous protein osteocalcin or **osteoid**. Interestingly, alkaline phosphatase has been found on osteoblast cell surfaces, which may play an important role in the mineralization of cartilage and bone matrix (Chan & Duque, 2002). Finally, the average life span of an osteoblast ranges from 3 months to 1.5 years (Porth, 2005). Note, however, that the aging process causes osteoblasts to decline in number and life span.

Osteoclasts are large cells formed in bone morrow that originate from macrophage-like cells. Osteoclastic cells are formed by the production of blood-derived monocytes. Osteoclasts are designed to absorb and remove unwanted bone tissue, causing the bone to be "remodeled" or "destroyed." After the osteoclasts resorb bone, they journey to the area of exposed bone and begin to put down osteoid. This protein mixture known as osteoid is secreted by the osteoblasts. When the osteoid is mineralized, new bone tissue has been formed. Unlike the osteoblasts, as individuals age there is an increase in the number of osteoclasts, resulting in a greater bone turnover rate and a decline in bone density (Chan & Duque, 2002).

Another cell that is found in bone tissue is the hematopoietic cell. These cells are found in the red marrow of the long and flat bones and are responsible for the production of blood cells. Bone marrow can be found in the sternum, spine, skull, hips, and ribs.

Bone has the ability to repair itself to meet the functional needs of the body (Beers & Porter, 2006). This dynamic process of forming bone and destroying bone is based on the remodeling–modeling process.

Bone Remodeling–Modeling Process

Bone is a dynamic structure that involves living tissue that continuously undergoes the physiological process of remodeling and modeling during the human life span. Remodeling is the process by which old bone is replaced by new bone (bone turnover). **Modeling** is the process by which bone growth occurs and where there is a higher rate of bone formation relative to bone loss. The osteoclast cells are the bone-remodeling cells and the osteoblasts are the bone-forming cells.

Bone growth is coordinated by polypeptides, steroids, thyroid hormones, and local factors such as growth hormones, cytokines, and prostaglandins (Chan & Duque, 2002). Bone resorption is highest during bone growth and occurs at the juncture between the diaphysis and the epiphysis. When peak bone mass is achieved, generally in the third decade of life, the rates of breakdown and formation are equivalent. As a result, bone mass is thought to re-

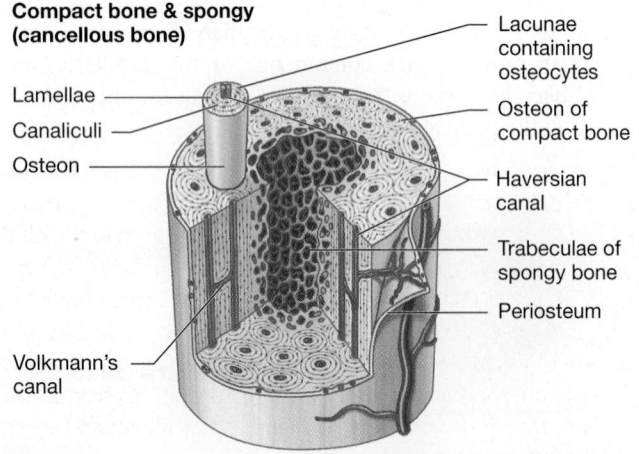

Compact bone & spongy (cancellous bone)

- Lamellae
- Canaliculi
- Osteon
- Volkmann's canal

- Lacunae containing osteocytes
- Osteon of compact bone
- Haversian canal
- Trabeculae of spongy bone
- Periosteum

FIGURE 55–3 ■ Compact and cancellous bone with Haversian canal.

main stable for a period of time. As we age, the rate of breakdown increases and exceeds the rate at which bone is formed, resulting in the skeleton becoming fragile (Copstead & Banaski, 2005).

Material Properties of Bone

Nurses care for a variety of patients with bone disorders, therefore it is important to know the mechanical properties of the bone. For example, when a patient has a fracture, it is important to understand the underlying etiology of the injury or trauma to establish quality nursing goals and objectives for care. The nurse must understand that the combination of collagen and mineral (calcium and phosphate) equips the bone to withstand mechanical force.

When considering the mechanical properties of bone, two concepts are important to remember: stress and strain. First, stress results when mechanical force is applied to a stretched or compressed bone and the bone resists the force with internal counterforce. Compressive stressors are those of the body weight pushing the bone down, and tensile stressors come from the muscles, pulling the bones away from each other. Strain, the second concept, is expressed in length/original length and results as a force that is applied causing an amount of deformation in the bone relative to its original length (Gupta et al., 2005). Bones that are stiffer can withstand higher strain rates than softer bones. In addition, there is an increased amount of stored energy at high strain rates. Therefore, bones that fracture under high strain rates suffer greater damage and more involvement of soft tissue than fractures with less strain or energy applied to the bone (Gupta et al., 2005).

Three types of loading can be applied to bones: compression, tensile, and shear strain. Compressive loading occurs when there is an application of equal and opposite forces toward the surface. For example, compression loadings occur when an individual is standing and there is a shortening and widening of the vertebrae. If the density of the bone has declined then a fracture can occur (e.g., vertebral compression fracture) with widening (Gupta et al., 2005).

Tensile loading occurs when there is an application of equal and opposite loads outward from the surface. Shear loading is the application of a load parallel to a surface and the deformation is angular (Gupta et al., 2005). For example, tensile strain results when a bone is pulled and gets longer, and shear strain results when layers of a material slide against another. For example, shear strain occurs when a load is applied to a bone that is twisted or bent at the same time (Gupta et al., 2005).

Both the collagen matrix and the orientation of fibers within the matrix are two influential properties of bone handling of stress and strain. The amount of stress and strain that a bone can withstand depends on the bone density resulting from the proportion of minerals, cells, vessels, and calcium compound. The bone density varies according to the bone type and region where the bone is located. For example, cortical bone is stiffer than trabecular bone; therefore, cortical bone fractures under less strain than trabecular bone (Gupta et al., 2005).

Bone Tissue and Hormones

The combination of collagen and mineral (calcium and phosphate) equips the bone to withstand mechanical force. Bone density is under the influence of hormones produced within the body. For example, estrogen is required in both genders for skeletal maturation. Calcium and phosphorus are key components of the collagen matrix and under the control of the parathyroid and renal system. Therefore, a brief discussion of the hormonal influences will be presented.

Through the process of remodeling and modeling, the human bone has the ability to grow and regenerate to meet the needs of the body. Several endocrine glands influence bone modeling and remodeling processes. Endocrine glands that produce hormones that influence bone growth include the pituitary gland, parathyroid gland, thyroid gland, and adrenal glands. Chart 55–2 (p. 1732) lists the glands and their actions on bone tissue; Chart 55–3 (p. 1732) lists organs that also produce hormones that act on bone tissue.

The remodeling–modeling processes result from a balance between the two processes. A number of polypeptide growth factors have significant effects on bone and cartilage metabolism. Growth hormone is produced by the pituitary gland. This hormone stimulates bone formation by promoting the production of insulin-like growth factors (IGFs) by the osteoblasts by stimulating longitudinal bone growth. When given to adults, growth hormone can increase bone mass (Copstead & Banaski, 2005).

The thyroid hormone is necessary for growth and maturation of the skeleton because of the production of the hormone calcitonin, a 32-amino-acid peptide hormone. The major factor controlling calcitonin secretion is the extracellular concentration of ionized calcium. Elevated blood calcium levels promote calcitonin secretion, and secretion is prevented when calcium concentration falls below normal. Therefore, calcitonin has been determined to influence calcium and phosphorous metabolism in the body. For example, in the bone, calcitonin appears to act as an antagonist to the parathyroid hormone by preventing resorption of bone by hindering the activity of the osteoclasts, resulting in calcium and phosphorus being released in the blood. Calcitonin inhibits tubular reabsorption of calcium and phosphorus, resulting in an increased rate of their loss in urine. Finally, calcitonin delays calcium absorption from the intestine. The role of calcitonin appears to be minor in controlling calcium and phosphorous homeostasis in the human body. Clinical manifestations of hypersecretion or hyposecretion are generally not recognized. However, calcitonin has been found to be beneficial in Paget's disease and some types of osteoporosis (Fajardo & Di Cesare, 2005; Takeda, Taketani, Sawada, Sato, & Yamamoto, 2004).

The parathyroid gland produces the parathyroid hormone (PTH) and is considered the major hormone in controlling calcium and phosphorous metabolism. For example, when the calcium level falls in extracellular fluid, it is the job of the parathyroid hormone to bring the calcium levels up and the phosphorus levels down. Calcium and phosphorous homeostasis is maintained by PTH via three processes: (1) increases calcium in the blood by stimulating the number of osteoclasts to reabsorb bone mineral; (2) assists in the absorption of calcium in the small intestines by indirectly stimulating production of the active form of vitamin D in the kidney; and (3) binds to the receptors in the kidney to enhance tubular resorption of calcium, limiting the amount of calcium loss in the urine and increasing the excretion of renal phosphate and bicarbonate (Fajardo & Di Cesare, 2005).

Glucocorticoids are produced by the adrenal glands and are essential to the human body. In normal physiological concentrations, glucocorticoids promote bone cells; however, when

---

CHART 55–2   **Hormonal Effects on the Bone**

Gland	Hormones	Actions on Bone Tissue
Anterior pituitary gland	Growth hormone and somatotropin	• Stimulate the production of IGFs by the osteoblasts by stimulating longitudinal bone growth. • Increases the rate of mitosis of chondrocytes and osteoblasts. • Increases the rate of protein synthesis (collagen, cartilage matrix, and enzymes for cartilage and bone formation).
	Thyroid-stimulating hormone (TSH)	• Controls the rate of thyroxine production from the thyroid gland.
	Gonadotropins: luteinizing and follicle-stimulating hormones	• Controls growth and reproductive activities of the gonads.
Thyroid gland	Thyroxine (T_4) and triiodothyronine (T_3)	• Regulates the body's metabolic rate. • Increases the rate of protein synthesis. • Increases energy production from all food types.
	Calcitonin	• Peptide hormone. • Acts on the kidneys and bones to lower serum calcium levels. • Antagonist to PTH, which leads to lowering of the number of osteoclasts absorbed. • Delays calcium absorption from the intestine and increases calcium in the urine.
Parathyroid gland	Parathyroid hormone (PTH)	• Maintains normal serum calcium levels by secreting PTH, which increases bone resorption of calcium from bones to the blood, thereby raising blood calcium levels. • Increases the absorption of calcium by the small intestine and kidneys.
Adrenal glands	Glucocorticoids: cortisol	• Assist in the body's response to stress; suppressing inflammation, increasing serum glucose, and regulating metabolism of carbohydrates, fat, and protein. • Enhances protein synthesis. • Increases the breakdown of protein and fatty acids.
	Mineralocorticoids: aldosterone	• Regulates electrolyte concentrations (Na^+, K^+) in the extracellular fluid.
	Androgens: dehydroepiandrosterone sulfate and androstenedione	• Produce and maintain secondary sexual characteristics.

CHART 55-3   **Other Organ Systems and Hormones That Influence Bone Growth**

Organ	Hormone	Actions on Bone Tissue
Kidney	Vitamin D	Produced in the kidneys and affected by PTH, dietary intake of vitamin D (fat-soluble vitamin), and skin exposure to sunlight.
Ovaries or testes	Estrogen or testosterone	• Promotes closure of epiphyses of long bones, thereby stopping growth. • Assists with the retention of calcium in the bones, thereby maintaining a strong bone matrix.

---

glucocorticoid levels exceed normal concentration they have deleterious effects on the skeletal system. Either by direct or indirect means, high levels of glucocorticoids can reduce bone mass by (1) decreasing calcium absorption from the intestines, (2) reducing bone formation, (3) increasing bone resorption, (4) excreting calcium from the kidneys, and (5) decreasing the production of sex steroid (Copstead & Banaski, 2005; Fajardo & Di Cesare, 2005; Takeda et al., 2004). For example, high-dose glucocorticoids for infection can cause osteoporosis through the combination of decreasing bone formation and increasing bone resorption.

Vitamin D (1,25-dihydroxyvitamin) is produced by the kidneys and is a hormone. This hormone is under the influence of three factors: (1) PTH, (2) dietary intake of vitamin D (fat-soluble vita-

min), and (3) skin exposure to sunlight, or ultraviolet-B (UVB) radiation. Receptors to vitamin D are located in the bone, kidneys, intestines, and other cells. Vitamin D hormone is necessary for bone mineralization by promoting gastrointestinal absorption of calcium and phosphorus. When given in high doses, vitamin D can increase bone resorption (Fajardo & Di Cesare, 2005).

 *Women in northern latitudes have been shown to have a decline in their vitamin D levels during the winter months.*

Gonadal steroids are produced in the ovaries and testes. These include estrogen in females and androgens in males. Both contribute to maintaining bone metabolism by regulating rates of bone formation and bone resorption. These hormones are necessary for bone strength and decrease with aging (see the Gerontological Considerations box). Chart 55–4 summarizes hormone function and action on bone tissue.

Bone Disorders

Bone disorders can result from disuse, genetic or environmental influences, and traumatic injuries or accidents. Loss of function and independence may be experienced by an individual with bone disease. As a result the nurse must have a clear understanding of the effects of bone disease and how the disorder or disease will influence the individual. The focus of this section of the chapter is on the care of individuals with bone disease.

Osteoporosis

Bone is a matrix-mineral–like substance with varying degrees of density at various points within the structure. **Osteoporosis** is a skeletal disease that is characterized by low bone mass and deterioration of the bone tissue. This continued deterioration results

GERONTOLOGICAL CONSIDERATIONS Related to Changes in Bone Tissue

Changes in bone tissue that occur with aging include:

- Decline in muscle mass and connective tissue
- Reduction in cancellous bone (volume, number of cells, and width)
- Decline in bone density
- Reduction in gonadal status
- Reduction in estrogen levels
- Increase in osteoclast numbers and life expectancy
- Increased adiposity of bone marrow
- Decrease in blood vessels
- Reduction in cortical bone tissue related to bone absorption on the endosteal surface
- Increased porosity and decline in ability to deposit new bone on the endosteal surface
- Decline in hormonal response.

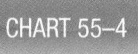

Hormone Function and Action on Bone Tissue

Hormone	Function	Clinical Manifestations
Anterior pituitary gland: growth hormone (somatropins)	Hypofunction	• *Children:* Delayed growth, fine features, and short stature proportionate • *Adult:* May be associated with hyposecretion of other pituitary hormones
	Hyperfunction	• *Children:* Increase linear growth and tall stature • *Adult:* acromegaly or giantism
Pituitary hyperstimulation of the adrenal cortex	Hypercortisolism or Cushing's syndrome	• Muscle weakness • Muscle wasting • Osteoporosis • Fractures
Thyroid-stimulating hormone (TSH)	Hyposecretion	• Retarded development • Dwarfism
Thyroxine (T_4) and triiodothyronine (T_3)	Hyposecretion	• Poor muscle tone • Growth retardation • Delayed bone development • Dwarfism • Loss of cortical and trabecular bone
	Hypersecretion	• Muscle weakness
Parathyroid	Hyposecretion	• Low serum calcium levels • Paresthesias, cramps, and spasms • Tetany • Chvostek's sign • Trousseau's sign
	Hypersecretion	• High serum calcium levels • Bone demineralization
Glucocorticoids		• Decline in bone formation and increased bone resorption • Osteoporosis • Fractures

in bone fragility and susceptibility to fractures (MacLean et al., 2008).

Epidemiology

Osteoporosis is the most common of the metabolic bone diseases (Frazier & Drzymkowski, 2009). It is estimated that 44 million people in the United States are affected by low bone mass and osteoporosis independent of race or ethnic background. More than 50% of women 50 years of age or older will have an osteoporotic fracture during their lifetime. Statistically, approximately 4% of patients more than 50 years of age who have a hip fracture die while hospitalized, and 24% die within 1 year after the injury (MacLean et al., 2008).

In the past osteoporosis was known primarily as a woman's disorder; however, research findings suggest that 19% of men over 50 years of age have been diagnosed with osteoporosis and 3.5 million men are at significant risk due to decreased bone mineral density. As with women, the changes in statistics are attributed to risk factors such as sedentary lifestyle, increased life expectancy, and history of fractures. In addition, advances in diagnostic screening in men have significantly improved. As a result, findings suggest that men are not immune to osteoporosis. The most recent statistics state that osteoporosis affects at least 25% of women and 12% of men over 50 years of age (Majumdar et al., 2008).

Risk factors for osteoporosis can serve as a guide for early detection; however, caution is advised because some individuals with osteoporosis do not demonstrate known risk factors. After the age of 30, when peak bone mass is reached and metabolic changes occur within the body, bone mass density begins to change. Loss of bone mass is a universal characteristic of humans; however, research findings suggest that genetic factors, body weight, smoking, alcohol, physical activity, and diet provide direct and indirect influences on the amount of bone mineral density loss (Raisz, 2005). See Chart 55–5 for a breakdown of risk factors for osteoporosis differentiated by gender.

Etiology and Pathophysiology

The disease process of osteoporosis is complex and insidious. Contributing factors such as genetic and environmental factors augment the complexity of the disease process (Cosman et al., 2005; Marcus & Gopalakrishnan, 2005). To understand the complicated etiology of osteoporosis, one must review the remodeling–modeling process of bone tissue.

Even under homeostatic conditions, bone remodeling appears to be intrinsically incompetent. As a result, the entire amount of bone replaced by formation does not always equal the amount removed earlier (Marcus & Gopalakrishnan, 2005). Genetic factors are linked to the maximal amount of bone mass a person has and correlate with the amount of skin pigmentation. Caucasians have the least bone mass, and African Americans have the most (Porth, 2005).

Unfortunately, over time and with the influence of extraneous variables (i.e., environmental factors, disease states), additional modification in the remodeling activity results in further loss of bone density and strength (Marcus & Gopalakrishnan, 2005). The age-related loss of bone occurs mainly in areas containing cancellous bone as in the spine and neck of the femur. This explains why these are common sites for fractures in patients with osteoporo-

CHART 55–5	Comparison by Gender of Risk Factors for Osteoporosis		
Risk Factor		**Women**	**Men**
Age: increased age is at greater risk		X	X
Small, thin-boned body frame		X	X
Ethnicity: Caucasian and Asian		X	X
Family history of fractures and osteoporosis		X	X
History of maternal hip fracture			X
Low body weight and low body mass index			X
Absence of estrogen (i.e., menopause)		X	
Unusually fast decline in testosterone (e.g., prostate cancer)			X
Decreased libido and impotence			X
Sedentary lifestyle or prolonged immobility		X	X
Anorexia		X	
Diet low in calcium and vitamin D		X	X
Malabsorption conditions (e.g., inflammatory bowel disease or gastric surgery)		X	X
Cigarette smoking		X	X
Excessive use of alcohol		X	X
Fractures after the age of 50 years		X	X
Decreased bone mineral density		X	X
Use of certain medications, such as corticosteroids and anticonvulsants		X	X
Presence of certain chronic medical conditions such as chronic renal failure or diabetes		X	X

sis. Osteoporosis may be primary or secondary to an underlying disease. Primary osteoporosis is the major category and includes three types: (1) idiopathic, (2) Type I postmenopausal, and (3) Type II (osteoporosis associated with the usual aging process). Idiopathic osteoporosis is uncommon and generally occurs in children and young adults with normal gonadal function. Idiopathic osteoporosis is a pediatric issue and is not discussed in this chapter. Type I osteoporosis, or postmenopausal osteoporosis, affects trabecular bone and occurs mainly in women ages 51 to 75 years old (Beers & Porter, 2006; Marcus & Gopalakrishnan, 2005). In Type II osteoporosis, osteoporotic changes are associated with the usual aging process (Beers & Porter, 2006).

In Type I or postmenopausal osteoporosis, there is an increase in the activity of the osteoclasts and a decline in the activity of the osteoblasts (bone formation), leading to increased bone resorption. Menopause is associated with the reduction of estrogen that is needed for the bone formation process, causing a decline in bone mineral density and strength that results in thin fragile bones. Bone loss generally stabilizes about 10 years after menopause (Hunter & Sambrook, 2000).

Type II osteoporosis is a result of the normal aging process. As an individual ages there is a decline in the number and activity of osteoblasts, which affects both trabecular and cortical bone. This type of osteoporosis is generally observed in adults who are 60 years of age or older. Both Type I and II osteoporosis can be observed in older women (McCance & Huether, 2006).

In some cases, osteopenias resulting from exercise-related amenorrhea and from prolactin-secreting tumors are considered to be primary osteoporosis (Marcus & Gopalakrishnan, 2005). Secondary osteoporosis is associated with bone loss resulting from clinical disorders (e.g., thyrotoxicosis and hyperadrenocorticism) and disorders of intestinal and renal function (Marcus & Gopalakrishnan, 2005). Research findings suggest there is a degree of bone loss related to the amount and duration of glucocorticoid use in humans. It appears that there is an increased rate of bone reabsorption (increasing osteoclastogenesis and decreasing the level of osteoprotegerin) and a slower rate of bone remodeling (decreasing the osteoblast population). In addition, glucocorticoids decrease calcium absorption by the gastrointestinal tract. Research findings suggest that postmenopausal women who have been diagnosed with rheumatoid arthritis and are taking steroids have a higher incident of generalized osteoporosis resulting in fractures, pain, and disability (Forsblad et al., 2003; Jochems et al., 2005). A few other causes of secondary osteoporosis include chronic obstructive pulmonary disease (COPD), immobilization, liver disease, rheumatoid arthritis, and sarcoidosis (Marcus & Gopalakrishnan, 2005). Chart 55–6 gives sources of secondary osteoporosis and their influence on bone.

Regardless of the cause, osteoporotic changes occur in both cortical and cancellous bone. The hard, outer surface of the cortex (diaphysis and metaphysis) in cortical bone begins to thin, and increased intracortical porosity occurs within the bone. As the disease progresses, there is a loss of the trabeculae of the cancellous bone (spongy bone containing the red bone marrow and located in the metaphysis of long bone). Further progress will result in thinning of the bone into the interior of the cancellous bone (spongy bone that contains both red and yellow marrow). Besides changes in the bone density there is also loss of trabecular connectivity.

Skeletal fragility is influenced by the ability of the bone cells to develop and includes (1) the inability to develop a skeleton that has sufficient mass and strength; (2) an imbalance resulting in bone resorption becoming greater than bone formation, leading to changes in the bone mass and structure; and (3) an insufficient formation reaction to improved resorption during bone remodeling (Raisz, 2005). Any change in the process of bone turnover will result in changes in bone structure. As a result, osteoporosis is a multifactorial and complex disease (Figure 55–4 ■).

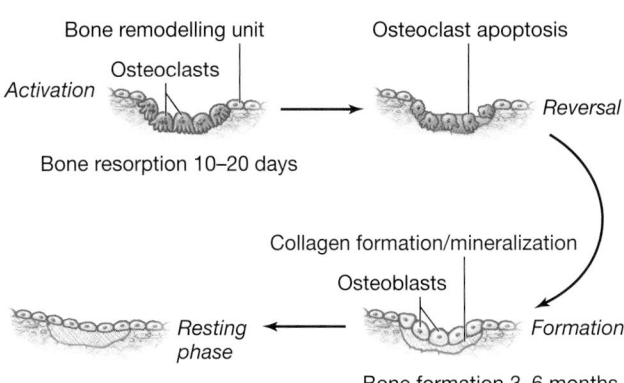

FIGURE 55–4 ■ Bone turnover cycle.

Clinical Manifestations

The clinical manifestations of osteoporosis may go undetected because individuals are often asymptomatic until the later stages. As the bone mass declines in both cortical and cancellous bone, the bone becomes fragile and has a higher risk of fracturing. Therefore, a fracture after minor trauma may be the first indication of having osteoporosis.

Common sites for osteoporosis involve the hand, wrist, spine, hip, knees, and feet. Fractures are common in the hip, vertebrae, and wrist. Osteoporosis is not only found in isolation but has been associated with rheumatoid arthritis, a side effect of glucocorticoid use, and in individuals with chronic renal failure. Regardless, a medical diagnosis of osteoporosis might not be determined until after the individual is hospitalized with a fracture (Lim et al., 2004). Signs and symptoms include fractures after a minor fall, kyphosis, loss of height, pain aggravated by movement or jarring, pathologic fractures of the spine and femur, spontaneous wedge fractures, and vertebral collapse producing pain that radiates around the trunk.

Laboratory and Diagnostic Procedures

Assessment of bone mass is the primary measurement for osteoporosis. Because osteoporosis results from a decline in bone density, low bone mass is the most important measurement to make a diagnosis and decide on the level of intervention. Therefore, bone mineral density tests are used to measure the bone density at various sites of the body. The DEXA is a dual-photon absorptiometry x-ray–based technique that allows measurement of any skeletal site as well as the entire skeleton because the technology corrects for soft tissue. Bone mineral content is measured and then compared to bone density values obtained in a reference population of the same race, gender, and age (Cosman et al., 2005).

Other studies that show a decline in bone mineral and bone structure include CT scan, ultrasound, regular x-rays, and, in rare cases, bone biopsy. Computed tomography (CT) is used to measure the spine. Peripheral CT units can be used to measure bone in the forearm or tibia. The results of the CT are based on a pure sample of trabecular bone because it measures true volumetric density (Cosman et al., 2005). The use of ultrasound provides additional information because it sends ultrasound crosswise through the bone and provides information on the amount of bone present. Radiologic examination will

| CHART 55–6 | Examples of Secondary Osteoporosis and Influence on Bone Resorption and Bone Formation |

Source	Bone Resorption	Bone Formation
Glucocorticoids	Normal to increased	Decreased
Hyperthyroidism	Increased	Increased
Immobilization	Increased then normal	Decreased
Heparin	Probably increased	Uncertain
Hypervitaminosis A	Increased	Uncertain
Anticonvulsants	Increased	Increased

Source: Marcus, R., & Gopalakrishnan, G. (2005). Secondary forms of osteoporosis. In F. L. Coe & M. J. Favus (Eds.), *Disorders of bone and mineral metabolism.* Philadelphia: Lippincott Raven Publishers.

demonstrate osteoporotic changes within the bone only after 30% to 60% loss of bone mass has occurred. Finally, bone biopsy will show thin, porous bone structure, and serum bone gal-protein (indicator of bone turnover) is elevated.

With regard to the diagnosis of osteoporosis, biochemical markers are now available that evaluate the process of bone modeling and remodeling. Biomarker response to therapy is useful for asymptomatic patients.

A general evaluation may be necessary to determine other problems and potential contributing factors to osteoporosis. A general evaluation may include (1) complete blood count (CBC), (2) serum calcium and phosphorus, (3) urine calcium, and (4) alkaline phosphatase (Cosman et al., 2005). For example, a CBC would provide information on infection, malnutrition, and anemias. A test of serum calcium and phosphorous levels would provide information on the level of calcium and phosphorus in relationship to malnutrition, osteomalacia, and abnormal levels in conjunction with hyper/hypo states. Urine calcium provides information on osteomalacia, malnutrition, and malabsorption as well as hyper/hypo states. Alkaline phosphatase will assess liver and bone isoenzymes. See Chart 55–7 for a summary of other labs that might be done and what contributing factors of osteoporosis are being assessed.

Screening for osteoporosis is relatively inexpensive. In addition, in 1998, the Bone Mass Measurement Act required Medicare to reimburse for bone mineral density tests. Anyone who has risk factors for osteoporosis is strongly encouraged to have a bone mineral density test. Testing for osteoporosis, especially in females, should start at age 50 and men ages 70 and

older. In the presence of fracture or history of fracture after the age of 45, both men and women are recommended to have a bone mineral density test. Men and women who have disorders or conditions that predispose them to low bone mineral density or who are on medications associated with bone loss (i.e., steroid therapy) are recommended to have their bone mineral density assessed on a regular basis. In general, bone mineral density tests are recommended to be done every 2 years but the frequency depends on the individual.

Medical Management

Management of osteoporosis is basically preventive in nature and begins in childhood. It is important to maintain an adequate supply of calcium and vitamin D throughout life in order to maintain peak bone mass. Exercise stimulates bone formation as a result of the mechanical load it places on bones. Preventing osteoporosis requires a multidisciplinary approach with members of the multidisciplinary team including a physician, nurse, exercise physiologist, physical therapist, occupational therapist, and nutritionist.

The goal of treatment is to prevent further bone loss and maintain independence and functionability of the individual. A holistic approach for medical management would involve screening, identification of underlying etiology, education, and pharmacologic and nonpharmacologic approaches (i.e., exercise and complementary alternative strategies) (National Institutes of Health [NIH], 2007). See Chart 55–8 for strategies for holistic patient management.

Pharmaceutical strategies may include medications to manage the osteoporosis and pain associated with the disease. A

CHART 55–7 Labs for Further Evaluation of Osteoporosis

Pertinent Labs	Normal Range	Contributory Disorders
TSH	2–10 µU/mL	
Free T$_4$	4–12 mcg/dL	• Thyroid function: hypo/hyperfunction
T$_3$	Varies with age	
Urinary cortisol	<100 mcg/24 hours	• Cushing's syndrome
Serum cholesterol	<200 mg/dL	• Bowel disease, malabsorption, or malnutrition
Serum albumin	3.5–5 g/dL	
Serum calcium	9–10.5 mg/dL	• Parathyroid gland (hypo/hypercalcemia), malignancy, or malnutrition
Serum PTH	10–65 pg/mL	• Parathyroid gland (hypercalcemia) or malignancy
Serum GLA-protein		• Rate of bone turnover
Hemoglobin	12–18 g/dL	• Anemia, malabsorption, or malnutrition
Hematocrit	37%–52%	
Antigliadin antibody test	negative	• Asymptomatic celiac sprue with selective malabsorption
Antiendomysial antibody test	negative	
Urine calcium, 24-hour	50–400 mg/24 hours	• <50 mg/day: osteomalacia, malnutrition, or malabsorption
		• >300 mg/day: hypercalcemia (Paget's disease), hyperparathyroidism, and hyperthyroidism
Serum immunoelectrophoresis	Subject to pathologist's interpretation	• Exclude the diagnosis of myeloma
Urine immunoelectrophoresis	Subject to pathologist's interpretation	
Bone biopsy	Rare	• Labeling and determination of rate of remodeling

CHART 55–8	Strategies for Holistic Management of Osteoporosis	
Pharmacologic	**Nonpharmacologic**	**Complementary Alternative Strategies**
Bisphosphates	Diet: total daily intake of 1,200–1,500 mg/day of calcium	Acupuncture
Estrogen	Exercise	Biofeedback
• Conjugated equine estrogens	• Aerobic: walking and jogging	Healing touch
• Estradiol	• Anaerobic: high impact exercises	Massage
• Estrone	• Stretching	Reflexology
• Esterified estrogen	• Yoga	Physiohelanics
• Ethinyl estradiol		
• Mestranol		
Calcitonin	Kyphoplasty	
Estrogen and progestin	Vertebroplasty	
PTH		
Other:		
• Selective estrogen response modulators		
• Tamoxifen		
• Raloxifene		
• Vitamin D		

health care provider may choose to treat the patient with a variety of medications: pain medication, anti-inflammatory medication (steroidal and nonsteroidal), bisphosphonates, calcitonin, calcium and vitamin D supplements, and PTH. In addition, the medication regimen might be aimed at suppressing bone resorption and increasing bone formation (NIH, 2007). For example, PTH is used to reverse the inhibitory effects of bone formation in secondary osteoporosis resulting from the use of glucocorticoids (Canalis, 2004).

Pharmacologic strategies include hormone replacement therapy for women who are postmenopausal and bisphosphonates to inhibit bone resorption. Calcium and vitamin D are important to bone mass. Adequate calcium intake is needed for peak bone mass and vitamin D is necessary for the absorption of calcium (Beers & Porter, 2006). See the Pharmacology Summary feature (p. 1738) for more information about medications to treat osteoporosis.

Nonpharmacologic strategies include diet and exercise. Diet and an adequate activity level can transform the genetic potential of an individual. Protein, vitamins, and minerals are important to the production of bone matrix. A diet that has less than the recommended dosage of protein, calcium, vitamins (C, D, and K), copper, manganese, and zinc will result in a lower bone mass density. Because bone responds to mechanical loading, an exercise behavior that includes high impact forces is recommended. Strength training is just one example of mechanical loading of the muscle and bone tissue (Marcus & Gopalakrishnan, 2005).

Complementary and alternative strategies are palliative in nature. These strategies can provide the individual with the ability to deal with pain (acute and chronic) and stress. Strategies such as biofeedback, yoga, massage, and reflexology can aid the individual in relief of pain, physical, emotional, and mental stress. These strategies can help increase the body's energy system to a state of well-being (NIH, 2007).

Nursing Management

Nursing care of the patient with osteoporosis is focused on the primary goals of maintaining independence and function, preserving bone mass, and preventing fractures. The majority of the strategies focus on education and behavioral changes.

Assessment

The initial step in the nursing process is assessment. In a patient with osteoporosis the focus of the assessment is identification of risk factors and problems that may be associated with the disease. Inquire regarding family history, previous fractures, dietary habits, exercise patterns, onset of menopause, use of alcohol, tobacco, corticosteroids, and caffeine consumption. Assessment of the individual's general appearance and posture can provide useful information about the structure and motion of the skeletal system. Therefore, the patient's height, weight, and body characteristics serve as objective data. In addition, assessing the spinal column for conditions of kyphosis, lordosis, and spinal deformity (dowager's hump) may suggest osteoporotic changes in the affected area.

The majority of patients with osteoporosis will be elderly. The nurse is responsible for identifying limitations not associated with the aging process and should differentiate from changes associated with osteoporosis. Older adults tend to have more than one medical condition, therefore, the nurse must expand her assessment to include other systems such as cardiovascular and neurological. Chart 55–9 (p. 1739) lists assessment summary and cues for osteoporosis.

PHARMACOLOGY Summary for Bone Disorders

Medication Category	Action	Application/Indication	Nursing Responsibilities
Bone Resorption Inhibitor			
Biphosphonates (Fosamax)	Reduces the activity of cells that cause bone loss, slow rate of bone loss after menopause, and increase the amount of bone mass	Prevention of postmenopausal osteoporosis	• Monitor serum calcium level before, during, and after treatment. • Ensure adequate dietary intake of calcium and vitamin D. • Teach patient to take medication in the morning with a full glass of water. Orange juice, coffee, and mineral water reduce the drug's effects. • To reduce esophageal irritation, teach patient not to chew or suck on the pill. • Teach patient to wait at least 30 minutes after taking the medication before eating, drinking, or taking another medication. • The patient should remain upright for 30 minutes after taking medication and until she has eaten the first food of the day.
Risedronate (Actonel)	Hinders excessive bone remodeling by binding to bone and reducing the rate at which osteoclasts are resorbed by bone	Treatment of Paget's disease of bone when serum alkaline phosphatase level is at least twice normal and patient is symptomatic	• Administer supplemental calcium and vitamin D. • Give calcium supplements and antacids at different times of day than risedronate to avoid impaired drug absorption. • Teach patient to take the medication at least 1 hour before first food or drink of the day while in an upright position and with a full glass of water. • Caution patient to remain upright for at least 30 minutes after taking medication.
Osteoporosis Prophylactic			
Raloxifene (Evista)	Prevents osteoporosis by binding to estrogen receptors, which decreases bone mineral density in postmenopausal women	Prevention of osteoporosis in postmenopausal women	• Assess distal extremities for impaired circulation and pain that may indicate thromboembolism. • Discontinue drug at least 72 hours before and during periods of prolonged immobilization. • Teach patient to avoid lengthy immobilization during travel due to the increased risk of thromboembolism.

Nursing Diagnosis

Nursing diagnoses for the patient with osteoporosis will be based on objective and subjective data collected during the assessment phase. Potential nursing diagnoses for osteoporosis include:

- *Pain* related to fracture and muscle spasm
- *Injury, Risk for* related to additional fracures due to osteoporosis
- *Constipation, Risk for* related to immobility and/or medications.

Outcomes and Evaluation Parameters

Outcomes for the patient with osteoporosis include relief from pain as verbalized by the patient. It is important for the patient to follow the treatment regimen to prevent further bone loss, increase strength and stability, and prevent additional fractures. The patient and family should institute preventive measures for safety in their environment. If they are sedentary, the patient may become constipated. Proper diet, mobility, and treatment regimen should improve bowel elimination with no signs of constipation or ileus.

Planning, Interventions, and Rationales

Educational interventions are focused on the following: (1) disease process, (2) risk factors, (3) medical management (pharmacologic interventions), (4) nonpharmacologic interventions, and (5) complementary and alternative strategies. It is very im-

| CHART 55–9 | **Nursing Assessment and Cues for Assessing a Patient with Osteoporosis** |

Assessment	Cues for Assessing
Cognitive ability	• Impairments: what, when, how, and current management
Current activity level	• Participation in activity: type, frequency, and duration
	• Activities of daily living
Environment	• Home environment
History of risk factors	• Identify the risk factors for osteoporosis
History of fractures	• When, how, and course of recovery
History of musculoskeletal disorders	• What, when, course of treatment, and current management
Location of discomfort	• When did it occur?
	• How did it occur?
	• Any precipitating factors?
Range of motion	• Ability and limitations
Neurological	• Dementia? Delirium?
	• Dizziness? Syncope? Orthostatic challenge
Impaired mobility	• Assess gait, balance, posture, and center of gravity
Medical history	• Past history of illnesses
Medications/recreational and prescribed	• List of medications, dosage, and frequency
Mood	• Verbalization of feelings
	• Ability to concentrate
Pain	• Verbalization of location, intensity, and description
	• Precipitating factors and factors that relieve
Posture and general appearance	• Observe for lordosis, scoliosis, and kyphosis
	• Height and weight

portant for the patient to understand the disease process. Identification of risk factors is needed so the patient can make an informed decision and modify any detrimental lifestyle behaviors. Depending on the clinical setting, monitoring the implemented strategies for changing behaviors may be achieved by asking the patient to keep a journal, followed by reinforcement of positive behavioral changes.

Teaching about the various prescribed medications is always essential to the educational component. Many of the medications prescribed for osteoporosis cause a variety of side effects. It is important for the patient to be knowledgeable about side effects and strategies for prevention. Therefore, the purpose, dosage, frequency, side effects, and special considerations should be reviewed with the patient. For example, some medications slow down gastrointestinal motility. As a result, individuals with osteoporosis have problems with constipation. It is prudent to educate the patient on monitoring the physiological response to new medications and combining medications. It is essential to assess the use of over-the-counter (OTC) drugs, vitamins, and minerals, because polypharmacy in the older adult is common. Refer to the Pharmacology Summary for a summary of pharmacologic agents.

Educational interventions for nonpharmacologic strategies include exercise and diet. The patient with osteoporosis can benefit from learning about the positive aspects of exercise on bone mass. If the patient with osteoporosis is active and wishes to remain active, an exercise physiologist can evaluate and prescribe an appropriate exercise program for the patient. However, if the patient has been sedentary for a significant period of time, consultation with a physical and occupational therapist may be the first step in intervening. Moderate exercise is best and can be achieved with walking, swimming, or riding a stationary bicycle.

Another lifestyle modification that may need to be implemented is a dietary modification. After assessing the patient's diet, the nurse may learn the patient may benefit from nutritional counseling and an adequate calcium and vitamin D intake. Good dietary sources of calcium include low-fat dairy products, spinach, kale, beans and legumes, broccoli, tofu, fortified orange juice, salmon, and sardines. Natural sources of vitamin D include cod liver oil, fatty fish, and eggs (Hogan, DeLeon, Gingrich, & Willcutts, 2007). Calcium nutrition is important during the adolescent growth spurt and in postmenopausal women. The surgeon general's report on *Bone Health and Osteoporosis* published recommendations for adequate calcium intake (U.S. Department of Health and Human Services [USDHHS], 2004). For adults the surgeon general recommends 1,000 to 1,200 milligrams of calcium depending on the age of the individual (NIH, 2007; USDHHS, 2004).

Immobility can be a result of osteoporosis. Slowing of the gastrointestinal tract function can result from immobility and the effects of the medication. The nurse should educate the patient about strategies to prevent constipation (diet high in fiber, exercise, and if prescribed, medication) and the potential risk of an ileus.

Other nursing interventions may include the following: administration of prescribed pain medication, advocating, and encouraging. Through education and encouragement, the nurse can promote understanding about adequate pain relief so the patient can focus on learning, participating, and maintaining functionability and self-care (see Chapter 15 ⊚).

The nurse can advocate for assistance in the home and self-care activities. If prescribed, the nurse can encourage the wearing of splints or braces to ensure proper musculoskeletal alignment. Education on protective pads worn on or around bony prominences can prevent fractures. The nurse promotes health by encouraging adherence to behavioral changes to promote peak bone mass and functionability.

Safety is an important consideration for patients with osteoporosis. Pain, weakness, and stiffness can place the individual at risk for falls resulting in fractures. Reviewing a patient's home environment may reveal dangerous situations (i.e., rugs and furniture within the traveled path) and may prevent falls that can lead to costly and debilitating bone fractures.

Osteoporosis is associated with the aging process but is not part of the normal aging process. Reduction of risk factors, adequate nutrition, and weight-bearing activities such as jogging, walking, jumping, and strength training can help preserve bone mass and strength. In addition, coordination and balance can be improved with endurance, strength, and flexibility training. If the goal is to maintain independence and the ability to function with daily activities, interventions aimed at improving muscle strength, coordination, and flexibility lowers the individual's risk for falling.

Fracture and Pathologic Fractures

A bone fracture is a major concern and a negative consequence of osteoporosis and cancer. Sustaining a fracture, especially in the aging population, is costly and renders the individual dependent and disabled (Hunter & Sambrook, 2000; Lim et al., 2004). A fracture is sustained when the individual experiences a complete or incomplete break in the continuity of bone or cartilage. A fracture can occur in any shape or size of bone in the body. In addition, a fracture can result from either direct or indirect trauma according to whether the forces are applied to the bone involved or at a distance from the affected bone and transmitted to it. The incidence of fracture is increased in patients who have low bone density.

The American Academy of Orthopaedic Surgeons (AAOS, 2008) estimates that there are about 7 million broken bones a year in this country. As a result, fractures are considered the most common orthopedic complaint facing the health care system. It has been estimated that one out of every two women and one out of every four men over the age of 50 will experience an osteoporosis-related fracture during their lifetime (NIH, 2007). Women ages 50 years and older are at risk for sustaining one of the following types of fractures: 17.5% risk for hip fracture, 16% for vertebral fractures, and 16% for Colles' fractures. For men the risk of sustaining a fracture is somewhat lower: 6% for hip fractures, 5% for vertebral fractures, and 2.5% for Colles' fractures (Hunter & Sambrook, 2000).

Etiology of Fractures

As an individual ages, there is a decline in muscle function, development of sarcopenia (decline in muscle mass), and slowing of the rate of bone resorption and remodeling. The decline in these three factors is observed in the aging process and contributes to the process of bone loss. For the older adult, common fracture sites relating to osteoporosis include hips, vertebrae, and wrists (Hunter & Sambrook, 2000; NIH, 2007). Fractures resulting from osteoporosis can leave the individual dependent and disabled, resulting in a decrease in their quality of life.

Fractures are costly, debilitating, and have long-term implications. For example, a fracture of the spine and hip can leave the individual physiologically, psychosocially, and economically disabled from the health costs and the recovery process. Not only can fractures negatively influence the quality of life of an individual, but morbidity is a detrimental outcome of sustaining a fracture (Hunter & Sambrook, 2000; Lim et al., 2004). For a detailed discussion regarding the pathophysiology, clinical manifestations, diagnosis and management of fractured bone, refer to Chapter 56 ⊚ .

■ Nursing Management

Acute care of musculoskeletal trauma is discussed in Chapter 56 ⊚ . Nursing care in the acute phase focuses on assessment, stabilization, and preparing the patient for surgery if necessary. Because fractures can be caused by a crushing force or direct blow, it is important during the initial assessment that the type of injury be communicated. Therefore, a historical account of the event may be helpful if the patient is conscious. Information that may be helpful includes type and time of injury, the environment in which the injury occurred, any concurrent injuries, past medical history and surgeries, and medications used. The majority of nursing care will focus on monitoring and prevention of complications. Therefore, monitoring the hemodynamics of the patient and using anticipatory strategies are essential.

Sustaining a fracture may interfere with the patient's ability to provide self-care. During the hospitalization the nurse may need to assist the patient with activities of daily living (ADLs). Family members may need to be educated on how to care for the patient, especially if the patient is discharged prior to rehabilitation.

The overall goal in the planning and implementation phase is to promote healing resulting in restored function of the affected body part. Recovery involves a multidisciplinary approach. In the older population, fractures can result in prolonged recovery periods and increase the risk for morbidity. A goal is to promote physical mobility; therefore, rehabilitation is begun as soon as possible to restore function. Physical therapy provides the patient with the knowledge and skills required to prevent muscle atrophy and enhance mobility with the use of assistive devices such as a walker and crutches. Because the hip is a common site for fracture in the elderly and patients with osteoporosis, the accompanying Nursing Process: Patient Care Plan for a Fractured Hip feature has been provided.

Health Promotion

Health promotion strategies can focus on education. For example, the community needs to be aware of safety measures that can be taken to prevent fractures while at home, work, or during leisure activities. Learning the importance of wearing seat belts and having airbags in automobiles can lessen a person's chances of experiencing blunt trauma during a car accident. An assessment of the home environment can reveal potential hazards for

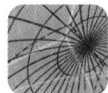

NURSING PROCESS: Patient Care Plan for a Fractured Hip

Assessment of Pain

Subjective Data:
Age/gender
Is the fracture communicating with the environment?
Cause of injury?
Vital signs
Pain: location, severity, description, and score

Objective Data:
Visual inspection of affected extremity:
Swelling
Joint limitation
Skin temperature changes
Observable deformities?
- Shortened
- Abducted/adducted?
- Rotation?

Vital signs
Overt and covert expressions of pain (i.e., grimacing)

Nursing Assessment and Diagnoses	Outcomes and Evaluation Parameters	Planning and Interventions with *Rationales*
Nursing Diagnosis: *Pain* related to fracture	**Outcome:** Comfort level maintained. *Evaluation Parameters:* Reports adequate pain control. Participates in ADLs without pain.	**Interventions and *Rationales:*** Assess for pain using a pain scale from 0–10. Additionally, description of the pain and location should be assessed. *To maintain consistency in assessing pain.* Assess cultural and religious beliefs about pain and pain relief. *In a dynamic system there is an interaction and transaction between one's physiological condition and one's cultural and religious beliefs. As a result, one's cultural and religious beliefs may impact how pain is treated. Treatment may involve strategies other than traditional Western medicine.*

Assessment of Impaired Physical Mobility

Subjective Data:
Do you experience pain that interferes with activity?
Are there activities you feel you are unable to do?

Objective Data:
Assess:
Strength and balance
Response to activity by taking vital signs at rest and then after they perform an activity
Coping strategies

Nursing Assessment and Diagnoses	Outcomes and Evaluation Parameters	Planning and Interventions with *Rationales*
Nursing Diagnosis: *Physical Mobility, Impaired* related to fractured hip	**Outcomes:** The patient will develop independence. The patient will be able to ambulate with minimal assistance. *Evaluation Parameters:* The patient will participate in physical therapy activities. The patient will be able to exercise without significant pain or activity intolerance.	**Interventions and *Rationales:*** While in bed maintain neutral positioning of hip with a trochanter roll and a pillow between the legs when turning. *Neutral positioning prevents stress on the fixation and minimizes external rotation. Supporting the legs with pillows during turning prevents adduction of the hip.* Teach the patient how to accomplish position changes by herself. Teach the patient isometric exercises to maintain and increase strength of the quadriceps and gluteal muscles. *Strengthening of muscles assists with ambulation. Teaching patients how to position themselves encourages their active participation in their care and prevents unwanted stress on the hip.*

Assessment of Nutritional Intake

Subjective Data:
Describe your usual intake pattern.
Is this intake sufficient?
Do you have religious dietary restrictions or practices?
How often do you exercise?
Who prepares your meals?
Do you feel you have enough energy?

Objective Data:
General appearance
Weight
Hair, nails, and skin
Muscle mass
Edema

(continued)

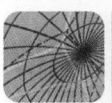

NURSING PROCESS: Patient Care Plan for a Fractured Hip—*Continued*

Nursing Assessment and Diagnoses	Outcomes and Evaluation Parameters	Planning and Interventions with *Rationales*
Nursing Diagnosis: *Nutrition, Imbalanced: Less Than Body Requirements*	**Outcome:** The patient will maintain adequate nutrition to assist with healing. **Evaluation Parameter:** Maintenance of weight without loss of muscle mass.	**Interventions and *Rationales:*** Facilitate education with a dietary consultant. *Consultation can ensure a diet that provides optimal caloric and nutrient intake.* Encourage frequent oral hygiene. *Poor oral hygiene leads to bad breath and a bad taste in the mouth, which decreases the appetite.* Provide the patient with printed material outlining dietary needs and restrictions. *Aids the patient in selecting the proper foods.* Promote the intake of protein foods with high biologic value: eggs, meats, and dairy products. *Complete proteins provide the positive nitrogen balance needed for growth and healing.* If the patient has osteoporosis, encourage intake of foods rich in calcium: Low-fat dairy products Spinach Kale Beans and other legumes Broccoli Tofu Salmon Sardines. Also encourage foods rich in vitamin D: Cod liver oil Fatty fish Eggs Fortified foods such as milk and cereals. *Calcium adds strength and stiffness to bones. Vitamin D is essential for calcium absorption and normal bone mineralization.*

Assessment of Skin Integrity

Subjective Data:
Is the discomfort in the area of your surgical incision decreasing?
Have you noticed any drainage from the surgical site?
Inquire if the patient is experiencing pain, itching, or discomfort to any area on the skin.

Objective Data:
Assess the patient's skin and surgical site for redness, swelling, or drainage.

Nursing Assessment and Diagnoses	Outcomes and Evaluation Parameters	Planning and Interventions with *Rationales*
Nursing Diagnosis: *Skin Integrity, Impaired: Risk for* related to immobility and surgical incision	**Outcome:** Patient will achieve wound healing and not develop a pressure ulcer. **Evaluation Parameters:** The patient will relate minimal discomfort at the surgical site, and the incision will remain without signs of infection. The patient will show no signs of redness over bony prominences.	**Interventions and *Rationales:*** Monitor vital signs and lab results. *Temperature, pulse, and white blood cell count may increase in response to infection.* Maintain use of aseptic technique. *Use of aseptic technique avoids the introduction of infectious organisms.* Assess surgical site for appearance and character of drainage. *Redness, edema, and drainage at the surgical site indicate infection.* Reposition the patient every 2 hours and assess skin for redness or change in sensation. Add padding to bony prominences. *Repositioning and adding padding relieves pressure on the bony prominences. Redness or a change in sensation on the skin may indicate the development of a pressure ulcer.*

falling, especially for the elderly population. It is recommended that pathways in the house be cleared of furniture, throw rugs, and clutter. For the older adult adequate lighting and proper footwear are essential in preventing unnecessary falls causing fractures.

Evidence-Based Practice

As stated earlier, screening for risk factors and falls assessment will identify those who are at risk for osteoporosis and/or falls

and fractures. The New Zealand Guidelines Group developed a best practice, evidence-based guideline that provides recommendations for appropriate and effective processes for assessment of personal, social, functional, and clinical needs in older people. The Evidence-Based Practice box includes the evidence-based guideline for the prevention of hip fractures in people ages 65 years and older.

Prevention of Hip Fracture in People Ages 65 Years and Older

Clinical Problem

Older people are at a high risk for falls and hip fracture. Guidelines for evaluation of risk factors and preventive strategies will decrease the prevalence of the problem.

The following guideline from the New Zealand Guideline Group provides an evidence-based summary of the clinical aspects of hip fracture prevention and preventive strategies for those older people at high risk of hip fracture.

Research Findings

The consequences of hip fractures in older people create a significant and increasing burden of illness in the community, and can precipitate a dramatic decline in physical function. Twenty percent of older people who sustain a hip fracture die within a year. Two years after the fracture, survivors are more than four times likely to have limited mobility than people of similar age without a fracture and are more than twice as likely to be functionally dependent. Evidence shows that women are at greater risk of hip fracture than men, and this risk increases steadily and substantially with age. In addition to gender, other factors that increase the risk of hip fracture are:

- Living in institutional care
- Significant cognitive impairment
- Certain medications (e.g., anticonvulsants, corticosteroids)
- Personal history and lifestyle factors
- Certain medical conditions (e.g., type II diabetes in women)
- Low bone mineral density.

The guideline makes recommendations on risk assessment and effective preventive strategies for reducing hip fractures. A second guideline has been developed for acute management and immediate rehabilitation after hip fracture in people ages 65 years and over and is available from the New Zealand Guideline Group.

Recommendations for Risk Assessment of Individuals at High Risk of Hip Fracture

Individuals at high risk of sustaining a hip fracture include the following:

- Women ages 80 years and older and men ages 85 years and older
- Women ages 70 years and older and men ages 75 years and older:
  - Living in institutional care OR
  - With significant cognitive impairment.
- Women ages 70 years and older and men ages 75 years and older with one or more of the following conditions:
  - Visual acuity 0.2 (6/30)
  - History of a fall with fracture in the previous year
  - History of frequent falling

- Type II diabetes (evidence available for women only)
- If currently using any of the following medications:
  - Anticonvulsant therapy
  - Opioids (including propoxyphene containing pain medication)
  - Corticosteroids (doses greater than prednisone 5 mg/day or equivalent)
  - Any psychotropic drug
  - Type Ia antiarrhythmics.
- Women ages 70 years and over with three or all of the following four personal history/lifestyle factors:
  - Smoking history
  - Personal history of any previous fracture
  - History of maternal hip fracture
  - Low body mass index.
- Women ages 65 years and older are at high risk if their bone mineral density (BMD) is 2 standard deviations (SDs) below normal for age (Z-score > −2.0), and 75 years and older if BMD is 1 SD below normal for age (Z-score > −1.0). The decision on prevention/treatment should take into account Z-score AND other risk factors.
- Men ages 75 years and older with any of the following personal history/lifestyle factors:
  - Low body mass index
  - Smoking history
  - History of spine, hip, or wrist fracture
  - History of stroke.
- Men ages 70 years and older are at high risk if their BMD is 2 SDs below normal for age (Z-score > −2.0), and 80 years and older if BMD is 1 SD below normal for age (Z-score > −1.0). The decision on prevention/treatment should take into account Z-score AND other risk factors.

Screening

- The available evidence does not support the use of BMD measurement for population screening of asymptomatic individuals.
- At present, there is only limited evidence that the use of BMD measurement in selected individuals is effective in reducing the risk of future fractures.

Recommendations for Preventive Strategies
Preventing Falls

- A program of muscle strengthening and balance training, individually prescribed by a trained health professional in a New Zealand primary health care setting, reduces the frequency of falls in high risk community-dwelling older people.

(continued)

RISK ASSESSMENT & PREVENTIVE STRATEGIES
FOR HIP FRACTURE IN OLDER PEOPLE

SUMMARY ALGORITHM

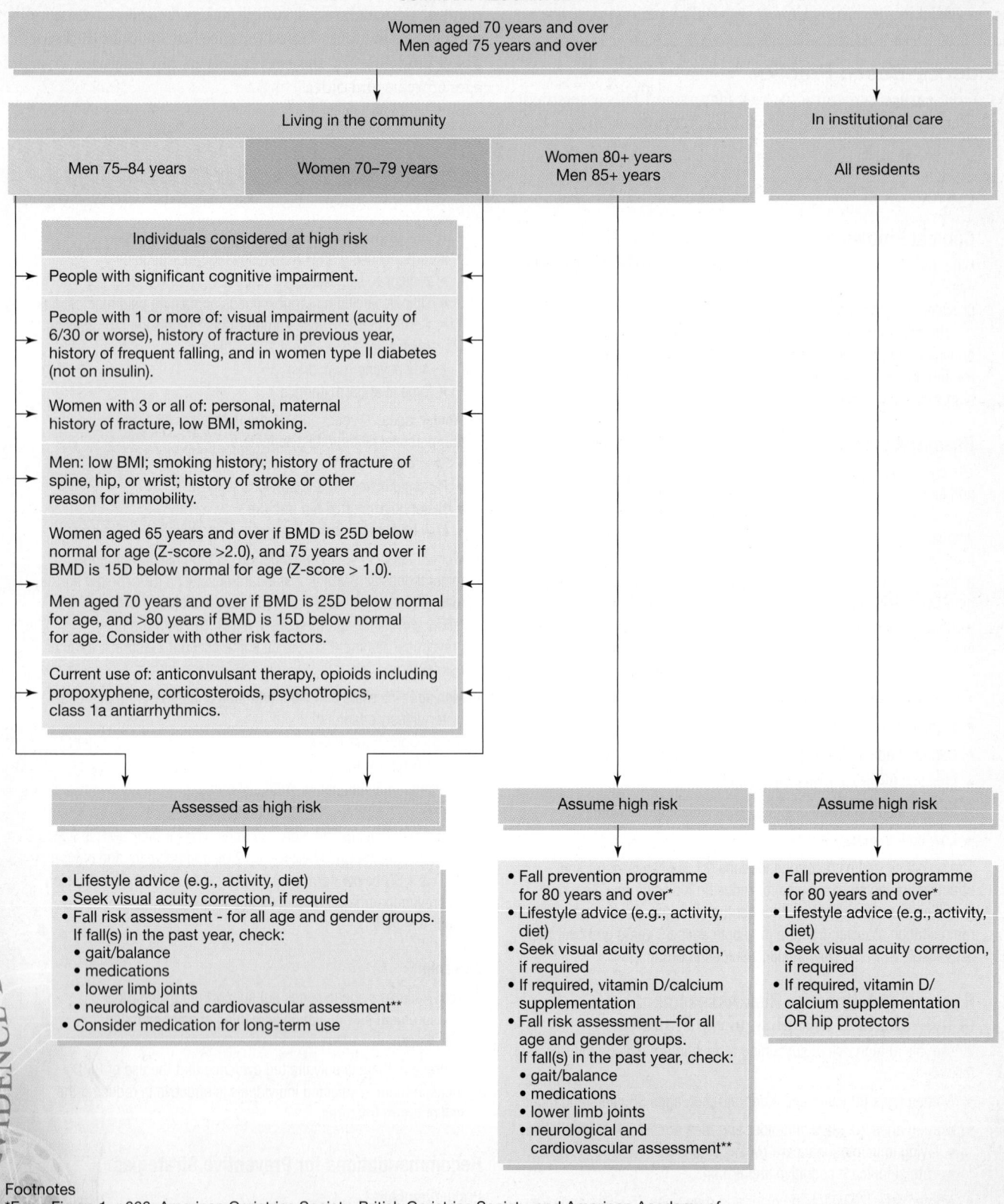

EVIDENCE-BASED PRACTICE

Footnotes

*From Figure 1, p666: American Geriatrics Society, British Geriatrics Society, and American Academy of Orthopaedic Surgeons Panel on Falls Prevention Guideline for the prevention of falls in older persons *Journal of the American Geriatrics Society 2001; 49:* 664-672.
**Refer.[24]

Source: This guideline was developed by William Gillespie (Convenor), John Campbell, Melinda Gardner, Lesley Gillespie, Jan Jackson, Clare Robertson, Jean-Claude Theis, and Raymond Jones. The consultation group included Marion Robinson, Heather Thomson, and Jim Reid. Published by New Zealand Guidelines Group Inc. Reproduced with permission from New Zealand Guidelines Group. Prevention of Hip Fracture amongst People aged 65 years and over. Guideline summary. Wellington: 2003.

- Multidisciplinary, multifactorial health/environmental screening/intervention programs reduce the frequency of falls in high-risk community-dwelling older people.
- Assessment, advice, and facilitation of home environment modification, when conducted in an experimental situation by a trained occupational therapist, reduces the frequency of falls in high-risk community-dwelling older people.

Medication for Bone Protection

- Daily supplementation with vitamin D and calcium reduces the hip fracture rates among high-risk older people in institutional care, or who have already sustained a hip fracture.
- Bisphosphonates (alendronate, risedronate) reduce hip and other fracture rates in community-dwelling older women under 80 years of age.
- Evidence for the effectiveness of hormone replacement therapy (HRT) in reducing hip fracture rates in women ages 65 years and older is conflicting. In view of more recent evidence on the risks of HRT, it is not recommended for first-line prevention of hip fracture. (Refer to Appendix C in full guideline or HRT Update Summary from the New Zealand Guidelines Group.)

Hip Protectors

- Hip protectors appear to reduce the incidence of hip fractures in older people in institutional care provided that compliance/adherence is achieved.

Choosing a Prevention Strategy—
Current Estimates of Cost Effectiveness

- In frail older people in residential or nursing home care, calcium and vitamin D supplementation appears more cost effective than the use of hip pads, although both approaches have similar efficacy.
- The cost effectiveness of bisphosphonates compared with HRT is sensitive to compliance and the incidence of adverse events, and is unclear. (Refer to Appendix C in full guideline for current advice on HRT from the New Zealand Guidelines Group.)
- The overall cost effectiveness of fall prevention programs, compared with other strategies used for hip fracture prevention, is not known.

Implications for Nursing Practice

Nurses should screen older patients for risk factors for falling and increased potential for fractures. Using the findings, the nurse will educate the patient and family regarding ways to decrease their risks and to increase mobility and safety within their environment.

Critical Thinking Questions

1. How does screening for risk factors help to prevent hip fractures?

2. Why is exercise important in preventing fractures of the hip?

Answers to Critical Thinking Questions appear in Appendix D.

Osteomyelitis

Osteomyelitis is an infection of the bone that requires aggressive early treatment to decrease the amount of bone or joint damage.

Epidemiology

Unlike the "silent" onset of osteoporosis, osteomyelitis can have an acute, subacute, or chronic onset. The acute and chronic forms can present the same clinical picture. The bones that are most commonly involved include the upper ends of the humerus and tibia and the lower end of the femur. Occasionally the spinal vertebrae may be affected (Frazier & Drzymkowski, 2009).

The first line of defense for the bone is the skin; however, bones can become infected through the bloodstream, direct invasion, and infections in adjacent bone or soft tissues. One in 5,000 children may experience acute osteomyelitis (King et al., 2006). In general, children tend to have a higher incident of acute osteomyelitis and adults tend to present with subacute and chronic osteomyelitis (King et al., 2006; Mayo Clinic, 2007). Individuals with diabetes have a 16% risk factor for acquiring osteomyelitis. The problem with osteomyelitis is that symptoms develop over time and may go unnoticed for several days to a week. Individuals who experience vertebral osteomyelitis have a 10% to 15% risk of developing neurological problems due to spinal cord compression from the inflammatory process (King et al., 2006).

Etiology and Pathophysiology

The cause of the inflammatory process results from pyogenic organisms such as *Staphylococcus aureus, Staphylococcus epidermidis, Escherichia coli, Mycobacterium tuberculosis, Neisseria gonorrhoeae,* Pseudomonas, Salmonella, fungi, and mycobacteria. These organisms are not age discriminate and can affect anyone at any age. *Staphylococcus aureus* is responsible for 90% of

the infections followed by streptococcal bacteria (Frazier & Drzymkowski, 2009). Individuals who are at risk for developing osteomyelitis include individuals having a compromised immune system, diabetes, peripheral vascular disease, malignancies, and the presence of prosthetic hardware within the bone (Frazier & Drzymkowski, 2009).

Acute osteomyelitis falls into two categories: hematogenous and direct contact. Hematogenous osteomyelitis is an infection caused by bacterial infection from a distant site migrating by way of the bloodstream to the bone. It is commonly seen in children. Two common bone sites provide a rich environment for organism growth: the vascular metaphysic of growing bones and the distal metaphysic. The pyrogenic organism finds the rich blood supply of the metaphysic of the growing bone an ideal environment for receiving needed nutrients for growth and proliferation. A sharp angle at the distal metaphysic structure slows the blood, causing stagnation and thrombosis formation. The thrombosis formation can result in ischemia, leading to necrosis and bacterial growth (King, et al., 2006).

The other category of acute osteomyelitis, direct contact, results from direct trauma or surgery. It is the direct contact of bacteria or the implanting of bacteria from the outside environment that can cause infection. For example, osteomyelitis can be diagnosed following a surgical procedure. In this case, the disease process is localized to a specific bone but can potentially spread to surrounding tissues. Osteomyelitis resulting from direct trauma, injury, or surgery involves many organisms and the clinical manifestations tend to be more localized than those of hematogenous osteomyelitis (King et al., 2006).

Chronic osteomyelitis is typically associated with other disease processes. It is the primary disease process that predisposes the individual to bone infections. For example, individuals with diabetes have a higher incidence of osteomyelitis because of the poor circulation in the lower extremities and high level of blood sugar. Peripheral vascular disease, sickle cell anemia, and immune deficiency syndrome are just a few examples of other primary disease processes that predispose an individual to osteomyelitis (King et al., 2006).

In summary, osteomyelitis is a complex bone disorder with the potential for chronic and long-term effects. Therefore, medical diagnosis must be on the accurate classification of the cause (direct or indirect) and the organism involved. In some cases, young, rapidly growing, normal cells and cells subjected to inflammation and change in their blood supply can exhibit characteristics that may indicate bone tumor.

Clinical Manifestations

Clinical manifestations of osteomyelitis include the following symptoms: fever, edema at involved site, warmth to touch, tenderness at site, and movement or joint limitations at the involved site (i.e., contractures). The patient may have generalized complaints of fatigue and malaise. As the infection progresses a subperiosteal abscess may develop. The purulent material causes pressure and eventual fracturing of small pieces of bone.

Laboratory and Diagnostic Procedures

Lab tests that will help in the diagnosis of osteomyelitis include CBC and blood cultures. For the CBC, the white blood cells and leukocytes (leftward shift with increased polymorphonuclear leukocyte) will be elevated and the hemoglobin will be decreased. The erythrocyte sedimentation rate is also elevated. Needle aspiration of bone with culture of material taken is essential to identifying the causative organism.

Radiographic images in the initial stages may not be helpful. Eventually, the x-rays will demonstrate a swelling of overlying tissues and about 40% to 50% focal bone loss. An MRI may be helpful in making the diagnosis. MRI will differentiate soft tissue from bone marrow involvement and is useful for surgical localization of the osteomyelitis. Other tests include a bone scan and ultrasonography. The ultrasonograph can demonstrate soft tissue abscess or fluid collection and periosteal elevation.

Medical Management

Medical management in the acute phase focuses on treating the underlying cause for full recovery with minimal loss of function. Pharmacologic and surgical interventions are possible strategies. Management is geared toward preventing nonhealing of the wound, sepsis, immobility, and amputation.

Medical intervention may include immobilization of the affected bone and prescribing medications such as pain medicines and antibiotics. Pharmacologic interventions include the use of broad-spectrum antibiotics until organism sensitivity is obtained. Generally, antibiotics will be administered intravenously and may extend over a course of 4 to 6 weeks. Oral antibiotics may be prescribed following the completion of the intravenous (IV) antibiotics.

Surgery may be considered to incise the site and drain the abscess. If it is chronic osteomyelitis, surgery is recommended to remove the dead bone. The wound may require repeated debridement followed by frequent sterile dressing changes. It is suggested that patients be placed on drainage and secretion precautions.

Physical therapy may be ordered to maintain the patient's activity level and teach the patient how to use assistive devices during the no-weight-bearing stage. Healing requires adequate nutrition. A nutritionist may be consulted to assess caloric and protein intake. Dietary planning is based on the patient's need for calories, protein, and vitamins to promote healing.

A social worker or case manager may be another key member of the multidisciplinary team providing coordination of appropriate inpatient and outpatient care. When the patient is discharged, the home health nurse becomes important for following medical treatment in the home environment. In this disease process, strict adherence to the medical regimen is imperative to prevent the chronicity of the disease. Therefore, it is essential for the home health nurse to reinforce education on medication and appropriate lifestyle changes.

■ Nursing Management

Nursing care focuses on rest, immobilization of the affected part, and administration of analgesics, antipyretics, and antibiotics. The affected extremity should be supported to facilitate adequate circulation and proper alignment to prevent contractures (Christensen & Kockrow, 2003). Preventive care will include monitoring the wound, performing prescribed wound care, preventing dehydration, reinforcing adherence to the antibiotic regimen, and regular follow-up. See the Nursing Process: Patient Care Plan for Osteomyelitis feature for more details.

Education focuses on information about the disease process, medications, signs of inflammation, and changes that might indicate worsening of the condition. If osteomyelitis is not treated properly, it can become chronic. In such cases the individual may go home with an indwelling catheter or PICC line for antibiotics. The patient and family members will need education on how to care for the intravenous types of lines. The Patient Teaching & Discharge Priorities for Osteomyelitis box (p. 1748) lists other aspects of patient education.

Osteitis Deformans (Paget's Disease)

Osteitis deformans is a chronic disorder that causes irregular bone breakdown and formation, which in turn causes the bones to weaken. This results in pain, bone deformities, fractures, and arthritis.

Epidemiology and Etiology

The cause of osteitis deformans is unknown. It can occur in only a portion of one bone, the entire bone, or many bones throughout the skeletal system. The most common sites are the pelvis and tibia. Other less affected areas include the femur, clavicle, skull, and spine. The disease usually presents in patients older than 40 years of age and becomes increasingly more common with age (Frazier & Drzymkowski, 2009).

Pathophysiology

With this disease, the affected areas of bone produce new bone faster than old bone can be broken down. The disease usually occurs in two stages: the vascular stage, in which bone tissue is broken down but the spaces are filled with blood vessels and fibrous tissue rather than new bone; and the sclerotic stage, in

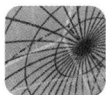

NURSING PROCESS: Patient Care Plan for Osteomyelitis

Assessment of Pain

Subjective Data:
On a scale of 1–10 with one being a little pain and 10 being the worst pain you have ever felt, at what level is your pain?
Do you routinely take pain medication at home? If yes, what is the name of the medication and why do you take it?
Are you allergic to any medications?

Objective Data:
Monitor patient for:
Facial grimacing
Change in breathing pattern
Change in blood pressure and/or pulse rate
Diaphoresis
Agitation

Nursing Assessment and Diagnoses	Outcomes and Evaluation Parameters	Planning and Interventions with *Rationales*
Nursing Diagnosis: *Pain, Acute* related to inflammation	**Outcome:** Pain level will be tolerable. *Evaluation Parameter:* Patient will not exhibit symptoms of pain and will verbalize pain control.	**Interventions and *Rationales:* Nonpharmacologic:** Reduce lighting and noise, and provide room for the patient's significant others. Cultural and spiritual factors such as prayer, ritual, and music can also increase the patient's comfort. *Promotes relaxation and comfort.* **Pharmacologic:** Medicate the patient with narcotics and nonsteroidal anti-inflammatory drugs as ordered. Assess for effectiveness. *Bone pain is usually severe.* Elevate and support the affected extremity. *Elevating the extremity reduces edema by enhancing venous return. Supportive positioning protects against muscle strain.* Teach the patient to report increasing or uncontrolled pain. *Increasing pain may indicate ineffective therapy or worsening infection.*

Assessment of Knowledge of Treatment Regimen

Subjective Data:
Do you understand which medications you are taking and when to take them?
Can you tell me what osteomyelitis is?
What is your weight-bearing status?

Objective Data:
Patient takes medications as prescribed.
Patient demonstrates proper wound care.
Patient reports no elevation of temperature or recurrence of pain or other symptoms at the site.

Nursing Assessment and Diagnoses	Outcomes and Evaluation Parameters	Planning and Interventions with *Rationales*
Nursing Diagnosis: *Knowledge, Deficient* related to treatment regimen	**Outcome:** The patient will comply with therapeutic plan. *Evaluation Parameters:* The patient will take medications on time, demonstrate proper wound care, and report signs or symptoms of complications quickly.	**Interventions and *Rationales:*** Teach the patient and family the importance of adhering to the therapeutic regimen. *Knowledge regarding the reasons for the therapeutic plan and the consequences that may occur if not followed will motivate the patient to adhere.*

Assessment of Nutritional Intake

Subjective Data:
Describe your usual intake pattern.
Is this intake sufficient?
Do you have religious dietary restrictions or practices?
How often do you exercise?
Who prepares your meals?
Do you feel you have enough energy?

Objective Data:
General appearance
Weight
Hair, nails, and skin
Muscle mass
Edema

(continued)

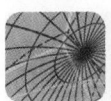

NURSING PROCESS: Patient Care Plan for Osteomyelitis—*Continued*

Nursing Assessment and Diagnoses	Outcomes and Evaluation Parameters	Planning and Interventions with *Rationales*
Nursing Diagnosis: *Nutrition, Imbalanced: Less Than Body Requirements*	**Outcome:** The patient will maintain adequate nutrition to assist with healing. **Evaluation Parameter:** Maintenance of weight without loss of muscle mass.	**Interventions and *Rationales:*** Facilitate education with a dietary consultant. *Consultation can ensure a diet that provides optimal caloric and nutrient intake.* Encourage frequent oral hygiene. *Poor oral hygiene leads to bad breath and a bad taste in the mouth, which decreases the appetite.* Provide the patient with printed material outlining the dietary needs and restrictions. *Aids the patient in selecting the proper foods.* Promote the intake of protein foods with high biologic value: eggs, meats, diary products. *Complete proteins provide the positive nitrogen balance needed for growth and healing.* Promote the intake of foods high in protein and vitamins A, B, and C. Common food sources include meat, fish, poultry, fortified cereals, dairy products, dark green and yellow vegetables, citrus fruits/juices, potatoes, cauliflower, and tomatoes. *Promotes cell regeneration.*

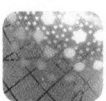

PATIENT TEACHING & DISCHARGE PRIORITIES for Osteomyelitis

Need	Teaching
Nutrition: • Patient and family	Work with dietitian to plan a high-protein diet rich in vitamins A, B, and C to promote cell regeneration.
Medications: • Patient	Stress importance of taking prescribed antibiotics as scheduled even if patient is feeling better.
	Teach the patient the signs and symptoms of any side effects that may occur.
Safety: • Patient and family	Stress importance of a safe environment to prevent falls and possible fractures.
	Teach the proper use of any assistive devices that may be required.
Avoidance of continued infections: • Patient and family	Stress the importance of reporting signs of infection.
	If patients require long-term antibiotics they will require a special intravenous line such as a PICC. Education for maintenance of the catheter and the importance of aseptic technique should be emphasized.
	Stress importance of follow-up appointments to assess therapeutic effectiveness.

which the vascular fibrous tissue hardens and is similar to bone but is fragile, leading to pathologic fractures (Frazier & Drzymkowski, 2009).

Clinical Manifestations

Osteitis deformans rarely causes symptoms. When symptoms do occur they usually include bone pain at the site. The pain can become disabling because it is constant and worse at night. Patients may experience edema or deformity at the affected site. If the ossicles of the ear are involved, hearing loss or deafness will occur. Complications of the disease include pathologic fractures, hypercalcemia, renal calculi, spinal cord injury, and occasionally development of bone sarcoma (Frazier & Drzymkowski, 2009).

Laboratory and Diagnostic Procedures

Radiographic imaging, bone scanning, and a bone marrow biopsy assist with diagnosis. Serum lab results will show an elevated alkaline phosphatase, and urinalysis will reveal an elevated

hydroxyproline concentration. Both results indicate a high rate of bone production.

Medical Management

Treatment of osteitis deformans is symptom based. Treatment goals are the relief of pain and prevention of bone loss. Injections of the hormone calcitonin may be given to regulate the level of calcium in the blood and help prevent bone loss. A diet high in protein, calcium, and vitamin D also helps to prevent bone loss, especially if the use of bisphosphonate medications has been added to the treatment plan (Frazier & Drzymkowski, 2009).

 Nursing Management

The goals of nursing management include education regarding the disease process and palliative treatment of symptoms. It is important to teach the patient that exercise is an important part of the treatment plan to stimulate bone growth and maintain flexibility and strength. Maintaining a healthy weight is also important to avoid undue stress on affected bones.

Benign Bone Tumors

Bone tumor is an abnormal growth of the bone cells and can be benign or cancerous. The tumors can be from cartilage (chondrogenic), from bone (osteogenic), or from fibrous tissue (fibrogenic). Benign bone tumors do not spread to other tissues or organs.

Epidemiology

Generally, adults over the age of 40 years and children ages 10 years or younger are at a higher risk for developing bone tumors. Examples of benign bone tumors include aneurysmal bone cyst, osteochondroma, fibrous dysplasia, chondroblastoma, and osteoid osteoma.

Etiology and Pathophysiology

Bone tumors can be classified according to their origins or as benign or malignant. Benign bone tumors generally are not life threatening, present few symptoms, and do not result in death. A tumor in the bone causes the normal bone tissue to react by osteolytic response (bone destruction) or osteoblastic response (bone formation). Bone tissue cells are very active and new bone is constantly forming and old bone is dissolving. Bone tumors result from an abnormal growth of cells that can originate from bone cells, cartilage, fibrous tissue, marrow, or vascular tissue.

Generally benign tumors illustrate the geographical pattern by having a slow symmetrical growth pattern. Slow erosion can cause bone destruction and may cause the adjacent normal bone to respond to the tumor by altering its normal pattern of remodeling. The bone's surface changes and the contours enlarge in the tumor areas. Because adjacent tendons and muscles provide structural support for the bone, as the adjacent tissues are displaced, the bone becomes weakened and fracture can result. A few examples of benign bone tumors include nonossifying fibroma, osteochondroma, osteoma, osteoblastoma, enchondroma (Ollier's disease), bone cyst, chondroblastoma, and giant cell tumor (McCance & Huether, 2006). Osteochondroma accounts for 35% to 50% of all benign tumors (Copstead & Banaski, 2005). Pathologic characteristics of bone tumors include bone destruction, attrition, or expansion of the cortex and also periosteal response to changes in underlying bone (McCance & Huether, 2006).

Clinical Manifestations

There are two predominant clinical manifestations for benign tumors: Pressure around surrounding tissues may cause pain, and range of motion may be affected if the tumor becomes too large. Pain is usually the presenting symptom and is often worse at night or after exercise. At times bone tumors produce no symptoms and are detected when the weakened bone fractures.

Diagnostic Procedures

Radiographs, CT scan, radionuclide bone scan, and/or MRI can be used to diagnose the tumor.

Medical Management

The treatment for bone tumors, whether benign or malignant, is surgical excision. Surrounding muscle and other tissue are of-

ten removed and bone grafting may be needed. Amputation may be required depending on the tumor site and extent. Surgical removal alone is enough to treat benign bone tumors.

Nursing Management

The care of patients with bone tumors is preventive in nature. Health promotion revolves around monitoring the size of the bone tumor. If the tumor is removed surgically, nursing and collaborative care will focus on preparing the patient for surgery followed by monitoring and prevention of postop complications. For the care of the patient undergoing orthopedic surgery, refer to Chapter 57 .

Bone Cancer and Bone Metastases

The most common types of primary bone cancer include osteosarcoma, chondrosarcoma, and Ewing's sarcoma (Frazier & Drzymkowski, 2009).

Epidemiology

In the year 2008 it was estimated that 2,380 new cases of bone and joint cancer would be diagnosed. Approximately 1,470 deaths are expected from these cancers. Osteosarcoma is the most common bone cancer (35% of the reported cases), followed by chondrosarcoma (26% of the reported cases) and Ewing's sarcoma (16% of the reported cases) (American Cancer Society [ACS], 2008).

Osteosarcoma usually presents in young people between the ages of 10 and 30. A small percentage of cases (10%) develop in people who are greater than 60 years of age (ACS, 2008). Osteosarcoma has a greater incidence in males than females and the tumor most often develops in the arm, leg, or pelvis.

Chondrosarcoma is a cancer of cartilage cells and is uncommon in people younger than 20 years of age. After the age of 20, the risk of developing the cancer continues to rise until the person reaches the age of 75. The incidence is equal for men and women (ACS, 2008). Chondrosarcoma may present anywhere in the body where there is cartilage, but the most common sites are the pelvis, leg, and arm bone. It will occasionally present in the trachea, larynx, and chest wall.

Ewing's sarcoma is a primary malignant bone tumor in the pediatric and adolescent population. It usually occurs in the second decade of life and approximately 80% of cases are in people younger than 20 years of age (Lahl, Fisher, & Laschinger, 2007). Although there is no significant difference between the races in the incidence of osteosarcoma, there is a significantly higher incident of Ewing's sarcoma in Caucasian children when compared to children of the same age from the African American population (Lahl et al., 2007). Ewing tumors form in the cavity of the bone and most often present in the long bones of the leg and arm.

Etiology and Pathophysiology

Bone metastasis and primary bone cancer are two separate disease processes and are treated differently. Secondary tumors arise from cells that have broken off from the original tumor site and enter the lymph system or bloodstream and travel to that specific area. Bone metastases are generally observed in patients who have had a relapse in their cancer. Approximately 75% of the bone metastases originate from carcinomas of the prostate, breast, kidney, and lung. To a lesser extent, other cancers that spread to the bone can come from the following cancers: thyroid, colon, and melanoma. The bones most commonly affected are the pelvis, vertebrae, ribs, femur, and humerus (Frazier & Drzymkowski, 2009).

Malignant bone tumors that are primary tumors are rare and typically emerge from connective and supportive tissue cells. Primary malignant bone tumors account for greater than 85% of bone tumors in the pediatric population, but are rarely seen after the age of 30 (Frazier & Drzymkowski, 2009).The exact cause of bone cancer is unknown.

Recent findings suggest that an individual's DNA can become defective or mutated. Oncogenes promote cell division and tumor suppressor genes cause cells to die or slow down cell division. DNA mutations can activate oncogenes or inactivate tumor suppressor genes. Also, it has been determined that individuals with bone cancer can inherit mutations from their parents. As a result, cancerous cells form a tumor and invade and destroy adjacent bone tissue. The rate of growth of the tumor and the response to treatment depends on the type of cancer involved. Most bone cancers are not inherited, but a result of mutations acquired. For instance, radiation is used as a treatment for some cancers, but can also cause cancer by damaging DNA. Bones that are exposed to radiation as a treatment are more likely to develop bone cancer later (ACS, 2008; see Chapter 11 ☉).

Bone destruction from the tumor can result in one of three different types of patterns: (1) geographic pattern, (2) moth-eaten pattern, or (3) permeative pattern. With the geographic pattern, the tumor edges have well-defined margins. In the moth-eaten pattern, the margins are less defined and are easily separated from the bone. When the margins are not clear and abnormal lytic bone merges with normal bone, this is suggestive of the permeative pattern (McCance & Huether, 2006). Bone tumors that are considered malignant include osteosarcoma, chondrosarcoma, chordoma, and Ewing tumor. Lymphoma and multiple myeloma also start in the bones, but are not considered bone cancer because they develop in the lymph nodes and in the plasma cells, respectively.

Osteosarcoma is the most common primary bone cancer and usually presents between the ages of 10 and 15 years old. It usually develops in the distal femur, followed by the proximal tibia and humerus. Most patients die within 2 years due to metastasis to the lung. Risk factors include Paget's disease, PTH injections for osteoporosis, and radiation therapy for other forms of cancer (Frazier & Drzymkowski, 2009).

Ewing's sarcoma involves the pelvis and lower extremity. The tumor usually presents between the ages of 4 and 25 years of age. The tumor is invasive and extends into the soft tissue. Metastasis occurs early and is usually to the lungs and other bones (Frazier & Drzymkowski, 2009). Chondrosarcoma also involves the pelvis and lower extremity, but usually presents between the ages of 30 and 60 years old. The tumor grows slowly and is locally invasive (Frazier & Drzymkowski, 2009).

Clinical Manifestations

Due to the destruction, erosion, and expansion of the tumor, pain is the primary symptom. The intensity of the pain can be mild to severe. If a fracture is sustained, the patient will have acute pain. As a result of swelling, the patient may experience range-of-motion (ROM) limitation and joint effusion. The area may be tender to palpation and warm to touch with superficial blood vessels noticeable. Osteosarcoma begins with pain and swelling and a "sunburst" appearance on radiograph. Ewing's sarcoma presents with pain and swelling, fever, fatigue, anemia, and leukocytosis. On radiograph the tumor has an "onion skin" appearance. Chondrosarcomas are slow growing so the pain is intermittent and dull. The tumor presents a lobular pattern on radiograph.

Laboratory and Diagnostic Procedures

Radiographs are useful in demonstrating tumor activity and will show increases and decreases in bone density. A bone scan can detect the extent of the malignancy and help follow the planned therapy. CT and MRI will demonstrate soft tissue involvement and the exact location of the tumor.

Lab tests will include chemistry and CBC. Serum alkaline phosphatase is generally elevated. In some situations, the hematologic lab values will be altered. Other tests include bone biopsy, arteriography, chest x-ray, and lung scan to detect metastasis.

Medical Management

The treatment of bone cancer is best achieved by a multidisciplinary team. The objective or the goal is to slow the growth of the tumor by destroying and removing the lesion. Depending on the specific type of bone tumor, chemotherapy, surgery, radiation, or a combination of these treatments may be used.

▇ Nursing Management

The care of the patient with bone cancer is challenging. Therapeutic management might include chemotherapy, radiologic therapy, surgery, and pharmacologic interventions. Chemotherapy may be administered prior to having surgery done and then to prevent metastases. A combination of therapies may be used to achieve optimal response and minimize potential drug resistance. Immunotherapy and hormone therapy may also be used. Supportive care may need to be given during the course of the disease and involves case workers, social workers, and hospice.

The primary focus of nursing care is relief of pain, prevention of pathologic fractures, and provision of a supportive environment. The nursing care will involve the patient's response to pain control measures, side effects of the pain medications, chemotherapy, and radiation therapy. Nursing care that focuses on preoperative and postoperative care may be implemented if a surgical procedure is indicated (see Chapter 57 ☉). If the stage of cancer is advanced, pathologic bone fractures may occur; therefore, inactivity would be encouraged. For a detailed discussion of care for the patient with cancer, refer to Chapter 64 ☉ .

▇ Muscular Disorders

This section of the chapter details various types of muscle diseases. Although several of these diseases are not very common, it is important for nurses to understand both the pathophysiology of the conditions and the associated nursing care considerations that are required to fully care for these patients. After completion of this section, the nurse will be able to formulate critical thinking skills associated with these uncommon but debilitating and sometimes chronic disorders.

Muscular Dystrophies

Muscular dystrophies are a group of genetic myopathies caused by a protein deficiency in muscle membranes. In other words, a person's DNA is not producing a particular protein named dystrophin that is required by muscles and muscle membranes to function properly. Therefore, a person with a muscular dystrophy has progressive muscle weakness leading to an inability to control any voluntary movement (Figure 55–5 ■). The muscles eventually atrophy from nonuse. Skeletal muscles are not the only muscles affected by muscular dystrophy. The cardiac muscle and diaphragm may be affected as well (Muscular Dystrophy Association [MDA], 2008).

Genetics

Genetics play the key role in whether a child develops muscular dystrophy (MD). Muscular dystrophy occurs when a gene on the X chromosome fails to make the protein dystrophin. Without dystrophin, muscle cells are unable to function properly, leading to skeletal muscle weakness or failure. Most children afflicted with muscular dystrophy are males, because male children have only one X chromosome (from the mother). If that X chromosome is not producing dystrophin, then the child will develop MD. Female children receive X chromosomes from both parents, so even if one X chromosome is flawed, it is likely that the other X chromosome can provide the dystrophin, and she will have few or no symptoms, but will be a carrier (Figure 55–6 ■). Even though the incidence of MD is mostly in males, MD weakness develops in 2.5% to 20% of females. The incidence in male children is about 1 in 3,500 live male births (Centers for Disease Control and Prevention [CDC], 2008a; MDA, 2008).

Duchenne Muscular Dystrophy

In children, especially male children, the most prevalent muscular dystrophy is Duchenne muscular dystrophy (DMD). In

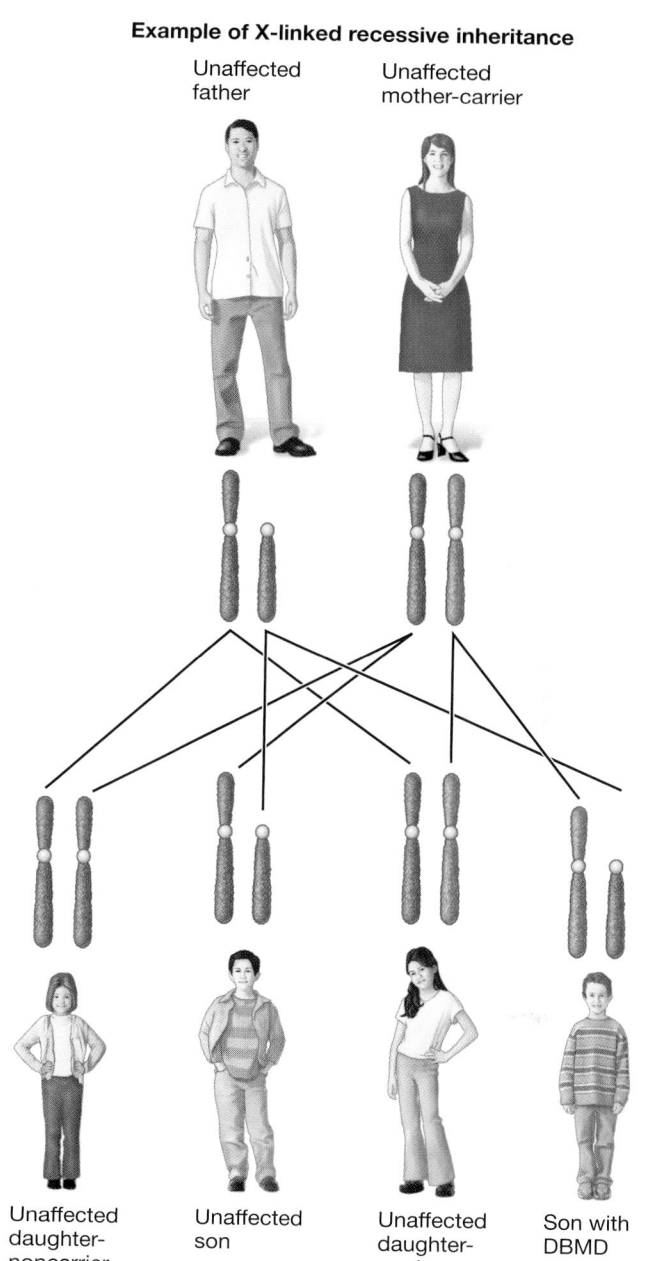

Example of X-linked recessive inheritance

Unaffected father — Unaffected mother-carrier

Unaffected daughter-noncarrier — Unaffected son — Unaffected daughter-carrier — Son with DBMD

FIGURE 55–6 ■ Muscular dystrophy inheritance pattern.

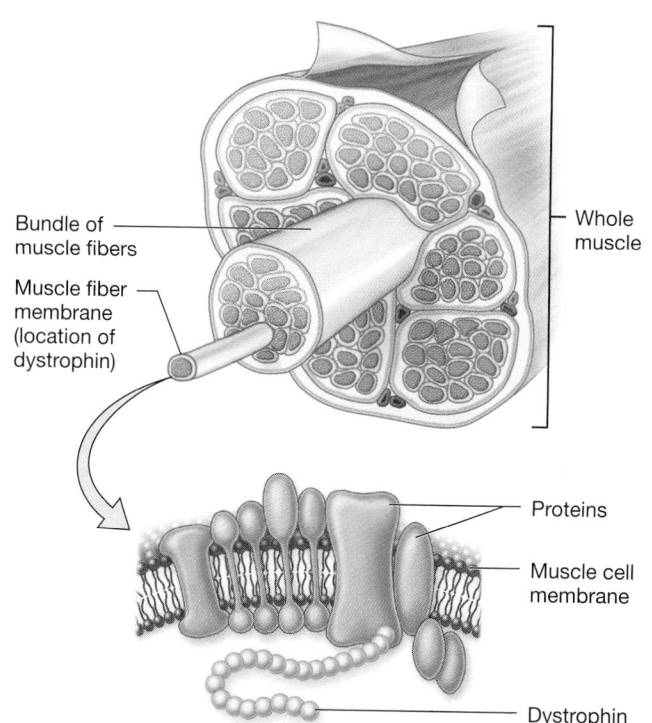

FIGURE 55–5 ■ Muscle fiber membrane.

Whole muscle

Bundle of muscle fibers

Muscle fiber membrane (location of dystrophin)

Proteins

Muscle cell membrane

Dystrophin

Duchenne muscular dystrophy, there is a complete absence of dystrophin. Muscle weakness and loss of muscle develop gradually, with signs usually first appearing when the child is 2 through 6 years old, but symptoms generally are exhibited about age 3 (CDC, 2008a). Weakness starts near the trunk then progresses to the extremities about 3 to 5 years after the initial weakness is experienced. Most commonly, the lower extremities are affected before the upper extremities (Figure 55–7 ■, p. 1752).

The weakness begins with the child having difficulty with simple tasks, such as maintaining his or her balance, and it leads to an inability to perform activities such as climbing stairs or getting up from a bed or chair. Children afflicted with DMD are late starters in learning to walk and as toddlers have enlarged calf muscles. By school age, the child has an unsteady gait and falls quite often, almost appearing clumsy. The child uses the Gowers' maneuver to rise up from the floor (Figure 55–8 ■, p. 1752). The

MyNursingKit | Muscular Dystrophy Association

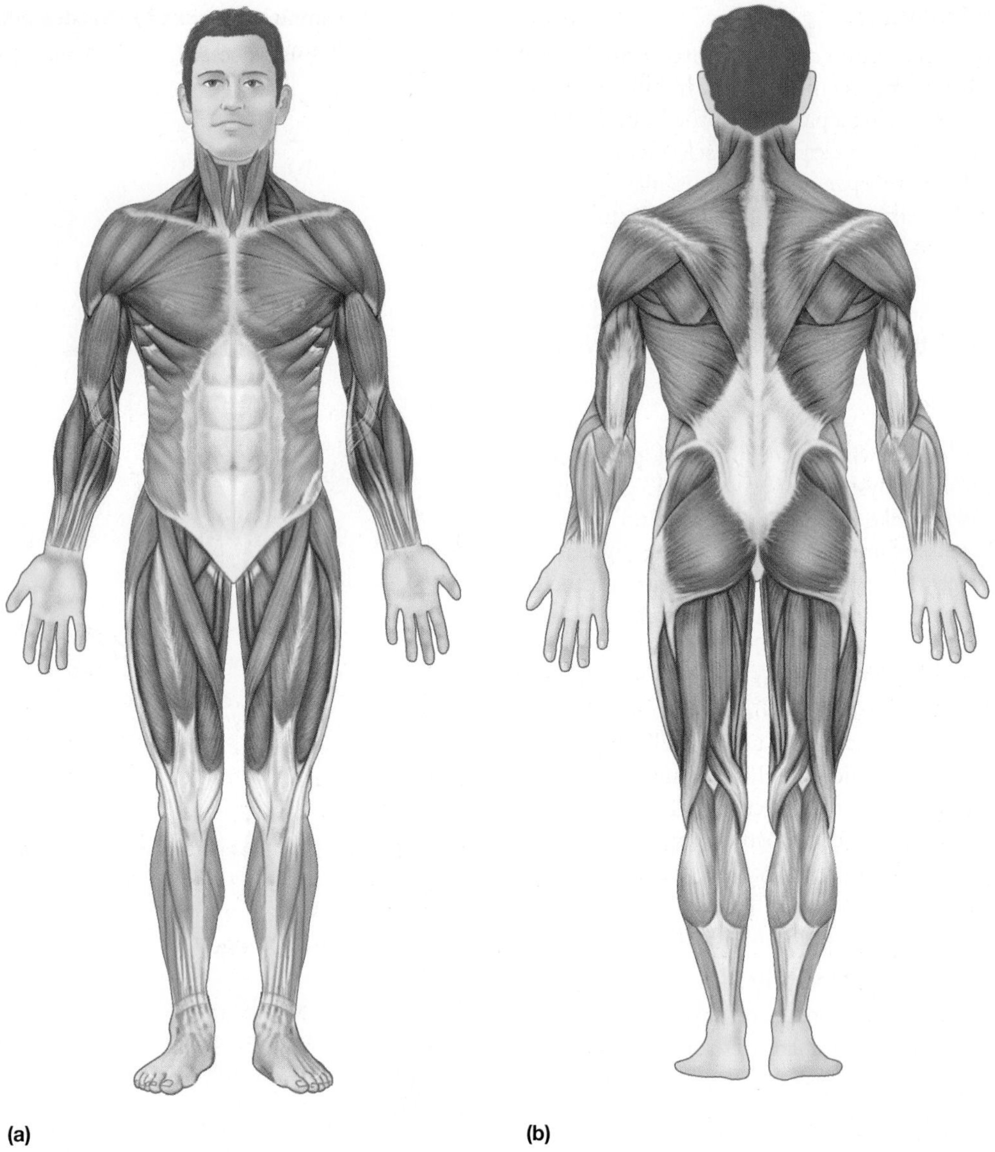

(a)   (b)

FIGURE 55–7 ■ Muscles affected by muscular dystrophy.

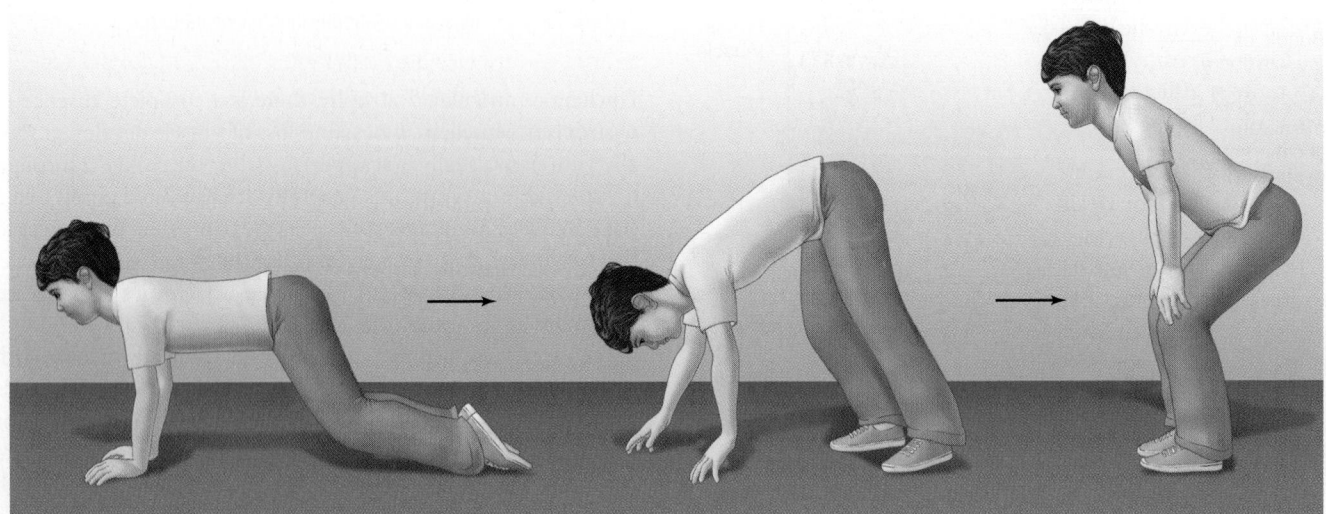

FIGURE 55–8 ■ Gowers' maneuver.

Gowers' maneuver involves the child getting on his hands and knees, then raising his rear end, which allows the child to walk on his hands and knees, and then achieving a standing position. The child often walks on the toes or balls of his feet with a waddling gait. To compensate for a lack of balance, the child sticks his abdomen out and puts his shoulders back (MDA, 2008).The child also has difficulty running, and generally is unable to jump or hop. Between the ages of 7 and 12, the child will no longer be able to walk and will use a wheelchair. Adolescents are usually unable to perform daily tasks, such as eating, with their arms, hands, or fingers. The course of the disease is progressive and usually fatal in the teens or early 20s. Death is usually due to respiratory or heart problems (CDC, 2008a).

Becker Muscular Dystrophy

Becker muscular dystrophy (BMD) is a less common type of MD, and the disease is generally milder than DMD. In BMD, some dystrophin is produced and it does not manifest itself until a person is in his teens or young adulthood when the person notices himself becoming weaker than usual when engaging in physical exercise or activities. This weakness is usually first noticed in the pelvic and hip area, the thighs, and the shoulders. The severity and progression of the disease vary depending on the amount of dystrophin that is being released. The child/adolescent generally has a normal IQ for age.

Complications Associated with Duchenne or Becker Muscular Dystrophy

Several serious and sometimes life-threatening complications may result from DMD or BMD.

Cardiomyopathy The most serious complications involve the cardiac and respiratory systems. As discussed in Chapter 41, cardiomyopathy is due to cardiac muscle weakening, a direct result of the absence or lack of dystrophin. Cardiomyopathy leads to heart failure, which is a major cause of death in patients with muscular dystrophy. Primary dilated cardiomyopathy and conduction abnormalities develop with DMD. Most MD patients usually do not become symptomatic until they are in their teens, probably due to their lack of ability to exercise. Approximately 70% of those with BMD develop cardiomyopathy. As discussed in Chapter 41, patients with cardiomyopathy have shortness of breath, fluid in the lungs characterized by crackles or rhonchi, and lower extremity edema due to the heart muscle's inability to pump. Boys afflicted with muscular dystrophy often die from heart failure by the time they are in their 20s (CDC, 2008a).

Respiratory Distress Children with muscular dystrophy have an increased risk for weakness of the diaphragm and other ancillary muscles that assist in ventilation (MDA, 2008). If the diaphragm and other muscles are weak, then the child will have trouble expanding the chest to allow for effective inspiration and expiration. These children also have trouble coughing. Difficulty coughing coupled with weak, poor inspiratory/expiratory effort places MD patients at high risk for respiratory infections. Simply being in a room with someone who has a mild rhinitis or cold can predispose these children to pneumonia. With progression of the disease, many of the children will require long-term assisted mechanical ventilation or a tracheostomy. In addition, because patients with muscular dystrophy are prone to respiratory infections, it is extremely important for them to be current with their pneumococcal and flu vaccinations.

Muscle Atrophy and Contractures When a muscle is weak and unused, it deteriorates and shortens, leaving the associated joint prone to a permanent flexed position called a *contracture*, the shortening of a muscle attached to a joint. Contractures can affect the knee, elbow, wrist, hip, and finger joints. If preventive measures are not taken, contractures can become permanent, causing total loss of mobility to the affected joint, as well as discomfort. To prevent such contractures, it is important for all joints to be passively exercised.

Cognitive Effects Around one-third of the boys affected with Duchenne muscular dystrophy have some form of a progressive learning disability (MDA, 2008). In addition, some children with DMD have some level of mental retardation. Researchers believe that the lack of dystrophin in the brain affects the child's cognitive, behavioral, and intellectual abilities. Specific cognitive and intellectual skills affected are verbal skills, memory, attention, and focusing skills. In addition, some boys have difficulty with emotional interaction (MDA, 2008). School counselors, psychologists, and neuropsychologists can educate the family in techniques that may assist with learning and interaction skills.

Spinal Abnormalities Exaggerated curvature of the spine is prevalent in young adults with Duchenne muscular dystrophy. The three types of curvatures are **lordosis**, or swayback, noticed mostly in those young men who are still able to ambulate; **scoliosis**, or a lateral curvature of the spine; and **kyphosis**, or hunchback. Scoliosis that is severe can lead to respiratory problems, sleeping problems, and the inability to sit straight or remain seated for prolonged periods of time.

Treatment for spinal curvatures consists of attaching metal rods to the spine to help keep the spine in straight alignment.

Osteoporosis Normally, muscles exert pressure on the bones they are attached to, which helps to maintain the strength of the bones. The weakening of muscles from muscular dystrophy can lead to weakening of bones, or osteoporosis. The bones become very thin and brittle, which can lead to pathologic fractures. In patients with muscular dystrophy, simple daily activities, such as lifting a heavy object or twisting, may cause a bone to break. Many patients in wheelchairs experience pathologic fractures due to their inability to bear weight.

Laboratory and Diagnostic Procedures

Diagnosis of muscular dystrophy is based on signs and symptoms noted specifically in toddlers in the prewalking or walking phase. Observance of the Gowers' maneuver is a telltale sign of muscular dystrophy. Other affirmation of the disease includes an elevated level of serum creatinine kinase (CK), an enzyme that is found in skeletal muscles. Normally there are high levels of CK in the muscle and low levels in the blood. With MD, there is a breakdown of the muscle membrane and CK leaks out into the blood. The patient with MD will have a CK level that is 20 to 200 times higher than normal and is increased from the time of birth (CDC, 2008a).

Genetic testing may be done to look for a mutation in the dystrophin gene. The test first looks for large pieces of the gene that are missing or duplicated. If a deletion or duplication is found in the dystrophin gene, the diagnosis is confirmed. Sixty-five to 70% of patients with DMD or BMD will have a deletion or duplication (CDC, 2008a).

Other diagnostic tests include a muscle biopsy of the involved muscle to document the absence of dystrophin. An **electromyelogram (EMG)** will differentiate between a myopathy and neuropathy. An electromyelogram is important in the diagnosis of muscular dystrophy because it measures electrical activity in muscles and can demonstrate the muscle damage that is associated with muscular dystrophy.

Pulmonary function tests and an electrocardiogram (ECG) may be done to evaluate degree of respiratory or cardiac involvement.

Medical Management

At this time there is no specific treatment for muscular dystrophy; however, modalities such as medications, exercise, and diet may enhance the mobility of the patient and ability to move and function independently as long as possible.

Medications A glucocorticoid such as prednisone, which has an anti-inflammatory effect, has been shown to delay the progression of the disease and to improve muscle mass (Frazier & Drzymkowski, 2009). Prednisone must be prescribed cautiously, however, due to its numerous side effects.

Exercise Exercise is important in people afflicted with muscular dystrophy. The function of ambulating should be encouraged because it maintains the motion of a joint and prevents the joint from contracting. Passive range-of-motion (PROM) exercises are helpful in preventing contractures of the joints if the patient cannot actively exercise. PROM exercises must be performed on each joint at least every 4 hours while the patient is awake to prevent the muscles and tendons associated with the joints from shortening or atrophying. A child who can walk should continue to walk, even if only short distances, for as many months or years as he is able. Walking is an exercise that helps to maintain muscle strength and mobility. If the child cannot or does not walk, the muscles will lose strength and atrophy more quickly.

An alternative exercise therapy method called Watsu is being utilized by people with physical disabilities. Watsu involves the person doing limb and muscle stretching while floating in warm water, either actively or passively. The stated benefits of Watsu include total relaxation and a calming effect, not only to the limbs and muscles but to the patient as well (Osborn, 2005). General aquatic therapy in warm water also maintains the muscle tone.

Diet The nurse should assess dietary considerations for patients with muscular dystrophy. Patients with muscular dystrophy have certain specific nutritional requirements for health maintenance. A well-balanced diet is imperative for several reasons. Because the muscles are in the process of breaking down, and because maintenance of muscle mass is necessary to keep MD patients in good health, the muscles have high energy requirements. Moreover, they require high protein intake. MD patients typically require 68% more protein in their diets than average healthy adults (Leighton, 2003).

It is also important for MD patients to maintain a reasonable body weight. Obesity can cause exacerbation or worsening of respiratory and cardiac dysfunction, whereas weight loss can signify muscle wasting and decreasing energy stores and can further complicate an already weakened cardiac and respiratory system. Constipation due to immobility is also a potential complication of muscular dystrophy. Therefore, it is important that people diagnosed with muscular dystrophy consume at least eight glasses of water a day (unless contraindicated by other health conditions) and eat a diet high in fiber, which may avoid constipation.

Nursing Implications Regarding Diet It is important for weight measurement and monitoring to be a part of the patient's care plan. When assisting a patient with meal planning, the nurse should encourage a diet high in protein, fiber, minerals, and vitamins. A referral to a dietitian may be warranted if weight loss or significant weight gain is noted. It is also important for the nurse to be cognizant of upper extremity involvement in a patient with MD, because the patient will need to be fed.

Physical Therapy Physical therapy is aimed at prolonging muscle strength and thus preventing contractures. Both active and passive ROM exercises are indicated, and walking is encouraged if possible to enhance strength and stamina. Physical therapy should also focus on gait training and transfer training. When ambulation is lost, the patient needs to see a physical therapist for customization of a wheelchair, for recommendations about devices that assist with ADLs, and for help accomplishing tasks.

Occupational Therapy Occupational therapy focuses on exercises that allow the patient with MD to perform ADLs such as eating, dressing, or brushing teeth. Whereas physical therapy focuses on gross motor movements, occupational therapy focuses more on the maintenance of fine motor movements.

Braces and Standing Walkers Braces may be used to support the ankles and feet of an ambulatory child with MD. Braces are also utilized to prevent plantar flexion, a type of contracture. A standing walker can assist the patient to stand, thus promoting circulation and allowing the patient to bear weight on her joints.

Research

Current medical research into muscular dystrophy is focusing on several areas:

- **Protein repair**—Boosting the functions of proteins may help repair damage to muscle cells.
- **"Gene-silencing"**—This research is aimed at attempting to "turn off" the cells that harbor an elongated stretch of DNA thought to cause a type of MD.
- **Miniaturized genes for dystrophin**—These types of genes have been shown to improve the muscles of mice with Duchenne muscular dystrophy.
- **DNA testing**—Better DNA testing might reveal mutations in the dystrophin gene (MDA, 2008).

Myotonic Muscular Dystrophy

Myotonic dystrophy or Steinert's disease is the most common adult form of muscular dystrophy. It, like Duchenne muscular dystrophy, is caused by a defective gene that is transferred from one generation to another. The manifestations of myotonic dystrophy involve muscle wasting of the distal extremities, including hands, forearms, and feet and also the face and neck. The *myotonic* part of the term myotonic dystrophy refers to a delay in the relaxation phase after muscle contraction. An example would be a person who is unable to release his hand after gripping something. Fifty percent of the cases of myotonic dystrophy are diagnosed by age 20; however, many cases are not diagnosed until 50 years of age (MDA, 2008).

Clinical Manifestations

Myotonic dystrophy is a multisystem disease because it affects organs and tissues other than muscles. Myotonic dystrophy can affect the eyes, specifically in the manifestation of cataracts; the muscles involved in swallowing, resulting in dysphagia; the respiratory system, involving weakness of the diaphragm and an adverse reaction to anesthesia; the gastrointestinal system, including decreased peristalsis; and the endocrine system, resulting in alteration or inappropriate insulin secretion, increased carbohydrate metabolism, and excessive sleeping (MDA, 2008). Unlike with other dystrophies that can usually be diagnosed based on muscle wasting symptoms alone, myotonic dystrophy is often diagnosed based on presentation of other symptoms. In some cases, the patient's initial complaint to her health care provider may be a change in vision or difficulty swallowing.

Laboratory and Diagnostic Procedures

Myotonic muscular dystrophy is diagnosed by a complaint of distal weakness and myotonia. A muscle biopsy will determine the diagnosis. DNA testing will also delineate a diagnosis of myotonic dystrophy by finding an abnormality on chromosome 19. Some patients in the early stages of the disease have the "classic" look of myotonic dystrophy: muscle wasting of the face, jaw, neck, hands, feet, and forearms.

Medical Management

Treatment is based on support of the wasting muscles. In addition, avoiding complications such as constipation from decreased gastric peristalsis, aspiration from difficulty swallowing, and decreased visual acuity from resulting cataracts should be addressed.

Medications used for myotonic dystrophy include phenytoin (Dilantin), mexiletine (Mexil), carbamazepine (Tegretol), quinine, and procainamide (Pronestyl). All of these medications may be useful in treating the delayed muscle relaxation that generally occurs in patients with myotonic dystrophy (Mayo Clinic, 2007).

Research

Medical research is focused on isolating and mapping the genetic defect. The defect for myotonic dystrophy is in the arm of chromosome 19. Knowledge of the exact chromosome may allow for better genetic testing and reveal avenues for further research for treatment modalities.

Limb Girdle Muscular Dystrophy

This type of muscular dystrophy primarily affects the pelvis and shoulder areas. Limb girdle muscular dystrophy generally has a slow progression rate, but it is not uncommon in some patients for it to progress rapidly. Muscle weakness and wasting may begin at the upper extremities and progress to the lower extremities or have just the opposite pattern of progression. The signs and symptoms are usually noted during childhood, but they can also begin during the teen years and into adulthood. The incidence of male-to-female cases is about equal.

Facioscapulohumeral Disease

Facioscapulohumeral disease (FSHD) is a rare type of muscular dystrophy that affects the face, shoulder girdle, and upper arms and is more common in females than males. Diagnosis is made based on specific symptoms, which include weakness in the muscles that open and close the eyes; the muscles that allow a person to purse the lips, to smile, and to whistle; and the muscles that stabilize the scapula. Other affected muscles include the muscles of the hip girdle, foot, and abdomen. The diagnosis of FSHD is usually made by the time a person is in her 20s. The progression of this type of muscular dystrophy is insidious, with extended periods where the disease seems to be arrested.

Oculopharyngeal Muscular Dystrophy

This type of muscular dystrophy generally strikes people who are in their 50s and 60s. The most prominent feature is bilateral ptosis, in which the eyelids droop to the level of the pupil or below the level of the pupil. The patient has a contraction of the occipitofrontal muscle (muscle at the forehead) that is evident on observation and he tends to tip the forehead back in order to compensate for the ptosis, which can impair vision. The patient also has ocular muscle weakness, which prevents lateral eye movement, and weakness of the pharyngeal muscles (ineffective gag reflex), leading to dysphagia for solid foods.

Patients with oculopharyngeal muscular dystrophy also have weakness in their leg muscles and proximal hip girdle. The long-term problems associated with oculopharyngeal muscular dystrophy have less to do with the muscle weakness than with the dysphagia and the resulting possibility of aspiration pneumonia. With supplemental nutrition, modification to food consistency, and proper positioning, patients with this type of muscular dystrophy can have a good quality of life. Chart 55–10 (p. 1756) summarizes the differences in the types of muscular dystrophies.

■ Nursing Management for the Patient with Muscular Dystrophy

Nursing care for patients with muscular dystrophy is aimed at supporting the patient's independence level, preventing complications, and preventing injury, as discussed in the Nursing Process: Patient Care Plan for Muscular Dystrophy feature (p. 1756).

■ Collaborative Management

Many aspects of care are required for patients with muscular dystrophies. For the patient, the care of a nurse, nutritionist, physical therapist, occupational therapist, and orthotics technician will assist the patient to maintain mobility for as long as possible. For the caregiver, assistance from a financial counselor, psychologist, home health nurse, and access to respite care will decrease the chance of severe caregiver role strain.

Gerontological Considerations

Some patients diagnosed with myotonic muscular dystrophy are over the age of 50 and patients diagnosed with oculopharyngeal muscular dystrophy are usually in their 50s or 60s. Nursing considerations for these patients include safety issues, because as a person ages, muscle mass and muscle tone decrease. In addition to the weakness caused by the muscular dystrophy, the nurse must be aware of the normal aging process. Referrals to physical therapy or the use of assistive devices, such as canes or walkers, may be necessary.

CHART 55–10 Differences in the Types of Muscular Dystrophies

Type of Dystrophy	Signs/Symptoms	Onset and Progression
Duchenne	Mostly males Late walkers Unsteady gait Gowers' maneuver	Noticeable at 2–6 years of age Wheelchair bound by 7–12 years of age Many develop respiratory and cardiac problems and die by the mid-20s
Becker	Weakness after engaging in physical exercise or activities Begins in pelvic area, thighs, hips, and shoulders	Teens or young adults Generally will require assistive devices
Myotonic	Muscle wasting in upper extremities, face, neck, hands, forearms, feet	Adults Multisystem effects with chronic problems
Limb-girdle	Muscle wasting in hips and shoulders	Childhood, teen, or adult Cardiopulmonary complications
Facioscapulohumeral	Muscle wasting in face, shoulder girdle, and upper arms	Young adulthood
Oculopharyngeal	Bilateral ptosis Patient tips the head back Dysphagia for solid food	50s–60s

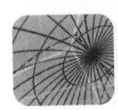

NURSING PROCESS: Patient Care Plan for Muscular Dystrophy

Assessment of Muscle Strength

Subjective Data:
Are you experiencing weakness in any muscle groups?
Are you having difficulty walking or feel off balance?

Objective Data:
Assess strength in upper and lower extremities.
Observe patient as she ambulates.

Nursing Assessment and Diagnoses	Outcomes and Evaluation Parameters	Planning and Interventions with *Rationales*
Nursing Diagnosis: *Activity Intolerance Impaired Physical Mobility*	**Outcome:** Ability to maintain enough muscle strength to ambulate as long as possible. **Evaluation Parameter:** Ability to stand with assistive devices.	**Interventions and *Rationales:*** Teach family to perform PROM exercises. Have them do the exercises three times a day. *Maintains joint mobility and prevents contractures.* Administer prednisone if prescribed. *May improve muscle mass and prolong ambulation.* Teach patient and family the need to maintain appropriate weight. *Obesity makes it difficult for the patient to move and support herself.* Teach patient/family the importance of maintaining safety in the home by keeping it uncluttered *to prevent injury.*

Assessment of Nutritional Status

Subjective Data:
Do you have difficulty swallowing?
What types of food do you eat?
Who prepares your meals?

Objective Data:
Assess patient's skin turgor and fragility.
Assess for excessive loss of hair.

Nursing Assessment and Diagnoses	Outcomes and Evaluation Parameters	Planning and Interventions with *Rationales*
Nursing Diagnosis: *Nutrition, Imbalanced: Less Than Body Requirements*	**Outcome:** The patient/family will be able to understand the rationale for and provide well-balanced meals three times a day. **Evaluation Parameters:** The patient will not experience weight loss of 2.5 kg in a 24-hour period. The patient will drink at least one supplement per day.	**Interventions and *Rationales:*** Ensure a well-balanced meal high in protein, carbohydrate, fiber, vitamins, and minerals *to promote healthy bones, muscles, and tissues and to provide energy.* Weigh daily, using the same scale and the same type of clothing. *Weight loss may indicate muscle-mass wasting, as well as possible malnutrition.* Provide carbohydrate and/or protein supplements as needed. *Supplements assist in maintaining adequate nutrition, which is required to maintain a healthy musculoskeletal system.*

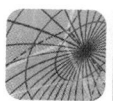

NURSING PROCESS: Patient Care Plan for Muscular Dystrophy—*Continued*

Assessment of Elimination
Subjective Data:
How often do you have a bowel movement?
Is it difficult for you to have a bowel movement?

Objective Data:
Document frequency and quality of bowel movements.

Nursing Assessment and Diagnoses	Outcomes and Evaluation Parameters	Planning and Interventions with *Rationales*
Nursing Diagnosis: *Constipation, Risk for*	**Outcome:** The patient will not be constipated. **Evaluation Parameter:** The patient will not have difficulty having a bowel movement.	**Interventions and *Rationales:*** Provide a high-fiber diet. *Fiber adds bulk to the stool.* Encourage the patient to drink 2,500 mL fluid per day (unless contraindicated by a medical condition). *Fluids help to maintain a soft stool.* Administer stool softener as ordered *to maintain a soft stool.* Reposition the patient every 2–4 hours *to facilitate peristalsis.*

Assessment of Self-Care
Subjective Data:
Are you able to bathe yourself?

Objective Data:
Observe ability to get in and out of the bath and wash body or body parts.

Nursing Assessment and Diagnoses	Outcomes and Evaluation Parameters	Planning and Interventions with *Rationales*
Nursing Diagnosis: *Self-Care Deficit: Bathing/Hygiene*	**Outcome:** The patient will participate in all aspects of care and ADLs. **Evaluation Parameters:** The patient will be able to wash body with minimal assistance.	**Interventions and *Rationales:*** Allow as much independence as possible, allowing the patient to assist in tasks that maintain or build self-esteem. *Maintenance of a positive attitude will allow for a better quality of life.*

Assessment of Swallowing Ability
Subjective Data:
Do you have difficulty swallowing?
Do you ever choke on your food?

Objective Data:
Depressed cough and gag reflexes
Impaired swallowing

Nursing Assessment and Diagnoses	Outcomes and Evaluation Parameters	Planning and Interventions with *Rationales*
Nursing Diagnosis: *Aspiration, Risk for*	**Outcome:** The patient will not aspirate. **Evaluation Parameters:** The patient will have an intact gag reflex. The patient will have clear lung sounds before and after eating and drinking.	**Interventions and *Rationales:*** Assess the patient's gag reflex prior to administering food or fluids. *A gag reflex that is not intact is a precursor to aspiration.* Assess lung sounds before and after meals/drinking. *A new onset of adventitious lung sounds may indicate aspiration.* Assess respiratory status before and after meals/drinking. *Shortness of breath, difficulty breathing, and increased respiratory rate may be indicative of aspiration.* Provide thickened liquids. *Thickened liquids are easier to swallow through esophagus and into stomach.* Teach the patient and family to eat small bites of food. *Patient is less likely to choke.*

Assessment of Cardiac Function
Subjective Data:
Do you experience shortness of breath with physical activity?

Objective Data:
Assess patient's activity tolerance by noting onset of shortness of breath or pain.

(continued)

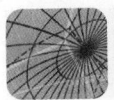

NURSING PROCESS: Patient Care Plan for Muscular Dystrophy—*Continued*

Nursing Assessment and Diagnoses	Outcomes and Evaluation Parameters	Planning and Interventions with *Rationales*
Nursing Diagnosis: *Cardiac Output, Decreased*	**Outcome:** Patient will demonstrate increasing tolerance for physical activity. **Evaluation Parameters:** The patient will have audible S_1 and S_2 heart sounds. The patient will not have any cyanosis or pallor. The patient's capillary refill will be 3 seconds or less.	**Interventions and *Rationales*:** Monitor heart sounds. *Muffled heart sounds may be indicative of cardiomyopathy.* Assess color. *Pallor, cyanosis may be indicative of decreased cardiac output.* Assess capillary refill. *Capillary refill greater than 3 seconds may indicate decreased cardiac output.* Schedule rest periods between activities *to decrease the workload of the heart.* Restrict fluids *to decrease the workload of the heart.*

Assessment of Breathing

Subjective Data:
Do you have difficulty breathing?
Do you feel short of breath?

Objective Data:
Ineffective chest excursion
Nasal flaring
Orthopnea
Use of accessory muscles to breathe

Nursing Assessment and Diagnoses	Outcomes and Evaluation Parameters	Planning and Interventions with *Rationales*
Nursing Diagnosis: *Breathing, Ineffective*	**Outcome:** The patient will demonstrate effective breathing patterns. **Evaluation Parameters:** The patient will have eupneic respirations and normal color and will breathe without the use of accessory muscles. The patient will have an oxygen saturation level of between 90% and 100%.	**Interventions and *Rationales*:** Observe for dyspnea (difficulty breathing), pallor or cyanosis, rate and depth of respirations, use of accessory muscles. *Tachypnea (rapid respiratory rate, usually greater than 24 per minute), bradypnea (slow respiratory rate, usually less than 10 per minute), and shallow respirations will indicate respiratory dysfunction.* Monitor oxygen saturation levels via pulse oximeter. *Levels below 90% may indicate hypoxia.* Encourage rest periods as needed *to allow for easier respirations.* Teach purse-lipped and deep breathing exercises *to expand lungs for maximum oxygen intake and expel carbon dioxide.*

Assessment of Caregiver Role

Subjective Data:
Are you having any difficulty with any of the caregiver tasks?
How is your health?
Are you having trouble sleeping?
Do you have any concerns regarding your loved one's care?

Objective Data:
The caregiver is:
Experiencing headaches
Has lost or gained weight
Is angry
Is feeling depressed

Nursing Assessment and Diagnoses	Outcomes and Evaluation Parameters	Planning and Interventions with *Rationales*
Nursing Diagnosis: *Caregiver Role Strain, Risk for*	**Outcome:** The caregiver will demonstrate emotional health. **Evaluation Parameters:** Free of anger. Free of depression. Less frustrated. Verbalizes a sense of control and self-esteem.	**Interventions and *Rationales*:** Refer patient/family to the Muscular Dystrophy Association and other local support groups. *Discussing concerns with others in the same situation provides a support network.* Allow the patient/family to verbalize fears/concerns. *Provides support.*

As people with muscular dystrophy age, they experience many associated symptoms that adults without muscular dystrophy also experience. Eyesight often decreases. Cataracts are more prevalent in older people, as is arcus senilis, a thin gray-white ring that surrounds the eye margin and may affect the vision. Peristalsis slows down and appetite and nutritional caloric needs decrease with age. Because protein is so important for maintenance of healthy muscles, especially in a patient with MD,

the nurse should take care to assist patients in meal planning or refer them to a dietitian. See the Patient Teaching & Discharge Priorities for Muscular Dystrophy box for more information.

Myopathies

Myopathy refers to any disease of the muscle (National Institute of Neurological Disorders and Stroke [NINDS], 2008). There are various forms of myopathies, which can be inherited or can

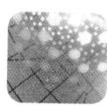

PATIENT TEACHING & DISCHARGE PRIORITIES for Muscular Dystrophy

Need	Teaching
Safety: • Setting (home)	Maintain a safe environment by not having clutter on the floor. Remove throw rugs, electrical wires, clutter toys, etc.
Proper nutrition: • Patient	Eat a well-balanced diet to include protein, carbohydrates, minerals, vitamins.
Self-care activities: • Patient and family	Provide as much of own care as possible to maintain independence, but rest when needed.
Maintain mobility: • Patient and family	Move joints as much as possible.
Prevent constipation: • Patient and family	Eat a diet high in fiber and drink at least 2500 mL fluid/day.

occur in later years (Chart 55–11). Myopathies can also be secondary complications due to endocrine disorders, metabolic disorders, muscle inflammation or infection, certain drugs, or gene mutations (NINDS, 2008).

Clinical Manifestations

The main sign of generalized myopathy is weakness of limbs. In some cases, exercise increases the weakness; in other cases, exercise improves the weakness or even causes it to disappear (NINDS, 2008). Affected muscle groups vary by patient.

Medical Management

Treatment varies according to the type of myopathy. Some patients may require symptomatic treatment only, whereas others may require supportive care, such as braces or other orthotic devices, medications, or physical therapy National Institute of Neurological Disorders & Stroke (2008). The prognosis for myopathies again varies depending on the type. Some patients do not have a disrupted quality of life, whereas to others the myopathy may be disabling.

Types of Myopathies

Following are descriptions of the types of myopathies, clinical presentation, and medical management. Nursing management for the patient with myopathies is presented at the end of the section.

Congenital Myopathy

This type of myopathy is due to a chromosomal defect leading to **hypotonia**, an absence of muscle tone resulting in flaccid, weak muscles in infancy and weakness and delayed motor activity in later childhood years. Diagnosis of a congenital myopathy is made by muscle tissue sampling, which indicates changes in the structure and morphology of the muscle. Treatment is supportive.

Hypokalemic Myopathy

Hypokalemic myopathy is common in the elderly and is due to a low serum potassium level caused by long-term diuretic use (Merck, 2003). Other causes of hypokalemic myopathy include potassium deficiency in the diet, excessive alcohol consumption, aldosteronism, intestinal wasting of potassium (malabsorption), and licorice intoxication (Merck, 2003). Hypokalemic paralysis can occur with diabetic ketoacidosis, after an amphotericin B treatment, chronic diarrhea, renal tubular acidosis, or other chronic conditions that cause hypokalemia.

Clinical Manifestations   Muscle weakness due to hypokalemic myopathy develops gradually and usually affects the proximal muscles of the legs, arms, trunk, and neck. In some cases the thoracic muscles and diaphragm are also affected (Merck, 2003). In patients with hypokalemic myopathy, the potassium level is less

CHART 55–11   Types of Myopathies

Type	Signs/Symptoms
Congenital	Chromosomal defect leading to hypotonia in infancy and weakness and delayed motor activity in later childhood years.
Hypokalemic	Common in the elderly and due to an electrolyte imbalance caused by long-term diuretic use. Affects proximal muscles of the legs, arms, trunk, and neck; may affect thoracic muscles and diaphragm.
Mitochondrial	Affects the ocular muscles; may cause encephalomyopathies.
Steroidal	Chronic use of prednisone can lead to muscle weakness, increased risk for pathologic fractures.
Inflammatory:	
• Polymyositis	Acquired diseases of the skeletal muscle.
• Dermatomyositis	Generalized muscle weakness.
• Inclusion body myositis	Identified by a heliotrope (bluish-purplish in color) rash and muscle weakness. Progressive inflammation of the muscles, usually in men over 50 years of age.

than 3 mEq/L (normal is 3.5 to 5.0 mEq/L). Deep tendon reflexes are less active than normal or may be inactive. The only complaint the patient has is of lethargy; there are no complaints of pain or discomfort (Merck, 2003).

Medical Management Potassium replacement therapy reverses hypokalemic myopathy within 1 month. Chronic hypokalemic myopathy may need to be treated with oral potassium supplements and the patient should be encouraged to eat foods rich in potassium such as avocado, banana, cantaloupe, dates, figs, orange juice, potato, prunes, and some salt substitutes.

Mitochondrial Myopathy

Mitochondrial myopathy is named for the part of the cell it affects, the mitochondria that are responsible for producing most of the energy that is needed for cells to function. A mitochondrial disease can shut down some or all the mitochondria, depleting the essential energy supply. Because muscle cells and nerve cells have especially high energy needs, muscular and neurological problems are common features of mitochondrial disease. Symptoms can include muscle weakness, exercise intolerance, hearing loss, trouble with balance and coordination, seizures and learning deficits (MDA, 2003).

Medical Management Treatments aim at fixing or bypassing the defective mitochondria. These treatments are dietary supplements based on three natural substances involved in the production of the energy molecule ATP. One supplement is creatine, which normally acts as a reserve for ATP by forming a compound called *creatine phosphate*. When a cell's demand for ATP exceeds the amount its mitochondria can produce, creatine can release phosphate to rapidly enhance the ATP supply. Another substance is carnitine, which improves the efficiency of ATP production by helping import certain fuel molecules into mitochondria, and cleaning up some of the toxic by-products of ATP production. Carnitine is available as an over-the-counter supplement called L-carnitine. The last supplement is coenzyme Q10 (coQ10), which is a component of the electron transport chain that uses oxygen to manufacture ATP. Some mitochondrial diseases are caused by coQ10 deficiency, and there is evidence that coQ10 supplementation is beneficial in these cases (MDA, 2003).

Steroid-Induced Myopathy

Long-term corticosteroid usage can lead to muscle weakness and increased risk for pathologic fractures. Patients on corticosteroids for more than 1 year are at risk for steroid myopathy. The manifestations of the muscle weakness are insidious, particularly with a daily dose for more than 6 months (Younger, 2003).

Medical Management Unless contraindicated, the patient should be changed to alternate-day usage of corticosteroids as soon as possible. If the weakness is primarily due to steroid usage, then the symptoms should subside in about 2 to 3 months after the steroid dosage is decreased, and complete recovery is expected (Merck, 2003). A daily exercise regimen is recommended to promote muscle tone.

Inflammatory Myopathies

The inflammatory myopathies are a group of acquired diseases of the skeletal muscle (Dalakas & Hohfield, 2003). These types of myopathies have in common moderate to severe muscle weakness, but all are treatable. The three types of inflammatory my-

opathies are polymyositis, dermatomyositis, and inclusion body myositis. See the Pharmacology Summary on Muscular Disorders.

Polymyositis

Polymyositis (PM) is a type of myopathy that occurs slowly over weeks and months. It is an autoimmune connective tissue disorder that causes damage to muscle fibers. Polymyositis usually affects proximal muscles and causes weakness to those muscles. Complaints include decreasing ability to perform simple tasks, such as combing hair or rising from a chair, or tasks involving fine motor movement (Dalakas & Hohfield, 2003).

Polymyositis affects predominantly women, and African Americans, ages 45 to 65 years old (Merck, 2003). The cause of PM is unknown, but may be triggered by viral, bacterial, or parasitic agents, drugs, vaccinations, or even stress.

Clinical Manifestations Symptoms that accompany polymyositis may be systemic, as well as muscular. Generalized muscle weakness is the main complaint from patients. The weakness is more prevalent in the hips and thighs and the weakness begins as an "ache." For most patients the initial complaint that brings them to see the health care provider is weakness in the upper and lower extremities. Patients with PM also may experience fatigue, weight loss, and changes in nails or skin, including a rash or redness. Systemic involvement includes dysphagia, cardiac involvement, and respiratory involvement. Polymyositis may also occur with another connective tissue disorder known as an overlap syndrome.

Laboratory and Diagnostic Procedures Diagnosis of polymyositis is based on symptomology, the exclusion of other neuromuscular diseases, muscle biopsy findings, elevated serum CK levels (muscle enzymes), and an abnormal electromyography. The confirmatory diagnosis is made with five criteria: proximal muscle weakness, elevated CK, EMG changes, positive muscle biopsy, and a typical skin rash.

Medical Management The treatment for polymyositis depends on the severity of the symptoms and involvement of other systems. The goal of treatment is to improve the patients' quality of life, thus allowing them to carry out their normal ADLs. Various medications are used to treat polymyositis, including prednisone and immunosuppressive drugs, such as methotrexate and azathioprine (Imuran).

The prognosis is poor if the muscle weakness is progressive and severe. This may lead to aspiration pneumonia, dysphagia, malnutrition, and respiratory failure. The patients benefit from physical therapy and a scheduled exercise routine. Frequent monitoring for progression of muscle weakness is warranted.

Dermatomyositis

Dermatomyositis is an autoimmune disease that affects the small blood vessels and capillaries in muscles. It is identified by a heliotrope (bluish-purplish in color) rash and muscle weakness. Degeneration of the skin and muscle ultimately occur, leading to bilateral muscle weakness and some muscle atrophy, mostly of the proximal limb muscles. The heliotrope rash is noted on the eyelids, while an erythematous rash is noted on the chest, face, and neck. Gottron's rash, a reddish raised rash or papules, is noted on the metacarpophalangeal joints and the interphalangeal joints. The nail beds are thick and cracked. Dermatomyositis affects women more than men, and approximately

PHARMACOLOGY Summary for Muscular Disorders

Medication Category	Action	Application/Indication	Nursing Responsibilities
Anticonvulsant			
Phenytoin: (Dilantin)	Helps stabilize the neurons by regulating voltage-dependent sodium and calcium channels, inhibiting calcium movement across neuronal membranes, and enhancing sodium-potassium ATP activity in neurons and glial cells.	To treat delayed muscle relaxation	• Preferred administration routes are oral and intravenous injection. • If patient has difficulty swallowing, open the rapid-release capsules and mix with food or fluid. • To minimize gastric distress, give medication with or just after meals. • If administering through a nasogastric tube, minimize drug absorption in tubing by diluting suspension threefold with sodium chloride or sterile water. After administration, flush tube with at least 20 mL of diluent. • Long-term therapy may increase the patient's requirements for folic acid or vitamin D supplements.
Class IB Antiarrhythmic			
Mexiletine: (Mexil)	Inhibits fast sodium channels in myocardial cell membranes.	To treat delayed muscle relaxation	• Assess for signs of thrombocytopenia, which can occur within a few days of starting mexiletine therapy. • Teach patient to take drug at evenly spaced intervals, to avoid missing doses. • To minimize gastric distress, give medication with food.
Analgesic, Anticonvulsant			
Carbamazepine: (Tegretol)	Slows nerve impulse transmission by blocking sodium channels thus preventing sodium from entering the cell.	To treat delayed muscle relaxation	• Drug is metabolized by the liver—use with caution in patients with impaired hepatic function. • Monitor white blood cell and platelet counts. Decreased counts may indicate bone marrow depression. • To minimize gastric distress, give medication with food. • Teach patient to wear sunscreen to prevent photosensitivity reactions. • Teach patient and family to notify health care provider if they experience unusual bleeding or bruising, fever, rash, or mouth ulcers.
Antiarrhythmic			
Procainamide: (Pronestyl)	Inhibits sodium influx through cell membranes.	To treat delayed muscle relaxation	• Teach patient to swallow extended release tablets whole, without crushing or chewing them. • If patient has difficulty swallowing, have patient crush regular-release tablets or open capsules and mix with food or fluid. • Teach patient to take medication 1 to 2 hours after meals with a full glass of water. • Teach patient and family to notify health care provider if patient experiences unusual bleeding or bruising, fever, rash, or diarrhea.
Antipsoriatic, Antirheumatic			
Methotrexate	Inhibits dihydrofolate reductase, the enzyme that reduces folic acid to tetrahydrofolic acid. Inhibition of the acid interferes with DNA synthesis and cell reproduction.	Immunosuppressant	• Follow policy for preparing and handling drug. Avoid skin contact. • Increase patient's fluid intake to reduce risk of gastric distress. • Assess patient for signs of bleeding and infection.

(continued)

PHARMACOLOGY Summary for Muscular Disorders—*Continued*

Medication Category	Action	Application/Indication	Nursing Responsibilities
Antimetabolite, Immunosuppressant Azathioprine: (Imuran)	May prevent proliferation and differentiation of activated B and T cells. Inteferes with DNA and RNA synthesis.	Immunosuppressant	• Teach patient to take oral drug with food or meals to minimize gastric distress. • Therapy increases risk of viral, fungal, bacterial, and protozoal infections. Monitor for signs of infection especially in patients with cardiac insufficiency or hepatic disease. • Administer oral dose 30 minutes prior to meals. • Warn patient to avoid alcohol, sedatives, and other CNS depressants. • Be aware of multiple IV drug incompatibilities and light sensitivity.

10% of the patients have some type of malignancy, with breast and lung tumors being the most common (Merck, 2003).

Clinical Manifestations   The patient presents with one or more of the following signs: the heliotrope rash; Gottron's papules, which are violet-colored plaques at the finger joints; or **Gottron's sign**, a reddened smooth, scaly rash at the finger joints; thickened fingernails; and muscle weakness. The rash, however, may be noted without muscle weakness. The weakness is a gradual process, usually developing over several months. The proximal limb muscles are affected and are weaker than the distal muscles. In addition, neck muscles are weak. Other muscles involved are those involved with swallowing, leading to possible dysphagia. Other complaints include myalgia and muscle tenderness. Other organs may also be involved, including the respiratory system, which may lead to interstitial lung disease; the cardiac system, which may lead to cardiomyopathy and conduction anomalies; and the gastrointestinal tract, leading to delayed emptying. Microvasculopathy (very small capillaries, veins, and arteries that do not allow for adequate perfusion) of the gastrointestinal tract occurs, leading to ulcerations and perforations of the intestine.

Laboratory and Diagnostic Procedures   Diagnosis of dermatomyositis is determined by signs and symptoms, elevated CK levels, an elevated eosinophil sedimentation rate, and an elevated antinuclear antibody titer. Muscle biopsy shows atrophy of muscle fibers, a decreased number of capillaries and **perivascular** (around blood vessels) infiltrates. An EMG shows muscle inflammation (Merck, 2003).

Medical Management   Treatment is the same as for polymyositis. The patient should be monitored for tumors, and additional tests to rule out breast and lung cancer should be anticipated.

Inclusion Body Myositis

Inclusion body myositis (IBM), like the other myopathies, is an autoimmune disorder that is characterized by a progressive inflammation of the muscles. It occurs mostly in men over age 50 and is a common inflammatory myopathy in the elderly.

Clinical Manifestations   The patient complains of asymmetric muscle weakness, usually beginning in the wrists, finger flexors, and knee extensors. Muscle atrophy usually develops early compared to the other myopathies. In some cases facial muscles are involved, as is dysphagia. Patients with IBM may remain ambulatory for many years, even after the symptoms begin (Merck, 2003).

Medical Management   Elevated CK levels and muscle biopsies that show eosinophilic and cytoplasmic inclusion bodies are the main two diagnostic tools for IBM. As of this writing, there is no known treatment for IBM, however, prednisone and immune globulin have been shown to be effective. Prevention of footdrop and wrist drop is an important aspect in the maintenance of quality of life. This is achieved by bracing and physical therapy.

■ Nursing Management

The object of nursing care is to encourage as much independence as the patient can tolerate, teaching safety measures and the importance of adhering to the prescribed medication regime.

Assessment

It is essential that the nurse listen and document the patient's complaints. Question the patient on:

- When the symptoms began
- Whether there are any accompanying symptoms
- Whether the symptoms have affected the patient's ability to maintain ADLs
- What type of medications the patient is taking, both prescription and OTC
- Whether the patient has noticed any change in his nutritional status
- Whether the patient has noticed any changes in the skin (i.e., rash, redness, etc.).

The nurse must assess the patient's condition by physical examination. Test muscle strength resistance of the affected limb, the unaffected limb, and compare both sides. Auscultate heart and lung sounds. Test deep tendon reflexes (biceps, triceps, patellar). Inspect the extremities for footdrop or wrist drop. Assess the skin for color and the presence of any rashes. Observe gait, balance, and the patient's ability to participate in the exam. For further nursing management, refer to the Nursing Process: Patient Care Plan for Muscular Myopathies.

Gerontological Considerations for Patients with a Myopathy

It is common for myopathies to develop in people in their 50s and 60s. As with all patients with muscle diseases, safety concerns are a priority. The older a person becomes, the more brittle the bones become. Muscle mass and tone decrease and combined with the effects of aging, the added muscle weakness associated with myopathy puts the patient at risk for falls and other injuries. In creating a plan of care for a patient diagnosed with a myopathy, safety must be a priority. For more information, see the Research Opportunities and Clinical Impact Related to Muscular Myopathies (p. 1765).

Many of these patients are diagnosed at an age when they might be contemplating retirement and future plans with their spouse. A medical diagnosis of a myopathy will alter their lifestyle and many may become depressed. Nurses should anticipate patients reacting negatively to this new diagnosis and need to be aware of mood swings that are typical for a patient with a myopathy. For more information, see the Patient Teaching & Discharge Priorities for Muscular Myopathies box (p. 1765).

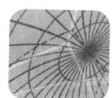

NURSING PROCESS: Patient Care Plan for Muscular Myopathies

Assessment of Muscle Strength

Subjective Data:
Have you experienced weakness in any extremity?
Have you had difficulty swallowing?

Objective Data:
Assess patient's ability to perform ROM on all limbs.
Assess patient's ability to perform resistance tests on all four limbs, flexion of the biceps and extension of the triceps:

- Hand grip
- Flexion of the hip
- Adduction at the hip
- Abduction at the hip
- Extension at the hips
- Extension at the knee
- Flexion at the knee
- Dorsiflexion and plantar flexion

Nursing Assessment and Diagnoses	Outcomes and Evaluation Parameters	Planning and Interventions with *Rationales*
Nursing Diagnosis: *Disuse Syndrome, Risk for*	**Outcome:** The patient is able to perform ROM on all extremities. **Evaluation Parameter:** The patient is able to perform resistance on all four limbs.	**Interventions and *Rationales:*** Provide a physical or occupational therapy referral as needed. *Physical therapists and occupational therapists are able to provide the patient with additional exercises for isotonic muscle movement.* Encourage the patient to eat a well-balanced diet (protein, carbohydrates, vitamins, and minerals) *to maintain a healthy musculoskeletal system.* Teach patient and family the need to maintain appropriate weight. *Obesity makes it difficult for the patient to move and support himself.* Teach patient/family the importance of maintaining safety in the home by keeping it uncluttered *to prevent injury.*

Assessment of Activity Tolerance

Subjective Data:
Do you become fatigued after performing simple tasks?

Objective Data:
Test patient's muscle strength before and after performing physical tasks.

Nursing Assessment and Diagnoses	Outcomes and Evaluation Parameters	Planning and Interventions with *Rationales*
Nursing Diagnosis: *Activity Intolerance*	**Outcome:** The patient is able to perform ADLs without extreme fatigue. **Evaluation Parameter:** The patient and family have implemented an activity/rest period schedule.	**Interventions and *Rationales:*** Instruct the patient and family to pace activities per patient tolerance by assisting in devising an exercise plan that is tolerable and does not cause fatigue. *To decrease muscle fatigue and patient exhaustion.* Encourage the patient to eat a well-balanced diet (protein, carbohydrates, vitamins, and minerals) *to maintain a healthy musculoskeletal system.*

Assessment of Ability to Perform Self-Care

Subjective Data:
What activities are difficult for you to perform?
Do you require assistance with activities?

Objective Data:
Observe patient and evaluate ability to perform ADLs.

(continued)

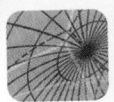

Nursing Assessment and Diagnoses	Outcomes and Evaluation Parameters	Planning and Interventions with *Rationales*
Nursing Diagnosis: If progressive, *Self-Care Deficit: Bathing/Hygiene* and *Dressing/Grooming*	**Outcome:** The patient is able to perform ADLs without extreme fatigue. ***Evaluation Parameters:*** The patient has developed a schedule for performing ADLs. The patient will perform active ROM exercises on all joints three times a day.	**Interventions and *Rationales:*** Teach patient/family to pace daily hygiene practices *to allow the patient to maintain independence.* Encourage active ROM exercises to all joints as prescribed *to maintain joint mobility.* Set up exercise plan with the patient, keeping in mind the patient's limitations. *Exercise helps maintain a healthy musculoskeletal system.*

Assessment of Fall Risk

Subjective Data:
Do you have difficulty with balance?
Have you fallen recently?

Objective Data:
Have the patient walk and observe for balance and muscle weakness.

Nursing Assessment and Diagnoses	Outcomes and Evaluation Parameters	Planning and Interventions with *Rationales*
Nursing Diagnosis: *Falls, Risk for*	**Outcome:** The patient will not fall. ***Evaluation Parameters:*** Patient/family understand the importance of safety and will ensure safety measures are taken in the home. Patient demonstrates slower ambulation and verbalizes understanding about taking designated rest periods in between ambulation, if required.	**Interventions and *Rationales:*** Discuss with the patient/family safety issues in the home, such as throw rugs or other obstacles that may precipitate falls. *Such obstacles can lead to more serious injury.* Discuss with the patient/family the importance of taking time when ambulating. *May prevent serious injury and maintain level of independence.*

Assessment of Swallowing

Subjective Data:
Do you ever choke on your food?
Do you have difficulty swallowing?

Objective Data:
Have speech pathology do a swallow study.
Observe patient swallowing liquid and watch for coughing.

Nursing Assessment and Diagnoses	Outcomes and Evaluation Parameters	Planning and Interventions with *Rationales*
Nursing Diagnoses: *Swallowing, Impaired* and/or *Aspiration, Risk for*	**Outcome:** The patient will not aspirate. ***Evaluation Parameters:*** If required, the patient will see a speech pathologist. The patient and family demonstrate cutting foods into smaller pieces.	**Interventions and *Rationales:*** Refer to speech pathology. *Speech pathologists are able to detect various types of swallowing abnormalities.* Teach the patient and family to eat small bites of food. *Patient will be less likely to choke.* Provide thickened liquids to prevent aspiration. *Thickened liquids are easier to swallow directly into esophagus and stomach.*

Assessment of Coping

Subjective Data:
Do you feel unusually fatigued?
Have you been able to communicate your concerns?

Objective Data:
Observe for:
Decreased use of social support
Destructive behavior toward self and others
Inability to meet basic needs
Inadequate problem solving
Lack of goal-directed behavior
Poor concentration

Nursing Assessment and Diagnoses	Outcomes and Evaluation Parameters	Planning and Interventions with *Rationales*
Nursing Diagnosis: *Coping, Ineffective*	**Outcome:** The patient demonstrates effective coping. ***Evaluation Parameters:*** The patient: Takes actions to manage stressors. Shows self-restraint regarding compulsive or impulsive behaviors. Seeks information concerning illness and treatment. Reports decrease in negative feelings.	**Interventions and *Rationales:*** Allow the patient/family to verbalize fears and concerns. *Provides a support network.* Refer to local and national support system. *Provide support of other people in similar situations.*

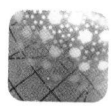

PATIENT TEACHING & DISCHARGE PRIORITIES for Muscular Myopathies	
Need	**Teaching**
Safety considerations	Pace exercise and performance of ADLs with rest periods.
Importance of maintaining joint flexibility	Perform active ROM exercises on all joints three times a day.
Eat a well-balanced diet	Eat foods high in protein, vitamins, minerals, and carbohydrates.
Regular checkups	If symptoms worsen, see primary care provider immediately. Maintain follow-up appointments.

Rhabdomyolysis

Rhabdomyolysis is defined as a syndrome involving muscle necrosis or breakdown. The injured muscle fibers release myoglobin into the bloodstream. The myoglobin then alters the filtration in the kidneys, causing damage and failure. The degree of illness ranges in severity from elevations in muscle enzymes without any symptoms noted by the patient to severe life-threatening symptoms such as electrolyte imbalances and acute renal failure. Some of the causes of rhabdomyolysis include trauma with muscle compression, surgical procedures in which there is a long period of muscle compression, immobilization due to a comatose or postictal state (usually occurring after seizure activity when the patient has been unconscious and unresponsive to stimuli) in which the patient is lying in one position for long periods of time, extreme physical exertion, snakebite, toxins, and viral, bacterial, or fungal infection (Bartelmo & Lockhart, 2008).

Clinical Manifestations and Diagnosis

The patient typically presents to the hospital with muscle pain (myalgia), fatigue, fever, nausea and vomiting, and dark-colored urine. The diagnosis of rhabdomyolysis is based on elevated serum CK levels, which typically are 100 times normal or higher. The high levels of CK come primarily from the necrosis of skeletal muscle. Myoglobinuria (the presence of myoglobin in the urine) results from muscle tissue breakdown and the muscle substances entering the urine and represents an extremely abnormal condition. Myoglobin may be detected in the urine when the serum level is 1,500 to 3,000 ng/mL.

Complications

Numerous complications are associated with rhabdomyolysis:

- Acute renal failure due to tubular obstruction secondary to the myoglobulin pigments
- Electrolyte imbalance:
  - Hyperkalemia (elevated potassium levels in the blood) and hyperphosphatemia (elevated phosphate levels in the blood) can result due to the release of potassium and phosphate from the damaged muscles.
  - Hypocalcemia (low serum calcium level) due to deposited calcium salts in the muscle tissue. This electrolyte imbalance can be severe and patients often show other symptoms associated with hypocalcemia, such as disturbances in cardiac conduction or blood coagulation.
  - Hyperuricemia (elevated uric acid level in the bloodstream) is a result of purine metabolism, resulting in an elevated serum uric acid concentration. Purines are present in nucleic acids, which are both obtained from endogenous and dietary sources.
  - Metabolic acidosis (electrolyte imbalance involving shift of the acid–base balance toward the acid side) can also occur.
  - Compartment syndrome (increased pressure in muscle compartment, may lead to permanent disability of the associated joint) due to edema of a limb and muscle.

Medical Management

The treatment of rhabdomyolysis involves identifying and addressing the underlying cause. Prompt management and prevention of acute renal failure related to the muscle breakdown that causes the myoglobinuria is essential. Increased fluids are administered to hydrate the patient, thereby avoiding or preventing obstruction of the renal filtration process by the myoglobin, which could result in acute renal failure.

◼ Nursing Management

Patients with acute or severe rhabdomyolysis are hospitalized and, due to the severity of the kidney involvement, may be closely monitored in an intensive care unit (ICU). Nursing care will focus on hydration, strict fluid management, and close attention to the impact of possible abnormal electrolyte levels. Bicarbonate is given intravenously to prevent myoglobin from breaking down into toxic compounds in the kidney. Refer to Chapter 47 😊 for

RESEARCH OPPORTUNITIES AND CLINICAL IMPACT RELATED TO MUSCULAR MYOPATHIES	
Research Area	**Clinical Impact**
If the patient maintains his regular regime (at a slower pace), could the disease progression be delayed?	Maintenance of the patient's "normal" routine may promote a better quality of life.
How does a patient's support system affect the progression of the disease?	A positive family support system may prevent depression or a lack of self-esteem related to the disease.

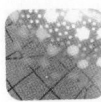

PATIENT TEACHING & DISCHARGE PRIORITIES for Rhabdomyolysis

Need	Teaching
Safety	Ensure home is free of obstacles.
	Take time with ADLs.
Monitor urine output	Inform primary care provider if urine output is low.
	If on a fluid restriction, explain to the patient the importance of maintaining the restriction, so as not to overload heart and lungs.
Follow-up care for kidney and electrolyte monitoring	Stress importance of notifying primary care provider if developing difficulty breathing, swelling, very dry skin, low urinary output, and discolored urine.

nursing management of the patient in acute renal failure. See the box titled Patient Teaching & Discharge Priorities for Rhabdomyolysis for more information.

Eaton-Lambert Syndrome

Eaton-Lambert syndrome is an autoimmune disease that affects muscular activity and function. It is usually associated with small cell carcinoma of the lung and affects men more often than women. Eaton-Lambert syndrome is caused by a decrease in acetylcholine release. In addition, serum from patients with this syndrome contains circulating immunoglobulin antibodies that block calcium channels. Calcium is required by motor nerve fibers to function (Merck, 2003).

Clinical Manifestations

Patients with Eaton-Lambert syndrome complain of muscle fatigue primarily in the leg and trunk muscles. Other symptoms include occasional hyporeflexia, or weak tendon reflex, but muscle contraction restores the tendon reflex. Autonomic symptoms are also present, such as dry mouth, impotence, decreased lacrimation and sweating, orthostatic hypotension, and decreased pupillary reaction to light accommodation (Merck, 2003).

Laboratory and Diagnostic Procedures

Diagnosis of Eaton-Lambert syndrome is made by electrophysiological responses to nerve stimulation. Affirmation of Eaton-Lambert syndrome is also determined by an elevated level of antibodies to the voltage-gated P/Q-type calcium channel. Elevations of these types occur in practically all cases due to lung cancer.

Medical Management

Patients with a diagnosis of lung carcinoma should be monitored frequently for muscle weakness. In some cases, the neuro-

muscular transmission improves after the tumor is removed. Drugs that increase acetylcholine release are also used as well as drugs that control immune-mediated diseases. These drugs include prednisone, azathioprine, and immune globulin.

■ Nursing Management

The object of nursing management is to teach patients safety measures and adherence to their medication regime. If the cause of Eaton-Lambert syndrome is lung cancer, then the nurse should provide symptomatic care and education. For more information, see the Patient Teaching & Discharge Priorities for Eaton-Lambert Syndrome box.

Muscle Cramps

Muscle cramps are sudden involuntary contractions in one or more muscle that last for a few seconds to minutes. Muscle cramps can be caused by a nerve that malfunctions, as in spinal cord injury, or from dehydration, lack of minerals in the body, overuse or straining of the muscle, and a decreased blood supply to the muscle (MedLine Plus, 2008).

The bundles of fibers that make up the muscle contract and expand to produce movement. It is important to keep the fibers stretched out so that they may respond vigorously during exercise. If the muscle is poorly conditioned, then it is more likely to become fatigued, which can change the spinal neural reflexes causing cramping. Overexertion of the muscle depletes the oxygen supply to the muscle cells, leading to waste products that cause muscle spasm (AAOS, 2008).

Exercise-induced muscle cramps are manifested by pain and involuntary muscle contractions that occur either during exercise or immediately after exercise (Dumke, 2003). The pain is often spasmodic and episodic. Exercise-induced muscle cramps

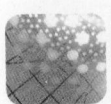

PATIENT TEACHING & DISCHARGE CONSIDERATIONS for Eaton-Lambert Syndrome

Need	Teaching
Safety	Ensure home is free of obstacles.
	Take time with ADLs.
Mobility	Maintain joint mobility by performing active ROM exercises on all joints three times a day.

CHART 55–12	Muscle Cramps	
Type	**Cause**	**Treatment**
Fatigue	Inadequate stretching prior to exercise Dehydration	Stretching of the affected muscle Adequate hydration with electrolyte-based beverage
Exercise	Inadequate training	Training with warm-up exercise, hydration, well-balanced diet
Hypocalcemia	Low calcium level	A diet that includes foods high in calcium or calcium supplements Monitor electrolytes
Idiopathic	Unknown; occurs during bedtime	Stretching exercise after cramps begin or before bedtime

occur more frequently during hot weather as sweat drains the body of fluid, sodium, and other minerals such as potassium and calcium. The lack of these nutrients may cause the muscle to spasm. It is also thought that muscle cramps primarily occur over muscles that span two joints (AAOS, 2008; Dumke, 2003).

Calcium plays an important role in the musculoskeletal system. One of its primary roles is in regulating muscle contraction and relaxation. A person who has hypocalcemia is at risk for muscle spasms of the face and extremities. Hypocalcemia also results in hyperactive deep tendon reflexes. Hypercalcemia, in turn, can cause generalized muscle weakness and flaccidity of the muscles.

Idiopathic muscle cramps are muscle cramps that occur with no particular etiology. The cramps are usually without accompanying weakness. Idiopathic muscle cramps generally affect healthy, middle-aged or elderly adults and generally occur during the nighttime or when the person is sleeping. The most common muscles affected are of the calf or foot muscles, causing plantar flexion to the afflicted foot. The various types of muscle cramps are summarized in Chart 55–12.

Medical Management

Diagnosis is made on the patient's subjective complaints and lack of any weakness or disability. The treatment is prophylactic, in that the patient is instructed to stretch prior to exercise and to maintain balanced nutrition and fluid intake. Patients who have night cramps should be encouraged to perform stretching exercises on the legs prior to falling asleep. When muscle cramps occur, the patient is instructed to stretch directly after the pain begins.

■ Nursing Management

The nursing plan of care involves education regarding safety issues and measures to prevent the occurrence of muscle cramps. Research into the efficacy of electrolyte-based drinks is addressed in the Research Opportunities and Clinical Impact Related to Muscle Cramps box.

Assessment

The nurse should assess the patient's condition through a physical examination. Observe the patient during ambulation. Test resistance on all four extremities. Monitor electrolyte levels. Obtain a daily "diary" of the patient's intake and output. Obtain a history regarding the cramps by asking do they only occur with exercise, are they relieved by stretching, is there a family history of muscle cramps? Although most muscle cramps are benign, they can be signs of underlying disease such as spinal nerve irritation or compression, thyroid disease, or liver disease (AAOS, 2008). Note that the elderly are prone to muscle cramps for reasons discussed in the Gerontological Considerations box.

Fibromyalgia

Fibromyalgia is a syndrome of chronic musculoskeletal pain. It is common in the elderly population and a major cause of disability. The exact cause is unknown, but one theory suggests that

GERONTOLOGICAL CONSIDERATIONS Related to Muscle Cramps

In addition to the decreased muscle mass and tone that are inherent to the aging process, many elderly people do not drink enough fluids due to the fear and embarrassment of incontinence. Therefore, it is imperative that the nurse teach the older patient the importance of hydrating, exercising in moderate temperatures to prevent the onset of muscle cramps, and performing some mild stretching exercises. Before suggesting electrolyte-based drinks, the nurse should know the patient's laboratory values of sodium and potassium. If a patient has a history of hypernatremia or hyperkalemia, then recommending these drinks on a daily basis may be detrimental to his health. The older patient needs to eat a well-balanced diet with vitamins and minerals to maintain bone and muscle integrity. Encourage the patient to have regular checkups in which electrolyte levels are monitored.

RESEARCH OPPORTUNITIES AND CLINICAL IMPACT RELATED TO MUSCLE CRAMPS

Research Need	Clinical Impact
In exercise-induced muscle cramps, will drinking one to two glasses of an electrolyte-based drink prior to exercising prevent muscle cramps?	A decreased incidence of muscle cramps due to dehydration, as well as longer endurance levels.

stress is responsible for fibromyalgia. Other theories suggest that the patient has an abnormal amount of pain-related chemicals in the nervous system; the patient has a conscious or subconscious tension, resulting in sleep disturbances; or the patient has a lowered pain threshold.

Recent studies have shown that patients with fibromyalgia have a "skewed" central pain processing function in their body (Peeke, 2003). Research has also shown that patients with fibromyalgia have elevated levels of a nerve growth factor and a chemical signal called *substance P* in the spinal fluid. Also, the amount of serotonin, the chemical produced in the brain that has an effect on nerves, is low (Frazier & Drzymkowski, 2009). These patients become extremely sensitive to even minor pain. Fibromyalgia is not associated with any type of musculoskeletal disorder, nor does it predispose a patient to a musculoskeletal disorder, but it may coexist with certain rheumatologic diseases such as lupus or arthritis.

Clinical Manifestations

The main signs and symptoms of fibromyalgia are pain in the back, neck, forearms, and knees. Besides joint and muscle pain, other symptoms are headaches, inability to sleep which leads to daytime fatigue, dizziness, alternating constipation and diarrhea, generalized weakness, depression, numbness and tingling of hands and feet, and memory loss. The onset of symptoms may be associated with psychological distress, trauma, or infection. The symptoms are aggravated by poor posture, strenuous exercise, and smoking (Frazier & Drzymkowski, 2009).

Laboratory and Diagnostic Procedures

The diagnosis of fibromyalgia is based on the patient's subjective symptoms, as well as a medical and surgical history. Patients with fibromyalgia do not have any other associated musculoskeletal disorder; therefore, arthritis, inflammations, and bursitis should be ruled out. Patients with this condition complain not only of muscle and joint aches but are extremely tender in these specific areas: at the antecubital area, below the clavicles, at the posterior neck, at the posterior top of the buttocks, and at the lateral pelvis. The American College of Rheumatology (2008) uses criteria for classification of fibromyalgia. This criteria includes widespread pain for a minimum of 3 months, and pain at 11/18 tender points on palpation. These points include the occipital, low cervical trapezius, supraspinatus, rib, epicondyle, and gluteal and knee areas.

Medical Management

The treatment of fibromyalgia is based on the severity of pain, stress level, and overall health of the patient. There is no cure for fibromyalgia but treatment will help to alleviate symptoms and restore function. The plan of care will involve patient education, stress reduction, physical exercise, and medications to reduce pain and improve the quality of sleep.

The federal Food and Drug Administration has approved the use of pregabalin (Lyrica) for patients with fibromyalgia. Two double-blinded studies indicated that people using the medication showed rapid and sustained pain reduction and improved sleep patterns for 6 months (Arthritis Foundation, 2008).

A scheduled exercise plan is important for increasing the blood supply, oxygen, and nutrients to joints and muscles. Recommended exercises include walking, bike riding, swim-ming, or aerobic exercise. Watsu, an exercise regimen performed in warm water, has been shown to be effective in patients with fibromyalgia (Osborn, 2005). The patient with fibromyalgia may require assistance in eliminating or controlling the stress that is causing symptoms. Anxiety and depression must be controlled in order to control fibromyalgia. Sometimes an antidepressant may be ordered to assist the patient through the "rough spots" and can promote the balance of pain-producing chemicals. A continuing medication regimen and an exercise plan are helpful in maintaining healthy muscles and joints.

■ Nursing Management

Nursing care should focus on assisting the patient to participate in a regimen that alleviates or minimizes the discomfort, as well as methods to deal with the patient's current stressors. Education about the illness, the importance of sleep, use of pain management strategies, adaptation to their illness, and promotion of regular exercise should be the nurse's role in assisting patients with this illness. See the Nursing Process: Patient Care Plan for Fibromyalgia feature and the Gerontological Considerations for Fibromyalgia box.

Alternative Treatments for Patients with Fibromyalgia

Massage therapy and relaxation techniques have been shown to help relieve the pain, stiffness, and sleep disturbances associated with fibromyalgia, as discussed in more detail in the Complementary and Alternative Therapies box (p. 1770).

Other alternative treatments used for patients with fibromyalgia include acupuncture, herbal products, reflexology, biofeedback, meditation and prayer, and **transcutaneous electrical nerve stimulation (TENS)** (pain relief via low-voltage electrical stimulation over a painful area).

Poliomyelitis

The onset of polio occurred in the 1950s with devastating outcomes for patients, such as flaccid paralysis of the legs. People contracted polio through a virus that is spread from infected

GERONTOLOGICAL CONSIDERATIONS for Fibromyalgia

As people get older, sleep patterns change and many people do not sleep soundly throughout the night. Inadequate sleep is exacerbated in patients diagnosed with fibromyalgia, and so, besides the usual safety issues related to pain in the joints, they are particularly at risk for falls because of fatigue.

Older patients need to be aware that as the liver function decreases with age, medications are not filtered as quickly, leading to a faster rate of toxicity. This is particularly important when taking nonsteroidal anti-inflammatory agents, which can lead to ulcerations of the stomach and intestinal wall. Tylenol can cause altered liver function, which is especially dangerous to a patient who already has decreased liver function.

Lastly, chronic or acute pain, coupled with stress, may cause an older patient to feel hopeless, helpless, and alone, which may lead to depression.

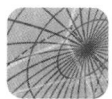

NURSING PROCESS: Patient Care Plan for Fibromyalgia

Assessment of Pain

Subjective Data:
On a scale of 1–10 with 1 being a little pain and 10 being the worst pain you have ever felt, at what level is your pain?
Do you routinely take pain medication at home? If yes, what is the name of the medication and why do you take it?
Are you allergic to any medications?

Objective Data:
Pain assessed during ROM to all joints. Pain greater when bending and turning the neck.
Monitor patient for:
Facial grimacing
Change in breathing pattern
Change in blood pressure and/or pulse rate
Diaphoresis
Agitation

Nursing Assessment and Diagnoses	Outcomes and Evaluation Parameters	Planning and Interventions with *Rationales*
Nursing Diagnosis: *Pain, Acute* or *Chronic*	**Outcome:** Pain level will be tolerable. **Evaluation Parameters:** Diminished or absent level of pain through patient's self-report. Absence of physiological indicators of pain.	**Interventions and *Rationales:*** Assess the patient's pain level on a scale of 1–10. Assess the pain level with bending the back, ROM of all joints. *Determining a specific pain level in relation to certain movements is helpful in devising an exercise plan, and prescribing a medication regime.* Assist the patient in developing an exercise plan that is not too strenuous. Teach medication regime and the importance of adherence to the medication plan, as well as reporting of side effects related to NSAIDs: gastric upset, rectal, or oral bleeding, bruising, abdominal discomfort. If on Tylenol, monitor liver enzymes. *Long-term Tylenol use or high-doses of Tylenol may cause liver damage.*

Assessment of Coping

Subjective Data:
Do you feel unusually fatigued?
Have you experienced altered sleep patterns?
Have you been able to communicate your concerns?

Objective Data:
Observe for:
Decreased use of social support
Destructive behavior toward self and others
Inability to meet basic needs
Inadequate problem solving
Lack of goal-directed behavior
Poor concentration

Nursing Assessment and Diagnoses	Outcomes and Evaluation Parameters	Planning and Interventions with *Rationales*
Nursing Diagnosis: *Coping, Ineffective*	**Outcome:** The patient will demonstrate effective coping. **Evaluation Parameters:** The patient: Takes actions to manage stressors. Shows self-restraint regarding compulsive or impulsive behaviors. Seeks information concerning illness and treatment. Reports decrease in negative feelings.	**Interventions and *Rationales:*** Allow the patient/family to verbalize fears and concerns. *Provides a support network.* Assist the patient in finding ways to cope with stress: Refer to social services or a therapist to assist the patient in managing stressful situations. *Social services and/or therapy can assist the patient in dealing with stress via several techniques.* Refer to local and national support system. *Provides support of other people in similar situations.* If the patient is placed on antidepressants, teach the patient the importance of maintaining the dose schedule and not to change or discontinue the medication without talking to her primary care provider. *Abruptly discontinuing antidepressants can exacerbate the symptoms of clinical depression.*

oropharyngeal secretions or fecal matter. Although polio has been fairly well eradicated in the United States, many Third World countries are struggling to control the onset and outbreak of polio (CDC, 2008b).

Epidemiology and Etiology

The polio virus infects the anterior horn cells of the gray matter of the spinal cord, which causes selective destruction of the motor neurons. The virus enters the body through the nasal and oral passages, crosses into the gastrointestinal tract, and enters the bloodstream traveling to the central nervous system. The incubation period is 7 to 21 days. It is highly infectious but up to 95% of patients who have the virus have no symptoms. Approximately 6% will have flu-like symptoms and fewer than 1% result in permanent paralysis. Of the patients who progress to paralysis, 5% to 10% die as a result of the virus affecting the respiratory muscles (CDC, 2008b; Frazier & Drzymkowski, 2009).

Clinical Manifestations

The poliovirus damages the nerves that control muscles. Because of the nerve damage, patients with polio have extreme muscle weakness and at times paralysis of an extremity. The patient will present with a low-grade fever, discharge from the sinuses, and malaise. As the disease progresses, the patient will complain of muscle weakness, stiff neck, nausea and vomiting, and flaccid paralysis of the muscles involved. The muscles affected atrophy and decreased tendon reflexes and joint deterioration evolve. Many patients with polio require assistive devices, such as canes, walkers, and crutches. In some cases, the paralysis affects the respiratory muscles, causing death.

Medical Management

The treatment for polio is immunization. Two forms of immunization are currently used against the polio virus: an injected polio vaccine (IPV) or a live, oral polio vaccine (OPV). Both vaccines are effective in preventing transmission of the disease from person to person, but in some cases the OPV can cause polio. For this reason, many health professionals recommend the IPV vaccine instead.

The vaccine schedule against polio varies for children and adults:

- **Children**—Children receive four doses of IPV at 2 months of age, 4 months of age, 6 to 18 months of age, and a booster at 4 to 6 years of age.
- **Adults**—For adults who have not previously received the vaccine, it is important to administer it if they (1) plan to travel to countries where polio is active, (2) work with the polio virus, or (3) care for patients with polio.

For the patient who actually has active polio, the treatment is supportive. Analgesics and moist heat application are administered for pain. In the acute phase bed rest is indicated followed by physical therapy and evaluation for the use of assistive devices such as braces.

Post-Polio Syndrome

Post-polio syndrome (PPS) is acquired by patients who previously had polio. In some patients who have had polio, some of the undamaged nerves grow branches that connect to muscles that have lost their nerve connection, allowing some movement to the muscle. However, it is now being noted that the nerve connections are

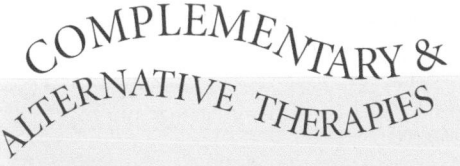

COMPLEMENTARY & ALTERNATIVE THERAPIES   **Massage**

Description:
The general definition of massage therapy is the use of one's hands, fingers, elbows, forearm, or feet on another's body to elicit relaxation, reduce stress, promote health, or to treat a specific condition of the musculoskeletal system. Most U.S. states require a massage therapist to be licensed in order to practice. Massage therapy has evolved during the twentieth century to become a well known, respected therapy.

Research Support:
One study examined the impact of massage applied after exercise on muscle soreness. The study involved 10 healthy participants who performed 10 sets of 6 arm exercises. Three hours later, each participant then received 10 minutes of massage on only one arm; the other arm received no treatment. Although researchers found that massage had no effect on muscle function, they did find a significant decrease in muscle soreness in the arm that received massage (Zainuddin, Newton, Sacco, & Nosaka, 2005).

Massage that is performed on the patient's hand (or hand massage) is a simple, nonintrusive nursing intervention that the nurse can incorporate into routine nursing care activities. The nurse who utilizes hand massage can convey caring, promote comfort, and facilitate nurse–patient communication. One study evaluated the effect of hand massage on older adults residing in a nursing home. Outcomes were measured in terms of comfort and satisfaction. Over specific time periods, researchers found significant group differences in comfort and satisfaction between control and intervention groups. However, researchers found no significant differences in comfort levels or satisfaction with care over time (Kolcaba, Schirm, & Steiner, 2006). This may, in part, be due to the prevalence of memory impairment in older adults.

A review of 13 published randomized and quasi-randomized studies aimed to examine the effect of massage therapy on low-back pain, which is one of the most common musculoskeletal problems. Many people seek relief of their low-back pain through massage therapy. These studies showed that massage may be beneficial for patients with low-back pain, particularly when combined with exercise and education. However, researchers felt that more studies are needed to confirm these conclusions (Furlan, Imamura, Dryden, & Irvin, 2008).

References
Furlan, A. D., Imamura, M., Dryden, T., & Irvin, E. (2008, October). Massage for low-back pain. *Cochrane Database Systematic Reviews, 8*(4), CD001929.

Kolcaba, K., Schirm, V., & Steiner, R. (2006). Effects of hand massage on comfort of nursing home residents. *Geriatric Nursing, 27*(2), 85–91.

Zainuddin, Z., Newton, M., Sacco, P., & Nosaka, K. (2005). Effects of massage on delayed-onset muscle soreness, swelling, and recovery of muscle function. *Journal of Athletic Training, 40*(3), 174–180.

not as strong as once thought and therefore start to break down again after a time. This breakdown causes renewed weakness of the muscle they control. The progressive weakness is not noted until 15 years or more after the initial disease and involves already affected muscles (Frazier & Drzymkowski, 2009; WebMD, 2007).

Clinical Manifestations

Manifestations include new muscle weakness, fatigue, and muscle and joint pain. Some patients may develop dysphagia, respiratory difficulty, and decreased ability to tolerate cold. Those at risk for developing PPS are patients who had polio as a teenager or adult, still have muscle weakness, are female, and have had respiratory difficulty related to damage to the nerves that control breathing (WebMD, 2007).

Medical Management

Continuation of an active lifestyle is important for patients with PPS. The goals of treatment are to learn ways to stay active despite muscle weakness and to control muscle and joint pain with analgesics, heat and cold, and a balanced diet. The patient may require the use of assistive devices in order to maintain their ADLs and normal routine.

 # Nursing Management

Nursing care is directed to supportive care, safety measures, and adherence to an exercise regimen.

Assessment

The nurse should listen to the patient's subjective complaints and ask about the following:

- The patient's medical–surgical history
- When the symptoms began
- Whether there are any accompanying symptoms
- Whether the symptoms have affected the patient's ability to maintain ADLs
- What type of exercise the patient engages in and how often the patient exercises
- Whether the patient has traveled to any Third World countries
- What type of medications the patient is taking, both prescription and OTC
- Whether the patient has had any respiratory difficulty, back pain, or dysphagia.

The nurse should objectively assess the patient by performing a physical examination. Observe the patient during ambulation. Test resistance of all four limbs. Auscultate lung sounds. Have the patient bend forward and backward (if able) to test the strength of the back muscles.

Nursing Diagnosis

The primary diagnoses for the patient with poliomyelitis or PPS include:

- *Physical Mobility, Impaired*
- *Fatigue*

- *Falls, Risk for*
- *Airway Clearance, Ineffective*
- *Disuse Syndrome, Risk for*

Outcomes and Evaluation

Outcomes include maintenance of a clear airway as exhibited by the patient's ability to swallow and cough, maintenance of current muscle use as exhibited by the patient's ability to perform scheduled exercises, and maintenance of functional alignment of all joints. Due to muscle weakness, the patient is at risk for falls. Outcome criteria would include no falls. Fatigue will be evaluated by the patient's ability to plan rest periods throughout the day to maintain strength.

Planning, Interventions, and Rationales

Patient education is key to the prevention of polio. Parents should be encouraged to have their children vaccinated and any adult who has not been vaccinated and is traveling to a Third World country is advised to receive the vaccine.

The patient with polio or PPS will be evaluated for factors that increase the risk of muscle and joint complications, such as preexisting conditions such as arthritis or surgery, that would reduce mobility. Muscle function depends on activity to maintain and increase muscle strength and maintain balance and muscle tone. Disuse will cause atrophy and lead to shortening of muscle fibers and reduce joint motion.

An active exercise program should be developed, as the patient's condition permits, including complete ROM to all joints at least four times daily. Active exercise promotes maximum muscle contraction and helps to maintain muscle strength and endurance. Full ROM exercises to all joints stretches the surrounding muscle fibers and maintains the coordinated function of the joint structures.

It is important to plan rest periods between activities to prevent fatigue. Rest periods assist with endurance and the ability to participate in the plan of care.

Administer analgesics and warm and cold compresses to areas of discomfort. Promoting comfort permits physical activity.

Instruct the patient on the use of mobility aids (canes, braces, walkers). Educating the patient regarding the importance of mobility aids helps her adjust to using them. Mobility aids help to prevent injury and can offer the patient a sense of security.

Evaluation

Prognosis for the patient with poliomyelitis is fair depending on the muscles that are involved. The prognosis for PPS is good. Evaluation of the plan of care will include the patient's statement that pain is controlled and an assessment of muscle strength along with the patient's ability to participate in the exercise regimen. If the patient requires mobility aids, evaluation will include proper use of the device as exhibited by the patient and a lack of falls or injury as reported by the patient. For more information, see Patient Teaching & Discharge Priorities for Post-Polio Syndrome (p. 1772).

Health Promotion for Patients with Musculoskeletal Disorders

All of the ailments discussed in this section have some type of permanent disability and/or an acute or chronic discomfort or

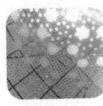

PATIENT TEACHING & DISCHARGE CONSIDERATIONS for Post-Polio Syndrome

Need	Teaching
Need for exercise regime	Maintain and plan a daily exercise regime that promotes bone and muscle activity, but is not physically exhausting, such as walking or bike riding.
Eat a well-balanced diet	Set up a dietary menu that includes, vitamins, minerals, protein, calcium, and carbohydrates.
Maintain body mass index for height (ideal body weight)	Weigh weekly. If gaining weight, modify diet to decrease carbohydrates.
Rest periods	Rest if tired or in between activities and exercise programs.

weakness associated with them. Healthy living, to include not being overweight, eating a healthy diet, and practicing some type of exercise plan, is mandatory for preventing further complications in patients with these conditions. A scheduled exercise program is prescribed in order to maintain joint mobility, to increase circulation and oxygenation to the muscles and tissues, and to strengthen bone. Patients should maintain a weight that is appropriate for their height, because added weight causes stress to an already impaired musculoskeletal system. Maintenance of weight is predicated on a good exercise plan, plus a diet low in fats.

The concept of the federal government's *Healthy People 2010* campaign is not just for healthy individuals but can benefit everyone, even those with chronic or disabling conditions. It is a framework of national health objectives designed to identify preventable threats to health and establish goals to reduce these threats. The leading health indicators that correlate with this chapter are as follows: Engage in an exercise program, abstain from tobacco use and substance abuse, maintain weight per body mass index (ideal weight), receive immunizations for polio if traveling to a Third World country, and maintain regular visits with a health care provider. Therefore, nursing responsibilities should include health teaching to include dietary management, weight control, abstinence from smoking, and a viable exercise program.

Clinical Preparation

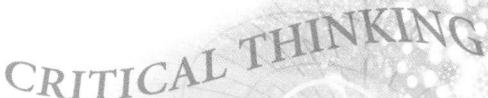

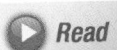

Read

- History of Current Illness
- Past Medical History
- Physical Exam
- Admitting Medical Orders
- Laboratory Study Results

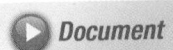

Document

- Summary of Hospitalization
- Pathophysiology Form
- Laboratory Values
- Laboratory Results Explanation

Apply

- List of Potential Nursing Diagnoses
- Concept Map
- Critical Thinking Questions

Log on to MyNursingKit.com to download forms you will need and to complete further steps in the Clinical Preparation assignment.

HISTORY OF PRESENT ILLNESS

You are the nurse on a medical–surgical unit. You have been notified that you will be receiving a patient from the emergency department (ED). The ED nurse calls the unit and gives report on the 72-year-old female being admitted. She was found by her daughter in her home on the floor of her bedroom approximately 12 hours after a fall. The patient states she does not clearly remember what led to the fall and is complaining of sharp, constant right hip discomfort.

Medical–Surgical History

The patient has a history of hypertension. She states she has never had an operation.

Social History

The patient states she has never smoked. She drinks alcohol occasionally. She walks for 20 minutes daily and takes a t'ai chi class on Tuesday afternoons.

Physical Exam

The patient is orientated to person, place, and time. Pupils are equal and react to light. Bilateral grasps are equal and strong. She rates her right hip pain at an 8 on a scale of 0 (no pain) to 10 (most pain ever). Vital signs: temp: 99°F; BP: 180/90 mmHg; heart rate: 104 bpm; 22 respirations per minute, even and relaxed. Bilateral breath sounds are present and clear in all lobes; however, bilateral breath sounds are slightly diminished in the lower lobes. Right leg is adducted and internally rotated, but patient denies numbness or tingling of her right foot. Right pedal pulses palpated less than left, but right pedal pulse strong by Doppler. She states that she takes high blood pressure medication and on occasion an aspirin for joint discomfort.

Admitting Medical Orders

Service: orthopedic surgery
Diagnosis: fracture right hip
Allergies: no known allergies
Vital signs: every 4 hours including oxygen saturation
Call house officer: temp > 38.5°C, HR > 110 or < 60, RR > 30 or < 12, BP sys > 160 or < 90, O_2 sat < 92%, urine output < 120 mL in 4 hours, change in neurological exam, any Hct result that is 5 less than the baseline ED Hct
Activity: bed rest
Diet: nothing by mouth
IVs: D5.45NS with 20 mEq of KCl at 100 mL/hr
I&O: every shift
Respiratory care: incentive spirometer every hour when awake
DVT prophylaxis: sequential compression device to lower extremities bilaterally
Treatments: skin traction to right lower extremity
Consent to be signed for open reduction and internal fixation of right trochanter

To the operating room tomorrow on call
Insert Foley catheter
Daily weight

Scheduled Medications

Atenolol 50 mg po every day
Preop medication per anesthesiologist

PRN Medications

Phenergan 25 mg IV every 6 hours prn nausea
Morphine 2–4 mg IV every 4 hours prn pain
Ativan 0.5 mg IV every 6 hours prn anxiety
Tylenol 650 mg PO every 4 hours for pain

Ordered Laboratory Studies

Complete blood count and Chem panel every morning

Ordered Diagnostic Studies

Chest x-ray every morning

LABORATORY STUDY RESULTS

Test	ED Initial	ED 2nd (4 hours)	On Admission to Floor
CBC			
Hemoglobin (Hgb)	10.5 g/dL	9.5 g/dL	9.5 g/dL
Hematocrit (Hct)	34%	33%	32%
RBC	3.2/mm³	3/mm³	3/mm³
Reticulocytes	2.0%	2.4%	2.4%
MCV	72 µm³	68 µm³	68 µm³
MCH	27 pg	25 pg	25 pg
Platelets	150/mm	146/mm³	146/mm³
Electrolytes			
Sodium	135 mEq/L	135 mEq/L	140 mEq/L
Potassium	3.6 mEq/L	3.6 mEq/L	3.9 mEq/L
Calcium	9 mg/dL	9 mg/dL	9 mg/dL
BUN	14 mg/dL	14 mg/dL	16 mg/dL
Creatinine	0.8 mg/dL	1 mg/dL	1.2 mg/dL
Glucose	150 mg/dL	148 mg/dL	140 mg/dL

CRITICAL THINKING QUESTIONS

1. What pertinent information can be assessed by the medical–surgical nurse?
2. What are the patient's risk factors for sustaining a fracture?
3. What other lab tests might the nurse anticipate?
4. What are the goals of medical management for this client?
5. What are two priority nursing diagnoses?
6. What are some postoperative instructions for this client?

Answers to Critical Thinking Questions appear in Appendix D.

NCLEX® REVIEW

1. The mechanical properties of bone are based on which of the following?
   1. Age and flexibility
   2. Nutritional status and body weight
   3. Stress and strain
   4. Gravity and circumference

2. A nurse is providing a preventive health care seminar related to ways to decrease the effects of osteoporosis. Which of the following risk factors does the nurse discuss which apply to both men and women?
   1. Anorexia
   2. Diet low in calcium and Vitamin D
   3. History of maternal hip fracture
   4. Low body weight and low body mass index

3. A nurse has provided an overview of evidence-based care for prevention of hip fracture in older people. Which statement made by a participant warrants further education?
   1. "Living at my own home increases my chance of a fracture."
   2. "Taking anticonvulsants may increase my possibility of falling."
   3. "Insulin-dependent diabetic patients are more at risk."
   4. "Women experience more hip fractures than men."

4. All forms of muscular dystrophies have what element in common?
   1. The cause of death is due to systemic infection.
   2. The average life expectancy is into the fourth decade.
   3. Muscle membranes have a protein deficiency or absence of dystrophin.
   4. Cognitive development and functioning are not at a full level.

5. A 75-year old male with long-term alcohol abuse would likely experience which of the following myopathies?
   1. Hypokalemic
   2. Polymyositis
   3. Steroid-induced
   4. Inclusion body myositis

6. The diagnosis of fibromyalgia is based on the patient's report of:
   1. long-term arthritis history.
   2. treatment for depression.
   3. familial tendency of the condition.
   4. subjective symptoms.

Answers for review questions appear in Appendix D

KEY TERMS

cancellous (trabecular) bone *p.1729*
compact (cortical) bone *p.1729*
dermatomyositis *p.1760*
electromyelogram (EMG) *p.1754*
endoskeletal *p.1728*
Gottron's sign *p.1762*
Haversian canals *p.1729*
hypotonia *p.1759*

kyphosis *p.1753*
lamellar bone *p.1729*
lordosis *p.1753*
modeling *p.1730*
osteoblasts *p.1730*
osteoclasts *p.1730*
osteocytes *p.1730*
osteoid *p.1730*

osteology *p.1728*
osteoporosis *p.1733*
periosteum *p.1728*
perivascular *p.1762*
scoliosis *p.1753*
subchondral bone *p.1729*
transcutaneous electrical nerve stimulation (TENS) *p.1768*

EXPLORE **PEARSON mynursingkit**™

MyNursingKit is your one stop for online chapter review materials and resources. Prepare for success with additional NCLEX®-style practice questions, interactive assignments and activities, web links, animations and videos, and more!

Register your access code from the front of your book at
www.mynursingkit.com

REFERENCES

American Academy of Orthopaedic Surgeons. (2008). *Muscle cramps.* Retrieved May 24, 2008, from http://orthoinfo.aaos.org/topic.cfm?topic=A00200#Cause

American Cancer Society. (2008). *Detailed guide: Bone cancer.* Retrieved May 17, 2008, from http://www.cancer.org/docroot/CRI/content/CRI_2_4_1X_What_Is_bone_cancer

American College of Rheumatology. (2008). *Fibromyalgia.* Retrieved May 24, 2008, from http://www.rheumatology.org/publications/classification/fibromyalgia/fibro.asp

Arthritis Foundation. (2008). *Fibromyalgia.* Retrieved May 24, 2008, from http://www.arthritis.org/new-fibro-treatment.php

Bartelmo, J. M., & Lockhart, A. (Eds.). (2008). *Nursing: Understanding diseases.* Philadelphia: Lippincott Williams & Wilkins.

Beers, M. H., & Porter, R. S. (Eds.). (2006). *The Merck manual of diagnosis and therapy* (18th ed.). Whitehouse Station, NJ: Merck Research Laboratories.

Canalis, E. (2004). Mechanisms of glucocorticoid induced osteoporosis. *Arthritis Research Therapy, 6*(Suppl. 3), 37.

Centers for Disease Control and Prevention. (2008a). *Duchenne and Becker muscular dystrophy.* Retrieved May 24, 2008, from http://www.cdc.gov/ncbddd/duchenne/

Centers for Disease Control and Prevention. (2008b). *Polio.* Retrieved May 25, 2008, from http://www.cdc.gov/vaccines/vpd-vac/polio/in-short-both.htm

Chan, G. K., & Duque, G. (2002). Age-related bone loss: Old bone, new facts. *Gerontology, 48*(2), 62–71.

Christensen, B., & Kockrow, E. (2003). *Adult health nursing* (4th ed.). St. Louis: Mosby.

Copstead, L. E., & Banaski, J. L. (2005). *Pathophysiology* (2nd ed.). St. Louis: Elsevier.

Cosman, F., Nieves, J. W., Zion, M., Woelfert, L., Luckey, M., & Lindsay, R. (2005). Daily and cyclic parathyroid hormone in women receiving alendronate. *New England Journal of Medicine 353,* 566–575.

Dalakas, M. C., & Hohfield, R. (2003). Polymyositis and dermatomyositis. *Lancet, 363.*

Dumke, C. L. (2003). Muscle cramps are not all created equal. *Athletic Therapy Today,* pp. 42–43.

Fajardo, M., & Di Cesare, P. E. (2005). Disease-modifying therapies for osteoarthritis: Current status. *Drugs and Aging, 22*(2), 141–161.

Forsblad D'Elìa, H., Larsen, A., Waltbrand, E., Kvist, G., Mellström, D., Saxne, T., et al. (2003). Radiographic joint destruction in postmenopausal rheumatoid arthritis is strongly associated with generalized osteoporosis. *Annals of Rheumatic Disease, 62*(7), 617–623.

Frazier, M. S., & Drzymkowski, J. W. (Eds.). (2009). *Essentials of human diseases and conditions* (4th ed.). St. Louis: Saunders.

Gupta, R., Caiozzo, V., Cook, S. D., Barrack, R. L., & Skinner, H. B. (2005). *Current diagnosis and treatment in orthopedics* (4th ed.). New York: McGraw-Hill Medical.

Hogan, M. A., DeLeon, E., Gingrich, M. M., & Willcutts, K. (2007). *Nutrition and diet therapy* (2nd ed.). Upper Saddle River, NJ: Pearson Prentice Hall.

Hunter, D. J., & Sambrook, P. N. (2000). Bone loss: Epidemiology of bone loss. *Arthritis Research, 2,* 441–445.

Jochems, C., Islander, U., Erlandsson, M., Verdrengh, M., Ohlosson, C., & Carlsten, H. (2005). Osteoporosis in experimental postmenopausal polyarthritis: The relative contributions of estrogen deficiency and inflammation. *Arthritis Research and Therapy, 7,* R837–R843.

King, R. W., Johnson, D., Stearns, D. A., Talavera, F., Weiss, E. L., Halamka, J., et al. (2006). *Osteomyelitis.* Retrieved January 22, 2007, from http://www.emedicine.com/emerg/topic349/htm

Lahl, M., Fisher, V. L., & Laschinger, K. (2007). Ewing's sarcoma family of tumors: An overview from diagnosis to survivorship. *Clinical Journal of Oncology Nursing, 12*(1), 89–97.

Leighton, S. (2003). Nutrition for boys with Duchenne muscular dystrophy. *Nutrition & Dietetics, 60,* 1.

Lim, S., Joung, H., Sin, C. S., Lee, H. K., Kim, K. S., Shin, E. K., et al. (2004). Body composition changes with age have gender-specific impacts on bone mineral density. *Bone, 35,* 792–798.

MacLean, C., Newberry, S., Maglione, M., McMahon, M., Ranganath, V., Suttorp, M., et al. (2008). Systematic review: Comparative effectiveness of treatments to prevent fractures in men and women with low bone density or osteoporosis. *Annals of Internal Medicine, 148,* 197–213.

Majumdar, S. R., Johnson, J. A., McAlister, F. A., Bellerose, D., Russell, A. S., Hanley, D. A., et al. (2008). Multifaceted intervention to improve diagnosis and treatment of osteoporosis in patients with recent wrist fracture: A randomized controlled trial. *Canadian Medical Association Journal, 178*(5), 569–575.

Marcus, R., & Gopalakrishnan, G. (2005). Secondary forms of osteoporosis. In F. L. Coe & M. J. Favus (Eds.), *Disorders of bone and mineral metabolism.* Philadelphia: Lippincott Raven Publishers.

Mayo Clinic. (2007). *Muscular dystrophy.* Retrieved May 25, 2008, from http://www.mayoclinic.com/health/muscular-dystrophy/DS00200

McCance, K., & Huether, S. (2006). *Pathophysiology: The biologic basis for disease in adults and children* (5th ed.). St. Louis: Mosby.

MedlinePlus. (2008). *Muscle cramps.* Retrieved May 24, 2008, from http://www.nlm.nih.gov/medlineplus/musclecramps.html

Merck. (2003). *Merck manual of geriatrics.* (2003). Whitehouse Station, NJ: Author.

Muscular Dystrophy Association. (2008). *Facts about Duchenne and Becker muscular dystrophies.* Retrieved August 17, 2008, from http://www.mda.org/publications/fa-dmdbmd-what.html

Muscular Dystrophy Association (MDA). (2003). *Facts about mitochondrial myopathies.* Retrieved August 27, 2008, from http://www.mda.org/Publications/mitochondrial_myopathies.html#whatare

National Institutes of Health. (2007). *Osteoporosis.* Retrieved May 25, 2008, from http://www.niams.nih.gov/Health_Info/Bone/Osteoporosis/default.asp

National Institute of Neurological Disorders and Stroke. (2008). *Myopathy.* Retrieved May 24, 2008, from http://www.ninds.nih.gov/disorders/myopathy/myopathy.htm

Osborn, K. (2005). *Water, watsu, and wellness.* Retrieved May 25, 2008, from http://www.massageandbodywork.com/Articles/OctNov2005/Water.html

Peeke, P. M. (2003). 90 days to fibromyalgia relief. *Prevention.* Retrieved August 17, 2008, from http://www.prevention.com/cda/article/90-days-to-fibromyalgia-relief/dff472e50d803110VgnVCM10000013281eac____/health/conditions.treatments/fibromyalgia

Porth, C. (2005). *Pathophysiology: Concepts of altered health states* (7th ed.). Philadelphia: Lippincott Williams & Wilkins.

Raisz, L. G. (2005). Pathogenesis of osteoporosis: Concepts, conflicts, and prospects. *Journal of Clinical Investigation, 115*(12), 3318–3325.

Seeman, E. (2002). Pathogenesis of bone fragility in women and men. *Lancet, 359,* 1841–1850.

Takeda, E., Taketani, Y., Sawada, N., Sato, T., & Yamamoto, H. (2004). The regulation and function of phosphate in the human body. *Biofactors, 21*(1–4), 345–355.

U. S. Department of Health and Human Services. (2004). *Bone health and osteoporosis: A report of the surgeon general.* Retrieved June 20, 2008, from http://www.surgeongeneral.gov/library/bonehealth

WebMD. (2007). *Post-polio syndrome.* Retrieved May 25, 2008, from http://www.webmd.com/brain/tc/post-polio-syndrome-topic-overview

Younger, D. S. (2003). The myopathies. *Medical Clinics of North America, 87,* 899–907.

Caring for the Patient with Musculoskeletal Trauma

Miki Patterson
Cheryl Wraa

Outcome-Based Learning Objectives

After studying this chapter, the learner will be able to:

1. Describe the incidence, prevalence, and prevention strategies for musculoskeletal trauma.
2. Explain the pathophysiological stages of bone healing.
3. Compare and contrast the various types of fractures and methods for fracture treatment.
4. Apply nursing diagnoses and the nursing process to the care of the patient with musculoskeletal trauma.
5. Discuss potential complications related to musculoskeletal trauma.
6. Identify research implications for nursing practice in caring for the musculoskeletally injured patient.

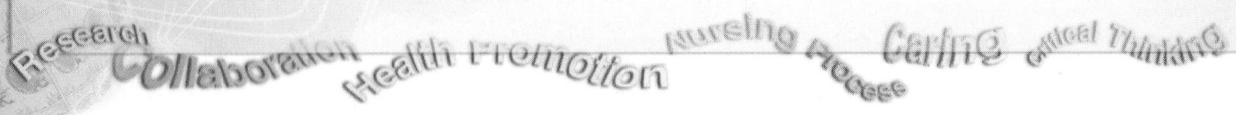

MUSCULOSKELETAL TRAUMA affects most people at some point in their lifetime. Musculoskeletal injuries are a frequent occurrence in blunt trauma, such as motor vehicle crashes, falls, crush injuries, sports injuries, and auto versus pedestrian collisions. Musculoskeletal injuries can also be a result of penetrating trauma such as gunshot or stab wounds (Bongiovanni, Bradley, & Kelley, 2005). Injuries to the musculoskeletal system occur in 85% of patients who sustain blunt trauma (American College of Surgeons (ACS), 2004). Prevention is the only method to decrease the effects of injuries to the muscles, tendons, ligaments, and bones. Whether at home, in the workplace, at play, or on the road, many strategies have been designed to reduce or prevent injuries. Helmets and seat belts; bike, gun, and water safety; and reduced alcohol consumption are major strategies addressed by the Centers for Disease Control and Prevention (CDC) and Emergency Nurses Association (ENA) to prevent injuries. Every 30 minutes someone in the United States dies in an alcohol-related crash (ENA, 2006). Public awareness and education can affect social change and help to decrease the incidence of alcohol-related injuries.

Half of all sports-related injuries are also preventable. Education and awareness surrounding protective equipment, safer playing environments, and rules designed to prevent injury are important in reducing the frequency and severity of sports in-

juries (National Safe Kids Campaign, 2003). Stretching, warm-up exercises, and strengthening and balance training regimens are key in preventing sports injuries.

Etiology

Musculoskeletal trauma results from injuries that are accidental and nonaccidental to a person's bones, joints, and soft tissues. "Accidental" trauma is caused by overuse, impact, sports injuries, and vehicle crashes. Motor vehicle crashes, bicycle and pedestrian injuries, and falls are the most common etiology for musculoskeletal trauma. Nonaccidental or inflicted trauma is seen as a result of domestic violence, child abuse, and altercations and may take the form of blunt trauma, whereby impact is made between the body and an object or force, or penetrating trauma, when an object such as a knife or bullet enters the body. The most common musculoskeletal injuries are strains, sprains, contusions, and fractures.

Health Promotion

The best cure for musculoskeletal trauma is prevention. For athletes, a proper warm-up, stretching, training, supervision, equipment, and surfaces help to prevent common sports injuries. Environmental factors may also play a role in sports safety. For instance, playing on wet or uneven turf may cause athletes to lose their footing and fall, injuring or twisting a joint or extremity. Properly trained coaches and trainers are important in preventing musculoskeletal trauma. They should understand the nutrition and hydration needs of athletes as well as developmental differences and norms. For example, children with open **physes** (growth plates) should perform very limited fastball pitching, because the movement involved with this type of pitching can permanently deform their elbows due to stress on the physis or growth plates.

It is also important not to allow athletes to compete with pain or injuries unless a clinician has evaluated them. Nurses united in the mission "to advance the quality of musculoskeletal health care by promoting excellence in research, education and nursing practice" have formed the National Association of Orthopedic Nurses (NAON) and provide information and educational materials on a wide variety of topics and issues.

Prevention of trauma related to motor vehicle crashes is a major health care issue. Health education that stresses prevention of the problems associated with alcohol consumption and driving is a common goal of public health and other groups such as MADD (Mothers Against Drunk Driving) and SADD (Students Against Destructive Decisions, founded as Students Against Driving Drunk). To fight the high incidence of teen crashes nationwide, the Recording Artists, Actors and Athletes Against Drunk Driving (RADD) Coalition and the National Highway Traffic Safety Administration (NHTSA), both members of the National Organizations for Youth Safety (NOYS), have joined forces with others to develop programs to educate teens regarding this issue.

■ Pathophysiology

Understanding the mechanism and physiological affect of an injury will assist the nurse in prioritizing the assessment and care of the patient with a musculoskeletal injury. Following are descriptions of common injuries found in musculoskeletal trauma.

Contusions

A **contusion** is an injury to soft tissue caused by trauma in which the skin is not broken. A contusion is characterized by pain, discoloration (bruising), and swelling. The initial treatment is ice for 48 hours to constrict the capillaries and impede blood and edema in tissue, later followed by warm moist applications to assist increasing circulation to resorb the edematous fluid.

Sprains and Strains

A **strain** is an injury to the muscle belly or its tendon attachment to bone, typically caused by excessive force or load on a joint or muscle. The associated pain may be described as dull or sharp pain that increases with movement of the muscle. With intramuscular bleeding, it can take up to 24 hours for any bruising to become visible because the blood remains primarily within the muscle sheath, causing pain and local swelling (Anscomb, 2007).

Sprains are similar in nature to strains, but they occur at the **ligaments** (strong fibrous bands of connective tissue) that attach bone to bone. Sprained ankles are one of the most common musculoskeletal injuries in people of all ages, athlete and sedentary alike (Harvard Women's Health Watch, 2007). The

most common type of ankle sprain occurs when the foot rolls inward, damaging the ligaments of the outer ankle (Figure 56–1 ■). Medial ankle sprains, which affect the ligaments of the inner ankle, occur most often in contact sports and are more likely to cause chronic ankle instability with subsequent sprains. The severity of the sprain depends on the degree of damage to the ligaments and how unstable the joint becomes. Chart 56–1 (p. 1778) describes the three grades for this type of injury. Oftentimes a Grade 3 sprain is accompanied by an **avulsion fracture** whereby the ligament breaks off a small piece of the bone at its attachment. The area may have an effusion, ecchymosis, and be very tender to palpation.

Both strains and sprains are diagnosed by a physical exam and history. A radiograph of the affected extremity may be used to rule out an associated fracture.

Medical Management

The initial treatment follows the acronym **PRICE**:

- **Protection**—Immobilize and prevent weight bearing. Grade 2 and 3 sprains are protected from further injury by splints, braces, or casts.

- **Rest**—This is important during the first 24 to 48 hours after the injury to prevent further damage.

- **Ice**—The use of ice has many benefits. Cold helps to relieve pain by reducing nerve conductivity, slowing metabolism of oxygen at the injury site, and reducing cell death and inflammation. An ice pack should be applied to the affected area with the limb elevated and remain in place for 10 to 15 minutes, three to four times a day for the first 3 to 4 days postinjury. Contraindications to ice therapy are cold sensitivity (Raynaud's disease), skin lesions, and peripheral vascular disease.

- **Compression**—Compression aids in the control of edema at the injury site by applying direct pressure and increasing venous return. The pressure should be graduated. When patients begin to bear weight on the extremity, they should wear a compression bandage only when the foot is on the floor and not when elevated. Patients should only need to use a compression bandage for the first 4 to 5 days because the acute inflammatory phase should be over.

- **Elevation**—Elevation is only effective if the affected limb is raised above the heart.

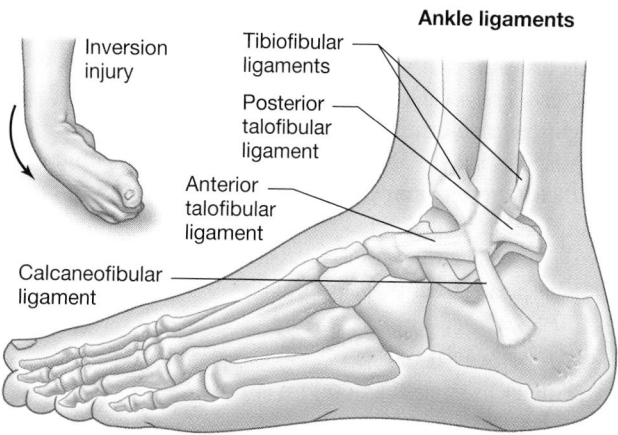

Ankle ligaments

Inversion injury

Tibiofibular ligaments

Posterior talofibular ligament

Anterior talofibular ligament

Calcaneofibular ligament

FIGURE 56–1 ■ Ankle ligaments and inversion injury.

CHART 56–1 **Grades of Sprain Severity**

Severity	Degree of Ligament Damage	Symptoms	Recovery Time	Treatment
Grade 1	Ligament stretched	Mild pain, swelling, and tenderness. Bruising uncommon. Joint stable with no difficulty bearing weight.	1–3 weeks	Mild injury PRICE
Grade 2	Partial tear 20–75%	Moderate pain, swelling, and tenderness. Some bruising. Joint may have mild to moderate joint instability. Patient will have some decreased ROM and function. Patient will experience pain with weight bearing and walking.	3–6 weeks	PRICE Restrict weight bearing Splint Cast Brace
Grade 3	Complete tear or rupture	Severe pain, swelling, tenderness, and bruising. Unstable joint with loss of function and ROM. Patient will be unable to bear weight or walk.	Several months	PRICE Restrict weight bearing Splint Cast Brace May require surgical intervention

Source: Adapted from Harvard Women's Health Watch. (2007). *Recovering from an ankle sprain.* Retrieved April 5, 2008, from http://www.health.harvard.edu.

The most commonly used analgesic for sprains and strains is a nonsteroidal anti-inflammatory drug (NSAID). Medical attention should be sought immediately for any loss of function, sensation, pallor, or pain that is disproportionate to the injury.

Nursing Management

The nursing management of strains and sprains initially focuses on protection of the limb and pain control. Patient teaching regarding exercises to help restore function and prevent injury are essential to the patient's recovery.

Assessment

The nurse should obtain a thorough history to help differentiate a soft tissue injury from a possible fracture. The circumstances leading up to and the mechanism of the injury should be explored. Strains and muscle ruptures usually occur from a sudden stretch on a muscle that is actively contracting, such as during a sport or when lifting a heavy object. A sprain is usually the result of a sudden trauma such as tripping. A pop or snap felt at the time of injury could indicate ligament rupture or fracture. Inquire regarding previous injury to determine if the joint may have weakness. During physical examination, compare both extremities to distinguish any deformity or asymmetry. Complete rupture of the muscle is identified by a break in the normal muscle outline, particularly with resisted movement. Evaluate the extremity for range of motion. It is normal to have decreased function as the swelling increases, so it is important to determine a baseline assessing the difference between active, passive, and resisted movement.

Nursing Diagnoses

The primary nursing diagnoses for sprains and strains include:

- *Pain, Acute*
- *Physical Mobility, Impaired*
- *Knowledge, Deficient* related to plan of care.

Outcomes and Evaluation Parameters

The desired outcomes for the patient with a strain or sprain are relief of pain, protection of the joint, and return of strength and mobility. Following the PRICE regimen described above will help to control pain and swelling. Rehabilitative range-of-motion (ROM), stretching, and strengthening exercises, as described in Figures 56–2 ■ and 56–3 ■, will help to strengthen and protect the joint. Evaluation parameters include pain control as described by the patient, resolution of edema, and return of strength and range of motion.

Planning, Interventions, and Rationales

Administration of anti-inflammatory medication, elevation, application of an elastic bandage for compression, and application of an ice pack for 15- to 20-minute intervals four to five times a day will assist in decreasing the swelling and pain. Teaching the patient ROM, stretching, and strengthening exercises like those shown in Figures 56–2 ■ and 56–3 ■ will help the patient regain strength and mobility to the joint, hence restoring function and preventing further injury.

Health Promotion

Health teaching for patients with contusions, strains, and sprains centers on restoration of function and prevention of further injury. Balance training is found to reduce injury to the ankle and the knee. Balance training in the form of t'ai chi improves balancing ability and muscular cocontraction around the ankle joint, which is helpful in reducing injury in older adults who are balance impaired. Balance training in conjunction with strength and agility training has been used to enhance the neuromuscular responses to stabilize the knee joint in female athletes, thus reducing injury (Hrysomallis, 2007). The Complementary and Alternative Therapies feature (p. 1780) discusses the use of chiropractic care for extremities.

Range of motion, stretching, and strengthening: First 1–2 weeks

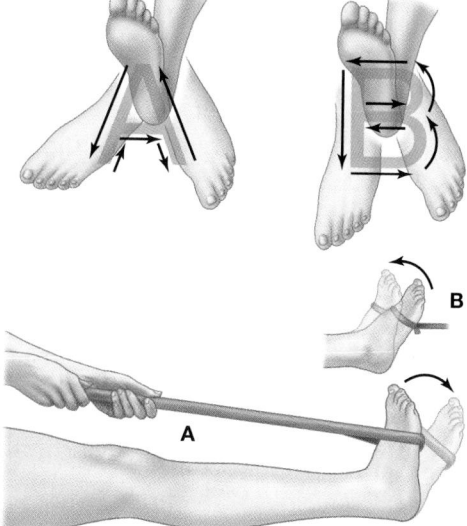
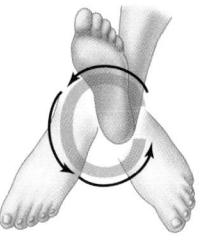

Ankle alphabet. With the heel on the floor, write all the capital letters of the alphabet with your big toe, making the letters as large as you can.

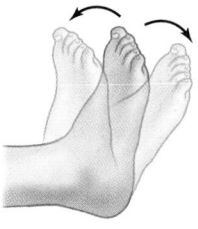
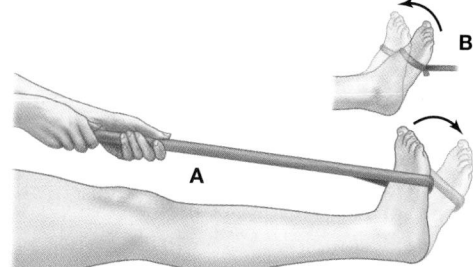

Flexes. Rest the heel of the injured foot on the floor. Pull your toes and foot toward your body as far as possible. Release. Then point them away from the body as far as possible. Release. Repeat as often as possible in the first week.

Press down, pull back. Loop an elasticized band or tubing around the foot, holding it gently taut (A). Press your toes away and down. Hold for a few seconds. Repeat 30 times. Tie one end of the band to a table or chair leg (B). Loop the other end around your foot. Slowly pull the foot toward you. Hold for a few seconds. Repeat 30 times.

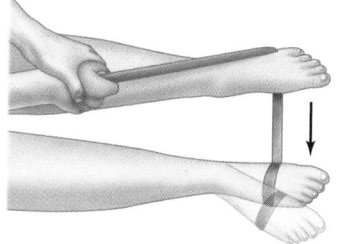

Ankle eversion. Seated on the floor, with an elasticized band or tubing tied around the injured foot and anchored around your uninjured foot, slowly turn the injured foot outward. Repeat 30 times.

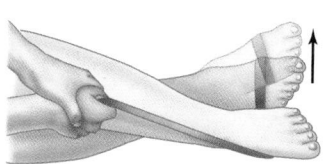

Ankle inversion. Seated on the floor, cross your legs with your injured foot underneath. With an elasticized band or tubing around the injured foot and anchored around your uninjured foot, slowly turn the injured foot inward. Repeat 30 times.

FIGURE 56–2 ■ Range of motion, stretching, and strengthening of the ankle. Perform the first 1 to 2 weeks after injury.
Source: Harvard Women's Health Watch. (2007). *Recovering from an ankle sprain.* Retrieved April 5, 2008, from http://www.health.harvard.edu

Stretching and strengthening: Weeks 3–4

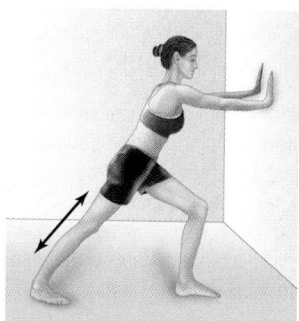

Standing stretch. Stand one arm's length from the wall. Place the injured foot behind the other foot, toes facing forward. Keep your heels down and the back knee straight. Slowly bend the front knee until you feel the calf stretch in the back leg. Hold for 15–20 seconds. Repeat 3–5 times.

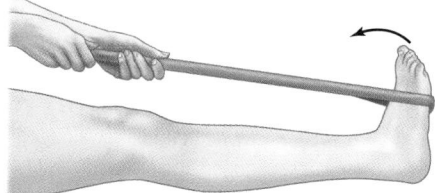

Seated stretch. Loop an elasticized band or tubing around the ball of the foot. Keeping the knee straight, slowly pull back on the band until you feel the upper calf stretch. Hold for 15 seconds. Repeat 15–20 times.

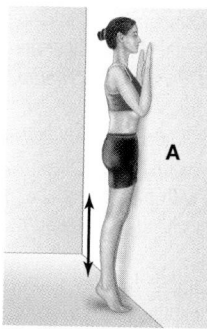

Rises. Stand facing a wall with your hands on the wall for balance (A). Rise up on your toes. Hold for 1 second, then lower yourself slowly to the starting position. Repeat 20–30 times. As you become stronger, do this exercise keeping your weight on just the injured side as you lower yourself down.

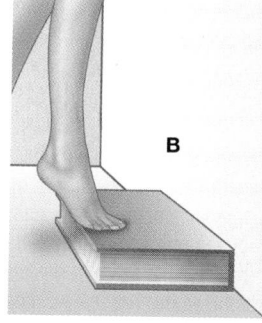

Stretches. Stand with your toes and the ball of the affected foot on a book or the edge of a stair (B). Your heel should be off the ground. Use a wall, chair, or rail for balance. Hold your other foot off the ground behind you, with knee slightly bent. Slowly lower the heel. Hold the position for 1 second. Return to the starting position. Repeat up to 15 times, several times a day. This exercise can place a lot of stress on the ankle, so get your clinician's go-ahead before trying it.

FIGURE 56–3 ■ Stretching and strengthening exercises for the ankle. Perform 3 to 4 weeks after injury.
Source: Harvard Women's Health Watch. (2007). *Recovering from an ankle sprain.* Retrieved April 5, 2008, from http://www.health.harvard.edu

Dislocations

A **dislocation** is a displacement of a bone from its normal position in a joint. With a dislocation, injuries to the ligaments and capsule of the joint are present. A compound dislocation occurs when soft tissue is torn and the joint is exposed to air, which can result in contamination and requires surgical intervention. The dislocation is very painful and requires reduction as soon as possible to reduce pain and avoid vascular and/or nerve damage. For example, a dislocated hip pulls against the soft tissue capsule that contains the vessels that feed the femoral head. This force can occlude the blood supply to the femoral head, which leads to severe complications such as **avascular necrosis (AVN)**, in which the bone tissue dies due to a temporary or permanent loss of blood supply to the bone. Dislocation may also cause significant neurological injury due to the proximity of the nerve to the joint. For example, an anterior shoulder dislocation may cause axillary nerve injury. As with vascular damage, reduction of the bone to its normal position in the joint is accomplished as soon as possible.

 A dislocation is considered an orthopedic emergency.

Etiology

The cause of a dislocation is usually an injury that exerts force great enough to tear the joint ligaments such as a fall, motor vehicle crash, or sports-related impact. A fracture may also be associated with the dislocation.

Clinical Manifestations

The patient will usually present with a deformity of the extremity. He will have severe pain and may have decreased sensation and or circulation distal to the injury.

Diagnostic Procedure

A radiograph of the joint and surrounding bones may be done to rule out an accompanying fracture.

Medical Management

Initial treatment consists of protection and reduction of the dislocation by a trained individual as soon as possible. Ideally, repositioning of the joint should occur within 15 to 30 minutes (Frazier & Drzymkowski, 2007). After that time frame, the joint may be so edematous and painful that the reduction may be impossible without general anesthesia.

COMPLEMENTARY & ALTERNATIVE THERAPIES — Chiropractic

Description:
Chiropractic is a health care profession that involves manual manipulation of the musculoskeletal system to correct vertebral subluxation (a misalignment) or joint dysfunction. Conventional chiropractic uses corrective thrusts of the hands that are called adjustments. Other forms of chiropractic may use an "activator," which is a small instrument that aligns bone positions with less force.

Research Support:
There is a scarcity of higher-level research designs in chiropractic studies, such as randomized controlled trials. The studies discussed below represent the best studies of chiropractic care to date.

One review of literature by a group of Australian researchers sought to document both the quantity and type of research on the use of chiropractic care for lower extremity conditions. All articles that the research team chose for inclusion were those with a lower extremity diagnosis, and those in which doctors of chiropractic performed the treatment. The research team conducted an analysis on the 1,652 articles identified to assess those that included peripheral and/or spinal treatment. The research team found that there were a large number of case studies and a smaller number of higher-level publications. The research team also found that there is a predominance of multimodal management of both spinal and peripheral components in the peer-reviewed literature (Hoskins, McHardy, Pollard, Windsham, & Onley, 2006).

One study focused on patients with chronic musculoskeletal pain, and compared the clinical outcomes of two chiropractic approaches for these patients. The two approaches included the most common approach, diversified spinal manipulation, and a nonmanipulative mind–body approach, the Bioenergetic Synchronization Technique. The study involved 81 patients, of which 74 were females, and the median age was 66 years. The patients were treated for 4 weeks, followed by a 3-week nontreatment interval. Results showed similar mean improvements in the Pain Disability Index for both the Bioenergetic Synchronization Technique group and the diversified technique group (Hawk, Rupert, Colonvega, Boyd, & Hall, 2006).

The goal of another study focused on attitudes regarding chiropractors and chiropractic care. The study involved two groups: persons who had used chiropractic services and those who had not. The first objective of the study was to determine whether there were differences in attitudes and other determinants of care-seeking behavior between the two groups of persons. This study also aimed to determine whether members of these two groups were interested in choosing nonmedical doctors (such as chiropractors) for providing routine services. The results showed different attitudes and preferences about health and health care in people who had seen a doctor of chiropractic before than in those who had never seen a doctor of chiropractic. However, researchers found that both groups preferred physician assistants and nurse practitioners to chiropractors to perform routine health care services (Gaumer & Gemmen, 2006).

References

Gaumer, G., & Gemmen, E. (2006). Chiropractic users and nonusers: Differences in use, attitudes, and willingness to use nonmedical doctors for primary care. *Journal of Manipulative and Physiological Therapy, 29*(7), 529–539.

Hawk, C., Rupert, R. L., Colonvega, M., Boyd, J., & Hall, S. (2006, September). Comparison of bioenergetic synchronization technique and customary chiropractic care for older adults with chronic musculoskeletal pain. *Journal of Manipulative and Ohysioliogical Theraphy, 29*(7), 540–549.

Hoskins, W., McHardy, A., Pollard, H., Windsham, R., & Onley, R. (2006). Chiropractic treatment of lower extremity conditions: A literature review. *Journal of Manipulative and Physiological Theraphy, 29*(8), 658–671.

Nursing Management

Nursing management consists of assessment and protection of the extremity, pain control, and education to regain strength and mobility of the affected joint.

Assessment

Complete a thorough examination of the extremity involved including a peripheral nerve assessment to determine neurological impairment and continual reassessment for any progression. Chart 56–2 describes common nerve involvement for specific dislocations. Assess capillary refill and pulses distal to the injury to determine vascular impairment.

Nursing Diagnoses

Primary nursing diagnoses for the patient with a dislocation include:

- *Acute Pain*
- *Risk for Injury*
- *Impaired Physical Mobility*.

Outcomes and Evaluation Parameters

The desired outcomes for the patient with a dislocation are relief of pain, prevention of damage to the nerves and vasculature, and restoration of strength and mobility of the affected joint. Evaluation parameters include control of pain as described by the patient, restoration of nerve and vascular function, and return of strength and mobility to the joint as exhibited by range of motion and strength assessment.

Planning, Interventions, and Rationales

As stated earlier, a dislocation is an orthopedic emergency. The nurse should quickly assess and immobilize the affected joint and extremity to prevent further damage and to recognize any vascular or nerve involvement. The patient will require intravenous pain medication because the pain is severe. The nurse should anticipate and prepare the patient for conscious sedation because this will most likely be needed for reduction. Postreduction, the patient will require a stabilization splint to prevent the joint from reinjury until the tissues have healed.

Health Promotion

Teaching the patient ROM exercises to maintain mobility and strengthening exercises for the muscles that surround the joint is essential for optimal outcome. Repeated dislocation is potentially damaging to the joint. Review with the patient the proper use of splinting devices and the plan of care for timing or resumption of activities.

Fractures

A quick review of bone basic anatomy is helpful to understand terminology use in the description of fractures and injuries. Long bones are found in the upper and lower extremities and are classified as such because they have certain anatomic features in common as shown in Figure 56–4 ■ (p. 1782). The shaft of the long bone is mainly compact bone hollowed out to form a marrow-filled medullary canal. All long bones have an **epiphysis**, the bone end beyond the physis; physis, growth plate; **metaphysis**, an area of widening between the diaphysis and physis; and **diaphysis**, the shaft between both metaphysis on each end. Bone ends typically form a joint with another bone end and are differentiated as the proximal (closest to a person's head or core) and distal.

Short bones are found in the wrist and ankle. They are irregularly shaped and, except for the compact bone on the surface, they are spongy throughout. Flat bones are found where protection of underlying structures is needed, such as the skull and ribs, or a large area for muscle attachment, such as the scapula. They consist of a layer of spongy bone between two layers of compact bone.

Healing of Fractures

Fractures are a discontinuity of the bone that may be complete or incomplete (Porth, 2005). A fracture or break in the bone causes a healing cascade beginning with the blood that leaks out at the fracture site. This hematoma is rich in osteoclasts, which make bone. Clotting factors that remain due to the hematoma initiate the formation of a fibrin meshwork that serves as a framework for the fibroblasts and new capillary buds. Granulation tissue is formed and gradually replaces the clot.

During cellular proliferation and callus formation, the osteoblasts, or bone-forming cells, multiply and differentiate into the fibrocartilaginous callus. This process begins distal to the

CHART 56–2	Peripheral Nerve Assessment		
Injury	**Nerve**	**Motor**	**Sensation**
Wrist dislocation	Median distal	Thenar contraction with opposition	Index finger
Anterior shoulder dislocation	Musculocutaneous	Elbow flexion	Lateral forearm
Distal humeral shaft, anterior shoulder dislocation	Radial	Thumb, finger MCP extension	First dorsal web space
Anterior shoulder dislocation, proximal humerus fracture	Axillary	Deltoid	Lateral shoulder
Knee dislocation	Posterior tibial	Toe flexion	Sole of foot
Fibular neck fracture, knee dislocation	Superficial peroneal	Ankle eversion	Lateral dorsum of foot
Posterior hip dislocation	Superior gluteal	Hip abduction	

Source: Adapted from American College of Surgeons. (2004). *Advanced Trauma Life Support Student Course Manual.* Chicago: American College of Surgeons.

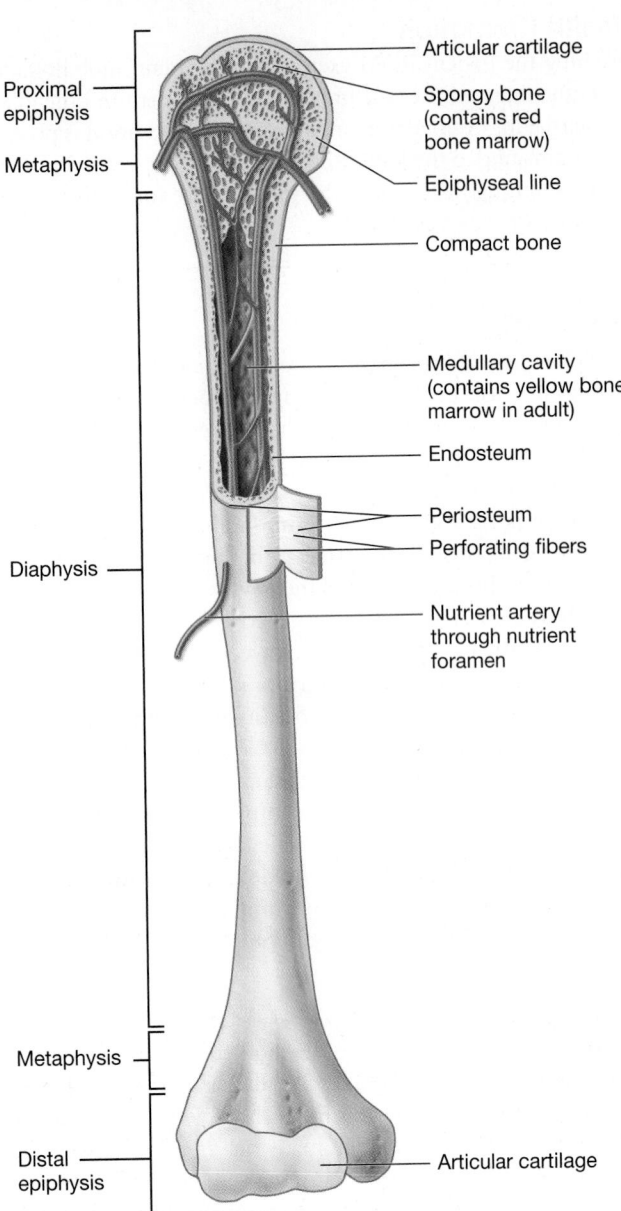

FIGURE 56–4 ■ Long bone.

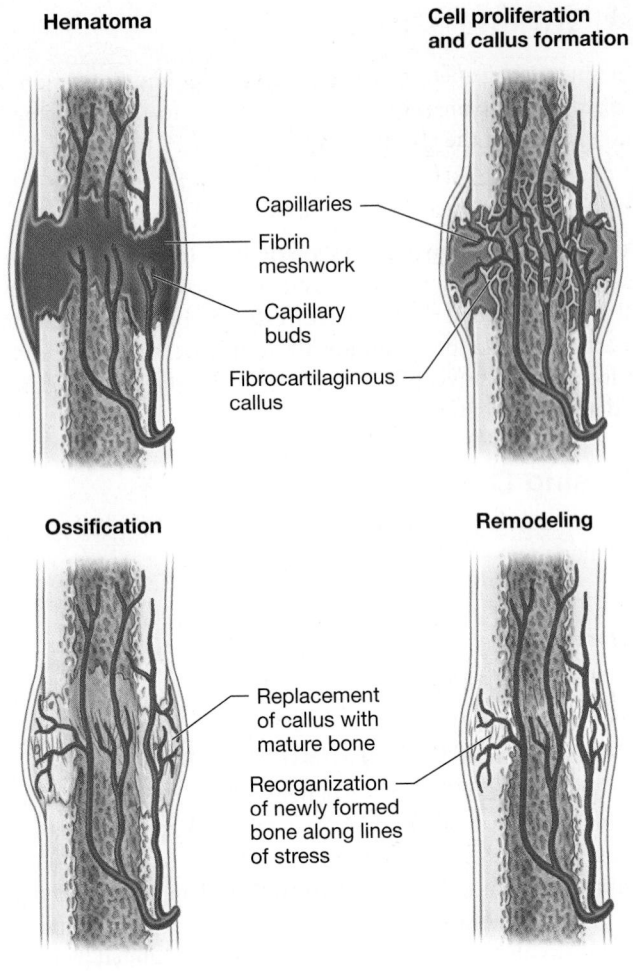

FIGURE 56–5 ■ Bone healing.

fracture where there is greater blood supply. Within a few days a cartilage "collar" is evident around the fracture site. The edges of the collar that are on either side of the fracture unite to form a bridge that connects the bone fragments. Initially the callus is soft but within the third to fourth week of fracture healing, the bone calcifies as mineral salts are deposited.

Ossification is the final lying down of bone after the fracture has been bridged and the fragments are united. Mature bone replaces the callus, and the fracture site feels firm and appears united on radiograph. It is at this point that a cast may be removed. The remodeling process involves resorption of the excess callus in the marrow space and the external aspect of the fracture. The process is directed by mechanical stress and weight bearing becoming stronger in relation to its function (Figure 56–5 ■). Healing time is dependent on the site and type of the fracture and on the underlying health of the patient. With long bones, displaced fractures, and fractures with less surface area, strength and function usually return within 6 months after bone union is complete. Small nondisplaced fractures require less time to heal and the patient will usually have full function within 2 to 4 weeks.

Classification of Fractures

Fractures are classified in various ways; the simplest is whether a fracture is open or closed. A closed fracture is when the soft tissue envelope, which may be damaged, does not communicate with the outside; in effect, there is no skin opening. An open fracture means there is a tear in the soft tissue, exposing the bone to the outside environment. The important concept is that all open fractures have the potential to be contaminated, and this increases the morbidity (or frequency of complications or poor outcome) and mortality (fatal outcome) of the injury. The time frames vary by institution but many consider 6 to 8 hours the maximum time that a contaminated fracture can wait to be taken to the operating room and "washed out," a process that is often referred to as an *inspection and debridement* (I&D) (Feliciano, Mattox, & Moore, 2008). During the I&D the fracture and soft tissue are washed out with a pulsed lavage, typically with antibiotic solution. The soft tissue is inspected, debris is removed, and any damaged or necrotic tissue is debrided to try to reduce the possibility of infection. Chart 56–3 shows a grading classification for open fractures.

Grade I is typically an "inside-out" fracture, that is, one in which the end of the fractured bone pokes through the skin and

	CHART 56–3	**Grading of Open Fractures**

Grade	Description
Grade I	Wound less than 1 cm with minimal soft tissue injury. Wound bed is clean. Bone injury is simple with minimal comminution.
Grade II	Wound is greater than 1 cm with moderate soft tissue injury. Wound bed is moderately contaminated. Fracture contains moderate comminution.
Grade III	Following fractures automatically results in classification as type III: • Segmental fracture with displacement • Fracture with diaphyseal segmental loss • Fracture with associated vascular injury requiring repair • Farmyard injuries or highly contaminated wounds • High-velocity gun shot wound (GSW) • Fracture caused by crushing force from fast moving vehicle.
Grade IIIA	Wound less than 10 cm with crushed tissue and contamination. Soft tissue coverage of bone is usually possible.
Grade IIIB	Wound greater than 10 cm with crushed tissue and contamination. Soft tissue is inadequate and requires regional or free flap.
Grade IIIC	Fracture in which there is a major vascular injury requiring repair for limb salvage.

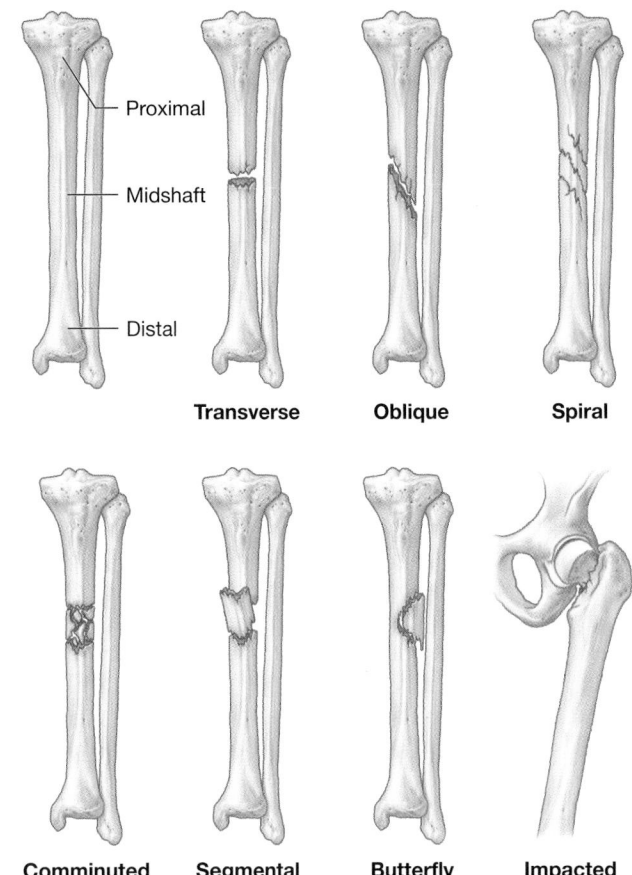

FIGURE 56–6 ■ Classification of fractures by direction of fracture.

returns. This is considered the cleanest fracture with limited risk for deep infection. A Grade II fracture occurs when a soft tissue wound is greater than 1 cm with moderate contamination and soft tissue injury. A Grade III fracture has a greater than 10-cm wound opening, is severely contaminated, and involves comminution of the bone, soft tissue loss, and vascular injury (*Gustillo classification of fracture*, 2004).

There are other ways to classify fractures such as by appearance, apposition angulation, and mechanism of injury. Long bone fractures may be described by their appearance, which also gives some indication of the mechanism of injury. Descriptors such as *transverse, oblique, spiral, comminuted, segmental, butterfly,* and *impacted* are commonly used (Figure 56–6 ■).

Transverse fractures are horizontal to the bone shaft and usually result from a direct blow. Healing of nondisplaced transverse fractures is usually uneventful because the muscle pulls and compresses the bone ends together, which is key in bone healing. Oblique fractures are diagonal in nature and may allow shortening of the bone due to the muscle pulls. The diagonal configuration may allow the bone ends to slide down on each other. A spiral fracture is as described: spiral, typically caused by rotatory torsion. These fractures are suspicious of inflicted injury in nonambulating children, because they typically occur as a result of limb twisting. Segmental fractures describe bone that is broken in more than one place. These fractures are difficult to

manage without surgical intervention to stabilize the bone fragments. In butterfly fractures, large pieces of the bone are shaped like a butterfly with one side longer than the other. Impacted fractures occur when broken ends of bone are forced together. These fractures have a high rate of healing and limited pain because most pain of fractures comes from the innervated periosteum portion of the bone ends rubbing against each other. Impacted fractures do not readily move but need to be protected from displacing until healing occurs.

Fracture apposition speaks to the relation of the bone ends to each other; for example, if half of each bone end is touching the other, it is considered 50% opposed. If the bones ends are not in contact at all, it may be referred to as 100% displaced or 0% apposition. Nondisplaced fractures keep anatomic alignment. Fracture angulation describes the angle at the apex of the fracture in relation to the proximal fragment of bone. Some fracture descriptions are specific to the particular bone such as spine and pelvis fractures.

Spinal fractures can occur in the 7 cervical vertebrae, frequently referred to as the C-spine, 12 thoracic vertebrae or T-spine, and 5 lumbar vertebrae or L-spine, and are classified as stable or unstable using a three column theory. This theory divides the vertebrae into three columns, the anterior, middle, and posterior columns. If any two of these columns are disrupted, the spine is considered to be unstable.

 CRITICAL ALERT *When two vertebral columns are disrupted, the spinal cord and nerve roots are no longer protected from serious neurological injury.*

An unstable spine is typically treated with complete bed rest with log rolling, a Roto Rest bed or Stryker frame bed, or surgical fixation. The special beds allow the patient to be turned without flexing the patient's spine. Changes in position are needed to avoid pressure areas and pooling of fluids. Some spine fractures are described by the mechanism of injury, such as a **burst fracture** that occurs when an axial load is placed on the spine and a vertebra explodes out in all directions. This form of fracture may push bone fragments into the spinal canal and has the potential for neurological damage. Burst fractures are unstable, and patients need to be watched for any neurovascular changes in the lower extremities.

 Any changes in exam should be reported to attending surgeons immediately, because deficits can become permanent.

A **chance fracture** is one through bony and or ligamentous portions of the spine caused by distraction of vertebrae. The most common scenario is a person in the back seat of a car with only a lap belt that has been involved in a motor vehicle crash. The impact forces the person's upper body forward, while the lap belt holds the person down, producing tearing through the spine. These injuries may not be visible on plain spine films so any trauma patient with back pain should be suspect for injuries.

Many C-spine fractures or ligamentous injuries are unstable and require surgical treatment and or treatment in cervical traction or a halo vest to prevent neurological compromise. Both halo vest and cervical traction rely on two, four, or more pins to be placed in a ring around the patient's head and torqued to 6 to 8 pounds of pressure, which enable the pins to penetrate the outer table of the skull, securing them in place. Care of the pin site includes watching for any drainage, erythema, or movement. For a detailed discussion of spine and spinal cord injuries, refer to Chapter 32 .

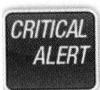 *Clear drainage from a pin site or ear could represent cerebrospinal fluid and must be reported to the attending surgeon immediately.*

Medical Management

Initial management of an extremity fracture consists of immobilization that includes the joint above and the joint below the fracture. After the extremity is splinted, neurological and vascular status is reassessed and a plan for definitive care is accomplished:

- Femoral fractures are temporarily immobilized with a traction splint that applies force distally at the ankle as the splint is pushed proximally into the perineum. Excessive traction for long periods of time may cause skin damage to the foot, ankle, or perineum.
- Tibia fractures are immobilized with padded cardboard long-leg splints or a splint made with plaster immobilizing the lower leg, knee, and ankle.
- Ankle fractures may be immobilized with a pillow splint or padded cardboard. It is important to avoid pressure over bony prominences.
- The hand is temporarily splinted in an anatomic functional position with the wrist slightly dorsiflexed and the fingers gently flexed. This can be done by placing the hand over a roll of gauze or rolled towel and then securing a short arm splint.

- Forearm and wrist fractures are immobilized flat on padded cardboard splints or a pillow.
- The elbow, upper arm, and shoulder are usually immobilized to the body in a flexed position using a sling.

Narcotics are generally needed for effective pain relief and should be given in small frequent doses. The patient will be further evaluated to determine the extent of the injury and if she will require simple casting or surgical intervention for open reduction and internal fixation.

There are typically five treatment options for fractures: closed treatment with casting, traction, surgical treatment with external fixation, open reduction with internal fixation, or intramedullary rod. A combination of these options may also be used. There are risk, benefits, and indications for each, which are discussed next.

Casting, Bracing, and Splinting

The easiest and sometimes most cost-effective treatment for fractures is the cast. A **cast** is a rigid circumferential encasement device made of plaster or fiberglass. Casting material (plaster or fiberglass and Webril/cotton padding) is relatively inexpensive and readily available. Casting does not completely keep bones from moving and it may allow shortening or displacement of fractures. Patients may complain of hearing or feeling crepitus, crunching or grinding of their bone ends moving in the cast.

A cast must include the joint above and the joint below a fractured long bone. This restricts joint motion for the length of time needed for fracture healing but renders those joints stiff when treatment is complete and frequently requires rehabilitation of atrophied muscles. However, this form of treatment is not optimal in the immediate postinjury period because it is rigid and does not allow for the swelling of tissues, which typically occurs for the first 3 days after a fracture. Fractures can be painful until the bone ends begin to granulate and get "sticky" around 10 to 14 days in the average, well-nourished, nonsmoking patient. Another problem with casting is there is no access to soft tissues to observe for pressure points or skin breakdown. Most cast material must stay dry so it is difficult for the patient to take a bath or shower. Fiberglass casting tape used with a waterproof Gortex liner is now used for certain applications allowing casts in showers or chlorinated swimming pools.

A splint or brace is manufactured or made by the caregiver with casting material. It allows the fractured bone to rest within a firm surface to decrease motion, but is not circumferential. The splint or brace is secured by straps or wrapped circumferentially with a bandage. This allows for adjustment if there is increased swelling and removal for visualization of the soft tissues.

Traction

Traction is a treatment option that is used in most underdeveloped countries but is not the treatment of choice in the United States due to the cost of long hospital stays and the complications associated with the immobilization involved with traction. The purpose of traction is to maintain alignment of the bone with an axial pull along the axis of the bone to counteract the pulls of the muscles. **Skin traction** or **Buck's boots traction** consists of straps or foam boots secured to lower extremities with a cord pulling no more than 6 pounds and is frequently used for comfort in patients with hip fracture. No more than 6 pounds should be placed on this kind of traction because pressure areas will develop. The nurse should examine the skin under the boot or bandage wrap every 4 to 6 hours looking for any reddened areas.

Skeletal traction entails placement of a skeletal pin that is drilled through the bone such as a distal femur or proximal tibia. The portions of the skeletal pin exiting the skin on either side of the limb are attached to a bail. A cord is secured to the bail and runs through pulleys to a weighted bag suspended at the end of the bed. The purpose of the weight is to pull along the axis of the bone to counteract the muscle forces (spasm) in an attempt to bring bones "out to length" and/or maintain anatomic alignment. A trapeze on the bed may help the patient move in the bed; however, it should not be used if the patient has a spine fracture.

Pin site care is an important nursing function. Skeletal traction pins are exposed to the environment where they protrude through the skin and can allow bacteria to travel down to the bone. Skeletal pins are generally not painful except when placed or removed or if the pin sites become infected. It is expected that the pin site will be red, tender, and have bloody or serosanguineous drainage for the first 24 to 72 hours. After that time any tenderness or drainage should be suspect for infection. Pin sites should also remain flat and not be allowed to tent on the pin. Pin releases are performed to keep the skin off the pin. The tent provides a warm moist dark area for bacteria (always present at the pin skin interface) to accumulate and grow. For more on pin site care, see the box titled Evidence-Based Practice.

Traction has high morbidity and mortality risks, especially in elderly patients. The problems with traction stem from the immobilization involved, which can produce complications such as skin breakdown, urinary tract infection, pneumonia, deep venous thrombosis (DVT), and pulmonary embolism (PE). The cost of hospitalization for traction in the United States far exceeds that of surgical treatment. Traction is labor intensive, from setting up traction beds, repeating x-rays frequently, and changing the axis of the pull to change the angulation of the fracture.

External Fixation

External fixation refers to a form of treatment in which the bones or bone ends of a fracture are held in place by skeletal pins, which are screwed into the bone and attached to a frame worn on

---

Pin Site Care

Clinical Problem

Infection of pin sites is one of the most common complications associated with the use of skeletal pins, wires, and external fixation (Walker, 2007). An infection at the pin site is painful and will delay mobilization of the patient. The infection may also lead to other severe complications including osteomyelitis, nonunion of the bone at the fracture site, delayed fracture healing, loss of fracture alignment, or systemic infection. All of these complications can result in long-term pain and possible disability. Due to the significance of pin site care, it is important to base the care and technique on evidence.

Research Findings

Hydrogen peroxide was commonly used in the past to cleanse pin sites, especially to remove crusts from around the pin site. Currently, the use of hydrogen peroxide is discouraged because it may cause damage to the healthy tissue surrounding the pin. It has also been associated with increased infection rates and the disruption of the skin's normal flora (Walker, 2007).

In 2005, the National Association of Orthopaedic Nurses completed a systematic analysis of the research literature on skeletal pin site care and sought opinions of an expert panel to develop guidelines for skeletal pin site care (Holmes & Brown, 2005). They found that there were two experimental studies regarding pin site care, but they explored different aspects: one study explored cleansing solutions and the other addressed frequency of site care. The panel also reviewed five case series studies in which one that reported comparison of two methods of site care was judged to be of high quality. Using the methodology of expert consensus, the panel developed the following major recommendations:

- Pins located in areas with considerable soft tissue should be considered at greater risk for infection.
- After the first 48 to 72 hours when drainage may be heavy, pin site care should be done daily or weekly for sites with mechanically stable bone–pin interfaces.

- Chlorhexidine 2 mg/mL solution may be the most effective cleansing solution for pin site care.
- Patients and their families should be taught pin site care before discharge from the hospital. They should be required to demonstrate whatever care needs to be done and should be provided with written instructions that include signs and symptoms of infection.

Implications for Nursing Practice

Guidelines reflect the state of current knowledge within the health care literature regarding the effectiveness of current practice. Clinical practice guidelines are developed by reviewing these findings and seeking the opinions of known experts in that field of practice. The expert consensus is vital in practice that has little or no research to review.

Although there was little research regarding care of the skin immediately surrounding the skeletal pin site, some of what had been done was judged to be of good quality and therefore useful. It is clear that (1) the solution used to cleanse pin sites should be chlorhexidine and (2) nurses should not use peroxide.

Critical Thinking Questions

1. What risks are involved if pin sites are not kept clean and dry?

2. Which assessment findings would the nurse expect a patient with an infected pin site to exhibit?

Answers to Critical Thinking Questions appear in Appendix D.

References

Holmes, S. B., & Brown, S. J. (2005). Skeletal pin site care: National Association of Orthopaedic Nurses guidelines for orthopaedic nursing. *Orthopaedic Nursing, 24*(2), 99–107. Retrieved August 5, 2008, from http://www.guidelines.gov/summary/summary.aspx?doc_id=7420&nbr=004379&string=pin+AND+site+AND+care.

Walker, J. A. (2007). Evidence for skeletal pin site care. *Nursing Standard, 21*(45), 70–76.

EVIDENCE-BASED PRACTICE

the outside of the body. External fixation devices (EFDs) have become the treatment of choice for many fractures, especially when soft tissues are damaged and access is needed for wound care.

Unlike casting, external fixation allows for greater mobility and joint motion above or below the fracture. External fixation may be used for emergent stabilization of fractures or as definitive treatment. Scars are minimal compared to open reduction internal fixation or intramedullary rodding. For some the pins may be removed in a clinic.

The most common complication of external fixation is pin site infection. Skeletal pins protrude though an opening in the skin, which creates a foreign body reaction. The body reacts by forming a bursal lining between the pin and skin. This protective membrane produces fluid to reduce the friction at the pin/skin interface. This fluid is easily contaminated by the bacteria skin flora and needs to be allowed to drain out at the pin site to reduce the concentration of microorganisms. (See the Evidence-Based Practice box, p. 1785.)

Another complication of external fixation or skeletal traction is a plantar flexion contracture of the foot. Without support the foot will rest in plantar flexion and this can result in Achilles tendon shortening or tightness. This deformity can be avoided with frequent stretching and the use of a foot plate.

Open Reduction Internal Fixation

A very common method of fracture fixation is **open reduction internal fixation (ORIF)**, in which a fracture is exposed by an incision in the skin directly over the fracture. Implants such as plates (strips of metal), screws, and wires are placed directly on or in the bone to anatomically stabilize a fracture (Figure 56–7 ■). This method of fracture fixation allows direct visualization of the fracture but can disrupt the circulation to the bone and leave large surgical scars.

Complications associated with this method are wound infection and hardware failure or breakage. It is not optimal for use with comminuted or osteoporotic bone or damaged or suboptimal soft tissues. Patients with conditions such as peripheral vascular disease, diabetes, and obesity frequently encounter healing problems. Screw heads may be prominent and irritate tissue, and hardware may need to be removed following healing.

Intramedullary Rod

Intramedullary (I-M) rodding refers to a method of fracture fixation that entails sliding a metal rod down the medullary canal of a long bone (Figure 56–8 ■). This form of fixation allows for anatomic alignment and is helpful for segmental fractures. I-M rods allow for early weight bearing because they share the load and leave joints free to move. They may need to be removed after healing is complete. The holes left by the screws are stress risers and fractures may occur through them when an I-M rod is removed.

The benefits of this fixation method include small surgical scars in less obvious places than with other methods. For example, the rod in Figure 56–8 ■ was placed through a 4-cm incision above the hip, and small stab incisions were made to place the screws. There is a slight increased risk of fat embolism with this method because of the pressure exerted in the canal by the reamer or from hammering the I-M rod down, which may force fat into the bloodstream.

■ Nursing Management

Nursing management of the patient with an extremity fracture involves relief of pain and frequent reassessment of neurovascular status. Patients with femur fractures require frequent monitoring of their vascular status because femoral shaft fractures are associated with significant blood loss of up to 1,500 to 2,000 mL and the patient can develop hypovolemic shock (Feliciano et al., 2008).

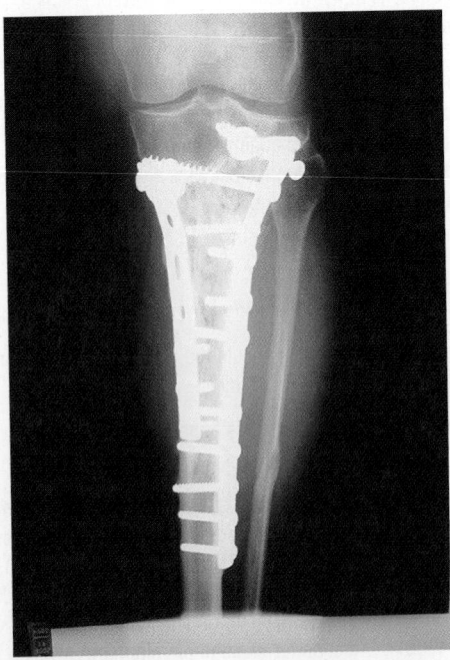

FIGURE 56–7 ■ Open reduction internal fixation.
Source: Cheryl Wraa

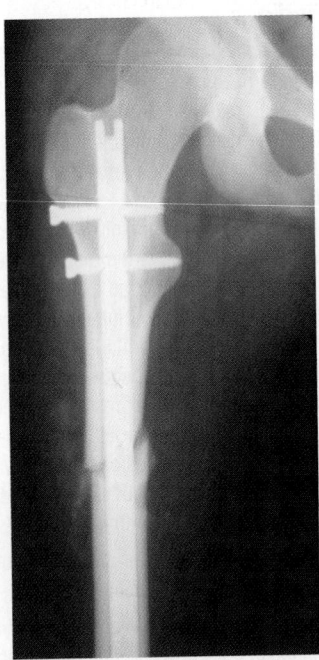

FIGURE 56–8 ■ Intramedullary rodding.
Source: Cheryl Wraa

Assessment

Initial assessment of an extremity fracture includes observation for deformities, breaks in the skin, and a thorough assessment of vascular and sensory status distal to the extremity. Frequent reassessment of neurovascular status is necessary to prevent complications.

Nursing Diagnoses

The primary nursing diagnoses for the patient with an extremity fracture include:

- *Pain, Acute*
- *Physical Mobility, Impaired*
- *Injury, Risk for*
- *Fluid Volume, Risk for Deficient*
- *Infection, Risk for.*

Outcomes, planning, intervention, and evaluation are discussed under pelvic fractures.

Pelvic Fractures

A large amount of force is required to fracture the pelvis. Therefore, the nurse should be anticipatory and assess for other serious injuries. The pelvis consists of two innominate bones and the sacrum, which form a ring of bone. The bones are held in a structural unit primarily by the ligaments of the pelvis (Figure 56–9 ■). The strongest ligamentous structures are in the posterior aspect of the pelvis at the sacroiliac (SI) joints. These ligaments have to hold up the weight-bearing forces from the lower extremities to the spine that are transferred to the SI joints. Major blood vessels are located on the inner wall of the pelvis (Figure 56–10 ■). Whenever the pelvis is fractured, these arteries and associated veins can be damaged and extensive bleeding will occur. The lumbar and sacral plexus of nerves run through the posterior pelvis and can be affected with pelvic trauma

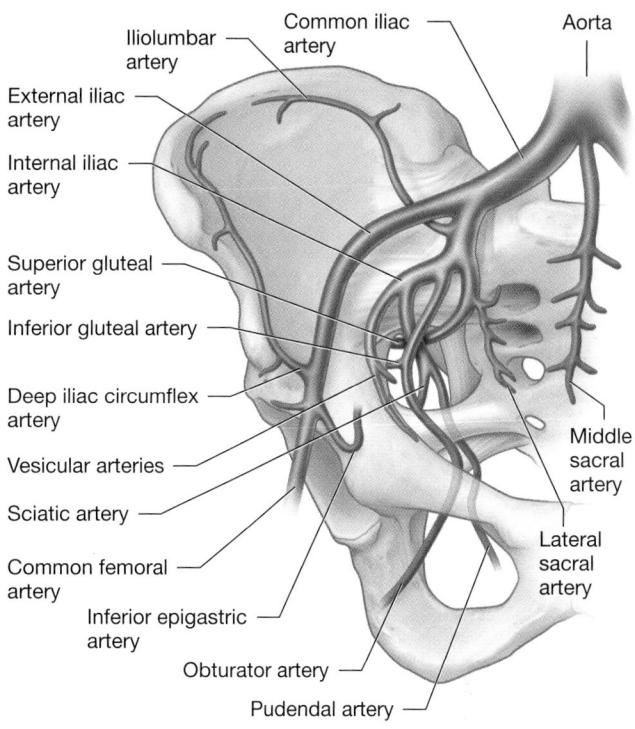

FIGURE 56–10 ■ Vascular anatomy of the pelvis.

(Figure 56–11 ■). Organs that can be injured during a trauma with pelvic fracture are the bladder and urethra, vagina, prostate, and gastrointestinal system.

Three types of forces cause damage to the pelvis. The first and most common is lateral compression (Figure 56–12 ■, p. 1788). Examples include a pedestrian hit on his side by a motor vehicle, a fall from a height where the patient lands on her side, and a motor vehicle crash where intrusion of the vehicle compresses the pelvis.

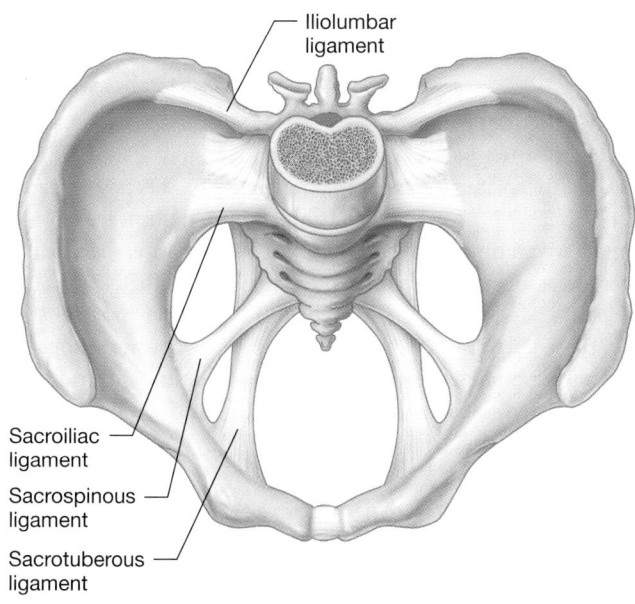

FIGURE 56–9 ■ Ligaments of the pelvis.

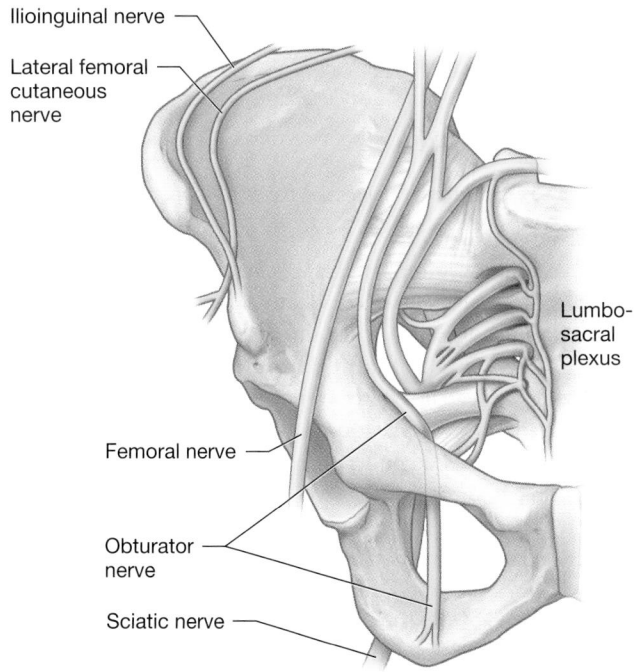

FIGURE 56–11 ■ Neuroanatomy of the pelvis.

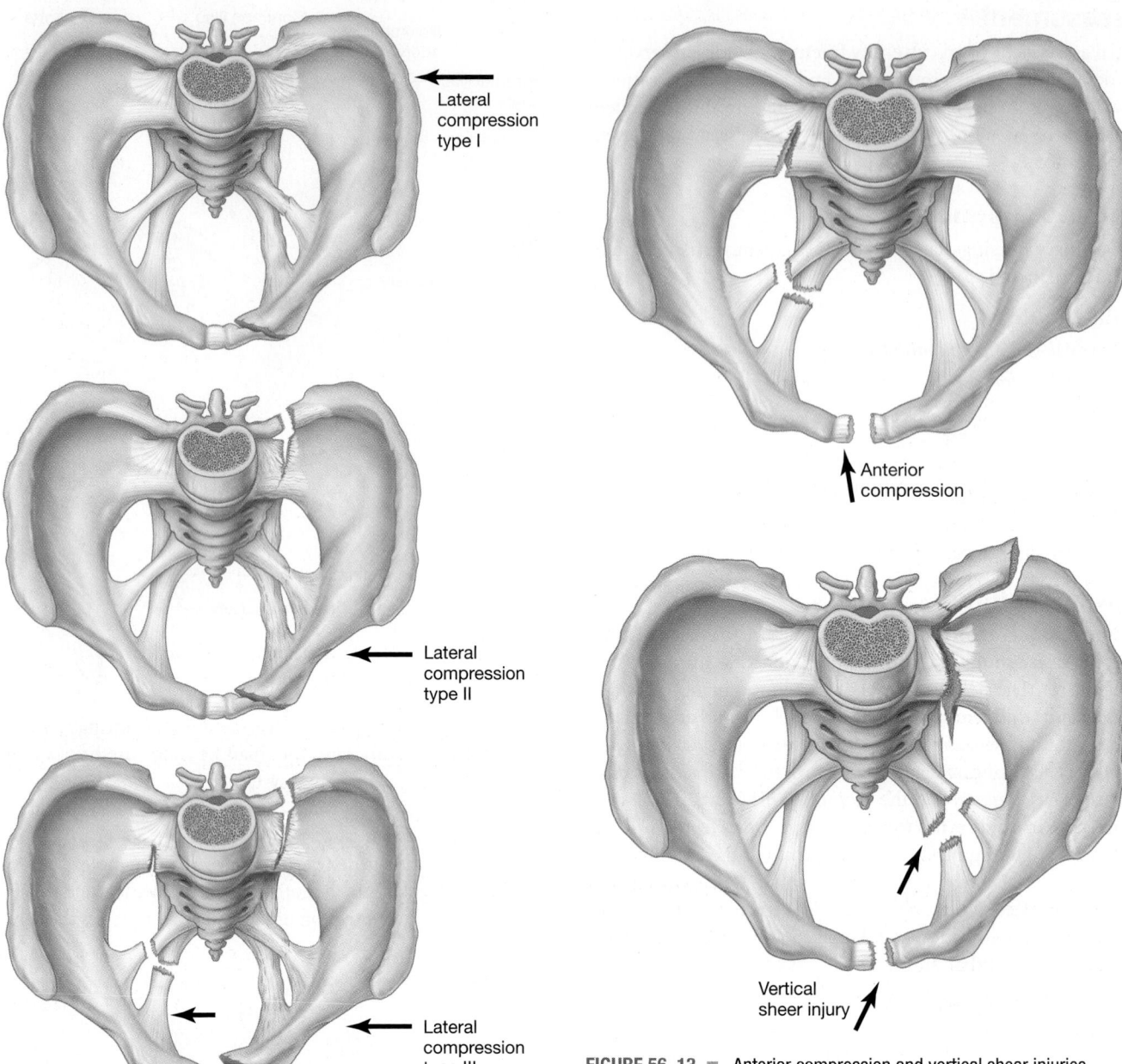

Lateral compression type I

Lateral compression type II

Lateral compression type III

FIGURE 56–12 ■ Lateral compression fractures.

Anterior compression

Vertical sheer injury

FIGURE 56–13 ■ Anterior compression and vertical shear injuries.

The second most frequent force is from an anterior or posterior (AP) direction. This occurs from either direct contact with the iliac spine or force transmitted from the femur (Figure 56–13 ■). An example of the mechanism would be when a person's legs are spread apart in a motorcycle crash. The injury can involve ligament disruption only and the injury usually manifests itself as a widened pubic symphysis and SI joints. The third type of force is vertical shear (see Figure 56–13 ■). This type of injury is most commonly seen in patients who jumped from a height and landed on an extended lower extremity. The vertical shear injury disrupts the restraining ligaments of the hemipelvis, rendering it mechanically unstable.

One or more of these forces may have injured patients at one time. It is important for the nurse to inquire as to the mechanism of injury to be anticipatory of the type of injury the patient may have sustained.

Epidemiology

Fractures of the pelvis comprise approximately 2% of all fractures. With isolated pelvic injury, mortality has been reported to be 1% to 2%. Almost 20% of multiple injured blunt trauma patients have an injury to the pelvic ring. When closed pelvic fractures are associated with multiple injuries, the mortality rises to 10% to 15%. Mortality associated with open pelvic fractures has been reported to be 30% to 50%, and pelvic fractures associated with intracranial hemorrhage or severe abdominal injuries have been reported to be as high as 50% (Mohanty, Musso, Powell, Kortbeek, & Kirkpatrick, 2005).

Clinical Manifestations

During physical examination, the nurse should inspect the pelvis to see if there is a rotation of the iliac crest and/or any difference in leg length. When palpating, exert gentle lateral compression and distraction of the iliac crests and inward compression of the symphysis pubis to determine pelvic stability.

CRITICAL ALERT *It is critically important to be careful when maneuvering the pelvis so as not to cause damage to the vasculature or neural bundles.*

If the pelvis feels unstable, alert the health care team so others will not attempt to manipulate the pelvis and cause further damage or increased bleeding. Inspect the skin and skin folds to identify any open fractures. Observe the meatus to check for blood signifying a possible urethral injury.

 CRITICAL ALERT *If there is blood at the meatus, do not attempt to insert a Foley catheter.*

The health care team will perform a digital rectal exam to evaluate for sensation, sphincter tone, presence of blood, and position of the prostate. Female patients will undergo a vaginal exam to look for tears in the vagina signifying an open fracture. The lower extremities should be evaluated for pulses, motor, and sensation.

Diagnostic Tests

Initially, an AP radiograph of the pelvis will show most fractures and associated dislocations. This view, however, does not allow the health care team to determine the degree of bone displacement and small factures may be missed. Additional views called inlet and outlet views may be obtained. The inlet view is taken at a 60-degree angle from the head toward the feet. This will show the posterior and cephalic displacement of fractures of the posterior arch, widening of the SI joint, and displacement of the anterior arch. The outlet view is a 45-degree angle taken from the foot of the bed directed toward the head. This helps in identifying a displacement or leg-length discrepancy, disruptions of the SI joints, and sacral factures.

Computed tomography (CT) of the pelvis assists with the diagnosis of crushing, shearing injuries, SI joint displacement, acetabular injuries, and posterior osseous ligamentous structure of the pelvis. The scan will also assist in diagnosing associated visceral injuries and bleeding.

Medical Management

The most important factors that direct management of pelvic injury are the patient's hemodynamic status and stability of the pelvic ring. In the patient who is both hemodynamically and mechanically unstable and the bleeding is thought to be from the pelvic fracture, external stabilization of the pelvis is a priority. The main sources of bleeding are the presacral venous plexus and fractured bony surfaces. External stabilization with a pelvic binder decreases the hemorrhage by reducing the volume of the pelvic basin and approximating the fracture ends. Pelvic binders are cloth and go around the pelvis circumferentially (Figure 56–14 ■). They are simple to apply, inexpensive, and can be placed in the prehospital setting. Potential complications of the binder include skin necrosis if left in place for a long period or applied too tightly. If a binder is applied too tightly with lateral compression injuries with sacral fractures, it may cause visceral or neural injury.

The source of bleeding from pelvic fractures is usually venous but arterial injury can occur and account for hemodynamic instability in 10% to 20% of patients (Mohanty et al., 2005). For the patients who remain hemodynamically labile after external stabilization, pelvic angiography may be performed for identification and embolization of the source of bleeding. Patients who are hemodynamically stable but exhibit an arterial

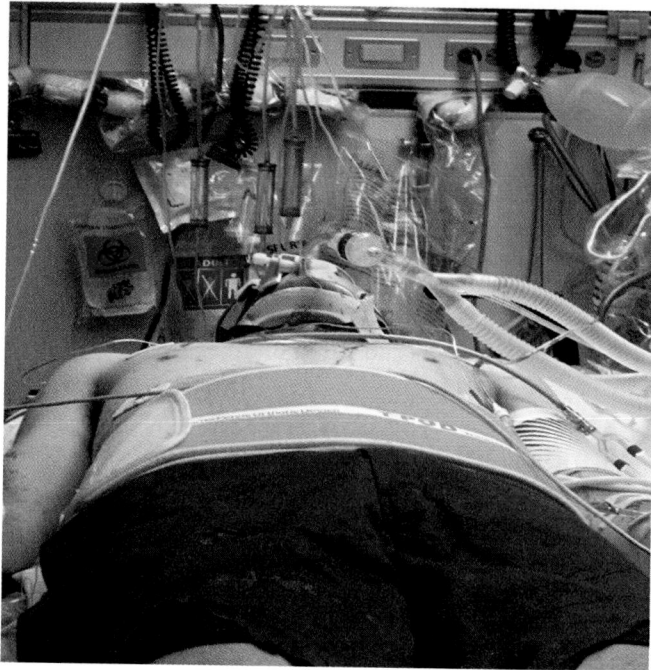

FIGURE 56–14 ■ Pelvic binder.
Source: Cheryl Wraa

blush on CT scan, signifying bleeding at the site, may also undergo angiography for embolization.

Minimally displaced pelvic fractures that have ligamentous stability of the pelvic ring are treated with protected weight bearing on the affected side and pain medication. If displacement at the fracture site occurs when the patient begins to bear weight, further surgical treatment may be necessary. Fractures that have marked displacement of the anterior ring without complete posterior ring disruption are usually treated with reduction and surgical anterior ring stabilization. Patients who have complete disruption of the posterior ring will require surgical stabilization of both the anterior and posterior pelvic ring.

■ Nursing Management

Initial nursing management of the patient with a pelvic fracture includes continued reassessment for potential complications, pain control, and keeping the patient still after a binder is applied. If the patient requires surgical stabilization, postfixation nursing management includes pain control, continued assessment for complications such as bleeding, infection at the incised site, DVT, PE, and pneumonia. For care of the orthopedic surgical patient, refer to Chapter 57 ☺.

Assessment

Initial nursing management of the patient with a pelvic fracture includes continued assessment of the patient for concomitant injuries, and signs and symptoms of potential complications.

Nursing Diagnoses

The primary nursing diagnoses for the patient with pelvic fracture include:

- *Pain, Acute*
- *Physical Mobility, Impaired*

- *Injury, Risk for*
- *Fluid Volume, Deficient, Risk for*
- *Infection, Risk for.*

Outcomes and Evaluation Parameters

The desired outcomes for the patient with a fracture of any type are relief of pain, prevention of damage to the nerves and vasculature, and restoration of strength and mobility. Evaluation parameters include control of pain as described by the patient, restoration of nerve and vascular function as demonstrated by exam, and return of strength and mobility as noted by assessment.

Planning, Interventions, and Rationales

With all fractures, the nurse should quickly assess and immobilize the affected extremity or pelvis to prevent further damage and to recognize any vascular or nerve involvement. Figure 56–15 ■ illustrates how to quickly assess for sensory and motor function.

The patient will require intravenous pain medication because fracture pain is severe. In the postresuscitative phase, pain control is critical to assist with rehabilitation to normal activities of daily living. Studies have shown that patients who receive adequate pain relief recover more quickly (Bongiovanni et al., 2005). Patients are better able to participate with physical therapy if their pain is appropriately managed.

If the patient presents with an open fracture, apply a sterile dressing immediately to help protect the open wound from further contamination. Postoperatively any wounds, dressings, or splints should be monitored for signs of infection such as warmth and redness, drainage with a foul odor, purulent drainage, increased pain, and fever. If signs of infection are noted, notify the health care team immediately.

For the patient who has an unstable pelvic fracture, the nurse should anticipate the need for a blood transfusion and ensure the patient has been typed and crossmatched for blood products. If the patient is placed in a pelvic binder, the nurse should assess position of the binder and ensure smooth, direct contact between the patient and binder to avoid skin breakdown. Chart 56–4 shows an example of a patient care standard for pelvic binder management.

The nurse is critical in monitoring the patient for signs that would indicate the onset of hypovolemic shock and the need for resuscitative measures. An orthopedic trauma patient who has experienced fractures of the pelvis or long bones is at risk for significant bleeding. The nurse should monitor the patient's hemodynamic status including vital signs and laboratory values. A patient may lose as much as 20% of his blood volume before exhibiting signs and symptoms of shock. The nurse should monitor the vital signs for an increase in heart rate, decrease in blood pressure, increase in respiratory rate, and a decrease in urine output. Laboratory results will show a decrease in the hemoglobin and hematocrit. Refer to Chapter 61 for a detailed discussion of shock.

Nerve	Sensory function		Motor function	
Peroneal	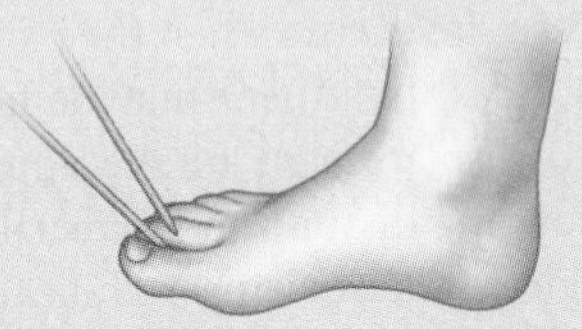	Prick the lateral surface of the big toe and the medial surface of the second toe.	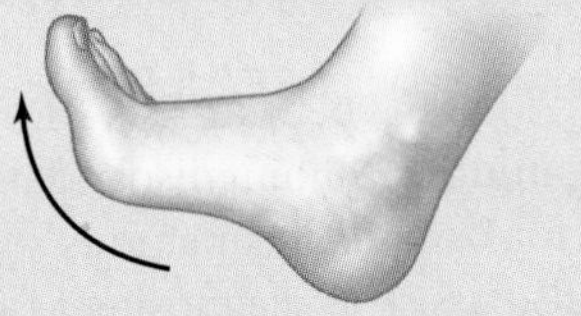	Ask the patient to dorsiflex his ankle and extend his toes.
Tibial	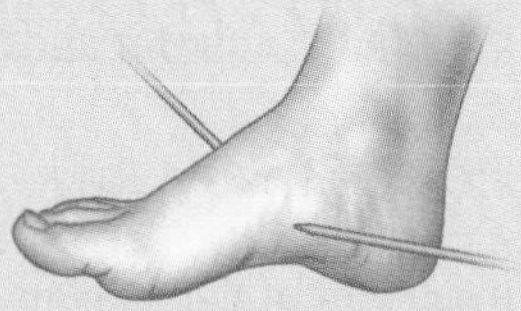	Prick the medial and lateral surfaces of the foot.	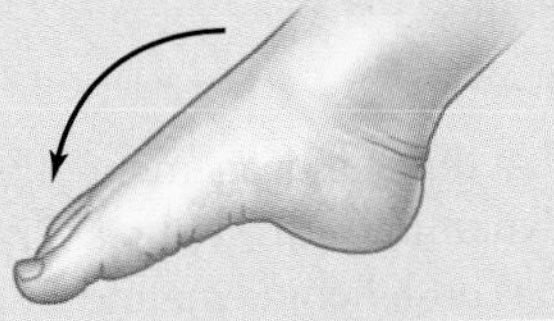	Ask the patient to plantarflex his ankle. Note whether the patient can flex his toes.
Radial	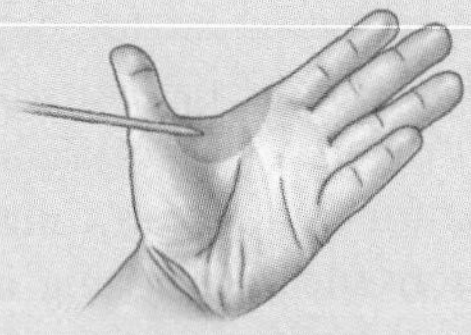	Prick the web space between the thumb and index finger.	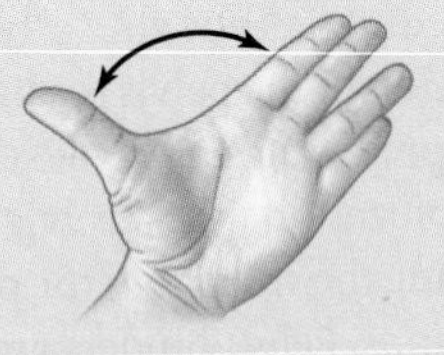	Ask the patient to hyperextend his wrist or thumb.
Ulnar	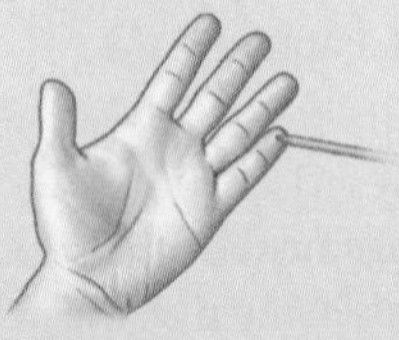	Prick the distal fat pad of the fifth (small) finger.	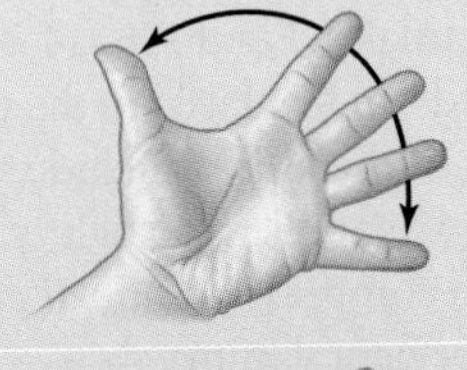	Ask the patient to abduct all his fingers.
Median	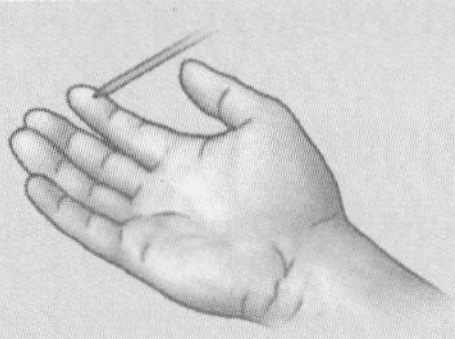	Prick the distal surface of the index finger.	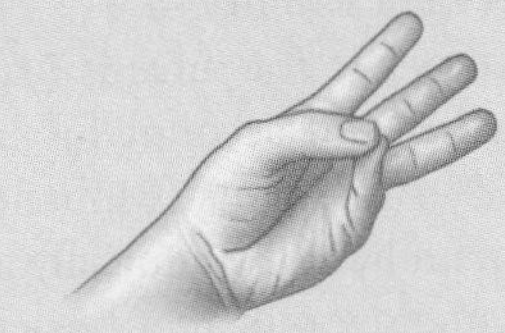	Ask the patient to oppose his thumb and fifth finger. Note whether patient can flex his wrist.

FIGURE 56–15 ■ Motor and sensory assessment.

CHART 56-4	Pelvic Binder Management

UC Davis Health System
Pelvic Binder Management
Patient Care Standards VI-10
Revised 2/11/07

I. SETTING

Emergency Department and Intensive Care Units
Performed by: Independent function by RN after binder has been placed by health care provider.

II. OUTCOME STANDARDS

A. Provide a quick, safe and effective method in initial treatment of pelvic fractures.

B. Lower mortality rate.

C. Aid in pain management due to disruption of pelvis.

D. The patient will not develop skin breakdown due to compressive nature of binder.

E. Patient will maintain alignment and hemodynamic stability as exhibited by: systolic blood pressure >90, will maintain integrity of distal pulses, warmth of distal extremitites.

III. SUPPORTIVE DATA

Unstable pelvic fractures in the poly-traumatized patient are a significant source of blood loss and mortality. Evidence supports the use of a stabilization device (pelvic binder), which applies anterior/posterior pelvic compression, for use in initial treatment to stabilize a suspected pelvic fracture to help prevent blood loss and aid in pain control. The pelvic binder is a temporary device until definitive treatment can be accomplished.

IV. PROCEDURE

A. Initial Placement

1. Initial Placement will typically occur in the Emergency Department and is placed by the MD.

2. Upon arrival to admitting unit and throughout the patient stay, assess position of the binder, ensure smooth, direct contact between patient and binder. Assure that there are no creases or wrinkles in binder, which could quicken skin breakdown.

B. Ongoing care:

1. Once the pelvic binder has been placed, it should not be removed or adjusted for 72 hours, unless the patient requires operative intervention for the region covered by the binder, or other contraindications are noted.

2. If, after 72 hours, the patient is hemodynamically stable, (SBP shall remain >90 mmHg, x 4 hours and hemoglobin remains stable) the health care provider should be at the bedside for the first release of compression, then the nurse shall:

a. Routinely release the pulley-tab by detaching the Velcro tab from the belt and allow the draw strings to relax 1cm, without losing compression of pelvis every 2 hours.

b. If visible, assess as much skin integrity as possible with each 1cm release as listed above. If the health care provider wishes to assess full circumference skin integrity of the pelvis/torso, the binder may be log-rolled, otherwise, the binder shall remain in place and the maximum release by the nurse will be as stated in #1 above.

3. Report any changes to the health care provider team.

4. Document on the appropriate department tool the following:

a. Time of pelvic binder application.

b. Initial status of skin integrity in pelvic region.

c. Every 2 hour release of pulley system.

d. Skin assessment with each release.

e. Notification of health care provider if patient condition changes or skin breakdown noted.

Source: UC Davis Health System, University of California, Davis (2007).

Health Promotion

Rehabilitation is an important aspect of the care of the patient with a fracture. The patient should be mobilized as soon as possible to prevent further complications. Physical therapy should begin early to prevent contractures and increase mobility and strength to the extremity.

Traumatic Amputations

Traumatic amputations are when part or all of a digit or limb is severed from the body. These are upsetting to patients as well as staff. Many emergency service members bring the amputated part to the hospital in hopes of possible reattachment.

Surgical reattachment of a severed limb is done only under certain circumstances because the surgery is difficult. It is not attempted with a digit of the hand unless it is a thumb or index finger needed for function and the wound has clean borders. Crush-type amputations are not attempted due to the poor outcome. Only cleanly separated traumatic amputations in patients without significant risk factors for impaired healing such as smoking are considered for reimplantation. For adults, it is nearly impossible for nerves to regenerate in the lower extremity, and the reattached limb may be painful and dysfunctional (Feliciano

et al., 2008). Complete amputation and a prosthesis could allow a patient to return to normal activities in days to weeks, whereas reconstruction of mangled limbs can span over years with a huge psychological strain and impact on function and occupation. For a complete discussion of amputation refer to Chapter 57 .

There are as many physical/mobility issues to deal with as there are emotional issues for the patient with an amputation. The patient may need to have wound care to the stump and have trouble just looking at it. The patient may have bizarre sensations such as feeling like her foot is cold or itchy when it is not there. These are called phantom limb sensations. Patients may need to retrain their brains to distinguish where their body ends. Most will also need to grieve the loss of their limb and counseling should be initiated prior to discharge. Prostheses will be made and a great deal of physical and occupational therapy may be needed to adapt to a missing limb or digit.

Complications of Musculoskeletal Trauma

Most all complications of musculoskeletal trauma are detected early by an accurate complete nursing assessment. Assessment of the injured patient begins with the ABC's of airway, breathing, and circulation. Orthopedic assessment consists of vital signs, pain assessment, inspection, palpation, and the extremely important neurovascular exam. Inspection is head to toe, appraising skin integrity and discoloration such as bruising.

Palpate for areas of tenderness, crepitus, or swelling. The neurovascular exam consists of assessing the color, temperature, capillary refill, pulses, edema, sensory and motor function, and pain level of an extremity such as a hand or foot. The neurovascular exam of the extremities should be performed and documented with each vital sign assessment (or as ordered), and changes need to be reported to the health care team. Many acute care centers have a neurovascular check sheet for patient assessment. Figure 56–16 ■, A–F, shows examples of the neurovascular documentation section of an electronic medical record. When assessing an extremity, comparison of the affected extremity to the nonaffected extremity is important.

Pulses are assessed at typical points such as the radial pulse at the wrist and the dorsalis pedis pulse on the mid-dorsum of the foot. Posterior tibial pulses can be felt just posterior to the medial malleolus.

Sensory and motor function of each nerve branch should be assessed. The upper extremity nerves are the radial, ulnar, and median nerves. Lower extremity nerves are the peroneal and tibial. Muscle strength (graded 5–0) and joint range of motion, both passive (the nurse moves the joint for the patient) and active (the patient moves the joint), are assessed and documented and expressed as a ratio such as 4/5 (4 out of 5).

Pain should be assessed frequently, and there are many methods to do this including observation of facial grimace, guarding postures, limp, and vital sign changes such as elevated blood pressure and pulse. Refer to Chapter 15 ⊘ for a complete discussion of pain assessment.

Orthopedic injuries are very painful. Broken bones hurt until they stop moving, which may be 14 days or longer. Pain management is paramount for injured patients for many reasons including comfort level, adequate ventilation, rehabilitation, and aiding with sleep. Most patients, including children, will require narcotics. Children have historically been undermedicated, which can have long-term implications. Physiological predictors of post-traumatic stress disorder (PTSD) in children have shown that the strongest of the physiological correlations appears to be patients' perception of their pain. The worse the degree of early pain, the more likely that they will exhibit PTSD after the injury (Norman, Stein, Dimsdale, & Hoyt, 2007). Orthopedic patients frequently have physical therapy ordered and will need to get out of bed as soon as possible to prevent the complications of bed rest and immobilization. It is helpful to have patients premedicated 30 to 60 minutes prior to physical therapy.

Mobility

Patients with musculoskeletal trauma may have mobility issues. Even a sports injury may require crutches and a change in weight-bearing status. Many assistive devices, such as wheelchairs, walkers, crutches, canes, or reachers, are available. Wheelchairs need to

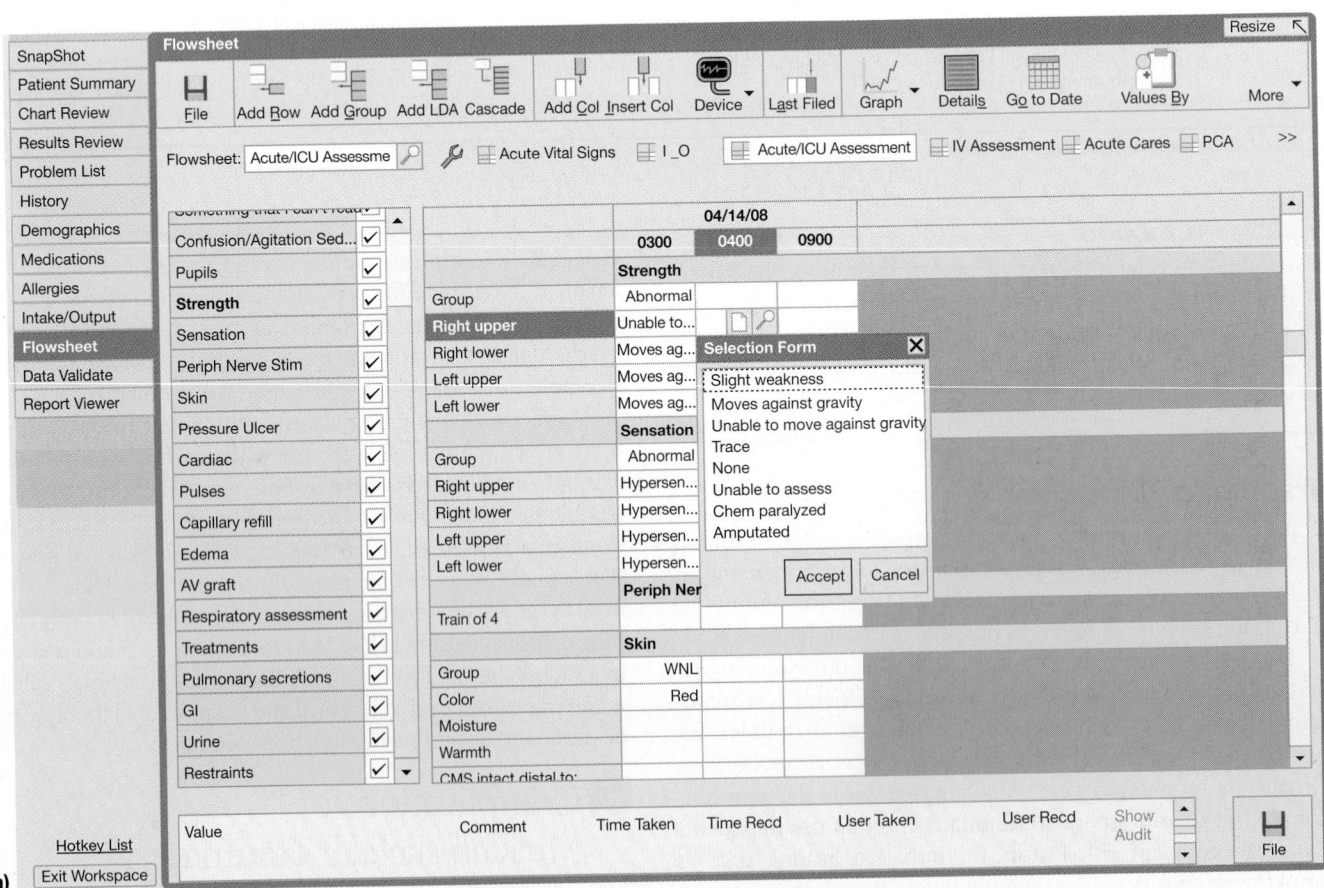

FIGURE 56–16 ■ Neurovascular assessment: (A) strength; (B) sensation; (C) skin; (D) pulses; (E) capillary refill; (F) edema.

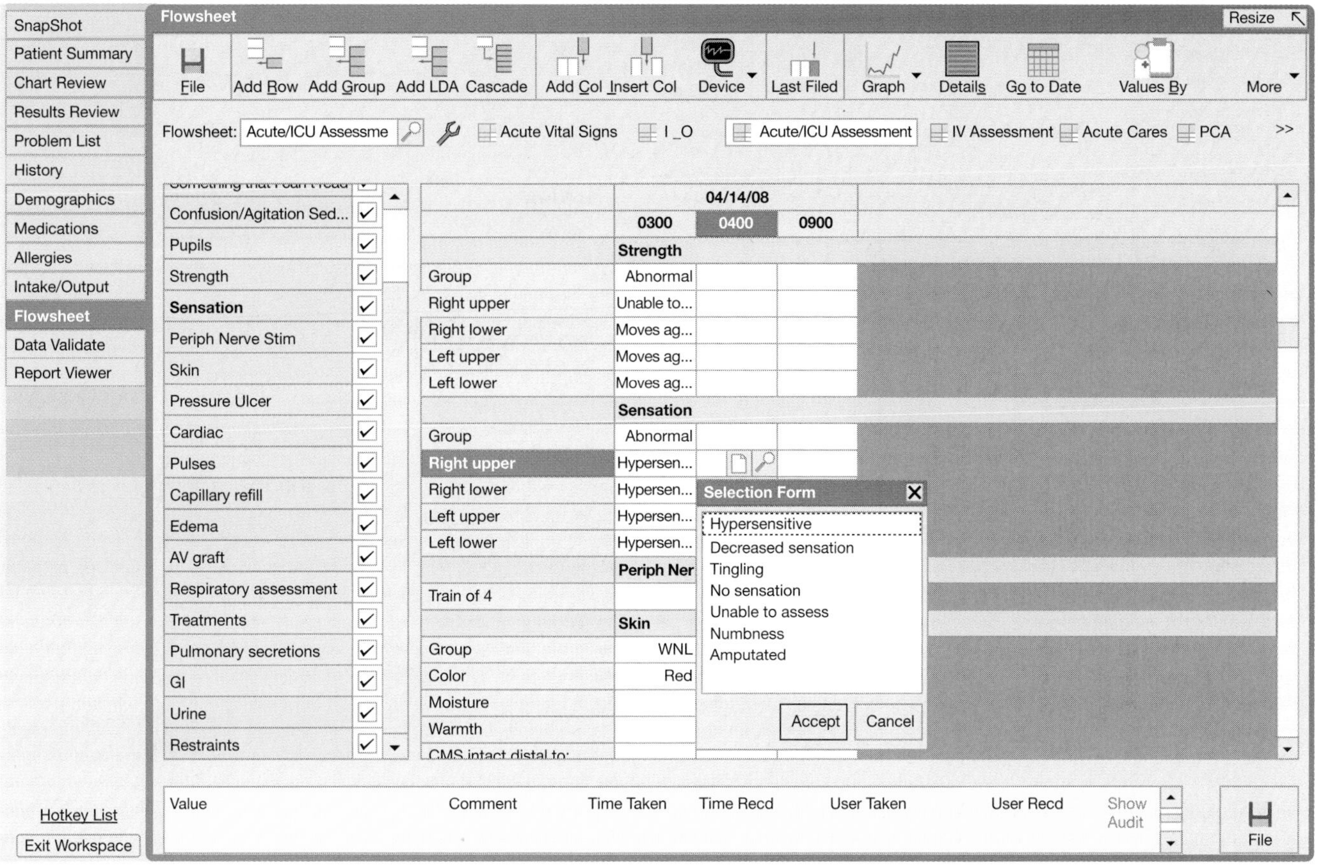

(b)

FIGURE 56–16 ■ Neurovascular assessment: (A) strength; (B) sensation; (C) skin; (D) pulses; (E) capillary refill; (F) edema.—*Continued*

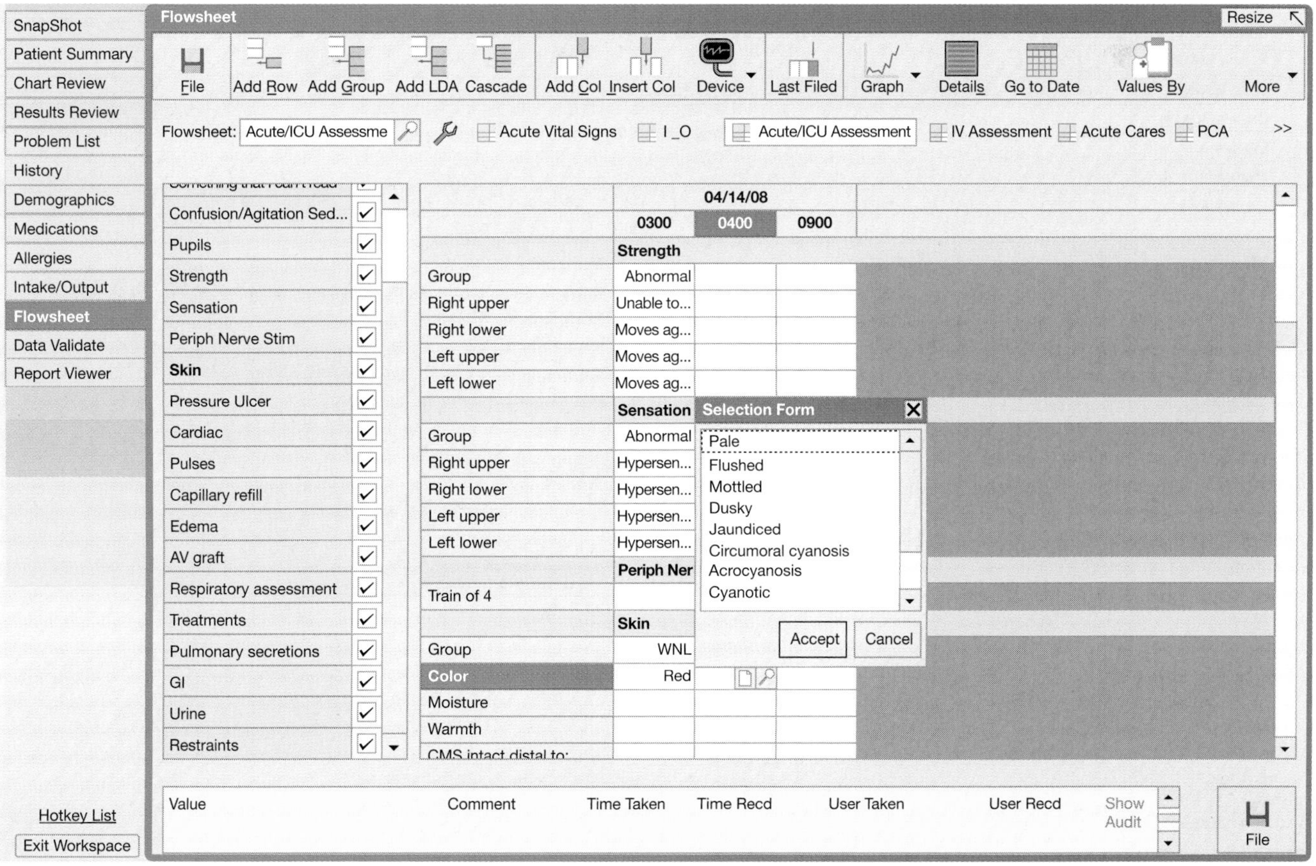

(c)

FIGURE 56–16 ■ Neurovascular assessment: (A) strength; (B) sensation; (C) skin; (D) pulses; (E) capillary refill; (F) edema.—*Continued*

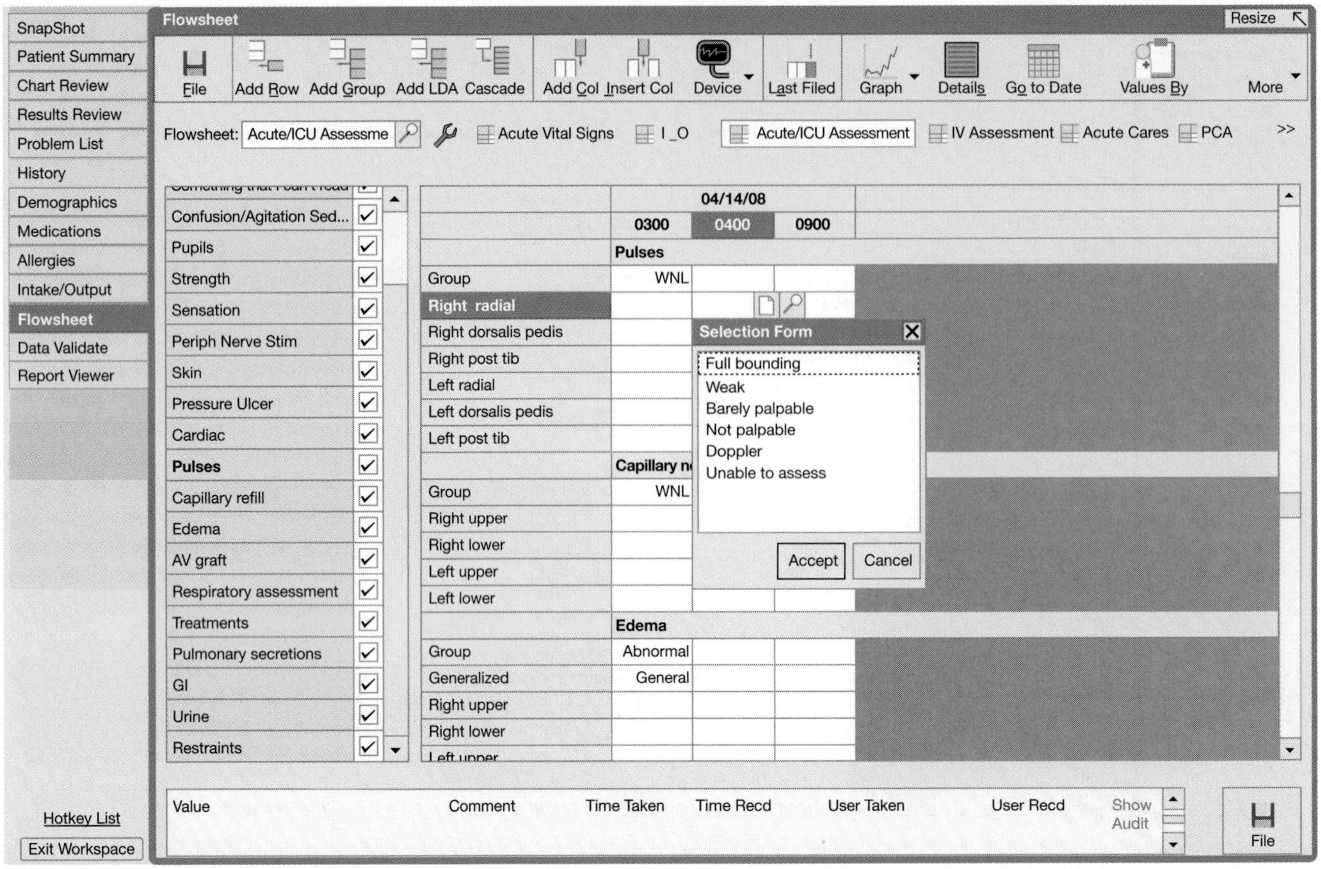

Flowsheet — (d)

SnapShot | Patient Summary | Chart Review | Results Review | Problem List | History | Demographics | Medications | Allergies | Intake/Output | **Flowsheet** | Data Validate | Report Viewer

File | Add Row | Add Group | Add LDA | Cascade | Add Col | Insert Col | Device | Last Filed | Graph | Details | Go to Date | Values By | More

Flowsheet: Acute/ICU Assessme | Acute Vital Signs | I_O | Acute/ICU Assessment | IV Assessment | Acute Cares | PCA | >>

	04/14/08		
	0300	0400	0900
Pulses			
Group	WNL		
Right radial			
Right dorsalis pedis			
Right post tib			
Left radial			
Left dorsalis pedis			
Left post tib			
Capillary re...			
Group	WNL		
Right upper			
Right lower			
Left upper			
Left lower			
Edema			
Group	Abnormal		
Generalized	General		
Right upper			
Right lower			
Left upper			

Left sidebar checklist: Confusion/Agitation Sed... ✓ | Pupils ✓ | Strength ✓ | Sensation ✓ | Periph Nerve Stim ✓ | Skin ✓ | Pressure Ulcer ✓ | Cardiac ✓ | **Pulses** ✓ | Capillary refill ✓ | Edema ✓ | AV graft ✓ | Respiratory assessment ✓ | Treatments ✓ | Pulmonary secretions ✓ | GI ✓ | Urine ✓ | Restraints ✓

Selection Form [X]
- Full bounding
- Weak
- Barely palpable
- Not palpable
- Doppler
- Unable to assess

[Accept] [Cancel]

Value | Comment | Time Taken | Time Recd | User Taken | User Recd | Show Audit | File

Hotkey List | **(d)** | Exit Workspace

FIGURE 56–16 ■ Neurovascular assessment: (A) strength; (B) sensation; (C) skin; (D) pulses; (E) capillary refill; (F) edema.—*Continued*

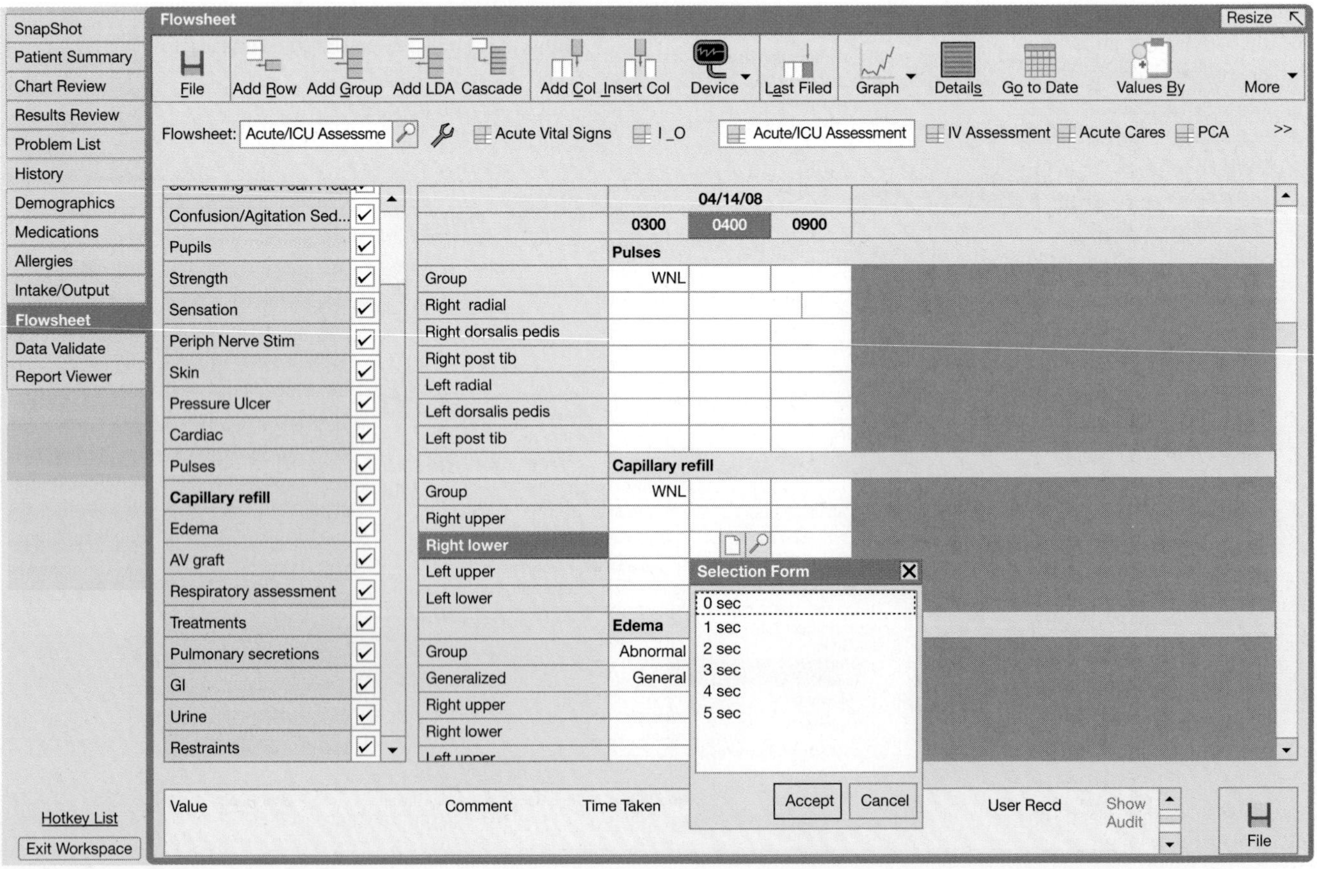

Flowsheet — (e)

SnapShot | Patient Summary | Chart Review | Results Review | Problem List | History | Demographics | Medications | Allergies | Intake/Output | **Flowsheet** | Data Validate | Report Viewer

File | Add Row | Add Group | Add LDA | Cascade | Add Col | Insert Col | Device | Last Filed | Graph | Details | Go to Date | Values By | More

Flowsheet: Acute/ICU Assessme | Acute Vital Signs | I_O | Acute/ICU Assessment | IV Assessment | Acute Cares | PCA | >>

	04/14/08		
	0300	0400	0900
Pulses			
Group	WNL		
Right radial			
Right dorsalis pedis			
Right post tib			
Left radial			
Left dorsalis pedis			
Left post tib			
Capillary refill			
Group	WNL		
Right upper			
Right lower			
Left upper			
Left lower			
Edema			
Group	Abnormal		
Generalized	General		
Right upper			
Right lower			
Left upper			

Left sidebar checklist: Confusion/Agitation Sed... ✓ | Pupils ✓ | Strength ✓ | Sensation ✓ | Periph Nerve Stim ✓ | Skin ✓ | Pressure Ulcer ✓ | Cardiac ✓ | Pulses ✓ | **Capillary refill** ✓ | Edema ✓ | AV graft ✓ | Respiratory assessment ✓ | Treatments ✓ | Pulmonary secretions ✓ | GI ✓ | Urine ✓ | Restraints ✓

Selection Form [X]
- 0 sec
- 1 sec
- 2 sec
- 3 sec
- 4 sec
- 5 sec

[Accept] [Cancel]

Value | Comment | Time Taken | User Recd | Show Audit | File

Hotkey List | **(e)** | Exit Workspace

FIGURE 56–16 ■ Neurovascular assessment: (A) strength; (B) sensation; (C) skin; (D) pulses; (E) capillary refill; (F) edema.—*Continued*

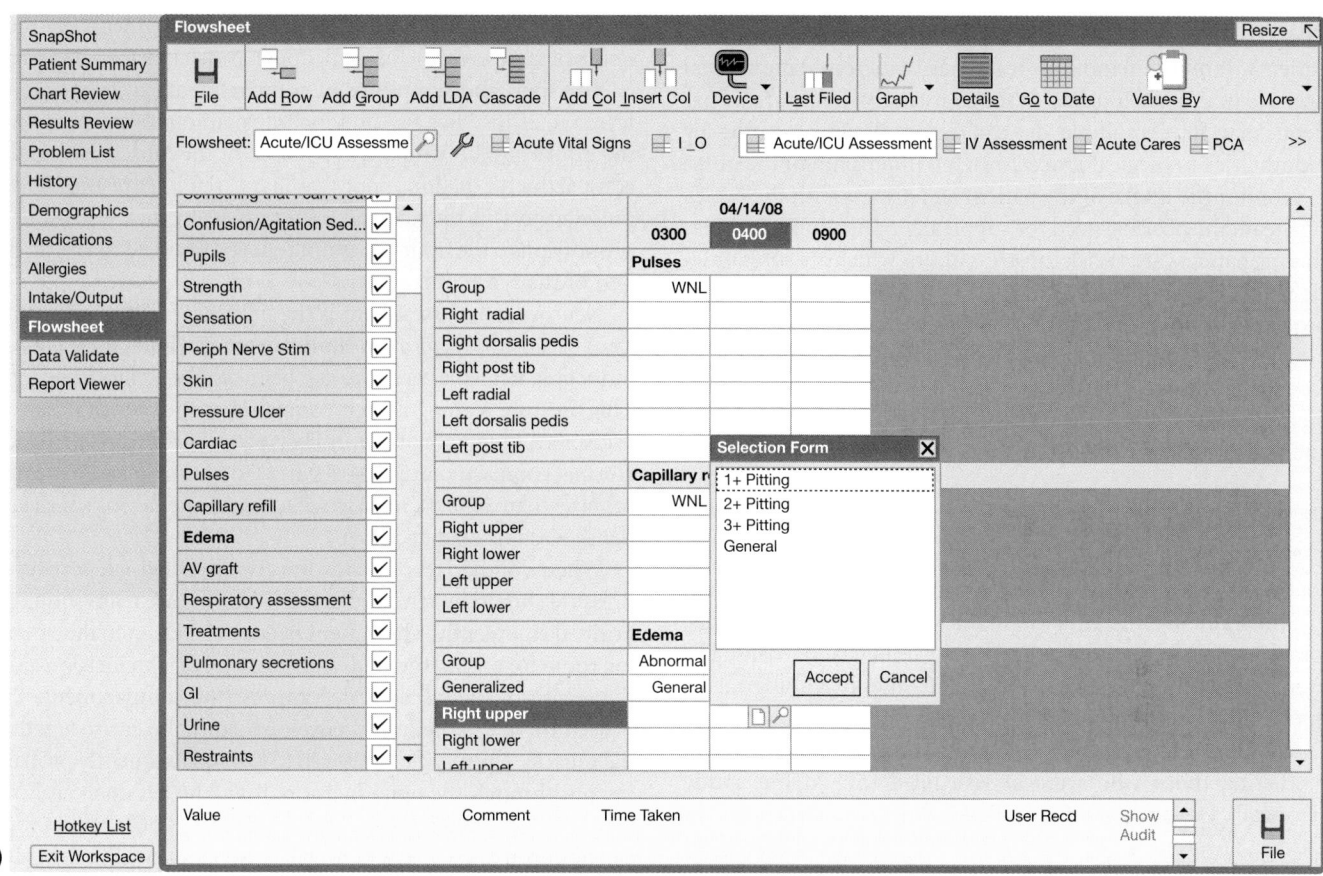

(f)

FIGURE 56–16 ■ Neurovascular assessment: (A) strength; (B) sensation; (C) skin; (D) pulses; (E) capillary refill; (F) edema.—*Continued*

be fit to the patient and can come with elevating leg rests and reclining backs. Manual, one-side drive, and electric wheelchairs are available depending on patients' abilities and the time they will be expected to use one.

Walkers are frames with four posts and handgrips usually made of aluminum. They may be required by elderly patients or those who are large or have difficulty with balance and need to have restricted weight bearing. Walkers may have wheels on the front legs for patients who cannot lift them.

Crutches are devices used in pairs to aid ambulation by transferring weight to upper extremities. Crutches come in two types—axillary crutches and forearm (also referred to as loftstrand or Canadian) crutches. The axillary crutches can be made of wood or aluminum. When patients are fitted for axillary crutches (allowing for four fingerwidths between axilla and crutch top) they should be encouraged not to rest their armpits

on the crutch. Most of the weight can be carried on the palms of the hand if there is no injury to hand or arm. If such an injury exists, a platform crutch may be more appropriate. The weight of a patient for these crutches is limited to 113 kg (250 pounds) for most manufacturers of wooden crutches. It is very important to teach the patient the proper use and to observe them using the crutches.

A cane is a wooden or metal stick with a curved graspable handle at the top. A cane should be used on the opposite side of the injury to "unload" an extremity or aid with balance. In addition, it should be measured to fit to the palm of a nearly fully extended arm when laterally placed 8 to 12 inches from the foot.

Many musculoskeletal conditions will require a specific weight-bearing status. This is a directive on how much weight the clinician would—or would not—like the patient to put on an extremity (Chart 56–5).

CHART 56–5   Weight-Bearing Status

NWB	Nonweight bearing	Should not put any weight on extremity (not even to push up in bed).
TDWB, TTWB	Touch down or toe touch	Allowed to let toe touch the ground for balance and allows leg to be rested on the ground but no weight should be placed on it.
PWB	Partial weight bearing	Usually a percentage of the person's weight, for example, 25–50%.
WBAT	Weight bearing as tolerated	The patient may begin to put weight on the extremity as pain recedes.
FWB	Full weight bearing	Allowed to walk normally on the extremity; does not require crutches.

Nutrition

Patients who sustain multiple trauma have increased nutritional needs to heal tissue injuries. In the resuscitative phase, many patients may have multiple days of being allowed nothing by mouth prior to surgical procedures. It is important for the nurse to monitor the intake of the patient and discuss with the health care team the possible need for supplement nutrition. Multiple-trauma patients are at risk for stress ulcers, which are sores or lesion on the lining of the stomach or duodenum and may be prophylactically treated with H_2-receptor antagonists, proton pump inhibitors, and sucralfate. Frequently patients involved in trauma have social issues such as drug or alcohol abuse and poor dietary habits. These will need to be taken into consideration and addressed individually.

Psychological Recovery

The psychological impact and sequelae of musculoskeletal trauma are not well known. There are more factors involved than just the trauma of the injury itself; there are medical treatments, loss of mobility or school or work time, financial burdens, and even changes in self-concept. PTSD and other psychological sequelae can be seen months after physical recovery.

Wishful thinking as a coping mechanism was distinctive in predicting those who were at risk for PTSD in one study (Dougall, Ursano, Posluszny, Fullerton, & Baum, 2001). A greater awareness of psychological repercussions from trauma, especially inflicted or disfiguring injuries, is needed. There are early identifiable risk factors for post-traumatic maladjustment: panic during or immediately after the trauma, reexperiencing symptoms, avoidance, sleep disturbance, injury from an assault, previous trauma and psychiatric history, and blaming someone else for the injury. Rusch, Gould, Dzwierzynski, and Larson (2002) discussed that any reexperiencing of symptoms, avoidance, trauma-related phobias, depression, irritability, and increased substance use suggests psychological impairment. Younger children may regress or exhibit changes in play or sleep including night terrors, aggression, irritability, avoidance, and emergence of new fears (Rusch et al., 2002).

Compartment Syndrome

Compartment syndrome is a common complication and the cause of poor outcomes and much litigation. **Compartment syndrome** is a condition whereby increasing pressure within the muscle compartments compromises circulation and the function of soft tissues, nerves, and vessels in that compartment, which leads to anoxia of the tissue and necrosis, which in turn leads to more edema in the compartment and a subsequent increase in pressure.

Compartment syndrome is cyclical and builds until a surgical release of the fascial envelope is performed. If pressure is not reduced, irreversible muscle damage and nerve damage can occur within hours and can also lead to life-threatening complications such a rhabdomyolysis and renal failure. Compartment syndrome can occur due to increasing internal pressure, for example, from bleeding into the compartment by fractured bone and torn muscle tissue or overhydration or from the external pressure applied by the trauma itself, casts, dressing, burns (tight eschar), or even clothing. The most commonly affected compartments are those of the tibia (lower leg), forearm, upper arm, hand, foot, and thigh.

The signs and symptoms of compartment syndrome are referred to as the "five Ps," and include pain out of proportion to the injury or pain with passive stretch of the muscle within that compartment, pallor, poor capillary refill, paresthesia, and pulselessness in the affected extremity. Pain that seems out of proportion to the injury or is not relieved by analgesia is the earliest of the symptoms.

Neurovascular assessment is the best way to note early symptoms because it is typically a clinical diagnosis, but if there is doubt intracompartmental pressure can be measured with a transducer. This pressure reading is then compared to the patient's diastolic pressure. A difference of 30 mmHg is essential for tissue perfusion. Normal compartment pressures are 0 to 8 mmHg and a pressure of more than 30 to 45 mmHg will cause tissue necrosis if the patient's diastolic reading is low.

When compartment syndrome is suspected, all sources of pressure should be removed and the health care team should be notified emergently. The patient needs to be taken to the operating room for an emergent **fasciotomy**, which is an incision along the length of the fascia to decompress the compartment. This procedure opens the fascial envelope along the entire length of the muscle. The muscle is allowed to expand, frequently protruding out through the open incision. It will be left open and covered with wet saline dressings for several days until the skin edges can be approximated again. Any necrotic tissue will be debrided. Skin grafts or amputations may be required for severe cases.

Rhabdomyolysis

Rhabdomyolysis occurs when the injured skeletal muscle fibers break down and leak inflammatory mediators, such as myoglobin and creatinine kinase, into the circulation. It is most commonly seen with crush injuries but can occur with any massive soft tissue injury.

Complications associated with rhabdomyolysis include acute renal failure. This occurs due to renal tubular obstruction from the filtration of the released myoglobin. The patient may also exhibit respiratory distress due to muscle weakness and fluid and electrolyte imbalances.

Signs and symptoms of rhabdomyolysis include pain, tenderness, swelling, bruising, and weakness within the affected muscles. Upon assessment the muscles involved may feel soft and flabby. The patient's urine will also become dark in color (referred to as myoglobinuria) as the renal system attempts to filter the myoglobin. Patients may also develop systemic symptoms including general malaise, fever, nausea and vomiting, confusion, agitation, and anuria as the acute renal failure progresses. Diagnosis is confirmed by a creatinine kinase level. The level will be increased to five times or more of the normal value.

Treatment consists of administration of IV fluids to maintain circulating blood volume and perfuse the kidneys while flushing the myoglobin from the kidneys. Creatinine kinase levels should be obtained and high rates of fluid continued until the levels decrease to 1,000 units/L. The patient's associated acidosis is treated with a sodium bicarbonate infusion to alkalinize the urine. Fifty percent to 70% of patients who develop acute renal failure will require dialysis to treat the electrolyte imbalances and fluid overload (Bongiovanni et al., 2005). Most patients have a complete recovery of renal function after treatment.

Deep Venous Thrombosis and Pulmonary Embolism

Deep venous thrombosis is a blood clot in the venous circulatory system typically in the lower extremity. Virchow's triad—venous stasis, intimal damage, and hypercoagulability—combines to a state of thrombogenesis. A recent analysis of 1,602 patients who developed DVT and PE identified in the American College of Surgeons National Trauma Data Bank revealed the following significant risk factors: age greater than 40; lower extremity fracture with an abbreviated injury scale (AIS) > 3 (scale is from 1 to 6, with 1 being lowest severity and 6 being highest severity); head injury with an AIS > 3; exceeding 3 ventilator days; venous injury; and a major operative procedure (Knudson, Ikossi, Khaw, Morabito, & Speetzen, 2004). Other risk factors have been identified that reflect the hypercoagulable state. Higher levels of homocysteine and plasminogen activator-1 levels correlate with DVT in a study of patients with spinal cord injury (Aito, Abbate, Marcucci, & Cominelli, 2007). Prophylaxis for DVT consists of early ambulation, use of serial compression devices (SCDs) of the lower extremities, and administration of low-molecular-weight heparin or unfractionated heparin for anticoagulation. If the clot extends proximally, a portion may break loose and cause a pulmonary embolism.

Pulmonary embolism is a blood clot that has broken free from a site that travels through venous circulation, through the right side of the heart to the lungs where it lodges in one or both branches of the pulmonary artery to obstruct or partially obstruct circulation. The most common signs and symptoms are anxiety or a feeling of impending doom coupled with dyspnea. For a detailed discussion of PE, see Chapter 35 🔗.

Fat Embolism Syndrome

Fat embolism syndrome (FES) occurs when fat globules released from long-bone fractures enter the circulatory system. Up to 90% of long-bone fractures have some release of fat emboli associated with the fracture, only 3% to 4% progress to FES (Feliciano et al., 2008). In the most severe cases, the emboli can produce multiple-organ failure from both a direct embolic effect and from activation of the inflammatory cascade. The most commonly noted triad of symptoms is acute respiratory failure, neurological dysfunction, and a petechial rash (Chart 56–6). Acute respiratory failure may be the only symptom in a large number of patients.

Cast Syndrome

Cast syndrome or superior mesenteric artery syndrome (SMAS) can be fatal. SMAS occurs when there is compression of the superior mesenteric artery at the duodenum, from anterior pressure such as a body cast or brace and posteriorly resisted by the descending aorta and spine (Shetty, 2004). This compression impedes the blood flow to the bowel, causing ischemia and eventually necrosis of the gastrointestinal tract and vessel walls that can result in hemorrhage and death. This is most often seen in children in body casts or hip spica casts; however, it also is seen in adults with casts or back braces especially if they have

CHART 56–6	Classic Triad for Signs and Symptoms of Fat Embolus	
Early Findings	**Later Findings**	**Last Component**
Hypoxemia Dyspnea Tachypnea	Neurologic abnormalities: Confusion Altered LOC Focal deficits Possible seizures	Petechial rash found most often on the head, neck, anterior thorax, subconjunctiva, and axillae.

Source: Weinhouse, G. (2008). Fat embolism syndrome. Retrieved August 10, 2008, from http://www.utdol.com/online/content/topic.do?topicKey=cc_medi/13397&selectedTitle=1~27&source=search_result.

had spine injury or surgery where there is any hyperextension of the lumbar spine or distraction injuries of the spine.

The first symptoms are vague abdominal pain, pressure, distention, and irritability; this is followed by nausea, projectile vomiting, and bowel obstruction. SMAS may occur postoperatively or days or weeks later especially with very young children growing larger in hip spica casts. Early treatment is essential, begun by bivalve (cutting both sides of the cast to relieve pressure), window (cutting a section of the cast away from a pressure point), or removal of the cast (or brace). Decompression of the stomach is achieved with a nasogastric (NG) tube to continuous intermittent suction.

Pressure Ulcers

Skin integrity and prevention of pressure areas is key to orthopedic nursing. Keeping heels off the bed is crucial, as is padding of bony prominences. Providing adequate nutrition and hydration and keeping the skin clean and dry are measures aimed at promoting good skin turgor.

Complex Regional Pain Syndrome

Complex regional pain syndrome (CRPS), formerly known as reflex sympathetic dystrophy (RSD), is a diffuse persistent pain usually associated with vasomotor, trophic, and bony changes and limited mobility of an extremity following a local injury. Early referral to physical therapy for movement and pain clinic personnel who specialize in this disorder is crucial.

◼ Gerontological Considerations

The nurse should be aware of specific gerontological considerations for musculoskeletal trauma. Hip and wrist fractures are the most common types of fractures in elderly patients. Conditions such as osteoporosis or tumor may predispose the elderly to a pathologic or insufficiency fracture. In such a fracture the bone is not strong enough for its function and it breaks through the weakened framework with little trauma. Fractures in the elderly may occur prior to, or as a result of, a fall. A high mortality rate is associated with hip fracture in the elderly; more than 4% die during hospitalization and 10% to 35% die within a year of the injury (Meehan, 2002; Morris & Zuckerman, 2002). Delay in surgical repair of hip fracture is associated with complications of bed rest including atelectasis, thromboembolism, urinary tract infection, and pressure ulcers (Orosz et al., 2004). Early weight bearing and return to preferred living situation with adequate services has been associated with better medical, psychosocial, financial, and cultural outcomes (Meehan, 2002).

Prevention of fractures is a key nursing initiative. Fall prevention, nutrition evaluation, and encouraging screening and osteoporosis treatment for elderly patients are essential for good quality-of-life outcomes.

Elderly patients have other considerations such as sensory and metabolic deficits and delays in medication absorption and healing. Constipation is a major concern for the elderly who sustain musculoskeletal fracture and are immobilized or who require narcotics or undergo surgery. There are psychosocial issues for the elderly such as fear of becoming infirm, being in pain, running out of money, having to be dependent on family, asking for help, appearance concerns such as assistive devices making them look old, sexuality, being alone, and that the road back to recovery may be too much. They may grieve over loss of function, friends, or lifestyle. Most will lose a functional level after a hip fracture; for example, if they were ambulatory within their community, they may only be ambulatory at home after the injury.

Research Opportunities

Both physiological and psychosocial opportunities exist for research in orthopedic nursing. The Research Opportunities chart includes a sample of topics for further nursing research.

Summary

Orthopedic injuries are a frequent occurrence because of blunt trauma and increasingly of penetrating trauma. The nurse plays a crucial role within the health care team in providing timely care for this population. The nurse will be the one to frequently assess and monitor the patient's orthopedic injury and is in the position to recognize and intervene when potential life- and limb-threatening conditions occur.

RESEARCH OPPORTUNITIES AND CLINICAL IMPACT RELATED TO ORTHOPEDIC NURSING

Research Area	Clinical Impact
Physiological Research	
The management of pin sites placed for skeletal traction and external fixation.	Nurses do not have sufficient evidence on which to base best care of pin sites to prevent infection.
Use of alternative methods to manage pain on the orthopedic unit.	Alternative methods of pain management such as acupuncture, acupressure, and massage could be used by nurses to help manage pain.
Development of guidelines to manage pain treatment when patients are transferred to rehab/extended care facilities or home.	There are no guidelines and reported poor pain control of patients after discharge from acute care.
Psychosocial, Ethical, and Legal Research	
Effectiveness of discharge teaching and plans of care and reality of resource availability in the home or community for postoperative patients or those with musculoskeletal injuries.	Many patients are discharged quickly without sufficient resources in place or without understanding plans of care. For example, what is ordered for home and what actually occurs may not be the same. Identify areas for improvement in teaching information and methods, as well as community resources for the postoperative or injured orthopedic patient, especially the elderly, uninsured, and underinsured.
	Prevent the return of underinsured patients who use the emergency department for their health care.
	Decrease return visits and get patients into the appropriate health care systems, decreasing costs.

Clinical Preparation

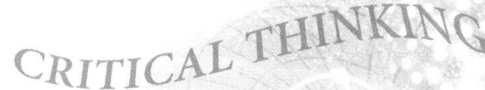

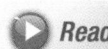 **Read**

- History of Current Illness
- Past Medical History
- Physical Exam
- Admitting Medical Orders
- Laboratory Study Results

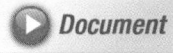 **Document**

- Summary of Hospitalization
- Pathophysiology Form
- Laboratory Values
- Laboratory Results Explanation

 **Apply**

- List of Potential Nursing Diagnoses
- Concept Map
- Critical Thinking Questions

Log on to MyNursingKit.com to download forms you will need and to complete further steps in the Clinical Preparation assignment.

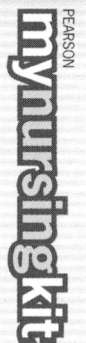

HISTORY OF PRESENT ILLNESS

The patient is a 17-year-old female who was involved in a high-speed, single-vehicle frontal crash and had a negative toxicology/drug screen. Multiple injuries include a concussion and a forehead laceration that has been sutured. She has had her right open tibia fracture washed out with application of an external fixator. She has had an IM rod placed in her right femur fracture. Head CT was negative. Her admitting diagnoses include multiple trauma, right femur fracture, right open tibia/fibular fracture with soft tissue loss, chest contusion, loss of consciousness at the scene, and a forehead laceration.

Medical–Surgical History

The patient takes no medications. Previous surgeries include an appendectomy at age 10.

Social History

The patient is a junior in high school and lives with her parents. The patient denies smoking, drinking, or use of illicit drugs.

Physical Exam

The patient opens her eyes to voice and is oriented. Pupils are equal, round, and reactive to light and accommodation. Suture line on forehead is clean, dry, and intact. Breath sounds are equal bilaterally with equal chest rise. The patient complains of pain to right chest wall with deep breath, no crepitus noted. Heart sounds are normal. Abdomen is soft and nontender with diminished bowel sounds in all quadrants. Right thigh is edematous; suture line is dry and intact. External fixator to right lower leg is intact; pin sites exhibit slight redness and small amount of serous drainage. Motor and sensory to extremities are intact. Peripheral pulses are slightly decreased in the right lower extremity. The patient complains of pain in the right leg at a 6 on a 0–10 scale.

Admitting Medical Orders

Service: trauma service with orthopedic consultation

Diagnosis: concussion, right femur fracture, right open tibia/fibular fracture with soft tissue loss, chest contusion, forehead laceration

Allergies: amoxicillin

Vital signs with oxygen saturations q4h × 24 hours

Call house officer: temp > 38.5°C, HR > 130 or < 60, RR > 30 or < 12, BP sys > 160 or < 90, O_2 sat < 92%, urine output < 120 mL in 4 hours, change in neurological or abdominal exam, any Hct result that is 5 less than the baseline ED Hct, any change in neurovascular exam of the right lower extremity

Activity: patient's weight-bearing status is touch down to right leg; up to chair with assistance

Diet: advance diet as tolerated

Intravenous fluids: D5/0.45 NS with 20 mEq of KCl at 100 mL/hr

Foley catheter to gravity drainage

I&O: every shift

Respiratory care: incentive spirometer every hour when awake

DVT prophylaxis: sequential compression device to left lower extremity

Wound care: pin site care tid, clean forehead laceration with half-strength H_2O_2 and apply bacitracin, elevate right lower extremity

Scheduled Medications

Hydromorphone PCA 0.2 mg/mL, incremental dose 0.4 mg, lock-out 10 minutes

Vancomycin 1 g IV q8h

Docusate capsule 100 mg by mouth twice daily

Enoxaparin 30 mg subcutaneously q12h

PRN Medications

Phenergan 25 mg IV q6h prn nausea

Morphine 2–4mg IV q4h prn pain

Ativan 0.5 mg IV q6h prn anxiety

Ondansetron 4 mg IV q12h if needed for nausea

Ordered Laboratory Studies

CBC every morning

Chem 7 panel every other day

LABORATORY STUDY RESULTS

Test	Preop	Postop, Immediate	Postop, 4 Hours
WBC	28.5/mm³	19.3/mm³	22.4/mm³
RBC	4.40/mm³	4.33/mm³	4.65/mm³
Hemoglobin	13.9 g/dL	12 g/dL	14.5 g/dL
Hematocrit	41%	40%	43%
Platelet count	412/mm³	357/mm³	399/mm³
APTT	20.3 seconds		
INR	0.98		
Sodium	140 mEq/L		
Potassium	3.6 mEq/L		
Chloride	109 mEq/L		
Carbon dioxide	23 mEq/L		
Urea nitrogen	11 mg/dL		
Creatinine blood	0.8 mg/dL		
Glucose	179 mg/dL		
Calcium	8.1 mg/dL		
Lipase	17 unit/dL		

CRITICAL THINKING QUESTIONS

1. On initial admission to the floor postoperatively, which complications should you assess for?

2. In what position should the right leg be placed?

Answers to Critical Thinking Questions appear in Appendix D.

NCLEX® REVIEW

1. The nurse is planning a health promotion program for sports injuries. Which of the following would be the most important for the nurse to emphasize in this program?

1. How to use new equipment
2. Prevention of injuries
3. Why sports need to be supervised
4. How injuries are related to the time of day

2. A patient with a fracture is able to have his cast removed. The nurse realizes this patient is in which phase of the fractured bone healing process?

1. Fibroblast framework
2. Callus formation
3. Bone calcification
4. Ossification

3. A victim of a motor vehicle crash has an open fracture of the left femur. Which of the following is a priority of care for this patient?

1. Provide pain relief.
2. Prevent damage to surrounding tissue.
3. Decrease the potential for contamination.
4. Cast the affected bone immediately.

4. The nurse is planning care for a patient with a fractured pelvis and femur. Which of the following would be a priority for this patient's care?

1. Monitoring hemodynamic status.
2. Arranging for a traction set-up.
3. Providing explanation of nursing care to follow.
4. Administering oral narcotic analgesics.

5. A patient sustained a crushing injury to both legs. Which of the following would indicate to the nurse that rhabdomyolysis has occurred?

1. Muscle spasms of the affected extremities
2. Dark colored urine
3. Excessive thirst
4. Double or blurred vision

6. The patient who had a right above-the-knee amputation tells the nurse "I keep wanting to scratch my right foot." Which of the following should the nurse respond to this patient?

1. It's a side effect of your pain medication.
2. You are experiencing something called phantom sensations.
3. Your leg was amputated and it isn't there anymore.
4. I can get a psychiatrist for you to talk with.

Answers for review questions appear in Appendix D

KEY TERMS

avascular necrosis (AVN) *p.1780*
avulsion fracture *p.1777*
Buck's boots traction *p.1784*
burst fracture *p.1784*
cast *p.1784*
chance fracture *p.1784*
compartment syndrome *p.1796*
contusion *p.1777*
diaphysis *p.1781*

dislocation *p.1780*
epiphysis *p.1781*
external fixation *p.1785*
fasciotomy *p.1796*
fractures *p.1781*
intramedullary (I-M) rodding *p.1786*
ligament *p.1777*
metaphysis *p.1781*

open reduction internal fixation
(ORIF) *p.1786*
physes *p.1777*
PRICE *p.1777*
skeletal traction *p.1785*
skin traction *p.1784*
sprain *p.1777*
strain *p.1777*

PEARSON

EXPLORE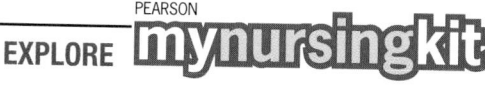

MyNursingKit is your one stop for online chapter review materials and resources. Prepare for success with additional NCLEX®-style practice questions, interactive assignments and activities, web links, animations and videos, and more!

Register your access code from the front of your book at
www.mynursingkit.com

REFERENCES

Aito, S., Abbate, R., Marcucci, R. & Cominelli, E. (2007). Endogenous risk factors for deep-vein thrombosis in patients with acute spinal cord injuries. *Spinal Cord, 45*(9), 627–631.

American College of Surgeons. (2004). *Advanced Trauma Life Support Course Manual.* Chicago: American College of Surgeons.

Anscomb, S. (2007). Managing sprains and strains. *Practice Nurse, 33*(5), 44–49.

Bongiovanni, M. S., Bradley, S. L., & Kelley, D. M. (2005). Orthopedic trauma critical care nursing issues. *Critical Care Nursing Quarterly, 28*(1), 60–71.

Dougall, A. L., Ursano, R. J., Posluszny, D. M., Fullerton, C. S., & Baum, A. (2001). Predictors of posttraumatic stress among victims of motor vehicle accidents. *Psychosomatic Medicine, 63*(3), 402–411.

Emergency Nurses Association. (2006). *Alcohol and injury facts.* Retrieved September 11, 2007, from http://www.ena.org/ipinstitute/fact/ENAIPFactSheet-Alcohol.pdf

Feliciano, D. V., Mattox, K. L., & Moore, E. E. (Eds.). (2008). *Trauma* (6th ed.). New York: McGraw-Hill.

Frazier, M. S., & Drzymkowski, J. W. (Eds.). (2007). *Essentials of human diseases and conditions* (4th ed.). St. Louis: W. B. Saunders.

Gustillo classification of fracture. (2004). Retrieved January 1, 2004, from http://www.wheelessonline.com/oa2/60.htm

Harvard Women's Health Watch. (2007). *Recovering from an ankle sprain.* Retrieved April 5, 2008, from http://www.health.harvard.edu

Holmes, S. B., & Brown, S. J. (2005). Skeletal pin site care: National Association of Orthopaedic Nurses guidelines for orthopaedic nursing. *Orthopaedic Nursing, 24*(2), 99–107.

Hrysomallis, C. (2007). Relationship between balance ability, training and sports injury risk. *Sports Medicine, 37*(6), 547–555.

Knudson, M. M., Ikossi, D. G., Khaw, L., Morabito, D., & Speetzen, L. (2004). Thromboembolism after trauma: An analysis of 1602 episodes from the American College of Surgeons National Trauma Data Bank. *Annals of Surgery, 240*(3), 490–498.

Meehan, A. J. (2002). National Consensus Conference on improving the continuum of care for patients with hip fracture. *Orthopaedic Nursing, 21*(1), 16–22.

Mohanty, K., Musso, D., Powell, J. N., Kortbeek, J. B., & Kirkpatrick, A. W. (2005). Emergent management of pelvic ring injuries: An update. *Canadian Journal of Surgery, 48*(1), 49–56.

Morris, A. H., & Zuckerman, J. D. (2002). National Consensus Conference on improving the continuum of care for patients with hip fracture. *Journal of Bone & Joint Surgery—American Volume, 84-A*(4), 670–674.

National Safe Kids Campaign. (2003, 7/2003). *Sports and recreation.* Retrieved September 1, 2003, from http://www.safekids.org/tier2_rl.cfm?folder_id=178

Norman, S. B., Stein, M. B., Dimsdale, J. E., & Hoyt, D. B. (2007). Pain in the aftermath of trauma is a risk factor for post-traumatic stress disorder. *Psychology Medicine, 10,* 1–10.

Orosz, G. M., Magaziner, J., Hannan, E. L., Morrison, R. S., Koval, K., Gilbert, M., et al. (2004). Association of timing of surgery for hip fracture and patient outcomes. *Journal of the American Medical Association, 291*(14), 1738–1743.

Porth, C. M. (Ed.). (2005). *Essentials of pathophysiology.* Philadelphia: Lippincott Williams & Wilkins.

Rusch, M. D., Gould, L. J., Dzwierzynski, W. W., & Larson, D. L. (2002). Psychological impact of traumatic injuries: What the surgeon can do. *Plastic and Reconstructive Surgery, 109*(1), 18–24.

Shetty, A. (2004). *Superior mesenteric artery syndrome.* Retrieved January 2, 2005, from http://www.emedicine.com/ped/topic2175.htm

Walker, J. A. (2007). Evidence for skeletal pin site care. *Nursing Standard, 21*(45), 70–76.

57 Caring for the Patient During Musculoskeletal Surgical Procedures

Karen Cooper
Kathleen Osborn

With contributions by:
Cheryl Wraa

Outcome-Based Learning Objectives

After studying this chapter, the learner will be able to:

1. List components of the neurovascular assessment appropriate for a patient who has had orthopedic surgery.
2. Discuss the types of precautions required to prevent hip dislocation in the postoperative hip replacement patient.
3. Describe the nursing actions appropriate for a patient with symptoms of complications, including compartment syndrome.
4. Describe the appropriate use of assistive devices utilized for orthopedic patients.
5. Discuss the importance of optimal pain control in the postoperative orthopedic patient.

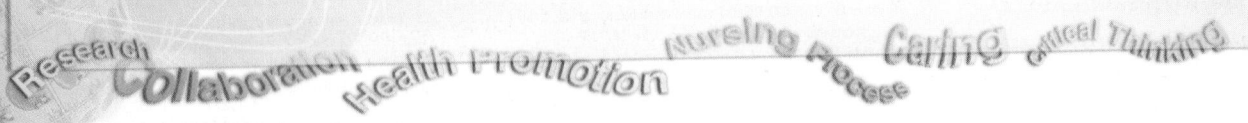

PATIENTS UNDERGOING musculoskeletal surgery generally fall into two categories: (1) those that have experienced increasing pain or disability over time causing them to seek a surgical resolution to their complaints, or (2) patients who have had a traumatic event. The patient who enters the hospital for an elective orthopedic procedure often has the benefit of preoperative teaching and preparation for the procedure. The patient who has experienced a traumatic event may present unique challenges for the nurse, both preoperatively and postoperatively. The nurse is in a unique position to recognize potential problems and prevent complications that have a direct impact on the ability of the patient to improve or maintain functional status and return to a productive lifestyle. Orthopedic surgical patients face recovery from both the sequelae of surgery and anesthesia as well as potential complications specific to the orthopedic problem encountered. The nursing process provides a systematic approach to the identification of actual or potential problems that impact the patient's recovery. These actual and potential problems are identified from assessment data and are utilized to develop a plan of care specific to the patient's needs.

The orthopedic surgeon performs a physical assessment and diagnostic testing to determine whether the diseased/traumatized bone or joint requires surgical replacement of the joint or simple repair. Repair may include removal of bone and ligament particles, smoothing of joint surfaces, reconnection of torn ligaments, or replacement of ligaments with allograft (cadaver) or autograft (tissue from another area to replace damaged ligaments or bone). Replacement of the joint may include repair as well as the implantation of a new joint.

Traumatic injuries play a large part in the need for orthopedic surgery in patients of all ages. Congenital deformities are generally repaired in the pediatric population. Spinal surgery for scoliosis is usually performed in the early adolescent period, whereas spinal surgery for disk repair or laminectomy is performed in young and middle adulthood. Hip fractures are a common traumatic injury for the elderly, as is joint replacement surgery. The life of an artificial joint and the surrounding bone tissue is shorter than that of a natural joint, with current artificial hips and knees lasting approximately 20 years. Knowledge of biographic and demographic data is important in planning appropriate care for the patient. Elder patients are at risk for postoperative delirium. Knowledge of the patient's prior experiences, abilities, and accomplishments can assist the nurse in providing patient-specific interventions to maintain orientation and prevent cognitive function alterations.

Preoperative Assessment of the Orthopedic Surgical Patient

The assessment of the preoperative orthopedic surgical patient must take into account both the health history as well as the history surrounding the surgical event. Knowledge of patient demographics, related to the injury, general health, and medical and social history, is often obtained from the preoperative history and physical exam. The nurse must be diligent in obtaining information regarding the presurgical status of the patient. The mechanism of injury is important for the nurse to know to be able to formulate a plan of care for the patient with appropriate attention to patient safety and necessary interventions and precautions for the patient. For example, did the patient fall because he had a stroke and now has residual weakness on one side of his body? Was the patient in a skilled nursing facility and fell from bed because she was confused? Did the patient trip and fall as an unpreventable accident? The time of injury to surgery also impacts the focus of nursing assessment and care planning. If the patient fell and fractured a hip, was taken to the emergency department, and was not allowed to eat or drink for many hours prior to surgery, closer attention to intake and output and potential hypovolemia is a greater concern. If the patient was injured in a motor vehicle crash, there may be other associated injuries that will complicate care. The type of surgery performed has inherent risks and complications that the nurse must anticipate and utilize in focusing the patient assessment specific to the patient and his needs.

Clinical Manifestations

Pain, loss of function, and deformity are the three major complaints associated with musculoskeletal conditions that cause the patient to seek surgical care. It is important to utilize a consistent pain scale when assessing the patient's pain level. Chapter 15 ☞ includes an in-depth discussion of pain. Loss of function may be directly related to the injury or indirectly related to nerve damage or pain.

The mechanism of injury is also an important factor because treatment may be necessary as an emergency procedure for a traumatic injury. Patients having elective surgical procedures, such as a total knee replacement for osteoarthritis or below knee amputation for peripheral vascular disease, may have very different expectations regarding the proposed surgery. The patient electing to have a knee replacement may see the surgery as desired to relieve chronic pain and deformity and to restore function. The patient facing an amputation may have unresolved issues regarding the decision to have surgery and fears loss of function. The psychological preparation, physical abilities, and function of the patient preoperatively are important to consider in providing care in the postoperative period.

Past Medical History

The past medical history gives important information regarding potential complications that may occur during the postoperative period. For example, patients with a history of cardiovascular disease may suffer perioperative myocardial infarction, dysrhythmias, or delay in surgical healing. Patients with diabetes may be more prone to postoperative infection and need for altered glucose control. Patients with a prior history of deep venous thrombosis (DVT) are at greater risk for developing postoperative DVT. If the patient has asthma or chronic obstructive pulmonary disease (COPD), she may be at greater risk for pulmonary complications.

Medications

All medications should be reviewed with the patient prior to surgery. Cardiac, pulmonary, and renal medications should alert the nurse to potential complications and the need for anticipatory planning in the care of the patient. In addition, medications that increase bleeding tendencies should be discontinued prior to surgery. Aspirin, heparin, and nonsteroidal anti-inflammatory drugs (NSAIDs), which are platelet inhibitors, need to be discontinued prior to surgery.

Oral bisphosphonates such as alendronate (Fosamax) are used to prevent bone loss from osteoporosis and may be discontinued during hospitalization. Hormone replacement therapy for postmenopausal females may increase the risk of postoperative deep venous thrombosis, so it is also frequently discontinued during hospitalization. Calcium supplements of 1,000 to 3,000 milligrams daily and calcitonin nasal spray may also be prescribed to prevent bone loss.

The nurse should ask the patient specifically about over-the-counter medications and dietary supplements. Ginseng, garlic, and *Ginkgo biloba* dietary supplements interact with platelets and may increase bleeding during surgery. Chart 57–1 (p. 1804) discusses herbal supplements that may impact surgery.

Allergies

The nurse must be knowledgeable of the patient's allergies to prevent potential anaphylactic reactions to medications administered pre- and postoperatively. Patients may also report prior negative reactions to medications as allergies. For example, if morphine causes gastric upset the patient may report this as an allergy. If a morphine patient-controlled analgesia (PCA) is ordered for the patient, the nurse must teach the patient that adverse reactions are not always present with decreased dosages of the medication. The nurse must also be aware of potential allergic reactions to medications that may have cross sensitivity, such as penicillin allergies possibly related to cephalosporin allergy. Patient allergies should be recorded on the health care provider order forms and medication administration record to prevent medication errors.

Prior Surgeries and Hospitalizations

The patient's prior hospital and surgical experiences should be explored with the patient. If the patient has had negative experiences in the past, the nurse should utilize knowledge of these problems in the care planning process to communicate patient needs and attempt a positive current hospital experience. Expectations of the current hospitalization should be elicited and clarified if necessary. The plan of care for the current hospitalization and surgery should be reviewed with the patient and specific daily goals should be negotiated.

Cardiovascular Disease

Knowledge of preexisting cardiovascular disease is an important consideration in planning the care of the orthopedic surgical patient. Many anesthetic agents cause myocardial suppression and increase the risk of surgical cardiac events. Preoperative

CHART 57–1 **Herbal Supplements and the Orthopedic Surgical Patient**

Herbal Supplement	Reported Use	Nursing Considerations
Garlic	Treat high blood pressure. Treat atherosclerosis.	Increases risk of bleeding especially if other anticoagulants, antiplatelet, or anti-inflammatory medications are administered. May affect glycemic control. Discontinue 1–2 weeks prior to surgery.
Ginkgo biloba	May decrease plaque formation in atherosclerosis to reduce peripheral vascular disease.	May increase effects of anticoagulants and antiplatelet medications to increase bleeding postoperatively. Discontinue 2 days–2 weeks prior to surgery.
Ginseng	Improve concentration and stamina.	Inhibits platelet aggregation and may potentiate bleeding especially if additional anticoagulants or antiplatelet medications are administered. Discontinue 1–2 weeks prior to surgery.
Glucosamine	Decrease joint discomfort, increase joint flexibility, and "rebuild" cartilage.	May affect serum glucose levels and interact with insulin effect. Monitor serum glucose. May increase blood pressure and heart rate, thereby masking signs of hypovolemia in the postoperative patient.

evaluation of chest pain should be carried out, and a 12-lead ECG is performed to determine whether the patient has signs of myocardial ischemia. Patients with a history of dysrhythmias may require telemetry monitoring before and after surgery. Antidysrhythmic medications should be continued during the postoperative period. If the patient has a pacemaker or implantable cardioverter defibrillator (ICD), magnetic resonance imaging (MRI) is contraindicated.

Pulmonary Disease

Patients with preexisting pulmonary disease are at greater risk of developing pulmonary complications in the postoperative period. Patients with chronic obstructive pulmonary disease (COPD) may have lower baseline arterial oxygen levels that may delay wound healing. This population may also be at greater risk for carbon dioxide retention and decreased respiratory drive. Frequent assessments of respiratory status including respiratory rate, depth, and oxygen saturation should be performed. Supplemental oxygen may be necessary to promote adequate oxygenation; however, low flow rates are generally prescribed to prevent suppression of the respiratory drive. Unit 7 ⬤ includes in-depth discussion of pulmonary disorders.

Diabetes

Surgical stress and alterations in a patient's normal eating patterns can affect blood glucose levels. Surgical stress may increase insulin needs in the postoperative period. Nothing by mouth (NPO) status increases the risk of hypoglycemia. The patient's capillary blood glucose levels should be assessed at regular intervals to monitor glucose levels. Patients may be placed on sliding scale coverage for blood glucose in addition to their regular insulin or oral hypoglycemic regimen, as elevated blood glucose levels increase wound healing time. Patients with diabetes may also be at greater risk for infection. Surgical wounds should be carefully inspected for signs and symptoms of infection.

Functional Status

The patient's previous functional status should be evaluated preoperatively and goals set for the postoperative period that are equal to or better than the preoperative functional status. Elders who undergo surgery are at risk for functional decline because they may be dependent on the nurse for all activities. Patients should be encouraged to engage in activities to their full potential. More time should be allotted for elder activities, as they frequently require more time to complete activities of daily living. Patients with a prior history of stroke may have residual weakness that impedes the patients' ability to perform postoperative rehabilitation exercises and activities of daily living. The stroke may have been the original cause of injury for the patient.

Genetic Factors

Osteogenesis imperfecta (OI), commonly called "brittle bone" syndrome, is an extremely rare genetic disorder affecting type I collagen formation. There are several types. Type I is the mildest form of the disease. Patients are prone to fractures, have collagen deficiency, and females have an increased risk of postmenopausal osteoporosis. Type II OI is nearly always fatal during the neonatal period due to birth injuries. Type III (severe) OI patients have severe bone deformities, have sufficient but abnormal collagen, and are prone to bone fractures. Respiratory insufficiency related to rib fractures and thoracic cage deformity is a major complication in this group. They may fracture a rib simply by coughing. Type IV, or "moderate OI with short stature" patients, is similar to type III, but has less skeletal deformity. With this disease the treatment of fractures is often complicated by delayed union.

Occupational History

Occupation is an important factor in musculoskeletal injuries in terms of both causation and recovery. Depending on the injury, the patient may be unable to return to work for weeks or months after injury or surgery. If injured at work and now unable to return to work on a permanent basis, the patient may need vocational rehabilitation. If the injury is unrelated to work, but the patient must now be off from work to recover, this may cause financial hardship.

Culture

Patients' cultural history should be included in the plan of care for the patients. If they have specific requirements for the gender of the nurses and caretakers assigned to them, these should be accommodated whenever possible. Knowledge of a patient's pain expression should be included in the plan of care. Cultural accommodations for activities of daily living (ADL) and cultural dietary accommodations may be necessary and should be communicated. The patient should be offered spiritual affiliation if desired.

Anesthetic

The anesthetic agents utilized for orthopedic surgery depend on the type of surgery planned and the duration of the surgery. General anesthesia usually involves a combination of inhaled anesthetic agents, paralytics, and narcotics. Epidural anesthesia may be utilized in the patient undergoing lower extremity or low back surgery. When epidural anesthesia is utilized, the administration of narcotics, sedatives, and hypnotics is generally restricted to prevent respiratory compromise. The type of epidural anesthetic should be reported and the time of the last dose clearly recorded so that patients do not receive opioid narcotics during the period specified for the epidural agent used.

Subcutaneous pain pumps may be used in some orthopedic procedures. These devices deliver a slow, continuous infusion of local anesthetic into the operative or suture site to prevent or relieve postoperative pain. The nurse and patient should anticipate that the area surrounding the insertion site will be numb. The goal of such pumps is to decrease the need for oral or intravenous postoperative pain medication, which may contribute to respiratory depression or drowsiness. Adverse reactions are related to sensitivity or allergy to the local anesthetic. A complete discussion of the various types of anesthesia, along with the medical and nursing management of the patient, is in Chapter 26 .

Surgical Procedures

Prior to surgery the surgical site, level, or digit should be marked by initialing the correct operative site with indelible pen or other means such as an adhesive strip according to hospital protocol. This is a Joint Commission requirement for patient safety (called the universal protocol) to prevent surgery at the wrong site. The marking may be part of a preoperative patient check at the time of admission or at the time that the surgical consent is signed. The nurse verifies the patient's understanding of the operative procedure as well as confirming the correct site or side, limb, or digit of the surgery. Chapter 26 outlines the Association of periOperative Registered Nurses (AORN) and the American College of Surgeons national standards for prevention of wrong-site surgery.

Preprocedure education should include the surgery itself, its inherent risks and benefits, and options for blood donation. Elective patients frequently are scheduled for same-day surgery, so that the responsibility for preoperative preparation falls on the outpatient or office nurse.

There are commercially available preoperative and surgery-specific films and pamphlets for patients to view prior to surgery that can be helpful in providing portions of preoperative education to the patient. Chapter 24 includes a complete discussion of blood administration. It is not within the scope of this chapter to review all types of orthopedic surgery. Selected orthopedic surgical approaches that require hospitalization will be covered.

Upper Extremity Surgery

Upper extremity surgeries include total shoulder or elbow joint replacement, rotator cuff repair, and open reduction or stabilization of fractures of the humerus, radius, or ulna. Most elective upper extremity surgeries below the elbow are performed on an outpatient basis. Shoulder and elbow surgery may require one or more inpatient hospital days to ensure that nerve entrapment does not occur from postoperative edema. Reduction and stabilization of fractures are discussed in detail in Chapter 56 .

The shoulder is a ball-and-socket joint that is made up of three bones: the upper arm bone (humerus), shoulder blade (scapula), and collarbone (clavicle). The top of the humerus fits into the small socket (glenoid) of the shoulder blade to form the shoulder joint (glenohumeral joint). The socket of the glenoid is surrounded by a soft-tissue rim (labrum). The articular cartilage and a thin inner lining (synovium) of the joint allow the smooth motion of the shoulder joint. The upper part of the shoulder blade (acromion) projects over the shoulder joint. One end of the collarbone is joined with the shoulder blade by the acromioclavicular (AC) joint, and the other end of the collarbone is joined with the breastbone (sternum) by the sternoclavicular joint. The joint capsule, which is a thin sheet of fibers that surrounds the shoulder joint, allows a wide range of motion, yet provides stability. The rotator cuff is a group of four muscles—the supraspinatus, infraspinatus, teres minor, and subscapularis—that along with the tendons attaches the upper arm to the shoulder blade. A saclike membrane (bursa) between the rotator cuff and the shoulder blade cushions and helps lubricate the motion between these two structures. The rotator cuff stabilizes the humeral head in the glenoid fossa. The muscles attached to the rotator cuff enable arm motion that allows an individual to take part in activities such as throwing or swimming.

Rotator Cuff Repair

Rotator cuff tears can occur from a single traumatic injury (Figure 57–1 , p. 1806). These patients often report recurrent shoulder pain for several months and can recall the specific injury that triggered the onset of the pain. A cuff tear may also happen at the same time as another injury to the shoulder, such as a fracture or dislocation. Of note, most tears are the result of overuse of the muscles and tendons over a period of years. People who are especially at risk for overuse are those who engage in repetitive overhead motions such as baseball, tennis, weight lifting, and rowing. Rotator cuff tears are most common in people over the age of 40 (American Academy of Orthopaedic Surgeons [AAOS], 2007a). Partial thickness or full-thickness tears may occur (Figure 57–2 , p. 1806). Partial thickness rotator cuff tears are associated with chronic inflammation and the development of spurs on the underside of the acromion or the acromioclavicular joint. Full-thickness tears are most often the result of impingement, partial thickness rotator cuff tears from heavy lifting or falls. Clinical manifestations include:

- Atrophy or thinning of the muscles about the shoulder
- Pain in the front of the shoulder that radiates down the arm when lifting the arm or when lowering the arm from a fully raised position
- Weakness when lifting or rotating the arm
- Crepitus or crackling sensation when moving the shoulder in certain positions

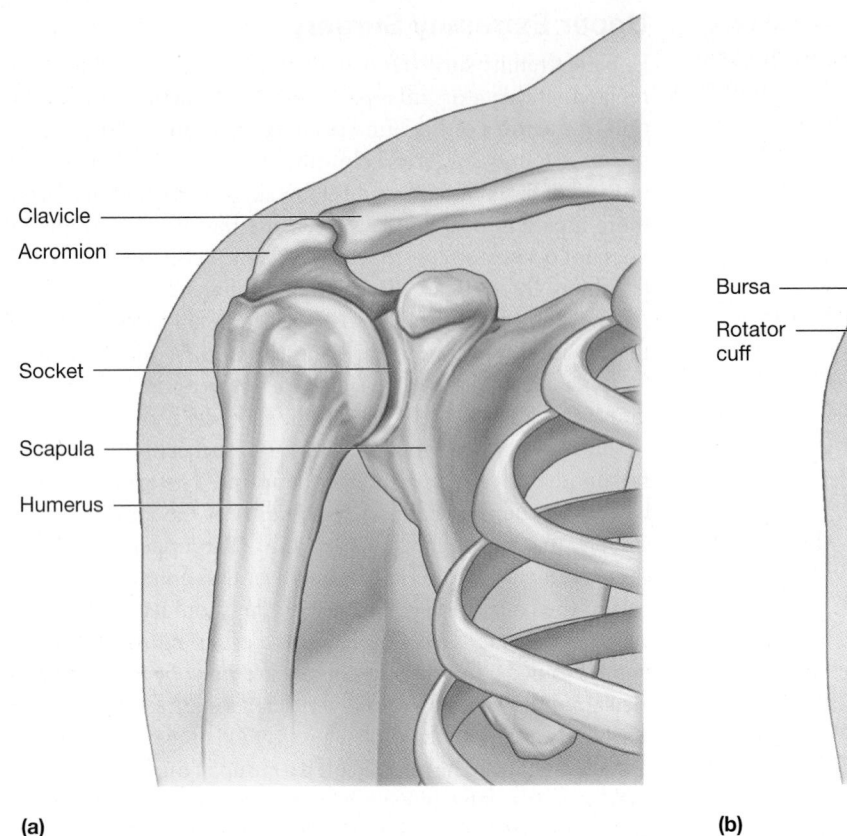

Clavicle
Acromion
Socket
Scapula
Humerus

(a)

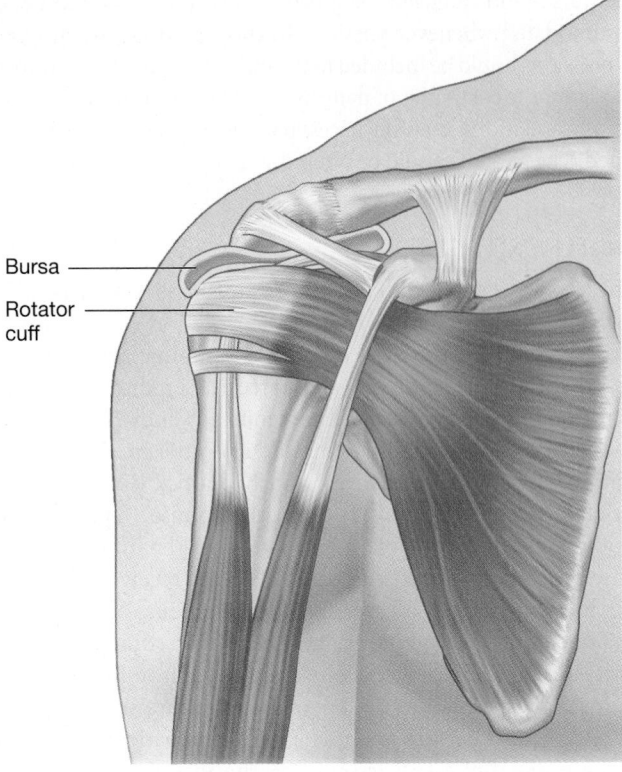

Bursa
Rotator cuff

(b)

FIGURE 57–1 ■ Shoulder anatomy.

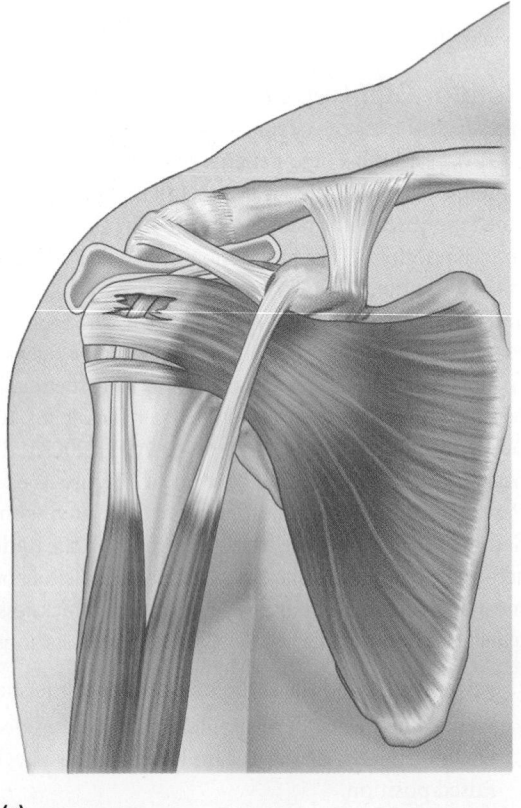

(a)

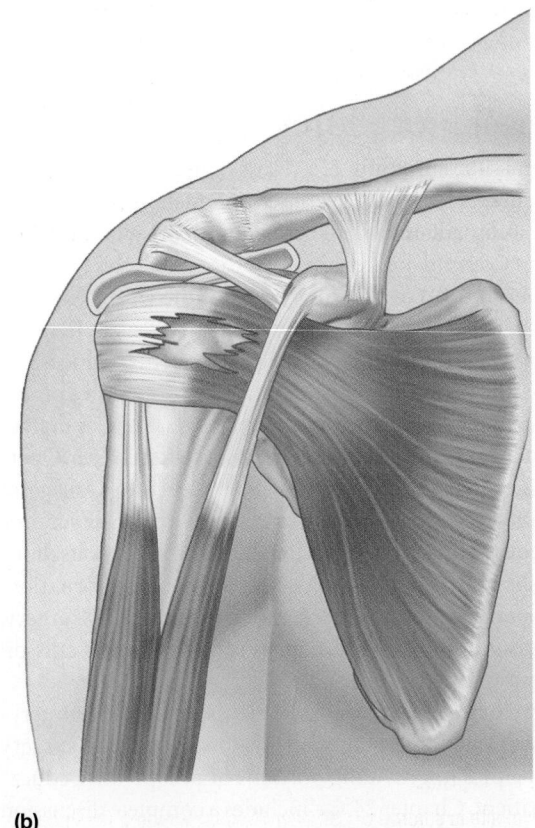

(b)

FIGURE 57–2 ■ (A) Impingement with partial tear. (B) Full-thickness tear.

- When the tear occurs with an injury, there may be sudden acute pain, a snapping sensation, and an immediate weakness of the arm.

Symptoms may develop right away after a trauma, such as a lifting injury or a fall on the affected arm, or they may develop gradually with repetitive overhead activity or following long-term wear.

The type of surgical repair depends on the size, shape, and location of the tear. A partial tear (see Figure 57–2A ■) may require only a trimming or smoothing procedure, called a *débridement*. A complete tear (see Figure 57–2B ■) within the thickest part of the tendon is repaired by suturing the two sides of the tendon back together. If the tendon is torn away from where it inserts into the bone of the humerus, it is repaired directly to bone (AAOS, 2007a). There are two approaches to the surgical procedure: open or arthroscopic. The open surgical approach is described in Chart 57–2. With an arthroscopy the orthopedic surgeon inserts a pencil-thin device with a small lens and lighting system into tiny incisions to look inside the joint. The images inside the joint are relayed to a TV monitor, allowing the surgeon to make a diagnosis. Other surgical instruments can be inserted to make repairs, based on findings. Many of these surgical repairs can be done on an outpatient basis.

Shoulder Arthroplasty

Arthroplasty refers to restoration of a joint either by **total joint replacement**, replacement of a joint with a prosthesis, or by resurfacing bone and removing damaged bone and cartilage. Total replacement of the shoulder and elbow is not as common as of the hip and knee. An indication for the surgery is severe pain resulting from rheumatoid arthritis, osteoarthritis, avascular necrosis, or post-traumatic arthritis. Osteoarthritis and rheumatoid arthritis can destroy the shoulder joint and surrounding tissue. Arthritis is discussed in detail in Chapter 58 ⊕.

Clinical manifestations include pain that progressively worsens and is aggravated by activity. When the glenohumeral shoulder joint is affected, the pain is centered in the back of the

shoulder and frequently intensifies with changes in the weather. If the acromioclavicular joint is involved, the pain is focused in the front of the shoulder. A person with rheumatoid arthritis of both shoulders may have pain in all these areas. Limited motion is another problem. It may become more difficult to lift the arm to comb hair or reach up to a shelf. A clicking or snapping sound (crepitus) may be heard with movement. As the disease progresses, any movement of the shoulder causes pain. Night pain is common and sleeping may be difficult. The involved arm is typically weak due to muscle atrophy, is tender to touch, and has limited range of motion. Crepitus (a grating sensation inside the joint) may be felt with movement. X-rays of an arthritic shoulder will show a narrowing of the joint space, changes in the bone, and the formation of bone spurs (osteophytes) (American Academy of Orthopaedic Surgeons, 2007b).

The surgical approach used to treat the arthritis of the glenohumeral joint is by replacing the entire shoulder joint with a prosthesis (total shoulder arthroplasty) or by replacing the head of the upper arm bone (hemiarthroplasty) (see Chart 57–2). The goal of surgery is to restore the best possible function to the joint by removing scar tissue, balancing muscles, and replacing the joint surfaces. Figure 57–3 ■ shows the artificial joint components including the humeral ball (which is made of metal) and the glenoid component (which is made of plastic). The humeral ball is fixed to the humerus with the humeral stem, and the glenoid component is attached to the shoulder blade using a small amount of bone cement. Shoulder range of motion is

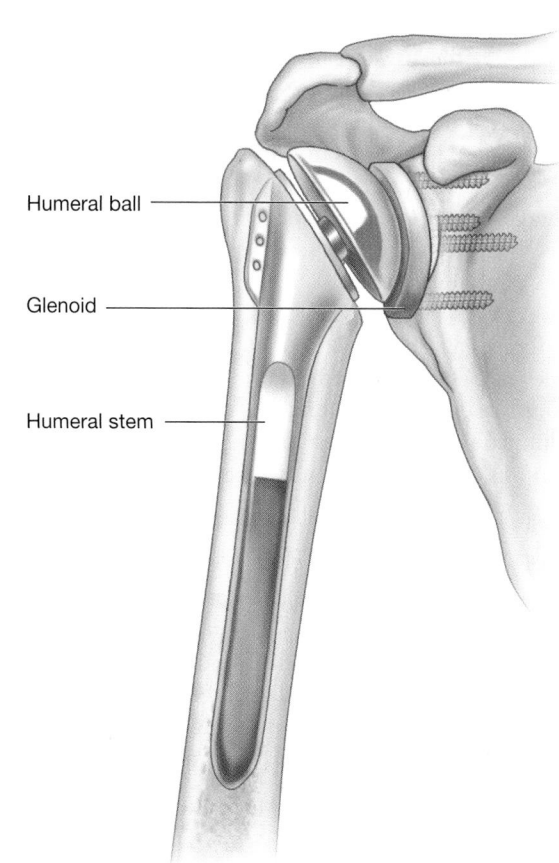

FIGURE 57–3 ■ Shoulder arthroplasty.

CHART 57–2   Shoulder Arthroscopy

- Incision is made approximately 6–10 inches in length to expose the shoulder joint.
- The humeral head is dislocated from the socket.
- The head of the humerus is shaved/removed to shape the bone to fit the implant, and the bone canal is drilled to prepare for the prosthesis implant.
- The implant is inserted into the humerus.
- The glenoid socket is shaved to create a smooth articular surface or is shaved and a concave disk implanted to replace the glenoid socket surface. Holes may be drilled into the glenoid surface to secure the implanted glenoid socket.
- Debris (torn ligaments, bone fragments, and clots) are removed, and ligaments are adjusted.
- The surgical site is sutured closed after the joint is tested for smooth motion.

started immediately after the procedure, and patients are usually discharged from hospital 3 days after surgery if they are comfortable and have a good range of passive motion. The recovery of strength and function may continue for up to 1 year after surgery (Matson & Warme, 2008). Hemiarthroplasty is a shoulder replacement wherein only the humeral head is replaced with an artificial joint.

The most common surgical procedure used to treat arthritis of the acromioclavicular joint is a resection arthroplasty. A small piece of bone from the end of the collarbone is removed, leaving a space that later fills with scar tissue. Surgical treatment of arthritis of the shoulder is generally very effective in reducing pain and restoring motion (American Academy of Orthopaedic Surgeons, 2007b).

Shoulder Subluxation and Dislocation Repair

Shoulder instability or subluxation and shoulder dislocation are potentially painful and disabling conditions. Subluxation and dislocation both represent problems that occur when the humeral head does not stay centered correctly in the socket (or *glenoid*). These problems may manifest themselves with pain from doing the normal activities of daily living, to the inability to lift the arm without dislocating the joint.

The treatments for these conditions vary widely depending on the severity of symptoms and signs. Many patients will improve with the appropriate bracing and physical therapy. However, for those patients who require surgery, arthroscopic surgery is used to diagnose the exact nature of the joint instability. The goal of surgery is to reestablish the stability of the humeral head in the shallow glenoid socket without compromising the shoulder motion. Using the scope, the surgeon can evaluate the entire shoulder joint and can usually treat the conditions leading to the instability with this approach. Infrequently, patients may require an open surgery, using an incision about 8–13 cm (3 to 5 inches) long to correct the problem. The procedure can usually be performed within a few hours under general (or nerve block) anesthesia.

Patients undergoing arthroscopic shoulder stabilization will require a sling for usually 2 to 3 weeks, and simple range-of-motion exercises may be performed daily. Outpatient physical therapy for reestablishing pain-free motion and strengthening the shoulder muscles will be needed for a few months. Normally, a person can return to most forms of normal activity within 6 weeks, limited athletics between 10 and 14 weeks, and all activities and even contact athletics can usually be accomplished between 14 and 24 weeks, depending on the sport (Wahl & Slaney, 2005).

Elbow Repair

The elbow is a hinge and ball-and-socket joint made up of the humerus, ulna, and radius. The positioning and interaction of the bones in the joint allow for a small amount of rotation as well as hinge action. The primary stability of the elbow is provided by the ulnar collateral ligament on the medial (inner) side of the elbow. As muscles contract and relax, two unique motions occur:

- The hinge joint allows the elbow to bend and straighten (flexion and extension, respectively).
- Rotation through the ball-and-socket joint allows the hand to be rotated palm down and palm up (pronation and supination, respectively).

Osteoarthritis of the elbow occurs when the cartilage surface is damaged or becomes worn. This can happen because of a previous injury such as elbow dislocation or fracture, or it may also be the result of degeneration of the joint cartilage. Osteoarthritis usually affects the weight-bearing joints, such as the hip and knees; therefore, the elbow is one of the least affected joints because of its well-matched joint surfaces and strong stabilizing ligaments. As a result, the elbow joint can tolerate large forces across it without becoming unstable. The most common cause of osteoarthritis is a previous injury, such as a fracture that involved the surface of the joint or an elbow dislocation. Injury to the ligaments resulting in an unstable elbow can also lead to osteoarthritis, even if the elbow surface is not damaged, because the normal forces across the elbow are altered, causing the joint to wear out more rapidly. Of note, one of the most common injuries to the elbow occurs on the lateral, or outer, side of the elbow, referred to as lateral epicondylitis (tennis elbow) (American Academy of Orthopaedic Surgeons, 2007c).

The most common clinical manifestations of elbow arthritis are pain and loss of range of motion. Patients also report a "grating" or "locking" sensation in the elbow. The grating is due to loss of the normal smooth joint surface caused by cartilage damage or wear. The locking is caused by loose pieces of cartilage or bone that dislodge from the joint and become trapped between the moving joint surfaces, blocking motion. As the disease progresses, joint swelling may also occur. The swelling may also cause numbness in the ring finger and small finger due to ulnar nerve pressure. Finally, if the elbow cannot be moved through its normal range of motion, it may stiffen into a position in which it is bent (flexion) (American Academy of Orthopaedic Surgeons, 2007c).

Arthroscopy, which removes loose bodies or inflammatory/degenerative tissue in the joint, provides symptom improvement at least in the short term. It also attempts to smooth out irregular surfaces. Multiple small incisions are used to perform the surgery. It can be done as an outpatient procedure, and recovery is reasonably rapid. If the joint surface has worn away completely, the most definitive treatment is joint replacement. For patients who are too young or too active to have prosthetic joint replacement, there are other surgical options. If loss of motion is the primary symptom, the surgeon can release the contracture and smooth out the joint surface. At times, a new surface made from the patient's own body tissues can be made. These procedures can provide years of symptom improvement (American Academy of Orthopaedic Surgeons, 2007c).

Elbow Dislocation

Elbow dislocations are a common injury that typically occurs when a person falls onto an outstretched hand. On impact the force is sent to the elbow, and usually there is a turning motion in this force that can rotate the elbow out of its socket. Because the elbow is stabilized with the combined effects of bone surfaces, ligaments, and muscles, when it dislocates, any or all of these structures can be injured to different degrees. There are three basic types of elbow dislocation: a simple, a complex, and a severe dislocation. A simple dislocation does not have any major bone injury. A complex dislocation can have severe bone and ligament injuries. With a severe dislocation, the blood vessels and nerves that travel across the elbow may be injured. If this happens, there is a risk of losing the arm.

A complete elbow dislocation is extremely painful, and the arm will look deformed and may have an odd twist at the elbow. A partial elbow dislocation can be harder to detect; because the elbow is only partially dislocated, the bones can spontaneously relocate and the joint may appear fairly normal. The elbow usually will move fairly normally, but it is painful. There may be bruising on the inside and outside of the elbow where ligaments may have been stretched or torn. Partial dislocations can continue to recur over time if the ligaments never heal. The pulses on the injured side must be checked. If the artery is injured, the hand will be cool to touch and may have a white or purple hue due to the diminished blood supply. If nerves were injured during the dislocation or from subsequent swelling, some or all of the hand may be numb and not able to move. Over time, following a dislocation, there is an increased risk for arthritis in the elbow joint if the alignment of the bones is not good; the elbow does not move and rotate normally; or the elbow continues to dislocate.

An elbow dislocation should be considered an emergency injury. The goal of immediate treatment is to return the elbow to its normal alignment, and the long-term goal is to restore function to the arm. With a complex elbow dislocation, surgery may be necessary to restore bone alignment and repair ligaments. Blood vessel or nerve injuries will also need surgical repair.

After surgery, the elbow may be protected with an external hinge. This device protects the elbow from dislocating again. Late reconstructive surgery can successfully restore motion to some stiff elbows. This surgery removes scar tissue and extra bone growth. It also removes obstacles to movement.

Carpal Tunnel Repair

The wrist is an extremely complex joint that provides the mobility to give the hand a full range of motion, while at the same time providing the strength for heavy gripping. There are 15 bones from the end of the forearm to the hand. The wrist has 8 small bones, called carpal bones. These bones are grouped in 2 rows across the wrist. The proximal row begins with the thumb side of the wrist and is made up of the scaphoid, lunate, triquetrum, and pisiform bones. The distal row of carpal tunnel bones is made up of the trapezium, trapezoid, capitate, and hamate bones.

The proximal row connects the radius and the ulna (forearm) to the bones of the hand. The bones of the hand are called the metacarpal bones. These are the long bones that lie within the palm of the hand. The metacarpals attach to the phalanges, which are the bones in the fingers and thumb (eOrthopod, 2003).

The carpal tunnel is a narrow, tunnel-like structure in the wrist (Figure 57–4 ■). The bottom and sides of this tunnel are formed by wrist (carpal) bones and the top of the tunnel is covered by the transverse carpal ligament. The median nerve and tendons travel from the forearm into the hand through this tunnel. With carpal tunnel syndrome, tendons in the wrist swell and put pressure on the median nerve, causing hand numbness and pain. Carpal tunnel syndrome is more common in women than in men and affects up to 10% of the entire population (American Academy of Orthopaedic Surgeons, 2007d). The causes of carpal tunnel syndrome include:

- Heredity
- Repetitive motions of the hands or wrist over a very long period of time

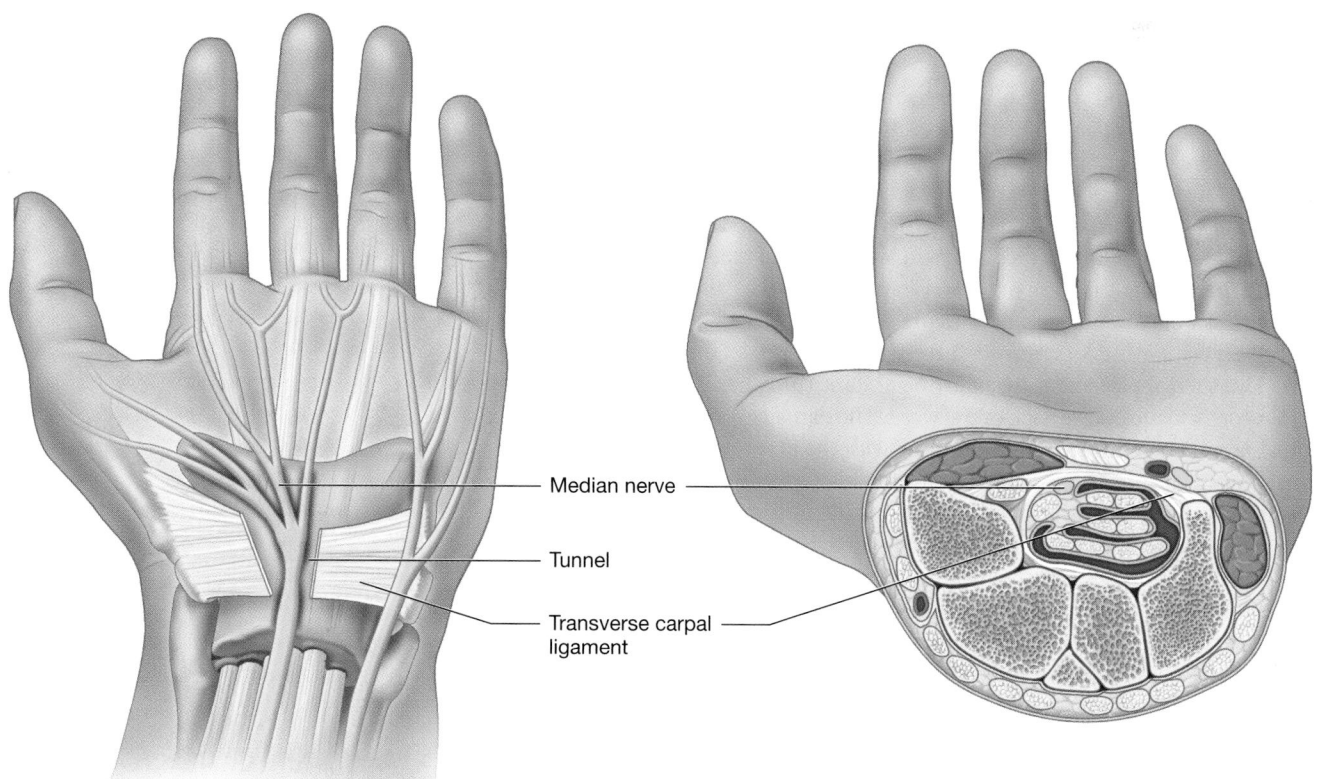

(a)   (b)

FIGURE 57–4 ■ Carpal tunnel syndrome.

MyNursingKit | Carpal Tunnel Syndrome Fact Sheet

- Hormonal changes related to pregnancy and menopause
- Diabetes, rheumatoid arthritis, and thyroid gland imbalance
- In some cases idiopathic

The clinical manifestations are pain, numbness, and tingling in the hand. Patients describe an electric-shock-type pain in the fingers or hand. The thumb side of the hand is usually most involved. Movement of the hand and wrist such as when holding an object like a phone, or when reading or driving makes the pain occur. Shaking the hand often helps decrease symptoms. Clinical manifestations initially are intermittent, but over time they may become constant. Fine motor coordination such as is needed to button a button can be difficult. When the condition is very severe, muscles in the palm may become visibly wasted.

Treatment begins with a brace or splint worn at night to keep the wrist in a natural position. Splints can also be worn during activities that aggravate symptoms. Anti-inflammatory medications such as ibuprofen help with pain relief. As the disease progresses and the individual becomes more disabled, surgery may become necessary. The decision whether to have surgery is primarily based on the severity of the symptoms. In more severe cases, surgery is considered sooner because other treatment options are less helpful. In very severe cases, surgery may be recommended to prevent irreversible damage. The surgeon uses an endoscope to access and open the top of the carpal tunnel, which increases the size of the tunnel and decreases pressure on the nerve. Typically the surgery is done on an outpatient basis under local anesthesia. Recovery is gradual; on average, grip and pinch strength generally return by about 2 months after surgery. Complete recovery may take up to 1 year, although it may be longer if the nerve is severely affected before treatment is attempted (American Academy of Orthopaedic Surgeons, 2007d).

Wrist Arthroplasty

Both osteoarthritis and rheumatoid arthritis affect the strength of the fingers and hand, making it difficult to grip or pinch. The typical candidate for wrist replacement surgery has severe arthritis. However, the surgery is limited to individuals who do not need to use the wrist to meet heavy demands in daily use. The primary reasons for wrist replacement surgery are to relieve pain and to maintain function in the wrist and hand. It may also improve the ability to perform daily living activities.

The surgery consists of removal of the worn-out ends of the bones and their replacement by an artificial joint (prosthesis). An incision is made on the back of the wrist. The damaged ends of the lower arm bones are removed, along with the first row of carpal bones. The radial component of the prosthesis is inserted into the center of the radius bone on the outside of the lower arm. The carpal component is then inserted into the center hand bone (third metacarpal) or screwed into the remaining row of carpal bones. Bone cement may be used to hold the components in place. Wrist arthroscopy surgery is often combined with other procedures to correct deformities or disorders in the tendons, nerves, and small joints of the fingers, and the thumb.

After surgery a cast is worn for the first several weeks, followed by a protective splint that will need to be worn for the next 6 to 8 weeks. Gradual exercises will need to be done for several weeks to restore movement and, eventually, to increase power and endurance. Wrist arthroplasty can improve motion to about 50% of normal. The physical demands that are placed on the wrist pros-

thesis will have an effect on how long the implant lasts. Use of a hammer or pneumatic tools may need to be avoided, and the amount of weight lifted must be limited. A fall on the outstretched hand may break the prosthesis, so activities such as roller sports, which could result in a fall, should be avoided. The average wrist replacement can be expected to last 10 to 15 years with careful use (American Academy of Orthopaedic Surgeons, 2007e).

Postoperative Assessment

Initial assessment during the initial postoperative period should focus on the potential problems of hypovolemia, bleeding complications, hypoxemia, and neurovascular compromise. After upper extremity surgery, the nurse must perform a neurovascular assessment that includes all digits of the hand, specifically the thumb and fourth and fifth fingers in order to test for ulnar nerve function (Figure 57–5 ■). Ask the patient to make an "OK" sign with his thumb and index finger to check motor integrity related to the ulnar nerve. The assessment of function of the operative extremity should be compared to that of a nonoperative/noninvolved site.

Upper extremity surgeries frequently utilize slings, immobilizing dressings, splints, and binders postoperatively. Slings may be used to elevate the extremity above the level of the heart to decrease edema formation. An elastic and Velcro shoulder immobilizer is generally used with rotator cuff repair surgery. The patient may remove the immobilizer for hygiene purposes or for performing the prescribed exercises with the affected arm until the formal physical therapy program is begun. The patient with a shoulder arthroplasty will have a shoulder immobilizer or sling after surgery. External fixator devices and splints may be utilized to immobilize and retain alignment of the arm. The length of immobilization depends on the severity of the type of surgery and the surgeon's preference. An exercise program will help regain motion and strength in the involved extremity. This program be-

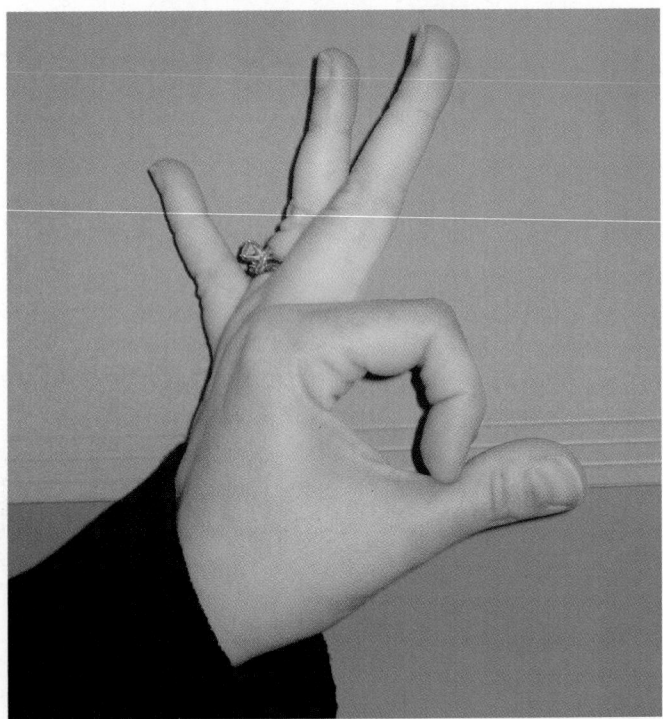

FIGURE 57–5 ■ OK sign for ulnar integrity.
Source: Cheryl Wraa

MyNursingKit | Journal of Bone and Joint Surgery

gins with passive motion, advances to active and resistive exercises, and is typically coordinated by the surgeon and the physical therapist. Complete recovery may take several months. A strong commitment to rehabilitation is important to achieve a good surgical outcome. The surgeon will examine the outcome to advise when it is safe to return to overhead work and sports activity.

Total Hip Arthroplasty

The most common cause of severe hip pain is arthritis. It is estimated that 40 million people in the United States have some form of arthritis (Arthritis Foundation, 2008). The three most common types of arthritis that cause joint pain are osteoarthritis, rheumatoid arthritis, and trauma-related arthritis, which is a result of joint injury causing inflammation and joint damage (Arthritis Foundation, 2008). Hip replacement is also used for patients with bone tumor or bone loss from insufficient blood supply to the bone (avascular necrosis).

The hip joint is formed where the top of the femur meets the acetabulum, or socket of the pelvic bone (Figure 57–6 ■). The top of the femur is ball shaped and fits into the socket formed by the acetabulum. The bones are covered by a layer of smooth cartilage that cushions and protects the bones and allows easy motion. Also surrounding the joint is the synovial lining, which produces a moisturizing lubricant. Ligaments connect the bones of the joint and hold them in place. The ligaments also add strength and elasticity for movement. Large muscles attached by tendons keep the joint stable.

Arthritis or inflammation causes the surfaces of the joint to become rough, causing the severe pain. When conservative treatment fails to provide adequate relief from pain, radiographs show destruction of the joint, and mobility is impaired, total hip replacement is considered. If the patient is active, the artificial hip joint may need to be replaced in 15 or 20 years. Revision total hip surgery, or redo, is a more complex procedure, and in general the surgery takes longer and there is greater blood loss.

Osteolysis is the term used to describe previously repaired joints whose components have worn out or become damaged.

Hip replacement surgery involves removal of the femoral head, creation of a "posthole" in the femur for the implant or femoral stem, acetabular repair with implant of cup and liner, and finally, placement of the femoral head on the stem (Figure 57–7 ■ and Chart 57–3). Hip replacement surgery may involve the use of cement, particularly if there is poor bone quality. Bone cement ingredients may include antibiotics, but are primarily polymers that improve adhesion. This is particularly useful for patients who have high potential for delayed healing or infection. The use of cement may decrease the healing time for surgery, as bone growth and regeneration to secure the joint are not necessary. If the patient has the potential for repeated surgery, however, the use of cement will require that a greater area of revision and removal of bone occur, and this must be considered in the decision of whether cement should be used. Elderly patients who will not require further surgery for repair or replacement are therefore more likely to receive surgery that includes the use of cement.

CHART 57–3   **Hip Replacement Surgical Procedure**

- Open surgical incision is 10–14 inches.
- Minimally invasive hip replacement incisions are made—one or two 1–2-inch incisions.
- The femoral head is dislocated from the acetabular socket.
- The acetabular socket is shaved to resurface and shape the bone to receive the shell implant (a dome-like surface, which may include a liner).
- The femoral head is removed and shaved to shape the bone. The femoral canal is drilled to receive the implant stem.
- The stem of the implant is inserted into the femur.
- A surgical drain is implanted and the surgical site closed with sutures.

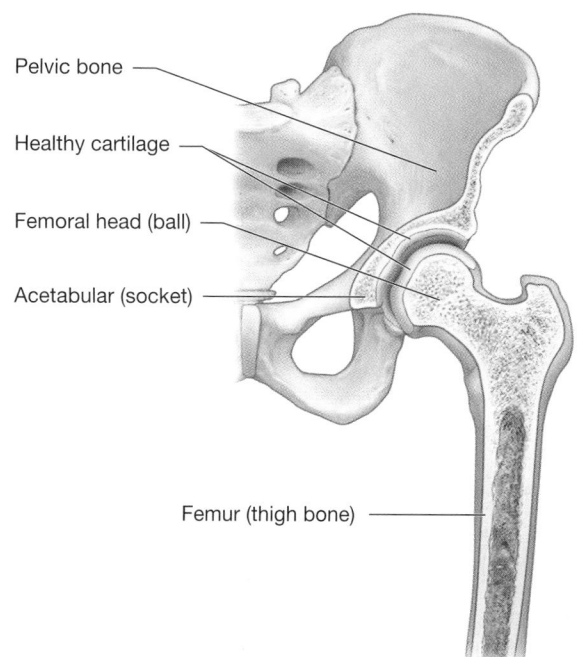

FIGURE 57–6 ■ Hip joint.

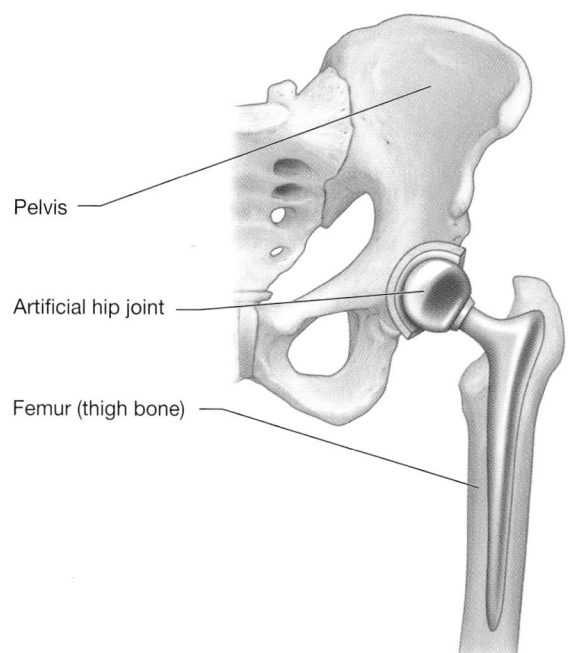

FIGURE 57–7 ■ Artificial hip joint.

Postoperative Assessment

Initial assessment during the postoperative period should focus on the potential problems of hypovolemia, bleeding complications, hypoxemia, and neurovascular compromise. After hip arthroplasty or closed reduction, the patient will be placed on hip precautions (Chart 57–4). The type of precautions required depends on the approach that was utilized. For instance, if a posterior approach was used, the patient will be placed on posterior hip precautions. The goal of the precautions is to prevent the hip from dislocating posteriorly. Anterior hip precautions involve avoiding activities that would allow the hip to dislocate anteriorly. Chart 57–4 outlines the specific precautions for both posterior and anterior approaches. The immediate postoperative nursing management of hip surgery patients is outlined in Chart 57–5, which

---

CHART 57–4   Hip Precautions

Posterior Hip Precautions	Anterior Hip Precautions
Hip abductor pillow while in bed.	Hip abductor pillow while in bed.
Do not bend hip greater than 90 degrees.	Take mini steps when walking.
Use an elevated toilet seat.	Do not assume a straddle position—like mounting a horse.
Do not sit in low chairs.	Do not twist or turn the body away from the operative side.
Do not twist or turn the body toward the operative side.	Do not turn leg and foot outward.
Do not turn leg and foot inward.	Do not lift operative leg up and out.
Keep operative leg straight when getting up and use one's arms to push up.	

CHART 57–5   Total Hip Arthroplasty Clinical Pathway

Activity	Operative Day	Postoperative Day 1	Postoperative Day 2	Postoperative Days 3–5
General	Admit to postoperative unit. Intake and output (I&O). Urinary catheter to gravity, surgical drain, empty prn; notify health care provider of drainage >200 mL/shift. Posterior hip precautions. Sequential compression device. Abduction pillow while in bed. Diet: clear liquids; progress to regular diet. Medications: patient-controlled analgesia (PCA); antinausea; stool softener; IV antibiotic every 8 hours for 6 doses. Nursing: neurovascular checks; monitor dressing drainage; monitor surgical drain output; vital signs every hour × 2 hours, then every 4 hours. Turn and position every 2 hours; pressure ulcer prevention.	Low-molecular-weight heparin (LMWH) 40 milligrams subcutaneous daily. Surgical drain discontinued by health care provider.	Discontinue urinary catheter. Oral pain medication. Discontinue PCA. Confirm surgical drain has been discontinued. Saline lock IV when taking 2,000 milliliters of fluids in 24 hours.	Laxative if no bowel movement (BM). Discontinue IV prior to discharge.
Physical Activity	Bed rest 8 hours. Out of bed (OOB) to chair in 8 hours. Incentive spirometry every 2 hours while awake.	OOB to chair. Meals tid. Ambulate bid.	OOB to chair tid. OOB to bathroom. Ambulate tid.	Independent ambulation with walker.
Diagnostic Tests	Hemoglobin and hematocrit.	Hemoglobin and hematocrit.		
Discharge Planning/Patient Education	Abduction pillow. Walker. Instruct patient on hip precautions and transfer technique.	Raised toilet seat. Reinforce patient education on hip precautions.	Discuss discharge plan with patient: skilled nursing facility (SNF) versus home.	Instruct patient/family on LMWH injection and wound care if home discharge.

describes a clinical pathway for hip arthroplasty. Discharge planning is complex for hip surgery patients. The general considerations for discharge planning and home modifications specific for hip surgery are discussed in Chart 57–6.

Refer to Chapter 55 🔗 for a complete discussion of the repair and management of fractured hips.

Pelvic Surgery

The pelvis is comprised of the iliac crest, ilium, sacrum, coccyx, ischial tuberosities, and acetabulum. The symphysis pubis is the anterior joint of the pelvis, and the sacroiliac joint is the posterior joint. Pelvic fractures are frequently associated with other traumatic injuries from motor vehicle crashes. It is essential to know the mechanism of injury because it assists the health care team in anticipating additional injuries, especially with motor vehicle crashes. Common additional injuries that are associated with pelvic fractures are femur fracture, bladder rupture, and risk for retroperitoneal bleed.

Simple fractures that are not displaced are considered to be stable fractures. Unstable fractures are fractures in which ligaments are torn, there are multiple fractures, or there is movement of the pelvic girdle with downward pressure with the patient in a supine position. If the pelvic fracture is unstable, it may be treated with external fixation or internal fixation. Pelvic fracture surgery, along with the nursing and medical management, is described in detail in Chapter 56 🔗 .

Knee Surgery

The knee is the largest joint in the body and one of the most easily injured. It is made up of four bones: the femur, the tibia, the fibula, and the patella (Figure 57–8 ◼). The knee contains four main ligaments: the inner medial collateral ligament (MCL); the outer lateral collateral ligament (LCL); the anterior cruciate ligament (ACL); and the posterior cruciate ligament (PCL). The function of the ligaments is to help control motion by connecting bones and by bracing the joint against abnormal types of motion. The knee muscles that go across the knee joint are the quadriceps (front of knee) and the hamstrings (back of knee). Another important structure, the meniscus, is a wedge of soft cartilage between the femur and the tibia that serves to cushion the knee and helps it absorb shock during motion.

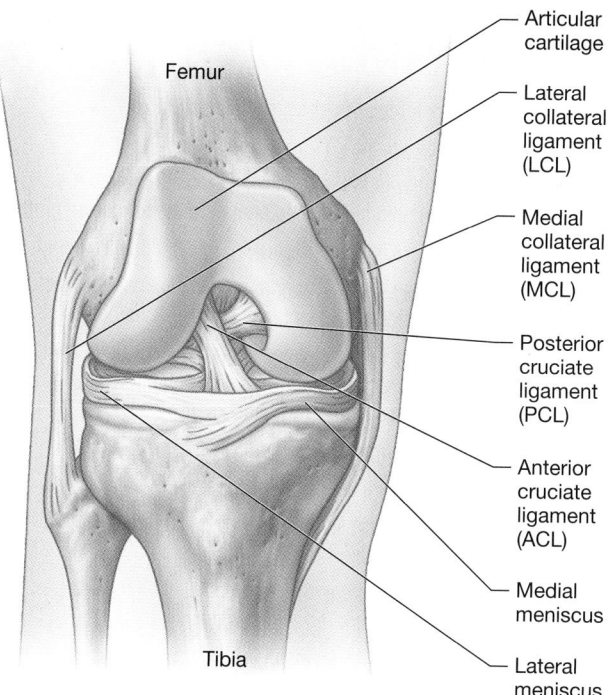

FIGURE 57–8 ◼ Knee anatomy.

Common sports injuries occur with the ligaments. Ligaments may be stretched predisposing the joint to dislocation. Ligaments may also be torn if overextension or trauma occurs. Ligaments do not regenerate. If they are torn and disability or frequent dislocations occur, they must be repaired or replaced. The anterior cruciate ligament (ACL) and the medial collateral ligament (MCL) are frequently injured in sports. The posterior cruciate ligament (PCL) may also be injured.

Anterior Cruciate Ligament (ACL) Repair

Changing direction rapidly, slowing down when running, and landing from a jump may cause tears in the ACL. Athletes who participate in skiing, basketball, and those who wear cleats, such as football players, are susceptible to ACL injuries. The goal of the ACL reconstruction surgery is to prevent instability and restore the function of the torn ligament, creating a stable knee. Patients treated with surgical reconstruction of the ACL have long-term success rates of 82% to 95%. Recurrent instability and graft failure are seen in approximately 8% of patients (American Academy of Orthopaedic Surgeons, 2007f). The ACL is not usually repaired because of failure over time with this approach. The ACL is generally replaced by a substitute graft made of tendon. The sources of tendon include patellar, hamstring, or quadriceps tendon autograft (from patient); or patellar tendon, Achilles tendon, semitendinosus, gracilis, or posterior tibialis tendon allograft (taken from a cadaver). There also are synthetic grafts available. The surgery procedure is described in Chart 57–7 (p. 1814).

Knee Arthroplasty

If osteoarthritis wears away a knee joint's articular cartilage, arthroplasty (replacement) is a common and successful procedure that improves knee motion and allows a patient to resume relatively normal activities without pain. The surgeon resurfaces

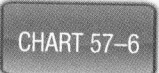

CHART 57–6 **Home Modifications for Hip Surgery Patients**

- Securely fastened safety bars or handrails for the bath and shower
- A stable armchair with a firm seat cushion allowing the knees to remain lower than the hips
- A raised toilet seat
- A shower bench or chair
- A sock aid and a long-handled shoe horn for putting on and taking off shoes and socks without excessively bending at the hip
- A "reacher" to access items without bending at the hip
- Removal of all loose carpets and electrical cords from walkways
- Food and household items up to waist level to prevent bending

CHART 57–7 Anterior Cruciate Ligament Repair Surgery

- May be done as open repair or endoscopic procedure.
- Open repair requires a 6-inch or greater incision.
- Endoscopic repair utilizes 2–3 one-inch incisions and utilizes a surgical drill inserted into incisions to prepare bone to receive graft.
- Debris is removed (torn ligaments, particles, clots, bone fragments).
- Meniscus and cartilage injuries are trimmed or repaired, and the torn anterior cruciate ligament (ACL) stump is then removed.
- Ligaments are typically replaced with allograft, autograft, or synthetic graft. If bone attachments are necessary, surgical drills may be utilized to prepare the bone for graft attachment.
- ACL graft is placed in almost the same position as the torn ACL.
- Graft may be secured with sutures or screws.
- Open repair entrance site is sutured closed, and a drain may be inserted for blood collection.
- Before the surgery is complete, the surgeon will verify that the knee has full range of motion.
- Elastic support or immobilizer may be used postoperatively for simple repairs, to contain movement, and to prevent surgical site stress.
- Continuous passive motion (CPM) devices may be used postoperatively for extensive repairs or anterior cruciate ligament surgeries to prevent shortening of the ligament and prevent joint stiffening and loss of range of motion.
- ACL repairs are usually done on an outpatient basis.

CHART 57–8 Knee Arthroplasty

- Thigh tourniquet is applied to decrease bleeding during surgery.
- Incision is made in anterior knee approximately 10 inches in length.
- Femoral head and tibia are surgically shaved to prepare for prosthetic implant.
- The patella is shaved or replaced to allow free movement after joint prosthesis is implanted.
- Debris in surgical site is removed.
- A drain may be inserted to remove blood from surgical area.
- Prosthesis is implanted.
- Surgical site is sutured closed.
- Continuous passive motion (CPM) may be utilized postoperatively utilizing progressive angles of flexion and extension as prescribed by the health care provider.

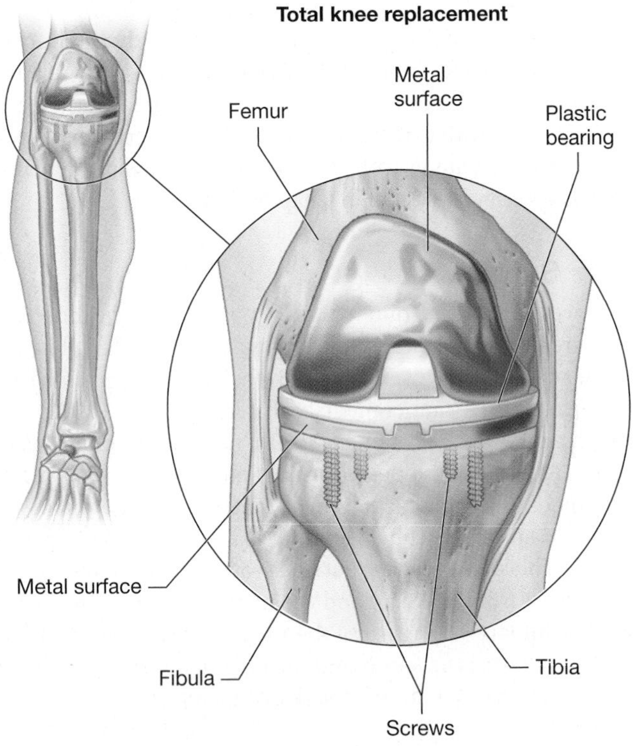

FIGURE 57–9 ■ Knee arthroplasty.

the knee joint, replacing damaged and worn weight-bearing surfaces with a prosthesis (implant) made of metal alloys, ceramic material, or high-density plastic parts that may be joined to bone by acrylic cement (Figure 57–9 ■). Up to three bone surfaces may be replaced during the total replacement of the knee: the lower condyles of the femur, the top surface of the tibia, and the back surface of the kneecap. Chart 57–8 presents the surgical procedure.

Postoperatively early mobilization is important. Initially, there is a bulky dressing around the knee and a drain to remove any fluid buildup. The drain will be removed in a day or two. A continuous passive motion exercise machine that will slowly and smoothly straighten and bend the knee is typically applied after surgery. Although pain after surgery is quite variable and not entirely predictable, it can be controlled with medication. The hospital stay may last from 3 to 7 days. The goal for discharge is to have the patient get in and out of bed independently, bend the knee up to approximately 90 degrees, extend the knee fully, walk with crutches or a walker, and demonstrate knowledge of the prescribed home exercises.

Nursing management of the patient with a total knee replacement is multifaceted and requires a comprehensive plan to ensure a return to pain-free function. General aspects of care for patients requiring orthopedic surgery are discussed in the Nursing Management of the Postoperative Patient section and outlined in the Nursing Process: Patient Care Plan feature later in this chapter (p. 1822). Use of a clinical pathway for the specific management provides the health care team with an organized, comprehensive approach to nursing management (Chart 57–9).

Meniscus Repair

The meniscus is a wedge-like rubbery cushion located where the femur and tibia meet at the knee joint (see Figure 57–8 ■, p. 1813). The meniscus helps the knee joint carry weight, glide, and turn in many directions. It also keeps the femur and tibia from grinding against each other. Meniscal tears can occur with twisting, pivoting, and decelerating motions of the knee. These injuries often occur in combination with other injuries such as a torn anterior cruciate ligament. As the cartilage weakens and wears

CHART 57-9   **Total Knee Arthroplasty Clinical Pathway**

Activity	Operative Day	Postoperative Day 1	Postoperative Day 2	Postoperative Day 3 Discharge
General	Admit to postoperative unit. Intake and output (I&O). Urinary catheter to gravity, surgical drain, empty prn; notify health care provider of drainage > 100 mL/shift. Continuous passive motion (CPM) machine while in bed; antiembolism stocking; sequential compression device to nonoperative leg. Diet: clear liquids; progress to regular diet. Medications: patient-controlled analgesic (PCA); antinausea; stool softener; IV antibiotic every 8 hours for 6 doses. Nursing assessment: neurovascular checks; monitor dressing drainage; monitor surgical drain output; vital signs every hour × 2 hours, then every 4 hours. No pillow under knees.	Discontinue urinary catheter. Saline lock IV. Low-molecular-weight heparin (LMWH) 40 milligrams subcutaneous daily. Health care provider to discontinue surgical drain.	Confirm surgical drain has been discontinued.	Laxative if no bowel movement (BM). Discontinue IV.
Physical Activity	Bed rest. Dangle at bedside.	Out of bed (OOB) to chair tid for meals. Ambulate with crutches bid.	OOB to chair tid for meals. Ambulate with crutches tid.	Independent ambulation with crutches.
Diagnostic Tests		Hemoglobin and hematocrit.		
Discharge Planning/Patient Education	Obtain crutches. Instruct patient on performance of foot pump exercises. Inform about CPM machine.	Crutch walking instruction. No weight bearing. Instruct in transfer technique.	Discuss discharge plan with patient: skilled nursing facility (SNF) versus home. Order home CPM machine for patient.	Instruct patient/family on LMWH injection and wound care if home discharge. Instruct on CPM application.

thin over time, a degenerative tear can occur without any significant trauma.

Clinical manifestations typically include a "popping" sensation when the tear occurs followed by inflammation, stiffness and swelling, pain, buckling, and fluid collection. Without treatment, a fragment of the meniscus may loosen and drift into the joint, causing it to slip, pop, or lock; and the knee may lock at a 45-degree angle, until it is manually moved or otherwise manipulated. Initially the treatment includes rest and pain medication. If the tear does not heal on its own and the knee becomes painful, stiff, or locked, a surgical repair may be necessary. The surgeon can examine the area arthroscopically and trim off damaged pieces of cartilage. A cast or brace is typically used to immobilize the knee after surgery. A course of rehabilitation exercises is necessary before resuming previous activities.

Postoperative Assessment

Initial assessment during the initial postoperative period should focus on the potential problems of hypovolemia, bleeding com-

plications, hypoxemia, and neurovascular compromise. After lower extremity surgery, the nurse must perform a neurovascular assessment that includes all toes on the affected side.

Lower extremity surgeries frequently utilize splints, slings, immobilizing dressings, and binders postoperatively. The extremity needs to be elevated above the level of the heart to decrease edema formation. The patient may remove the immobilizer for hygiene purposes or for performing the prescribed exercises with the affected joint until the formal physical therapy program is begun. The length of immobilization depends on the severity of the type of surgery and the surgeon's preference. An exercise program will help regain motion and strength in the involved extremity. This program begins with passive motion, advances to active and resistive exercises, and is typically coordinated by the surgeon and the physical therapist. Complete recovery may take several months. A strong commitment to rehabilitation is important to achieve a good surgical outcome. The surgeon will examine the outcome to advise when it is safe to return to overhead work and sports activity.

Amputation

Amputation is the surgical removal or traumatic loss of a part. In the upper extremities amputation is rare and often associated with trauma, meningococcemia, and osteosarcoma. Osteosarcoma necessitates the removal of the bone in which the cancer is present. Chapter 55 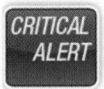 discusses osteosarcoma and other types of bone cancer. In the lower extremities, peripheral vascular disease, diabetes, and gangrene are the frequent causes for elective amputation. Below knee amputation (BKA) is preferred to above knee amputation because balance and coordination are more stable, gait is more natural, and there is a better potential for revisions, if needed. Above knee amputation (AKA) requires more energy to ambulate. The AKA patient must raise the hip and swing the prosthesis/leg forward for clearance because the leg plus prosthesis must remain straight. In the elderly this may be a safety risk, and wheelchair mobility is a safer practice.

Traumatic amputation is a sudden loss of the part and may require more extensive removal of tissue, bone, and muscle than amputation due to vascular insufficiency. Traumatic amputation is discussed in Chapter 56 . Traumatic amputation may be associated with increased potential for phantom limb pain, body image disturbance, and grief/loss disturbance than amputation resulting from chronic disease processes.

Chart 57–10 describes the surgical procedure for amputation. The Evidence-Based Practice feature provides information regarding stump and phantom limb pain.

Postoperative Assessment

Because many amputations are the result of peripheral vascular insufficiency, the patient must be monitored closely for skin integrity and with particular care given to prevent pressure ulcer development. The remaining heel should be floated off of the mattress with pillows or a heel protection device. In the immediate postoperative period, stump care usually involves elevation of the stump and compression wrapping of the extremity to prevent edema. A figure-of-eight method beginning at the distal stump is utilized to wrap the stump.

Phantom limb pain is a common complication of amputation. Current research is attempting to define characteristics and causative factors of phantom limb pain and to determine whether specific treatments may be performed prior to and during surgery to prevent phantom limb phenomena. Current treatments for phantom limb pain include pain medication, antiseizure medication, antidepressants, nerve block, spinal stimulation, use of transcutaneous electrical nerve stimulation (TENS) units, and biofeedback or other cognitive pain-relief modalities. Pain management is discussed in Chapter 15 .

CRITICAL ALERT *The stump should be elevated for the first 24 hours to prevent postoperative edema. After 24 hours, keep the stump flat while in bed or extended while out of bed in a chair to prevent contracture of the nearest joint.*

Spinal Surgery

Back pain is the cause of more lost work hours than any other medical condition and is the second leading cause of work absences. Most back pain occurs between the ages of 45 and 64, and it is more common among men than women (eMedicineHealth, 2008). The spine can be divided into three categories: the vertebral bony column, intervertebral disks, ligaments, and muscles; spinal cord and nerves; and the spinal cord vasculature. The bony vertebral column consists of 33 vertebrae separated and cushioned by the intervertebral disks. The bony vertebrae and disks are joined together by ligaments. The disks allow a degree of flexibility to the spine. They temporarily flatten out and bulge when compressed, acting as shock absorbers. If the disk is under an extreme load, the central nucleus can rupture through the surrounding cartilaginous fibers resulting in a herniated disk, which places pressure on the nerve root. Approximately 25% of people who have back pain have a herniated disk (eMedicineHealth, 2008). The most common site of back pain is in the lower back with more than 95% of operations being performed on the fourth and fifth lumbar vertebrae.

Discectomy refers to surgery in which the diseased disk is removed. **Laminectomy** refers to surgery in which only part of the disk, usually only the herniated portion, is removed. It is called a laminectomy because the surgeon must cut through the lamina to access the herniated disk. During the procedure, the surgeon will make an incision over the vertebrae and down to the bony arches of the vertebrae. The ligament joining the vertebrae along with all or part of the lamina is removed to see the involved nerve root. The surgeon will then pull the nerve root back toward the center of the spinal column and remove part of or the entire disk. The incision will be closed, and the large back muscles will protect the spine and nerve roots. Traditional discectomy or laminectomy surgical procedures usually involve 3- to 4-day hospital admissions. Patients are generally placed on a patient-controlled analgesia (PCA) machine to control their pain postoperatively. Initially patients are kept flat in bed for 24 hours and logrolled, ensuring that spinal alignment is maintained, every 2 hours to prevent pressure ulcers.

Minimally invasive surgery can be done through arthroscopic procedures and with the use of lasers. Procedures done arthroscopically include:

- **Foraminotomy**—This procedure is used to relieve pressure on nerves being compressed by the intervertebral foramen, the space where a nerve root exists in the spinal canal. The compression can be caused by bone, bulging disk, or scar tissue. A small incision is made and the scope is placed. With the use of small surgical instruments and or a laser, the bone or tissue that is compressing the nerve is removed. The patient is ambulated within 2 hours of the procedure.

- **Laminotomy**—This procedure is used to relieve the pressure on the spinal canal for the exiting nerve roots and spinal cord by increasing the amount of space available. The pressure

---

CHART 57–10 Surgical Amputation

- A tourniquet (pneumatic or other restrictive device) is applied above the area to be amputated.
- A skin flap is prepared by excising the skin from the muscle and folding it back (away from the area to be amputated).
- A guillotine device or saw is used to perform the amputation.
- The skin flap is utilized to close the surgical wound.

Stump and Phantom Limb Pain

Clinical Problem

A significant problem following amputation is acute stump pain and phantom limb pain. Phantom limb pain during the first year following surgery is reported by up to 70% of amputees (Lambert et al., 2001). Pain in the affected limb prior to surgery is correlated to the degree of stump and phantom limb pain postoperatively.

Research Findings

Lambert et al. (2001) completed a randomized prospective study comparing preoperative epidural and intraoperative perineural analgesia. Preoperative epidural patients received epidural bupivacaine and diamorphine 24 hours before surgery, during surgery, and 3 days postoperatively. The intraoperative perineural patients received an intraoperatively placed perineural catheter for intra- and postoperative administration of bupivacaine. During the surgery all of the patients received general anesthesia. Their results showed that, during the first 3 days postoperatively, pain scores were significantly higher in the perineural group. After 3 days, 29% of the patients in the epidural group and 44% of patients in the perineural group reported phantom pain. In 6 months phantom pain was reported in 63% of the epidural group and 88% of the perineural group. In 1 year phantom pain was reported in 38% of the epidural group and 50% of the perineural group. When comparing the two groups, the study did not show a significant difference in limb pain but did show that the epidural group had significantly better pain control immediately postoperatively.

Another study (Jahangiri, Jayatunga, Bradley, & Dark, 1994) looked at the combination of drugs that were used in the epidural infusion. Because the infusion of morphine and bupivacaine can cause hypotension, it can make the patient difficult to manage on a ward and may require a higher level of care for monitoring. The study compared the effectiveness in reducing stump and phantom limb pain with epidural infusion containing bupivacaine, clonidine, and a lower dose of diamorphine. The control group received opioid analgesia on demand. There were 13 patients in the study group and 11 patients in the control group. Pain was assessed postoperatively at 7 days, 6 months, and 1 year. At 1 year, 1 patient in the study group and 8 patients in the control group had phantom limb sensation. The researchers concluded that perioperative epidural infusion of bupivacaine, clonidine, and diamorphine is safe and effective in reducing phantom pain after amputation.

In 2003, Gehling & Tryba conducted an analysis of factors contributing to the results of phantom limb pain prophylaxis. They analyzed all published articles on phantom limb pain prophylaxis from 1966 to 1999. Their results found an association between regional analgesia via epidural infusion pre-, intra-, and postoperatively and a significant reduction of phantom limb pain 12 months after amputation.

Implications for Nursing Practice

Studies show a significant reduction in acute postoperative stump pain and the development of phantom limb pain with pre-, intra-, and postoperative analgesia via epidural infusion. Patient education regarding epidural infusion and knowledge regarding the effects and side effects of the medication used is of great importance. Advocating having the infusion started preoperatively appears to benefit the patient especially with regard to phantom limb pain 12 months following surgery.

Critical Thinking Questions

1. What is the reasoning for beginning the epidural infusion prior to surgery and continuing 3 days after surgery?

2. Why is it important to prevent or decrease the incidence of phantom limb pain?

Answers to Critical Thinking Questions appear in Appendix D.

References

Gehling, M., & Tryba, M. (2003). Prophylaxis of phantom pain: Is regional analgesia ineffective? *Der Schmerz, 17*(1), 11–19.

Jahangiri, M., Jayatunga, A. P., Bradley, J. W., & Dark, C. H. (1994). Prevention of phantom pain after major lower limb amputation by epidural infusion of diamorphine, clonidine, and bupivacaine. *Annals of the Royal College of Surgery in England, 76*(5), 324–326.

Lambert, A. W., Dashfield, A. K., Cosgrove, C., Wilkins, D. C., Walker, A. J., & Ashley, S. (2001). Randomized prospective study comparing preoperative epidural and intraoperative perineural analgesia for the prevention of postoperative stump and phantom limb pain following major amputation. *Regional Anesthesia Pain Medicine, 26*(4), 316–321.

EVIDENCE-BASED PRACTICE

---

may be caused by bone spurs, spinal stenosis, arthritis, a bulging or herniated disk, or scar tissue. The procedure is done in the same manner as the foraminotomy. The patient is able to ambulate within 2 hours of the procedure.

- **Percutaneous arthroscopic discectomy**—This procedure is the removal of a bulging or herniated disk that is pressing on a nerve root or the spinal cord. The procedure is done in the same manner as the foraminotomy. The patient is able to ambulate within 2 hours of the procedure.

Spinal fusion (fusing vertebrae together with bone graft or plates and screws so that an area of the spine cannot move) surgery may be performed after traumatic, unstable injuries to stabilize the spine and prevent further injury and loss of function

(Figure 57–10 ■, p. 1818). In some cases it may also be performed to treat vertebral fractures, kyphosis, or scoliosis. Bone grafts are used like cement to weld the vertebrae together, or the bones are held together by plates and screws so that they can no longer move. If an autologous bone graft is used, the piece of bone is generally taken from the iliac crest during the back surgery. Allograft bone donations are obtained from donor banks or stored in the operating room in a refrigerator or freezer. Allograft bones are obtained from cadavers and are sterilized and frozen, or stored in sterile packaging. There are several types of spinal fusion surgery options, including:

- **Posterolateral gutter fusion**—The procedure is done through the back.

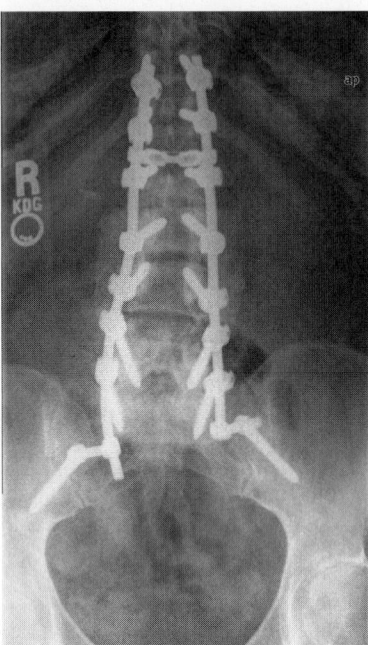

FIGURE 57–10 ■ Spinal fusion with plates and screws x-ray.
Source: Karen Cooper RN, MSN, CCRN, CNS

- **Posterior lumbar interbody fusion (PLIF)**—The procedure is done from the back and includes removing the disk between two vertebrae and inserting bone into the space created between the two vertebral bodies.
- **Anterior lumbar interbody fusion (ALIF)**—The procedure is done from the front and includes removing the disk between two vertebrae and inserting bone into the space created between the two vertebral bodies.
- **Anterior/posterior spinal fusion**—The procedure is done from the front and the back.

Postoperative Assessment

After surgery, until the bones fuse, the patient may need to wear a brace to maintain alignment of the spine. The operative site must remain in strict anatomic alignment. For example, if the patient with back surgery is to be turned, the back must remain in a straight line during turning so there is no torque or twisting of the operative site. The surgeon may order the patient to be flat in bed after surgery for a specified amount of time. Prior to getting the patient out of bed, a back brace must be placed on the patient while lying flat. This is done by logrolling the patient, applying the pieces of the brace, and securing the Velcro straps. A thoracolumbosacral orthosis (TLSO) is the type of brace generally utilized (Figure 57–11 ■). It is specially created from a mold of the patient and made of durable plastic, using Velcro straps to hold the two sides together. The TLSO is also used as the postoperative brace for other types of back surgery. In order to ensure that the patient can achieve a standing position without bending, the patient should be assisted from the flat-in-bed position in the raised bed to the erect position with two-person support.

Postoperative complications after spinal surgery may include transient bowel and bladder dysfunction due to edema of the spine causing compression of the sympathetic and parasympathetic nerve tracts. The nurse will monitor the pa-

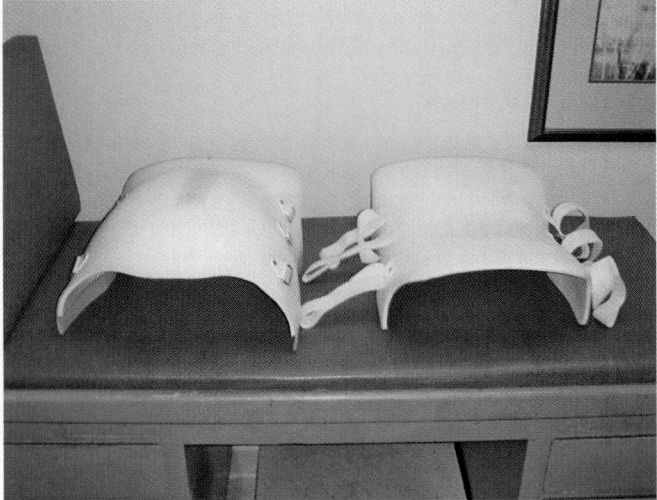

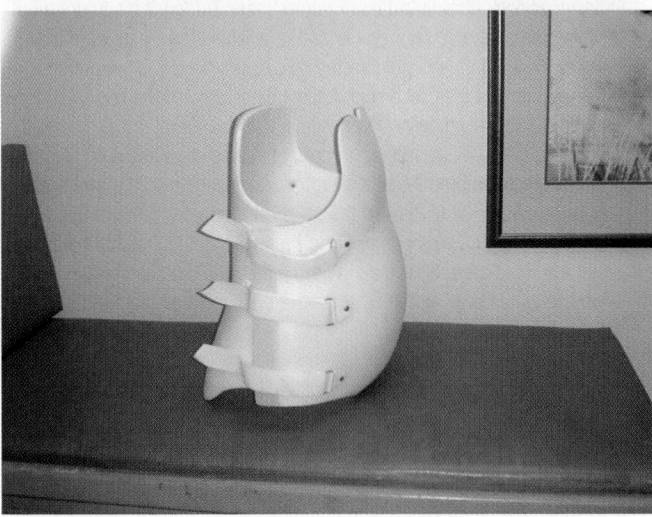

FIGURE 57–11 ■ Thoracolumbosacral orthosis brace (TLSO).
Source: Karen Cooper RN, MSN, CCRN, CNS

tient for return of bowel sounds, and the patient should not receive a diet until bowel sounds return. If the patient has difficulty emptying her bladder after surgery, she may require intermittent urinary catheterization. The spinal dressing must be monitored for both bleeding and possible cerebrospinal fluid (CSF) leak.

A CSF leak may occur if the dura is opened during the surgical procedure. During spinal surgery, the dura of the spinal cord is invaded and there is a potential for the surgical site to leak CSF. CSF leaks appear as a clear fluid that forms a halo around any serous drainage on the dressing. CSF leaks increase the potential for development of meningitis and often cause a postoperative headache that is worse when the patient is upright. The surgeon should be notified if a CSF leak is present or suspected. A blood patch may be used to treat the CSF leak from the surgical site. An anesthesiologist injects 5 to 20 milliliters of unclotted blood into the surgical site (into the epidural space). After the blood patch is performed, the patient should remain flat in bed for 2 hours to ensure that the blood does not migrate and is allowed to clot and prevent further CSF leakage.

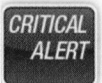 *Cerebrospinal fluid leak in the spinal surgery patient should be reported immediately and precautions to prevent meningitis instituted.*

COMPLEMENTARY & ALTERNATIVE THERAPIES

Healing Touch

Description:

Healing touch is an energy healing technique in which practitioners use their hands to therapeutically affect the patient's energy field. Despite the name, healing touch practitioners never actually touch the patient; instead, they keep their hands about 3 inches above the patient's skin, tapping into—and aligning and balancing—the energy field that surrounds the body. Although the body is never physically touched, patients report an improvement in musculoskeletal conditions. Therapeutic effects can include relieving pain, accelerating wound healing, preventing illness, promoting relaxation, and easing the dying process. Healing touch, which emerged in the 1970s from other energy healing techniques such as therapeutic touch, is now performed by practitioners all over the world, including nurses.

Research Support:

One article cited a patient's improvements after trauma, including improvements in physiological and psychological complaints, health perception, and well-being (Burr, 2005). A clinical study involved 56 patients who received healing touch and completed the Healing Touch Comfort Questionnaire. Of the 56 patients, 51 were women, and 5 were men, with an average age of 51. Study results showed that participants who received more than four healing touch treatments had higher comfort levels than those with fewer than four treatments (Dowd, Kolcaba, & Steiner, 2006).

A pilot study assessed the effect of healing touch on chronic neuropathic pain in patients with spinal cord injury. The study involved the administration of both healing touch as well as guided progressive relaxation on 12 veterans over the course of six weekly home visits. The instruments used to assess outcomes showed sensitivity, such as the Diener Satisfaction with Life Scale, which showed increased well-being in the healing touch group and no change in the control group. However, there was a large variation among the groups. Researchers concluded that healing touch may benefit chronic pain (Wardell, Rintala, Duan, & Tan, 2006).

References

Burr, J. P. (2005, September-October). Jayne's story: Healing touch as a complementary treatment for trauma recovery. *Holistic Nurse Practitioner, 19*(5), 211–216.

Dowd, T., Kolcaba, K., & Steiner, R. (2006, May-June). Development of the healing touch comfort questionnaire. *Holistic Nurse Practitioner, 20*(3), 122–129.

Wardell, D. W., Rintala, D. H., Duan, Z., & Tan, G. (2006). A pilot study of healing touch and progressive relaxation for chronic neuropathic pain in persons with spinal cord injury. *Journal of Holistic Nursing, 24*(4), 231–240.

If the patient has had back pain for many years, it may be difficult to manage his pain postoperatively. Chronic pain follows different neural pathways. Refer to Chapter 15 ⊙ for an indepth discussion of pain assessment and treatment. Control of the environment to encourage relaxation and alternative therapies such as healing touch, described in the Complementary and Alternative Therapies box, are interventions the nurse can use to help relieve the patient's pain.

Ankle and Foot Surgeries

The act of walking can put up to 1.5 times one's body weight on one's foot. During 1 hour of strenuous exercise, the feet will cushion up to 1 million pounds of pressure (American Academy of Orthopaedic Surgeons, 2005). The foot has 26 bones. The ankle joint is comprised of the talus and the ends of the tibia and fibula. It is supported by three groups of ligaments. The movement of the foot and ankle is supported by the muscles and tendons. Most injuries of the foot and ankle are caused by overuse, poor conditioning, and improperly fitting shoes.

Ankle pain is most commonly due to a sprain but also can be caused by arthritis, gout, bone fracture, tendonitis, infection, poor structural alignment of the leg or foot, or chronic ankle joint instability from a severe injury or multiple injuries. The most common injury of the ankle is a sprain. During a fall or jump, the foot is likely to turn inward (inversion) and stretch or tear ligaments. Every day approximately 25,000 people sprain their ankle (American Academy of Orthopaedic Surgeons, 2005). The ankle joint is held together and protected from abnormal movement by the ligaments. Normally, a ligament will stretch within its limits and then return to normal position. When a ligament is forced to stretch beyond its limits, a sprain occurs. A severe sprain will actually cause tearing of the elastic fibers of the ligament. The ligament that is most commonly injured is the lateral ligament on the lateral aspect

of the ankle. For a detailed discussion of sprains, refer to Chapter 56 ⊙.

Tendon Injuries

Tendons connect muscle to bone. Two tendons run along the outer aspect of the ankle and foot to help stabilize the ankle joint. These tendons are called the peroneal tendons (Figure 57–12 ■). Peroneal tendon injuries can be acute or chronic and occur most often in patients who participate in sports that involve repetitive ankle motion. The tendon may have an acute tear or fray from overuse. The tendons can also sublux out of their normal position.

The largest and strongest tendon of the lower leg is the Achilles tendon. The tendon connects muscles in the lower leg with the calcaneus bone. A complete or partial tear of the Achilles tendon is called a rupture (Figure 57–13 ■, p. 1820). Jumping, pivoting, or sudden acceleration to a run can stretch the tendon beyond its capacity and cause a tear.

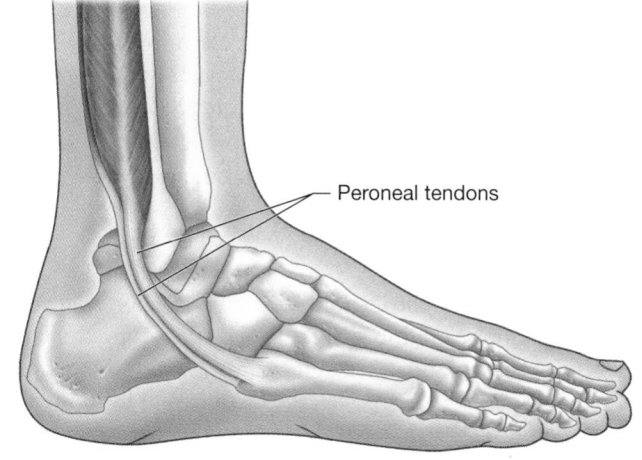

FIGURE 57–12 ■ Peroneal tendons.

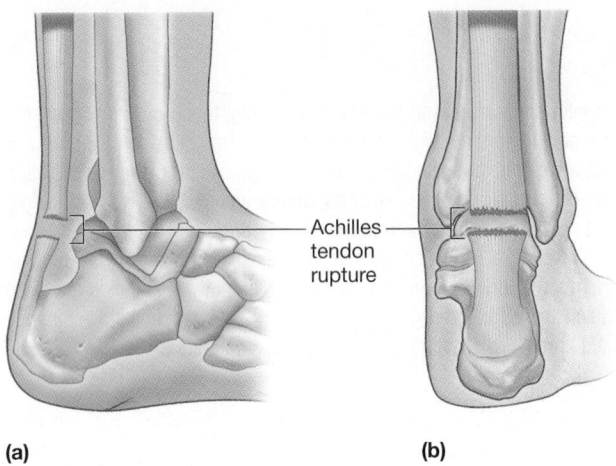

(a)   (b)

FIGURE 57–13 ■ Achilles tendon rupture.

Injury to the tendons or ligaments of the ankle will cause severe pain, swelling, and difficulty with mobilization, because weight bearing will increase the pain. Without proper healing, the joint will become unstable, injury will reoccur, and the patient will develop chronic ankle pain. Other causes of chronic ankle pain include arthritis of the joint, synovitis (inflammation of the joint lining), an injury to the nerves that pass through the ankle, and development of scar tissue after a sprain, which takes up space in the joint and places pressure on the ligaments.

Symptoms of chronic ankle pain include pain on the lateral side of the ankle, swelling, stiffness, difficulty walking on uneven ground or high heels, tenderness, and repeated ankle sprains.

Nonsurgical management for minor sprains and strains is covered in Chapter 56 🖜. If conservative treatment does not bring relief, then surgery may be required. Surgical treatment for ankle injuries is rare, but it is used for injuries that fail to respond to nonsurgical treatment and for persistent instability after months of rehabilitation and nonsurgical treatment.

Surgical options include:

- **Arthroscopy**—A surgeon examines the joint to see whether there are any loose fragments of bone or cartilage, or part of the ligament caught in the joint, and cleans debris and makes repairs.
- **Reconstruction**—A surgeon repairs the torn ligament or tendon with suture, or uses other ligaments and/or tendons found in the foot and around the ankle to repair the damaged ligaments.
- **Arthroplasty**—A surgeon replaces the joint with an artificial joint.

Ankle Arthroscopy

Arthroscopy of the ankle includes surgical evaluation and treatment for multiple conditions. During the arthroscopy, small incisions are made and fiber-optic cameras with very small surgical tools are placed through the incision into the joint and used to perform the repair. Arthroscopy is used to remove debris in the ankle joint from torn cartilage or from a bone chip. It can also be used to repair or reattach tendons and ligaments damaged during a severe sprain.

Ankle Reconstruction

Ankle reconstruction is the repair of the torn ligament or tendon with sutures, or the use of other ligaments and/or tendons found in the foot and around the ankle to repair the damaged ligaments. The procedure may be done through arthroscopic surgery or as an open procedure.

Ankle Arthroplasty

Ankle arthroplasty is the replacement of the joint with an artificial joint (Figure 57–14 ■). Although ankle arthroplasty is done much less frequently than knee or hip replacement, it can reduce the pain from arthritis. To fit the metal socket in place, the ends of the tibia and the fibula are shaped first. Following that, the top of the talus is shaped so the metal talus component can be inserted. After the bones are prepared, all the different pieces of the artificial ankle joint are put into place. To make sure that the ankle socket or the tibial component fits tightly, two screws are placed through the fibula and the tibia just above the artificial ankle joint. To prevent any motion that could loosen the artificial joint, bone is grafted between the fibula and the tibia to fuse them. The bone graft is taken from the bone that was removed earlier during the shaping procedure.

Postoperative Assessment

Weight-bearing status will be determined by the surgeon and will depend on the extent of the repair. Some patients will be allowed to bear weight with crutches; others will be placed in an immobilizer for as long as 6 weeks. If the surgery was extensive, such as remodeling of the ankle, a cast may be applied to prevent the patient from moving the joint too early and to promote healing. The nurse should instruct the patient to keep the incisions clean and dry and to observe for any signs of infection such as redness, increased pain, and drainage. The ankle should be elevated and iced to minimize swelling and prevent increased pain.

Surgical Management for the Foot

The most common foot surgeries are for the treatment of bunions and hammer toes. A bunion, also called hallux valgus, is a turning outward of the big toe (Figure 57–15 ■). The first metatarsal be-

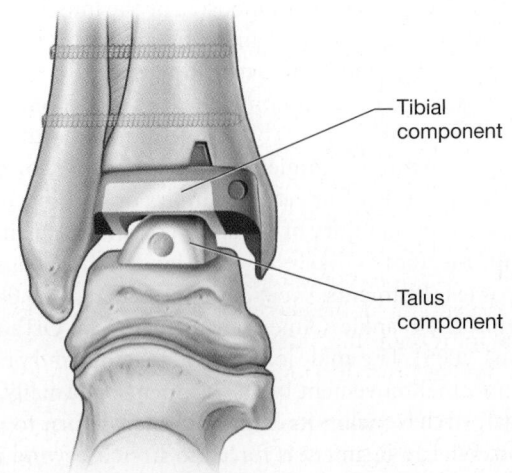

FIGURE 57–14 ■ Ankle arthroplasty.

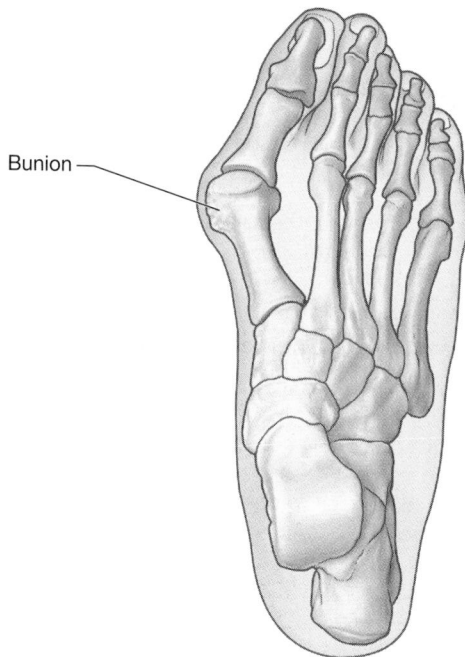

FIGURE 57–15 ■ Bunion.

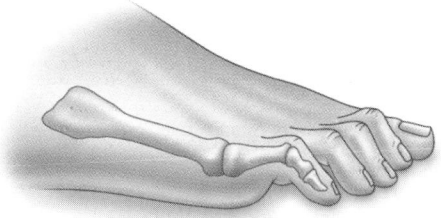

Hammer toes

FIGURE 57–16 ■ Hammer toe.

comes prominent on the inner border of the foot. This bump is the bunion and is made up of bone and soft tissue. The larger the bunion becomes, the more pressure is exerted on the joint while walking and the more pain develops. The big toe may angle toward and even move under the second toe. The deformity may even progress to force the second toe out of alignment, at times overlapping the third toe, and the foot will appear deformed. As the bunion progresses, arthritis may develop in the joint.

The bunion is painful and can make it difficult to wear shoes and affect mobility. Bunions can be caused by polio or arthritis, but most commonly are caused by ill-fitting shoes and heels that squeeze the toes into an unnatural position. A study by the American Orthopaedic Foot & Ankle Society found that 88% of women in the United States wear shoes that are too small, and 55% have bunions. Bunions are nine times more common in women than in men (American Academy of Orthopaedic Surgeons, 2001).

A hammer toe is a deformity of the second, third, fourth, or fifth toe. The toe is bent at the middle joint and resembles a hammer (Figure 57–16 ■). Initially, hammer toes are flexible and can be corrected with simple measures but, if untreated, they become fixed and require surgery. Hammer toe results from shoes that do not fit properly or a muscle imbalance. Muscles work in pairs to straighten and bend the toes. If the toe is bent and held in one position for a long period of time, muscles tighten and cannot stretch out.

Multiple surgical procedures may be done alone or in combination depending on the degree of deformity. The goal of surgery is to realign the joint, relieve pain, and correct the deformity. The procedures include:

- **Repair of the tendons and ligaments around the toe**—With a bunion, the tissues may be too tight on one side and too loose on the other, creating an imbalance that causes the big toe to drift toward the others. This procedure shortens the loose tissues, lengthens the tight ones, and is usually combined with an osteotomy.
- **Osteotomy**—The surgical cutting of bone and realignment of the joint.
- **Exostectomy**—Removal of the excess bone on the toe joint; used only for an enlargement of the bone with no drifting of the big toe.
- **Arthrodesis**—Removal of the damaged joint surfaces, followed by the insertion of screws, wires, or plates to hold the surfaces together until it heals.
- **Resection arthroplasty**—Removal of the damaged portion of the joint to create a flexible "scar" joint.

■ Nursing Management

The plan of care for the orthopedic patient is formulated by the registered nurse in conjunction with the patient. The nursing process provides the framework to ensure that all aspects of patient management are being addressed. The nurse caring for the patient after surgery must consider the time since surgery (postoperative days since surgery) in setting priorities and determining patient progress toward discharge. Pain control in the postoperative period is a major focus, because it can indicate potential problems or prevent the patient from completing necessary exercises and reaching goals that are necessary to recover and rehabilitate. (See the Pain Management section later in this chapter.) General postoperative assessment is discussed in Chapter 27 ⬤.

The nursing assessment of the patient is both holistic and focused. The nurse must rely on the patient's self-report to provide the necessary information to determine the patient's current status accurately. The Nursing Process: Patient Care Plan feature (p. 1822) provides examples of subjective and objective assessment and evaluation data for the patient with a musculoskeletal disorder as a foundation for providing care to this population. The nurse collects this assessment data to evaluate factors such as pain, neurovascular status, wound appearance, and drains and dressings, specific therapeutic modalities, and exercising.

Neurovascular Assessment

The neurovascular assessment is a requirement in the assessment of patients with musculoskeletal injury and surgery. The neurovascular assessment should be performed bilaterally so

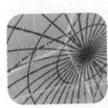

NURSING PROCESS: Patient Care Plan for the Orthopedic Surgical Patient

Assessment of Airway and Gas Exchange

Subjective Data:
Are you having difficulty breathing?
Can you take a deep breath and cough for me?
Do you feel like you are getting enough air?
Do you use an inhaler or have a history of lung problems?

Objective Data:
Lung sounds
Oxygen saturation, arterial blood gas analysis
Respiratory rate, depth, effort
Mental status

Nursing Assessment and Diagnoses	Outcomes and Evaluation Parameters	Planning and Interventions with *Rationales*
Nursing Diagnosis: *Gas Exchange, Impaired* related to anesthetic or narcotic effect, fluid overload, pulmonary or fat emboli, pneumonia, or preexisting pulmonary or cardiovascular disease exacerbation	**Outcomes:** Airway open. Adequate gas exchange. **Evaluation Parameters:** Breath sounds clear, without evidence of snoring or stridor. Oxygen saturation > 94% or as ordered by health care provider. Arterial blood gas demonstrates $PaO_2 > 80$ mmHg and $PaCO_2$ 35–45 mmHg. Respiratory rate 12–20 per minute, unlabored with good chest expansion. Alert and oriented to person, place, time, and situation.	**Interventions and *Rationales:*** Initially a jaw thrust maneuver may be necessary to maintain an open airway if the patient has snoring breath sounds indicating airway obstruction from tongue. If this maneuver is necessary, the patient may require additional reversal agents such as naloxone or flumazenil. The anesthesiologist or surgeon may need to be contacted for orders for these medications. *To maintain open airway.* Assess patient for adequacy of respiratory rate and depth, auscultate breath sounds, and monitor oxygen saturation. Analyze arterial blood gas when results are available. *Indicates gas exchange is adequate.* Assess patient's level of consciousness and orientation to person, place, time, and situation. *Confusion, agitation, restlessness, or difficult arousal may indicate hypoxia.* Encourage patient to perform incentive spirometry (ICS) every 1–2 hours for 10 breaths while awake. Have patient cough and deep breathe after utilizing ICS. Assist patient out of bed (OOB) to chair and ambulating at least three times a day. *To promote adequate gas exchange, promote airway clearance, and prevent atelectasis.*

Assessment of Neurovascular Status

Subjective Data:
Can you move your (name part distal to surgery)?
Where do you feel me touching you? Is this sharp or dull?
Are you in pain? Can you describe your pain using a scale of 0 to 10?
Do you have any numbness or tingling?

Objective Data:
Strength of movement   Color of skin
Sensation   Skin temperature
Pulses   Capillary refill time

Nursing Assessment and Diagnoses	Outcomes and Evaluation Parameters	Planning and Interventions with *Rationales*
Nursing Diagnosis: *Neurovascular Dysfunction, Peripheral: Risk for* related to edema, vascular insufficiency, nerve damage, or surgical complication	**Outcomes:** Absence of neurovascular deficits. Skeletal structures in alignment. **Evaluation Parameters:** Full strength. Sensation intact. No numbness, tingling, or pain. Pulses 2–3+ palpated. Skin warm, pink, and dry. Capillary refill time < 3 seconds.	**Interventions and *Rationales:*** Perform neurovascular assessment every 2–4 hours. Assess bilateral extremities. *To give indication of normal findings for patient.* Elevate limb above level of heart in position of function. *To decrease edema formation and prevent contracture.* Evaluate sensation using a dermatome chart for patients with epidural anesthesia/catheters and patients with spinal surgery. *Dermatome chart describes level of anesthesia or deficit.* Evaluate strength and range of motion during planned postoperative activities. *Postoperative exercise improves circulation, improves healing, and prevents contractures and deconditioning.*

Assessment of Volume Status

Subjective Data:
Are you thirsty?
Do you need to urinate?
Do you feel cold?
How is your breathing?
Do you feel anxious? Or that your heart is beating faster than normal?

Objective Data:
Urine output, color, specific gravity
Blood loss from surgical drains/dressing
Intake and output balance
Heart rate, blood pressure, respiratory rate (RR)
Blood urea nitrogen (BUN)/creatinine
Hemoglobin (Hgb) and hematocrit (HCT)
Skin turgor, capillary refill

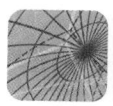

NURSING PROCESS: Patient Care Plan for the Orthopedic Surgical Patient—*Continued*

Nursing Assessment and Diagnoses	Outcomes and Evaluation Parameters	Planning and Interventions with *Rationales*
Nursing Diagnoses: *Fluid volume, Deficient* related to blood loss and inadequate fluid intake *Fluid volume, Imbalanced: Risk for* due to impaired renal function and fluid intake in excess of output	**Outcome:** Adequate and balanced intake and output. *Evaluation Parameters:* Vital signs within normal limits. Intake and output balance. Lungs clear. Urine output adequate. BUN and creatinine normal. Hgb and HCT stable. Drainage from wound < 50 milliliters in 24 hours.	**Interventions and *Rationales:*** Strict intake and output (I&O) to include all po liquids, IV fluid intake and urine, gastric, and wound drainage output. Maintain shift and ongoing totals. Assess wound drainage. Frankly bloody drainage may be present on the first postoperative day, but should change to serosanguinous after that. Notify health care provider of excessive blood loss. *To give an accurate reflection of fluid balance.* Obtain vital signs as ordered. *Tachycardia and low blood pressure may indicate hypovolemia. Increased respiratory rate or adventitious breath sounds may indicate volume overload.* Monitor laboratory studies for signs of hypo-/hypervolemia. *The hemoglobin and hematocrit, BUN, and creatinine levels provide information on volume status.*

Assessment of Pain

Subjective Data:

Can you describe your pain for me using a 0–10 scale with 0 being no pain and 10 being the worst pain you have ever had?
Using that 1–10 scale, what is your comfort level?

Objective Data:
Patient pain score
Type of pain-relief modality

Nursing Assessment and Diagnoses	Outcomes and Evaluation Parameters	Planning and Interventions with *Rationales*
Nursing Diagnosis: *Pain, Acute* related to surgical procedure, compartment syndrome, osteoarthritis, or cerebrospinal fluid (CSF) leak (in spinal surgery patient)	**Outcomes:** Patient will have pain controlled and will be able to participate in all aspects of rehabilitation program. *Evaluation Parameter:* Pain scale score at or below predetermined comfort level score.	**Interventions and *Rationales:*** Medicate patient for pain score greater than comfort level. Notify health care provider if symptoms unrelieved by ordered medication. *Patients have a right to pain control within their described comfort level. Pain that is not relieved may indicate development of complications such as compartment syndrome.* Place spinal patient in supine position if he complains of headache. *CSF leak headache increases with drainage, upright position.*

Assessment of Wound Status and Potential for Infection

Subjective Data:

Are you having more or less pain in your (name surgical site) today?
Do you feel as though you have fever or chills?
Are you having urinary frequency or urgency?

Objective Data:
Temperature and vital signs
Wound drainage appearance, odor
Suture site redness, edema, warmth
Urine appearance, odor
Wound/urine culture results
White blood count (WBC) results

Nursing Assessment and Diagnoses	Outcomes and Evaluation Parameters	Planning and Interventions with *Rationales*
Nursing Diagnosis: *Infection, Risk for* and delayed wound healing related to age, open surgery, compound fracture, and comorbid condition	**Outcomes:** Wound/bone healing within expected time frame. No evidence of infection. *Evaluation Parameters:* Surgical incision is clean, dry, and approximated, without redness. Urine clear, no odor. Vital signs within normal limits (WNL). WBC count < 11,000/mcL.	**Interventions and *Rationales:*** Obtain vital signs as ordered or every 4 hours, including temperature. *To provide early indication of changes indicating infection.* Assess surgical site and drainage each shift. *To provide early indication of changes indicating infection.* Monitor lab values, especially WBC count. *Elevations in WBC indicate infection.*

Assessment of Functional Status

Subjective Data:

How do you feel today?
Are you able to bathe and perform your postoperative exercises unassisted, or do you need some help?
How far did you walk yesterday?

Objective Data:
Amount in feet that patient is able to ambulate
Time in hours that patient is out of bed
Amount of persons needed to get patient out of bed or to assist with ambulation
Assistive devices needed for mobility

(continued)

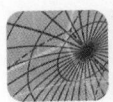

NURSING PROCESS: Patient Care Plan for the Orthopedic Surgical Patient—*Continued*

Nursing Assessment and Diagnoses	Outcomes and Evaluation Parameters	Planning and Interventions with *Rationales*
Nursing Diagnosis: *Self-Care, Readiness for Enhanced* related to surgery, pain, immobility, or decreased mental status	**Outcome:** Patient able to care for self. ***Evaluation Parameters:*** Able to perform postoperative exercises including transfers, ambulation, and pulmonary toilet at prescribed intervals. Able to ambulate with walker 50 feet with steady gait; able to ambulate unassisted for 50 feet with steady gait. Able to complete toilet and hygiene functions unassisted.	**Interventions and *Rationale:*** Patient should be assisted out of bed as soon as feasible. Follow health care provider orders/clinical pathway instructions for mobility and activities. If health care provider does not order progressive mobilization of the patient, notify health care provider to obtain activity orders. *To prevent deconditioning and maintain or improve functional status.*

Assessment of Skin Integrity
Subjective Data:
Are you able to turn and position yourself?
Do you have any painful areas while you are in bed?
Do you have any reddened areas that you are aware of?

Objective Data:
Skin appearance
Patient position
Presence of pressure relief device

Nursing Assessment and Diagnoses	Outcomes and Evaluation Parameters	Planning and Interventions with *Rationales*
Nursing Diagnoses: *Skin Integrity, Risk for Impaired* related to decreased sensorium and immobility.	**Outcome:** Patient will have no evidence of skin breakdown. ***Evaluation Parameters:*** Skin surface clean, dry, pink, and intact. Patient position change is performed or observed at least every 2 hours while in bed or every 15 minutes while seated.	**Interventions and *Rationales:*** Turn and position patient every 2 hours while in bed (logroll, maintaining spinal alignment if patient with spinal surgery). Float heels off of bed with pillows or heel lift device. Follow hospital protocol for use of pressure relief mattresses and overlays. *To prevent pressure ulcer development.* Assess skin integrity and document each shift and with each change in position. Assess areas over bony prominences, where prostheses, casts, traction, or splints contact. *To provide early detection of potential for skin breakdown.*

Assessment of Patient's Understanding of Treatment Plan and Continuing Care Needs
Subjective Data:
Do you have any questions about your plan of care?
What are your goals for today?
Do you have anyone at home to assist you?
Tell me about your home so that I have a good picture of it.

Objective Data:
Observation of activities
Verbalization of continuing care plan

Nursing Assessment and Diagnoses	Outcomes and Evaluation Parameters	Planning and Interventions with *Rationales*
Nursing Diagnoses: *Knowledge, Deficient* of self-care needs and treatment plan related to postoperative delirium *Therapeutic Regimen Management, Ineffective* related to postoperative exercises, administration of deep venous thrombosis (DVT) prophylaxis, and self-care activities without assistance related to age, obesity, decreased functional capacity, and lack of home support	**Outcome:** Patient is able to discuss a realistic plan for self-care after hospital discharge. ***Evaluation Parameters:*** Patient verbalizes knowledge of plan of care and goals. Patient demonstrates ability to perform postoperative exercises correctly in the appropriate frequency. Patient verbalizes a plan for assistance with activities of daily living (ADL) and ongoing therapeutic requirements if needed. Demonstration of ability to ambulate at least 100 feet and perform self-care activities.	**Interventions and *Rationales:*** Assess patient's readiness to learn and provide patient education regarding patient procedures, activities, medications, and care needs. *Assessment of patient readiness enables the nurse to provide education at appropriate times.* Begin discharge planning on admission. Encourage significant other/family participation in plan. Evaluate care needs compared with patient abilities. Patient/significant other should be able to verbalize/demonstrate essential activities prior to discharge. *To ensure that sufficient time is allotted to provide education and training so that patient/family are able to perform activities after discharge.* Prior to discharge, ensure that patient understands plan of care and is able to verbalize important aspects in her own words and to verbalize a plan for obtaining medications, equipment, and assistance in the home environment. *To help ensure compliance with treatment plan.*

that the affected extremity can be compared to the unaffected extremity. If the patient undergoes spinal surgery, the neurovascular assessment is performed on the parts of the body distal to the surgical site. The neurovascular assessment includes assessment of the five Ps: pain, pulse, paresthesia, paralysis, and pallor. A complete assessment of circulation, motor, and sensory functions must be performed. Neurovascular compromise or deterioration should be reported to the surgeon immediately. The nurse should anticipate performing the neurovascular assessment in conjunction with vital signs.

The neurovascular assessment should proceed systematically. Activities that may cause pain should be performed last. The nurse should first inspect the extremities for general appearance including color and presence of edema. Skin color should be described as pink or normal, pale, or cyanotic. Red or ruddy skin may indicate venous engorgement. Skin temperature and presence of moisture should be assessed. Normally the skin is warm and dry. Coolness of the skin may indicate decreased circulation. Excessive warmth or heat may indicate an early sign of infection or cellulitis. Moist skin is frequently found in the skin folds of obese persons and may require interventions to prevent fungal infection or skin maceration. Moist skin may also indicate venous insufficiency, excessive effort, or fever.

The pulse strength provides information regarding blood supply to the affected extremity and surgical site. Pulses most distal to the surgical site should be palpated. If no pulse is present, the nurse should obtain Doppler pulses and systematically attempt to palpate the presence of a pulse in a proximal direction. For example, if no dorsalis pedis or posterior tibial pulse is present, the nurse should next palpate for a popliteal pulse. Pulses in the lower extremities include the dorsalis pedis, posterior tibial, and popliteal. Pulse points in the upper extremities include the radial and brachial. The pulse should be described as grade 0–4 or as a Doppler pulse (Chart 57–11).

Skin turgor indicates hydration status and also helps describe the fullness of tissue in the operative extremity. After surgery, the inflammatory process causes vasodilation of vessels supplying the site, which results in tissue swelling. Because the part may be immobilized after surgery, venous return is decreased because of decreased muscle pump action. Skin turgor may be described as normal/brisk, slow, or tense. The skin of the distal extremity should be compressed between the nurse's thumb and index finger to a tent-like projection and released to test turgor. The skin should return to its normal state briskly. Slowed skin turgor indicates low volume status or dehydration. Tense skin cannot be tested. Edema in the surgical area is assessed regularly. Right after surgery, edema is a normal occurrence due to tissue manip-

ulation during surgery, and it gradually diminishes over time. If skin is tense or the extremity edematous, the patient should be instructed to elevate the part above heart level and perform appropriate exercises to increase muscle pump action and venous return. Patients with shoulder or arm surgery should perform finger exercises or hand squeezes with a rubber ball. Patients with lower extremity surgery should perform dorsiflexion and plantar flexion (foot pumps). The reoccurrence of edema may indicate infection.

Capillary refill testing is used to evaluate arterial filling in the small vessels supplying the skin. It can be assumed that if the capillary refill is normal, the circulation in the larger vessels is also intact. Capillary refill is described in seconds. Either a nail bed or distal skin may be tested. The nail bed or skin is depressed with one finger until the skin blanches and then is released. The test site is then observed for the time it takes for skin color to return to normal. Normal capillary refill time is less than 3 seconds. Delayed capillary refill (greater than 3 seconds) indicates decreased tissue perfusion.

The sensory and motor assessments evaluate nerve function. Prior to testing sensation, the nurse should have the patient close her eyes, or the area to be tested should be obstructed from view with the bedsheets. This will prevent the patient from giving information based on what she sees instead of what she actually feels. If the patient underwent extremity surgery, testing of sensation distal to the surgical site is required. If the patient underwent spinal surgery or epidural anesthesia, a more comprehensive evaluation utilizing dermatomes should be performed. Nerve impulses may be delayed due to surgical complications or from compression of nerves by postoperative edema. When assessing sensation, the nurse should apply light touch and ask the patient "where" she feels the touch. If the patient is repeatedly asked, "Do you feel this?" the patient may reply yes because she feels that is the expectation and therefore gives inaccurate responses.

Motor strength is assessed by asking the patient to perform specific activities. These activities involve testing the patient's ability to move the part, the strength of the part in moving against gravity, and the strength of the part against resistance. Motor strength should be graded on a scale of 0 to 5. If the patient is unable to move the part, he receives a score of zero. If full strength is demonstrated and is equal to the unaffected part, the patient should receive a score of 5.

Pain Management

Patients are entitled to be in their "comfort zone" at all times. The nurse must assess the patient for the specific cause of pain and provide appropriate interventions. Knowledge of the medications administered during surgery and the timing of the last dose of pain medications is important for the nurse accepting the patient in the postanesthesia care unit (PACU) and the orthopedic unit. Pain medication may be administered via the epidural, oral, intramuscular, cutaneous, or intravenous route. Patient-controlled analgesia (PCA) or around-the-clock pain medication is often utilized in the early postoperative period. The PCA can be set to deliver a constant or basal rate in addition to the patient's being able to self-administer a preset dose at prescribed intervals to achieve pain control.

CHART 57–11	Pulse Strength Chart
0	No palpable pulse
1+	Weak, barely palpable, or easily obliterated
2+	Palpable
3+	Strong, easily palpable
4+	Bounding

Surgical pain is concentrated at the surgical site and is generally described as sharp and nonradiating. Pain assessment should be based on a consistent scale. Many scales are available for use using a numeric scale or pictures to help the patient describe her pain level. Each patient has a particular comfort level or pain tolerance level. Pharmacologic and nonpharmacologic interventions should be utilized to ensure that the patient's pain score is maintained within the comfort range. Pain may be anticipated prior to physical therapy or other activities and the patient offered pain medication prior to these activities. Pain is assessed with each set of vital signs and after administering pain medications.

Atypical pain requires a comprehensive assessment. The nurse should have the patient describe the location and quality of pain with each assessment. It should not be assumed that all pain is related to the surgical site. Chest pain, pain at sites other than the operative site, and increased pain should be evaluated to determine the cause. The underlying cause should be corrected to relieve the pain. For example, if the pain is cardiac in origin, interventions to relieve myocardial ischemia should be performed. Chapter 15 includes an in-depth discussion of pain management.

Appearance of Surgical Site and Dressing

The surgical dressing should be inspected for the presence of blood and drainage. In the immediate postoperative period, oozing of blood may be expected. The area of drainage should be marked using a pen or indelible marker so that the rate of bleeding can be objectively assessed. Excessive bleeding may indicate that a blood vessel has not been sufficiently contained during surgery. The surgeon should be notified if there is excessive bleeding. The surgeon may order additional reinforcement of the dressing, or it may require pharmacologic therapy such as vitamin K, cryoprecipitate, or discontinuation of anticoagulant therapy. In some cases, the patient may need to be returned to the operating room. Surgical wound drainage should be described as sanguineous if it is frankly bloody or serosanguineous if it is pinkish or blood mixed with plasma. Wound drainage may increase with patient movement, and the nurse should assess the patient's activity to determine whether the activity is causing strain on the suture line. Activities and positions that place stress or strain on the suture line should be avoided. The dressing of a spinal surgery patient should be assessed for the presence of cerebrospinal fluid (CSF). If CSF is present, the surgeon should be notified.

The surgeon is frequently the first person to change the primary surgical dressing. Symptoms of wound infection generally appear within 3 days of surgery and should be assessed within this time period. The suture line should be assessed to determine whether the skin is approximated and the sutures and staples are intact. Purulent or malodorous drainage should be reported to the surgeon. Infection is discussed later in this chapter in the Complications section.

Surgical Tubes and Drains

Postoperative orthopedic patients will frequently have surgical drains and urinary catheters. The urinary catheter should be discontinued as soon as the patient is able to get out of bed and ambulate, to reduce the risk of a urinary tract infection. The patient should be able to urinate within 8 hours after the urinary catheter is discontinued. Surgical drains may be discontinued 24 hours after surgery if output is less than about 50 milliliters in 24 hours. Many surgical drains use suction to withdraw blood and fluid. The nurse should ensure that the suction device used is activated. For example, a Hemovac or Jackson Pratt drain must be compressed to create suction. Chapter 67 includes an in-depth description of the various surgical drains.

Therapeutic Modalities

Many therapeutic modalities are commonly ordered for patients undergoing orthopedic surgery. **Continuous passive motion devices** (machines into which the affected extremity or joint is placed to perform slow, continuous passive range of motion to avoid stiffness and prevent a decrease in range of motion) may be utilized for patients who have knee surgery to prevent loss of range of motion of the joint. Sequential compression devices or compression stockings may be utilized in patients at risk for DVT. Cryotherapy units or ice bags may be utilized to decrease pain and swelling in the joint after surgery. Physical therapy as well as active and passive range of motion may be required to prevent loss of function and to maintain strength and range of motion in the orthopedic patient.

Exercise

Planned exercise is an important part of the recovery plan for the orthopedic surgical patient. Specific exercises, often called therapeutic exercises, will be prescribed to promote and maintain range of motion and function. The plan of care for the patient should include specific measurable goals for the patient. Because orthopedic surgery is generally performed to improve function or repair a defect, typical goals include range of motion, the strength of the limb, or ability to participate in the rehabilitation exercise program. Specificity and measurability of the goal are important so that it is clear whether the patient has attained it or not. For example, if the goal for a patient is that he will be able to ambulate independently 50 feet by day 2 after surgery is not met and the patient ambulates with assistance for only 20 feet, there is an objective starting point for the analysis of why the goal was not accomplished. The patient should be encouraged to continue the exercises prescribed in the hospital after discharge. An overall general health exercise program should be encouraged as well to ensure cardiovascular and bone health.

Discharge Planning

Knowledge of where the patient resides, the physical aspects of the residence such as number of stairs or size of bathrooms (is the bathroom large enough for the patient to turn around in with a walker?), is information necessary to plan for the patient's safe discharge. Presence of children or significant others who are willing to assist the patient after hospitalization will influence the discharge plan. Elder patients who have had joint replacement surgery frequently require skilled nursing care beyond hospitalization. If the hospitalized elder is a primary caregiver for a spouse now left at home without assistance, the patient will need to make arrangements to provide care for the spouse during the current hospitalization. Anxiety related to home and financial concerns can impede the patient's recovery and rehabilitation.

Postoperative precautions and exercises may also be taught prior to surgery. Precautions and exercises to be performed depend on the surgical site (back, lower extremity, upper extremity, and pelvis). In some cases the patient may be asked to perform exercises such as walking to build endurance, specific exercises to improve circulation, or exercises to increase strength and range of motion.

Environment

The physical environment of the home should be discussed with the patient. Specific accommodations may be necessary, and the patient should plan for these prior to discharge. For example, the patient may require a hospital bed after surgery, and friend or family assistance should be elicited to configure the environment for this. Throw rugs should be removed, if necessary, to prevent falls. Postoperative equipment such as cryotherapy, hospital bed, elevated toilet seat, or continuous passive motion (CPM) devices should be ordered and their presence in the home assured prior to discharge. If the patient will have activity restrictions or precautions after surgery, the physical environment in the home may need simple alterations such as the movement of articles for activities of daily living to an accessible area. If the patient resides in a physical environment that prevents activity prescribed for recovery or ability to obtain access to health care appointments or supplies, the nurse must assist the patient to develop an alternate plan for home care. If friends or family are unable to assist with an alternate living situation for the recovery period, assistance from discharge planning or social work may be needed to assist patient placement in a rehabilitation, assisted living, or skilled nursing facility.

Complications

The nurse should be knowledgeable regarding not only potential complications related to general surgery but also complications specific to orthopedic surgery. The nurse must be alert to subtle, early signs and symptoms of complications and respond quickly to prevent permanent disability, decompensation, or delays in recovery.

Respiratory Insufficiency

Pulmonary complications in the orthopedic surgical patient may be related to a variety of causative factors. **Fat embolus** is a complication specific to orthopedic injuries involving long bone fracture. Fat globules from the bone marrow travel into the venous system and to the pulmonary vessels. Fat blocks the pulmonary vessels and inactivates surfactant, which promotes the development of acute respiratory distress syndrome (ARDS). The patient will develop respiratory distress: tachypnea, air hunger, and hypoxia. Other signs and symptoms associated with fat embolus are fever, tachycardia, restlessness, decreased mental status, and petechiae. Arterial blood gas findings demonstrate an initial decrease in $PaCO_2$ followed by increased $PaCO_2$ and low PaO_2. Other diagnostic tests such as chest x-ray and ventilation/perfusion scan are nonspecific for fat embolus. Patients with suspected fat embolus should be intubated and placed on mechanical ventilation with positive end-expiratory pressure (PEEP). Treatment is largely supportive until the condition resolves. A detailed discussion of the diagnosis and management of ARDS is in Chapter 36 .

Pulmonary embolus may also cause respiratory insufficiency and is usually associated with deep venous thrombosis. Signs and symptoms are similar to fat embolus, but pulmonary embolus is not generally associated with the development of ARDS.

After arrival to the medical–surgical floor, the patient should be monitored closely for the first 4 to 12 hours to ensure that the vital signs remain stable and the respiratory rate and effort appropriate. Routine vital signs and respiratory status are then observed for the remainder of hospitalization. Incentive spirometry is typically ordered for the postoperative period to promote lung expansion and prevent respiratory complications such as atelectasis and pneumonia. Typically, the patient is encouraged to perform incentive spirometry every 1 to 2 hours while awake. Coughing and deep breathing should follow use of the incentive spirometer to assist in the removal of secretions from smaller airways. Patients are now assisted out of bed as soon as they are able, depending of the type of surgery. Sitting in a chair enables the patient to expand the thorax to a greater degree than while in bed and also acts to promote respiratory function. Pneumonia is a serious complication, particularly for the gerontological postoperative patient. The patient may be at risk for aspiration pneumonia related to decreased mental status, use of nasogastric (NG) tubes, or preexisting medical conditions such as stroke or dysphagia. Elevations in temperature should alert the nurse to the potential that the patient has atelectasis or pneumonia. Aggressive pulmonary toilet is needed to remove secretions and improve airway exchange.

Venous Thromboembolism

Venous thromboembolism (VTE) includes both deep venous thrombosis (DVT) and pulmonary embolism. Risk factors in the orthopedic surgical population include immobility of a limb, long surgical times in a single position, hypercoagulablity of blood due to activation of the clotting cascade from surgical stimulation and from being NPO, as well as endothelial disruption from the surgery or trauma itself. The three factors of venous stasis, hypercoagulability, and vessel injury make up Virchow's triad for VTE risk. Virchow's triad is discussed in Chapter 43 .

Patients undergoing total hip and total knee repair/replacement surgery are at high risk for DVT, and current standards of practice include providing DVT prophylaxis in these patient populations. Prevention strategies to decrease the incidence of DVT include the administration of heparin (unfractionated or low molecular weight), the use of antiembolism stockings, and the use of sequential compression devices. Most pulmonary emboli occur as the result of DVT. Additional risk factors for VTE include obesity, use of oral contraceptives, old age, varicose veins, prior VTE, and Factor V Leiden (FVL) gene mutation. Factor V Leiden disorder is the most common blood coagulation disorder. Approximately 4% to 7% of the population is heterozygous for Factor V Leiden disorder. The risk of VTE in a heterozygous patient is increased in the presence of other risk factors such as obesity or use of oral contraceptives. Homozygous Factor V Leiden disorder severely increases the risk of thromboembolic event, and these patients are placed on anticoagulants (Edmonds, Crichton, Runciman, & Pradhan, 2004; Folsom et al., 2002; Ornstein & Cushman, 2003).

In spite of appropriate therapy, the incidence of DVT in orthopedic patients is still prevalent, and nurses must be diligent in assessing patients for signs and symptoms of DVT. DVT symptoms may be nonspecific. The patient may complain of pain in an extremity. The extremity may become swollen, edematous, and tender at or distal to the clot. Although the legs are the most common site for DVT, immobile arms are also at risk to develop clots. Pain associated with DVT may increase with exercise of the part. A positive Homans' sign is associated with lower leg DVT. Homans' sign is considered positive when plantar and dorsiflexion on the affected side cause calf pain. DVT is discussed in detail in Chapter 43 ☺ .

Symptoms of VTE may range from dramatic to nonspecific. The patient with pulmonary embolism may have acute onset of chest pain, shortness of breath, decreased sensorium, and pink, frothy sputum. Typically, the patient with pulmonary embolism will demonstrate tachycardia and tachypnea. Arterial blood gases may be normal or demonstrate hypoxia. Oxygen saturation may be normal or decreased in pulmonary embolism. Pulmonary embolism is discussed in detail in Chapter 36 ☺ .

Compartment Syndrome

Compartment syndrome is a rare condition occurring when swelling within an anatomical compartment restricts blood flow. An anatomical compartment is one in which the fascia or an external device such as a cast prohibits expansion of the compartment as edema and engorgement increase. This causes compression of vascular and nervous system structures. As edema and engorgement increase, pain increases and is unrelieved by narcotic pain medication administration. The area affected will be swollen and tense. Pain significantly increases with extension or flexion of the affected part. There may be changes in the neurovascular assessment of the patient indicating that compartment syndrome is present. The patient may have pain, paresthesia, pulselessness, paralysis, and/or pallor of the part. If compartment syndrome in an extremity is suspected, the extremity should not be elevated, but should be maintained at the level of the heart to improve perfusion. Normal tissue pressure is less than 15 mmHg. Numerous devices may be utilized to determine tissue or compartment pressure. If the tissue or compartment pressure is greater than 30 mmHg, compartment syndrome should be suspected. Treatment of compartment syndrome requires release of the constriction to accommodate swelling. If a cast is causing the restriction, it should be bivalved (cut down both sides). If the constriction is at the fascial level, the patient will require surgery. There are devices available that can be inserted through the skin to measure the actual compartment pressure. If the nurse suspects compartment syndrome is present, the surgeon should be notified immediately to prevent permanent disability or loss of limb.

Pressure Ulcers

Patients with orthopedic injuries are also at particular risk for the development of preventable pressure ulcers. For example, patients with hip surgery are at particular risk for heel pressure ulcers. The heels should be floated off of the mattress utilizing pillows. If the pillows are insufficient to maintain the heels off of the bed, assistive devices such as heel lift boots or specialty pressure relief beds or mattresses may be utilized. The best tool to prevent pressure ulcer development is repositioning the patient

at least every 2 hours. Frequent assessment of the skin allows early detection of potential impairments in skin integrity requiring more aggressive interventions. The orthopedic patient may also develop pressure ulcers in areas where prosthetic devices, casts, splints, or traction causes friction. If there is evidence of friction, extra padding may be needed, or adjustment of the splint, prosthesis, or cast may be necessary.

Infection

Patients with traumatic injuries such as open fractures, preexisting infection, cardiovascular disease or diabetes, and extremes of age are at risk of developing postoperative infections. Postoperative infection will increase the duration of hospitalization and may precipitate sepsis. Prior to surgery the skin over the surgical site is prepped with an antibacterial solution such as povidone-iodine; or if there is an existing wound, it is irrigated copiously with normal saline. Although prophylactic antibiotic therapy, typically a cephalosporin, is given preoperatively and postoperatively, infection may occur. The nurse should be alert to the signs and symptoms of postoperative surgical site infection. Signs of surgical infection include redness, erythema, warmth, edema, purulent drainage, dehiscence of the suture site, and fever. A wound culture may be obtained to determine the organism responsible for the infection and appropriate antibiotic coverage. The sutures or staples may be removed to promote local therapy with wound dressings.

Osteomyelitis is infection of the bone itself. The incidence of osteomyelitis is highest in patients who have had compound fractures, external fixator devices, and open orthopedic procedures. This infection may be related to invasion by bacteria, fungus, or virus. Tuberculosis infection may occur in the bone tissue as a result of exposure to tuberculosis. The patient may complain of deep bone pain. Failure of the surgical site or pressure ulcer to heal may be the first indication that osteomyelitis is present. Confirmation that osteomyelitis is present may be obtained from MRI, CT, x-ray, bone biopsy, or bone scan. Treatment for osteomyelitis requires long-term, generally 6 weeks of, antibiotic therapy.

Late complications of orthopedic surgery include infection of the surgical hardware. The decision to remove the hardware is dependent on the impact on patient mobility, pain level, age, and potential complications such as neurovascular injury, deformity, and inability to replace the implant, which may have significant impact on the patient's mobility and ability to continue working in her current occupation. In cases of external fixator devices or screw implants, removal of hardware is less complicated and does not necessarily impact the patient's activities of daily living. If bone has healed and the screws or plates are no longer necessary for joint or bone stability, the surgery has far less impact on patient mobility and ability to carry out activities of daily living or occupational activities.

Joint Dislocation

Dislocation may occur due to overextension of the joint. Complications of dislocation include pain, decreased range of motion, and neurovascular compromise. Strict adherence to joint precautions can prevent complications of dislocation. Signs and symptoms of joint dislocation include swelling, pain, immobility, and shortening (the extremity appears shorter than the unaffected extremity).

Heterotrophic Ossification

Heterotrophic ossification (HO) is the development of bone tissue in areas where bone tissue is not normally present. Myositis ossificans progressiva develops in childhood and is the progressive development of bone tissue (ossification) in soft tissues throughout the body. The life span of patients with myositis ossificans progressiva is severely shortened, and patients frequently die from complications of compression of vital organs from lesions in the second or third decade. Heterotrophic ossification is a late complication that may be seen in musculoskeletal and spinal cord injury. The exact mechanism of bone formation is not known, but it is thought to be an inflammatory reaction of intramuscular and connective tissue after injury or surgery. Sepsis or infection may predispose the patient to the development of HO. Symptoms associated with heterotrophic ossification depend on the site and size of the lesion. In spinal cord injury, the site of the anomalous bone lesion is always lower than the level of injury. Frequent sites of post-traumatic heterotrophic ossification are the soft tissues surrounding the hips, knees, shoulders, or elbows. Patients may be asymptomatic if the lesion is small; or they may experience pain, decreased range of motion, and signs of inflammation or infection if the lesion is large or interferes with joint motion. Signs and symptoms in an extremity with a heterotrophic lesion may include pain, swelling, rubor, pain, and fever. Because these signs and symptoms are similar to those of venous thrombosis, the patient will have radiologic studies such as a bone scan and x-rays to determine whether the patient has heterotrophic ossification, as well as testing for VTE such as D-dimer and ultrasound flow studies of the extremity.

Treatment of heterotrophic ossification includes administration of nonsteroidal anti-inflammatory medications and indomethacin for pain, in addition to focused radiation to the joint. These medications may decrease the development of heterotrophic ossification as well. Etidronate disodium may be administered to patients prone to the development of heterotrophic ossification to prevent lesion formation, and is administered preoperatively and postoperatively when the HO lesions are surgically excised.

Osteonecrosis or Avascular Necrosis

Osteonecrosis (avascular necrosis) is the death of bone tissue and may occur at any time after injury to bone due to impairment of circulation. Patients at high risk of osteonecrosis include patients taking steroids, receiving radiation therapy, or with alcohol dependence. Many medical conditions such as sickle cell anemia, HIV, gout, and osteoporosis may be predisposed to osteonecrosis.

▉ Collaborative Management

A multidisciplinary team approach is necessary to optimize care for the orthopedic surgical patient. The surgeon determines the activity prescription for the patient, and the nurse works collaboratively with the physical therapists to enable the patient to perform activities to the level of his capabilities. It is important that any required restrictions to activity and precautions to prevent hip dislocation or spinal torque be taken. Because many patients will have comorbid conditions, this collaboration ensures patient safety. Adequate nutrition is necessary for wound healing and to maintain patient strength. The clinical dietician is a valuable team member to provide input regarding adequate caloric intake that adheres to dietary restrictions that may be present for patients with cardiovascular, endocrine, or renal disease. Because many hip replacement and amputation patients may require home care assistance and assistive devices, or skilled care after discharge, discharge planners and/or social work assistance is helpful. Individual patients may also require psychiatric consultation depending on their response to their surgery or the event that caused the surgery to be necessary. Spiritual support for patients during hospitalization may also assist the patients in adapting successfully to their current situation and maintaining a positive outlook necessary to participate fully in rehabilitation efforts.

Health Promotion

The greatest impact that nurses can have regarding musculoskeletal injuries and surgery is that of prevention. Patients who have musculoskeletal surgery generally receive explicit instructions on how to prevent the recurrence of their injury. It would be a great service to elders to provide information on home safety before they become injured and have surgery. Safety devices to prevent injury such as bathroom safety bars should be made available to elders by their health plans or should be a requirement for installation by landlords.

Another method in which health care providers can improve eldercare is by reviewing medications at each visit and in pharmacies. Over-the-counter medications should be included in the pharmacy medication lists so that better prevention of polypharmacy reactions is achieved.

Health promotion includes regular exercise. Walking not only is an excellent cardiovascular exercise but also maintains bone mass. Obesity is increasing in the United States, and education on the effects of obesity on knee and hip joints may assist in promoting the maintenance of appropriate weight maintenance.

Hormone replacement therapy to prevent osteoporosis remains controversial. Women who are postmenopausal should be encouraged to perform exercises and maintain calcium levels with supplements, or oral bisphosphonates may assist in preventing bone loss. Women should receive education by their health care providers on the options available.

The nurses in the presurgical clinic, the postanesthesia care unit, and the surgical unit, the home care nurse, and the skilled nursing facility all play a pivotal role in the care of the patient undergoing musculoskeletal surgery. The nurse who is knowledgeable about the patient's history, needs, preferences, and available resources is in a unique position to promote a positive surgical experience for the patient. Holistic and focused assessments and early intervention act to prevent postoperative complications and ensure that the patient receives prompt treatment to prevent permanent disability or prolonged rehabilitation times. A comprehensive knowledge of the potential complications associated with particular injuries and surgeries enables the nurse to focus on prevention and early detection of potential problems. The nurse who understands the importance of postoperative activities such as turning and positioning, exercise, and assessment of neurovascular status will provide vigilant care that assists the patient in achieving care goals. Through interaction with the patient in obtaining the history and assisting the patient with activities, the nurse can obtain data and utilize information to create and implement a plan of care specific to the patient as an individual.

Research

There are multiple opportunities for research available in the realm of musculoskeletal surgical complications and therapies.

It is an exciting time in nursing research, and important practice changes are beginning to rely on new evidence. Any of the questions listed in the Research Opportunities and Clinical Impact box lend themselves to study that may impact the future of orthopedic nursing care.

RESEARCH OPPORTUNITIES AND CLINICAL IMPACT RELATED TO MUSCULOSKELETAL SURGICAL PROCEDURES

Research Opportunities	Clinical Impact
Prophylactic antibiotic therapy is commonplace for orthopedic surgical procedures. Studies could be performed comparing the infection rates in low-risk patients, comparing the use of prophylactic antibiotics versus placebo.	Is the use of prophylactic antibiotic therapy necessary, or should it be reserved for patients who are at high risk of infection?
Which therapy is more effective in preventing deep venous thrombosis (DVT): sequential compression devices or elastic compression stockings? Many institutions utilize both. Is this overkill or an added expense? Research studies could compare the use of sequential compression devices alone versus the use of elastic compression stockings alone versus the use of both.	Possible cost savings for the institution and the patient.
Is there a difference in discharge date or ability to participate in postoperative activities in patients who receive regional/epidural anesthesia versus those who receive general anesthesia? Are there differences in the perceived ability to participate in postoperative activities between the two groups? Are there differences in the postoperative pain scores between the two groups? Is there a difference in the pain scores reported between patients receiving pain-controlled analgesia (PCA) versus those who received epidural anesthesia?	Possibility of decreased hospital stay for the patient.
Is there a difference in the range of motion, distance ambulated between patients who receive preoperative exercise counseling prior to elective joint replacement and those who do not?	Possibility of decreased hospital stay for the patient. Decreased rehabilitation time.

Clinical Preparation

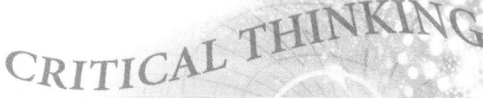

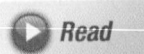 **Read**

- History of Current Illness
- Past Medical History
- Physical Exam
- Admitting Medical Orders
- Laboratory Study Results

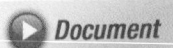 **Document**

- Summary of Hospitalization
- Pathophysiology Form
- Laboratory Values
- Laboratory Results Explanation

 **Apply**

- List of Potential Nursing Diagnoses
- Concept Map
- Critical Thinking Questions

Log on to MyNursingKit.com to download forms you will need and to complete further steps in the Clinical Preparation assignment.

HISTORY OF PRESENT ILLNESS

Mrs. T. is a 72-year-old patient who was admitted to the hospital for right total hip replacement. She has right hip osteoarthritis as the result of osteonecrosis secondary to prednisone use for polymyalgia rheumatica. She has painful right knee arthritis and end-stage right hip osteoarthritis not responding to conservative management and was scheduled for right total hip replacement. A posterior approach total hip replacement was performed under general anesthesia. Estimated blood loss during the procedure was 1,000 mL. Cell Saver was utilized during the procedure and shed blood returned to the patient as was planned preoperatively. The patient was sent to the recovery room in stable condition.

Medical–Surgical History

The patient has a history of hypertension, mild cardiovascular disease, obesity, polymyalgia rheumatica, and right knee arthritis. Her surgical history includes a hysterectomy at age 50 due to fibroid tumors, and removal of her gallbladder at age 35 due to gallstones.

Social History

Mrs. T. is a retired teacher who lives alone in a retirement community. She has two daughters and one son who all live in the area. She has never smoked and has a glass of wine each evening.

Physical Exam

You receive the patient on day 1 postoperatively from her right total hip replacement. She is awake, alert, and oriented. Her vital signs are within normal limits. Breath sounds are equal bilaterally, diminished at the bases with rales. Her abdomen is slightly distended, soft, nontender with minimal bowel sounds. The patient states that she has not passed flatus or had a bowel movement since the surgery. The patient has a Foley catheter that is draining clear, yellow urine. Motor and sensory of all extremities are intact. Her surgical site is clean, dry, and intact. She complains of pain to the right hip at a 6 on the scale of 1–10.

Admitting Medical Orders

Service: orthopedic surgery
Diagnosis: right hip replacement
Allergies: none
Vital signs: every 4 hours including oxygen saturation, and neurovascular checks to right lower extremity
Call house officer: temp > 38.5°C, HR > 110 or < 60, RR > 30 or < 12, BP sys > 160 or < 90, O_2 sat < 92%, urine output < 120 mL in 4 hours, change in neurovascular exam to right lower extremity, any Hct result that is 5 less than the baseline postoperative Hct
Activity: up to chair 4 times per day with assistance; ambulate with physical therapy twice daily
Posterior hip precautions:
- Hip abductor pillow while in bed
- Do not bend hip greater than 90 degrees
- Use an elevated toilet seat
- Do not sit in low chairs
- Do not twist or turn the body toward the operative side
- Do not turn leg and foot inward
- Keep operative leg straight when getting up and use your arms to push up

Diet: low-sodium, low-fat diet
IV: D5/.45NS with 20 mEq KCl IV at 100 mL/hr
Foley to gravity drainage
I&O: every shift
Respiratory care: use incentive spirometer hourly when awake
DVT prophylaxis: low-molecular-weight heparin, sequential compression devices to lower extremities

Scheduled Medications

Atenolol 50 mg po daily
Nifedipine 30 mg po daily
Lisinopril 10 mg po daily
Cefazolin sodium 1 g IV q8h for 6 doses
Enoxaparin 30 mg subcutaneously q12h
Oxycodone HCl 10 mg po q12h around the clock (hold for delirium)
Docusate sodium 100 mg po bid

PRN Medications

Magnesium hydroxide (laxative) oral 2,400 mg po prn
Morphine sulfate 1–3 mg IV q2h prn for severe pain
Metoclopramide hydrochloride (Reglan) 10 mg IV q6h prn for nausea and vomiting

Ordered Laboratory Studies

CBC and electrolyte panel every morning

LABORATORY STUDY RESULTS

Test	Preop	Postop, Immediate	Postop Day 1
WBC	8/mm³	12/mm³	9 K/mm³
RBC	4.55/mm³	4.27/mm³	4.30/mm³
Hemoglobin	11 g/dL	9.8 g/dL	9.5 g/dL
Hematocrit	32%	29%	28%
Platelet count	221/mm³	196/mm³	196/mm³
APTT	30 seconds	31 seconds	
INR	1.2	1.0	1.0
Sodium	135 mEq/L	140 mEq/L	138 mEq/L
Potassium	3.4 mEq/L	3.1 mEq/L	3.5 mEq/L
Chloride	102 mEq/L	105 mEq/L	103 mEq/L
Carbon dioxide	23 mEq/L	25 mEq/L	24 mEq/L
Urea nitrogen	11 mg/dL	12 mg/dL	12 mg/dL
Creatinine blood	0.8 mg/dL	1.0 mg/dL	1.0 mg/dL
Glucose	130 mg/dL	140 mg/dL	120 mg/dL
Calcium	8.1 mg/dL	8.1 mg/dL	8.3 mg/dL
Lipase	17 unit/dL	20 unit/dL	19 unit/dL

CRITICAL THINKING QUESTIONS

1. How can you distinguish the difference between expected postoperative pain and the pain caused by compartment syndrome?

2. What areas of assessment must be performed immediately upon a patient's admission to the nursing unit after orthopedic surgery?

3. What types of precautions are necessary for a patient who has had a total hip replacement?

4. How are pulmonary complications prevented during the postoperative period?
What assessments and actions do you perform for a confused elderly postoperative patient?

Answers to Critical Thinking Questions appear in Appendix D.

NCLEX® REVIEW

1. A patient has undergone surgery for a fractured tibia. The nurse plans to complete a neurovascular assessment. Which of the following aspects will be included? Select all that apply.
   1. Pain level
   2. Pulse quality
   3. Sensation and movement
   4. Color of extremity
   5. Level of consciousness
   6. Use of muscles

2. A nurse is reviewing home care with a patient following a hip replacement procedure. Which of the following instructions would be included?
   1. Slightly bend the operative leg when getting up from the chair or bed.
   2. Exercise the affected extremity by turning the leg inward 5–10 times.
   3. Progressively increase the amount of bending at the waist daily.
   4. Use an elevated toilet seat in the main bathroom at home.

3. The nurse strongly suspects the occurrence of compartment syndrome in a patient wearing a long-leg cast. In preparation for the health care provider to come and perform the necessary treatment; the nurse would gather what supplies or equipment?
   1. Ace bandages to wrap around the bivalved cast
   2. Extra pillows to elevate the casted leg above the heart
   3. Syringe, needle and topical anesthetic to aspirate the hematoma
   4. A percussion hammer to physically assess reflexes for damage

4. Of the following assistive devices, which would be the most appropriate for home use for a patient who has undergone a total hip replacement procedure?
   1. Heel lift boot
   2. A "reacher" tool
   3. Continuous passive motion (CPM) machine
   4. Wheelchair

5. A nurse is serving as a preceptor for a new graduate on an orthopedic unit. As they enter a patient's room using patient's-controlled analgesia (PCA), the nurse states, "This pump is delivering a 2 mg basal rate of morphine sulfate, along with prn doses." The new graduate reflects understanding of the order through which statement?
   1. "The patient receives 2 mg of the drug when he pushes the delivery button."
   2. "Every hour 2 mg of morphine is delivered continuously."
   3. "The maximum amount of morphine to be received is 2 mg per hour."
   4. "The pump administers a beginning dose of 2 mg and increases the amount hourly."

Answers for review questions appear in Appendix D

KEY TERMS

amputation p.1816
arthrodesis p.1821
arthroplasty p.1807
compartment syndrome p.1828

continuous passive motion device p.1826
discectomy p.1816
fat embolus p.1827
heterotrophic ossification (HO) p.1829

laminectomy p.1816
osteolysis p.1811
osteonecrosis p.1829
total joint replacement p.1807

PEARSON
EXPLORE mynursingkit™

MyNursingKit is your one stop for online chapter review materials and resources. Prepare for success with additional NCLEX®-style practice questions, interactive assignments and activities, web links, animations and videos, and more!

Register your access code from the front of your book at
www.mynursingkit.com

REFERENCES

American Academy of Orthopaedic Surgeons (AAOS). (2001). *Bunion surgery.* Retrieved May 28, 2008, from http://orthoinfo.aaos.org/topic.cfm?topic=A00140

American Academy of Orthopaedic Surgeons (AAOS). (2005). *Sprained ankle.* Retrieved May 27, 2008, from http://orthoinfo.aaos.org/topic.cfm?topic=A00150

American Academy of Orthopaedic Surgeons (AAOS). (2007a). *Rotator cuff tears.* Retrieved May 29, 2008, from http://orthoinfo.aaos.org/topic.cfm?topic=A00064

American Academy of Orthopaedic Surgeons (AAOS). (2007b). *Arthritis of the shoulder.* Retrieved May 30, 2008, from http://orthoinfo.aaos.org/topic.cfm?topic=A00222

American Academy of Orthopaedic Surgeons (AAOS). (2007c). *Osteoarthritis of the elbow.* Retrieved May 31, 2008, from http://orthoinfo.aaos.org/topic.cfm?topic=A00421

American Academy of Orthopaedic Surgeons (AAOS). (2007d). *Carpal tunnel syndrome.* Retrieved June 2, 2008, from http://orthoinfo.aaos.org/topic.cfm?topic=A00005#Anatomy

American Academy of Orthopaedic Surgeons (AAOS). (2007e). *Wrist joint replacement (wrist arthroplasty).* Retrieved June 2, 2008, from http://orthoinfo.aaos.org/topic.cfm?topic=A00019

American Academy of Orthopaedic Surgeons (AAOS). (2007f). *ACL injury: Does it require surgery?* Retrieved June 2, 2008, from http://orthoinfo.aaos.org/topic.cfm?topic=A00297

Arthritis Foundation. (2008). *Arthritis and related diseases.* Retrieved August 29, 2008, from http://www.arthritis.org/faq.php

Edmonds, M. J., Crichton, T. J., Runciman, W. B., & Pradhan, M. (2004). Evidenced-based risk factors for postoperative deep vein thrombosis. *ANZ Journal of Surgery, 74,* 1082–1097.

eMedicineHealth. (2008). *Lumbar laminectomy.* Retrieved June 10, 2008, from http://www.emedicinehealth.com/lumbar_laminectomy/article_em.htm

eOrthopod. (2003). *Wrist anatomy.* Retrieved June 2, 2008, from http://www.eorthopod.com/public/patient_education/6607/wrist_anatomy.html

Folsom, A. R., Cushman, M., Tsai, M. Y., Aleksic, N., Heckbert, S. R., Boland, L. L., et al. (2002). A prospective study of venous thromboembolism in relation to Factor V Leiden and related factors. *Blood, 99*(8), 2720–2725.

Matson, F. A., III, & Warme, W. J. (2008). *Total shoulder joint replacement for shoulder arthritis: Surgery with a dependable, time-tested conservative prosthesis and accelerated rehabilitation can lessen pain and improve function in shoulders with arthritis.* Retrieved May 30, 2008, from http://www.orthop.washington.edu/uw/shoulderreplacement/tabID__3376/ItemID__62/Articles/Default.aspx

Ornstein, D. L., & Cushman, M. (2003). Factor V Leiden. *Circulation, 107,* e94–e97.

Wahl, C. J., & Slaney, S. L. (2005). *Arthroscopic shoulder surgery for shoulder dislocation, subluxation, and instability: Why, when and how it is done.* Retrieved May 30, 2008, from http://www.orthop.washington.edu/uw/arthroscopic/tabID__3376/ItemID__162/Articles/Default.aspx

Caring for the Patient with Arthritis and Connective Tissue Disorders

Kathy Riccosa

With contributions by:
Cheryl Wraa
Kathleen Osborn

Outcome-Based Learning Objectives

After studying this chapter, the learner will be able to:

1. Differentiate autoimmune disease from connective tissue disease.
2. Utilize the nursing process when planning care for each autoimmune disease.
3. Compare and contrast the etiology, pathophysiology, clinical manifestations, nursing management, and prevention of the various types of arthritis.
4. Identify the four highest priority nursing diagnoses for rheumatoid arthritis and osteoarthritis.
5. Describe nursing management for patients experiencing gout.
6. Compare and contrast the clinical manifestations and nursing management of each of the following connective tissue diseases: (a) myositis, (b) polymyositis, and (c) dermatomyositis.

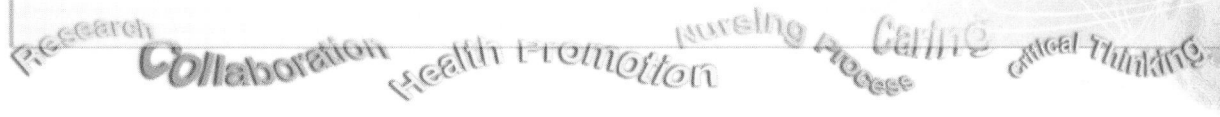

CONNECTIVE TISSUE consists of cells surrounded in an extracellular matrix of fibers, which serves to add strength and support, bind, and protect the various organs of the body. Three types of fibers make up the various connective tissues found in the body: collagen fibers, reticular fibers, and elastic fibers. Any inflammation of these tissues in joints can cause connective tissue disorders. Common connective tissue disorders include lupus erythematosus, gout, and Lyme disease. It is frequently very difficult to make a definitive diagnosis because signs and symptoms are often vague. It is projected that 37% of the population in the United States, or 1 million people, have a heritable connective tissue disorder (WrongDiagnosis.com, 2008). Connective tissue disorders are not just one disease, but a collection of more than 100 unique conditions that can destroy the connective tissue of the joints and have results ranging from daily pain to complete immobility.

Arthritis

Arthritis is a common descriptive term that applies to the collection of rheumatic diseases that can be localized, self-limiting conditions or systemic, autoimmune processes (Porth, 2005). It is estimated that by the year 2030, 67 million Americans 18 years of age and older will be diagnosed by a health care provider as having arthritis (Centers for Disease Control and Prevention [CDC], 2007).

Osteoarthritis: Epidemiology and Etiology

Osteoarthritis (OA), the most common form of arthritis, is a chronic condition that accompanies aging, most commonly affecting weight-bearing joints. OA is a leading cause of pain and disability in the elderly. Seventy percent of people age 40 and older and 80% of those age 65 and older are afflicted with this chronic condition (FamilyPracticeNotebook.com, 2008; Porth, 2005). Osteoarthritis (OA) was previously thought to be a normal consequence of aging; however, it is now realized that osteoarthritis results from a complex interplay of multiple factors, including joint integrity, genetic predisposition, local inflammation, mechanical forces, and cellular and biochemical processes. The disease can occur as a primary idiopathic disorder that is localized or generalized (involves more than three joints). Secondary OA is due to an underlying cause such as congenital defects of joint structure, single severe trauma or multiple traumas, inflammatory diseases, or metabolic disorders. The disease is usually diagnosed by an overall clinical impression based on the patient's age, history, findings on physical examination, and radiographic findings (Kalunian, 2007; Porth, 2005).

Pathophysiology

Joint degeneration with OA occurs on the articular surfaces of the cartilage with bony formations at the edges of weight-bearing joints, such as the knees and hips. OA also involves the joints of the fingers at the proximal interphalangeal joints (Figure 58–1 ■), and can affect the wrists, elbows, ankles, spinal vertebrae and joints of the pelvis. OA results in significant changes in both the composition and the mechanical properties of cartilage. Early in the disease the cartilage contains more water and fewer concentrations of proteoglycans, the large molecules that afford elasticity and stiffness and allow cartilage to

resist compression. There is also a decrease in local synthesis of new collagen and an increase in the breakdown of existing collagen. It is thought that the changes are a result of the release of cytokines that stimulate production and the release of enzymes that are destructive to joint structures. This damage predisposes the cartilage tissue to more injury and impairs the cells' ability to repair the damage by producing new collagen and proteoglycans (Porth, 2005).

Clinical Manifestations

Patients will complain of a brief interval of morning stiffness, pain on motion with overuse of affected joint, and over time the possibility of joint bone deformity (FamilyPracticeNotebook.com, 2008). Joints most frequently affected are the knees, hips, cervical and lumbar vertebrae, proximal and distal joints of the hand, and the first metatarsophalangeal joints of the feet (Porth, 2005).

Laboratory and Diagnostic Procedures

According to the Hospital for Special Surgery (2005) three different radiologic techniques are used to determine the diagnosis of arthritis: plain radiographs of the affected joint, computed tomography (CT), and magnetic resonance imaging (MRI). See the Diagnostic Tests box for these diagnostic tests as well as the radiologic tests used to identify OA and the expected abnormalities that would be found.

Medical Management

Initially, the best treatment for weight-bearing joints is rest. As the condition becomes more progressive, then nonsteroidal anti-inflammatory agents may be taken to alleviate discomfort of the affected joints. Medications used would include classifications such as nonsteroidal anti-inflammatory drugs (NSAIDs), cyclooxygenase-2 (COX-2) inhibitors, and antimalarials to relieve symptoms. The Pharmacology Summary feature on page 1839 outlines medications used to treat arthritis and connective tissue disorders. A multidisciplinary approach may include a nutritionist to help with weight reduction and a physical therapist to develop an exercise program to include range-of-motion exercises.

Once the patient exhausts previous options and the patient's quality of life is further compromised, surgical intervention

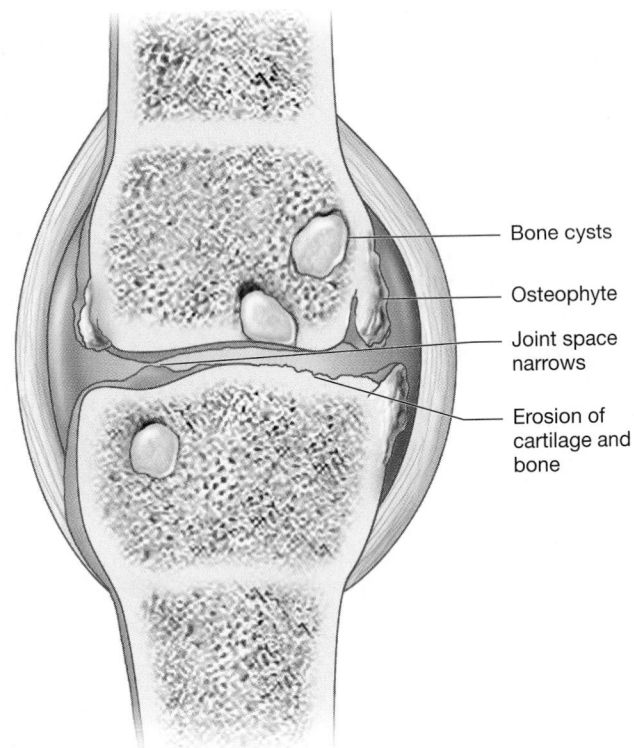

Bone cysts
Osteophyte
Joint space narrows
Erosion of cartilage and bone

FIGURE 58–1 ■ Joint degeneration with OA.

DIAGNOSTIC TESTS for Osteoarthritis

Test	Expected Abnormality	Rationale for Abnormality
DIAGNOSTIC TEST		
Bone density	Increased. Asymmetrical joint cartilage loss.	Subchondral sclerosis. Confirmation of bone on bone contact.
Erythrocyte sedimentation rate (ESR)	Increased.	Presence of inflammatory disease.
Rheumatoid factor	Negative.	No rheumatoid arthritis.
RADIOLOGIC TEST		
X-ray	Degenerative changes. Narrowing of bone space.	Articular surfaces are worn where bone rubs against bone.
Computed tomography (CT)	Bone spurs.	Bone cyst and sclerosis are common with disease progression.
Magnetic resonance imaging (MRI)	Reactive bone edema. Soft tissue swelling. Bone fragments within the joint.	Very sensitive test to bony and soft tissue changes. Able to identify early degenerative changes.

should be considered. There are three kinds of surgical procedures that can improve the health of patients suffering from osteoarthritis: synovectomy, arthrodesis, and reconstructive surgery. A synovectomy is the removal of the swollen synovial casing prior to damage to the bone and cartilage taking place. Fusion of the joint is called arthrodesis. An arthrodesis is done when there is severe destruction of the surfaces of the joint. Joint replacements, usually total knee or total hips, are done when these weight-bearing joints have been completely damaged. It is important that the patient be aware of options in order to make an informed decision about the care received. For a detailed discussion regarding orthopedic surgery, refer to Chapter 57 ⊙.

Nursing Management

The nursing process provides a framework to create a comprehensive plan of care for the patient with OA. The nursing process will lead the nurse in utilizing the problem-solving approach in caring for patients with OA. The nurse begins with the general assessment and then concentrates on the clinical manifestations specifically related to OA.

Assessment

When assessing the patient with osteoarthritis, subjective symptoms include pain, tenderness in joints, fatigue, generalized weakness, anorexia, cold intolerance, and parasthesia. Objective symptoms include joint changes such as being enlarged, limited movement, stiffness, swelling, redness, localized heat around the joint, shiny stretched skin over and around the joint, and **subcutaneous nodules**. Other objective assessments are weight loss, elevated temperature, crepitus of joints, deformities or contractures, and cold and clammy extremities. Decreased hemoglobin and elevated white blood count (WBC) could support the diagnosis of osteoarthritis.

Nursing Diagnoses

For the patient with OA, the following are the highest priority nursing diagnoses. Based on these nursing diagnoses, plans and expected outcomes can be generated.

1. *Pain, Chronic* related to bone rubbing against bone, inflammation, or deformity
2. *Mobility: Physical, Impaired* related to stiffness
3. *Falls, Risk for* related to malaise and weakness
4. *Body Image, Disturbed* related to arthritic changes in joints
5. *Readiness for Enhanced Self-Care* related to inability to perform activities of daily living independently
6. *Imbalanced Nutrition: More than Body Requirements* related to obesity
7. *Powerlessness* related to changes in disease process, financial status, and role of the family.

Planning

The interdisciplinary team is critical to the success of treating the patient with OA because the collaborative method will provide assistance to the patient in a holistic approach. Based on the degree and severity of symptoms, the nurse should assist the patient with comfort, exercise, and pharmacologic therapies to reduce pain with a variety of medication choices, such as nonsteroidal anti-inflammatory drugs (NSAIDs). Discussing other options will be helpful in regard to surgical intervention to ease discomfort and improve mobility. See the Gerontological Considerations box on page 1836 for additional information.

Outcomes and Evaluation Parameters

The desired outcomes for the patient with OA include control of pain and stiffness, maintenance of quality of life, and ability to perform self-care activities. Evaluation parameters include the patient's expression that the pain is controlled, the patient reports no falls, and the patient is able to perform daily self-care activities.

Interventions and Rationales

With OA, pain relief from spasms, inflammation, or swelling is of the highest priority. Medications are instituted to help with the relief of the symptoms. The nurse needs to teach the patient to read the adverse effects of the medication and take precautions to prevent gastrointestinal upset, such as having food in one's stomach before taking the drug. See the Pharmacology Summary feature on page 1839 for specific drugs for treating OA.

Nonpharmacologic interventions include the use of heat to reduce muscle spasms and cold to reduce inflammation and pain. In addition, there are multiple alternative therapies, as described in the Complementary and Alternative Therapies box (p. 1836). For the prevention of contractures, the patient should be active in exercise, sleep on a firm mattress, and use splints to maintain alignment. Elevation of the extremity and rest will reduce swelling, and splints will maintain alignment to prevent contractures. A physical activity program should range from passive and active range of motion to swimming, which is critical in minimizing the complications of immobility. Also, the use of splints and/or supportive devices may be useful in maintaining alignment and promoting function.

If a patient is at risk for falls, it is critical that that be identified on admission. A fall protocol should be implemented with frequent observation of the patient, toileting often, offering nourishments, and responding quickly to the patient call light. Review the hospital's policy and procedure to ensure patient safety. This practice will assist in keeping the patient safe while hospitalized. The family should also be made aware of the risk and taught how to keep the patient safe while at home, such as by removing scatter rugs, removing clutter, and providing assistance when the patient is ambulatory.

If the patient is unable to perform activities of daily living, there might be issues related to care. Encourage the patient to be as independent as possible, and offer assistance when needed. Provide support and positive feedback each time the patient makes an effort to perform activities.

Managing weight loss can be challenging. Consulting a nutritionist will help provide a low-calorie, balanced, appealing diet plan to reduce weight. It is important to realize that weight reduction is a slow process, and weight loss may take a long period of time depending on the amount the patient needs to lose. Incorporate ethnic foods when possible.

As a person loses function, powerlessness may follow. Empowerment is critical to the patient's well-being. Encourage the patient to verbalize any concerns, and listen actively. Utilize reflective communication, as it will assist the patient to discover how best to function. In fact, it is important to encourage the patient to be as independent as possible and be proud of accomplishments made. Because OA is a chronic disease, discharge instructions are important to ensure compliance with the health care plan. For more details, see the Patient Teaching & Discharge Priorities box for the patient with osteoarthritis.

Evaluation

Explore the implications of having this debilitating disease and its effects on the patient's life, such as living with pain and creating an environment where the patient is safe. Encourage weight reduction in patients who are obese as well as promoting exercise. Promote independence and offer assistance when needed. Allow the patient to become empowered to take control by keeping informed about the latest therapeutic, pharmacologic, and surgical interventions.

Rheumatoid Arthritis: Epidemiology and Etiology

Rheumatoid arthritis (RA) is a chronic inflammatory process that affects the peripheral joints and surrounding muscles, liga-

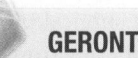

GERONTOLOGICAL CONSIDERATIONS

Because a large number of baby boomers are reaching an average age of 55 and older, and obesity continues to increase, it seems likely that more patients will be experiencing osteoarthritis and become inactive because it is difficult to move. Teaching health promotion is critical to maintaining well-being: Diet and exercise should be the priorities of education.

ments, tendons, and blood vessels. It is thought to be an autoimmune disorder that not only involves tissue hypersensitivity but also has a genetic component. Antiglobulin antibodies combine with immunoglobulin in the synovial fluid and form complexes. Neutrophils are then attracted to the joint space and cause destruction.

RA most commonly affects women between ages 20 and 40, and is present in 2% to 3% of the population. One out of every 6 people, or 2.1 million Americans, have RA (InnerVibrance, 2006). As the baby boomers age, it is estimated that 60 million people will be affected with RA by the year 2020 (InnerVibrance, 2006). RA is noted worldwide as affecting three times more women than men, although it can occur at any age, with the peak incidence being between ages 25 and 55 (Frazier & Drzymkowski, 2009).

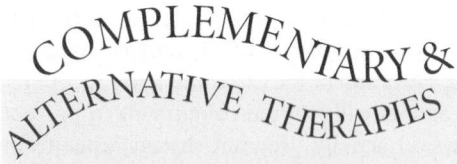

COMPLEMENTARY & ALTERNATIVE THERAPIES for Osteoarthritis and Rheumatoid Arthritis

Description:
Some conditions have shown improvement from many different CAM therapies. Therefore, nurses would be remiss to recommend only one CAM therapy to their patients. Osteoarthritis (OA) and rheumatoid arthritis (RA) are conditions for which multiple approaches have benefit.

Research Support:
A study by an English research team aimed to better understand CAM use among patients with RA. The researchers identified three goals of the study: to assess the impact of a patient's use of CAM therapy on the patient's perspective of health and well-being, to understand why a patient chooses a CAM therapy, and to learn which forms of CAM therapies were most commonly used by patients. Researchers found that the most commonly used CAM therapies were herbal remedies and supplements, and aromatherapy massage. Results showed that, compared to conventional treatments, CAM therapies had advantages due to a lower incidence of adverse reactions, greater patient choice, psychological comfort, and an increased quality in the patient–therapist relationship. Researchers concluded that the high incidence of CAM use by patients with RA indicates a need for more evidence-based information about its use and safety (Rose, 2006).

Guided imagery with relaxation (GIR) is a commonly used CAM therapy by patients with OA. A randomized pilot study tested the effect of GIR on health-related quality of life in women with OA. Study participants used GIR for 12 weeks. Results showed that GIR significantly increased participants' health-related quality of life in comparison to the control group (Baird & Sands, 2006). Results of other studies suggest that acupuncture, several herbal medicines, and capsaicin cream have an encouraging risk-benefit profile (Ernst, 2006).

Another study assessed the Benson Relaxation Technique (BRT) used concurrently with medication to determine its effect on disease activity in patients with RA. The experimental group received BRT combined with medication and the control group received medication only. The two groups showed a significant difference in anxiety, depression, and feeling of well-being. Although the two groups' clinical symptoms and laboratory findings were not statistically significant, they did indicate a decline in disease progress. Researchers concluded that BRT can be an effective technique in improving symptoms in patients with RA (Bagheri-Nesami, Mohseni-Bandpei, & Shayesteh-Azar, 2006). Another study examined the impact of a nurse-led rheumatology clinic on patients with RA. Researchers concluded that such clinics can be not only a source for empowering patients with RA to adopt new stances to alternative actions, but they can also help patients achieve a higher level of faith in their own abilities (Arvidsson et al., 2006).

References
Arvidsson, S. B., Petersson, A., Nilsson, I., Andersson, B., Arvidsson, B. I., Petersson, I. F., et al. (2006). A nurse-led rheumatology clinic's impact on empowering patients with rheumatoid arthritis: A qualitative study. *Nursing and Health Sciences, 8*(3), 133–139.
Bagheri-Nesami, M., Mohseni-Bandpei, M. A., & Shayesteh-Azar, M. (2006). The effect of Benson Relaxation Technique on rheumatoid arthritis patients: Extended report. *International Journal of Nurse Practitioners, 12*(4), 214–219.
Baird, C. L., & Sands, L. P. (2006). Effect of guided imagery with relaxation on health-related quality of life in older women with osteoarthritis. *Research in Nursing and Health, 29*(5), 442–451.
Ernst, E. (2006). Complementary or alternative therapies for osteoarthritis. *Nature Clinical Practice Rheumatology, 2*(2), 74–80.
Rose, G. (2006). Why do patients with rheumatoid arthritis use complementary therapies? *Musculoskeletal Care, 4*(2), 101–115.

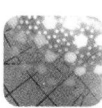

PATIENT TEACHING & DISCHARGE PRIORITIES for Osteoarthritis

Need	Teaching
Because the joints affected are weight bearing, it is important not to contribute to stress of those joints by additional weight.	Encourage patients who are obese to reduce weight.
Increase mobility.	Promote the patient to participate in an exercise program (stretching, passive and active range of motion, swimming, t'ai chi)
Maintain range of motion.	
Do not exacerbate symptoms.	
Joint protection.	Modify work or home environment to accommodate limited weight bearing.
Reduce pain and avoid complications of drug therapy.	Pharmacologic therapy: Teach about each drug classification, how to take the medication, drug interactions, adverse effects, and reporting any complications to health care provider.

Pathophysiology

RA begins with an inflammatory process in the synovial membrane and joint capsule with swelling causing the infiltration of lymphocytes, macrophages, and neutrophils that perpetuate the inflammatory response. These cells produce enzymes that cause the destruction of cartilage, which then becomes fibrous, causing calcification of the fibrous tissue (InnerVibrance, 2006). The inflammatory response has four signs: redness, heat, swelling, and pain. In some RA patients, pannus (development of an extensive network of new blood vessels in the synovial membrane that is destructive) is experienced (Figure 58–2 ■). Pannus is a feature that differentiates RA from other forms of inflammatory arthritis (Porth, 2005).

Clinical Manifestations

An assessment is critical in making a diagnosis of RA. Assessment of the joints is to observe inflammation and deformity in affected joints. With RA, patients experience remissions and ex-acerbations of the disease. Remissions are periods of time that the disease process is inactive, and exacerbations are flare-ups or when the disease becomes active. During exacerbations, patients may experience the following: fatigue, low-grade fever, anorexia, joint pain and swelling due to inflammation, and symmetrical joint deformity. Most often the joints of the hands are affected (MedicineNet.com, 2008a).

RA not only affects the joints but also may affect organs of the entire body. Glands may become swollen, and the patient's mouth may become dry. Other organs affected may include the lungs, blood, and spleen. RA can cause rheumatoid nodules in the lungs, causing pleuritis. There is a decrease of red blood cells, causing anemia, and a decrease of white blood cells due to spleen enlargement (MedicineNet.com, 2008a). Frequently, vasculitis may occur, which results in an impairment of blood supply and potentially causes necrosis of tissues of the nail beds and dermal ulcers (MedicineNet.com, 2008a).

Laboratory and Diagnostic Procedures

Diagnostic imaging is important for patients to undergo to determine the presence and severity of rheumatoid arthritis (MedicineNet.com, 2008a). The Diagnostic Tests box (p. 1838) outlines the laboratory and diagnostic tests commonly used to diagnose rheumatoid arthritis.

Medical Management

RA is a chronic condition without a cure. However, certain measures are used to control this disease and treat symptoms, such as pain control, maintaining joint function, reducing damage to joints and reducing deformity (MedicineNet.com, 2008a). Early intervention will improve outcomes, so patients should be seen as soon as possible to reduce complications. Treatment includes the following: pharmacologic interventions, rest, exercises, safeguarding joints, and patient teaching. Sometimes it is more effective to use a blend of medications to treat the discomfort associated with RA such as NSAIDs and corticosteroids. Other drugs may be considered based on the patient's severity of disease and the response to the disease. Common medications given would include antineoplastics (methotrexate) or antimalarials (Plaquenil). Patient education regarding medication should include information about its actions, adverse effects, and interactions with food or other medications in order to ensure proper medication administration. Some of these medications are long acting, and the patient

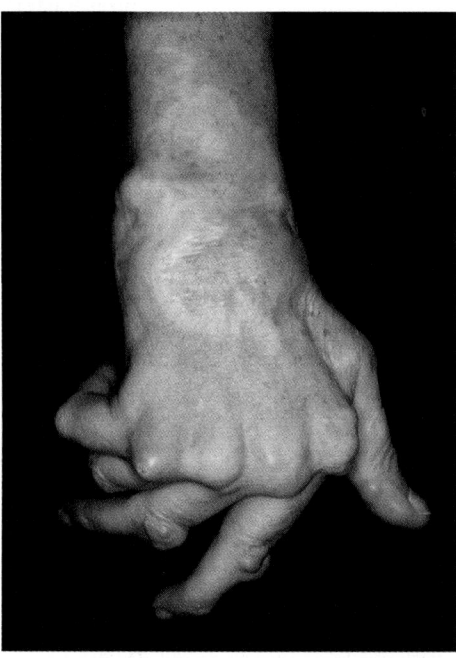

FIGURE 58–2 ■ In some RA patients, pannus (development of an extensive network of new blood vessels in the synovial membrane that is destructive) is experienced.
Source: Princess Margaret Rose Orthopaedic Hospital/Photo Researchers, Inc.

DIAGNOSTIC TESTS for Rheumatoid Arthritis

Test	Expected Abnormality	Rationale for Abnormality
LABORATORY TEST		
Rheumatoid factor	Positive or can be negative	Indicates presence or absence of rheumatoid arthritis (RA)
Anticitrulline antibody	Positive	Indicates presence of RA in the absence of rheumatoid factor
Antinuclear antibodies	Positive	Indicates presence of RA
Sedimentation rate	Increased	Presence of inflammation in joints
DIAGNOSTIC TEST X-ray	Abnormal joint space with erosion of articular surface	Presence of RA in affected joints

needs to be compliant and take the medications as directed to maximize their effect. See the Pharmacology Summary of Medications used to treat arthritis and connective tissue disorders feature.

Nursing Management

The nursing process provides a framework to create a comprehensive plan of care for the patient with RA. The nursing process will lead the nurse in utilizing the problem-solving approach in caring for patients with RA. The nurse begins with the general assessment and then concentrates on the clinical manifestations specifically related to RA. Nursing management for the patient with RA also includes education to assist the patient with progression of the disease and maintenance of quality of life.

Assessment

During a subjective assessment, the patient may complain of joint stiffness, pain, and swelling. Also, there may be complaints of being tired and fatigued. Some patients experience weight loss due to anorexia. An objective assessment includes subcutaneous nodules over bony prominences and symmetrical, bilateral involvement of joints, which can cause creaking or crackling in the affected joints called crepitus. Over time, some patients experience contractures and muscle atrophy.

Nursing Diagnoses

The highest priority nursing diagnoses for the patient with RA are:

1. *Pain, Chronic* related to bone rubbing against bone, inflammation, or deformity
2. *Mobility: Impaired Physical* related to stiffness
3. *Falls, Risk for* related to malaise and weakness
4. *Body Image, Disturbed* related to arthritic changes in joints
5. *Activity Intolerance* related to fatigue
6. *Self-Care, Readiness for Enhanced* related to inability to perform activities of daily living independently
7. *Nutrition: Imbalanced, Less than Body Requirement* related to anorexia
8. *Powerlessness* related to changes in disease process, financial status, or role of the family

Planning

During the planning stage, goals are to prevent contractures/deformities and provide health teaching. A multidisciplinary team is critical for the success of treating a patient with RA. Health care team members would include health care providers, nursing staff, occupational therapists, physical therapists, and dietitians. Collaborative and coordinated care is essential for the patient to meet both short- and long-term goals.

Outcomes and Evaluation Parameters

The desired outcomes for the patient with RA include control of pain and stiffness, maintenance of patient's quality of life, and ability to perform self-care activities. Evaluation parameters include the patient's expression that the pain is controlled, the patient reports no falls, and the patient is able to perform daily self-care activities.

Interventions and Rationales

Maintaining joint mobility is critical. Active range of motion may promote maximum function in the joints. Encouraging patients to participate in passive range of motion also encourages independence and active patient participation to promote independence. Water exercise works well with this disease as it allows the body to move easily and does not put stress on the joints. Therefore, the patient will be able to optimize joint function.

For RA it is necessary to provide rest during times when the disease process flares up. Encourage the patient to perform active range of motion, as well as providing passive range of motion to prevent contractures. Provide scheduled activities with planned rest periods to prevent fatigue. Offer heat to reduce the inflammatory process and encourage motion. Offer medications to control pain, such as nonsteroidal anti-inflammatory drugs, corticosteroids, high dosages of acetylsalicylic acid, or narcotics.

This debilitating disease causes visible deformities most often in the hands. Patients may experience issues with the appearance evident with body changes and limited movement. The nurse needs to provide an atmosphere in which a rapport can be built with the patient. Time must be made for the patient to feel comfortable to verbalize feelings or concerns by listening actively. Assist the patient in making realistic short- and long-term goals; support the patient by providing referrals to local chapters of the American Arthritis Association and other organizations.

PHARMACOLOGY Summary of Medications Used to Treat Arthritis and Connective Tissue Disorders

Medication Category	Action	Application/Indication	Nursing Responsibility
Nonsteroidal Anti-Inflammatory Drugs Ibuprofen (Motrin, Advil) Diclofenac (Voltaren) Naproxen (Naprosyn)	Exerts anti-inflammatory, analgesic action by inhibition of prostaglandin synthesis; antipyretic effects by action on hypothalamus.	Rheumatoid arthritis, osteoarthritis, mild to moderate pain. Off-label use: psoriatic arthritis, systemic lupus.	• Monitor for adverse effects: nausea, vomiting, diarrhea, constipation, blurred vision, and tinnitus. • Monitor for exacerbation in patients with asthma or existing renal, liver, or hematopoietic dysfunction. • Be aware of multiple drug interactions (aminoglycosides, anticoagulants, beta-blockers, and others). • Warn patient that alcohol and smoking increase incidence of gastrointestinal (GI) bleeding. • Be aware of increased risk of myocardial infarction, stroke, and cardiovascular thrombosis, especially in the presence of existing cardiovascular disease.
Cyclooxygenase-2 (COX-2) Inhibitor Celecoxib (Celebrex)	Exerts anti-inflammatory, analgesic, and antipyretic effects by inhibiting prostaglandin synthesis.	Rheumatoid arthritis, osteoarthritis, ankylosing spondylitis, postoperative pain.	• Monitor for adverse effects: dyspepsia, abdominal pain, nausea, and headache. • Monitor for signs of hepatotoxicity (nausea, vomiting, itching, abdominal pain), and GI bleeding (tarry stools, upper GI distress). • Be aware of drug interactions (diuretics, aminoglycosides, warfarin, angiotensin-converting enzyme [ACE] inhibitors, and others). • Monitor for altered drug efficacy or toxicity. • Monitor hematocrit (HCT), hemoglobin (Hgb), electrolytes, and liver and renal function. • Be aware of increased risk of myocardial infarction, stroke, and cardiovascular thrombosis, especially in the presence of existing cardiovascular disease. • Give 2 hours before or after antacids.
Disease-Modifying Antirheumatic Drugs (DMARDs): **Antineoplastic** Methotrexate (MTX, Rheumatrex)	Exerts immunosuppressive effect by inhibiting T lymphocytes and depleting folate needed for DNA, RNA, and protein synthesis.	Severe, disabling rheumatoid arthritis. Off-label use: psoriatic arthritis, systemic lupus.	• Monitor for adverse effects: headache, rash, nausea, vomiting, diarrhea, stomatitis, and alopecia. • Observe for signs of severe adverse effects: bone marrow suppression; liver, lung, kidney, or GI toxicities. Monitor complete blood count (CBC), renal and hepatic function, metabolic profile, and chest x-ray at regularly scheduled intervals. • Be aware of multiple drug interactions (acetylsalicylic acid [ASA], NSAIDs, digoxin, phenytoin, and others). Observe for altered drug efficacy or toxicity. • Advise patient of increased toxicity with alcohol and caffeine consumption. Contact health care provider before using over-the-counter (OTC) drugs. • Warn patient of photosensitivity and to use sun block.

(continued)

PHARMACOLOGY Summary of Medications Used to Treat Arthritis and Connective Tissue Disorders—*Continued*

Medication Category	Action	Application/Indication	Nursing Responsibility
Immunosuppressants Cyclosporine (Sandimmune, Neoral) Mycophenolate (CellCept) Azathioprine (Imuran)	Suppresses immune response by inhibiting lymphocyte replication or disrupting helper T cells.	Treatment of rheumatoid arthritis unresponsive to conventional therapy, systemic lupus.	• Monitor for adverse effects: hirsutism, hypertension, nausea, vomiting, and infection. • Observe for signs of toxicity: tremors, seizures, altered mental status, visual disturbances, nephrotoxicity, and neurotoxicity. • Monitor CBC, magnesium, potassium, blood sugar, liver, and renal function tests. • Be aware of multiple drug interactions (digoxin, NSAIDs, erythromycin, verapamil, cimetidine, allopurinol, and others). Monitor for altered drug levels, nephrotoxicity, or leukopenia.
Cyclophosphamide (Cytoxan)	Blocks DNA, RNA, and protein synthesis.	Off-label use: treatment of severe rheumatoid arthritis.	• Monitor for adverse effects: dizziness, nausea, vomiting, alopecia, hyperkalemia, and hyponatremia. • Monitor for severe adverse effects: leukopenia, pulmonary emboli, interstitial pulmonary fibrosis, nephrotoxicity, and hemorrhagic cystitis. • Monitor leukocyte and platelet counts, HCT, electrolytes, and renal function including urinalysis.
Sulfonamide Antibiotic Sulfasalazine (Azulfidine)	Reduces inflammation by decreasing production of arachidonic acid metabolites.	First line treatment for rheumatoid arthritis.	• Monitor for adverse effects: rash, headache, nausea, vomiting, and bloody diarrhea. • Observe for serious adverse effects (bone marrow suppression, hepatitis). Monitor CBC, and renal and liver function tests.
Tumor Necrosis Factor (TNF) Inhibitors Etanercept (Enbrel) Infliximab (Remicade)	Reduces inflammation by preventing TNF mediated cellular response.	Rheumatoid arthritis management, psoriatic arthritis, ankylosing spondylitis.	• Monitor for adverse effects: infection, nausea, headache, and injection/infusion site reactions. • Monitor for signs of severe adverse effects: blood dyscrasia, demyelinating diseases, sepsis, especially in poorly controlled diabetes and other predisposing diseases. • Monitor CBC, chest x-ray, urinalysis, and C-reactive protein. • Be aware of drug interactions (methotrexate, azathiopine, leflunomide, and others). Monitor for increased risk of blood dyscrasia.
Antimalarials Hydroxychloroquine (Plaquenil) Chloroquine (Aralen) Quinacrine	Exerts anti-inflammatory effect by inhibiting prostaglandin synthesis.	Treatment of rheumatoid arthritis.	• Monitor for adverse effects: hypotension, nausea, diarrhea, pruritus, irritability, headaches, weakness, hair loss, or bleaching. • Monitor electrocardiogram (ECG), CBC, and liver and kidney function. • Observe for potential exacerbation of disease when given in presence of blood, liver, GI, or neurological disorders. • Monitor for irreversible retinal damage. Warn patient of importance of regular eye exams. • Be aware of multiple drug interactions (antacids, cimetidine, methotrexate, and others). • Give with food to decrease adverse GI effects.

PHARMACOLOGY Summary of Medications Used to Treat Arthritis and Connective Tissue Disorders—*Continued*

Medication Category	Action	Application/Indication	Nursing Responsibility
Glucocorticoids			
Prednisone (Meticortin) Prednisolone (Delta-Cortef)	Anti-inflammatory, immunosuppressant activities due to inhibition of prostaglandin synthesis, histamine release, and phagocyte and lymphocyte function.	Acute exacerbation of rheumatoid arthritis, pulse therapy.	• Monitor for adverse effects: mood swings, anxiety, insomnia, nausea, vomiting, weight gain, acne, and delayed wound healing. • Observe for increased risk of GI bleeding and, in rheumatoid arthritis patients, pneumonia. • Monitor blood count, glucose, and electrolytes. • Be aware of drug interactions (theophylline, warfarin, and others). Monitor for toxicity or decreased efficacy. • Warn patient of potential need for dose adjustment if ill or if stress increases. Do not abruptly stop drug.
Chelating Agent			
D-penicillamine	Antirheumatic effect likely due to inhibition of collagen formation and depression of immunoglobin M (IgM), rheumatoid factor, and immune complexes.	Rheumatoid arthritis. Off-label use: scleroderma.	• Monitor for adverse effects: rash, pruritus, fever, arthralgia, nausea, vomiting, abdominal pain, and diarrhea. • Monitor for severe adverse effects: ptosis, diplopia (myasthenia gravis syndrome), exertional dyspnea, cough, wheezing (bronchiolitis obliterans), hematuria, proteinuria (nephritic syndrome), or decreased platelets or leukocytes (bone marrow depression). • Observe for reactivation of previous peptic ulcer, hepatic dysfunction, or pancreatitis. • Monitor CBC and urine tests monthly. • Give 1 hour before or 2 hours after eating. Avoid antacids or iron preparations. • Advise patient to increase fluid intake.

Because many of the patients with RA are young, surgical intervention may be appropriate when dialoguing about different treatment options for maintaining or improving the quality of life. Surgical treatment options for those with RA such as the following may be discussed: synovectomy, arthrodesis, and/or reconstructive surgery. Information is critical when considering all of the alternatives for treatment. Because this is a chronic disease, discussing discharge priorities is essential. For more information, see the Patient Teaching & Discharge Priorities box (p. 1842) about rheumatoid arthritis.

Evaluation

When evaluating the patient's status, the goal is to have the patient become as independent as possible by having minimal loss of mobility and increased ability to perform the activities of daily living. The installation of safety devices in the home, such as guardrails in the bathrooms and shower areas will assist the patient in living independently, as well as in gaining confidence in his abilities. The patient is to remain adverse-effect free from the use of medications to treat this disease. Finally, if there is no sign of recovery, provide the patient with information on ways to have the best quality of life possible using adaptive equipment or information regarding joint surgery. Examine the ability to

continue working or the ideas of retirement, financial status, and changes in the role of the family.

Health Promotion

Health teaching should include education regarding the adverse effects of NSAIDs because gastrointestinal upset, as well as gastric bleeding, is common. Signs of gastric bleeding are black tarry stools.

 Ringing in the ears (tinnitus) is a toxic side effect of aspirin use. Be sure to monitor these adverse effects with patients taking a high dosage of aspirin.

Encourage patients to remain as independent as possible. This is achieved by using assistive devices such as splints, walkers, or canes for performing activities of daily living and ambulation. Encourage patients to pace activities with rest in order to prevent fatigue. Teach patients to use body mechanics for body posture. Allow patients to verbalize frustrations and encourage them to adapt to their disabilities. Self-determination should also be encouraged to achieve the highest level of function with the patient with rheumatoid arthritis. Knowledge is power when making critical decisions about all types of treatment choices. See the Gerontological Considerations box on page 1842 for more information.

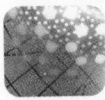

PATIENT TEACHING & DISCHARGE PRIORITIES for Rheumatoid Arthritis

Need	Teaching
Pain control	Teach the patient about medications that assist the patient's pain.
Maintaining joint function	Active range of motion.
	Passive range of motion.
	Gentle exercise, such as swimming or moving joints in a Jacuzzi.
Rest	Alternate activities with period of rest.
	Elevate affected joint to optimize circulation.

GERONTOLOGICAL CONSIDERATIONS for Rheumatoid Arthritis

Rheumatoid arthritis is a debilitating condition that affects the whole person. The goal of treatment is to treat the patient holistically and attempt to control the signs and symptoms of the disorder. The patient's safety is critical and assisting her with activities of daily living is important while maintaining her dignity. Families may need to be involved in caregiving as a patient becomes incapacitated.

Psoriatic Arthritis: Epidemiology and Etiology

Psoriatic arthritis is an inflammatory process associated with psoriasis. For a detailed explanation of psoriasis, refer to Chapter 66 🔗. Initially psoriatic arthritis was considered a variant of rheumatoid arthritis, but it is now recognized as a distinct clinical entity (Gladman, 2007).

Psoriatic arthritis does not favor either gender. Among patients with psoriasis, estimates of prevalence vary from 4% to 6% up to 30% (Gladman, 2007). Psoriatic arthritis carries an incidence of approximately 6 per 100,000 per year, and a prevalence of approximately 1 to 2 per 1,000 (Gladman, 2007). The exact cause of psoriatic arthritis and of psoriasis itself is not known. It is thought that certain genetic, immunologic, and environmental factors contribute to the disease. It is known that psoriasis occurs in families, with approximately 40% of patients having a family history of the disease in first-degree relatives (Gladman, 2007).

Psoriatic arthritis had not been considered an autoimmune disease, but a number of immune abnormalities have been identified in patients with psoriasis and psoriatic arthritis. Included are:

- Elevated serum levels of immunoglobulins and antinuclear antibodies.
- T cell expression of HLA-DR molecules and receptors for interleukin-2 with a variety of adhesion molecules and the secretion of proinflammatory cytokines.
- Fibroblasts from the synovium show enhanced proliferative activity and platelet-derived growth factors (Gladman, 2007).

Environmental factors that have been associated with the development of psoriasis and psoriatic arthritis include both bacterial and viral infections, and trauma (Gladman, 2007). Patients that develop psoriatic arthritis have given a history of trauma to that joint prior to the onset of the disease. It is not clear how the trauma is related to psoriatic arthritis.

Pathophysiology

Psoriatic arthritis is an autoimmune disease with a known human leukocyte antigen (HLA)–associated risk factor. Psoriatic arthritis affects the ligaments, tendons, fascia, and joints. This disease occasionally develops even in the absence of detectable psoriasis. Psoriatic arthritis may occur at higher frequencies when skin involvement is more severe, especially when pustular psoriasis is present; however, recent studies suggest that this may not be valid (Hammadi, 2008).

Clinical Manifestations

Patients present with pain and stiffness in the affected joints. The stiffness worsens with prolonged immobility and is alleviated with physical activity. The affected joints will be tender, painful when the joint is stressed, and present with effusions. Most frequently the patients present with polyarthritis, followed by oligoarthritis. Distal arthritis and arthritis mutilans are considered most specific for psoriatic arthritis (Gladman, 2008). Other common features include soft tissue inflammation at the site of tendon insertion into the bone of the Achilles tendon, the plantar fascia, and the pelvic bones; tenosynovitis of the flexor tendons of the hands, the extensor carpi ulnaris tendon, or other sites; and **dactylitis**, a uniform swelling of the soft tissues between the metacarpophalangeal and interphalangeal joints. With dactylitis, there is diffuse swelling of the entire digit, which is often referred to as "sausage digit." Dactylitis occurs in approximately one-half of patients with psoriatic arthritis and is associated with an increased risk of progressive joint damage (Gladman, 2008). The patient may also have nail involvement characterized by pits in the nail plate and onycholysis (separation of the lateral edges of the nail plate from the nail bed).

Laboratory and Diagnostic Procedures

There is no specific diagnostic laboratory test for psoriatic arthritis. In approximately one-third of patients there is an elevated sedimentation rate and leukocytosis showing an inflammatory response. Rheumatoid factor (RF) is found in only 2% to 10% of cases of psoriatic arthritis. The presence of joint damage radiologically is seen in two-thirds of patients on diagnosis. Radiologic findings show both erosive changes and new bone formation in the distal joints. Magnetic resonance imaging (MRI) reveals inflammation in the adjacent bone marrow and soft tissues with the appearance of inflammation of entheses in joints that may not be clinically inflamed. These findings suggest that **enthesitis** (inflammation at the site of tendon insertion into bone) is the primary lesion in psoriatic arthritis. Psoriatic arthritis is also associated with decreased bone mineral density, which may lead to osteoporosis and increased risk of fractures.

Medical Management

The first line of treatment for psoriatic arthritis is usually the administration of nonsteroidal anti-inflammatory medications (NSAIDs). The use of both selective cyclooxygenase-2 (COX-2) inhibitors and nonselective NSAIDs is noted, and the choice is usually a health care provider or patient preference. This class of drug controls the mild inflammatory features of psoriatic arthritis. The combination of nonselective NSAIDs with an antiulcer drug may reduce the risk of gastroduodenal damage from the drug. Antiulcer drugs are discussed in Chapter 45 .

If the arthritis does not respond to NSAIDs and the patient exhibits polyarticular involvement, the patient may benefit from early use of disease-modifying antirheumatic drugs (DMARDs). Also, patients whose psoriasis and arthritis are of equal severity may benefit from medications used for control of psoriasis. Although there is a lack of evidence in regards to its efficacy, methotrexate has been the drug of choice for psoriatic arthritis (Gladman, 2008). The most serious potential side effects of methotrexate include liver toxicity, bone marrow suppression, and interstitial lung disease. Because of the liver toxicity, patients must not consume alcohol when taking methotrexate. If the patient refuses to give up alcohol, sulfasalazine may be used as long as there is no known allergy to sulfa drugs. If the disease does not improve after 3 months of treatment with a DMARD, then an anti–tumor necrosis factor (anti-TNF) agent may be introduced. Etanercept and infliximab have received regulatory approval for the treatment of psoriatic arthritis. See the earlier Pharmacology Summary for Arthritis and Connective Tissue Disorder on p. 1839.

Any patient with psoriasis with the complaint of joint discomfort should be evaluated for psoriatic arthritis. The patient's goals include relief of pain, treatment of the infection, rehabilitation of the joint after the infection subsides, and knowledge of treatment regimen. Evaluation parameters include control of pain as expressed by the patient, decrease in the signs and symptoms of infection, and the ability of the patient to articulate the plan of care. Patients may obtain complete relief of joint tenderness and swelling and, with continued use of medication, avoid a relapse. Patients who present with mild disease, less disability, and male gender are associated with a greater likelihood of achieving remission (Gladman, 2008). Assessment and protection of the affected joint are important to the success of treatment.

■ Nursing Management

Nursing management focuses on the same issues as with all types of arthritis: early recognition, pain relief, and protection of the joint from further damage. The nurse may support and immobilize the affected joint in a splint. Because the inflammatory process can cause scar tissue within the joint, it is important to splint the joint in a functional position. Analgesics are prescribed to control pain and anti-inflammatory medication such as NSAIDs may be used to control joint inflammation.

The nurse instructs the patient on the process of psoriatic arthritis so he may understand the therapeutic regimen. Of importance is the adherence to the therapeutic regimen, support of

the affected joint, and adherence to weight-bearing and activity restrictions during the inflammatory process to prevent permanent damage to the joint. If assistive devices are to be used, the nurse will help the patient in learning safe use of the devices. Evaluation includes decreased pain and swelling. The patient will report adequate pain relief and an increase in physical mobility with demonstrated safe use of assistive devices.

Gouty Arthritis: Epidemiology and Etiology

Gouty arthritis is a condition in which there is an imbalance in purine metabolism, which increases uric acid in the joints with the formation of uric acid crystals (MedlinePlus Medical Encyclopedia, 2007). Gout can affect any joint but most commonly affects those of the feet, especially the great toe. According to the National Institutes of Health, approximately 275 people out of 100,000 are affected (MedlinePlus Medical Encyclopedia, 2007). Based on all of the different types of arthritis, gouty arthritis accounts for 5% (National Institute of Arthritis and Musculoskeletal and Skin Diseases, 2008). Primary gout most commonly occurs in men over age 30 and postmenopausal women. Secondary gout occurs in the elderly (Frazier & Drzymkowski, 2009).

The cause of primary gout is unknown but is thought to have a hereditary component with a defect in purine metabolism. This disease is more common in men than in women and those who are overweight. Onset of an acute attack of gout sometimes follows excessive eating or drinking (MedlinePlus Medical Encyclopedia, 2007). Risk factors include heredity, an enzyme defect, and exposure to lead (MedlinePlus Medical Encyclopedia, 2007).

Pathophysiology

With gouty arthritis, there is an imbalance with purine metabolism. Instead of the uric acid crystals being excreted through the kidneys, they accumulate in the joints. These crystals are needle-like causing excruciating pain, usually in the joints of the elbows, wrist, fingers, knees, ankles, and toes, with 75% of patients affected in the great toe (Figure 58–3 ■) (National Institute of Arthritis and Musculoskeletal and Skin Diseases, 2008). Gout

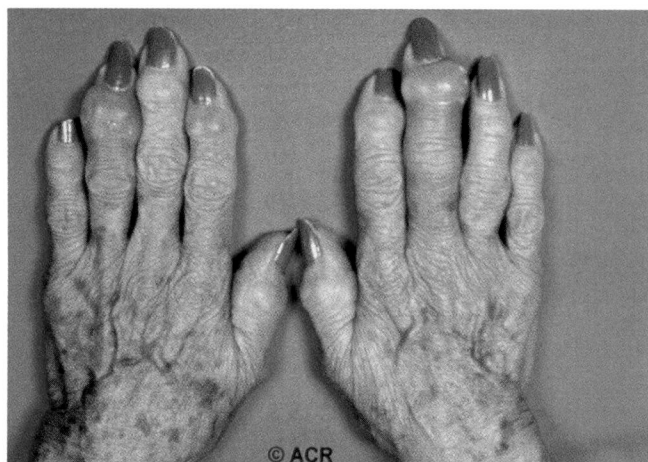

FIGURE 58–3 ■ Instead of the uric acid crystals being excreted through the kidneys, they accumulate in the joints. These crystals are needle-like causing excruciating pain, usually in the joints of the elbows, wrists, fingers, knees, ankles, and toes, with 75% of patients affected in the great toe.
Source: © 1972–2004 American College of Rheumatology Clinical Slide Collection. Used with permission.

follows an intermittent course and a patient can be free from symptoms for years between attacks.

Clinical Manifestations

According to Meiner (2001), gout has a four-stage progression: asymptomatic, acute gout episode, interval gout, and chronic tophaceous gout. During the asymptomatic phase, there is an elevation of uric acid in the blood, but no symptoms (MedlinePlus Medical Encyclopedia, 2007). In the second stage, called acute gout episode, there is an increase of uric acid crystals accumulating in the space of the joints. These uric acid crystals can also settle in cartilage in the earlobes. This is called **tophi**. During this stage, the patient experiences a sudden onset of severe pain, usually in the night. Other manifestations include increased swelling and inflammation, which cause the affected part to feel hot. Some will experience knife-like pain in the earlobe, elbow, or feet. This sudden attack can be triggered by stress, illness, or the consumption of alcohol or drugs. Without treatment, this phase can last from 3 to 10 days. Interval gout is the period of time this condition is in remission. Finally, the fourth stage, called chronic tophaceous gout, occurs when the illness is not treated, which results in disabling effects such as permanent damage to the joints and kidneys (Meiner, 2001).

Laboratory and Diagnostic Procedures

Elevated blood levels of uric acid occur in some individuals, but are normal in approximately 10% of people during an acute attack of gouty arthritis. Moreover, uric acid levels are elevated in 5% to 8% of the general population, so the presence of an elevated level does not necessarily mean that gout is the cause of an inflamed joint. X-ray examination of the joint is primarily used to assess underlying joint damage, especially in patients who have had multiple episodes of gouty arthritis. The most useful and accurate test is joint aspiration. A needle is inserted into the joint to withdraw a sample of fluid, which is examined to see whether there are gout crystals or bacterial infection present. Sometimes other crystals can be found in the joint fluid, such as calcium pyrophosphate, which is caused by an entirely different condition called pseudogout ("like gout"). Joint aspiration is the ultimate method of being certain of a diagnosis of gouty arthritis, as opposed to other causes such as an infection in the joint (eMedicineHealth, 2008).

Medical Management

Medical management focuses on mitigating the clinical manifestations of gouty arthritis. Medications used specifically for gout include colchicine and allopurinol. These drugs reduce uric acid production, thus reducing the inflammatory process. It is important to monitor uric acid levels while on medication (Frazier & Drzymkowski, 2009).

Patients with gout must adhere to a dietary regimen to reduce the consumption of purines. Foods that should be avoided are dried beans and peas, organ meats, wheat germ, anchovies, and seafood. Patients should consume a moderate amount of protein. The recommendation is to eat only 200 grams of meat, poultry, or fish twice weekly and to eliminate organ meats. Alcohol consumption should be limited to 1 drink 3 times a week, whereas beer ingestion should be completely discontinued, as it has a high purine count and increases gout risks regardless of amount (Hogan, 2007). It is not recommended for individuals to follow a high-protein, low-carbohydrate diet because this can worsen the symptoms. Because fat intake should also be limited, patients should select low-fat meats and use nonsaturated oils. Increasing fluid intake is critical to dilute urinary uric acid crystals. Patients should consume between 2 and 3 liters of fluid daily (Hogan, 2007). See the Pharmacology Summary of medications used to treat gouty arthritis.

PHARMACOLOGY Summary of Medications Used to Treat Gouty Arthritis

Medication Category	Action	Application/Indication	Nursing Responsibility
Antigout Agents Colchicine Allopurinol (Aloprim, Zyloprim) Probenecid (Benemid)	Exerts anti-inflammatory effect; decreases pain and swelling by interrupting the inflammatory response. Reduces uric acid; has no direct anti-inflammatory or analgesic action.	Treatment of acute gout, prophylaxis, and recurrent gouty arthritis. Off-label use: scleroderma. Treatment of chronic gout.	• Observe for early signs of toxicity (colchicine): weakness, anorexia, nausea, vomiting, diarrhea, especially in presence of cardiac, renal, or hepatic disease. • Observe for severe adverse effects: nausea, sore throat or mouth, fever, fatigue, unusual bleeding, or bruising (bone marrow depression). • Monitor serum uric acid, CBC, electrolytes, urinalysis, and renal and hepatic function. • Monitor IV site to prevent extravasation when colchicine given IV. • Monitor for drug interactions (vitamin B_{12}, erythromycin, NSAIDs, and others with colchicine; theophylline, ampicillin, thiazide diuretics, and others with allopurinol; some antibiotics, vitamin C, and cranberry juice with probenecid). • Advise patient to increase fluid intake. • Give after a meal to reduce gastric distress.

Nursing Management

Utilization of the nursing process will guide the nurse in understanding the method for organizing critical thinking skills when providing patient care in the presence of specific illness. When planning care, the short-term goals should be directed at pain reduction or comfort based on the causative factors. Because gouty arthritis is a chronic disease and there are interventions that help control the clinical manifestations, developing a health plan is essential. See the Evidence-Based Practice for the Treatment of Gouty Arthritis feature for a discussion of the literature regarding the treatment of gouty arthritis. Long-term goals should be focused on patients becoming compliant to medication and dietary regimens. The Nursing Process: Patient Care Plan feature (p. 1846) outlines the nursing management of the patient with gouty arthritis.

Health Promotion

Because gouty arthritis is caused by indulging in foods high in purines, it can be controlled by eating a well-balanced, low-calorie, low-purine diet and by reducing alcohol consumption. Foods to be avoided are alcohol, organ meats, and rich foods such as gravies, dried legumes, and anchovies. These foods will increase uric acid in the blood and can lead to uric acid crystal buildup most often resulting in uric acid crystals located in the joint of the great toe. Pain medications are not the treatment of choice, rather antigout medications and dietary therapy to reduce the uric acid level.

Compared to other connective disorders, gouty arthritis has been noticeably understudied in the literature (Mikuls & Saag, 2005). On reviewing the literature, it is determined that there are no formal national guidelines for the *risks* of gouty arthritis. It is important to determine that the main vulnerability factor for acquiring gouty arthritis is an increased uric acid level in the blood. However, based on a review of many articles and websites, the National Guidelines box (p. 1847) offers guidelines for *reducing* the incidence of gouty arthritis.

Collaborative Management

To achieve optimal functioning, patients with gouty arthritis need a multidisciplinary team approach, including health care providers, nurses, social workers, physical therapists, pharmacists,

---

Treatment of Gouty Arthritis

Clinical Problem

An acute attack of gouty arthritis is very painful. The drug colchicine has been used to decrease the symptoms related to gout but has gastrointestinal side effects that may increase the patient's distress.

Research Findings

A comparison was done to determine whether the effectiveness of colchicine was preferred over that of the placebo with a sample size of 43 patients (Schlesinger, Schumacher, Catton, & Maxwell, 2006). For those patients who had taken colchicine, there was a reduction of the following symptoms: pain (34%) and tenderness on palpation, swelling, redness (30%). However, all patients on colchicine (100%) developed gastrointestinal (GI) symptoms: vomiting and/or diarrhea.

Implications for Nursing

The actual medication improved acute gout attacks, but caused GI adverse effects with all who took this medication due to the frequency necessary to reduce pain, swelling, and other symptoms causing the gout attack. Encouraging patients to maintain a low purine diet and avoid excessive use of alcohol in order to prevent an acute attack may be a better alternative for the patient.

Critical Thinking Questions

1. How can you maximize the effect of antihyperuremic medications and reduce the gastrointestinal side effects?

2. Are there other classifications of medications other than antihyperuremics that could work in the treatment of gout?

Reference

Schlesinger, N., Schumacher, M. C., Catton, M., & Maxwell, L. (2006). Colchicine for acute gout. *Cochrane Database of Systematic Reviews*, 2006, Issue 4. Retrieved June 20, 2007, from http://mrw.interscience.wiley.com/cochrane/clsysrev/articles/CD006190/frame.html.

Clinical Problem

There is no consensus among rheumatologists about the standardized treatment of patients who have gouty arthritis.

Research Findings

On a literature search, 310 potential articles for review were identified. Many articles were eliminated due to their not being relevant or being written in a language other than English. Thus, 120 articles were included in the database. Finally, twenty-three (19%) articles that were randomized controlled trials were used in this study (Mikuls et al., 2004). In a breakdown of these pharmaceutical studies, 48% discussed nonsteroidal anti-inflammatory drugs (NSAIDs) in treatment of gouty arthritis, 8% studied colchicines, and 43% discussed urate-lowering medications for long-term therapy. The expert panel in this study examined both articles on medication (urate-lowering medications and NSAIDs) as well as on other process indicators (lifestyle modifications). The literature suggested that the topic of gouty arthritis was understudied as a connective tissue disorder, compared to other connective tissue disorders that have been studied and reported in the literature.

Implications for Nursing Practice

The topic of gouty arthritis is understudied and presents as an opportunity to nurses to explore ways to improve patient plans of care in regards to gouty arthritis.

Critical Thinking Question

1. What type of research can be conducted by nursing in the area of gout?

Answers to Critical Thinking Questions appear in Appendix D.

Reference

Mikuls, T. R., MacLean, C. H., Olivieri, J., Patino, F., Allison, J., Farrar, J. T., et al. (2004). Quality of care indicators for gout management. *Arthritis & Rheumatism, 50*(3), 937–943.

EVIDENCE-BASED PRACTICE

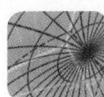

NURSING PROCESS: Patient Care Plan for Gouty Arthritis

Assessment of Pain

Subjective Data:
Do you have pain?
Is it constant or intermittent?
What brings it on and what makes it go away?
What intensity is it (numeric, colors, or faces), including location, character?

Objective Data:
Monitor:
Uric acid levels
Onset of pain
Relieving factors

Nursing Assessment and Diagnoses	Outcomes and Evaluation Parameters	Planning and Interventions with *Rationales*
Nursing Diagnoses: *Comfort, Readiness for Enhanced Pain, Acute* related to uric acid crystal deposits in affected joints	**Outcome:** Comfort level maintained. **Evaluation Parameters:** Uric acid levels are within normal limits. Pain controlled with or without nonpharmacologic therapies or with or without medication. Joint swelling decreased.	**Interventions and *Rationale:*** Assess pain on a scale. Monitor uric acid levels. Alternative pain interventions: position, elevation, ice, distraction. Medicate as ordered by the health care provider. *As there is an increase in blood uric acid levels, uric acid crystals form in joints causing discomfort, usually affecting one affected joint: warm and swollen.*

Assessment of Nutrition

Subjective Data:
What kinds of foods do you eat on a daily basis?
Have you gained or lost weight in the last year?
Do you eat at home or in restaurants?
Who prepares the meals?
What is your knowledge of foods containing purines?

Objective Data:
Monitor:
Weights at specified interval
Meal selections
Verbalizing foods consumed high in purines

Nursing Assessment and Diagnoses	Outcomes and Evaluation Parameters	Planning and Interventions with *Rationales*
Nursing Diagnosis: *Nutrition: Imbalanced, More than Body Requirements* related to increased intake of foods high in purine and increased calories	**Outcome:** Patient adherence to a low-purine diet. **Evaluation Parameters:** Patient will be able to verbalize appropriate meal planning with foods low in purine. Weight loss at reasonable amount weekly based on baseline weight (about 1–2 pounds per week).	**Interventions and *Rationales:*** Obtain a sample of patient's meal choice selections in a week to determine baseline purine intake. Create low-purine weight loss meal plan to include cultural foods in order to decrease uric acid, such as grains, fruits, vegetables, and beans. Teach the patient to avoid the following foods high in purines: cheese, wine, organ meats, and shellfish. Encourage the patient to drink plenty of liquids, about 2,000–3,000 milliliters daily, *to reduce potential creation of kidney stones.* Encourage the patient to have alkaline-ash diet *to increase the urine pH and decrease the precipitation of uric acid, and to improve the action of gouty medications, such as probenicid.*

Assessment of Therapeutic Regimen

Subjective Data:
Explain your dietary needs.
Explain why and when you take your medications.

Objective Data:
Patient is able to verbalize low-purine foods and the incorporation of these foods into low-calorie diet plan
Weight loss
No joint discomfort

Nursing Assessment and Diagnoses	Outcomes and Evaluation Parameters	Planning and Interventions with *Rationales*
Nursing Diagnosis: *Therapeutic Regimen Management, Effective*	**Outcome:** Patient will adhere to therapeutic regimen to control exacerbations. **Evaluation Parameter:** Verbalizing compliance to the prescribed therapeutic regimen.	**Interventions and *Rationale:*** Patient will verbalize compliance with the following: Foods low in purine and calories Compliance to medication Comfort Management of weight loss Exercise: passive and active range of motion. *Compliance to the above therapeutic regimen will empower the patient to take control of this disease by providing knowledge about therapeutic treatment.*

NATIONAL GUIDELINES for Health Promotion for Gouty Arthritis

Healthy People 2010 is a set of government objectives that encourages a healthy lifestyle in order to promote health. Its two main goals are (1) increasing the quality of years of a healthy life and (2) eliminating health disparities (DHHS, 2000). It is important when caring for a patient with gouty arthritis to provide the proper education that will enhance his health promotion. With gout, there is an increase of uric acids from purine metabolism. It has been discussed that diets high in purine can cause gout. Two of the health indicators identified by *Healthy People 2010* are overweight/obesity and substance abuse. Most often, people who are overweight are typically consuming foods high in purines, thus making this population of people more at risk for gouty arthritis. It is imperative for the patient to understand that behavioral changes will reduce, if not eliminate, this disease process and thus promote a healthy lifestyle. By consuming an increased amount of alcohol, uric acid will be metabolized from the liver and passed in the bloodstream to be excreted in the kidneys. However, excretion can be inhibited with gouty arthritis, causing the uric acid crystals to remain in the tissues (Chemocare.com, 2005).

Thus, it is important to remember two factors when caring for a patient with gout. One is that the increased consumption of foods high in purines results in high uric acid in the blood. Second, the decreased ability to excrete uric acids from the kidneys causes a buildup of uric acid crystals in the tissues. Healthy lifestyle choices can make the difference between one acute attack of gouty arthritis and a lifetime of gout attacks. Educating the patient is powerful, but having the patient incorporate behavioral changes can be life altering by promoting healthy choices.

Sources: Chemocare.com. (2005). *Hyperuricemia.* Retrieved July 30, 2007, from http://www.chemocare.com/managing/hyperuricemia-high-uric-acid.asp; and U.S. Department of Health and Human Services (DHHS). (2000). *Healthy People 2010.* Retrieved July 30, 2007, from http://www.healthypeople.gov.

occupational therapists, psychologists/psychiatrists, and dieticians. Ongoing physical therapy will help increase range of motion in the joints. The occupational therapist assists the patient with exercises that will enhance fine motor movements, whereas the social worker and a psychologist/psychiatrist are used to help the patient adjust to a chronic illness. Finally, a comprehensive plan for nutrition is important for teaching the patient and family about dietary restrictions. The pharmacist helps the team coordinate the medication regimen.

Reactive Arthritis

Reactive arthritis is caused by a reaction to an infection somewhere else in the body (National Institute of Arthritis and Musculoskeletal and Skin Diseases, 2002). This disease has several other names, such as Reiter's syndrome or undifferentiated spondylarthropathy. Many conditions refer to a spectrum of diseases that share certain clinical manifestations; among the most common is the spondyloarthropathy family, called undifferentiated spondylarthropathy, whereas reactive arthritis and Reiter's syndrome encompass a small amount of cases (Yu, 2008). Reactive arthritis characteristically causes inflammatory response in the genitourinary tract, the joints, and the eyes (National Institute of Arthritis and Musculoskeletal and Skin Diseases, 2002).

Epidemiology

This disease is more common in men than in women. Men between ages 20 and 40 more frequently develop reactive arthritis. When the trigger is a sexually transmitted infection, men still outnumber women by 9%. Food-borne infections do not discriminate between genders in transmitting reactive arthritis. However, women experience a milder case with remissions and exacerbations (National Institute of Arthritis and Musculoskeletal and Skin Diseases, 2002).

Etiology

This is a noncontagious disease. On the other hand, for this disease to be communicable, one must pass the bacterium that triggers the disease from person to person (National Institute of Arthritis and Musculoskeletal and Skin Diseases, 2002). Reactive arthritis usually begins between 1 and 3 weeks after becoming infected. One organism, called *Chlamydia trachomatis*, is spread through sexual contact and without treatment can cause reactive arthritis and respiratory infection, called *Chlamydia pneumoniae* (National Institute of Arthritis and Musculoskeletal and Skin Diseases, 2002).

Gastrointestinal infections, such as *Salmonella, Shigella, Yersinia,* and *Campylobacter,* also are responsible for causing reactive arthritis (National Institute of Arthritis and Musculoskeletal and Skin Diseases, 2002).

Pathophysiology

A patient develops a bacterial infection as identified earlier. Spondyloarthropies cause inflammation and bone destruction at the site of insertion (Yu, 2008). Reactive arthritis most commonly causes secondary conditions, such as arthritis, uveitis, and urethritis (Yu, 2008). However, a variety of symptoms can occur affecting the following: musculoskeletal system, enthesopathy, inflammatory spine pain, genital lesions, skin lesions, inflammatory eye disease, inflammation of the bowel mucosa, cardiac disease, amyloidosis, and evidence of preceding infection (Yu, 2008).

Clinical Manifestations

Asymmetrical joint swelling often occurs, especially in the lower extremities (knees and ankles). Enthesopathy is the inflammation around the insertion of ligaments, tendons, joint capsule, or fascia near the bone (Yu, 2008). Other symptoms that may occur are dactylitis, inflammation of the neck and low back, painless skin lesions called **circinate balanitis**, unilateral uveitis, Crohn's-like bowel inflammation, aortic regurgitation, amyloidosis, and rheumatic infections.

Laboratory and Diagnostic Procedures

Confirmation of this disease examines both laboratory data and diagnostic imaging. Laboratory tests that can confirm reactive arthritis are as follows: (1) HLA-B27, (2) alpha E beta 7 in T lymphocytes (for patients with spondylarthropathy and Crohn's), (3) epithelial E-cadherin, (4) CD163-positive macrophages, (5) lymphocytes with T helper-2 phenotype, (6) immunoglobin A (IgA) antibodies, (7) proteinuria, (8) erythrocyte sedimentation rates, (9) ligase chain reaction, (10) polymerase chain reaction, and (11) stool cultures for the presence of diarrhea (Yu, 2008). Diagnostic tests that also can confirm reactive arthritis include MRI for bone confirmation, slit lamp examination for eye involvement, x-ray, and computed tomography (Yu, 2008).

Accurate diagnosis tends to occur in the advanced stage, because the glomerular filtration is greatly reduced, leading to increased uremia, electrolyte abnormalities, and metabolic acidosis. More information is provided in the Diagnostic Tests box for undifferentiated spondylarthropathy.

Medical Management

Treatment is symptomatic control and prevention. The medications most commonly used are as follows: (1) nonsteroidal anti-inflammatory drugs to reduce joint inflammation, (2) glucocorticoids to reduce severe joint inflammation, (3) topical glucocorticoids to reduce skin lesions and promote healing, (4) anti-infectives to rid infections, (5) immunosuppressants to suppress the immune system when previous medications have not been effective, and (6) tumor necrosis factor inhibitor drugs to reduce a protein involved with inflammation when other medication therapies are again ineffective (National Institute of Arthritis and Musculoskeletal and Skin Diseases, 2002). See the earlier Pharmacology Summary for Arthritis and Connective Tissue Disorders featured on p. 1839.

Physical activity is needed to promote range of motion in the affected joints. Range-of-motion exercises reduce stiffness and promote flexibility. Using hydrotherapies also assists the patient in maximizing movement of the joints of the body, especially the limbs and spine.

■ Nursing Management

The nursing process provides the framework for a nurse to offer knowledgeable and sound patient care. The *assessment* includes evaluating the clinical manifestations associated with reactive arthritis, as described earlier. It is also important to complete a head-to-toe assessment when evaluating the patient's current condition. The nurse needs to question the patient and family about their knowledge of the disease, the associated risk factors, and necessary treatments. Identifying the *nursing diagnoses* pro-

vides a method to analyze the priorities in providing patient care. These include:

1. *Pain, Acute* related to joint and spine inflammation
2. *Knowledge, Deficient* related to lack of information about pathophysiology, difficulty to confirm diagnosis, and treatment options
3. *Activity Intolerance* related to polyarthritis
4. *Skin Integrity, Impaired* related to skin lesions
5. *Diarrhea* related to bowel inflammation
6. *Sensory Perception: Disturbed Visual* related to uveitis.

The *outcome* goals of treatment are to have the patient symptom free and compliant with therapy. *Evaluation parameters* include to treat infection, keep the condition in remission by complying with the therapeutic regimen and avoiding risk factors, and to avoid exacerbations.

Nursing planning and interventions include teaching the patient about the risk factors, medications, and supportive treatments; for example, the importance of exercise because it is essential to maintain or promote joint function of the lower extremities and the spine. Finally, reactive arthritis is difficult to diagnose, so the nurse needs to encourage the patient to have patience during the diagnosis phase of the illness and utilize the multidisciplinary team. The *outcome* is to improve the quality of life by mitigating and preventing symptoms with the treatment plan. The goals for *evaluation* include no infection, the patient complies with the therapeutic regimen to remain in a state of remission, and absence of exacerbation.

■ Collaborative Management

Specialists must be incorporated in caring for a patient with reactive arthritis based on symptoms, Those participating, for example, would be an ophthalmologist for eye disease, gynecologist for female genital disease, urologist to treat genitourinary disease in both males and females, dermatologist for skin lesions, orthopedist for surgical intervention with joint

---

DIAGNOSTIC TESTS for Undifferentiated Spondylarthropathy

Test	Expected Abnormality	Rationale for Abnormality
Urinalysis	Presence of red blood cells, red blood cell casts Low specific gravity (1.010) Low osmolality (less than 400 mOsm/kg)	Impaired filtration Decreased ability to concentrate urine
Serum creatinine	Rising serum creatinine	Indicates advanced renal insufficiency
Blood urea nitrogen (BUN)	Rising serum BUN	Indicates advanced renal insufficiency
Arterial blood gases (ABGs)	Metabolic acidosis pH < 7.35 HCO_3 < 24 mEq/L	Impaired filtration
Electrolytes	Hyperkalemia Hyperphosphatemia Hypocalcemia	Impaired filtration

disease, rheumatologist for arthritis, and physical therapist for promoting joint function.

Ankylosing Spondylitis

Ankylosing spondylitis (AS) is a type of arthritis that affects the spine and the sacroiliac joints. This systemic inflammatory disease is usually progressive and affects primarily the spinal column (Figure 58–4 ■). The patient may also experience fatigue, weight loss, fever, diarrhea, and eye pain and photophobia due to uveitis (Frazier & Drzymkowski, 2009).

Epidemiology and Etiology

In the United States, AS affects 129 out of 100,000 people, mainly adolescents and young adults. It is most common among Native Americans but also affects other ethnicities (American College of Rheumatology, 2008). It is more common in men and typically begins in the sacroiliac area and adjacent soft tissues (Frazier & Drzymkowski, 2009).

It is not certain how a patient gets AS. There is a common genetic marker, called HLA-B27, in affected individuals. Some individuals become predisposed after exposure to bowel or urinary tract infections (American College of Rheumatology, 2008).

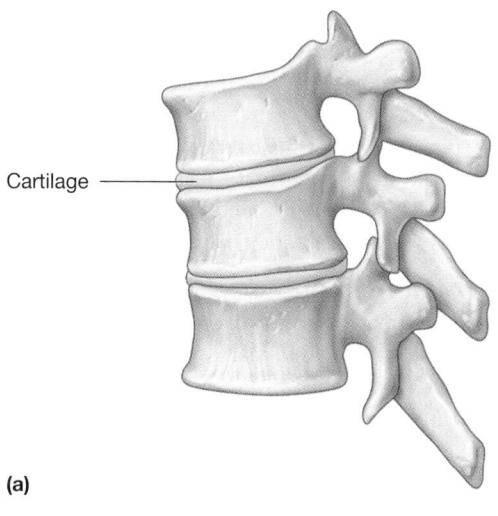

Cartilage

(a)

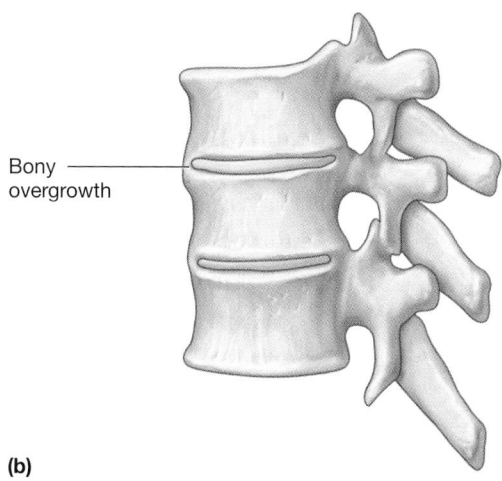

Bony overgrowth

(b)

FIGURE 58–4 ■ Bony overgrowth of ankylosing spondylitis. (A) Normal vertebrae (B) Vertebrae with bony overgrowth typical of ankylosing spondylitis.

Clinical Manifestations

Ankylosing spondylitis usually occurs first in the sacroiliac area. The patient may experience low back pain and stiffness in the morning that improves with activity. An early sign is that a patient will have a loss of flexibility in the lumbar spine. Arthritis can occur in attaching joints, tendons, and ligaments as in the shoulder, hips, and feet. As the inflammation increases and healing occurs, new bone growth fuses the bones together such as in the ribs and vertebrae (American College of Rheumatology, 2008). With restriction of the ribs, lung capacity may be impaired as well as normal functioning with activities of daily living. As the condition advances, there can be involvement of the eye inflammation and the valves of the heart can be affected (American College of Rheumatology, 2008). The patient may also have a history of inflammatory bowel disease or a family history of arthritis (Frazier & Drzymkowski, 2009).

Laboratory and Diagnostic Procedures

Laboratory data include the following tests: sedimentation rate indicating inflammation, hemoglobin and hematocrit to determine anemia, and HLA-B27 assay, indicating an increase to confirm the diagnosis of AS. Diagnostic tests that are helpful to confirm the diagnosis are x-rays and bone scans (American College of Rheumatology, 2008).

Medical Management

Early detection, diagnosis, and treatment are the best plan in controlling AS (American College of Rheumatology, 2008). Medications that are helpful in treating AS include nonsteroidal anti-inflammatory medications and methotrexate (an oncology chemotherapeutic agent). See the earlier Pharmacology Summary for Medications Used to Treat Arthritis and Connective Tissue Disorders on p. 1839.

Rest is just as important as having physical activity. The patient needs to plan rest periods. The patient needs to sleep an ample amount of time during the night as well (American College of Rheumatology, 2008).

■ Nursing Management

The use of the nursing process will assist the nurse in being able to understand the disease and provide appropriate patient care. The specific disease process will be featured under each stage of the nursing process.

Assessment

Nursing assessment includes evaluating the specific joint and back manifestations described earlier. The assessment also needs to include an in-depth assessment of the other organs such as the heart valves. Chapter 9 ◉ includes a description of an in-depth nursing assessment.

Nursing Diagnoses

The priority nursing diagnoses for the patient with AS include:

1. *Pain, Chronic* related to arthritic joint discomfort
2. *Activity Intolerance* related to musculoskeletal changes
3. *Breathing Pattern, Ineffective* related to changes in rib cage affecting lungs
4. *Fatigue* related to anemia.

Outcomes, Planning, and Evaluation

Outcomes for the patient with AS include relief of pain as expressed by the patient; relief of edema as noted on assessment; and maintenance of posture and mobility through physical therapy and moderate exercise. When planning care, it is important to treat joint symptoms as they present themselves. Utilizing the multidisciplinary team to assist the patient in maintaining function is essential. Physical therapy and occupational therapy can assist the patient in remaining functional. Encourage the patient to remain as independent as possible with therapeutic and non-therapeutic measures, such as understanding of and compliance with the medication regimen and balancing the therapeutic regimen of physical activity. Exercise programs can maintain posture and joint flexibility (American College of Rheumatology, 2008). Respiratory therapy will assist the patient in maintaining lung function. The patient can enhance lung capacity by swimming or aerobic activities. Because ankylosing spondylitis is a progressive condition, it is critical that the patient maintain a program of continuing care (American College of Rheumatology, 2008). The goals for the evaluation are to have the pain managed effectively and the patient able to continue to perform activities of daily living, breathe effectively, and have decreased fatigue.

Septic Arthritis: Epidemiology and Etiology

Nongonococcal bacterial arthritis (**septic arthritis**) is the most destructive form of acute arthritis and can result from trauma, from direct inoculation of bacteria during joint surgery, from spread of infection from another part of the body (hematogenous), or when an infection from an adjacent bone extends through the cortex into the joint space (Goldenberg & Sexton, 2007).

The incidence of septic arthritis is estimated to be 2 to 5 per 100,000 persons (Kherani & Shojania, 2007). Predisposing factors include being over age 80, rheumatoid arthritis, diabetes, skin infection, recent joint surgery or a prosthetic joint, and oral carriage of *Staphylococcus aureus* (Goldenberg & Sexton, 2007; Kherani & Shojania, 2007). Each of the predisposing factors has a modest impact on the risk, but combinations of the factors lead to a substantially increased risk.

Pathophysiology

In the majority of cases, septic arthritis arises from hematogenous spread of bacteria to the joint. Common sources of the infection include intravenous drug use, indwelling catheters, and an underlying immunocompromised state such as HIV infection. Bacteria are more likely to localize in a joint with preexisting arthritis, with patients with rheumatoid arthritis being especially susceptible (Goldenberg & Sexton, 2007). Any microbial pathogen can cause septic arthritis, but organisms such as *Staphylococcus aureus* and *Streptococcus* more commonly cause joint infections than do gram-negative bacilli. Most joint infections are monomicrobial with rare polymicrobial infections occurring in patients with penetrating trauma that involves the joint space. Initially the bacteria deposit in the synovial membrane and produce an acute inflammatory response. The bacteria quickly enter the synovial fluid, creating purulent joint inflammation. Within 1 week the synovial membrane develops hyperplasia, and the cytokines and proteases that were released cause cartilage degradation and inhibit cartilage synthesis. With large effusions, pressure necrosis can result in further cartilage and bone loss. Chart 58–1 outlines causes of infectious arthritis with clinical clues.

Clinical Manifestations and Laboratory and Diagnostic Procedures

Patients with septic arthritis present with a single swollen and painful joint. Common joints affected are the knee (>50%), wrist, ankles, and hips (Goldenberg & Sexton, 2007). Systemic chills, fever, and leukocytosis are usually present. There may also be evidence of an associated skin, urinary, or respiratory infection. The definitive diagnostic test is the identification of bacteria via a culture of the synovial fluid obtained from joint aspiration.

Medical Management

The infection is treated with broad-spectrum intravenous antibiotics initially and then organism-specific antibiotics after the culture results are available. Intravenous antibiotics are continued until symptoms disappear. A typical duration of therapy is 3 to 4 weeks with approximately 2 weeks of intravenous antibiotics and the remainder with oral antibiotics. Progressive range-of-motion exercises will be needed once the infection has subsided. The patient also is treated with antipyretics and pain medication as necessary.

CHART 58–1 **Causes of Septic Arthritis**

Organism	Clinical Clues
Staphylococcus aureus	Healthy adult with skin breakdown, previously damaged joint, or prosthetic joint
Streptococcus	Healthy adult, splenic dysfunction
Neisseria gonorrhoeae	Healthy sexually active adult, associated tenosynovitis, vesicular pustules, and negative synovial fluid culture and gram stain
Aerobic or anaerobic gram-negative bacteria	Immune-compromised patients, gastrointestinal infection
Mycobacterium species	Immune-compromised patient with recent travel to or residence in an endemic area
Fungal	Immune-compromised patients
Spirochete	Exposure to ticks

Source: Adapted from Goldenberg, D., & Sexton, D. (2007). Bacterial (nongonococcal) arthritis in adults. *UpToDate.* Retrieved October 23, 2007, from http://www.uptodate.com/patients/content/topic.do?topicKey=~hcmhzYL2SL2ACJ&selectedTitle=7~147&source=search_result.

Nursing Management

Nursing management focuses on early recognition, pain relief, and protection of the joint from further damage. The nursing process provides a framework for organizing and managing the care of patients with septic arthritis.

Assessment

Patients with septic arthritis present with a warm, painful, and swollen joint with decreased range of motion. Patients at risk are those who are elder, are diabetic, have RA, or have preexisting joint disease or joint replacement. Elderly patients and those taking immunosuppressive or steroid medications may not exhibit as dramatic a reaction to the infection. If there is a risk of infection, the patient must have ongoing assessment to detect it as early as possible.

Nursing Diagnoses

The highest priority nursing diagnoses for the patient with septic arthritis are:

1. *Pain, Acute* related to inflammation and swelling
2. *Mobility: Physical, Impaired* related to pain and swelling of joint
3. *Falls, Risk for* related to pain and swelling of joint
4. *Infection, Risk for*
5. *Knowledge, Deficient* related to treatment regimen.

Outcomes and Evaluation Parameters

The patient's goals include relief of pain, treatment of the infection, rehabilitation of the joint after the infection subsides, and knowledge of treatment regimen. Evaluation parameters include control of pain as expressed by the patient, decrease in the signs and symptoms of infection, and the ability of the patient to articulate the plan of care.

Planning, Interventions, and Rationales

The nurse must support and immobilize the affected joint in a splint. Because the inflammatory process can cause scar tissue within the joint, it is important to splint the joint in a functional position. Analgesics are prescribed to control pain; and after the infection has responded to antibiotic therapy, anti-inflammatory medication such as NSAIDs may be used to limit joint damage.

Evaluation

Evaluation includes absence of infection exhibited by decreased pain and swelling, normal temperature, normal white blood cell count, and negative wound cultures. The patient will report adequate pain relief and an increase in physical mobility with demonstrated safe use of assistive devices. The patient will also be able to articulate an understanding of the continued therapeutic regimen and demonstrate compliance by taking medications as prescribed, demonstrating proper wound care, and reporting signs and symptoms of complications promptly.

Septic joints that are diagnosed and treated early usually recover normal function. Assessment and protection of the affected joint are important to the success of treatment. If the articular cartilage is damaged during the inflammatory response to the infection, joint fibrosis and decreased function may result.

Health Promotion

The nurse instructs the patient on the process of septic arthritis so the patient may understand the therapeutic regimen. Of importance is the adherence to the antibiotic regimen, support of the affected joint, and adherence to weight-bearing and activity restrictions during the inflammatory process to prevent permanent damage to the joint. If assistive devices are to be used, the nurse will help the patient in learning safe use of the devices.

If joint fluid was surgically drained, the nurse teaches the patient aseptic techniques for dressing changes and wound care. The patient should be given instruction for range-of-motion exercises and encouraged to perform them after the infection subsides to maintain optimal joint function.

Systemic Lupus Erythematosus: Epidemiology and Etiology

Systemic lupus erythematosus (SLE) is a chronic inflammatory autoimmune disease that attacks connective tissue or organs. SLE is characterized by remissions and exacerbations, which are common during the spring and summer months. SLE affects mostly women from 30 to 40 years old (Frazier & Drzymkowski, 2009). The etiology is unknown, but it is thought that there is a defect in the body's immunologic mechanism, a predisposition genetically, or an environmental stimulus. Chapter 60 🌐 includes a complete discussion of the immune mechanisms related to SLE.

Pathophysiology

Certain immune complexes deposit in blood vessels, among collagen fibers, and on organs that cause necrosis and inflammation in the major organs, such as the kidneys, brain, eyes, lymphatic system, gastrointestinal (GI) tract, lungs, and skin. A significant feature with SLE is the body's ability to form antibodies against many different tissue components. For a patient who is genetically susceptible, there are multiple predisposing factors associated with SLE. These include physical or mental stress, exposure to sunlight or ultraviolet light, viral or streptococcal infections, pregnancy, and abnormal estrogen metabolism. SLE can also be aggravated or triggered by specific medications such as procainamide, anticonvulsants, hydralazine, and, less commonly, sulfa drugs, penicillins, and hormonal contraceptives.

Clinical Manifestations

Subjective assessment includes weakness, sensitivity to light, and pain in the joints. Objective assessment may reveal elevated temperatures; butterfly rash on the face and the palms of the hands, a type of Raynaud's disease; loss of weight; and dysfunction in one or any of the organs of the renal, gastrointestinal, cardiac, respiratory, or neurological system. Raynaud's disease is discussed in Chapter 43 🌐. With gastrointestinal involvement, patients often experience ulcers in the mouth and nasopharyngeal areas, with 90% of patients experiencing joint pain similar to that of RA. In addition, renal complications are common such as glomerulonephritis. Central nervous system changes occur, such as headaches, irritability, and depression.

Laboratory and Diagnostic Procedures

Two specific tests are used to confirm the diagnosis of SLE: lupus erythematosus preparation (LE prep) and antinuclear antibodies (ANAs). Other laboratory tests would include the following: anti-DNA, anti-Sm antibody, serum complement test, and complement proteins C3 and C4. For more details, see the Diagnostic Tests box for SLE.

Medical Management

There is no permanent cure for SLE; therefore, the goal of treatment is to relieve symptoms and protect organs by decreasing inflammation and/or the level of autoimmune activity in the body. Many patients with mild symptoms may need no treatment or only intermittent courses of anti-inflammatory medications. Those individuals with more serious illness involving damage to internal organs may require high doses of corticosteroids in combination with other medications that suppress the body's immune system (MedicineNet.com, 2008d). See the earlier Pharmacology Summary feature of Medications Used to Treat Arthritis and Connective Tissue Disorders on p. 1839.

Patients with SLE need more rest during periods of active disease. Lack of sleep has been found to be a significant factor in developing fatigue in these patients. The health care provider needs to work with the patient and family to develop a plan that addresses sleep quality and the effects of underlying depression, lack of exercise, and self-care coping strategies on overall health. During these periods, carefully prescribed exercise is still important to maintain muscle tone and range of motion in the joints.

Nonsteroidal anti-inflammatory drugs (NSAIDs), such as aspirin, ibuprofen (Motrin), naproxen (Naprosyn), and sulindac (Clinoril), are effective in reducing inflammation and pain in muscles, joints, and other tissues. Corticosteroids are more potent than NSAIDs; therefore, they are used to restore function when the disease is active and are particularly helpful when internal organs are involved. Corticosteroids can be given by mouth, injected directly into the joints and other tissues, or administered intravenously. Unfortunately, corticosteroids have serious side effects when given in high doses over prolonged periods, and the health care provider must monitor the activity of the disease in order to use the lowest doses that are safe (MedicineNet.com, 2008d).

Hydroxychloroquine (Plaquenil) is an antimalarial medication found to be particularly effective for SLE patients with fatigue, skin, and joint disease. It has been found to be significantly effective in reducing the frequency of abnormal blood clots in SLE patients. For resistant skin disease, other antimalarial drugs, such as chloroquine (Aralen) or quinacrine, are considered and can be used in combination with hydroxychloroquine (MedicineNet.com, 2008d).

Immunosuppressive medications are used for treating patients with more severe manifestations of SLE with damage to internal organs. Examples of immunosuppressive medications include methotrexate (Rheumatrex, Trexall), azathioprine (Imuran), cyclophosphamide (Cytoxan), chlorambucil (Leukeran), and cyclosporine (Sandimmune). All immunosuppressive medications can seriously depress blood cell counts and increase risks of infection and bleeding. Most recent research is indicating benefits of rituximab (Rituxan) in treating lupus. Rituximab is an intravenously infused antibody that suppresses a particular white blood cell, the B cell, by decreasing their number in the circulation. B cells have been found to play a central role in lupus activity, and when they are suppressed, the disease tends toward remission (MedicineNet.com, 2008d).

Recently, mycophenolate mofetil (CellCept) has been used as an effective medication for lupus when it is associated with kidney disease. It helps reverse active lupus kidney disease (lupus renal disease) and helps maintain remission after it is established. Additionally, it has fewer side effects than the traditional immunosuppressive medications (MedicineNet.com, 2008d).

In SLE patients with serious brain or kidney disease, plasmapheresis is sometimes used to remove antibodies and other immune substances in order to suppress immunity. Some SLE patients develop seriously low platelet levels, thereby increasing the risk for spontaneous bleeding. Because the spleen is believed to be the major site of platelet destruction, surgical removal of the spleen is sometimes performed to improve platelet levels. Plasmapheresis has also been used to remove proteins (cryoglobulins) that can lead to vasculitis. End-stage kidney damage from SLE requires dialysis and/or a kidney transplant (MedicineNet.com, 2008d).

DIAGNOSTIC TESTS for Systemic Lupus Erythematosus

Test	Expected Abnormality	Rationale for Abnormality
Lupus erythematosus (LE) prep	Elevated	Presence of systemic lupus erythematosus (SLE).
Antinuclear antibody (ANA)	Elevated	Presence of autoantibodies in blood.
Anti-DNA	Present	Conclude whether there are antibodies in the genetic materials in the cell.
Anti-Sm antibody	Present	Antibodies present on the ribonucleoprotein on the cell nucleus.
Serum complement test	Present	Presence of total group proteins, which can be consumed in immune reactions.
Complement proteins C3 and C4	Present	Examine specific levels of proteins present.
Urinalysis (UA)	Hematuria Proteinuria	Evidence of kidney involvement.

Nursing Management

The goals of nursing management are to limit complications from the disease which vary with each patient. The nursing process provides the framework for the development of the plan of care.

Assessment

Nursing management of the patient with SLE includes ongoing assessments for signs of infection and any dysfunction of the renal, gastrointestinal, cardiac, respiratory, and neurological systems. It is essential to observe patients for signs or symptoms of organ complications. Watch for signs of cardiac involvement such as tachycardia. With respiratory involvement, a patient may experience increased respirations, dyspnea, tachypnea, or orthopnea. Diarrhea, abdominal pain, or distention may indicate gastrointestinal disturbances. Renal involvement may manifest itself as weight gain, scanty urine, and decreased specific gravity; ataxia or ptosis may also indicate neurological involvement. Notify the health care provider immediately about any hematologic signs such as malaise, weakness, chills, and/or epistaxis.

Nursing Diagnoses

Nursing diagnoses related to the patient with SLE are listed in priority order:

1. *Injury, Risk for* related to weakness
2. *Comfort, Readiness for Enhanced* related to joint and/or nerve pain
3. *Activity Intolerance* related to weakness and anemia
4. *Skin Integrity, Impaired* related to photosensitivity
5. *Oral Mucous Membrane, Impaired* related to mouth and nasopharyngeal ulcers
6. *Nutrition: Imbalanced, Less than Body Requirements* related to anorexia and weight loss
7. *Fluid Volume, Excess* related to kidney dysfunction and/or corticosteroid use
8. *Anxiety* related to fear of the disease process
9. *Therapeutic Regimen Management, Readiness for Enhanced* related to exacerbation of disease process.

Outcomes and Evaluation Parameters

Outcomes for the patient with SLE include adaptation to the physical and psychological changes brought about by the disease. The goal is to reduce or limit complications of SLE. The evaluation parameters include the patient's verbalizing an understanding of the changes that are occurring and identifying strategies to cope. The patient should also be able to explain the current therapeutic regimen and identify strategies to prevent complications and reduce side effects of medications.

Planning, Interventions, and Rationales

Planning includes developing a comprehensive health maintenance plan. Interventions include teaching the patient about ways to reduce injuries, controlling discomfort, balancing rest with activity, maintaining skin integrity, reducing oronasopha-ryngeal ulcers, improving diet, restoring fluid volume, reducing anxiety, and complying with the medication regimen.

When implementing care, one of the most important measures to promote is rest. Patients should try to sleep between 8 and 10 hours a night. Encourage the patient to pace activities and plan rest. Stress should be avoided and an unhurried environment is preferred. Teaching the patient and family the importance of rest and decreased stress is paramount.

It is important to provide passive or active range of motion to promote joint movement. Ensure that the patient has not sustained any injuries or falls. Determine whether the patient experiences pain normally or while on medications, and if he remains physically active within his ability to do so. Additionally, the nurse needs to promote proper skin care, which includes hygiene, use of mild soap, use of sunscreen when outdoors, and avoidance of exposure to the sunlight. Observe the skin and oropharyngeal cavities to determine whether they are intact and without lesions. Encourage mouth care a couple times a day if the patient has mouth ulcers, and encourage the patient to change the consistency of his diet to reduce irritation and promote nutritious meals while he has stomatitis.

The diet should be balanced with all of the food groups, which will promote nutritional status, as well as counteract nutritional interactions with corticosteroids. A diet low in sodium is encouraged for patients who have edema, which could indicate renal involvement. Patients should have daily weights, intake, and output to determine fluid volume balance. Encourage the intake of vitamin C, as it is essential in the biosynthesis of collagen and increases total collagen synthesis. Ascertain whether the patient maintains her weight, maintains fluid balance, and can tolerate her diet of choice. Keep the patient calm and allow her to verbalize concerns about the disease process. With the proper diet and precautions, the patient should remain in a state of remission, while simultaneously keeping the organs intact and healthy. The Patient Teaching & Discharge Priorities box (p. 1854) outlines discharge planning for the patient with SLE.

Health Promotion

Providing adequate health teaching is also a goal in the plan of care. It is critical that the patient understand about medications, such as the different classifications, actions, adverse effects, and any interactions with food or other medications. Common medications used for SLE are analgesics, nonnarcotic analgesics, corticosteroids, oncologic drugs, and antimalarials. In addition to understanding about medications, it is important that the patient understand the disease process, diagnosis, prognosis, and treatments available. Teach the patient ways to avoid sun, changing doses of medications, fatigue, infections, and pregnancy without approval from her health care provider. Promote regular exercise and prevent fatigue. Medic alert bracelets should be worn.

Scleroderma: Epidemiology and Etiology

Progressive systemic sclerosis or scleroderma is a progressive autoimmune disease that affects women four times more than men, with peak incidence between ages 35 and 50 (Frazier &

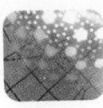

PATIENT TEACHING & DISCHARGE PRIORITIES for Systemic Lupus Erythematosus

Need	Teaching
Safety	Stress the need to reduce injuries. Teach the patient and family ways to reduce risks in their environment to prevent falls.
Integrity of oral mucosa	Explain the importance of reducing irritation of the nose, mouth, and throat to reduce oronasopharyngeal ulcers.
Rest	Encourage the patient to balance rest with activity.
Skin integrity	The patient should maintain skin integrity to prevent integumentary involvement.
Diet	Provide the patient with plan for a balanced diet to maintain health.
Adequate fluid volume	Stress the importance of restoring fluid volume to prevent dehydration.
Low stress	Encourage the patient to reduce stress to prevent a flare-up of systemic lupus erythematosus (SLE). Encourage support groups.
Medications	Teach the patient and family the importance of the patient's medications and the need to comply with medication regimen to prevent further organ damage.

Drzymkowski, 2009; Porth, 2005). Scleroderma crosses all ethnic backgrounds. However, those of European descent are afflicted more than African Americans (National Institute of Arthritis and Musculoskeletal and Skin Diseases, 2006; Porth, 2005). Again, as with other diseases covered in this chapter, the cause is unknown and believed to be autoimmune. With scleroderma, the immune system stimulates the production of an excess of fibroblasts, the cells that produce collagen. In limited scleroderma the hardening of the skin is limited to the hands and face. Diffuse scleroderma also involves the trunk and proximal extremities. The diffuse scleroderma is a severe and progressive disease with early onset of organ involvement including the gastrointestinal tract, heart, lungs, and kidneys (Frazier & Drzymkowski, 2009; Porth, 2005).

Pathophysiology

Scleroderma causes fibrotic changes in connective tissue throughout the body. It can involve any of the following systems: integumentary, circulatory, joints, alimentary canal, cardiac, respiratory, renal, and/or gastrointestinal tract. As the disease becomes more involved, the acronym CREST syndrome identifies a group of symptoms affiliated with the disease's getting advanced with a poor recovery or chance of remission. C stands for calcium deposits in organs; R stands for Raynaud's type symptoms; E stands for esophageal dysfunction; S stands for sclerodactyly, meaning scleroderma of the fingers and toes; and T stands for telangiectasia, which is a vascular lesion formed by dilation.

Clinical Manifestations

The disease is characterized by inflammatory and then degenerative and fibrotic changes in the skin, blood vessels, synovial membranes, skeletal muscles, and internal organs.

Subjective clinical findings are verbalized by the patient who complains of joint pain and muscle weakness. Objective clinical findings note hard skin that fixes to underlying structures. The affect becomes flat and general body movements are rigid. Telangiectases are noted on the lips, fingers, face, and tongue. Some patients develop dysphagia and Raynaud's-type symptoms.

Laboratory and Diagnostic Procedures

Initially, the diagnosis of the scleroderma syndrome is based on the clinical manifestations of the illnesses. Laboratory data would consist of positive LE prep with elevated gamma globulin levels, and the presence of antinuclear antibodies. A particular antibody, the anticentromere antibody, is found almost exclusively in the CREST form of scleroderma. Anti-Scl-70 antibody (antitopoisomerase I antibody) is most often seen in patients with the diffuse form of scleroderma. Other tests that help evaluate the presence or extent of any internal disease include upper and lower gastrointestinal examinations; chest x-rays, lung function testing, and CAT scanning to examine the lungs; and ECG, echocardiograms, and sometimes heart catheterization to evaluate the pressure in the arteries of the heart and lungs.

Medical Management

Because this is a chronic disease, medical management focuses on symptom control and improving the patient's quality of life. Medications are utilized to assist the patient with symptoms of the disease. Corticosteroids help with the inflammation, and salicylates or narcotics are used for joint discomfort. For Raynaud's-type symptoms, vasodilators are used to increase circulation. Most commonly, immunosuppressants and D-penicillamine are also administered. Hand warming and protection from cold temperatures may be all that is necessary for mild Raynaud's disease. Low-dose aspirin is frequently prescribed to prevent tiny blood clots in the fingers, especially in patients with a history of fingertip ulcerations. Medications that dilate the arteries, such as nifedipine (Procardia, Adalat) and nicardipine (Cardene), or topical nitroglycerin applied to the side of the affected digit is frequently used to treat moderate Raynaud's disease. Gently applied finger splints can protect tender tissues. A class of medications that is typically used for depression, the selective serotonin reuptake inhibitors, such as fluoxetine (Prozac), can sometimes improve the circulation of the affected digit. In cases of severe Raynaud's disease, surgical procedures, such as those used to interrupt the nerves of the finger that stimulate constriction of the blood vessels (digital sympathectomy), may be necessary. Ulcerations of the fingers can require topical or oral antibiotics (MedicineNet.com, 2008b).

Medications used to treat esophagus irritation and heartburn are omeprazole (Prilosec), esomeprazole (Nexium), and lansoprazole (Prevacid). Antacids can also be helpful. Elevating the head of the bed can reduce the backflow of acid into the esophagus that causes inflammation and heartburn. Avoiding caffeine and cigarette smoking also helps. Constipation, cramping, and diarrhea are sometimes caused by bacteria that can be treated with tetracycline or erythromycin. Increased fluid intake and fiber intake are good general measures to help with constipation (MedicineNet.com, 2008b).

Medications that are used to suppress the overly active immune system include penicillamine, azathioprine, and methotrexate. Serious inflammation of the lungs (alveolitis) can require immune suppression with cyclophosphamide (Cytoxan) along with prednisone. Approximately 10% of patients with the CREST variant that develop scleroderma have pulmonary hypertension (Chapter 36), which is often treated with calcium antagonist medications, such as nifedipine, and anticoagulation (MedicineNet.com, 2008b).

Irritated, itchy dry skin can be helped by emollients such as Lubriderm, Eucerin, or Bag Balm. Colchicine may be helpful in decreasing the inflammation and tenderness that periodically accompany the calcinosis nodules in the skin. Telangiectasias, such as those on the face, can be treated with local laser therapy. Sun exposure should be minimized as it can worsen telangiectasias (MedicineNet.com, 2008b). Medications used to treat scleroderma are addressed in the earlier Pharmacology Summaries on p. 1839.

Nursing Management

The nursing process provides the framework necessary to develop a comprehensive health care plan. The goals of nursing care involve control of pain and support of the patient and family.

Assessment

As with all of the joint diseases, nursing assessment focuses on the extent of joint range of motion and pain. With scleroderma, the nurse must also assess for organ involvement. The lungs, heart, skin, and gastrointestinal system must be assessed for involvement. Chapter 9 outlines the essential components of the nursing assessment for each of these organs.

Nursing Diagnoses

The highest priority nursing diagnoses for the patient with scleroderma are as follows:

1. *Pain, Chronic* related to joint pain
2. *Skin Integrity, Impaired* related to skin lesions
3. *Body Image, Disturbed* related to flat affect, skin lesions, and telangiectases
4. *Falls, Risk for* related to limited motion and rigidity
5. *Therapeutic Regimen Management, Ineffective* related to noncompliance with medications
6. *Mobility: Physical, Impaired* related to rigidity and limited movement
7. *Anxiety* related to poor prognosis.

Planning, Interventions, Rationales, and Evaluation

When planning the treatment for the patient with scleroderma, the goal is to support the patient and family and improve the quality of life, because there is no cure. When implementing the care, the nurse must be knowledgeable about which organs are involved and the associated clinical manifestations. The nurse must continually monitor function of all vital organs, such as the heart, lungs, and kidneys, to determine the perfusion. Explain the purpose of each medication and the importance of compliance. Advise the patient about the adverse effects of all of the medications.

Engage in regular inspection of skin and oropharyngeal areas to maintain skin integrity. Because skin manifestations are common, it is essential that the patient be taught to use mild soap and lotion on the skin. The use of emollient lotions is helpful as is strict adherence to sunscreens. The nurse should stress to avoid exposure to the cold due to vasoconstriction of vessels, thereby decreasing peripheral circulation. If there is lung involvement, provide education on the importance of not smoking, and deep breathing exercises should be encouraged to improve oxygenation.

Include the multidisciplinary team in assisting the patient to be independent for as long as possible. Physical therapy can usually provide assistance to keep the patient moving and aid with mobility. Ensure joint pain is managed with or without medication, and combine with physical therapy in order to improve physical mobility. Occupational therapy can provide assistance with activities of daily living. Evaluate the patient for signs of increased muscle weakness and rigidity. Make certain the patient is compliant with medications and understands the importance of the treatment regimen. The patient needs to be reminded to keep himself away from situations that may lead to falls or high levels of anxiety.

Finally, have discussions with the patient about the physical changes that are occurring to help her be better able to cope with changes in her body image as the disease progresses. Explain which symptoms need to be reported to the health care provider, and stress the importance of regular medical examinations. Evaluation of the health plan includes an assessment of the patient's knowledge of the disease, the importance of compliance with the treatment plan, and limitations.

Lyme Disease

Lyme disease is a bacterial infection that affects the organs and joints that is transmitted from black-legged ticks. In the city of Lyme, Connecticut, a group of children spontaneously developed a debilitating arthritis. The Centers for Disease Control and Prevention (CDC) was alerted to this phenomenon, and research into the progression of illness and disease vectors was underway. In 1977, at the conclusion of the investigation, it was found that deer ticks were transmitting a degenerative disease to humans, which was subsequently named Lyme disease, after the city that had brought medical attention to it (Centers for Disease Control and Prevention, 2008).

Epidemiology

In 2006, 19,931 cases of Lyme disease were reported, showing a national average of 8.2 cases per 100,000 persons (Centers for Disease Control and Prevention, 2008). The deer tick bites the host (human) and transmits the disease. In the United States, Lyme disease is heavily concentrated in the areas of the Northeast, Southeast, and West Coast (Centers for Disease Control and Prevention, 2008).

Etiology

Lyme disease is caused by bacteria, called *Borrelia burgdorferi*, which are found in infected black-legged ticks. There are two species of black-legged ticks: *ixodes scapularis* located in the Northeast and north central United States and *ixodes pacificus* in the western parts of the United States. These ticks are much smaller than the ticks that animals such as dogs and cattle carry. Ticks feed by placing their mouth on the human and sucking the blood. The bacteria are transferred slowly by transmitting the infection over a couple of days of feeding (Centers for Disease Control and Prevention, 2008).

Those individuals who live in rural areas near trees and overgrown shrubs may be at risk for Lyme disease. Outdoor activities, such as hiking, camping, gardening, working in forestry, and wildlife/parks management in specified areas, expose participants to a higher risk of being infected (Centers for Disease Control and Prevention, 2008).

Pathophysiology and Clinical Manifestations

An infected tick attaches to a human, sucks the person's blood, and transfers the disease. There are three stages of the disease, which can affect many systems of the body.

1. Early localized disease, occurring a few days to 1 month after the tick bite.
   - Erythema chronicum migrans (reddened area where the tick bite occurred) occurs in 70% to 80% of patients.
   - Associated symptoms and signs may include fatigue, malaise, lethargy, headache, stiff neck, myalgias, arthralgias, and regional or generalized lymphadenopathy.
2. Early disseminated disease occurring days to 10 months after the tick bite.
   - Carditis. Occurs in approximately 5% of untreated patients. Manifestations include conduction defects, mild cardiomyopathy, or myopericarditis.
   - Neurological disease. Occurs in approximately 15% of untreated patients. Manifestations include lymphocytic meningitis; encephalitis; cranial neuropathy (most often facial, can be bilateral), peripheral neuropathy, or radiculoneuropathy; or myelitis.
   - Musculoskeletal involvement. Occurs in approximately 60% of untreated patients. Manifestations include migratory polyarthritis and/or polyarthralgias.
   - Skin involvement. Multiple erythema chronicum migrans lesions, erythema nodosum.
   - Lymphadenopathy. Regional and/or generalized.

   - Eye involvement. Conjunctivitis, iritis, choroiditis, vitritis, retinitis.
   - Liver disease. Liver function test abnormalities, hepatitis.
   - Kidney disease. Microhematuria, asymptomatic proteinuria.
3. Late or chronic disease, occurring months to years after the tick bite.
   - Musculoskeletal symptoms. Approximately 60% of untreated patients develop intermittent monoarticular or oligoarticular arthritis; approximately 10% of untreated patients develop persistent monoarthritis, usually affecting the knee.
   - Neurological disease. Incidence is rare but may be exhibited by chronic, often subtle, encephalopathy, encephalomyelitis, and/or peripheral neuropathy (Sexton, 2008).

Laboratory and Diagnostic Procedures

It is important to obtain the correct diagnosis before treating this condition. Be sure that the patient obtains a blood test that can be used to detect the presence of antibodies from the bacterium to corroborate the diagnosis. Antibiotics can be given to cure the disease if caught early. The most common classifications of anti-infectives are tetracyclines and penicillins. Another goal is to prevent this disease for further progression. It is important to talk to patients about prevention and health promotion.

Medical Management

For early-stage Lyme disease, oral antibiotics are the standard treatment. These usually include doxycycline for adults and children older than 8, or amoxicillin or cefuroxime axetil for elder adults, younger children, and pregnant or breast-feeding women. These drugs often clear the infection and prevent complications. A 14- to 21-day course of antibiotics is usually recommended. If the disease has progressed, intravenous antibiotic for 14 to 28 days is an effective treatment plan for eliminating infection, although it may take some time to recover symptomatically (MayoClinic.com, 2008).

The flu-like symptoms are treated with supportive measures, depending on the presenting symptoms. For example, fever is treated with antipyretics and rest, and the joint pain is treated with NSAIDs and rest.

◼ Nursing Management

The nursing process provides the framework for the management of patients with Lyme disease. Nursing management focuses on treatment of the infection and education of the patient and family on ways to avoid exposure to ticks and possible reinfection.

Assessment

Assessment of the early localized disease, the first stage, which occurs between days 7 and 10, includes evaluating for a growing rash called erythema chronicum migrans (ECM). ECM looks like a bull's eye on the affected part. Assess for flu-like symptoms: headache, confusion, forgetfulness, stiff neck, irregular heartbeat, achy and swollen joints, and swollen lymph glands

(Frazier & Drzymkowski, 2009). During the second stage, which occurs a couple of weeks to months after being infected, the nurse needs to focus the assessment on the neurological system. Assessment findings could include severe headaches, poor motor balance, and temporary facial paralysis. During the late stage of the disease, which can occur from months to years after being infected, the musculoskeletal system is attacked. Arthritis is a complication of this disease. Approximately 5% of the people infected will develop chronic arthritis (Centers for Disease Control and Prevention, 2008).

Nursing Diagnoses

The following are the high-priority nursing diagnoses for the patient with Lyme disease:

1. *Infection, Risk for* related to tick contamination
2. *Pain, Acute* related to neurological symptoms of the disease
3. *Knowledge, Deficient* related to unfamiliarity of Lyme disease.

Interventions, Outcomes, and Evaluation Parameters

Nursing interventions are dependent on the stage of the disease and the patient's clinical manifestations. For example, early in the disease process, the management would focus on treating the flu-like symptoms. The later stages of the disease are more complex, and the nursing care is dependent on what systems are involved. For example, if there is neurological involvement and muscle weakness, the nurse must focus on protection of the airway and prevention of patients falling or injuring themselves. The outcome of care is to have the patient free of infection as exhibited by a decrease in symptoms. It is imperative that the patient and family understand ways to protect themselves from exposure and reinfection. During this phase of the nursing process, the evaluation parameters would include educating the patient about the disease and its cause, signs, symptoms, treatment, and prevention by examining discharge priorities. For more information, see the Patient Teaching & Discharge Priorities box about Lyme disease.

Health Promotion

It is important to teach individuals about ways to prevent disease. Many things can be done to promote protection from Lyme disease. During the summer months, avoid areas where ticks are contaminated. Be sure to wear long sleeve shirts, long pants, and socks. Tuck socks into pants and tuck shirts into pants to minimize exposure of the skin. By wearing light color clothing, ticks

are easily seen and can be removed before getting bit. It is important to use tick repellents, such as DEET. Be careful not to overuse these products. Avoid high grassy trails when walking. Once individuals are finished being outdoors, they should remove their clothing and wash it. Also, they should examine their body thoroughly and remove any attached ticks. Use tweezers to carefully remove them. Once the tick is removed, be sure that antiseptic is used to clean the area. Check pets to be certain that they do not have ticks. Tick collars can be put around the neck of the pets.

Sjögren's Syndrome: Epidemiology and Etiology

Sjögren's syndrome (SS) is an autoimmune disease. SS immune cells attack and destroy the glands that produce tears and saliva (Frazier & Drzymkowski, 2009). In the United States, SS affects 1 million to 4 million people. Usually the ratio of women to men is 9 to 1 (Borenstein, 2007). Sjögren's syndrome is found more commonly in patients with a family history of other autoimmune illnesses.

Pathophysiology

SS is an inflammatory disease that can affect different parts of the body. SS features inflammation in the glands of the body resulting in dryness in the affected areas. SS is characterized by the increased production of more antibodies in the blood that are directed against various tissues of the body. This particular autoimmune illness is caused by inflammation of the glands that produce tears (lacrimal glands), leading to decreased water production for tears and eye dryness. Inflammation of the glands that produce the saliva in the mouth (salivary glands, including the parotid glands) leads to mouth dryness (MedicineNet.com, 2008c). SS is not considered a connective tissue disease when it involves the glands affecting the eyes and mouth only. However, when SS is associated with RA, then it is considered a connective tissue disease (MedicineNet.com, 2008c).

Clinical Manifestations

The two symptoms that are the hallmark of Sjögren's syndrome are dry eyes and dry mouth (Sjögren's Syndrome Foundation, 2008). The disease can also cause dryness in other body organs including the kidneys, gastrointestinal tract, lung, and blood vessels. Many patients have debilitating joint pain and fatigue. The symptoms can wax and wane and go into remission. Some

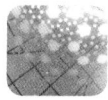

PATIENT TEACHING & DISCHARGE PRIORITIES for Lyme Disease

Need	Teaching
Knowledge of disease process	Encourage understanding of the infectious process of Lyme disease. Early detection is critical for early treatment and prevention of complications.
Prevention	Those who live in highly infected areas should be taking precautions to reduce the risk of getting infected. Teach patient the importance of using insect repellant when out of doors in high risk areas.
Medications	Encourage compliance with medication regimen. If infected, it is imperative to continue to take entire prescription as ordered by health care provider.

patients may have only mild symptoms where others are severely affected and experience a poor quality of life.

Laboratory and Diagnostic Procedures

According to Sjögren's Syndrome Foundation (2008), 70% of individuals with SS will have an elevated antibody (ANA), which measures antibodies that react against normal components of the cell nucleus. Sjögren's syndrome antigens (SSA and SSB) are also elevated; with 70% of the population having SS, the rheumatoid factor is elevated, measuring positive. The erythrocyte sedimentation rate is also elevated, indicating an active inflammatory process. Immunoglobulins measure normal blood proteins and are also elevated with SS (Sjögren's Syndrome Foundation, 2008).

Other tests that may be used are the following: the Schirmer's test, measuring tear production; Rose Bengal and Lissamine green, using dyes to observe abnormal cells on the surface of the eye; slit lamp exam, magnifying the volume of tears of the eye by viewing it in its resting state; parotid gland flow, measuring the amount of saliva produced over a certain period of time; salivary scintigraphy, measuring salivary gland function; sialography, an x-ray of the salivary duct system; and lip biopsy, used to confirm lymphocytic infiltration of the minor salivary glands (Sjögren's Syndrome Foundation, 2008).

Medical Management

There is no cure for SS at this time. However, symptoms can be treated. Patients can use moist replacement therapies for symptoms of dryness. Increasing fluid intake, using oral sprays, and chewing sugarless gum may help oral dryness. Wearing sunglasses to protect the eyes and using artificial tears are recommended (Frazier & Drzymkowski, 2009). Many classifications of medications are helpful, such as nonsteroidal anti-inflammatory drugs for musculoskeletal symptoms, and corticosteroids and immunosuppressive therapies for severe complications (National Institute of Neurological Disorders and Stroke, 2008d).

Nursing Management

When utilizing a nursing problem-solving approach, the nursing process will lead the nurse to understand the disease process while prioritizing care for those with SS.

Assessment

For subjective assessments, patients will complain of feeling dryness in the following locations: mouth, mucous membranes, and skin. Objective assessments include irritation, a gritty feeling, or painful burning in the eyes; dry mouth; dysphagia; swelling of saliva glands; and dryness of nasal passage or throat, or vagina or skin (National Institute of Neurological Disorders and Stroke, 2008d). There are periods of remissions and exacerbations. Exacerbations usually occur after an illness.

Patients also may experience blurred vision, recurrent mouth infections, swollen parotid glands, hoarseness, dysphagia, debilitating fatigue, and joint pain (National Institute of Neurological Disorders and Stroke, 2008d).

Nursing Diagnoses

The following is a list of high-priority nursing diagnoses for the patient with Sjögren's syndrome:

1. *Nutrition: Imbalanced, Less than Body Requirements* as related by dysphasia
2. *Pain, Chronic* related to dried secretions in mucous membranes and joint pain
3. *Knowledge, Deficient* related to unfamiliarity of educational resources
4. *Communication: Verbal, Impaired* related to hoarseness
5. *Self-Care, Readiness for Enhanced* related to debilitating fatigue.

Interventions, Outcomes, and Evaluation Parameters

Interventions include protecting the affected tissues, assisting in preventing complications, avoiding irritation to the tissues, monitoring for signs and symptoms of infection, and assessing for the development of complications. Outcomes for the patient with SS include relief of symptoms of dryness in the oral cavity and eyes. Evaluation parameters include adequate nutritional status, pain abatement, awareness of educational resources, ability to communicate effectively, and care for self.

■ Myositis: Epidemiology and Etiology

Myositis is an uncommon disease wherein the immune system inflames the body's own healthy muscle tissue. There are four kinds of myositis: polymyositis (PM), dermatomyositis (DM), inclusion body myositis (IBM), and juvenile myositis (JM) (National Institute of Neurological Disorders and Stroke, 2008a, 2008b, 2008c). PM can occur at any age, but affects those between ages 40 and 50. DM, like PM, can arise at any age, but is more prevalent between ages 40 and 60 and between ages 5 and 15. Both are more common in African Americans than in Caucasians and affect more women than men (Frazier & Drzymkowski, 2009; National Institute of Neurological Disorders and Stroke, 2008a, 2008c). Myositis occurs more readily with patients who have lupus. IBM typically begins after age 50 and is more common in women than in men. Globally, DM and PM together affect 5 to 10 people out of 100,000 (MayoClinic.com, 2007). Theses conditions are usually caused by an injury, infection, or autoimmune condition (Ariel & Teitel, 2007).

Pathophysiology

Myositis is a disease where the immune system causes chronic inflammation of the voluntary muscles of the body. Voluntary muscles are consciously controlled to help move the body. Myositis may be triggered by an injury, infection, or an autoimmune disease. PM consists of muscle weakness. DM has the same symptoms as PM; but DM differs because of the skin involvement with a distinctive rash over the face, shoulders, arms, and bony prominences (MayoClinic.com, 2007).

Clinical Manifestations

Symptoms for PM include muscle weakness especially proximal to the trunk, such as in the hips and shoulders. Patients have difficulty getting up out of chairs, climbing stairs, lifting objects, and reaching overhead (National Institute of Neurological Disorders and Stroke, 2008c). As the condition advances, some patients have dysphasia.

With DM, patients have the same symptoms as PM, but a rash exists. This rash is purplish blue discolorations on the face, eyelids, bridge of nose, neck, shoulders, elbows, knees, knuckles, upper chest, and back (American Association of Orthopedic Surgeons, 2008; National Institute of Neurological Disorders and Stroke, 2008a). Some patients develop calcium deposits under the skin that manifest as bumps under the skin. IBM has a gradual onset of muscle weakness all over the body. Atrophy of the muscles can occur in wrists or fingers, forearms, and thighs. Some people may develop dysphagia. JM is a combination of the three other kinds of myositis: PM, DM, and IBM.

Laboratory and Diagnostic Procedures

A laboratory test that can assist with the diagnosis of myositis is the creatine kinase. This test measures autoantibodies and the muscle enzymes. Two diagnostic tests that also can confirm the diagnosis are the electromyogram and magnetic resonance imaging to identify the inflamed muscles (MayoClinic.com, 2007).

Medical Management

The health care provider needs to reassure the patient that there are treatments available, but no cure. Prompt treatment consists of reducing inflammation and restoring strength. Some methodologies can curb muscle atrophy. First, medications may improve myositis. Corticosteroids act to suppress the immune system and slow the attack on healthy muscles (MayoClinic.com, 2007). Nonsteroidal anti-inflammatory medications are given to reduce pain. Physical therapy will help the patients strengthen muscles. An exercise program may be beneficial to prevent muscle atrophy and promote range of motion. Utilizing a whirlpool bath, heat, and gentle massage may be beneficial (MayoClinic.com, 2007). Rest can assist this condition. Pacing activities and planning rest are valuable in reducing inflammation of muscles (MayoClinic.com, 2007).

Nursing Management

Utilization of the nursing process will provide the nurse with the tools necessary to provide safe and sound patient care. The nurse must assess for muscle weakness, as this is the most common symptom. Varying degrees of loss of muscle strength may cause difficulty in getting up from a sitting position, climbing stairs, or lifting an object above the shoulders. Some patients may complain of muscle aches and tenderness to touch.

Nursing Diagnoses

Nursing diagnoses that are a priority for a patient with myositis include:

1. *Self-Care, Readiness for Enhanced* related to muscle weakness
2. *Activity Intolerance* related to muscle atrophy
3. *Body Image, Disturbed* related to rash
4. *Falls, Risk for* related to inability to support body's weight
5. *Pain, Chronic* related to muscle atrophy.

Interventions, Outcomes, and Evaluation Parameters

Nursing interventions include assisting the patient with activities of daily living and spacing care to allow for periods of rest. Outcomes for the patient with myositis include restoring strength and reducing muscle weakness in order to prevent atrophy of muscles. Promote independence by encouraging the patient to perform activities of daily living to the fullest extent while balancing rest and physical activity. Evaluation parameters are that the patient is able to provide own self-care, report activity tolerance, accept body image changes, have no falls, and have no pain with or without medications.

Research

Many clinical trials are taking place on a variety of connective tissue diseases, such as arthritis and lupus. Several connective tissue diseases are also inherited. These trials examine the effects of medication on the disease itself, whereas others examine the issue of stem cells to correct the condition. Many of these disorders can be controlled by changes in behavior or lifestyle changes in which diet and exercise play a critical role. For specific information about research that is being conducted, go to the National Institutes of Health's website to search for the most up-to-date information and research on specific diseases.

MyNursingKit | National Institute of Health

Clinical Preparation

CRITICAL THINKING

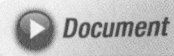 **Read**

- History of Current Illness
- Past Medical History
- Physical Exam
- Admitting Medical Orders
- Laboratory Study Results

 **Document**

- Summary of Hospitalization
- Pathophysiology Form
- Laboratory Values
- Laboratory Results Explanation

Apply

- List of Potential Nursing Diagnoses
- Concept Map
- Critical Thinking Questions

Log on to MyNursingKit.com to download forms you will need and to complete further steps in the Clinical Preparation assignment.

HISTORY OF PRESENT ILLNESS

E A is a 48-year-old Caucasian male who works as a pastry chef at one of the most prestigious hotels in San Francisco. He is married and has 13 children. He weighs 378 pounds and has a history of kidney stones on the left side. He came into the emergency department when he had completed work after the dinner crowd. He presented symptoms of an elevated temperature of 101°F, chills, malaise, and excruciating pain in his right great toe.

Medical–Surgical History

Upon interview: The patient revealed that his father and grandfather had gout.

Physical Exam

Patient verbalized, "I feel real tired and have had a temperature of 100 degrees for two days." His toe was swollen, red, and hot. On a pain scale, the patient indicated his pain was an "11." Laboratory tests were collected and the only elevations were a serum uric acid level and a low pH in the urine. Tophi are located in the following places: (1) his ear lobes bilaterally, (2) right elbow, and (3) bilateral knees. The physician ordered the patient to have the following medications: allopurinol and colchicine and a diet low in purines.

CRITICAL THINKING QUESTIONS

1. What risk factors presented in this scenario indicate gout?
2. What types of food may cause an acute attack of gouty arthritis?
3. What are three objective assessments that lead you to believe the patient may have gout?

4. What is a complication of having too much serum uric acid and low pH? Which organ is most commonly involved?

Answers to Critical Thinking Questions appear in Appendix D.

NCLEX® REVIEW

1. A patient was told she has lupus erythematosus. Which of the following should the nurse instruct this patient?
   1. It's a term to describe rheumatic disease.
   2. It's a chronic inflammatory process that affects joints.
   3. It's a common connective tissue disorder.
   4. It's an inflammation associated with psoriasis.

2. Which of the following should the nurse include when planning the care of a patient with rheumatoid arthritis?
   1. Increase activity
   2. Maximize activities of daily living
   3. Restrict calories
   4. Prevent deformities

3. A patient is admitted with circinate balanitis and uveitis. The nurse realizes this patient is most likely experiencing:
   1. Reactive arthritis.
   2. Rheumatoid arthritis.
   3. Osteoarthritis.
   4. Septic arthritis.

4. The nurse has completed the assessment of a patient with osteoarthritis. Which of the following nursing diagnoses would be applicable to this patient?
   1. *Knowledge Deficit*
   2. *Ineffective Coping*
   3. *Imbalanced Nutrition: More than Body Requirements*
   4. *Fluid Volume Deficit*

5. A patient is diagnosed with gout. The nurse should instruct this patient to avoid which of the following foods?

1. Lettuce
2. Gravies
3. Broccoli
4. Chicken

6. A patient is admitted with muscle weakness and a blue-tinted rash on his face, neck, and back. The nurse realizes this patient is most likely experiencing:

1. Myositis.
2. Polymyositis.
3. Dermatomyositis.
4. Inclusion body myositis.

Answers for review questions appear in Appendix D

KEY TERMS

ankylosing spondylitis *p.1849*
circinate balanitis *p.1847*
dactylitis *p.1842*
enthesitis *p.1842*
gouty arthritis *p.1843*
Lyme disease *p.1855*

myositis *p.1858*
osteoarthritis (OA) *p.1833*
psoriatic arthritis *p.1842*
reactive arthritis *p.1847*
rheumatoid arthritis (RA) *p.1836*

septic arthritis *p.1850*
Sjögren's syndrome *p.1857*
subcutaneous nodules *p.1835*
systemic lupus erythematosus *p.1851*
tophi *p.1844*

PEARSON
EXPLORE **mynursingkit™**

MyNursingKit is your one stop for online chapter review materials and resources. Prepare for success with additional NCLEX®-style practice questions, interactive assignments and activities, web links, animations and videos, and more!

Register your access code from the front of your book at
www.mynursingkit.com

REFERENCES

American Association of Orthopedic Surgeons (AAOS). (2008). *Myositis.* Retrieved September 1, 2008 from http://orthoinfo.aaos.org/topic.cfm?topic=A00198

American College of Rheumatology. (2008). *Ankylosing spondylitis.* Retrieved May 24, 2008, from http://www.rheumatology.org/public/factsheets/as.asp

Ariel, D., & Teitel, M. D. (2007). Myositis. *Healthline.* Retrieved July 23, 2007, from http://www.healthline.com/adamcontent/myositis

Arthritis-FAQ.com. (2007). *Gout overview.* Retrieved July 18, 2007, from http://www.arthritis-faq.org/gout.html

Borenstein, D. (2007). Epidemiology, diagnostics and management. *Medscape Today.* Retrieved July 23, 2007, from http://www.medscape.com/viewarticle/423760

Centers for Disease Control and Prevention (CDC). (2007). *Prevalence of arthritis.* Retrieved May 24, 2008, from http://www.cdc.gov/arthritis/data_statistics/arthritis_related_statistics.htm#1

Centers for Disease Control and Prevention (CDC). (2008). *Lyme disease.* Retrieved May 24, 2008, from http://www.cdc.gov/ncidod/dvbid/lyme/ld_statistics.htm

Chemocare.com. (2005). *Hyperuricemia.* Retrieved July 30, 2007, from http://www.chemocare.com/managing/hyperuricemia-high-uric-acid.asp

eMedicineHealth. (2008). *Gout.* Retrieved May 23, 2008, from http://www.emedicinehealth.com/gout/article_em.htm

FamilyPracticeNotebook.com. (2008). *Osteoarthritis.* Retrieved August 25, 2008, from http://www.fpnotebook.com/Rheum/Osteoarthritis/Ostrthrts.htm

Frazier, M. S., & Drzymkowski, J. W. (Eds.). (2009). *Essentials of human diseases and conditions* (4th ed.). St. Louis: Saunders Elsevier.

Gladman, D. (2007). Pathogenesis of psoriatic arthritis. *UpToDate.* Retrieved October 23, 2007, from http://www.uptodate.com/patients/content/topic.do?topicKey=~nKkKMlvosxl56.&selectedTitle=1~78&source=search_result

Gladman, D. (2008). Clinical manifestations and diagnosis of psoriatic arthritis. *UpToDate.* Retrieved August 21, 2008, from http://www.uptodate.com/patients/content/topic.do?topicKey=~FFX.7DwCxZDGbF&selectedTitle=2~150&source=search_result

Goldenberg, D., & Sexton, D. (2007). Bacterial (nongonococcal) arthritis in adults. *UpToDate.* Retrieved October 23, 2007, from http://www.uptodate.com/patients/content/topic.do?topicKey=~hcmhzYL2SL2ACJ&selectedTitle=7~147&source=search_result

Hammadi, A. A. (2008). Psoriatic arthritis. *eMedicine.com.* Retrieved May 23, 2008, from http://www.emedicine.com/MED/topic1954.htm

Hogan, M. A. (2007). *Nutrition & diet therapy* (2nd ed.). Upper Saddle River, NJ: Pearson Prentice Hall.

Hospital for Special Surgery. (2005). *Osteoarthritis.* Retrieved May 1, 2006, from http://www.imaginghss.org/imaging-of-orthopaedic-conditions/osteoarthritis.htm

InnerVibrance. (2006). *Rheumatoid arthritis.* Retrieved February 28, 2006, from http://www.innervibrance.com/rheumatoid_arthritis.html

Kalunian, K. C. (2007). *Pathogenesis of OA: Diagnosis and classification of OA.* Retrieved August 28, 2008, from http://www.utdol.com/online/content/topic.do?topicKey=osteoart/3785&selectedTitle=1~150&source=search_result

Kherani, R., & Shojania, K. (2007). Septic arthritis in patients with preexisting inflammatory arthritis. *Canadian Medical Association Journal, 176*(11), 1605–1608.

MayoClinic.com. (2007). *Polymyositis.* Retrieved May 24, 2008, from http://www.mayoclinic.com/health/polymyositis/DS00334

MayoClinic.com. (2008). *Lyme disease: Symptoms.* Retrieved May 23, 2008, from http://www.mayoclinic.com/health/lyme-disease/DS00116/DSECTION-2

MedicineNet.com. (2008a). *Rheumatoid arthritis.* Retrieved May 23, 2008, from http://www.medicinenet.com/rheumatoid_arthritis/article.htm

MedicineNet.com. (2008b). *Scleroderma.* Retrieved May 21, 2008, from http://www.medicinenet.com/scleroderma/article.htm

MedicineNet.com. (2008c). *Sjogren's syndrome.* Retrieved May 23, 2008, from http://www.medicinenet.com/sjogrens_syndrome/article.htm

MedicineNet.com. (2008d). *Systemic lupus erythematosus (SLE or lupus).* Retrieved May 23, 2008, from http://www.medicinenet.com/systemic_lupus/article.htm

MedlinePlus Medical Encyclopedia. (2007). *Acute gouty arthritis.* Retrieved May 23, 2008, from http://www.nlm.nih.gov/medlineplus/ency/article/000422.htm

Meiner, S. (2001). Gouty arthritis: Not just a big toe problem. *Geriatric Nursing, 22*(3), 132–134.

Mikuls, T. R., MacLean, C. H., Olivieri, J., Patino, F., Allison, J., Farrar, J. T., et al. (2004). Quality of care indicators for gout management. *Arthritis & Rheumatism, 50*(3), 937–943.

Mikuls, T. R., & Saag, K. G. (2005). Gout treatment: What is evidence-based and how do we determine and promote optimized clinical care? *Current Rheumatology Reports, 7*(3), 242–249.

National Institute of Arthritis and Musculoskeletal and Skin Diseases (NIAMS). (2002). *Reactive arthritis.* Retrieved December 18, 2004, from http://www.niams.nih.gov/hi/topics/reactive/reactive.htm

National Institute of Arthritis and Musculoskeletal and Skin Diseases (NIAMS). (2006). *Scleroderma.* Retrieved August 21, 2008, from http://www.niams.nih.gov/hi/topics/scleroderma/scleroderma.htm

National Institute of Arthritis and Musculoskeletal and Skin Diseases (NIAMS). (2008). *Arthritis: Causes and risk factors—Gout.* Retrieved August 21, 2008, from http://nihseniorhealth.gov/arthritis/causesandriskfactors/01.html

National Institute of Neurological Disorders and Stroke. (2008a). *Dermatomyositis information page.* Retrieved August 21, 2008, from www.ninds.nih.gov/disorders/dermatomyositis/dermatomyositis.htm

National Institute of Neurological Disorders and Stroke. (2008b). *Inclusion body myositis information page.* Retrieved August 21, 2008, from http://www.ninds.nih.gov/disorders/inclusion_body_myositis/inclusion_body_myositis.htm

National Institute of Neurological Disorders and Stroke. (2008c). *Polymyositis information page.* Retrieved August 21, 2008, from http://www.ninds.nih.gov/disorders/polymyositis/polymyositis.htm

National Institute of Neurological Disorders and Stroke. (2008d). *Sjögren's syndrome information page.* Retrieved August 28, 2008, from http://www.ninds.nih.gov/disorders/sjogrens/sjogrens.htm

Porth, C. (2005). *Pathophysiology: Concepts of altered health states* (7th ed.). Philadelphia: Lippincott Williams & Wilkins.

Schlesinger, N., Schumacher, M. C., Catton, M., & Maxwell, L. (2006). Colchicine for acute gout. *Cochrane Database of Systematic Reviews,* 2006, Issue 4. Retrieved June 20, 2007, from http://mrw.interscience.wiley.com/cochrane/clsysrev/articles/CD006190/frame.html

Sexton, D. H. (2008). Clinical manifestations of Lyme disease. *UpToDate.* Retrieved April 30, 2008, from http://www.uptodate.com/patients/content/topic.do?topicKey=~9197/aelfkcit3&selectedTitle=2~133&source=search_result

Sjögren's Syndrome Foundation. (2008). *Sjögren's syndrome.* Retrieved September 1, 2008, from http://www.sjogrens.org/syndrome/diagnosis.html

U.S. Department of Health and Human Services (DHHS). (2000). *Healthy People 2010.* Retrieved July 30, 2007, from http://www.healthypeople.gov

WrongDiagnosis.com (WD.com). (2008). *Prevalence and incidence of connective tissue disorders.* Retrieved June 30, 2008, from http://www.wrongdiagnosis.com/c/connective_tissue_disorders/prevalence.htm

Yu, D. (2008). *Reactive arthritis.* Retrieved September 1, 2008, from http://www.utdol.com/online/content/topic.do?topicKey=spondylo/7349&selectedTitle=1~86&source=search_result

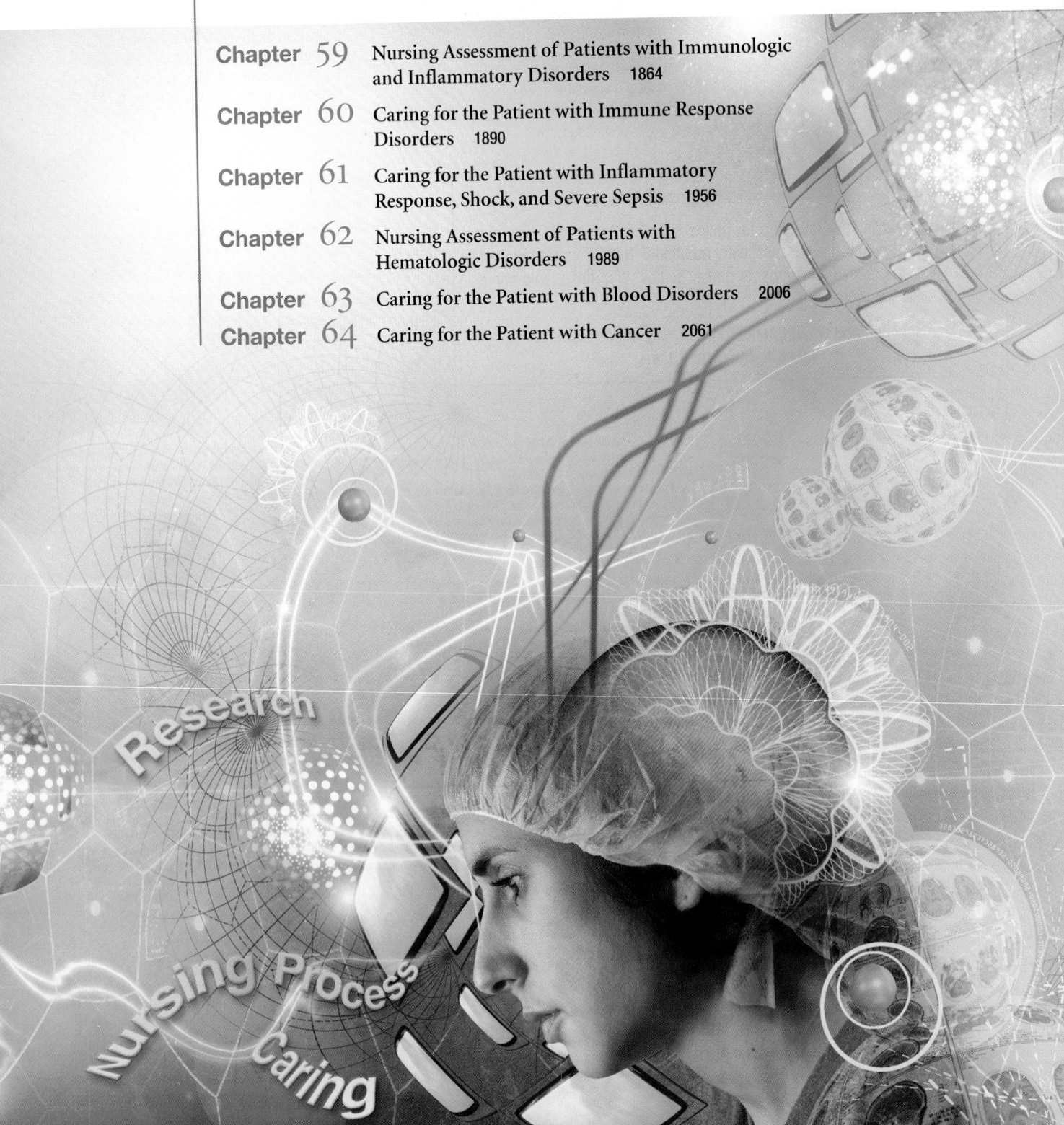

UNIT 13

Nursing Management of Patients with Immunologic, Inflammatory, and Hematologic Disorders

Research

Nursing Process

Caring

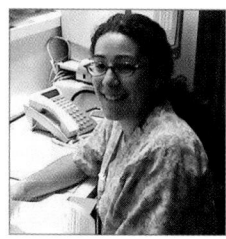

SOLEDAD SANCHEZ My name is Soledad Sanchez and I always knew I wanted to be a nurse. This feeling came from my mother who left an indelible mark on my career choice. She cared for her children and others with a calming, warm sense that easily transmitted to other people. Trained as a nurse by religious sisters in her native country, she continued to use those skills in the United States as she helped others in need. Before attending nursing school, I did not really understand what it meant to be a nurse. Through my education, I soon developed a love for physiology and pathophysiology and gained a deeper understanding of the full scope of the healing process from a biological and humanitarian perspective. In 2001 I received my associate degree in nursing from Cerritos College. Later I attended Cal State Long Beach for a BS degree. I have been a registered nurse for 7 years, the last two of which I have been employed at a large medical center in Northern California. My experience has challenged me and nurtured a deeper understanding and compassion for people's most vulnerable moments in life.

"My experience has challenged me and nurtured a deeper understanding and compassion for people's most vulnerable moments in life."

I work on a 27-bed unit caring for patients from a number of specialties including oncology and neuroscience. I care for a wide diversity of oncology patients. For example, there are the young adults with new diagnoses of cancer whose emotional state is very fragile. Virtually every aspect of their lives as well as that of their families is affected. It is essential to establish a rapport with them and to assess their coping mechanisms. Only then will they open themselves up to you, making the patient–nurse relationship more comfortable, which allows for better communication and the implementation of optimal care delivery options. It becomes easier to discuss their fears and show compassion—just the mere action of sitting by their bedside and talking to them at eye level shows that we care. **Compassion** is a powerful healing tool.

As a registered nurse, I am part of a collaborative team of health care providers that includes physicians, social workers, dieticians, and pharmacists who strive to deliver quality patient care with the patient's desired goals in mind. As a certified chemotherapy and biotherapy provider, I am able to provide curative and palliative care to our patients who have cancer. Patient education is vital to this role, as is evaluating and understanding the orders. The integrity of the therapy is maintained by two independent checks of the dosages and assessment factors. This **confidence** is one facet of the six components of caring; having confidence not just in oneself, but in one's fellow colleagues helps create an environment of teamwork, trust, and dependability.

My approach to nursing is framed by the six components of caring: **compassion**, **competence**, **confidence**, **conscience**, **commitment**, and **comportment**. While the daily routine of oncology nursing centers on assessing and administering chemotherapy to patients, one key aspect is examining and assessing the side effects of chemotherapy and patients' tolerance. For example, a male patient in his early thirties with sarcoma in his second cycle of chemotherapy reported that with his last cycle he developed severe nausea, vomiting, and constipation. After discussing his previous medication regimen and past history, I developed a clear image of a possible regimen. After consulting with the chemotherapy pharmacist, a treatment plan was established that was very effective in treating his side effects. **Competence** was demonstrated by obtaining a detailed history of the patient, knowledge of the medication, and collaboration with the interdisciplinary team.

Another example of incorporating the components of caring is that of an elderly patient admitted for generalized weakness and subsequently diagnosed with non-Hodgkin's lymphoma. Knowing the prognosis was poor and the patient was in a frail state, I was concerned and uncomfortable with the oncologist's orders for chemotherapy. I proceeded to call the patient's partner and physician. After explaining the chemotherapy agents and possible side effects, a social worker was called to conduct a family conference. The patient was later discharged home with hospice care. I could not in good **conscience** blindly follow the initial orders. Ultimately, my professional **commitment** to the patient was demonstrated by advocating for the best possible quality of life.

Clinical reasoning is achieved after collecting and evaluating all pertinent patient assessment data. During initial report of the day, you begin using critical thinking and clinical reasoning to establish a plan of care for the patient and with your assessment you refine your plan on an ongoing basis.

Oftentimes, nursing is bittersweet because you enter people's lives when they are most vulnerable. Through that vulnerability you can encounter immense strength, which is the sweetest part for me. I see my role as using my abilities to access and foster that strength, and being humbled by it. Strength is found in the most extraordinary places. Helping someone during their time of suffering is an art in itself.

59

Nursing Assessment of Patients with Immunologic and Inflammatory Disorders

Debra Brady
Kathy Yeates

With contributions by:
Kathleen Osborn

Outcome-Based Learning Objectives

After studying this chapter, the learner will be able to:

1. Describe the function of the organs, tissues, and cellular components of the immune system.

2. Compare and contrast the significance of self antigens versus non-self antigens and immune tolerance.

3. Compare and contrast cell-mediated and humoral immunity in relationship to the type of lymphocytes involved, response to antigens, and role in immune protection.

4. Compare and contrast the actions of cytokines, lymphokines, interleukins, interferons, complement, and tumor necrosis factor on immune function.

5. Explain the action and significance of acquired immune response through immunizations.

6. Explain the action and significance of antigen presentation in B-cell activation, stimulation of immunoglobulin production, and secondary immune response.

7. Discuss the effects of aging on the immune system.

8. Apply the assessment skills of inspection, palpation, percussion, and auscultation in evaluating body systems and determining the status of immune function.

9. Interpret and relate immune-related laboratory tests when assessing immune function.

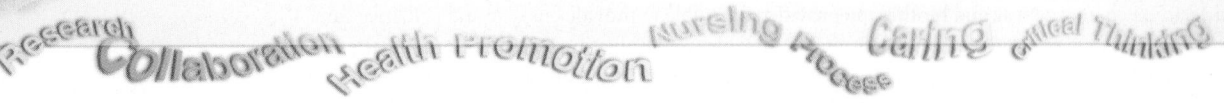

AN INTACT and functioning immune system is critical for survival. The immune system functions to protect the body from invasion of microorganisms and foreign substances, in addition to eliminating damaged or mutant cells such as cancer cells. The protective process of response to a foreign substance is referred to as **immunity**. To function appropriately, it is essential that the immune system be able to differentiate between "self" cells and an infinite number of "non-self" substances and foreign cells such as bacteria, viruses, or tumor proteins. Any substance that the immune system recognizes as foreign is referred to as an **antigen**. The ability to differentiate self from non-self is referred to as **immune tolerance**. Loss of immune tolerance is the basis for numerous immune abnormalities, which are discussed in Chapter 60 🔗.

The immune system includes central and peripheral lymphoid tissues and immune cells that function to defend the body against disease through natural and acquired immunity as well as the inflammation process. Chart 59–1 provides an overview of the immune response.

Natural immunity is accomplished through specific organs, cells, and chemicals that are present at birth or shortly after, as discussed below. Acquired immunity includes antibodies, immunocompetent T cells and B cells, and cytokines that act to remove antigens that are considered non-self (Rote, 2006). Immune cells also include a variety of white blood cells such as macrophages, neutrophils, and eosinophils. This chapter focuses on the anatomy and physiology of normal immune function and assessment of the immune system. A complete description of inflammation is available in Chapter 61 🔗.

Genetic factors play a key role in immune function. Abnormalities in gene development that affect the immune system will be discussed in Chapter 60 🔗 as they relate to the development of specific disease processes.

Anatomy of the Immune System

The major components of the immune system include the bone marrow, the lymphatic system including lymph nodes and lymphatic circulation, and the spleen. These organs and tissues are located throughout the body in order to provide systemic immune response.

CHART 59–1	**Overview of Inflammation and Natural and Acquired Immunity**
	Key Features
INFLAMMATION	Initial response to injury of any kind. Includes cells, such as neutrophils and macrophages, and chemical mediators, such as histamine, complement, and clotting cascade. Inflammation produces the symptoms of redness, swelling, heat or fever, pain, and loss of function.
NATURAL IMMUNITY	Organs such as skin, lymphatic system as well as immune tolerance to self antigens. Mechanical processes such as cough can help remove debris from the body. Gastric pH helps protect the stomach from bacteria. Mucous membranes wash debris away and may have lysozyme secretions that can eliminate debris and bacteria.
ACQUIRED IMMUNITY	System of cells such as B and T cells that protect through immunoglobulins and cell-mediated immune response. Antibodies produced by B cells can attach to antigens and stimulate phagocytosis. T cells regulate the production of antibodies and release other lymphokines that direct immune cells to eliminate antigens or destroy mutant cells.

Sources: DeFranco, A. L., Locksley, R., & Robertson, M. (2007). *Immunity: The immune response in infectious and inflammatory disease.* Sunderland, MA: Sinauer Associates; McCance, K., & Heuther, S. (2006). *Pathophysiology: The biological basis for disease in adults and children* (5th ed.). St. Louis: Mosby; Porth, C. (2007). *Essentials of pathophysiology* (7th ed.). Philadelphia: Lippincott Williams & Wilkins.

Bone Marrow

Knowledge of the functions of bone marrow is important in understanding the development of the immune system. As demonstrated in Figure 59–1 ■ (p. 1866), bone marrow is rich in *stem cells*, cells that can differentiate into a variety of cell lines that are critical for immune function. Stem cells have the capacity to produce any type of cell that they are chemically directed to make. For example, stem cells differentiate into white blood cells such as granulocytes, lymphocytes, and monocytes. Granulocytes become neutrophils, eosinophils, and basophils. Lymphocyte precursors in bone marrow become B- and T-cells lines. Monocytes differentiate from white blood cell precursors. Monocytes circulate in the blood and mature into macrophages. Bone marrow stem cells also differentiate into red blood cells (erythrocytes) and platelets (thrombocytes) (Twite & Gaspard, 2007).

Granulocytes

Granulocytes are the line of white blood cells that differentiate into neutrophils, basophils, and eosinophils. They are named granulocytes because their cell cytoplasm contains granules of chemicals such as histamine. These granules can be seen on Gram stain, and are used to identify and count the cells microscopically.

Neutrophils

Neutrophils are important phagocytic cells. Their function is to consume cellular debris, immune complexes, and bacterial and viral particles. Neutrophils are the first group of white blood cells to arrive at the site of injury or cell death. They have a short life span, approximately 72 hours or less.

Basophils

Basophils migrate from the bloodstream into tissue and mature into mast cells. Mast cells are filled with granules of histamine and are important in initiating the inflammatory response following injury. When a body cell is injured, mast cells in the immediate vicinity release large quantities of histamine, stimulating the inflammatory response (DeFranco, Locksley, & Robertson, 2007).

Eosinophils

Eosinophils comprise a very small portion of the total number of white blood cells. They are stimulated to increase their numbers in the presence of parasites. The number of eosinophils also increases in the presence of allergies. Eosinophils are responsible for increasing the immune and inflammatory response.

Nongranulocytes

The **nongranulocyte** cell lines include lymphocytes and monocytes. These cells are identified microscopically by their large nucleus and the lack of granules in their cytoplasm. Nongranulocytes are highly effective phagocytic white blood cells that can engulf large numbers of foreign antigen, such as bacteria.

Monocytes

Monocytes circulate in the blood and migrate into tissue to mature as macrophages. The primary function of monocytes and macrophages is phagocytosis. They arrive at the site of cell injury hours to days after neutrophils. Macrophages have a longer life span, have a higher tolerance for an acidic environment, and are capable of consuming larger amount of debris for an extended period of time than other monocytes (Rote, 2006).

Lymphocytes

Lymphocytes differentiate into T lymphocytes and B lymphocytes. Microscopically T and B lymphocytes appear similar, with a large nucleus and no granules in the cytoplasm. T lymphocytes, also known as CD4 cells, are responsible for regulating and initiating the immune response. The primary function of B cells is the production of antibodies such as immunoglobulins (Ig): IgE, IgG, IgA, IgM, and IgD (DeFranco et al., 2007).

Deficiencies in functional bone marrow and stem cells can lead to immune deficiency disorders. Primary immune dysfunction such as an IgG deficiency is an example of the incorrect maturation of B cells that cannot produce immunoglobulin G (Twite & Gaspard, 2007).

Lymphatic System

The **lymphatic system** is comprised of the vessels, lymph nodes, and lymph tissue. This system of vessels drains lymph fluid, referred to as chyle, through the entire body and returns it to venous circulation in the chest. The vessels drain **chyle** (a milky fluid comprised of serous fluid, white cells, and fatty acids) into the thoracic and lymphatic ducts in the mediastinum. The

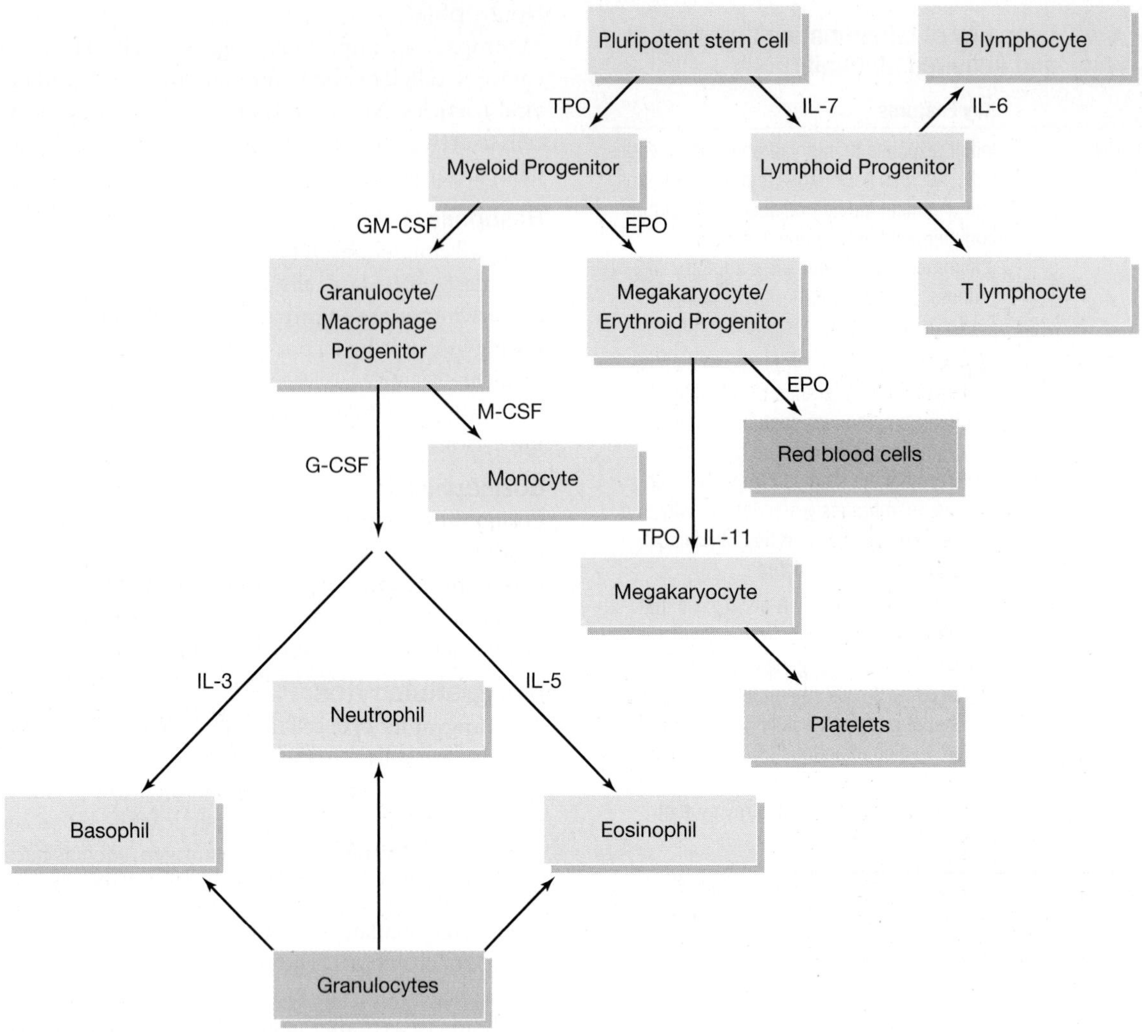

Pluripotent stem cell
B lymphocyte
TPO
IL-7
IL-6
Myeloid Progenitor
Lymphoid Progenitor
GM-CSF
EPO
Granulocyte/ Macrophage Progenitor
Megakaryocyte/ Erythroid Progenitor
T lymphocyte
EPO
M-CSF
Red blood cells
G-CSF
Monocyte
TPO
IL-11
Megakaryocyte
IL-3
IL-5
Neutrophil
Platelets
Basophil
Eosinophil
Granulocytes

FIGURE 59–1 ■ Cell line differentiation in bone marrow.

lymph vessels follow the same route as veins and arteries and run parallel to veins. Chyle then drains from the mediastinum into the heart through the superior vena cava.

Lymph nodes and lymph tissue filter debris from the breakdown of cells, bacteria, virus, and fungal antigens. Lymphocytes such as T and B cells are found in lymph nodes. Lymph nodes and tissue contain or house macrophages that ingest cells, bacteria, and debris. Two-thirds of fixed lymph tissue is located in the abdomen surrounding the intestinal tissue, and is referred to as Peyer's patches. This is important because the vessels that deliver blood to the intestines facilitate the entry of large molecules of digested materials into the circulatory system. Vessels able to absorb large food particles may also allow the entry of viral and bacterial particles. Hence, immune protection by Peyer's patches is vital (Twite & Gaspard, 2007). A high concentration of lymph tissue also is located in the lungs. Alveolar macrophages function with lymph tissue to protect the lungs from bacteria, virus, and debris from the outside environment (DeFranco et al., 2007).

Lymph nodes are consolidated groups of lymph tissue and are found throughout the body. Lymph nodes located in the neck, axilla, and groin may be palpated. Like lymph tissue, they contain macrophages and lymphocytes, and are able to filter and remove dead cells, bacteria, and other debris from the system as well as assist in mounting the immune response (Figure 59–2 ■).

MyNursingKit | Video: Health and Physical Assessment: Lymphatic—Lymph Nodes: Anatomy

During infection, inflammation, or injury, lymph nodes in the area of injury will become swollen. An example of this is the swelling of lymph nodes in the axilla and neck during pneumonia (Rote, 2006).

CRITICAL ALERT *Patients with compromised immune function such as HIV/AIDS or cancer patients on chemotherapy need to have lymph nodes examined even if no other complaint is present. Nodes swollen by cell debris of any kind warrant further investigation.*

Tonsils and Adenoids

Tonsils and adenoids are consolidated lymph tissue located in the throat. They function to remove and filter debris, bacteria, and viruses from the upper airways and mouth. Like all consolidated lymph tissue, they contain B and T cells as well as macrophages (DeFranco et al., 2007).

Spleen

The spleen plays a significant role in immune function as part of the lymphatic system. It is comprised of white and red pulp and is involved in hematologic filtration, sequestering of red and white cells, and immune response. The white pulp of the spleen is rich in lymphocytes that can be activated in an immune response. The red pulp is responsible for filtering out

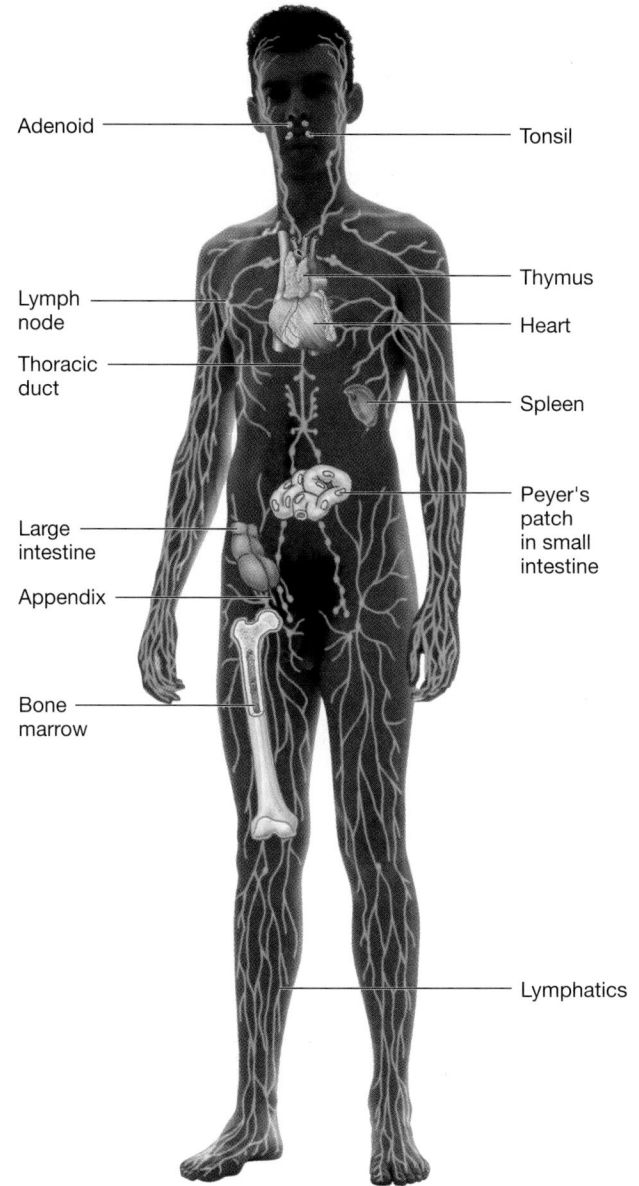

Adenoid
Tonsil
Lymph node
Thymus
Heart
Thoracic duct
Spleen
Peyer's patch in small intestine
Large intestine
Appendix
Bone marrow
Lymphatics

FIGURE 59–2 ■ Lymphatic system with lymph nodes.

old or damaged red blood cells. The spleen may also sequester red and white blood cells and platelets, and thereby decrease these levels in the circulating blood volume. The spleen may become enlarged in acute inflammatory or infectious disease processes because of the stimulation of the immune response. An enlarged spleen (splenomegaly) can be involved in a plethora of disease processes such as trauma, cancer, infection, portal hypertension, thrombosis, cysts, and mononucleosis, and this assessment finding warrants further investigation (Twite & Gaspard, 2007).

To assess the spleen, place the patient on the right side, and percuss down the midaxillary line from an area of resonance over the lung to dullness over the spleen. The spleen is normally not detected on palpation. If detected, the spleen should not be percussed more than 6 to 8 cm (about 2 to 3 in.) above the left costal margin. An enlarged spleen is diagnosed if there is a greater than 8-cm finding above the costal margin (Dillon, 2007).

Physiology of the Immune System

The physiology of the immune system includes the function of the lymphatic tissues, cells, and chemicals that provide protection from infectious agents, antigens, and mutated cells and enable the body to differentiate self from non-self. The immune response includes both natural and acquired immunity.

Natural Immunity

Natural immunity is the responsibility of a group of body organs, cells, and chemicals that are present at birth or shortly after. These include the cells and chemicals of the inflammatory response, barriers such as skin, and chemicals such as complement. **Natural immunity** is defined as the organs, cells, and secretions of the body that provide protection from foreign proteins, chemicals, and other non-self particles. Natural immunity includes the integumentary system, the lymphatic system, and secretions such as lysozymes, immunoglobulins, and subcellular receptors such as toll-like receptors. The white blood cells and chemicals of the inflammatory response are an important part of natural immunity. All of these components of natural immune function are present at birth (Figure 59–3 ■, p. 1868).

Physical and Chemical Barriers

Anatomic and chemical barriers provide the first line of defense in immune protection. Physical barriers include the skin and the mucous membranes. Natural immune system chemical barriers include lysozymes, acidic pH of the stomach, and toll receptors, all of which are discussed below.

Skin

Natural immunity starts with the skin. Skin is physically the largest organ of the human body. It acts as a barrier to debris, bacteria, and other organisms. It protects soft organs and tissue from changes in the environment. Skin is capable of inhibiting bacterial growth. Bacteria are always present on the surface of the skin in varying quantities. The small amount of moisture and pH of the skin protect it from bacterial growth. Therefore, intact skin is critical to the survival of the organism. Even small breaks in the integrity of skin can lead to large wounds or infections locally or systemically because organisms are able to enter the body (Rote, 2006).

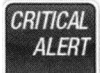 *Careful examination of the skin is an essential part of every physical assessment of patients. Patients may require education about maintaining skin integrity. When a rash or skin breakdown occurs, patients need to be educated to report to their health care provider the onset of the symptoms, where on the body it is occurring, and any attempted home treatment.*

Mucous Membranes

Mucous membranes also form part of the first line of defense in natural immunity. Mucous membranes assist in protecting the body from attack by washing dirt and debris from the body. Ciliated cells in the trachea move bacteria and dirt from the trachea through a wavelike motion. In addition, mucous membranes in the mouth secrete lysozymes and immunoglobulins that are mildly antibiotic and assist in protecting the

The immune system

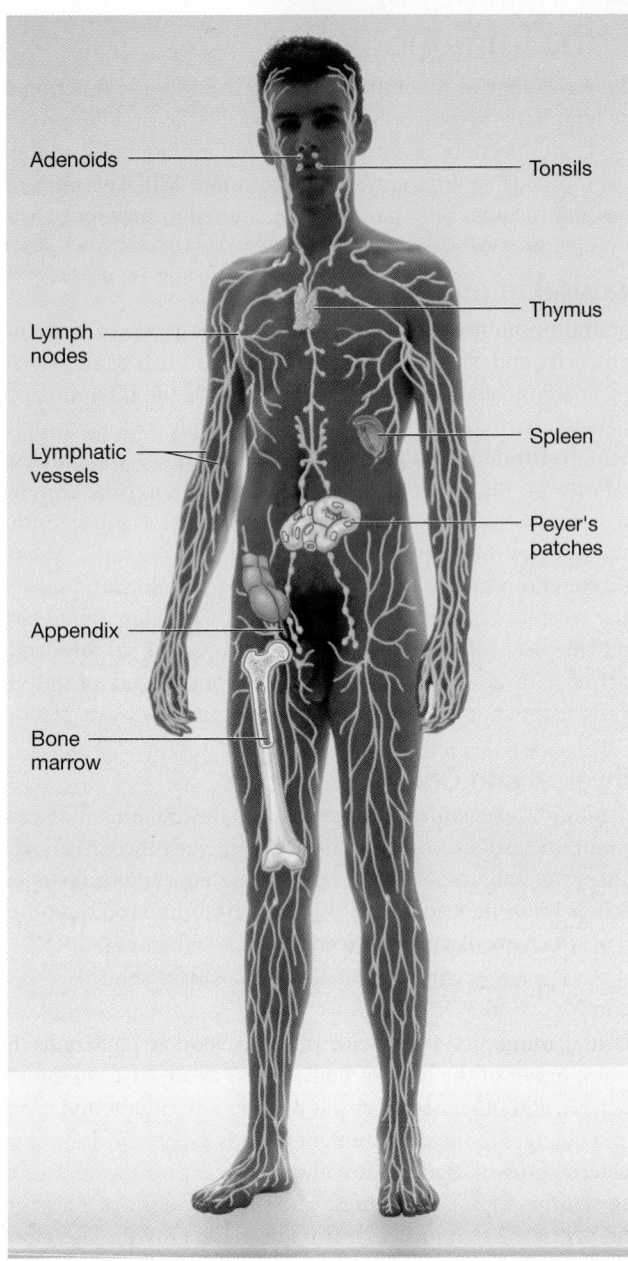

FIGURE 59–3 ■ Immune system with organs.
Source: Michael Freeman/Phototake NYC

mouth from bacterial infection (Sommer, 2007). Oral care is essential in preventing infections in the oral cavity.

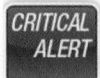 **CRITICAL ALERT** *Patients who are receiving supplemental oxygen by mask or ventilator need frequent oral care. Although oxygen by mask and ventilator can be humidified, patients may not be able to keep oral mucosa moist and clean. Gentle swabbing with soft swabs and water or mouthwash can help keep the mouth moist. Patients receiving oxygen by mask may require assistance with brushing their teeth. Patients on a ventilator are dependent on the nurse for oral care. There is growing evidence that oral bacteria can lead to nosocomial pneumonia (Tablan et al., 2004).*

Gastric pH

Immune protection is also provided in the stomach. The pH of the stomach ranges from approximately 1.0 to 3.0. This pH is so acidic most bacteria, fungi, and viral particles are unable to survive.

Toll Receptors

Finally, **toll receptors** present at the cellular level are small receptors on the surface of many types of immune and tissue cells that are able to initiate immune responses when pieces of bacterial cell walls attach to them. Humans are born with these toll receptors and they comprise an important innate protection for the body because they act as a gate or point of initiation of certain cell functions (Figure 59–4 ■). Toll receptors are shaped to accept the lipopolysaccharide portion of the cell wall of bacteria, while others are shaped to accept the wall of a fungal cell (De-Franco et al., 2007).

Toll receptors not only stimulate the immune system, they also can signal a cell to start **apoptosis**, or programmed cell death. Infected cells can often be induced to undergo apoptosis and destroy themselves (Rote, 2006). Additionally, cells stimulated by the attachment of a lipopolysaccharide piece of bacterial wall are able to stimulate the release of tumor necrosis factor, a key chemical in initiating immune and inflammatory responses. This response is critical in alerting the system to the presence of non-self antigens such as bacteria (DeFranco et al., 2007).

Toll-like receptors

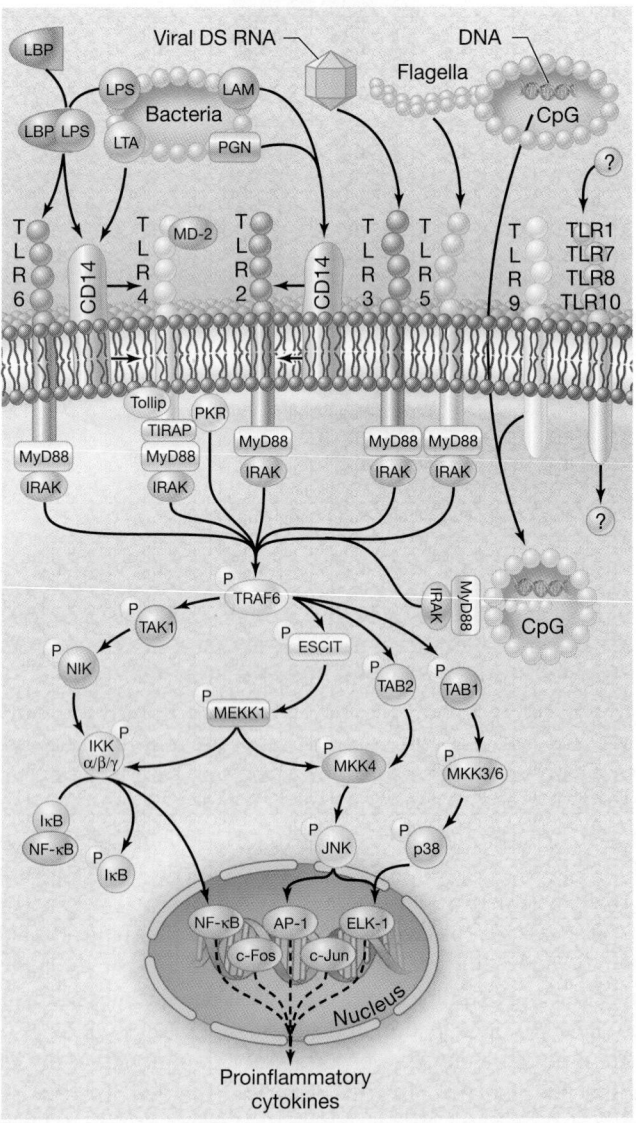

FIGURE 59–4 ■ Toll receptors.

Self Versus Non-Self

Self is defined as all cells of the body and the receptors on those cells that are recognized as unique to that individual. Major histocompatibility complex (MHC) receptors on cells are an example of a marker used by the immune system to determine if a cell belongs to the organism or not. Additionally, **human leukocyte antigens (HLAs)** are protein markers on the cell wall of white blood cells that alert the immune system to the appropriateness of a cell belonging to the system. These are the markers that are tested for matching in organ transplant because an exact HLA match will minimize the immune response and the risk of transplant rejection (Rote, 2006).

Non-self is any protein, antigen, or the stimulatory part of any foreign cell that the immune system does not recognize as self. Antigens are small proteins that can signal the immune system to mount a response and eliminate the foreign cell, bacteria, virus, or fungus (DeFranco et al., 2007).

Bacteria, virus, fungi, and amoebic parasites are major threats to the survival of the human body. The immune system is constantly looking for cells and proteins that are not self. Cancer cells frequently lack specific markers, thus, the immune system may or may not recognize the mutant cell as non-self (Figure 59–5 ■). If the immune system does not identify the mutated malignant cells, a tumor may develop. Chapter 64 ⊙ discusses the development of a cancerous tumor in detail.

Immune Tolerance

Immune tolerance is defined as the ability of the immune system to tolerate all **self antigens** while retaining the ability to mount an immune response to **non-self antigens**. Immune tolerance begins during embryonic development of the immune system. Lymphocytes that react with self antigens are selectively eliminated as the immune system develops. This leaves the newborn with B-cell and T-cell lines that do not attack self antigens. Self antigens include HLAs and MHC, as well as several other antigenic particles that are often cell receptors. When the body reacts to self receptors or other cell parts as an antigen, autoimmune disease may result (DeFranco et al., 2007). Chapter 60 ⊙ discusses autoimmune diseases.

Inflammatory Response

The inflammatory response is an important part of the body's response to any injury and an integral part of the immune response. White blood cells such as neutrophils and macrophages travel to the site of injury in response to the chemicals of inflammation such as histamine, complement, and bradykinin. Inflammation presents with symptoms of redness, edema, pain, and heat from increased blood flow to the area of injury (Sommer, 2007).

The inflammatory response is seen in cell injury, allergy reactions, anaphylaxis, and many disease processes. Cells and chemicals of the inflammatory response also stimulate the activity of T cells and B cells to mount an immune response. For a complete discussion of inflammation see Chapter 61 ⊙.

Acquired Immunity

Acquired immunity occurs after birth and includes antibodies, immunocompetent T cells and B cells, and cytokines that act to remove antigens that are considered non-self. Acquired immunity also includes immunizations received as a child or an adult. Acquired immunity can be described as the ability of the immune cells to correctly produce antibodies, regulate the immune response, and respond only to non-self antigens (DeFranco et al., 2007). **Active acquired immunity** involves the production of antibodies by the immune system in response to specific foreign antigens, such as bacteria. This immunity is considered acquired because the body develops the ability to regulate the immune system and produce antibodies after birth and after exposure to antigens in the environment. Active immunity is acquired by either contracting the disease or through a vaccination. Acquired immunity involves lymphocyte cells and chemicals that can confer long-term permanent protection against the disease for which the antibodies have been produced. Figure 59–6 ■ (p. 1870) describes immune cell differentiation from precursor cells.

Lymphocytes include **T cell** and **B cells**. **T lymphocytes** are involved in the cellular immune response and are responsible for stimulating and regulating the immune response. The **B lymphocytes** are involved in the humoral immune response and are responsible for the creation and release of antibodies and development of long-term immune protection.

Cellular Immune Response

The cellular immune response is initiated by white blood cells called T cells. T cells are vital in regulating immune function (Figure 59–7 ■, p. 1870). T-cell lymphocytes are responsible for stimulating or decreasing the immune response through the production of chemicals called cytokines that can directly destroy cells, help macrophages find the antigen and consume it, and protect cells from viral attachment (Twite & Gaspard, 2007).

T Lymphocytes

T-cell precursors in the bone marrow differentiate into types of T lymphocytes. Immature T cells travel from the bone marrow via the bloodstream to the thymus gland and other lymphatic tissues. T cells mature and differentiate primarily in the thymus during childhood. Following puberty the thymus gland shrinks, and T-cell differentiation and maturation predominantly occurs in other lymphatic tissue such as the white pulp of the spleen and the lymph nodes.

T lymphocytes are the regulatory cells of the immune system whose function is to start and stop the immune processes. These processes include phagocytosis, cytokine secretion, and activation of B cells (Sommer, 2007). As a consequence, the functions

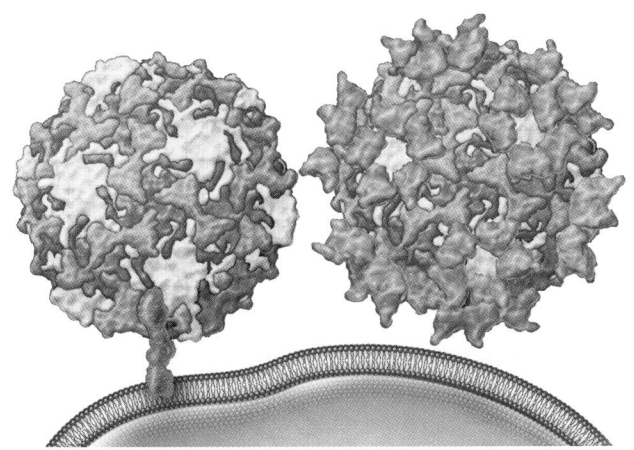

FIGURE 59–5 ■ (A) Self versus (B) non-self.

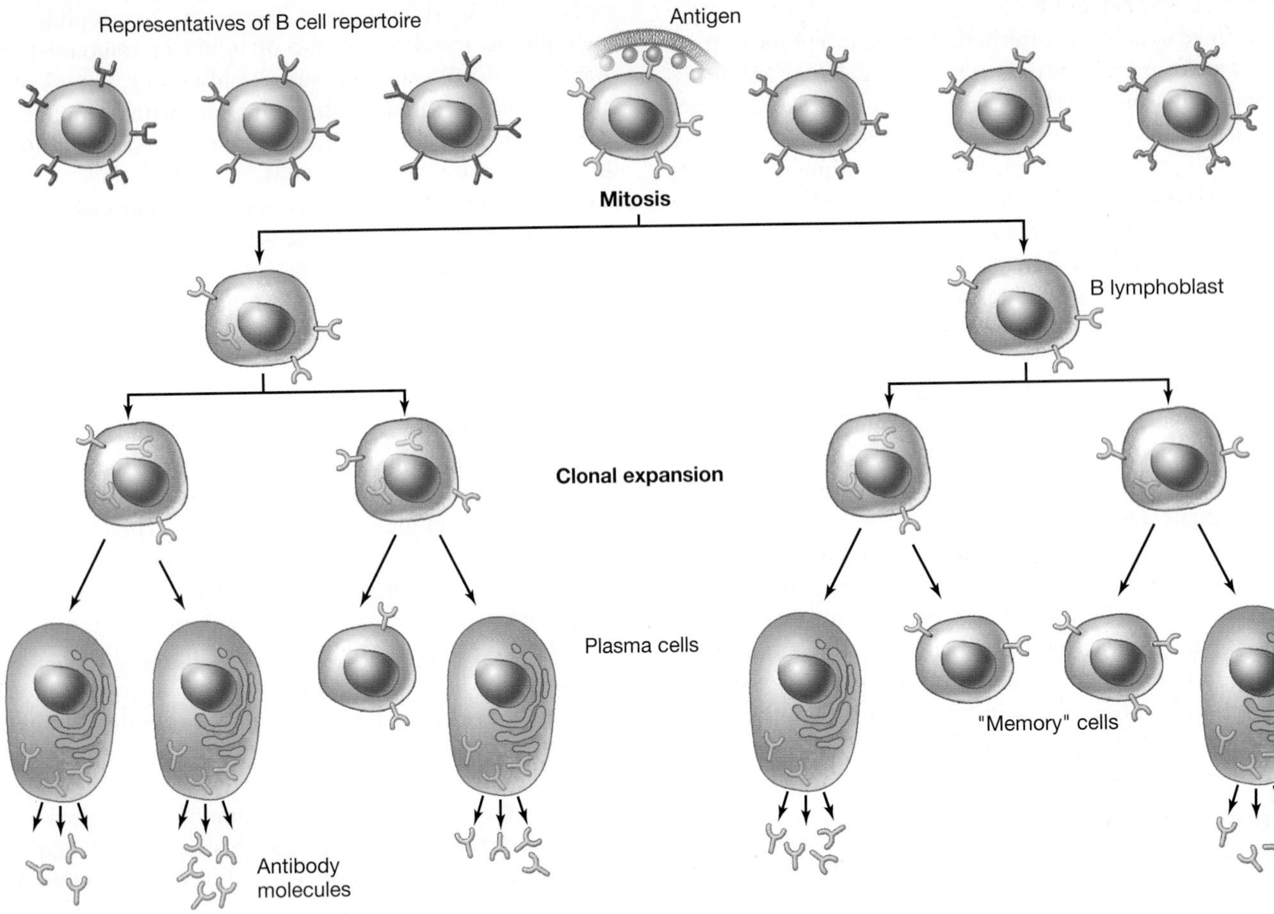

Representatives of B cell repertoire   Antigen

Mitosis

B lymphoblast

Clonal expansion

Plasma cells

"Memory" cells

Antibody
molecules

FIGURE 59–6 ■ Immune cell differentiation from precursors.

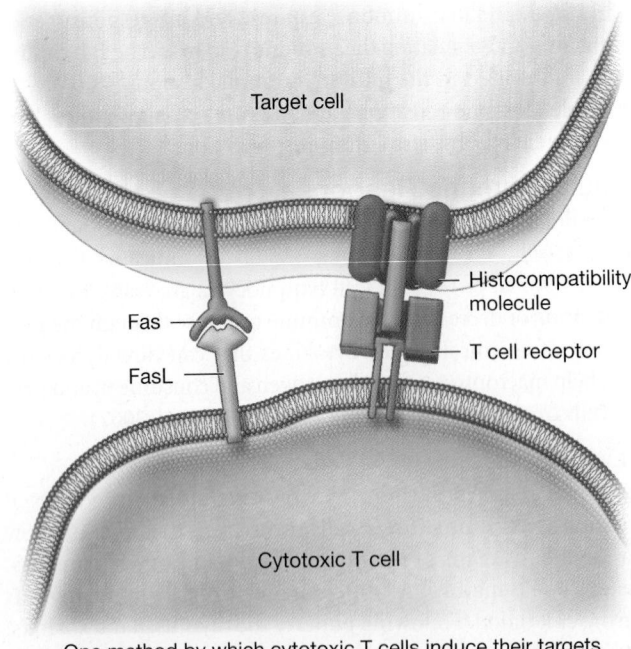

One method by which cytotoxic T cells induce their targets
(e.g., virus-infected cells) to commit suicide (apoptosis)

Target cell

Histocompatibility
molecule

Fas

T cell receptor

FasL

Cytotoxic T cell

FIGURE 59–7 ■ T cell.

of T cells are called the **cell-mediated immune response**. There
are an extensive number of T-cell types. T cells are named by
their function or by the identifying markers on the cell membrane (DeFranco et al., 2007). The most significant T cells and
their role in immune function are discussed next.

T-Helper Cells   **T-helper cells** are also called CD4 cells because of
the CD4 receptors on the surface of this group of T cells. T-helper
cells are divided into T-helper 1 and T-helper 2 cell lines. T-helper
1 cells help upregulate immune activity and produce chemicals
called cytokines that stimulate cytotoxic cells to destroy mutant
and cancer cells. T-helper 1 cells produce cytokines that are
chemotactic (that is, they tell cells to come to the area of infection). CD4 receptors have been identified as the receptor that the
human immunodeficiency virus (HIV) attaches to and uses to enter the T cell, thereby severely affecting immune function, which
is discussed in detail in Chapter 60 🌐 (Sommer, 2007).

T-helper 2 cells stimulate B cells to make antibodies to specific antigens. This is accomplished through the release of
chemicals such as interleukins and the antigen presentation
process (DeFranco et al., 2007). Memory T cells function to retain a "chemical memory" of virus particles encountered by the
memory cells. The next exposure to the "remembered" virus results in a quick immune response to the virus. For example,
memory T cells are responsible for protection against virus infections such as rhinovirus, one group of cold viruses. The first
exposure to a rhinovirus usually results in cold symptoms such

as sore throat, sneezing, and cough. The memory T cells retain a memory of that specific rhinovirus which lasts for a lifetime. On second exposure to that same virus, the memory T cells are able to stimulate an immune response much more quickly, thus minimizing or preventing symptoms of infection. Frequent infections with rhinovirus occur because the virus mutates rapidly, creating a new virus antigen. Thus, the memory T cells must go through the process of developing a memory for each new rhinovirus. More than 200 rhinoviruses have been identified. Children have greater numbers of colds than adults because they have not been exposed to as many virus antigens as adults and subsequently have not developed the same immune memory as adults (Sommer, 2007).

Suppressor T Cells Suppressor T cells, also called CD8 cells, slow or stop the immune response. This downregulation is the primary role of suppressor T cells, and is an important part of regulation of the immune system because the ability to stop the production of antibodies and cell destruction is important once the threat of infection has been overcome (DeFranco et al., 2007).

Natural Killer Cells Natural killer cells, also referred to as "null cells," are types of T cells that lack CD4 or CD8 external receptors, but are able to directly kill cells or send cytokine messages to start the process of programmed cell death (apoptosis). Natural killer cells are usually directed to initiate cell death by T-helper 1 cells (Rote, 2006). Chart 59–2 describes lymphocyte function in greater detail.

CHART 59–2 Lymphocyte Functions

Lymphocyte	Functions
B cell	Antibody production.
Plasma cell	Antibody production, responsible for primary antibody response.
Memory cell	Antibody production, responsible for secondary antibody response.
T-cell lines	Regulation, stimulation, downregulation of immune function through the use of chemical mediators. Null cells and natural killer cells may destroy infected cells directly.
T-helper cells (CD4) T-helper 1 T-helper 2 Memory T-helper cells	Stimulate and upregulate immune function. Assist in antigen presentation. Activate B cells to make antibodies (T-helper 2); stimulate natural killer cells (T-helper 1); nonspecific immune memory function (memory T cells).
Suppressor T cells (CD8)	Can slow or downregulate immune function. Slow release of inflammatory cytokines.
Natural killer cells	T-cell line able to chemically kill infected cells and tumor cells.

Sources: DeFranco, A. L., Locksley, R., & Robertson, M. (2007). *Immunity: The immune response in infectious and inflammatory disease.* Sunderland, MA: Sinauer Associates; McCance, K., & Heuther, S. (2006). *Pathophysiology: The biological basis for disease in adults and children* (5th ed.). St. Louis: Mosby; Porth, C. (2007). *Essentials of pathophysiology* (7th ed.). Philadelphia: Lippincott Williams & Wilkins.

Cytokines and Lymphokines

Cytokines are chemical messages produced by cells to communicate with other cells in the body. Cytokines have a plethora of functions such as chemotaxis and opsonization. **Chemotaxis** is the movement of additional white blood cells to an area of inflammation in response to the release of chemical mediators by neutrophils, monocytes, and injured tissue. **Opsonization** is the chemical coating of an antigen or cell that makes that cell more attractive to phagocytes. Cytokines that are made by lymphocytes are called **lymphokines** and include interleukins and interferons. Other examples of cytokines are tumor necrosis factor, tissue factor, and growth inhibitory factor (DeFranco et al., 2007). A variety of cytokines and their functions are described in Chart 59–3 (p. 1872) (McCance & Heuther, 2006).

Interleukins

Interleukins are lymphokines, chemical mediators released by lymphocytes, that enable the cells of the immune system to communicate and coordinate the immune response. Interleukins are crucial to the immune response. Interleukin-1 and interleukin-6 are pro-inflammatory and stimulate the release of chemicals such as tumor necrosis factor and tissue factor that begin the inflammatory response, as discussed in Chapter 61 . Interleukin-12 slows and helps stop the immune and inflammatory responses (Sommer, 2007).

Interferons

Interferons are proteins made and released by T cells when the invading organism is a virus. This group of lymphokines functions to protect other cells from viral attack. They inhibit the production of the virus within infected cells, prevent the spread of the virus to other cells, and enhance the activity of macrophages, natural killer cells, and cytotoxic T cells. Interferons also inhibit the growth of certain tumor cells. Interferons made by recombinant technology are used to treat a variety of disease states. One example of this is alpha interferon, which is used to slow the growth of new blood vessels in some cancerous vascular tumors (Rote, 2006).

Tumor Necrosis Factor

Tumor necrosis factor (TNF) is a small peptide that is produced by a variety of cells, including granulocytes and lymphocytes. TNF is critical in the stimulation of the initial inflammatory response, specifically the activity of macrophages and granulocytes. It also is important in telling cells to initiate programmed cell death or apoptosis when mutations occur. This function is important in inhibiting tumor development and growth because chronic inflammation has been implicated in the development of some types of cancerous tumors due to cell changes that occur with a long-term inflammatory response (DeFranco et al., 2007).

Tissue Factor

Tissue factor (TF) is another cytokine that is important in immune function and inflammation. Tissue factor can be released by a variety of injured tissue cells, macrophages, and platelets. The function of TF is to stimulate platelets to stick together and form the beginning of a clot. This is critical in stopping blood loss from injured blood vessels. Formation of a stable clot and initiation of the clotting cascade are important aspects of the inflammatory response, which is regulated by cells of the immune

CHART 59–3   Cytokines and Their Functions

Cytokine	Functions
Tumor necrosis factor (TNF)	Stimulates immune and inflammatory responses. Is capable of killing cancer cells. Can activate macrophages and granulocytes. Is responsible in part for wasting seen in cancer. Can stimulate apoptosis.
Interleukin (IL)	
IL-1	Activates T cells, induces fever, is an inflammatory mediator, assists in upregulating immune function.
IL -2	Promotes T-cell growth and replication. Can activate T cells and natural killer cells.
IL-3 (multiple colony-stimulating factor)	Stimulates the proliferation of hematopoietic precursor cells.
IL-4	Stimulates growth of T cells, B cells, mast cells, eosinophils.
IL-5	Stimulates growth of B cells, eosinophils.
IL-6	Acts synergistically with IL-1 and TNF to increase inflammation. Stimulates growth of B cells and differentiation into plasma, memory cells. Can induce fever.
IL-7	Stimulates growth of T and B cells.
IL-8	Chemotactic factor for neutrophils and T cells.
IL-9	Some stimulation of precursor cells of the T-cell line and red blood cell.
IL-10	Stimulates B cells and antibody production. Slows cytokine release by T cells and natural killer cells.
IL-12	Stimulates gamma-interferon production. Promotes cell-mediated immune response.
IL-16	Chemotactic factor for T cells, monocytes, and eosinophils.
IL-17	Stimulates release of IL-6, IL-8, and granulocyte colony stimulating factor.
IL-18	Upregulates natural killer cell function. Stimulates the release of gamma Interferon.
Interferons	
Alpha-interferon	Can slow and inhibit viral replication. Also activates natural killer cells.
Beta-interferon	Blocks viral replication.
Gamma-interferon	Blocks viral replication, activates macrophages, can enhance natural killer cell function; differentiation of B cells.
Colony-stimulating factors	All colony-stimulating factors enhance differentiation and activation of white blood cell lines. Cells stimulated include macrophages and granulocytes. Erythropoietin stimulates differentiation and growth of red blood cells.

Sources: DeFranco, A. L., Locksley, R., & Robertson, M. (2007). *Immunity: The immune response in infectious and inflammatory disease.* Sunderland, MA: Sinauer Associates; McCance, K., & Heuther, S. (2006). *Pathophysiology: The biological basis for disease in adults and children* (5th ed.). St. Louis: Mosby; Porth, C. (2007). *Essentials of pathophysiology* (7th ed.). Philadelphia: Lippincott Williams & Wilkins.

system. Tissue factor is a very significant cytokine that contributes to the body's protective inflammatory response (Sommer, 2007). Chapter 61 ☞ provides a detailed examination of the inflammatory process.

Complement Proteins and Function

Complement is a group of small proteins made in the liver and present in blood that can interact with cells and each other for a variety of functions. Complement proteins are important in the inflammatory and immune responses. Complement 3b is an opsonin or chemical that coats or attaches to an antigen or cell. After attachment the cell or antigen is especially attractive to neutrophils and macrophages. This stimulates the phagocytic cells to approach and consume the cell or antigen. Complement 3a and 5a are chemotactic and can chemically call phagocytic cells such as neutrophils as well as T cells and B cells to the area of infection (DeFranco et al., 2007).

Complement can be activated by immune complexes attached to cell membranes or antibodies attached to cell membranes. When this occurs, complement fragments form a complex either around an attached antibody or directly to re-

ceptors on the cell membrane or wall. This complex of complement is capable of directly lysing a cell wall and killing the organism or cell (Rote, 2006). Figure 59–8 ■ diagrams the classic complement pathway and the alternate pathway. Both pathways end in cell lysis or death.

Humoral Immune Response

The **humoral immune response** is defined as the antibodies or immunoglobulins and the B lymphocytes that produce them. Antibodies are proteins that bind to antigens and immobilize or destroy them. The attachment of the antibody to the antigen is called an immune complex. The immune complex helps stimulate the immune response and can provide long-term protection from bacterial, viral, and fungal antigens.

B Lymphocytes

B-lymphocyte cells (B cells) are white blood cells that differentiate in bone marrow and enter the blood (Figure 59–9 ■, p. 1874). B lymphocytes are responsible for the production of antibodies. **Antibodies**, which are also called **immunoglobulins**, are proteins made by B cells that are capable of attaching to antigens

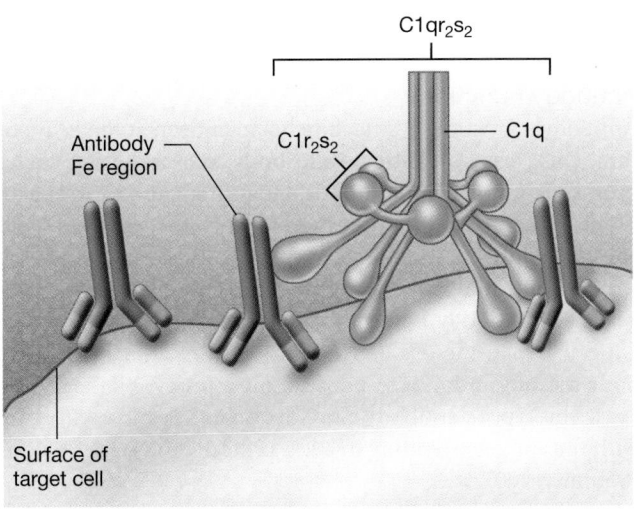

(a)

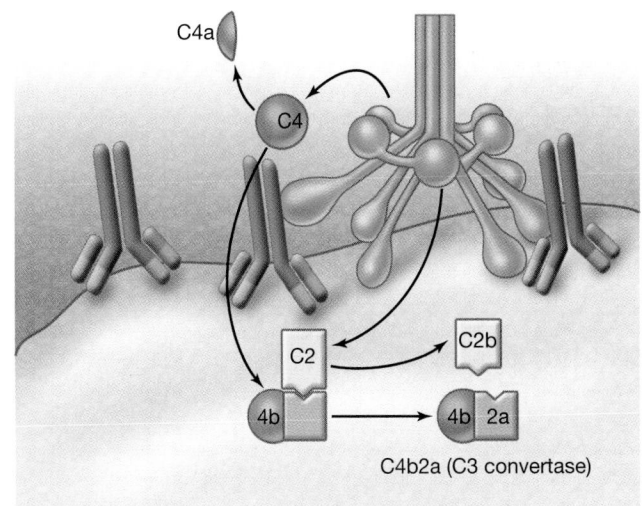

(b)

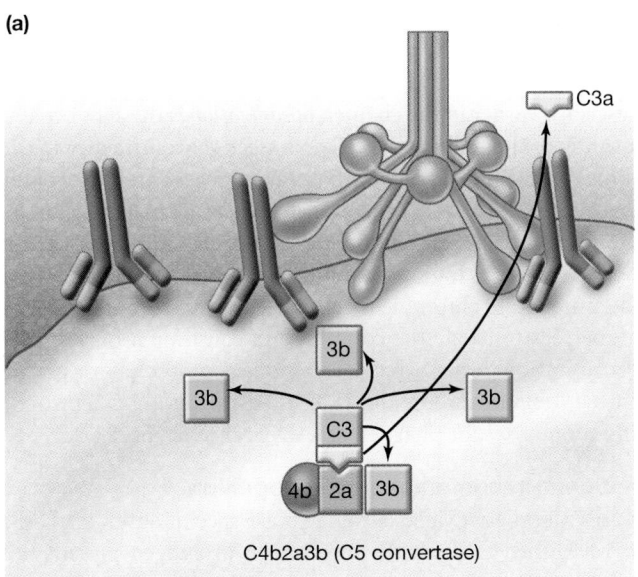

(c)

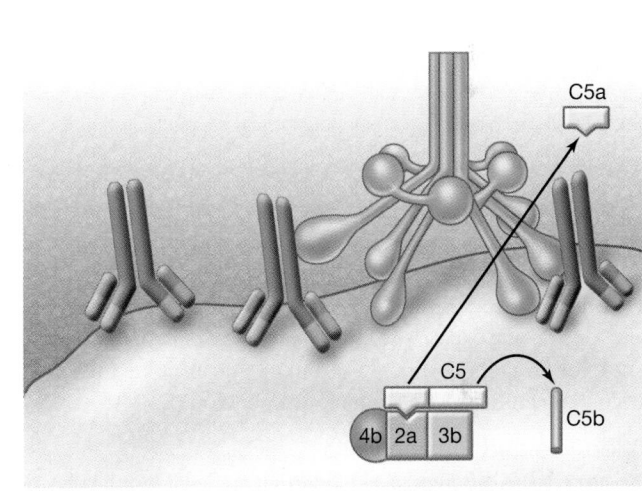

(d)

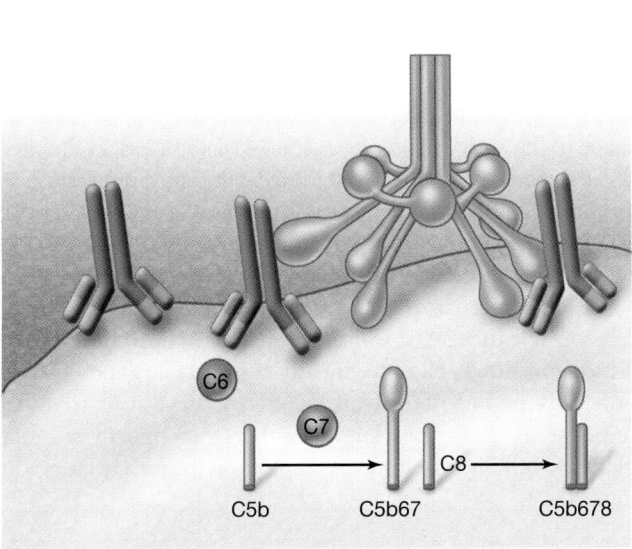

(e)

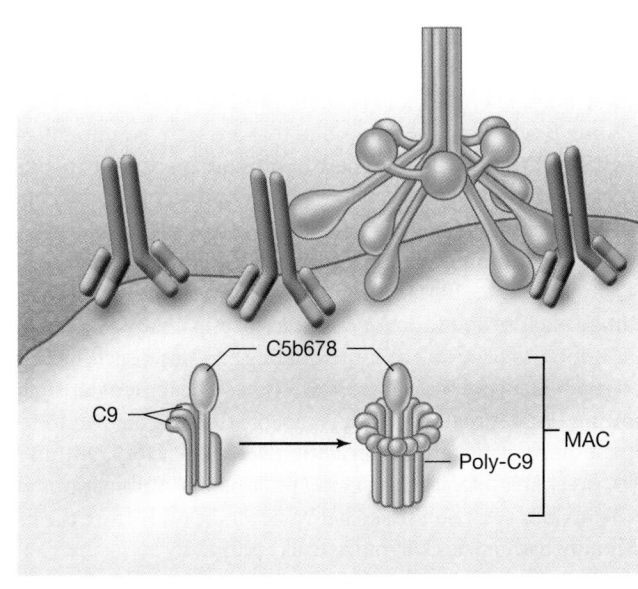

(f)

FIGURE 59–8 ■ Complement cascade.

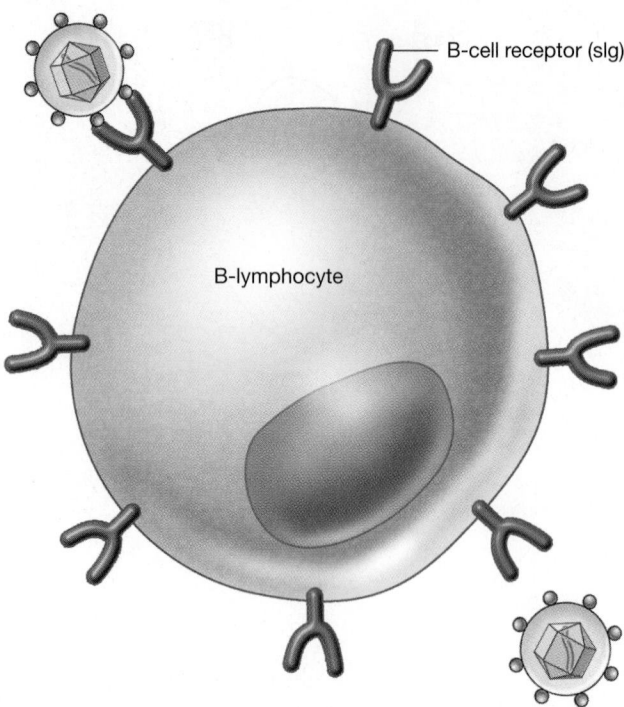

FIGURE 59–9 ■ B cell.

and stimulating immune responses. B cells differentiate in the blood into either plasma B cells or memory B cells. B cells may be stimulated directly by some antigens or by T cells to make antibodies. Once stimulated, B cells make antibodies during their entire life span. Memory B cells can produce immunoglobulins more quickly and in greater numbers when an antigen is seen the second time (Sommer, 2007).

Antibodies and Plasma Cells

Plasma cells are differentiated B cells that are found in the plasma and are responsible for production of specific antibodies. Plasma cells produce the antibodies in response to a primary or initial exposure to an antigen. The most common groups of antibodies, also known as immunoglobulins, include immunoglobulin G (IgG), immunoglobulin A (IgA), immunoglobulin M (IgM), immunoglobulin D (IgD), and immunoglobulin E (IgE).

Some B cells produce antibodies that are secreted into saliva, lung, and intestinal tissue. These antibodies are usually of IgA and are referred to as secretory antibodies because they are found in secretions such as tears and saliva. Secretory antibodies provide immune defense at the portal of entry of a pathogen (DeFranco et al., 2007). Antibodies (immunoglobulins) have multiple shapes and functions as described in Chart 59–4.

Antibodies have one or more binding sites for attachment to antigens. The antibody is composed of a **fragment antigen binding (FAB) portion**, which is capable of being shaped to receive a specific antigen. **Deoxyribonucleic acid (DNA)** within B cells is capable of creating many millions of combinations of FAB portions of antibodies to help protect the body from the invasion by pathogens (DeFranco et al., 2007).

The **fragment crystalline (FC) portion** of the antibody is capable of attaching to the membrane of infected cells, mutant cells, or foreign pathogens (bacteria or viruses) and assisting macrophages to eliminate them (Rote, 2006). Figure 59–10 ■ (p. 1876) provides

a visual representation of an immunoglobulin and the FAB and FC binding sites.

Antibody Functions

Antibodies function by attaching to an antigen at the FAB portion. This creates an **antigen– antibody complex** (also called an **immune complex**) and is important in stimulating a strong immune response and destruction of the antigen. The antibody–antigen complex can attract other phagocytic cells such as neutrophils and macrophages to help eliminate the antigen. Each antibody is specifically shaped for only one type of antigen. When there is an exact fit between antigen and antibody, a strong antibody response results. However, if the fit is not exact, this type of antibody may not be able to bond as effectively with the antigen, resulting in a less profound immune response (Sommer, 2007).

Antibodies clustered around an antigen block its activity by neutralization, opsonization, agglutination, and precipitation. **Neutralization** is the process of changing the charge or shape of the antigen and blocking its ability to attach to another cell. As described earlier in the chapter, *opsonization* is the act of coating an antigen and making the cell or antigen more attractive to consume for phagocytic cells such as macrophages and neutrophils. Figure 59–11 ■ (p. 1876) demonstrates the formation of an immune complex that utilizes the process of opsonization. **Agglutination** is the surrounding and attaching of antibodies to the antigen and clumping together. Again, this stimulates the immune cells to locate the complex and consume it or destroy it. **Precipitation** occurs when an immune complex falls or precipitates out of circulation and is more easily found by neutrophils and monocytes for phagocytosis (DeFranco et al., 2007).

Antigen Presentation and Recognition

B cells must be activated or told to make specific antibodies; this is accomplished through the mechanism of antigen presentation. When a foreign antigen enters a host, the macrophages found in tissue, or monocytes found in blood, ingest the bacterium or virus and then digest the antigen. The macrophage expresses a portion of the digested antigen on its cell surface in the form of a small protein receptor with a part of the bacterial wall attached. T cells are often found near macrophages and can chemically bind to the receptor and accept the antigen onto their surface. T cells then present the antigen to the B cells that have a receptor to match the shape of the antigen. Linking of the T cell and B cell at the site of the antigen activates the B cell to make the appropriately shaped antibody to attach to the antigens (Rote, 2006). Figure 59–12 ■ (p. 1876) depicts the process of antigen presentation by a T cell to a B cell and the creation of antibodies.

Another mechanism of antigen recognition occurs when B cells are able to recognize antigens that may attach to surface receptors on the B cells and directly stimulate antibody production. This method of recognition often occurs during secondary response. It is also possible for antigens to directly stimulate plasma B cells by attaching to receptors on the cell surface (Sommer, 2007).

Memory B Cells

The first exposure to a specific antigen is known as a **primary immune response**. A primary immune response results in evidence of immunoglobulin production in 4 to 8 days after the initial ex-

CHART 59–4	**Immunoglobulins and Their Functions**	
Class of Immunoglobulin	**Primary Function**	**Structure**
IgG	Majority of circulating immunoglobulins are IgG. Capable of most immune functions, such as agglutination, opsonization, neutralization, activation of complement, precipitation. Can cross the placenta; major Ig found in neonatal blood.	
IgM	First antibody produced in primary immune response. This antibody is first produced during embryonic development.	
IgA	Most commonly found in secretions such as saliva. Major function is to protect eyes, mouth, nose, gut, and lung from colonization and disease caused by viruses and bacteria. Secretory immunoglobulin, class. IgA2 most often found in lacrimal, saliva, gut, lung, nose secretions. Neutralizes bacterial and viral antigens.	
IgD	Least understood. Attaches to B cells and acts as an antigen. Present in small quantities in blood.	Monomer (see IgG)
IgE	Primary antibody in allergic responses. Least concentration of IgE in serum.	Monomer (see IgG)

Sources: DeFranco, A. L., Locksley, R., & Robertson, M. (2007). *Immunity: The immune response in infectious and inflammatory disease.* Sunderland, MA: Sinauer Associates; McCance, K., & Heuther, S. (2006). *Pathophysiology: The biological basis for disease in adults and children* (5th ed.). St. Louis: Mosby; Porth, C. (2007). *Essentials of pathophysiology* (7th ed.). Philadelphia: Lippincott Williams & Wilkins.

posure to an antigen. During this period some B cells differentiate into memory B cells that retain the ability to quickly recognize and produce antibodies to the antigen. The second time the host encounters the same antigen it produces antibodies in greater numbers, and more quickly than during the primary exposure. This stronger immune response is referred to as the **secondary immune response** and occurs in 1 to 3 days.

The presence of memory B cells often means the host will have a milder set of symptoms or no response to the pathogen. An example of a member B-cell response is primary and second exposure to cold or rhinovirus. During the first exposure to the antigen, cold and flu symptoms are at their peak for the first 4 to 5 days. The primary immune response requires 7 to 10 days to produce sufficient lymphokines and antibodies to eliminate the

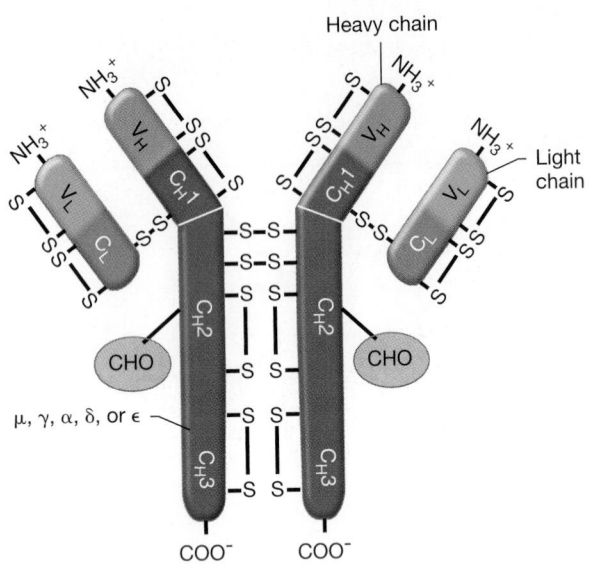

(a)

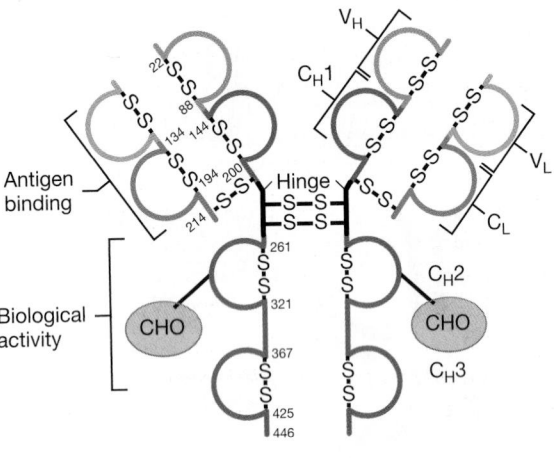

(b)

FIGURE 59–10 ■ Immunoglobulin with FAB and FC binding sites.

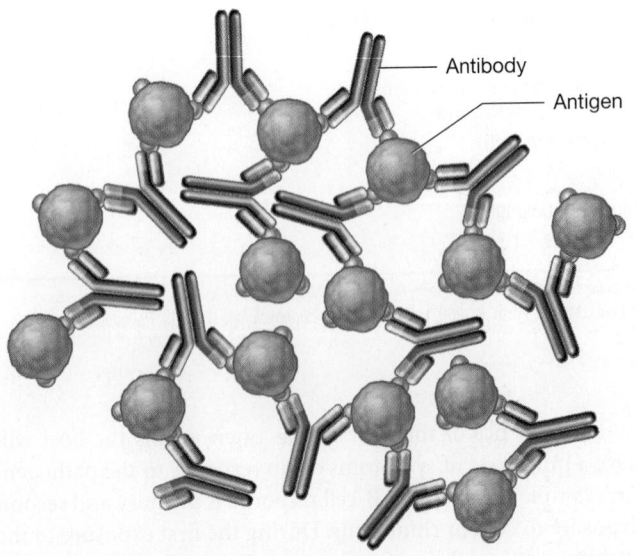

FIGURE 59–11 ■ Immune complex and the process of opsonization.

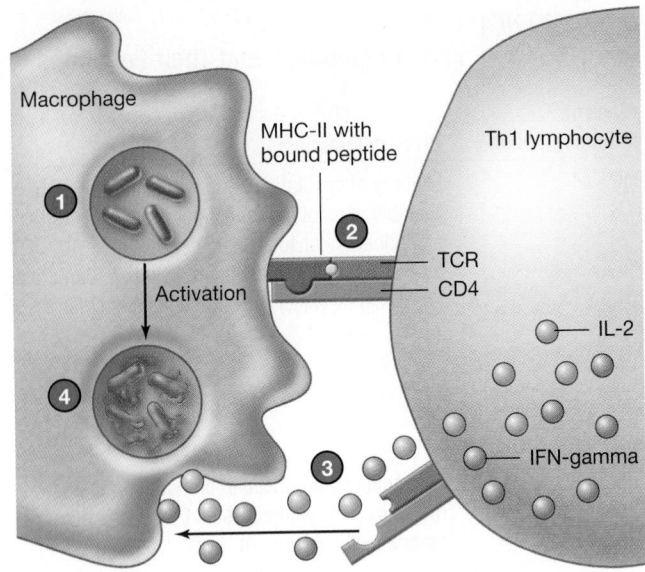

FIGURE 59–12 ■ Antigen presentation (sequential graphic).

virus and the symptoms that accompany it because the level of antibodies in the blood is lower with the primary response. The next exposure of the same rhinovirus activates memory B cells, and the production of antibodies specific to that antigen is quicker and greater in the secondary response. The consequence for the patient is mild or no cold symptoms (Figure 59–13 ■) (Porth & Sweeney, 2007).

Ongoing research regarding the body's production of antibodies in response to specific antigens has resulted in significant developments in the diagnosis and treatment of diseases that affect the immune system. Chart 59–5 discusses the history and development of monoclonal antibodies, which represent one application of these research advancements.

Immunizations

Immunization is a term often used interchangeably with *vaccination* or *inoculation* and involves the process of stimulating the immune system to create active immunity for protection against a disease. A **vaccine**, a preparation that contains an infectious agent or its components, is administered to stimulate the production of antibodies that can prevent infection or create resistance to infection from that agent (Rote, 2006).

Antigens used in vaccines to stimulate an immune response may be inactivated (whole-killed microorganisms or purified products derived from them), live-attenuated (live virus weakened through chemical or physical processes), or recombinant (artificially manufactured from segments of DNA from different sources). Vaccines against influenza, diphtheria, and tetanus use inactivated antigens. Attenuated vaccines include vaccines for measles, mumps, rubella, polio, yellow fever, and varicella. Genetically engineered recombinant antigens are currently being developed and are the basis for research in developing an HIV vaccine (Centers for Disease Control and Prevention [CDC], 2007b). Vaccines are most commonly administered by needle injections, but also can be given by mouth and by aerosol.

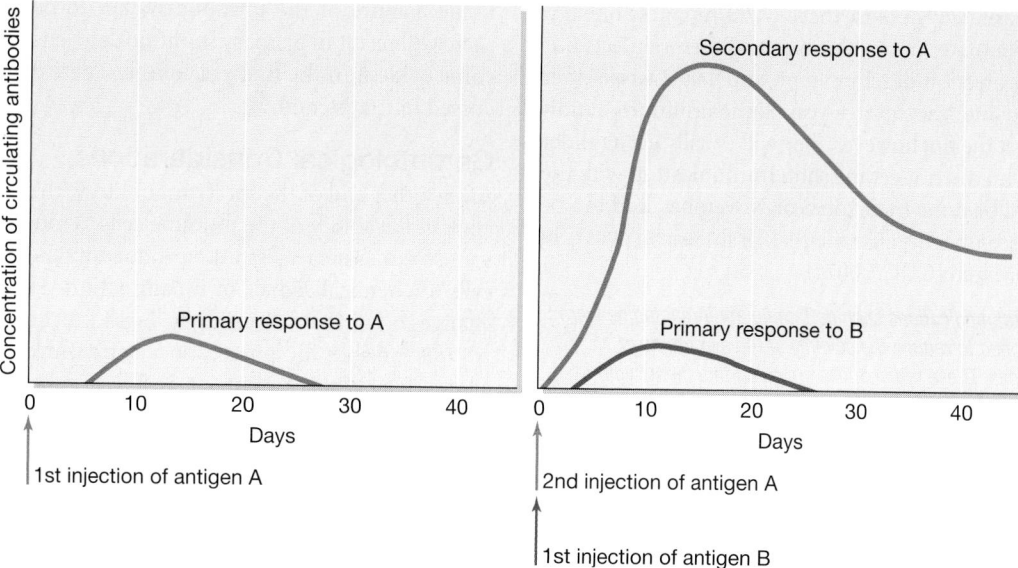

FIGURE 59–13 ■ Primary and secondary immune response curves.

CHART 59–5 Monoclonal Antibodies

When antibody production begins in response to an antigen, B cells become plasma cells and start to make antibodies. The normal antibody response includes variations in the antibodies produced because the multiple antigenic properties on the antigen cause a spectrum of B cells to proliferate. This results in more than one clone of the initial B cells, even though all the B cells were stimulated to proliferate by the same antigen. This is called the polyclonal response (Rote, 2006). However, in the 1970s researchers Kohler and Milstein (1975) developed a B-cell clone that produced a single antibody capable of binding with only one antigen called a monoclonal antibody. The monoclonal antibodies are antigen specific and can be produced in large quantities in a laboratory. Monoclonal antibodies are created by fusing antibody-producing B cells from the spleen of animals (usually mice) that have been injected with a specific antigen with rapidly growing plasma cells. One example of rapidly growing plasma cells is malignant myeloma cells. These are used because they proliferate rapidly and can live for a very long period of time in culture medium. This fusion process results in a hybridoma cell that produces a large quantity of monoclonal antibodies that are able to target a single antigen involved in a disease process (Dunne, 2007).

The development of monoclonal antibodies has had a profound effect on disease research, diagnosis, and treatment approaches. In cancer research, monoclonal antibodies are continually being developed to react against specific antigens on cancer cells and enhance the patient's immune response (Wilkes, 2005). They have been used extensively in cancer drug therapy to inhibit specific tumor growth factor (Franson, 2005). For example, Cetuximab is a monoclonal antibody used to treat metastatic colorectal cancer in combination with chemotherapy or when a patient is nonresponsive to chemotherapy treatment (Thomas, 2005; Wilson, Shannon, Shields, & Stang, 2007).

Monoclonal antibodies are also a vital part of early detection of viral infections. Monoclonal antibodies can be labeled with a fluorescent dye or enzyme and targeted for a specific viral pathogen, which allows visualization and identification of the pathogen with fluorescent microscopy (Dunne, 2007). Thus, monoclonal antibody technology enables the clinician to order tests for viral antigens to detect a disease early in its course and diagnose and treat it appropriately to realize the goal of improving patient outcomes (Rote, 2006).

National Guidelines for Immunization

All individuals should have their immunization status evaluated regularly. Recommended immunization schedules vary slightly by country. In the United States, the CDC conducts a national immunization program and publishes extensive information related to vaccines and recommended immunizations. The National Guidelines box summarizes immunizations for adults.

The CDC encourages annual immunization of the general population with the influenza vaccine, and strongly recommends it for adults 50 years and older, residents of long-term care facilities, individuals with chronic illnesses, immunosuppressed individuals, health care workers, and any other individuals coming in close contact with people at risk of contracting influenza. Inactive influenza vaccine has been used in the United States for many

NATIONAL GUIDELINES for Immunizations for Adults in the United States

Vaccines Needed by All Adults

1. Varicella (chickenpox) vaccine
2. Hepatitis B vaccines (adults at risk, i.e., health care workers, child care workers, military)
3. Measles-mumps-rubella (MMR) vaccine
4. Tetanus-diphtheria vaccine

Vaccines Needed for Those 50 Years of Age and Older

1. Influenza vaccine (for the flu) annually

Vaccines Needed for Those 65 Years of Age and Older

1. Pneumococcal vaccine (to prevent pneumonia caused by *Streptococcus pneumoniae*)

Vaccines Needed by All Health Care Workers

1. Influenza vaccine (for the flu) annually
2. Hepatitis B vaccine

Source: Centers for Disease Control and Prevention. (2007). *Immunizations.* Retrieved January 2, 2007, from http://www.cdc.gov/vaccines

years and is given annually because the flu virus mutates annually. The virus usually mutates in birds or pigs and then reinfects humans. Immune protection develops approximately 2 weeks after the immunization and lasts up to a year. Some immunized individuals will still get the flu; however, they will usually get a milder case than those who did not get the shot. Immunization with the flu vaccine should be done in October or November, and can be given as late as December because the peak of flu season occurs in January through March (CDC, 2007c).

 Antiviral medications such as Tamiflu and Amantadine were developed to reduce the severity of the symptoms of influenza. These medications are given to patients with influenza to block viral infection and decrease the length of illness. Treatment of influenza is especially important for immunosuppressed patients or older adults who may not have a fully competent immune system (CDC, 2007c).

Immunization with the pneumococcal vaccine to protect against *Streptococcus pneumoniae* diseases is strongly recommended by the CDC for individuals 65 years of age or older. Pneumococcal vaccine is also recommended by the CDC for individuals with high risk such as those who are immunocompromised, children under age 2, and children in day care situations. Pneumococcal infection results in serious disease such as pneumonia, bacteremia, meningitis, sinusitis, and otitis media. The CDC reports that pneumococcal disease kills more people in the United States each year than all other vaccine-preventable diseases combined (CDC, 2007d).

 The smallpox vaccine that many people received up to 50 years ago is now conferring only a percentage of the protection initially available. A bioterrorism attack using smallpox could potentially infect a large part of the population. As an individual ages, the cells that make the antibodies age as well and this can affect immune response to disease (DeFranco et al., 2007).

Effects of Age on the Immune System

The major protection of the newborn against antigens occurs through the transfer of maternal IgG antibodies across the placenta during fetal development, especially during the last weeks of pregnancy (Rote, 2006). Hence, infants born prematurely may be significantly immune deficient. Immunoglobulin G antibodies remain active in the newborn for the first several months while the infant's production of immunoglobulins, specifically IgM, rises rapidly and attains adult levels by approximately 1 year of age (Sommer, 2007). Infant serum IgA levels are first detected approximately 2 weeks after birth and attain adult levels by 7 years of age. Further immune protection can be attained through the transfer of maternal IgA in the colostrum of milk during breast-feeding. Research has indicated that these antibodies provide local immunity for the intestinal system and decrease diarrheal infections in underdeveloped countries (Sommer, 2007).

The thymus is also a major contributor to immune development because it generates mature immunocompetent T lymphocytes during infancy and childhood. By puberty, when the mature immune cells are sequestered in the peripheral lymphoid tissues, the thymus atrophies and is replaced by adipose

tissue. Failure of the immune system to develop normally *in utero* will result in primary immune deficiencies that usually become evident in the first year of life. These deficiencies are discussed in Chapter 60 .

Gerontological Considerations

At the other end of the spectrum of life, with aging, there is a decline in the ability of the immune cells to mount an immune response and a decrease in the production and response of these cells to chemical signals of inflammation. The most significant changes occur in relationship to T-cell function, which is primarily responsible for protection against infections and tumors (Rote, 2006; Wojda & Witt, 2003). The number and percentage of T cells, both T-helper and suppressor T cells, decrease with age. Additionally, the ability of lymphocytes to produce interleukins is diminished as the body ages (Burns, 2004). The decline in T-cell numbers and function with aging results in greater susceptibility to infection. Influenza and pneumococcal pneumonia are two examples of diseases that most adults are relatively protected from until they reach age 55 to 60. After that time, the slower response of T cells and B cells can result in severe infections.

An additional effect of aging on the adult immune system is a delayed or decreased hypersensitivity reaction. When allergy testing is done in older adults, there may be a depressed ability to mount an inflammatory response to the antigen injected. This is referred to as **anergy**, and results from the diminished ability of the T-cell line to produce chemical mediators of inflammation. Individuals who show evidence of anergy are at greater risk of developing cancer and have higher rates of mortality in general (Sommer, 2007).

Aging also results in a decreased ability on the part of immune cells to identify self antigens, while at the same time there is an increase in the number of auto-antibodies produced. This results in higher incidences of autoimmune disease with aging (Rote, 2006; Wojda & Witt, 2003). Research also indicates that there is increased DNA mutation with aging that results in higher numbers of abnormal cells, and that the immune system fails to recognize and eliminate these problem cells. This in part accounts for the greater incidence of tumors and cancers in older adults (Camplejohn et al., 2003; Sommer, 2007). The Gerontological Considerations box summarizes the clinical effects of aging on the immune system.

 *Older adults may not demonstrate the classic symptoms of infection and inflammation such as fever. As a result of decreased immune function, older adults may become hypothermic when they have a systemic infection. The white blood cell count is usually elevated, but may not be as noticeable a response as that seen in a younger person. Symptoms such as altered level of consciousness and confusion should be carefully assessed and evaluated in any patient who is older and especially in patients from settings such as skilled facilities where the incidence of urinary tract infections may be higher (Porth, 2007).*

Genetic Implications

Nurses need an ongoing knowledge of the discoveries of genetic research to be able to identify and assess individuals at risk. Nurses also need an adequate understanding of the genetic research to be able to teach patients and families about the risk factors, tests, and

GERONTOLOGICAL CONSIDERATIONS of the Effects of Aging on the Immune System

Effect on Immune System	Clinical Signs
Decreased percentage of T cells	Risk of infection, tumor.
Decreased percentage of T-helper cells	Cannot initiate immune response as quickly.
Decreased percentage of suppressor T cells	Cannot downregulate immune system as quickly.
Decreased interleukin production	Slows inflammatory and immune responses to infection.
Decreased number of interleukin receptors on cells	Slows inflammatory and immune responses.
Delayed stimulation of T cells and B cells	Slows inflammatory response and may decrease ability to recognize cancer cells.
Decreased primary and secondary production of antibodies	Reduced response to infectious organisms, more severe infection, i.e., pneumonia.
Delayed hypersensitivity response	Decreased allergic response, increased severity of infections.
Increased auto-antibody production	More exacerbations of autoimmune disease.

Sources: Burns, E. A. (2004). Effects of aging on immune function. *Journal of Nutrition Health and Aging, 8*(1), 9–17; McCance, K., & Heuther, S. (2006). *Pathophysiology: The biological basis for disease in adults and children* (5th ed.). St. Louis: Mosby; Porth, C. (2007). *Essentials of pathophysiology* (7th ed.). Philadelphia: Lippincott Williams & Wilkins.

treatment of diseases with a familial or genetic association. Patients with high risk for inherited diseases such as cancer or immune abnormalities will benefit the most from this information.

DNA is the building block that forms genes. Genes are present in the nucleus of every cell and confer all of the inherited characteristics. Genes also regulate cell activity and determine how the cell develops and functions. The Human Genome Project identified and mapped all of the genes of the human body (Khoury, 2006). One result of this work has been a better understanding of the fundamental role that DNA and genes play in the development of the majority of diseases. Research has focused on discovering which genes are linked to the development of specific diseases such as immune disorders like asthma, systemic lupus erythematosus (SLE), and cancer. The major task ahead is to create the bridges from genomic discoveries to disease prevention and improved treatment (Tranin, 2006).

Alterations of specific genes on immune cells are a focus of ongoing immunologic genetic research. An example of this is the overproduction of IgE and leukotrienes and the development of asthma (Meurer, Lustig, & Jacob, 2006). Asthma is known to be a complex disorder with genetic and familial association. Specific genes are now being identified that have links to increased risk for developing asthma (Postma et al., 2005). Research has also linked variation in genotypes to how patients respond to common asthma medications such at albuterol, which supports the significance of genotyping in determining the most effective drug treatment to improve patient outcomes (U.S. Food and Drug Administration, 2005).

Currently genotyping is done at only a few research centers, but it is not unrealistic to envision this becoming a common aspect of the clinical work-up for patients with immune alterations (Steinke & Borish, 2006). DNA mutations and alterations in gene functioning have major ramifications for identifying and treating disease processes that affect the immune system and all other body systems. Genetics is discussed in Chapter 11 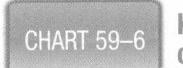.

ASSESSMENT OF THE IMMUNE SYSTEM

Immune function assessment begins with a thorough health history and physical examination because disorders of the immune system can affect any system in the body. Listening carefully to the patient's complaints about current and past medical problems provides valuable clues to immune function. It also gives direction for physical assessment and diagnostic testing that is completed in collaboration with the health care provider or other members of the health care team. Chart 59–6 outlines essential information about the immune system assessment.

Patient History

A thorough assessment of a patient should include biographic data, demographic data, risk factors for illness, and focused

CHART 59–6 Key Criteria for Assessment of the Immune System

Assessment	Nursing Implications
Complete health history	Current complaint, prior diseases, immunizations, chronic disease, known immune disease, nutritional status, functional status.
Family health history	Genetic association with many diseases including some cancers, heart disease, some autoimmune diseases.
Social history	Abuse of alcohol or drugs, smoking, diet, sexual behaviors, and occupation can all impact immune function and likelihood of transmission of infectious diseases.
Medications	Drugs affect immune function. Drugs may interact with each other. Side effects may affect assessment (e.g., corticosteroids suppress immune function).
Physical Assessment	
Inspection	Skin and mucous membranes intact, examine all rashes, wounds, note any exudate.
Palpation	Palpate lymph nodes in neck, groin, axilla. Palpate abdomen and kidneys.
Percussion	Thorax, abdomen.
Auscultation	Lung sounds can give clue to infection. Auscultate for heart murmurs.

Sources: D'Amico, D., & Barbarito, C. (2007). *Health and physical assessment in nursing.* Upper Saddle River, NJ: Pearson Prentice Hall; DeFranco, A. L., Locksley, R., & Robertson, M. (2007). *Immunity: The immune response in infectious and inflammatory disease.* Sunderland, MA: Sinauer Associates; Porth, C. (2007). *Essentials of pathophysiology* (7th ed.). Philadelphia: Lippincott Williams & Wilkins.

inquiry into the patient's current problem. The most common complaints related to the immune system and lymphatic tissues involve infection, allergy response, enlarged lymph nodes, and lymphedema (Wilson & Giddens, 2005). Assessment should include recent exposure to any infectious diseases. Risk factors that impact immune function would include a genetic familial history of immune-related diseases as well as lifestyle choices and habits that increase exposure to communicable diseases. Sexually transmitted infections are discussed in Chapters 49 and 50 ☉. Substance abuse behaviors that may alter immune function are discussed in Chapter 16 ☉.

Inflammation is often the first step in stimulating the immune system. Indicators of inflammation should be assessed including questions about fever, malaise, swelling, redness, cough with or without pain, and decreased function of a limb or part of the body. Inquire about the presence of rashes, skin cracks, or open wounds with serous drainage, bleeding or pus that may indicate infection. Inquire if the patient is experiencing night sweats or cough with or without sputum. If sputum is present, what color is it? Various colors of sputum indicate infection with different types of organisms. For example, infections involving pseudomonas are usually a green color, whereas rust-colored sputum is associated with *Klebsiella* (Porth & Sweeney, 2007). It also is important to gain information about the duration and frequency of infections. Incurable or recurrent infections are often the first indicator of significant impaired immune function. An example of this is frequent and recurrent oral or vaginal candida infections, as seen in patients with HIV infection.

Pain

The integration of the immune system throughout the body's other systems means that alterations in immune function can present themselves in a variety of manifestations. Pain is one of the most common first complaints with immune abnormalities due to the presence of inflammation. For example, enlarged lymph nodes in the presence of viral or bacterial infection may be very tender and painful. Detailed assessment of pain is a vital aspect of the history and physical examination and should be quantified using a specific pain scale. Chapter 15 ☉ includes examples of pain assessment scales.

Past Medical History

Information gathered should include a history of childhood diseases, prior hospitalizations, and diagnostic and surgical procedures. Question the patient regarding a medical history of chronic disease such as hepatitis, diabetes, chronic obstructive pulmonary disease, or renal failure. This is significant because chronic diseases can impair immune function. Inquire about a history of diseases specifically related to immune disorders such as cancer or autoimmune diseases such as SLE or rheumatoid arthritis. Additionally, all patients should be assessed for allergies to medications, food, and environmental antigens such as pollen or pet dander (D'Amico & Barbarito, 2007).

It also is important to know if the patient has had surgeries that involved removing lymph nodes due to malignancy or trauma, or any organ transplant. Loss of lymph nodes will alter lymphatic drainage and decrease immune function. Organ transplant requires lifelong immunosuppressive medications that result in immune suppression and a significantly increased risk for contracting an infection. A history of any blood transfusions should also be obtained because blood products contain foreign antibodies that can alter normal immune response. Also, blood transfusions prior to 1985 were not screened for HIV. Subsequent screening has almost eliminated this risk (CDC, 2007a). Blood administration safety is discussed in extensive detail in Chapter 23 ☉.

Knowledge of the patient's immunization status also is important in preventing illness and promoting optimal health. Inquire about childhood diseases such as chicken pox, measles, mumps, whooping cough, or immunizations against these diseases, as well as a current tetanus vaccine, which must be updated every 10 years. Ask adult patients if they have received the annual influenza vaccine. Any adult with a history of pneumonia should receive the pneumococcus vaccine. Additionally, the CDC recommends that all adults over the age of 65 receive a pneumococcus vaccine if they have not already been immunized (CDC, 2007b). Inquire about past or present exposure to tuberculosis and the dates and results of tuberculin tests such as a tine test or purified protein derived (PPD) test, as well as any follow-up chest x-ray results. Obtain information on recent travel to another country or history of living in another country, especially developing countries, because a traveler is at risk of being exposed to multiple strains of resistant organisms (D'Amico & Barbarito, 2007).

Medication History

Medications can significantly affect the immune system. It is essential to obtain a complete list of all medications, including over-the-counter (OTC) medications, that the patient is currently taking. Common OTC medications such as nonsteroidal anti-inflammatory drugs (e.g., ibuprofen, cyclooxygenase-2 inhibitors, and aspirin) that are taken in large quantities can cause significant decreases in leukocytes and neutrophils. Prescription medications the patient is taking to treat ongoing medical problems can result in profound immune suppression. Drugs such as corticosteroids or cytotoxic agents such as cyclophosphamide are immunosuppressive and significantly increase the patient's susceptibility to infection. Antibiotics in large doses or administered over a prolonged period of time can also affect immune function and result in hemolytic anemia, leukopenia, and neutropenia as well as agranulocytosis (Shannon, Wilson, & Stang, 2004).

Interactions between various medications need to be considered before patients are treated with additional medications for the current complaint. Some medications, such as antibiotics, interfere with the action of others. Herbal supplements can also have significant drug interactions and patients should be questioned regarding herbal supplement use. Addition of new medications to the patient's treatment regime should prompt discussion with a consulting pharmacist to identify any possible medication interactions and an examination of laboratory values to identify possible immune alterations.

Family History

Many of the diseases that affect the immune system are related to specific gene alterations that predispose members of the same family to the development of similar immune disorders. Examples of this are certain types of malignancies such as breast cancer, autoimmune diseases such as SLE, and development of allergies (Porth & Sweeney, 2007). Inquire if any members of the patient's family have been diagnosed with cancer and what type, as well as any other diseases involving the immune system such as rheumatoid arthritis or allergic asthma. It is important to know if members of the patient's immediate family (parents, grandparents, siblings) are deceased and the cause of death. Genetic predisposition plays a critical role in the development of many diseases in addition to those that affect the immune system, such as heart disease, emphysema, and diabetes. This information helps identify the patient's risk factors for disease development and can direct the physical examination and diagnostic work-up.

Social History

It is important to ask about the patient's occupation. Exposure to certain environmental substances can effect the action of the immune system. For example, asbestos and coal dust are known to result in cell changes that can lead to cancerous tumor (Porth & Sweeney, 2007). Additionally, the risk of development of occupational allergies is directly related to the frequency of exposure to certain products, as exemplified by the increased incidence of latex allergies among individuals who have daily exposure to latex products (National Institute for Occupational Safety and Health, 2007). Issues of importance when attending to patients from various cultures or ethnic groups are discussed in the Cultural Considerations box.

Inquire about lifestyle habits such as smoking, alcohol and drug use, and sexual practices, all of which place the patient at an increased risk for development of diseases that impact immune function. Illicit injection drug use and multiple sexual partners are high-risk behaviors associated with transmission of infections of hepatitis and HIV, as discussed in Chapter 60 ☟.

 *Questions about lifestyle habits such as alcohol and drug use and sexual practices are sensitive. These issues should be addressed in a private setting, without other family or friends present. It is also helpful to ask sensitive questions toward the end of the patient history after the nurse has had an opportunity to establish rapport with the patient.*

It is also important to obtain information related to the patient's social support system. The availability of family and friends to provide psychological and physical care during illness and as-

CULTURAL CONSIDERATIONS for Treating Patients from Various Cultures

Cultural factors also can impact the patient's concept of health, comfort with the medical exam, and choices of medical treatment. For some cultural groups decision making related to health care is not autonomous, and the patient may prefer that the head of the family or clan be present when the patient's diagnosis, treatment, or prognosis is discussed (Jarvis, 2004). Knowledge about the patient's cultural attitudes can facilitate taking the history and completing the physical examination. For example, concerns about modesty may be an issue during examination of lymph nodes in the breast and groin area for women in Asian, Hispanic, American Indian, or Alaskan Native cultural groups, and may be sensitively addressed by having a same-gender health care provider and covering the perineum during the exam (Wilson & Giddens, 2005).

sist the patient in managing medications and follow-up treatment is essential for compliance with the prescribed treatment regime. Diagnosis of diseases related to the immune system, such as cancer or HIV infection, are frequently devastating and provoke high anxiety related to the issue of dying. Chronic diseases, such as SLE or rheumatoid arthritis, can dramatically alter the patient's lifestyle and occupational choices. Nurses are in an ideal position to identify issues related to lack of social support and to provide resources and referrals to address this issue, in an effort to decrease the risk of depression and isolation that can result.

▉ Physical Assessment

Lymphatic tissues and cells of the immune system are located throughout the body. The immune system affects every other body system. Often signs of immune abnormalities are subtle. Therefore, a thorough physical examination involves inspection, palpation, percussion, and auscultation of various body systems to identify any abnormal function. Careful examination and palpation of immune tissue, especially the lymph nodes, are particularly important because enlarged and painful lymph nodes may indicate infection, inflammation, or malignancy. Figure 59–2 ▉ (p. 1867) describes the location of lymph nodes and the tissues that are drained by part of the lymph system.

Inspection

Inspection is always the first step in a physical examination. Look globally at the patient. Does the patient look fatigued, feverish, or pale? Is the patient well nourished, thin, or obese? Fever indicates an acute infection. Fatigue and weight loss may be associated with chronic disease processes. Inadequate nutrition affects the ability of the immune cells to function normally and causes immunosuppression. Rapid and significant weight loss that is unintentional is a serious concern because it is a symptom of malignancy. An unintentional weight loss of 10 pounds or more in a month is also an indicator of a need for a nutritional consult. Optimal nutrition is essential for immune function. Loss of protein reserves results in atrophy of lymphoid tissue and decreased antibody and T-cell response. Decreased vitamin and mineral intake affects the proliferation and maturation of immune cells and suppresses immune function. Malnutrition lowers the body's resistance to disease and increases morbidity and mortality from infection (Scrimshaw, 2003; Urden, Stacy, & Lough, 2006). An extensive discussion on the importance of nutrition for body function can be found in Chapter 14 ☟. General inspection also includes careful examination of the intactness of the skin and mucous membranes because they are the first line of defense in protecting the body from invasion by microorganisms.

Inspection should be directed to the area of complaint. For example, if the complaint is related to symptoms of a persistent cough and sore throat, inspect the mucous membranes of the throat and the lymph nodes of the neck (see Figure 59–2 ▉, p. 1867). Superficial lymph nodes should not be visible, thus the presence of edema, erythema, and red streaks is indicative of inflammation and infection (Wilson & Giddens, 2005).

Additionally, observe for edema of the extremities and at lymph node sites. Edema may be localized and related to a wound or infectious process that causes swelling in an extremity or related changes in normal circulatory flow. Areas of edema that are red and warm indicate inflammation. Note any signs of lymphedema, nonpitting edema at the site of lymph nodes that indicates inadequate drainage from lymphatic vessels and excessive accumulation of fluid in the interstitial spaces around the lymph vessels. This can occur for a variety of reasons including congenital abnormalities in the development of the lymphatic system (Milroy's disease), blocked lymphatic channels due to infection or malignancy, or surgical removal of lymph nodes related to trauma or prior malignancy. The presence of lymphedema should prompt questions related to the onset and duration of the swelling because this is a symptom associated with the development of malignancies (D'Amico & Barbarito, 2007).

Palpation

Palpate lymph nodes for size, tenderness, warmth, and mobility (see Figure 59–2 ■, p. 1867 for lymph node locations) and note if any are edematous. Ask the patient if it is painful to have the nodes palpated. Normally superficial lymph nodes are pain free and nonpalpable. Enlarged lymph nodes from acute infection are tender, slightly firm, and move freely. In contrast, malignancy is indicated when enlarged nodes are nontender, hard, asymmetrical, and nonmobile (attached to the underlying tissues) (Wilson & Giddens, 2005). If the nodes are enlarged or tender, focus assessment on the structures from which they drain. For example, if lymph nodes in the neck are bilaterally edematous, tender, firm, and freely movable, infection of the head and throat may be indicated. If the complaint is in the lower extremities, the groin lymph nodes should be palpated for edema and tenderness. Additionally, any edema in extremities should be palpated to determine the extent and level of pitting. A thorough examination also involves palpation of the abdomen, which contains a large number of immune tissues, for assessment of and pain or identification of a mass.

Percussion

Percussion is helpful in determining if there is inappropriate fluid or a mass in an organ, indicating disease. For example, percussion over the lung is done to determine if fluid is present that would change the normal resonant sound of the lung tissue to a dull sound, which may indicate infection. Kidneys are percussed to determine if there is tenderness in the area, indicating possible infection or tumor (Jarvis, 2004). Abnormalities in percussion sounds warrant further investigation and collaborative discussion with the health care provider for follow-up with more in-depth diagnostic testing of the body system involved.

Auscultation

Lung sounds such as coarse and fine crackles indicate fluid from infection or edema. Heart sounds such as valve sounds and murmurs give indications about the function of the organ. Cardiac valve dysfunction with murmurs is not uncommon in autoimmune diseases such as SLE or rheumatoid disease (Jarvis, 2004). Abdominal auscultation is done to assess bowel sounds. For example, a loss of bowel sounds may indicate an ileus or infarcted bowel.

Integumentary Assessment

Skin should be assessed with each evaluation of the patient. Normal skin is intact and free from areas of redness, swelling, rashes,

purpura, or lesions that may indicate inflammation, an allergic reaction, or infectious processes. Examine the skin and identify any nodules, lumps, or wounds that are present. Evaluate these abnormalities for symptoms of infection such as redness, inflammation, streaking lines, edema, or drainage. Signs of rash or petechiae indicate an allergic response or infection. A variety of autoimmune diseases have signs or symptoms seen on the skin. Scleroderma is one example of autoimmune disease that affects the quality of the skin. Patients with scleroderma often have firm, hard skin and may have a somewhat immobile facial expression. Chapter 60 ☺ includes discussions of allergies and autoimmune diseases. Information on skin abnormalities is extensively discussed in Chapters 66 and 67 ☺.

While examining the skin, give special attention to bony prominences where redness can indicate the first stage of skin breakdown, and to skinfolds under the breast and in the groin where small cracks in the skin may go undetected. Inspect the mucous membranes, which should be pink, moist, and free of lesions.

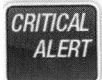 **CRITICAL ALERT** *A patient who is obese may have difficulty cleansing skinfolds especially on the back, the thighs, and under a pendulous abdomen. Skinfolds that are not cleaned regularly place the patient at increased risk for development of candidiasis (yeast) infection or the development of boils that can go undetected. The patient may also be embarrassed by lack of cleanliness and feel very uncomfortable with a skinfold examination. A caring and nonjudgmental attitude on the part of the nurse is vital in helping the patient feel accepted and building a therapeutic relationship.*

Neurological Assessment

The brain is protected from injury and invasion by the bones of the cranium. Protection from birth also includes the blood–brain barrier, which is the mechanism of tight connections between endothelial cells in blood vessels that prevent many particles from diffusing into the brain. The brain does not have lymph tissue, but protection is provided by lymph nodes in the neck (Rote, 2006). Examination of the head and neck involves inspection and palpation of the lymph nodes of the head located in front of and behind the ear and extending along the jaw and under the chin, the anterior and posterior neck, and the supraclavicular area. Palpation of the periauricular lymph nodes is done to assess lymph nodes that drain lymph fluid from the head (Figure 59–14 ■). The technique for palpation of the lymph nodes of the neck can be seen in Figure 59–15 ■. Swollen, tender, red nodes in these areas may reflect infection in the face, neck, or head.

Many autoimmune diseases have a neurological component. Physical examination of immune function in the neurological system includes assessment of the symmetry of the face. Examine the face for presence of facial droop or a facial expression that is frozen or not responsive to emotion. Disorders of the immune system that affect the neurological system include Guillain-Barré, myasthenia gravis, and cerebral vascular accident. Additionally, Bell's palsy also can present with an asymmetrical facial expression. Patients presenting with fever and stiffness of the neck should be assessed for meningitis. Extremities should be assessed for numbness, tingling, or unilateral or bilateral paralysis. Chapter 28 ☺ provides information on neurological abnormalities and a description of a full neurological assessment.

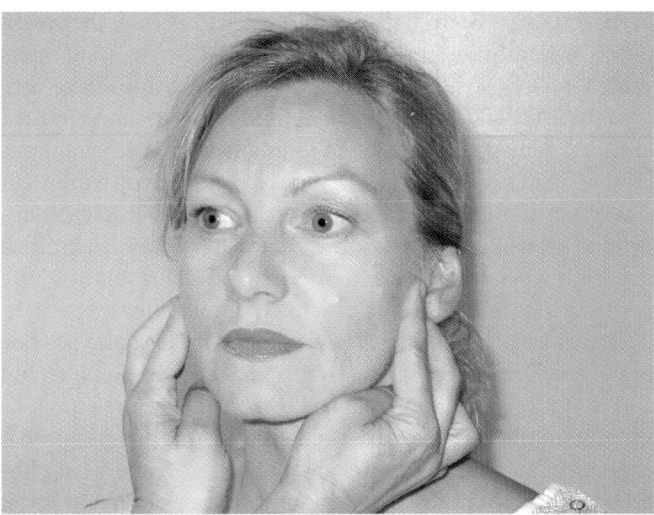

FIGURE 59–14 ■ Palpation of the periauricular lymph nodes.

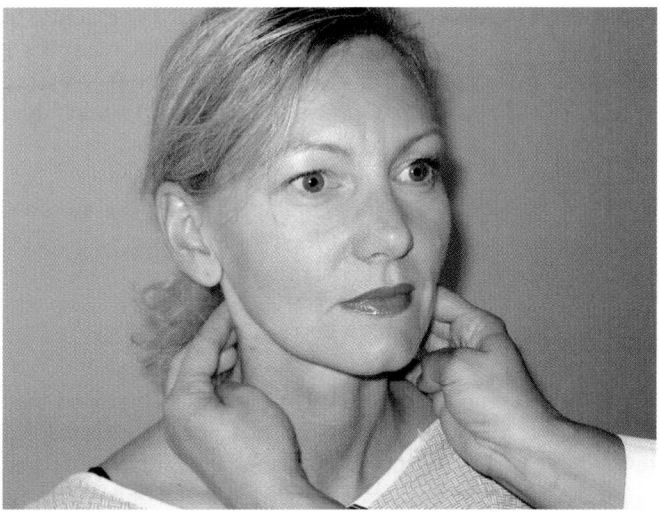

FIGURE 59–15 ■ Palpation of the posterior superficial cervical chain lymph nodes.

Cardiovascular Assessment

The heart and vascular system are closely associated with lymphatic vessels. A lymphatic vessel is located next to each combination of artery and vein. Chyle drains into the right atrium from the lymphatic and thoracic ducts. Chyle mixes with blood and is delivered from the heart into circulation. Protection is also provided by the presence of immune cells, including B cells, T cells, macrophages, neutrophils, and basophils. Immunoglobulin is also circulating in the blood. The vascular system allows rapid delivery of immune cells and chemicals to all areas of the body (Sommer, 2007). A functioning cardiovascular system is essential for proper immune function.

Assessment of immune function in the cardiovascular system itself primarily focuses on laboratory data and the clinical presentation of the patient. Elevated white blood cell counts often occur with inflammation from an ischemic cardiac event such as acute myocardial infarction or an infectious process such as endocarditis. See Unit 8 ☮ for a full discussion of cardiac abnormalities.

Respiratory and Chest Assessment

The respiratory system utilizes several natural mechanisms of protection to support immune function. The upper airway contains the tonsils, which are made up primarily of lymphoid tissue and help trap and process antigens. The cough reflex helps remove debris from the bronchial airways. Ciliated cells in the trachea and airways move cells, debris, and bacteria toward the mouth and away from alveoli. Fixed macrophages are present in lung tissue to phagocytize bacterial cells and debris. The lungs also are rich in vascular tissue, and immune cells are present in circulation to help protect against debris, virus, and bacteria (Rote, 2006). Situations that damage the cilia and alter pulmonary tissue such as smoking or inhalation burn injuries place the patient at increased risk for infection. Medical treatment for acute respiratory failure that requires mechanical intubation bypasses all of the natural defense mechanisms and is one of the primary reasons that extubation as early as is safe for the patient is strongly recommended (Tablan, Anderson, Besser, Bridges, & Hajjeh, 2004).

Competent immune function is critical in the respiratory system because of the variety and quantity of microorganisms that the pulmonary tissues are exposed to on a daily basis. Lung sounds should be auscultated. Patients with infectious processes may have coarse or fine crackles or a friction rub of the pleura. A friction rub indicates inflammation of the pleura, which may be associated with infection (D'Amico & Barbarito, 2007). Patients who present with a complaint of pain with cough or difficulty breathing should be evaluated for elevated white blood cell counts. Because the lungs' ability to clear debris and bacteria is so important, the quality and quantity of secretions must be assessed. Secretions that are green, yellow, or brown should be evaluated by laboratory culture to detect an infectious process.

Assessment of the respiratory system and structures of the chest involves inspection and palpation of the nodes in the supraclavicular area, the axilla, and the breast. Figure 59–16 ■ demonstrates the appropriate hand position for examining supraclavicular lymph nodes. Palpation and detection of enlarged supraclavicular nodes are of particular concern because these nodes are at the end of a chain of ducts, such as the thoracic duct, that drain the upper abdomen, lungs, breasts, and

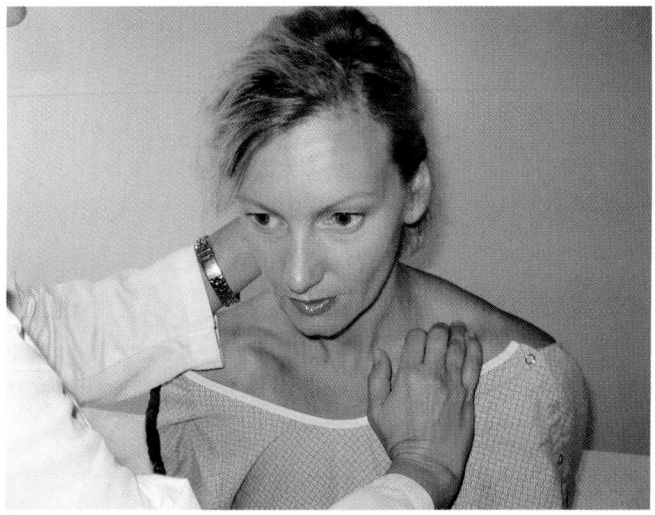

FIGURE 59–16 ■ Palpation of the supraclavicular lymph nodes.

arms and are often the site of metastatic disease (Wilson & Giddens, 2005).

The majority of the drainage from the breast flows into the axillary nodes. Palpation of axillary nodes is shown in Figure 59–17 ■. Lymph nodes of the breast are located deep in the tissue and are rarely palpable. Axillary nodes that are enlarged, painful, and mobile indicate infection located in the breast or arm or systemic disease such as systemic syphilis. In contrast, axillary lymph nodes that are enlarged, painless, asymmetrical, and fixed to underlying tissue are indicative of malignant diseases such as breast cancer and Hodgkin's lymphoma (D'Amico & Barbarito, 2007).

Gastrointestinal Assessment

Immune function is supported through a variety of natural protective mechanisms within the gastrointestinal system (GI). The act of emesis can rid the stomach of toxins and bacteria. The stomach produces hydrochloric acid and maintains a pH of approximately 3.00. This is so acidic that only a few organisms can exist in the stomach. An example of one of the few organisms that can tolerate an acidic environment is *Helicobacter pylori*, which is the cause of many gastric ulcers. *H. pylori* can withstand the acidic environment and start to grow on the cell walls of the stomach. This growth is followed by acid secretion that further stresses the cells such that the cell walls in the stomach break down and an ulcer is formed (Rote, 2006). Gastric ulcers also may occur due to the secretion of additional acid as part of the stress response with illness. It is important to address this potential problem area.

CRITICAL ALERT *A critical assessment of the protection of the entire gastrointestinal system is essential for all patients hospitalized for greater than a day or two. The stress of illness, as well as immobility, places the gastric mucosa at risk of degradation. The consequence of loss of protection can be GI bleed and/or stress ulcer. Proton pump inhibitors or H2-receptor blockers are necessary for many patients.*

The intestines have a rich vasculature. The vessels of the small and large intestine are responsible for absorption of large molecules of digestion. Large numbers of bacteria are always present in the intestines. Some bacteria are needed to assist in the breakdown of food molecules. The structure of the intestine offers protection for the body's internal environment from these bacteria. In addition, two-thirds of all fixed lymph tissue is located in the abdomen and is referred to as gut-associated lymphatic tissue (GALT) (Sommer, 2007). Specific clusters of lymph tissues are the Peyer's patches, which are not palpable, and the appendix, which produces pain in the right lower abdominal quadrant when inflamed and infected and can result in severe peritonitis if rupture occurs prior to surgical removal.

Accessory organs of the GI tract such as the liver also provide protection from antigens. Fixed macrophages in the liver filter out and consume bacteria and cellular debris. The liver also is responsible for the filtering of toxins. The spleen, located in the upper left abdominal quadrant, houses a large network of B and T lymphocytes and macrophages that filter antigens from the blood and it is important in immune function for fighting systemic infection.

Assessment of immune function of the GI system should include inspection, auscultation, percussion, and palpation of all four abdominal quadrants. Inspection assesses symmetry of the abdomen and quality of the skin. Lack of symmetry or taunt skin can indicate a mass or infection. Auscultation of abdomen occurs prior to percussing or palpating the abdomen, so that the presence or absence of bowel sounds or pain is not affected. Auscultation enables identification of bowel abnormalities, such as absent bowel sounds with paralytic ileus or mechanical obstruction. Percussion of the abdomen focuses on areas of tympany and dullness. Tympany usually indicates the presence of gas. Dullness is usually present over tissue or fecal material in the gastrointestinal tract and is also the sound with presence of a tumor. All four quadrants of the abdomen should be percussed. Chapter 44 ⊙ demonstrates appropriate hand position for percussion of the abdomen. Areas of dullness should then be palpated for a mass. Pain upon palpation should be further assessed for quality, degree, duration, and other occurrences of the same pain. Pain can be related to infection or a disease process affecting the underlying tissue (Jarvis, 2004). Additional information on GI assessment can be found in Chapter 44 ⊙ .

Genitourinary System

Organs of the genitourinary system provide natural immune protection for the body by several mechanisms. Mechanical flow of urine can wash debris from the urethra. The kidneys also filter out drug metabolites. Vaginal secretions contain immunoglobulins and other immune cells that can provide some protection from bacteria, fungi, and virus (Rote, 2006).

Immune assessment of the genitourinary system includes inspection, percussion, and palpation to identify the presence of infection or malignant tumors. External genitalia should be free from swelling and drainage. Skin should be intact and free from lesions and redness around the anus and upper inner thigh area. Percussion of the kidneys and bladder is not usually necessary unless the patient complains of specific flank pain, difficulty emptying the bladder, or an urge to urinate without being able to do so. Palpation of the bladder should be pain free and the bladder should be soft. Kidneys may be palpated by pressing one hand on the anterior surface of the abdomen below the ribs and pushing gently with the other hand from the back in the same

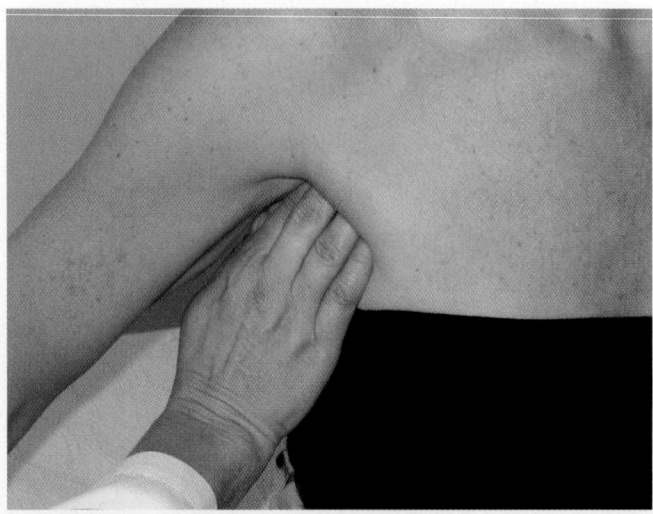

FIGURE 59–17 ■ Palpation of axillary lymph nodes.

location below the ribs. Chapter 44 👁 demonstrates palpation of the kidneys. Abnormalities of the genitourinary system are addressed in Chapter 47 👁.

Lymph nodes in the groin should also be inspected and palpated with either the genitourinary or musculoskeletal system exam. Figure 59–18 ■ demonstrates appropriate patient draping of the groin area and hand position for palpation during the inguinal lymph nodes examination. Normally, inguinal nodes are small and mobile and difficult to palpate. The superior and inferior inguinal lymph nodes receive drainage from the upper and lower leg, the vulva, and lower third of the vagina in females, and the penis and scrotal surface in males. Enlarged, tender, firm, and freely movable nodes indicate an infection or inflammatory process in any of these tissues and warrant further investigation. Additionally, assessment for the presence of lymphedema should be included.

Musculoskeletal Assessment

Musculoskeletal assessment that focuses on immune function should include inspection and palpation of joints and limbs for evidence of swelling, inflammation, or infection. Assess for the presence of pain with range of motion and any limitation of joint motion. Autoimmune diseases such as rheumatoid arthritis and SLE include joint pain and swelling as a significant symptom. An extensive discussion of musculoskeletal assessment can be found in Chapter 54 👁.

Common Laboratory and Diagnostic Exams of the Immune System

In addition to physical examination of immune tissues and various body systems, laboratory tests are required to evaluate the phagocytic, cellular, and antibody functions of the immune system. These tests are generally ordered when an abnormality such as an infection or a specific complaint related to an organ function is identified.

Laboratory Tests

An initial complete blood count (CBC) with manual differential is essential for identifying immune system abnormalities and providing a basis for determining the need for other forms of testing. Elevated total white blood counts (total WBC) can indi-

cate infection, inflammation, or in some cases blood disease such as leukemia. Low white blood cell counts indicate immunosuppression, as seen with various cancers or infections such as HIV and warrant full investigation. For example, a patient with symptoms of an undiagnosed HIV infection may have a low total WBC and a very low total lymphocytes count on the CBC differential. This would prompt the health care provider to follow up with further tests to determine the level of T lymphocytes called CD4 cells, and HIV antibody testing as described in Chapter 60 👁. Chapter 62 👁 includes an in-depth discussion of the complete blood count.

White blood counts are differentiated into total lymphocytes, monocytes, neutrophils, bands (immature neutrophils), basophils, and eosinophils. All specific cell types are described as a percentage of total white cells. Neutrophils comprise approximately 70% of the total WBC and are the first cells on the scene of trauma, infection, or inflammation. Immature neutrophils are called bands. An increase in the number of bands in the serum circulation (>7%), indicates that the body is mounting a major inflammatory response, or fighting an infection, such as an abscess, because it is depleting the number of mature neutrophils and starting to use immature neutrophils that are less capable of ingesting antigens (Rote, 2006).

The CBC also includes information on platelets that are important in identifying immune abnormalities. Diseases such as systemic lupus erythematosis (SLE) may first be seen as thrombocytopenia on the CBC and prompt further testing. Another example is autoimmune thrombocytopenia, an autoimmune disease process in which the body identifies its own platelets as foreign and destroys them. Platelet abnormalities are of special concern because patients with platelet counts that are significantly decreased (<100,000 mm³) have an increased risk of bleeding. Decreased hemoglobin and hematocrit levels also occur in immune abnormalities. Anemia can result from autoimmune diseases. One of the first indications of a tumor can be decreased hemoglobin or hematocrit in the presence of no evidence of gross bleeding (Lefever-Kee, 2006). Abnormalities of lymphocyte counts on the CBC can be further evaluated by tests that examine specific T-cell and B-cell counts and immune function. This information is summarized in Chart 59–7 (p. 1886). Chapter 62 👁 includes an in-depth discussion of laboratory data.

Immune Function Tests

Specific serum tests examine the function of the immune system. Erythrocyte sedimentation rate (also known as a "sedimentation rate" or "sed rate"), C-reactive protein, antinuclear antibody tests, anti-IgG, IgG levels, IgM levels, enzyme-linked immunosorbent assay, and Western blot are all examples of serum tests designed to look at one specific chemical or antigen and the body's response to it.

The erythrocyte sedimentation rate (ESR) is a serum test that is used to diagnose acute and chronic inflammation, as well as rheumatoid and autoimmune diseases. In the presence of inflammatory mediators, blood proteins are altered and red blood cells stick together and then fall out of solution when the blood sample is spun. This results in an elevated sedimentation rate. The test does not diagnose a specific disease, but is a sensitive and early indicator of a widespread inflammatory, autoimmune, or

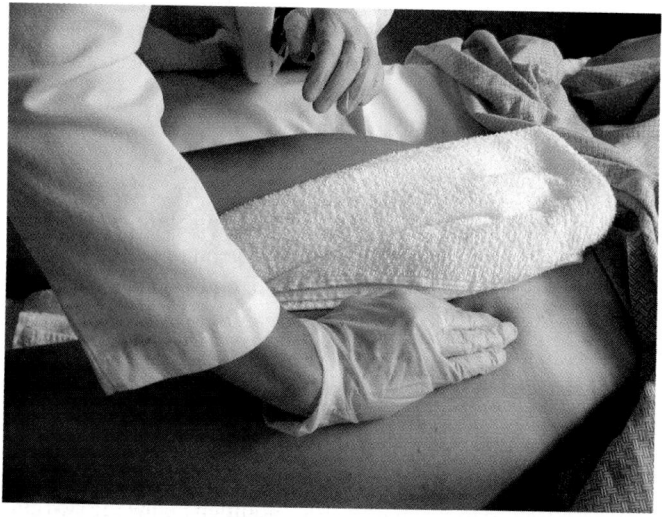

FIGURE 59–18 ■ Palpation of inguinal lymph nodes with draping.

Reading the White Blood Cells on a Complete Blood Count Differential

Reading the WBC Differential	Test Result Implications
Neutrophils (55–65% of WBC count)	Largest group of granulocytes, first on the scene. High counts of >67% of total WBC indicate inflammation or infection. Low counts may indicate systemic infection or abscess. If neutrophils are low and bands are very high, abscess or systemic infection is likely. Usually lives only about 72 hours.
Bands (immature neutrophils) (should be less than 10% of the total percentage of neutrophils)	Immature neutrophils with banded rather than segmented nuclei. An elevation in this count (more than 10% of total WBC count) may indicate a large bacterial infection such as an abscess, pneumonia, or sepsis.
Basophils (0.3–0.5% of WBC count)	Basophils are granulocytes that migrate out of circulation to become mast cells. Mast cells can release histamine in response to injury or cell death, a key first step in inflammation. Usually basophils comprise 0.75% of total WBC.
Eosinophils (1–3% of WBC count)	Eosinophils are granulocytes and comprise about 1–4% of total white blood cells. Eosinophils are elevated with allergies and parasite infestation.
Lymphocytes (20–30% of WBC count)	Lymphocytes are not usually more specifically identified. Lymphocytes usually comprise about 25–33% of total WBC. However, if very elevated, they may indicate infection or lymphoma. If very low, they may indicate infection or malignancy.
Monocytes (3–8% of WBC count)	Monocytes are nongranulocyte white blood cells that migrate out of circulation to become macrophages. Total monocytes are important for their potential to phagocytize cell debris, bacteria, virus, and fungal cells.

Sources: DeFranco, A. L., Locksley, R., & Robertson, M. (2007). *Immunity: The immune response in infectious and inflammatory disease.* Sunderland, MA: Sinauer Associates; McCance, K., & Heuther, S. (2006). *Pathophysiology: The biological basis for disease in adults and children* (5th ed.). St. Louis: Mosby; Porth, C. (2007). *Essentials of pathophysiology* (7th ed.). Philadelphia: Lippincott Williams & Wilkins.

malignant disorder. In SLE, for example, an ESR test is a standard part of a diagnostic work-up and is most often elevated. The ESR also is ordered when an autoimmune disease is suspected such as rheumatoid arthritis. A protein called rheumatoid factor is often present in the serum of patient's with rheumatoid disease in greater quantities than individuals without autoimmune diseases (Lefever-Kee, 2006).

A test often ordered in conjunction with the ESR is the C-reactive protein (CRP) test. CRP is a glycoprotein produced by the liver in response to acute inflammation. It is a more rapid and sensitive indicator of acute inflammation than the ESR and indicates the presence of inflammation but not the cause. CRP levels decline rapidly from serum when inflammation has subsided (Van Leeuwen, Kranpitz, & Smith, 2006). Increased levels of CRP can be found in immune-related diseases such as SLE, rheumatoid arthritis, Crohn's disease, and inflammatory bowel disease, but are not always consistently elevated for unknown reasons. The test has proven most helpful in diagnosis of acute flare-ups of inflammatory immune diseases and in monitoring response to therapy (Peng, 2005). Elevated levels are also found in acute bacterial infection, rheumatic fever, during the second half of pregnancy, and in acute myocardial infarction (Lefever-Kee, 2006). The major focus of recent research related to CRP has centered on its role in acute myocardial infarction. Chapter 40 contains an in-depth discussion to CRP as related to coronary artery disease.

Most immune function tests also look for the presence of an antibody to a specific antigen. Antigens are often destroyed by the time a test has been ordered or may be present in only small quantities or hidden inside cells. Antibody activity is much easier to measure and test. Diagnosis for specific autoimmune diseases such as SLE, scleroderma, or rheumatoid arthritis involves testing for a variety of antibodies. Antinuclear antibodies (ANAs) are immunoglobulins (IgG, IgM, IgA) that react with the nuclear portion of leukocytes, forming auto-antibodies against the host's DNA and ribonucleic acid (RNA). The presence of these antibodies is indicative of SLE and warrants further testing for anti-DNA antibodies, which are further diagnostic of SLE. Total ANA levels can also be elevated in scleroderma, rheumatoid arthritis, cirrhosis, leukemia, and malignancy (Porth & Sweeney, 2007; Van Leeuwen et al., 2006).

Other antibody tests evaluate infection with a specific bacterium or virus such as hepatitis or HIV. An example of this is the enzyme-linked immunosorbent assay (ELISA) and the Western blot tests, which detect the presence of antibodies created in response to infection with the HIV antigen. Many of the tests currently used to assess immune function utilize monoclonal antibodies as the mechanism to bind the auto-antibodies present in the patient's blood (Lefever-Kee, 2006). The Diagnostic Tests box describes the diagnostic laboratory tests used for assessment of the immune system and related nursing implications.

Computerized Axial Tomography

Immune system diseases can affect any body system. As a result computerized axial tomography (CT) scans are frequently used in the process of diagnosis of immune system abnormalities because they are able to provide detailed images of body structures. The CT scan uses a narrow x-ray beam that examines body sections from different angles and creates and a three-dimensional image of the organ or structure being studied. CT scans are 100 times more sensitive than two-dimensional x-rays and also show the shape, size, and sites of bleeding as well as mass effects in organs (Lefever-Kee, 2006). CT scans are most often used to identify areas of gross morphology and sites of possible tumors. Good-quality CT scans provide important information about organs and vascular function and enable identification of disease abnormalities.

DIAGNOSTIC TESTS to Assess Immune Function

Test and Normal Value	Expected Abnormality	Rationale for Abnormality

Blood count with differential
WBC count:
RBC:
  Males: 4.5–6 µL
  Females: 4–5 µL
HBG:
  Males: 13.5–18 g/dL
  Females: 12–16 g/dL
HCT:
  Males: 40–54%
  Females: 36–46%
WBC 5,000–10,000 µL
  Neutrophils: 55–65%
  Basophils: 0.3–0.5%
  Lymphocytes: 20–30%
  Monocytes: 3–8%
  Basophils: 0.3–0.5%
	RBC count, hemoglobin/hematocrit (HBG/HCT) are important in determining the presence of anemia, blood loss, and hydration status, and the number of red blood cells and white blood cells, including neutrophils, basophils, and monocytes.
	The differential white blood count (WBC) total percentages will equal 100%. The percentages vary depending on the type of disease process. For example, with acute bacterial infection the percentage of neutrophils will be elevated, whereas in acute allergy or parasite infection basophils will have an increased percentage.
		The blood count with differential is a routine part of hospital admission. Nursing assessment includes monitoring lab trends to determine the presence of a disease process and the effectiveness of treatment.

CD4 count 450–1,400/mm³	Total T-helper lymphocytes. Low numbers (<500) may indicate HIV or other immunodeficiencies.	A low CD4 is sensitive information and should not be shared casually.
Antinuclear antibodies (ANA): negative	Measures the number of antibodies made to parts of the patient's cells' nuclei. Indicates autoimmune disease.	Anticipate additional serum exams for immune function. Few autoimmune diseases are diagnosed with one serum exam.
Enzyme-linked immunosorbent assay (ELISA/ EIA): negative	Serum exams able to detect antibodies in blood. HIV is an example of an ELISA test.	It is important to know what antibody is being tested.
Western blot: negative	Another exam used to test for HIV. This exam is more sensitive to HIV. It is done if the initial ELISA for HIV is positive.	Western blot exams are also done for other immune related diseases.
Assays of IgG, IgA, IgM, IgD, IgE *Adult:* IgG: 650–1,700 mg/dL IgA: 770–400 mg/dL IgM: 40–350 mg/dL IgD: 0–8 mg/dL IgE: 1–120 mg/dL	Serum assays of level of IgG in the blood can help identify patients with deficiencies. IgG deficiency is relatively common.	Many immune diseases begin with multiple infections, fatigue, or vague symptoms. Immunoglobulin testing is an indication that immune function may be impaired. Care to reduce risk of infection is important.
Erythrocyte sedimentation rate (ESR or sed rate), Westergren method: *Males <50 years:* 0–15 mm/hour *Females <50 years:* 0–20 mm/hour	Test measures the time it takes red cells to precipitate out of serum. An increased rate implies inflammation, a common problem in many immune diseases.	Sed rate may be elevated in inflammatory diseases such as rheumatoid arthritis, chronic infection, cancer, and other immune problems. Care should be taken to assess patients for increased risk of infection.
C-reactive protein (CRP) Titer: >1:2	Measures acute inflammation 6–10 hours postinjury and tissue destruction. Nonspecific test for inflammation that rises early.	CRP may be elevated early in acute inflammatory process and tissue destruction related to bacterial infection, tissue ischemia, tissue necrosis, and flare-ups in autoimmune diseases.

Sources: Lefever-Kee, J. (2006). *Laboratory and diagnostic tests: Nursing implications* (6th ed.). Upper Saddle River, NJ: Pearson Prentice Hall; Van Leeuwen, A., Kranpitz, T., & Smith, L. (2006). *Davis's comprehensive handbook of laboratory and diagnostic tests with nursing implications* (2nd ed.). Philadelphia: F. A. Davis; Porth, C. (2007). *Essentials of pathophysiology* (7th ed.). Philadelphia: Lippincott Williams & Wilkins.

Specific CT tests may require a contrast agent to enhance the films and help identify small tumors or abnormalities. The nurses must have an understanding of why the test is ordered and any preparation of the patient that is required to ensure optimal testing. Patient teaching about the process is essential to alleviate fears about the unknown testing process, because all CT scans require the patient to lie still on the testing table. The CT scanner is shaped like a large donut and the testing table moves through the center hole of the structure. Feeling enclosed in the CT scanner can provoke anxiety in some patients. Patients may require sedation or the presence of the nurse to safely and successfully complete the exam.

Additional laboratory and diagnostic tests such as skin allergy testing and diagnostic testing for various autoimmune diseases,

HIV infection, and bone marrow biopsies are discussed in detail along with the specific disease processes in Chapter 60 .

Health Promotion

Health promotion related to the immune system is focused on risk factor identification and management of allergies and infections. Education needs to include information on lifestyle choices and habits that increase the risk for communicable disease transmission. For example, there are more than 18 million cases of newly diagnosed sexually transmitted infections each year that are preventable with education and compliance with risk factor prevention such as condom use (CDC, 2006). Identification of genetic risk factors for allergies such as food allergies can prevent mild to life-threatening allergic reactions.

Immunization education is a critical element in disease prevention and can help save precious health care dollars spent on preventable infections. Immunization education is especially important for vulnerable populations such as infants and children because of their incompletely developed immune system, the elderly due to the slowing effects of aging on immune response, and individuals with suppressed immune response due to disease or medications.

Summary

A fully competent immune system is essential to protecting the human body from disease and disability. An alteration in the ability of the immune system to eliminate pathogens, distinguish self from non-self, or identify and eliminate the proliferation of mutant cells results in immune associate diseases. Immune tissues and cells are intricately associated with all body systems; therefore, a thorough assessment of immune function involves assessment of multiple body systems, as well as evaluation of cellular components of the immune system such as neutrophils and B and T lymphocytes and the development of specific antibodies. Abnormalities of the immune system can affect any system in the body, and they are frequently first evidenced by an inflammatory response. Chapters 60, 61, and 64 provide information on immune abnormalities including immune hypersensitivity responses, immune deficiency, inflammation, and cancer.

NCLEX® REVIEW

1. A patient is diagnosed with an immune deficiency disorder. The nurse realizes this patient is demonstrating a malfunction of which of the following body structures?
   1. Lymph nodes
   2. Spleen
   3. Bone marrow
   4. Adenoids

2. A patient is diagnosed with an autoimmune disorder. The nurse realizes this disease process was caused by:
   1. The body reacting to self receptors as an antigen.
   2. The body's ability to tolerate all self antigens.
   3. The body's ability to respond to non-self antigens.
   4. Adequate B and T cells that do not attack self antigens.

3. A patient is receiving a transfusion of plasma cells. The nurse realizes these cells will contribute to which of the following:
   1. Produce antibodies in response to exposure to an antigen
   2. Stop or slow the immune process
   3. Send messages to start the process of programmed cell death
   4. Stimulate cells to destroy cancer cells

4. A patient is diagnosed with liver cirrhosis. The nurse realizes that which of the following elements of immunity might be altered in this patient?
   1. Tumor necrosis factor
   2. Interferons
   3. Complement
   4. Interleukins

5. A patient tells the nurse that she does not want a flu shot because she doesn't want the live flu virus in her body. Which of the following should the nurse respond to this patient?
   1. The live flu virus is weakened so it won't cause the flu.
   2. The vaccine is made from killed flu organisms.
   3. The vaccine is made artificially so you won't get the flu from the shot.
   4. You can take the vaccine by mouth instead.

6. The nurse is caring for a patient with an infection. Which of the following explains how the patient's body will create antibodies to fight the infection?
   1. T-cell activation
   2. Antigen presentation
   3. Linking of T cells
   4. Linking of B cells

7. An elderly male doesn't understand why "just a little cold" developed into pneumonia. Which of the following should the nurse explain to this patient?
   1. Delayed hypersensitivity response
   2. Decreased primary and secondary production of antibodies
   3. Increased auto-antibody production
   4. Decreased percentage of suppressor T cells

8. A patient appears fatigued and tells the nurse he has no appetite even though he knows he can eat more because he's losing so much weight. Which of the following does this information suggest to the nurse?
   1. The patient has blocked lymph glands.
   2. The patient has an infection within an organ.
   3. The patient has a skin infection.
   4. The patient is at risk for malnutrition.

9. A patient is being assessed for rheumatoid arthritis. Which of the following diagnostic tests might be ordered to aid in this patient's diagnosis?
   1. Erythrocyte sedimentation rate
   2. Antinuclear antibodies
   3. Enzyme-linked immunosorbent assay
   4. Western blot test

Answers for review questions appear in Appendix D

KEY TERMS

acquired immunity *p.1869*
active acquired immunity *p.1869*
agglutination *p.1874*
anergy *p.1878*
antibody *p.1872*
antigen *p.1864*
antigen–antibody complex *p.1874*
apoptosis *p.1868*
B cells *p.1869*
B lymphocytes *p.1869*
cell-mediated immune response *p.1870*
chemotaxis *p.1871*
chyle *p.1865*
complement *p.1872*
cytokines *p.1871*
deoxyribonucleic acid (DNA) *p.1874*

fragment antigen binding (FAB) portion *p.1874*
fragment crystalline (FC) portion *p.1874*
human leukocyte antigens (HLAs) *p.1869*
humoral immune response *p.1872*
immune complex *p.1874*
immune tolerance *p.1864*
immunity *p.1864*
immunization *p.1876*
immunoglobulin *p.1872*
interferon *p.1871*
interleukin *p.1871*
lymph nodes *p.1866*
lymphatic system *p.1865*
lymphokines *p.1871*
natural immunity *p.1867*

neutralization *p.1874*
nongranulocyte *p.1865*
non-self antigen *p.1869*
opsonization *p.1871*
plasma cells *p.1874*
precipitation *p.1874*
primary immune response *p.1874*
secondary immune response *p.1875*
self antigen *p.1869*
T cells *p.1869*
T-helper cells *p.1870*
T lymphocyte *p.1869*
tissue factor (TF) *p.1871*
toll receptors *p.1868*
tumor necrosis factor (TNF) *p.1871*
vaccine *p.1876*

EXPLORE mynursingkit™

PEARSON

MyNursingKit is your one stop for online chapter review materials and resources. Prepare for success with additional NCLEX®-style practice questions, interactive assignments and activities, web links, animations and videos, and more!

Register your access code from the front of your book at
www.mynursingkit.com

REFERENCES

Burns, E. A. (2004). Effects of aging on immune function. *Journal of Nutrition Health and Aging, 8*(1), 9–17.

Camplejohn, R. S., Gilchrist, R., Easton, D., McKenzie-Edwards, E., Barnes, D. M., Eccles, D. M., et al. (2003). Apoptosis, ageing and cancer susceptibility. *British Journal of Cancer, 88*(4), 487–490.

Centers for Disease Control and Prevention. (2006). Sexually transmitted diseases treatment guidelines, 2006. *Morbidity and Mortality Weekly Reports, 55*(RR-11), 1–96. Retrieved July 21, 2008, from http://www.cdc.gov/std/treatment/2006/rr5511.pdf

Centers for Disease Control and Prevention. (2007a). *How safe is the blood supply?* Retrieved January 2, 2007, from http://www.cdc.gov/hiv/resources/qa/qa15.htm

Centers for Disease Control and Prevention. (2007b). *Immunizations.* Retrieved January 2, 2007, from http://www.cdc.gov/vaccines

Centers for Disease Control and Prevention. (2007c). *Key facts about flu.* Retrieved January 2, 2007, from http://www.cdc.gov/flu/keyfacts.htm

Centers for Disease Control and Prevention. (2007d). *Pneumococcal disease.* Retrieved January 2, 2007, from http://www.cdc.gov/vaccines/vpd-vac/pneumo/default.htm

D'Amico, D., & Barbarito, C. (2007). *Health and physical assessment in nursing.* Upper Saddle River, NJ: Pearson Prentice Hall.

DeFranco, A. L., Locksley, R., & Robertson, M. (2007). *Immunity: The immune response in infectious and inflammatory disease.* Sunderland, MA: Sinauer Associates.

Dillon, P. M. (2007). *Nursing health assessment: A critical thinking, case studies approach* (2nd ed.). Philadelphia: F. A. Davis.

Dunne, J. (2007). Infection, inflammation, and immunity. In C. M. Porth (Ed.), *Essentials of pathophysiology* (pp. 229–246). Philadelphia: Lippincott Williams & Wilkins.

Franson, P. (2005). Antivascular endothelial growth factor monoclonal antibody therapy: A promising paradigm in colorectal cancer. *Clinical Journal of Oncology Nursing, 9*(1), 55–60.

Jarvis, C. (2004). *Physical examination and health assessment* (4th ed.). St. Louis: W. B. Saunders.

Khoury, M. (2006). *The human genome project: "Gene sequencing and discovery are only the beginning."* Retrieved January 8, 2006, from

the Centers for Disease Control and Prevention website: http://www.cdc.gov/genomics/training/file/print/perspectives/AfterHGP.pdf

Kohler, G., & Milstein, C. (1975). Continuous cultures of fused cells secreting antibody of predefined specificity. *Nature, 256,* 495–497.

Lefever-Kee, J. (2006). *Laboratory and diagnostic tests: Nursing implications* (6th ed.). Upper Saddle River, NJ: Pearson Prentice Hall.

McCance, K., & Heuther, S. (2006). *Pathophysiology: The biological basis for disease in adults and children* (5th ed.). St. Louis: Mosby.

Meurer, J., Lustig, J., & Jacob, H. (2006). Genetic aspects of the etiology of asthma treatment. *Pediatric Clinics of North America, 53*(4), 715–725.

National Institute for Occupational Safety and Health. (2007). *Latex allergy: A prevention guide.* Retrieved July 21, 2008, from http://www.cdc.gov/niosh/98-113.html

Peng, S. (2005). C-reactive protein. *Medline Plus Medical Encyclopedia.* Retrieved January 4, 2007, from http://www.nlm.nih.gov/medlineplus/ency/article/003356.htm

Porth, C. (2007). *Essentials of pathophysiology* (7th ed.). Philadelphia: Lippincott Williams & Wilkins.

Porth, C., & Sweeney, K. (2007). Alterations in immune response. In C. M. Porth (Ed.), *Essentials of pathophysiology* (pp. 293–319). Philadelphia: Lippincott Williams & Wilkins.

Postma, K., Meyers, D., Jongepier, H., Howard, D., Kippelman, G., & Bleecker, E. (2005). Genomewide screen for pulmonary function in 200 families ascertained for asthma. *American Journal of Respiratory & Critical Care Medicine, 172*(4), 446–52.

Rote, N. (2006). Immunity. In K. L. McCance & S. E. Heuther (Eds.), *Pathophysiology: The biological basis for disease in adults & children* (5th ed., pp. 168–227). St. Louis: Mosby.

Scrimshaw, N. S. (2003). Historical concepts of interactions, synergism and antagonism between nutrition, and infection. *Journal of Nutrition, 133*(1), 316S–321S.

Shannon, M. T., Wilson, B. A., & Stang, C. L. (2004). *Health professional's drug guide.* Upper Saddle River, NJ: Pearson Prentice Hall.

Sommer, C. V. (2007). The immune response. In C. M. Porth (Ed.), *Essentials of pathophysiology* (pp. 134–149). Philadelphia: Lippincott Williams & Wilkins.

Steinke, J., & Borish, L. (2006). Genetics of allergic disease. *Medical Clinics of North America, 90*(1), 1–15.

Tablan, O., Anderson, L., Besser, R., Bridges, C., & Hajjeh, R. (2004). Guidelines for preventing health-care–associated pneumonia, 2003. *Morbidity and Mortality Weekly Reports, 53*(RR03), 1–36. Retrieved January 4, 2006, from http://www.cdc.gov/mmwr/preview/mmwrhtml/rr5303a1.htm

Thomas, M. (2005). Cetuximab: Adverse event profile and recommendations for toxicity management. *Clinical Journal of Oncology Nursing, 9*(3), 322–338.

Tranin, A. (2006). The bridge from genomic discoveries to disease prevention. *Oncology Nursing Forum, 334,* 891–910.

Twite, K., & Gaspard, K. (2007). Disorders of the white blood cells and lymphoid tissues. In C. M. Porth (Ed.), *Essentials of pathophysiology* (pp. 247–266). Philadelphia: Lippincott Williams & Wilkins.

Urden, L., Stacy, K., & Lough, M. (2006). *Thelan's critical care nursing: Diagnosis and management* (5th ed.). St. Louis: Mosby.

U.S. Food and Drug Administration. (2005). Genetics play role in response to asthma drug. *Food and Drug Administration Consumer Magazine, 39*(1), 36.

Van Leeuwen, A., Kranpitz, T., & Smith, L. (2006). *Davis's comprehensive handbook of laboratory and diagnostic tests with nursing implications* (2nd ed.). Philadelphia: F. A. Davis.

Wilkes, G. (2005). Therapeutic options in the management of colon cancer. *Clinical Journal of Oncology Nursing, 9*(1), 31–44.

Wilson, B. A., Shannon, M. T., Shields, K. M., & Strang, C. L. (2007). *Nurse's drug guide.* Upper Saddle River, NJ: Pearson Prentice Hall.

Wilson, S., & Giddens, J. (2005). *Health assessment for nursing practice* (3rd ed.). St. Louis: Elsevier Mosby.

Wojda, A., & Witt, M. (2003). Manifestations of aging at the cytogenetic level. *Journal of Applied Genetics, 44*(3), 383–399.

60

Caring for the Patient with Immune Response Disorders

Debra Brady
Kathy Yeates

With contributions by:
Kathleen Osborn

Outcome-Based Learning Objectives

After studying this chapter, the learner will be able to:

1. Differentiate the nursing management for patients with immune hypersensitivity responses and immune deficiencies.

2. Compare and contrast the immune hypersensitivity response related to allergy, autoimmune, and alloimmune disorders.

3. Compare and contrast the pathophysiology, clinical manifestations, and laboratory data for the human immunodeficiency virus (HIV) and acquired immune deficiency syndrome (AIDS).

4. Prioritize the nursing management of the patient with HIV/AIDS to decrease the incidence of opportunistic infections.

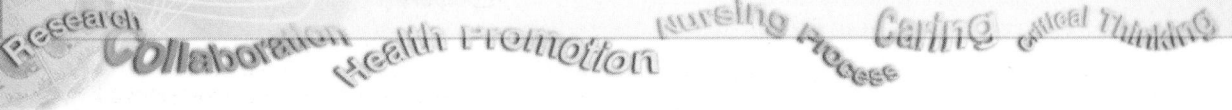

Research Collaboration Health Promotion Nursing Process Caring Critical Thinking

IMMUNE DISORDERS result from a loss of regulation of some aspect of the immune system. Immune disorders fall into two general categories: immune hypersensitivities and immune deficiencies. **Immune hypersensitivity** occurs when the immune system overresponds to an antigen, either from the environment, from the individual himself, or from another individual. Hypersensitivity disorders fall into three broad categories based on the type of triggering antigen, and include allergic, autoimmune, and alloimmune reactions. An **allergic response** occurs when the antigen is from the external environment, as opposed to an **autoimmune response**, which is triggered by a self-antigen. An **alloimmune response** occurs when the antigen is from another human. Within each of these categories are four specific mechanisms by which the immune system overresponds, referred to as **type-specific hypersensitivity reactions**.

Immune deficiencies occur when all or some part of the immune system fails to develop or is damaged through disease processes. The end result is an inability to mount an appropriate immune response. The two types of immune deficiencies are primary and secondary. **Primary immune deficiencies** result from genetic abnormalities. **Secondary immune deficiencies** occur for a variety of reasons including normal aging, malnutrition, malignancies, immunosuppressive drug therapy, and infections such as the human immunodeficiency virus (HIV).

Immune Hypersensitivities: Allergic, Autoimmune, and Alloimmune Responses

An **immune hypersensitivity response** occurs when the immune system does not maintain self-tolerance, in other words, when it overreacts to the presence of a foreign antigen. This process also initiates the mechanisms of inflammation that result in destruction of healthy tissue. Hypersensitivity reactions can be categorized according to the type of antigen (allergy, autoimmune, alloimmune), the time sequence of the reaction (immediate or delayed), and the mechanism of immunologic response. When an antigen is environmental or external in origin it is referred to as an **allergy**. An example of this type of hypersensitivity reaction is "hay fever," or allergies to common weeds and pollen. In autoimmune reactions the body fails to recognize self-antigens and begins to destroy its own proteins. Multiple clinical disorders are associated with autoimmune diseases such as multiple sclerosis and systemic lupus erythematosus. An alloimmune response occurs when the immune system reacts against the antigens in or on the tissue from another individual, as seen with grafted tissue.

A hypersensitivity response that occurs within seconds to hours is categorized as an **immediate hypersensitivity reaction**.

An anaphylactic reaction is a prime example of this type of response. A **delayed hypersensitivity reaction** can take several hours to days, as exemplified by a contact dermatitis reaction. The way in which the immune system responds to an antigen and the time sequence of the reaction is determined by the mechanism of immunologic response. These are categorized as types I and IV and are discussed next.

Mechanism of Hypersensitivity Immune Response

Four distinct mechanisms or types of immunologic reactions are involved in allergic, autoimmune, and alloimmune reactions and can cause damage to body tissues: **type I (IgE-mediated allergic reactions)**, **type II (tissue-specific–mediated reactions)**, **type III (immune complex–mediated reactions)**, and **type IV (cell-mediated reactions)**. The type I, II, and III hypersensitivity responses involve antigen–antibody interactions and are known as immediate hypersensitivity reactions. The type IV response is an antigen–lymphocyte interaction and involves a delayed hypersensitivity reaction. Chart 60–1 provides an overview of these categories and specific clinical examples.

Type I IgE-Mediated Hypersensitivity

Type I IgE-mediated hypersensitivity, also known as anaphylactic hypersensitivity, is the most common of the hypersensitivity disorders and involves the production of antigen-specific IgE antibody after exposure to a foreign antigen or **allergen**. Examples include plant pollen, pet dander, foods, and drugs. **IgE antibodies** are produced by the plasma cells in response to the foreign antigen. The process of creating antibodies that match the antigen is called **sensitization**. The IgE antibodies connect to receptors on mast cells in the connective tissue. The process of sensitization may take only one exposure or several exposures to the allergen depending on the level of IgE production. This explains why many allergic responses take time to develop.

When a hypersensitivity reaction occurs, the allergen binds to IgE antibodies on the mast cell and causes degranulation of mast cells and release of histamine. **Histamine** causes smooth muscle contraction, vasodilatation, and increased vascular permeability

and primarily affects the skin, mucous membranes, and lung. The histamines are responsible for the clinical symptoms associated with type I reactions such as redness, itching, mucous production, and bronchial constriction. The reactions can be localized in tissue, or systemic as with an anaphylactic response. The severity of the clinical symptoms is dependent on the sensitivity of the individual, the amount of allergen exposure and mediator release, and the entry route of the allergen. For example, an injected allergen from an insect sting elicits a very rapid hypersensitivity response (Porth & Sweeney, 2007; Rote, 2006).

Type II Cytotoxic Specific Reaction

Type II hypersensitivity reactions involve **tissue-specific antigens**, which are proteins located in the cell membrane of some tissues such as blood, nerves, lungs, and kidneys. Type II reactions are mediated by IgG or IgM antibodies and occur when the immune system fails to recognize a host's self-antigen or antigens on donated red blood cells. IgG or IgM antibodies interact with the tissue-specific antigen on a target cell's plasma membrane to form antibody–antigen complexes. Type II reactions can occur in several ways. This explains the variety of clinical signs and symptoms observed in this type of reaction.

The hallmark of type II hypersensitivity reactions is that they are limited to those tissues or organs that have tissue-specific antigens. One example is Goodpasture's syndrome. Antibodies are formed against the tissue-specific antigen found in the basement membrane of the glomeruli in the kidneys and the alveoli in the lungs. The result is destruction of these tissues and the associated clinical symptoms of renal failure and lung damage. In myasthenia gravis the immune system fails to recognize the tissue-specific antigen on nerve ending receptor sites and binds to acetylcholine receptors on the muscle, causing faulty muscle enervation. Type II hypersensitivity reactions are responsible for Rh-hemolytic disease of the newborn and antibody–antigen reactions involving red blood cell (RBC) destruction such as incompatibility reactions in blood transfusions (Porth & Sweeney, 2007; Rote, 2006).

Blood Transfusion Reactions

Blood transfusion reactions are an example of a type II hypersensitivity antibody–antigen reaction that results in activation

---

CHART 60–1   Types of Immune Hypersensitivity Reactions

| TYPE I
IgE-Mediated Reaction | TYPE II
Tissue-Specific-Mediated Reactions | TYPE III
Immune Complex-Mediated Reactions | TYPE IV
Cell-Mediated Reactions |
|---|---|---|---|
| • Antibody–antigen mediated
• IgE production after exposure to an antigen
• Release of histamine and inflammatory mediators
• Clinical examples: allergy, anaphylaxis | • Antibody–antigen mediated
• Occurs at tissue-specific sites by interaction of antibody with tissue cell antigen
• Clinical examples: blood transfusion reaction, Goodpastures | • Antibody–antigen mediated
• Immune complexes form in circulation and travel to various tissues
• Clinical examples: serum sickness, SLE | • T-lymphocyte mediated
• Cytotoxic T cells attack and destroy cellular targets directly
• Clinical examples: latex allergies, PPD reactions |

Note: An antibody–antigen reaction is an immune complex reaction.

Sources: DeFranco, A. L., Locksley, R., & Robertson, M. (2007). *Immunity: The immune response in infectious and inflammatory disease.* Sunderland, MA: Sinauer Associates; Rote, N. (2006). Immunity. In K. L. McCance & S. E. Huether (Eds.), *Pathophysiology: The biological basis for disease in adults and children* (5th ed., pp. 168–227). St. Louis: Mosby; Sommer, C. (2007). The immune response. In C. M. Porth (ed.), *Essentials of pathophysiology* (pp. 247–268). St. Louis: Lippincott Williams & Wilkins.

of the complement cascade and initiation of a systemic inflammatory response. Inflammatory cascades and the systemic inflammatory response result in the lysis of target cells and are discussed in great detail in Chapter 61 ⊚. All RBCs have type-specific antigens on their surface except type O. The B lymphocytes produce antibodies specific to all other blood antigens. If the patient has type A blood, each blood cell is coated with antigen A and carries B antibodies. An individual with type B blood has B antigens on the surface of each red blood cell and carries A antibodies. If a patient with type A blood is erroneously given type B blood, the individual receives A antibodies that attach to the A antigen and form an immune complex (Figure 60–1 ■). This immune complex stimulates the complement cascade that produces lysis of the cell, resulting in cell death.

The major clinical problems with blood transfusion reactions relate to the stimulation of an overwhelming systemic inflammatory response and shock state. Oxygen carrying capacity is lost because the patient's own red blood cells are destroyed, as are the RBCs in the transfused blood. Additionally, the cellular debris following cell lysis contains large proteins that may block the tubules of the glomeruli in the kidney and can produce acute tubular necrosis (Rote, 2006).

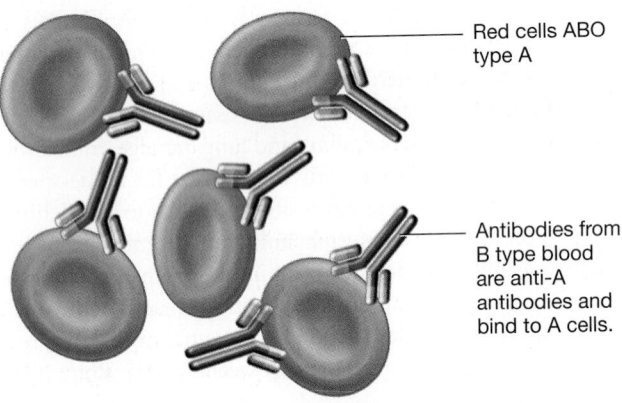

Red cells ABO type A

Antibodies from B type blood are anti-A antibodies and bind to A cells.

Step one transfusion reaction - ABO blood groups
Patient with A type blood received B type blood. B type blood has anti-A antibodies. These antibodies attach to the A type red cells.

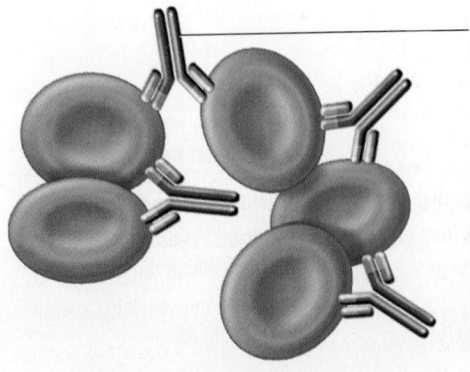

Type A red blood cells with antibodies from B type blood cross link and clump together. The immune system then sends phagocytes to ingest the clumped cells.

Step two transfusion reaction
Anti-A antibodies crosslink the cells together. This is agglutination. This makes it much easier for the immune system to send phagocytes to ingest the cells.
(From University of Michigan, Madison, 2002)

FIGURE 60–1 ■ Red blood cell immune complex.

The ABO blood antigen is only one example of many antibodies and antigens that blood is tested for prior to blood transfusion. Another important factor is the Rhesus (Rh) factor. This factor, along with the ABO factor, is the most significant because of the severity of the clinical response such as anaphylactic reaction and refractory shock. An extensive discussion of blood products, testing, and key safety factors in blood administration can be found in Chapter 23 ⊚.

Type III Immune Complex–Mediated Reaction

Type III hypersensitivity reactions also involve IgG and IgM antibody–antigen immune complexes. However, they differ from type II reactions because the antigen in type III reactions is soluble and released into circulation, instead of staying localized at a specific cell surface. The antigen can travel and deposit in extravascular tissue, such as joints, and then an antibody–antigen reaction can occur. In other instances, the antibody–antigen reaction can happen in the circulation, which results in the immune complex being deposited in tissue, such as the glomeruli. In either case, damage to the tissues results because the immune complex stimulates the complement cascade and the mediators of inflammation. Neutrophils attempt to phagocytize large immune complexes, and in the process lysosomal enzymes are released at the tissue site, further stimulating the inflammation process and damaging the surrounding tissues.

As a result of the mobility of the type III antigen–antibody complex, systemic or local responses also can occur although the reactions are not organ specific. Serum sickness is an example of a systemic response. Immune complexes are produced in the circulation in response to a foreign antigen and in response to some drugs such as sulfonamides and penicillin. The clinical symptoms of serum sickness include rash, fever, lymphadenopathy, arthralgias, and myalgias, and they result from the immune complexes being deposited in the walls of small blood vessels, kidneys, and joints throughout the body (Porth & Sweeney, 2007).

Type IV Cell-Mediated Reactions

Type IV reactions differ from the other three types of hypersensitivity reactions in that the response is delayed, instead of immediate, with onset 24 to 48 hours after antigen exposure. Secondly, the T cells of the immune system mediate these reactions, instead of antibodies. Type IV reactions occur as a result of an overreaction between normal cell-mediated mechanisms and an antigen that triggers the T cells to destroy the target cell directly or to release cells to produce lymphokines. The lymphokines activate phagocytic cells, especially macrophages at the inflammatory site. Examples of these types of reactions are seen with exposure to poison ivy, poison oak, and purified protein derivative (Rote, 2006).

Immune Hypersensitivity

The four mechanisms of immune response described above can be seen in all three categories of antigen reaction: allergic, autoimmune, and alloimmune. These categories account for the variety of clinical manifestations seen with hypersensitivity response.

Allergy Etiology and Epidemiology

The hallmark of allergy reactions is the IgE-mediated antibody–antigen response. An allergic reaction involves a type I hypersensitivity response in which an environmental antigen stimulates an overproduction of IgE antibodies that attach to mast cells. The interaction of these antibodies with an **allergen**, such as a type of environmental or foreign antigen, stimulates the release of histamine and proinflammatory mediators from mast cells. This release results in the irritating and uncomfortable symptoms associated with allergies including itching eyes, nose, and throat, cough, congestion, runny nose, watery eyes, and often bronchospasm. If the hypersensitivity reaction is severe, as with an anaphylactic reaction, the allergic response can be life threatening.

Allergic disease affects millions of people in the United States and the incidence is increasing on an annual basis (Asthma and Allergy Foundation of America, 2007). Evidence indicates that a large portion of this increased prevalence is among children who are developing allergic diseases in childhood (Brandtzaeg, 2007). Research has shown that the development of a food allergy in early childhood is associated with an increased risk of respiratory allergies (James, 2003; Wong, 2007). Current research is focused on risk factors that may be responsible, including those listed in the Risk Factors for Respiratory Allergies box. Studies to date have been disappointingly inconclusive (Bochner & Hamid, 2003; Halken, 2003; Zutavern & Brockow, 2006). Clear evidence of a single causative factor has not been identified and it is most probable that the occurrence of allergic diseases will be found to be a result of multiple factors (Asher et al., 2006; O'Connell, 2003).

The most consistent factor appears to be evidence of a genetic predisposition to hypersensitivity reactions. In the general population, the risk of developing an allergy is approximately 25%. This risk doubles when one parent has allergies (50% risk) and triples if both parents have allergies (75% risk) (Asthma and Allergy Foundation of America, 2007). The focus of allergy treatment is identification of the triggering allergen so that plans can be made to minimize or eliminate exposure to allergens and to manage symptoms.

Pathophysiology of Allergy Reactions

Normally, millions of IgE molecules of different specificities are attached to each mast cell. It is thought that individuals who are **atopic** (produce a hypersensitivity response) have a genetic predisposition to have greater than normal levels of IgE production (Dunne, 2007). With each reexposure to a triggering antigen, there is increased IgE production, increased mast cell degranulation, and increased release of histamine. The histamine causes vasodilation in local blood vessels. Additionally, endothelial cells pull apart and localized swelling occurs. This process can allow the allergen to enter the bloodstream. If this occurs a systemic

allergic response can result because basophils in the bloodstream also are stimulated to release histamine. This is the basis for an anaphylactic reaction (Rote, 2006).

Clinical Manifestations of Allergic Response

Clinical manifestations of the allergic response occur in tissues such as skin, mucous membranes, the lungs, and the gastrointestinal tract because they are highly vascular and have an abundance of mast cells as part of a fully competent immune system. There are a wide variety of allergic hypersensitivity reactions and clinical manifestations. Chart 60–2 (p. 1894) describes some of the common allergens and their associated symptoms.

Skin Allergies

Allergic responses are commonly manifested on the skin. This in fact is the basis for skin testing for allergies. A wheal and flare response is typical of a localized allergic response on the skin from exposure to an allergen, such as the resin of a star thistle plant, which binds with IgEs and causes immediate degranulation of the mast cells in the subcutaneous tissue. The clinical manifestation is a **wheal** or small, round, serous-filled raised blister, which is surrounded by a **flare** or round area of redness. This reaction occurs from the release of histamine, which causes local vasodilatation, redness, swelling, itching, and heat (Porth & Sweeney, 2007).

Other skin reactions, such as allergic contact dermatitis or a poison ivy reaction, are cell-mediated type IV delayed hypersensitivity reactions (Figure 60–2 ■, p. 1894). On first exposure the protein in poison ivy (which is the allergen), stimulates immune and memory T cells, which is an example of sensitization. A second contact with the poison ivy resin stimulates sensitized T cells. The reaction reaches maximum intensity in 24 to 72 hours and results in clinical symptoms of blistering vesicles and red, scaled areas (Rote, 2006).

Latex Allergy

Latex allergies can occur as both a type I allergic reaction or as a type IV cell-mediated reaction in response to contact with products containing natural latex. Type I reactions occur rapidly after exposure, usually within minutes. The release of IgE antibodies is responsible for the symptoms, which can include redness of the exposed skin, urticaria, asthma, itching, and conjunctivitis, which also may progress to anaphylactic shock (Rote, 2006). Exposure to the proteins that act as antigens in latex can occur through use of gloves on skin or IV catheters into the bloodstream. The antigens can also be inhaled through ventilator and handheld nebulizer tubing, and internal tissue can be exposed when surgical equipment and Foley catheters are used (Urden, Stacy, & Lough, 2006). Type I reactions can be life threatening because of their bronchial constrictive effect on the airway and vasodilation of blood vessels, which decreases perfusion pressure (American College of Allergy, Asthma and Immunology, 2007).

 **CRITICAL ALERT** *Latex reaction can occur during a surgical procedure. Symptoms of reaction in the anesthetized patient include flushing, facial edema, wheezing, bronchospasm, laryngeal edema, tachycardia, hypotension, and in extreme cases cardiac arrest.*

Latex reactions also can be a type IV delayed reaction, much like contact dermatitis, which present symptoms between 4 and 48 hours after exposure. Symptoms include dryness at the site of

---

RISK FACTORS for Respiratory Allergies

- Genetic predisposition
- Frequency of viral infections
- Increased use of antimicrobial cleansing products in the home
- Early childhood exposure to allergens
- Dietary factors
- Air pollution
- Immunizations

CHART 60–2	Common Allergens	
Common Allergen	**Characteristics**	**Symptoms**
Pollen	Allergen is the dry pollen that is present in the air. Early spring: tree pollen (oak, elm, poplar) Early summer: rose pollen, grass pollen (Timothy, red-top) Early fall: weed pollen (ragweed)	Sneezing, runny nose, congestion, itching of the noses, eyes, ears, throat, and mouth
Animal dander	Allergen is the protein found in the saliva, dander, or urine of an animal with fur, not the "hair" of the animal.	Sneezing, itching, runny nose, swollen itchy eyes and throat
Dust mites	Allergen is the microscopic droppings of mites found in bedding, upholstery, carpets. Most common trigger of year-round allergies and asthma.	Congested or runny nose, sneezing (especially in the morning), itchy watery eyes, coughing, wheezing
Mold	Allergen is the spores that are disseminated by the fungi. Molds thrive in humid areas such as bathrooms and basements.	Sneezing, runny nose, congestion, itching of the noses, eyes, ears, throat, and mouth
Insect stings	Allergen is to the protein in the venom of the insect sting. Majority of sting reactions in the United States are caused by yellow jackets, honeybees, paper wasps, hornets, and fire ants.	Flushing, itching, hives, swelling at site of bite *Potential anaphylactic reaction:* light-headedness, feeling of impending doom, swelling in the throat, wheezing, severe bronchoconstriction, nausea, vomiting, drop in blood pressure, shock = medical emergency
Medications Common: antibiotics	Allergen is the protein in the medication or the substance with which the medication is made.	Rash, hives, general itching, tingling or itching of the mouth/pallet, potential anaphylactic reaction as described above
Food allergies Most common: nuts, fish, shellfish, milk, chicken eggs, kiwi, seeds	Allergen is to the protein in the food particle. Majority of reactions develop within the first hour. Generally, the longer it takes for symptoms to develop, the less severe the reaction.	Oral itching or tingling in the mouth/pallet, lip swelling, swelling of the face, generalized flushing, itching, nausea, vomiting, and potential anaphylactic reaction as described above

Sources: American Academy of Allergy, Asthma and Immunology. (2006). *Why is the incidence of allergy increasing?* Retrieved February 23, 2007, from https://www.aaaai.org/aadmc/inthenews/wypr/2006archive/increasing_allergies.html; American College of Allergy, Asthma and Immunology. (2007). *Be S.A.F.E.: Managing allergic emergencies.* Retrieved February 19, 2007, from http://www.acaai.org/public.

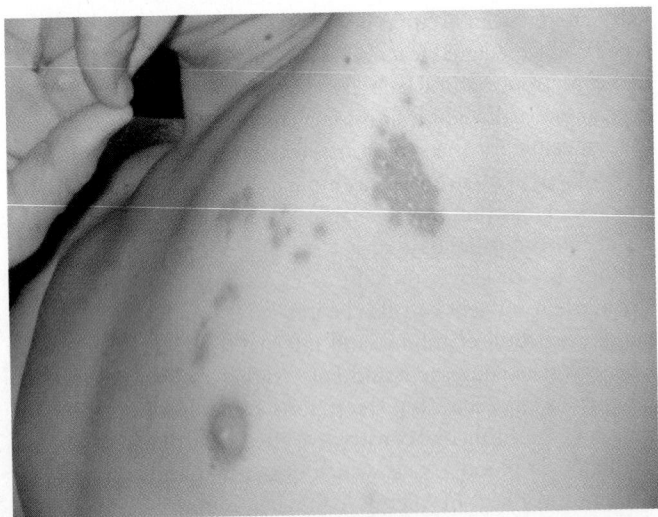

FIGURE 60–2 ■ Skin allergy type IV response.

exposure, itching, and cracking of the skin. These symptoms are followed by redness, swelling, and scabbing of the fissures and cracks in the skin. This usually occurs within a day or two of the initial symptoms. This type of reaction is often seen in health care workers who handle latex equipment and use latex gloves. All hospitals now provide latex-free gloves and most institutions provide latex-free disposable products of all kinds, such as IV tubing, blood tubing, ventilator equipment, and aerosol tubing. The increase in incidence of type IV latex reactions has coincided with the advent of standard precautions, which increased the use of gloves. Increased glove use has primarily been implicated as the foremost point of exposure for heath care workers. Estimates of the number of sensitized health care workers range from 8% to 17%. As with any antigen, the more often an individual is exposed to the antigen, the more likely the individual will become sensitized to that antigen. Powder in gloves has been removed in hospital settings to reduce the risk of aerosolized exposure to latex. These exposures can be dangerous to the sensitized individual and result in a life-threatening anaphylactic response (National Institute for Occupational Safety and Health [NIOSH], 2007).

Identifying individuals at risk for latex allergy is essential to preventing the allergic response. Factors such as working in any industry using latex or rubber components (health care workers, housekeepers, hairdressers) increases the risk, as does a history of hay fever or asthma, and/or allergies to certain foods such as bananas, avocado, kiwi, and strawberry. The proteins found in these foods have a similar structure to latex proteins and can trigger an allergic response. Patient populations with increased risk factors include those with neural tube defects such as myelomeningocele or spina bifida, those who require chronic bladder catheterization such as patients with spinal cord trauma or neurogenic bladders, and those who have had multiple surgeries. All of these factors involve multiple contacts with latex products, which enhance the risk of developing latex allergies. Any individual who is identified as part of the high-risk groups just listed or someone who can describe a contact dermatitis type reaction after exposure to latex should be considered at risk for a latex allergy (Ahmed, Sobczak, & Yunginger, 2003; NIOSH, 2007).

 Patients with neural tube deficits have a high risk of developing latex allergies (estimated 28% to 67% increased risk). They frequently also undergo multiple surgeries, which increase their risk factor. Latex-free products should always be used when caring for patients with neural tube deficits, even when prior latex allergy has not been identified (Urden et al., 2006).

As mentioned, latex-free products are now available and are to be used in all hospital settings with latex-sensitive individuals. These products are usually provided on special carts containing disposable equipment that is entirely latex free. The patient's room should have a latex allergy alert sign posted. Health care workers with latex sensitivity must stringently adhere to the same precautions. Powder-free and latex-free gloves must be used. In addition, special barrier creams are available to use on the hands for added protection. Symptoms of latex allergy need to be reported per agency protocol to the employee health center.

Food Allergies

Food allergy reactions most commonly involve mucous membranes and the gastrointestinal (GI) tract, but can quickly lead to an anaphylactic response. Food allergies are now the leading known cause of anaphylactic reactions treated in emergency departments in the United States. It is estimated that there are 30,000 food-related anaphylactic reactions that result in 150 to 200 deaths per year (Food Allergy & Anaphylaxis Network, 2006; Sampson, 2003). One example is the individual who is sensitive to peanuts. The peanut protein antigen attaches to the IgE antibody, causing the mast cells to degranulate and release histamine. The sensitive individual experiences early symptoms of allergy such as tracheal and oral itching, swelling, redness, nausea, and vomiting. The response can be limited to itching on the interior of the mouth and the GI tract, it or can be as profound as a severe anaphylactic reaction.

 One of the most common early symptoms of an allergic reaction is itching in the mouth and palate. It is important to assess this in individuals complaining of allergy symptoms or who are receiving a new drug such as an antibiotic or vaccine.

Anaphylactic Reaction

Anaphylaxis can be a localized or systemic hypersensitivity response to an antigen that can quickly progress to a medical emergency if not recognized and treated appropriately. The continuum of symptoms in anaphylaxis can range from itching, erythema, vomiting, and breathing difficulties to severe laryngeal edema, respiratory distress, vascular collapse, shock, and death (Figure 60–3 ■, p. 1896)

Combinations of presenting symptoms may vary in an individual experiencing an anaphylactic reaction depending on the number of IgE antibodies on the mast cells, the number of mast cells that degranulate and release histamine, and the release of other proinflammatory mediators such as bradykinin and sero-

tonin. Symptoms of anaphylactic response are usually immediate (less than 30 minutes), although the oral route of allergen exposure can have a 2-hour delay. A secondary response or biphasic reaction is seen in approximately 20% of patients with anaphylaxis and can occur 4 to 8 hours after the initial remission of symptoms due to secondary mediators of inflammation such as bradykinin. In general, the anaphylactic reaction is more life threatening if the hypersensitivity response is immediate (Rote, 2006).

The result of a severe systemic anaphylactic reaction is a form of shock called *distributive shock* that results in massive vasodilatation, loss of blood pressure, and inadequate distribution of blood supply and oxygen to all body tissues. Chapter 61 🌐 provides an in-depth description of distributive shock. Concurrent smooth muscle bronchoconstriction and laryngeal edema initially cause inspiratory and expiratory wheezing and difficulty breathing, which may progress to complete airway obstruction. Death can result from full circulatory collapse or severe bronchial constriction, or a combination of both. Nursing care focuses on early recognition of anaphylactic symptoms, airway management, and collaborative aggressive medication treatment to stem the continuum of anaphylactic response and prevent death.

 *Patients can be in extreme danger when breath sounds diminish after wheezing because the airways are completely constricted and no air is being inspired or expired due to edema.*

Treatment focuses on immediate administration of intramuscular adrenaline. Adrenaline's alpha-receptor agonist activity reverses vasodilation and decreases edema. Its beta-receptor activity relaxes smooth muscle thus dilating bronchioles, suppresses histamine release, and increases myocardial contractility. Administration of supplemental oxygen, establishment of intravenous (IV) access, and administration of IV fluid to support intravascular volume in patients with hypotension are also essential. Corticosteroids are a key aspect of ongoing drug therapy and work to control inflammatory mediators. Other medications that may be included in treatment are antihistamines and inotropic and antiarrhythmic agents.

Medical Management of the Allergic Hypersensitivity Response

The goal for successful medical treatment for individuals with allergic hypersensitivity is focused on avoidance of triggering allergens, prevention of a hypersensitivity response, and relief of allergy symptoms. Therefore, identifying the causative allergens is primary to effective management of allergic disease. This involves obtaining a thorough patient history and diagnostic studies, followed by creation of a drug therapy and treatment regime for allergy symptom management. For severe allergy problems this treatment plan may include allergy desensitization shots.

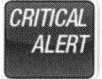 *A thorough history of allergies is essential prior to the start of any medications. Individuals with a family history of hypersensitivity response are at greater risk for allergic response. The nurse must be aware of a patient's allergies prior to administering any medication. This is especially crucial with IV medications, such as antibiotics, because the antigen is given directly into the bloodstream, bypassing the local response delay, and can result in stimulation of an immediate severe anaphylactic reaction.*

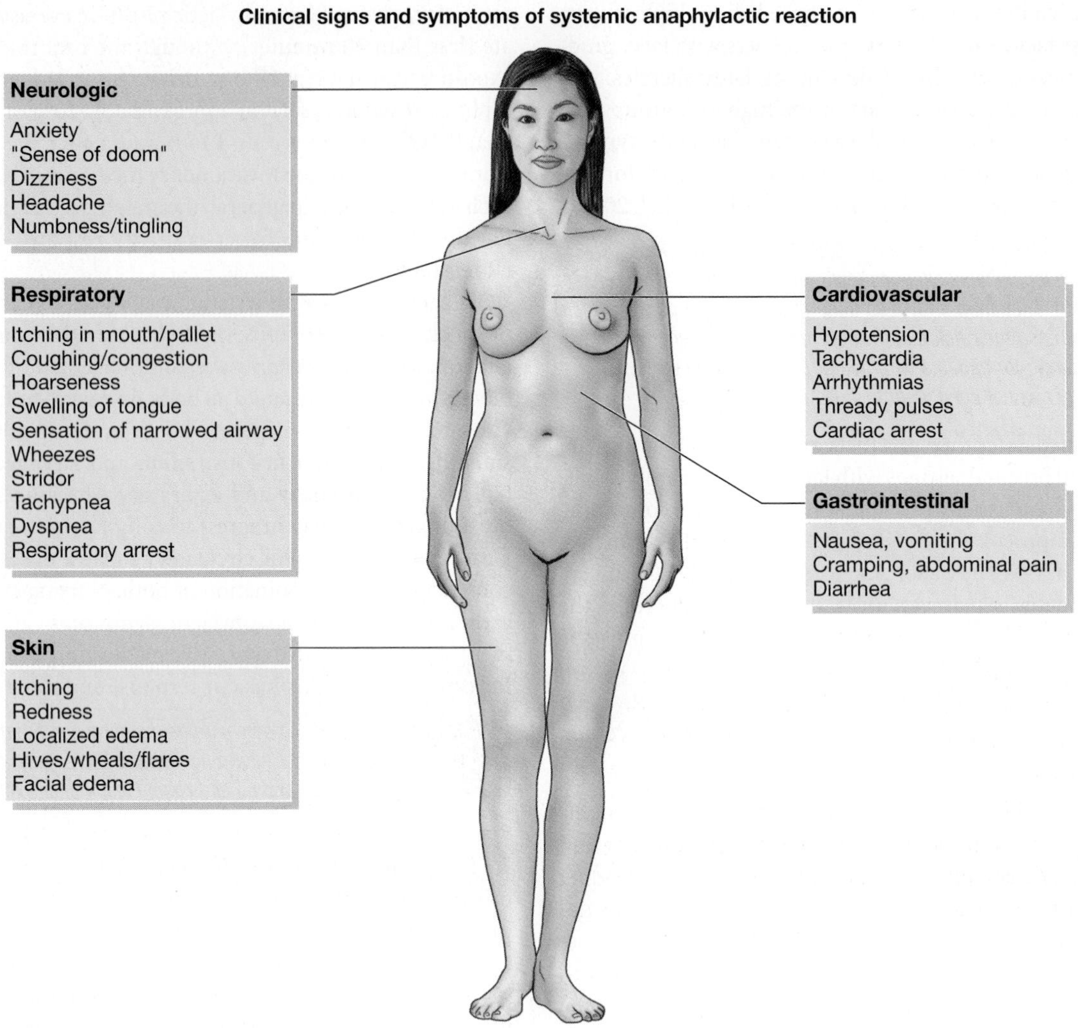

Clinical signs and symptoms of systemic anaphylactic reaction

Neurologic

Anxiety
"Sense of doom"
Dizziness
Headache
Numbness/tingling

Respiratory

Itching in mouth/pallet
Coughing/congestion
Hoarseness
Swelling of tongue
Sensation of narrowed airway
Wheezes
Stridor
Tachypnea
Dyspnea
Respiratory arrest

Skin

Itching
Redness
Localized edema
Hives/wheals/flares
Facial edema

Cardiovascular

Hypotension
Tachycardia
Arrhythmias
Thready pulses
Cardiac arrest

Gastrointestinal

Nausea, vomiting
Cramping, abdominal pain
Diarrhea

FIGURE 60–3 ■ Anaphylaxis symptoms.

Laboratory and Diagnostic Procedures

Allergy symptoms are very disruptive, uncomfortable, and can be expensive to treat. In the extreme they can be life threatening. Therefore, it is important to identify the specific triggering allergen(s) to which the atopic individual may be sensitized so that contact with the allergen can be avoided and a plan developed to treat the symptoms most effectively. Allergy testing includes blood and sputum laboratory tests to determine total IgE and allergen-specific IgE, as well as skin tests with small amounts of allergens to evaluate sensitivity.

Blood Tests

Initial laboratory tests to detect lymphocyte, eosinophil, and immunoglobulin abnormalities commonly include a complete blood count (CBC) with white blood cell differential (WBC). This provides a total lymphocyte and eosinophil count. The eosinophil count is usually elevated with type I hypersensitivity reactions and is one of the indicators used to confirm a diagnosis of allergy. Nasal smears, sputum, and bronchial secretions may also be tested for the presence of eosinophils, which indicate probable allergy.

Tests for measuring immunoglobulins include the radioimmunosorbent test (RIST), which measures circulating levels of total IgE. A more specific test is the radioallergosorbent test (RAST), which provides a sensitive measurement of the specific IgE antibodies that are elevated in response to many allergens. Ongoing testing research has resulted in the development of a RAST that detects specific IgE antibody to approximately 15 allergens that evoke the large majority of pollen- and food-related allergic disorders (American Academy of Allergy, Asthma and Immunology, 2007).

The major advantage of RAST testing is the decreased risk of systemic reaction. However, it is more costly and results are not as readily available as with skin tests. Therefore, RASTs are generally reserved for individuals in which skin testing is not possible due to skin conditions that may interfere with the results, concerns about severe anaphylaxis, or because of medications that the individual is taking (American Academy of Allergy, Asthma and Immunology, 2007).

Skin Tests

Skin testing involves introducing small amounts of various allergens into the skin of allergic individuals through either intradermal injection or a scratch, or "prick test," technique on the individual's back. The scratch or prick test is the least sensitive of the two tests, but it also carries a lower risk of systemic reaction. It is performed by placing small drops of allergen onto the skin, then pricking through it to introduce the allergen. If the individual is sensitive to a specific allergen, IgE antibodies activate mast cells to degranulate, histamine is released, and a localized reaction is produced causing a wheal (swelling) and flare (redness) within 15 minutes. The diameter of the flare is usually indicative of the level of sensitivity to the allergen. Allergy medications may suppress skin reaction and result in a false-negative reading. Therefore, allergy medications including antihistamines and corticosteroids are generally held for 48 to 96 hours prior to allergy testing (American Academy of Allergy, Asthma, and Immunology, 2007).

The profound danger with skin testing is that in severely allergic individuals even a small amount of skin test allergen can cause a systemic anaphylactic response, which requires immediate and emergent attention. Therefore, skin testing should never be performed if the individual is experiencing respiratory abnormalities such as bronchospasm.

 Nursing care for the patient in the outpatient allergy testing clinic focuses on assessment for symptoms of anaphylactic response, respiratory assessment, airway management, and rapid treatment of anaphylactic emergency. Skin tests should never be undertaken if emergency equipment and medications to treat anaphylactic reaction are not available.

Pharmacologic Management of Allergies

Drug therapy is the primary focus of allergy management. The vast majority of allergies are mediated by an IgE interaction between an allergen and receptors on the IgE antibody that stimulate the release of histamine. The goal of medications that relieve allergy symptoms is to decrease histamine release and its effects on the mucosa, skin, and tissues. A wide variety of allergy medications are available. Health care providers may suggest over-the-counter (OTC) products or write specific drug prescriptions. Frequently, the medication the patient uses is determined by insurance coverage. The Pharmacology Summary of Medications to Treat Allergy Symptoms (p. 1898) describes common allergy medications for symptom management. Major categories of drugs that provide symptomatic relief include antihistamines, sympathomimetic and decongestant drugs, corticosteroids, mast cell stabilizers, and antipyretic drugs.

The wide variety of allergy medications available often leads to confusion regarding which medication to take to alleviate symptoms or how to dose the medications correctly. Therefore, a primary role for members of the health care team is providing patient education on the appropriate dosing of allergy medication and the potential adverse effects that can occur if medication directions are not followed.

Desensitization Immunotherapy

Desensitization, or giving "allergy shots," involves introducing small amounts of the triggering allergen to the sensitive individual in increasing amounts over a long period of time, with the goal of decreasing the severity of the allergic reaction. The exact mechanism of how desensitization occurs is not fully understood. It is thought that desensitization may work by inducing the production of blocking antibodies that bind with the allergen and neutralize it so that it cannot bind with IgE and degranulate mast cells. Desensitization injections also may stimulate the production of suppressor T lymphocytes, which suppress the production of IgE

and inhibit hypersensitivity (Rote, 2006). However, this form of treatment does have a significant risk of systemic anaphylaxis.

Nursing Management

Nursing care of patients with allergies is focused on helping patients and families identify and avoid allergy triggers, education about medication for symptom relief, and instruction regarding strategies to prevent a severe allergy hypersensitivity response. Nursing care also involves early recognition and emergent treatment of anaphylactic reaction. Application of the nursing process will facilitate a comprehensive approach to the assessment and care of the patient with allergies. The Nursing Process: Care Plan for the Patient with Anaphylactic Response feature (p. 1899) provides information and sample questions to be used in obtaining a thorough assessment and history of the allergies. Nursing diagnoses are developed from the assessment data. The care plan also provides detailed outcome goals and evaluation parameters, and the nursing interventions (with rationales) used to achieve these outcomes.

Health Promotion

The health care team can further promote patient health and safety by encouraging patients with a history of anaphylactic reactions to wear a medical alert bracelet or other form of medical identification tag that identifies allergies to medications, foods, or other substances. This type of ID alerts members of the health care providers to potential problems in the event of an emergency. Additionally, instructing patients with a history of anaphylactic reaction to carry a self-administered epinephrine kit to use in the event of an anaphylactic reaction is essential. Kits, such as the EpiPen (Figure 60–4 ■, p. 1903), are easy to use and can save lives in an anaphylactic emergency (American College of Allergy, Asthma and Immunology, 2007).

Collaborative care related to hypersensitivity response is focused on:

- Identifying allergens and preventing exposure and further reactions
- Appropriate use of allergy medications to relieve symptoms
- Prompt identification and treatment for patients experiencing anaphylactic response
- Follow-up care with an allergy specialist.

Collaborative Management

Optimal care of the patient with an allergic hypersensitivity response involves a collaborative approach among the health care provider, the nurse, and the pharmacist. Allergy diagnosis and development of an effective treatment plan are done by the health care provider. Nursing care involves extensive patient education on avoiding allergy triggers and teaching about allergy symptoms that require immediate medical attention. The nurse also educates the patient on medications, monitors the effectiveness of the treatment, and ensures that the patient's medical records reflect current allergy status. The pharmacist is an important member of the team who can advise patients about medication treatment options and provide extensive patient education on drug effects.

PHARMACOLOGY Summary of Medications to Treat Allergy Symptoms

Medication Category	Action	Application/Indication	Nursing Responsibility
Antihistamines			
First generation: • Diphenhydramine (Benadryl) • Clemastine (Tavist)	First-generation histamine receptor blocks the effects of histamine at H$_1$ receptors.	Treatment of allergies to provide symptomatic relief of itching eyes, nose, throat; runny nose; and watery eyes; and to decrease swelling. Used in combination with decongestants and for cold and sinus treatment.	Causes significant sedation. Monitor patient for drowsiness. Instruct patients to avoid alcohol and other Central nervous system (CNS) depressants when taking antihistamines to avoid cumulative effects of sedation.
Second generation: • Fexofenadine (Allegra) • Cetirizine (Zyrtec) • Desloratadine (Clarinex) • Loratadine (Claritin)	Less sedating. Longer half-life.		Second-generation antihistamines are contraindicated in patient with dysrhythmias because the drug prolongs the Q-T interval. Use with caution in patients with liver and/or renal impairment because these drugs are metabolized in the liver and excreted in the kidneys.
Intranasal Corticosteroids • Fluticasone (Flonase) • Beclomethasone (Beconase)	Applied directly to nasal mucosa. Does not have systemic side effects of steroids given orally or parenterally.	First-line treatment of allergic rhinitis to decrease local inflammation, swelling of tissues, and irritation of mucosa.	Instruct patient to clear nose, shake inhaler thoroughly, and assess for broken mucous membranes that will allow medication into bloodstream causing systemic effects prior to administration. May cause burning and dryness of nasal passages. Instruct patient to use preservative-free saline spray or petroleum jelly to decrease dryness.
Decongestants and Sympathomimetics • Pseudoephedrine (Sudafed, Actifed) PO • Phenylephrine (Neo-Synephrine, Sinex) Intranasal	Stimulates alpha-adrenergic receptors in the sympathetic nervous system, causing nasal passages to constrict.	Treatment of congestion. Dries mucous membranes and decreases drainage.	Assess for nasal excoriation and bleeding. Monitor the patient for psychosocial/emotional changes; may cause agitation. Monitor vital signs; can increase heart rate, and/or blood pressure. Oral sympathomimetics are contraindicated in patients with hypertension. Monitor blood glucose in patients who are diabetic because oral dose can increase glucose levels.

Sources: Adams, M., Josephson, D., & Holland, L. (2005). *Pharmacology for nurses: A pathophysiologic approach.* Upper Saddle River, NJ: Pearson Prentice Hall; Deglin, J., & Vallerand, A. (2007). *Davis's drug guide for nurses.* Philadelphia: F. A. Davis; Wilson, B. A., Shannon, M., Shields, K., & Stang, C. (2007). *Nurse's drug guide.* Upper Saddle River, NJ: Pearson Prentice Hall.

All members of the health care team have a role in identifying patients with allergies, providing appropriate education on allergy triggers and medications for symptom relief, and preventing anaphylactic response in multiple health care settings. Providing patient education to promote self-care regarding signs and symptoms of anaphylactic reaction is essential and is addressed in Chart 60–3 (p. 1904).

Research Topics Related to the Allergic Hypersensitivity Response

Research in the area of allergic hypersensitivity responses is multifaceted. The fact that allergies affect such a large section of the population makes identification of genetic and environmental factors that contribute to the development of allergies a major priority (see the Genetic Considerations box, p. 1904).

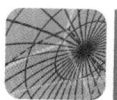

NURSING PROCESS: Patient Care Plan for Anaphylactic Response

Assessment of Airway and Gas Exchange

Subjective Data:

Are you allergic to any medications, food, or other substances?
Did you come in contact with something you are allergic to?
How much of the substance were you exposed to?
How long ago did you first notice itching or swelling or breathing changes?
Has this ever happened to you before?
Did you take anything to treat your allergies?

Objective Data:

Edema (e.g., face, eyes, tongue, extremities)
Work of breathing (e.g., increased rate, use of accessory muscles, gasping, loudness, grunt)
Lung sounds (e.g., strider, wheezes, absent breath sounds)
Oxygen saturation (e.g., <94% on room air)
Vital signs (HR > 100, RR > 22 < 8, SBP < 90, or mean arterial pressure [MAP] < 60)
Skin (e.g., red, rash, wheal and flare)

Nursing Assessment and Diagnoses	Outcomes and Evaluation Parameters	Planning and Interventions with *Rationales*
Nursing Diagnoses: *Ineffective Airway Clearance* related to bronchial and/or laryngeal spasm and edema *Alteration in Gas Exchange* related to bronchial and/or laryngeal spasm and edema	**Outcomes:** Clear airway. Adequate gas exchange. ***Evaluation Parameters:*** Patent airway. Even, unlabored respirations < 22/minute. Clear breath sounds. O₂ saturation > 94% on room air. IV access available. Emergency medications available and administered as prescribed. No alteration in level of consciousness. Alert and oriented to person, place, and time. Pulse oximetry and ABGs within normal limits.	**Interventions and *Rationales:*** Assess for airway edema, stridor, wheezes, and decreased breath sounds. *Maintaining open airway is the highest priority.* Position for comfort, high semi-Fowler's. *Promotes lung expansion and respiratory effort.* Assess respiratory rate, pattern, work of breathing, chest wall movement. *Rapid, shallow respiratory rate and increased work of breathing indicate hypoxemia from airway obstruction and the need for ventilatory support.* Auscultate lungs for wheezes, stridor, decreasing or absent breath sounds. *Stridor indicates narrowing airway. Decreased breath sounds are ominous and indicate airway obstruction. Absence of breath sounds indicates complete airway obstruction.* Report respiratory distress to the health care provider. *Medical intervention may be indicated to prevent respiratory failure.* Administer humidified oxygen (O₂) as prescribed. *Supplemental O₂ increases the alveolar gas concentration and diffusion of O₂ to the cells and tissues of the body.* Establish intravenous (IV) access with large-bore IV. *To enable administration of emergency medications and fluid.* Do not delay administration of emergency medications by non-IV route while establishing IV access. *Many emergency medications can be given SQ or IM if IV access is not available and are crucial for controlling airway edema and enabling gas exchange.* Administer medications as prescribed: subcutaneous epinephrine 1:1,000, 0.3–0.5 mL as ordered, repeat every 20–30 minutes as needed. *A potent bronchodilator and vasoconstrictor to counteract the effects of histamine.* Diphenhydramine (Benadryl) 50 mg IV or IM. *Blocks the bronchial constrictive effects of histamine released from mast cells.* Corticosteroid: Solu-Medrol 120 mg IV. *Blocks the proliferation of inflammatory mediators that increase airway obstruction.* Assess for changes in level of consciousness (agitation, confusion, delirium, stupor, and coma). *Cerebral function is very sensitive to decreases in oxygenation, indicates tissue hypoxemia.* Frequent respiratory assessment, continuous monitoring of pulse oximetry, and arterial blood gases (ABGs). *Status can deteriorate quickly. A secondary or delayed response can also result from secondary mediators of inflammation such as bradykinin several hours after the initial incident.*

(continued)

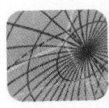

NURSING PROCESS: Patient Care Plan for Anaphylactic Response—*Continued*

Nursing Assessment and Diagnoses	Outcomes and Evaluation Parameters	Planning and Interventions with *Rationales*
	Intubation equipment available and functioning.	Prepare for possible endotracheal intubation, gather intubation supplies, and collaborate with respiratory therapy (RT) for ventilator setup. *Intubation requires a team approach; gathering and checking equipment early prevents delay in intubation.* If intubation is required, collaborate with health care provider and RT to monitor ventilator and maintain ventilator settings. *To maximize oxygenation and ventilation, support cellular oxygenation, and prevent tissue hypoxemia and ischemia.* Assess respiratory function. *To verify bilateral breath sounds post intubation.*
	Endotracheal tube appropriately placed. Equal chest wall expansion and breath sounds. ABGs within normal limits. Transfer to the appropriate level of care.	Obtain chest x-ray postintubation. *To verify appropriate placement of endotracheal tube (ETT) in trachea 1–2 cm above the carina.* Test arterial blood gases (ABG). *To evaluate oxygenation.* Patients with severe anaphylactic response requiring intubation will be cared for in the intensive care unit (ICU) setting. The focus of care is controlling airway edema, normal ABGs, and extubation as soon as is safe for the patient.

Assessment of Cardiac Output

Subjective Data:
Do you feel dizzy or weak?
Have you fainted?

Objective Data:
Blood pressure (SBP < 90, mean arterial pressure (MAP) < 60)
Heart rate > 100
Are peripheral pulses present?
Is skin color pale or red or mottled?

Nursing Assessment and Diagnoses	Outcomes and Evaluation Parameters	Planning and Interventions with *Rationales*
Nursing Diagnosis: *Risk for Decreased Cardiac Output* related to vasodilation with anaphylactic shock	**Outcome:** Tissue perfusion maintained. *Evaluation Parameters:* Blood pressure and heart rate within normal limits, mean arterial pressure (MAP) >60 mmHg. (Chapter 25 🔗 explains MAP)	**Interventions and *Rationales:*** Assess blood pressure, MAP, and heart rate frequently. Evaluate for a drop in blood pressure and increased heart rate (HR). *Indicates shock.* *Histamine and inflammatory mediators cause peripheral vasodilation, and capillary membrane permeability results in decreased volume of blood to the heart, drop in blood pressure, and decreased tissue perfusion. HR increases to try and meet cellular oxygen needs and compensate for tissue hypoxia.*
	Capillary refill < 3 seconds; skin pink, warm and dry; palpable peripheral pulses.	Assess peripheral perfusion for weak thready pulses, pale or mottled skin color, decreased skin temperature, slow capillary refill. *Indicates decreased blood flow in the capillaries, a sign of impaired tissue perfusion as shock progresses and cardiac output decreases.* Absence of circulatory failure. Report abnormal vital sign changes and assessment findings to the health care provider. *Medical intervention with IV fluids and medications may be immediately necessary to prevent circulatory failure.* Administer IV fluids. *To increase cardiac output and promote circulation and tissue perfusion.* Administer vasoactive IV medications (e.g., Levophed) as prescribed. *To vasoconstrict peripheral blood vessels, increase MAP > 60, support perfusion of vital central organs.*

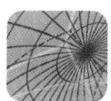

NURSING PROCESS: Patient Care Plan for Anaphylactic Response—*Continued*

Assessment of Pain and Anxiety

Subjective Data:
What is your pain level on the 1–10 scale, where a 1 is very little pain and 10 is the worst pain imaginable?
Are you feeling anxious?
Do you take pain or antianxiety medications routinely at home?
What helps when you have anxiety?
Do you have any medication allergies?
Do you have cultural or religious practices that impact your pain or anxiety?

Objective Data:
Facial grimaces with movement
Taut or anxious facial expression
Restlessness and irritability
Vital signs (HR > 100, BP > 140)

Nursing Assessment and Diagnoses	Outcomes and Evaluation Parameters	Planning and Interventions with *Rationales*
Nursing Diagnoses: *Pain* and *Anxiety* related to air hunger/hypoxia and emergency treatment procedures	**Outcomes:** Comfort level maintained. Anxiety controlled. **Evaluation Parameters:** Patient reports pain level < 3 or at acceptable level. States anxieties. Cooperative with emergency medical treatment. Premedicated for procedures as prescribed.	**Interventions and *Rationales:*** Assess pain and anxiety levels using an objective scale. *Increases consistency in quantifying pain.* Remain with patient, provide calm reassurance, and explain all treatments. *Air hunger is extremely frightening to the patient; anxiety will increase respiratory rate and oxygen demand and hinder patient's ability to cooperate with treatment.*
		Advocate for pain and sedation medications for intubation procedure if blood pressure is stable. *Endotracheal intubation is uncomfortable; anxiety increases sympathetic nervous system stimulation and oxygen demands.*
	Pain and anxiety assessed and treated while intubated.	Assess pain and anxiety while intubated using objective scales and alternative communication techniques (pointing to scale, writing board, and hand signs). *Endotracheal tube can cause pain at the back of the throat. Breathing through a small ETT can induce anxiety. Pain and anxiety will increase oxygen demands. The ETT prevents the patient from communicating verbally, but the nurse must still be able to address the patient's needs.* Administer medication as prescribed. *To maintain comfort and decrease anxiety.*

Nursing Assessment of Fluid/Volume Status

Subjective Data:
Do you feel dizzy, tired, or thirsty?

Objective Data:
Blood pressure (SBP < 90, MAP < 60 mmHg)
Heart rate > 100
Urine output < 30 mL/hr

Nursing Assessment and Diagnoses	Outcomes and Evaluation Parameters	Planning and Interventions with *Rationales*
Nursing Diagnosis: *Deficient Fluid Volume* related to anaphylactic shock	**Outcome:** Fluid volume and tissue perfusion maintained. **Evaluation Parameters:** Blood pressure normal. MAP > 60 mmHg.	**Interventions and *Rationales:*** Assess and continuously monitor blood pressure, MAP, HR, and urine output. *Anaphylactic shock results in vasodilation of blood vessels and decreased intravascular fluid volume that is clinically evident as decreased blood pressure, MAP, and urine output. Heart rate increases to compensate for decreased volume status. Patients with severe anaphylactic response and fluid volume deficits will need ICU level care.*
	Urine output = or > 30 mL/hr.	Place Foley catheter and monitor hourly urine output and fluid intake. *Decrease in blood pressure and MAP < 60 will decrease glomerular filtration rate and place patient at risk for prerenal failure. The kidneys receive 25% of the cardiac output. A urine output of less than 30 mL/hr indicates decreased perfusion to the kidneys and fluid volume deficit. Trending hourly fluid volume intake and output is essential with fluid resuscitation therapy.* Administer IV fluids as prescribed. *To increase intravascular volume and tissue perfusion.* Report decreased blood pressure, MAP, and urine output to the health care provider. *Medical intervention may be indicated to correct fluid volume deficit.*

(continued)

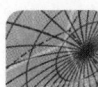

NURSING PROCESS: Patient Care Plan for Anaphylactic Response—*Continued*

Assessment of Potential Allergy Response

Subjective Data:

Do you have any allergies to medication, food, plants, animals, or other materials (such as latex)?

Do you have any history of previous allergy reactions such as rash, itching, tingling, or swelling in your mouth, or breathing difficulties?

Have you undergone allergy testing?

Does anyone in your family have allergies?

Do you take any allergy medications?

Objective Data:

Gather baseline data on:

Airway

Vital signs

Rash

Itching

Edema

Lung sounds

Nursing Assessment and Diagnoses	Outcomes and Evaluation Parameters	Planning and Interventions with *Rationales*
Nursing Diagnosis: *Risk for Injury* related to allergy hypersensitivity response	**Outcome:** Identification of allergy triggers and prevention of anaphylactic response. ***Evaluation Parameters:*** Allergies identified in patient's medical record.	**Interventions and *Rationales:*** Obtain a thorough patient and family allergy history at the time of admission and prior to administering new medications to the patient. *To prevent administering a medication or treatment, or using equipment to which the patient has an allergy. Safe nursing practice requires allergy assessment prior to medication administration.*
	Allergy triggers communicated to health care team and avoided.	Document patient allergies and inform other members of the health care team (health care provider, pharmacy, nursing staff). *To facilitate communication and prevent prescribing of medication or treatments or use of equipment to which the patient is allergic.* Follow agency protocol for placing allergy alerts in medical record, electronic patient database, the nursing Kardex (Rand), and on the patient's arm band. *To alert members of the health care team to the patient's allergies.*
	No allergy hypersensitivity reactions.	Assess for symptoms of hypersensitivity reaction when administering any medications to patient. *A history of allergy response increases the risk of future hypersensitivity responses.*

Assessment of the Patient's and Family's Education Needs Regarding Allergy Response

Subjective Data:

What causes your allergy symptoms?

How do you avoid triggering your allergies?

What can you do to alert health care providers about your allergies?

What should you carry with you if you have experienced an anaphylactic reaction?

Objective Data:

Verbalizes education needs

Identifies mode of receiving educational material

Participates in education discussion

Nursing Assessment and Diagnoses	Outcomes and Evaluation Parameters	Planning and Interventions with *Rationales*
Nursing Diagnosis: *Deficient Knowledge* regarding allergies and prevention of anaphylactic response	**Outcome:** Patient avoids allergy trigger and has no further anaphylactic reactions. ***Evaluation Parameters:*** Verbalizes understanding of allergy signs and symptoms, anaphylactic allergen triggers.	**Interventions and *Rationales:*** Assess the patient's and family's learning needs, readiness to learn, and preferred method of education (verbal, written, audiovisual). *To present information at a time and in a manner the patient and family can understand. Hypersensitivity reactions have a genetic link; therefore, families must be informed about potential hypersensitivity and how to prevent them.*
	Consistently follows plan to avoid allergy triggers.	Provide information on allergy management self-care as presented in Chart 60–3 (p. 1904), and assist the patient and family in developing a plan to eliminate exposure to the triggering allergen and decrease symptoms and progression of allergy sensitivity. *To promote self-care and help the patient and family eliminate allergy triggers.*
	Identifies symptoms of allergy response.	Instruct patient to monitor response to medications, foods, and insect stings by self-assessing for mouth/pallet itching, swelling, rash, itching of skin or eyes. *To identify symptoms of allergy response.*

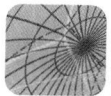

NURSING PROCESS: Patient Care Plan for Anaphylactic Response—*Continued*

Nursing Assessment and Diagnoses	Outcomes and Evaluation Parameters	Planning and Interventions with *Rationales*
	Seeks appropriate medical attention for allergy symptoms. Informs health care providers of allergy status.	Instruct patient to seek immediate medical attention for airway swelling or shortness of breath with exposure to triggering allergen. *Promotes seeking early medical treatment of potential life-threatening anaphylactic response.* Instruct patient to inform future health care providers of allergy and anaphylactic response. *Prevents future exposure to allergen and anaphylactic response.*
	Purchases and wears medical alert tag.	Instruct patient to purchase and wear a medic alert bracelet that lists the triggering allergen and history of anaphylactic response. *Alerts health care providers to allergen and anaphylactic response, especially in an emergency situation when patient may not be able to speak for herself.*
	Carries epinephrine self-medication emergency syringe.	If anaphylactic triggering allergen is an insect, plant, or food, instruct the patient to carry emergency epinephrine at all times. *To self-administer epinephrine for an anaphylactic reaction.*
	Keeps appointments and completes allergy testing if indicated.	Encourage follow-up appointments with primary care health care provider to determine need to see allergist and undergo IgE allergen-specific diagnostic testing. *To determine triggering allergens so that exposure to them can be eliminated.*

Sources: Adams, M., Josephson, D., & Holland, L. (2008). *Pharmacology for nurses: A pathophysiologic approach.* (2nd ed.) Upper Saddle River, NJ: Pearson Prentice Hall; American College of Allergy, Asthma and Immunology. (2007). *Be S.A.F.E.: Managing allergic emergencies.* Retrieved February 19, 2007, from http://www.acaai.org/public; Carpenito-Moyet, L. (2008). *Nursing care plans and documentation* (5th ed.). Philadelphia: Lippincott Williams & Wilkins.

A greater understanding of the association between allergies and the development of other pulmonary diseases also is a major priority. Additional areas of current medical and nursing research related to allergies are presented in the Research Opportunities and Clinical Impact box (p. 1905).

■ Autoimmune Hypersensitivity Response

The ability to differentiate self-antigens from foreign antigens is referred to as *immune tolerance*. Recognition of self-antigens is vital for normal immune function because it prevents the immune system from destroying the host. When the immune system fails to recognize self-antigens an autoimmune response occurs. This is the basis for **autoimmune diseases,** which can affect any tissue in the body. The triggering mechanisms for a breakdown of tolerance are varied among autoimmune diseases. In most instances, the exact mechanism that stimulates an autoimmune response is unknown, although several theories have been supported by research and multiple others are currently being investigated (Rote, 2006).

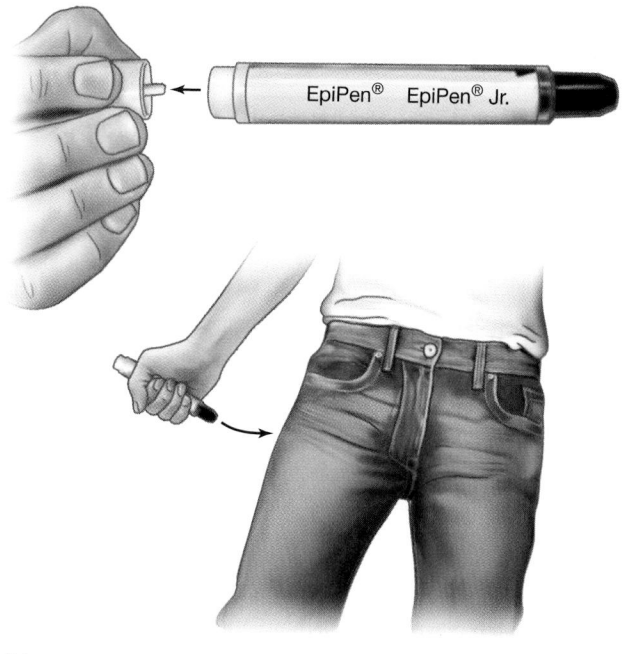

(b)

FIGURE 60–4 ■ EpiPen.

CHART 60-3 Self-Care Allergy Management

Allergens and Education Goal for Self-Care	Actions for Self-Care
Allergen: Pollen and mold *Goal:* Minimize exposure to pollens and molds.	• Remain inside on days when pollen counts are high. • Wear a mask when during high-exposure times (windy days, when grass is being cut). • Avoid contact with freshly cut grass, dry leaves, and weeds. • Avoid damp, moist structures like basements. • Clean showers and tubs several times a week. • Avoid sprays and perfumes.
Allergen: Dust mites and animal dander *Goals:* Reduce dust in the home, school, and work environment. Eliminate animal dander from home environment.	• Replace window coverings with pull shades. • Use hypoallergenic mattress and pillow. • Replace carpet with wood, tile, or linoleum. • Wash floor, dust, and vacuum several times a week. • Wear a mask when cleaning. • Minimize upholstered furniture, throw pillows/rugs, and tufted bedspreads. • Change air filter frequently on air conditioning/heating system. • Choose a pet that does not have fur or feathers such as fish or reptile.
Allergen: Insect stings *Goal:* Minimize exposure to insect venom.	• Quickly leave an area where bees, wasps, or yellow jackets are present. • Carefully check grass areas before sitting to avoid ants or other insects. • Carry an EpiPen when picnicking, hiking, or camping.
Allergen: Foods *Goal:* Eliminate foods from diet that may cause allergy symptoms.	• Identify specific foods to avoid by keeping an allergy food journal noting triggering foods and allergy symptoms. • Develop a list of foods to avoid and share this with anyone who cooks in the household. • Read labels when buying food and avoid allergy-triggering substances. • Ask questions regarding ingredients in food when eating out to avoid allergy triggers.
Allergen: Medication *Goal:* Avoid allergy-triggering medications.	• Make of list of medication allergies and inform any health care providers of allergies. • Wear a medical alert tag for history of anaphylactic medication response. • Review over the counter (OTC) medications with pharmacists to check for potential allergy.

Sources: American Academy of Allergy, Asthma and Immunology. (2006). *Why is the incidence of allergy increasing?* Retrieved February 23, 2007, from https://www.aaaai.org/aadmc/inthenews/wypr/2006archive/increasing_allergies.html; American College of Allergy, Asthma and Immunology. (2007). *Be S.A.F.E.: Managing allergic emergencies.* Retrieved February 19, 2007, from http://www.acaai.org/public.

GENETIC CONSIDERATIONS for the Allergic Hypersensitivity Response

The National Heart, Lung, and Blood Institute (NHLBI) of the National Institutes of Health is currently working on a study to examine the role of genetic factors in the development of lung disease including asthma. A large portion of the money spent on treating asthma is associated with the treatment of allergic asthma. The NHLBI study is working to define the distribution of abnormal genes seen in a number of lung diseases. The hope is that greater knowledge of genetic components of lung disease will lead to new clinical treatments. A second outcome for this study is a better understanding of the development of lung diseases such as allergic asthma (Steinke, Borish, & Rosenwasser, 2003).

Epidemiology and Etiology

Approximately 5% of the U.S. population is affected by autoimmune disorders (American Academy of Allergy, Asthma and Immunology, 2006). A genetic predisposition to autoimmune disease is supported by the association of various autoimmune abnormalities within family groups. The peak time of development of autoimmune disease is ages 15 to 45. Sex hormones appear to have some relationship to the frequency and manifestation of the autoimmune disease systemic lupus erythematosus because it occurs 10 times more frequently in women than men (Porth & Sweeney, 2007).

Pathophysiology of Autoimmune Diseases

Normally, immunologic tolerance is formed in humans during embryonic development. During this developmental period, some lymphocytes can be created that are not able to differentiate between self-antigens and non–self-antigens, referred to as autoreactive lymphocytes. To attain immune tolerance, the immune system must suppress or eliminate these autoreactive lymphocytes.

The loss of immune tolerance is the basis for all autoimmune diseases. Multiple mechanisms may be involved in the loss of tolerance, but in most instances the exact process is unknown. Research has centered on the following theories: (1) exposure to a previously sequestered antigen, (2) develop-

RESEARCH OPPORTUNITIES AND CLINICAL IMPACT RELATED TO THE ALLERGY HYPERSENSITIVITY RESPONSE

Research Area	Clinical Impact
Pursue development of new classes of allergy medication.	Decrease IgE stimulation and the inflammatory response; symptom control and improved functional ability.
Identify genetic factors associated with development of allergies.	Development of new therapies that more specifically target the allergy trigger and overproduction of IgE.
Identify environmental factors associated with development of allergies.	Development of new therapies that more specifically target the allergy trigger and overproduction of IgE.
Identify genetic and environmental links between allergies and the development of asthma.	Control of IgE stimulation to prevent development of asthma.
Determine pharmacologic action of herbal and complementary therapy in the treatment of allergy.	Identifying the effective or harmful action of herbal medications in treatment of allergy response to promote new treatments and deter use of unproven therapies.

ment of a neoantigen, (3) complications of an infectious disease, (4) emergence of a forbidden clone, and (5) alteration of a suppressor T cell (DeFranco, Locksley, & Robertson, 2007). Current research indicates that development of autoimmune disease is probably multifactorial and involves a combination of the multiple mechanisms described below, as well as the effect of an original insult, environmental influences, and genetic factors (Embry, 2004; Gomez-Peurta et al., 2005; Kuwabara, 2004). Chapter 59 ⊕ provides a discussion about immune assessment.

Sequestered Antigens

Sequestered antigens are normal self-antigens found in cells that have not come in contact with the immunologic tissue during fetal development. Therefore, the immune system does not recognize it as a self-antigen. These are tissues that are not drained by the lymphatic system and therefore do not usually come in contact with immunologic cells. Examples of these include receptors on the cornea of the eye and the testicles. These are referred to as immunologic privileged sites. Although these tissues lack lymphatic tissues, they are vascular. Therefore, if trauma occurs immunologic cells will be delivered to the site. This can initiate an autoimmune response because the immune system has not recognized these antigens by previous exposure (Porth & Sweeney, 2007).

Neoantigens

Neoantigens are created by the developing fetal immune system while it is in the process of eliminating autoreactive lymphocytes. During the process of eliminating these autoreactive lymphocytes, pieces of the lymph receptors may not be destroyed. These small bits of immune garbage are neoantigens and they can hide in lymph tissues. They may attach at a later time to receptors on normal cells, triggering an autoimmune response (DeFranco et al., 2007).

Complications of Infectious Disease: Molecular Mimicry

When a foreign antigen invades the body and is destroyed by the immune system, small pieces of the cell wall of the bacterial or viral invader can remain in the circulation. If these foreign antigen proteins attach to a normal cell, the complex makes the host cell look like the cell of the foreign antigen and this triggers the autoimmune response. Group A streptococcus bacteria are the most commonly studied bacteria that can initiate this response. An example of this is the streptococcal bacteria that attach to the cells of heart valves and stimulate the immune system to attack and destroy the heart valve tissue (Rote, 2006). Chapter 41 ⊕ discusses the impact of this process on heart valve function.

Forbidden Clone

A clone is a second cell produced by replication of a cell. A *forbidden clone* is a mutant cell that is a type of autoreactive lymphocyte that should be eliminated. The theory about forbidden clones revolves around the concept that during normal embryonic development the original autoreactive lymphocyte is eliminated by the embryo's immune system, but a copy (clone) remains hidden (usually in lymphoid tissue). These cells can emerge at a later date and attach to self-antigens, thereby triggering an autoimmune response and destroying normal self-cells. This is an important area of research, because the exact triggering mechanisms of many autoimmune diseases, such as systemic lupus erythematosus or rheumatoid arthritis, are unknown (DeFranco et al., 2007).

Suppressor Cell Dysfunction

A major function of suppressor T cells is to control inappropriate immune responses. There are many different lines of suppressor T cells. If a single group of these T cells is dysfunctional, a tissue-specific autoimmune response can occur. If several lines of suppressor T cells are dysfunctional, generalized autoimmune disease can occur. An example of this is systemic lupus erythematosus (SLE). It is thought that T cell dysfunction is partly responsible for the large variety of autoantibodies seen in SLE because the T cells do not suppress the production of antibodies created by B cells against normal cells (DeFranco et al., 2007).

Superantigens

Normally, antigens ingested by macrophages are "presented" to T-helper cells to initiate the stimulation of B cells to make antibodies to that antigen. Chapter 59 ⊕ discusses this concept in detail. Usually only a small number of T-helper cells are activated by one antigen. Some gram-positive bacteria such as Staphylococcus and Streptococcus can make chemicals called exotoxins that are capable of circumventing the normal antigen presentation process. Referred to as superantigens these exotoxins are capable of activating far greater numbers of T-helper cells. Toxic shock syndrome related to staphylococcus infection is one example of a superantigen-mediated disease (Porth & Sweeney, 2007). Chapter 49 includes an in-depth discussion of toxic shock syndrome.

Original Insult

The actual mechanism of some autoimmune responses is known to be the result of exposure to an identifiable insult, referred to an "original insult." For example, the allergy or type I hypersensitivity response is stimulated by the presence of a foreign protein such as pollen. The administration of certain drugs such as quinidine and methyldopa has been associated with an autoimmune lupus-like syndrome in susceptible elderly patients that dissipates when the medication is stopped (Rizzo & Gunta, 2007). In many autoimmune diseases, the original insult is not traceable. Research is examining areas such as viral infections, in which aspects of the viral particle remain on the plasma membrane of cells or are introduced permanently into the host's DNA (DeFranco et al., 2007).

Specific genetic markers may also play a role in autoimmune disease, as discussed in the Genetic Considerations for Autoimmune Disease box.

Clinical Manifestations

Autoimmune disorders can affect any tissue in the body, and are manifested in a variety of clinical symptoms depending on the system that is the target. The initiation of an autoimmune disorder is commonly associated with the onset of another illness or profound physical or psychological stressor, such as severe flu, pregnancy, or death of a significant other. It also is significant to note that once individuals have developed one autoimmune disorder, they are at increased risk for developing manifestations of other autoimmune diseases (Rote, 2006). Chart 60–4 lists the most common autoimmune disorders, target antigens, and symptoms.

Medical Management

Medical management involves determining the diagnosis, medication treatment plan, and symptom management for disease complications. The difficulty in differentiating autoimmune diseases is that many of them have multiple self-antigens and re-

---

GENETIC CONSIDERATIONS for Autoimmune Disease

Research indicates that genetic factors play a major part in autoimmune disease. Specific genetic markers have been associated with some autoimmune diseases, such as myasthenia gravis and SLE. Genetic markers, called **human leukocyte antigens (HLAs),** can be tested within families to determine if the individual tested is at risk for developing an autoimmune disease (Rizzo & Gunta, 2007). It is believed that an original insult in combination with genetic factors is responsible for stimulation of autoimmune response. Future research in this area is focusing on genome sequences that could contribute to the later development of autoimmune disease.

---

quire a significant number of tests prior to making a diagnosis with confidence.

Laboratory and Diagnostic Procedures

The focus of the diagnostic workup is serum tests. These tests include autoantibody testing, complement levels, and protein electrophoresis. **Autoantibody tests** evaluate the level of autoantibodies in the blood to specific self-antigens. One of the primary tests is the antinuclear antibody (ANA). This is a monoclonal antibody (see Chapter 59) that attaches to **autoantibodies** that are made in response to self-antigens from the nucleus. A positive ANA test indicates that autoantibodies to nuclear proteins are present and increases the likelihood of a diagnosis of autoimmune disease. For example, patients with SLE often have high levels of ANA and high levels of anti-DNA autoantibodies. A differential diagnosis of an autoimmune disease is usually based on cumulative evidence from several test results (see the Diagnostic Tests for Autoimmune Disease box, p. 1908) (Rote, 2006).

Drug Therapy

The wide variety of autoimmune disorders presents a challenge in drug therapy. The goals of drug therapy are to suppress the immune system in general and control symptoms related to specific self-antigens if possible. One of the mainstays of therapy is the use of **corticosteroids,** a class of drugs that decrease the inflammatory response and suppress immune activity by controlling T-cell response. As previously noted, T cells are responsible for the regulation of the immune system and stimulating B cells to produce antibodies. Decreasing T-cell stimulation of B cells and subsequent antibody production is essential to the control of autoimmune disease. Additional drugs such as cyclophosphamide (Cytoxan, a chemotherapy drug) are also used in autoimmune diseases such as SLE to control or moderate symptoms and decrease autoantibody activity. Cyclophosphamide acts to decrease antibody production by suppression of bone marrow activity, specifically B- and T-cell suppression (Adams, Josephson, & Holland, 2005). Other treatments to decrease autoantibody production include the use of monoclonal antibodies (Chapter 59) and **plasmapheresis,** which is discussed in Chart 60–5 (p. 1909).

Systemic Lupus Erythematosus

Systemic lupus erythematosus (SLE) is an example of a systemic type III hypersensitivity autoimmune disease characterized by damage to joints and soft organs as a result of the effects of autoantibodies and antibody–antigen activity (immune complex responses). Patients with SLE have symptoms as varied as joint pain, fever, malaise, recurrent infections, renal failure, and endocarditis with valve dysfunction. Cardiac valve disease is discussed in Chapter 41 . Renal failure is discussed in Chapter 47 .

Epidemiology and Etiology

The cause of SLE is unknown, but research indicates that the development of autoantibodies most likely results from a combination of factors including genetics, hormonal influences, immune abnormalities, and environmental factors (Rote, 2006). A genetic predisposition is clearly involved in that certain families show a larger number of SLE members than the population at large and there is evidence of SLE development in identical twins (Anaya, Tobon, Vega, & Castiblanco, 2006). It is possible that as many as

CHART 60–4 Autoimmune Disorders by Body System

Disease/System	Probable Antigen	Organ or Tissue	Symptoms
Blood			
Immune thrombocytopenic purpura	Platelet surface	Blood	Bruising, purpura, bleeding
Antiphospholipid antibody syndrome	Platelet membrane phospholipids	Blood	Bleeding, purpura, bruising
Respiratory System			
Goodpasture's syndrome	Septal membrane of alveoli (basement membrane)	Lungs, alveoli	Shortness of breath, respiratory failure, decreased gas exchange
Renal System			
Immune complex glomerulonephritis	Various immune complexes	Glomeruli, kidney	Acute renal failure, inflammation, fever, pain
Goodpasture's disease	Glomeruli basement membrane	Glomeruli, kidney	Decreased renal function, anuria, oliguria, pain
Connective Tissue/Systemic Diseases			
Systemic lupus erythematosus	Antigens from DNA, organelles, cytoplasm, and possible extracellular sites	Joints, muscle, skin, kidney, heart, lung	Rash, joint pain, arthralgias, fatigue, fever, impaired renal function, increased risk of infection, heart valve disease
Rheumatoid arthritis	Immunoglobulin G, collagen	Joints	Pain and swelling in joints
Scleroderma	Nuclear antigens, immunoglobulin G	Multiple organs, including skin, joints	Hard, shiny painful skin, immobile masklike face
Endocrine System			
Graves' disease (hyperthyroidism)	TSH receptors on membrane of thyroid cells	Thyroid, metabolic	Myxedema, exophthalmos, increased metabolic rate
Insulin-dependent diabetes	Islet cells, insulin, receptors on pancreatic cells	Pancreas, metabolic	Hyperglycemia, polyuria, thirst, weight loss, ketosis
Addison's disease	Surface antigen on steroid producing cells in adrenal gland	Adrenal gland	Hypotension, fatigue
Primary myxedema	Microsomes	Thyroid	Orbital and facial edema, fatigue

Sources: DeFranco, A. L., Locksley, R., & Robertson, M. (2007). *Immunity: The immune response in infectious and inflammatory disease.* Sunderland, MA: Sinauer Associates; Rote, N. (2006). Immunity. In K. L. McCance & S. E. Huether (Eds.), *Pathophysiology: The biological basis for disease in adults and children* (5th ed., pp. 168–227). St. Louis: Mosby; Sommer, C. (2007). The immune response. In C. M. Porth (Ed.), *Essentials of pathophysiology* (pp. 247–268). St. Louis: Lippincott Williams & Wilkins.

four genes are involved in SLE development (Rizzo & Gunta, 2007). The disease is known to affect women more often than men and researchers are exploring the role of hormones in expression of SLE (National Institute of Arthritis and Musculoskeletal and Skin Diseases [NIAMSD], 2003) because the greatest incidence of the disease occurs in women ages 15 to 45.

Cultural factors may also play a role in SLE development because it occurs more frequently in African American, Hispanics, and Caucasians. Additionally, researchers have found that Hispanics and African Americans have a higher incidence of kidney damage and death rates when compared to Caucasians (NIAMSD, 2003).

Furthermore, environmental factors that may act as triggers for autoantibody production include ultraviolet light from the sun as well as interior lights, thermal burns, drugs, and possibly some viral triggers (Rizzo & Gunta, 2007; Medem, 2003). It has also been shown that drug-induced SLE syndrome can occur with exposure to certain medications such as procainamide, hydralazine, isoniazid, quinidine, methyldopa, and phenytoin (NIAMSD, 2003).

Pathophysiology

As mentioned earlier, the development of SLE is characterized by the formation of autoantibodies or antigen–antibody complexes that can damage a variety of tissues by identifying them as foreign cells and attempting to destroy them. This results from hyperactivity of B cells that are polyclonal and produce different types of autoantibodies (Rizzo & Gunta, 2007). Several autoantibodies have been identified in SLE including ANAs, such as anti-DNA, and antibodies against surface antigens on RBCs and platelets. Autoantibodies produced against these blood cells cause their destruction and lead to the clinical conditions of anemia and thrombocytopenia.

Clinical Manifestations

SLE may present with a variety of symptoms that do not point to a specific, easily identified disease process. This is what makes diagnosis of SLE very time consuming and challenging This difficulty in diagnosis is related to the potential number of autoantibodies and the wide range of organs that can be affected.

DIAGNOSTIC TESTS for Autoimmune Disease

Autoimmune Test	Expected Abnormality	Rationale for Abnormality
IgG levels	Measures levels of IgG in the blood. IgG is elevated in autoimmune diseases.	IgG levels are elevated in autoimmune diseases such as rheumatoid arthritis (RA) and Systemic Lupus Erythematosus (SLE). Individuals with autoimmune disease generally produce too many IgGs that can form antibody complexes with host cells and stimulate destruction of the host's cells.
Anti-IgG levels	Measures level of autoantibodies to IgG. Elevated levels of anti-IgG indicate the immune system is making antibodies to self proteins.	Patients with autoimmune disease such as RA often have elevated levels of anti-IgG antibodies. The immune system is responding to the rheumatoid factor and IgG complexes.
Antinuclear antibody (ANA)	Measures level of autoantibody to protein found in the cell nucleus. Elevated levels of ANA and specific patterns of staining indicate the body is making antibodies to self proteins. Individuals with negative tests do not have SLE or RA.	Patients capable of making antibodies to self proteins in elevated quantities are exhibiting signs of autoimmune disease.
Anti-DNA antibody (Tests for anti–double-strand DNA or anti–single-strand DNA)	Measures level of autoantibody to patient's own DNA. This is an enzyme-linked immunosorbent assay (ELISA)-type test. Positive tests indicate an individual is making IgG antibodies to the individual's own DNA. Individuals with negative tests do not have SLE or RA.	Patients with SLE and other collagen-associated autoimmune diseases make IgG antibodies that attack a variety of host or self proteins or markers.
Antiphospholipid antibody (Actually a group of antibodies including anticardiolipin antibodies)	Measure level of autoantibody to part of the cell wall. Platelet malfunction. Increased level of antiphospholipid antibodies indicates a risk of increased clotting. Increased levels are also see in SLE, RA, and antiphospholipid syndrome.	Patients with SLE, RA, and antiphospholipid syndrome have increased levels of the antiphospholipid antibody. The antibodies attach to phospholipids (one example is the IIB) on the platelet surface and stimulate clotting activity at the platelet level. Patients with SLE are at increased risk of clotting abnormalities such as thromboembolism.
Rheumatoid factor	Measures an autoantibody to the FC portion of IgG. These antibodies bind to synovial tissue and with complement stimulate phagocytosis of joint and bone tissue. High levels are found in patients with RA and Sjögren's syndrome.	Patients with autoimmune diseases such as RA, sarcoidosis, syphilis, and SLE, as well as viral infections, liver disease, and other chronic inflammatory diseases, all stimulate a positive test.
IgE antibodies (RAST)	A group of six respiratory and food allergies that promoted immediate allergic responses. RAST is radioallergosorbent. IgE in serum attaches to test antigens. Positive is 400% greater than normal IgE.	Patients with high IgE levels usually exhibit indications of allergic response. The individual capable of attaching IgE to test antigens will exhibit symptoms of allergy to triggers.
Erythrocyte sedimentation rate (ESR or sed rate)	Measures amount of settling of RBCs over 1 hour. Often first indicator of an acute inflammatory process or chronic inflammatory diseases.	Autoimmune diseases such as RA, inflammatory diseases, infections, carcinomas, and SLE all have increased sed rates. Chronic inflammation occurs in autoimmune disease when the host's immune system consumes or attacks cells that it views as non-self.
Complement 4 (C4) level	Level of C4 is decreased in patients with SLE and inborn C4 deficiency. Complement is a necessary part of a competent immune system.	Inborn C4 deficiency, SLE. Patients with inborn C4 deficiency do not make enough C4. In SLE and RA, patients make C4, but it is consumed in the phagocytic process of the immune system attacking self-antigens.
Total hemolytic complement (CH50)	CH50 is decreased in autoimmune diseases and increased in some carcinomas and acute inflammatory responses.	Patients with SLE, serum sickness, and severe RA are able to make adequate complement, but it is consumed in the autoimmune process of the host immune system inappropriately phagocytizing self cells such as collagen in joints and renal tubules.

DIAGNOSTIC TESTS for Autoimmune Disease—*Continued*

Autoimmune Test	Expected Abnormality	Rationale for Abnormality
Radioimmunoassay (ELISA/EIA for specific enzyme-linked diseases)	Positive results indicate autoimmune disease and are usually validated with second test.	ELISA tests allow labs to look for specific antibodies in autoimmune diseases such as Graves', Addison's, and HIV. A positive exam is repeated. A second positive triggers the next more sensitive test, i.e., Western blot for HIV.

Sources: Kee, J. L. (2005). *Laboratory and diagnostic tests with nursing implications* (7th ed.). Upper Saddle River, NJ: Pearson Prentice Hall; National Institute of Arthritis and Musculoskeletal and Skin Diseases. (2006). *Lupus: A patient care guide for nurses and other professionals* (3rd ed.). Retrieved September 2, 2008, from http://www.niams.nih.gov/hi/topics/lupus/lupusguide/chp7.htm; Van Leeuwen, A., Kranpitz, T., & Smith, L. (2006). *Laboratory and diagnostic tests with nursing implications* (2nd ed.). Philadelphia: F. A. Davis.

CHART 60–5   Plasmapheresis: A Treatment for Autoimmune Disease

Plasmapheresis refers to the technique of removing only the plasma portion of the blood. Plasmapheresis is usually a voluntary blood product donation process. The blood donor has her blood circulated through a machine that removes plasma and returns normal saline and RBCs back to the donor. Donated plasma contains clotting factors that can be used to help patients who have massive hemorrhage and are unable to clot their own blood effectively. The plasma also contains antibodies that are withdrawn during the pheresis process. Hence, plasmapheresis can also be used as a treatment in a number of autoimmune diseases. Plasmapheresis withdraws the immunoglobulins, immune complexes, and autoantibodies that are present in plasma, thereby decreasing the immune factors stimulating the autoimmune response.

Myasthenia gravis is an example of an autoimmune disease that can be treated with plasmapheresis. The process of filtering off the plasma also filters out large numbers of autoantibodies that are believed to be stimulating the myasthenia crisis. Plasmapheresis is usually only used to treat myasthenia crisis. Drug therapy remains the mainstay of therapy for patients not in crisis.

Plasmapheresis has also been indicated for patients with Guillain-Barré syndrome and rapidly progressing acute glomerulonephritis.

Nursing care of the patient receiving therapeutic plasma exchange or plasmapheresis includes patient education about the process of pheresis itself and the rationale that is applicable for treatment of the patient's specific disease process. The patient has a needle and catheter inserted into a vein and the blood is drawn from the vein and saline and red cells returned through the same catheter. Potential complications include hematoma at the needle insertion site, dizziness following donation, nausea, and hypotension. Specially trained nurses at major blood centers operate the pheresis machines and complete the treatment as ordered by the health care provider.

Sources: Porth, C., & Sweeney, K. (2007). Alterations in immune response. In C. M. Porth (Ed.), *Essentials of pathophysiology* (pp. 293–319). St. Louis: Lippincott Williams & Wilkins.

Laboratory tests to diagnose SLE are described in the Diagnostic Tests for Systemic Lupus Erythematosus box (p. 1910).

Symptoms often seen early in the disease include swollen joints, fatigue, unexplained fever, red rash (commonly a "butterfly" shape over the cheeks), arthritis, arthralgias, unexplained hair loss, photosensitivity, swollen lymph nodes, and edema in the legs or around the eyes. As the disease progresses, SLE can affect several organ systems. Although many patients have symptoms only in joints or skin, as many as 40% will have renal symptoms. Patients with SLE may develop nephritis or inflammation of the kidneys. The effect of this inflammation may temporarily or permanently reduce the ability of the kidney to filter nitrogenous wastes such as blood urea nitrogen and creatinine. Some patients with SLE will require short- or long-term hemodialysis related to the damage to their kidneys (Rote, 2006). Chapter 47 discusses hemodialysis.

Other organ systems that can become involved include the blood, blood vessels, lungs, or the neurological system. Anemia, leukopenia, and thrombocytopenia have all been noted in patients with SLE. These blood disorders are discussed in Chapter 63. Vasculitis and inflammation of blood vessels also occur in SLE. Swelling in blood vessels may affect the ability of blood to circulate and place the patient at risk for developing blood clots. Development of endocarditis, myocarditis, or pericarditis is also a potential risk for SLE patients. Valves may be damaged or destroyed in the patient with endocarditis. Patients with valve damage may present with chest pain or shortness of breath (Chapter 41).

Neurological manifestations of SLE include headache, memory loss, visual changes, changes in behavior, and stroke. The difficulty of evaluating neurological symptoms may be related to some of the side effects of medications used to treat the disease. Additionally, the stress of living with a complex disease such as SLE may add to some neurological symptoms (NIAMSD, 2003).

Medical Management

There is no cure for SLE; however, many patients have fewer exacerbations with adequate drug therapy. The key to therapy is reducing inflammation and immune response. Primary therapy for SLE is pharmacologic with the mainstay of therapy being corticosteroids. Drugs such as prednisone, dexamethasone, methylprednisolone, and hydrocortisone have all been used to treat SLE. Side effects have often interfered with patient compliance. Short-term side effects of corticosteroids include weight gain, increased appetite, edema, and emotional liability.

Patients with only joint pain and arthritis pain may be treated successfully with nonsteroidal anti-inflammatory drugs (NSAIDs) such as ibuprofen, naproxen, indomethacin, sulindac, piroxicam, and oxaprozin. These drugs reduce the pain, swelling, and immobility of joint arthralgias by blocking various chemicals of inflammation. To treat neurological symptoms, immunosuppressive drugs may be used. Drugs such as cyclophosphamide (Cytoxan) or azathioprine (Imuran) have been

DIAGNOSTIC TESTS for Systemic Lupus Erythematosus

Test	Expected Abnormality	Rationale for Abnormality
Antinuclear antibody (ANA) (a primary test for SLE)	Increased level of autoantibodies, usually IgG. Increased ANA in the serum indicates autoimmune activity. Specific staining patterns help differentiate SLE from other collagen diseases such as RA.	Autoantibodies to nuclear proteins increase because patients with SLE produce IgGs to a variety of self-antigens, including nuclear proteins. The immune system stimulates B cells to make antibodies to self proteins.
Anti-DNA antibody	Increased level of autoantibodies to patient's own DNA indicates a positive test.	The patient produces increased autoantibodies to own DNA because the T and B cells in patients with SLE are reacting to antigens that are normally viewed as self, in this case DNA.
Erythrocyte sedimentation rate (ESR or sed rate)	Elevated sed rate can indicate chronic inflammation. Elevated sed rate is often the first test done when patients are being worked up for general symptoms that could indicate autoimmune disease.	Sed rate is elevated in SLE because immune complexes continually stimulate the immune system, especially macrophages, to consume the IgG and the cell to which it is attached. This further stimulates inflammation.
Complement levels	Decreased due to presence of immune complexes that have used up complement factors.	Part of inflammation process related to abnormal antibody production.
Biopsy of skin and/or kidney	Changes in the kidney tissue.	Antibodies adversely affect the tissue.
Complete blood count (CBC)*	Decreased platelets, increased risk of bleeding and/or leukopenia.	Decreased platelets occur because immunoglobulins can attach to the antigens on the surface of the platelet and stimulate phagocytosis and activation of complement. Platelets can decrease in patients with SLE to less than 100,000 /mm^3 leading to development of bleeding abnormalities such as prolonged clotting time, purpura, petechiae, or oozing from invasive line insertion sites.
Chemistry panel (renal panel)*	Increased creatinine levels.	Increased creatinine indicating renal injury can occur in SLE because IgG attaches to renal cell surfaces, creating an immune complex that is then attacked by macrophages. This leads to decreased renal function at the tubular and cellular level and is evidenced by increasing creatinine levels.
Urinalysis*	The presence of protein and/or sodium in urine may indicate renal impairment.	Damage to the kidneys occurs with SLE when IgG attaches to renal tubule cells and this immune complex stimulates macrophages to phagocytize the renal cells leading to abnormal glomerular basement membrane function and the inability of the glomeruli to appropriately reabsorb sodium and proteins. Decreased renal function can eventually lead to renal failure, a major complication of SLE.

*This test is also a common laboratory abnormality seen in patients with complications related to SLE.

Sources: Kee, J. L. (2005). Laboratory and diagnostic tests with nursing implications (7th ed.). Upper Saddle River, NJ: Pearson Prentice Hall; National Institute of Arthritis and Musculoskeletal and Skin Diseases. (2006). Lupus: A patient care guide for nurses and other professionals (3rd ed.). Retrieved September 2, 2008, from http://www.niams.nih.gov/hi/topics/lupus/lupusguide/chp7.htm; Van Leeuwen, A., Kranpitz, T., & Smith, L. (2006). Laboratory and diagnostic tests with nursing implications (2nd ed.). Philadelphia: F. A. Davis.

used to decrease the action of some immune cells and block the growth of immune cells.

Another class of drugs used to treat SLE is antimalarial drugs. Hydroxychloroquine (Plaquenil), chloroquine (Aralen), and quinacrine (Atabrine) are all antimalarial drugs that have been effective in treating SLE. The exact mechanism of action for these drugs in SLE is unknown and research has centered on the effect of these drugs on suppressing immune function (DeFranco et al., 2007). When taken continuously, antimalarial drugs have been helpful in preventing "flares" or exacerbations of SLE.

Nursing Management

Nursing care of the patient with autoimmune disease focuses on educating patients and families regarding the disease process and medications, as well as providing interventions to promote symptom control and management. The goal of nursing care is to provide an individualized plan of care that promotes patient comfort and maximizes patient independence and self-care activities. The nursing process provides an excellent template for accomplishing this goal. An example of how the nursing process is applied in autoimmune disease is provided in the following discussion of SLE, with diagnoses for autoimmune diseases listed in Chart 60–6.

Nursing care of the patient with SLE presents numerous challenges. Attempts at diagnosis may be lengthy and difficult. Generalized and often vague symptoms of SLE can increase the patient's sense of loss of control and perception that health care professionals may not take them seriously. Flares of the disease may add to the patient's feelings of loss of control or depression.

Assessment

Nursing assessment begins with listening carefully to the patient's concerns and developing a supportive therapeutic relationship. The nursing assessment includes a thorough history of symptoms with focus on patient reports of fatigue, rashes, pain including headaches, and swollen joints. The history will guide the nurse in performing an in-depth physical examination of all systems because of the varied organs and tissues that can be affected by SLE.

Nursing Diagnoses

Common nursing diagnoses associated with SLE include:

- *Pain*
- *Fatigue*
- *Impaired Mobility*
- *Ineffective Tissue Perfusion*

CHART 60–6 — Nursing Diagnoses for Patients with Autoimmune Disease

- *Deficient Knowledge* related to therapeutic regimen, self-care, and immunosuppressive medications
- *Deficient Knowledge* related to signs/symptoms of autoimmune disease exacerbation
- *Risk for Infection* related to immune suppression medications and alterations in immune function
- *Fatigue* related to autoimmune disease
- *Chronic Pain* related to autoimmune disease
- *Impaired Oral Mucous Membrane* related to immune suppression medications
- *Risk for Impaired Skin Integrity* related to immunosuppressive medications
- *Sexual Dysfunction* related to immunosuppressive medications and fatigue
- *Risk for Imbalanced Nutrition: Less Than Body Requirements* related to decreased appetite with chronic disease process
- *Risk for Activity Intolerance* and *Self-Care Deficit* related to disease exacerbation
- *Coping Ineffective,* related to chronic disease process lifestyle alteration and fatigue
- *Risk for Social Isolation* related to chronic fatigue, autoimmune disease exacerbations.

Sources: Carpenito-Moyet, L. (2008). *Nursing care plans and documentation* (5th ed.). Philadelphia: Lippincott Williams & Wilkins; National Institute of Arthritis and Musculoskeletal and Skin Diseases. (2006). *Lupus: A patient care guide for nurses and other professionals* (3rd ed.). Retrieved September 2, 2008, from http://www.niams.nih.gov/hi/topics/lupus/lupusguide/chp7.htm; University of California Davis Health System. (2001). *Living with your kidney transplant.* Sacramento: UC Davis Transplant Center.

- *Urinary Elimination Impaired*
- *Decreased Cardiac Output*
- *Coping. Readiness for enhanced coping ineffective*

Planning, Interventions, and Outcome and Evaluation Parameters

Planning nursing care of patients with SLE should focus on the specific problems the patient describes as well as assessment findings. Frequent reassessment to identify potential problems such as joint or renal impairment is done on an ongoing basis. Patient teaching regarding the importance of adhering to medication regimens, reporting side effects, and assisting the patient to identify flares of the disease early are vital nursing interventions. The remainder of nursing care centers around symptom control and psychosocial support. Outcome and evaluation parameters to determine the effectiveness of the treatment plan include symptom control, effective medication regime, and prevention of disease flares.

Health Promotion

It is important for individuals with SLE to understand the importance of obtaining regular health care, not just during disease flares. The patient needs to be taught to receive regular physical examinations, blood pressure checks, and laboratory work to enable the health care team to identify problems early and help prevent disease exacerbation. Annual gynecological and breast exams for women and prostate specific antigen (PSA) tests for men are recommended, as are annual influenza vaccines. An eye exam should also be done yearly if the patient is taking corticosteroids or antimalarial medications to screen for visual changes.

Learning to recognize the early warning signs of an SLE crisis is also vital in preventing it or reducing the intensity. Warning signs include increased fatigue, pain, rash, fever, abdominal discomfort, headache, and dizziness (NIAMSD, 2003). Maintaining a healthy lifestyle by eating well, exercising daily, and controlling stress is important in preventing SLE exacerbations. Developing an effective support system for emotional support, to improve coping skills, and to boost morale is an essential part of this process.

Collaborative Management

Accurate diagnosis, early treatment, patient education on medications and disease management, and development of an individualized plan of care designed to empower the patient are critical for successful living with an autoimmune disease such as SLE. A team approach that involves health care providers or various specialties, nurses, and social workers is essential in creating an effective treatment plan that enables the patient to have a productive and rewarding life in spite of the devastating impact of an autoimmune disease.

Health care providers specifically manage the multiple phases of the diagnosis and medical treatment plan. This involves medication management, laboratory testing, and monitoring and treatment of disease progression. Nursing care, described earlier, includes symptom management, patient and education medications for symptom control, and education on early signs and symptoms of disease exacerbation. The social worker assists with home management, respite care for caregivers, and financial concerns.

Research Topics Related to the Autoimmune Hypersensitivity Response

Research related to the autoimmune hypersensitivity response is focused primarily on molecular genetic studies to determine genetic links in the development of allergic and autoimmune responses and advancement of new drug therapies to treat the diseases associated with these responses. As studies progress to clinical trials, nurses play a significant role in study coordination, gathering of data, and analysis of patient response to new treatments. Immunosuppressive drug therapy to treat autoimmune disease is an area of extensive research. There are multiple drug studies currently in the clinical trial phase that nurses are involved in coordinating (NHLBI, 2004b).

Research in autoimmune diseases also focuses on improving quality of life for patients with specific disease processes. For example, scleroderma is a systemic autoimmune disease that can result in the development of pulmonary fibrosis, the primary cause of mortality in these patients. Traditionally, treatment has focused on suppression of the immune system largely through the use of corticosteroids. Now a new approach using cyclophosphamide, which has been used to treat neoplasms of the immune system and SLE, is in clinical trials at 13 major university hospitals in the United States (NHLBI, 2004b).

Research in controlling the autoimmune hypersensitivity response also focuses on the development of monoclonal antibodies to treat specific diseases such as SLE. Additional information on current medical and nursing research related to autoimmune hypersensitivity is provided in the Research Opportunities and Clinical Impact box.

◼ Alloimmune Hypersensitivity Response

The alloimmune response is a type of immune reaction in which the antigen, the host's immune system, responds to an antigen from another human or another species. This is the type of response that occurs when tissues or organs are transplanted. This is a normal immune response, because the immune system is reacting to foreign antigens. Therefore, matching the antigens between the donor and recipient of transplanted cells and suppressing the immune response are the key concepts in preventing organ and tissue transplant rejection.

Epidemiology and Etiology

The advancements in surgical technique and immunosuppressive medications have substantially improved the success of organ and tissue transplants. There is a growing shortage of available organs for transplant. Approximately 89,000 people in the United States are currently on the waiting list for an organ transplant, and another 4,000 are added annually (National Kidney Foundation, 2005). Organs that can currently be transplanted include the kidneys, liver, pancreas, heart, and lungs. Blood and numerous other body tissues including skin, bone, cartilage, corneas, veins, and bone marrow also can be transplanted. An autograft is a transplant of tissue or whole organ from one part of an animal to the same animal. Transplants between two identical twins are isograft. A transplant that occurs from one animal to another or one human being to another is called an allograft. When the graft occurs from a lower animal to a human it is a xenograft. The goal with any graft is to minimize the risk of alloimmune response that results in rejection of the transplanted tissue or organ (Rote, 2006).

Different mechanisms of hypersensitivity immune response are involved in alloimmune reactions. The type IV cell-mediated

RESEARCH OPPORTUNITIES AND CLINICAL IMPACT RELATED TO THE AUTOIMMUNE HYPERSENSITIVITY RESPONSE

Research Area	Clinical Impact
Development of monoclonal antibodies for treatment of autoimmune diseases	Control of autoimmune disease progression and clinical symptoms
Stem cell cloning to develop new methods for delivery of monoclonal antibodies	Improved drug therapy by reducing side effects of monoclonal antibody therapy
Identification of genetic factors that contribute to development of autoimmune diseases such as myasthenia gravis and Goodpasture's syndrome	Enable gene alteration to prevent and treat autoimmune disease
Identification of viral triggers of autoimmune dysfunction such as Epstein-Barr virus and autoimmune-associated migraine headaches	Prevention of disease progress and development of effective treatment
Identification of environmental triggers such as pesticides or radiation exposure that contribute to the development of autoimmune disease	Control of exposure to environment triggers to prevent altered immune function
Drug therapy for treatment of symptoms of autoimmune disease such as digital ulcers in scleroderma. For example, bosentan is an endothelin-1 antagonist that causes relaxation of the smooth muscle of the blood vessel and decreased pressures and is in current clinical trials in 21 U.S. test sites	New drug treatments to control pain and improve patient's quality of life. The bosentan study is evaluating improved blood flow and healing in finger ulcers of patients with scleroderma. Goal is a reduction of digital ulcers, improved healing of digital ulcers, and increased hand function (Korn & Seibold, 2004)

response is the type of alloimmune reaction involved in transplant rejection. The T cells are primarily responsible for this type of response. Antibody-mediated responses and complement also play a significant role in alloimmune reaction.

Pathophysiology

The antigen system primarily responsible for alloimmune reaction is the HLA system. There are six different HLA markers: HLA-A, HLA-B, HLA-C, HLA-D, HLA-DR, and HLA-DQ. These create identifying protein markers that are on cell surfaces throughout the body and differentiate self from non-self. Each of these markers is capable of creating multiple different gene subtype combinations that are the basis for HLA inheritance in families. Identical twins will have the same HLA markers; family members will have similar HLA markers. HLA matching is critical in organ transplant and is the ideal marker for genetic study of diseases (Rote, 2006).

To maximize the potential for graft acceptance, there must be a donor–recipient match between HLA subtypes. This match is vital because an organ that is transplanted (kidney, lung, or heart) is rich in donor vascular tissue, white blood cells, and lymphatic tissue, all of which carry HLA subtype antigens and, thus, are able to trigger an alloimmune response. An exact or extremely close HLA match is essential to prevent the host's immune system from reacting against the donor's graft. Tissues such as corneas, cartilage, and veins have minimum concentrations of immune tissue with specialized HLA antigens; therefore, only blood typing and crossmatching is required when matching a donor and recipient.

Graft Rejection

Host versus graft disease (HVGD) occurs when the recipient's immune system reacts against the foreign antigens on the cells of the graft. This can occur in allograft tissues or organs such as kidney, lung, and heart, and is classified as hyperacute, acute, and chronic. Type II and type IV hypersensitivity reactions occur in most types of rejection. The T cells involved in rejection are T-helper cells (CD4) and T-cytotoxic cells (CD8). Consequently, T-cell activity must be suppressed in order to prevent rejection. T-cell suppression is the primary target of immunosuppressive therapy for transplant recipients.

Hyperacute rejection is rare and occurs when the recipient has a preexisting antibody to the antigen in the graft tissue. The graft may turn white immediately or during the next several hours as vascular stasis occurs in the transplanted tissue. This is a result of the antigen–antibody complexes that stimulate the release of proinflammatory mediators and of complement. Complement, a primary mediator in the antigen–antibody reactions, attracts tissue-destroying neutrophils and macrophages, and stimulates the coagulation cascade, which results in coagulation in the microvasculature of the graft tissue (Rote, 2006). Hyperacute rejection occurs because of previous exposure to an antigen, such as with prior blood transfusions, organ transplants, or multiple pregnancies (Urden et al., 2006).

Acute graft rejection is a type IV cell-mediated immune response that occurs approximately 2 weeks to a month after transplant. This type of delayed hypersensitivity response occurs when the recipient's T cells are activated against the unmatched HLA antigens on the transplanted donor tissue. The result is destruction of the transplant tissue by T cells and inflammatory mediators. Immunosuppressive drugs may delay the response.

The symptoms exhibited during acute rejection are consistent with an inflammatory response and include fever, swelling, tenderness, and redness over the graft site. The result will be progressive organ failure evidenced in laboratory findings such as elevation in creatinine with kidney transplant rejection or increase in liver enzymes with liver transplant rejection. Acute rejection can be slowed or reversed with changes in immunotherapy treatment. Research to develop new and improved immunosuppressive drug therapies is ongoing (Food and Drug Administration [FDA], 2003b).

Chronic graft rejection occurs a few months to years after transplant and involves a slow progressive failure of the transplanted organ. Although improvements in immunotherapy have made significant strides in prevention or slowing of acute tissue rejection, chronic graft rejection continues to be a major problem. The exact mechanism of chronic graft rejection is not well understood. It is thought to involve T-cell-mediated cytotoxic cells and macrophages that damage the endothelial cell lining of blood vessels causing thickening and fibrosis of the microvasculature (Rote, 2006). Over time the organ slowly fails as evidenced by clinical symptoms and elevation of laboratory values that reflect organ function.

Graft Versus Host Disease

In **graft versus host disease (GVHD)** donor-grafted tissue contains functional immune cells that respond to the recipient's tissue antigens. As a result, the grafted tissue supersedes the immune function of the recipient and produces antibodies against the host tissue, initiates cytotoxic responses, and begins to attack tissue in the host. Patients who experience this type of immune reaction are usually severely immunocompromised.

GVHD is most often seen in bone marrow transplants (see Chapter 64 ⬤ for a complete description of bone marrow transplant). This occurs because prior to bone marrow transplant, the host's immune system is reduced or eliminated by radiation and/or chemotherapy. When donor marrow is introduced, T lymphocytes in the donor marrow recognize that the recipient's HLA antigens are foreign and initiate an immune attack against cells rich in HLA antigens. Sites of initial GVHD symptoms include skin, liver, intestines, and, of course, the recipient's immune system cells. The response may be as mild as a rash on the skin or as severe as liver failure. GVHD can be prevented through the elimination or destruction of T cells in donated tissue with immunosuppressive therapy (Porth & Sweeney, 2007).

Clinical Manifestations

The clinical manifestations of alloimmune hypersensitivity response can occur through two different mechanisms. The most common mechanism is graft disease (HVGD) and involves the recipient's immune system reacting against the donor tissue. As discussed earlier, graft rejection is classified as hyperacute, acute, or chronic based on various symptoms and the amount of time that has elapsed since transplant. The second mechanism of alloimmune hypersensitivity response, GVHD, occurs when the immune cells in the donor's tissue mount a reaction against the host.

Medical Management

Medical management of the patient with alloimmune response is targeted at preventing graft rejection and early identification and suppression of immune activity that could lead to graft failure. As with other forms of autoimmune diseases, this involves depressing immune function. Immunosuppressive drug therapy is the focal point of alloimmune medical treatment.

Immunosuppressive Therapy

Immunosuppressive therapy will vary according to the type of organ or tissue being transplanted and institutional/health care provider protocols. For information on specific organ transplants, refer to the chapters related to the organ being transplanted such as heart, lungs, liver, and kidney. The goal of immunotherapy is to suppress the activity of the T-helper and T-cytotoxic cells and interfere with the secretion of interleukins (see Chapter 59 ◉) that stimulate the inflammatory and immune response. Another focus of the treatment is to minimize the toxic effects of these drugs, which include nephrotoxicity, electrolyte abnormalities, hypertension, hepatoxicity, hyperglycemia, and the hematologic effects of leukopenia, thrombocytopenia, and anemia (Adams et al., 2005; Wilson, Shannon, Shields, & Stang, 2007). Therefore, patients must have frequent laboratory tests to evaluate blood chemistry, liver function, kidney function, and hematology cell production in order to monitor the effects of medication and allow for dose adjustments.

Initial immunotherapy begins prior to the transplantation procedure. High doses of immunosuppressive agents are used initially and for a short time after surgery. These doses are then tapered to maintenance levels. Common drugs used and the implications for nursing care are found in the Pharmacology Summary of Medications to treat Autoimmune and Immunosuppressive Drug Therapy feature. If rejection develops, high-dose steroids and antilymphocyte therapy such as monoclonal antibodies are frequently used.

■ Nursing Management

The goal of nursing management for the patient with alloimmune response is prevention of transplant rejection and promotion of optimal quality of life and independence. Nursing care of the patient with tissue transplant must focus on educating patients and families regarding the importance of immunosuppressive therapy including the side effects and precautions and also the signs and symptoms of transplant rejection. The nurse monitors for adherence to prescribed medications, and side effects of drug therapy such as alteration in renal and hepatic function, alteration in skin integrity, and possible opportunistic infection. The nursing process provides an excellent template to assess, treat, and evaluate patients with tissue transplant and subsequent alloimmune response. The Nursing Process: Care Plan for the Patient with an Organ Transplant feature (p. 1917) applies the nursing process to the most common nursing diagnosis associated with alloimmune response and graft rejection.

■ Collaborative Management

The essence of collaborative care is exemplified in the care of transplant patients. A strong multidisciplinary team approach and a committed family support system are essential to help prepare the patient for transplant and monitor the patient's medications, treatments, and follow-up care after transplant. Prior to transplant the patient is interviewed by a health care provider from the transplant team to determine appropriateness for transplant. An additional screening is done by a psychologist to determine if the patient is mentally prepared to receive a transplant and understand and comply with the required treatment regime. A pretransplant nurse coordinator is also involved, and is responsible for scheduling all of the required preliminary tests and appointments.

At the time of transplant and immediately following, other members of the multidisciplinary team become involved. These include a team of transplant surgeons and other health care provider specialties depending on any complicating factors. Transplant unit nurses care for the patient immediately after surgery and educate and prepare the patient and family for the responsibilities associated with discharge home. These include teaching about monitoring vital signs and preventing infection, medication administration and compliance, laboratory tests trending, and follow-up appointments.

The pharmacist also has a crucial role in medication education and working with the health care provider to tailor the medication treatment plan. Additionally, a dietitian provides teaching on nutritional needs and dietary restrictions specific for the organ being transplanted. For example, patients with renal transplant would receive teaching regarding a low-sodium diet. The social worker and discharge planner nurse assist in helping the family with financial concerns, arranging any home care needs, and connecting with community resources.

Post-transplant care involves the addition to the team of a post-transplant nurse coordinator. This nurse provides the patient and family with continual support and is the primary point of contact for them regarding questions, medications, any symptoms or complications, and follow-up appointments. The post-transplant coordinator functions as a very specialized case manager to triage any patient problems and determine what members of the transplant team the patient needs to see. Additionally, the patient continues to be followed on a regular basis by the transplant surgeon and several other members of the team to optimize successful transplant.

Research Topics Related to the Alloimmune Hypersensitivity Response

Research in the area of alloimmune hypersensitivity response is primarily focused on preventing transplant rejection. Areas of research involve development of new immunosuppressant medications with minimal side effects that promote optimal immune suppression and quality of life for the transplant patient. Information related to some of the current research in this area is presented in the Research Opportunities and Clinical Impact box (p. 1921).

■ Immunodeficiencies

Immune deficiencies occur when the immune system experiences abnormalities in function that result in a decreased or compromised ability to appropriately respond and protect the host from an antigenic attack. Primary immune deficiencies are the result of genetic abnormalities in the embryonic development of the immune system.

PHARMACOLOGY Summary of Medications to Treat Autoimmune and Immunosuppressive Drug Therapy

Drug	Action	Application/Indication	Nursing Responsibility
Nonsteroidal Anti-Inflammatory Drugs (NSAIDs) • Ibuprofen • Naproxen • Indomethacin • Sulindac • Piroxicam • Oxaprozin	Reduce the pain, swelling, and immobility of joint arthralgias by blocking release of prostaglandins and leukotrienes responsible for inflammation and pain.	Drug of choice for patients with autoimmune disease such as lupus with little or no organ involvement. Patients with serious organ involvement or disease flares will require steroid anti-inflammatory drugs and immunosuppressive medications.	Assess pain level. Various NSAIDs effect people differently and after a time they may develop a tolerance, requiring a change to a new drug in the class. Monitor for bleeding, GI upset, and decreased renal function. Instruct patient to take NSAIDs with food or milk to decrease GI symptoms. Salicylates (including ASA) are contraindicated in persons under age 19 due to Reye's syndrome.
Antimalarial Drugs • Hydroxychloroquine sulfate (Plaquenil) • Chloroquine (Aralen) • Quinacrine (Atabrine)	The exact mechanism of action for these drugs in SLE is unknown. They are effective in suppressing some immune function related to lupus and controlling mild inflammatory symptoms.	Low doses are used to manage mild symptoms of lupus including arthritis, skin rashes, mouth ulcers, fatigue, and fever. May enable reduction of total daily dose of corticosteroids.	Instruct the patient that medications may take several weeks to become effective in controlling symptoms. Monitor for vision changes; can cause retinal damage.
Glucocorticosteroids • Steroids: prednisone, dexamethasone, methylprednisolone, and hydrocortisone	Interfere with inflammatory response and antigen presentation. Block cytokine genes, thereby impairing synthesis of IL-1, -2, -3, and -6. Inhibit TNF.	Used to control exacerbations of autoimmune diseases. For transplant patients used in combination with calcineurin inhibitors such as cyclosporine, and antimetabolites and cytotoxic agents such as azathioprine as triple-drug immunosuppressive therapy to prevent transplant rejection.	Monitor laboratory tests: serum glucose, lipid levels. Administer insulin as prescribed. Monitor wound healing. Promote skin integrity (change position frequently, avoid adhesive tape). Provide patient education on diet and body changes: low-fat, low-cholesterol diet with low calories between meal snacks. Monitor changes in strength; provide a physical therapy consult as needed. Administer medication with food; collaborate with health care provider for orders for hydrochloric acid (H2) receptor blockers or antacids for gastric complaints. Monitor for signs and symptoms of infection. Instruct patient on techniques to avoid infection (perform hand hygiene frequently, avoid crowds and ill individuals).

(continued)

PHARMACOLOGY Summary of Medications to Treat Autoimmune and Immunosuppressive Drug Therapy—*Continued*

Drug	Action	Application/Indication	Nursing Responsibility
Calcineurin Inhibitor • Cyclosporine (Sandimmune and Neoral) • Tacrolimus (Prograf)	Reduce transcription of IL-2. Impair cytokines that are required for T-cell activation (more potent than cyclosporine).	The mainstay of immunosuppressive therapy; used as part of triple-drug immunosuppressive therapy to prevent transplant rejection. Now also commonly used to treat autoimmune diseases such as lupus.	Monitor and report abnormal laboratory tests: serum creatinine, BUN, potassium, serum transaminases, bilirubin, and glucose levels. Administer insulin as prescribed. Administer antiemetic and antidiarrhea agents as prescribed. Monitor and report serum cyclosporine trough levels and changes in neurological status for dose adjustments. Provide patient education on frequent oral care, such as dental cleaning every 6 months or more frequently if gingival hyperplasia occurs.
Antimetabolites • Azathioprine (AZA, Imuran) • Cyclophosphamide (Cytoxan) • Methotrexate (Rheumatrex) • Sirolimus (Rapamune) • Mycophenolate Mofetil (CellCept)	Inhibit aspects of lymphocyte replication, which decreases leukocytes. Inhibit proliferation of B- and T-cell lines. Decrease leukocytes. Selectively inhibit proliferation of B and T lymphocytes.	Used in combination with cyclosporine and steroids as triple-drug immunosuppressive therapy to prevent transplant rejection. Azathioprine is one of the most widely used immunosuppressive drugs for lupus. Cytoxan is reserved for treating lupus with kidney disease or other internal organ involvement. Rheumatrex is predominantly used for lupus arthritis. Sometimes used as an alternative to cyclophosphamide for lupus with kidney involvement.	Monitor and report symptoms of infection (hyper- or hypothermia, chills, malaise) and/or jaundice. Monitor and report abnormal labs: CBC, serum transaminases, and bilirubin. Monitor fluid intake and urine output daily. Assess gastrointestinal disturbances and administer antiemetics and antidiarrhea agents as ordered.
Monoclonal and Polyclonal Antibodies • Alemtuzumab (Campath) • Basiliximab (Simulect) • Daclizumab (Zenapax) • Infliximab (Remicade) • Muromonab-CD3 (Orthoclone OKT3) • Rituximab (Rituxan) • Lymphocyte immunoglobulin (Antithymocyte Globulin: Equine, Atgam)	Monoclonal antibody targeting CD3 receptor on T cells. Downregulates T-cell activity. A specific lymphocyte immunoglobulin that is a lymphocyte-selective immunosuppressant agent. Composed of sterile, purified, concentrated immunoglobulin G (IgG) from serum of horses immunized with human thymus lymphocytes. The immune globulin lymphocytes bind with the patient's antigen reactive T lymphocytes and decrease or alter killer T-cell function.	Organ and tissue transplant immune suppression. Used in combination with cyclosporine and corticosteroid therapy to prevent transplant rejection. To prevent or delay onset or to reverse acute renal allograft rejection.	Monitor and report fever, chills, nausea and vomiting, headache. Administer antiemetics and antipyretics as ordered. Monitor and report abnormalities in respiratory status (dyspnea, increased respiratory rate, decrease in pulse oximetry readings, abnormal breath sounds). Administer oxygen as ordered. Monitor pulse oxygen saturation and arterial blood gases (ABGs); report abnormalities. Monitor for signs/symptoms of infection.

Sources: Adams, M., Josephson, D., & Holland, L. (2008). *Pharmacology for nurses: A pathophysiologic approach.* (2nd ed.) Upper Saddle River, NJ: Pearson Prentice Hall; National Institute of Arthritis and Musculoskeletal and Skin Diseases. (2006). *Care of the lupus patient.* Retrieved February 19, 2007, from National Institute of Health website: http://www.niams.nih.gov/hi/topics/lupus/lupusguide/chp7.htm; University of California Davis Medical Center Transplant Center. (2001). *Living with your kidney transplant.* Sacramento: Author; University of California Davis Health System. (2003). *Atgam IV administration. Patient care standard A-7.* Sacramento: Author.

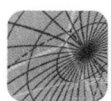

NURSING PROCESS: Patient Care Plan for Organ Transplants

Assessment of Knowledge

Subjective Data:

Do you have a way in which you best learn information (e.g., reading, watching a video on the subject, or having 1:1 instruction)?

Who in your family is going to help you at home with your medications, vital sign monitoring, and follow-up appointments?

Is this a good time to do some of your teaching or are you too tired or in pain?

Objective Data:

Patient is awake, alert, oriented.

Patient does not show signs of pain or discomfort (e.g., pain level assessed at tolerable for patient, VS stable).

Appropriate person from family is present.

Patient and family verbalize readiness to learn.

Nursing Assessment and Diagnoses	Outcomes and Evaluation Parameters	Planning and Interventions with *Rationales*
Nursing Diagnosis: *Deficient Knowledge* related to therapeutic regimen and self-care, immunosuppressive medications, signs/symptoms of transplant rejection, and discharge follow-up	**Outcomes:** Successful recovery without graft rejection or complications. Patient and family demonstrate self-care activities to prevent graft rejection. ***Evaluation Parameters:*** Participates in learning sessions and asks questions. Verbalizes education needs to reduce risk of graft rejection and maintain health. Develops plan to meet follow-up care needs and initiates lifestyle changes.	**Interventions and *Rationales:*** Assess patient's and family's level of understanding of information, participation in teaching sessions, initiation of self-care activities, and medication administration technique. Assess knowledge level and lifestyle expectations of patient and family. *To determine educational needs and clarify expectations.*
	Verbalizes understanding to notify transplant coordinator immediately for any health problems.	Provide information via multiple modalities including written, video, presentations by transplant team, demonstration/return demonstration. *Provides individualized learning plan, enhances learning experience, and provides resources postdischarge.* Instruct patient and family about the importance of adhering to medical treatment regime including follow-up appointments, frequent need for laboratory testing draws to assess effectiveness of immunosuppressive drug therapy. *To prevent complications of graft rejection or medication side effects.*
	Verbalizes rationale for and doses of specific immunotherapy medications and follow-up lab tests and appointments. Accurately self-doses all immunosuppressive therapy drugs prior to discharge. Demonstrates self-care by adhering to treatment regime including immunosuppressive drug therapy. Verbalizes signs and symptoms of transplant rejection.	Review immunosuppressive medication doses, side effects, and administration schedule. *To provide information about why and how immunosuppressive drugs are administered.* Observe patient self-administering medications appropriately. *To assess appropriate medication administration.*
	Reports any symptoms of transplant rejection early to transplant coordinator.	Instruct about signs and symptoms of rejection: fatigue/general malaise, "flu-like" feeling, fever, sudden weight gain, delayed wound healing, pain in or around specific organ transplanted or changes in normal function. *To identify early signs of rejection.* Instruct to notify transplant coordinator immediately for any of the above symptoms. *To initiate prompt medical treatment.*

Assessment of Infection

Subjective Data:

Do you have any pain?

Do you have a temperature?

Are you having any "flu-like" symptoms (body aches, fatigue, cough, sore throat, stiff neck)?

Do you have any rashes?

Do you have any burning with urination?

Do you have any redness or tenderness anywhere?

Do you have any sores anywhere?

Do you have any unusual or foul-smelling drainage (e.g., from vagina, penis, rectum, ears)?

How long have the symptoms been going on?

What have you done to treat the symptoms?

Have you taken any over the counter (OTC), prescription, or herbal medications for symptom relief?

Objective Data:

Head-to-toe assessment with focus on the specific area of patient complaint; report any abnormal findings (e.g., abnormal vital signs, pain, "flu-like" symptoms, rashes, redness, discharge, sores, drainage, bloody stools, and urinary discomfort).

(continued)

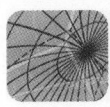

NURSING PROCESS: Patient Care Plan for Organ Transplants—*Continued*

Nursing Assessment and Diagnoses	Outcomes and Evaluation Parameters	Planning and Interventions with *Rationales*
Nursing Diagnosis: *Risk for Infection* related to immune suppression medications	**Outcome:** No infection. ***Evaluation Parameters:*** Patient and family verbalize understanding of signs/symptoms of infection and notify transplant coordinator immediately of any health problems.	**Interventions and *Rationales:*** Instruct patient and family to monitor and report any symptoms of infection. *To facilitate prompt medical treatment and minimize risk of rejection.* Instruct patient and family about signs and symptoms of infection: fever, chills, "flu-like" feeling, cough with or without sputum, sore throat, shortness of breath, rashes, burning with urination, foul discharge from penis, vagina, loose or bloody stools, any redness/tenderness or drainage from incision; swollen lymph nodes; any new or unusual pain, stiff neck, sores in mouth or on tongue. *To identify early signs/symptoms of infection, facilitate early medical treatment, and minimize risk of rejection.* Instruct to notify transplant coordinator immediately. *To initiate prompt medical treatment.*
	Patient and family demonstrate understanding of self-care by following plan to minimize infection risk.	Instruct patient and family on ways to minimize risk of infection including performing hand hygiene frequently, avoid crowded areas, and avoid contact with people who are sick. *To minimize exposure to infectious organisms.* Perform weekly self-exam to assess for swelling of lymph nodes. *To detect symptoms of infection early.* Drink 6–8 glasses of water a day and empty your bladder frequently, avoid bubble baths, urinate after sex, wear cotton crotch underwear. *To prevent urinary tract infections.* Wear a mask and gloves when working in the garden. *To avoid fungi and bacteria in soil.* Do not handle pet waste or litter box. *Cat litter can transmit infectious organisms.* Swim only in pools with chlorine. *Lakes and ponds have multiple infectious organisms.* Cook all meats thoroughly before eating and wash fruits/vegetables well. *To decrease bacteria.*
	Daily log completed and brought to follow-up appointments.	Instruct in self-care practices to monitor for complications and documenting in daily log: temperature, weight before breakfast, blood pressure, pulse, changes in medications, changes in health status. *To identify early signs of complications and provide trend information to transplant team.*
	Performs vital sign monitoring accurately and records information in daily log appropriately.	Observe patient taking own temperature, pulse, blood pressure, and weight and recording these prior to discharge. *To assess skill and ensure accuracy of readings and need for additional teaching.*

Assessment of Skin and Oral Mucosa

Subjective Data:
Do you have any red, sore, or open areas on your skin?
Do you have any redness or drainage from your surgical incision?
Do you have any sores in your mouth?
Are you able to bathe and do oral care daily?
Do you have acne?
Do you use a sun block?

Objective Data:
Assess:
Redness on pressure points (coccyx, heals, elbows)
Skin tears: around wound site, IV sites, lab draw sites where tape has been applied
Incision site: redness, drainage, foul odor, proximity of suture line, intact staples/sutures
Skinfolds, especially with patients who are obese: redness, breakdown
Oral membrane: open sores in mouth, white coating on tongue indicating possible candidiasis infection

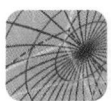

NURSING PROCESS: Patient Care Plan for Organ Transplants—*Continued*

Nursing Assessment and Diagnoses	Outcomes and Evaluation Parameters	Planning and Interventions with *Rationales*
Nursing Diagnosis: *High Risk for Impaired Skin Integrity* related to opportunistic infections of the mucus membranes	**Outcome:** Intact mucous membranes. **Evaluation Parameters:** Verbalizes importance of oral care. Practices self-care by performing oral care according to plan. Takes antibiotics prior to any dental work.	**Interventions and *Rationales:*** Inspect gums, mouth, and tongue daily and report abnormalities. *To facilitate appropriate medical treatment.* Provide frequent oral care. *To keep mucous membranes moist and promote patient comfort.* Instruct in importance of oral care; encourage frequent oral care during the day and regular dental checkups and inspection of gums, mouth, and tongue daily. *Immunosuppression increases risk of opportunistic infections. Medication side effects can cause hypertrophy of the gums.* Patient to inform dentist of immunosuppressed status. *To facilitate prescription of antibiotics prior to any dental work.* Patient to always take antibiotics prior to dental work. *To minimize risk of blood infection from dental work.*

Assessment of Post-Transplant Self-Care

Subjective Data:

Are you taking your medications, and are you able to keep your clinic appointments?

Are you able to eat a balanced, nutritious diet?

Have you gained or lost weight?

Are you easily fatigued or can you participate in daily light, low-impact exercise, such as walking?

Are you experiencing any sexual difficulties you would like to discuss?

Are you seeing family and friends regularly?

Are you planning to travel anywhere out of the area?

Objective Data:

Keeps follow-up lab and medical appointments

Weight (above or below goal weight)

Contacts transplant coordinator with travel plans

Nursing Assessment and Diagnoses	Outcomes and Evaluation Parameters	Planning and Interventions with *Rationales*
Nursing Diagnoses: *High risk for Impaired Skin Integrity* related to post-transplant status and necessity for lifelong immunosuppressive medication	**Outcome:** Intact skin and oral mucous membranes. **Evaluation Parameters:** No evidence of pressure ulcers, skin tears, or sores on mucous membranes. Verbalizes instructions for post-op wound care. Practices self-care by following post-op care instructions. Verbalizes importance of skin care. Practices self-care by performing skin care daily.	**Interventions and *Rationales:*** Assess for alteration in skin integrity and reposition frequently. *To promote skin integrity. Broken skin provides entry for bacteria.* Avoid the use of adhesive tape. *To minimize the risk of skin tears.* Instruct in postoperative home care: care of wound site, monitoring for redness and drainage. *Indicates infection.* Gently clean skin around incision daily with soap and water. *To decrease bacteria and risk of infection.* Do not apply lotion over wound. *Increases risk of infection.* Avoid heavy lifting/strenuous exercise. Do not lift more than 20 pounds for 6–8 weeks. *To prevent damaging suture/incision.* Get adequate rest and fluids. *To promote healing.* Discuss importance of bathing daily, using a mild soap, and applying lotion to dry skin. *To decrease bacteria on skin and, hence, risk of infection and to maintain skin integrity.* Discuss care of acne that can develop as a side effect of medication: no picking at acne, use of acne soap, use of over the counter (OTC) benzyl peroxide lotion in 5% or 10% if acne persists. *To maintain skin integrity and decrease risk of infection.* Instruct in necessity of treating skin carefully, avoiding strong sunlight, wearing sun block with an SPF of 15 or higher. *Steroid medications result in fragile skin that tears and burns easily. Broken skin provides entry for bacteria.* Assist as needed with oral care every 2–4 hours, keep mucous membranes moist, brush teeth with soft brush three times daily. *To maintain moist oral mucosa and decrease risk of infection. Brushing teeth removes the bacteria much more effectively than oral swabs.*

(continued)

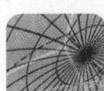

NURSING PROCESS: Patient Care Plan for Organ Transplants—*Continued*

Nursing Assessment and Diagnoses	Outcomes and Evaluation Parameters	Planning and Interventions with *Rationales*
		Assist as needed with lip care and application of lip balm. *To prevent drying and cracking and promote patient comfort.* Discuss and help problem solve difficulties with medication compliance and scheduling of appointments or laboratory tests. Provide referrals to collaborative services (dietary, social services, and transplant coordinator) as needed. *To promote compliance and optimal post-transplant care.* Discuss importance of selecting nutritious foods. Collaborate to create healthy menu options to make at home. *To promote healthy food choices and wound healing and maintain health.*
Imbalanced Nutrition: Less than Body Requirements related to decreased or inappropriate nutritional intake	Maintains optimal weight.	Determine optimal weight and plan to attain weight goal. *Medications can result in weight loss, or weight gain (especially prednisone, which stimulates appetite). Malnutrition impairs immune function; excessive weight places additional strain on all body organs.* Collaborate with dietitian if patient has special diet needs. *To promote optimal nutrition.*
	Lifestyle adapted to prevent transplant rejection and maintain optimal quality of life. Verbalizes and demonstrates lifestyle changes to adhere to medication and treatment regime, prevent infection, and promote optimal physical and mental health. Develops dietary plan and follows it at home.	Discuss importance of gradually increasing daily exercise and allowing rest periods between activities. *To promote increasing mobility and avoid excessive fatigue.* Collaborate with patient to develop a low-impact exercise plan that can be implemented when cleared by health care provider. *To encourage activity, promote overall health, decrease sedentary lifestyle, and prevent osteoporosis.*
Activity Intolerance related to postoperative transplant status	Practices self-care by participating in appropriate daily exercise.	Discuss risks of contact sports and strenuous exercises with new transplant. *To provide rationale for low-impact exercises and promote health.*
Risk for Sexual Dysfunction related to immunosuppressive medications and fatigue	Verbalizes concerns and questions regarding sexual function.	Offer information on possible sexual dysfunction related to immunosuppression medications and encourage discussion if patient has questions. *Medications can cause erectile dysfunction, decreased libido, and impaired orgasmic ability.*
Social Isolation related to decreased social interaction during transplant process, feelings of being "different"	Develops/maintains social support system.	Encourage family/friends to visit, call, and send cards and pictures. Encourage patient to phone and write notes to family/friends. *To decrease social isolation.*
Deficient Knowledge related to travel planning	Communicates travel plans, identifies transplant center closest to destination, and continues with scheduled medication regime.	Provide information on community resources including support groups/transplant clubs. *To provide support and guidance with problem solving.* Discuss importance of notifying transport team of travel plans. *To facilitate communication, plan for missed appointments, coordinate with transplant center at point of destination for any care needs.* Instruct patient to always hand-carry immunosuppressive medications if traveling by plane. *To avoid missing medication doses if luggage is lost.*

Sources: Carpenito-Moyet, L. (2008). *Nursing care plans and documentation* (5th ed.). Philadelphia: Lippincott Williams & Wilkins; Porth, C., & Sweeney, K. (2007). Alterations in immune response. In C. M. Porth (Ed.), *Essentials of pathophysiology* (pp. 293–319). St. Louis: Lippincott Williams & Wilkins.

Symptoms of primary deficiencies usually appear shortly after birth. Secondary immunodeficiency occurs when the immune system is damaged and unable to mount an appropriate immune response due to a variety of factors that range from normal aging to infections that eliminate immune cells and severely impair function as in HIV. The immunodeficiency section will briefly review the abnormalities related to primary immune deficiency and related disorders. The focus of this section will be on secondary immunodeficiencies and specifically the pathophysiology, clinical manifestations, and treatment of HIV.

Primary Immune Deficiencies

Primary immune deficiencies are categorized according to the type of immune cell that is genetically malformed or dysfunctional. These categories include phagocytic cell dysfunction, B-cell (humoral) deficiencies, T-cell (cell-mediated) deficiencies, and combined B-cell and T-cell deficiencies.

RESEARCH OPPORTUNITIES AND CLINICAL IMPACT RELATED TO THE ALLOIMMUNE HYPERSENSITIVITY RESPONSE

Research Area	Clinical Impact
Development of medications, such as monoclonal antibodies for use in preventing transplant rejection	Improved ability to transplant organs and reduce incidence of rejection
Identification of additional antibodies and markers to better match tissue and organs for transplant	Reduced transplant rejection through improved matching of host and recipient
Method of delivery of antirejection medication so that these medications are delivered directly to the transplant site rather than administered systemically	Reduced complications of systemic administration of antirejection drugs such as weight gain and increased risk of infection
Investigation into controlling immune cells through manipulation of newly identified cytokines	Regulation of the immune system to divert activity away from transplanted tissue, thus decreasing incidence of rejection
Trial of use of oral autoantigens to induce tolerance of transplanted pancreatic islet cells	Reduced transplant rejection of pancreatic islet cells in diabetic patients to improve quality of life and reduce comorbidities of diabetes
The role of B-cell deficiencies in reducing the risk of transplant rejection of pancreatic islet cells	Ability to better control and decrease B-cell activity to improve antirejection therapy for pancreatic transplant patients
Examination of HLA markers and the importance of a maximal match versus optimal match to prevent transplant rejection.	To better predict which transplants have higher risk of rejection and optimize antirejection drug therapy treatment.

Sources: American Academy of Allergy, Asthma and Immunology, http://www.acaai.org; Centers for Disease Control and Prevention, http://www.cdc.gov; DeFranco, A. L., Locksley, R., & Robertson, M. (2007). *Immunity: The immune response in infectious and inflammatory disease.* Sunderland, MA: Sinauer Associates.

Phagocytic Dysfunction

Several primary immune deficiencies have been identified related to abnormal function of phagocytic cells, most commonly neutrophils. For genetic reasons, neutrophils may not develop in adequate numbers or they may be dysfunctional. If an individual is unable to make an appropriate number of neutrophils, then she is unable to mount an adequate immune response. If the neutrophil DNA is dysfunctional, adequate numbers of neutrophils are unable to migrate and travel to the site of injury or infection and appropriately protect the host from foreign antigens (Rote, 2006).

B Cell (Humoral) Deficiencies

There are two different kinds of B-cell deficiencies. In the first group of disorders, B-cell precursors are unable to differentiate into plasma cells. This deficiency results in inadequate immunoglobulin levels (IgG, IgA, IgM, IgD, IgE) and recurrent infection. Immunoglobulins are discussed in Chapter 59 🔗. The second type of B-cell disorder is the more serious one. In this disease, also known as Brutton's disease, the B cells are unable to differentiate into mature B cells. As a result no plasma cells can be found in circulation, and no immunoglobulins are produced causing major immune deficits including lack of immunologic memory (Rote, 2006).

T-Cell (Cell-Mediated) Deficiencies

The function of T cells is to regulate the immune response. T-cell deficiencies most commonly result in opportunistic infections. Therefore, these abnormalities do not commonly manifest themselves immediately after birth. This type of deficiency is suspected when an infant has repeated opportunistic infections such as candidiasis of the oral, vaginal, or rectal mucosa. There are a wide variety of T-cell-mediated deficiencies, which are differentiated by the type of T cells affected. One extreme example of T-cell-mediated dysfunction is the rare disorder called DiGeorge syndrome. In this disease the thymus does not develop properly and, therefore, T cells are unable to mature and appropriately stimulate an immune response to a foreign antigen. The result is susceptibility to opportunistic infections, symptoms of which begin to appear shortly after birth (Porth & Sweeney, 2007).

Combined B-Cell and T-Cell Deficiencies

Several variations of combined immunodeficiency syndrome have been identified and involve a mutation in one or more of the many genes that involve lymphocyte development and response. This results in low or absent levels of B lymphocytes and T lymphocytes in serum, as well as low or absent levels of IgG and IgA. Subsequently, the diseases that result from these deficiencies range from moderate to fatal in severity. The most severe form of congenital B- and T-cell deficiencies is severe combined immunodeficiency (SCID). This deficiency results from multiple genetic abnormalities that cause all white blood cell lines to fail to develop normally from a stem cell, leading to absence of all immune function. Infants with this genetic defect have failure to thrive, chronic diarrhea and multiple opportunistic infections that usually result in death before 2 years of age. More recently, bone marrow transplant has been used with success to treat infants identified with SCIDS at birth or within the first 3 months of life (Sommer, 2007). Bone marrow transplant is discussed in Chapter 64 🔗.

Secondary Immune Deficiencies

Multiple factors contribute to secondary immune deficiencies; the most significant of these are listed in Chart 60–7 (p. 1922). Immunosuppressive therapy for treatment of autoimmune diseases and prevention of organ transplant rejection and also chemotherapy agents are the most prevalent medications that contribute to secondary immune deficiencies. Suppression of the

---

CHART 60–7 | **Common Causes of Secondary Immunodeficiency**

- *Drug-induced immunodeficiency:* chemotherapy drugs, corticosteroids
- *Age:* infants and older adults
- *Malnutrition:* dietary deficiency, cirrhosis, cachexia
- *Stress*
- *Medical treatments:* surgery, anesthesia, radiation
- *Injury:* trauma, burns
- *Diseases:* AIDS, diabetes mellitus, chronic renal disease, malignancies, alcoholic cirrhosis, SLE

---

immune system places these patients at a high risk for **opportunistic infections (OIs)**, which are infections from microorganisms that are not usually considered pathogens, but cause disease if the immune system is impaired. Therefore, a primary focus of nursing care for patients who are immune suppressed is prevention of infection.

Other factors that can contribute to immune suppression are age and malnutrition. The effect of aging on the immune system is discussed in Chapter 59 ☺. Aging results in decreased thymus and T-cell functioning, which contribute to increased levels of autoimmune disease and malignancies in the older adult. Infants have decreased function because the immune system is still in the process of maturing.

Nutrition also plays a key role in immune function. Prolonged malnutrition with low protein intake contributes to decrease in lymphatic tissue, atrophy of the thymus gland, and altered cell-mediated immune response. Without appropriate nutritional intake, general cell function is impaired and increases the susceptibility to infection (Rote, 2006).

Major injuries such as trauma and burns destroy immune tissues such as the skin and can result in shock states that damage cell function. Medical treatment requiring surgery that removes immune organs such as the lymph nodes, the spleen, or the thymus also impairs immune response. Additionally, radiation suppresses immune function by destroying the lymph tissue directly or by causing atrophy of bone marrow function and depressing stem cell production of lymphocytes.

Numerous diseases significantly impact immune function by altering immune tissue or cells and leaving the individual susceptible to secondary infections. A primary example of the impact of disease on the immune system is evident in human immunodeficiency virus (HIV) infection, which is discussed in the remainder of the chapter.

Human Immunodeficiency Virus and Acquired Immunodeficiency Syndrome

Acquired immunodeficiency syndrome (AIDS) is the syndrome of opportunistic infections that occurs as the final stage of infection with the human immunodeficiency virus. AIDS was first recognized as a new disease entity in 1981, when previously healthy, young homosexual males in Los Angeles and New York were diagnosed with *Pneumocystis carinii* pneumonia (PCP) and a rare cancer, Kaposi's sarcoma. The diagnoses were extremely disturbing because these disease entities had previously only been seen in individuals who were severely immunosuppressed, elderly, or debilitated, and indicated an unknown disease that caused profound immune impairment (Centers for Disease Control and Prevention [CDC], 1981a, 1981b).

During the course of the next few years, thousands of cases were primarily diagnosed among homosexual males and illicit injection drug users. Research, initially stymied because of the social stigma associated with homosexuality and illicit drug use, began to accelerate at a rapid rate as other population groups were diagnosed with AIDS. These individuals included hemophiliacs and other blood transfusion recipients, women through heterosexual contact with infected individuals, and finally infants of infected mothers. An understanding of the epidemic proportions of AIDS was beginning to dawn as cases were reported in multiple countries and almost all continents by the mid-1980s (CDC, 1995; Johnsen, 2003).

Etiology

The **human immunodeficiency virus (HIV)**, the virus that infects CD4 T cells and is the agent responsible for causing AIDS, was identified in 1984. It became apparent that AIDS was the most severe and final stage in a continuum of illnesses associated with HIV infection, which fatally impairs immune function. Subsequent research has identified two specific strains of HIV: HIV type 1 (HIV-1) and HIV type 2 (HIV-2). Virtually all of the cases in the United States are HIV-1. This strain is associated with acute and rapid progression from HIV infection to a diagnosis of AIDS. HIV-2 was identified in West Africa in 1986 and may have been present decades earlier. It is the dominant strain in Africa. HIV-2 involves a slower, milder progression to AIDS than HIV-1, with increased infectiousness at the end of the disease process. Both HIV-1 and HIV-2 have the same modes of transmission and are associated with the same opportunist infections (CDC, 1998).

Epidemiology

The severity of the HIV/AIDS epidemic has exceeded all initial predictions. As of December 2003, an estimated 20 million people worldwide had already died of AIDS, and another 38.6 million people, ages 15 to 45, were living with HIV/AIDS at the end of 2005 (United Nations Program on HIV/AIDS [UNAIDS], 2006). Of the 38.6 million people living with HIV/AIDS worldwide, 37 million are adults. Infected women comprise 47% of this population.

Resource-poor countries have been especially devastated by HIV/AIDS. Sub-Saharan Africa is home to 70% of the world's HIV/AIDS population and is the most affected region in the world (World Health Organization [WHO], 2007). This spread has primarily been attributed to heterosexual transmission, migration patterns, and limited condom use as well as significant mother-to-infant transmission. These factors have been fueled by poverty, lack of health care resources to diagnose HIV infection, lack of HIV prevention education, and limited access to antiretroviral treatment (Johnsen, 2003). The WHO's *AIDS Epidemic Update* estimates that in the year 2005 alone, there were 4.1 million people worldwide newly infected with HIV (13,000 new cases daily), and another 2.8 million deaths due to AIDS (UNAIDS, 2006). This represents a slight decline of about 10% since the peak HIV infection rate in the late 1990s. This is attributed to international efforts between 2001 and 2005 to provide antiretroviral therapy and prenatal screening, treatment, and education to pregnant women infected with HIV in resource-poor countries, specifically sub-Saharan African countries (UNAIDS, 2006).

In the United States, according to the CDC, as of December 2005, there was an estimated 1,039,000 to 1,185,000 people living with HIV infection, one-fourth of whom were unaware they were HIV positive. Approximately 40,000 new HIV infections are added to this number on an annual basis in the United States, half of which occur in people under 25 years of age. Seventy percent of new infections occur among men, and 30% among women (CDC, 2005c). The prevailing means of new HIV infection among men in the United States continues to be homosexual sex (60%), followed by injection of drugs with a contaminated needle (25%). New HIV infections in women in the United States continue to occur primarily through having unprotected heterosexual sex (75%), and approximately 25% are due to injection drug use with contaminated equipment (National Institute of Allergy and Infectious Diseases, 2004).

A cumulative total of 9,300 cases of AIDS have been reported in children ages 12 and under in the United States. Approximately 7% of these cases are attributed to exposure to infected blood products or tissue prior to 1985. The vast majority (about 91%) of cases are a result of prenatal exposure and infected mother-to-infant transmission (CDC, 2003a). The predominance of infected mother-to-infant transmission is consistent with global HIV/AIDS data for children, which estimates that 3 million children are now living with HIV/AIDS, the vast majority of whom are in resource-poor countries (WHO, 2002).

The face of HIV/AIDS is changing in the United States. Currently, 10% of the individuals diagnosed with HIV/AIDS are over 50 years of age. This percentage is expected to increase as effective antiretroviral medications increase life expectancy and the baby boom generation ages (Ress, 2003). HIV/AIDS in the United States also is changing in relationship to race and gender. There is an increase in the proportion of cases being reported among African Americans and Hispanics, as opposed to Caucasian males at the onset of the epidemic. More than half of new HIV infections occur among African Americans, though they represent only 13% of the population. Hispanics are also disproportionately represented (CDC, 2003a). Additionally, women account for an increasing proportion of AIDS cases. This is evidenced by the fact that from 1985 to 2002, the proportion of HIV/AIDS cases among women increased from 7% to 27% (National Institute of Allergy and Infectious Disease, 2004). It also is disturbing to note that women are diagnosed later and begin treatment at a later stage than men and, consequently, have higher morbidity and mortality rates (Branson et al., 2006).

The sad reality of HIV/AIDS infection in the 21st century is that in countries with limited economic resources it continues to be a devastating and rapidly fatal illness, predominantly affecting individuals 15 to 45 years of age in the prime of life and reproductive capacity. In economically stable countries, where there is access to antiretroviral treatment and public health resources, HIV/AIDS is transitioning to a chronic disease process that is involving an increased proportion of elderly, nonwhite, and female victims.

Transmission

While the devastation HIV can wreak is catastrophic, HIV transmission is limited to contact with infected body fluids that have lymphocytes that can harbor HIV. These fluids include blood, semen, vaginal secretions, and breast milk. There also must be a sufficient viral load and a susceptible host for transmission to occur. An infected individual with a high viral load (first months after initial infection, or during an AIDS illness) has an increased ability to transmit HIV. Additionally, prolonged or repeated exposure to infected fluids will greatly increase the risk of transmission (Rote, 2006).

It is important to understand that HIV is not spread through casual contact such as working with someone, shaking hands, hugging, dry kissing, or sharing eating utensils. Repeated studies have failed to demonstrate transmission of the virus through sweat, tears, saliva, urine, emesis, sputum, respiratory droplets, or feces. Studies on vector transmission by insects have also been negative (CDC, 2005c). The Risk Factors box lists the high risk factors associated with HIV transmission.

Sexual Transmission

The most common method of HIV transmission is through sexual contact with an HIV-infected partner. Sexual activity enables exposure to blood, semen, and vaginal secretions, which contain lymphocytes that harbor HIV. Breaks in the skin caused by sexual trauma, such as anal intercourse or the presence of genital lesions from other sexually transmitted infections (STIs), will increase the risk of infection.

The majority of reported HIV infections in the United States are in men who have sex with men, including homosexuals, bisexuals, and prison population groups (CDC, 2005c). The incidence of HIV infection among men who have sex with men declined in the 1990s due to intense AIDS awareness and education campaigns and an emphasis on safer sex practices. However, current data indicate an increased incidence of unsafe sexual practices, and rising HIV infection rates in some urban areas among men who have sex with men. Recent data from the CDC indicates that number of HIV/AIDS diagnoses among men who have sex with men increased 85% between 2003 and 2004 (CDC, 2005c). This may be attributed in part to the association between the knowledge of the benefits of antiretroviral therapy in deterring HIV progression to AIDS and a relapse in high-risk sexual behaviors. The National Guidelines box (p. 1924) lists CDC guidelines for antiretroviral therapy.

Heterosexual HIV transmission is the most common method of infection in developing countries such as Africa and Asia, where approximately 90% of all new HIV infections occur worldwide (Johnsen, 2003). The rate of infection among women is rising steadily. The majority of women do not engage in high-risk behavior and practice monogamy, but are being infected

---

RISK FACTORS for HIV Infection

- Unprotected sex (sex without a male or female condom) with an HIV-infected male or female
- Sharing of injection equipment
- Blood product recipient (especially prior to screening in 1985)
- Infants born to mothers with HIV infection

Sources: Centers for Disease Control and Prevention. (2007, July). *HIV and AIDS: Are you at risk?* Retrieved September 3, 2008, from http://www.cdc.gov/hiv/resources/brochures/at-risk.htm; Kirton, C. D., Talotta, D., & Zwolski, K. (Eds.). (2001). *Handbook of HIV/AIDS nursing.* St. Louis, Mosby; Shaw, J. K., & Mahoney, E. A. (Eds.). (2003). *HIV/AIDS nursing secrets.* Philadelphia: Hanley & Belfus.

NATIONAL GUIDELINES for Antiretroviral Therapy in HIV Infections

Population	Guideline	Summary
Adults and adolescents	Guidelines for the Use of Antiretroviral Agents in HIV-1-Infected Adults and Adolescents (2006)	Guidelines for treating HIV-infected adults and adolescents, including utilization of resistance testing, initiation of HIV treatment, preferred first-line regimens, adverse events to antiretroviral medications, managing treatment-experienced patients, and considerations for special populations.
Pregnant women and infants	Recommendations for the Use of Antiretroviral Drugs in Pregnant HIV-1-Infected Women for Maternal Health and Interventions to Reduce Perinatal HIV-1 Transmission in the United States (2006)	Guidelines for treating HIV-infected pregnant women and interventions to prevent perinatal transmission, including information on drug regimens, safety and toxicity of medications, delivery options, and care of infants born to HIV-infected mothers.
Pediatric	Guidelines for the Use of Antiretroviral Agents in Pediatric HIV Infection (2006)	Guidelines for treating HIV-infected infants, children, and adolescents, including clinical monitoring, initiation of treatment, pediatric-specific drug information, and managing complications.
Health care workers exposed to HIV on the job	Updated U.S. Public Health Service Guidelines for the Management of Occupational Exposures to HIV and Recommendations for Postexposure Prophylaxis (2005)	Guidelines for the procedures and prevention measures that should be followed when workers are exposed to HIV on the job.
HIV-infected individuals	Guidelines for the Prevention of Opportunistic Infections in Persons Infected with Human Immunodeficiency Virus (2002)	Public Health Service and Infectious Diseases Society of America guidelines for the prevention of opportunistic infections in persons infected with HIV.
HIV-positive adults, adolescents, and children with infections	Treating Opportunistic Infections Among HIV-Infected Adults and Adolescents (2004) and Treating Opportunistic Infections Among HIV-Exposed and Infected Children (2004)	Guidelines for treatment of infections in individuals who are HIV infected or HIV exposed.
Individuals with TB and HIV	Treatment of Tuberculosis (2003)	Guidelines for the treatment for and management of people with tuberculosis.
HIV-positive individuals and partners	Incorporating HIV Prevention into the Medical Care of Persons Living with HIV (2003)	Recommendations of the CDC, NIH, Health Resources and Services Administration, and the HIV Medicine Association of the Infectious Diseases Society of America, including risk screening, behavior interventions, partner counseling and referrals, legal issues, partner notification.
HIV testing in the general population	Revised Recommendations for HIV Testing of Adults, Adolescents, and Pregnant Women in Health-Care Settings (2006)	Recommendations on HIV testing procedures for health care providers working in hospital emergency departments, urgent care clinics, inpatient services, substance abuse treatment clinics, public health clinics, community clinics, correctional health care facilities, and primary care settings. Recommendation for general HIV screening, with ability to "opt-out" instead of screening only high-risk or symptomatic individuals.

Note: All of the guidelines listed in this chart are available from http://aidsinfo.nih.gov.

Source: Bartlett, J. G., & Lane, H. C. (2007). *Guidelines for the use of antiretroviral agents in HIV-1-infected adults and adolescents. Developed by the DHHS Panel on Antiretroviral Guidelines for Adults and Adolescents—A working group of the Office of AIDS Research Advisory Council.* Retrieved January 10, 2008, from http://aidsinfo.nih.gov/contentfiles/AdultandAdolescentGL.pdf.

through unsafe sex practices with their HIV-infected male partners (UNAIDS, 2006). HIV-infected male-to-female transmission occurs more frequently than infected female-to-male transmission. This occurs because the risk of infection is greater for the partner who receives the semen and has a prolonged exposure to contact with the HIV-infected fluid.

Contaminated Needle Transmission

A major factor in the spread of HIV has been transmission by sharing of injection equipment. Used needles contain only a small amount of blood, but this can be contaminated with HIV. Drug preparation equipment used in mixing drugs can also be contaminated. If individuals are consistently sharing needles and equipment, as is common with illicit drug use, the potential for repeated exposure exists, which increases the risk of transmission. Sharing equipment to inject drugs is the major means of transmission in Eastern and Central Europe, East Asia, and the Pacific Islands (UNAIDS, 2006).

Contaminated Blood Products

Blood products prior to 1985 were not screened for HIV antibodies. As a result HIV-contaminated blood has been the cause of 2% of the adult and 8% of the reported AIDS cases in the United States (CDC, 2006a). Since 1985, with the use of HIV antibody screening on all blood transfusion products, this risk has been significantly reduced. The blood supply in the United States is among the safest in the world. More recently, blood screening tests have become available to detect for the virus through DNA testing prior to the production of antibodies. The risk of infection (estimated to be 1 in 2,000,000 transfusions) does still exist because of the **window period**, the time between actual HIV infection and when the tests can detect the presence of the virus or antibodies to the virus in blood. The length of the window period is currently 12 to 16 days (American Red Cross, 2003). Further discussion on blood product testing can be found in Chapter 23 .

Perinatal Transmission

HIV infection can be transmitted from an infected mother to her infant during pregnancy, at the time of delivery through exposure to the mother's blood, or after birth via breast-feeding. Multiple factors influence this potential for transmission. Blood is a highly infectious substance and the fetus receives oxygen, nutrients, antibodies, and other substances via the placental circulation. HIV antibodies are transmitted from an HIV-infected mother to the infant via placental circulation. This is why infants born to HIV-infected mothers will test positive for HIV antibodies immediately after birth. However, transmission of the virus may not have occurred.

The process of HIV-infected mother-to-infant transmission is not clearly understood. Researchers currently believe that the placenta actually plays a protective role, creating a barrier to HIV transmission, and that 60% of HIV mother-to-infant transmissions may occur at the time of delivery (Anderson, 2004). It is known that the risk of HIV mother-to-infant transmission is significantly increased if the mother has a high amount of HIV in circulation, an advanced AIDS disease, and/or breast-feeds. Research has clearly indicated that treatment of the mother during pregnancy with antiretroviral therapy and a short-term treatment of the infant postdelivery substantially reduce the risk of HIV mother-to-infant transmission (Branson et al., 2006). It is estimated that without maternal antiretroviral treatments 14% to 40% of infants born to HIV-infected mothers would be infected (Averitt & Sowell, 2003). The rate of perinatal infection is related to the mother's access to health care and antiretroviral therapy. In economically poor countries such as South Africa, where there is limited antiretroviral treatment and health care, infection rates are among the highest (UNAIDS, 2006).

The mode of delivery for HIV-infected women is an area of ongoing research and clinical debate. Increasing evidence supports the theory that use of cesarean sections in clinical situations where there is prolonged labor, or rupture of membranes greater than 4 hours before delivery, or a high viral load may help prevent prenatal transmission (Averitt & Sowell, 2003). Others argue that for women who have undetectable viral loads or who are on antiviral medications and have received adequate prenatal care a vaginal delivery may be a viable option. The Public Health Service Task Force (2006) recommends scheduled cesarean section for HIV-1 RNA (viral load) > 1,000 copies/mL. Because a cesarean section is a surgical procedure and also may present risks to the mother and infant, the Public Health Service Task Force (2006) recommends that viral load levels be evaluated at 34 to 36 weeks' gestation to enable discussion between the mother and her clinician as to the optimal delivery mode. There is general consensus that a cesarean section helps minimize the risk of perinatal transmission when viral loads are high. However, more research is needed in relationship to the benefits of cesarean section in specific clinical situations before it is deemed the accepted mode of delivery for all HIV-infected women.

Transmission to Health Care Workers

Health care workers, especially laboratory technicians and nurses, have a very small but real risk of occupational exposure to HIV transmission through needlestick injuries and mucous membrane exposure of infected patient body fluids. The CDC (2001) estimates that the average risk of HIV infection following a cut exposure or needlestick exposure to HIV-infected blood is 0.3%. The key factors in HIV infection of health care workers has been exposure to a large volume of blood delivered by a deep puncture, or extended contact with infected bloody dressings to open cuts on the health workers' hands, arms, or face (NIOSH, 1999).

To address these issues, the CDC together with the Hospital Infection Control Practices Advisory Committee (HICPAC) developed and mandated standard precautions to reduce the risk of blood and body fluid exposure and transmission of pathogens. Additionally, the Needlestick Safety and Prevention Act became law in 2000 and it mandates the use of needleless devices by all health care facilities to protect against sharps injuries. The nurse needs to remain vigilant in the use of standard precautions when working with any blood and body fluids. Appropriate use of needle guards and needleless medication administration systems and disposal of sharps in designated containers are essential.

In the event of a blood or body fluid exposure, the CDC in *Management of Occupational Blood Exposures* (2001) recommends that specific steps be taken. These include immediately washing the exposed site with soap and water and repeated flushing of exposed mucous membranes with water. The process of determining the risk of exposure, HIV testing of the source of contamination, and baseline HIV testing of the health care worker should also occur immediately. To facilitate this process, most health care facilities require urgent reporting of blood exposure incidents to the health care workers' supervisors and follow-up with employee health services for treatment and any additional testing.

The CDC recommends that health care workers who have had a significant blood or body fluid exposure be offered antiretroviral medications postexposure because some data suggest that such prophylaxis may significantly reduce the risk of HIV infection. However, the adverse effects of antiretroviral therapy can be substantial and this must be considered when evaluating the exposure risk and use of prophylactic antiretroviral therapy. The course of antiretroviral therapy is 4 weeks and should be started immediately or within 72 hours of exposure to be maximally effective (CDC, 2005a).

Pathophysiology

HIV belongs to a class of viruses made up of ribonucleic acid (RNA). Every virus is an obligate parasite that requires a living cell as the host. RNA viruses also are called retroviruses because they must be transcribed back into DNA through the action of an enzyme called **reverse transcriptase** in order to reproduce. In the process of infection, the virus first enters a cell with a specific type of receptor found on the surface of some cells called a CD4 receptor. Lymphocytes, called **CD4+ T cells**, are T-helper cells that have more CD4 receptor sites than other types of cells; therefore, they are the primary targets of infection (Rote, 2006). HIV entering the host stimulates a humoral and cell-mediated response that activates the immune system and recruits CD4+ T cells to the area of infection in the blood. As a result HIV is able to infect many CD4+ T cells in a short period (Porth & Sweeney, 2007). Other cells such as monocytes, macrophages, astrocytes (cells in the brain), and

oligodendrocytes (cells in the central nervous system) also have CD4 receptors, which explains why HIV may infect these cells.

After the viral particle enters the cell, reverse transcriptase creates a DNA particle from the RNA. The DNA particle enters the nucleus and inserts itself into the host's DNA. HIV DNA can then direct proteins and enzymes to replicate the HIV portion and create more HIV particles. Figure 60–5 ■ describes this process. It is important to understand the viral replication process because medications to control HIV infection are directed at different aspects of HIV replication. The human immunodeficiency virus is devastating to the host's immune system, specifically the CD4+ T cells. As previously discussed under normal immune function in Chapter 59 🔗, CD4+ T cells exist to help regulate the immune system. If an individual is unable to initiate an immune response because of the loss of T cells, even the most benign infection can be deadly.

HIV is a highly infective virus for several reasons. It replicates easily and rapidly and mutates frequently. These mutations make it extremely difficult to create a consistently effective drug or a vaccine because the shape of the HIV molecules changes frequently (Rote, 2006). Additionally, the normal number of CD4+ T cells is 800 to 1,200 microliter of blood, and competent T-helper cells live approximately 100 days. CD4+ T cells that

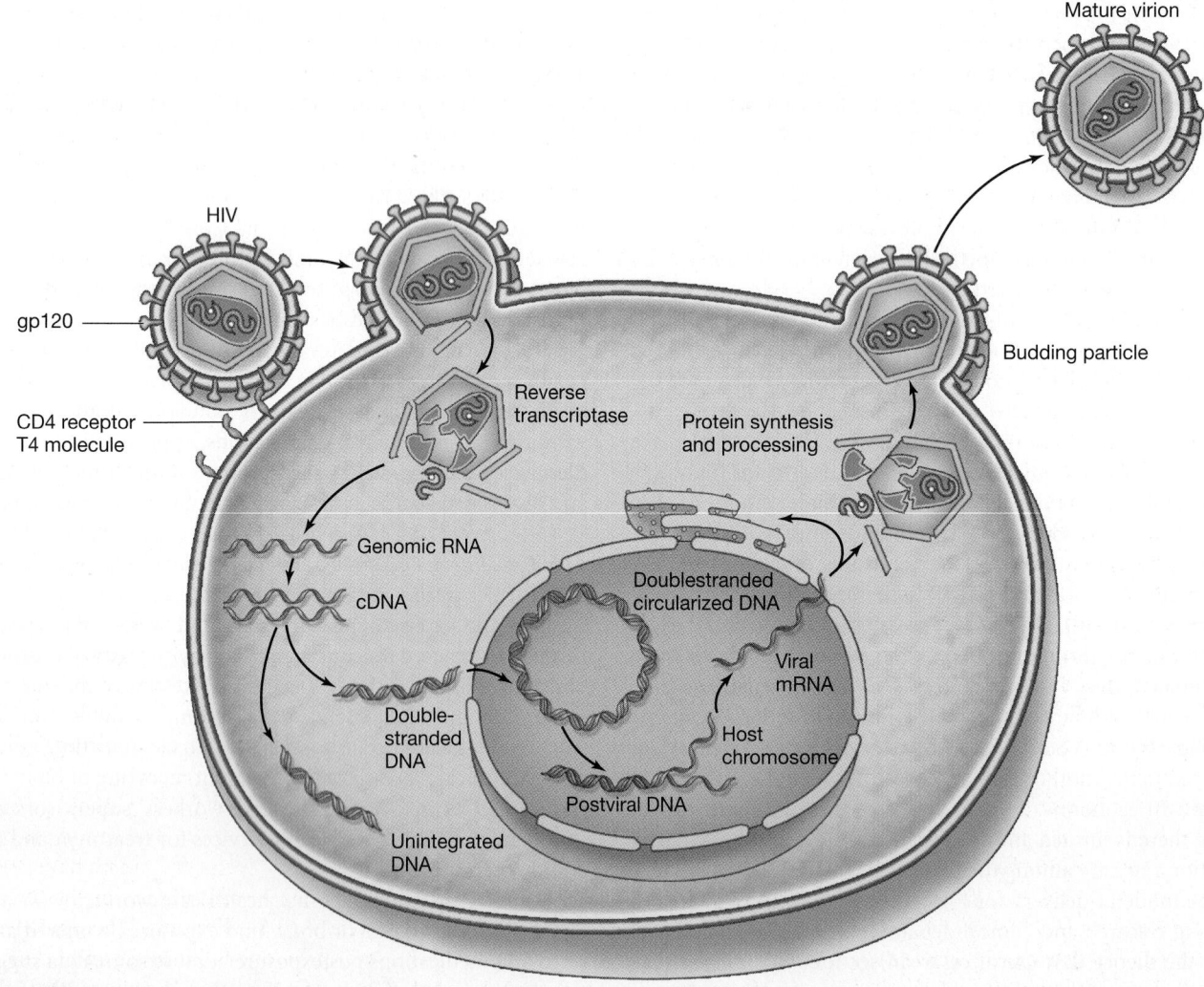

FIGURE 60–5 ■ HIV infecting CD4+ T cell.

have been infected with HIV are now known to live only 2 days (Fauci, 1996). It also is known that the infected host can adequately compensate for the loss of CD4+ T cells for several years. Research has shown the bone marrow to be capable of producing adequate cells despite the HIV infection destroying up to 1 billion CD4+ T cells per day for many years (Fauci, 1996).

Eventually, the immune system function and CD4+ T cells are overwhelmed by the virus and destroyed through several mechanisms. Every new HIV particle attaches to the cell membrane and buds outward as it breaks free of the host cell. When many HIV particles are released, holes develop in the plasma membrane. Cytoplasm and organelles can leak out, killing the cell. Lymphoid tissue also can house infected T cells and viral particles. Over time the degradation of the lymph system by HIV sheds additional virus into the blood. This has been shown to be a factor in the progression of the disease. Also, macrophages and monocytes can be infected with HIV. Macrophages become a reservoir for HIV because the molecule can replicate within the cell. Trauma, inflammation, and infection at the site of the macrophage can cause rupture of the macrophage and the release of HIV into surrounding tissue (DeFranco et al., 2007; Fauci, 1991). Additionally, as part of the normal immune response, antibodies to HIV attach to infected T-helper cells and stimulate the activation of the complement cascade. This results in the direct lysis of the cell membrane and death of the infected cell. Cell lysis by complement as explained in Chapters 59 and 63 ☺ also releases any completed viral particles into the host's system, further adding to the viral load.

Research is continuing to explore other mechanisms about how HIV destroys infected cells. Apoptosis or programmed cell death of infected cells is one theory currently being researched. Additionally, increased production of cytokines may be implicated in destruction of infected T-helper cells. Finally, superantigen and autoimmune responses also are being studied as possible mechanisms of cell destruction in HIV infection (DeFranco et al., 2007).

Stages of HIV/AIDS

The classification system of HIV infection and progression to AIDS was expanded and redefined by the CDC in 1993 to emphasize the significance of CD4+ T-cell counts as a marker of HIV-related immunosuppression. The subsequent classification system is based on two categories: clinical conditions associated with HIV infections and laboratory CD4+ T-cell counts. There are three major classifications that are differentiated by the clinical symptoms: A (asymptomatic), B (symptomatic, but not AIDS defining), and C (symptomatic AIDS indicator conditions). Three classifications also differentiate the CD4+ T-cell laboratory tests and are based on the declining number of CD4+ T cells per microliter of blood: category 1: >500 cells/μL; category 2: 200 to 400 cells/μL; and category 3: <200 cells/μL. Chart 60–8 (p. 1928) describes the CDC classification system. This classification system is important because it tracks the progression of the disease, helps determine the type and effectiveness of antiretroviral therapy, and determines if changes in therapy are required. It also provides clear definitions of AIDS diseases for research purposes, the results of which will facilitate more effective disease treatments.

Immediately following infection with HIV, the virus proliferates rapidly and the immune system begins to make antibodies against the virus. However, the viral replication of HIV increases more rapidly than the immune system is able to respond, resulting in a high **viral load** (the number of viral particles in a sample of blood). During the period of primary infection (1 to 3 weeks) the individual may by asymptomatic or display symptoms of **acute retroviral syndrome**, which is characterized by malaise, fever, lymphadenopathy, and skin rash. The fact that an infected individual can be asymptomatic or have only vague, flu-like symptoms makes early diagnosis of HIV infection difficult (Porth & Sweeney, 2007).

Additionally, the first months after infection encompass the "window period" in which the infected individual has not produced sufficient HIV antibodies that can be measured by an HIV antibody test. The window period usually lasts up to 3 months, but can extend to 6 months in some individuals. During the window period HIV antibody tests are negative, even in the presence of HIV infection. HIV antigen tests are now available that can detect the presence of viral particles as early as 2 weeks after infection; however, a window period still remains. These facts coupled with the initial high viral load are major contributing factors to the spread of HIV among those engaging in high-risk behaviors (Branson et al., 2006).

In the months following initial infection, proliferation of the virus, and stimulation of the immune responses, the viral load stabilizes. During this period of time, immune responses slow replication, but the virus is not completely eliminated. The infected individual in this first stage of HIV infection may show signs of an acute infection such as fatigue, fever, and generalized lymphadenopathy. It is during this time (usually between 3 weeks to 3 months after initial infection) that the individual converts to **HIV antibody positive status**, also referred to as *seropositive status*. This indicates that there is infection with HIV that is resulting in the production of HIV antibodies (Shaw, 2003). In some individuals conversion to HIV seropositive antibody status may take as long as 6 months. The individual may remain in category A, a relatively symptom-free stage for as long as 8 to 10 years, although the viral replication is active and will increase substantially as the immune system deteriorates (Porth & Sweeney, 2007).

Progression to category B HIV is defined by a transition from asymptomatic status to generalized symptoms. These symptoms may include but are not limited to fever of unknown origin, oral or vaginal candidiasis, herpes zoster, shingles, peripheral neuropathy, or pelvic inflammatory disease.

Category C is **AIDS indicator conditions**. A diagnosis of AIDS is made when the HIV-infected individual is diagnosed with an opportunistic infection or an AIDS defining cancer or when the CD4+ T-cell count falls below 200 cells/μL. Examples of AIDS defining diseases include PCP, toxoplasmosis, cytomegalovirus, non-Hodgkin's lymphoma, and Kaposi's sarcoma.

It is important that nurses understand the pathophysiology of HIV/AIDS and the specific stages of HIV disease and progression to AIDS because of the significant role nurses have in patient education about HIV/AIDS, transmission of the disease, and purpose of the prescribed medications. This knowledge base will also enable the nurse to identify issues and necessary nursing interventions specific to the different categories of HIV/AIDS. For example, an infected individual in category A

CHART 60–8 **Classification System for HIV Infection and Expanded AIDS Surveillance Case Definition for Adolescents and Adults**

Clinical Category A Asymptomatic, Acute HIV	Clinical Category B Symptomatic, But Not Category C Conditions	Clinical Category C AIDS-Defining Conditions
One or more of the conditions listed below in an adolescent (≥13 years) with documented HIV infection and no conditions in categories B or C: • Asymptomatic HIV infection • Persistent generalized lymphadenopathy • Acute HIV infection with accompanying illness (acute retroviral syndrome) or history of acute infection **CD4+ T-Cell Count Categories** A1 ≥ 500 cells/µL A2 ≥ 200–499 cells/µL A3 ≤ 200 cells/µL	Examples of conditions in category B include but are not limited to: • Candidiasis: oropharyngeal (thrush) • Candidiasis: vulvovaginal (persistent, frequent, or resistant to therapy) • Cervical dysplasia/cervical carcinoma *in situ* • Constitutional symptoms: persistent fever (38.5°C) or diarrhea lasting for more than 1 month • Hairy leukoplakia (oral) • Herpes zoster involving two distinct episodes, or more than 1 dermatome • Idiopathic thrombocytopenic purpura • Pelvic inflammatory disease • Peripheral neuropathy **CD4+ T-Cell Count Categories** B1 ≥ 500 cells/µL B2 ≥ 200–499 cells/µL B3 ≤ 200 cells/µL	• Candidiasis of bronchi, trachea, lungs, or esophagus • Cervical cancer (invasive) • Coccidioidomycosis • Cryptococcosis • Cryptosporidiosis with chronic diarrhea for more than 1 month • Cytomegalovirus disease (other than liver, spleen, or nodes) • Encephalopathy (HIV related) • Herpes simplex: chronic ulcers, bronchitis, pneumonitis, or esophagitis • Histoplasmosis • Isosporiasis with diarrhea for more than 1 month • Kaposi's sarcoma • Lymphoma: Burkitt's, immunoblastic, primary brain • *Mycobacterium avium* complex • *Mycobacterium tuberculosis* • *Pneumocystis carinii* pneumonia • Pneumonia (recurrent) • Wasting syndrome due to HIV **CD4+ T-Cell Count Categories** C1 ≥ 500 cells/µL C2 ≥ 200–499 cells/µL C3 ≤ 200 cells/µL

Note: As of January 1, 1993, individuals with category C conditions and those in categories A3 and B3 were considered to have AIDS.

Sources: Adapted from Centers for Disease Control and Prevention. (1993). Revised classification system for HIV infection and the expanded surveillance case definition of AIDS among adolescents and adults. *Morbidity and Mortality Weekly Report, 44* (RR-17). Retrieved February 23, 2007, from http://www.cdc.gov/mmwr/preview/mmwrhtml/00018871.htm; Centers for Disease Control and Prevention. (1999). Appendix: Revised surveillance case definition for HIV infection. *Morbidity and Mortality Weekly Report, 45* (RR-13), 29–31; Porth, C., & Sweeney, K. (2007). Alterations in immune response. In C. M. Porth (Ed.), *Essentials of pathophysiology* (pp. 293–319). St. Louis: Lippincott Williams & Wilkins.

---

with a latent infection will need educational information focused on avoiding transmitting the disease and new medications, whereas care for the individual with a declining CD4 count in category B will focus more on infection prevention, symptom management, and medication adherence.

Clinical Manifestations of HIV/AIDS

The clinical manifestations of HIV/AIDS are varied and may affect almost any organ in the body. Nurses need to understand the causes, signs and symptoms, diagnostic tests, and possible medical interventions in order to plan collaboratively for patient care. This will enable the nurse to provide appropriate nursing interventions and promote comfort measures that enhance the quality of life for patients with HIV/AIDS throughout the course of the disease. The specific clinical manifestations related to the opportunistic infections are outlined next.

Opportunistic Infections and Malignancies

Opportunistic infections (OI) occur in HIV-infected individuals as the virus destroys sufficient numbers of CD4+ T cells and the body is not able to protect itself. As CD4+ counts drop to <200 cells/µL the incidence of opportunistic infection accelerates rapidly. Malignancies occur due to impairment in the immune system's ability to recognize and destroy abnormal cells that are regulated, in part, by T-cell function.

Diseases associated with HIV/AIDS are a result of impairment of the immune system that leaves the HIV-infected individuals susceptible to OIs and malignancies. Diseases also can be the direct result of the effects of HIV on specific tissue, as seen in AIDS-related GI and neurological dysfunction. Chart 60–9 describes the clinical manifestations of the most common opportunistic diseases associated with HIV/AIDS, as well as the diagnostic tests and medical treatment the nurse needs to anticipate coordinating as part of collaborative care.

CHART 60–9 HIV/AIDS: Common Opportunistic Diseases

Clinical Manifestation by Body System	Possible Opportunistic Infection or Disease	Diagnostic Tests and Findings	Medical Treatment	Nursing Critical Assessments
Respiratory				
1. Increased respirations, nonproductive cough, dyspnea on exertion, adventitious breath sounds, increased, hypoxemia	1. *Pneumocystis carinii* pneumonia (PCP)	1. CD4 < 200 cells/μL Chest x-ray (bilateral patchy infiltrates), sputum culture or bronchoalveolar lavage (+ culture growth for PCP)	1. Antibiotic therapy (trimethoprim-sulfamethoxazole [TMP-SMZ]), bronchodilator therapy	1 & 2 & 3 Respiratory rate, work of breathing, auscultate breath sounds, pulse oximetry saturation, sputum color/amount, monitor arterial blood gases (ABGs), to determine need for oxygen and ventilation support
2. Dyspnea, productive cough, blood-tinged sputum 1 & 2 General body system: fever, night sweats, fatigue, weight loss are common to almost all respiratory opportunistic infections	2. *Mycobacterium tuberculosis* (TB)	2. TB skin test, chest x-ray, sputum for AFB stain and culture	2. Isoniazid (INH), ethambutol (Myambutol), rifampin (Rifadin), pyrazinamide	
3. Increasing shortness of breath eventually progressing to respiratory failure	3. Kaposi's sarcoma	3. Chest x-ray, bronchoscopy examination and biopsy	3. Chemotherapy, radiation, alpha-interferon to decrease tumor size	
Gastrointestinal (GI)				
1. Inflamed oral mucosa, GI pain/cramping, bloody diarrhea, weight loss	1. Cytomegalovirus (CMV)	1. Stool specimen for examination and culture, endoscopy exam, biopsy, and culture	1. Medications: foscarnet (Foscavir), ganciclovir (Cytovene), cidofovir (Vistide)	1 & 2 Daily fluid intake and output, diarrhea, daily weight, oral intake (calorie count) Laboratory tests: complete blood count (CBC), electrolytes, blood urea nitrogen (BUN), serum albumin and transferrin levels
2. Anorexia, diarrhea, nausea, vomiting, weight loss, abdominal pain	2. *Mycobacterium avium* complex (MAC)	2. Stool specimen and culture, small bowel biopsy with AFB stain and culture	2. Antibiotic treatment when T cells < 100 cells/μL clarithromycin, (Biaxin), azithromycin (Zithromax), ciprofloxacin (Cipro), rifampin (Rifadin)	
3. White patches in mouth, throat, tongue that bleeds if scraped, redness in oral cavity, → pain and difficulty swallowing, progressing to esophagus	3. Oral candidiasis	3. Microscope exam and culture of lesion scraping	3. Antifungals: Clotrimazole troches or Nystatin topical, po/IV fluconazole (Diflucan), clotrimazole (Lotrimin), itraconazole, amphotericin B (Fungizone)	3. Oral cavity, pain with swallowing, po intake ability
4. Anorexia, weight loss >10%, chronic diarrhea, fever >30 days unknown origin, chronic weakness, decreased muscle mass	4. HIV wasting (HIV causes changes to GI cells)	4. Rule out other causes: stool specimen and culture, endoscopy exam biopsy and culture	4. Symptom management • Diarrhea: octreotide acetate (Sandostatin) • Skin breakdown: barrier creams • Nutrition: appetite stimulant (Megestrol) • NV: antiemetic, Dronabinol • Oral nutritional supplement: Advera	4. Daily fluid I&O, diarrhea, daily weight, po intake (calorie count) Laboratory tests: CBC, electrolytes, BUN, serum albumin and transferrin levels

(continued)

CHART 60–9 **HIV/AIDS: Common Opportunistic Diseases—*Continued***

Neurological

1. Forgetfulness, decreased attention and concentration, progressive impaired motor function	1. HIV encephalopathy (virus causes dysfunction of neuro cells)	1. Rule out opportunistic infections or malignancy: cultures of blood, CSF; CT scan, MRI	1. Antiretroviral therapy, comfort measures, symptom management for any other clinical manifestations	1. Orientation, ability to remember medications, level of self-care with ADLs, gait, and risk of falling
2. Headaches, sensory and visual deficits, dizziness, aphasia, seizures, personality changes	2. Primary brain lymphoma	2. Tests listed above	2. Chemotherapy/ radiation	2. Same as above
3. Headache, decreased level of consciousness, fever, stiff neck, visual changes, seizures	3. Cryptococcal meningitis	3. CT scan, CSF analysis, serum antigen test	3. Antifungal medications: amphotericin B (Fungizone), fluconazole (Diflucan), flucytosine (Ancobon), itraconazole (Sporanox)	3. Level of consciousness, neurological function, symptoms of infection (fever, stiff neck, WBC)
4. Pain, numbness in extremities, general weakness, decreased deep tendon reflexes, impotence	4. HIV peripheral neuropathy (caused by HIV demyelinating disorder)	4. Rule out other potential causes by above tests	4. Neurontin for pain	4. Neurological function, pain, changes in sexual patterns

Skin

1. Nonblanching, flat or raised purple-brown lesions Progression of various shapes and sizes	1. Kaposi's sarcoma	1. Biopsy of lesion	1. Liquid nitrogen or cryotherapy to skin lesions, radiation of lesions, chemotherapy, alpha-interferon to decrease tumor size	1. Inspect skin for raised or flat purple-brown lesions of various sizes, pain or discomfort, changes in any other body system such GI and respiratory
2. Ulcer lesions of oral and nasal mucosa or ulcer lesions of the genital and perianal mucosa	2. Herpes simplex virus type 1 (HSV1) oral, herpes simplex virus type 2 (HSV2)	2. Viral culture	2. Antiviral medications: acyclovir (Zovirax), famciclovir (Famvir), valacyclovir (Valtrex), foscarnet (Foscavir)	2. Ask patient regarding pain/discomfort of mouth or perianal area. Inspect mucous membranes of the mouth, nose, and perianal area

Eyes

Visual changes: "seeing spots," unilateral visual loss → bilateral loss → blindness	Cytomegalovirus (CMV)	Ophthalmoscope examination	T-cell counts < 50 cells/μL = antiviral (ganciclovir or foscarnet), not curable infection, medication must be taken for life. Side effects of medications are significant and can interfere with HAART	Decreased vision ability, visual fields, presence of "spots," ability to read medication labels and identify drug and dose to take

CHART 60–9 HIV/AIDS: Common Opportunistic Diseases—*Continued*

Female Genitalia/ Sexual Health

1. Genital itching, bleeding between menses, redness/swelling of external genitalia, white or yellow cheeselike discharge	1. Vaginal candidiasis	1. Microscopic examination and culture of lesion scraping	1. Antifungal medications: fluconazole (Diflucan), clotrimazole (Lotrimin), severe/incurable infection with above medications = amphotericin B (Fungizone)	1. Sexual health risk factors including multiple sex partners, unprotected sex, changes in genitalia or new discharge. Color of genitalia and presence of redness, vaginal discharge
2. Bleeding between menses or after intercourse; foul-smelling, blood-tinged vaginal discharge	2. Cervical intraepithelial neoplasia or cervical cancer	2. Cervical colposcopic examination and cone biopsy	2. Chemotherapy and radiation	2. Sexual health risk factors as above. Changes in menses bleeding or unusual vaginal discharge

Sources: Carpenito-Moyet, L. (2008). *Nursing care plans and documentation* (5th ed.). Philadelphia: Lippincott Williams & Wilkins; Corless, I. B., & Nicholas, P. K. (2003). Nursing care of patients with HIV/AIDS. In J. K. Shaw & E. A. Mahoney (Eds.), *HIV/AIDS nursing secrets* (pp. 33–39). Philadelphia: Hanley & Belfus; Crowe, S., Hoy, J., & Mills, J. (Eds.). (2002). *Management of the HIV-infected patient.* London: Taylor & Francis; Kirton, C. D., Talotta, D., & Zwolski, K. (Eds.). (2001). *Handbook of HIV/AIDS nursing.* St. Louis, Mosby; Porth, C., & Sweeney, K. (2007). Alterations in immune response. In C. M. Porth (Ed.), *Essentials of pathophysiology* (pp. 293–319). St. Louis: Lippincott Williams & Wilkins.

The last column lists critical assessment issues that need to be the focus of nursing assessment. This information provides more detail on specific AIDS-related diseases to enhance the nurse's understanding of these clinical manifestations.

Pneumocystis carinii Pneumonia

***Pneumocystis carinii* pneumonia (PCP)** is an opportunistic fungal respiratory infection that can develop in severely immunosuppressed individuals. In the early years of the AIDS epidemic, 75% of HIV-infected patients developed PCP at some point in their illness. Advances in disease understanding and treatment with prophylactic antibiotic therapy and corticosteroids have resulted in a decrease in the incidence of PCP. PCP is a fungal infection that proliferates in the alveoli causing bronchial consolidation. Chest x-ray results will indicate bilateral patchy infiltrates. PCP results in symptoms of acute respiratory failure with decreasing arterial oxygen levels to less than 70%, and increased work of breathing, which, if left untreated, will result in respiratory arrest and death (Judd & Mijch, 2002).

Mycobacterium Tuberculosis *Mycobacterium tuberculosis* (TB) is another prevalent bacterial disease that is predominantly associated with infection, but also can be manifested in blood and cerebrospinal fluid (CSF). Unlike PCP respiratory infections, TB usually occurs early in continuum of HIV infection, often preceding a diagnosis of HIV infection. The CDC estimates that approximately 30% of TB cases among people ages 25 to 44 are occurring in HIV-infected individuals. Additionally, because the HIV infection impairs the immune system so severely, people infected with HIV and TB have a 100 times greater risk of developing active TB and becoming infectious, compared to people not infected with HIV (CDC, 2003b).

In patients who have TB, purified protein derivative (PPD), the laboratory test for detecting TB, will test positive early in HIV infections. As the immune system fails with progressing HIV disease, patients who have TB will usually have negative PPD tests because the appropriate immune response cannot be mounted to the PPD antigen. Conclusive diagnostic testing for TB is done by chest x-ray and acid-fast bacillus testing of sputum, blood, or CSF.

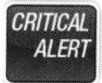 *Individuals who present with a persistent cough, night sweats, and fever should be tested for TB. If they have a positive TB test and the individual engages in high-risk behaviors, HIV testing should be discussed and encouraged.*

Hepatitis Virus B and C Hepatitis virus B (HVB) and hepatitis virus C (HVC) are common opportunist infections in HIV-infected individuals because both are transmitted through shared body fluids such as blood, semen, and vaginal secretions, and high-risk behaviors promote the spread of both infections. Hepatitis is more easily transmitted because fewer hepatitis viral particles are required to initiate an infection than with HIV. Transmission by large or repeated exposures to contaminated blood by skin punctures is the most common mode of infection. Hence, the CDC estimates that 50% to 90% of HIV-positive injection drug users are also infected with HVC. Co-infection with HVC is present in approximately one-quarter of HIV-infected persons in the United States (CDC, 2005b).

The hepatitis virus affects liver function including metabolism of drugs, production of clotting factors, production of glucose and albumin, and filtering of waste, all of which contribute to the wasting syndrome in HIV. A combined HIV/HVB infection will increase morbidity and mortality due to the diminished function of both the immune system and the liver (CDC, 2005b). Therefore, the current U.S. Public Health Service/ Infectious Diseases Society of America guidelines recommend HVB screening of all HIV-infected persons to promote early identification and treatment of HVB co-infection to reduce risk of chronic liver disease (Workowski & Berman, 2006).

***Mycobacterium Avium* Complex** Another leading opportunistic infection is *Mycobacterium avium* complex (MAC), which includes a group of organisms (*M. avium, M. intracellulare,* and *M. scrofulaceum*). These organisms are usually found in food, water, and soil. They can cause respiratory infections, but most often are found in the GI tract, bone marrow, and lymph nodes. MAC infections are a major cause of severe weight loss and chronic diarrhea. Severe weight loss in persons with AIDS and a MAC infection is associated with T-cell counts less than 100 and high mortality rates.

In addition to MAC infections, other opportunistic pathogens such as cytomegalovirus (CMV) and candidiasis also affect the GI tract. CMV and MAC infections result in changes to the gastrointestinal lining that cause anorexia, chronic diarrhea, GI malabsorption, and significant weight loss. These are all symptoms of wasting syndrome, which is associated with a category C case definition of AIDS and is discussed next.

Wasting Syndrome **Wasting syndrome**, one of the hallmark clinical manifestations of AIDS-related diseases, is defined as:

- A loss of lean body tissue from increased protein metabolism
- Changes in metabolic rates
- Anorexia and diarrhea.

Diagnostic criteria include chronic diarrhea for more than 30 days, weight loss of greater than 10% from baseline, and chronic weakness. Antiretroviral therapy and the production of lactic acid can be contributing causes (Bartlett, 2003). Tumor necrosis factor (TNF) and other cytokines have been implicated in research as a contributing factor that increases metabolic rate, anorexia, and metabolism of proteins. TNF and cytokines are described in detail in Chapter 59 . However, no conclusive studies have shown a direct effect from cytokine levels. Wasting syndrome is associated with severe debilitation in the advanced stages of AIDS.

Candidiasis Candidiasis is a fungal opportunist infection that affects virtually all patients with AIDS. Oral candidiasis creates white patches in the mouth that can extend into the esophagus and stomach. This can make swallowing difficult and painful and significantly decrease oral intake due to discomfort. This places the patient at even greater risk for malnutrition and fluid and electrolyte imbalance. Also of concern is the fact that oral lesions can allow dissemination of the candidiasis into the bloodstream, causing a fungal sepsis that is life threatening.

 **CRITICAL ALERT** *Frequent and thorough oral assessment and care by the nurse is essential for the patient with oral candidiasis to maintain intact mucous membranes and prevent the spread of systemic infection by oral lesions.*

Candidiasis infection in skinfolds can lead to extensive skin breakdown. This is extremely uncomfortable for the patient and can lead to the development of a systemic fungal infection (see Figure 60–6). Vaginal candidiasis in HIV-infected women is a frequent and recurrent problem. Women with AIDS also have a higher incidence of pelvic inflammatory disease (PID). The diagnosis and treatment of PID are discussed in Chapter 49 . As result of their immune-suppressed state, HIV-infected women with PID frequently require inpatient treatment with IV antibiotics.

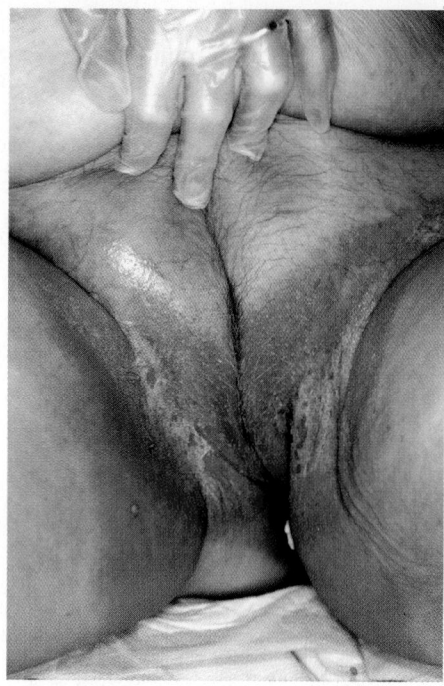

FIGURE 60–6 ■ Candidiasis in skinfolds.
Source: ISM/Phototake NYC

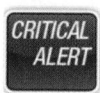 **CRITICAL ALERT** *Frequent and persistent vaginal candidiasis may be the first sign of HIV infection in a woman.*

Herpes Zoster and Herpes Simplex Herpes zoster and herpes simplex viral infections are common in patients with HIV or AIDS. Herpes infections recur in any individual who has been infected because the virus remains in human DNA neurons. Stress, infections, and surgery can all stimulate a recurrence of shingles (herpes zoster) and/or cold sores (herpes simplex). For HIV-positive individuals, the risk of repeated exacerbations of herpes is increased due to the decreased ability to mount an immune response.

Other Infectious Organisms and Disease Processes
Opportunistic infections also are responsible for many of the neurological changes associated with AIDS. The majority of individuals with AIDS have neurological alterations at some point during the disease process. Cryptococcus is a fungus that causes a meningitis infection, mental changes, and seizures. TB and CMV infections are also implicated in neurological alteration. Additionally, CMV causes retinitis, which is the leading cause of blindness in patients with AIDS.

AIDS dementia complex is a major factor in decreased neurological function. Approximately 20% of patients with AIDS have the disorder (Brew, 2002). AIDS dementia is not caused by an opportunistic pathogen, but by actual changes to the neuro cells due to the HIV infection. The brain cells infected by HIV are predominantly the monocyte-macrophage CD4 cells. It is believed that HIV causes the release of chemicals that result in destruction of the cell and interfere with the neurotransmission needed for normal cerebral function (Porth & Sweeney, 2007). The clinical manifestations of these changes are a progressive decline in cognitive, motor, and behavioral functions. Initially memory deficits will occur, progressing to confusion, hallucinations, seizures, coma, and death.

Oncologic Manifestations

Patients with HIV/AIDS have an increased incidence of cancer. As cell-mediated immunity declines, malignant cells are not identified and destroyed internally, as they would be by an intact immune system. This leads to the development of the secondary cancers included in the CDC's classification of AIDS diseases: Kaposi's sarcoma, B-cell lymphoma (non-Hodgkin's), primary lymphoma of the brain, and invasive cervical carcinoma.

Kaposi's sarcoma is a malignancy involving the endothelial layer of the blood and lymphatic vessels and is the most common AIDS-related cancer. This is not surprising given the fact that lymphatic tissues are an integral part of the immune system where HIV infection resides and replicates. Raised or flat cutaneous lesions can appear anywhere on the body and are deep purple to brown and/or pink in color. The lesions can progress rapidly and cause extensive disfigurement, disruption in skin integrity, venous stasis, lymphedema, and pain. Lesions also can develop in internal organs rich in lymphatic tissue, such as the lining of the GI tract, and the lungs. This can lead to extensive tissue damage, organ failure, and death.

 *Kaposi's sarcoma often develops on the face, resulting in extensive disfigurement and increasing feelings of social isolation and depression in the patient with AIDS. Nursing interventions are focused on addressing issues of altered body image and social isolation to maximize self-acceptance and support and decrease the risk of depression.*

Lymphomas are malignancies of the lymphoid tissue that can be located anywhere in the body. The two lymphomas commonly associated with AIDS are non-Hodgkin's lymphoma and primary lymphoma of the brain. AIDS-related lymphomas differ from lymphomas found in the general population in that they are more aggressive tumors and tend to develop outside the lymph nodes, most commonly in the brain. Primary brain lymphoma is rapidly growing and is highly resistant to treatment. Common sites of non-Hodgkin's lymphomas are found in the bone marrow, liver, GI tract, mucous membranes, and the skin. Chemotherapy is frequently not successful in AIDS-associated non-Hodgkin's lymphoma because of prevalent immunosuppressive status and the complications that occur with opportunistic infections.

Invasive cervical carcinoma is a major complication for HIV-infected women. HIV-infected women have a 10 times greater prevalence of cervical dysplasia, which is a precursor lesion for cervical cancer, than women not infected with HIV (Kaplan, Masur, & Holmes, 2002). To promote early treatment and prevent the development of invasive cervical cancer, it is recommended that HIV-infected women have Papanicolaou (Pap) smears every 6 months and aggressive treatment with cone biopsy if pap smears are abnormal (see Chapter 49). To emphasize the importance of integrating gynecologic care into medical services for HIV-infected women, the CDC included invasive cervical cancer in the 1993 *Revised Classification System for HIV Infection.* HIV-infected women with cervical malignancy most commonly die of cervical cancer as opposed to other opportunistic diseases. Chapter 49 discusses STIs and the associated treatments.

Medical Management

There is no cure for HIV infection. Development of an HIV vaccine to prevent HIV infection or control HIV progression to AIDS has not been successful thus far. However, advancements in antiviral medication treatments have slowed the progression of HIV infection and have provided new opportunities and challenges for medical treatment of the patient with HIV/AIDS. Initial medical treatment involves identification of patients at risk, followed by diagnostic testing and counseling. Individuals who are positive for HIV infection may be started on antiretroviral therapy. Medical management also involves identification and treatment of OIs and symptom control that optimizes comfort and quality of life for the patient with HIV/AIDS.

Laboratory and Diagnostic Procedures

Tests that screen for HIV antibodies in the blood have a high degree of reliability and are used in diagnosing HIV infection. Testing for HIV antibodies also can be done on oral fluids and urine. The issue with antibody testing is the window period discussed earlier, in which infection is present, but antibodies are not detected by current test technology. The HIV antibody testing process described in the Diagnostic Tests box (p. 1934) produces highly accurate results that take 1 to 2 weeks to complete and involves pretest and post-test counseling.

Tests that determine the presence of a viral load (i.e., the number of copies of HIV antigens in a sample of blood) also have been developed. However, these tests are labor intensive and expensive and not used for routine HIV screening. The exception to this is the presence of clinical symptoms consistent with acute retroviral syndrome, which occurs during the window period where antibody testing will be negative (Bartlett & Lane, 2007). Viral load levels are routinely monitored on patients with confirmed HIV infection to determine antiretroviral medication needs.

In 2002 the FDA approved the OraQuick Rapid HIV-1 Antibody test and has subsequently approved three other rapid HIV tests that screen for HIV antibodies and return results in 15 to 60 minutes (CDC, 2006b). The benefit of this testing is that test results are immediately discussed with the individual, and he or she is informed that all positive tests are sent for confirmation by further antibody testing. The rapid HIV tests have a high degree of specificity (99%) and can be used in routine screening in emergency departments and labor and delivery suites.

Rapid HIV tests also have been studied as an outreach screening tool for high-risk groups such as those in chemical dependency programs, homeless shelters, gay youth drop-in centers, or prostitute support programs. The benefit of this type of screening is that it provides immediate results and increased rates of post-test counseling, which can potentially help prevent HIV transmission and initiate appropriate early treatment. The major disadvantage of rapid HIV testing is that there is a slightly higher rate of false-positive tests, and all positive tests must be confirmed with more HIV-sensitive and specific **Western blot (WB)** tests (Greenwald, Burstein, Pincus, & Branson, 2006).

HIV testing is confidential. Most states require written informed consent documentation prior to testing. However, in 2006 the CDC released revised recommendations for HIV testing of adults, adolescents, and pregnant women in health care settings that represents a radical departure from current testing practices, which focus on testing at-risk populations only.

DIAGNOSTIC TESTS for HIV and Patient Counseling

Test	Expected Abnormality	Rationale for Abnormality and Patient Counseling and Education
The following tests are for diagnostic screening of HIV antibodies:	CDC current recommendations call for HIV screening in all health care settings for adults, adolescents, and pregnant women once they are notified of testing, unless the individual declines (opt-out screening). This represents a change from HIV testing based on individuals with risk factors to HIV testing as a routine part of medical care. Many health care facilities are in the process of implementing these guidelines. Pretest counseling is not required in the current recommendations for acute care settings because the time-consuming nature of such counseling may decrease screening recommendation implementation. However, individuals being tested for HIV are often afraid to find out the test results. Providing a supportive open environment for counseling and education is an important aspect of nursing care.	*Screening Rationale:* Increase screening, foster earlier detection of HIV infection, identify and counsel persons with unrecognized HIV infection to enable treatment and reduce transmission of HIV. Routine screening as part of diagnostic work-up for illness can facilitate earlier diagnosis and treatment with HAART. *Pretest counseling:* • Establish a therapeutic relationship. • Inform of the benefits of testing. • Provide information about the test and testing procedures. Include the fact that all positive tests are confirmed with a second test. • Inform that obtaining results may require returning for a second visit, or may be available same day depending on the type of testing. • For individuals with identified risk factors, encourage annual screening. • Provide education regarding preventing of HIV transmission.
Enzyme immunoassay (EIA; previous test was the ELISA): Detects the presence of serum antibodies that bind to HIV antigens. Test requires two visits, testing, and then discussion of results/counseling process. Results take 2–3 days.	EIA results that are negative for antibodies are reported as negative tests. EIA tests that are positive are repeated. If the second EIA test is positive, a Western blot test is ordered.	*Rationale for EIA abnormality:* Positive antibodies indicate infection with HIV antigen that has caused the immune system to produce HIV antibodies. Negative test results do not need to be confirmed with a second test. Post-test counseling for the individual with risk factors who is HIV negative or who has an indeterminate test should include: • Discussion of risk behaviors and the possibility of false-negative tests during the window period. • If recent risk behaviors are identified, encourage follow-up testing at 3 weeks, 6 weeks, 3 months, and 6 months. • Reinforcement education regarding prevention of HIV transmission.
Western blot (WB) test: Antibody test with great sensitivity and specificity used to confirm presence of HIV antibodies. Results take 1–3 days.	Western blot results that are negative for antibodies are reported as negative tests; positive tests are reported as positive for HIV infection. Blood that tests positive is reported as HIV-antibody positive (seropositive) and confirms a diagnosis of HIV infection.	*Rationale for Western blot:* Confirms HIV antibodies. Has a lower false-positive rate than the EIA. Negative results indicate no infection with HIV antigen. Post-test counseling for the individual with an HIV-antibody positive test should include: • Provide emotional support. • Inform that test results indicate HIV infection, but that this does not necessarily indicate AIDS and further testing is needed. • Provide referrals and discuss options for treatment including antiretroviral treatment, HIV clinic referrals, and need for baseline testing on CD4+ T-cell counts and HIV viral load levels. • Discuss the variety of effective treatments to encourage hope. Discuss follow-up lab tests. • Determine the level of social support available. • Help the individual identify partners who need testing. • Provide information on HIV support groups and community resources. • Reinforce education information on prevention of HIV transmission.

DIAGNOSTIC TESTS for HIV and Patient Counseling—*Continued*

Test	Expected Abnormality	Rationale for Abnormality and Patient Counseling and Education
Rapid HIV antibody tests: Immunoassay screening tests for HIV antibodies that provide results in 10–60 minutes. OraQuick (OraQuick Advance) rapid 1. HIV-1/HIV-2 antibody test 2. Reveal G2 rapid HIV-1 antibody test 3. Uni-Gold Recombigen HIV test 4. Multispot HIV-1/HIV-2 rapid test	All rapid HIV tests detect antibodies with sensitivities similar to EIAs, do not require instruments, and are interpreted visually. HIV antigens are fixed to the reagent strip; if HIV antibodies are present in the blood specimen, they affix to the antigen. The kit's colorimetric reagent binds to these antibody–antigen complexes to create a color change that is a visual indicator positive for antibodies. Results are available in approximately 20 minutes. A negative test requires no further confirmation test. A positive test is then confirmed by a Western blot test.	*Rationale for rapid HIV antibody tests:* Provides results in same visit as test to decrease rate of patients failing to return for confirmatory HIV test results, reduces barriers to early diagnosis of HIV, and increases access to treatment and prevention services. • Initially used predominately in community-based programs, and sex-worker outreach clinics for rapid identification of HIV, and in labor and delivery in acute care settings to minimize risk of perinatal transmission. Increased use in all health care settings encouraged as part of CDC recommendations to increase HIV screening (CDC, 2006c). • Inform patient that results will be available the same visit and that confirmatory testing is needed if the rapid test result is reactive. • Be supportive and prepared to give results along with counseling and referrals. • If result is negative inform patient that he/she is not infected, unless there was risk of exposure in the last 3 months. Then retesting is recommended at 3 and 6 months. • For positive results discuss confirmation testing with Western blot test. • Provide appropriate education and counseling based on initial test results as described above under EIA conventional testing.
Ongoing tests: CD4+ T cells and viral load tests are recommended at the time of initial HIV diagnosis to monitor the progression of HIV infection in seropositive patient and determine initiation or changes in antiretroviral therapy. *CD4+ T-cell count test:* Measures the total number of CD4 T-helper cells per microliter of blood.	CD4 low (<500 cells/µL) indicates decreased T-cell numbers and increased risk for opportunistic diseases.	*Rationale for CD4+ T-cell count test:* HIV attaches to CD4+ T cells, infecting them, destroying them, and decreasing the number of CD4+ cells, which impairs immune response; provides measurement of HIV progression to AIDS and effectiveness of HAART (p. 1937). • Provide patient with information on cell count levels, encourage follow-up lab tests and monitoring to determine treatment regime.
Viral load test: Done via polymerase chain reaction (PCR), HIV RNA, or bDNA tests to measure the actual amount of viral particles present in a blood sample.	Viral load levels of less than 10,000 copies/mL are considered "low" and copies greater than 100,000 are considered "high."	*Rationale for viral load test:* High levels indicate rapidly multiplying HIV, one marker of progression of HIV to AIDS; if patient on HAART indicates ineffective HAART treatment (p. 1937) due to drug resistance and/or lack of compliance with treatment regime. • HIV-infected individuals with viral load levels of less than 20,000 copies/mL have a low risk of disease progression. *Provide education on the following:* • Initial testing and follow-up testing: • Every 3–4 months in patients not on antiretroviral therapy. • Two to 8 weeks after initiation of antiretroviral therapy. • Every 3–4 months in patients on therapy. • When there is a decline in the clinical condition decisions need to be made to continue or change treatment.

Sources: Dybul, M., Fauci, A. S., Bartlett, J. G., Kaplan, J. E., & Pau, A. K. (2002). CDC Guidelines for Using Antiretroviral Agents Among HIV-Infected Adults and Adolescents Recommendations of the Panel on Clinical Practices for Treatment of HIV. Retrieved on September 5, 2008 from http://www.cdc.gov/mmwr/preview/mmwrhtml/rr5107a1.htm; Centers for Disease Control and Prevention. (2006c). Revised recommendations for HIV testing of adults, adolescents, and pregnant women in healthcare settings. *Morbidity and Mortality Weekly Report, 55*(RR-14), 1–17; Greenwald, J., Burstein, G., Pincus, J., & Branson, B. (2006). A rapid review of rapid HIV antibody tests. *Current Infectious Disease Reports, 8,* 125–131.

The revised CDC recommendations advocate HIV screening as a routine part of medical care for patients, similar to screening for other treatable conditions (CDC, 2006c). Individuals would be notified that testing will be performed unless the patient declines, a process that is referred to as opt-out screening. Persons at high risk for HIV should be screened annually. The guidelines also recommend that general consent for medical treatment be considered sufficient, and a separate written HIV testing consent not be required. Additionally, prevention counseling should not be required with diagnostic testing or HIV screening in health care settings. The ethical considerations surrounding HIV testing are discussed in the Ethical Issues box.

The rationale for the recommendations is that undiagnosed HIV-infected individuals frequently visit health care settings such as hospitals or acute care clinics years prior to a diagnosis, but are not tested for HIV in all health care settings. This results in a delay in effective antiretroviral treatment. Additionally, individuals aware of their positive HIV status significantly reduce sexual behavior that might transmit HIV, so early screening has the potential to substantially decrease the number of new HIV infections in the United States (Marks, Crepaz, Senterfitt, & Janssen, 2005). Routine prenatal HIV screening with streamlined counseling and consent procedures has substantially increased the number of pregnant women tested and contributed to significant declines in perinatal HIV transmission rates (CDC, 2002). This success has not been mirrored in the general population where HIV screening is rarely performed and the number of new

HIV infections has remained stable at approximately 40,000 annually in the United States (Branson et al., 2006).

Furthermore, prevention efforts need to address each succeeding generation of adolescents ages 13 to 19 years. Forty-seven percent of high school students report they have had sexual intercourse at least once, and 37% indicated they did not use protection during their last sexual intercourse experience. This is despite the fact that 89% stated that they learned about HIV/AIDS in their high school curriculum (CDC, 2005d). It is estimated that over half of HIV-infected adolescents have not been tested and are not aware of their infected status (Branson et al., 2006). The goals of the recommendations are to increase HIV screening of patients, including pregnant women, in health care settings; promote early detection of HIV infection; identify and counsel HIV-infected individuals and connect them to clinical and prevention services; and further reduce HIV transmission in the United States.

Currently, testing is focused on high-risk individuals who self-identify the need for testing or are encouraged by health providers to be tested because of identified risk factors. Testing is funded and performed by the state public health departments. At the anonymous public testing site, the individual receives a test code, a name is not associated with the test results, and results do not become part of the medical record. Pretest and posttest counseling is available at testing sites or by phone (Corbett, 2004). Approximately 2.1 million tests are conducted annually in publicly funded testing and referral programs alone. However, the CDC reports that a large percentage of individuals, 60% to 70%, do not return for test results (CDC, 2006b). The recent development of rapid HIV tests with comparable sensitivity and the specificity of enzyme immunoassays (EIAs), which provide testing and results in the same visit, can help address this issue. Anonymous testing also can be done at home with HIV antibody test kits. However, home tests raise concerns about lack of availability of counseling and prevention education that are an integral part of HIV testing. Anonymous testing may be preferred by individuals who fear discrimination or placement of the test result in their medical record where insurance companies may have access to the information (Johnsen, 2003).

Counseling regarding HIV encompasses two components: provision of information and prevention counseling. Counseling should be presented in an open, nonjudgmental manner and in the language that the individual is best capable of understanding. Verbal as well as written information or audiovisual materials that the individual can take home and review should be included. The CDC's revised recommendations for HIV testing released in 2006 change some of the previous recommendations for prevention counseling for individuals who take rapid HIV tests in a health care setting. The recommendations indicate that prevention counseling should not be required with HIV diagnostic testing or as part of an HIV screening program in health care settings such as emergency departments, urgent care clinics, inpatient services, substance abuse treatment clinics, public health and community clinics, correctional facilities, and primary care settings (CDC, 2006b). This is an effort to remove barriers to HIV screening in busy health care settings. However, the CDC continues to support prevention counseling in all settings for persons at high risk for HIV and in nonmedical settings such as community-based organizations, outreach settings, or mobile vans (CDC, 2006b).

ETHICAL ISSUES Related to HIV Infection

A significant ethical issue that the nurse in the acute care setting may encounter when caring for a patient with a newly diagnosed HIV-positive antibody status is the issue of sexual or needle-sharing partners at high risk for HIV infection. The HIV-infected patient may be very hesitant, embarrassed, or fearful about disclosing an HIV-positive test result to partners. This creates an ethical dilemma in that it places partners at risk for undiagnosed HIV infection, limits their choices for testing and potential treatment if needed, and violates their rights to know their risk for infection.

The nurse must abide by the ethical principle of respect for autonomy and confidentiality, while at the same time encouraging the patient to employ the ethical principle of veracity (truthfulness) in informing partners. The nurse may encourage the patient in making this ethical choice by developing a therapeutic relationship, asking about support systems and partners, listening to concerns, reviewing benefits of early screening for partners, and obtaining a social service referral to access resources for partner notification. State legislation requires health departments to offer anonymous HIV partner notification services to newly reported HIV-infected persons. The HIV partner counseling services inform persons of their possible exposure, and offer counseling, testing, and referral services (CDC, 2003a).

The importance of notifying sexual and needle-sharing partners of their exposure to HIV is also enforced by Federal Ryan White CARE Reauthorization act of 1996, which requires health departments show "good faith" in notifying marriage partners of HIV-infected persons. The nurse can provide emotional support and obtain referral resources to help newly diagnosed HIV-infected patients and spouses communicate and address this difficult situation.

The CDC still recommends that patients in all settings receive information regarding HIV testing, HIV infection, and the meaning of results. Patients must be informed of the HIV screening in a face-to-face discussion or through written or audiovisual material. Information provided should include the testing process, the meaning of test results, ways HIV is transmitted and how to prevent it, and where to obtain further testing and services. Ongoing HIV counseling is vital for individuals who test positive for HIV. Overwhelming feelings of fear, anxiety, depression, and social isolation frequently occur with an HIV diagnosis. Nurses are in an optimal position to develop therapeutic relationships that support the HIV-positive patient, to review risk factors for transmitting HIV infection, and to encourage compliance with follow-up testing and antiretroviral therapy. Nurses also can help facilitate referrals to social services for assistance with financial concerns, and community and psychological support services.

Tests that monitor the progression of HIV infection include the CD4+ T-cell counts and viral load assay tests. CD4+ T-cell counts, as previously discussed, are essential in assessing for decreased immune function and the diagnosis of AIDS. Equally important are viral load tests such as the HIV RNA, polymerize chain reaction (qPCR), or the branched chain DNA (bDNA) tests, which measure the viral activity and are reported as the number of "copies" per milliliter. Viral load testing is done at the time of HIV diagnosis and as a baseline, and then every few weeks to months depending on the initiation or type of drug treatment therapy. Viral load levels of less than 10,000 copies/mL are considered "low" and copies greater than 100,000 are considered "high" (Corbett, 2004). HIV-infected individuals with HIV RNA levels of less than 20,000 copies/mL have a low risk of disease progression (Bartlett & Lane, 2007). As the HIV progresses the CD4+ T-cell counts decline and the viral load increases, resulting in susceptibility to OIs and malignancies.

Testing for HIV resistance to antiretroviral drugs in patients being treated for HIV infection is currently possible. This is an important tool in determining antiretroviral therapy. Genotyping and phenotyping assays are available. Genotyping assays detect drug resistance mutations present in reverse transcriptase and protease genes. Phenotyping assays measure the ability of the virus to grow in different antiretroviral drug concentrations. Information on drug resistance is important in identifying patients who are not responding to their antiretroviral medication regime and in guiding decisions regarding changes in therapy (Bartlett & Lane, 2007).

Antiretroviral Drug Therapy for HIV Infection

Antiretroviral drugs are pivotal in delaying the progression of HIV to AIDS. The goal of drug therapy is to decrease the viral load (HIV RNA level < 55,000 copies/mL), increase or maintain CD4+ T-cell counts at greater than 200 cells/mL (greater than 500 cells/µL preferred), and delay the onset of HIV symptoms and opportunistic infections. A variety of antiretroviral agents are now available for use in treatment.

The complexity of the medications involved and concerns about appropriate treatment for patients who are asymptomatic with low HIV RNA levels and an adequate CD4+ T-cell count has created some confusion on when to initiate antiretroviral therapy. Antiretroviral drugs have serious adverse effects and

drug resistance can develop with prolonged use or nonadherence, requiring changes in therapy that limit future treatment options. To address these concerns, the U.S. Department of Health and Human Services published guidelines for the use of antiretroviral agents in HIV-1-infected adults and adolescents in July 2003, with subsequent revisions in 2006 (Bartlett & Lane, 2007). Viral load and CD4+ T-cell levels are essential parameters in deciding to initiate or change antiretroviral therapies. In general, treatment should be offered to persons who have HIV RNA levels > 55,000 copies/mL or <350 CD4+ T cells/µL.

Treatment for HIV involves combinations of various antiretroviral drugs that interfere with different aspects of the HIV replication cycle, and the treatment is referred to as **highly active antiretroviral drug therapy (HAART)**. Combination therapy has the greatest effect in controlling HIV proliferation and minimizing the development of drug resistance. Antiretroviral drugs are grouped according to the mechanism of action against HIV (see Figure 60–7 ■, p. 1938).

Nucleoside reverse transcriptase inhibitors are a group of drugs that prevent viral replication by blocking the attachment of the nucleoside to the replicated DNA molecule. The nonnucleoside reverse transcriptase inhibitors make up another group of drugs that also prevent viral replication, but through a different mechanism. These drugs prevent the bond between a nucleotide and the growing DNA molecule of HIV. An additional group of drugs, the protease inhibitors, stop the replication of new RNA by inhibiting the action of protease enzymes, which are responsible for the synthesis of reverse transcriptase. A more recent class of medication, fusion inhibitors, is also available and works by preventing HIV from binding to CD4+ T cells and infecting healthy cells. Chart 60–10 (p. 1939) provides additional information on specific medication and adverse effects that can be used in patient teaching.

Central to the treatment of HIV/AIDS is adherence to the prescribed antiviral medication regime. If antiviral medications are not taken properly or consistently, CD4+ T-cell counts will decrease and viral loads of HIV will significantly increase, leading to greater risk of opportunistic infection (Branson et al., 2006; Dybul et al., 2002; Kaplan et al., 2002). Furthermore, resistance to these medications can develop if the treatment regime is not followed (Branson et al., 2006; Little et al., 2002). Essential to creating strategies to improve adherence is a supportive therapeutic relationship between the patient and the provider, and a negotiated treatment plan that the patient commits to that considers his daily routines, meal schedules, and medication side effects (Bartlett & Lane, 2007).

The lack of adherence to medication treatment is a major concern in HIV treatment. The focal issue has been the complexity of dosing schedules, the volume of pills that the patient must manage, and the serious adverse effects of these medications, including fatigue, loss of appetite, diarrhea, and nausea and vomiting (Bartlett & Lane, 2007). Other issues that have been identified include socioeconomic factors such as homelessness, lack of insurance or finances, or lack of transportation to clinic appointments. Psychological factors also have been implicated including mental illness, poor coping skills, and failure to understand that self-care is a priority (especially for HIV-infected women balancing multiple caregiver roles) (Shaw & Mahoney, 2003).

MyNursingKit | Animation: Drugs: Infectious Drugs—Antiviral Agent: Zidovudine

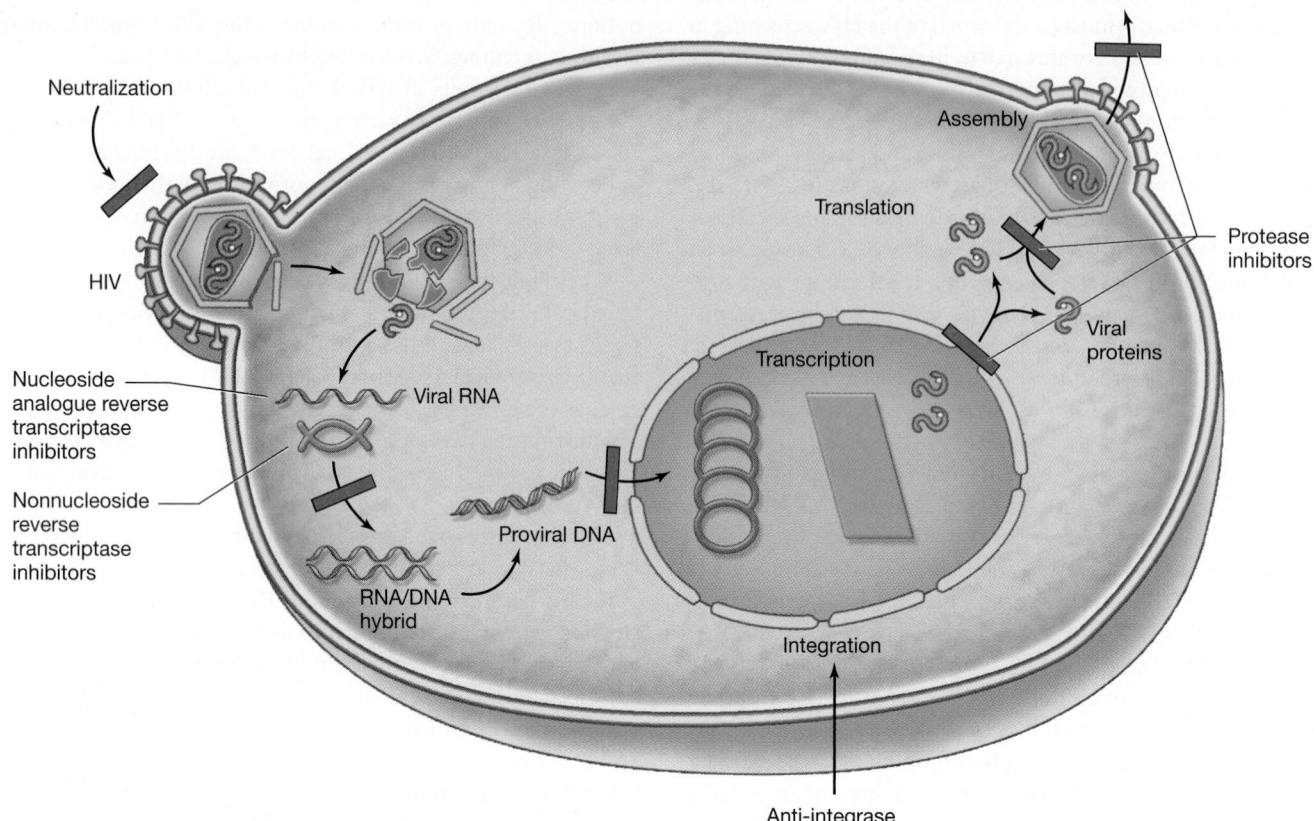

FIGURE 60-7 ■ HIV replication and targets of antiretroviral therapy.

Pharmaceutical companies have responded to these issues by developing combination antiviral medications to decrease the volume of pills patients must manage, and therefore simplifying medication schedules. Research is ongoing in this area. Another area of significant research involves antiretroviral therapy during pregnancy (Dabis, Bequet, & Ekouevi, 2005; Tasha, Kumwenda, & Gibbons, 2003). HIV-infected mother-to-fetus transmissions are responsible for more than 90% of HIV infection in children, and antiretroviral therapy during pregnancy has demonstrated significant declines in this transmission rate (Public Health Service Task Force, 2006).

Nurses play a pivotal role in medication adherence through extensive patient and family education and follow-up regarding medication side effects and concern. Additionally, nurses can facilitate the coordination and development of a patient-centered plan of care that addresses the socioeconomic, psychological, and physiological factors effecting medication adherence.

Treatment of Opportunistic Infections and Symptom Management

The medical treatment for opportunistic infections and symptom management was summarized earlier in Chart 60-9 (p. 1929). Drug therapy is the mainstay of treatment of opportunistic infections (OIs). The development of resistant organisms in an immunosuppressed individual is challenging and frequently involves treatment with new and innovative combinations of antibiotic therapy. Symptoms requiring treatment may be the result of antiretroviral drugs, treatment of opportunistic infection, or

proliferation of HIV resulting in greater loss of immune function. In addition to infection, commonly treated symptoms include diarrhea, anorexia and weight loss, skin breakdown, pain, and depression. Nurses have an essential role in ongoing assessment of the patient's response to treatment and facilitating symptom management in order to promote optimal patient outcomes.

Nursing Management

The nursing care of the patient with AIDS involves multiple physical as well as psychological and social support issues. Because of the impairment to the immune system, any body organ can be the target of an opportunistic infection or cancer, making nursing care especially challenging. To date there is no cure for HIV. A diagnosis of HIV/AIDS is psychologically devastating to patients, the vast majority of whom are 15 to 45 years of age and have not previously confronted issues of mortality. HIV/AIDS also carries a social stigma that may result in rejection by family and friends and social isolation at a time when the patient faces issues of grief and fear of dying. Nurses have a primary role in addressing these needs, and providing skilled, compassionate nursing care that is respectful to the individual's values, culture, and right to make individual choices (American Nurses Association, 2004).

The nursing process provides a template to assess, treat, and evaluate patients with HIV/AIDS. Use of the nursing process will facilitate creation of individualized care plans that optimize symptom management, patient comfort, and family support.

CHART 60–10   HIV/AIDS Infection Antiretroviral Agents

Drug Therapy	Drug Action	Application/Indication	Nursing Responsibilities
Protease Inhibitors • Nelfinavir (Viracept) • Ritonavir (Norvir) (keep refrigerated) • Lopinavir and ritonavir (Kaletra) • Saquinavir (Fortovase) • Indinavir (Crixivan) (Take 1 hour before or 2 hours after eating.) • Amprenavir (Agenerase)	Stop the replication of new RNA by inhibiting the action of protease enzymes, which are responsible for the synthesis of reverse transcriptase.	One of the three categories of drugs that are combined to treat HIV and are referred to as HAART (p. 1937).	Monitor the patient for anemia, anorexia/nausea, diarrhea, headache, fever, malaise. Monitor labs: triglycerides, ALT, AST, alkaline phosphatase, CK and uric acid levels, thrombocytopenia. • Instruct patient to take with food due to bitter taste, and not to mix with juice because it increases the bitterness. • Inform patient of potential redistribution of body fat centrally (the "protease paunch"), facial atrophy, breast enlargement, "buffalo hump."
Non-Nucleoside Reverse Transcriptase Inhibitors • Delavirdine (Rescriptor) • Nevirapine (Viramune) • Efavirenz (Sustiva) (Not to be used during pregnancy or breast-feeding. Women of childbearing years need pregnancy test prior to taking drug.)	Prevent viral replication, but through a different mechanism than protease inhibitors. These drugs prevent the bond between a nucleotide and the growing DNA molecule of HIV.	One of the three categories of drugs that are combined to treat HIV and are referred to as HAART (p. 1937).	• Monitor patient for fatigue, rash, headache, painful peripheral neuropathy (reversible with lower doses), insomnia, nightmares (usually resolve in 2 weeks) retinal changes (eye exam recommended every 6–12 months). • Monitor for increase in ALT, AST, alkaline phosphatase. • Monitor creatinine levels of patient with renal insufficiency. • Instruct patient to maintain adequate hydration and not to take with antacids.
Nucleoside Reverse Transcriptase Inhibitors • Zidovudine (AZT, ZDT, Retrovir) (Take 1 hour before or 2 hours after meals.) • Lamivudine (3TC, Epivir) • Combivir (lamivudine and zidovudine combination) • Didanosine (ddl, Videx) (Take 1 hour before or 2 hours after meals. Two tablet doses, of which 1 is a buffer, must be chewed or dissolved to ensure adequate buffer for absorption.) • Stavudine (d4T, Zerit) • Zalcitabine (ddC, HIVID) • Tenofovir Disoproxil Fumarate (DF, Viread) • Adefovir dipivoxil (Preveon) • Abacavir (Ziagen) (Alcohol increases abacavir levels 41%. Some reported fatal hypersensitivity reactions.)	Prevent viral replication by blocking the attachment of the nucleoside to the replicated DNA molecule.	One of the three categories of drugs that are combined to treat HIV and are referred to as HAART (p. 1937).	• Monitor for bone marrow suppression: neutropenia, anemia, granulocytopenia. • Monitor ALT, AST. • Monitor creatinine clearance in patient with renal impairment. • Monitor for malaise, insomnia, nightmares (subside in about 2 weeks), painful peripheral neuropathy (reversible with lower medication doses), visual changes (eye exam recommended every 6–12 months), GI intolerance, and nausea/vomiting.

(continued)

CHART 60–10	HIV/AIDS Infection Antiretroviral Agents—*Continued*		
Drug Therapy	**Drug Action**	**Application/Indication**	**Nursing Responsibilities**
Fusion Inhibitor • Enfuvirtide (Fuzeon) (subcutaneous injection twice daily)	Interferes with entry of HIV-1 into host cells by inhibiting the fusion of the virus and cell membranes.	Treatment of advanced HIV disease with evidence of resistance to other therapies.	• Monitor for irritation at injection site, nausea, insomnia, peripheral neuropathy. • Instruct patient to keep medication refrigerated, reconstitute according to directions, rotate injection sites.

Sources: Adams, M., Josephson, D., & Holland, L. (2005). *Pharmacology for nurses: A pathophysiologic approach.* Upper Saddle River, NJ: Pearson Prentice Hall; Shaw, J. K., & Mahoney, E. A. (Eds.). (2003). *HIV/AIDS nursing secrets.* Philadelphia: Hanley & Belfus; Shannon, M., Shields, K., & Stang, C. (2007). *Nurse's drug guide.* Upper Saddle River, NJ: Pearson Prentice Hall.

Because of the complexity of HIV infection multiple nursing diagnoses apply. An extensive list of potentially applicable diagnoses is provided in Chart 60–11. Some of the most common nursing diagnoses that impact patients with HIV/AIDS, outcome goals, evaluation parameters, and appropriate nursing interventions are found in the Nursing Process: Care Plan for the Patient with HIV/AIDS. Alternative treatments for HIV/AIDS are addressed in the Complementary and Alternative Therapies box (p. 1947).

Treatment Choice Issues

Diagnosis of a disease process such as HIV/AIDS that has no cure is devastating. The highest prevalence of HIV infection is found in a very young population (15 to 45 years), the vast majority of whom have not faced issues of terminal illness or chronic treatment. This may prompt a desire to explore issues of spirituality, concepts of the soul, and life after death. It may result in feelings of overwhelming fear that result in a search for a higher power. The nurse needs to be sensitive to these issues and assess the patient's feelings regarding spiritual needs so that appropriate referrals can be made. The patient also may choose to explore alternative therapies. It is imperative that the nurse remain open minded about these options and respectful of the treatment choices that the patient makes.

Discharge Priorities

Due to the chronic nature of HIV/AIDS, the process of discharging a patient from the hospital is complex. The nurse must address the medication schedule, physical care needs, and emotional issues surrounding the diagnosis. If followed carefully, current treatments can prolong and give quality to the person's life. Additionally, caregiver considerations must be addressed. The Patient Teaching & Discharge Priorities box (p. 1947) and Chart 60–12 (p. 1948) outline the important information that is essential for patients with HIV/AIDS and their partners and caregivers that must be provided on discharge.

Ongoing Care

For patients who have been diagnosed with HIV/AIDS, collaborative care includes assessment of physical status as well as the knowledge level of the patient, partner, family, and friends in order to address education needs. The promotion of self-care, independence, and adherence to the prescribed treatment plan is the primary goal in the care of the patient with AIDS. With antiretroviral therapy, HIV infection is transitioning to a chronic disease. Many HIV-infected individuals are able to maintain home and work functions for several years and are regularly followed by their health care provider or an AIDS outreach clinic. As the disease progresses care needs increase and the patient becomes increasingly dependent on family and friends to provide support. Social workers, community support services, home care nurses, community health nurses, and hospice nurses are often able to provide complex in-home nursing care that enables patients to remain comfortable at home.

Nurses are pivotal in providing ongoing patient and family education and making appropriate referrals to a variety of community-based organizations that can also supply support such as meals, housekeeping, transportation, or shopping. They also have additional information on national resources that the patient or family can access. Such organizations include the National Association of People with AIDS, CDC National AIDS Hotline, and the National Association on HIV over Fifty. (For a discussion of AIDS in people over age 50, see the Gerontological Considerations box, p. 1948.) At the point where the patient's symptoms cannot be managed at home or a caregiver is not available, a transfer to skilled nursing care or an acute care facility is needed to ensure patient comfort.

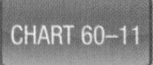 CHART 60–11   **Nursing Diagnoses for the Patient with HIV/AIDS**

- *Acute/Chronic Pain* related to opportunistic infections/malignancies
- *Impaired Skin Integrity* related to malnutrition, altered metabolic state, immobility, alerted sensation, skeletal prominence
- *Fatigue* related to malnutrition, hypermetabolic state with infection, fluid/electrolyte imbalance
- *Deficient Fluid Volume* related to copious diarrhea, profuse sweating, vomiting, hypermetabolic state, fever
- *Confusion* related to neurological opportunistic infections/malignancies and altered metabolic processes
- *Deficient Knowledge* related to disease, transmission, prognosis, treatment, and self-care
- *Ineffective Therapeutic Regimen Management* related to complexity of medications and socioeconomic limitations
- *Ineffective Coping* related to fear, grief, and despair with life-threatening disease process
- *Anxiety* related to anticipatory fear of physical decline and the dying process

Note: These are the most common potential nursing diagnoses for the patient with HIV/AIDS.

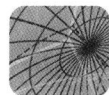

NURSING PROCESS: Patient Care Plan for HIV/AIDS

Assessment of Infection

Subjective Data:

Have you been running a temperature?

Have you had chills or periods of sweating?

Are you having any "flu-like" symptoms (body aches, fatigue, cough, sore-throat, stiff neck)?

Have you been coughing up any sputum? What color is it?

Have you noticed any rashes?

Do you have pain anywhere?

Do you have any burning with urination?

Do you have any redness or tenderness anywhere?

Do you have any sores anywhere?

Do you have any unusual or foul-smelling drainage (e.g., from vagina, penis, rectum, ears)?

How long have the symptoms been going on?

What have you done to treat the symptoms?

Have you taken any over the counter (OTC), prescription, or herbal medications for symptom relief?

Have you been taking your antiviral medications as prescribed?

Objective Data:

Abnormal vital signs (e.g., temp > 101 or < 97, HR >100, BP < 90 or MAP < 60)

Skin: rashes, wounds, sores, redness, heat, or edema

Oral cavity: sores, white patches, poor dental hygiene

Drainage: color, amount and foul smell from any wounds, incisions, mucous membranes

Urine: amber, cloudy, amount of time Foley catheter in place

Pain with palpation

Invasive lines/catheters: amount of time they have been in place, redness, drainage at insertion site

Laboratory Tests: CBC with differential to evaluate WBC count (neutrophils < 4,000 or > 12,000/mm^3; bands > 10%

CD4 T-cell count: <500/cells/uL

HIV viral load count: >25,000 copies/mL

Cultures: blood, sputum, stool, urine, wound (+ for bacterial or viral pathogens)

Nursing Assessment and Diagnoses	Outcomes and Evaluation Parameters	Planning and Interventions with *Rationales*
Nursing Diagnosis: *Risk for Infection* related to immunodeficiency from HIV infection	**Outcome:** No infection. ***Evaluation Parameters:*** Vital signs within normal parameters. Alert and oriented. Clear lungs. Intact skin or mucous membrane without edema, pain, redness, or drainage. Wounds/incisions healing. No discomfort with urination. Invasive line and catheter sites are not red or draining. Symptoms of infection identified early and prompt treatment initiated.	**Interventions and *Rationales:*** Assess for symptoms of infection: fever, chills, diaphoresis; tachycardia, tachypnea, hypotension; decline in neurological status; dyspnea, cough, adventitious breath sounds; white patches in oral cavity or painful swallowing; redness, swelling, or drainage from wounds or vaginal or perianal area; open lesions on face, lips, or perianal area; urinary frequency, urgency, or burning sensation; pain in any location. *Promotes early detection of infection.*
		Notify health care provider of symptoms of infection. *Early detection and treatment help prevent progression to refractory sepsis. Infections increase patient mortality.*
	WBC within normal limits.	Monitor WBC count and differential. *Elevated or abnormally low WBC counts indicates possible infection.*
	Cultures negative for organisms.	Obtain cultures of blood, sputum, urine, wound drainage, skin lesions, mouth, and stool as ordered prior to the start of the first dose of antibiotic. *Assists in identifying infecting organisms and targeting appropriate treatment. Obtaining culture prior to starting antibiotics increases the potential to capture the organism in the culture. Do not delay the antibiotics if some cultures such as sputum cannot be obtained.*
	Medications given on time. Antibiotic therapy sensitive to infecting organism as evidenced by decreasing fever, WBC, and sputum production. Patient continues HAART regime.	Administer antimicrobial medications as prescribed. *Treats current infection or prevents additional opportunistic infections (OI).* Administer HAART as prescribed and stress adherence to medication regime. *Decreases rate of HIV replication and increases CD4 counts.*
	Health care providers and family perform hand hygiene frequently prior to and following patient contact.	Prevent infection by washing hands before and after all patient contacts; instruct patient/family to perform hand hygiene frequently, especially after toileting, prior to eating or handling medications. *Reduces risk of OI cross-contamination.*
	Intake & output (I&O) balanced; patient maintaining or gaining weight.	Maintain fluid and nutritional intake; strict I&O, calorie count. *Dehydration and malnutrition impair immune function and wound healing.*

(continued)

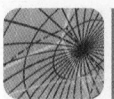

NURSING PROCESS: Patient Care Plan for HIV/AIDS—*Continued*

Nursing Assessment and Diagnoses	Outcomes and Evaluation Parameters	Planning and Interventions with *Rationales*
	No new skin or mucous membrane breakdown.	Maintain skin and mucous membrane integrity with frequent turning and oral care every 2 hours. *Skin and mucous membranes are the first line of immune defense; lesions allow OI portal of entry.*
	Invasive lines and catheters secured. No invasive line or catheter-induced infections. Catheters and invasive lines removed promptly when no longer of benefit in patient treatment.	Maintain sterile technique during all invasive procedures (urinary catheterization, IV line placement). Perform meticulous care of any invasive lines or catheters; change out catheters according to agency policy.
	Patient performs activities of daily living (ADLs).	Maintain closed system for drains. Discontinue catheters/invasive lines as soon as possible. *Prevents hospital-acquired infections.* Anchor catheters/tubes (IV lines, urinary catheters) securely. *Reduces trauma to tissue and decreases risk of introducing pathogens from in and out movement of catheter.*
	Patient out of bed (OOB) and turned every 2 hours.	Assist with mobility, out of bed three or more times a day unless contraindicated or turning every 2 hours. *Prevents skin breakdown, deep venous thrombosis, constipation, and pulmonary stasis, which may increase length of hospitalization and infection risk.*
	Lungs clear.	Assist with inspirometer, coughing, and deep breathing every 1–2 hours when awake. *To prevent pulmonary stasis, which increases risk of OI.*
	Patient and family can verbally identify signs and symptoms of infection. Patient and family report early symptoms of infection to health care providers.	Instruct patient and family about signs and symptoms of infection and infection prevention and the need to report possible infection. *Enables early detection and treatment.*
	Patient environment is clean.	Maintain cleanliness/personal hygiene. Clean household surfaces with disinfectant. *Decreases presence of potentially infective organisms.*
	Has others handle pet cleanup.	Avoid handling animal waste or cleaning cages. *Infectious organisms such as CMV are in animal feces.*
	Uses recommendations for food handling.	Clean and cook foods thoroughly (scrub skins of fruits and vegetables, cook meat and eggs). *To eliminate pathogens.* Avoid exposure to others' body fluids and do not share eating utensils. *Patient/family teaching to minimize exposure to OI is essential to preventing infection.*

Assessment of Airway and Gas Exchange

Subjective Data:
Are you having difficulty breathing?
Have you been coughing?
What color is the sputum you are coughing up?

Objective Data:
Respiratory rate:
Use of substernal and/or intercostals muscles with inspiration/expiration
Unequal chest wall movement
Oxygen saturation:
Adventitious breath sounds: wheezes, fine or course crackles
Decreased level of consciousness (LOC) (lethargy→confusion→stupor)
Skin changes: mottled extremities, central cyanosis
Arterial Blood Gases (ABG)

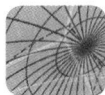

NURSING PROCESS: Patient Care Plan for HIV/AIDS—*Continued*

Nursing Assessment and Diagnoses	Outcomes and Evaluation Parameters	Planning and Interventions with *Rationales*
Nursing Diagnoses: *Ineffective Airway Clearance* related to (1) opportunistic pulmonary infection, increased bronchial secretions or (2) stasis of secretion from decreased ability to cough from general weakness	**Outcomes:** Clear airway. Adequate gas exchange. ***Evaluation Parameters:*** Respiratory rate 12–20 breaths/min. Unlabored breathing without use of accessory muscles.	**Interventions and *Rationales:*** Assess for rapid shallow respirations. *Indicates hypoxia and poor gas exchange.* Assess for use of accessory muscles. *Indicates increased work of breathing and progression to respiratory failure.* Assess for abnormal or absent breath sounds. *Indicates pulmonary infiltrates or consolidation that decreases gas exchange.*
Risk for Impaired Gas Exchange related to pulmonary secretions from opportunistic infections	Clear breath sounds. Alert and oriented. Skin is pink, warm. Normal ABG values. Pulse oximetry saturation > 94%. Appropriate medical treatment as needed. Patient cooperative with oxygen administration. Sputum culture obtained. Antibiotic therapy sensitive to infecting organism as evidenced by decreasing fever, WBC, and sputum production. Patient able to cough and clear secretions. Patient verbalizes understanding and performs pulmonary self-care. Patient reports decreased breathing problems. Patient has energy to cough and clear secretions. Secretions cleared. Airway and ventilation maintained.	Assess for cough and sputum; note amount, color and consistency of sputum. *A yellow, green, or tan color indicates presence of infecting organism.* Assess level of consciousness (restless, confused, somnolence). *Altered level of consciousness is an early indicator of hypoxia and decreased perfusion to the brain.* Assess dusky, cyanotic skin color. *Indicates tissue hypoxia.* Monitor ABGs and pulse oximetry oxygen saturation. *To assess adequacy of gas exchange.* Report respiratory distress to health care provider. *Enables prompt initiation of appropriate medical treatment.* Administer humidified oxygen as prescribed. *Supplemental oxygen increases the alveolar gas concentration and diffusion of oxygen to the cells and tissues of the body. Humidification helps loosen secretions and promote airway clearance.* Obtain sputum sample for culture. *To identify specific infecting organism so appropriate antibiotic is prescribed.* Administer antibiotic therapy as prescribed. *To treat infectious organism.* Maintain fluid intake of 3 L/day unless contraindicated. *To decrease viscosity of secretions.* Administer mucolytics and bronchodilators as prescribed. *To thin secretions and dilate airways, thus increasing gas exchange.* Maintain the head of the bed >30% at all times unless contraindicated. Instruct patient to turn, cough, deep breathe, and use the inspirometer every 1–2 hours when awake. *Facilitates breathing, increases gas exchange, and prevents atelectasis and pulmonary secretion stasis.* Encourage adequate rest periods. *Prevents excessive fatigue, which impairs ability to breathe.* Perform tracheal suctioning as needed. *Removes secretions if patient is unable to do so, clears airway, improves gas exchange.* Assist with endotracheal intubation; maintain ventilator settings as prescribed. *Maintains airway and gas exchange.*

Assessment of Nutrition

Subjective Data:
Do you have an appetite?
What are you eating and how often do you eat?
Are you losing weight?
Are you experiencing nausea or vomiting?
Are you having any difficulty chewing or swallowing?

Objective Data:
Daily weight
Laboratory tests: serum protein, albumin, transferrin levels, Hbg/Hct, electrolytes
Oral cavity: edema, white patches indicating *Candida* infection, open lesions, loose or decaying teeth

(continued)

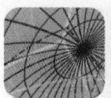

NURSING PROCESS: Patient Care Plan for HIV/AIDS—*Continued*

Nursing Assessment and Diagnoses	Outcomes and Evaluation Parameters	Planning and Interventions with *Rationales*
Nursing Diagnosis: *Imbalanced Nutrition: Less than Body Requirements* related to decreased oral intake associated with anorexia, nausea/vomiting, and impaired absorption and utilization of nutrients from effects of HIV infection	**Outcome:** Maintained or improved nutritional status. *Evaluation Parameters:* Gains weight. Adequate hydration. Normal electrolytes, albumin, hemoglobin/hematocrit, transferring levels.	**Interventions and *Rationales:*** Assess for significant weight loss or weight below normal for patient's height, weight, and age. *Indicates malnutrition.*
		Assess diet weight loss and diet history, food likes, dislikes, and intolerances. *Identifies education needs and allows for individual dietary plan.*
	Oral and esophageal opportunistic infections treated appropriately, as evidenced by no pain with swallowing, pink nonedematous mucous membranes. Laboratory values improving and trending toward normal ranges.	Assess and report abnormalities of oral cavity, mucous membranes, and swallowing. *To identify treatable OIs (oral candidiasis, esophagitis) that interfere with intake and facilitate medical treatment oral candidiasis.*
		Monitor fluid and electrolytes, serum protein, albumin, transferrin levels, hemoglobin/hematocrit energy level. *Low levels indicate inadequate intake/malnutrition, which places patient at increased risk for infection.*
	Intake of daily calories is nutritious and meets or exceeds body requirements.	Consult with dietician to determine patient's nutritional needs. *To obtain information on calorie needs and facilitate meal planning.* Monitor daily intake with calorie count. *To provide data on total daily calorie intake.*
		Consult with health care provider and dietitian on high-calorie supplements. *To increase calorie intake when larger volumes of food cannot be tolerated.*
	Patient and family use diet plan, report increased intake and weight is increased. Nutritious food available to patient.	Collaborate with patient/family to create a plan to increase intake:
		1. Eat 6–7 small protein-rich foods. *To decrease nausea from feeling "over full" and to increase calorie intake.*
		2. Select soft foods if patient has difficulty swallowing (eggs, ice cream, cooked vegetables, pureed meats). *To decrease swallowing pain.*
		3. Rest prior to meals. *To conserve energy for eating.*
		4. Hold liquids 1 hour prior to eating. *To reduce satiety.*
	Eats meals with others weekly.	5. Encourage patient to eat meals with family/friends. *To increase social interaction and provide encouragement to eat.*
		Assess need for community resources and consult social worker or community liaison regarding financial assistance if patient cannot afford food. *To provide resources on nutritious foods.*
	Decreased nausea and increased intake.	Administer prescribed medications:
		1. Antiemetics. *To decrease nausea.*
		2. Appetite stimulants (dronabinol, megestrol acetate). *To counteract anorexia effects of disease and medications.*
		3. Cytokine inhibitors (thalidomide). *To improve appetite by suppressing TNF-α production (used only in cases of severe wasting syndrome).*
	Decrease in rate of weight loss.	Consult with health care provider and dietitian about enteral or parenteral nutrition if patient unable to gain weight. *Provides additional nutritional support (used with severe wasting syndrome).*

Assessment of Diarrhea

Subjective Data:

How many bowel movements are you having a day?
What is the consistency and color of the stool?
Are you taking any medications to stop diarrhea?
How many glasses of water/liquid are you drinking per day?
Are you experiencing abdominal pain or cramping?
Is the area around your rectum sore or bleeding?
What type of foods do you typically eat during the day?

Objective Data:

Vital signs (low BP, rapid HR may indicate dehydration)
Measurement of the number, volume, and consistency of bowel movements per day
Perianal area: red, excoriated
Skin turgor: tenting
Urine output: < 700 mL/day
Laboratory tests: abnormalities in electrolytes, phosphorus, magnesium, Hbg, RBCs
Stool culture: pathogens

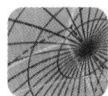

NURSING PROCESS: Patient Care Plan for HIV/AIDS—*Continued*

Nursing Assessment and Diagnoses	Outcomes and Evaluation Parameters	Planning and Interventions with *Rationales*
Nursing Diagnoses: *Bowel Incontinence* and *Diarrhea* related to HIV infection and/or opportunistic infections in the GI tract	**Outcome:** Normal bowel habits. ***Evaluation Parameters:*** One to two soft, formed stools/day. Fluid and electrolyte status maintained. Factors contributing to acute episodes of diarrhea identified and avoided. Weight increasing. Opportunistic infection treated appropriately as exhibited by decreasing incidence of diarrhea, normal stool cultures. Adequate fluid status maintained as evidenced by urine output > 700 mL/day, good skin turgor, stable blood pressure. Normal electrolytes, hemoglobin (Hgb), Red blood cells (RBC). Decreased abdominal cramping and acute episodes of diarrhea. Perianal skin intact. Patient and family use diet plan, report decreased episodes of diarrhea, and weight is increased.	**Interventions and *Rationales:*** Assess for frequency and volume of loose stools and for abdominal cramping. *To determine the amount of diarrhea, fluid volume loss, and level of abdominal discomfort.* Identify factors that cause and alleviate diarrhea. *To help individualize care and create an effective plan.* Weigh daily and document amount. *To trend weights as part of intervention assessment.* Obtain stool cultures. *Identifies opportunistic infections.* Administer antimicrobial therapy as prescribed. *To eliminate or control infecting organisms.* Instruct patient to have fluid intake of >3 L/day unless contraindicated. *To prevent hypovolemia.* Monitor and report abnormal laboratory values (potassium, sodium, calcium, phosphorus, magnesium, Hbg, RBCs). *Chronic diarrhea and small intestinal inflammation may impair electrolyte absorption and absorption of vitamins necessary for Hbg and RBC formation.* Administer anticholinergics, antispasmodics, and opioids as prescribed. *To decrease intestinal motility and spasms.* Assess for perianal excoriation. *To determine need for skin barrier creams or application of external drainage bag to protect skin.* Instruct patient/family in diet measures to decrease bowel hyperactivity. *To help rest bowel and possibly decrease diarrhea.* Eliminate bowel-irritating foods such as raw vegetables, nuts, and fried or fatty foods. *To reduce stimulation to the bowel.* Avoid coffee and nicotine. *Bowel stimulants.* Encourage nonspicy, bland diet (BRAT diet = bananas, rice, applesauce, toast). *Carbohydrates are easier to digest and cause less stimulation of the bowel.*

Assessment of Oral Mucous Membranes

Subjective Data:
Are you having any difficulty or pain with chewing and swallowing?
Do you have any sores in your mouth?
Are you brushing your teeth at least twice a day?
Do you use a lip balm to protect your lips?

Objective Data:
Oral cavity: edema, white patches, open lesions, loose or decaying teeth, purple lesions

Nursing Assessment and Diagnoses	Outcomes and Evaluation Parameters	Planning and Interventions with *Rationales*
Nursing Diagnosis: *Impaired Oral Mucous Membrane* related to immunologic deficit and presence of opportunistic infection/malignancy such as candidiasis, herpes, Kaposi's sarcoma; malnutrition and/or dehydration; side effects of drugs and chemotherapy; ineffective oral hygiene	**Outcome:** Integrity of mucous membranes maintained. ***Evaluation Parameters:*** Patient reports no oral discomfort. Mucous membranes pink, moist, intact.	**Interventions and *Rationales:*** Assess patient for oral pain and difficulty with chewing or swallowing. *Indicates problem in oral cavity that affects patient comfort and impacts oral intake.* Assess oral cavity for ulcerations, redness, white patches, especially on the side of the tongue. *Indicates probable oral candidiasis or progressing esophagitis.*

(continued)

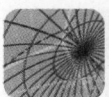

NURSING PROCESS: Patient Care Plan for HIV/AIDS—*Continued*

Nursing Assessment and Diagnoses	Outcomes and Evaluation Parameters	Planning and Interventions with *Rationales*
	Oral and esophageal opportunistic infections treated appropriately and effectively.	Report symptoms of candidiasis. *To initiate medical treatment.*
		Obtain cultures or oral lesions as prescribed. *To identify opportunistic pathogens and target medical treatment.*
	Identified dental problems treated appropriately.	Assess for swelling of gingiva, loose or decaying teeth. *Indicates poor oral hygiene; increases risk of infection from dental source.*
	Medications effective as evidenced by decreasing symptoms of infection.	Refer to dental consultation if necessary. *To treat oral decay.*
		Administer medications as prescribed: antifungals, antibiotics. *To treat infections.*
	Lips and surrounding skin intact.	Assess for cracks or fissures at corners of mouth and on lips. *Indicates sources of oral discomfort.*
	Tumors or growths in oral cavity treated appropriately as evidenced by decreased size of lesion and increased patient comfort.	Assess for purple lesions or tumors. *Indicates possible Kaposi's sarcoma or lymphoma.*
		Prepare patient for treatment with radiation, chemotherapy, and excision of lesions as prescribed. *To provide emotional support and coordinate care needs.*
	Patient reports decreasing oral discomfort, participates in oral care. Practices oral hygiene self-care instructions.	Assist with oral care every 2 hours. Rinse oral mucosa with saline and dilute hydrogen peroxide solution. *Decreases spread of lesions.*
		Use a soft toothbrush or sponge-tipped swab, nonabrasive toothpaste, and lip moisturizer.
		Brush teeth a minimum of twice a day. *Decreases acid formation from retained food, moistens mucous membranes, prevents infection, and promotes comfort.*
		Avoid lemon glycerin swabs and alcohol-based mouthwashes. *Acid irritates lesions and alcohol-based products dry mucous membranes.*
		Encourage use of commercial salivary product or hard candy or gum. *Neutralizes acids by increasing saliva flow and protects mucous membranes.*
		Instruct patient and family in aspects of oral hygiene. *To promote comfort and self-care.*
	Family/friends support oral hygiene self-care practices.	Collaborate with patient/family to plan menu that avoids salty, spicy, acidic, or abrasive foods. *To decrease aggravation of oral lesions.*
	Patient has decreased oral pain.	Avoid extremely hot or cold foods. *Mucous membranes are sensitive to temperature extremes.*
	Moist pink mucous membranes.	Instruct patient to have fluid intake of >2,500 mL/day if not contraindicated. *To maintain hydration and keep mucous membranes moist.*
		Encourage patient to avoid smoking. *To decrease drying and irritation to mucous membranes.*

Sources: Carpenito-Moyet, L. (2008). *Nursing care plans and documentation* (5th ed.). Philadelphia: Lippincott Williams & Wilkins; Corless, I. B., & Nicholas, P. K. (2003). Nursing care of patients with HIV/AIDS. In J. K. Shaw & E. A. Mahoney (Eds.), *HIV/AIDS nursing secrets* (pp. 33–39). Philadelphia: Hanley & Belfus; Porth, C., & Sweeney, K. (2007). Alterations in immune response. In C. M. Porth (Ed.), *Essentials of pathophysiology* (pp. 293–319). St. Louis: Lippincott Williams & Wilkins.

The HIV/AIDS epidemic means that nurses throughout all aspects of the health care system will be called on to care for patients with HIV infection. Foundational to nursing is providing care in a compassionate, committed, and nonjudgmental manner. Care for the patient with AIDS involves a wide spectrum of activities from a gentle touch that communicates compassion, to education on a complex medication regimen and multiple interventions to treat opportunistic infections and malignancies. Nurses also play a central role in providing emotional support to patients and families during the dying process and facilitating the discussions on end-of-life care. The complexity of HIV infection presents multiple care needs that nurses, using the nursing process, are well equipped to address. Nurses are an essential part of a collaborative care approach to optimizing treatment for the patient with AIDS.

Health Promotion

The primary mode of HIV/AIDS prevention is education and lifestyle modification for at-risk groups. Nurses, other health care providers, social workers, and community health educators, and schools play a central role in providing education about HIV/AIDS and infection prevention. Instructing individuals and communities on safer sex practices and ways to decrease disease transmission with injection drug use is essential. Chart 60–12 (p. 1948) provides a teaching guide for individuals and

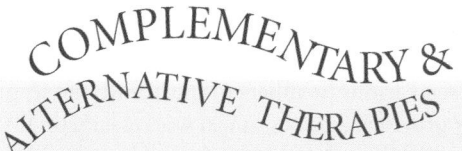

COMPLEMENTARY & ALTERNATIVE THERAPIES for Patients with HIV/AIDS

THERE IS growing support among HIV-infected patients for the use of complementary and alternative treatments in symptom management. Alternative therapies focus on the interaction of the mind, body, and spirit and the concept of treating the whole person. Alternative therapies used in conjunction with traditional Western medicine therapies may improve the patient's overall well-being (Swanson et al., 2000). The four basic categories of alternative therapies are listed here along with examples of the therapies used most frequently:

1. *Nutritional therapies:* vegetarian or microbiotic diets, Chinese herb mixtures, vitamin C or beta-carotene substances

2. *Physical treatments:* acupressure, acupuncture, reflexology, therapeutic touch, crystals, and yoga

3. *Spiritual or psychological therapies:* humor, faith healing, guided imagery, hypnosis

4. *Biological therapies and drugs:* oxygen, zone, and urine therapy; non–FDA-approved drugs (*N*-acetylcysteine, pentoxifylline).

Source: Swanson, P., Harris, B., Holzmayer, V., Devare, S., Schochetman, G., and Hack J. (2000). Quantification of HIV-1 group M (subtypes A–G) and group O by the LCx HIV RNA quantitative assay. *Journal of Virological Methods, 89*(1, 2), 97–108.

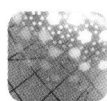

PATIENT TEACHING & DISCHARGE PRIORITIES for the HIV-Infected Individual with AIDS

Need	Teaching
Knowledge of disease process	Provide verbal and written instructions on ways HIV can be transmitted to avoid infecting other persons (unprotected sex, sharing of needles, exposing others to blood or body fluids).
Understanding of medications	Have patient administer medications on schedule and verbalize importance of compliance with HAART therapy to control disease progression and decrease risk of developing drug resistance.
	Teach the purpose, dose, and possible side effects of all medications to increase compliance and prevent over- or underdosing.
	Explain the importance of a follow-up laboratory appointment schedule to monitor medication effectiveness.
Prevention of opportunistic infections	Teach signs and symptoms of infection and strategies to avoid exposure to opportunistic infections.
	Encourage avoidance of people with communicable diseases such as colds or flu.
Reportable clinical manifestations	Instruct patient/family to report: • Symptoms of infection (fever, malaise, aching joints) • New or worsening rash or sores • Difficulty eating or swallowing • Nausea, vomiting, diarrhea that lasts for more than 2 days • New or worsening pain • Weight loss.
Ongoing care	Explain the purpose of clinic and laboratory follow-up appointments for ongoing monitoring of medication effectiveness and assessment of CD4+ T-cell and viral load counts.
	Provide schedule and contact information for appointments following discharge.
	Explain value of regular health screenings including checkups with monitoring of weight and dental care.
Family/support system	Assess availability of support system to provide emotional support, and assist with medications and transportation to appointments.
	Collaborate with discharge planner/case manager RN (if available) and assess discharge needs to home or extended care.
	Assess need for home assistive devices.
	Assess need for home health care provider.
Emotional adjustment of patient/family due to chronic nature of disease	Answer questions honestly.
	Encourage verbalization of feelings, fears.
	Discuss possibility of depression and encourage discussion of this with health care provider.

---

partners regarding practices to decrease HIV transmission risk that can be used by a variety of HIV/AIDS prevention educators.

It is important that HIV-infected patients and their families and friends understand the routes of transmission of HIV to prevent infection and alleviate fears of casual transmission. The information provided can address these issues and alleviate fears that may interfere with social support for the patient with HIV/AIDS.

Collaborative Management

A multidisciplinary collaborative approach to preventing HIV infection and transmission and providing treatment for patients with HIV/AIDS is essential. A variety of individuals using different educational approaches in varied settings can most effectively communicate the facts about HIV/AIDS. Effective treatment of individuals with HIV infection and AIDS requires

GERONTOLOGICAL CONSIDERATIONS Related to HIV/AIDS

In the United States, 10% of all reported AIDS cases occur in adults over 50 years of age. Older adults are at increased risk for contracting HIV/AIDS because of declining immune system function with aging. Additionally, AIDS is associated with youth, sexual activity, and IV drug use, factors that are generally not linked with the elderly population. Sexual contact is the most common form of HIV transmission, yet there is a prevalent misconception that older adults are not sexually active. Older adults are beyond childbearing years, so they often fail to use condoms when engaging in sexual activity. Additionally, older adults may have had a history of IV drug use that results in latent HIV infection. They also can be current IV drug users, but given the more conservative nature of their social group and the socially unacceptable nature of this addiction, this issue may be denied. As a consequence there is denial on the part of older adults and the health care community that this group is at risk for HIV infection, and the potential for misdiagnosis and subsequent failure to treat with antiretroviral therapy is significant (Ress, 2003).

Nurses must be aware that the older adult is also at risk for HIV/AIDS and assess the risk factors by means of a thorough nursing history. It is essential to advocate for the patient by asking the medical team about possible HIV antibody testing when a diagnosis is unclear and the patient has risk factors and symptoms consistent with an AIDS-related illness.

coordination between various members of the health care team such as health care providers, nurses, social workers, dietitians, and community workers at various levels of care from clinics, to home care, to acute care.

The health care provider is primarily responsible for diagnosis and development of the medical treatment plan. The role of the nurse is centered on providing emotional support and monitoring and managing disease symptoms. Nurses also provide education on medications and the importance of compliance with the medication regimen, ongoing laboratory tests and appointments, and minimizing the risk of opportunistic infections. Social workers offer assistance in addressing financial concerns, managing personal care needs, and accessing community referrals and social networks in the community and acute care setting. Dietitians also have a significant role in monitoring nutritional needs and developing specialized nutritional plans that may include supplements in light of HIV complications and wasting syndrome. For more on nutrition and how it affects patients with HIV/AIDS, see the Evidence-Based Practice feature.

Collaborative care of HIV-infected patients also involves extensive education of patients, family, and friends regarding antiretroviral medications and prevention of opportunistic infections as discussed earlier in Chart 60–9 (p. 1929). Collaborative care also involves identifying potential risk factors for HIV

CHART 60–12 | Patient and Partner Teaching Guide on Preventing HIV Transmission

- Practice abstinence or mutual monogamy or limit the number of sexual partners.

- Do not have unprotected sex. Use latex condoms (animal skin condoms do not prevent HIV transmission). For latex allergies use female condoms that are latex free.

- Do not lubricate the condom with spermicidal agent nonoxynol-9 or use spermicidal agent nonoxynol-9 because this may increase vaginal tissue damage and the risk of HIV infection.

- Do not use oil-based sex lubricants because this can damage the condom. Water-based lubricants are safe to use.

- Do not reuse male or female condoms.

- Always use a condom with other methods of birth control. Cervical caps or diaphragms will decrease the risk of pregnancy, but not HIV transmission.

- Always use dental dams for oral female genital or anal stimulation.

- Avoid anal intercourse or manual anal intercourse "fisting" to prevent injury to tissues.

- Use safer sex practices, such as mutual masturbation, to decrease damage to mucous membranes.

- If entering a mutually exclusive monogamous relationship, both partners should undergo HIV testing. There is a window period of up to 6 months before HIV antibody testing is positive, so the above guidelines should be followed during the window period when HIV status is unknown.

- If you are HIV antibody positive, inform previous, current, and prospective sex partners and drug-using partners of your HIV status. Follow the above guidelines.

- If you are HIV antibody positive, inform health care providers of HIV status. Laws protect the confidentiality of this information. This information helps direct your medical treatment.

- If you are HIV antibody positive, do not share items that may be contaminated with blood such as needles, drug works, sex toys, razors, or toothbrushes.

- If you are HIV antibody positive, do not donate blood, plasma, sperm, or body organs.

GUIDELINES FOR SAFER USE OF INJECTION EQUIPMENT

If you use injection drugs, consider stopping and entering a treatment program. If you cannot make that choice, use the following guidelines to limit your risk of HIV and other disease transmission.

- Use sterile needles and syringes.

- Do not share your needles, syringes, or drug preparation equipment ("works").

- Access needle and syringe exchange programs, when available, to exchange used needles and syringes and obtain sterile ones.

- If injection equipment is shared, clean it thoroughly before use: Rinse the syringe and needle twice with tap water, fill the syringe with full-strength household bleach for 30 seconds, shake and squirt out, repeat bleaching process a second time, then rinse again twice with tap water.

- Do not share your drug preparation equipment. If it is shared, clean it thoroughly with bleach and water.

- Do not share your bleach or rinse water.

Sources: Centers for Disease Control and Prevention. (2007, July). *HIV and AIDS: Are you at risk?* Retrieved September 3, 2008, from http://www.cdc.gov/hiv/resources/brochures/at-risk.htm; Shaw, J. K., & Mahoney, E. A. (Eds.). (2003). *HIV/AIDS nursing secrets.* Philadelphia: Hanley & Belfus; Workowski, K. A., & Levine, W. C. (2002). Sexually transmitted diseases treatment guidelines. *Morbidity and Mortality Weekly Report, 51*(RR-06).

Healthy Nutrition and the Patient with HIV/AIDS

Clinical Problem

The relationship between nutrition and HIV/AIDS is complex and not fully understood. It is known, however, that healthy nutrition plays a role in alleviating common symptoms of HIV such as diarrhea, anorexia, sore mouth, and muscle wasting. There are many gaps in current knowledge about the impact of malnutrition on management and progression of HIV. It is known that HIV causes increased energy requirements, nutrient malabsorption and loss, complex metabolic alterations, and frequently a loss of appetite that culminates in weight loss and muscle wasting. The effect of HIV on nutritional status begins early in the course of infection, at times even before the patient is aware of being infected (Bogden et al., 2000).

Vitamins and minerals needed for the immune system to fight infections include A, B-complex, C, and E, and selenium and zinc. These substances are commonly found to be deficient in people living with HIV in all settings. In addition, deficiencies of antioxidant vitamins and minerals contribute to oxidative stress, which may accelerate immune cell death and increase the rate of HIV replication (Allard et al., 1998; Banki, Hutter, Gonchoroff, & Perl, 1998).

Research Findings

Fawzi and colleagues (2004) conducted a study to evaluate the impact of micronutrient supplements (vitamin A alone, multivitamins including vitamin B-complex and vitamins C and E, and multivitamins plus vitamin A) on the risks of clinical disease progression, HIV-related complications, CD4+ cell counts, and viral load in HIV-positive women. The researchers followed 1,078 HIV-infected pregnant women over a 2-year period. The women were randomly assigned in blocks of 20 to receive a daily oral dose of one of four regimens of vitamins for the duration of the study.

The results of the study indicate that multivitamin supplementation with vitamin B-complex, vitamin C, and vitamin E significantly delayed the progression of disease among HIV-infected women, as reflected by the relative risk of progression to WHO stage 4 or death from AIDS-related causes. Supplementation with vitamin A alone had weaker effects that for the most part were not significantly different from those produced by placebo. The study also found that supplementation with multivitamins also reduced the incidence of complications including:

- Oral thrush
- Oral ulcers
- Difficulty swallowing
- Nausea
- Vomiting
- Diarrhea.

The researchers concluded that micronutrients may protect the integrity of oral and gastrointestinal epithelia and enhance local and systemic immunity.

Implications for Nursing Practice

This study clearly indicates the efficacy of vitamin supplements for HIV patients for retarding the progress of the disease. When teaching the patient and caregivers about the complex nutritional issues associated with the disease, the nurse needs to include information about the type, amount, and administration schedule of vitamins. It is essential that nurses stress the importance of a continued course of micronutrient supplements. These supplements are readily available and typically inexpensive, which makes it easier for patients to comply with the therapy.

Critical Thinking Questions

1. Which of the following interventions would be effective in increasing medication compliance for patients with HIV/AIDS?
   a. Education about the impact of the medication on disease progression
   b. Ease of availability and financial resources
   c. Caregiver compliance
   d. Show patient laboratory results that support stabilization of the disease

2. Which of the following clinical manifestations would you as the nurse assess for vitamin efficacy?
   a. Diminished or absent diarrhea
   b. Stabilization or increase in CD4+ counts
   c. Absence of candidiasis
   d. No painful swallowing

Answers to Critical Thinking Questions appear in Appendix D.

References

Allard, J. P., Aghdassi, E., Chau, J., et al. (1998). Effects of vitamin E and C supplementation on oxidative stress and viral load in HIV-infected subjects. *AIDS, 12,* 1653–1659.

Banki, K., Hutter, E., Gonchoroff, N. J., & Perl, A. (1998). Molecular ordering in HIV-induced apoptosis. Oxidative stress, activation of caspases, and cell survival are regulated by transaldolase. *Journal of Biological Chemistry, 273*(19), 11944–11953.

Bogden, J. D., Kemp, F. W., Han, S., et al. (2000). Status of selected nutrients and progression of human immunodeficiency virus type 1 infection. *American Journal of Clinical Nutrition, 72*(3), 809–815.

Fawzi, W. W., Msamanga, G. I., Spiegelman, D., Wei, R., Kapiga, S., Villamor, E., et al. (2004). A randomized trial of multivitamin supplements and HIV disease progression and mortality. *New England Journal of Medicine, 351*(1), 23–32.

EVIDENCE-BASED PRACTICE

---

infection in patients who have not been diagnosed with HIV and patient knowledge of how HIV is transmitted. Key questions to determine the level of HIV infection risk are a vital aspect of assessment. It is also important to apply an understanding of HIV/AIDS epidemiology in identifying increasingly at-risk populations including women, non-Caucasians, and people over 50 years of age.

The complexity of HIV antiretroviral treatment, the psychologically devastating nature of the disease, and the various body systems that are affected by AIDS mandate a collaborative care approach to maximize patient treatment, and promote comfort and quality of life.

CRITICAL ALERT *HIV key risk assessment questions to ask include the following: Have you had a blood transfusion of any type? If so, was it before 1985? Have you ever had a vaginal, anal, or oral sexual experience without a condom or barrier device? Have you ever had a sexually transmitted infection? Have you ever shared needles, syringes, or other injecting equipment with another person?*

Research Topics Related to the Immune Deficiencies

Research related to immune deficiencies is multifaceted. Nurses are involved in many areas of study including coordinating clinical research sites, data collection, drug studies, and clinical outcomes research. The Research Opportunities and Clinical Impact box provides information on some of the current areas of medical and nursing research under investigation.

The development of a vaccine for HIV is a primary focus of continuing research related to HIV and AIDS. In 1987 The National Institute of Allergy and Infectious Diseases (NIAID) began the first clinical trial of an experimental vaccine. Since that time 23 potential vaccines and 10 adjuvants (substances that might enhance the vaccine's effects) have been tested. The development of a vaccine has been particularly challenging because

HIV mutates rapidly and lives within the cell and hides from antibodies. The NIAID began a phase II vaccine study in 1997 to determine if combining two experimental vaccines can safely stimulate an immune response. To accelerate vaccine development, in September 2003 the NIAID awarded $81 million to four companies researching different strategies for creating a vaccine. NIAID Director Anthony S. Fauci stated at the time of the awards, "A safe and effective HIV vaccine is critical to the control of HIV globally. These awards will speed the development of promising HIV vaccine candidates that are based on recent advances in HIV vaccine design and on the latest discoveries of HIV virology and immunology" (NIAID, 2003). There is a continual hope that at some point in the not-too-distant future, HIV infection will be preventable and AIDS a disease of the past.

RESEARCH OPPORTUNITIES AND CLINICAL IMPACT RELATED TO IMMUNE DEFICIENCIES

Research Area	Clinical Impact
Gene research to identify DNA factors associated with development of genetic immune deficiencies	Develop gene therapy that will help with prevention and treatment of genetic immune deficiencies.
	Provide information to promote informed decision making for couples in genetic counseling.
Development of a vaccine to protect against infection after exposure with HIV	Reduce active cases of HIV and AIDS through prevention with vaccine.
Epidemiologic studies that focus on areas of the world where the incidence of HIV is increasing and the risk factors noted in those areas	Reduce cases of HIV through education of populations at greatest risk worldwide.
Development of new classes of antiretroviral medications	Improve survival, slow progression of HIV infection, maximize development of antiretroviral medications.
Development of a DNA bank of genes, HIV genes, and enzyme codes	Promote research and development of better therapies and vaccines.
Clinical trials of patient compliance with a self-injectable medication (Enfuvirtide)	Provide new route of delivery of drug that may reduce side effects. However, an injectable form requires more extensive patient education.
Clinical trial of calcium carbonate to treat diarrhea in HIV patients receiving protease inhibitors	Reduce side effects and improve quality of life for patients taking multiple antiretroviral medications.
Clinical trials of high-dose combination therapy to extend life in advanced AIDS patients	Improve quality and delay further progression of disease for advanced AIDS patients, and decrease development of resistance.
Comparative studies on HIV viral loads, initiation of antiretroviral therapy, and development of drug resistance	Guide the appropriate initiation of antiretroviral therapy to help prevent development of drug resistance.
Study of adherence, quality of life, and satisfaction with combination drug therapy among patients with multiple years of HIV diagnosis	Improve teaching of medication therapy and increase compliance for newly diagnosed HIV patients starting therapy. Prevent drug resistance.
Comparative studies on viral loads and perinatal transmission for vaginal versus cesarean delivery modes	Develop clear guidelines on the safest method of delivery for HIV-infected pregnant women that also limits perinatal HIV transmission.
Comparative studies on effectiveness of complementary therapies for HIV disease progressive management	Provide new drug treatments to control pain and improve the patient's quality of life.

Clinical Preparation

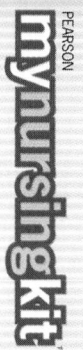

 Read

- History of Current Illness
- Past Medical History
- Physical Exam
- Admitting Medical Orders
- Laboratory Study Results

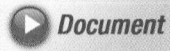 **Document**

- Summary of Hospitalization
- Pathophysiology Form
- Laboratory Values
- Laboratory Results Explanation

 **Apply**

- List of Potential Nursing Diagnoses
- Concept Map
- Critical Thinking Questions

Log on to MyNursingKit.com to download forms you will need and to complete further steps in the Clinical Preparation assignment.

HISTORY OF PRESENT ILLNESS

Mr. B is a 42-year-old Spanish-speaking, thin, anxious-appearing male in moderate discomfort due to abdominal pain that he first noticed 2 weeks ago and described as dull. He does not have a regular doctor and presented to the emergency department (ED) with abdominal pain. Patient requests a Spanish-speaking interpreter. He states, via an interpreter, that he has had increased abdominal pain during the past 5 days, has lost more than 20 pounds during the last 3 months, does not have an appetite, and is having increasing difficulty swallowing because of "sores" in his mouth. He has been unable to take solid

foods for the past 3 days due to painful swallowing, and has taken very little juice or water during the past 24 hours. Denies nausea, vomiting.

He is being admitted by internal medicine to the medical–surgical unit. States he did not want to come to the doctor earlier because he does not have the money to pay the bill. Came to the ED today "because the pain was getting very bad, and I am afraid something is wrong with me." Upon admission to the floor, the patient is awake and alert. He states he is continuing to have pain in his abdomen despite medication.

Medical–Surgical History

No known allergies
Medications: none
Denies history of cancer or family history of cancer
Denies history of abdominal trauma or injuries, gastric reflux disease, hernia, or colitis
Positive history of fatigue, intermittent fever, chills, and night sweats during the past 6 months
Genital herpes onset age 19, intermittent recurrence, most recent occurrence 1 year prior
Surgeries: appendectomy at age 22 in Mexico

Social History

Immigrated to the United States 2 years prior, unmarried, lives with his brother and his brother's family; employed in lawn care and home maintenance business
Drinks 1–2 beers daily
Smokes 1/2 pack of cigarettes per day × 25 years
Prior IV drug use; none in the past 7 years
Intermittently sexually active with various partners

Physical Exam

Vital signs: BP 101/45, HR 108, RR 22, temp 36.8°C, oxygen saturation 95% on room air
Pain: 6/10
Neurological: alert and oriented × 3, worried expression on face, neurological exam normal, communicates with minimal English, primary language is Spanish

HEENT: oral mucous membranes are red and inflamed, multiple white lesions present on oral mucosa and extending to the posterior oral pharynx. Tonsils slightly enlarged, poor dental care, four teeth missing on anterior and left lateral upper jaw. Submandibular lymph nodes bilaterally enlarged and tender to palpations. Ears and eyes normal
Neck: cervical lymph nodes enlarged bilaterally, right greater than left, tender to palpation; full range of neck motion present
Respiratory: denies shortness of breath; unlabored respirations; equal chest wall expansion; no chest deformities evident or palpated; lungs clear
Cardiovascular: tachycardia with occasional irregular beat, S_1, S_2, no murmur, pulses palpable in all extremities, capillary refill WNL
GI/GU: abdomen slightly distended but soft, palpable mass lower quadrants, bowel sounds present in all quadrants, abdomen painful to light palpation in all quadrants, greatest area of pain in lower quadrants. Denies painful urination, normal size genitals, uncircumcised, no drainage from penis, with no evidence of lesions
Skin: intact, dry; poor skin turgor; no evidence of discoloration, rash, or bruising
12-lead ECG: showed sinus tachycardia, occasional PVCs and no other abnormalities
Abdominal CT: results indicate a pelvic mass in the retroperitoneal space above the bladder; size estimated at 20 cm by 15 cm

Admitting Medical Orders

Medical service

Consults: Surgical, Social Services, Oncology

Admit to medical–surgical floor with telemetry monitoring

Admitting diagnosis: abdominal pain, pelvic mass, r/o abdominal malignancy, oral and esophageal candidiasis

Allergies: none

Full code status

Strict I&O

Vital signs and oxygen saturation q4h

Daily weight

Diet: clear liquids

Ambulation ad-lib

Incentive spirometer q1–2h

Sequential compression devices (SCDs) to lower extremities when in bed

Call house officer: BP < 90 systolic or diastolic > 90; HR >120 and < 60, RR >30; temp > 38.2°C: oxygen saturation < 92%

IV: 0.9% saline with 20 mEq of KCl via infusion pump at 500 mL/hr × 1 liter, then decrease rate to 125 mL/hr

Scheduled Medications

Diflucan 200 mg po daily

Protonix 40 mg po daily

Nystatin 5 mL q6h, swish & swallow

PRN Medications

Morphine sulphate 2–4 mg IV push q2h prn for severe pain

Vicodin 1–2 tabs (5/500) po q6h prn for moderate pain

Ativan, 0.5 mg po q4h prn anxiety

Zofran 4 mg IV q4h prn nausea

Ordered Laboratory Studies

CBC with differential on admission

Blood count daily

Complete metabolic panel (CMP), amylase, lipase, PO_4, PT/INR/PTT, UA, CD4 cell count

HIV antibody test (health care provider has completed consent for testing with patient and this is documented on chart)

Ordered Diagnostic Studies

12-lead ECG

Abdominal CT

LABORATORY STUDY RESULTS

Test	Day 1	Day 2	Day 3
Sodium	148 mEq/L	142 mEq/L	138 mEq/L
Potassium	2.9 mEq/L	3.9 mEq/L	4.2 mEq/L
Chloride	113 mEq/L	99 mEq/L	99 mEq/L
Venous carbon dioxide	22 mEq/L	25 mEq/L	25 mEq/L
Blood urea nitrogen (BUN)	42 mg/dL	22 mg/dL	19 mg/dL
Creatinine	1.1 mg/dL	0.9 mg/dL	0.7 mg/dL
Blood glucose	143 mg/dL	124 mg/dL	133 mg/dL
Calcium	7.9 mg/dL	7.8 mg/dL	7.9 mg/dL
Total protein	5.2 g/dL		
Amylase	72 units/L		
Lipase	27 units /L		
Magnesium	1.9 mEq/L	2.0 mEq/L	2.1 mEq/L
Phosphorus	3.1 mg/dL		
Albumin	2.9 g/dL	2.9	2.9
Alkaline phosphatase	225 units/L	197 units/L	192 units/L
Total bilirubin	1.2 mg/dL		
AST (SGOT)	64 units/L	99 units/L	104 units/L
ALT (SGPT)	52 units/L	80 units/L	92 units/L
WBC	1700/mm³	1600/mm³	1600/mm³
Hemoglobin	10.1 g/dL	9.8 g/dL	9.8 g/dL
Hematocrit	30.2%	29.8%	29.8%
RBCs	4.0/mm³	3.9/mm³	3.9/mm³
Neutrophils	88%		
Lymphocytes	2%		
Monocytes	3%		
Platelets	227,000/mm³	208,000/mm³	87,000/mm³
PTT	34 seconds		
PT	13.1 seconds		
INR	1.22 seconds		
CEA		> 11 ng/mL	
CD4 count	170 cells/uL		
HIV antibody	Positive		
ABGs			
PO_2	92 mmHg		
Oxygen saturation	95%	94%	
pH	7.34		
PCO_2	39 mmHg		

CRITICAL THINKING QUESTIONS

1. What information was obtained that suggested the need for HIV testing?

2. Review the laboratory findings from the ED. Which ones are abnormal, what is the possible rationale for these abnormalities, and how are these abnormalities evidenced in physical assessment findings?

3. EIA and Western blot tests are ordered to confirm the diagnosis. The CD4 count results are 187 cells/μL. What is the rationale for ordering this test and what is the significance of the result?

4. Mr. B is HIV positive, but does he have AIDS according to the CDC guidelines?

5. What additional treatment should you anticipate for Mr. B based on his HIV test results and CD4 results?

Answers to Critical Thinking Questions appear in Appendix D.

NCLEX® REVIEW

1. The nursing management and collaborative care for patients with an immune hypersensitivity response differs from those who have immune deficiencies. When the nurse suspects the patient has developed an immune hypersensitivity response, the clinical picture may be based on which of the following characteristics?

   1. The immune system loses self-tolerance and immune deficiencies result.
   2. Hypersensitive reactions are determined by the type of antigen, the time sequence of the reaction, and the immunological response.
   3. The primary mechanism of a hypersensitive response is a genetic disorder that occurred during the embryonic development of the immune system.
   4. Hypersensitive responses are usually the result of opportunistic infections which activate a primary response from the T and B cells.

2. Which of the following describes processes that differentiate the immune hypersensitivity response resulting from an autoimmune mechanism from those resulting from an allergic or alloimmune mechanism?

   1. The primary trigger for a hypersensitive reaction is a genetic defect.
   2. The origin for an alloimmune reaction is from the host's DNA.
   3. The trigger for an autoimmune response is a self-antigen.
   4. Once activated, the hypersensitive response is identical regardless of trigger.

3. Which of the following differentiate the pathophysiology and clinical manifestations of Acquired Immune Deficiency Syndrome (AIDS) from Human Immunodeficiency Virus (HIV)? Select all that apply.

   1. HIV is the end disease manifestation of AIDS.
   2. AIDS is a syndrome of opportunistic infections that occurs as a final stage in patients infected with HIV.
   3. HIV transmission is limited to contact with infected body fluids that have lymphocytes that can harbor HIV.
   4. AIDS precedes HIV and allows for the progression of the virus' entry into the host's lymphocytes.

4. Nursing management of the HIV/AIDS patient to decrease the incidence of opportunistic infections may involve which of the following? Select all that apply.

   1. Subjective assessment to promote the early detection of infection from any body region.
   2. Start antibiotics prior to obtaining cultures to ensure the appropriate therapy is initiated in a timely manner.
   3. Health care providers and family members wash hands before and after patient contact to reduce the risk of opportunistic infection cross-contamination.
   4. Encourage hydration and maintenance of weight to support the immune system.

Answers for review questions appear in Appendix D

KEY TERMS

acquired immunodeficiency syndrome
   (AIDS) *p.1922*
acute graft rejection *p.1913*
acute retroviral syndrome *p.1927*
AIDS indicator conditions *p.1927*
allergen *p.1891*
allergic response *p.1890*
allergy *p.1890*
alloimmune response *p.1890*
anaphylaxis *p.1895*
atopic *p.1893*
autoantibodies *p.1906*
autoantibody tests *p.1906*
autoimmune diseases *p.1903*
autoimmune response *p.1890*
CD4+ T cells *p.1926*
chronic graft rejection *p.1913*
corticosteroids *p.1906*
delayed hypersensitivity reaction *p.1891*
desensitization *p.1897*
flare *p.1893*

graft versus host disease (GVHD) *p.1913*
highly active antiretroviral drug therapy
   (HAART) *p.1937*
histamine *p.1891*
HIV antibody positive status *p.1927*
host versus graft disease (HVGD) *p.1913*
human immunodeficiency virus
   (HIV) *p.1922*
human leukocyte antigen (HLA) *p.1906*
hyperacute rejection *p.1913*
IgE antibodies *p.1891*
immediate hypersensitivity reaction *p.1890*
immune deficiencies *p.1890*
immune hypersensitivity *p.1890*
immune hypersensitivity response *p.1890*
Kaposi's sarcoma *p.1933*
neoantigens *p.1905*
opportunistic infections (OIs) *p.1922*
plasmapheresis *p.1906*
Pneumocystis carinii pneumonia
   (PCP) *p.1931*

primary immune deficiency *p.1890*
reverse transcriptase *p.1926*
secondary immune deficiencies *p.1890*
sensitization *p.1891*
skin testing *p.1896*
systemic lupus erythematosus (SLE) *p.1906*
tissue-specific antigens *p.1891*
type-specific hypersensitivity
   reactions *p.1890*
type I (IgE-mediated) allergic
   reaction *p.1891*
type II (tissue-specific–mediated)
   hypersensitivity reaction *p.1891*
type III (immune complex–mediated)
   reaction *p.1891*
type IV (cell-mediated) hypersensitivity
   reaction *p.1891*
viral load *p.1927*
wasting syndrome *p.1932*
Western blot (WB) *p.1933*
wheal *p.1893*
window period *p.1925*

REFERENCES

Adams, M., Josephson, D., & Holland, L. (2008). *Pharmacology for nurses: A pathophysiologic approach.* (2nd ed.) Upper Saddle River, NJ: Pearson Prentice Hall.

Ahmed, D. D., Sobczak, S. C., & Yunginger, J. W. (2003). Occupational allergies caused by latex. *Immunology and Allergy Clinics of North America, 23*(2), 205–219.

Allard, J. P., Aghdassi, E., Chau, J., et al. (1998). Effects of vitamin E and C supplementation on oxidative stress and viral load in HIV-infected subjects. *AIDS, 12,* 1653–1659.

American Academy of Allergy, Asthma and Immunology. (2006). *Why is the incidence of allergy increasing?* Retrieved February 23, 2007, from https://www.aaaai.org/aadmc/inthenews/wypr/2006archive/increasing_allergies.html

American Academy of Allergy, Asthma and Immunology. (2007). *Tips to remember: What is allergy testing.* Retrieved February 16, 2007, from http://www.aaaai.org

American College of Allergy, Asthma and Immunology. (2007). *Be S.A.F.E.: Managing allergic emergencies.* Retrieved February 19, 2007, from http://www.acaai.org/public

American Nurses Association. (2004). *Position statement: AIDS/HIV Disease and socio-culturally diverse populations.* Retrieved January 19, 2004, from http://www.nursingworld.org/readroom/position/blood/bldvrs.htm

American Red Cross. (2003). *What happens to every blood donation.* Retrieved October 10, 2003, from http://www.redcross.org/services/biomed/blood/supply

Anderson, J. (Ed.). (2004). *A guide to the clinical care of women with HIV.* Retrieved February 23, 2007, from the Department of Health and Human Services Health Resources and Services Administration website: http://hab.hrsa.gov/publications/womencare05

Anaya, J., Tobon, G., Vega, P., & Castiblanco, J. (2006). Autoimmune disease aggregation in families with primary Sjogren's syndrome. *Journal of Rheumatology, 33*(11), 2227–2234.

Asher, M., Montefort, S., Bjorksten, B., Lai, C., Strachan, D., Weiland, S., et al. (2006). Worldwide time trends in the prevalence of symptoms of asthma, allergic rhinoconjunctivitis, and eczema in childhood: ISAAC phases one and three repeat multicountry cross-sectional surveys. *Lancet, 368*(9537), 733–748.

Asthma and Allergy Foundation of America. (2007). *Allergy facts and figures.* Retrieved February 19, 2007, from http://www.aafa.org

Averitt, S. A., & Sowell, R. L. (2003). Pregnancy and HIV/AIDS. In J. K. Shaw & E. A. Mahoney (Eds.), *HIV/AIDS nursing secrets* (pp. 133–143). Philadelphia: Hanley & Belfus.

Banki, K., Hutter, E., Gonchoroff, N. J., & Perl, A. (1998). Molecular ordering in HIV-induced apoptosis. Oxidative stress, activation of caspases, and cell survival are regulated by transaldolase. *Journal of Biological Chemistry, 273*(19), 11944–11953.

Bartlett, J. G. (2003). *Wasting [HIV] antibiotic guide.* Accessed December 25, 2003, from Johns Hopkins Division of Infectious Diseases website: http://hopkins-abxguide.org/terminals/diagnosis_terminal.cfm?id=622

Bartlett, J. G., & Lane, H. C. (2007). *Guidelines for the use of antiretroviral agents in HIV-1-infected adults and adolescents. Developed by the DHHS Panel on Antiretroviral Guidelines for Adults and Adolescents—A working group of the Office of AIDS Research Advisory Council.* Retrieved January 10, 2008, from http://aidsinfo.nih.gov/contentfiles/AdultandAdolescentGL.pdf

Bochner, B. S., & Hamid, Q. (2003). Advances in mechanisms of allergy. *Journal of Allergy and Clinical Immunology, 111*(3 Suppl.), S819–S823.

Bogden, J. D., Kemp, F. W., Han, S., et al. (2000). Status of selected nutrients and progression of human immunodeficiency virus type 1 infection. *American Journal of Clinical Nutrition, 72*(3), 809–815.

Brandtzaeg, P. (2007). Why we develop food allergies: Coached by breast milk and good bacteria, the immune system strives to learn the difference between food and pathogens before the first morsel crosses our lips. *American Scientist, 95*(1), 28.

Branson, B., Handsfield, H., Lampe, M., Janssen, R., Taylor, A., Lyss, S., & Clark, J. (2006). Revised recommendations for HIV testing of adults, adolescents, and pregnant women. *MMWR* 55 (RR-14): 1-17 Retrieved on September 5, 2008 from http://www.cdc.gov/mmwr/pdf/rr/rr5514.pdf.

Brew, B. J. (2002). Neurological manifestations of HIV infection. In S. Crowe, J. Hoy, & J. Mills (Eds.), *Management of the HIV-infected patient.* London: Taylor & Francis.

Carpenito-Moyet, L. (2008). *Nursing care plans and documentation* (5th ed.). Philadelphia: Lippincott Williams & Wilkins.

Centers for Disease Control and Prevention. (1981a). Opportunistic infections and Kaposi's sarcoma in homosexual men. *Morbidity and Mortality Weekly Report, 30.* Retrieved September 22, 2003, from http://aids-info.net/micha/hiv/aids/cdc81.htm

Centers for Disease Control and Prevention. (1981b). Pneumocystis pneumonia—Los Angeles. *Morbidity and Mortality Weekly Report, 30,* 250. Retrieved September 22, 2003, from http://aids-info.net/micha/hiv/aids/cdc81.htm

Centers for Disease Control and Prevention. (1993). Revised classification system for HIV infection and the expanded surveillance case definition of AIDS among adolescents and adults. *Morbidity and Mortality Weekly Report, 44*(RR-17). Retrieved February 23, 2007, from http://www.cdc.gov/mmwr/preview/mmwrhtml/00018871.htm

Centers for Disease Control and Prevention. (1995). First 500,000 AIDS cases, United States, 1995. *Morbidity and Mortality Weekly Report, 44,* 46. Retrieved January 19, 2004, from http://www.thebody.com/cdc/mmnov24.html

Centers for Disease Control and Prevention. (1998). *Human immunodeficiency virus type 2.* Retrieved January 19, 2004, from http://www.cdc.gov/hiv/pubs/facts/hiv2.htm

Centers for Disease Control and Prevention. (2001). Appendix B: Management of occupational blood exposures. *Morbidity and Mortality Weekly Report, 50*(RR-11), 45–46. Retrieved February 27, 2007, from http://www.cdc.gov/mmwr/preview/mmwrhtml/rr5011a3.htm

Centers for Disease Control and Prevention. (2002). HIV testing among pregnant women in the United States and Canada 1998–2001. *Morbidity and Mortality Weekly Report 51,* 1013–1016. Retrieved February 27, 2006, from http://www.cdc.gov/search

Centers for Disease Control and Prevention. (2003a). *HIV partner counseling and referral services guidance.* Retrieved February 27, 2007, from http://www.cdc.gov/hiv/pubs/pcrs/pcrs-doc.htm

Centers for Disease Control and Prevention. (2003b). *TB education and training resource guide—TB and HIV/AIDS co-infection.* Retrieved February 23, 2007, from CDC National Prevention Information Network website: http://www.cdcnpin.org/scripts/tb/guide/co_inf.asp

Centers for Disease Control and Prevention. (2005a). Appendix B: Updated U.S. Public Health Service guidelines for management of occupational exposures to HIV and recommendations for postexposure prophylaxis. *Morbidity and Mortality Weekly Report, 54*(RR-09), 1–17. Retrieved February 25, 2006, from http://www.cdc.gov/mmwr/preview/mmwrhtml/rr5011a3.htm

Centers for Disease Control and Prevention. (2005b). *Co-infection with HIV and hepatitis C virus.* Retrieved February 23, 2007, from http://www.cdc.gov/hiv/resources/factsheets/coinfection.htm

Centers for Disease Control and Prevention. (2005c). *HIV/AIDS update basic statistics.* Retrieved February 23, 2007, from http://www.cdc.gov/hiv/stats.htm

Centers for Disease Control and Prevention. (2005d). Youth risk behavior surveillance in the United States, 2005. CDC Surveillance Summaries, 2006. *Morbidity and Mortality Weekly Report, 55*(SS-5). Retrieved February 27, 2006, from http://www.cdc.gov/search

Centers for Disease Control and Prevention. (2006a). *How safe is the blood supply in the United States?* Retrieved February 23, 2007, from http://www.cdc.gov/hiv/resources/qa/qa15.htm

Centers for Disease Control and Prevention. (2006b). *Important updates on OraQuick procedures.* Retrieved February 23, 2007, from http://www.cdc.gov/hiv/resources/qa/prevention.htm

Centers for Disease Control and Prevention. (2006c). Revised recommendations for HIV testing of adults, adolescents, and pregnant women in healthcare settings. *Morbidity and Mortality Weekly Report, 55*(RR-14), 1–17.

Corbett, J. V. (2004). *Laboratory tests and diagnostic procedures.* Upper Saddle River, NJ: Pearson Prentice Hall.

Corless, I. B., & Nicholas, P. K. (2003). Nursing care of patients with HIV/AIDS. In J. K. Shaw & E. A. Mahoney (Eds.), *HIV/AIDS nursing secrets* (pp. 33–39). Philadelphia: Hanley & Belfus.

Crowe, S., Hoy, J., & Mills, J. (Eds.). (2002). *Management of the HIV-infected patient.* London: Taylor & Francis.

Dabis, F., Bequet, L., Ekouevi, D., & ANRS 1201/1202 DITRAME PLUS Study Group. (2005). Field efficacy of zidovudine, lamivudine and single-dose nevirapine to prevent peripartum HIV transmission. *AIDS, 19*(3), 309–318.

DeFranco, A. L., Locksley, R., & Robertson, M. (2007). *Immunity: The immune response in infectious and inflammatory disease.* Sunderland, MA: Sinauer Associates.

Deglin, J., & Vallerand, A. (2007). *Davis's drug guide for nurses.* Philadelphia: F. A. Davis.

Dunne, M. (2007). Infection, inflammation, and immunity. In C. M. Porth (Ed.), *Essentials of pathophysiology* (pp. 229–246). St. Louis: Lippincott Williams & Wilkins.

Dybul, M., Fauci, A. S., Barlett, J. G., Kaplan, J. E., Pau, A. K., & Panel on Clinical Practices for Treatment of HIV. (2002). Guidelines for using antiretroviral agents among HIV-infected adults and adolescents. *Annals of Internal Medicine, 137*(5 Part 2), 381–433.

Embry, A. (2004). The multiple factors of multiple sclerosis: A Darwinian perspective. *Journal of Nutritional & Environmental Medicine, 14*(4), 307–317.

Fauci, A. S. (1991). Immunopathogenic mechanisms in human immunodeficiency virus infection. *Annals of Internal Medicine, 114,* 678–693.

Fauci, A. S. (1996). Immunological mechanisms of HIV infection. *Annals of Internal Medicine, 124,* 654.

Fawzi, W. W., Msamanga, G. I., Spiegelman, D., Wei, R., Kapiga, S., Villamor, E., et al. (2004). A randomized trial of multivitamin supplements and HIV disease progression and mortality. *New England Journal of Medicine, 351*(1), 23–32.

Food Allergy & Anaphylaxis Network. (2006). *Anaphylaxis.* Retrieved February 19, 2007, from http://www.foodallergy.org/anaphylaxis/index.html

Food and Drug Administration. (2003b). New regimen for kidney transplants. *FDA Consumer 37*(4), 1–4. Retrieved October 10, 2003, from http://www.fda.gov/FDAC/departs/2003/403_upd.html#kidney

Gomez-Peurta, J., Martin, H., Amigo, H., Aguirre, M., Camps, M., Cuardrado, M., et al. (2005). Long-term follow-up in 128 patients with primary antiphospholipid syndrome: Do they develop lupus? *Medicine, 84*(4), 225–230.

Greenwald, J., Burstein, G., Pincus, J., & Branson, B. (2006). A rapid review of rapid HIV antibody tests. *Current Infectious Disease Reports, 8,* 125–131. Hamilton, R. G., & Adkinson, N. F., Jr. (2003). Clinical laboratory assessment of IgE-dependent hypersensitivity. *Journal of Allergy and Clinical Immunology, 111*(2), 687–701.

Halken, S. (2003). Early sensitization and the development of allergic airway disease: Risk factors and predictors. *Pediatric Respiratory Review, 4*(2), 128–134.

James, J. M. (2003). Respiratory manifestations of food allergies. *Pediatrics, 111*(6), 1625–1631.

Johnsen, C. (2003). Epidemiology of HIV. In J .K. Shaw & E. A. Mahoney (Eds.), *HIV/AIDS nursing secrets* (pp. 1–8). Philadelphia: Hanley & Belfus.

Judd, F., & Mijch, A. (2002). In S. Crowe, J. Hoy, & J. Mills (Eds.), *Management of the HIV-infected patient.* London: Taylor & Francis.

Kaplan, J., Masur, H., & Holmes, K. (2002). Guidelines for prevention of opportunistic infections among HIV infected persons 2002. Recommendations of the U.S. Public Health Service and the Infectious Diseases Society of America. *Morbidity and Mortality Weekly Report, 51*(RR-8). Retrieved February 27, 2007, from http://www.cdc.gov/mmwR/PDF/rr/rr5108.pdf

Kee, J. L. (2005). *Laboratory and diagnostic tests with nursing implications* (7th ed.). Upper Saddle River, NJ: Pearson Prentice Hall.

Korn, J., & Seibold, J. (2004). *RAPIDS-2: A randomized, double-blind, placebo-controlled, multi-center study to assess the effect of bosentan on healing and prevention of ischemic digital ulcers in patients with systemic sclerosis.* Retrieved January 19, 2004, from http:www.sctc-online.org/studies/rapids2.htm

Kuwabara, S. (2004). Guillain-Barré syndrome: Epidemiology, pathophysiology and management. *Drugs, 64*(6), 597–610.

Little, S. J., Holte, S., Routy, J. P., Daar, E. S., Markowitz, M., Collier, A. C., et al. (2002). Antiretroviral-drug resistance among patients recently infected with HIV. *New England Journal of Medicine, 347*(6), 438–439.

Marks, G., Crepaz, N., Senterfitt, J., & Janssen, R. (2005). Meta-analysis of high-risk sexual behavior in persons aware and unaware they are infected with HIV in the United States: Implications for HIV prevention programs. *Journal of Acquired Immune Deficiency Syndrome, 39*(138), 620–629.

Medem. (2003). *Care of the lupus patient.* Retrieved January 16, 2004, from http://www.medem.com/search

National Heart, Lung and Blood Institute. (2004b). *Scleroderma lung study.* Retrieved January 19, 2004, from http://sclerodemalungstudy.medsch.ucla.edu/title.htm

National Institute of Allergy and Infectious Diseases. (2003). *NIAID awards $81 million to HIV vaccine development.* Retrieved October 21, 2003, from http://www.niaid.nih.gov/newsroom/releases/HVDDTTeams2.htm

National Institute of Allergy and Infectious Diseases. (2003c). *NIAID initiative addresses primary immune deficiency diseases.* Retrieved September 22, 2003, from http://www.niaid.nih.gov/newsroom/releases/pirc.htm

National Institute of Allergy and Infectious Diseases. (2004). *Facts and figures: HIV/AIDS statistics.* Retrieved January 11, 2004, from http://www.niaid.nih.gov/factsheets/aidsstat.htm

National Institute of Arthritis and Musculoskeletal and Skin Diseases. (2003). *Handout on health: Systemic lupus erythematosus.* Retrieved February 19, 2007, from National Institute of Health website: http://www.niams.nih.gov/hi/topics/lupus/slehandout/index.htm#Lupus_3

National Institute of Arthritis and Musculoskeletal and Skin Diseases. (2006). *Care of the lupus patient.* Retrieved February 19, 2007, from National Institute of Health website: http://www.niams.nih.gov/hi/topics/lupus/lupusguide/chp7.htm

National Institute for Occupational Safety and Health. (1999). *NIOSH alert: Preventing needlestick injuries in health care settings* (NIOSH Publication No. 2000-108). Retrieved October 10, 2003, from http://www.cdc.gov/niosh/2000-108.html

National Institute for Occupational Safety and Health. (2007). *Latex allergy: A prevention guide* (NIOSH Publication No. 98-113). Retrieved February 16, 2007, from http://www.cdc.gov/niosh/98-113.html

National Kidney Foundation. (2005). *25 facts about organ donation and transplantation.* Retrieved February 23, 2007, from http://www.kidney.org

Needlestick Safety and Prevention Act. (2000). One Hundred Sixth Congress of the United States of America. Signed into law by President Clinton November 6, 2000. Retrieved October 10, 2003, from http://www.afscme.org/publications/2736.cfm

O'Connell, E. J. (2003). Pediatric allergy: A brief review of risk factors associated with developing allergic diseases in childhood. *Annals of Allergy Asthma Immunology, 90*(6 Suppl. 3), 53–58.

Porth, C., & Sweeney, K. (2007). Alterations in immune response. In C. M. Porth (Ed.), *Essentials of pathophysiology* (pp. 293–319). St. Louis: Lippincott Williams & Wilkins.

Public Health Service Task Force. (2006). *Recommendations for the use of antiretroviral drugs in pregnant HIV-1-infected women for maternal health and interventions to reduce perinatal HIV-1 transmission in the United States.* Retrieved February 23, 2007, from http://AIDSinfo.nih.gov

Ress, B. (2003). HIV disease and aging: The hidden epidemic. *Critical Care Nurse, 23*(5), 38–42.

Rizzo, D., & Gunta, K. (2007). In C. M. Porth (Ed.), *Essentials of pathophysiology* (pp. 1015–1045). St. Louis: Lippincott Williams & Wilkins.

Rote, N. (2006). Immunity. In K. L. McCance & S. E. Heuther (Eds.), *Pathophysiology: The biological basis for disease in adults and children* (5th ed., pp. 168–227). St. Louis: Mosby.

Sampson, H. (2003). Anaphylaxis and emergency treatment. *Pediatrics, 111*(6) ,1601–1608.

Shaw, J. K. (2003). Opportunistic infections. In J. K. Shaw & E. A. Mahoney (Eds.), *HIV/AIDS nursing secrets* (pp. 9–13). Philadelphia: Hanley & Belfus.

Shaw, J. K., & Mahoney, E. A. (Eds.). (2003). *HIV/AIDS nursing secrets.* Philadelphia: Hanley & Belfus.

Sommer, C. (2007). The immune response. In C. M. Porth (Ed.), *Essentials of pathophysiology* (pp. 247–268). St. Louis: Lippincott Williams & Wilkins.

Steinke, J. W., Borish, L., & Rosenwasser, L. J. (2003). Genetics of hypersensitivity. *Journal of Allergy and Clinical Immunology, 111*(2 Suppl.), S495–S501.

Tasha, T., Kumwenda, N., & Gibbons, A. (2003). Short postexposure prophylaxis in newborn babies to reduce mother-to-child transmission of HIV1: NVAZ randomized clinical trial. *Lancet, 362*(9391), 1171–1177.

United Nations Program on HIV/AIDS. (2006). *Report on the global AIDS epidemic: Executive summary.* Retrieved February 27, 2007, from http://www.unaids.org/en/hiv_data/2006GlobalReport/default.asp

Urden, L., Stacy, K., & Lough, M. (2006). *Thelan's critical care nursing: Diagnosis and management* (5th ed.). St. Louis: Mosby.

Van Leeuwen, A., Kranpitz, T., & Smith, L. (2006). *Laboratory and diagnostic tests with nursing implications* (2nd ed.). Philadelphia: F. A. Davis.

Wilson, B. A., Shannon, M., Shields, K., & Stang, C. (2007). *Nurse's drug guide.* Upper Saddle River, NJ: Pearson Prentice Hall.

Wong, G. (2007). Symptoms of asthma and atopic disorders in preschool children: Prevalence and risk factors. *Clinical and Experimental Allergy, 37*(2), 174–179.

Workowski, K., & Berman, S. M. (2006). Sexually transmitted diseases treatment guidelines 2006. *Morbidity and Mortality Weekly Report, 55*(RR-11), 76–78. Retrieved February 27, 2006, from http://www.guideline.gov

World Health Organization. (2007). *Global HIV prevalence has leveled off.* Retrieved January 6, 2009, from http://www.wpro.who.int/sites/hsi/ documents/epi_updates.htm

Zutavern, A., & Brockow, I. (2006). Timing of solid food introduction in relationship to atopic dermatitis and atopic sensitization: Results from a prospective birth cohort study. *Pediatrics, 117*(2), 401–412.

Caring for the Patient with Inflammatory Response, Shock, and Severe Sepsis

Renee Holleran

Outcome-Based Learning Objectives

After studying this chapter, the learner will be able to:

1. Compare and contrast the etiologies of anaphylactic, cardiogenic, hypovolemic, neurogenic, and septic shock.
2. Describe the cellular alterations that occur in shock.
3. Describe the body's response to shock.
4. Identify the factors that place a patient at risk of developing shock.
5. Discuss the emergency care of the patient in shock including identification of the underlying cause, management of the patient's airway, breathing, and circulation, and selected pharmacologic interventions.
6. Describe the acute care of the patient in shock, including oxygen management, circulatory management, nutritional management, skin care, and pain and sedation management.
7. Compare and contrast systemic inflammatory response syndrome (SIRS), sepsis, and severe sepsis based on the definitions used by the American College of Chest Physicians/Society of Critical Care Medicine.
8. Prioritize the treatment of the patient with SIRS and identify strategies to prevent the development of SIRS.
9. Understand the etiologies, epidemiology, and management of multiple organ dysfunction syndrome (MODS) as an end result of shock and severe sepsis.
10. Prioritize the treatment of the patient with MODS and identify strategies to prevent the development of MODS.

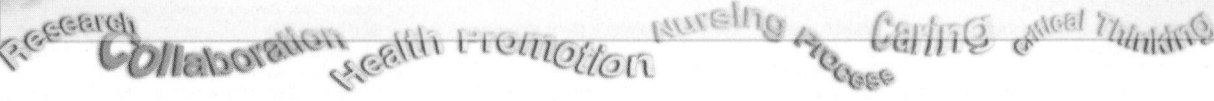

Shock

Shock has been described as the "rude unhinging" of the machinery of life. Shock in and of itself is not a disease, but a clinical manifestation of the body's inability to perfuse tissues adequately (McCance & Huether, 2006). Shock has multiple etiologies, including alterations in the circulating volume of blood or plasma in the body, alterations in the heart's capability to pump, and alterations in peripheral vascular resistance. Regardless of the cause of shock, the systemic response is detrimental and often leads to multiple organ dysfunction syndrome (MODS) and death. It is important to have an understanding about the causes of shock, so it can be prevented or rapidly recognized to prevent life-threatening complications.

Epidemiology

Explaining what shock was and how to treat it did not really begin until the late 19th and early 20th centuries. During World War I surgeons and physiologists thought that a toxin was released from traumatized tissues that caused shock. In 1964, shock was diagnosed when the patient had acute circulatory insufficiency that was characterized by a cardiac output inadequate to provide perfusion to major organs. Nurses and health care providers waited for specific clinical manifestations such as a systolic blood pressure less than 90 mmHg or an increase in heart rate before shock management began. Research was conducted to see how much volume needed to be lost before the patient was considered to be in "shock." Shock was looked at in "pieces" instead of as a systemic response to a particular insult to the body whether from an injury, disease, or infection (Grenvik, Ayres, Holbrook, & Shoemaker, 2000).

In recent years the definition and management of shock has been challenged. In 1992 and again in 2003, the American College of Chest Physicians and Society of Critical Care Medicine developed a consensus definition for sepsis and multiple organ failure. One of these definitions described **systemic inflammatory response syndrome (SIRS)**, a systemic response of the immune system that can be triggered by both infectious and noninfectious causes. Originally associated with sepsis, other researchers, particularly those who dealt with critically injured patients, recognized that SIRS is probably the first phase of shock (Ertel et al., 1995; Levy et al., 2003; Moore et al., 1996).

Mortality from shock is difficult to calculate because shock is generally not classified as a cause of death. Death usually results from multiple organ dysfunctions. For example, each year 660,000 to 750,000 people are hospitalized with an infectious process that causes sepsis, which leads to acute organ dysfunction (Micek, Shah, & Kollef, 2003). About 50% of these patients will die. Risk factors such as age, preexisting illness, and inappropriate antibiotic use can increase patient mortality (Martin et al., 2003). These risk factors are explained in more detail later in this chapter.

Etiology

The etiologies of shock have been classified in various ways. The most common classification is by the cause of the shock syndrome, for example, sepsis from infection is referred to as septic shock (McCance & Huether, 2006). Another classification is related to the amount of circulating volume in the body and how it is affected by the shock syndrome, for example, low-volume shock or absolute hypovolemia (Campbell, 2004; Chapman, 2003). This type of classification is outlined in Chart 61–1. The following subsections describe the etiology of shock based on the cause.

Anaphylactic Shock

Anaphylactic shock results from an antigen–antibody reaction. The body becomes hypersensitive to a specific agent such as a medication like penicillin. When this happens, vasodilatation of blood vessels occurs, causing pooling of blood. Because the blood has pooled in the periphery, perfusion to the tissues is markedly diminished or absent. In addition, other body systems will react to the toxin. In particular, the pulmonary system will respond with vasoconstriction, causing respiratory distress and potential respiratory arrest (McCance & Huether, 2006). Chart 61–2 lists causes of anaphylactic shock. Chapter 60 ⊛ includes a more detailed discussion of anaphylaxis.

Cardiogenic Shock

When the heart is unable to pump effectively, cardiogenic shock will develop. Myocardial infarction is one of the most common causes of damage to the heart that may lead to the development of the heart's inability to function and eventually cause cardiogenic shock. Refer to Chapter 40 ⊛ for a detailed description. Despite advances in technological care, the mortality rate of cardiogenic shock remains high. Chart 61–2 lists causes of cardiogenic shock.

CHART 61–1 Shock Syndromes

Shock Syndrome	Etiology
Low-volume shock (absolute hypovolemia)	Major loss of blood or circulating body fluid such as plasma.
High-space shock (relative hypovolemia)	Injury or toxin affects the blood vessels, which results in the redistribution of blood and fluid. For example, in spinal shock, damage to the sympathetic nervous system causes vasodilation and alteration in blood distribution.
Mechanical (obstructive) shock	A condition that slows or obstructs blood flow in or out of the heart. Examples include cardiac tamponade, tension pneumothorax, vena cava obstruction.

CHART 61–2 Causes of Specific Shock Syndromes

Shock Syndrome	Causes
Anaphylactic shock	Insect bites Medication allergies Food allergies Latex allergies Idiopathic reactions
Cardiogenic shock	Myocardial infarction Myocardial contusion Ruptured ventricles Ruptured papillary muscles Cardiomyopathy
Hypovolemic shock	Traumatic injury (abdominal trauma, chest trauma, orthopedic trauma) Gastrointestinal bleeding Vomiting and diarrhea Osmotic diuresis Diabetic ketoacidosis Thermal injuries
Neurogenic shock	Spinal cord or medulla trauma Anesthetic agents Severe emotional stress Severe pain
Septic shock	Bacterial infections Viral infections Immunosuppression Technology (indwelling urinary or intravenous catheters, feeding tubes) Antibiotic misuse

---

Hypovolemic Shock

Hypovolemic shock results from significant fluid loss that alters the amount of circulating volume in the body. Fluid loss can include loss of blood, plasma, or other body fluids. Hemorrhagic shock is the most common type of shock encountered when a person has suffered multiple system traumas. Hemorrhagic shock can also be the result of upper and lower gastrointestinal bleeding, ruptured aortic aneurysm, hemorrhagic pancreatitis, and long-bone fractures. Fluid loss that is not hemorrhagic can be caused by diarrhea, vomiting, and inadequate repletion of fluid losses as in heat stroke, burn wounds, and leaking of plasma into the interstitial or "third spacing," which can occur with intestinal obstruction, pancreatitis, and cirrhosis. Chapter 68 ⊛ discusses "third spacing" of fluid.

The loss of intravascular volume causes a reduction in preload. *Preload* refers to the force that stretches the ventricles to an initial length. The resting force on the heart is determined by pressure in the ventricles at the end of diastole. Factors that affect preload include muscle fiber length, stretch, volume, and wall stress (Chapman, 2003). Because of these factors, blood volume returning to the heart is inadequate, which affects the amount of the blood returning to the circulation. When blood is lost, or unavailable because of sequestration, the ability to carry oxygen to the cells is also lost because of the decrease in hemoglobin. Chart 61–2 contains a summary of the most common causes of hypovolemic shock.

Neurogenic Shock

Neurogenic shock results from an imbalance between the sympathetic and parasympathetic stimulation of vascular smooth muscle, which results in vasodilation (McCance & Huether, 2006). The body's circulating blood volume generally remains unchanged. However, injury or medications that affect the spinal cord or medulla will cause an imbalance between the sympathetic and parasympathetic nervous systems. Because of this imbalance, clinical symptoms usually associated with shock are different. For example, the patient may be hypotensive, but not tachycardic. Chart 61–2 (p. 1957) contains a list of the causes of neurogenic shock. Chapter 32 ⊕ includes an in-depth discussion of spinal cord injuries and neurogenic shock.

Septic Shock

Septic shock is defined as sepsis that is refractory to fluid resuscitation (McCance & Huether, 2006). Septic shock results in hypotension and perfusion abnormalities. Impaired perfusion will cause lactic acidosis, oliguria, and alterations in mental status. Septic shock occurs when an infectious agent or infection-induced mediator causes systemic decompensation. Because of the body's response to the mediators, there is decreased **systemic vascular resistance (SVR)** (arterial systolic pressure; normal SVR is 900 to 1,400 dyn·s/cm⁵), as well as maldistribution of the blood into the microcirculation, causing compromised tissue perfusion and cellular dysfunction (McCance & Huether, 2006; Society of Critical Care Medicine, 1999). Chapter 24 ⊕ includes a detailed discussion regarding SVR. Despite advances in antibiotic and antiviral therapies, the cases of septic shock, particularly in hospitals, continue to rise. The mortality rate from septic shock is about 50% and increases when the patient has other comorbid risk factors such as immunosuppression, age, or preexisting diseases such as diabetes (Micek et al., 2003; Russell, 2006). Chart 61–2 (p. 1957) outlines the causes of septic shock.

In summary, there are multiple etiologies that may place the patient at risk for developing shock. It is important to be cognizant of any or all of these when a patient presents with symptoms that may indicate the initiation of the "rude unhinging of the machinery of life." Critical interventions must begin as early as possible to prevent irreversible shock, and death.

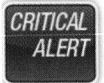 *The primary treatment for all shock syndromes is early recognition of factors that may place the patient at risk for developing shock. Be aware of specific risk factors that may cause particular shock syndromes. For example, patients with an indwelling urinary catheter are at risk for becoming septic and predisposes them to septic shock.*

Pathophysiology

Shock is a syndrome that results from inadequate tissue perfusion. As previously discussed, there are multiple causes of shock that will produce alterations in circulating volume, alterations in cardiac pump function, or alterations in peripheral vascular resistance (PVR), resulting in impairment of cellular metabolism. This results in both impaired oxygen and glucose use.

The amount of oxygen available for tissue consumption per unit of time is defined as oxygen delivery (DO_2). The body generally does have some oxygen reserve available in order to respond to stress. However, if the patient has any preexisting illnesses or injury, this will strain the body and decrease or eliminate the additional oxygen cushion. The amount of oxygen extracted from the tissues for metabolism is known as oxygen consumption (VO_2). Oxygen consumption is calculated by determining the difference between the amounts of oxygen returned to the right side of the heart. It is dependent on the patient's cardiac output, hemoglobin concentration, and the arterial and venous oxygen saturation. When the patient has suffered an injury or illness that has caused an alteration in the blood flow for any of the above reasons, an oxygen debt will occur. This can be exaggerated by the patient's preexisting medical condition as well as by the patient's age, for example, the patient with chronic obstructive pulmonary disease whose oxygen level is lowered due to the disease process (Selfridge-Thomas, 1995).

Sodium moves from outside the cell to increase water into the cell. This causes potassium to exit the cell, thereby altering nervous, cardiovascular, and muscular cell function. These systems then become impaired. Additionally, water is drawn from the vascular space to compensate for water drawn into the cells, further reducing circulating blood volume. Cells will shift from aerobic to anaerobic metabolism to compensate for oxygen loss. This causes metabolic acidosis, which affects enzyme activities and cellular functions such as repair and division. Cellular damage causes enzymes to be released, which will destroy noninjured cells.

Glucose metabolism is impaired in a manner similar to that of oxygen metabolism. The result of this impaired metabolism is insulin resistance. This phenomenon has been observed in patients with sepsis and those who are critically ill or injured. The stress response that is initiated by an illness or injury triggers gluconeogenesis to supply glucose energy to heal. The liver and kidneys produce more glucose in response to epinephrine, norepinephrine, glucagons, and cortisol, which are part of the body's stress response (Cartwright, 2004). **Insulin resistance (IR)** has been described as unresponsiveness of anabolic processes to the normal effects of insulin and possibly tissue insensitivity to insulin. The severity of IR is thought to be the result of an increased production of serum cytokines (Ball, de Beer, Gomm, Hickman, & Collins, 2007; Zauner et al., 2007). Insulin resistance and glucose toxicity impair cellular growth metabolic processes. IR has been associated with multiple organ failure, nosocomial infections, and renal injury (Ball et al., 2007).

Overall the pathophysiology of sepsis has a profound effect on all of the body systems. This is well illustrated in Figure 61–1 ■. Because of inadequate tissue perfusion, the body turns to anaerobic metabolism to produce energy. In addition, other pathophysiological pathways are initiated that affect all body systems due to the release of toxins as well as the body's inability to effectively manage these toxins. If not stopped, these toxins will cause multiple organ failure and death.

As previously discussed and illustrated in Figure 61–1 ■, inadequate perfusion and a reduction in available oxygen will trigger cellular and systemic responses. Alteration in cellular metabolism causes alteration in ATP production, failure of the sodium-potassium pump, redistribution of cellular ions, and interstitial fluid shifts. Blisters or blebs develop on cell walls and eventually rupture, which will release cellular enzymes and cause further damage to other cells.

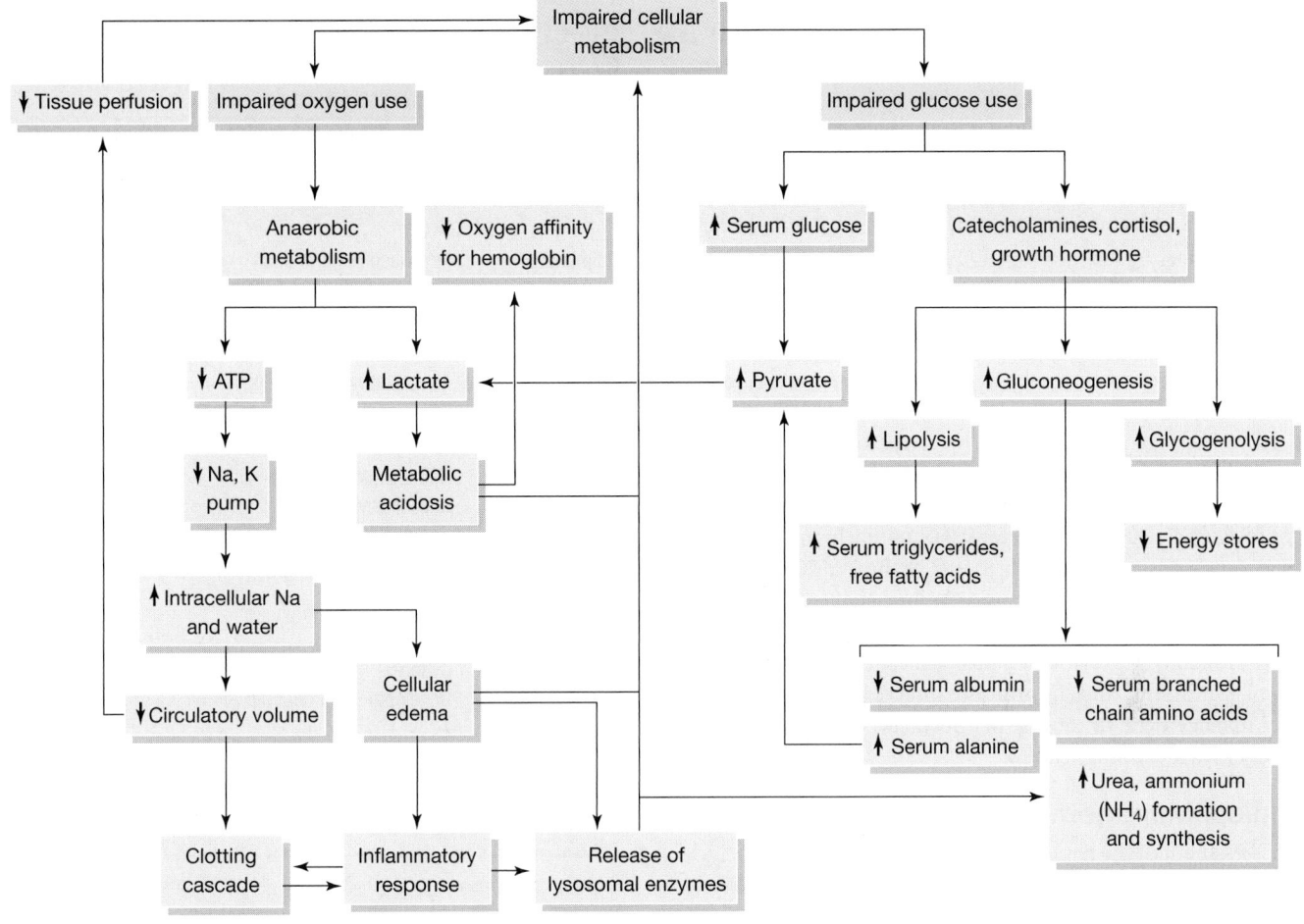

FIGURE 61–1 ■ A network of cascading events in response to inflammation.

Research continues to demonstrate that specific triggers such as infection, illness, and injury trigger a systemic inflammatory response syndrome (Johnson, Brunn, & Platt, 2004; Levy et al., 2003; Rangel-Frausto, 2005). In response, the immune system activates a complement cascade system that causes macrophages to respond. When macrophages respond to an "insult," they cause the release of substances that contribute to platelet aggregation causing clot formation, which "plugs" the vessel and at times causes vasodilation. Examples of these substances include cytokines, thromboxane, prostaglandins, and a slow-reacting substance of anaphylaxis. The end result is further tissue damage due to inadequate perfusion.

The brain is dependent on both oxygen and glucose. When either of these is not sufficient, an alteration in cerebral perfusion occurs. The patient will suffer an altered mental status, which will eventually lead to coma and even death.

Cardiac output declines because of an alteration in both preload and afterload. Afterload is the initial resistance that must be overcome by the ventricles in order to develop enough force to open the semilunar valves and propel the blood into the systemic and pulmonary systems. In addition, specific toxins such as myocardial depressant factor are released from damaged cardiac cells and a hypoperfused pancreas, causing further myocardial dysfunction and hypoxia. These result in cardiac dysrhythmia, which will further impair cardiac function. The

pulmonary system suffers acute lung injury eventually leading to acute respiratory distress.

Urinary output is decreased because of the shift of sodium, which pulls water into the cells for conservation of fluid. Decreased blood flow to the kidneys impairs their ability to detoxify the toxic substances that result from anaerobic metabolism. Inadequate blood flow to the gastrointestinal (GI) tract causes the activation of circulating neutrophils that provoke multiple organ failure. The integumentary system responds by diverting blood from the skin. Pale, fragile skin affords little protection and places the patient at risk for hypothermia and further system disruptions.

A change in blood flow to the vital organs (brain, heart, and kidneys) triggers baroreceptors, which cause the release of catecholamines, increasing the heart rate and cardiac output and causing further vasoconstriction and tissue injury. See Chapter 21 ☞ for an explanation of the normal regulation of blood pressure. Skeletal muscle, which is a major reservoir of amino acids, begins to break down and release these acids from their stores. Muscle weakness and eventual wasting result.

The "unhinging of the machinery of life" continues until irreversible changes and eventually death occur. What is unfortunate is that many of the interventions used for the treatment of shock actually contribute to the development of further complications such as third spacing, ischemia-reperfusion injury, ventilator-associated pneumonia (VAP), Multiple Organ Dysfunction Syndrome (MODS), and in some cases death. VAP is the most common hospital-acquired infection among patients who are mechanically ventilated.

Ischemia reperfusion injury is a multifactorial process that occurs when anaerobic metabolism is initiated by hypoperfusion and hypoxia that leads to an oxygen deficit in endothelial, parenchymal, or immune competent cells (Krau, 2007). The energy deficit that results from prolonged ischemia can lead to irreversible tissue damage through apoptosis or necrosis of parenchymal cells. In addition, reperfusion can also cause secondary tissue damage and organ dysfunction.

During the reperfusion phase, superoxide anions are generated from available oxygen. Superoxide anions are further reduced to hydrogen peroxide and hydroxyl ions, referred to as free oxygen radicals. These free oxygen radicals induce lipid peroxidation, membrane disintegration, and DNA damage, causing apoptosis and necrosis of endothelial, parenchymal, and immune cells (Kaszaki, Wolfard, Szalay, & Boros, 2006; Keel & Trentz, 2005). Ischemia-reperfusion injury is one of the major triggers of MODS (Krau, 2007).

In summary, as previously stated, prevention, early recognition of symptoms, and appropriate interventions are the primary management strategies for shock (McCance & Huether, 2006; Selfridge-Thomas, 1995).

Medical Management

The assessment of the patient who may be in shock must include a high index of suspicion because the body's initial ability to compensate may mask the clinical signs of shock. Patient risk factors such as significant injuries, catastrophic illness, age, and allergies must be quickly acknowledged. It is interesting that both the very young and aged share similar risk factors for developing shock including compromised immune systems due to age; fluid shifts; and an integumentary system that may not afford needed protection. Inadequate tissue perfusion and hypoxia will manifest itself in a variety of ways, as summarized in Chart 61–3.

 *Even though some specific clinical manifestations, such as hypotension and tachycardia, are associated with shock, physical fitness, preexisting illness, certain injuries (spinal cord trauma), and medications (beta-blockers) may mask the anticipated symptoms.*

The Emergency Period of Shock Care

The emergency period of care for the patient in shock begins as soon as the risk for shock has been identified. The primary goal of shock management is to identify the cause and intervene to prevent the pathophysiology that results from ischemic and anoxic cell injury (Arabi, Shirawi, Memish, Venkatesh, & Al-Shimemeri, 2003). The care of the patient will be directed at identifying and correcting the cause of the shock, maintaining oxygen perfusion, controlling active bleeding, supporting the patient's circulatory status, maintaining the patient's body temperature, managing pain, and providing emotional support.

Prehospital Care and Transport

Patients who are in shock have been identified as "load and go situations," which means that they must be transported as

CHART 61–3	Clinical Manifestations of Inadequate Tissue Perfusion and Hypoxia
System	**Clinical Manifestation**
Neurological	Altered mental status
	Irritability
	Seizures from hypoxia
	Coma
Pulmonary	Increased respirations
	Crackles from fluid shifts
	Decreased oxygen saturation despite an increase in oxygen administration
Cardiovascular	Increased heart rate
	Decreased or absent peripheral pulses
	Cardiac dysrhythmia
Gastrointestinal	Nausea and vomiting
	Absent bowel sounds
Genitourinary	Decreased urinary output
	Increased specific gravity
Integumentary	Cool clammy skin
	Mottling
	Cyanosis
	Development of decubiti
Musculoskeletal	Generalized weakness
	Wasting
	Inability to wean from ventilator due to muscle wasting

quickly as possible to the nearest hospital (Campbell, 2004; McSwain, Salomone, & Pons, 2007). The prehospital care provider needs to focus care on the critical interventions that need to be performed to save the patient's life while preparing for and initiating rapid transport (Figure 61–2 ■). A brief primary assess-

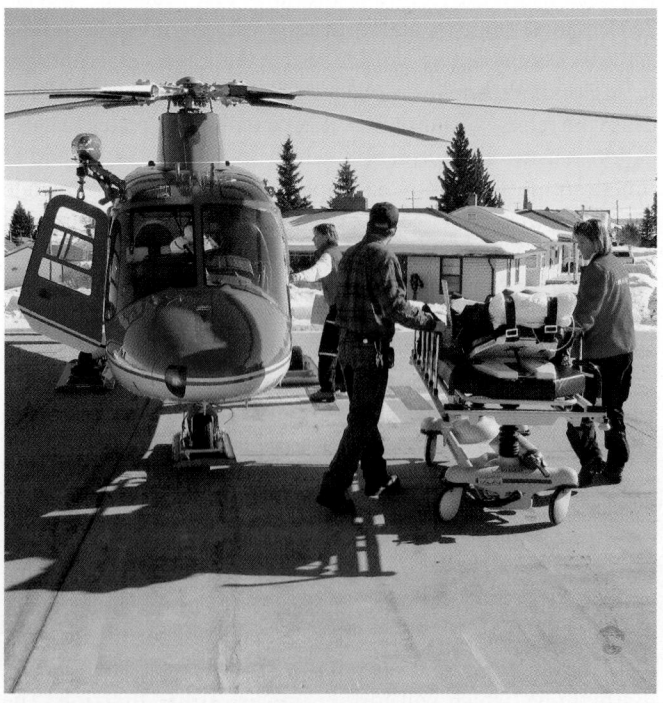

FIGURE 61–2 ■ Rapid transport for a patient in shock.

ment includes evaluating the patient's A = airway with cervical spine protection if trauma is suspected, B = breathing, C = circulation, D = disability, and performing E = exposure and environmental management. Only critical interventions such as airway management should be executed before transport. Additional interventions such as obtaining intravenous (IV) access, immobilization measures (such as the application of a traction splint), warming the patient, and performing a secondary assessment should be accomplished during transport (McSwain et al., 2007). Chapter 74 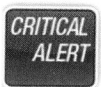 discusses the rapid primary and secondary assessment for the patient at risk for shock.

If an active source of blood or fluid loss is identified, it should be managed as much as possible before and during transport. (Fluid resuscitation is discussed in the next section.) Pelvic and long-bone fractures can cause enormous blood loss. Pneumatic antishock garments (PASGs), though controversial, may be of use for the patient in shock during transport. Chart 61–4 contains a summary of the indications and contraindications for use of PASGs in the prehospital setting (Campbell, 2004; McSwain et al., 2007). Another device that has been used to stabilize pelvic fractures is the trauma pelvic orthotic device (T-POD). It has been found to be effective in maintaining pelvic cross-sectional area and pelvic volume (Carrigan, Born, Fitzpatrick, & Reilly, 2004).

In summary, the prehospital care of the patient in shock involves early recognition of the risk of shock and rapid transport of the patient to definitive care. A primary assessment should be performed and critical interventions initiated. There should not be any additional delays in getting the patient to a center that can provide appropriate and life-saving care.

> **CRITICAL ALERT** *The patient in shock should be rapidly transported to a facility that can provide the definitive care required. For example, a trauma patient in shock should be transported to a trauma center when possible.*

Emergency Department Care

The care of the patient in shock in the emergency department depends on a collaborative approach. It begins with performing a primary assessment and initiating critical interventions to support the patient's A = airway, B = breathing, and C = circulation. Interventions that were performed in the prehospital environment need to be reevaluated and considered when resuscitating

the patient, for example, how much fluid the patient received during transport. A secondary assessment is then performed including exposing the patient to identify any obvious signs of illness or injury that may be the source of the shock. An in-depth discussion of the primary and secondary assessments is contained in Chapter 74 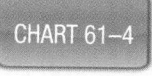. The Risk Factors box contains a summary of the most common risk factors for the development of shock.

The source of the clinical insult needs to be immediately identified. When there is no obvious indication, other pieces of patient history and risk factors must be considered, for example, the age of the patient or medications that the patient may be prescribed. For example, certain medications may place a patient at risk of shock, particularly septic shock. These include medications that cause immunosuppression and antibiotic and antiviral therapies. Additionally, the elderly and young are at greatest danger of developing shock because of changes in their immune system and body surface area related to age. An in-depth discussion of these differences and the potential risks the elderly pose are contained in Chapters 59 and 60 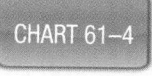.

The pathophysiological changes initiated by the body's response to shock cause the patient to become hypoxic. Therefore, the patient will require airway and ventilatory support. This may be as simple as administering oxygen by 100% nonrebreather mask or it may require endotracheal intubation. A chest radiograph can reveal a possible infection or source of blood or other fluid loss or even an obstructive reason for shock such as a cardiac tamponade. Chapter 33 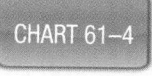 discusses respiratory assessment and management.

The patient's circulatory status needs to be assessed. Peripheral and central pulses should be palpated to determine perfusion. Remember, the body will divert blood from the periphery to enhance oxygenation of the brain, heart, and kidneys. The patient's skin will be pale, cold, and clammy. The patient will need to be kept warm by increasing the room temperature, covering with warm blankets, or using a commercial device to deliver heat. The skin is friable and at risk of additional injury so the patient should be handled and moved as gently as possible.

CHART 61–4 Indications and Contraindications for the Use of Pneumatic Antishock Garments with Shock

Indications	Contraindications
Suspected pelvic fractures with hypotension	Penetrating thoracic trauma
Profound hypotension (systolic blood pressure less than 60 mmHg)	Stabilization of an isolated lower extremity fracture
Suspected intraperitoneal hemorrhage	Evisceration of abdominal organs
Suspected retroperitoneal hemorrhage	Impaled objects in the abdomen
	Pregnant abdomen
	Traumatic arrest

RISK FACTORS for the Development and Source of Shock

Indication	Source of Shock
Active bleeding anywhere on the body	Hemorrhage
Abdominal bruising	
Long-bone deformities	
Open fractures	
Amputations	
"Coffee-stain" emesis	
Penetrating trauma	
Purpura	Sepsis
Rashes	
Decubitus	
Gangrene	
Indwelling urinary catheters	
Indwelling IV ports	
Feeding tubes	
Burns	Hypovolemia
Dehydration	

A 12-lead ECG should be obtained to rule out myocardial injury as the source of shock. Prolonged ischemia related to hypotension can also place the patient at risk of a myocardial infarction. Chapter 38 🔗 discusses the 12-lead ECG and Chapter 40 🔗 discusses myocardial infarction. Blood studies are obtained to provide baseline assessment data, identify the physiological effects of the shock state, identify a source of infection, and evaluate the effects of specific treatments. Blood studies should include complete blood count (CBC) with a differential, serum electrolytes, whole blood glucose, blood urea nitrogen (BUN), serum creatinine, coagulation studies, liver function studies, and lactate levels. For the patient with suspected hemorrhagic shock, a type and screen or type and cross should be obtained.

When sepsis is suspected, specific laboratory tests should be performed to identify the source of the sepsis. Examples of these include blood cultures, urine cultures, cultures of any suspected wounds or appliances, and cerebrospinal fluid cultures. The Diagnostic Tests for Shock box contains a description of these tests. Additional radiography studies are required for diagnosis and may include computed tomography (CT) scans, magnetic resonance imaging (MRI), and angiography.

Because shock involves alterations in circulating volume, cardiac function, or peripheral vascular resistance (PVR), the primary purposes of circulatory resuscitation are as follows:

- Restore oxygen transport and cellular uptake of oxygen.
- Mitigate against oxygen debt accumulation and decrease the use of anaerobic metabolism to supply cellular energy.
- Restore pre-resuscitation oxygen deficit.
- Prevent the metabolic derangements that lead to SIRS and eventual MODS and eventually multiple organ system failure (MOSF). These complications are discussed later in the chapter.

What is important to remember is that circulatory resuscitation may involve both volume resuscitation as well us the use of va-

DIAGNOSTIC TESTS for Shock

Test	Expected Abnormality	Rationale for Abnormality
Complete blood count with a differential	Increased white blood cell count	An increased white blood cell count may indicate a stress response as well as an infection.
	Increase in neutrophils	An increase in neutrophils will help differentiate an infection as the cause of the shock.
Hemoglobin concentration	Decreased with fluid	Adequate hemoglobin is needed to ensure adequate oxygen delivery.
	Increased with fluid loss	
Platelet count	Increase in number of platelets	Platelets increase as a stress response.
Serum electrolyte levels	Decreased sodium levels	Movement of sodium into the cell displaces potassium from the cell.
	Increased potassium levels	
Whole blood glucose	Increased glucose levels	Glucose metabolism is impaired.
Blood urea nitrogen Creatinine	Increase in both	Renal dysfunction occurs.
Arterial blood gases	Respiratory alkalosis	Increase respirations to blow off CO_2 to decrease metabolic acidosis.
	Metabolic acidosis	Metabolic acidosis results from anaerobic metabolism.
	Hypoxia	Hypoxia results from inadequate tissue perfusion.
Serum lactate levels	Elevated	Reflect tissue perfusion. An increased level indicates inadequate tissue perfusion and anaerobic metabolism. A higher lactate level indicates a higher degree of shock and potential for death.
Coagulation studies PT and PTT	Prolonged	Due to cellular dysfunction and abnormal clotting cascade. More profound if disseminated intravascular coagulation (DIC) is present.
Blood cultures	Presence of bacteria	Blood cultures should not be used without a good reason. Patients who are febrile, elderly patients, IV drug abusers, and patients with neutropenia, prosthetic heart valves, or indwelling devices are examples of those who should have blood cultures drawn.
Urinalysis	Presence of white blood cells, bacteria, increased specific gravity	Identify source of infection. Indicates the level of the body's response to shock.
Gram stains	Specific sites recognized as a source of infection	Immediate test that would indicate the presence of bacteria from a specific source such as an indwelling urinary catheter.
Type and crossmatch		Identify specific blood type for infusion of blood and blood products.
Cardiac enzymes	Normal or abnormal	Identify myocardial injury as source of shock.

soactive medications to maintain adequate **end-organ perfusion**, the perfusion of the end organs such as the integumentary system.

Large-bore intravenous (IV) lines need to be inserted. Central IV access may be obtained with a catheter that will also allow the insertion of devices for hemodynamic monitoring. It is imperative to ensure aseptic technique to prevent the possibility of introducing infection and increasing the risk of sepsis. Chapter 22 🔗 discusses the various types of intravenous catheters and their indications for use.

Fluid Resuscitation

During the last 20 years, the common methods once used for fluid resuscitation in shock have been challenged by research. Researchers have discovered many pertinent issues that must be considered when resuscitating the patient in shock. First, hypotension may actually be a protective mechanism, especially in the patient who has sustained a penetrating injury. Increasing a patient's blood pressure multiplies the chances that clots that have been formed will dislodge and, depending on the resuscitation fluid, dilutes circulating volume and in turn increases clotting time (Jacobs, 1994; Keel & Trentz, 2005; Kowalenko, Stern, Dronen, & Wang, 1992; Martin, Bicknell, Pepe, Burch, & Mattox, 1992). Chart 61–5 contains a summary of some of the complications of massive fluid resuscitation (Ackerman, 1994; Alexander, 1996; Edelman, White, Tyburski, & Wilson, 2007; Fernandes et al., 2007; Rueden & Dunham, 1994).

Fluids that are used for resuscitation include lactated Ringer's solution or normal saline. The type of fluid used will depend on the provider's preference, because at present the research has not clearly defined one more favorably over the other. The initial amount of fluid will range from 2 to 3 liters for an adult if the cause of the shock is unknown. If the patient has sustained blood loss, then administration of blood and blood products will be needed. Infusion therapy and blood administration are discussed in depth in Chapters 22 and 23 🔗, respectively. It is important to remember that patients who have sustained blood loss greater than 2 liters should not receive excessive fluid resuscitation from either colloids or crystalloids until surgical management of bleeding has been initiated because it dilutes the existing volume and further diminishes oxygen-carrying capacity. In contrast, a patient who is septic and hypotensive may require early fluid boluses to maintain a systolic blood pressure greater than 90 mmHg (Keel & Trentz, 2005; Russell, 2006).

Because of the complications of massive fluid resuscitation as noted in Chart 61–5, the effects of fluid resuscitation must be closely monitored. A urinary catheter should be inserted to measure urinary output. Adequate hydration in an adult should yield a urinary output of 30 to 50 mL/hr or 0.4 to 1.0 mL/kg of body weight. Adequate fluid resuscitation is also evaluated by a decrease in heart rate, presence and strength of the patient's central and peripheral pulses, patient's improving level of consciousness, and return of bowel sounds.

Hemodynamic monitoring can be used to monitor the effectiveness of resuscitation. This may include the insertion of a pulmonary artery catheter (PAC). However, any additional invasive procedures may leave the patient at risk of infection and sepsis. An in-depth discussion of the use of hemodynamic monitoring is included in Chapter 24 🔗.

Pharmacologic Support

Shock resuscitation may also include the need for pharmacologic support. Different medications may be used for different shock states. The purpose of the medication may be to augment blood flow to the brain, heart, and kidneys or to fight the infection that caused the sepsis leading to shock. The medications that are typically used in selected shock states are listed in the Pharmacological Summary feature (p. 1981) (Kline, 2002; McCaffery & Sinclair, 2006; Russell, 2006).

Pain Management

Pain management for the patient in shock is oftentimes neglected. One of the major reasons is that analgesics and sedation agents can cause hypotension and respiratory depression, furthering complications. However, research has adequately demonstrated the consequences of poor pain management, which include increased peripheral vascular resistance, increased consumption of myocardial oxygen, increased metabolic rate, increased levels of circulating stress hormones, hypercoagulability, decreased gastric motility, and hopelessness (Semonin Holleran, 2002). Pain management should never be neglected when providing care for the patient in shock.

Appropriate use of analgesics and sedative agents can only serve to support patients. Chapter 15 🔗 provides an in-depth discussion of the assessment and management of pain.

Additional Interventions

Depending on the cause of the shock, other interventions may be indicated. For example, the patient who has suffered a spinal cord injury will need to be appropriately immobilized during transport and in the emergency department. Chart 61–6 (p. 1964) contains a summary of additional interventions that may be indicated to manage shock based on the source of the clinical insult.

Acute Care Period of Shock

The unstable patient in shock will generally be admitted to the critical care unit. The care initiated will be continued including support of the patient's oxygenation and circulatory status.

CHART 61–5	**Complications of Massive Fluid Resuscitation**

- Hypothermia
- Coagulopathy
- Metabolic derangements
  - Acidosis
  - Hypocalcemia
  - Hypomagnesia
  - Hypophosphatemia
  - Hypokalemia
- Organ dysfunction and extravascular fluid shifts
- Adult respiratory distress syndrome
- Sepsis
- Acute renal failure
- Pneumonia
- Ventilator-assisted pneumonia
- Increased length of stay

CHART 61–6	Additional Interventions for the Management of the Patient in Shock

Shock State	Additional Interventions
Hypovolemic	Direct pressure for active bleeding Surgery to control bleeding Immobilization of any long bones to decrease bleeding Ultrasound of chest and abdomen to discover bleeding For the patient with traumatic injury, may perform a FAST (focused abdominal ultrasound for trauma) exam to discover abdominal bleeding CT of abdomen or chest Endoscopy or colonoscopy to discover blood loss
Cardiogenic	Obtain cardiac enzymes Fibrinolytic therapy Angioplasty Intra-aortic balloon pump (IABP) insertion
Neurogenic	Spinal immobilization Spinal stabilization using halos or tong devices Warming measures to maintain body temperature
Obstructive	Tension pneumothorax Needle decompression Chest tube insertion Cardiac tamponade Pericardiocentesis Cardiac window

Some type of shock monitoring should be established. This may include monitoring of the patient's central venous pressure (CVP), pulmonary artery pressure monitoring with PACs, monitoring of oxygen transport and consumption, cardiovascular indices, and respiratory monitoring. CVP and PACs are discussed in Chapter 24 .

The complications related to the body's response to shock pose additional problems in the acute period. Nutritional support is an important intervention during the acute care period for the management of the patient in shock from injury, illness, or infection. This is discussed further later in the chapter (also see Chapter 14). Skin care and promoting and maintaining mobility are important in the acute period. Skin breakdown and immobility can lead to further risk of the development of sepsis. Pain management and sedation will be required by the patient (see Chapter 15).

In addition, the psychosocial needs of patients and their family must be anticipated and dealt with. Depending on the cause of the shock state and the progression of clinical manifestations, both the patient and the family may have to face death or long-term disabilities. End-of-life issues are discussed in more depth in Chapter 17 .

In conclusion, the medical management of the patient in shock is directed at early recognition of the risk factors that threaten the development of the "rude unhinging of the machinery of life." Once the clinical manifestations of shock are evident, it is imperative that the source of the clinical insult be found and critical interventions initiated to prevent the complications that come from impaired cellular and glucose metabolism. Prevention is the primary way to keep patients from suffering the potential irreversible consequences of shock.

Nursing Management

The nursing management of the patient in shock begins with an in-depth assessment of the patient, including identifying any current and past medical history that would place the patient at risk for developing shock. Mechanisms of injury that may place the patient at risk for hemorrhagic or hypovolemic shock or an infection should be quickly identified so that the systematic compensatory response of the body can be decreased or eliminated. Frequent monitoring and assessment of trend changes in vital signs and clinical manifestations of inadequate tissue perfusion and hypoxia, especially level of consciousness, skin color and temperature, and urinary output, can provide the most reliable information in the early identification of shock.

Once the source of shock or clinical insult has been identified, nursing care is focused on the specific cause. Fluid resuscitation and administration of blood and blood products will be required in the management of a patient in hemorrhagic or hypovolemic shock. This will require careful monitoring of organ perfusion including the presence of peripheral pulses, maintenance of a perfusing blood pressure, and correction of acid–base balance.

Many patients experiencing shock may have suffered injuries that limit their mobility and place them at risk for skin breakdown and deep venous thrombosis (DVT). Range-of-motion (ROM) exercises, turning, and meticulous skin care are needed to prevent sources of infection.

Vasopressor medications that may be used to maintain end-organ perfusion will also place the patient at risk for injury to the extremities due to the vasoconstrictive properties of these medications, which markedly diminish blood flow distally. Careful monitoring and early recognition of decreased blood flow can assist in early intervention and prevention.

Emotional and spiritual support of the patient and the family is essential for the patient in shock. If the patient has sustained severe enough injury, death may be imminent and the family must be allowed time to be with the patient. End-of-life decisions may need to be made in a limited period of time (see Chapter 17).

Pain management can be very challenging in the shock patient. Hypotension is a common clinical manifestation of inadequate tissue perfusion and may impede adequate pain management because of fear that medications may make the patient's symptoms worse. The nurse must play an advocacy role that ensures that the patient's pain and anxiety is sufficiently managed. The Nursing Process: Patient Care Plan feature contains a summary of the nursing care of the patient in shock. The Ethical Issue feature (p. 1967) describes ethical issues in the care of the patient in shock.

Evidence-based practice has suggested some specific guidelines for the resuscitation and management of the patient in shock. The Evidence-Based Practice feature (p. 1967) contains a summary of some this evidence.

Collaborative Management

To achieve optimal recovery and return to society, the patient in shock requires a multidisciplinary team that includes health care providers, nurses, pharmacists, social service personnel, physical therapists, and nutritionists. To prevent the complications related to shock and its sequelae, nurses and health care providers must be alert to the risk factors that can contribute to the development of shock.

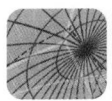
Assessment of Circulation and Perfusion

Subjective Data:

How did you get injured?

When did your symptoms begin?

Do you have any other preexisting health problems such as heart, lung, or kidney disease?

Do you take any medications that may affect your blood pressure?

Do you take any medications that affect your immune system?

Do you take any medications that may make you bleed?

Objective Data:

Oxygen saturation

Work of breathing

Peripheral and central pulses, presence, rate and quality

Blood pressure, respiratory rate, and temperature

Skin color and temperature

Diaphoresis

Nursing Assessment and Diagnoses	Outcomes and Evaluation Parameters	Planning and Interventions with *Rationales*
Nursing Diagnoses: *Tissue Perfusion Ineffective* related to alterations in circulating volume *Fluid Volume Deficient* related to alterations in circulating volume *Cardiac Output, Decreased* related to alterations in circulating volume and cardiac pump function	**Outcome:** Improved tissue perfusion. **Evaluation Parameters:** Presence of peripheral pulses by palpation or Doppler. Capillary refill <2 seconds. Maintenance of a perfusing blood pressure. Improved mental status. Glasgow Coma Scale (GCS) 15. Follows commands. No restlessness/fatigue. Oxygen saturation within normal limits. Control of blood and fluid loss. Adequate hydration. Corrected acid–base balance. Improved core body temperature. Adequate cardiac output and blood pressure.	**Interventions and *Rationales:*** Assess peripheral pulses and compare to central pulses. *Decrease in or loss of peripheral pulses indicates decreased tissue perfusion.* Assess skin color, temperature. *Capillary refill indicates body's attempt to compensate for decreased perfusion by diverting blood flow from the periphery to the central circulation.* Assess patient's GCS and ability to follow commands. Monitor restlessness and confusion *as an indication of decreased cerebral perfusion and worsening shock state.* Assess for obvious signs of bleeding, *which will cause blood loss and alter circulating volume.* Apply direct pressure and pressure dressings, assist with clamping of bleeding vessels, and prepare patient for operative intervention *to prevent blood and volume loss.* Apply PASG to manage large-volume loss from such injuries as a pelvic fracture *to prevent blood and volume loss.* Initiate large-bore IV catheters. Assist with insertion of central venous access. Insert or assist with insertion of intraosseous needles *to replace volume and blood loss to maintain adequate circulation and improve perfusion.* Administer appropriate isotonic solution at 20 mL/kg and increase as indicated by patient's urinary output of 0.5 mL/kg/hr *to maintain adequate circulation and improve perfusion.* Prepare for administration of blood and blood products *to replace lost blood and increase oxygen to the tissues.* Administer O-negative blood if needed immediately. Administer blood components such as fresh frozen plasma and platelets *to maintain adequate circulation and improve perfusion.* Place warm blankets on the patient. Use a commercial warming device. Warm fluids and blood *to prevent hypothermia and maintain adequate circulation and improve perfusion.* Obtain 12-lead ECG to assess the status of the myocardium. Increase cardiac contractility by administering a fluid bolus. Initiate medications to improve contractility: • Dopamine hydrochloride • Dobutamine hydrochloride • Amrinone lactate. Initiate medications to decrease afterload: • Nitroprusside sodium • Nitrates. Initiate medications to increase afterload: • Norepinephrine bitartrate • Epinephrine. *To improve cardiac output.* Prepare the patient for interventions that may increase reperfusion to an injured myocardium, e.g., percutaneous transluminal coronary angioplasty (PCTA) or insertion of an intra-aortic balloon pump *to improve cardiac output.*

(continued)

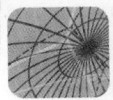

Assessment of Airway

Subjective Data:
Are you feeling short of breath?
Are you having difficulty breathing?

Objective Data:
Assess breath sounds.
Assess respiratory rate, rhythm, depth, and symmetry.
Monitor oxygen saturation.
Monitor Arterial Blood Gas (ABG) values.

Nursing Assessment and Diagnoses	Outcomes and Evaluation Parameters	Planning and Interventions with *Rationales*
Nursing Diagnosis: *Airway Clearance, Ineffective* related to altered level of consciousness, obstruction by secretions, and aspiration of foreign matter	**Outcome:** Patient will maintain a patent airway. **Evaluation Parameters:** Regular rate, depth, and pattern of breathing. Bilateral chest expansion. Effective cough and gag reflex.	**Interventions and *Rationales*:** Open and clear airway. *Patient may have secretions in mouth.* Insert oro- or nasopharyngeal airway. *Patient may have adequate respiratory drive but needs support to keep airway open.* Prepare to assist with endotracheal intubation. *Level of consciousness too low to protect and maintain airway.*

Assessment of Nutrition

Subjective Data:
How is your appetite?
Has it changed recently?
Have you experienced any weight loss?

Objective Data:
24-hour caloric intake
Daily weight
Presence of bowel sounds
Nausea and vomiting
Flatus

Nursing Assessment and Diagnoses	Outcomes and Evaluation Parameters	Planning and Interventions with *Rationales*
Nursing Diagnosis: *Imbalanced Nutrition Risk for: Less than Body Requirements* related to decreased appetite secondary to treatments, fatigue, environment, and increased protein and vitamin requirements for healing	**Outcome:** Patient will ingest daily nutritional requirements for activity level and metabolic needs. **Evaluation Parameters:** Patient maintains adequate weight. Patient maintains adequate caloric intake.	**Interventions and *Rationales*:** Communicate the need for adequate caloric intake of carbohydrates, fats, protein, vitamins, minerals, and fluids. *Adequate nutrition can reduce the risk of complications and promote healing.* Consult with the nutritionist to establish appropriate daily caloric requirements. *Consultation helps to ensure optimal intake.* Offer small frequent meals *to help prevent gastric distention.* Determine the patient's food preferences and arrange to have those foods provided. Encourage family to bring allowed foods from home. Eliminate any offensive odors. Control pain and nausea. Provide a relaxed atmosphere during meals. *These interventions can improve appetite and lead to increased intake.*

Assessment of Anticipatory Grieving

Subjective Data:
Do the patient and/or family realize the gravity of the illness or injury?
Do the patient and/or family have any support systems?
Do the patient and/or family have any spiritual beliefs that may assist them at this time?
Are there any cultural practices that are important to them at this time?

Objective Data:
Observe family interaction with the patient.
Observe how the patient reacts to the illness or injury.
Observe how the staff is interacting with the patient and family.
Observe for anger, crying, physical threatening, or inability to cope with the situation.

Nursing Assessment and Diagnoses	Outcomes and Evaluation Parameters	Planning and Interventions with *Rationales*
Nursing Diagnosis: *Coping, Readiness for Enhanced Grieving*	**Outcome:** Patient and/or family are able to make decisions about care. **Evaluation Parameters:** Patient and family verbalize realistic perception of the patient's condition and chances of survival. Spiritual care is provided as identified by the patient and family. End-of-life decisions are made by the patient and/or family to ensure a painless and dignified death.	**Interventions and *Rationales*:** Provide the patient and the family with information about their illness or injury especially related to outcomes *to assist the patient and family with grieving.* Allow the family to see the patient as soon as possible, especially if the patient is near death. Explain to the family what the patient looks like and how comfort has been provided for the patient *to assist the patient and family with grieving.* Provide requested spiritual care by contacting appropriate personnel. Respect cultural rituals related to the patient and family beliefs. Consult with personnel such as the ethics committee when problems arise with end-of-life decisions *to assist the patient and family with grieving.* Help the staff to recognize signs and symptoms of their own grief and provide them with resources *to assist them with the grieving process.*

ETHICAL ISSUES Related to Patients in Shock

Identification of end points in the resuscitation of patients in shock is difficult. Guidelines for futile resuscitation are limited and the concept of palliative care in the resuscitation of trauma patients is now being proposed. Mosenthal and Murphy (2003) pointed out the need for trauma surgeons to consider the integration of palliative care and trauma care. Two issues in particular make it important to consider this issue. First, despite aggressive resuscitation, research continues to demonstrate that 10% to 15% of all trauma patients will die. Others may suffer disabling effects that may greatly challenge their quality of life. Secondly, a severe injury in the elderly has a greater mortality than in a similarly injured young person. Technology and the availability of health care resources make it mandatory that resuscitation end points and guidelines be developed to ensure that compassionate care is given at the end of life for these patients.

Once the source of shock has been identified, care is directed at managing that source and assisting the body to maintain physiological functions such as cerebral and renal perfusion. This may be done through such interventions as fluid resuscitation or pharmacologic management. Because a patient in a shock state has compromised body systems, the assistance of pharmacist is necessary to ensure that the appropriate medications are correctly prescribed and administered.

The critical nature of shock places patients at risk of death or long-term complications that require the teamwork of nursing and social services personnel to help both the patient and family face and manage the changes that death or disability may bring. Family dynamics are often impacted by prolonged hospitalization and change in role function within the family structure. In addition, there are times when end-of-life decisions must be made and social service personnel will play an important role in supporting

Management of Bleeding Following Major Trauma

Clinical Problem

The management of bleeding following major trauma to prevent hemorrhagic shock is a worldwide challenge. The time elapsed from injury to operation or method to manage the bleeding such as embolization needs to be minimized. Recognition and resuscitation of the trauma patient with uncontrolled bleeding must be early and managed appropriately to prevent the sequelae of shock such as sepsis and MODS.

Research Findings

Spahn and colleagues (2007) developed evidenced-based guidelines for the management of bleeding following major trauma. The authors reviewed numerous papers and developed guidelines based on clinical evidence.

Recommendations include the following:

- Minimize the time from injury to surgical intervention.

- Clinically assess the extent of hemorrhage using an established grading system such as the American College of Surgeons' Advanced Trauma Life Support Classification of Hemorrhage.

- For patients who are actively bleeding and in shock, perform an immediate bleeding control procedure such as surgery if the source of the bleeding has been identified and resuscitation measures have not been successful.

- Quickly identify the source of bleeding through the uses of such measures as sonography, FAST, CT, and hematocrit.

- Implement surgical interventions such as pelvic fracture stabilization, embolization, cross-clamping, and damage control as needed to control hemorrhage.

- Coagulopathy should be managed with blood products and the administration of rFVIIa (recombinant activated coagulation Factor VII).

Implications for Nursing Practice

These guidelines point out the need for nurses to quickly recognize a patient at risk of bleeding based on mechanism of injury or past medical history, for example, a patient who is taking an anticoagulant such as warfarin or aspirin for cardiovascular disease. Ongoing nursing assessment needs to include identification of uncontrolled bleeding, clinical manifestations of hemorrhagic shock such as altered mental

status, hypotension, tachycardia, and decreased urinary output. The nurse must be prepared to assist the health care provider with clinical assessment as well as prepare the patient for further testing. In some cases, the nurse must recognize the need for the patient to be transferred to a center where definitive care can be provided and assist the patient and family in the transfer and transport process. The management of hemorrhagic shock requires a collaborative approach by both nursing and health care provider colleagues.

Critical Thinking Questions

1. Which of the following would be a clinical manifestation of uncontrolled bleeding in an injured patient?
   a. Hypotension after infusion of 2 liters isotonic crystalloid infusion
   b. Presence of a fractured femur managed with a traction splint
   c. Negative abdominal computerized tomography examination
   d. Urinary output of greater than 50 mL per hour in an adult patient

2. Identify a nursing measure that may decrease the risk of complications from hemorrhagic shock
   a. Preparing the injured patient for transfer to definitive care
   b. Infusing 7 liters of crystalloid solution through a central line
   c. Administering intravenous antibiotics to decrease the risk of infection
   d. Hyperventilating the intubated patient with 100% oxygen

3. In order of priority, what are the most important interventions that should be performed for the injured patient who is actively bleeding?
   a. Suctioning blood from the patient's airway
   b. Stabilizing the patient's pelvis with a sheet
   c. Applying 100% oxygen by mask to the patient
   d. Initiating a large-caliber intravenous for fluid resuscitation

Answers to Critical Thinking Questions appear in Appendix D.

Reference

Spahn, D. R., Cerny, V. Coats, T. J., Duranteau, J., Fernandez-Mondejar, E., Gordini, G., et al. (2007). Management of bleeding following major trauma: A European guideline. *Critical Care, 11*(1). Retrieved April 21, 2007, from http://www.medscape.com/viewarticle/554058.

EVIDENCE-BASED PRACTICE

the nursing and medical staff with implementing difficult decisions. Physical therapy is begun as soon as possible to decrease complications such as muscle wasting that can contribute to additional healing problems.

Finally, a comprehensive plan for nutrition is important in enhancing healing, regaining strength, and preventing additional complications such as infection. The nutritionist works with the health care team from the time of admission through discharge to ensure proper nutritional support. The primary focus of nutritional support is providing exogenous energy and protein to minimize gluconeogenesis, catabolism (protein oxidation), and the loss of lean tissue associated with injury (Reid & Campbell, 2004). Patients in shock are in a hypermetabolic state. This requires nutritional support that prevents malnutrition and its consequences (Cartwright, 2004). Before nutritional support can be initiated, a nutritional assessment must be completed. This assessment includes the patient's social, medical, and dietary history before the illness, injury, or infection. Additional factors such as the patient's normal appetite, medications, and food allergies and the use of supplements or special diets must also be included in the nutritional assessment. The "culture" of the patient should also be considered. Currently, various prescribed regimes are available to provide nutrition to patients who are severely ill, injured, or septic (Bertolini, Luciani, & Bioli, 2007; Cartwright, 2004). Nutrition is discussed further in Chapter 14 .

Gerontological Considerations

The changes related to age can present additional challenges for the care of the elderly patient in shock. A decrease in cardiac output by almost half as well as a decreased response to endogenous catecholamines will impair an elderly patient's ability to respond to the redistribution of blood and fluids. Changes in blood pressure and heart rate are different from that seen in other age groups. Many of the prescribed medications for the elderly, such as beta-blockers, will also affect physiological responses. Age causes diminished perfusion to all organs. This may manifest itself in a normal altered mental status and an inability to concentrate urine. Both are important subtle signs of the early stages of shock. As age advances, the immune system becomes less able to provide protection from diseases (Kaplow & Hardin, 2007). In the elderly, sepsis can result from diseases such as pneumonia or urinary tract infections.

Shock resuscitation in the elderly must be closely monitored. These patients are prone to develop complications such as congestive heart failure and pulmonary edema. Also, nutrition and skin care are important areas of focus for the elderly patient in shock. Preexisting medical problems, appliances such as indwelling catheters, and feeding tubes are all things that can contribute to problems in the care of the elderly patient in shock, as listed in the Gerontological Considerations box.

Systemic Inflammatory Response, Sepsis, and Severe Sepsis

In 1991 the American College of Chest Physicians (ACCP) and the Society of Critical Care Medicine (SCCM) organized a conference to provide a conceptual and practical framework for defining the systemic inflammatory response to infection (ACCP/

GERONTOLOGICAL CONSIDERATIONS Related to Shock

Pulmonary
- Decreased blood flow to the lungs so elderly already have a preexisting oxygen deficit
- Decreased elasticity and strength for ventilation and less able to compensate for metabolic acidosis by increasing ventilations

Cardiac
- Decrease in cardiac output related to age, which will decrease the body's ability to compensate for alterations in volume from shock
- Baroreceptor sensitivity decreases, decreasing the body's ability to compensate for fluid volume changes
- Diminished perfusion to all organ systems
- Medications such as beta-blockers will alter the heart's response to shock

Neurological
- Normal mental status may be altered due to decreased blood flow to the brain
- Previous disease such as a stroke will alter patient's level of consciousness

Renal
Age decreases blood flow to the kidneys, decreasing the kidney's ability to concentrate urine and detoxify

Integumentary
- Skin is less elastic
- Less fat and more easily injured
- Less able to maintain normothermia and at greater risk of becoming hypothermic

Medications
Numerous medications can alter the body's response to a clinical insult as well as leave the patient at greater risk of developing shock: beta-blockers, steroids, antibiotics, antivirals

---

SCCM Consensus Conference Committee, 1992). The members of this conference developed and introduced definitions of sepsis, SIRS, and septic shock. In 2001, these groups reconvened to include additional representation from European intensive care societies (Levy et al., 2003). This group concluded the following:

- The current concepts of sepsis, severe sepsis, and septic shock remain useful.
- An expanded list of signs and symptoms of sepsis is needed.
- The diagnostic criteria for SIRS published in 1992 are overly sensitive and nonspecific.
- A method of staging sepsis is needed to ensure more effective management.

The group suggested the use of the PRIO system (predisposition, insult, response, and organ dysfunction) for the staging of sepsis, as outlined in Chart 61–7.

The consensus definitions begin with SIRS and culminate in a description of multiple organ dysfunction syndrome. It is important to note that just because a patient may have SIRS or sepsis, she may or may not progress to septic shock and/or MODS.

CHART 61–7	The PRIO System of Staging Sepsis
Domain	Present
Predisposition	Premorbid illness with reduced probability of short-term survival; cultural or religious beliefs, age, gender
Insult (infection)	Culture and sensitivity of infecting pathogens; detection of disease amenable to source control
Response	SIRS, other signs of sepsis, shock, C-reactive protein
Organ dysfunction	Organ dysfunction as number of failing organs or as a composite score using a specific formula such as the Pediatric Logistic Organ Dysfunction formula

SIRS is an organized immune response that can be triggered by infectious or noninfectious clinical insults including burns, pancreatitis, acute respiratory distress syndrome, surgery, and trauma (Robertson & Coppersmith, 2006). The incidence of SIRS has been estimated to occur in more than half of all patients who are in the intensive care unit (ICU) and greater than 80% of surgical patients who are in the ICU (Robertson & Coppersmith, 2006).

Sepsis is a clinical syndrome defined as the presence of SIRS associated with a confirmed infectious process (King, 2007; Rangel-Frausto, 2005). Septic shock is a state of acute circulatory failure characterized by persistent hypotension unexplained by other causes, for example, despite the fact that adequate fluids have been administered. It is important to remember the differences between a pediatric and adult patient when describing septic shock. Septic shock in pediatric patients is manifested by tachycardia with signs of decreased perfusion including altered peripheral pulses, altered mental status, and capillary refill greater than 2 seconds. Chart 61–3 earlier in the chapter (p. 1960) outlines the clinical manifestations of shock in the adult patient.

 CRITICAL ALERT *Hypotension is a late and ominous sign of decompensated shock in the pediatric patient.*

Severe sepsis is defined as sepsis (the presence of a confirmed infection and a systemic inflammatory response), but there is now single or multiple organ failure (Kaplow & Hardin, 2007). The patient is hypotensive, which causes hypoperfusion abnormalities such as arterial hypoxemia, acute oliguria, and coagulation abnormalities.

Epidemiology and Etiology

Each year, throughout the world, thousands of patients die from sepsis. Sepsis is the 10th leading cause of death in the United States and the leading cause of death in noncardiac care units (Gupta & Jonas, 2006; Miniño, Heron, & Smith, 2006). Since the time of Hippocrates, medicine has observed the consequence of sepsis and sought treatments to alleviate its deadly consequences (Porter, 1997).

There are approximately 400,000 to 500,000 septic cases in the United States each year. This increase is multifactorial and related to an increased numbers of patients who are elderly and immuno-

compromised (Porth, 2005). Many factors have contributed to this including an immunosuppression from medications such as chemotherapy and diseases such as human immunodeficiency virus (HIV). Chronic health problems (e.g., renal and liver disorders), traumatic injury, bone marrow suppression, surgical or invasive procedures, and sequential infections treated with multiple antibiotics are other examples of significant risk factors for the development of SIRS and severe sepsis. Substance abuse and malnutrition may also contribute to SIRS and sepsis (King, 2007).

Pathophysiology

The innate and adaptive immune systems both respond to a clinical insult. The innate immune system is the first line of defense and it can be activated within minutes. The adaptive immune system is more specific in defending the body from microbes, but takes longer to be initiated. When the immune system suffers a clinical insult, such as a devastating injury or exposure to a pathogen or pathogens, a chain of events is initiated that is intended to activate receptors. These receptors, in turn, activate intracellular signaling pathways and transcription factors, resulting in expression of the gene immune response (McCance & Huether, 2006; Robertson & Coppersmith, 2006). These defense mechanisms initiate an inflammatory response to the intruder. Research has observed that there are specific host immune responses to each pathogen that are mediated by various sets of pathogens associated with molecular patterns and pattern recognition receptors. In other words, there is not one particular medication or medical management strategy that can treat all patients with SIRS and sepsis (Bochud & Calandra, 2003; McCance & Huether, 2006).

A comprehensive theory that helps explain the body's response to a critical illness or injury encompasses the hypothesis that the body starts out "fighting" an invader or responding to an insult such as an injury by having a hyperinflammatory response. A second response may occur due to infection or the degree of the injury that has occurred. If the event that initiated the response resolves quickly, the patient typically recovers. However, comorbid factors such as age, disease, extensive injury, and sometimes even the management of the infection or injury can cause a hypoinflammatory state. This state may be reversed, taking weeks or months, or it may progress to MODS (Robertson & Coppersmith, 2006).

Three principal actions occur within the body with sepsis: inflammation, coagulation, and fibrinolysis. Inflammation is a complex systemic response to mechanical, ischemic, chemical, or microbial triggers that activate an immediate inflammatory and immune response. The purpose of the inflammatory response is to protect the body from further injury and promote rapid healing. When the infection occurs, endotoxins and exotoxins are produced that initiate a cellular response. This cellular response sparks a cascade of events that results in inflammation and cellular injury (King, 2007; Tazbir, 2004). As a result of the release of histamine, prostaglandins, bradykinin, C-reactive proteins, and other mediators, vasodilation occurs near the injured area with vasoconstriction of arterioles. This results in increased microvascular permeability, allowing exudate to form at the site. Neutrophil activation and adhesion are initiated, which promotes phagocytosis in order to clean the area and prepare for healing. Inflammation is further increased by the activation of the antigen–antibody response to the infectious agent, resulting in the release of cytokines including tumor necrosis factor (TNF) and interleukins 1, 6, and 8 (Rangel-Frausto, 2005). Inflammation normally localizes an infection and kills the invading organism, but when inflammation is extreme it results in vascular congestion, endothelial injury and dysfunction, and overstimulation of the coagulation system (Tazbir, 2004).

The coagulation cascade is activated by the endothelial injury described above, leading to clot formation. The cytokines activate TNF and the endothelial injury activates Factor XII resulting in the activation of clotting factors that cause thrombin generation. Normally this cascade is helpful in the healing process because it helps repair damaged vessels. To prevent the proinflammatory mediators from damaging the normal tissues and organs, anti-inflammatory mediators are released to keep the infection at a local level. Normally with infection the body suppresses fibrinolysis (clot breakdown) to allow time to destroy the antigen. In sepsis, coagulation produces thrombi that become emboli, which ultimately block microvasculature throughout the body, causing cellular death and organ dysfunction. Another reason for increased formation of thrombi with sepsis is the decrease in circulating activated protein C (APC). When thrombin binds with thrombomodulin, protein C becomes activated. **Protein C** is a normal component of the anticoagulant system and in the presence of sepsis it attempts to achieve homeostasis by decreasing inflammation and coagulation and increasing fibrinolysis. A low serum level of APC is associated with sepsis, coagulopathy, multiple organ dysfunction, and increased mortality (Tazbir, 2004). Figure 61–1 ■ (p. 1959) provides an illustration of this process. Chapter 62 ⊚ discusses the normal clotting cascade, the function of these factors, and their relationship to the normal immune function.

When sepsis occurs, the regulatory mechanisms have failed and uncontrolled inflammation overwhelms the body's normal protective responses. Excess coagulation, exaggerated inflammation, and abnormal fibrinolysis spread beyond the isolated area of infection. This leads to systemic vasodilation, hypotension, and a generalized increase in vascular permeability, extravascular sequestration, and increased cellular aggregation with microvascular obstruction and greatly accelerated coagulation. The accelerated coagulation and suppressed fibrinolysis increase the disposition of fibrin clots, causing microvascular hypoperfusion and resulting in decreased blood flow to vital organs such as the lungs and kidneys. When blood flow is compromised to more than one organ system, severe sepsis develops. This may lead to multiple organ failure and death. In a healthy state, the body will "break up" these clots through fibrinolysis. Chapter 62 ⊚ discusses the normal function of clotting.

Cellular dysfunction that occurs in sepsis results from multiple causes. The mechanisms that contribute to cellular dysfunction include cellular ischemia, disruption of cellular metabolism due to the effects of inflammatory mediators such as cytokines, and the toxic effects of free radicals. Unfortunately, in an effort to compensate for the shock state, cells undergo changes that reduce cellular energy, damage cell walls, and release other toxic substances, leading to irreversible shock despite the eradication of the underlying cause of the clinical insult (Hollenberg et al., 2004).

When the body suffers a clinical insult from such things as traumatic injury or infection, the immune system will respond.

When there is an imbalance in this immune response, a devastating inflammatory response can occur that will result in tissue injury, vascular collapse, multiple organ failure, and eventually, in some patients, death.

Infection causes a generalized inflammatory response system that initiates the continuum of sepsis to severe sepsis (sepsis with organ dysfunction), leading to septic shock. Systemic mediators, which are bloodborne communicators, are activated in this hyperinflammatory response and lead to microcoagulation, consumption of platelets, and inhibition of clot lyses (fibrinolysis). A secondary problem includes uncontrolled alterations in vascular tone, vasodilation in large vessels (where pressure is measured), and both vasodilation and vasoconstriction in small vessels where oxygen delivery takes place. This alteration along with microvascular clotting limits oxygen delivery and may lead to ischemia of distant organs. This evolution may eventually lead to multiple organ dysfunction syndrome. MODS is diagnosed when two or more organ systems fail (Bochud & Calandra, 2003; Chettle, 2003; McCance & Huether, 2006). Recent research has demonstrated that certain infectious agents interact with specific receptors (toll-like) in the body. Toll receptors are discussed in Chapter 59 ⊚. In addition, severe gene polymorphisms have been associated with increased susceptibility to sepsis. Controlling both of these discoveries should assist in the direction of the management of sepsis and septic shock (Bochud & Calandra, 2003; Gupta & Jonas, 2006).

Clinical Manifestations

The clinical manifestations of shock were discussed earlier in the chapter. However, because septic shock results from the body's response to an infectious agent, it is important to keep in mind that septic shock may initially manifest with different clinical manifestations from other forms of shock. The patient may be febrile and chilling; the skin may be flushed and warm to the touch; peripheral pulses may be bounding as the body attempts to "fight" the causative agent although patients who are in advanced stages of sepsis, immunocompromised, or have an immature immune system may not be able to activate an adequate response to "fight" the infectious agent. Such patients quickly deteriorate as described earlier in Chart 61–3 (p. 1960).

The recent 2004 information from the SCCM describes septic shock as sepsis with signs of hypoperfusion (Gupta & Jonas, 2006; Hollenberg et al., 2004). As the shock syndrome progresses, and hypoperfusion becomes more profound, the patient will become hypotensive, develop a weak and thready pulse, cool and clammy skin, increased capillary refill, especially in the pediatric patient, altered mental status, decreased or absent urinary output, hypoactive bowel sounds, and rapid shallow respirations. About one-half of the patients with decompensated septic shock will die of multiple organ failure (King, 2007).

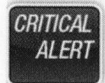 *A patient who is suspected of being in septic shock who is hypothermic is in an advanced stage of sepsis and at great risk of dying.*

Laboratory and Diagnostic Procedures

The Diagnostic Tests for SIRS and Septic Shock box contains a summary of the laboratory tests that can be used to diagnose SIRS and septic shock.

Medical Management

The challenges associated with the medical management of the patient with SIRS, sepsis, or septic shock prompted an international conference. In 2003, critical and infectious disease experts across the world developed management guidelines that could be used by all providers who come in contact with patients who may be at risk for sepsis (Dellinger et al., 2008). This consensus group affirmed the definitions of sepsis and septic shock and developed national guidelines for the initial management of sepsis. These guidelines (see the National Guidelines box, p. 1972) contain evidence-based and consensus recommendations for the initial resuscitation, diagnosis, and management of sepsis and severe sepsis.

In addition, the consensus group began an educational campaign that has been adopted worldwide to prevent and promote earlier recognition of risk factors and provide a universal evidenced-based approach to the management of sepsis (Dellinger et al., 2008). The Surviving Sepsis Campaign describes the management of a patient with suspected or confirmed sepsis beginning with recognition by the patient or the family and management in the emergency department and the critical care unit. Early, goal-directed therapy is the cornerstone of the initial management of the patient with sepsis (Russell, 2006).

The management of the patient in severe sepsis or septic shock should begin before the patient is admitted to the critical care unit. Just as with any patient in shock, the patient's airway, breathing, and circulation need to be assessed and critical interventions initiated. The major focus during the resuscitation of these patients is to prevent the consequences of tissue hypoperfusion and hypoxia. In addition, the source of the infection must be quickly identified and appropriately treated in order to stop the cause of the sepsis. Chart 61–8 (p. 1973) contains a summary of guidelines for the ongoing management of severe sepsis and septic shock from the SCCM (Dellinger et al., 2008).

Another important responsibility is the surveillance and application of guidelines for the use of antimicrobial agents that are used to manage sepsis and prevent development of antimicrobial resistance. Antibiotic use should be reevaluated every 48 to 72 hours to ensure that the correct medications are being administered and that no toxic side effects are occurring. (See the Pharmacology Summary on p. 1981)

◼ Nursing Management

Nurses play a key role in the prevention and early recognition of sepsis. It is important to be aware of potential sources of infection such as the presence of urinary catheters, central venous or arterial catheters, and continuous ventilator support. Meticulous

DIAGNOSTIC TESTS for SIRS and Septic Shock

Test	Expected Abnormality	Rationale for Abnormality
White blood cells	Leukocytosis Leukopenia Normal white blood cell count with immature forms	Leukocytosis and leucopenia occur as part of the body's inflammatory response. White blood count will reflect an inflammatory process in order to fight the infectious agent.
Blood glucose	Hyperglycemia	In infection, glucose production is increased to provide additional energy. This will continue to occur until the liver fails.
Blood cultures	Evidence of an infectious cause of the sepsis. These will require time for growth. Antibiotic therapy should be held until appropriate cultures have been obtained.	Blood cultures will optimize the identification of the causative agent.
Culture and antibiotic sensitivity of suspect infection sites such as urine, sputum, invasive lines	Source of infection	Allows for identification of source of infection and appropriate antibiotic to treat it.
Arterial blood gases	Respiratory alkalosis Metabolic acidosis Hypoxia	Increased respirations to decrease CO_2, which is how the lungs compensate for metabolic acidosis, which results from anaerobic metabolism because of the lack of energy substrates to the cells. Hypoxia results from inadequate tissue perfusion.
Serum lactate levels	Elevated	Reflects tissue perfusion; increased level indicates inadequate tissue perfusion that results in lack of energy substrates and anaerobic metabolism.
Coagulation studies	Decrease in platelet numbers as shock progresses Increased prothrombin time (PT), increased partial thromboplastin (PTT), increased INR, and increased fibrin split products	These reflect activation of the clotting cascade and signal development of disseminated intravascular coagulation (DIC). Chapter 63 ⊙ contains a complete discussion of DIC.

NATIONAL GUIDELINES for the Initial Management of Sepsis

Initial Resuscitation	Guideline
Goal directed during the first 6 hours	Maintain with fluids and vasopressors: • Central venous: 8–12 mmHg • MAP > 65 mmHg • Urine output > 0.5 mL kg^{-1} hr^{-1} • Central venous (superior vena cava) or mixed venous oxygen saturation > 70%
Diagnosis	Appropriate cultures of suspected sources of infection.
Antibiotic therapy	Antibiotic therapy should be initiated within 1 hour of recognition of severe sepsis, after appropriate cultures are obtained. The antibiotic regimen should be reassessed every 48–72 hours on the basis of microbiological and clinical data with the aim of using the appropriate antibiotic to prevent the development of resistance and toxicity.
Source control	Drainage of abscesses. Debridement of necrotic tissue. Removal of infected devices.
Fluid therapy	Fluid resuscitation may consist of colloids or crystalloids. No evidence is available to support one over the other. Fluid challenge over 30 minutes of 500–1,000 mL monitoring vital signs and urinary output. May be repeated.
Vasopressors	When appropriate fluid challenge fails and there is a need to restore end-organ perfusion, therapy with vasopressors may be started. Norepinephrine or dopamine are preferably given through a central catheter. Arterial line should be placed for monitoring.
Inotropic therapy	Use in patients with low cardiac output despite adequate fluid resuscitation. Dobutamine may be used to increase cardiac output.
Steroids	IV stress dose corticosteroids are recommended only in patients with adequate volume replacement and who require vasopressors to maintain an adequate blood pressure.
Recombinant human activated protein C (rhAPC)	Recommended for patients who are at high risk of death and with no absolute contraindication related to bleeding risk or a relative contraindication that outweighs the risk of the treatment.
Mechanical ventilation of sepsis-induced acute lung Injury (ALI) and ARDS	Low tidal volume 6 mL/kg predicted based on body weight. Avoid high plateau pressures. To decrease days of mechanical ventilation and ICU length of stay, a conservative fluid strategy for patients with established ALI/ARDS who are not in shock. For patients with ALI/ARDS, application of at least a minimal amount of positive end-expiratory pressure. Use protocols for weaning.
Sedation, analgesia, neuromuscular blockade in sepsis	Protocols should be used to manage the patient and ensure adequate sedation and pain management, but avoid the consequences of immobility and too much medication.
Glucose control	Maintain blood glucose < 150 mg/dL after initial stabilization.
Bicarbonate therapy	Not recommended for treatment of hypoperfusion-induced lactic acidemia with pH > 7.15.
Deep venous thrombosis	Medical and mechanical treatment based on the severity of the patient's condition.
Stress ulcer prophylaxis	H$_2$ receptors have been found to be more effective in severe sepsis.
Consideration for limitation of support	Advance care planning and end-of-life issues must be considered and addressed.

Source: From Dellinger, R. P., Carlet, J. M., Masur, H., Gerlach, H., et al. (2008). Surviving Sepsis Campaign guidelines for management of severe sepsis and septic shock. *Critical Care Medicine,* 32(3), 858–873.

hand hygiene and the use of strict aseptic technique when managing any break in skin integrity such as wounds or invasive lines can help prevent infection. Patients who take steroids or other immunosuppressive medications must be taught how to recognize signs and symptoms of infection such as spiking a fever and chilling.

Nurses should also ensure the use of standard precautions, especially excellent hand hygiene, to prevent the transmission of microorganisms in the areas in which they work (Smith & McInnis, 2007).

Nursing care of the patient with sepsis is summarized in the Nursing Process: Patient Care Plan for Severe Sepsis (p. 1974).

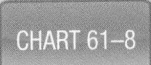 **CHART 61–8**   Management of Severe Sepsis and Septic Shock

Intervention	Rationale
During the first 6 hours resuscitation is directed at: • Central venous pressure 8–12 mmHg • Mean arterial pressure (MAP) >65 mmHg • Urine output >0.5 mL/kg/hr • Central venous or mixed oxygen saturation >70%. Obtain vascular access. Aggressive fluid resuscitation of natural or artificial colloids or crystalloids may be used to achieve outlined parameters, vasopressors are used to maintain adequate perfusion and in some cases blood transfusions are done.	Goal-directed therapy has been shown to improve patient outcomes. Fluid resuscitation, use of vasopressors, and in some cases blood transfusions may be used to obtain the goals of adequate perfusion and oxygenation to compromised tissues.
Appropriate cultures of blood or any other potential infection site should be obtained before initiation of antibiotic therapy.	Diagnostic studies (e.g., blood cultures, radiographs, and CT exams) should be performed promptly to identify the source of the infection or causative agent organism. Sources such as abscesses need to be drained.
Antibiotic therapy is based on the patient history, underlying diseases, clinical syndrome, and susceptibility patterns in the patient's community and in the health care facility.	Failure to initiate appropriate antibiotic therapy promptly has adverse consequences. Inappropriate antibiotic therapy can lead to the development of a superinfection and the development of resistance.
Vasopressors should be started after an appropriate fluid challenge has failed. Vasopressors may also be indicated in the instance of a life-threatening hypotension along with fluid resuscitation.	Beyond a certain MAP, autoregulation in various vascular beds is lost. Vasopressors will be needed to maintain perfusion.
Provide inotropic support.	Supplements low cardiac output.
IV corticosteroids for 7 days in three or four divided doses are recommended in patient in septic shock, not responding to fluid replacement and vasopressor therapies.	Decreases stress response and may reverse shock states.
Use of recombinant human activated protein C is recommended in patients with a high risk of death such as patients who are in sepsis-induced organ failure, septic shock, or sepsis-induced respiratory distress. Patient must have a low risk of bleeding and the benefits of treatment must outweigh the risks.	The inflammatory response in severe sepsis is linked to procoagulant activity and endothelial activation. This drug has been shown in some cases to improve survival. It needs to be administered as early as possible.
Red blood cell administration should only be administered when hemoglobin decreases to < 7.0 g/dL.	Research has suggested that patients with severe sepsis can tolerate lower hemoglobin. Blood transfusions may actually worsen sepsis by initiating an additional inflammatory response.
Keep glucose < 150 mg/dL	Nutrition is important for the septic patient.
Mechanical ventilations should be closely monitored to prevent VAP, pulmonary injury, and adequate oxygenation.	Mechanical ventilation has been associated with multiple complications and an increased mortality. A weaning protocol should be in place and mechanically ventilated patients should undergo a spontaneous breathing test so that the patient can come off the ventilator as soon as possible.
Sedation, analgesia, and neuromuscular blockade should be goal driven.	Predetermined end points with the use of these medications prevent additional stress and harm to a compromised patient and also provide comfort and pain management.
Provide bicarbonate therapy for management of hypoperfusion-induced lactic acidemia.	There is no evidence to support this treatment.
Deep venous prophylaxis should be started to prevent the risk of emboli. This can be done with either low-dose unfractionated heparin or low-molecular-weight heparin. For patients with bleeding risk, mechanical devices should be used. In some patients, a combination of both may be required.	Prevents complications of deep vein thrombosis (DVT).
Stress ulcer prophylaxis should be initiated.	Stress ulcers cause additional complications in severe sepsis.
Consideration of limitation of support should be discussed with patient (when possible) and family. This should include: • Advanced care planning • Realistic goals of treatment • Withdrawal of support • Comfort care.	Aggressive management may not be in the patient's best interest. There may be no difference in outcome based on the cause of the severe sepsis and septic shock. Underlying quality of patient's life before the onset of severe sepsis and septic shock must be examined.

Source: From Dellinger, R. P., Carlet, J. M., Masur, H., Gerlach, H., et al. (2008). Surviving Sepsis Campaign guidelines for management of severe sepsis and septic shock. *Critical Care Medicine,* 32(3), 858–873.

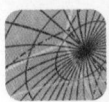

NURSING PROCESS: Patient Care Plan for Severe Sepsis

Assessment of Airway and Gas Exchange

Subjective Data:

Are you short of breath?

Are you getting enough air?

Do you breathe better sitting up?

Have you had a cough?

Are you coughing anything up and, if so, what color is it and how much?

Have you had a fever or chills?

Objective Data:

Work of breathing

Increased rate, use of accessory muscles, retractions

Lung sounds

Oxygen saturation

Skin color

Capillary refill

Nursing Assessment and Diagnoses	Outcomes and Evaluation Parameters	Planning and Interventions with *Rationales*
Nursing Diagnoses: *Gas Exchange, Impaired Risk for* related to inadequate tissue perfusion *Airway Clearance, Ineffective* related to altered mental status from inadequate tissue perfusion	**Outcome:** Adequate gas exchange. ***Evaluation Parameters:*** Normal arterial blood gases. Decreased respiratory rate because of a decreased need to compensate for metabolic acidosis; 12–20 breaths per minute. Adequate perfusion for the patient to become alert and oriented. Clear breath sounds.	**Interventions and *Rationales:*** Assess for symptoms of increased work of breathing, which indicate inadequate tissue perfusion: oxygen saturation, length of capillary refill, skin temperature, and color *to assess tissue perfusion.* Monitor ABGs and oxygen saturation to assess adequacy of gas exchange and level of shock state. *When the body responds to shock, it will divert blood from the periphery and direct it to the brain, lungs, and kidneys.* Monitor for changes in mental status such as restlessness and confusion. *Indicators of inadequate gas exchange with resultant cerebral hypoxia.* Observe for pallor and cyanosis, especially in the mucous membranes. *Indicators of inadequate gas exchange with resultant tissue hypoxia.* Administer 100% oxygen by nonrebreather mask. *To increase available oxygen and decrease tissue hypoxia.* Report respiratory distress and hypoxia to the health care provider. *Intubation and mechanical ventilation may be needed to deliver greater amounts of oxygen and maintain adequate tissue perfusion.*

Assessment of Fluid Volume Deficit

Subjective Data:

Are you thirsty?

How much fluid have you taken in?

What kind of fluids have you been drinking?

When was the last time you urinated?

Do you have any appetite?

Objective Data:

Decreased or absent peripheral pulses

Weak central pulses

Cool and clammy skin

Pale skin

Decreased or absent urinary output

Altered mental status

Alterations in vitals signs

Tachycardia, increased pulse pressure, decreased mean arterial pressure

Poor skin turgor

Nursing Assessment and Diagnoses	Outcomes and Evaluation Parameters	Planning and Interventions with *Rationales*
Nursing Diagnosis: *Fluid Volume, Deficient* related to alterations in circulating blood volume due to impaired vascular function from the effects of endotoxins on vasomotor tone	**Outcome:** Adequate circulating fluid volume. ***Evaluation Parameters:*** Adequate peripheral perfusion. Normal capillary refill time. Normal urinary output (minimum of 30 mL/hr). Improvement in mentation. Heart rate 60–100 beats per minute with normal sinus rhythm. Blood pressure systolic greater than 100 mmHg.	**Interventions and *Rationales:*** Insertion of large-bore intravenous catheters *to provide fluid resuscitation.* Insert central venous catheter *to measure pressure and monitor central pressure.* Insert a urinary catheter *to measure hourly urinary output. These measures help with assessment of adequacy of fluid resuscitation.* Monitor effectiveness of the use of prescribed vasopressors, *which are used to improve blood pressure and support circulation.* Monitor heart rate, blood pressure, and quality of central and peripheral pulses *to assess adequacy of fluid resuscitation.* Report signs of inadequate perfusion (e.g., hypotension, tachycardia, and low urinary output) to the health care provider *so that additional interventions such as administration of other vasopressor agents can be started to improve circulation.*

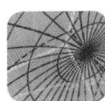

NURSING PROCESS: Patient Care Plan for Severe Sepsis—*Continued*

Assessment of Infection

Subjective Data:

Have you had an infection in the last 2 weeks?

How often do you urinate? Do you feel you completely empty your bladder with each urination?

Have you been running a fever?

Do you have a cough?

Do you have burning on urination?

Do you have a history of infections? If so, what kind? How were they treated?

Are you taking any medications such as steroids, antibiotics?

Have you had an organ transplant?

Have you recently traveled outside of the country? If you have, where? Were you told of possible diseases such as avian flu where you traveled?

Objective Data:

Fever	Presence of a urinary catheter
Chills	Feeding tube
Flushed skin	Decubitus
Presence of purpura, petechiae	Presence of wounds
Abscess	Urinary catheter?
Open wound	Feeding tube?
Burns	White blood count

Nursing Assessment and Diagnoses	Outcomes and Evaluation Parameters	Planning and Interventions with *Rationales*
Nursing Diagnoses: *Infection* related to a focus of infection	**Outcomes:** Identification of focus of infection. Infection resolved. ***Evaluation Parameters:*** Decrease or absence of fever. Removal of source of the infection, for example, draining of an abscess or removal of an invasive catheter. Normal white blood cell count and differential.	**Interventions and *Rationales:*** Measure and monitor the patient's body temperature using the most appropriate method. For example, rectal, esophageal, or bladder so the most accurate temperature is measured. *Effects of treatment can also be monitored.* Perform measures to decrease the patient's fever such as administration of an antipyretic or application of a cooling blanket. *To prevent side effects of fever such as dehydration.* Note the presence of a source of an infection, for example, urinary catheter, draining wound, rigid abdomen, and colored sputum. *To determine cause and infection site.* Obtain blood cultures by drawing blood from two sites. At least one should be drawn percutaneously and one drawn through each vascular access device unless the device was recently inserted to identify infectious agent. *To diagnose the presence of sepsis.* Obtain cultures from other sites such as urine, CSF, or other body fluids to identify source and infectious agents. *To identify source of infection.* Use aseptic technique when changing dressings or drawing blood from invasive lines *to prevent introduction of further sources of infection.* Perform hand hygiene frequently and use infection control measures when indicated *to prevent introduction of further sources of infection.* Instruct the patient's family about hand hygiene *to prevent further introduction of infection.* Report to the health care provider changes in temperature as prescribed *so appropriate interventions and medications can be given to manage a fever.* Administer antibiotics per health care provider's orders.

Assessment of Tissue Perfusion

Subjective Data:

Is it getting harder to breathe?

Are you more tired than before?

Is your chest hurting?

Are you having pain anywhere?

Objective Data:

Lung congestion	Abdominal distention and tenderness
Oxygen saturation	
Work of breathing	Bowel sounds
Central and peripheral pulses	Jaundice of eyes and skin
Cardiac rhythm	Enlarged liver
Urinary output	Muscle strength
Urine color	Mobility
Level of consciousness	

(continued)

NURSING PROCESS: Patient Care Plan for Severe Sepsis—*Continued*

Nursing Assessment and Diagnoses	Outcomes and Evaluation Parameters	Planning and Interventions with *Rationales*
Nursing Diagnosis: *Tissue Perfusion, Ineffective* related to organ dysfunction	**Outcome:** Prevention of further organ failure and treatment instituted. ***Evaluation Parameter:*** Effective prevention of MODS.	**Interventions and *Rationales:*** Initiate prescribed treatments including fluid resuscitation and vasopressor and antibiotic administration. *To hemodynamically stabilize the patient and treat the cause of infection.* Carefully monitor intake and output. *To evaluate for adequate fluid resuscitation.* Turn and position patient frequently *to prevent skin breakdown and development of DVT.* Monitor for bleeding that may occur due to altered clotting mechanisms. *To prevent hemorrhage.* Prepare patient and family for end-of-life decisions. *To prepare the family for possible death.*

It is based on the management of the patient's airway and breathing to improve oxygenation and circulation. Circulatory support may include fluids as well as vasopressors to maintain a perfusing blood pressure and prevent additional complications.

Collaborative Management

The care of the patient with sepsis requires a multidisciplinary approach in order to increase the patient's chances of survival. The nurse plays an important role in the early recognition of the risk of sepsis occurring as well as recognizing its early signs when it does. Health care providers who participate in the management of the patient with sepsis include specialty health care providers such as a critical care intensivist, surgeons, and infectious disease specialists; nurses; pharmacists; and respiratory and physical therapists.

The health care providers who care for the patient with sepsis are responsible for identifying the cause of the sepsis. This may involve taking the person to surgery to drain an abscess or remove an injured organ. The intensivist is responsible for managing the patient's cardiovascular and pulmonary systems. Nurses are responsible for the continuous monitoring and administration of medications and fluids as well as the emotional and spiritual support of the patient and his family. Pharmacists participate in the evaluation of the appropriate antibiotics and vasoactive medications to fight the cause of the sepsis and maintain the patient's vital sign. Because many of these patients require intubation and mechanical ventilation, the respiratory therapist will assist in the management of the patient's oxygenation. Finally, the physical therapist will be responsible for supporting the nursing staff in providing range of motion (ROM) exercises for sedated patients and moving patients out of bed when possible to prevent further complications from immobility.

Multiple Organ Dysfunction Syndrome

Multiple organ dysfunction syndrome is the end result of severe sepsis. A critical injury or a disease process that initiates a mas-

sive systemic inflammatory response can also activate it. It does not require an infectious process to trigger it. Despite recognition of this disease process since the mid-1970s, mortality from MODS remains high, ranging from 60% to 100% (McCance & Huether, 2006).

Etiology

Multiple organ dysfunction syndrome (MODS) is a spectrum of organ dysfunction in a patient who has SIRS or septic complications. One or more organ systems may be involved (Bumbasirevic, Karamarkovic, Lesic, & Bumbasirevic, 2005; Gupta & Jonas, 2006). Triggers that can initiate MODS include multiple injuries, burns, hemorrhagic or hypovolemic shock, acute pancreatitis, acute respiratory distress syndrome (ARDS), and acute renal failure. Examples of patients who are at risk for the development of MODS include patients with chronic diseases; persons of advanced age; patients who have diabetes, cancer, pulmonary contusions, and widespread necrosis; and those with chronic infections who are being treated with immunosuppressant therapies. It remains a mystery why not all patients with these risk factors develop MODS. Research is now being directed at identifying biomarkers that place patients at greater risk of developing both sepsis and MODS (McCance & Huether, 2006).

Pathophysiology

Multiple organ dysfunction ranges from organ impairment to failure. MODS is classified into primary or early MODS and secondary or late MODS. In primary or early MODS, there is local and generalized hypoperfusion. This triggers both the inflammatory and stress responses discussed previously in this chapter. As a result, microphages and neutrophils are "primed or ready to fight" by cytokines and when any additional insult occurs, such as further tissue injury, the primed cells trigger an even greater response and start progressive organ dysfunction and secondary or late MODS.

Secondary or late MODS results from an excessive inflammatory response after a latent period following the initial insult that is manifested in organs distant from the original site of the injury (Krau, 2007; McCance & Huether, 2006). Just as in sepsis, three primary mechanisms are activated: the inflammatory response, coagulation, and fibrinolysis. It is the body's own defense mechanisms that ultimately contribute to organ compromise and failure (Krau, 2007).

The inflammatory response in MODS leads to hypermetabolism and maldistribution of blood flow. Maldistribution of blood results in tissue hypoxemia, further organ injury, and eventual cell death. Hypermetabolism that results from the stress response causes catabolism, further straining major organs such as the heart and eventually impeding cardiac output. Catabolism causes loss of lean muscle mass and depletion of oxygen and fuel supplies (McCance & Huether, 2006). Oxygen reserves are depleted in MODS because of the body's initial inflammatory response to the primary insult and resulting hypermetabolism. Myocardial depressant factor, which is secreted because of pancreatic hypoperfusion, causes further depression of the myocardium, thus contributing to further hypoxia.

Reperfusion injury, which results from the reestablishment of blood flow after ischemia, causes conversion of the enzyme xanthine dehydrogenase to xanthine oxidase to form oxygen free radicals with oxygen when hypoperfused tissues are reperfused. These oxygen radicals attack already damaged tissues. As discussed earlier in this chapter, reperfusion injury can lead to MODS (McCance & Huether, 2006). Figure 61–3 ■ (p. 1978) summarizes the pathophysiology of MODS. The treatment and management continues to challenge those who provide critical care and continues to be responsible for mortality that is generally the end result of MODS.

Clinical Manifestations and Diagnosis

The clinical manifestations of MODS depend on the area or areas of the body affected. Primary or early MODS is difficult to monitor. Examples of primary MODS in a trauma patient may include the primary cerebral edema seen in a head injury or ARDS that develops after a thoracic injury (Keel & Trentz, 2005). Secondary or late MODS has a specific pattern of injury that can be observed and measured. Several scoring systems exist that describe the progress of MODS. The sequential organ failure assessment (SOFA) score describes the degree of organ failure and how it changes over time. SOFA is summarized in Chart 61–9 (p. 1979). Secondary or late MODS generally evolves over 14 days to a period of weeks.

In summary, the clinical manifestations of MODS are the result of inflammatory mediator damage, tissue hypoxia, and hypermetabolism. The clinical manifestations of organ dysfunction are summarized in Chart 61–10 (p. 1979) (McCance & Huether, 2006).

Laboratory and Diagnostic Procedures

The laboratory and diagnostic tests used to evaluate MODS are specific to the organ systems that are failing. For example, hyperbilirubinemia and increased serum aspartate transaminase, serum alanine aminotransferase, lactic dehydrogenase, alkaline phosphatase, and ammonia levels are indicative of liver failure. Patchy infiltrates on a chest radiograph are seen with ARDS. Decreased or absent urinary output reflects renal failure. The Diagnostic Tests for MODS box (p. 1980) contains information on laboratory tests that are monitored in the patient with MODS.

Medical Management

The primary focus for the management of MODS is to prevent it from occurring. Rapid recognition of the source of infection or management of the cause of shock or sepsis is one way to decrease the risk of the secondary insult. Nosocomial infections from invasive lines or catheters as well as poor hand hygiene must also be managed. After the initial injury or infection has been treated, care is directed at controlling infection, providing adequate tissue oxygenation, restoring and maintaining vascular volume, and supporting individual organ function. Antibiotics must be chosen carefully and closely monitored (McCance & Huether, 2006). Because tissue hypoxia is a major problem, intubation and mechanical ventilation may be required. Oxygen saturation should be maintained between 88% and 92%. However, mechanical ventilation can lead to additional problems such as VAP, which may lead to the secondary assault triggering the onset of MODS.

Adequate volume resuscitation and vascular support need to be ongoing. Volume resuscitation decreases the risks of complications from hemoconcentrated blood due to shifts in interstitial spaces. Replacing and maintaining volume also improves the supply and demand imbalance that occurs with hypermetabolism. Vasopressors such as epinephrine or norepinephrine may be used to increase systemic vascular resistance and improve cardiac output and oxygenation. Any problem that increases oxygen demand such as fever needs to be managed. Excessive body temperatures may require cooling measures such as hypothermia blankets as well as medications such as acetaminophen. Patients may require analgesia and sedation to decrease pain and anxiety thus decreasing oxygen demand. Nutrition through enteral feeding helps maintain the gut barrier and reduces the translocation of bacteria, thus reducing the incidence of infection and other complications. Glucose levels are tightly controlled due to the effect of high glucose levels on tissue/organ function. Individual organs will require support and this management will be based on the organ or organ systems that have been affected.

■ Nursing Management

Nursing care for the patient with MODS includes early recognition of the risk factors for the development of MODS, and close monitoring of interventions initiated to treat the patients such as invasive lines and catheters. Meticulous skin care and aseptic technique must be used to insert and change any lines. The nurse should ensure that all who come in contact with the patient use meticulous hand hygiene and aseptic technique to prevent the risk of infection.

Frequent monitoring and assessment to trend changes in vital signs and clinical manifestations will provide the most reliable information about early signs of MODS. Nursing care needs to be focused on decreasing oxygen demand, which includes pain and anxiety management as well as spacing activity to allow for long periods of rest. The nurse should assess for signs of pain and anxiety and medicate as needed. Tachycardia related to pain and anxiety increases oxygen consumption due to the stress imposed on the body by pain. Positioning of the patient is important to prevent the complications that occur with immobility such as skin breakdown, pulmonary congestion, and pooling of blood and secretions. Hypermetabolism causes loss

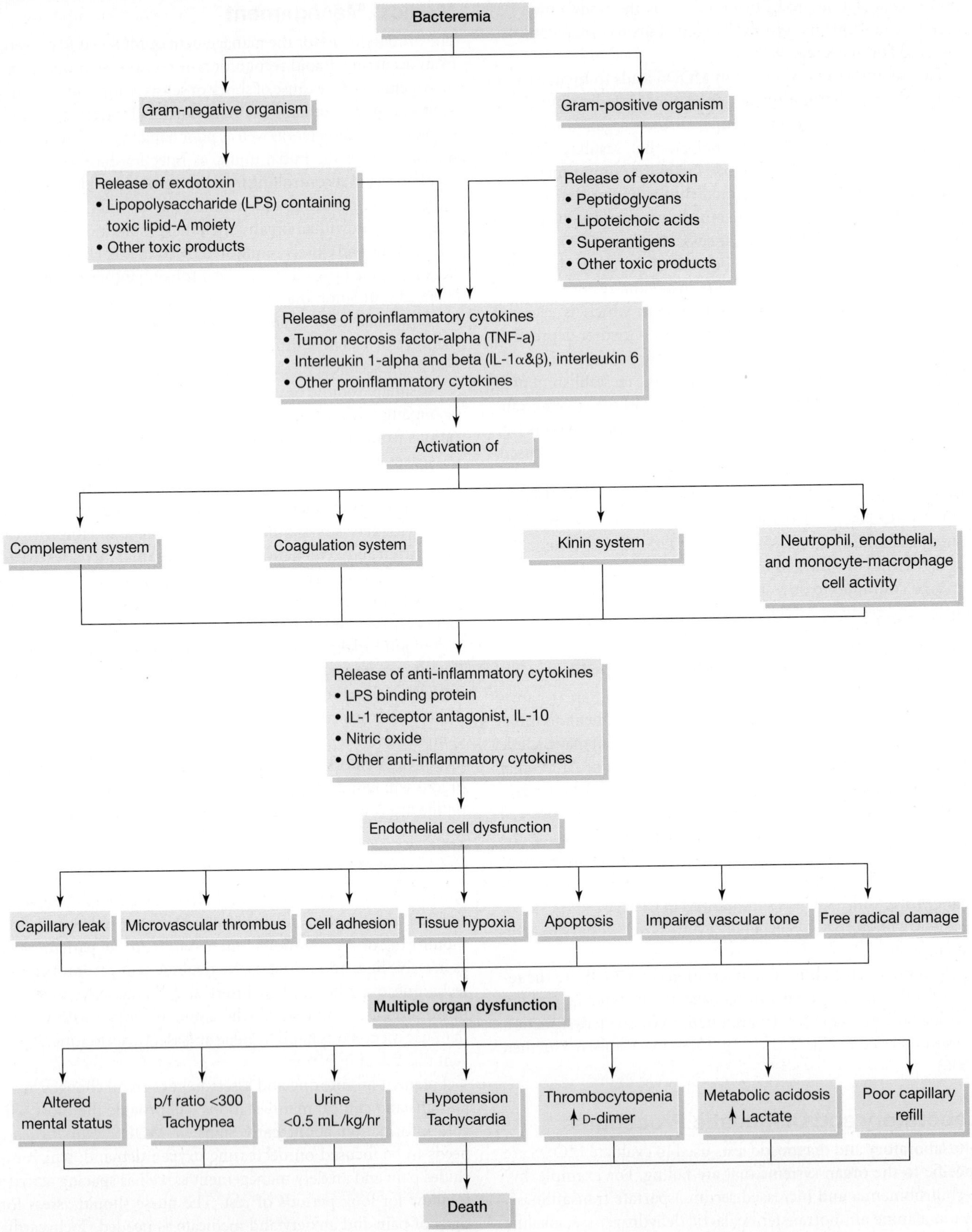

FIGURE 61–3 ■ Pathophysiology of MODS.

CHART 61-9   **Sequential Organ Failure Assessment (SOFA) Score**

	1	2	3	4
Respiration PaO$_2$/FiO$_2$(kP$_a$)	<53	<40	<26	<13
Coagulation platelets (10^3/μL)	<150	<100	<50	<20
Liver bilirubin (μmol/L)	20–32	33–101	102–204	>204
Cardiovascular Inotrope	MAP <70	Dopamine ≤ 5 μg/kg/min or dobutamine any dose	Dopamine >5 μg/kg/min or adrenaline < 0.1 μg/kg/min or noradrenalin < 0.1 μg/kg/min	Dopamine > 15 μg/kg/min or adrenaline > 0.1 or noradrenalin > 0.1
CNS		10–12	6–9	<6
GCS	13–14			
Renal Creatinine (μmol/L)	110–170	171–299	300–440	>440

Note: Key: MAP, mean arterial pressure; GCS, Glasgow Coma Scale.

CHART 61-10   **Clinical Manifestations of MODS**

PULMONARY

Dyspnea, patchy infiltrates, refractory hypoxemia, respiratory acidosis, and abnormal O$_2$ indices

Pulmonary hypertension

GASTROINTESTINAL

Abdominal distention and ascites

Intolerance of enteral feedings

Paralytic ileus

Gastrointestinal bleeding

Mucosal ulceration

Bacterial overgrowth in stool

LIVER

Increased bilirubin level

Increased liver enzymes

Increased serum ammonia level

Jaundice

Hepatomegaly

METABOLIC/NUTRITIONAL

Decreased lean body mass

Muscle wasting

Severe weight loss

Negative nitrogen balance

Hyperglycemia

Hypertriglyceridemia

Increased serum lactate levels

Decreased serum albumin

RENAL

Increased serum creatinine level and BUN

Oliguria, anuria, or polyuria related to acute tubular necrosis

CARDIOVASCULAR

HYPERDYNAMIC

Decreased:
  Pulmonary capillary wedge pressure
  Systemic vascular resistance
  Right atrial pressure

Increased:
  Oxygen consumption
  Cardiac output
  Cardiac index
  Heart rate

HYPODYNAMIC

Increased:
  Systemic vascular resistance
  Right atrial pressure
  Left ventricular stroke work index

Decreased:
  Oxygen delivery and consumption
  Cardiac output
  Cardiac index

CENTRAL NERVOUS SYSTEM

Lethargy

Altered level of consciousness

Fever

Hepatic encephalopathy

COAGULATION AND HEMATOLOGIC

Thrombocytopenia

Disseminated intravascular coagulation

IMMUNE

Infection

Decreased lymphocyte count

Anergy

Source: Adapted from McCance, K. L., & Huether, S. (2006). *Pathophysiology: The biologic basis for disease in adults and children* (5th ed.). St. Louis: Mosby.

DIAGNOSTIC TESTS for MODS

Test and Normal Values	Expected Abnormality	Rationale for Abnormality
Lactate level 1–2 mmol/L	4–5 mmol/L	Metabolic acidosis results from inadequate tissue perfusion and anaerobic metabolism.
D-dimer Negative	Positive	Indication of coagulopathy that is present in MODS.
Liver function tests	Increased	Liver is frequently one of the first organs to fail in MODS.
Arterial blood gases	pH acidosis PO_2 decreased	Acidosis and hypoxia result because of damage to the lungs and poor end-organ perfusion.

of muscle, so it is important to prevent additional loss of movement. Patients should receive active and passive ROM exercises to retain strength and joint motion.

Emotional support for both the patient and the family is essential. The high mortality rate associated with MODS points out the need to assist the family with preparing for difficult decisions about end of life. As discussed in Chapter 17 🔗, the nurse needs to be aware of any religious or cultural needs related to death and dying.

Administration of vasopressors will place the patient at risk of injury to fingers, hands, toes, and feet due to peripheral vasoconstriction. Frequent assessment of peripheral circulation is needed. Additionally, fluid resuscitation and shunting of blood and nutrients can lead to edema. Therefore, skin impairment can occur and is another source of infection. Positioning and use of special beds may improve the risk of these complications.

Health Promotion

The primary emphasis in the treatment for shock is prevention. Early recognition of factors that place a patient at risk for the development of a shock syndrome may greatly reduce patient morbidity and mortality. See the Complementary & Alternative Therapies box (p. 1982) for a discussion of the use of T'ai Chi Chun to strengthen the immune system. Traumatic injury contributes to the risk for all types of shock because of organ system injury. Injury prevention strategies may add to decreasing the incidence of shock. Examples of injury prevention and control strategies can be found in the Emergency Nurses Association's Trauma Nursing Core Course (ENA, 2007). Examples include:

- Engineering and technologic interventions (e.g., high-mounted rear brake lights)
- Enforcement and legislative interventions (e.g., state seat belt and helmet laws)
- Placing children in properly fitted and located car seats
- Education and behavioral interventions (e.g., school- and hospital-based education programs).

Sepsis and septic shock have become a serious problem in the United States. Prevention strategies to reduce the incidence of septic shock include (Masur, 2003):

- Age-appropriate vaccinations
- Reduction of the incidence of antibiotic-resistant pathogens in ICUs

- Aseptic management of invasive lines
- Aseptic management of indwelling catheters, feeding tubes, and central lines
- Frequent hand hygiene (Hand hygiene has become a major quality indicator in hospitals, clinics, and any place patient care is given.)
- Efforts to limit antibiotic resistance through policies to prescribe them and surveillance of their use.

Chart 61–11 contains a summary of an action plan that is being implemented to combat antimicrobial resistance.

■ Research

Research related to shock management is needed (1) to identify areas where practice could improve and (2) to evaluate and test selected interventions. Resuscitation end points and the identification of genetic markers that assist in the identification of patient's at risk to develop sepsis are needed (Gupta & Jonas, 2006). As pointed out earlier in this chapter, research continues to challenge how shock has been managed. The Research Opportunities and Clinical Impact Related to Shock Management box (p. 1983) provides a list of some of the research topics related to shock management that are under investigation. Keeping up with the constant changes in the literature is important to ensure that the patient is receiving the best and most effective care.

CHART 61–11 | **Summary of Action Plan to Combat Antimicrobial Resistance**

- Conduct a national public health education campaign to promote appropriate antimicrobial use as a national health priority.
- Develop and facilitate the implementation of educational and behavioral interventions that will assist clinicians in appropriate antimicrobial prescribing.
- Evaluate the effectiveness (including cost effectiveness) of current and novel infection control practices for health care and extended care settings and in the community.
- Promote adherence to practices proven to be effective.
- Support demonstration projects to evaluate comprehensive strategies that use multiple interventions to promote appropriate drug use and reduce infection rates, in order to assess how interventions found effective in research studies can be applied routinely and most cost effectively on a large scale.

PHARMACOLOGY Summary of Medications to Treat Shock, Severe Sepsis, and MODS

Medication Category	Action	Application/Indication	Nursing Responsibility

Antibiotics
 	
Broad-spectrum antibiotics are used initially because the infectious agent is generally not known.
Antibiotics should be chosen using the following guidelines:
 	
• What community the patient lives in or has come from
 	
• Epidemiology of sepsis in the hospital or community
 	
• Suspected agents:
  Fungi
  Gram-positive bacteria
  Highly resistant gram-negative bacilli
  Methicillin-resistant *Staphylococcus aureus*
  Vancomycin-resistant enterococcus
  Penicillin-resistant pneumococcus
	Will depend on the type of antibiotic that is prescribed by the clinician.	Choice of antibiotic should be based on the epidemiology of sepsis in the hospital and the community.
		Identification of the site of source or site of infection will direct the type of antibiotic approved.
		Only one antibiotic at a time, or monotherapy, is recommended.
			Assess history of drug allergies.
			Assess clinical manifestations of allergic reaction.
			Assess relief of clinical manifestations to determine drug effectiveness 48–72 hours after initiation of the antibiotic therapy.

Recombinant
 	
Human-Activated Protein C
	Antithrombotic:
	Irreversible inactivation of Factors V and VIII.
	Anti-inflammatory:
	Reduces formation of TNF, IL-8, IL-6, and thrombin; limits the rolling of monocytes and neutrophils on injured endothelium. Also may reduce apoptosis.
	Profibrinolytic:
	Inhibits plasminogen activator inhibitor-1 (PA-1).
		The following criteria should be used for the administration:
		
		• Severe sepsis of greater than 48 hours
		
		• High risk of death
		
		• Experienced medical care of the patient has not improved the condition
		
		• Static or deteriorating clinical condition
		
		• No evidence of:
		  Morbid obesity
		  Major surgery < 12 hours
		  Intracranial surgery or stroke < 3 months
		  Previous intracranial lesion
		  Epidural congenital bleeding diathesis
		  Gastrointestinal bleeding requiring intervention < 6 weeks
		  Trauma with bleeding risk
		  Pancreatitis
		  Chronic renal failure
		  Varices
		  Cirrhosis
		  Chronic jaundice or ascites
		  Platelets $< 30,000 \times 10^6$/L
		  Antithrombotic medication
		  Recent DVT or PE
		  Hypercoagulable
		  Immunocompromised
			Assess history that may contradict the administration of this medication.
			Carefully assess any indications of bleeding or coagulation disorders.
			Carefully assess relief of clinical manifestations to determine drug effectiveness or worsening of the patient's condition.

(continued)

PHARMACOLOGY Summary of Medications to Treat Shock, Severe Sepsis, and MODS—*Continued*

Medication Category	Action	Application/Indication	Nursing Responsibility
Corticosteroids			
Hydrocortisone Methylprednisone	Stimulates ACTH to increase cortisol. Stabilizes leukocyte lysosomal membrane. Inhibits phagocytosis and release of allergic substances. Reduces capillary dilation and permeability. Modifies immune response to various stimuli.	Treat adrenal insufficiency associated with septic shock. Treat inflammatory response related to spinal cord injury.	Assess relief of clinical manifestations. Carefully assess side effects: • Infection due to depressed immune response • Blood glucose • Gastric bleeding • Problems with wound healing.
Vasopressors			
Norepinephrine Dopamine Vasopressin	Reverse the vasodilation and reduced systemic vascular resistance. Promote alpha and beta sympathetic activity. Increase inotropy and chronotropy. Stimulate vasopressor receptors.	Vasopressors should not be used until appropriate fluid challenge fails to restore adequate blood pressure and organ perfusion. Vasopressin may be considered when fluid resuscitation and high-dose vasopressors have not worked.	Assess relief of clinical manifestations by monitoring MAP and urinary output. Assess the potential side effects of the medications such as peripheral vasoconstriction.
Insulin therapy	Inducts euglycemia, and anti-inflammatory effect. Protects endothelial and mitochondrial function.	Controls hyperglycemia, improves lipid levels, and has anti-inflammatory, anticoagulant, and anti-apoptic actions.	Assess patient glucose to maintain glucose level <150 mg/dL (8.3 mmol/L).
Recombinant			
Activated Coagulation Factor VII (rFVIIa)	Promotes coagulation.	Facilitates cell membrane binding.	Assess for bleeding.

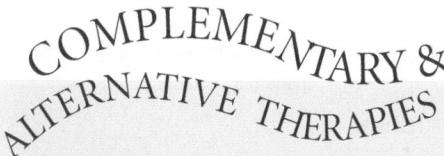

COMPLEMENTARY & ALTERNATIVE THERAPIES   T'ai Chi Chun

Description:
T'ai chi chun (TCC) is a CAM therapy that has multiple applications. Originating in Asia, TCC is a form of exercise that is used to improve balance, build muscle strength, and improve coordination. TCC uses a series of 20 slow, regular movements that many refer to as "moving meditation," and can be easily performed by older and medically compromised individuals.

Research Support:
A review of literature examined the quantity and quality of research evidence regarding the therapeutic benefits of Taiji, which is also known as tai chi chun (TCC). The research team examined more than 200 published reports, of which 17 controlled clinical trials met a high standard of methodological rigor. Evidence in these studies confirmed the following therapeutic benefits of TCC: improved quality of life, improved physical function including activity tolerance and cardiovascular function, improved pain management, improved balance, reduced risk of falls, enhanced immune response, and improved flexibility, strength, and kinesthetic sense. Researchers concluded that, according to preliminary research, TCC can be implemented in a variety of clinical populations (Klein & Adams, 2004).

A study conducted in Taiwan involved 37 middle-aged participants (14 men and 23 women) who engaged in 12 weeks of TCC exercises. Researchers investigated the effect of TCC on participants' functional mobility, beliefs about benefits of exercise on physical and psychological health, and immune regulation. Results showed that the participants experienced significant positive effects on functional mobility and beliefs about the health benefits of exercise after engaging in the 12 weeks of TCC. Immune system response was also positive: There was a significant decrease in monocyte count (although total white blood cell and red blood cell count did not change significantly); a significant increase in the ratio of T helper to suppressor cells (CD4:CD8); and a significant increase in CD4CD25 regulatory T cells (Yeh, Chuang, Lin, Hsiao, & Eng, 2006).

One paper discussed the results of a study that examined the effects of TCC on older adults' response and immunity to herpes zoster/shingles and varicella zoster virus. The study results showed that TCC improved health functioning and immunity to varicella zoster virus in older adults as compared to a control group (Irwin, Pike, & Oxman, 2004).

References
Irwin, M., Pike, J., & Oxman, M. (2004). Shingles immunity and health functioning in the elderly: T'ai chi chun as a behavioral treatment. *Evidence-Based Complementary and Alternative Medicine, 1*(3), 223–232.

Klein, P. J., & Adams, W. D. (2004). Comprehensive therapeutic benefits of Taiji: A critical review. *American Journal of Physical and Medical Rehabilitation, 83*(9), 735–745.

Yeh, S. H., Chuang, H., Lin, L. W., Hsiao, C. Y., & Eng, H. L. (2006). Regular t'ai chi chun exercise enhances functional mobility and CD4CD25 regulatory T cells. *British Journal of Sports Medicine, 40*(3), 239–243.

The death from sepsis that progresses to septic shock continues to increase each year. Research must be focused at multiple methods of prevention and management. Current research ideas and their clinical impact are discussed in the Research Opportunities and Clinical Impact Related to Sepsis, SIRS, and Severe Sepsis box (p. 1984).

new methodologies to measure the effects of sepsis, and the increased admissions to critical care units, approximately 50% of the patients who succumb to septic shock will die. The health care costs are in the billions of dollars each year.

Nurses need to realize that in order to manage this grave problem, care must first focus on prevention strategies, and that when a septic syndrome has begun, the best evidenced-based treatments must be used to improve patient outcomes and stop unnecessary morbidity and mortality.

◼ Summary

Sepsis, severe sepsis, and septic shock continue to cost more human lives every year. Despite the creation of new medications,

RESEARCH OPPORTUNITIES AND CLINICAL IMPACT RELATED TO SHOCK MANAGEMENT

Research Area	Clinical Impact
Physiological Research	
The role of apoptosis or programmed cell destruction in shock	Developing methods to intervene in the programmed destruction of cells
Role of heat-shock proteins in shock	Heat-shock proteins may play a role in the stress response initiated by the body in the shock state
Identity of specific markers that indicate a systemic shock response	Earlier diagnosis and identification of high risk patients
Development of an international definition of shock, SIRS, and sepsis	To standardize name and its significance related to research findings
Identification of the most appropriate solution for initial and continued fluid resuscitation: hypertonic saline, Ringer's lactate, or normal saline	Development of collaborative pathways for appropriate fluid resuscitation for the type of shock and nursing interventions to mediate the progression
Determination of whether fluid resuscitation should be controlled based on the source of the clinical insult. Theory that hypotensive may actually be a protective mechanism	
Hypothermia and minimal fluid resuscitation	Development of nursing guidelines for monitoring the patient's response to fluid resuscitation
Blood substitutes	
Recombinant hemoglobin solution	
Medications effective against bacteria and viruses without causing additional systemic damage, for example, ketolides, which bind to two sites on bacteria preventing the development of resistance	Antibiotic resistance is a growing problem, with an expanding number of resistant organisms occurring. Preventing resistance would help mitigate this issue.
Development of synthetic catecholamines to increase end-organ perfusion	Organ hypoperfusion causes complications and increase morbidity and mortality
Inhalation of nitric oxide (NO) inhibition by the use of methylene blue	NO has been found to increase in sepsis, which further contributes to vasodilation and decreased MAP
Staging of shock to guide clinical management	Development of nursing guidelines to monitor the stages of shock and progression of clinical manifestations
Development of guidelines for a universal approach to shock management so that better data can be collected about outcomes	Collaborative pathway for shock management
Shock monitoring: recent research questions the early use of invasive monitoring	Development of nursing guidelines for noninvasive monitoring
Use of extracorporeal membrane oxygenation therapy (ECMO)	ECMO can potentially remove mediators that initiate destructive cascades in such shock states as sepsis
Ethical Issues	
Identification of futile resuscitation parameters	Development of guidelines for the end points of resuscitation
Staging of shock and sepsis to identify irreversible futile resuscitation parameters	Development of nursing guidelines for withdrawal of support

RESEARCH OPPORTUNITIES AND CLINICAL IMPACT RELATED TO SEPSIS, SIRS, AND SEVERE SEPSIS

Research Area	Clinical Impact
Physiological Research	
Identification of how to implement guidelines for the management of severe sepsis and septic shock and measure patient outcomes	Implementation of a specific set of evidence-based guidelines should improve patient outcomes and control health care costs
Development of drugs that neutralize the inflammatory process	Drugs may be used to block the effects of specific toxins on the body
	Medications that neutralize the effects of the body's inflammatory response to infectious agents may improve the outcome of decompensated shock
Genetic studies that identify a person's predisposition to developing sepsis	Several gene polymorphisms have been associated with an increased susceptibility to sepsis
Vaccinations	Development of a vaccination that prevents SIRS when a patient has been exposed to an infectious agent
Ethical Issues	
Identification of end points that indicate that additional resuscitation would be futile	Development of guidelines for the end points of resuscitation
Development of guidelines for humane withdrawal of support	Development of nursing guidelines for withdrawal of support

Clinical Preparation

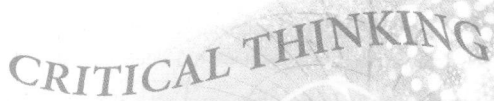

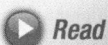 **Read**
- History of Current Illness
- Past Medical History
- Physical Exam
- Admitting Medical Orders
- Laboratory Study Results

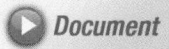 **Document**
- Summary of Hospitalization
- Pathophysiology Form
- Laboratory Values
- Laboratory Results Explanation

 **Apply**
- List of Potential Nursing Diagnoses
- Concept Map
- Critical Thinking Questions

Log on to MyNursingKit.com to download forms you will need and to complete further steps in the Clinical Preparation assignment.

HISTORY OF PRESENT ILLNESS

You are a nurse in a critical care unit and you have been notified that you will be receiving a new patient from the emergency department (ED). The ED nurse calls the following report: David is a 19-year-old college student who is brought to the ED by his friends. His friends said that he has been vomiting for the past 24 hours. This morning he was confused. The patient states that he does not feel well and has been "hot and cold." According to the patient's friends, there has been a recent outbreak of a viral infection on campus. They do not know what the name of the infection is, only that they had heard that it was occurring. The patient is awake and alert, but complaining of a headache. The ED nurse states that he has a petechial rash on his lower extremities and he has received a dose of ceftriaxone 2 grams intravenously.

His blood pressure is 100/70; heart rate 120; respiratory rate 28; his temperature is currently 100.8 orally.

Procedures Since Admission

Within a few hours of admission in the critical care unit, David's mental status begins to deteriorate. You notify the critical care resident and provide him with the following information. David's level of consciousness continued to deteriorate. The critical care resident elected to intubate David using sedation and neuromuscular blocking agents. David was placed on a ventilator. A second large-bore IV line was inserted to administer 2 liters of normal saline since David's blood pressure is staying around 90 systolic and his pulse is in the 130s to 150s. The resident also inserts an arterial line.

Medical–Surgical History

No known allergies
Taking no medications
No prior medical history other than normal childhood illnesses

Social History

David is a freshman at college; he is on the swimming team
States that he drinks beer on the weekend with his friends
Denies the use of illicit substances
Denies cigarette smoking

Physical Exam

Vital signs: BP 88/40; P 130; RR 36; T 104.0°F
Oxygen saturation: 90% on room air initially and then dropped to 86% on room air
HEENT: normal, braces on both upper and lower teeth
Heart: rapid rate; normal S_1, S_2
Lungs: bilateral basilar crackles
Abdomen: flat, soft nontender

Neurological exam: David is lethargic, but can be aroused with minimal stimulation. He is not able to answer simple questions, but will raise his arms and legs when asked. His pupils are 4 mm, equal, round and reactive. Complains of pain with neck movement
Skin: flushed and hot to the touch
Chest radiograph: basilar infiltrates
ECG: sinus tachycardia
Weight: 180 lbs (80 kg) Height 6'
Extremities: petechial rash on both lower extremities that does not blanch
DP and PT pulses 2+

Admitting Medical Orders

Medical ICU service
Floor: Medical Intensive Care Unit
Diagnosis: meningitis and septic shock
No known allergies

LABORATORY STUDY RESULTS

Test	Day 1	Day 2	Day 3
Sodium	141 mEq/L	139 mEq/L	138 mEq/L
Potassium	4.0 mEq/L	3.5 mEq/L	3.8 mEq/L
Chloride	100 mEq/L	113 mEq/L	113 mEq/L
Venous carbon dioxide	17 mEq/L	18 mEq/L	22 mEq/L
Calcium	6.6 mg/dL	7.0 mg/dL	8.6 mg/dL
Blood urea nitrogen	30 mg/dL	25 mg/dL	18 mg/dL
Creatinine	2.0 mg/dL	1.5 mg/dL	1.0 mg/dL
Blood glucose	150 mg/dL	138 mg/dL	120 mg/dL
Total Proteins	4.5 g/dL		
Magnesium	2.0 mg/dL	2.0 mg/dL	2.0 mg/dL
WBC	22, 000/mm^3	10,000/mm^3	10,500/mm^3
Hemoglobin	14.0 gm/dL	13.4 gm/dL	14.7 gm/dL
Hematocrit	40.8%	38.7%	43.1%
RBC	4.69 m/mm^3	4.49 m/mm^3	4.97 m/mm^3
Platelets	128 K/mm^3	137 K/mm^3	269 K/mm^3
ABGs			
PO$_2$	78 mmHg	100 mmHg	150 mmHg
O$_2$ saturation	88%	94%	98%
pH	7.27	7.30	7.35
PCO$_2$	36.5 mmHg	30 mmHg	28 mmHg
HCO$_3$	24 mEq/L	22 mEq/L	24 mEq/L
CSF	Positive for group B streptococcus		
CT scan	Cerebral edema		
ELISA	Antiviral immunoglobulin		
INR	1.18	1.2	1.25
PTT	32 seconds	32.6 seconds	33 seconds
Sputum culture		Negative	
Nasopharyngeal culture		Positive for group B streptococcus	
CSF culture		Positive for group B streptococcus	
Latex agglutination	Certain antibodies in body fluids		
UA	Within normal limits		

Foley
NG tube to low wall suction
Bed rest
Intake and output
Isolation: respiratory isolation
Ventilator settings:
TV 480
RR: 16
Oxygen: 60%
Mode: Assist/control
Peep: 5
Vital signs: every 15 minutes until stable then every 1 hour
Neurological checks every 30 minutes
IV: lactated Ringer's at 100mL/hr. Maintain systolic blood pressure at 100 mmHg with normal saline fluid bolus of 500 mL × 1
NPO until further notice
Call house officer: pulse < 60 and > 100/minute; BP < 90 and > 160 systolic; temperature > 38.5; urine output < 30 mL/hr for 2 hours; respiratory rate > 30/minute; oxygen saturation <92%
Sequential compression devices (SCDs) to lower extremities

Scheduled Medications

Ceftriaxone 2 grams IV once a day
Lansoprazole 30 mg NG once a day
Levophed drip (4 mg/250 mL of normal saline) at 2–12 micrograms per kilogram to maintain a systolic blood pressure at 100 mmHg

PRN Medications

Fentanyl 20–50 micrograms IV q2h for sedation and analgesia
Ativan 2–4 milligrams IV q4h for sedation
Acetaminophen suppositories q4h for fever greater than 102°F

Ordered Laboratory Studies

STAT blood cultures were obtained in the emergency department
CSF studies: cell count, protein, glucose levels sent from the ED
Cultures: sputum, nasopharyngeal, cerebrospinal fluid (CSF)
Latex agglutination
Enzyme-linked immunosorbent assay (ELISA)
CBC, INR/PTT, Ca, Mg, phosphorous, electrolyte panel daily
UA

Ordered Diagnostic Studies

CT scan of head; repeat with changes
Lumbar puncture

CRITICAL THINKING QUESTIONS

1. Upon initial admission to the critical care unit, what complications should you assess David for?

2. How is meningitis transmitted and how can you protect yourself?

3. Why would a medication such as Levophed be started to maintain David's blood pressure?

Answers to Critical Thinking Questions appear in Appendix D

NCLEX® REVIEW

1. A patient is diagnosed as being in shock after starting a new medication. The nurse realizes this patient is most likely experiencing which of the following types of shock?

1. Cardiogenic
2. Anaphylactic
3. Neurogenic
4. Septic

2. A patient in shock is demonstrating signs of insulin resistance. The nurse realizes this is because of:

1. The stress response.
2. Undiagnosed diabetes mellitus.
3. Excessive body weight.
4. Undiagnosed metabolic syndrome.

3. A patient in shock is demonstrating an alteration in level of consciousness. The nurse realizes that this is most likely due to:

1. Respiratory acidosis.
2. Low circulating blood volume or hypoglycemia.
3. Renal failure.
4. Hypertension.

4. The nurse is triaging victims of a multi-vehicular collision. Which of the following patients would be the most prone to developing shock?

1. 45-year-old male with a fractured femur
2. 86-year-old female with abdominal injuries
3. 55-year-old male with an injured arm and shoulder
4. 38-year-old male with cervical spine injuries

5. A patient in shock has lost more than two liters of circulating blood volume. Which of the following should be provided to this patient?

1. Normal saline
2. Packed red blood cells
3. Fresh frozen plasma
4. Dextrose 5% and water

6. The nurse is providing care to a patient in shock with an alteration in tissue perfusion and an increased afterload. Which of the following should be provided to this patient?

1. Dopamine hydrochloride
2. Nitroprusside sodium
3. Epinephrine
4. Norepinephrine bitartrate

7. A patient is diagnosed with pancreatitis. The nurse realizes this patient is prone to developing:
   1. Systemic inflammatory response syndrome.
   2. Sepsis.
   3. Septic shock.
   4. Severe sepsis.

8. A patient with systemic inflammatory response is demonstrating a fluid volume deficit. Which of the following would indicate an adequate fluid status for this patient?
   1. Urine output 0.25 mL/kg per hour
   2. Oxygen saturation 65%
   3. Mean arterial pressure 55 mm Hg
   4. Central venous pressure 10 mm Hg

9. The nurse suspects a patient is demonstrating signs of a reperfusion injury. Which of the following can this lead to?
   1. MODS
   2. SIRS
   3. Septic shock
   4. ARDS

10. A patient has severe sepsis. Which of the following should the nurse do to detect the early signs of MODS?
   1. Provide pain management
   2. Maintain on strict bed rest
   3. Reduce stress
   4. Frequent assessment of vital signs and clinical status

Answers for review questions appear in Appendix D

KEY TERMS

end-organ perfusion *p.1963*
insulin resistance (IR) *p.1958*
ischemia reperfusion injury *p.1960*
multiple organ dysfunction syndrome (MODS) *p.1976*

protein C *p.1970*
sepsis *p.1969*
septic shock *p.1958*
severe sepsis *p.1969*

systemic inflammatory response syndrome (SIRS) *p.1956*
systemic vascular resistance *p.1958*

EXPLORE PEARSON mynursingkit™

MyNursingKit is your one stop for online chapter review materials and resources. Prepare for success with additional NCLEX®-style practice questions, interactive assignments and activities, web links, animations and videos, and more!

Register your access code from the front of your book at
www.mynursingkit.com

REFERENCES

Ackerman, M. (1994). The systemic inflammatory response, sepsis and multiple organ dysfunction. *Critical Care Nursing Clinics of North America, 6*, 243–250.

Alexander, D. (1996). New concepts in shock management. *Air Medical Journal, 15*(2), 85–91.

American College of Chest Physicians/Society of Critical Care Medicine Consensus Conference Committee. (1992). Definitions for sepsis and organ failure and guidelines for the use of innovative therapies in sepsis. *Critical Care Medicine, 20*(6), 864–874.

Arabi, Y., Shirawi, N. A., Memish, Z., Venkatesh, S., & Al-Shimemeri, A. (2003). Assessment of six mortality models in patients admitted with severe sepsis and septic shock to the intensive care unit: A prospective cohort study. *Critical Care, 7*(6), R116–R122.

Ball, C., de Beer, K., Gomm, A., Hickman, B., & Collins, P. (2007). Achieving tight glycaemic control. *Intensive and Critical Care Nursing, 23*(3), 137–144.

Bertolini, G., Luciani, D., & Bioli, G. (2007). Immunonutrition in septic patients: Philosophical view of the current situation. *Clinical Nutrition, 26*, 25–29.

Bochud, P., & Calandra, T. (2003). Pathogenesis of sepsis: New concepts and implications for future treatment. *British Medical Journal, 326*(1), 262–266.

Bumbasirevic, V., Karamarkovic, A., Lesic, A., & Bumbasirevic, M. (2005). Trauma-related sepsis and multiple organ failure: Current concepts in the diagnosis and management. *Current Orthopaedics, 19*, 314–321.

Campbell, J. E. (2004). *Basic trauma life support for paramedics and other advanced providers* (5th ed.). Upper Saddle River, NJ: Brady/Prentice Hall Health.

Carrigan, R. B., Born, C. T., Fitzpatrick, M. K., & Reilly, P. M. (2004). Temporary stabilization of pelvic fractures with the trauma pelvic orthotic device in the polytrauma patient. Poster Presentation at the American Association for the Surgery of Trauma Annual Meeting, Orlando, FL, September 2003; also presented at the 71st Annual meeting of the AAOS, San Francisco, March 2004.

Cartwright, M. M. (2004). The metabolic response to stress: A complex nutrition support management. *Critical Care Nursing Clinics of North America, 16*, 467–487.

Chapman, C. (2003). Shock emergencies. In L. Newberry (Ed.), *Sheehey's emergency nursing* (5th ed., pp. 505–515). St. Louis: Mosby.

Chettle, C. (2003, February 10). Sepsis. *NurseWeek.* Retrieved December 7, 2004, from http://www.nurseweek.com

Dellinger, R. P., Carlet, J. M., Masur, H., Gerlach, H., et al. (2008). Surviving Sepsis Campaign guidelines for management of severe sepsis and septic shock. *Critical Care Medicine, 32*(3), 858–873.

Edelman, D., White, M., Tyburski, J., & Wilson, R. (2007). Post-trauma hypotension: Should systolic blood pressure of 90–109 mmHg be included? *Shock, 27*, 134–138.

Emergency Nurses Association. (2007). *Trauma nursing core course.* Des Plaines, IL: Author. Retrieved from http://www.ena.org

Ertel, W., Keel, M., Bonaccio, M., Steckholzer, U., Gallati, H., Kenny, J. S., et al. (1995). Release of anti-inflammatory mediators after mechanical trauma correlates with severity of injury and clinical outcome. *Journal of Trauma, Injury, Infection and Critical Care, 39*(5), 879–887.

Fernandes, T., Pontieri, V., Loretti, A., Teixeira, D., Abatepaulo, F., Soriano, F., et al. (2007). Hypertonic saline solution increases the expression of heat shock protein 70 and improves lung inflammation early after reperfusion in a rodent model of controlled hemorrhage. *Shock, 27*, 172–178.

Grenvik, A., Ayres, S., Holbrook, P., & Shoemaker, W. (Eds.). (2000). *Textbook of critical care* (4th ed.). Philadelphia: W. B. Saunders.

Gupta, S., & Jonas, M. (2006). Sepsis, septic shock and multiple organ failure. *Anesthesia and Intensive Care Medicine, 7*, 143–146.

Hollenberg, S., Ahrens, T., Annane, D., Astiz, M., Chalfin, D., Dasta, J., et al. (2004). Practice parameters for hemodynamic support of sepsis in adult patients: 2004 update. *Critical Care Medicine, 32*(9), 1928–1948.

Jacobs, L. (1994). Timing of fluid resuscitation in trauma. *New England Journal of Medicine, 331*(17), 1153–1154.

Johnson, G. B., Brunn, G. J., & Platt, J. L. (2004). Cutting edge: An endogenous pathway to systemic inflammatory response syndrome (SIRS)–like reactions through Toll-like receptor 4. *Journal of Immunology, 172*, 20–24.

Kaplow, R., & Hardin, S. R. (2007). *Critical care nursing: Synergy for optimal outcomes.* Boston: Jones and Bartlett.

Kaszaki, J., Wolfard, A., Szalay, L., & Boros, M. (2006). Pathophysiology of ischemia-reperfusion injury. *Transplantation Proceedings, 38*, 826–828.

Keel, M., & Trentz, O. (2005). Pathophysiology of polytrauma. *Injury, 36*(6), 691–709.

King, J. (2007). Sepsis in critical care. *Critical Care Clinics of North America, 19*, 77–86.

Kline, J. (2002). Shock. In J. Marx (Ed.). *Rosen's Emergency Medicine* (5th ed., pp. 33–47). St. Louis: Mosby.

Kowalenko, T., Stern, S., Dronen, S., & Wang, X. (1992). Improved outcome with hypotensive resuscitation of uncontrolled hemorrhagic shock in a swine model. *Journal of Trauma, 33*(3), 349–353.

Krau, S. D. (2007). Making sense of multiple organ dysfunction syndrome. *Critical care Nursing Clinics of North America 19,* 87–97.

Levy, M. M., Fink, M. P., Marshall, J. C., Abraham, E., Angus, D., Cook, D., et al. (2003). 2001 SCCM/ESICM/ACCP/ ATS/SIS International Sepsis Definition Conference.*Intensive Care Medicine, 29*(4), 530–538.

Martin, G. S., Mannino, D. M., Eaton, S., et al. (2003). The epidemiology of sepsis in the United States from 1979 through 2000. *New England Journal of Medicine, 348,* 1546–1554.

Martin, R., Bicknell, W., Pepe, P., Burch, J., & Mattox, K. (1992). Prospective evaluation of preoperative fluid resuscitation in hypotensive patients with penetrating truncal injury: A preliminary report. *Journal of Trauma, 33*(3), 354–362.

Masur, H. (2003). *Strategies to reduce the incidence of antibiotic-resistant pathogens in the ICU.* Retrieved December 10, 2003, from http://www.medscape.com

McCaffery, K., & Sinclair, J. (2006). Special considerations in pediatric intensive care. *Anaesthesia and Intensive Care Medicine, 7*(1), 22–28.

McCance, K. L., & Huether, S. (2006). *Pathophysiology: The biologic basis for disease in adults and children* (5th ed.). St. Louis: Mosby.

McSwain, N. E., Salomone, J. P., & Pons, P. (2007). *PHTLS: Prehospital trauma life support.* St. Louis: Mosby.

Micek, S. T., Shah, R. A., & Kollef, M. H. (2003). Management of severe sepsis: Integration of multiple pharmacologic interventions. *Pharmacotherapy, 23*(11), 1486–1496.

Miniño, A. M., Heron, M., & Smith, B. L. (2006, April 19). *Deaths: Preliminary data for 2004.* Retrieved September 6, 2008 from National Center for Health Statistics website: http://www.cdc.gov/nchs/products/pubs/pubd/hestats/prelimdeaths04/preliminarydeaths04.htm

Moore, F., Sauaua, A., Moore, E., Haenal, J., Burch, J. M., & Lezotte, D. C. (1996). Post injury multiple organ failure: A bimodal phenomenon. *Journal of Trauma, 40*(4), 501–512.

Mosenthal, A. C., & Murphy, P. A. (2003). Trauma care and palliative care: Time to integrate the two? *Journal of the American College of Surgeons, 197*(3), 509–516.

Porter, R. (1997). *The greatest benefit to mankind.* New York: W. W. Norton.

Porth, C. M. (2005). *Essentials of pathophysiology: Concepts of altered health states.* Philadelphia: Lippincott Williams & Wilkins.

Rangel-Frausto, M. S. (2005). Sepsis: Still going strong. *Archives of Medical Research, 36,* 672–681.

Reid, C. L., & Campbell, I. T. (2004). Nutritional and metabolic support in trauma, sepsis and critical illness. *Current Anaesthesia and Critical Care, 15,* 336–349.

Robertson, C. M., & Coppersmith, C. M. (2006). The systemic inflammatory response syndrome. *Microbes and Infection, 8,* 1382–1389.

Rueden, K., & Dunham, C. M. (1994). Sequelae of massive fluid resuscitation in trauma patients. *Critical Care Nursing Clinics of North America, 6,* 463–472.

Russell, J. A. (2006). Management of sepsis. *New England Journal of Medicine, 355*(16), 1699–1713.

Selfridge-Thomas, J. (1995). Shock. In S. Kitt, J. Selfridge-Thomas, J. Proehl, & J. Kaiser (Eds.), *Emergency nursing: A physiological approach* (2nd ed., pp. 37–53). Philadelphia: W. B. Saunders.

Semonin Holleran, R. (2002). The problem of pain in emergency care. *Nursing Clinics of North America, 37*(1), 67–78.

Smith, M. A., & McInnis, L. A. (2007). Antimicrobial resistance in critical care. *Critical Care Clinics of North America, 19,* 53–60.

Society of Critical Care Medicine. (1999). Practice parameters for hemodynamic support of sepsis in adult patients. *Critical Care Medicine, 27*(3), 639–660.

Spahn, D. R., Cerny, V., Coats, T. J., Duranteau, J., Fernandez-Mondejar, E., Gordini, G., et al. (2007). Management of bleeding following major trauma: A European guideline. *Critical Care, 11*(1). Retrieved April 21, 2007, from http://www.medscape.com/viewarticle/554058

Tazbir, J. (2004). Sepsis and the role of activated protein C. *Critical Care Nurse, 24*(6), 40–45.

Zauner, A., Nimmerrichter, P., Anderwald, C., Bischof, M., Schiefermeier, M., Ratheiser, K., et al. (2007). Severity of insulin resistance in critically ill medical patients. *Metabolism, 56,* 1–5.

Nursing Assessment of Patients with Hematologic Disorders

Janyce Cagan Agruss
Annita Watson

Outcome-Based Learning Objectives

After studying this chapter, the learner will be able to:

1. Explain how the hematologic system functions in an adult.
2. Describe the types, characteristics, and functions of blood cells.
3. Explain how the process of coagulation works in the event of an injury.
4. Describe appropriate nursing assessment/responsibilities related to the hematologic system in the adult patient.
5. Describe laboratory tests used to evaluate the hematologic system.
6. Distinguish between normal and abnormal test results for the hematologic system.
7. Discuss the meaning of "shift to the left."

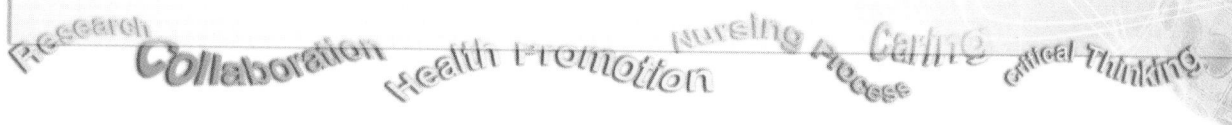

Research   Collaboration   Health Promotion   Nursing Process   Caring   Critical Thinking

THE HEMATOLOGIC SYSTEM is a very complex body system. Just as cardiology is the study of the heart, **hematology** is the study of blood, and just as the tissue of the heart comprises the cardiovascular system, blood is the tissue that makes up the hematologic system. The hematologic system can have problems inherent to itself, but it can also be a valuable source of information that reflects problems in other organ systems. Whether the gathering of hematologic data is for the purpose of evaluating the hematologic system itself or assessing other body systems, the nurse has to understand the functions, structure, diagnostic tests, terminology, and nursing responsibilities that are pertinent and relevant to the hematologic system. The nurse gathers this information through the assessment process and is reliant on both subjective and objective data.

Subjective assessment is accomplished by interviewing the patient or someone accompanying the patient (e.g., family member, friend) to obtain data regarding the patient's illness or reason for being seen by the health care provider. Objective assessment is that obtained by means other than a patient interview, for example, laboratory tests, x-rays, vital signs. In an objective assessment, the data are retrievable without being dependent on the patient providing the information.

Anatomy and Physiology of the Hematologic System

The anatomy of the hematologic system can be understood best by describing its components. Most obvious is blood, comprised of a wide variety of cells and supportive fluids. Additionally, there are other organ systems that both contribute to the conceptual understanding as well as to the overall function of the hematologic system. These include the lymphatic system, the spleen (a lymphatic organ), the liver, and the reticuloendothelial/mononuclear phagocyte system.

To best understand the physiology of the hematologic system, the reader should understand that blood is considered to be a type of connective tissue with two important responsibilities. First, blood and its associated vessels and organs provide a transport system that delivers nutrition, oxygen, and secretory products such as hormones throughout the body, as well as wastes to the kidneys and liver for disposal. Second, the immunologic products of the hematologic system are critical to the defense of the body against infections and other foreign materials. In performing the two primary responsibilities related to being a transport system, blood also functions to maintain body temperature, control pH (to maintain a range of 6.8 to 7.4), remove toxins from the body, and regulate body fluid electrolytes. The contribution of each component of the hematologic system to these functions is discussed below.

Bone Marrow

Any discussion about the hematologic system should begin with the bone marrow. Bone marrow is the soft material found in the center of bones and it is the origin of all blood cells. Bone marrow, one of the largest organs of the body, makes up about 4% to 5% of a person's total body weight. It consists of islands of cellular components (red marrow) separated by fat (yellow marrow). The **stem cell**, the precursor cell of all blood components (red blood cells, white blood cells, and platelets), resides in the bone marrow. When the proper stimulating signal is received, the stem cells undergo a series of cell division and differentiation resulting in the release of mature or nearly mature cells into the systemic circulation as depicted in Figures 62–1 ■, 62–2 ■, and 62–3 ■. This process is called **hematopoiesis**. See Chapter 63 for a thorough discussion of hematopoiesis.

Stem cell to erythrocyte
Stem cell
Erythroblast
Normoblast
Reticulocyte
Erythrocyte/
Red blood cell

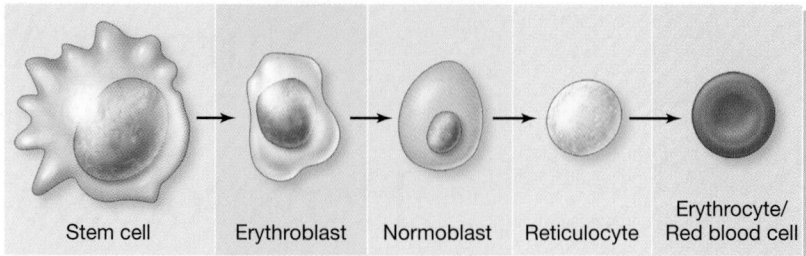

FIGURE 62–1 ■ Stem cell to erythrocytes.

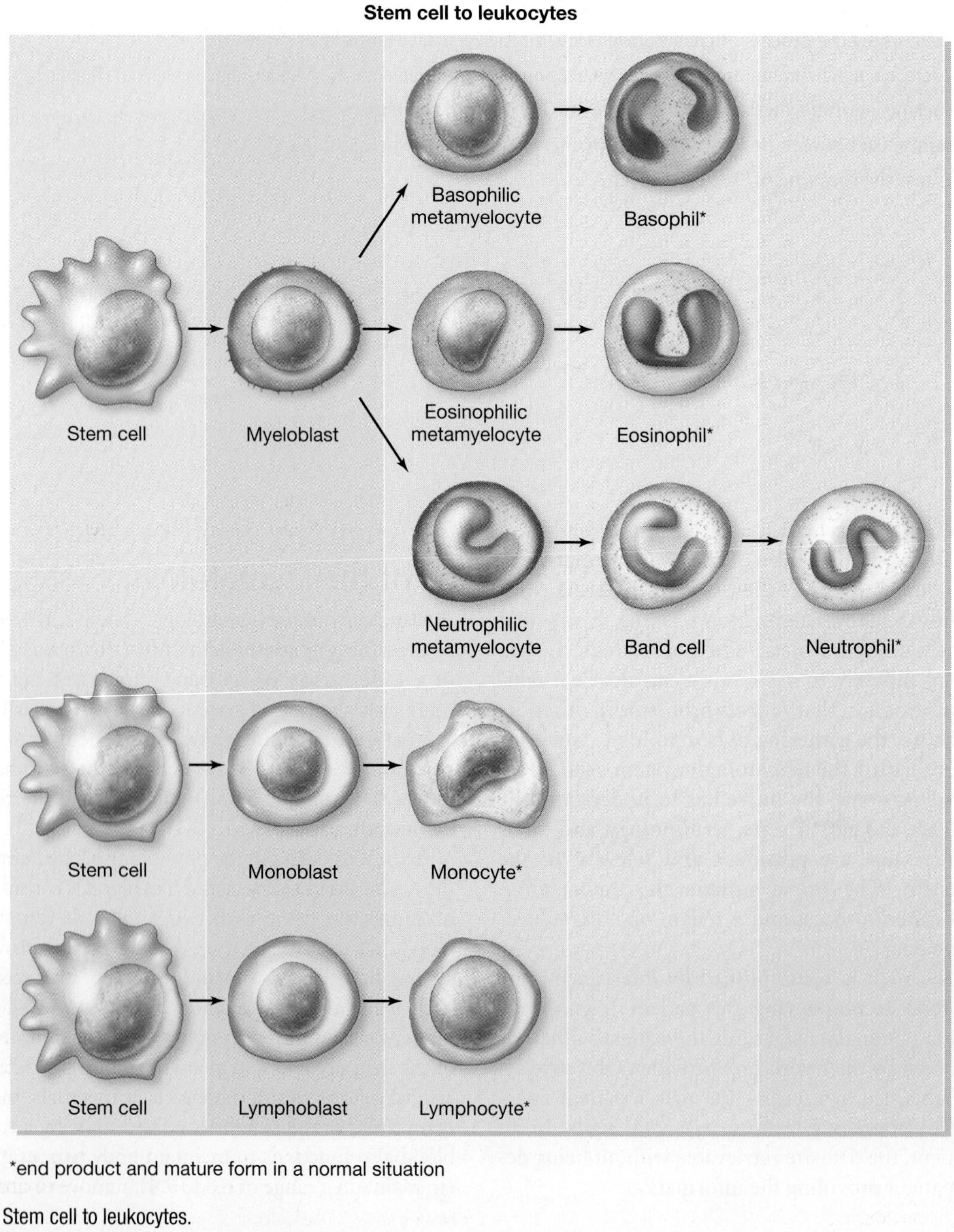

Stem cell to leukocytes
Basophilic metamyelocyte
Basophil*
Stem cell
Myeloblast
Eosinophilic metamyelocyte
Eosinophil*
Neutrophilic metamyelocyte
Band cell
Neutrophil*
Stem cell
Monoblast
Monocyte*
Stem cell
Lymphoblast
Lymphocyte*
*end product and mature form in a normal situation

FIGURE 62–2 ■ Stem cell to leukocytes.

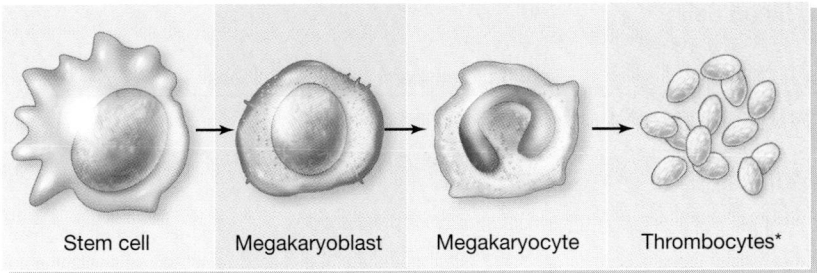

Stem cell to thrombocytes

Stem cell → Megakaryoblast → Megakaryocyte → Thrombocytes*

*end product and mature form in a normal situation

FIGURE 62–3 ■ Stem cell to thrombocytes (end product and mature form in a normal situation).

In children, all skeletal bones are involved in the production of stem cells. With aging, marrow activity decreases and usually is limited to the pelvis, ribs, sternum, and vertebrae. As a person ages, the proportion of red marrow diminishes and is replaced by yellow marrow (fat); however, in the healthy individual the fat can again be replaced by active (red) marrow if more blood cell production is required. In adults with diseases that cause bone marrow destruction, the liver and spleen also can produce blood cells by a process known as *extramedullary hematopoiesis.* Figure 62–4 ■ shows a picture of bone marrow. Nurses must always include bone marrow function when considering any disease related to the hematologic system.

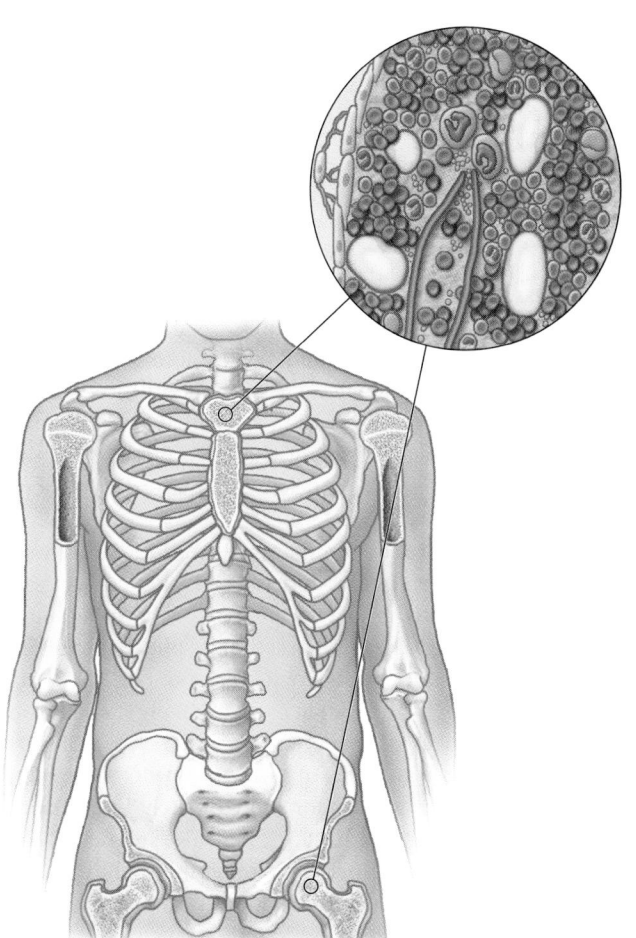

FIGURE 62–4 ■ Bone marrow.

Types of Blood Cells

Blood is a fluid tissue that has both function and structure. Blood contributes about 7% to the total body weight of a person with a volume (in an average-sized adult) of about 4 to 6 liters. It is composed of 55% plasma and 45% blood cells. **Plasma** is the straw-colored liquid in which the blood cells are suspended, and consists of approximately 90% water, with the remaining 10% being proteins, carbohydrates, electrolytes, and vitamins. A microscopic analysis of blood reveals a wide variety of blood cells that are broadly categorized into three major cell lines: **erythrocytes**, or **red blood cells (RBCs)**; **leukocytes**, or **white blood cells (WBCs)**; and **thrombocytes**, or **platelets**. Each cell line has its own characteristics and functions, as summarized in Chart 62–1 (p. 1992). Note that reticulocytes are immature red blood cells, typically composing about 1% of the red cells in the human body. Also note that *leukocyte* is a broad term applied to the various cells of the immune system, including granulocytes (basophils, eosinophils, and neutrophils), monocytes, and lymphocytes (T cells, B cells, and natural killer cells). Leukocytes are discussed below and in more detail in Chapters 59 ∞ and 60 ∞.

Erythrocytes (Red Blood Cells)

Erythrocytes, or red blood cells, make up about 40% of the total blood volume. The RBC is produced in the bone marrow and its function is to become filled with hemoglobin, maintain the chemical integrity of hemoglobin, and carry and distribute hemoglobin to the body's tissues. **Hemoglobin** is an iron-containing protein in RBCs that transports oxygen around the body. When oxygen combines with hemoglobin, the resulting oxyhemoglobin is bright red.

The normal shape of the red blood cell, a biconcave disk, is the optimal shape to perform this function. A biconcave disk can best be described as a donut or lifesaver shape. The cell has a diameter of approximately 8 μm and is very flexible, thus, allowing it to pass easily through capillaries that may be as small as 2.8 μm. RBCs also have a very thin membrane, which allows the oxygen and carbon dioxide to easily diffuse. A photograph of RBCs is shown in Figure 62–5 ■ (p. 1992). Their disk shape allows for optimal filling by the hemoglobin and ideal transport to body tissues through the circulatory system. The shape also provides a large surface that facilitates the absorption and release of oxygen molecules. With age, RBCs become increasingly fragile and are damaged by passing through narrow capillaries.

Red blood cells are terminally differentiated; that is, they can never divide. They live about 120 days and then are ingested by phagocytic cells (those that engulf and ingest foreign particles, cell waste material, and bacteria) in the liver and spleen. They are eventually broken down by the spleen into the blood pigments bilirubin and iron. These components are then transported to the liver where the iron is recycled for use by new erythrocytes. The remainder of the heme portion of the molecule is degraded into bile pigments and excreted by the liver. Approximately 3 million RBCs die and are scavenged by the liver each second.

There are approximately 4.5 to 5.8 million erythrocytes per microliter of healthy blood (although there are variations between males and females and racial groups). In the laboratory

MyNursingKit | Animation: Types of Blood Cells

CHART 62–1	**Characteristics and Functions of Blood Cells**	
	Function(s)	**Characteristic(s) and/or Conditions**
Erythrocytes	Transport oxygen and carbon dioxide to and from cells.	Lifesaver-shaped disk.
Reticulocytes	Synthesize hemoglobin after loss of the nucleus so new RBCs continue to be released into the circulation.	Immature, non-nucleated RBCs that contain RNA.
Leukocytes (WBCs)	Protect the body against foreign matter.	Different types of leukocytes. Leukocytosis: increase in the total number. Leukopenia: decrease in the total number.
Granulocytes:		Characterized by granules within their cytoplasm.
Neutrophils	The most abundant leukocyte, neutrophils may be increased or decreased in systemic infection. Work via phagocytosis.	Segmented neutrophil: nucleus has at least two lobes separated by a filament; this is the more mature version. Band neutrophil: nucleus without visible filament separating the lobes.
Eosinophils	Usually increased in allergic diseases.	Make up 3% of the leukocytes in adults. Cytoplasm contains larger round or oval granules.
Basophils	Function not exactly known, but may be present in hypersensitivity reactions.	Resemble neutrophils, except nucleus is indented. Least numerous of the leukocytes.
Monocytes/macrophages	Back up the neutrophils; may be increased in infections and/or hematologic disorders. Work via phagocytosis; they do cleanup work after neutrophils and may circulate for a longer period of time than the neutrophils.	Monocytes give rise to macrophages. Largest cell of normal blood.
Lymphocytes	Function to fight viral infection; may be increased or decreased in infectious illness.	T- and B-cell subsets.
Thrombocytes	Prevent blood loss by forming a platelet plug at the site of injury until a stable clot forms. May be increased in times of stress. May be decreased (thrombocytopenia) in bone marrow failure, autoimmune disease (idiopathic thrombocytopenia purpura), disseminated intravascular clotting (DIC)	Formed in the bone marrow. Have no nuclei.

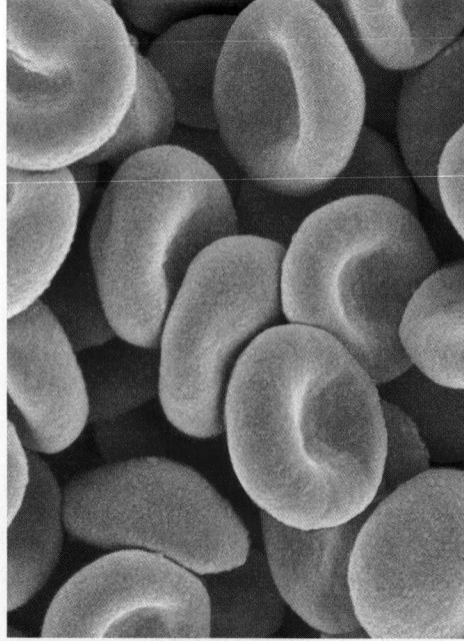

FIGURE 62–5 ■ Red blood cells (erythrocytes).
Source: © Micro Discovery/CORBIS All Rights Reserved

RBCs are counted as the total number of RBCs in 1 mm³ of blood. The typical red blood cell count is 4,600,000 to 6,200,000 per cubic millimeter for males and 4,500,000 to 5,100,000 cells per cubic millimeter for females. The number of RBCs is a measure of the blood's oxygen-carrying capacity. Hemoglobin accounts for approximately 95% of mature RBC composition. Immature erythrocytes have a nucleus, but mature erythrocytes have no nucleus.

The bone marrow releases immature forms of RBCs into circulation that are referred to as **reticulocytes**. Reticulocytes are juvenile RBCs produced by erythropoiesis that spend about 24 hours in the marrow before entering the peripheral circulation. They contain some nuclear material—remnants of RNA—that appears faintly blue (basophilic) in conventionally stained blood smears. When measured in the laboratory, the percentage of reticulocytes provides an index of the rate of RBC production. Normally reticulocytes account for approximately 1% of the circulating red blood cells (Porth, 2007). Reticulocytes persist for a few days in the circulation before forming the slightly smaller, mature red cell. The release of reticulocytes occurs as a normal response to an increased demand for RBCs, such as is the case with bleeding or possibly with disease.

In certain disorders such as sickle cell anemia the RBC has a different shape and is more rigid than normal cells, causing difficulty transporting hemoglobin to the tissues. Two major consequences occur when red blood cells sickle: hemolysis (destruction) of the sickled cells and vessel occlusion. The rigidity of the cells causes the obstruction of the microcirculation and ischemic injury to the tissues. This rigidity also makes the cells more prone to hemolysis or destruction while circulating through the spleen. The pain associated with sickle cell disease is due to vessel occlusion, resulting from ischemia. This can occur anywhere in the body (Porth, 2007). (See Chapter 63 to learn more about sickle cell anemia).

Leukocytes (White Blood Cells)

As mentioned, the principal cells of the immune system are the leukocytes, or white blood cells. WBCs generally are not present, except in a very small amount, in the bloodstream unless they are needed for defense against an infecting organism. They remain in the bone marrow, lungs, liver, spleen, and lymph nodes as developing and mature cells. They are separated into two major categories: **granulocytes** (or polymorphonuclear leukocytes [PMN]) and agranulocytes. Granulocytes are further divided into neutrophils, basophils, and eosinophils as determined by their staining properties in the laboratory. Agranulocytes are made up of monocytes and lymphocytes. Leukocytes have longevity of a few hours to a few days. There are approximately 5,000 to 10,000 leukocytes per microliter of blood.

Lymphocytes

Leukocytes are composed of approximately 24% to 35% **lymphocytes**, whose purpose is to recognize and respond to foreign antigens. Lymphocytes that produce antibodies include the T cells, B cells, and natural killer cells.

Approximately 60% to 70% of blood lymphocytes are T cells and 10% to 20% are B cells. A commonly shared misconception holds that the "B" in B cells refers to bone marrow, since these cells arise from bone marrow tissue. In actuality, the "B" stands for "bursa of Fabricius," a gland in birds where the cells mature and the first such tissue found in vertebrates. Immature B cells are produced by the bone marrow and released into the bloodstream. Upon interacting with an antigen, or protein, the B cells become activated into plasma cells, which are responsible for the production of antibodies, or immunoglobulins. All antibodies formed by the plasma cell are programmed to recognize only one unique protein structure: the antigen that stimulated the original B cell. (See Chapter 60 on immune response disorders for further discussion.) The process, referred to as the **humoral immune response**, is the mechanism in which organisms gain immunity to previously encountered substances.

T cells (lymphocytes) complete their maturation in the thymus gland and function in the peripheral tissues to produce cell-mediated immunity, as well as aiding in antibody production. Both T-cell and B-cell activation are triggered by the recognition of the antigen by unique surface receptors.

Both T cells and B cells destroy antigens (a foreign substance that is not naturally present and should not be in the body) and produce "memory cells" and antibodies. Memory cells attack disease-causing organisms if there is a subsequent invasion. This second response is much quicker than the first, thus preventing symptoms of the disease from occurring (Porth, 2007).

Natural killer cells (NK cells) are a type of lymphocytes that are functionally distinct from T and B cells. Like cytotoxic T cells they contain granules filled with potent chemicals; however unlike cytotoxic T cells, they do not need to recognize a specific antigen before being activated. They are a major component of the innate immune system and play a major role in the rejection of tumors and cells infected by viruses.

Basophils

Basophils make up approximately 0.3% to 0.5% of the total white blood count. Along with the mast cells, basophils release heparin (anticoagulant) and histamine (vasodilator) and other inflammatory mediators into the bloodstream. They participate in the destruction of bacteria with lysozyme and strong oxidants and play an exceedingly important role in allergic reactions (Porth, 2007). An increased or higher percentage of basophils in the blood may indicate an inflammatory condition somewhere in the body.

Neutrophils

Neutrophils compose approximately 55% to 65% of leukocytes and because their nuclei are divided into three to five lobes they are typically referred to as polymorphonuclear leukocytes. Neutrophils are primarily responsible for maintaining a normal host defense against pathogens and are the first leukocytes to respond to organisms that invade the body. They act by carrying out the process of phagocytosis and also by releasing enzymes such as lysozyme that destroy certain bacteria. Neutrophils respond quicker to infection than do monocytes. However, when monocytes reach the site of infection they arrive in much larger numbers and, therefore, can phagocytize many more microbes than neutrophils are able to. They also clear up cellular debris after an infection. Chapters 59 and 60 discuss the immune response.

Eosinophils

Eosinophils comprise approximately 1% to 3% of the leukocytes. They liberate heparin, histamine, and serotonin in allergic reactions, intensifying an inflammatory response. The current belief is that they release enzymes or chemical mediators that detoxify agents associated with allergic reactions (Porth, 2007). An increased or higher than usual percentage of eosinophils in the blood may indicate a parasitic infection somewhere in the body. Eosinophils attach themselves to the parasite by special surface molecules and release hydrolytic enzymes and other substances that kill the parasite.

Monocytes and Tissue Macrophages

Monocytes and tissue macrophages arise from a common precursor in the bone marrow. **Monocytes** are the largest of the white blood cells and make up about 3% to 8% of the total leukocyte count. Monocytes and macrophages are a part of the **reticuloendothelial** (or mononuclear phagocytic) **system (RES)**, whose function is to engulf and digest microbes and other foreign substances. The RES also removes senescent cells from circulation, and provides phagocytic cells for both inflammatory and immune responses. Monocytes migrate from the blood to various tissues where they mature into macrophages. Macrophages, also known as scavengers, can either stay in one tissue or migrate from an organ via lymphoid tissues. Examples of tissue macrophages include Kupffer cells in the liver, alveolar macrophages in the lung, and microglial cells of the central nervous system. Macrophages are activated when their membrane comes in contact with an antigen. Once the microbe is ingested, the cell generates digestive enzymes and toxic oxygen and nitrogen products, thus killing the invading antigen.

The phagocytic white cells have a life span of about 2 to 4 months, which allows the macrophages to remain at the affected site longer, sometimes until the antigen is destroyed. The macrophage response time works in concert with that of the first responders, neutrophils, which can rapidly surround and identify sources of infection, but only live for approximately 12 hours (Dailey, 1998; McPherson & Pincus, 2006).

Thrombocytes (Platelets)

Thrombocytes, or platelets, are large cell fragments that are disk shaped and approximately 2 to 4 μm in diameter. They have many granules but no nucleus, and they live for 5 to 9 days. There are approximately 150,000 to 400,000 platelets per microliter of blood. The platelet membrane is covered with a glycocalyx, consisting of glycoproteins, glycosaminoglycans, and several coagulation factors absorbed from the plasma (Ross, 2003). Glycoproteins act as a receptor in platelet function. Specifically, glycoprotein IIb/IIIa binds fibrinogen and forms bridges between adjacent platelets when activated, a process referred to as *aggregation*. Platelet activation and its role in hemostasis are discussed below.

Figure 62–6 ■ shows a Wright-stained smear of normal blood in which normal blood cells are shown.

Lymphatic System

The **lymphatic system**, consisting of organs, ducts, and nodes, is responsible for removing excess fluid, proteins, and large particles from the interstitial (between cells) spaces back to the bloodstream. The ducts (called lymph vessels) are thin tubes, which run throughout the body in much the same way as blood vessels and with a similar structure to the capillary walls; however, instead of blood, they transport lymph fluid. Lymph fluid is formed from the natural diffusion of fluid across the semipermeable cell membranes of blood vessels and peripheral tissues into the interstitial space. The main functions of the lymphatic system are to:

- Collect and return interstitial fluid, and thus help maintain fluid balance.
- Defend the body against disease by producing lymphocytes.
- Absorb lipids from the intestine and transport them to the blood.

Essentially, the lymphatic system is the highway and delivery system of the body. Blood volume is maintained in every organ of the body as a result of the presence of lymph vessels. Lymph fluid is carried via the lymphatic system to every system in the body and then is returned to the circulatory system. Foreign objects such as bacteria and viruses also are carried through the body by the lymphatic system. When interstitial fluid volume rises, the increasing pressure drives the fluid into the lymphatic capillary walls. The walls of the capillaries are very permeable, allowing fluid to drain easily from the tissue into the lymphatic capillaries. The lymphatic capillaries, the entry point into the lymphatic vascular system, join to form the larger diameter lymphatic vessels, which ultimately drain into the subclavian veins of the neck. Once incorporated into the bloodstream, the lymphatic fluid can be appropriately processed by the liver, spleen, kidneys, and other organs.

Lymph nodes are small aggregates of lymphoid tissue located along the lymphatic vessels throughout the body. Each node processes lymph fluid from a discrete, adjacent anatomic site (Porth, 2007). The human body has hundreds of clusters of lymph nodes placed strategically in the axillae, groin, and along the great vessels of the neck, thorax, and abdomen. The functions of the lymph nodes include removing foreign material from lymph before it enters the bloodstream and acting as the center for proliferation of immune cells. The lymph nodes are encapsulated structures where the lymph or chyle is juxtaposed (in proximity) to capillary blood vessels. According to Swartz (2001), the lymph nodes function as filters and reservoirs, acting as incubators for white blood cells. White blood cells, particularly B cells and T cells, mature and proliferate in the lymph nodes as they gain exposure to antigens absorbed from the interstitial fluid. During times of infection, these nodes can become swollen and tender as active lymphocytes, phagocytes, and invading bacteria and viruses initiate inflammation and the immune response; hence, the term "swollen glands." Swollen glands can be palpated in the neck, axilla (armpit), or groin. There also are lymph nodes that cannot be palpated in the abdomen, pelvis, and chest. The lymph fluid distributes immune cells and other factors throughout the body.

The lymphatic system also contains certain hormones, protein, and gastrointestinal fat depending on the original location of the interstitial fluid. For instance, interstitial fluid, and consequently lymph fluid, surrounding the gastrointestinal tract is milky and turbid with a high percentage of fat. This lymphatic fluid is known as **chyle**. Microscopic evaluation of lymph fluid reveals a close resemblance to blood, but lymph fluid is much more dilute.

Spleen

The spleen is a large, ovoid secondary lymphoid organ located in the upper left corner of the abdominal cavity. It generally cannot be palpated because it is under the ribs. The spleen stores blood (20 to 40 mL of RBCs), removes old blood cells, and, as one of its primary roles, filters and destroys antigens before they

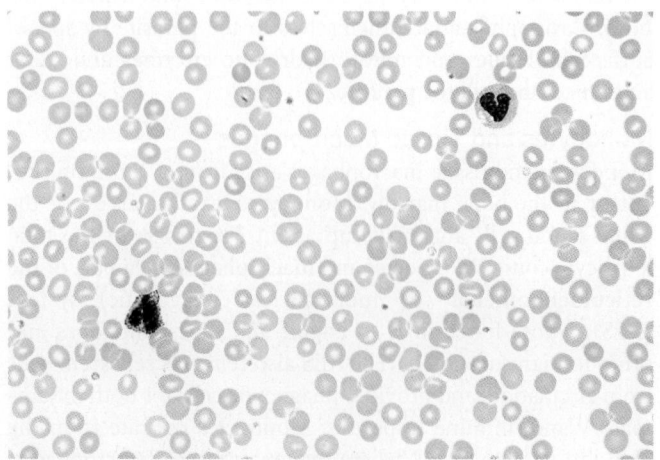

FIGURE 62–6 ■ Wright-stained smear of normal blood.
Source: © Visuals Unlimited/CORBIS All Rights Reserved

can enter the systemic circulation (Young, Gerson, & High, 2006). The spleen is able to remove defective or old erythrocytes from circulation. Most notably, the spleen is able to catabolize the hemoglobin released from decaying erythrocytes and return the iron component (heme) back to the bone marrow. Patients suffering from hematologic disorders that result in high turnover of erythrocytes frequently present with an enlarged spleen (splenomegaly). Additionally, the spleen stores approximately one-third of the total volume of platelets.

Liver

The liver is the largest visceral organ of the body that performs multiple functions. (See Chapter 46 🔗 for further discussion on the physiology and associated disorders of the liver.) Briefly, the liver produces bile; metabolizes hormones and drugs; synthesizes proteins, glucose, and blood clotting factors; stores vitamins and minerals; changes ammonia produced by deamination of amino acids to urea; and converts fatty acids to ketones. As it relates to hematology, the liver stores blood and plays an important role in the clotting mechanism of blood (discussed below). The liver produces the coagulation factors that are necessary for fibrin clot formation, and the liver can produce anticoagulants so there is not too much clotting. Disorders of the liver are discussed in depth in Chapter 46 🔗.

Normal Clotting Mechanism: Hemostasis

Hemostasis is defined as the stopping of blood flow. Under normal conditions hemostasis is regulated by a complex array of activators and inhibitors that maintain blood fluidity and prevent blood loss from the vascular space. The balance between the forces that cause blood to solidify or to remain fluid is very delicate and involves several interacting systems.

Intact blood vessels are central to moderating blood's tendency to clot. The endothelial cells of intact vessels prevent thrombus formation by secreting tissue plasminogen activator (t-PA) and by inactivating thrombin and adenosine diphosphate (ADP). Injury to vessels overwhelms these protective mechanisms and hemostasis occurs. A blood vessel must incur an injury in order for hemostasis to be initiated. Hemostasis then proceeds in two phases: primary and secondary hemostasis. Figure 62–7 ■ shows the normal sequencing of hemostasis, starting with the injury called the vascular phase.

Primary Hemostasis

Primary hemostasis is characterized by vascular contraction, platelet adhesion, and formation of a soft aggregate plug. It begins immediately after endothelial disruption. After the injury occurs there is an initial, temporary response of vasoconstriction. This is the body's adaptive mechanism that tries to stop or at least minimize blood loss following injury to a vessel. Vasoconstriction slows blood flow, enhancing platelet adhesion and activation. This vasoconstriction promotes the ability of platelets to gather at the site of injury. First, the platelet is attracted to the exposed subendothelial layer of collagen and adheres to it. To accomplish this, the platelet undergoes a shape change. Second, the platelets release ADP, which stimulates other platelets to stick together at the wound site, and then aggregation occurs. Aggregation occurs when the platelets adhere to each other to form a

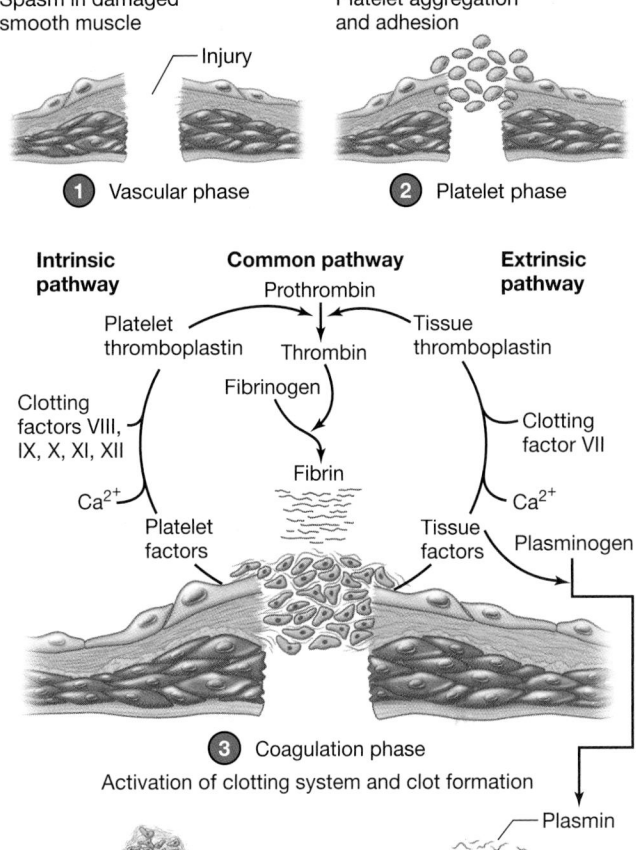

FIGURE 62–7 ■ Hemostasis progression.

beginning plug. Finally, coagulation occurs and fibrin forms around the platelet aggregate to initiate repair (Porth, 2007).

Primary hemostasis is short lived. The immediate postinjury vascular constriction abates quickly. If flow is allowed to increase, the soft plug could be sheared from the injured surface, possibly creating emboli.

Secondary Hemostasis

Secondary hemostasis is responsible for stabilizing the soft clot and maintaining vasoconstriction. This phase is initiated when the cascade system of coagulation is activated by substances released at the time of injury. Based on the type of stimulus or injury to the vessel, one of two clotting pathways is followed. These are referred to as intrinsic and extrinsic pathways, with the end result from either pathway being the conversion of prothrombin to thrombin. Thrombin is necessary for fibrinogen to be converted into fibrin, the stabilizing protein that anchors the fragile platelet plug to the site of injury; thereby, preventing further bleeding and allowing the injured vessel to heal. Primary and secondary hemostasis are summarized in Chart 62–2 (p. 1996).

Coagulation Factors and the Cascade System

Coagulation factors circulate in the plasma as cofactors or as procoagulants and, when activated, some of the components are

CHART 62–2	**Sequential Steps of Hemostasis**

A. Blood Vessel Spasm
   1. Cutting a blood vessel causes a release of neural reflexes and humoral factors that result in muscle spasm.

B. Platelet Plug Formation
   2. Platelets come in contact with the injured vessel wall, causing adhesion of the exposed edges of damaged blood vessels, forming a net with spiny processes protruding from their membranes.
   3. Platelet aggregation occurs soon after adhesion, resulting in a platelet plug to stop the bleeding.
   4. Platelet adhesion and aggregation stimulate the activation of the clotting cascade.

C. Blood Coagulation
   5. Damaged tissues release tissue thromboplastin, which activates the first in a series of factors leading to the production of prothrombin activator.
   6. Prothrombin activator converts prothrombin into thrombin, which, in turn, catalyzes a reaction that converts fibrinogen into fibrin. Fibrin forms a meshwork that cements the platelets and other blood components together. The amount of prothrombin activator formed is proportional to the amount of tissue damage.
   7. Once a clot forms, it promotes still more clotting through a positive feedback system. Fibroblasts invade the area and produce fibers throughout the clots.
   8. A clot that forms abnormally in a vessel is a thrombus; if it dislodges, it is an embolus.
   9. Within 20–60 minutes after a clot has formed, clot retraction begins, causing the edges of the broken blood vessel to pull together, thus assisting with hemostasis.
   10. Shortly after the formation of a clot, dissolution begins. Clots dissolve by fibrinolysis. The process involves the activation of plasmin by plasminogen, which then digests the fibrin strands of the clot. This allows blood flow to be reestablished and permanent tissue repair to take place.

needed for clot formation. The coagulation factors are generated in the liver cells, except for Factor VIII (or at least the von Willebrand's portion), which is produced in multiple organs, possibly the endothelial cells and megakaryocytes. The coagulation cascade system, as shown in Figure 62–8 ■, is the model typically referred to when describing the mechanism of coagulation.

Damaged tissue releases Factor III, which with the aid of Ca^{2+} will activate Factor VII, thus initiating the extrinsic mechanism. Factor XII from active platelets will activate Factor XI, thus initiating the intrinsic mechanism. Both active Factor VII and active Factor XI will promote cascade reactions, eventually activating Factor X. Active Factor X, along with Factor III, Factor V, Ca^{2+}, and platelet thromboplastic factor (PF_3), will activate prothrombin activator. Prothrombin activator converts prothrombin to thrombin. Thrombin converts fibrinogen to fibrin. Fibrin initially forms a loose mesh, but then Factor XIII causes the formation of covalent cross links, which convert fibrin to a dense aggregation of fibers. Platelets and RBCs become caught in this mesh of fibers, thus forming a blood clot.

As described above, coagulation is actually a cascade of events. In the normal scenario, one enzyme activates the follow-ing proenzyme until the mesh fibrin network is developed, established, and functioning, and a blood clot is formed and the bleeding stops.

Hereditary bleeding disorders, such as hemophilia, are caused by deficiencies in the factors involved in the coagulation cascade. Also, identification of the intrinsic versus the extrinsic pathway and what factors are involved in each of the pathways as described earlier is important because this information has implications for laboratory tests and medications that are ordered for patients.

History

Much of the evaluation of the hematologic system is based on a complete health history. When assessing a patient for hematopoietic system status it is important to be thorough and to consider presenting symptoms, chief complaint, and family history. Many hematologic conditions cause few symptoms, therefore, the use of extensive laboratory tests often is required to diagnose a hemotologic disorder. Hematologic disorders are discussed in depth in Chapter 63 .

A thorough history will help the nurse identify symptoms related to abnormalities with the hematologic system as well as current or potential problems. Information learned from a thorough history and physical exam could help prevent undesirable responses to current therapies and treatment plans. The essential assessment is contingent on obtaining both subjective and objective data as previously defined.

Biographic and Demographic Data

Assessment of biographic and demographic data includes information regarding age, race, gender, and ethnicity, all of which can impact the susceptibility to some hematologic disorders. For example, African Americans have a higher incidence of sickle cell anemia than Caucasians, and a family history of coagulation disorders increases the risk for the individual. A patient may not know she has a "hematologic" problem, but she may know that she tends to have problems stopping bleeding.

Chief Complaint

The current issue is the focus of why the patient is being evaluated currently. Unless the patient already has some knowledge of his hematologic system from previous evaluations, he usually will not know that he has a hematologic problem. He will merely know that he does not feel well. From the questions asked during the history taking, nurses can begin to determine whether or not they think that the patient is having a problem that arises from the hematologic system.

The chief complaint tells the health care provider, in the patient's own words, what problem(s) she is currently experiencing. The chief complaint focuses the history-taking process and prioritizes treatment regimens. When the chief complaint is documented, the health care provider actually writes the words that the patient has used to describe the complaint. For example, the patient may state, "I always feel tired, no matter how early I go to bed" or "It is all I can do to get through the day."

It also is important to determine the patient's own perception of his health status in order to assist the patient with developing a plan for future health promotion. Risk factors such as smoking and alcohol intake should be assessed as should the

THE COAGULATION CASCADE

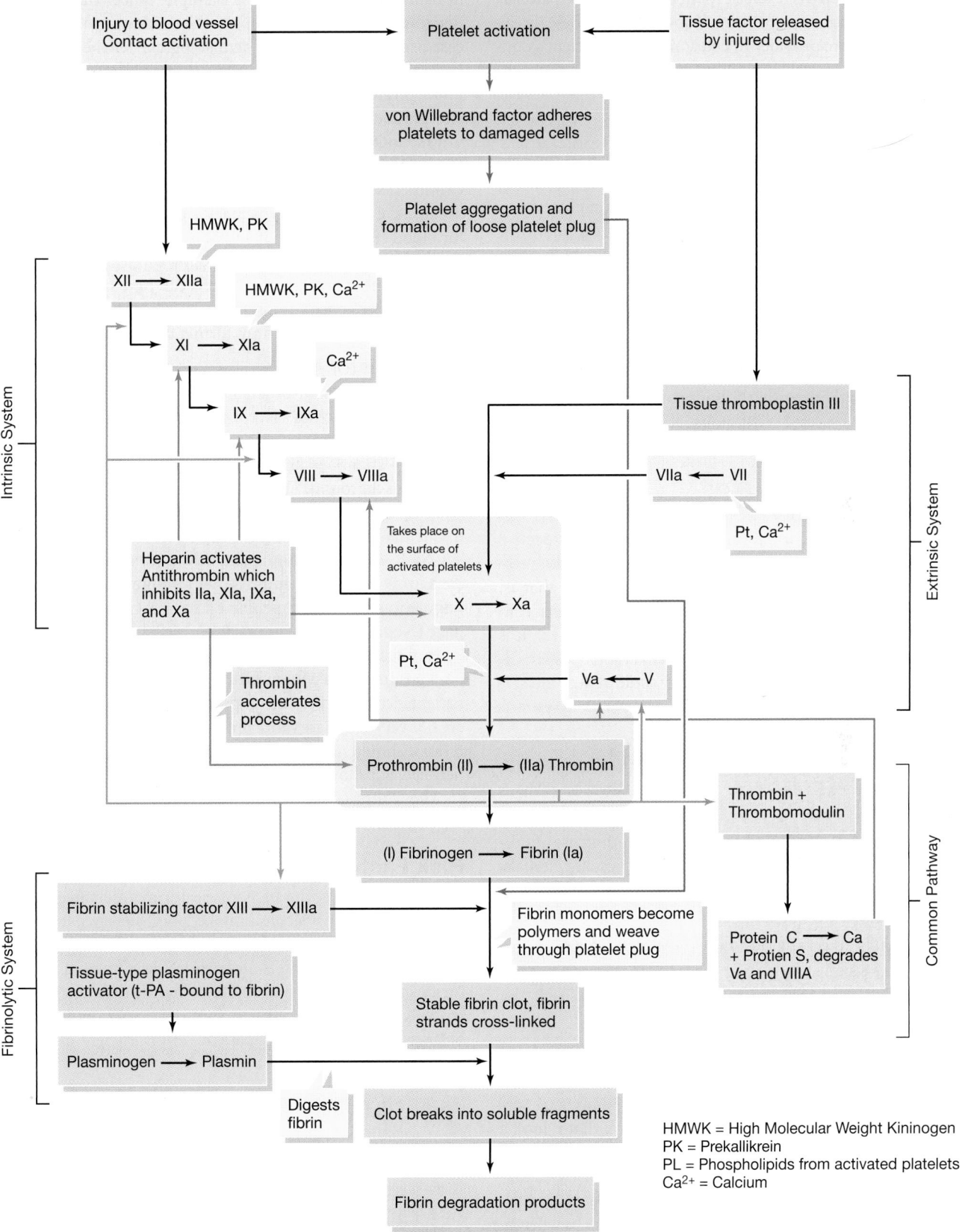

FIGURE 62–8 ■ Coagulation cascade.

patient's dietary history. Other assessment factors include elimination pattern, activity-exercise pattern, sleep–rest pattern, and cognitive-perceptual pattern. Knowledge of these areas helps the health care provider in determining the patient's current health status as well eliminating risk factors and promoting health restoration.

Presenting Symptoms

If patients are having problems with the erythrocyte, or RBC component, of their hematologic system, the usual presenting symptom is fatigue or weakness. The patient may say "I used to be able to make my bed in the morning after I got up, but now I am too tired to even do that." Another common presenting symptom of a hematologic problem is shortness of breath. In this situation patients may complain that they get tired and short of breath just walking around their own house.

If patients are having problems with the leukocytes, neutrophils, or WBC component of their hematologic system, they usually present with increasing episodes of illness and fevers. Finally, patients who present with unusual bleeding may be having problems with their platelets or thrombocytes or with their clotting mechanism.

Past Medical History

The history provides information from the patient's perspective and understanding. In assessing the patient, the nurse asks questions to determine what is happening to the patient, that is, what the patient is feeling and experiencing. In comparison to other systems (e.g., cardiovascular, nervous, reproductive), it is very unusual to ask questions about the hematologic system directly. Generally questions are asked that would reflect the status of the hematologic system. Several such specific questions are as follows:

1. Have you ever had any prior hematologic problems, such as anemia, bleeding disorders, and blood diseases such as leukemia?
2. What medicines have you been taking, including use of prescription and over-the-counter (OTC) drugs and herbals, many of which can interfere with clotting?
3. Have you been feeling fatigued?
4. Have you been getting sick more often than usual?
5. Have you been having fevers?
6. Have you had any bloody or black stools?
7. Have you ever vomited brown or red liquid?
8. Have you had surgery or a major injury requiring medical intervention, for example tumor removal, prosthetic heart valve placement, surgical excision of duodenum, and partial or total gastrectomy? Did anyone tell you that it took a long time to stop the bleeding?

    All of these procedures affect functioning of the hematologic system. For example, iron absorption occurs in the duodenum, and vitamin B_{12} is absorbed in the ileum. Wound healing complications and bleeding should be discussed as response to past surgeries and injuries.
9. Have you had your spleen removed?

These questions are suggestive of changes in the composition and characteristics of the blood cells.

Diseases that involve any of the hematologic organs will result in hematologic disorders. For example, cancer suppresses bone marrow, and liver disease impacts the clotting factors. Kidney disease also greatly impacts the hematologic system because it results in poor production of erythropoietin. Erythropoietin is a hormone produced by the kidney that promotes the differentiation and production of red blood cells in bone marrow. It starts the production of hemoglobin, the molecule within red blood cells that transports oxygen. Gastrointestinal (GI) disorders such as Crohn's disease also impact blood cell production and function because the GI tract is the primary source of the nutrients needed for blood cell development and because GI diseases carry a high propensity for bleeding. Similarly, any surgical manipulation of the component hematologic organs can have deleterious consequences. Assessment findings of previous gastrectomy, colectomy, or splenectomy warrant further diagnostic workup.

Family History

Many hematologic disorders have familial patterns. Genetic information offers clues as to possible hematologic problems that are known to be common in specific populations. For example, sickle cell anemia is known to be found in individuals with an African background. Thalassemia often can be found in patients with a Mediterranean background. Hemophilia is found more frequently in Caucasian males than in African American males. Tay-Sachs disease is found primarily in Jews of central and eastern European descent, and it is now also prevalent in non-Jewish populations, including people of French-Canadian/Cajun heritage (Nemours Foundation, 2008).

Familial patterns also can be the result of similar environmental exposure or behavior modeling within the family. For example, patients with families who engage in smoking, eat poor diets, or are not very active are more prone to engage in similar behaviors. A nurse should never make an assumption about patients' genetic heritage, but should always ask patients about their background.

The Cultural Considerations box discusses how culture can affect the function of the hematologic system.

Risk Factors

The traditional profile of poor health maintenance behaviors (smoking, excessive alcohol intake, poor dietary pattern, and a sedentary lifestyle) has an extremely negative impact on the hematologic system and is the basis for development of risk factors. Excessive alcohol use results in vitamin deficiencies and potentially GI damage that can suppress hematopoiesis. Poorly balanced diets also subject patients to insufficient quantities of

CULTURAL CONSIDERATIONS Related to the Hematologic System

Nurses should be prepared to care for diverse groups of people as the number of patients from other cultures entering the health care system increases. A great deal of variation is seen in the cultural habits of different demographic areas. Beliefs and values related to health, illness, and death, as well as daily habits, nutritional preferences, and health practices, may exist that are culturally important to patients and a part of their daily lives. For example, certain cultures only eat vegetarian foods, which can impact the amount of iron available to produce adequate RBCs.

iron, protein, vitamin B$_{12}$, and folate, all of which are critical in the production of blood cell lines.

Alterations in the hematologic system can come from a variety of sources including medications, diseases, behavior patterns, family history, and surgical interventions. Examples of risk factors associated with drugs and medications are given in the Risk Factors box. The presence of any of these risk factors places the patient at risk of hematologic system derangement. Many risk factors have only a temporary effect with the derangement subsiding once the risk factor is eliminated or resolved (e.g., temporary dietary deficiency), whereas others can result in permanent damage (bone marrow disease). When a patient presents with hematologic system risk factors, the interdisciplinary health team should provide appropriate assessment of existing alterations and education to prevent further damage.

Physical Examination

A complete physical examination is required to thoroughly assess the effects of hematologic system dysfunction. Because blood cells affect every major organ and body system, only a comprehensive examination can ensure that all possible derangements are identified. Generally, early indicators of hematologic derangement such as fatigue or bleeding can be identified during inspection. Although these signs can also be indicative of temporary and benign situations, keen health care providers will often act on these early indicators to progress toward more definitive diagnostic workups. If further physical examination, such as auscultation or palpation,

yields additional evidence of hematologic derangement, the health care provider would again move toward more definitive diagnostic tools such as laboratory and or radiologic assessments.

Inspection

Simple observation allows the health care provider to observe the patient's general appearance and exertional effort, both of which yield clues in an assessment of the hematologic system. Patients who are short of breath, fatigued, or exhibit poor stamina and poor mental acuity may be at risk of anemia or infection. Fever is a very serious sign that warrants prompt attention even in the absence of other clinical signs. For patients who are neutropenic (decreased neutrophil supply), oftentimes fever is the only observable indicator of infection in this very vulnerable population.

Skin

Changes in skin color often indicate erythrocyte disorders such as anemia (pale, loss of pallor), liver failure (yellow, jaundice), polycythemia vera (pink, flushed), or rapid breakdown of erythrocytes (brown, dark). Platelet and/or clotting derangements often produce tiny capillary bleeds manifesting as petechiae, purpura, or ecchymosis. The appearance of these skin changes, especially in the absence of recent identifiable injury, should be reported immediately so that a laboratory analysis can be performed. In patients with known hematologic deficiencies, assessment of the skin must be included during all routine assessments and whenever laboratory values or assessments of other body systems suggest hematologic derangement.

Head and Neck

The structures of the head, particularly the eyes and mouth, provide useful evidence in the evaluation of the patient with known, potential, or suspected hematologic derangement. Using a penlight, gloved hand, and tongue depressor, the nurse should thoroughly assess the gums, lips, tongue, and teeth. Symptoms warranting further collaboration and intervention include tenderness, increased or decreased saliva, inflammation, reddening, ulcerations, and bleeding. These symptoms are most worrisome in patients with neutropenia because they indicate signs of infection. See Chapter 64 🔗 for further discussion. Pernicious and iron deficiency anemia also produce a characteristic symptom of smooth tongue texture and pale gums.

With respect to the eyes, health care providers should assess the sclera for color and swelling. The appearance of yellow, jaundiced sclera warrants immediate reporting to the health care provider because this indicates an accumulation of bile pigment due to rapid or excessive hemolysis and also is a sign of liver disease. The neck should be inspected for signs of lymph node enlargement or tenderness, especially in the submaxillary, tonsillar, or supraclavicular regions.

Chest

Structures in the chest that yield clues to hematologic system health include the heart and the lymph nodes. The heart is a sensitive indicator of most abnormalities; for example, the heart rate will increase (tachycardia) in response to both infection and anemia. A widening pulse pressure is another compensatory mechanism to counteract inefficient oxygen delivery. The lymph nodes in the mediastinum or the axilla will become enlarged and tender in the presence of infection, lymphoma, and other metastatic cancers.

RISK FACTORS of Drugs and Medications

Many drugs have a deleterious effect on the hematologic system. Mechanisms of action include bone marrow suppression, which stunts the development of all three cell lines; suppression of the clotting cascade; and inflammatory process suppression, which affects WBC efficacy. Of particular concern are any drugs that are specifically termed as *myelosuppressive,* or suppressive of the bone marrow function. Drugs in this category, most notably chemotherapy drugs, will result in *pancytopenia,* or suppression of all three blood cell lines. Examples of more common drugs affecting blood function, specifically platelets, are salicylic acid (aspirin), clopidogrel (Plavix), eptifibatide (Integrilin), and ibuprofen (Advil).

Additionally, a patient can have an idiosyncratic reaction to any medication that may affect blood studies. For example, some individuals develop prolonged clotting times while taking antibiotics. Patients also may not understand the interactions when taking multiple medications or the impact of complementary drugs and/or diet. For example, when a patient is placed on warfarin, the amount of vitamin K taken needs to be minimized because it is an antidote for warfarin and will impact its ability to prolong clotting.

Social History

It is necessary to obtain a social history in order to identify potentially harmful habits and activities. For instance does the patient smoke and drink; if so how much and how often? Is he exposed to potentially traumatic events through his occupation and//or leisure activities? Does he live alone or with others, and if so, whom? These factors are important to determine as they may be risk factors which makes the patient more prone to homological disorders or complications from other disease factors.

CHART 62–3 **Use of Hematologic Testing to Determine Normal/Abnormal Conditions**

Body System	Normal Conditions	Abnormal Conditions
Hematologic	• CBC for work or school physicals • CBC for preoperative screening • CBC to monitor for side effects of medications	• Anemias/leukemias • RBC abnormalities • Infection
Gastrointestinal	• CBC for preoperative screening • CBC to monitor for side effects of medications	• Gastrointestinal bleeding • Appendicitis • Vitamin B_{12} deficiency
Cardiac	• CBC for preoperative screening	• Tachycardia-related anemia • Infection
Pulmonary	• CBC for preoperative screening	• Diffusing capacity of lung for carbon monoxide (D_LCO) • Infection
Renal	• CBC for preoperative screening	• Anemia • Infection
Musculoskeletal	• CBC for preoperative screening	• Infection

Abdomen

Abdominal tenderness is a general complaint, the appearance of which warrants a more detailed work-up. The first task is to isolate (if appropriate) the source of the tenderness, so as to identify which organ is involved. Enlarged spleens (splenomegaly) or livers (hepatomegaly) are general indicators of increased blood cell destruction, the cause of which must be identified. Additionally liver tenderness may be associated with clotting system abnormalities. Further blood studies are warranted whenever a complaint of abdominal tenderness is found.

Laboratory and Diagnostic Procedures

A variety of laboratory tests provide a thorough analysis of blood component status. Health care providers should evaluate laboratory tests not only for the relative quantity of components, but also for the size and character of each cell type. Most commonly, health care providers of any specialty rely on automated blood counts of peripheral cells (i.e., the complete blood count); however, microscopic evaluation of either peripheral blood or bone marrow aspirate yields additional information about size, character, and quality of blood cells. Chart 62–3 shows types of hematologic testing that can be conducted to determine normal and abnormal conditions.

Automated Blood Cell Analysis: Complete Blood Count

The automated blood count provides a highly accurate report of the number of blood cells (RBCs, WBCs, and platelets) in a given volume of peripheral blood. This section discusses each component of the complete blood count including normal/abnormal values and clinical implications. Chart 62–4 shows a listing of complete blood count (CBC) components and normal values. The normal values reflect the national standards for normal CBC values.

For further discussion, please refer to Chapter 63 🔗 on blood disorders and Chapter 60 🔗 on immune response disorders. Additionally, each of the disorder chapters discusses the laboratory values associated with the particular disorder.

Erythrocyte Evaluation

With regards to erythrocytes, the CBC provides a total number, morphologic analysis of blood cells, and hemoglobin analysis. The total RBC count is reported as RBC $\times 10^6/\mu L$ with normal values ranging from 3.6 to 5.2 depending on gender and ethnicity. Physiological increases in the RBC count occur with living in

CHART 62–4 **Complete Blood Count (CBC) Components and Normal Values**

Parameter	Normal Values
Red Blood Cell Indices	
Erythrocyte	*Men:* $4.6–6.2 \times 10^6$ cells/mm³ *Women:* $4.2–5.4 \times 10^6$ cells/mm³
Hemoglobin	*Men:* 13–18 g/dL *Women:* 12–16 g/dL
Hematocrit	*Men:* 45–54% *Women:* 36–46%
Mean corpuscular volume (MCV)	*Men:* 81–98 µmm³ *Women:* 81–98 µmm³
Mean corpuscular hemoglobin (MCH)	*Men:* 27–32 pg/dL *Women:* 27–32 pg/dL
Mean corpuscular hemoglobin concentration (MCHC)	*Men:* 32–36% *Women:* 32–36%
White Blood Cell Count Differential	
WBC count	4,500–11,000/µL
Polymorphonuclear neutrophils	1,800–7,800/µL (50–70%)
Band neutrophils	0–700/µL (0–10%)
Lymphocytes (MCV)	1,000–4,800/µL (15–45%)
Monocytes	0–800/µL (0–10%)
Eosinophils	0–450/µL (0–6%)
Basophils	0–200/µL (0–2%)
Platelet Function	
Platelets	150,000–400,000/µL

high altitude or after increased physical training, as a response to an increased need for oxygen. Pathologic reasons for an increase in the RBC count (polycythemia vera) are chronic obstructive lung disease and, in children with congenital heart disease who are cyanotic, as a response to chronic hypoxia. A decreased RBC count can be due to:

- Abnormal loss of erythrocytes (bleeding)
- Abnormal destruction of erythrocytes
- Lack of needed hormones and elements for production of erythrocytes
- Bone marrow suppression.

However, quantity alone is not a reliable indicator of red blood cell adequacy and function. For that reason, the RBC count is almost always evaluated in conjunction with hemoglobin analysis and morphologic indices (Corbett, 2008).

Recall that hemoglobin is the functional protein of the red blood cell that enables RBCs to carry out their primary function of oxygen transport. Hemoglobin (Hgb or Hb), measured in grams per deciliter, varies from 10 to 17 g/dL. Hemoglobin is reduced in cases of nutritional deficiency, bleeding, anemia, or hemodilution. Volume depletion (dehydration) or polycythemia vera, in turn, causes hemoglobin increases. The **hematocrit** value represents the percentage of hemoglobin in a given volume of whole blood that is occupied by packed RBCs, or the concentration of hemoglobin. However, this value is highly susceptible to fluid status changes such as dehydration; therefore, when making determinations about anemia, most clinicians tend to rely on hemoglobin. If a hematocrit value is not reported, it can be estimated by multiplying the hemoglobin by 3.

RBC indices reflect volume, color, and character of individual red blood cells, thus providing valuable data about the quality of these cells. The indices include these measurements: mean corpuscular volume, mean corpuscular hemoglobin, mean corpuscular hemoglobin concentration, and red cell distribution width.

The **mean corpuscular volume (MCV)** is a measure of the size of the RBCs. If the MCV is less than 78 μm³, the erythrocytes are microcytic, or smaller than normal. This occurs with iron deficiency anemia, lead poisoning, and thalassemia major and minor. An MCV of greater than 100 μm³ indicates that the erythrocytes are larger than normal (macrocytic). Macrocytic RBCs occur with liver disease, pernicious anemia, and folic acid deficiencies. The MCV can be used as a predictor of mortality in advanced cirrhosis. If the MCV is in the normal range the term *normocytic* is used. Anemia due to acute blood loss results in normocytic anemia (Corbett, 2008).

The **mean corpuscular hemoglobin (MCH)** measurement is the amount of Hgb present in one cell, whereas the **mean corpuscular hemoglobin concentration (MCHC)** is the proportion of each cell that is occupied by hemoglobin, indicating efficacy of interaction of the hemoglobin molecule with the erythrocyte. These two indices are discussed together because both are tests to determine whether the erythrocytes have a normal amount of Hgb (are normal color or *normochromic*), less Hgb (decreased color or *hypochromic*), or more Hgb (increased color or *hyperchromic*). Iron deficiency anemia is the most common cause of hypochromic anemia. Refer to Chapter 63 for further discussion of the clinical implications of variations in RBC indices.

The **red blood cell distribution width (RDW)** is a direct measurement of the homogeneity, or consistency, of red blood cell size. Immature cells are larger than mature cells and will result in RBC size variations. Additionally, the shape of red blood cells is highly influenced by the configuration of the hemoglobin molecule. Diseases such as sickle cell anemia and thalassemia, both diseases of hemoglobin, result in size variations. An increased RDW indicates a relatively heterogeneous population of red blood cells, indicating the presence of either abnormal or immature cells. The RDW is used to differentiate the various types of anemias.

The MCV, MCH, and MCHC measurements are primarily used in the classification of anemia. As discussed in Chapter 63 , *anemia* is a broad term applied to any situation resulting in a decrease in hemoglobin or erythrocytes. Anemia can be classified further (substantially) according to the underlying etiology, whether it is blood loss, iron deficiency anemia, or sickle cell anemia, for instance. These RBC indices are most useful in delineating the likely cause.

> **CRITICAL ALERT** A drop in hemoglobin level below 10 or a serial decrease in hemoglobin on consecutive reports may indicate anemia and should be reported to the health care provider immediately.

Leukocyte Evaluation

Leukocyte evaluation can be summarized by the white blood cell count value, which has a normal value of 4,500 to 10,000 cells per microliter. Normal values suggest that a patient has a sufficient number of cells to support host immune defense systems. However, the distribution of those WBCs is of significant clinical importance. White blood cells, or leukocytes, are a large heterogeneous group of cells, each with a unique role in host defenses as described earlier. Of these, the neutrophils are the first responder cells responsible for the initial detection of foreign antigens and initiation of the immune response cascade. However, the total neutrophil count is a summary value that combines immature (blasts), juvenile (bands), and fully mature stages of the neutrophils.

Only the fully mature neutrophils, and to some degree the juvenile subpopulations, are useful in defense. The bone marrow may be stimulated to release a large number of relatively immature cells and juvenile cells as a compensatory mechanism to combat severe infection. During this situation, the total WBC count increases, but the rise is due to the proliferation of juvenile cells. This phenomenon is termed a *shift to the left* and should be reported to the health care provider. In an otherwise healthy individual, this shift to the left may be an early sign of an otherwise undetected infection. If, however, the total WBC count remains within normal limits or even slightly below normal, and a shift to the left occurs, the patient may be left with insufficient host defenses. This can occur with bone marrow disease, immune system insufficiencies, or immunosuppressive therapies such as chemotherapy.

The **absolute neutrophil count (ANC)** is a useful measurement that reveals that proportion of the white blood cells that can be utilized in first response immune interactions. To calculate the ANC, add the bands to the neutrophils and multiply by the total WBC count. Values greater than 1,500 indicate normal immune defense. Some laboratories provide this number directly; however, it can be easily calculated from the white blood cell differential.

The WBC differential is a determination of each of the five types of WBCs in 100 WBCs. This is a separate test from the CBC and generally must be specifically ordered by the health care provider. In contrast to the automated CBC, the CBC with manual differential must be performed by a laboratory scientist who conducts a microscopic analysis of a blood smear. Bands and neutrophils (also called polymorphonuclear cells or stabs depending on the nomenclature used by the laboratory) are reported as a percentage of the total WBC count. See Chapters 60 and 64 on immunology and cancer, respectively, for further discussion.

 *ANC values below 1,000 indicate that the patient is at severe risk of infection and without sufficient defenses to prevent sepsis. Immediately assess the patient for signs of infection, initiate appropriate interventions, and report to the health care provider immediately.*

Platelet Evaluation

The platelet count is a useful indicator of bleeding risk because platelets are responsible for initiation of the clotting cascade. Fortunately, the platelet count requires little further calculation because its final value reported on the CBC can be used as an immediate indicator of platelet activity. Normal values range from 150,000 to 400,000. Increased platelet counts (thrombocytosis) occur with malignant tumors, especially if they are metastatic lesions, and with polycythemia vera and splenectomy. Low platelet counts (thrombocytopenia) may be idiopathic, related to cancer, due to an autoimmune disease, or the result of a viral infection. Low platelet counts are also common with acquired immunodeficiency disease (AIDS) (Corbett, 2008).

 Platelet levels below 30,000 indicate that the patient may be at imminent risk of internal bleeding, especially cranial bleeds. In this event, report to the health care provider immediately and implement bleeding precautions.

Coagulation Studies

As discussed when the clotting cascade was described earlier in the chapter, numerous components interact in a complex sequence of steps in response to endothelial injury (refer to Figure 62–8 ■, p. 1997). Insufficiencies in activity or supply in any of the components will result in abnormal bleeding. A variety of coagulation studies are utilized to identify individual insufficiencies. Chart 62–5 provides a description of each test and its normal values. Generally, longer time values indicate insufficient clotting factors or overactivity of clot-inhibiting therapy (such as heparin, Coumadin, or aspirin).

Bone Marrow Examination

Examination of the bone marrow may be required for several clinical scenarios, including these:

- Evaluation of unexplained peripheral blood cytopenias (decreased blood cell counts)
- Evaluation of unexplained excessive peripheral blood cell counts
- Evaluation of suspicious cells in the peripheral blood
- Staging or further analysis of leukemia or lymphoma
- Evaluation of fever of unknown origin
- Evaluation of patient iron stores when other tests are ambiguous.

Bone marrow aspiration removes a small amount of bone marrow *fluid* through a needle inserted into a bone. A bone marrow biopsy removes *bone* with the marrow inside and is obtained with a visual inspection of the marrow structure. Bone marrow samples are acquired by a health care provider using local anesthesia from the posterior superior iliac spine of the pelvis or the sternum.

Although there may be variations in technique among health care providers, if the biopsy is obtained from the iliac spine, the patient generally is placed into the lateral decubitus position with the top leg flexed and the lower leg straight. This position allows for optimal exposure of the iliac crest while providing stabilization with the lower leg. Oftentimes, nurses can assist the patient and health care provider in maintaining this optimal position.

Once the site is sterilized and anesthetized with local anesthetic, a small skin incision is made through which the bone marrow aspiration and biopsy needles are inserted. The bone marrow needle is comprised of an outer shell surrounding a stylet. Once the stylet has penetrated the marrow, it is removed and a syringe is attached to the shell allowing for aspiration of 2 to 3 mL of bone marrow. The bone marrow biopsy is done in much the same fashion with a specialized needle that is able to extract small amounts of bone. After the procedure, a small gauze square is applied with mild pressure to prevent bleeding. After the procedure patients should be assessed for pain and bleeding. Presence of either should be reported to the health care provider.

Bone marrow examination specifically evaluates the specimen for adequacy of volume and appropriate production of bone marrow cells. Specific results include:

- Evaluation of the adequacy of marrow development of each hematopoietic cell line.

CHART 62–5	**Coagulation Studies**	
Study	**Measures**	**Normal Value**
Prothrombin time (PT)	Extrinsic coagulation Factors I, II, V, VII, and X	12–15 seconds
Activated partial thromboplastin time (aPTT)	Intrinsic coagulation Factors I, II, V, VII, IX, X, XI, and XII	30–45 seconds
Bleeding time	Reflects platelet interaction and capillary constriction. A highly insensitive study, consequently use of this test is not favored	1–6 minutes
Thrombin time	Thrombin sufficiency	8–12 seconds
Fibrinogen	Fibrinogen sufficiency	200–400 mg/dL
Fibrin split products	Useful in detection of DIC. Reflects degree of fibrinolysis, which releases fibrin split products into bloodstream	<10 mg/dL

- Morphologic examinations of the cells to ensure that structures are consistent with normal cells.
- Infiltration of the bone marrow by inappropriate cells. Normally, only early precursors of blood cell lines should be observed in the marrow. Presence of other cells may indicate disease, most likely some type of malignancy.
- Fibrosis.

Gerontological Considerations

The effects of aging on the hematologic system currently are under study. It is thought, however, that the amount of red marrow and the number of stem cells decrease with aging, but the marrow is not completely depleted even in very old adults. The remaining stem cells retain their functional capacity to divide, but as they decrease in number they are gradually replaced by nonfunctional fat cells. This, in turn, potentially decreases the ability of the marrow to respond to the body's need for blood cells in the advent of injury or disease (Lichtman & Williams, 2001). The elderly patient is more vulnerable to possible problems with clotting, oxygen transport, and fighting infection, especially during periods of increased demand.

Laboratory parameters as they relate to the hematologic system of aging patients usually are not much different than those of a younger patient (Kane, Ouslander, & Abrass, 2004; McPherson & Pincus, 2006; Young et al., 2006). Although it is recognized that hemoglobin levels tend to decrease after middle age, more so in men than women (Guyton, 2006), aging changes do not usually occur with the WBC count or platelet count. It has been suggested that there may be some T-cell function loss and this may account for the poor response to immunizations in the elderly population (Young et al., 2006). The effect of anemia on the elderly is discussed in the Gerontological Considerations box.

Implications for Health Promotion

The hematologic system, without exception, affects every organ in the body. Its pivotal role dictates that its maintenance must be incorporated into any health promotion strategy. One need only review the risk factors of hematologic disorders to determine what health promotion activities should be taken. Individuals can do much to maintain and optimize the health of their hematologic system. Patients should be advised to examine their genetic history to determine whether there is any family history of bleeding disorders. Eating a well-balanced diet rich in iron, vitamin B_{12}, and proteins ensures that the bone marrow is supplied

with the requisite building blocks for blood cells. Direct patient teaching by nurses or referral to a registered dietitian can be of tremendous benefit to patients trying to navigate a plethora of food choices. The effect of nutrition on the hematologic system is discussed in detail in Chapter 63.

Exercise is critical for a healthy hematologic system both because it encourages production of blood cells from the marrow (resulting in reduced fatigue and shortness of breath) and it reduces the risk of cardiovascular disease. With increased exercise the patient is at decreased risk of coagulation disorders.

Excessive alcohol consumption damages the hematologic system on several fronts: (1) impaired nutrition, because beneficial calories are substituted with alcohol; (2) damage to the GI tract, resulting in bleeding and impaired absorption of vitamin B_{12}, iron, and folate; and (3) damage to the liver, resulting in decreased coagulation factors and erythrocyte processing. Nurses play a critical role in identifying opportunities to promote lifestyles that ensure the health of the hematologic system. Patients should be advised that diet may be a contributing factor for anemia. Refer to Chapter 63 on blood disorders for additional information on health promotion.

Critical Thinking Related to the Hematologic System

It is imperative that the nurse become familiar with the components of the laboratory tests and other examination tests that are used to evaluate the hematologic system. The nurse must:

- Be able to explain the purpose of the tests to patients and/or their family.
- Be able to explain to the patients and/or their family why the hematologic system is being evaluated for a patient in a particular situation.
- Be able to identify normal and abnormal values of a complete blood count.
- Be able to differentiate normal versus abnormal laboratory values according to the reference ranges for the laboratory performing the test. These reference points must be available; if they are not provided on the laboratory report, the nurse can call the laboratory and ask for the normal reference ranges for that particular test.
- Identify situations where evaluation of the hematologic system would be appropriate or inappropriate.

Tracking laboratory values over a time period to determine trending in abnormalities is an essential nursing measure and requires critical thinking. An isolated abnormal finding may not be significant, but if the value continues to trend toward abnormality, it becomes significant.

The nurse must rely on critical thinking skills when interpreting patients' symptoms and assessment findings to determine possible and potential patient diagnoses and to consider the appropriate action(s) to take. Analysis of these data allows the nurse to make a diagnosis and then follow up with any required interventions. It is imperative that the nurse communicate and collaborate with other members of the health care team in developing and implementing a plan of care for patients with any hematologic findings outside of the normal range.

GERONTOLOGICAL CONSIDERATIONS Related to Anemia

If an elderly person is anemic, often it is due to disease processes, such as GI bleeding or malnutrition, in other systems as opposed to the hematologic system. Abnormal values in these areas need to be brought to the health care provider's attention because further evaluation may be necessary. Thinking that changes in these parameters are solely due to aging may result in an incorrect interpretation of the laboratory test, which could then lead to incorrect management of the problem. It often is the duration of the disease process, not the person's age, that results in illness, morbidity, and mortality.

Summary

As presented in this chapter, the hematologic system is deeply integrated with every body system. Thus, alterations in the hematologic organs or cells can manifest virtually anywhere and, conversely, damage in a peripheral organ can impact the function of the blood system. For these reasons a thorough knowledge of the anatomy and physiology of the hematologic system is a critical tool in the nurse's arsenal. Appropriate assessment skills, including physical examination and diagnostic study evaluation, should be core skills for all nurses.

NCLEX® REVIEW

1. As it relates to the hematologic system in the adult patient, the nurse understands that:
   1. The stem cell is a primitive cell located in the bone marrow that is the precursor of red blood cells, white blood cells, and platelets.
   2. The liver and spleen can produce blood cells during intramedullary hematopoiesis when disease has caused bone marrow destruction.
   3. The blood is considered to be a type of connective tissue with one primary function, to transport oxygen, hormones, and waste products.
   4. The proportion of yellow bone marrow diminishes and is permanently replaced by red bone marrow as the healthy patient ages.

2. The nurse educator is teaching a class of new nurses regarding the functions of the hematologic system in the adult. Which of the following statements made by one of the participants indicates the need for further instruction?
   1. "White blood cells usually remain in the bone marrow, lungs, liver, spleen, and lymph nodes, unless they are needed."
   2. "Immature reticulocytes will persist for several days in the circulation before becoming a small, mature red blood cell."
   3. "The cells of the reticuloendothelial system facilitate blood clotting and initiate the inflammatory and immune responses."
   4. "Erythrocytes are responsible for transporting, maintaining, and distributing hemoglobin to the body's tissues."

3. The nurse is planning the care of the patient who is newly diagnosed with anemia. The nurse anticipates performing which of the following laboratory tests to better classify the anemia?
   1. PT, aPTT, PLT
   2. HGB, HCT, ANC
   3. RBC, RDW, WBC
   4. MCH, MCV, MCHC

4. Which of the following laboratory test results should the nurse immediately report to the health care provider?
   1. HCT 28%
   2. PLT 400,000/μL
   3. WBC 10,000/μL
   4. MCH 30pg/dL

5. During shift report the nurse is told a patient's laboratory values indicate a shift to the left. The receiving nurse understands that this phenomenon indicates:
   1. The measurement of the proportion of white blood cells that are available for use in a first response immune reaction.
   2. An increase in the total white blood cell count because of the proliferation of juvenile band and immature blast cells.
   3. A quantitative method of indicating the efficacy of interaction between the hemoglobin molecule and the erythrocyte.
   4. That there are insufficiencies in either activity or supply in one or more of the components of the clotting cascade.

6. Which of the following statements describes the correct sequence of events within the normal hemostasis mechanism?
   1. Soft aggregate plug formation, vasoconstriction, fibrin conversion into fibrinogen, initiation of the intrinsic coagulation mechanism
   2. Vascular contraction, intrinsic adenosine diaphosphate release, prothrombin conversion into thrombin, fibrinogen conversion into fibrin
   3. Platelet adhesion, onset of primary hemostasis pathway, Factor XI activates Factor XII, initiation of the extrinsic coagulation mechanism
   4. Start of intrinsic clotting pathway, Factor III and Factor V release, platelet thromboplastic factor release, Factor X activates Factor XI

7. A patient presents to the primary care clinic complaining of increasingly worsening fatigue over the last two months. Which of the following questions should the nurse ask in order to better differentiate the source of the patient's complaint?
   1. "Are you allergic to shellfish or IV dye?"
   2. "Have you had your gallbladder removed?"
   3. "What medications are you currently taking?"
   4. "Is there a family history of heart disease?"

Answers for review questions appear in Appendix D

KEY TERMS

absolute neutrophil count (ANC) *p.2001*
basophil *p.1993*
chyle *p.1994*
eosinophil *p.1993*
erythrocyte *p.1991*
granulocyte *p.1993*
hematocrit *p.2001*
hematology *p.1989*
hematopoiesis *p.1990*
hemoglobin *p.1991*
hemostasis *p.1995*

humoral immune response *p.1993*
leukocyte *p.1991*
lymphatic system *p.1994*
lymphocyte *p.1993*
mean corpuscular hemoglobin
    (MCH) *p.2001*
mean corpuscular hemoglobin
    concentration (MCHC) *p.2001*
mean corpuscular volume (MCV) *p.2001*
monocyte *p.1993*
neutrophil *p.1993*

plasma *p.1991*
platelet *p.1991*
red blood cell (RBC) *p.1991*
red blood cell distribution width
    (RDW) *p.2001*
reticulocyte *p.1992*
reticuloendothelial system (RES) *p.1993*
stem cell *p.1990*
thrombocyte *p.1991*
white blood cell (WBC) *p.1991*

PEARSON

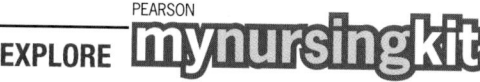
EXPLORE

MyNursingKit is your one stop for online chapter review materials and resources. Prepare for success with additional NCLEX®-style practice questions, interactive assignments and activities, web links, animations and videos, and more!

Register your access code from the front of your book at
www.mynursingkit.com

REFERENCES

Corbett, J. V. (2008). *Laboratory tests and diagnostic procedures: With nursing diagnosis.* Upper Saddle River, NJ: Pearson Prentice Hall.

Dailey, J. (1998). *Blood.* Arlington, MA: Medical Consulting Group.

Department of Health and Human Services, Agency for Toxic Substances & Disease Registry. (2005). Top 20 hazardous substances. Retrieved October 10, 2008 from http://www.atsdr.cedc.gov/cxcx3.html

Guyton, A. C. (2006). *Textbook of medical physiology* (11th ed.). St. Louis: Elsevier.

Kane, R., Ouslander, J., & Abrass, I. (2004). *Essentials of clinical geriatrics* (5th ed.). New York: McGraw-Hill.

Lichtman, M. A., & Williams, W. J. (2001). Hematology in the aged. In E. Beutler, M. A. Lichtman, B. S. Coller, T. J. Kipps, & U. Seligsohn (Eds.), *Williams hematology* (6th ed.). St. Louis: Mosby.

McPherson, R., & Pincus, M. (2006). *Henry's clinical diagnosis and management by laboratory methods* (21st ed.). Philadelphia: W. B. Saunders.

Nemours Foundation. (2008). *Tay-Sachs disease.* Retrieved March 24, 2008, from http://www.kidshealth.org/parent/medical/genetic/tay_sachs.html

Porth, C. (2007). *Essentials of pathophysiology: Concepts of altered health states.* St. Louis: Lippincott Williams & Wilkins.

Ross, M. H. (2003). *Histology: A text and atlas* (4th ed., pp. 229–231). Philadelphia: Lippincott William & Wilkins.

Swartz, M. A. (2001). *Advanced Drug Delivery Reviews, 50*(1–2), 3–20.

Young, N., Gerson, S., & High, K. (2006). *Clinical hematology.* Philadelphia: Mosby.

63

Caring for the Patient with Blood Disorders

Kristine Abueg

Outcome-Based Learning Objectives

After studying this chapter, the learner will be able to:

1. Describe the physiology of hematopoiesis, thrombopoiesis, and hemostasis.

2. Explain the pathophysiological alterations in erythropoiesis, thrombopoiesis, and hemostasis that give rise to specific hematologic disorders.

3. Compare and contrast the causes, the therapeutic management, and clinical presentation of the various types of anemias and hemostasis disorders.

4. Analyze laboratory values, correlating to physical signs and symptoms, and distinguish between various hematologic disorders.

5. Explain appropriate nursing interventions for the management of thrombocytopenia.

6. Compare and contrast the hallmark clinical presentation of bleeding disorders versus clotting disorders.

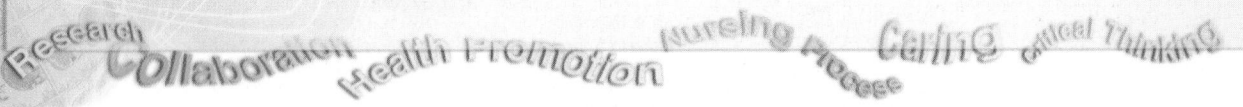

Research   Collaboration   Health Promotion   Nursing Process   Caring   Critical Thinking

Hematology involves the study of blood and blood, or hematologic, disorders. Blood actually contains both plasma and blood cells (as explained in Chapter 62 ☺). Plasma, comprised of water, proteins, salts, lipids, glucose, and other organic compounds, makes up 55% of blood volume. Its main purpose is to act as a liquid transport system between tissues. Hematology, however, involves the study of the cellular components of blood, specifically erythrocytes (red blood cells), leukocytes (white blood cells), and thrombocytes (platelets). Normal function of the cellular components is described in Chapter 62 ☺. Hematologic disorders arise when the normal functioning of these cell lines is disrupted either by disease, genetics, or environmental factors. The study of hematology and blood disorders is best approached by a systematic review of different blood components. This chapter focuses specifically on two cell lines: thrombocytes and erythrocytes. Refer to Chapters 59 and 60 ☺ for an in-depth review of the nursing care of patients with leukocyte disorders.

Some hematologic disorders are chronic, resulting in the need for permanent lifestyle adjustments, whereas others are acute medical conditions requiring immediate medical attention. Chronic hematologic diseases include sickle cell disease, thalassemia, and hemophilia. Acute hematologic disorders include acute anemia, thrombocytopenia, and disseminated intravascular coagulation. These acute disorders usually are not

independently occurring disease states, but serious side effects that result when another underlying disease process is present.

Most medical–surgical nurses are likely to care for patients with acute blood disorders, because most chronic diseases are well managed in the outpatient setting. However, patients with chronic hematologic disorders often are hospitalized for other illnesses such as infection, trauma, or cardiac problems. Physiological stressors can severely exacerbate chronic diseases potentially leading to "acute attacks." Such attacks, however, often can be prevented by diligent initial assessment paired with continual observation for deviation from the baseline. In the event an acute attack occurs, the nurse must ensure that immediate intervention and coordination with the interdisciplinary health team occur to prevent serious injury. For all of these reasons, it is critically important for the nurse to include any existing or potential hematologic disorder in a patient's care plan.

■ Hematopoiesis: Development of Blood Cells

Hematopoiesis is the process of blood cell development, beginning with the immature hematopoietic stem cell in the bone marrow and extending through to complete cellular maturation in the peripheral bloodstream. Problems that can occur during hematopoiesis account for many of the hematologic disorders discussed in this chapter; therefore, a review of the normal physiological processes involved in hematopoiesis is a useful foundation for the study of hematology.

As mentioned earlier, blood contains many specialized cell lines including erythrocytes (red blood cells), leukocytes (white blood cells), and platelets. Despite their variation in appearance and function, all of these cell types are generated from the hematopoietic stem cells. **Hematopoietic stem cells (HSCs)** reside largely in the spongy bone marrow of the femurs, hips, ribs, sternum, and other long bones, while a small volume of HSCs circulates in the peripheral blood. HSCs may be thought of as the common ancestor cell of all blood cell lines. Although HSCs eventually give rise to mature red blood cells (RBCs), platelets, and white blood cells (WBCs), they themselves do not possess the full capabilities of oxygen transportation, clotting, or immune response associated with their more mature progeny, the erythrocytes, platelets, and leukocytes. These *pluripotent* HSCs found in the bone marrow and the blood should not be confused with embryonic *totipotent* stem cells, which are found in developing embryos and can develop into any cell in the human body.

The goal of hematopoiesis is not only to produce large numbers of cells when needed, but also to produce well-differentiated cells. **Differentiation** is the process by which immature precursor cells (such as the hematopoietic stem cells) produce generations of increasingly more specialized cells, ultimately resulting in a fully functioning, mature cell (such as a mature erythrocyte or thrombocyte). Differentiation also is associated with increasing morphologic distinction, acquisition of a specialized cellular structure, and membrane proteins, and narrowing of the variety of blood cells that can be produced by a given cell. The hematopoietic cascade, as shown in Figure 63–1 ■, is a common and useful illustration of this process.

From the HSCs, the next level of specificity is the lymphoid or myeloid **progenitor cells**, or blood line–specific stem cells. The common lymphoid progenitor cell eventually gives rise to

the lymphoid cells of the immune system, specifically the natural killer cells, the T cells, and the B cells. Refer to Chapter 60 🔗 for a discussion of disorders related to these cell lines. The common **myeloid progenitor cell** further differentiates into the granulocyte-macrophage stem cell, the megakaryocytic stem cell, or the erythropoietic stem cell (proerythroblast). The granulocyte-macrophage stem cell will eventually give rise to the granulocytes (neutrophils, eosinophils, basophils) or the monocytes (monocytic cells of the immune system and macrophages). Immune system disorders related to these cell lines are discussed in Chapter 60 🔗. Of interest to this chapter are the **megakaryocytic stem cells**, which eventually will develop the platelets, and the **erythropoietic stem cells (proerythroblasts)**, which will develop into mature erythrocytes or red blood cells.

The process of hematopoiesis is stimulated on an "as-needed basis." Cellular and chemical signals, generated when the body requires increased production of blood cells, interact with cells undergoing hematopoiesis, beginning with the HSCs. An HSC receives a chemical signal to produce a particular cell line, to self-replicate to increase available HSCs, or even to undergo apoptosis, programmed cell death. Conversely, the absence of these chemical signals or the presence of inhibitory signals is associated with decreased levels of hematopoiesis. This elegant system of feedback regulation ensures that energy reserves are allocated efficiently and not wasted on production of already abundant cells. Common types of chemical signals responsible for the regulation of hematopoiesis include soluble factors such as cytokines, direct cell-to-cell interaction, and contact with the extracellular matrix of the blood-forming organs. Specific signals include hormones such as erythropoietin in the case of RBC production, and thrombopoietin and interleukins in the case of platelet cell production.

Research has expanded our understanding about the complexity, variety, and intricate interplay that exists among these cellular and chemical signals. A major field of research is directed at understanding these signals in an effort to expand the production of small numbers of highly pluripotent HSCs for clinical transplantation and for other scientific studies. Currently, exogenous administration of hematopoiesis-stimulating chemicals is already a cornerstone of treatment for many diseases. Future treatment options will almost certainly evolve to incorporate medications derived from a growing understanding of these chemical signals. Specialized hematopoiesis of the RBC line (erythropoiesis) and platelet-forming cell lines (thrombopoiesis) are discussed later in the chapter as they relate to anemia and thrombocytopenia. As illustrated throughout this chapter, problems during hematopoiesis account for a large proportion of hematologic disorders. Successful hematopoiesis requires precise interaction and a delicate balance between numerous cells, chemical factors, and the physiological environment. Because hematopoiesis plays a pivotal role during the most primitive stages of embryonic and cellular development, even minor disruptions can have far-reaching amplified consequences. These consequences thus become the focus of hematology. This chapter builds on the pathophysiological foundation of hematopoiesis just outlined, highlighting alterations in the process that give rise to clinical disorders.

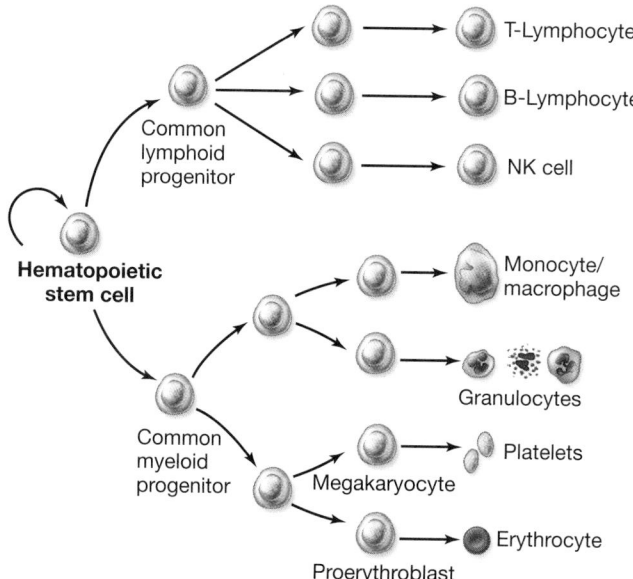

FIGURE 63–1 ■ The hematopoetic cascade.

Labels in figure: T-Lymphocyte; B-Lymphocyte; NK cell; Common lymphoid progenitor; Hematopoietic stem cell; Monocyte/macrophage; Granulocytes; Platelets; Megakaryocyte; Common myeloid progenitor; Erythrocyte; Proerythroblast

Anemia

Anemia is defined as a decrease in the total body erythrocyte volume, usually measured by a decrease in hemoglobin protein, a decreased hematocrit, and/or a decreased RBC count. The primary function of the erythrocytes is the transportation of oxygen on the hemoglobin molecules; thus, insufficiencies in the erythrocytes translate into an inability to maintain sufficient oxygen delivery to the tissues.

Etiology and Classifications of Generalized Anemia

According to data published by the National Center for Health Statistics in 2002, iron deficiency anemia, the most common form of anemia, was responsible for 4,614 deaths in America. Comprehensive mortality and morbidity for all causes of anemia is difficult to ascertain for two reasons. First, anemia is considered to be widely underdiagnosed, because patients often fail to seek diagnostic evaluation for symptoms of fatigue and shortness of breath, both hallmark signs of anemia. Second, anemia is not a disease in and of itself, but rather a clinical side effect that results from some underlying pathologic disease process that often complicates a statistical tabulation. Anemia can be triggered either by (1) loss of blood volume, (2) altered production of erythrocytes (hypoproliferative disorders), or (3) altered (increased) destruction of red blood cells. The various underlying etiologies have unique clinical presentations, which trigger a differential diagnostic workup. After resolution of immediate life-threatening situations such as hypoxia or blood loss, treatment is tailored to address the primary hematologic disorder causing the anemia.

Normal Physiology of Red Blood Cell Development

A detailed overview of erythrocyte development, or erythropoiesis, is described next as a foundation for discussing various causes of anemia. Understanding the root causes of these diseases illuminates not only the cause, but also aids in patient education and the judicious application of treatment options.

Erythropoiesis

Erythropoiesis, the process of hematopoiesis of erythrocytes (red blood cells), is stimulated primarily by the presence of erythropoietin, which acts on HSCs to produce the myeloid progenitor cell, thus starting the cascade toward RBC production. **Erythropoietin** is a hormone produced by the juxtaglomerular cells of the kidneys during periods of **hypoxia,** or decreased blood oxygen levels. Erythropoietin production also is modulated by other factors including thyroid-stimulating hormone, adrenal cortical steroids, adrenocorticotropic hormone, and human growth hormone (HGH). All of these factors are produced during periods of increased growth and their promotion of erythropoietin ensures sufficient supplies of oxygen will be available to growing tissues.

As discussed earlier, hematopoiesis results in cellular differentiation. During erythropoiesis, the pluripotent hematopoietic stem cell undergoes increasing differentiation, producing first the myeloid stem cell, then the pronormoblast, then the basophilic normoblast, the polychromatophilic normoblast, the orthochromatic normoblast, and then the reticulocyte (Figure 63–2 ■). The reticulocyte, or juvenile erythrocyte, is morphologically identifiable by its distinct reticulum in the cytoplasm. The reticulocyte circulates for approximately 3 days in the bone marrow before being released into the peripheral bloodstream where, after approximately 24 hours of undergoing changes in its cytoplasm, the reticulocyte will mature into a fully developed erythrocyte. Note, however, that high levels of erythropoietin, which occurs, for example, during hypoxic states or infection, may stimulate early release of reticulocytes from the bone marrow into the peripheral bloodstream, which is reflected on a complete blood count.

At the end of its designated life span (approximately 120 days), the aging erythrocyte (*senescent* erythrocyte) begins to display cell surface proteins, which trigger phagocytosis in the reticuloendothelial system. As described in Chapter 59 ⓒ, the reticuloendothelial system is comprised of phagocytic cells in the lymph nodes, spleen, and liver that clear the body of waste. Circulating macrophages consume the senescent erythrocyte and the hemoglobin, recycling the precious iron molecule by transporting it back to the body's iron stores.

Dietary elements play a key role in RBC production. Deficiencies in any of these dietary elements can negatively affect erythropoiesis. RBC development is highly dependent on sufficient quantities of metals (iron, cobalt, and manganese), vitamins (B_{12}, B_6, C, E, folate, riboflavin, pantothenic acid, and thiamin), amino acids, and carbohydrates. Although cellular growth requires all of these elements, vitamin B_{12}, folate, and iron play particularly pivotal roles in erythropoiesis. Folate and vitamin B_{12} are required for the extensive DNA synthesis that occurs with erythropoiesis. All proliferating cells require iron,

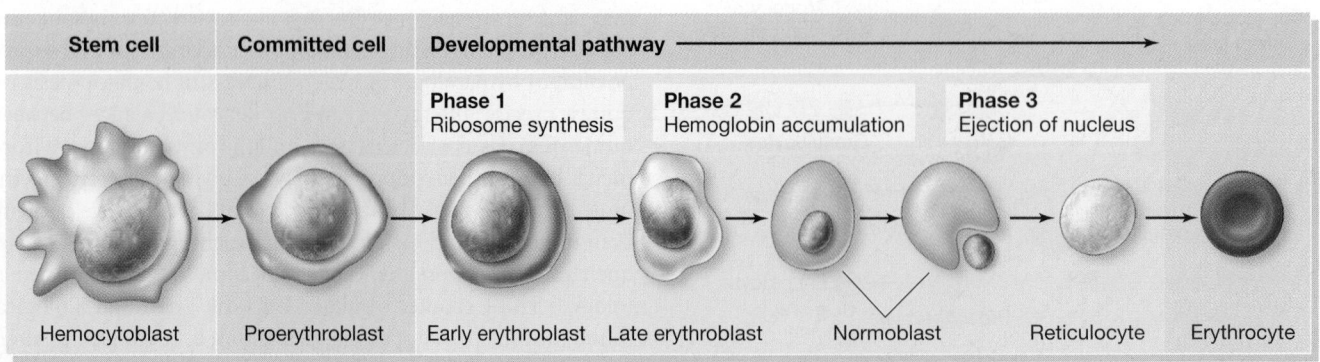

FIGURE 63–2 ■ Erythropoiesis.

but the iron requirements of erythroid cells in the late basophilic erythroblast through reticulocyte stages, when hemoglobin is synthesized and accumulates, are much greater than that for all other cell types (Koury & Ponka, 2004). Diseases such as megaloblastic anemia and iron deficiency anemia result when sufficient supplies do not exist to support erythropoiesis.

Hemoglobin Development

Hemoglobin is the core functional protein of the red blood cell, shuttling oxygen between tissues, allowing blood to transport 100 times more oxygen than could be transported in plasma alone. In erythropoiesis, hemoglobin first becomes detectable in the myeloid progenitor cell, with each subsequent cell generation gaining more and more hemoglobin molecule. Ultimately, the mature erythrocyte contains approximately 250 million hemoglobin molecules. Hemoglobin fulfills its oxygen-carrying function by binding iron to the four heme regions of the molecule. Closer observation of hemoglobin reveals that hemoglobin protein actually is comprised of four parts: two identical hemoglobin alpha chains and two identical hemoglobin beta chains. Iron binding is achieved when the hemoglobin alpha and beta chains form precise geometric configurations that allow iron to sit tightly in a lock-and-key style fit on the heme groups.

Healthy, functional hemoglobin conforms to one of two configurations. Which configuration it takes on depends on whether an O_2 molecule is bound to the heme, the pH of the environment, and the amount of a mediating chemical, 2,3-diphosphoglycerate. The combination of these factors varies in hypoxic states versus well-oxygenated states. This interaction is the foundation of the oxygen-release or oxygen-carrying mechanism of hemoglobin. An alteration to the geometric shape of hemoglobin is the underlying cause of many hematologic disorders such as thalassemia and sickle cell disease, which are discussed in detail later. The amount of hemoglobin in blood is a common clinical test used to diagnose disease. Although there are variations due to altitude, accepted values for hemoglobin for adult males are13.8 to 18 g/dL, and for adult females 12 to 16 g/dL (g/dL = grams per deciliter).

Clinical Presentation of Generalized Anemia

Decreased erythrocyte volume results in **anemic hypoxia**, or decreased oxygen availability to the tissues specifically due to decreased concentration of functional hemoglobin or a reduced number of red blood cells. Anemic hypoxia should be distinguished from **hypoxic hypoxia**, in which oxygen deprivation occurs from defective oxygenation in the lungs, as caused by abnormal pulmonary function, airway obstruction, or a right-to-left shunt in the heart (Pearson, 2000). For the purposes of this chapter, anemic hypoxia will be referred to as hypoxia. The clinical presentation of the patient with anemia primarily is due to the effects of hypoxia.

Laboratory and Diagnostic Procedures

An assessment of the patient with anemia involves an analysis of laboratory studies. Common laboratory tests used in the diagnosis of anemia are the complete blood count (CBC) to detect hematologic alterations and arterial blood gases (ABGs) to detect acid–base disturbances used in the evaluation of hypoxia.

Complete Blood Count   The complete blood count typically includes the following laboratory values pertinent to the study of red blood cells: hemoglobin (Hgb), hematocrit (Hct), red blood cells, reticulocyte mean corpuscle volume (MCV), and mean corpuscle hemoglobin (MCH). Normal values for these tests are summarized in Chart 63–1.

Hemoglobin values, as described in Chapter 62 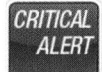, reflect the amount of hemoglobin protein measured in a volume of blood. Hemoglobin is decreased in cases of anemia of any etiology, hemorrhage, and hemodilution. Hemodilution occurs when excessive fluid (i.e., water and plasma) significantly dilutes a volume of blood, which can occur in situations such as water toxicity and excessive intravenous (IV) infusion. A significant drop in hemoglobin values (>3 g/dL) over a short time period (<24 hours) may indicate active bleeding.

> **CRITICAL ALERT** *A significant drop in hemoglobin values (>3 g/dL over a short period of time [<24 hours]) should be reported immediately to the health care provider. This may indicate active blood loss. This finding is of particular concern if blood loss is not readily visible (i.e., from gums, emesis, or stool) suggesting internal bleeding. Patients should be immediately assessed for level of consciousness, lung sounds, and acute areas of pain.*

The hematocrit, as described in Chapter 62, is the ratio of erythrocyte volume to a volume of whole blood, or the concentration of red blood cells. Hematocrit values follow the same pattern established by hemoglobin values: They decrease with excessive hydration (hemodilution), anemia, and hemorrhage.

The total RBC count reflects total volume of erythrocytes in a volume of blood. Total RBC values also tend to follow the directional patterns of hemoglobin and hematocrit. However, the total RBC value does not adequately indicate the quality or

---

CHART 63–1   **Summary of Common Complete Blood Count Findings in Anemia**

Lab Value	Normal Value	Expected Abnormality in Anemia	Rationale for Abnormality
Hemoglobin	*Women:* 12–16 g/dL *Men:* 13.5–18 g/dL	Decreased	Decreased hemoglobin production due to decreased erythrocyte production
Hematocrit	*Women:* 38–47% *Men:* 40–54%	Decreased	Decreased concentration of hemoglobin protein due to decreased erythrocyte production
Total RBC count	4.0–5.0 10^6/μL	Decreased	Reflects decreased total erythrocyte volume
Reticulocytes	0.5–1.5% of RBC count	Depends on etiology	Varies according to underlying etiology (acute or chronic, bone marrow involvement)

morphology of the erythrocytes. For these reasons, the morphologic RBC indices are often used in determination of anemia etiology, whereas the hemoglobin/hematocrit (H/H) ratio is more commonly used in the monitoring of anemia. Morphologic indices, as described in Chapter 62 ☯, including MCV, MCH, MCHC (mean corpuscular hemoglobin concentration), and average concentration of hemoglobin in each red blood cell are useful tools in describing the blood cell structures characteristic of each type of anemia.

Reticulocytes reflect the number of juvenile erythrocytes present in peripheral blood. Reticulocytes increase in most types of sustained anemia as erythropoiesis accelerates as a compensatory mechanism. Decreases in reticulocytes are associated with bone marrow suppression or deficient production of erythrocytes. If a finding of decreased reticulocytes accompanies decreased total WBC count and decreased platelet count, a further examination including a bone marrow aspiration may be warranted in the work-up for leukemia, aplastic anemia, or some other life-threatening bone marrow failure.

 If decreased reticulocyte values accompany a global decrease in all cell lines (RBCs, WBCs, and platelets) the patient should be immediately assessed for bone marrow failure.

Severity of Anemia

The severity of anemia symptoms generally is in direct proportion to the erythrocyte depletion as measured by the hemoglobin volume and hematocrit in the CBC. Delineating between severity states of anemia is somewhat arbitrary because a review of the literature reveals little agreement as to the exact hemoglobin values that constitute mild, moderate, or severe anemia states. Additionally, nurses should not rely solely on laboratory tests but must always incorporate physical and subjective findings when developing nursing interventions. Nonetheless, such delineation is a useful tool for discussion. Normal hemoglobin volume is defined at greater than 12 g/dL. Mild anemia is measured by a hemoglobin value of 10 to 12 g/dL. Moderate anemia is measured by a hemoglobin volume of 7 to 11 g/dL. Severe anemia is commonly defined by a hemoglobin volume of <7 g/dL and a hematocrit of less than 25%. Body system changes typically become more pronounced with increasing severity of anemia (Montoya, Wink, & Sole, 2002).

Physical Manifestations

The most common sign of anemia is generalized fatigue, as measured by patient self-report. The severity, pattern, and quality of fatigue are clinically significant findings that can contribute to the identification of an underlying etiology. In mild anemia, fatigue such as exertional dyspnea or lack of endurance may only manifest upon activity. With increasing severity of fatigue as hemoglobin levels drop, patients may report an inability to engage in activities of daily living (ADLs). Several fatigue severity scales that provide a rapid assessment of fatigue-related impairments have been validated in numerous research studies and are readily available for clinicians (Meek et al., 2000; Naschitz et al., 2004; Stouten, 2005). An example of one such fatigue scale, the Brief Fatigue Inventory, is shown in Figure 63–3 ■.

In addition to fatigue, physical manifestations of anemia can be grossly attributed to two major processes (Chart 63–2, p. 2012). The primary insult (hypoxia due to low erythrocyte volume) inflicts its own symptoms, whereas a secondary group of symptoms may arise from the body's attempt to compensate for the hypoxia. While every body system requires oxygen and, thus, is affected by anemia, the most notable evidence of hypoxia due to low erythrocyte volume can be observed in the cardiovascular system, the respiratory system, and in severe cases the neurological system (Lewis, Wallis, Leya, Hursting, & Kelton, 2003. Montoya et al., 2002):

1. **Cardiovascular system manifestations of anemia**—With mild anemia most patients may not report noticeable cardiovascular changes other than mildly increased fatigue. In moderate cases, the heart and vasculature system will attempt to compensate for decreased oxygen density by increasing the pulse rate (tachycardia). Sustained hypoxia or severe anemia can overcome the cardiovascular system, resulting in angina or even acute myocardial infarction.

2. **Respiratory system manifestations of anemia**—Anemic patients may present with varying degrees of respiratory difficulty. With mild cases of anemia, patients may experience exertional dyspnea or orthopnea.

3. **Neurological system manifestations of anemia**—Mild anemia typically does not result in neurological compromise. However, as hemoglobin levels drop and hypoxia increases (as in severe hemoglobin deficiency), patients may report headache, difficulty concentrating, vertigo, irritability, and eventually confusion.

Compensatory Mechanisms

In addition to the clinical presentation that results from hypoxia directly, nurses also must be aware of the manifestation of compensatory mechanisms. Biochemical detection of hypoxia in the bloodstream triggers a series of adaptive physiological compensatory mechanisms designed to slow organ damage. Despite the efficacy of these compensatory mechanisms, the reader should note that the oxygen requirements of tissues do not decrease over time. Hence, prolonged anemia and hypoxia can result in irreversible tissue damage if left unresolved. Immediately upon the detection of hypoxia, the body adapts with the following four processes:

1. **Decreased hemoglobin oxygen affinity**—Oxygen-starved, hypoxic peripheral tissues extract hemoglobin-bound oxygen from blood at high rates. Recall from the hemoglobin discussion earlier in the chapter that the configuration of the hemoglobin chains determines oxygen-binding capacity. Furthermore, the geometric configuration is driven by a number of environmental factors. Hypoxia creates an environment that causes the hemoglobin to form into an arrangement referred to as the **deoxyhemoglobin** configuration (Figure 63–4 ■, p. 2012).

   The result of this configuration is twofold. First, the heme iron atoms have a low binding affinity for oxygen, meaning that an oxygen (O_2) molecule is less likely to remain bound to the hemoglobin of an RBC. Secondly, the deoxyhemoglobin configuration stimulates the production of **2,3-diphosphoglycerate (2,3-DPG)**, which ultimately works to sustain the deoxyhemoglobin configuration. Both processes result in increased oxygen release to surrounding tissues. This process results in a *shift to the right,* a phrase used to summarize a graphical illustration of hemoglobin oxygen

Brief Fatigue Inventory

STUDY ID# _____   HOSPITAL # _____

Date: _____/_____/_____   **Time:** _____

Name: _____   _____   _____
                     Last   First   Middle Initial

Throughout our lives, most of us have times when we feel very tired or fatigued. Have you felt unusually tired or fatigued in the past week?   Yes [   ]   No [   ]

1. Please rate your fatigue (weariness, tiredness) by circling the one number that best describes your fatigue right now.

0	1	2	3	4	5	6	7	8	9	10
No Fatigue										As bad as you can imagine

2. Please rate your fatigue (weariness, tiredness) by circling the one number that best describes your usual level of fatigue during the past 24 hours.

0	1	2	3	4	5	6	7	8	9	10
No Fatigue										As bad as you can imagine

3. Please rate your fatigue (weariness, tiredness) by circling the one number that best describes your worst level of fatigue during past 24 hours.

0	1	2	3	4	5	6	7	8	9	10
No Fatigue										As bad as you can imagine

4. Circle the one number that describes how, during the past 24 hours, fatigue has interfered with your:

A. General activity

0	1	2	3	4	5	6	7	8	9	10
Does not interfere										Completely Interferes

B. Mood

0	1	2	3	4	5	6	7	8	9	10
Does not interfere										Completely Interferes

C. Walking ability

0	1	2	3	4	5	6	7	8	9	10
Does not interfere										Completely Interferes

D. Normal work (includes both work outside the home and daily chores at home)

0	1	2	3	4	5	6	7	8	9	10
Does not interfere										Completely Interferes

E. Relations with other people

0	1	2	3	4	5	6	7	8	9	10
Does not interfere										Completely Interferes

F. Enjoyment of life

0	1	2	3	4	5	6	7	8	9	10
Does not interfere										Completely Interferes

FIGURE 63–3 ■ Brief Fatigue Inventory scale.

saturation as a function of oxygen partial pressure (Figure 63–5 ■, p. 2012). In cases of decreased hemoglobin oxygen affinity, any given partial pressure of oxygen is associated with less oxygen saturating the hemoglobin molecule. This translates to more unbound oxygen available to tissues, an effective short-term compensatory mechanism against hypoxia.

2. **Cardiovascular compensation**—In cases of severe anemia (measured by hemoglobin <7 g/dL), the resulting tissue hypoxia triggers cardiovascular compensation. First the cardiac output increases in an effort to circulate more blood. This increased heart rate is matched by a decrease in peripheral vasculature resistance to first allow blood to flow

CHART 63–2 **Common Signs of Anemia**

- Abnormal paleness or lack of color of the skin
- Increased heart rate (tachycardia)
- Increased respiratory rate (tachypnea)
- Breathlessness, or difficulty catching a breath (dyspnea)
- Lack of energy, or tiring easily (fatigue)
- Dizziness, or vertigo, especially when standing
- Headache
- Irritability
- Decreased hemoglobin, decreased hematocrit, decreased RBCs

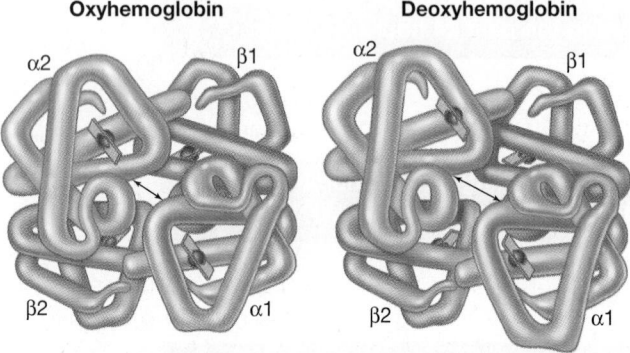

Oxyhemoglobin   **Deoxyhemoglobin**

FIGURE 63–4 ■ Hemoglobin and deoxyhemoglobin, the oxygen transporter.

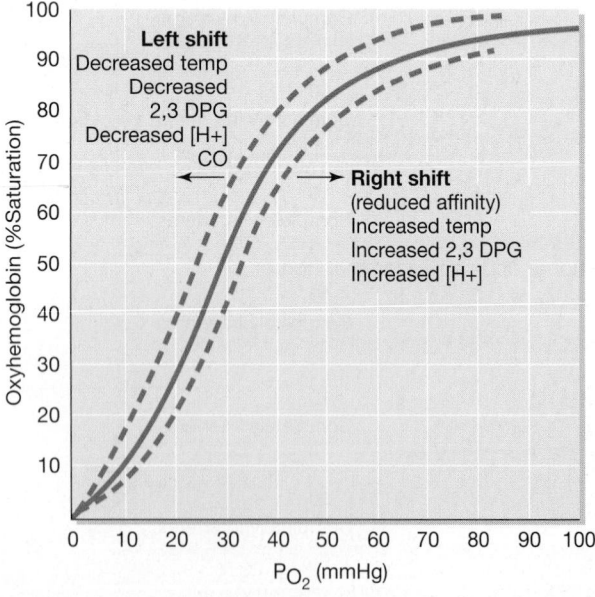

FIGURE 63–5 ■ Deoxyhemoglobin curve.

more quickly and then to reduce the oxygen demands of the heart muscle.

3. **Redistribution of blood flow**—Another compensatory mechanism is redistribution of blood flow. In hypoxic anemic states, the body selectively vasoconstricts blood vessels to reroute oxygenated blood toward certain vital organs and away from less critical areas. Blood is shunted away from skin and toward the heart and brain and other critical organs. While this shunting preserves "critical organs" as long as possible, oxygen deprivation in the "less critical" organs can result in intermittent claudication and pain.

4. **Increased erythropoietin to stimulate RBC production**—Of interesting note, during the redistribution of blood flow, selective vasoconstriction shunts blood away from the kidneys, which are hardly noncritical organs. However, detection of hypoxia by the kidneys results in increased production of erythropoietin. Recall from the earlier discussion that erythropoietin is the critical cytokine that triggers erythropoiesis, which ultimately increases RBC mass. Thus, the shunting of blood away from the kidneys is an adaptive attempt at long-term resolution of anemia.

Care of the patient with anemia first requires resolution of hypoxia. Left unresolved, hypoxia can become a life-threatening medical emergency as critical organs are deprived of oxygen, instigating a cascade of cellular breakdown, tissue damage, organ failure, and possibly death. (See Chapter 35 ⊘ for care of acute hypoxia.) If the hypoxia is associated with active and significant blood loss, an additional emergent priority is often the replacement of blood volume to attain erythrocyte levels sufficient to sustain oxygen delivery, as discussed later in the Anemia from Acute Blood Loss section.

In otherwise healthy patients without underlying hematologic disorders, these emergency interventions resolve not only the hypoxia, but the anemia as well. After stabilizing the cardiovascular, respiratory, and neurological risks of emergent hypoxia and blood loss, the focus shifts to determining the underlying cause of the anemia, usually via laboratory studies and a thorough history. Specific treatments and nursing interventions then are tailored to the underlying disease process. These specific treatments and nursing interventions are discussed later in relationship to each classification of anemia. However, some signs and symptoms and their correlating nursing interventions are common to all forms of anemia. These are discussed in the Nursing Process: Patient Care Plan for Generalized Anemia. When elderly patients are involved, the nurse should be aware of additional considerations, as outlined in the Gerontological Considerations box (p. 2015). The use of herbal supplements for the treatment of the fatigue that accompanies anemia is discussed in the Complementary and Alternative Therapies box (p. 2014).

Nursing Management

Nursing care for the patient presenting with anemia focuses on two goals: prevention of complications secondary to decreased oxygen-carrying capacity and thorough assessment to identify underlying etiologies. Decreased oxygen-carrying capacity carries the immediate risks associated with hypoxia: neurological and cardiac insults. Patients also frequently report activity intolerance and fatigue with sustained hypoxia, both of which must be addressed to prevent cardiovascular, respiratory, musculoskeletal, and digestive side effects.

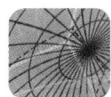

NURSING PROCESS: Patient Care Plan for Generalized Anemia

Assessment of Fatigue

Subjective Data:
Have you been short of breath? How long?
Do you have difficulty with energy throughout your day?
What makes it worse? What makes it better?
Do you have difficulty tolerating activity? Do you have difficulty with everyday chores?

Objective Data:
General: pallor, malaise, fatigue (preferably use validated scale)
Neurological: level of alertness, mental acuity
Respiratory: dyspnea, ventilation depth, tachypnea
Cardiovascular: tachycardia
Laboratory values: alterations to CBC

Nursing Assessment and Diagnoses	Outcomes and Evaluation Parameters	Planning and Interventions with *Rationales*
Nursing Diagnoses: *Activity Intolerance* related to decreased oxygen delivery to neuromuscular and cardiovascular systems	**Outcomes:** Free of shortness of breath. Able to perform ADLs. *Evaluation Parameters:* Patient self-report of lack of dyspnea upon exertion. Patient report of subjective decrease in bothersome fatigue effects as measured by fatigue scale scores. Unlabored respirations <24/min.	**Interventions and *Rationales:*** Assess normal activity pattern throughout day *in preparation for activity modification techniques (see below).* Provide assistance with activities *to minimize shortness of breath.*
Self-Care Deficit related to fatigue and weakness impacting ability to participate in ADLs	**Outcome:** Patient reports appropriate self-care techniques. *Evaluation Parameters:* Patient/family verbalizes or demonstrates plan for accommodating self-care activities. Patient able to perform ADLs at a developmentally appropriate level. Patient demonstrates energy conservation techniques such as activity planning, appropriate exertion levels, and assistive devices as needed.	**Interventions and *Rationales:*** Modify activities to coincide with patient's biologic energy cycles. *Patients should maintain a minimum level of activity to prevent cardiovascular and muscoskeletal decompensation. However, patients may be discouraged by fatigue. Planning activities at points in the day with normally higher energy levels maintains patient participation in activity.*
Deficient Knowledge related to dietary causes, underlying etiologies, and patient self-management techniques	**Outcome:** Patient demonstrates knowledge of appropriate dietary modifications if indicated, lifestyle changes, and self-management techniques. *Evaluation Parameters:* Patient reports knowledge of diet modification (increased iron, folate, vitamin B_{12}) if appropriate. Patient demonstrates plan to incorporate appropriate activity level into daily care. Patient verbalizes understanding of underlying causes of anemia and fatigue.	**Interventions and *Rationales:*** Determine patient's previous knowledge of or skills related to his or her diagnosis and the influence on willingness to learn. *New information is assimilated into previous assumptions and facts and may involve negotiating, transforming, or stalling.* Provide developmentally appropriate patient education that addresses underlying disease process, diet modification, medications, and activity modification. *Symptoms of anemia may require long-term management that is optimized by patient compliance.*

Assessment of Hypoxia

Subjective Data:
Do you feel short of breath? Do you have chest pain?
Do other areas of your body ache? How often?
Do you feel dizzy?

Objective Data:
Dyspnea
Decreased O_2 saturation
Tachycardia
Tachypnea

Decreased hemoglobin and hematocrit
Dizziness
Cyanosis
Hepatomegaly/splenomegaly

(continued)

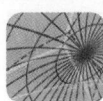

NURSING PROCESS: Patient Care Plan for Generalized Anemia—*Continued*

Nursing Assessment and Diagnoses	Outcomes and Evaluation Parameters	Planning and Interventions with *Rationales*
Nursing Diagnoses: *Impaired Gas exchange* related to insufficient hemoglobin oxygen delivery system, which can progress to cardiovascular, respiratory, neurological, and metabolic alterations	**Outcome:** Blood morphology and chemistry return to patient baseline. **Evaluation Parameters:** Hematocrit: • *Males:* 40.7–50.3% • *Females:* 36.1–44.3%. Hemoglobin: • *Males:* 13.8–17.2 g/dL • *Females:* 12.1–15.1 g/dL. RBC count: • *Males:* 4.7–6.1 million cells/µL • *Females:* 4.2–5.4 million cells/µL. ABG PaO_2: <90 ± 10. ABG pH: 7.35–7.45. Spot O_2 sat: <90% (depending on concurrent respiratory disease and age).	**Interventions and *Rationales:*** Monitor oxygen saturation levels and ABGs *as indicators of hypoxemia.* Administer supplemental oxygen when indicated *to maximize hemoglobin delivery of oxygen. However, use only when indicated by lab values. Hyperoxygenation suppresses erythropoiesis.* Administer blood transfusions for severe cases of anemia when ordered *to correct emergency deficiencies in oxygen delivery capacity.* Monitor for signs such as a falling hematocrit level, pain, pulmonary edema, fever, hypotension, hemolysis *as indicators of transfusion reactions (hemolysis and fluid overload).*
Risk of Injury: Falls related to weakness, dizziness, and possible compromised mental acuity	**Outcome:** Patient remains free of injury from falls. **Evaluation Parameters:** Patient experiences no injuries from falling. Environment is adjusted to minimize risk of falls. Patient verbalizes understanding of and demonstrates compliance with fall risk reduction plan.	**Interventions and *Rationales:*** Monitor for risk factors from falls such as unsteady gait, difficulty with transfers, orthopnea *to identify physiological and behavioral indicators of fall risk.* Adjust environment to minimize risk of falls by placing necessary items within reach of patient, positioning bed in low and locked position, frequent observation in an effort *to reduce additional risks of falls.* Reinforce patient instruction to call for assistance with ambulation if indicated *to avoid injury.* Assess vital signs (pulse, respirations, and BP) prior to ambulation *to identify possible need to alter mobility plan.*

Thorough assessments provide insight into the underlying etiology of anemia. Nurses are responsible for close monitoring of patient symptoms, alterations in laboratory values, and physical changes that may indicate the source of decreasing erythrocyte volume. Once these etiologies have been identified, the nurse, as part of the interdisciplinary health care team, is responsible for initiating interventions unique to that diagnosis.

The Nursing Process: Patient Care Plan for Generalized Anemia summarizes the interventions and rationales appropriate for patients presenting with initial signs and symptoms of anemia. This care plan is then enhanced with the nursing care indicated for specific underlying etiologies, which are discussed throughout the chapter.

COMPLEMENTARY & ALTERNATIVE THERAPIES

Herbal Supplements

Patients frequently seek out herbal supplements for the treatment of fatigue. The benefits of "energy boosters" are highly touted in the advertising for over-the-counter (OTC) preparations. Some patients who seek a more judicious integration of herbal and complementary medicine may enlist the care of a certified practitioner in complementary medicine, whereas others may rely solely on the advertising associated with OTC preparations.

Common herbs used for anemia include Spirulina, or blue-green algae (Mao, Van De Water, & Gershwin, 2000), alfalfa (*Medicago sativa*), dandelion (*Taraxacum officinale*) root or leaf, burdock (*Arctium lappa*), yellowdock (*Rumex crispus*), and dong quai (*Angelica sinensis*) (Blumenthal, 1999). If patients seek out homeopathic therapy, they may be prescribed ferrum phosphoricum or calcarea phosphorica. In addition to herbs, many patients may self-administer vitamins and minerals such as vitamin B_{12}, folic acid, and, most commonly, iron.

Many patients hold the common perception that herbs are natural and, therefore, inherently benign, however, many herbs can interact with traditionally prescribed medications or, if taken inappropriately, inflict untoward effects. The use of herbs, supplements, and vitamins should always be included and integrated into a thorough patient care plan.

References

Blumenthal, M. (1999). Twenty-seven major botanicals and their uses in the United States. In D. Eskinazi, M. Blumenthal, N. Farnsworth, & C. W. Riggins (Eds.), *Botanical medicine* (pp. 18–19). Larchmont, NY: Mary Ann Liebert.

Mao, T. K., Van De Water, J., & Gershwin, M. E. (2000). Effect of Spirulina on the secretion of cytokines from peripheral blood mononuclear cells. *Journal of Medicinal Food, 3*(3), 135–139.

GERONTOLOGICAL CONSIDERATIONS for Anemia

The frail elderly adult is at increased risk of anemia for several reasons ranging from the physiological changes associated with aging and the prevalence of comorbidities to nutritional deficiencies and sometimes the psychosocial consequences of aging. Agreement surrounding the prevalence of anemia in the older adult varies greatly, perhaps due to inconsistencies in the reporting of anemia. The most comprehensive study to date has been the third *National Health and Nutrition Examination Survey (NHANES) 1988–1994* (National Center for Health Statistics, 2008), which evaluated anemia in the community-dwelling adult. In persons 65 years and older, anemia was present in 11.0% of men and 10.2% of women, with the prevalence rising to more than 20% in people 85 years and older.

Nutritional deficiencies account for a large portion of anemia seen in older adults due in part to decreased appetite and difficulty in chewing. However, social processes such as meal preparation and financial constraints also may negatively impact an older adult's ability to consistently consume a well-balanced diet. Comorbidities such as cardiovascular disease, lung disease, cancer, and kidney failure can also negatively impact anemia by their effects on the organs of erythropoiesis, namely, the bone marrow and the erythropoietin-stimulating system of the kidneys. Perhaps most damaging to the effective treatment of anemia in the older adult is the unfortunate practice of dismissing patient reports of decreasing activity intolerance as a "normal part of aging." Although some decline in endurance and cardiovascular capacity may occur with age, symptoms such as ataxia, worsening angina, severe dyspnea, and certainly abnormal laboratory studies warrant further evaluation.

The consequences of anemia in the older adult have been associated with significant morbidities, further highlighting the need for vigilance. Anemia late in life has been correlated with increased rate of falls (Penninx et al., 2005), decreased muscle strength (Penninx et al., 2005), and a higher rate of hip fractures requiring surgery and increased length of stay (Dharmarajan, Pais, & Norkus, 2005). Tachycardia due to the compensatory mechanisms in sustained anemia also has been correlated with increased mortality. In chronic kidney failure in the older adult, sustained decreased hematocrit levels have been associated with left ventricular hypertrophy, increased morbidity and mortality, and poor quality of life (Lipschitz, 2003). The nurse plays a vital role in patient advocacy as part of providing adequate and unbiased care to the older adult.

Discharge Priorities

Management of anemia needs to continue after hospital discharge and may require long-term lifestyle and dietary change. It is essential that the patient and family be given the necessary information to make these changes. The Patient Teaching & Discharge Priorities box (p. 2016) outlines important information that should be conveyed to patients with generalized anemia.

Health Promotion

Treatment of anemia often involves lifestyle alterations to diet and activity level. Part of the assessment of the patient with anemia must include an evaluation of nutrition intake, especially iron, folate, vitamin B_{12}, and proteins because these are all required for erythropoiesis. Nurses play a critical role in helping patients identify dietary sources of these vital nutrients. The sections on iron deficiency anemia, folate deficiency anemia, and vitamin B_{12} anemia provide specific information about a diet that will provide these nutrients.

Activity level also must be addressed as part of a complete patient care plan. Anemia frequently is associated with fatigue and dyspnea, which may suppress a patient's ability to participate in ADLs or to maintain prior physical activity levels. However, mobility and exercise should be maintained to prevent cardiovascular and musculoskeletal deconditioning. If either of these two processes occurs, patients may run the risk of further exacerbating their fatigue and dyspnea. Nurses again play a pivotal role in assisting patients in identifying appropriate activity goals and incorporating activity into the daily patient care plan.

Collaborative Management

Comprehensive care of the patient with anemia requires the collaboration of an interdisciplinary team including registered dieticians, physical and occupational therapists, respiratory therapists, pharmacists, health care providers, and nurses. Registered dieticians can provide excellent resources to patients on how to identify and treat dietary deficiencies that exacerbate anemia and how to conserve energy when preparing meals. Additionally, the scientific grounding of the registered dietician can help patients evaluate the numerous health benefits claimed in food advertising.

Respiratory therapists are identified experts in the diagnosis of hypoxia, especially in delineating anemic hypoxia from hypoxia of respiratory etiology. Their expertise is particularly valuable when evaluating the judicious use of oxygen therapy. Physical and occupational therapists play a key role in mobility preservation. Consultation with a physical and occupational therapist should be made early (within a few days of admission) so that exercise techniques can be incorporated early on before debilitating severe anemia takes hold. Some studies have even indicated that early mobility can actually act as a preventive measure, increasing the need for collaboration with physical and occupational therapists (Mock, 2004). The pharmacist's knowledge of pharmacokinetics and drug–drug and drug–food interactions is of tremendous benefit to a patient care plan and their guidance should be sought whenever medications are to be evaluated or prescribed.

Anemia from Acute Blood Loss

Anemia from acute blood loss describes the loss of RBC volume due to RBCs leaving the circulating vascular space. Anemia from blood loss comprises a heterogeneous group of disorders ranging from "slow bleeds" to rapid trauma. Appropriate care of these patients focuses on determination of the underlying cause, prevention of immediate cardiovascular and hematologic emergencies, and, if appropriate, attenuation of underlying disease.

Pathophysiology and Etiology

When discussing the mechanisms responsible for anemia due to blood loss, three parameters should be included: underlying cause, rapidity of onset, and volume lost. Underlying causes include obvious bleeding such as trauma or menorrhagia (excessive menstrual bleeding) as well as less visible causes such as disorders of the gastrointestinal mucosa, slow cranial bleeding, and internal hemorrhage. Nurses should not rely solely on visible blood as an indication of bleeding, and instead should be aware of the system clinical presentation of blood loss, as discussed later. Bleeding that

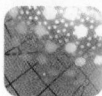

PATIENT TEACHING & DISCHARGE PRIORITIES for Generalized Anemia

Need	Teaching
Knowledge of dietary modifications	Of particular importance in iron deficiency anemia and megaloblastic anemias. Consult with registered dietitian to provide patient and family with effective tools and resources regarding meal planning, appropriate foods, and guidance on food label reading.
	Teach patients to eat frequent small meals to prevent fatigue.
Fatigue management	Reinforce teaching regarding daily fatigue scale.
	Teach patients to discuss results and trends of fatigue scale self-assessment with health care provider.
	Reinforce teaching regarding activity modification to maintain and preserve energy levels.
	Reinforce teaching that energy levels may decrease as a physiological response to disease process, and that asking for assistance and/or adjusting previous work/home activity schedules may be necessary.
	Suggest appropriate exercise activities for patient status including brief walks, chair exercises, bed exercises.
	Reinforce education regarding mobility as an effective means of prevention of cardiovascular and musculoskeletal deconditioning.
Understanding of medications	For iron supplementation, teach patients correct timing of administration and possible side effects (constipation). Reinforce key teaching points regarding hydration, constipation management, and iron absorption (see Chart 63–7, p. 2022).
	For hematopoietic growth factors, reinforce administration schedule for subcutaneous injections, which may include appointments with health care provider.
	Reinforce education regarding possible side effects of subcutaneous hematopoietic growth factors including bone pain and injection site soreness.
Disease prevention	Explain the need for maintenance of hemoglobin levels to ensure adequate oxygenation to tissues, thus decreasing risk of cardiac disease and infection.
Safety	Stress the importance of a medic alert bracelet to identify a heart problem to health care providers.
Reportable clinical manifestations	Instruct patient/family to report: • Change in exercise tolerance • Change in activity tolerance • Onset of new pain especially chest pain, headaches, or abdominal pain.

results from chronic conditions including Crohn's disease, diverticulitis, and rheumatoid arthritis frequently is associated with inflammation; this causes a functional iron deficiency and thus anemia. This syndrome is discussed in the Anemia of Chronic Disease section.

The rapidity of the blood loss impacts the body's ability to respond with compensatory mechanisms, which, in turn, relates to clinical presentation. With slow bleeds, which occur over the course of days to weeks, baroreceptors in the peripheral vascular system detect decreased pressure and respond by increasing plasma volume to preserve cardiovascular status. With this increase in volume, the heart and vascular system can generate enough blood pressure to maintain peripheral perfusion in the critical organs of the heart, lungs, brain, and kidneys. This process can result in a form of dilution anemia, in which the RBC mass is diluted by the increase in plasma volume. Hypoxia from this dilutional anemia is prevented by the compensatory mechanisms discussed earlier, including decreased hemoglobin oxygen affinity (shift to the right) and increased erythropoietin to stimulate RBC production. When the blood loss is rapid, occurring over the course of hours to days, total blood volume (including both RBCs and plasma) can decrease so severely as to cause hypovolemic shock. Hypovolemic shock is a medical emergency associated with high mortality and requires immediate emergency management interventions (see Chapter 61).

The third consideration is the total volume lost. With blood losses of up to 20% of total blood volume (Adamson, 2005), the compensatory mechanism of peripheral vasoconstriction initiates to shift blood flow to organs responsible for maintaining cardiovascular function and preventing hypoxia and hypovolemia. When blood loss becomes more pronounced, the body lacks sufficient circulating blood volume to support the vascular system or maintain adequate hydration and oxygenation of vital organs. The body's first attempt is to intensify cardiovascular compensatory mechanisms (tachycardia). However, with blood loss of at least 40% or more, all compensatory mechanisms become rapidly overwhelmed and symptoms of shock are imminent.

Clinical Presentation

Clinical presentation of the patient with blood loss is directly correlated to the *rapidity, location,* and *volume* of blood loss. Thorough assessment must include laboratory hematologic findings as well as cardiovascular measurements (pulse, blood pressure, and respiratory rate), integumentary signs (pallor, temperature, and diaphoresis), and renal and neurological changes. The action of multiple compensatory mechanisms may mask signs of anemia unless a multifaceted assessment is completed.

Physical Manifestations

Patients suspected of acute blood loss should be thoroughly monitored for changes in cardiovascular, integumentary, renal, and neurological status. These changes are summarized in the Nursing Process: Patient Care Plan for Generalized Anemia (p. 2013) and include tachycardia, tachypnea, decreased level of alertness, pallor, decreased urinary output, and diaphoresis. These start to become apparent with acute, rapid blood loss or when slow blood loss exceeds 20% of baseline. Additionally, bleeds of relatively small volume (i.e., less than 20%) into closed spaces can cause severe pain, swelling, tenderness, sudden changes in neurological status, and eventually death. Bleeding into the cranial vault, the pericardium, the pleural space, or musculoskeletal compartments is a medical emergency that requires prompt attention by the medical team. Please refer to specific chapters addressing these systems for a full discussion.

Bleeding into the gastrointestinal (GI) tract is often first detected via an observation of fecal occult blood, or hidden blood, in the stool. Fecal occult blood tests are cost-effective and rapid indicators of GI bleeding and, thus, are widely used as screening tools. **Melena**, or black tarry stools, appears when bacteria have had enough time to break down blood into component chemicals. In the case of lower GI bleeding, blood may not be in the colon long enough for bacterial breakdown; therefore, the presence of melena should not be the only indicator used to detect GI bleeding.

Alterations in Laboratory Values

For sudden blood loss, hematocrit values may not accurately indicate the severity of the problem because RBC mass is lost at the same rate as total blood volume; thus, the percentage of RBCs in the blood is unaffected. (Recall that hematocrit measures the percentage of RBCs in a volume of blood.) However, after 2 to 3 days when the body is able to initiate the compensatory mechanism of increasing plasma volume, RBCs become diluted, as reflected by decreasing erythrocyte, hemoglobin, and hematocrit values (Chart 63–3).

 CRITICAL ALERT *Any patient reporting with sudden pain in the abdominal area, retroperitoneal area, or musculoskeletal fascial compartments or a change in level of consciousness should be immediately assessed for blood pressure, pulse, and respiratory rate changes. These may indicate bleeding into a closed space, which requires immediate medical intervention. Do not rely on changes in laboratory values because these may not accurately reflect blood loss.*

Medical Management

The immediate goal of treatment for acute blood loss is prevention of cardiovascular collapse and hypoxia. Most patients presenting with slow bleeds also have normal kidney function, normal bone marrow function, and an adequate supply of iron. For these patients, the increased erythropoietin production is sufficient to compensate for lost RBCs; thus, additional treatment with blood products is unwarranted. Attention then turns to identification of the underlying disease process and attenuation of the blood loss. A thorough history will assist the clinician in identifying possible causes such as GI bleeding from intake of nonsteroidal inflammatory drugs (NSAIDs). Transfusion of red blood cells may be indicated for some patients to prevent cardiovascular system collapse. These patients are identified by a sudden decrease in hematocrit by more than 3%, significant observable hemorrhage, a hematocrit of <25%, or severe impending hypovolemia.

■ Nursing Management

Nursing priorities in the care of patients suspected of acute blood loss are multifaceted, evolving with the degree of blood loss and stage of treatment. The first goal is careful observation for early indicators of blood loss, especially in patients who present with high-risk diagnoses. Postoperative patients are at particular risk

---

CHART 63–3 Signs and Symptoms of Acute Blood Loss

% Blood Loss	Approximate Volume in Adult (5,000 mL [79 kg])	Symptoms	Physical Syndrome	Measurable Signs
<20	<1,000	Possible restlessness	Vasovagal reaction (peripheral vasoconstriction)	BP may be normal HR may be normal Urine output may be normal
20–30	1,000–1,500	Anxiety, dyspnea on exertion	Orthostatic hypotension, tachycardia on exertion	BP > 90 mmHg systolic HR 100–120 bpm RR > 24 Urine output 25–30 mL/hr
30–40	1,500–2,000	Syncope on sitting and standing	Orthostatic hypotension, tachcarydia at rest	BP 70–90 systolic HR > 120 beats/min Cool, pale skin RR increased Urine output 5–15 mL/hr
40	>2,000	Confusion, shortness of breath	Shock	BP < 90 systolic HR > 140 beats/min Cold, clammy skin RR increased/hyperventilation Urine output minimal

Sources: Adapted from Gosch, S., Watts, D., & Kinnear, M. (2002). Management of gastrointestinal hemorrhage. *Postgraduate Medical Journal, 78*(915), 4; Green, B. T., & Rockey, D. C. (2003). Acute gastrointestinal bleeding. *Seminars in Gastrointestinal Disease, 14*(2), 44. Kasper, D. L., Fauci, A. S., Longo, D. L., Braunwald, E., Hauser, S. L., & Jameson, J. L. (Eds.), *Harrison's principles of internal medicine* (16th ed.). New York: McGraw-Hill.

of bleeding from new incisions (both internal and external) and should be carefully monitored for changes in level of consciousness, cardiovascular changes from baseline, excessive blood loss from incision sites, and reports of pain.

Other high-risk populations include but are not limited to patients presenting with abdominal pain of known or unknown etiology, patients with musculoskeletal trauma, and patients with deficient platelet function. Monitoring of these patients should involve comprehensive assessment of hematologic laboratory studies, trends in urine output, trends in cardiovascular indicators (blood pressure, pulse, and respirations), integumentary changes, pain descriptions, and musculoskeletal changes.

If transfusions are administered, nursing goals revolve around the safe administration of blood products and monitoring for signs and symptoms of fluid overload or a transfusion reaction, both of which are discussed later in this chapter in the section on transfusion therapy (also see Chapter 23). Once the source of the blood loss is identified, nursing interventions, including patient education, assessment, and treatment administration, become specific to the underlying disease process. Generally, once the source of blood loss is identified and resolved, no further treatment of anemia due to acute blood loss is warranted.

Iron Deficiency Anemia

Iron deficiency anemia (IDA) is the most common underlying cause of anemia worldwide. Although iron deficiency is more common in developing countries, a significant prevalence was observed in the United States during the early 1990s among certain populations, such as toddlers and females of childbearing age. One of the national *Healthy People 2010* objectives is to reduce iron deficiency in these vulnerable populations by 3% to 4% (U.S. Department of Health and Human Services, 2000).

Recall from the discussion on hematopoiesis that iron is required for the heme portion of the hemoglobin protein. Thus, erythrocyte production is slowed when iron-dependent hemoglobin supplies are depleted or insufficient. The erythrocytes that are produced are morphologically distinct because of their small size (**microcytic**) and pale color (**hypochromic**). Signs and symptoms of anemia appear when iron supplies are depleted to the point that the physiological needs of erythropoiesis cannot be met. Depletion of iron stores can be a result of a variety of underlying causes including dietary intake insufficiency,

blood loss, or malabsorption disorders. The responsibilities of the health care provider are to first address any immediate needs of anemia such as hypoxia, then to determine and correct the underlying cause of the iron deficiency.

Iron Metabolism

Alterations in iron metabolism have consequences in many forms of anemia, including iron deficiency anemia, anemia of chronic disease, thalassemia, and hemolytic spherocytosis. Estimates of total iron body stores in healthy adults vary from 2.5 to 4.5 grams in women, to 3.5 to 5.5 grams in men. International differences in body size and normal values account for the variation in commonly reported values.

Iron is distributed throughout the body in both active metabolic forms and storage forms. Hemoglobin typically houses 2,100 mg of iron, representing the most significant active metabolic form. Other active forms include myoglobin (200 mg); metabolic tissues of the liver, spleen, and bone marrow (150 mg); and the iron transportation system (3 mg). Iron also exists in two "storage forms" within cells, as **ferritin** (700 mg) and **hemosiderin** (300 mg). These storage forms are metabolically inactive, meaning they do not directly contribute to erythropoiesis, oxygen transport, or immune or neurological function; rather they act like iron reservoirs.

Approximately 1 mg of iron is lost on a daily basis from a variety of mechanisms, namely, via cell **desquamation**, or the shedding of the outer epidermal layer. To maintain bodily functions, the body requires about 25 mg daily, which is partially derived through dietary absorption (1 mg) via the intestines. However, the majority of the daily iron requirement is supplied from the storage forms (Koury & Ponka, 2004; Miret, Simpson, & McKie, 2003; Umbreit, 2005; Weiss, 2002). For this reason, serum ferritin is commonly included in the analysis of IDA.

As iron is consumed, it is absorbed via the intestinal cells of the duodenum and jejunum and immediately forms a complex with iron transport proteins, namely, **transferrin**, which delivers the iron molecule to the target cells (growing erythrocytes, placenta cells, liver cells, spleen, and bone marrow). The amount of transferrin-bound iron is commonly used for measurement of iron levels. Iron molecules that will not be immediately used for erythropoiesis are converted to the storage forms ferritin and hemosiderin (Chart 63–4).

The rate of intestinal cell absorption is regulated by physiological needs. Absorption *increases* with decreased iron stores,

CHART 63–4	**Key Chemicals of Iron Metabolism**	
Chemical	**Function**	**Physiological Consequences**
Ferritin	Storage form	Used as measurement of iron status. High ferritin level indicates adequate status.
Hemosiderin	Storage form	Measurement of iron status. High hemosiderin level indicates adequate status, although test is rarely performed due to prevalence of ferritin.
Transferrin	Delivers iron to target cell	High levels of iron-bound transferrin indicate adequate iron status.
Hepcidin	Hormone that regulates iron absorption	Inhibits iron absorption. Increases macrophage consumption of iron. Increases (stimulated by infection, inflammation, and malignancy) result in decreased iron available for erythropoiesis. Decreases cause iron overload.

detection of a low peripheral erythrocyte count, increased erythropoietic activity in the bone marrow (i.e., pregnancy, growth spurts), or hypoxemia. Conversely, intestinal iron absorption *decreases* in the presence of inflammation, a process that contributes to the "anemia of inflammation" or "anemia of chronic diseases" (Weiss, 2002). The body produces a variety of systemic signals (neurotransmitters, hormones, and cytokines) in response to these stimuli. **Hepcidin**, produced by the liver, has been identified as the key regulatory hormone of iron absorption, adjusting the rate of iron absorption in response to total iron body reservoirs. Although the exact molecular mechanism remains to be elucidated, an emerging current body of research suggests that these systemic signals act on the intestinal cells of the duodenum and jejunum to alter iron absorption through regulation of the iron transport proteins (Koury & Ponka, 2004; Miret et al., 2003).

Pathophysiology

Iron deficiency anemia results from a combination of one or more processes: (1) excess iron loss, (2) iron absorption abnormalities, (3) reallocation of iron stores, and (4) insufficient dietary intake. Excess iron loss, iron absorption abnormalities, and insufficient dietary intake are classified as **absolute iron deficiencies** indicating insufficient amounts of total body iron. Reallocation of iron stores is referred to as a **functional iron deficiency**, which is a condition in which there is a failure to supply enough iron to the bone marrow for erythropoiesis, despite adequate total body iron stores. Each of these etiologies is associated with some underlying behavioral or pathologic process:

1. **Excess iron loss**—Blood loss, and the iron housed in the hemoglobin, is the leading cause of iron deficiency (Ponka, 2001). Chronic blood loss is most commonly attributed to gastrointestinal bleeding. Causes of GI bleeding include peptic ulcer disease, diverticulitis, hemorrhoids, esophageal varices, tumors, steroids, small tears along the rectum, and use of NSAIDs (see Chapter 45 💿). Many of these processes can exist for long periods of time, evading detection by the patient and cumulatively allowing for a substantial loss of blood and iron. One milliliter of blood contains about 0.5 mg of iron. A steady blood loss of as little as 3 to 4 mL per day, which often goes undetected by the patient, results in 1.5 to 2 mg of lost iron daily. This loss places excess demand on daily iron needs, resulting in a negative iron balance. Menstrual bleeding, which typically results in 40 to 80 mL of daily blood loss, also is associated with iron deficiency anemia, in part explaining the prevalence of iron deficiency anemia (IDA) among women.

2. **Iron absorption abnormalities**—Iron absorption abnormalities refer to any clinical situation that decreases the rate of intestinal absorption. As discussed earlier, absorption relies on the intricate interplay between intestinal cells, systemic cell signals, the iron transport system, and the storage forms of iron. Gastrointestinal tract abnormalities, such as surgical manipulation, Crohn's disease, and celiac disease, reduce the intestinal wall surface available for iron absorption. Liver disease also can result in IDA because transferrin is synthesized in the liver and the storage forms (ferritin and hemosiderin) partially reside in the hepatic cells of the liver. Additionally, several studies are beginning to examine

IDA that stems from genetic alterations in the iron transport proteins and intestinal absorption systemic signals, specifically hepcidin (Koury & Ponka, 2004; Miret et al., 2003; Umbreit, 2005; Weiss, 2002).

3. **Reallocation of iron stores**—Reallocation of iron stores refers to situations in which total body iron supplies are at normal levels, but the iron molecule is unavailable for erythropoiesis. In chronic inflammatory conditions, available iron is preferentially allocated to increased macrophage production. Again, hepcidin has been identified as the key hormone regulating macrophage consumption of iron. In fetal development, iron also is preferentially delivered to the developing fetus; however, maternal erythropoiesis may be impacted.

4. **Insufficient dietary intake**—When any of the preceding situations occurs, demand for iron can exceed iron intake. Initially, the storage forms act as buffers to adequately supply the active metabolic needs of the body. The efficiency of the storage forms means that early iron deficiency often is asymptomatic and therefore goes unreported by the patient. Hemoglobin and erythrocyte values are only mildly decreased, if at all. However, serum ferritin values may decrease from normal. Eventually, however, depletion of the storage forms can quickly outpace dietary intake, and the serum ferritin concentration falls. Erythropoiesis is impaired, producing pale (hypochromic), small (microcytic) erythrocytes. The decreased oxygen delivery capacity of these impaired erythrocytes results in the signs and symptoms of anemia.

Clinical Presentation

Iron deficiency anemia can have an insidious progression, often with no reportable symptoms despite falling iron stores. As iron depletion proceeds, IDA produces the signs common to all anemias and eventually manifests with morphologic, neurological, and integumentary symptoms unique to iron depletion. A laboratory analysis will reveal both qualitative and quantitative changes to RBC components. Oftentimes, IDA is first detected in the primary care setting during routine physicals or when patients seek evaluation for bothersome symptoms. The U.S. Preventive Services Task Force (2006) and the Centers for Disease Control and Prevention (CDC) (1998) have both issued national guidelines to assist practitioners in the early identification and treatment of these patients in an effort to prevent severe negative outcomes related to iron deficiency (see the National Guidelines box, p. 2020). In the acute care setting, iron deficiency most often presents as a consequence of bleeding, decreased oral intake, or chronic disease.

Physical Manifestations

Because the body's highly efficient iron storage system provides a rich reservoir for active metabolic needs, early IDA often does not produce bothersome symptoms. As with all anemia, the severity of the symptoms correlates to the degree of hemoglobin deficiency, which, in turn, correlates to volume of total iron body stores. As erythropoiesis becomes increasingly hampered, the patient may present with the general manifestations of anemia such as fatigue, pallor, shortness of breath, cold intolerance, headache, and activity intolerance. When iron stores fall critically low such that epithelial cell production is affected, the patient may present

NATIONAL GUIDELINES for Screening for Iron Deficiency Anemia

Source	Recommended Guideline
U.S. Preventive Services Task Force (2006) Centers for Disease Control and Prevention (1998)	*Recommendation:* Routine screening for iron deficiency anemia in asymptomatic pregnant women *Recommendation:* Routine iron supplementation for asymptomatic children ages 6 to 12 months who are at increased risk for iron deficiency anemia *Recommendation:* Periodic screening for anemia among high-risk populations of infants and preschool children, pregnant women, and nonpregnant women of childbearing age *Recommendation:* Universal iron supplementation to meet the iron requirements of pregnancy.

with symptoms uniquely indicative of IDA including pica (clay eating), glossitis (tongue inflammation), gastric atrophy, stomatitis, ice eating (pagophagia), and leg cramping (Montoya et al., 2002). Presentation of any of these symptoms beginning with mild activity intolerance warrants further evaluation of iron status.

Alterations in Laboratory Values

Laboratory tests in IDA reveal decreased erythrocytes common to all anemias. Hemoglobin and hematocrit levels also decrease in accordance with the severity of anemia. Additionally, low iron in the heme produces morphologically distinct erythrocytes. The MCV, MCHC, and MCH morphological indices are all decreased indicating a microcytic (small), hypochromic (light) cell suggestive of IDA. These erythrocyte changes are shown in Figure 63–6 ■.

Definitive diagnosis requires bone marrow aspiration revealing absent marrow stores of iron. However, other laboratory findings are sufficient to begin treatment of IDA, most notably low serum iron, serum ferritin, and serum transferrin and an elevated total iron binding capacity (TIBC). Serum iron levels fall as total body iron decreases; however, this value is highly sensitive to recent changes in diet. A decrease in serum ferritin is a more accurate indicator of iron stores. Serum transferrin (also referred to as TIBC) increases as a compensatory attempt to harvest more iron from the intestines, thus its value *increases* in IDA. These laboratory findings are summarized in the Diagnostic Tests box.

Medical Management

Treatment of iron deficiency anemia addresses three goals: alleviation of immediate distress caused by anemia, identification of the underlying etiology, and replacement of iron, if indicated. Immediate distress of anemia includes hypoxia and activity intolerance as discussed in the earlier section on generalized ane-

mia. A comprehensive patient assessment should include GI symptoms, menstrual patterns, or dietary changes because these will assist the practitioner in identifying the underlying etiology.

Because the majority of chronic blood loss is due to GI bleeding, a fecal occult stool is often ordered especially in the absence of adolescent growth spurts, menses, and pregnancy. A fecal occult stool test is an important and cost-effective first step in early detection of GI bleeding, particularly since melena (dark tarry stool) requires a relatively large blood loss of 50 to 75 mL from the intestinal tract. More invasive exploratory procedures may be indicated to first determine the source of the bleeding (cancerous tumors, polyps, ulcers), and also to stop hemorrhage if detected.

Dietary Modifications

Replacement of iron stores is first attempted with dietary alterations (Chapter 14). Dietary iron is consumed in one of two forms: **heme iron**, which is available in red meats and fish, and **nonheme iron**, which is available in vegetables, cereals, and fortified foods. A significant chemical difference exists between the two forms that impact their utility in dietary medication. Heme iron is considered readily **bioavailable**, meaning that its molecular configuration is readily used in erythropoiesis. More importantly perhaps, heme iron is much better absorbed (15% absorption rate) in the intestinal tract than nonheme iron (<5% absorption rate). Lastly, heme iron is rarely reduced by the presence of other substances in the intestinal tract. Nonheme iron absorption, however, is reduced by tannins (found in tea), calcium, polyphenols, and phytates (found in legumes and whole grains). Ascorbic acid is the only common food element known to increase nonheme iron bioavailability.

Consideration of bioavailability and food–food interactions should be included in patient education about dietary modifications (Grinder-Pederson, Bukhave, Jensen, Hojgaard, & Hansen, 2004; Hunt, 2003; Lopez & Martos, 2004; Umbreit, 2005). A major focus of nutrition research is the study of the interaction between various food groups and iron absorption.

Oral Iron Supplementation

Iron supplementation may be indicated if dietary modification alone is insufficient to correct iron stores, especially in severe cases of iron deficiency anemia (serum ferritin level that falls >10 from baseline). Supplemental iron is available in two forms: ferrous and ferric. Ferrous iron salts (ferrous fumarate, ferrous sulfate, and ferrous gluconate) are the best absorbed forms of iron supplements (Hoffman et al., 2000). For adults who are not pregnant, the CDC

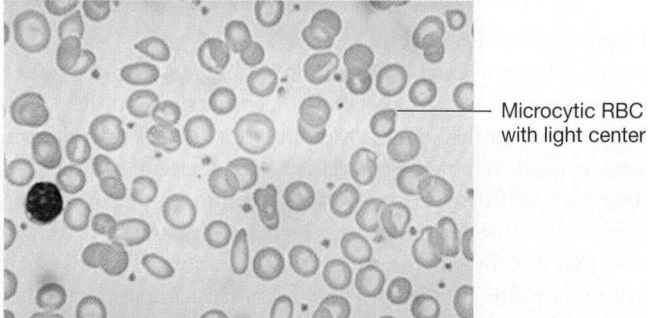

Microcytic RBC with light center

FIGURE 63–6 ■ Peripheral smear showing microcytic erthrocytes of IDA.
Source: Annita B. Watson

DIAGNOSTIC TESTS for Iron Deficiency Anemia

Test and Normal Values	Expected Abnormality in IDA	Rationale for Abnormality
Hemoglobin *Women:* 12–16 g/dL *Men:* 13.5–18 g/dL	Decreased	Early stages of IDA, hemoglobin will not be affected. In severe cases, low iron stores decrease hemoglobin production.
Hematocrit *Women:* 38–47% *Men:* 40–54%	Decreased	Decreased concentration of hemoglobin.
Serum Iron (Fe) *Women:* 63–140 µg/dL (11–25 µmol/L) *Men:* 75–150 µg/dL (13–27 µmol/L)	Decreased	Indicates decreased serum iron concentration. However, may be artificially increased by recent dietary ingestion or hemolytic states.
Serum ferritin 30–300 ng/mL *Average woman:* 49 *Average man:* 88	Decreased	Highly sensitive measurement of total body iron stores. The plasma ferritin value often falls to under 10% of its baseline level with significant iron deficiency.
Serum transferrin (also referred to as total iron binding capacity [TIBC]) 250–460 µg/dL	>8.5 µg/mL	Iron transport protein. Production is increased in response to low iron stores or increased iron needs.

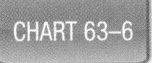

CHART 63–5 Common Oral Iron Supplement Formulations

Generic Name	Tablet (mg) (Elemental Iron Content [mg])	Elixir Iron Content (mg in 5 mL)
Ferrous sulfate	325 mg (65 mg elemental iron)	300 mg (60 mg elemental iron)
	195 mg (39 mg elemental iron)	90 mg (18 mg elemental iron)
Extended-release ferrous sulfate	525 mg (105 mg elemental iron)	
Ferrous fumarate	325 mg (107 mg elemental iron)	
	195 mg (64 mg elemental iron)	100 mg (33 mg elemental iron)
Ferrous gluconate	325 mg (39 mg elemental iron)	300 mg (35 mg elemental iron)

Source: Adamson, J. W. (2005). Iron deficiency and other hypoproliferative anemias. In D. L. Kasper, A. S. Fauci, D. L. Longo, E. Braunwald, S. L. Hauser, & J. L. Jameson (Eds.), *Harrison's principles of internal medicine* (16th ed., pp. 587–593). New York: McGraw-Hill.

recommends taking 50 to 60 mg of oral elemental iron (the approximate amount of elemental iron in one 300-mg tablet of ferrous sulfate) twice daily for 3 months for the therapeutic treatment of IDA. **Elemental iron** is the amount of iron in a supplement that is available for absorption (Chart 63–5).

Iron supplements can cause several gastrointestinal side effects, including constipation and upper epigastric pain, which contribute to patient noncompliance. Patient education should include techniques that can avoid such complications and also enhance iron absorption (see Chart 63–6). Switching to milder oral preparation such as ferrous gluconate tablets (325 mg with 39 mg of elemental iron) of carbonyl iron (Ircon) may be indicated if these techniques continue to prove unsuccessful.

Response to oral iron supplementation may be measured by an increase in peripheral reticulocytes as soon as 4 days after initiation of therapy, and by a rise in hemoglobin, hematocrit, and serum ferritin within 2 to 3 weeks. Patients should be advised to continue therapy for 2 to 3 months to fully restore depleted iron storage reservoirs (National Institutes of Health, 2005).

Parenteral Iron Supplementation

Parenteral iron supplementation may be indicated for patients who require more rapid correction of depleted iron stores or pa-

CHART 63–6 Patient Education Regarding Oral Iron Supplements

- Supplemental iron tablets should be taken 3 to 4 times daily per your health care provider's prescription.
- Some patients experience heartburn, nausea, or constipation when taking iron supplements. To help avoid these side effects, take iron tablets with a snack or full meal and at least 8 ounces of fluids.
- Do not lie down for at least 1 hour after taking iron pills.
- Your health care provider may prescribe a stool softener for you to help with constipation.
- Taking iron tablets with vitamin C (i.e., orange juice, strawberries) will help your body better absorb the iron.

tients with chronic kidney disease. However, significant side effect profiles of parenteral preparations have been reported including nausea, congestive heart failure, anaphylaxis, liver necrosis, and severe headache. Aronoff (2004) published a comprehensive meta-analysis of the literature surrounding parenteral IV therapy and found that rates of side effects such as anaphylaxis and infection were related to dose size and method of administration. Nonetheless, he also concluded that to be judged safe, IV iron therapy must show hematologic benefit (such as an increase in hemoglobin, decrease in erythropoietin dose, or both) without risking an increase in mortality or morbidity. A number of different IV preparations are currently available and each carries with it specific administration recommendations. Monitoring and test dose guidelines are listed in Chart 63–7.

 **CRITICAL ALERT** *During any administration of IV iron supplementation, if the patient reports any signs and symptoms of hypersensitivity or allergic reaction, stop the infusion, stay with the patient, monitor the airway, and call the health care provider immediately.*

■ Nursing Management

Nursing care of the patient with iron deficiency anemia focuses on management of symptomatic hypoxia consistent with all anemias. This includes providing patient education regarding prevention, detection, and management of iron deficiency and monitoring of possible complications from iron supplementation. Management of hypoxia related to anemia is a collaborative process and is addressed in the Nursing Process: Patient Care Plan for Generalized Anemia feature presented earlier in the chapter (p. 2013). Once IDA has been identified, nurses must provide patient education that can prevent recurrence. Because chronic GI blood loss is a major culprit, patients should be taught about the risk factors for GI bleed and early signs and symptoms (see Chapter 45 ⊘).

Nursing care also must focus on promotion of safe and effective iron supplementation. As discussed earlier, the efficacy of oral and IV iron supplementation is dependent on a variety of factors including timing of administration and management of bothersome side effects. To prevent noncompliance, patients should be advised about these risks prior to beginning iron supplementation and taught the management techniques listed in Chart 63–6 (p. 2021). Particularly with regard to oral supplementation, nurses should perform thorough abdominal assessments for heartburn and constipation. Encouraging proper positioning (high Fowler's or sitting), mobilization, and fluid intake will help minimize the occurrence of digestive problems. Patient education also should include dietary recommendations that will reinforce postdischarge behavior. Although a registered dietitian should be consulted whenever providing dietary recommendations, nurses should also reinforce dietary teaching whenever possible.

■ Collaborative Management

The comprehensive care of the patient with IDA benefits from the collaboration of nurses, pharmacists, and registered dietitians. Pharmacists should be consulted to prevent drug–drug and drug–food interactions that may inhibit iron absorption. In the acute care setting, registered dietitians coordinate inpatient meal planning to ensure that sufficient quantities of iron are supplied. Their planning efforts, however, require nursing staff to accurately assess and document patient intake of meals and snacks. Oftentimes, dietary intake is negatively impacted by financial and social limits such as shopping and meal preparation challenges. Long-term comprehensive care must then involve social workers and discharge planners who can assist the family with financial concerns and identification of community resources.

Anemia of Chronic Disease

Anemia is a common consequence of chronic diseases. The most common chronic diseases associated with anemia are cancer, chronic kidney failure, autoimmune disorders, and infectious diseases such as acquired immunodeficiency syndrome (AIDS). The prevalence of anemia of chronic disease (ACD) varies significantly depending on the underlying chronic disease and tends to increase with severity of the disease and age of the patient. Weiss and Gordeuk (2005) published a meta-analysis of anemia and chronic disease and reported prevalence ranges from 8% to 95%. In rheumatoid arthritis, anemia is the most common nonmusculoskeletal side effect, reported in 30% to 60% of patients. In cancer, anemia is reported in 30% to 90% of patients (Knight, Wade, & Balducci, 2004), and estimates in chronic kidney disease report a prevalence as high as 80% (National Kidney Foundation [NKF], 2001).

Recognition of ACD contributes to difficulties in statistical analysis. Fatigue and general malaise indicative of anemia are

CHART 63–7	Recommendation for Parenteral Infusion of Iron Supplementation			

Name (Generic and Trade)	Comments	Test Dose	Infusion Guidelines
Iron dextran injection (INFeD, DexFerrum)	Appropriate for single-dose administration. Intramuscular route available.	25 mg slow IV push, then 1 hour monitoring required on first infusion	100 mg over 2–5 minutes IV push *OR* Dilute dose in 250–1,000 mL 0.9%NS over 1–6 hours
Sodium ferric gluconate in sucrose (Ferrlecit)	Recommendation by National Kidney Foundation for 125 mg repeated in 8 doses. Suggested as alternative for patients hypersensitive to iron dextran	Not required; at health care provider's discretion 25 mg IV slow push or 25 mg in 50 mL of NS IV over 60 minutes	100 mg over 2–5 minutes IV push *OR* Dilute dose in 250–1.000 mL 0.9%NS over 1–6 hours
Iron sucrose injection (Venofer)		Not required; at health care provider's discretion 25 mg IV slow push	100 mg IV over 5 minutes *OR* Dilute dose in 100 mL 0.9%NS over 15 minutes

sometimes dismissed by health care providers as psychosocial consequences of chronic disease. However, numerous studies report decreased side effects and increased quality of life and survival rates when hemoglobin levels are vigilantly monitored and maintained at therapeutic levels above 10 g/dL, the criteria recommended by both the National Kidney Foundation's Kidney Disease Outcomes Quality Initiative (KDOQI) (National Kidney Foundation, 2001) and the National Comprehensive Cancer Network's clinical practice guidelines (Gillespie, 2003; National Comprehensive Cancer Network, 2008; Weiss & Gordeuk, 2005).

Pathophysiology

As mentioned earlier, anemia results from the inflammatory or infectious processes of chronic diseases including chronic kidney disease, cancer, rheumatoid arthritis, and chronic inflammatory bowel disease. Chemical signals produced by invading bacteria or a virus, a tumor, or the body itself attack erythropoietic cells and organs to negatively impact erythrocyte production and iron metabolism through a variety of mechanisms. These mechanisms can be categorized as follows:

1. **Decrease in iron absorption**—Iron availability is diminished by a decrease in the rate of intestinal iron absorption. Chronic disease also can trigger decreased appetite, further diminishing iron absorption. This process contributes to absolute iron deficiency.
2. **Diversion to macrophages**—As the body attempts to fight infection, cytokines divert available iron to the production of macrophages characteristic of chronic disease, resulting in a functional iron deficiency.
3. **Increased hemolysis of erythrocytes**—An increase in RBC hemolysis is stimulated by cytokines produced during inflammation and infection. Circulating macrophages then scavenge the liberated iron, again contributing to a decrease in circulating erythrocytes and functional iron deficiency.
4. **Decreased erythropoietin production and response**—Erythropoiesis also is impacted by a blunting of erythropoietin in chronic kidney disease or secondary to malignancy or infection. These diseases result in decreased production of erythropoietin and in the desensitization of the myeloid progenitor cell to the stimulating effects of erythropoietin. As a result, erythropoiesis rates fail to increase to meet the increased physiological demands imposed by disease and infection.
5. **Impaired erythropoiesis in the bone marrow**—Malignant tumors and infections first deplete iron and vitamin supplies and then crowd the bone marrow, leaving few resources for erythropoiesis. They also trigger apoptosis of the myeloid progenitor cells.

The simultaneous actions of these mechanisms ultimately result in measurable decreases in erythrocytes, hemoglobin, and hematocrit, along with hypoxia, activity intolerance, and fatigue.

Clinical Presentation

The physical signs and symptoms associated with ACD generally are indistinguishable from these associated with generalized anemia because both result directly from decreased circulating erythrocytes. Anemia also can exacerbate symptoms unique to the underlying disease process. In both cancer and chronic kidney disease, hematocrit and hemoglobin levels maintained below 10 mg/dL for more than 6 weeks are associated with increased myelosuppression, infection, left ventricular hypertrophy, and congestive heart failure. Cognitive and emotional complications include headaches, loss of concentration, depression, and impaired memory (Balducci, 2004; Gillespie, 2003; Ouellette, 2005).

Alterations in Laboratory Values

Anemia of chronic disease is distinguished by its etiology (association with an underlying chronic disease process) and its presentation in laboratory studies. ACD generally presents as mild anemia with hemoglobin levels typically between 8 and 9.5 g/dL. The CBC will show decreased total erythrocytes and decreased reticulocytes, indicating diminished erythropoiesis. The morphology of erythrocytes and iron status laboratory values will vary between ACD with absolute iron deficiency and ACD with functional iron deficiency. Typically, erythrocytes in ACD present first as normochromic and normocytic, then with increasing iron depletion progress to hypochromic and hypocytic, reflected by the MCHC, MCV, and MCH morphology indices. Ferritin levels in ACD with functional iron deficiency are increased, but decrease from baseline with absolute iron deficiency. Transferrin levels are decreased in all iron deficiency stages of ACD. These laboratory trends are summarized in Chart 63–8.

CHART 63–8   Laboratory Value Trends in Anemia with Chronic Disease and Variations for Iron Status

	ACD with Functional Iron Deficiency	ACD with Absolute Iron Deficiency
Complete blood count: hemoglobin	Decreased: Hgb < 10	Decreased
Complete blood count: hematocrit	Decreased	Decreased
Complete blood count: RBCs	Decreased	Decreased
Complete blood count: reticulocytes	Normal or decreased	Decreased
Morphology studies	Normochromic, normocytic; MCHC, MCV, MCH normal	Hypchromic, hypocytic; mean corpuscular hemoglobin concentration (MCHC), mean corpuscular volume (MCV), mean corpuscular hemoglobin (MCH) decreased
Iron studies: ferritin	Normal or increased	Decreased
Iron studies: transferrin	Decreased	Decreased
Iron studies: total body iron	Normal	Decreased

Medical Management

The goal of therapy in ACD is maintenance of hemoglobin and hematocrit at sufficient levels to promote disease healing and prevent systemic complications. The target range for hemoglobin and hematocrit are Hgb 11 g/dL (Hct 33%) to Hgb 12 g/dL (Hct 36%) as prescribed by the National Anemia Action Council, National Comprehensive Cancer Network, and NKF practice guidelines. Maintenance of hemoglobin and hematocrit values at these ranges has been correlated with decreased mortality and morbidity (National Anemia Action Council, 2008; National Comprehensive Cancer Network, 2008; National Kidney Foundation NKF, 2001).

The ultimate resolution of anemia in chronic disease, however, can be accomplished only with resolution of the underlying disease, such as cancer, chronic inflammation, or chronic kidney disease. Unfortunately, most of these diseases currently do not enjoy definitive options for permanent cure, implying that management of anemia becomes a lifelong challenge. Three primary options are implemented to maintain optimal hemoglobin and hematocrit values: blood transfusion, iron supplementation, and exogenous application of erythropoietin. Each option along with indications and monitoring guidelines is discussed next.

The judicious use of blood transfusion is an option in correcting acute anemia associated with chronic disease. Blood transfusion is reserved for patients with severe anemia (Hgb <8) or with obvious signs of bleeding such as visible loss of blood or a significant drop in hemoglobin/hematocrit in a relatively short period of time. The risks of blood transfusion, especially repeated transfusions over the course of many months to years, may outweigh the benefits to the patient. Repeated blood transfusions place the patient at risk for fluid overload and iron overload. Patients also can become sensitized to the proteins found in donated blood, increasing their risk for transfusion-related allergic reactions. See Chapter 23 😊 for a complete discussion of transfusion-related side effects.

Iron supplementation for ACD is reserved for patients with absolute iron deficiency. When ferritin levels indicate sufficient iron stores (greater than 100 ng/mL), as is the case in functional iron deficiency, with iron supplementation the patient is exposed to the possible effects of iron overload including tissue damage and acute cardiovascular events. When ferritin and transferrin levels show iron depletion, iron supplementation has shown some benefit in maintaining hemoglobin levels at the target range of <10. Iron supplementation may also be indicated for patients being treated with erythropoietic agents.

Erythropoietic agents are medications composed of the exogenous forms of erythropoietin, the primary stimulating hormone of erythropoiesis produced in the kidneys. The use of erythropoietic agents for the correction of ACD is reserved for patients with chronic kidney disease and patients undergoing chemotherapy or immunosuppressive therapy. These medications work much the same way that natural erythropoietin does, by stimulating differentiation and proliferation of the hematopoietic cascade. In chronic disease, erythropoietic agents also have been found to preferentially stimulate iron absorption by the erythroid progenitor cell over macrophages. Guidelines for use vary among diseases; refer to the chapters on kidney failure (Chapter 47 😊) and cancer (Chapter 64 😊) for guidelines.

Nursing Management

Anemia complicates an already difficult diagnosis of chronic disease. Conversely, prevention, detection, and early treatment of anemia can improve the patient's quality of life and clinical outcomes. Nurses play a key role in recognizing early signs of anemia, especially in the acute hospitalized patient. Nursing priorities for the care of the patient with any chronic disease should include assessment of activity tolerance and assessment of integumentary signs such as pallor, respiratory difficulty, and cognition, as described in the Nursing Process: Patient Care Plan for Generalized Anemia feature presented earlier in the chapter (p. 2013). Detection of any such signs indicates the need for immediate implementation of nursing interventions to reduce risk of falls and hypoxia.

Frequent analyses of laboratory values also assist the nurse in detecting underlying bleeding and/or iron deficiency. Patient education and establishment of the therapeutic patient–nurse relationship is particularly important for these patients who may be experiencing depression and exhaustion already brought on by their underlying disease process. Patient education priorities include proper medication administration, increasing awareness of side effects of therapy, safety interventions, and signs and symptoms of worsening anemia.

Megaloblastic Anemias: Folate Deficiency, Vitamin B$_{12}$ Deficiency, and Pernicious Anemias

Megaloblastic anemia results from impaired DNA synthesis of the erythrocyte RBC precursors. The impaired DNA synthesis results in production of large, immature red blood cells termed **megaloblasts**. Due to their immaturity and large size, these megaloblasts are often sequestered in the bone marrow rather than released into the periphery. If released into the peripheral bloodstream, megaloblasts are subject to an increased rate of hemolysis due to structural defects in their membranes. Both processes—bone marrow sequestration and increased hemolysis—result in a decreased total RBC count, or anemia. Most commonly, megaloblastic anemia is caused by deficient dietary intake of folic acid or vitamin B$_{12}$ (cobalamin) or by malabsorption of vitamin B$_{12}$ (pernicious anemia). These processes account for the vast majority of megaloblastic anemias; however, other causes have been implicated, as summarized in Chart 63–9.

Etiology and Pathophysiology

The exact chemical roles of vitamin B$_{12}$ and folate in erythropoiesis are still under investigation, although a great deal of research is being focused on the subject. What is known, however, is that **folate** plays a critical role in the biochemical reactions involved in cell development, especially erythropoiesis. Folate is the natural form, whereas folic acid is the synthetic form found in supplements and fortified food. Laboratory studies show that an absence of folate suppresses the proliferation of maturing erythrocytes. Furthermore, it also is known that folate is absorbed as an inactive dietary form and must be converted to an active form before being used in DNA synthesis.

Vitamin B$_{12}$ (cobalamin), an essential nutrient found in animal proteins, is responsible for this conversion of inactive folate

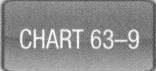

CHART 63-9 Common Causes of Megaloblastic Anemia

Major Causes

- Insufficient dietary intake of folic acid
- Insufficient dietary intake of vitamin B_{12} (cobalamin)
- Deficiencies in gastric intrinsic factor leading to malabsorption of vitamin B_{12} (pernicious anemia)

Other Causes

- Intestinal malabsorption due to chronic GI inflammatory processes or surgical shortening
- General malnutrition
- Liver disease
- Chronic hemolytic anemias
- Anticonvulsant medications such as phenytoin that interfere with folate absorption
- Drugs that have antifolate activity including methotrexate and trimethoprim
- Chemotherapies with DNA suppression activity
- Alcohol abuse

to active folate. This inextricable relationship is the reason vitamin B_{12} deficiency and folate deficiency have similar clinical presentations and often occur simultaneously. Once absorbed, vitamin B_{12} and folate are either transported directly to the bone marrow for erythropoiesis or stored in the liver and, to a small degree, in the pancreas.

Vitamin B_{12} requires the action of gastric **intrinsic factor (IF)** before being absorbed into the intestinal mucosa and bloodstream. Intrinsic factor is a substance secreted by the gastric parietal mucosa. Megaloblastic anemias that result from deficiencies in IF are termed **pernicious anemias**.

Clinical Presentation

Folate deficiency anemia, vitamin B_{12} deficiency anemia, and pernicious anemia typically progress slowly with symptoms manifesting gradually over years and months rather than days. In addition to the clinical signs common to all anemias, megaloblastic anemias also present with characteristic signs and symptoms and laboratory test results.

Physical Manifestations

The Nursing Process: Patient Care Plan for Generalized Anemia (see feature earlier in chapter, p. 2013) delineates the most common signs of anemia including fatigue, activity intolerance, exertional dyspnea, tachycardia, and hypoxia. Although this chapter focuses on the pivotal role of vitamin B_{12} and folate in erythropoiesis, both substances also are required for *all* DNA synthesis. In the absence of sufficient folate and vitamin B_{12} (either from dietary insufficiency or pernicious anemia), the patient can manifest gastrointestinal and integumentary signs and symptoms. These result from the absence of these vitamins in the production of epithelial cells. GI symptoms include a swollen and sore tongue (classically described as "smooth and beefy red"), anorexia, and nausea. Integumentary signs include hyperpigmentation over the hands and knuckles. Neurological symptoms

occurring with vitamin B_{12} deficiencies include peripheral neuropathy, unsteadiness, lack of coordination, ataxia, confusion, and memory loss. Reflexes may also be diminished, and a positive Babinski's sign may be observed. (Refer to Chapter 28 🔗 for a discussion neurological assessment.) These result from loss of myelination of nerve cells, of which vitamin B_{12} plays a critical role. Unfortunately, these symptoms often are permanent and irreversible.

Folate deficiency is clinically indistinguishable from vitamin B_{12} deficiency with the exception of neurological insults, which are not common in folate deficiency. Because nervous system findings are atypical, their appearance is clinically significant and warrants analysis for vitamin B_{12} deficiency or overlying neurological disease processes. The most common problem specifically associated with folate deficiency is neural tube defects, such as spina bifida, in newborns of mothers who had inadequate folate intake during pregnancy. Folate deficiency has also been linked to increased homocysteine (an amino acid found in the blood) levels, which in turn increases risk of cardiovascular disease and thrombosis. See Chapter 40 🔗 for a complete discussion of homocysteine and cardiovascular disease.

Alterations in Laboratory Values

Megaloblastic anemias result in changes to the CBC and RBC morphology studies. The hallmark diagnostic finding indicating megaloblastic anemia is macrocytosis or MCV (typically over 110 μm^3). Patients present with the decreased hemoglobin value typical of anemia as well as decreased reticulocytes count. Increased hemolysis can result in decreased erythrocyte levels. To specifically diagnosis megaloblastic anemia and its etiology, vitamin B_{12} and/or folate levels may need to be evaluated. An analysis of vitamin B_{12} and folate levels assists in establishing a definitive diagnosis. A serum vitamin B_{12} level of <100 pg/mL and a serum folate level of <5 ng/mL is diagnostic of vitamin B_{12} and folate deficiency, respectively.

The next task then is to determine the cause of the vitamin B_{12} and/or folate deficiency. A thorough nutritional history assists in isolating dietary causes; however, problems with absorption can be identified using a **Schilling test**. The patient is first given an *oral* dose of radioactively labeled vitamin B_{12}, and a 24-hour urine collection is measured for vitamin B_{12} excretion. Normally urinary excretion is at least 8% to 40% of total radioactively labeled vitamin B_{12}, indicating that the substance was absorbed and metabolized. If urinary excretion is lower than 8%, this may indicate an inability to absorb vitamin B_{12}, and a second stage of the test is performed. In this stage, the patient again is given an oral dose of radiolabeled vitamin B_{12}, but now with a parenteral dose of intrinsic factor. A 24-hour urine collection is repeated and results are compared with the first urine collection results. An increase in urinary excretion of radiolabeled vitamin B_{12} with the addition of IF suggests pernicious anemia.

Analysis then turns to identifying the cause of pernicious anemia. Radiologic examinations, histories, endoscopies, and occasionally surgical exploration may reveal conditions such as celiac disease, tropical sprue, gastric shortening, Crohn's disease, blind loops, and diverticuli, all of which contribute to decreased intestinal production of intrinsic factor. Another diagnostic exam involves the insertion of a nasogastric tube to measure gastric acid secretion. Insufficiencies in gastric acids point to gastric parietal cell problems, which also contribute to insufficient IF and vitamin B_{12} malabsorption.

Medical Management

The first task of medical management is to remove or alter any contributing factors to folate and/or vitamin B_{12} deficiency such as suppressive medication regimes. Dietary causes of both folate and vitamin B_{12} deficiency can be effectively treated with counseling, diet modifications, or vitamin supplementation. Recommended doses of folate supplements start with daily oral administration of 1 mg of folic acid for 4 months, and maintenance with 0.4 mg in a multivitamin for patients with an underlying cause or inadequate diet. Folate deficiencies due to malabsorptive processes require treatment of the underlying cause. Intravenous folate should always be considered in the management of alcoholism to help minimize some of the painful side effects of recovery.

Vitamin B_{12} supplementation usually is achieved via dietary modifications rather than pill form. The latest Recommended Dietary Allowance (RDA) for vitamin B_{12} is 2.4 mcg/day for persons aged 14 to 70 years; the average diet in the United States contains about 5 mcg daily. The prevalence of foods fortified with vitamin B_{12} means that increased intake can be readily achieved. However, the assistance of a registered dietitian is extremely valuable to ensure proper intake of recommended doses (see the Collaborative Management section that follows).

Vitamin B_{12} deficiency in the patient with absorption problems usually is managed with parental supplementation of the vitamin. The treatment schedule begins with parenteral 1,000 mcg vitamin B_{12}, followed by 1,000 mcg intramuscularly once a month for the rest of the patient's life. The efficacy of this approach is well documented. Patients report increased strength and stamina soon after institution of regular doses. Blood cell morphology begins to show normal red blood cells within hours of treatments with subsequent remission of the anemia during the next several weeks (Babior, 2000).

Oral supplementation has been available since 1968, however, it is not widely used for two reasons: for fear of noncompliance and a lack of understanding of alternate biochemical pathways for vitamin B_{12} absorption. However, there is growing evidence that oral administration may be just as effective as parenteral administration given appropriate doses (Nilsson et al., 2005; Nyholm et al., 2003).

■ Nursing Management

Nurses caring for the patient with megaloblastic anemias have the following priorities:

- *Continued assessment for signs and symptoms of hypoxic distress in severe cases.* The Nursing Process: Patient Care Plan for Generalized Anemia (see feature earlier in chapter, p. 2013) provides assessment guidelines and nursing interventions appropriate for use in megaloblastic anemia.
- *Prevention of mechanical injury from neurological changes.* In addition to the harm caused by hypoxia, these patients are at increased risk of falls and injury secondary to ataxia and lack of balance coordination. Patients with peripheral neuropathy secondary to vitamin B_{12} deficiency have diminished periph-

eral sensations, which increase their risk of injury. Nurses must include an assessment of progressive nerve damage and sensation and most importantly ensure the patient's environment is safe so as to limit injury.

- *Identification of high-risk populations.* Because vitamin B_{12} primarily is found in meats, vegetarians, especially vegans, are at particularly higher risk for vitamin B_{12} deficiency. The rate of folate deficiency is also particularly a concern in women of childbearing age and in the elderly. With this knowledge in hand, nurses may emphasize assessment of dietary histories and patient education to target these high-risk groups.
- *Patient education and reinforcement regarding dietary modifications and/or supplementation.* Patient education regarding dietary modifications is discussed in the next section. For patients requiring supplementation, nursing reinforcement and encouragement can be pivotal to ensuring compliance with a lifelong regime. Nurses should assess patients for compliance, efficacy, and safety of the intramuscular vitamin B_{12} injections and provide feedback as to its action. This can be accomplished by reviewing hematologic studies with the patient and indicating improvements when indicated.
- *Collaboration with the interdisciplinary team.* Collaboration with the health care team is important to ensure a comprehensive multifaceted approach to correction of underlying causes.

■ Collaborative Management

A major discharge priority for patients with megaloblastic anemia is verbalization of an understanding of dietary modifications and, if indicated, safe performance of medication self-administration techniques. To accomplish these goals, the nurse should collaborate with the health care provider, the registered dietitian, the pharmacist, and the discharge planner.

Dietitians play a critical role in providing accurate and appropriate patient education. Patients can become easily confused with food labels, such as "excellent" or "good" designed for advertising purposes. Handouts and food plans should be provided for clarification. Charts 63–10 and 63–11 (p. 2028) summarize selected food sources of vitamin B_{12} and folate, respectively. Information such as this, when discussed with a dietitian and patient, can help address concerns about adequate food sources. Family members should always be included in the patient education plan, both for support, but also to identify family members' risk of nutritional deficiency and to address familial behavioral patterns such as meal planning habits.

Collaboration with the pharmacist also should not be overlooked. A number of drugs can interfere with vitamin B_{12} or folate absorption and metabolism. The pharmacist is able to monitor drug regimens to prevent such deleterious drug–food interactions. Additionally, the pharmacist can provide materials to help with the administration of parenteral supplements.

Hemoglobinopathies

Hemoglobinopathy is a term used to describe a class of red blood cell disorders characterized by abnormal hemoglobin, which can

CHART 63–10 Selected Food Sources of Vitamin B_{12}

Food	Micrograms per Serving	Percent Daily Value
Mollusks, clam, mixed species, cooked, 3 ounces	84.1	1400
Liver, beef, braised, 1 slice	47.9	780
Fortified breakfast cereals (100% fortified), 3/4 cup	6.0	100
Trout, rainbow, wild, cooked, 3 ounces	5.4	90
Salmon, sockeye, cooked, 3 ounces	4.9	80
Trout, rainbow, farmed, cooked, 3 ounces	4.2	50
Beef, top sirloin, lean, choice, broiled, 3 ounces	2.4	40
Fast-food cheeseburger, regular, double patty and bun, 1 sandwich	1.9	30
Fast-food taco, 1 large	1.6	25
Fortified breakfast cereals (25% fortified), 3/4 cup	1.5	25
Yogurt, plain, skim, with 13 grams protein per cup, 1 cup	1.4	25
Haddock, cooked, 3 ounces	1.2	20
Clams, breaded and fried, 3/4 cup	1.1	20
Tuna, white, canned in water, drained solids, 3 ounces	1.0	15
Milk, 1 cup	0.9	15
Pork, cured, ham, lean only, canned, roasted, 3 ounces	0.6	10
Egg, whole, hard boiled, 1	0.6	10
American pasteurized cheese food, 1 ounce	0.3	6
Chicken, breast, meat only, roasted, 1/2 breast	0.3	6

Source: U.S. Department of Agriculture, Agricultural Research Service. (2003). *USDA nutrient database for standard reference, release 16.* Retrieved February 1, 2006, from the Nutrient Data Laboratory website: http://www.nal.usda.gov/fnic/cgi-bin/nut_search.pl.

result in a variety of clinical problems including hypoxia, accelerated RBC destruction, and decreased RBC production. All of these diseases result from genetic mutations in the coding sequences controlling the component hemoglobin chains. Classification of these diseases is often based on the type of genetic alteration (either point mutation, base pair, or deletion). They also are commonly classified on the basis of the molecular and chemical effect of the alteration. Alterations include decreased oxygen-binding capacity and structural defects that decrease the life span.

As with most genetic disorders, the severity of clinical symptoms depends on the role of the gene involved and on the inheritance pattern, with homozygous patients frequently presenting with severe debilitating disease, whereas heterozygous patients can often live asymptomatically unless presented with acute illness or environmental stress. More than 800 distinct diseases have been attributed to hemoglobinopathy, of which thalassemia and sickle cell disease are the most prominent. Both of these diseases are discussed in the following sections.

Thalassemia

The term **thalassemia** refers to a group of hematologic disorders characterized by the genetic inheritance of a mutated hemoglobin-coding gene that appears most frequently in persons of Southeast Asian, African, and Mediterranean descent. The hallmark characteristic of thalassemia is a structural change in the hemoglobin molecule that subjects affected red blood cells to increased rates of hemolysis. The thalassemias are

chronic disease states that are usually detected during infancy or adolescence. Cure of these anemias is not the goal for the acute care nurse. The focus instead becomes prevention of disease complications and treatment of symptom exacerbation.

Pathophysiology

Recall from the earlier discussion on hemoglobin synthesis that oxygen binding occurs when alpha and beta chains form precise geometric configurations that allows iron to sit tightly in a lock-and-key style fit on the heme groups. Thalassemia arises when the alpha and beta chains are of unequal proportions, which ultimately reduces the rate of RBC maturation in the bone marrow. Cells that do survive bone marrow development and enter the bloodstream are recognized in the spleen as structurally abnormal and are subject to higher rates of hemolysis.

The thalassemias are broadly divided into two groups: alpha thalassemia or beta thalassemia, depending on the type of inherited gene mutation. Beta thalassemia results from reduced beta chains, whereas the alpha thalassemias result from reduced alpha chains. Diseases are also characterized by their gene inheritance pattern: homozygous carriers, defining the inheritance of two defective genes, or heterozygous carriers, defining the inheritance of only one defective gene. Each combination of gene inheritance is associated with distinct clinical features.

Clinical Presentation

Alpha thalassemias are generally milder than the beta thalassemias and often present without symptoms or very mild

CHART 63–11 **Selected Food Sources of Folate and Folic Acid**

Food	Micrograms per Serving	Percent Daily Value as Developed by the Food and Drug Administraton
Breakfast cereals fortified with 100% of the DV (fortified with folic acid) 3/4 cup*	400	100
Beef liver, cooked, braised, 3 ounces	185	45
Cowpeas (blackeyed), immature, cooked, boiled, 1/2 cup	105	25
Breakfast cereals, fortified with 25% of the Daily Value 3/4 cup*	100	25
Spinach, frozen, cooked, boiled, 1/2 cup	100	25
Great Northern beans, boiled, 1/2 cup	90	20
Asparagus, boiled, 4 spears	85	20
Rice, white, long-grain, parboiled, enriched, cooked, 1/2 cup*	65	15
Vegetarian baked beans, canned, 1 cup	60	15
Spinach, raw, 1 cup	60	15
Green peas, frozen, boiled, 1/2 cup	50	15
Broccoli, chopped, frozen, cooked, 1/2 cup	50	15
Egg noodles, cooked, enriched, 1/2 cup*	50	15
Broccoli, raw, 2 spears (each 5 inches long)	45	10
Avocado, raw, all varieties, sliced, 1/2 cup sliced	45	10
Peanuts, all types, dry roasted, 1 ounce	40	10
Lettuce, Romaine, shredded, 1/2 cup	40	10
Wheat germ, crude, 2 tablespoons	40	10
Tomato juice, canned, 6 ounces	35	10
Orange juice, chilled, includes concentrate, 3/4 cup	35	10
Turnip greens, frozen, cooked, boiled, 1/2 cup	30	8
Orange, all commercial varieties, fresh, 1 small	30	8
Bread, white, 1 slice*	25	6
Bread, whole wheat, 1 slice*	25	6
Egg, whole, raw, fresh, 1 large	25	6
Cantaloupe, raw,1/4 medium	25	6
Papaya, raw, 1/2 cup cubes	25	6
Banana, raw, 1 medium	20	6

*Items marked with an (*) are fortified with folic acid as part of the Folate Fortification Program.

Source: U.S. Department of Agriculture, Agricultural Research Service. (2003). *USDA nutrient database for standard reference, release 16.* Retrieved February 1, 2006, from the Nutrient Data Laboratory website: http://www.nal.usda.gov/fnic/cgi-bin/nut_search.pl.

symptoms that respond well to supportive care when indicated. The severity of symptoms in patients with beta thalassemias depends heavily on the inheritance pattern (see the Genetic Considerations box). The term *beta-thalassemia minor* describes the inheritance of only one defective gene and one normal gene (heterozygous), whereas the term *beta-thalassemia major* is used for the inheritance of two defective genes (homozygous).

GENETIC CONSIDERATIONS for Thalassemia

Persons of Southeast Asia, Africa, and Mediterranean descent bear a genetic predisposition to thalassemia. Patients with alpha-thalassemia and beta-thalassemia minor are often asymptomatic and not identified; however, patients with beta-thalassemia major usually require transfusions beginning early in life (Forget, 2000).

Beta-thalassemia minor patients are able to produce small amounts of normal hemoglobin and, thus, are frequently asymptomatic due to long-term physiological adaptation. These patients are carriers for the genetic trait; therefore, genetic counseling may be offered for patients of reproductive age. Beta-thalassemia major (also called Cooley's anemia) results from complete lack of the beta protein in the hemoglobin chain manifesting as severe, life-threatening anemia. Symptoms that result from the increased rate of hemolysis include jaundice, hepatomegaly (enlarged liver), and splenomegaly (enlarged spleen). Pronounced pallor, tachycardia, and lethargy result from a critical lack of oxygen-binding capacity. The bone marrow is constantly in a state of increased erythropoiesis in an attempt to compensate for hemolysis and hypoxia, resulting in bone marrow expansion, recognized as thickening of facial bones and abnormal skeletal growth (Forget, 2000). The physiological demands imposed by beta-thalassemia major often can be so serious that many children who acquire the disease do not survive into adulthood. *3Beta-thalassemia intermedia* was a term coined by Sturgeon and colleagues in 1955 to describe a small group of patients who do not fit neatly into either the beta-thalassemia major or beta-thalassemia minor paradigms. These patients are hematologically too severe to be called "minor" and too mild to be called "major." These individuals are homozygous for thalassemia genes, but maintain hemoglobin levels of 7 to 10 g/dL without regular transfusions.

Alterations in laboratory values for thalassemia patients depend again on the form of the inherited mutation and the inheritance pattern. In addition to alterations in hemoglobin and red blood cells, clinicians should monitor for alterations in bilirubin, which provide indications of hemolytic effects in the liver. Chart 63–12 summarizes the changes in laboratory values and clinical symptoms relative to the type of thalassemia (Benz, 2003).

In addition to clinical presentation directly related to thalassemia, the constant need for transfusion to maintain adequate RBCs often results in transfusion-related complications and iron overload, as discussed next. Excessive iron comes from the patient's own hemolyzed red blood and the transfused blood, as well as increased iron absorption from food as a compensatory mechanism to combat anemia. The excess iron is stored in the spleen, liver, endocrine organs, and heart causing splenomegaly, hepatomegaly, cirrhosis, hormone imbalances, and cardiomyopathy, which can all eventually become fatal.

Medical Management

Patients with alpha thalassemias and beta-thalassemia minor are usually asymptomatic and usually do not require medical intervention. Patients with thalassemia major, however, often require frequent transfusions of packed RBCs to correct falling hematocrit and hemoglobin levels that result from rampant hemolysis. Transfusion doses are titrated to maintain therapeutic hemoglobin levels between 7 and 10 g/dL or to correct severe symptoms.

However, the leading cause of death among patients with thalassemia has shifted from hemoglobin-deficient anemia to iron overload associated with chronic blood transfusion therapy (Vichinsky, 2005). Thus, iron levels must be carefully monitored to prevent iron overload. Two common methods used to monitor iron are the serum ferritin test and liver biopsy. Iron chelation therapy with drugs such as desferrioxamine (Desferal) is administered intravenously or subcutaneously in an effort to bind and neutralize excessive iron from patients' bodies. Hydration and oxygenation complement transfusion and chelation therapy in an effort to rid the body of excess erythrocyte waste and maintain oxygen levels (Hoffbrand, 2005; Vichinsky, 2005).

Nursing Management

Nursing assessment of patients with thalassemia focuses on the hemolytic and hypoxic effects manifested in the integumentary, gastrointestinal, lymphatic, and cardiovascular systems. Patients should be observed for jaundice in the skin and eyes due to RBC destruction, and pallor from hemoglobin-deficient anemia. Abdominal pain and liver and spleen tenderness are indicators of thalassemia and should be included in a comprehensive assessment. Cardiovascular signs and symptoms of activity intolerance and hypoxia should also be assessed as indicators of both hemoglobin deficiency and iron accumulation in the cardiac muscle.

Nursing interventions based on the preceding assessments should prioritize activity alterations, pain management, and collaboration with the multidisciplinary team. The Nursing Process: Patient Care Plan for Generalized Anemia (see feature earlier in chapter, p. 2013) should be implemented in the care of these patients. If transfusion therapy is warranted, the nurse plays a critical role in managing the administration of blood products including assessing for signs of a transfusion reaction such as fluid overload, fever, and anaphylaxis.

Sickle Cell Disease

Sickle cell anemia is perhaps the most well known of the chronic erythrocyte disorders. In the United States it is estimated that more than 70,000 people suffer from sickle cell disease with about 1,000 babies born annually with the disease. Sickle cell occurs most frequently in African Americans and Hispanic Americans. About 1 in every 500 African Americans has sickle cell disease. It also affects people of Arabian, Greek, Maltese, Italian, Sardinian, Turkish, and Indian ancestry (see the Genetic Considerations box, p. 2030). **Sickle cell anemia** is the term given to a group of genetically based RBC diseases all characterized by misshapen "sickle-shaped" red blood cells. The source of the sickling is a malfunctioning hemoglobin molecule that twists the entire RBC from a soft, pliable, round donut shape into a long, hard, sticky elongated cell (Figure 63–7 ■, p. 2030).

Pathophysiology

Patients with sickle cell anemia acquire the sickle hemoglobin (HbS), a mutated version of the normal form of hemoglobin A.

CHART 63–12	**Laboratory Values and Clinical Presentation of the Thalassemias**

	Alpha Thalassemia	Beta-Thalassemia Minor	Beta-Thalassemia Intermedia	Beta-Thalassemia Major
Hemoglobin	Normal	>10 g/dL (normal)	7–10 g/dL	<7 g/dL
Red blood cell appearance	Microcytic and Hypochromic			
Red blood cells		Usually normal	Usually normal or decreased	Severely decreased
Jaundice	Usually absent	Usually absent	Usually absent or mild	Severe
Splenomegaly	Usually absent	Usually absent	Usually absent or mild	Severe
Skeletal changes	Absent	Usually absent	Usually absent or mild	Severe

GENETIC CONSIDERATIONS for Sickle Cell Disease

Sickle cell disease is acquired through genetic inheritance in families of African American, Hispanic American, Arabian, Greek, Italian, Sardinian, Maltese, Turkish, and Indian ancestry. Patients who inherit the sickle cell gene from one parent (heterozygous HbS/HbA) usually do not exhibit symptoms and are termed sickle cell carriers. Patients who inherit the sickle cell gene from both parents (homozygous) are subject to severe sickle cell crises. Because both homozygous and heterozygous patients can pass their genes onto their children, sickle cell carriers typically undergo some type of genetic counseling prior to childbearing (Armandola, 2002, Ramsey et al., 2001).

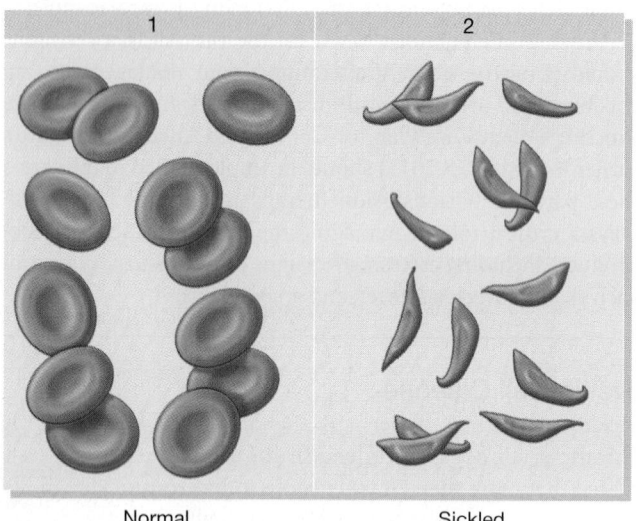

Normal   Sickled

FIGURE 63–7 ■ Red blood cells from sickle cell anemia.

Recall from the discussion on hemoglobin development and function earlier in the chapter that oxygen binding results in a geometric alteration of the hemoglobin molecule. In normal hemoglobin the oxygenated state and the deoxygenated state coexist without deleterious side effects. HbS, however, causes affected cells to transform into a rigid, elongated sickle shape upon release of the oxygen molecule, rather than the normal, flexible round configuration. Under normal circumstances, deoxygenated sickled cells make up only a small proportion of total blood volume, with minimal physical effects. However, any stress that results in oxygen deprivation increases the proportion of sickled cells.

Sickle cells possess "sticky membranes" and unusual shapes that occlude small blood vessels (a condition called *erythrostasis*), which serve to further potentiate oxygen deprivation. Sickled cells also are trapped by the spleen, further reducing circulating red blood cells and contributing to hypoxia. Initially, the hypoxia will stimulate increased erythropoiesis, thus reversing the cycle. However, if the hypoxia becomes extreme, widespread vessel occlusion leads to a syndrome termed *sickle cell crisis*. These crisis states are responsible for the severe pain of sickle cell disease. Pain, in turn, increases the demand for oxygen, hinders mobility and respiration, and taxes the cardiovascular system. Together the sequence of events escalates into a cycle of deoxygenation and RBC sickling. Gone unchecked, the resultant thrombosis and acidosis progress to organ failure and eventually death.

Crisis Syndromes of Sickled Red Blood Cells   The following critical situations may be seen in patients with sickle cell anemia:

- **Vaso-occlusive crisis**—Vaso-occlusive crisis is the occlusion of small vessels by long, hard chains of stacked sickled cells. This occlusion prevents oxygenation of surrounding tissues and tissue downstream of the occlusion. Oxygen deprivation in arterial vessels causes ischemic attacks and infarction. Oxygen deprivation to venous vessels leads to swollen, tender tissues as a result of the buildup of fluids and wastes. Both arterial and venous occlusions are hallmarked by severe pain.

- **Sequestration crisis**—Sequestration crisis occurs when sickled RBCs overwhelm and clog the spleen. As a result, circulating blood volume decreases, manifesting as decreased blood pressure, which in turn stagnates blood flow and causes deoxygenation. Sequestration crisis manifests as a painful, tender, grossly enlarged spleen.

- **Aplastic crisis**—The large numbers of RBCs destroyed in the spleen by sickle cell anemia places an extraordinarily high demand on the amount of bone marrow available to replenish available circulating erythrocytes into the bloodstream. This extraordinary demand overwhelms the bone marrow regulatory feedback mechanism, resulting in complete bone marrow shutdown, akin to a system overload. This complete bone marrow shutdown is referred to as aplastic crisis. As a result of aplastic crisis, reticulocytes (juvenile RBCs) are not produced, causing a severe drop in hemoglobin, up to 1 g/dL per day manifesting in severe lethargy, malaise, and deoxygenation.

- **Hyperhemolytic crisis**—Hyperhemolytic crisis is a rare complication. As the name implies, hyperhemolytic crisis is hallmarked by a massive increase in RBC destruction. Like aplastic crisis, hemoglobin rates drop rapidly. However, if the bone marrow is still intact, reticulocyte production is increased.

Clinical Presentation

The extent and severity of the disease depends on two criteria: the inheritance pattern (homozygous for HbS or heterozygous HbS/HbA) and the presence of deoxygenating triggering factors. Patients who are heterozygous HbS/HbA (termed sickle cell carriers) often live asymptomatic lives because the normal hemoglobin produced by HbA sufficiently prevents sickling crisis. Homozygous patients also usually live asymptomatic lives unless subjected to stressors such as infection, pain, blood loss, or high altitudes. Sickle cell crisis appears when the patient is subjected to such stressors or prolonged hypoxia. Peripheral tissue and organ damage become more apparent, and oxygen deprivation and blood stagnation increase with prolonged sickle cell crisis. Although every body system eventually can become affected, certain signs and symptoms are most frequently observed. These are:

- Persistent, usually painful, erection of the penis due to veno-occlusion causes both severe pain and embarrassment for male patients.

- Acute renal failure results primarily from arterial occlusion in the renal capillaries, which, in turn, leads to focal areas of hemorrhage or necrosis. Additionally, myoglobin and RBC waste products from extremely high RBC destruction can overload renal tubules, causing renal failure.

- Acute chest syndrome (ACS) results from a variety of causes. Causes directly pertaining to sickle cell crisis include pulmonary tissue infarction due to capillary occlusion and hypoventilation secondary to rib/sternal bone infarction. Treatment of sickle cell crisis can also exacerbate acute chest syndrome. Examples include hypoventilation secondary to narcotic administration and pulmonary edema induced by narcotics or fluid overload. Regardless of the cause, the resultant hypoxia severely increases hemoglobin sickling, making the appearance of ACS an ominous sign in the sickle cell patient. See Chapters 33, 34, and 36 ⓔ for complete discussion of ACS.
- Splenomegaly (enlarged spleen) results from splenic sequestration.
- Avascular necrosis (AVN), also known as ischemic necrosis, osteonecrosis, or aseptic necrosis of the large joints, results from interruption of the arterial supply of the femoral head. Patients with AVN have severe chronic joint pain, decreased weight-bearing ability, and joint malformation.
- Hemolytic anemia, or acute anemia caused by the accelerated breakdown of red blood cells, is characterized by splenomegaly, jaundice, and decreased urine output. Hemolytic anemia is discussed in greater detail later in this chapter.

As the microvasculature becomes increasingly occluded, major organs begin to suffer irreversible damage from hypoxia and thrombosis. Evidence of organ failure includes decreased level of consciousness (decreased cerebral tissue perfusion), decreased urine output and increased serum creatinine (decreased renal tissue perfusion), chest pain (decreased cardiopulmonary tissue perfusion), and abdominal pain (decreased liver, colon, and spleen perfusion).

Alterations in Laboratory Values

Laboratory studies analyzing RBC morphology are used to monitor for the prevalence of sickle cell hemoglobin. Hemoglobin electrophoresis analysis can reveal the presence of HbS in patients with sickle cell disease. Slide smears of peripheral blood samples can reveal partially or completely sickled cells with the proportion of sickled cells to normal cells increasing during crisis states. Hemoglobin values will be normal in patients with the sickle cell trait, but decreased below 7 g/dL during deoxygenation states or in homozygous patients. As sickling progresses the patient also will display evidence of increasing RBC breakdown manifested by decreased RBCs and increased bilirubin.

Medical Management

The cornerstone of sickle cell disease management is prevention of sickle cell crisis by ensuring adequate oxygenation via avoidance of triggering events at all times. Because patients are usually diagnosed as children, prevention of sickle cell crisis states should always involve collaboration with the parent. Any patient presenting to the acute care setting with a known history of sickle cell disease warrants particular attention to oxygenation and hydration status. In the unfortunate event that sickle cell crisis develops, supportive care must be implemented to prevent severe pain, organ failure, and death.

Treatments should include administration and monitoring of supplemental oxygen, analgesics for vaso-occlusive crisis, hydration, and, if indicated, blood cell transfusions to reverse hypoxia. Pharmacologic treatments to prevent sickle cell crisis are

currently being researched. Avenues for investigation include drugs such as hydroxyurea, butyrate, and arginine that stimulate the body to make normal types of hemoglobin, drugs to increase oxygenation to small blood vessels (Poloxamer 188, Flocor), drugs that make sickled cell membranes less "sticky," and gene therapies (Armandola, 2002; Marlowe & Chicella, 2002; Solovey, Solovey, Harkness, & Hebbel, 2001; Wang et al., 2002). Complementary and alternative therapy options are presented in the box on page 2034.

Nursing Management

Prevention of sickle cell crisis is a primary goal for any patient admitted with sickle cell disease, regardless of the primary admitting diagnosis. Situations that are most likely to cause HbS chains to sickle and stack include dehydration, blood stagnation, decreased pH (acidosis), and decreased PaO_2. Disease management thus focuses on:

- Maintenance of adequate hydration
- Maintenance of oxygenation to prevent acidosis and decreased PaO_2
- Prevention of hypercoagulability.

Effective management of these patients involves first identifying high-risk factors and then implementing effective preventive nursing and medical interventions. In the event that sickle cell crisis occurs, the medical team must quickly mobilize to treat pain and eliminate the triggering factors. Finally, all patients with sickle cell disease must be regularly assessed for evidence of organ and tissue dysfunction. In addition to the Nursing Process: Patient Care Plan for Generalized Anemia presented earlier (p. 2013), the Nursing Process: Patient Care Plan (p. 2032) for Sickle Cell Disease outlines specific nursing interventions aimed at preventing these sickling crisis states, addressing sickle cell crisis, and continued assessment of long-term sequelae.

Collaborative Management

Nursing collaboration with the multidisciplinary team is an effective means to address the multifactorial, complex needs of the patient with sickle cell disease. Interdisciplinary team members should include pharmacists, physical and occupational therapists, respiratory therapists, medical specialists such as hematologists, and the patient's primary health care provider.

Because pain is a major factor in sickle cell crisis, analgesia is certain to play a role in the acute hospitalization. Pharmacologic expertise can help ensure that appropriate and effective options are readily available and implemented (Buchanan, Woodward, & Reed, 2005). Emerging trends in the management of sickle cell disease suggest that nonpharmacologic interventions and long-term physical exercise plans can help prevent many of the complications related to sickle cell disease.

Physical, occupational, and rehabilitation therapists can provide assistance both in the acute care setting, but more importantly can provide patient education and referrals in preparation for discharge (see the Patient Teaching & Discharge Priorities box, p. 2034) (Bodhise, Dejoie, Brandon, Simpkins, & Ballas, 2004; Ramsey et al., 2001). Respiratory therapy, particularly during

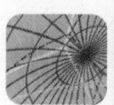

NURSING PROCESS: Patient Care Plan for Sickle Cell Disease

Assessment of Tissue Perfusion

Subjective Data:

Have you been short of breath?

Are you dizzy?

Are you having chest pain?

Have you had any nausea or vomiting or abdominal pain?

Do any of your extremities hurt?

Objective Data:

Integumentary: skin temperature cool, pale

Pulses: diminished, weak peripheral pulses

Renal: decreased urinary output, concentrated

Cerebral: restless, anxious, decreased level of alertness

Cardiopulmonary: tachypnea, tachycardia, angina, oxygen saturation decreased

Gastrointestinal: pain and tenderness with or without palpation

Laboratory values: hemoglobin <7, positive HbS, RBCs decreased, bilirubin elevated

Nursing Assessment and Diagnoses	Outcomes and Evaluation Parameters	Planning and Interventions with *Rationales*
Nursing Diagnosis: *Risk for Ineffective Tissue Perfusion: Cerebral, Renal, Cardiopulmonary, and Abdominal Organ* related to vaso-occlusive crisis	**Outcome:** Free of injury due to peripheral hypoxia. ***Evaluation Parameters:*** Cerebral: Patient remains alert and oriented. Cerebral: Pupil response remains unchanged from baseline. Cerebral: Gross reflex assessment remains unchanged from baseline. Renal: Urinary output remains adequate for patient (at least 30 mL/hr for nondialysis patients). Renal: Electrolyte blood studies and urinalysis remain within normal limits. Renal: Patient remains free of edema. Cardiopulmonary: Peripheral pulses remain intact compared to baseline. Cardiopulmonary: Patient remains free of chest pain. Cardiopulmonary: Lung and chest auscultation do not reveal adventitious or irregular sounds. Cardiopulmonary: Oxygenation status remains within normal limits as measured by spot O_2 saturation above 90% or within normal baseline parameters for patient and ABGs pH 7.3–7.5, $PaCO_2$ 35–45 mmHg. Abdominal: Gastric motility remains intact. Abdominal: Patient remains free of nausea, vomiting, severe cramping, and diarrhea.	**Interventions and *Rationales:*** Frequently monitor neurological signs including level of consciousness, Glasgow Coma Scale, papillary changes, and cranial nerves *to detect changes in level of consciousness and nerve damage.* Assess for signs of edema, urine output (color, amount) *as indicators of renal function.* Monitor blood studies (renal function tests, electrolytes) and urine tests (creatinine, protein) *as indicators of renal function.* Encourage oral fluid intake and administer intravenous fluid (as ordered) *to maintain fluid balance, hydration, and renal cell perfusion.* Administer hypotonic fluids such as dextrose 5% in water or in 0.45% normal saline. *Hypotonic fluids entering RBCs will reduce tendency of hemoglobin to crystallize into sickle shape and will promote dilution of already sickled cells and occluded vessels.* Report changes and trends in renal output and renal lab studies immediately to health care provider *to ensure timely interventions are implemented.* Assess peripheral pulses *as indicators of peripheral tissue perfusion.* Assess cardiac sounds *to detect irregular heart rhythms.* Assess jugular vein distention and peripheral edema *as indicators of cardiac muscle status.* Encourage patient to avoid strenuous activity t*o decrease cardiac workload and oxygen demands.* Assess for adventitious or diminished breath sounds. *Indicates decreased gas exchange and hypoxia.* Monitor respiratory rate and depth *to assess for respiratory distress.* Collaborate with respiratory therapist to administer high-flow oxygen therapy as ordered *to maximize oxygen availability in peripheral tissues.* Collaborate with health care provider to obtain ABGs when spot O_2 sat falls below 80% *as a more accurate analysis of acid–base balance.* Provide incentive spirometry every hour *to prevent atelectasis and acute chest syndrome.* Collaborate with health care provider for administration of oxygen for spot O_2 states of less than 80% *to prevent acidosis. However, do not administer O_2 for patients who are not hypoxic, because this may suppress bone marrow production of RBCs.* Assess for abdominal pain and tenderness *as indicators of gastric perfusion.* Perform abdominal auscultation *as indicators of gastric perfusion.* Monitor for nausea, appetite, vomiting, and diarrhea *as indicators of gastric function.* Offer small frequent meals *to minimize distention.*

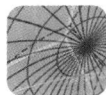

NURSING PROCESS: Patient Care Plan for Sickle Cell Disease—*Continued*

Assessment of Pain of Sickle Cell Disease
Subjective Data:
Are you feeling any pain? If so, where?
What makes it worse? What makes it better?
Can you describe it?
How have you treated sickle cell pain in the past?

Objective Data:
General: pallor, malaise, fatigue
Fever: assess for possible sites of infection
Neurological: level of consciousness (ominous sign of intracranial bleeding)
Lung sounds: crackles, diminished lung sounds
Respiratory: cough, dyspnea, ventilation depth
Cardiovascular: poor capillary refill, tachycardia, hypotension
Pain: location, quality, onset, and alleviating factors
Abdominal: painful, swollen left upper quadrant
Genitourinary: priapism
Neuromuscular: painful swollen joints, especially hips
Renal: renal lab values, urinary output volume and character
Lab values: hemoglobin (presence of sickle cell disease) A2 and F hemoglobin
Full blood count (FBC) to detect anemia, and reticulocyte count

Nursing Assessment and Diagnoses	Outcomes and Evaluation Parameters	Planning and Interventions with *Rationales*
Nursing Diagnosis: *Pain* related to vaso-occlusive crisis	**Outcomes:** Maintenance of adequate oxygenation and acid–base balance. Maintenance of comfort level. **Evaluation Parameters:** Able to communicate pain level and therapies that help alleviate it. Pain reduced and/or absent as evidenced by patient report and no pain behaviors: grimacing. Nonpharmacologic method of control is effective as evidenced by patient report and no pain behaviors. Reports satisfaction with pain management program.	**Interventions and *Rationales:*** Collaborate with patient to determine preferred pain control modalities. *Patients with chronic sickle cell disease are most familiar with personalized effective treatment options. Collaboration also promotes trust and therapeutic relationships.* Assess pain including rating and character frequently and reassess after any pain intervention *to provide early detection of pain and to measure effectiveness of interventions.* Administer pain medication on fixed schedule *to maintain consistent blood levels.* Administer RBCs per health care provider order in specific situations such as symptomatic anemia, a hematocrit reading 7 points below baseline, orthostasis, and a reticulocyte count of zero. *RBC transfusions provide nonsickled oxygen-carrying hemoglobin, increase oxygenation, and treat aplastic crisis.* Monitor for signs such as a falling hematocrit level, pain, pulmonary edema, fever, hypotension, and hemolysis *as indicators of transfusion reactions (hemolysis and fluid overload).*

acute chest syndrome, can help mitigate hypoxia and pain via the application of oxygen therapy. Finally, the patient's primary health care provider may benefit from consultation with a hematologist who specializes in sickle cell disease. The Evidence-Based Practice feature (p. 2035) discusses other interventions that can be used with patients who have sickle cell disease.

Hemolytic Anemias

Hemolytic anemia is a term applied to wide range of diseases characterized by increased RBC destruction, or hemolysis. Hemolysis begins in the peripheral bloodstream with the recognition by phagocytes of dying or damaged red blood cells. The spleen, liver, and reticuloendothelial system then completes degradation. Normally, the rate of hemolysis is balanced by the rate of erythropoiesis, thus maintaining a consistent volume of oxygen-carrying red blood cells in the peripheral circulation.

Infection, toxins, certain medications, injury, and other environmental stressors can all trigger minor increases in hemolysis,

which then result in a decrease in circulating red blood cells, triggering hypoxia. In healthy patients, this hypoxia stimulates increased erythropoietin production, accelerated erythropoiesis, and compensation of hypoxia. Clinically significant hypoxia, characterizing hemolytic anemia, results when the hemolysis persists or is so extensive that erythropoiesis cannot sufficiently compensate. Hemolytic anemia should be distinguished from anemia due to bone marrow disorders (Chart 63–13, p. 2035). In the latter, clinically significant hypoxia results from sluggish erythropoiesis; this cannot compensate for normal hemolysis.

Pathophysiology

Several pathophysiological processes can ultimately result in the anemia of hemolytic etiology just described. Commonly, causes of hemolytic anemia are grouped according to such processes. Certain causes are due to intrinsic defects in the erythrocyte, which decreases its ability to survive the normal RBC life span of 120 days. Deficiencies in metabolic, protective enzymes are the

PATIENT TEACHING & DISCHARGE PRIORITIES for Sickle Cell Anemia

Need	Teaching
Disease process	Discuss cause of disease.
Patient/family	Discuss triggers and risks of sickle cell crisis.
Prevention/management of sickle cell crisis	Discuss activities/scenarios that can exacerbate hypoxic state emphasizing oxygenation and hydration.
Patient/family	
	Teach family to recognize key physical symptoms of sickle cell crisis.
	Discuss appropriate use of oxygenation.
	Discuss appropriate use of pain medication to control pain.
Pharmacologic management	Discuss appropriate use of pharmacologic treatments including side effects and recommended dosing schedule.
Patient/family	
	Consult with pharmacist for drug-specific teaching.
Nutrition	Discuss role of balanced nutrition emphasizing need for key elements: vitamin B_{12}, folate, and iron.
Patient/family	Refer patient to dietitian for assistance in meal planning.
Physical exercise	Discuss and explore appropriate physical exercise options that would maintain muscle/bone/cardiovascular strength but limits risks of hypoxia.
Patient/family	
	Refer patient/family to physical, rehabilitation, and occupational therapy for outpatient consultation.

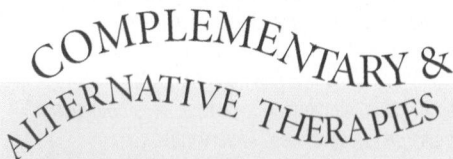

COMPLEMENTARY & ALTERNATIVE THERAPIES   Multiple Therapies

Description:
Several CAM therapies may be appropriate and effective for a specific ailment. For example, there are several CAM therapies that may be effective for sickle cell anemia.

Research Support:
Oxidation plays a significant role in the pathophysiology of sickle cell anemia. Studies have shown in-vitro antioxidant actions from aged garlic extract. One subsequent study examined the antioxidant effect of AGE on sickled red blood cells (RBCs). Study participants included 5 patients with sickle cell anemia (two men and three women, aged 24 to 58) who received a dose of 5 mL AGE daily. Whole blood samples collected from the participants at baseline and after the 4-week treatment period were analyzed for Heinz bodies. Results showed that, in all patients, there was a decrease in the number of Heinz bodies, which suggests that AGE has a significant antioxidant activity on sickled RBCs (Takasu, Uykimpang, Sunga, Amagase, & Niihara, 2006).

A Johns Hopkins University study identified CAM therapies that families of children with sickle cell anemia use and their interest in CAM. The study involved a telephone survey of 57 parents of children with sickle cell anemia. Study results were as follows:

- 54% used CAM therapies.
- 42% used bioenergetic therapies (prayer, spiritual, and energy healing).
- 28% used CAM that related to lifestyle, mind, and body (relaxation techniques, exercise, imagery, and diet).
- 12% used biochemical therapies (herbal medicines, megavitamins, and folk remedies).
- 5% used biomechanical therapy (massage).
- 83% felt that CAM was helpful.

Researchers concluded that use of CAM therapies, especially prayer, relaxation techniques, and spiritual healing is common for children with sickle-cell anemia (Sibinga, Shindell, Casella, Duggan, & Wilson, 2006).

Another study examined Qigong (pronounced "CHEE-kung") therapy, which is a form of energy healing, on breast cancer patients undergoing chemotherapy. White blood cells, platelets, and hemoglobin were measured in blood samples obtained from the study participants. The study involved 67 women, 32 in the experiment group who received a 21-day qigong therapy, and 35 in the control group who received no therapy. Researchers measured patients' blood counts the day before chemotherapy and during chemotherapy on days 8, 15, and 22. The 3-week qigong therapy resulted in significant differences in white blood cells, platelets, and hemoglobin between the experiment and control groups. Although researchers concluded that qigong therapy may improve blood counts in breast cancer patients undergoing chemotherapy, they recommended that more studies be conducted on Qigong before it can be introduced in clinical nursing practice (Yeh, Lee, Chen, & Chao, 2006).

References
Sibinga, E. M., Shindell, D. L., Casella, J. F., Duggan, A. K., & Wilson, M. H. (2006). Pediatric patients with sickle cell disease: Use of complementary and alternative therapies. *Journal of Alternative and Complementary Medicine, 12*(3), 291–298.

Takasu, J., Uykimpang, R., Sunga, M. A., Amagase, H., & Niihara, Y. (2006, March). Aged garlic extract is a potential therapy for sickle-cell anemia. *Journal of Nutrition, 136*(3 Suppl), 803S–805S.

Yeh, M. L., Lee, T. I., Chen, H. H., & Chao, T. Y. (2006, March-April). The influences of Chan-Chuang qi-gong therapy on complete blood cell counts in breast cancer patients treated with chemotherapy. *Cancer Nursing, 29*(2), 149–155.

Sickle Cell Crisis

Clinical Problem

Painful sickle cell crisis is not only a dreaded consequence of the disease but also presents a host of medical management problems to the health care team. Uncontrolled sickle cell crisis places the patient at risk of stroke, heart attack, and organ ischemia, as well as unrelenting pain. Numerous interventions have traditionally been applied in an attempt to control pain and increase oxygenation, thus reversing erythrocyte sickling and decreasing blood viscosity. Nurses and health care providers should be armed with treatment options that have demonstrated rapid effectiveness so that pain is relieved and to minimize the risk of long-term organ damage.

Research Findings

Two meta-analyses (Lottenberg & Hassell, 2005; Mehta, Afenyi-Annan, Byrns, & Lottenberg, 2006) specifically weighed the evidence regarding commonly implemented interventions used to treat painful sickle cell crisis including pharmacologic pain management, incentive spirometry, and hydration with IV fluid. With regard to oxygenation, both reports cite a randomized controlled study (38 hospitalizations) examining the impact of incentive spirometry. Each patient in the spirometry group took 10 maximal inspirations using an incentive spirometer every 2 hours while awake until the chest pain subsided. Of the 19 patients assigned to the spirometry group, only 1 developed pulmonary complications compared to 8 patients assigned to the nonspirometry group. Pulmonary complications included atelectasis, thoracic bone infarction, and infiltration.

Implications for Nursing Practice

These studies clearly provide strong evidence supporting incentive spirometry (IS) to reduce the risk of severe pulmonary complications during sickle cell crisis. Nurses play a very crucial role in providing education about the appropriate use of the incentive spirometer. Patients should be taught to use IS frequently and to maximal volume.

Nurses should include IS observation as part of their regular assessment and documentation. Barriers to effective incentive spirometry include pain, short duration of inspiration, and frustration since beneficial effects may take many days to appear. Nurses should assess for pain in relationship to IS and provide adequate pain management to ensure full chest expansion.

Encouragement and progress tracking should also be offered frequently as a motivational factor. Nurses can enlist family members in these motivational efforts by teaching them to read and report the intake volume of the incentive spirometry to the patient. When appropriate, chest auscultation results and general assessment observations should also be shared with patients to ensure them that their incentive spirometry efforts are in fact effective. Changes in IS volumes should be reported immediately, especially in connection with chest pain and changes in oxygenation.

Critical Thinking Questions

1. Identify the common barriers to effective incentive spirometry in the patient with sickle cell disease.

2. Discuss nursing measures that would increase the use of incentive spirometry in the patient with sickle cell disease.

3. List critical elements that should be included in a respiratory assessment of a patient experiencing sickle cell crisis.

Answers to Critical Thinking Questions appear in Appendix D.

References

Lottenberg, R., & Hassell, K. L. (2005). An evidence-based approach to the treatment of adults with sickle cell disease. *ASH Education Book,* pp. 58–65.

Mehta, S. R., Afenyi-Annan, A., Byrns, P.J., & Lottenberg, R. (2006). Opportunities to improve outcomes in sickle cell disease. *American Family Physician, 74*(2), 313–314.

EVIDENCE-BASED PRACTICE

CHART 63–13   Differences in Hemolysis in Hemolytic Anemia and Bone Marrow Disorders

Normal Hemolysis and Bone Marrow Function	Hemolytic Anemia	Anemia Due to Bone Marrow Disorders
Hemolysis matched by erythropoiesis	Increased hemolysis, normal erythropoiesis	Normal hemolysis, decreased erythropoiesis

---

first intrinsic cause of hemolytic anemia. The most common defect of this type is glucose-6-phosphate dehydrogenase deficiency. A second intrinsic defect results from fragility and instability in the membrane structure, which is the hallmark of hereditary spherocytosis. A third type of intrinsic defect, which results in increased hemolysis, is the hemoglobinopathies, such as those that occur in sickle cell anemia and thalassemia. However, the primary clinical effects are more closely attributed to hemoglobin rather than hemolysis and were thus discussed separately.

Extrinsic causes include situations where the red blood cell is structurally and chemically normal but an unfavorable external environment leads to increased hemolysis. These types of causes include infections, certain medications, autoimmune processes, toxins, and malignancies. Hemolytic anemias from these extrinsic causes are classically grouped together as the acquired hemolytic anemias. The hemolytic anemias also are commonly classified as being intravascular or extravascular, referring to the primary site of hemolysis. In intravascular hemolysis, damaged RBCs are destroyed in the peripheral circulation, and are associated most commonly with mechanical trauma and toxins. In extravascular hemolysis the primary site of destruction is in the spleen and liver. Normally, a red blood cell has enough flexibility to maneuver through the spleen and liver several times throughout the course of its life span. However, membrane defects (including antibody binding) cause some red blood cells to get trapped and eventually become phagocytosed and destroyed. The clinical signs and symptoms, pathophysiology, and treatment unique to each of the underlying etiologies are discussed on the next page.

Clinical Presentation

In addition to unique signs and symptoms associated with individual disease processes, the hemolytic anemias share common physical findings. Consistent with hypoxia of anemias, the patient may complain of fatigue, activity intolerance, and shortness of breath. Severity of hypoxic symptoms correlates with severity of hemolysis. Patients with chronic disorders such as enzyme deficiencies may present only with hypoxic symptoms during periods of acute exacerbation. Jaundice, hemoglobinuria (red-brown urine), splenomegaly, and hepatomegaly (particularly in combination with poor liver function) are additional indicators of persistent hemolysis. Decreased, concentrated urine output is an indication of acute renal failure due to occlusion by lysed red blood cells and is an emergent sign requiring immediate intervention.

Alterations in Laboratory Values

Although the initial cause may vary, hemolytic anemias share some common trends in laboratory studies. Early stages of hemolytic anemia may reveal reticulocytosis (elevated reticulocyte count) in response to accelerated erythropoiesis. RBC counts will be decreased according to the severity of the hemolysis. Plasma haptoglobin levels also may be decreased (especially in intravascular hemolytic anemias) as liberated globin from lysed red blood cells binds all available haptoglobin. As haptoglobin molecules become overwhelmed, a large portion of the hemolyzed hemoglobin is excreted as unconjugated bilirubin. The level of unconjugated bilirubin in hemolysis is typically 70 to 85 μmol/L (4 to 5 mg/dL), or higher if liver function is impaired. If the marrow cannot compensate to replace the RBCs (as indicated by a *decreased* reticulocyte count), the anemia will worsen. Other indicators supporting a diagnosis of hemolytic anemia are increased lactate dehydrogenase (LDH), and serum AST (SGOT) both due to accelerated RBC destruction (Chart 63–14) (Bunn & Rosse, 2003).

Medical Management

The first goal in the emergent management of the patient presenting with symptomatic hemolytic anemia is the stabilization of oxygenation status. Oxygen is administered to prevent critical organ hypoxia, however, administration should be carefully titrated to prevent suppression of erythropoiesis. Intravenous infusions serve to both maintain fluid volume for cardiovascular status and to preserve renal function by flushing the body of excess waste and unconjugated bilirubin. Another goal is the amelioration of rampant hemolysis. If appropriate, triggering agents such as drugs or toxins should be immediately removed. If the cause is extravascular and the patient presents with splenomegaly, a splenectomy, or surgical removal of the spleen, may be indicated (Dhaliwal, Cornnett, & Tierney, 2004). Splenectomy, however, usually is only indicated for certain forms of hemolytic anemia without identifiable triggering agents or in severe cases of acquired hemolytic anemia.

Once the patient is stabilized and risk of imminent organ failure has subsided, attention turns to identification of the underlying pathophysiological process. A CBC and RBC morphology can help rule out or point to bone marrow involvement. Liver function tests can assist in distinguishing hemolytic anemia from nonhematologic causes such as liver failure. A thorough patient history that emphasizes family history and possible toxin and drug exposure also provides important diagnostic clues.

■ Nursing Management

Nursing care of the patient with hemolytic anemia has three main goals: avoidance of triggering factors in susceptible patients and prevention and treatment of complications. High-risk patients such as those with enzyme deficiencies, membrane deficiencies, hemoglobinopathies, or patients with a history of autoimmune hemolytic anemia may initially arrive into the acute care setting without symptoms of rampant hemolysis. To minimize risk of hemolysis, the nurse should carefully review patient histories to identify high-risk persons.

Once identified, collaboration with the interdisciplinary team can help ensure that potential triggering agents are removed from the environment, if appropriate. These high-risk patients should be monitored closely for signs of generalized anemia including increasing fatigue, activity intolerance, and hypoxia, as described earlier in the Nursing Process: Patient Care Plan for Generalized Anemia (p. 2013). Assessments revealing decreased urinary output, hemoglobinuria, left flank pain (from splenomegaly), and fever suggest hemolytic anemia in particular. Analysis of laboratory values revealing reticulocytosis, decreased RBCs, increased bilirubin, and increased lactate dehydrogenase will further confirm hemolytic anemia.

Nursing interventions should then focus on minimizing the effects of blood cell hemolysis. The patient is at high risk for renal failure, thus, the nurse should prioritize interventions to maintain renal blood flow. These include encouraging oral intake and administration of IV fluid and blood component therapy as ordered. Frequent monitoring of urinary output, skin turgor, peripheral edema, and lung sounds will assist the nurse in determining fluid needs. Uncomfortable itching from excessive bilirubin, decreased oxygenation, and activity intolerance all increase the patient's risk for skin breakdown. Nurses should implement aggressive wound prevention protocols such as frequent turning, alleviation of pressure, and frequent skin lubrication to prevent skin breakdown. A third high-risk area of concern is pain related to splenomegaly and intravascular occlusion from lysed

CHART 63–14	**Signs and Symptoms of Hemolytic Anemia**
Physical Assessment	**Laboratory Values**
• Fatigue	• Reticulocytes: increased (reticulocytes decrease in severe hemolytic anemia or with failing bone marrow)
• Activity intolerance	
• Shortness of breath	
• Tachycardia	• Red blood cells: decreased
• Tachypnea	• Serum erythropoietin: increased
• Jaundice (severe cases)	
• Hemoglobinuria (severe cases)	• Serum haptoglobin: decreased
• Decreased urine output	• Unconjugated bilirubin: increased
• Splenomegaly	
• Hepatomegaly	• Lactate dehydrogenase: increased
	• Serum AST: increased

red blood cells. The nurse must perform frequent pain assessments and offer comfort measures, antipyretics, and analgesics (as ordered) to minimize increasing pain.

Glucose-6-Phosphate Dehydrogenase Deficiency

Glucose-6-phosphate dehydrogenase (G6PD) deficiency is the most common enzyme deficiency contributing to hemolytic anemia. Deficiencies in the enzyme are genetically encoded and relatively common especially in persons of African American and Mediterranean descent. Pyruvate kinase deficiency also results in hemolytic anemia, but occurs less frequently. Enzymatic deficiencies in erythrocytes increase the red blood cell's sensitivity and susceptibility to oxidative stress. Normal metabolism is associated with oxidative stress and produces an accumulation of free radicals and other substances that can disrupt function and growth. Enzymes such as G6PD and pyruvate kinase neutralize such free radicals, thus protecting the RBCs. Free radical accumulation is accelerated by a variety of situations that cause oxidative problems including exposure to certain drugs (malarial drugs, sulfonamides, nitrofurantoins, and chloramphenicol), dehydration, sepsis, and diabetic ketoacidosis. Therapeutic management involves removal of the triggering agent and supportive care until the hemolysis subsides. Due to the relatively high occurrence in certain ethnic groups, susceptible patients should be screened for G6PD deficiency before being administered oxidant drugs. Once a patient has been diagnosed and triggering agents identified, most patients with G6PD can live asymptomatically.

Hereditary Spherocytosis

Another cause of hemolytic anemia is defects in the red blood cell membrane. The RBC membrane is a specialized lattice structure of proteins arranged to produce strength, resilience, elasticity, and durability as the red blood cell navigates the peripheral bloodstream. Survival of the 120-day life span of the RBC is highly enhanced by this strong exoskeleton. Genetic disorders including hereditary spherocytosis, hereditary elliptocytosis, hereditary pyropoikilocytosis, and hereditary stomatocytosis all encode proteins that weaken the lattice structure and produce malformed erythrocyte membranes. For example, in **hereditary spherocytosis (HS)**, RBCs lack spectrin, a key membrane protein, which then forces the RBCs into an unstable spherical shape rather than the normal, more stable concave form. HS is a genetic disorder appearing in individuals of northern European descent, affecting approximately 1 in 1,000 to 2,500 patients. The mutated spherical shape of HS cells increases their rate of splenic destruction, resulting in higher rates of hemolysis. Figure 63–8 ■ shows grouped RBCs shown in profile and normal RBCs compared to a sickle RBC (Gallagher, 2005).

Clinical Presentation

Clinical presentation of HS varies with disease severity and inheritance pattern. Autosomal dominant forms and homozygous gene patterns produce persistent anemia, jaundice, and splenomegaly beginning early in life, thus, patients are frequently diagnosed as children. Heterozygous gene patterns can produce carrier states, in which patients are able to develop sufficient compensatory mechanisms and remain asymptomatic. Pallor, activity intolerance, and hypoxia may appear only when

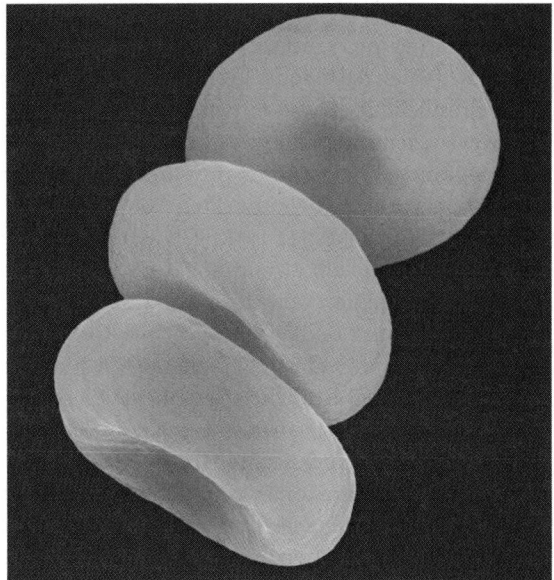

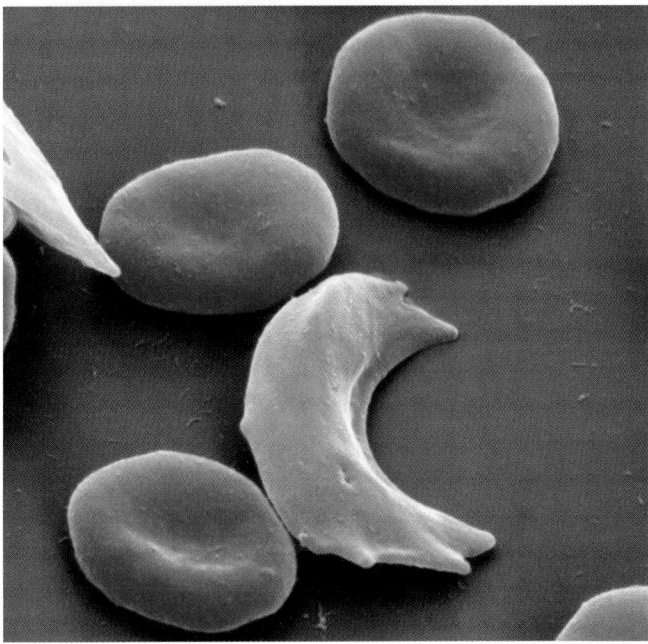

FIGURE 63–8 ■ (top) RBCs in profile, forming rouleaux and (bottom) Normal RBCs compared to a sickled RBC.
Source: (top) © Visuals Unlimited/CORBIS All Rights Reserved; (bottom) Oliver Meckes & Nicole Ottawa/Photo Researchers, Inc.

erythropoiesis is unable to compensate for hemolysis, such as occurs in severe infections, the presence of certain toxins, renal involvement, or bone marrow involvement. Rampant hemolysis of HS red blood cells will be indicated by splenomegaly and jaundice. These may be accompanied by biliary disease and cholecystitis.

Acquired Hemolytic Anemias

Acquired hemolytic anemias develop when an unfavorable external environment leads to increased hemolysis of structurally and chemically normal red blood cells. Such an environment can be mediated by three distinct pathophysiological processes: mechanical causes, infectious agents and toxins, and autoimmune reactions. Mechanical causes of hemolytic anemia describe any situation where normal red blood cells are subjected to extreme or repeated shearing forces, heat, or osmotic attack. Such forces can be generated when red blood cells are exposed to foreign bodies such as prosthetic heart valves, hemodialysis filters, shunts, and cell savers (used during surgery). Mechanical trauma such as prolonged high-impact exercise or pressure also can result in RBC destruction, particularly in the extremities. Prolonged heat exposure above 49°C can also cause RBC lysis, underscoring the potential dangers behind blood-warming devices.

Certain toxins and infectious agents also can cause chemical reactions within the red blood cell, or within the RBC membrane causing premature lysis and hemolytic anemia. Drugs known to contribute to shortened RBC life spans include lead, copper, interferon-alpha, nitrites, dapsonea, and arsenic. Infectious agents cause acquired hemolytic anemia through several different mechanisms including direct invasion by parasites (malaria), release of bacterial toxins (*Clostridium perfringens* and *Haemophilus influenzae* type B), and promotion of splenic sequestration.

Immune-mediated hemolytic anemia is one of the most common causes of acquired hemolytic anemia, and is further divided into autoimmune hemolytic anemia and alloimmune hemolytic anemia. **Autoimmune hemolytic anemia** describes any situation where the patient's own healthy immune system generates antibodies against proteins on his or her own red blood cells (autoantibodies). These autoantibodies are generally divided into two types, warm antibody hemolytic anemia and cold antibody hemolytic anemia. In the warm antibody type, the autoantibodies attach to and destroy red blood cells at temperatures equal to or in excess of normal body temperature. In the cold antibody type, the autoantibodies become most active and attach red blood cells only at temperatures well below normal body temperature. The warm antibody hemolytic anemia accounts for more than 80% of all disease cases. In either type of anemia, the mechanisms that trigger the generation of autoantobodies remain unclear. Possible causes include alteration to immune system development or stimulation by the microbial infections. Alloimmune hemolytic anemia occurs most commonly after prolonged exposure to donated RBC transfusion or after pregnancy. Other causes include malignancy, drugs, autoimmune disorders, systemic lupus erythematosus, and viral infection.

 *Correct crossmatching of blood involves ensuring that the RBC antibodies from donors will not stimulate autoimmune reactions in the recipient. Nurses must very carefully monitor blood cell transfusions checking for correct crossmatch prior to infusion and watching extremely closely for signs and symptoms of hemolytic anemia.*

Treatment must first address identification and removal of triggering agents. If immune-mediated reactions are suspected, Coombs' test will be ordered. Coombs' test detects the presence of circulating antibodies against RBC surface proteins. The presence of any antibodies is an abnormal result indicative of immune-mediated hemolytic anemia. Any of the alterations to laboratory values listed earlier in Chart 63–14 (p. 2036) also will support a diagnosis of hemolytic anemia.

Supportive care should focus on mitigating the immune response by use of immunosuppressive agents and corticosteroids. If mechanical forces are suspected, peripheral blood smears will reveal ruptured blood cells. Treatment for these cases is tailored

to the unique trauma involved. Nursing management is consistent with that presented earlier for hemolytic anemia and generalized anemia. Additionally, nurses should include an assessment for hemolytic anemia whenever a patient presents with history of the risk factors presented above. The Pharmacology Summary feature for anemia lists medications used to treat this disorder and their actions, applications, and nursing responsibilities.

Hemostasis: Regulation of Bleeding and Thrombosis

Hemostasis is the critical biologic process that mitigates blood loss due to injury to any blood vessel. Hemostasis is achieved via very complex and tightly controlled interactions among regulatory mechanisms, cellular components, vessel structures, hormones, plasma proteins, and other chemicals. Although it may appear that hemostasis would only be activated occasionally (i.e., with visible injuries), in actuality the microvasculature is constantly subjected to "mini-traumas" from normal changes in blood pressure and seemingly insignificant physical contact with the environment. Failure of any of the hemostasis mechanisms leads to abnormal clotting, abnormal bleeding, or in some cases both. A review of the normal processes of hemostasis assists the health care provider in understanding diseases that result from deviations in normal hemostasis.

Hemostasis Concepts

The process of hemostasis is a very tightly regulated and elaborate system of interacting proteins, cellular components, and chemical reactions. A discussion of some of the key concepts involved in hemostasis is a useful introduction to the chemical pathways that utilize them.

Cascades

The term *cascade* is an appropriate and important concept throughout hemostasis. In the absence of injury, the chemical components of hemostasis (factors, protein receptors) normally exist in an "inactivated" state in the bloodstream or on cell surfaces. However, injury sets off a chain of events that activates these chemical components. This activation process proceeds in a very specific sequence in which the activation of one chemical component in turn triggers the activation of the next chemical component. For instance, tissue factor transforms Factor VII into Factor VIIa. When Factor VIIa reaches sufficient quantities, it triggers the activation of Factor X into Factor Xa. Each step in the cascade can only proceed if the prior step produced sufficient quantities of activated factors. This concept helps to explain the bleeding (or insufficient clotting) tendencies that accompany certain diseases, such as liver failure, hemophilia, and von Willebrand's disease, which result in insufficient production of factors.

Factors

Factors are proteins present in the bloodstream that, when activated, help facilitate the next step of the coagulation cascade. Most factors are synthesized in the liver in a chemically inactive form. When the chemically inactive form comes into contact with its very specific catalyst, chemical and structural changes occur that convert the inactive form to the active form. Classically, the suffix *a* has been used to designate the active form of

PHARMACOLOGY Summary of Medications to Treat Anemia

Medicine Category	Action	Application/Indication	Nursing Responsibility
Erythropoietic agents	Provides exogenous source of erythropoietin, which stimulates differentiation and proliferation of the hematopoetic cascade. Also, stimulates iron absorption by the erythroid progenitor cells.	Anemia of chronic disease, renal failure, or cancer. Indicated with hemoglobin less than 20.	Assessment of laboratory values to assess efficacy of treatment. Assessment of side effects such as bone pain related to therapy. Patient education regarding self-administration techniques, if appropriate.
Oral iron supplementation	Provides additional iron supply to increase amount of elemental iron available for hemoglobin synthesis.	Iron deficiency anemia when dietary modification is insufficient.	Assessment of drug allergy history prior to administration. Assessment of clinical manifestations of complications such as upper epigastric pain, constipation. Patient education regarding techniques to enhance iron supplement absorption and prevent or treat constipation.
Parenteral iron supplementation	Stimulates release of iron from plasma, which replenishes depleted iron stores in bone marrow.	Severe iron deficiency anemia requiring rapid correction or for patients with chronic kidney disease.	Assessment of drug allergy history. Patient education regarding infusion procedure and potential/expected reactions. Monitoring for signs and symptoms of hypersensitivity and anaphylaxis during and after infusion.
Vitamin supplementation: folates and vitamin B_{12}	Corrects deficiency in key elements required for hemoglobin synthesis.	Serum vitamin B_{12} level less than 100 pg/mL and serum folate level less than 5 ng/mL.	Patient education regarding necessity for vitamin supplementation. Referral to dietary consult to identify additional sources of bioavailable vitamins in foods. Assessment of vitamin therapy efficacy such as patient report of energy.

the factor from the inactive form, and roman numerals used as a consistent label for all factors. Once in the active form, the factor can now act as a very specific catalyst for the activation of the next step of the cascade. Deficiencies in any of the clotting factors either from liver disease, vitamin K deficiency, or genetic causes manifests as a disorder of hemostasis. Chart 63–15 (p. 2040) lists the major factors central to hemostasis. The role of each factor is addressed in the discussion about the clotting cascades.

Hemostasis Pathways

Maintenance of normal blood flow requires hemostasis mechanisms to accomplish four critical goals: (1) recognition of the injury, (2) clot formation, (3) cessation of bleeding, and (4) clot lysis. Injuries to blood vessels are detected simultaneously by a number of body systems including the autonomic nervous system (which controls pain and vasoconstriction) and the hematologic system. Vasoconstriction in the target area serves to reduce the chance of blood loss from the injured site. More importantly perhaps, the mechanical (squeezing) action also helps to release chemicals that initiate clot formation. The clot begins as a soft, pliable plug that typically is used to slow minor bleeding (pri-

mary hemostasis), but then it progresses to a strong meshlike cover, encasing the injured vessel while it heals (secondary hemostasis). Once the injured vessel is healed, the clot must be removed in order to maintain a smooth surface on the blood vessel. The following section describes the hemostasis pathways beginning with formation of the soft plug (mediated by platelets), continuing onto the formation of the meshlike cover (accomplished via the clotting cascade), and finally termination of the clot (a process termed fibrinolysis). Figure 63–9 ■ (p. 2040) provides a graphic illustration of the stages of hemostasis.

Platelet Plug Formation: Primary Hemostasis

Under normal circumstances, circulating platelets neither stick to each other or to vessel walls. When injury to a vessel occurs, injured blood vessels interact with circulating platelets, ultimately leading to the formation of a clump of platelets, called the soft platelet plug, in a process known as *primary hemostasis*. The catalyst for primary hemostasis is the release of substances from the exposed subendothelial layer that interact with protein receptors on platelet's surfaces, inducing chemical and configurational changes, a process termed *activation*.

CHART 63–15	Major Factors Central to Hemostasis	
Factor	**Also Known As**	**Clotting Cascade Pathway***
I	Fibrinogen	Both
II	Prothrombin	Both
III	Tissue factor	Tissue factor (extrinsic)
IV	Calcium	Both
V	Proaccelerin	Both
VI	Accelerin	Both
VII	Proconvertin, cothromboplastin	Tissue factor (extrinsic)
VIII	Antihemophilic factor A	Contact activation (intrinsic)
IX	Christmas factor	Contact activation (intrinsic)
X	Stuart–Power factor	Both (common pathway)
XI	Plasma thromboplastin	Contact activation (intrinsic)
XII	Hegman factor	Contact activation (intrinsic)
XIII	Fibrin stabilizing factor	Both

*Refer to discussion on clotting cascade in the text.

Sources: Moran, T., & Viele, C. (2005). *Normal clotting. Seminars in Oncology Nursing, 21*(4), 1–11; Porth, C. M. (2007). *Essentials of pathophysiology: concepts of altered health states* (2nd ed.). Philadelphia: Lippincott Williams & Wilkins.

Once activated individual platelets undergo geometric and chemical changes that allow them to form a soft platelet plug. Formation of the platelet plug occurs rapidly via four distinct actions:

1. **Adhesion**—Adhesion refers to the sticking of platelets onto the injured vessel wall. Adhesion is initiated when von Willebrand's factor forms a bridge between exposed collagen from the subendothelial layer of the vessel wall and proteins (glycoprotein Ib) on the platelet surface. Patients afflicted with von Willebrand's disease lack sufficient quantities of the factor and can suffer uncontrolled bleeding.

2. **Aggregation**—On activated platelets, protein receptors (specifically IIb and IIa) seek out and bind to neighboring platelet membranes. Additionally, activated platelets adhere to fibrinogen, a chemical secreted into the bloodstream by the liver. Fibrinogen has the ability to form fibrous meshlike networks between platelets.

3. **Secretion**—The third function of activated platelets is the secretion of substances (a process called degranulation). Adenosine diphosphate (ADP) and serotonin recruit additional platelets to the site of injury and also stimulate more vasoconstriction. Other substances, including fibronectin, thomboxane A_2, thrombospondin, arachidonic acid, and platelet Factor V, stimulate the platelet membrane to form pseudopods (elongated shapes) and interact with fibrinogen, which help to stabilize the platelet plug. This soft platelet plug can form within seconds in the individual not lacking any of the required chemical factors. Its primary goal is the immediate abatement of minor bleeding; however, the temporary plug can be easily sheared off unless stabilized. Intracellular calcium, which is required for factor activation in the clotting cascade, also is released from the platelets.

4. **Assembly**—Finally activated platelet cell surfaces promote the assembly of enzymes necessary for the initiation of the

Normal

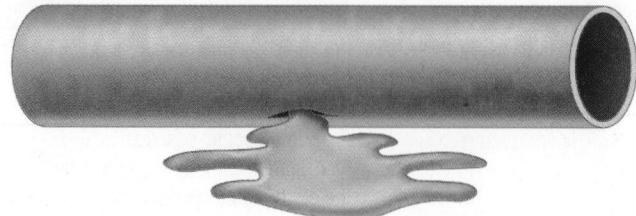
1 Bleeding starts

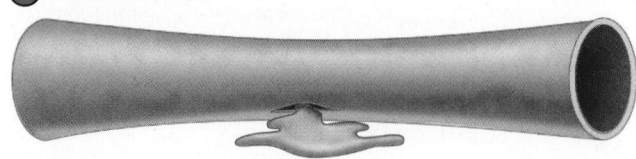
2 Vasoconstriction

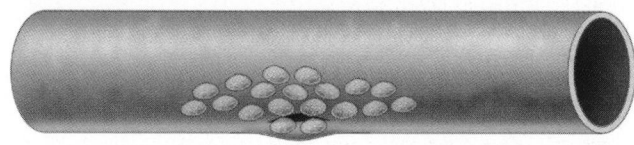
3 Soft platelet plug - primary hemostasis

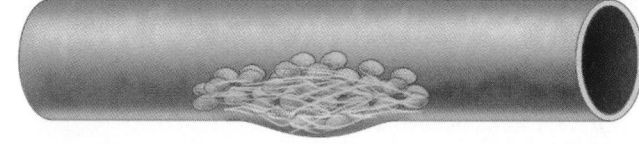
4 Fibrin clot formation - secondary hemostasis

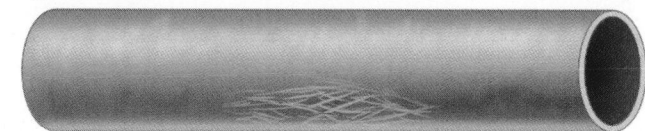
5 Clot lysis

FIGURE 63–9 ■ Stages of hemostasis.

clotting cascade. For example, von Willebrand's factor bound to the platelet can also bind coagulation factor VIII, a component of the clotting cascade (discussed next).

Clotting Cascade: Secondary Hemostasis

While vasoconstriction and platelets act rapidly to minimize blood loss, sustained turbulent blood flow at the site of injury can shear the platelet plug. The clotting cascade describes the sequential activation of factors ultimately leading to the formation of a fibrin sheath, which stabilizes the platelet plug. Rather than being a single cascade of events, the term *clotting cascade* actually describes two distinct series of events: the contact activation (or intrinsic) pathway and the tissue factor (or extrinsic) pathway. If successful, each pathway results in the activation of Factor X to Factor Xa, which begins the final stage of clotting, the common pathway.

The molecular mechanisms underlying the clotting cascade have been the focus of intense research for several years, most likely due to the role of clotting and hemostasis in diseases such as cardiovascular disorders, thrombosis, and stroke. Scientific advancements have reshaped the classic understanding of and terminology used with the clotting cascade process. Traditionally, it was thought that the two pathways acted independently to form the fibrin net. Now, however, it is widely recognized that deficiencies in one pathway cannot be compensated for by the other pathway, suggesting some degree of interaction. Second, the terms *intrinsic pathway* and *extrinsic pathway* have been replaced by the terms *contact activation* and *tissue factor*, respectively, describing the discovery of the initiating events of each pathway.

Contact Activation: The Intrinsic Pathway

The contact activation pathway describes the clotting cascade branch initiated by the contact between circulating plasma proteins and the negatively charged surface of the injured subendothelial layer. Figure 63–10 ■ describes the activation steps. Hageman factor (Factor XII) sets off the cascade by contacting the subendothelial layer, which causes it to become Factor XIIa (activated factor), setting off the series of activations culminating with Factor VIIa, which then leads to the common pathway (Hoffman & Monroe, 2005).

Tissue Factor: The Extrinsic Pathway

The extrinsic pathway describes the branch of the clotting cascade pathway initiated by tissue factor (TF) also called tissue thromboplastin, a substance released from injured cells of the subendothelial layers. In the presence of calcium and lipids released from platelets, tissue factor first activates Factor VII into Factor VIIa. Then tissue factor interacts with the newly activated Factor VIIa to activate Factor X into Factor Xa, the beginning step of the common pathway (Figure 63–11 ■).

The Common Pathway

Both the contact activation and tissue factor pathways converge with the activation of Factor X into Factor Xa (Figure 63–12 ■, p. 2042). In the presence of calcium and lipids from activated platelets, Factor Xa converts prothrombin (Factor II) to throm-

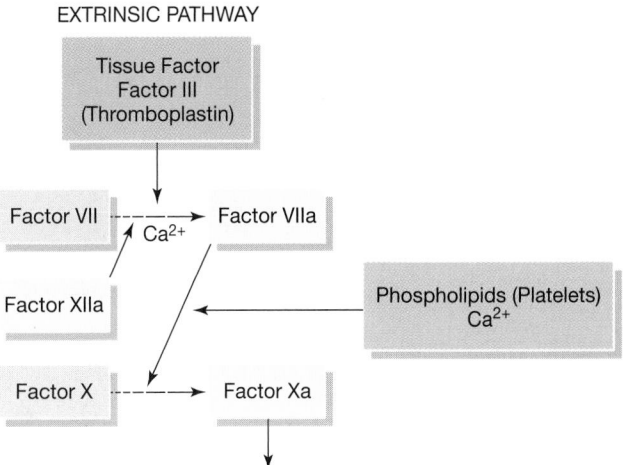

FIGURE 63–11 ■   The tissue factor activation (extrinsic) pathway.

bin (Factor IIa). Thrombin is an extremely powerful component in coagulation, playing three main roles. First, thrombin interacts and amplifies the contact activation (intrinsic) and tissue factor (extrinsic) pathways to form a positive feedback loop ensuring that coagulation continues. Second, thrombin interacts with fibrinogen to make fibrin strands (polymers). Last, thrombin also activates fibrin stabilizing factor (Factor XIII). In the presence of calcium, again released from platelets, Factor XIIIa and the fibrin strands weave through the platelet plug, forming a strong mesh (termed the fibrin mesh) and effectively sealing the site of injury and halting bleeding.

Termination of Clotting

The processes of platelet plug formation (primary hemostasis) and coagulation (secondary hemostasis) ultimately result in the formation of a fibrin mesh that effectively halts bleeding. However, left unchecked, continued fibrin formation can lead to vessel occlusion by expanding clots, thrombosis, blood stasis, and embolism. These molecular processes are the underlying causes behind serious diseases such as embolic stroke, cardiovascular disease, and deep venous thrombosis (DVT). To prevent such damage and to maintain smooth, adequate blood flow, hemostasis must include a process to regulate and eventually terminate clotting when no longer required. This termination phase of coagulation hinges on the action of three inhibitors: antithrombin, tissue factor pathway inhibitor, and protein C.

Antithrombin is a naturally occurring protein circulating in the bloodstream that neutralizes the actions of thrombin and activated Factors Xa, Xia, XIIa, and IXa. As injuries heal and vasoconstriction begins to subside, blood flow begins to return to normal levels, bringing antithrombin to the site of coagulation. Antithrombin is a key target in the pharmacologic treatment of thrombosis, because its activity is significantly accelerated by the anticoagulant heparin (Bajaj, Birktoft, & Steer, 2001).

Tissue factor pathway inhibitor (TFPI) neutralizes Factor X, halting progression of the common pathway and production of thrombin. Increased TFPI levels have been observed in the presence of heparin and low-molecular-weight heparin, and new drug therapies that enhance the action of TFPI are currently being developed (Bajaj et al., 2001).

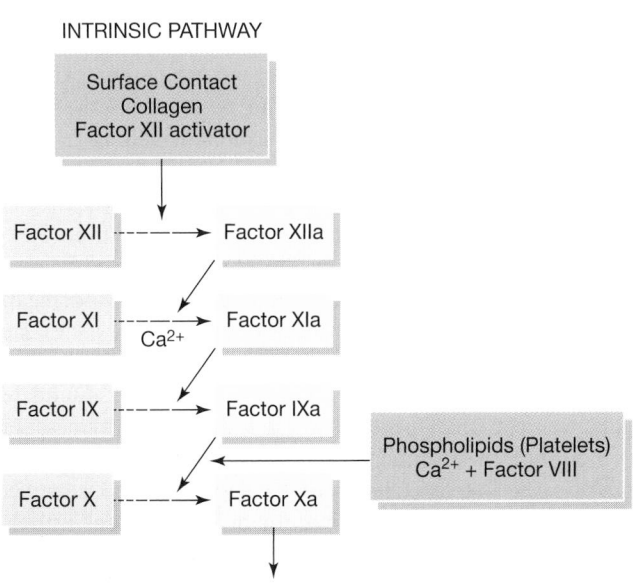

FIGURE 63–10 ■   The contact activation (intrinsic) pathway.

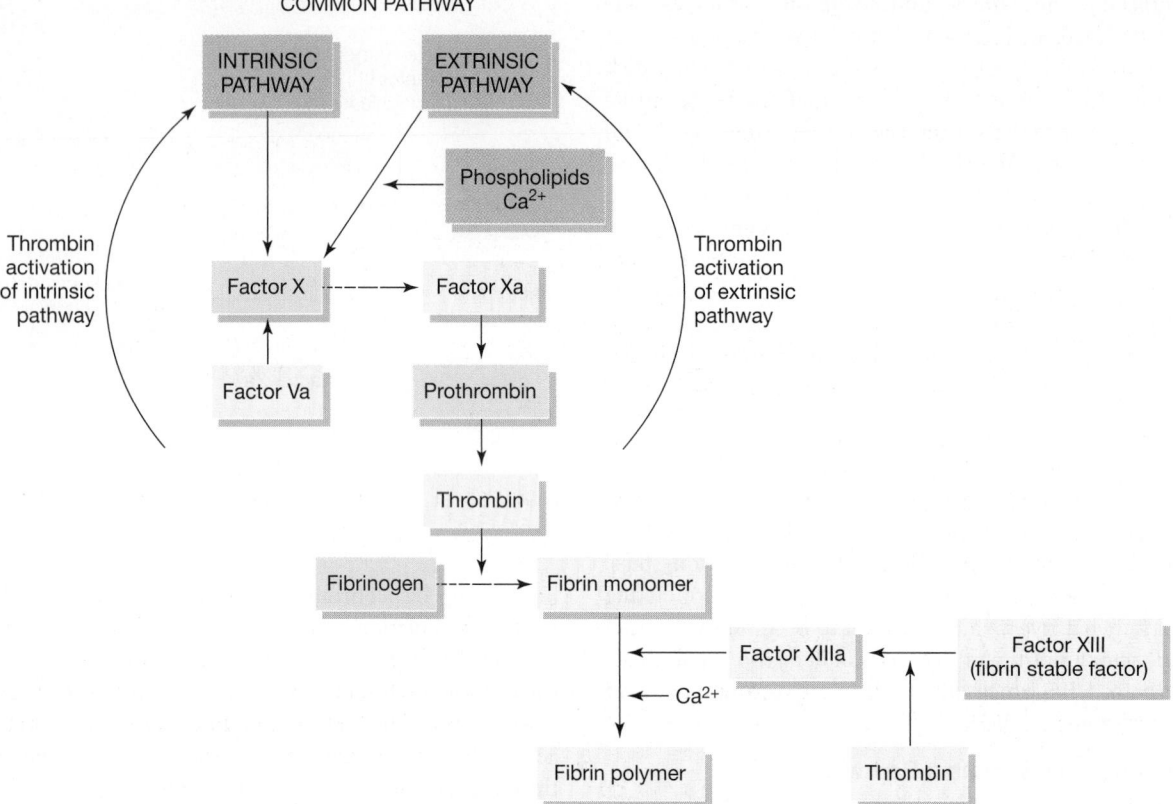

FIGURE 63–12 ■ The common pathway.

Activated protein C neutralizes Factor V of the tissue factor (extrinsic) pathway and Factor VIII of the contact activation (intrinsic) pathway. The activation of protein C occurs with the binding of thrombin to the subendothelial layer of the vessel wall; thus, accelerated thrombin production results in accelerated protein C activation and an effective braking mechanism for coagulation. Activated protein C therapy plays an important role in the therapeutic management of thrombosis especially in the management of septic shock (Chapter 61 ⊙).

Additional chemicals such as nitric oxide, prostacyclin, and thromboxane also limit excessive contributions to coagulation control by limiting platelet aggregation, activation, adhesion, and vasoconstriction. Activation of these components is the target of many anti-inflammatory drugs including non-steroidal anti-inflammatory drugs (NSAIDs), aspirin, and Cox-1 inhibitors.

Fibrinolysis: Clot Elimination

Once the endothelial layers of the blood vessel membrane have healed, the fibrin clot should be removed to optimize blood flow. The last phase of hemostasis is fibrinolysis, or the dissolution of the fibrin strands. Tissue plasminogen activator (t-PA), released by the endothelial cells during coagulation, and urokinase cause the activation of plasminogen to plasmin. Plasmin is a powerful enzyme that first digests fibrin strands into fibrin degradation products (FDPs), themselves extremely powerful promoters of fibrinolysis. FDPs are able to inhibit thrombin activity to slow clot formation and to accelerate plasmin production. As with most of the chemical elements in the coagulation cascade, medical research has developed drug treatments that exploit the natural activity of t-PA and urokinase in the management of thrombosis.

Laboratory and Diagnostic Procedures

Several blood tests are available to measure the efficacy of platelet plug formation (primary hemostasis), coagulation (secondary hemostasis), and fibrinolysis. The platelet count, usually part of the CBC, describes the number of circulating platelets in a volume of blood. Normal values range from 150,000 to 400,000 per microliter of blood. Values of less than 150,000 define thrombocytopenia and imply impaired clotting by platelets. However, spontaneous bleeding rarely occurs at levels above 50,000. Values greater than 400,000 are labeled thrombocytosis and imply excessive platelet clotting.

Bleeding time measures the efficacy of vasoconstriction and platelet response. In the bleeding time test, a blood pressure cuff is inflated around the arm to a specific pressure and then small incisions are made in the patient's arm. Normally, clot formation begins within 3 to 7 minutes.

Clotting time studies measure the amount of time required for a volume of blood to form a stable clot. Prothrombin time (PT) is measured in seconds and reflects the amount of time it takes to form a clot after the addition of tissue factor, thus measuring the tissue factor (extrinsic) pathway. Due to variations in tissue factor batches among laboratories, the International Normalized Ratio (INR) value was developed and is now widely used as a standardized interpretation of the test. Many of the components measured by the prothrombin time require vitamin K for their synthesis, thus diseases or dietary alterations that affect vitamin K also affect PT values. The activated partial thromboplastin time (aPTT), also expressed in seconds, measures the efficacy of the contact activation (intrinsic) pathway in clot formation. The normal values for these tests are listed in Chart 63–16.

CHART 63–16	Blood Tests/Values Indicative of Hemostasis	
Lab Value	**Normal Value**	**Rationale**
Platelets	150,000–400,000/mm³	Measures number of platelets in volume of blood. Reduction indicates thrombocytopenia.
Bleeding time	<12 minutes	Measures primary hemostasis efficacy.
Prothrombin time (PT)	10–20 seconds (significant variation in normal values between laboratories)	Measures efficacy of extrinsic pathway. Increased values indicate thrombotic tendencies. Reduction indicates bleeding tendencies.
International Normalized Ratio (INR)	0.8–1.2 INR	Used in conjunction with PT. Elevated in Coumadin therapy.
Partial thromboplastin time (aPTT)	Varies (compare with control); 35–45 seconds	Measures efficacy of intrinsic pathway. Increased values indicate thrombotic tendencies. Reduction indicates bleeding tendencies.
Fibrin degradation products (FDP)	<10 µg/mL	Measures efficacy of fibrinolytic system.
D-dimer	<0.5 mg/L	Measures efficacy of fibrinolytic system.

Fibrin degradation products (FDPs), especially D-dimer, measure the volume of these powerful fibrinolysis activators. Values are increased during sepsis, disseminated intravascular coagulation (or any coagulation event), and pregnancy.

Disorders of Hemostasis

When the tight regulation of hemostasis is disrupted by disease, drugs, or environmental factors, the affected patient can present with abnormal bleeding, abnormal clotting, or in some cases both. Like all blood disorders, disorders of hemostasis can be either acquired (as in response to sepsis or bone marrow suppression therapy) or chronic (as in genetic disorders of hemophilia and von Willebrand's disease). Disorders of hemostasis also can be categorized according to the deficient or errant component. Disorders of the platelet and vessel wall can be categorized as disorders of primary hemostasis and include thrombocytopenia, hemolytic uremic syndrome, and von Willebrand's disease. Disorders involving factor deficiencies affecting coagulation can be categorized as secondary hemostasis disorders and include liver disease, vitamin K deficiency, and hemophilia.

Disorders of Primary Hemostasis

Disorders of primary hemostasis include any problems affecting platelets or platelet interaction with the subendothelial vessel layer. All of these disorders result in prolonged bleeding times, resulting from slowed platelet plug formation. Qualitative problems or reduction of platelets from normal values are classified as the various thrombocytopenias and represent a significant portion of all disorders of hemostasis. Diseases resulting from abnormal interaction between the subendothelial layer of the vessel, although less common, also result in abnormal bleeding times and describe any disease process that affects platelet aggregation, adhesion, or secretion. Hemolytic uremic syndrome and von Willebrand's disease are discussed below as exemplars of this class of primary hemostasis disorders.

Thrombocytopenia

Thrombocytopenia is defined as a decrease in the number of circulating platelets from the normal value of 150,000/µL. Although significant, spontaneous bleeding usually is not observed until levels fall below 50,000/µL. It is one of the most common hematologic problems experienced by patients and warrants a thorough understanding by nurses and other health care providers. The causes of thrombocytopenia are numerous but, like most hematologic disorders, can be divided into two broad categories: thrombocytopenia due to impaired or suppressed production of platelets and thrombocytopenia due to accelerated destruction of platelets. The major patient care issue associated with thrombocytopenia is an increased tendency for bleeding.

Normal Physiology of Platelets

An understanding of the normal physiology of platelet development provides an effective foundation for a discussion about platelet disorders. Platelets are not cells with independently functioning nuclei and cytoplasmic structures like white blood cells and red blood cells; rather, they are shed fragments of the megakaryocyte. Platelet development proceeds in much the same fashion as that of red blood cells and white blood cells. Recall from the discussion at the beginning of the chapter about hematopoiesis that all cellular elements of the blood arise in the bone marrow from the hematopoeitic stem cell before undergoing differentiation, maturation, and release into the peripheral bloodstream (see Figure 63–1, p. 2007).

The complete pathway from HSC to fully mature platelet release into the periphery is called *thrombopoiesis.* The primary regulating substance in thrombopoiesis is thought to be the hormone **thrombopoietin**, produced by the liver and kidneys. Thrombopoietin directs the HSC to produce the megakaryocyte, the precursor to fully functioning platelets. Thrombopoietin additionally stimulates the megakaryocyte to undergo mitosis and reproduce itself (thus exponentially increasing the potential for platelet quantities), and most importantly triggers the fragmentation of the megakaryocyte into small particles. These particles are platelets, which are then released into the periphery and generally survive an 8- to 12-day life span. Senescent (aging) platelets begin to express cell surface proteins, which trigger its destruction by macrophages in the spleen and reticuloendothelial system. Alterations to thrombopoiesis can have deleterious effects on hemostasis ranging from increased bleeding to increased thrombosis.

Pathophysiology of Thrombocytopenia

Thrombocytopenia has been attributed to several underlying causes, which can be broadly divided into suppressed production or accelerated destruction. The pathophysiology of each class and representative disease processes are discussed below.

Impaired Production of Platelets

A number of disease processes as well as environmental factors impede thrombopoiesis and result in thrombocytopenia. Diseases such as leukemia, lymphoma, multiple myeloma, metastatic cancers, and aplastic anemia are associated with global suppression of hematopoiesis, which will thus include suppressed platelet production. Additionally, most of the treatment approaches (chemotherapy and radiation) used in cancer and other bone marrow diseases independently suppress thrombopoiesis. Exposures to viruses have resulted in selective suppression of the megakaryocyte and include human immunodeficiency virus (HIV), Epstein–Barr, rubella, and mumps exposure. A third mechanism for impaired platelet production is liver disease resulting in insufficient quantities of thrombopoietin, vitamin B_{12}, and vitamin K (Rios, Sangro, Herrero, Quiroga, & Prieto, 2005). Finally, exposure to certain drugs, especially large quantities of alcohol and thiazide diuretics, can suppress megakaryocyte production.

Accelerated Destruction of Platelets

Thrombocytopenia due to accelerated destruction can be subdivided into two categories: autoimmune causes and nonautoimmune causes. Autoimmune-accelerated destruction of platelets describes any situation in which the patient appropriately develops antibodies against invading pathogens, which then inappropriately attach to surface proteins of circulating platelets. When these antibody-bound platelets reach the spleen they are prematurely removed, causing thrombocytopenia. This autoimmune response has been observed following exposure to systemic lupus erythematosus, rheumatoid arthritis, HIV, and excessive transfusions, as well as certain drugs including depakote and heparin (Davoren & Aster, 2006; Gesundheit, Kirby, Lau, Koren, & Abdelhaleem, 2002).

Nonautoimmune processes contributing to early platelet destruction include exposure to prosthetic heart valves, thrombotic thrombocytopenic purpura (TTP), sepsis, and hemolytic uremic syndrome. In these situations, the thrombocytopenia can be attributed to increased utilization of platelets by the underlying disease process. As the platelets (appropriately) respond to vessel damage caused by these processes, they are removed from circulation, manifesting as a decreased platelet count.

Clinical Presentation

A diagnosis of thrombocytopenia often is made after observation of active bleeding, underscoring the need for vigilant assessment. Figure 63–13 ■ provides a graphical representation of bleeding sites throughout the body. Increased bleeding and a decreased platelet count are the primary diagnostic indicators of thrombocytopenia.

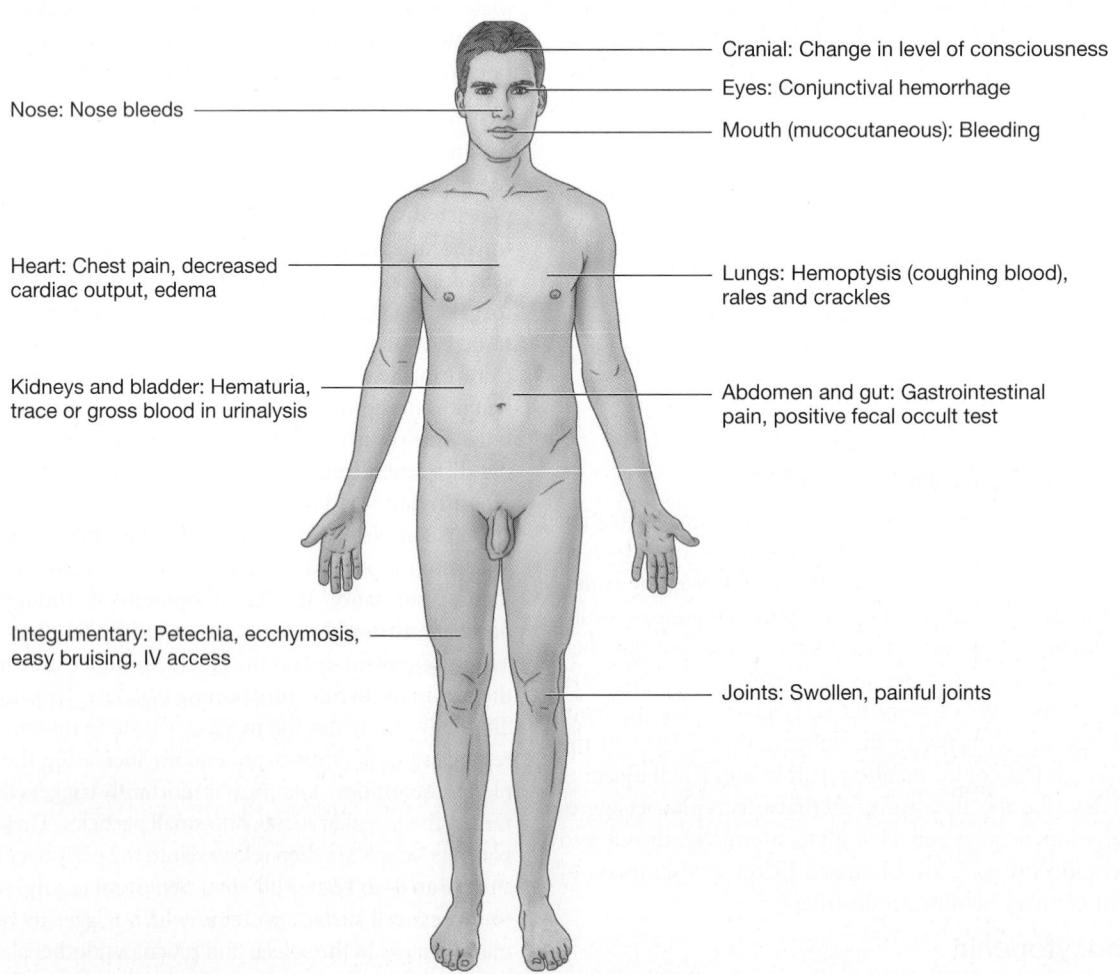

Nose: Nose bleeds

Cranial: Change in level of consciousness

Eyes: Conjunctival hemorrhage

Mouth (mucocutaneous): Bleeding

Heart: Chest pain, decreased cardiac output, edema

Lungs: Hemoptysis (coughing blood), rales and crackles

Kidneys and bladder: Hematuria, trace or gross blood in urinalysis

Abdomen and gut: Gastrointestinal pain, positive fecal occult test

Integumentary: Petechia, ecchymosis, easy bruising, IV access

Joints: Swollen, painful joints

FIGURE 63–13 ■ Assessment of bleeding sites.

Patients who present with platelet counts of less than 20,000 µL are at imminent risk of internal bleeding. A drop in the platelet count below this level should be immediately reported to the health care provider as part of a comprehensive assessment including neurological, respiratory, cardiovascular, and abdominal symptoms. Prepare for possible platelet transfusion.

Physical Manifestations   The primary physical manifestations of thrombocytopenia are the appearance of mucosal and cutaneous bleeding, and prolonged bleeding after invasive procedures. Degree of symptom severity correlates with platelet count. Below 100,000/mm³ patients may experience prolonged bleeding after surgery or any invasive procedure such as IV catheterization or dental treatments. Patients do not typically present with mucosal or cutaneous bleeding until platelet values reach 50,000/mm³ or lower. Mucosal bleeding can be observed in the gums especially following aggressive brushing or flossing, in the urinary tract, or from the nares. Patients also may report blood-tinged sputum after coughing or blood in the stool. Cutaneous bleeding appears as discoloration of the skin and can often be mistaken for rash. Cutaneous bleeding can be described as a continuum from small pinpoint lesions (petechiae), to larger group patches (purpura), to ecchymosis, or large (centimeters) patches of active bleeding into the skin.

At 20,000/mm³ the patient is considered at risk for spontaneous bleeding. Although anemia due to acute blood loss should be addressed, a greater concern is bleeding into closed spaces such as the cranium, pleural space, pericardial space, or abdomen. At critically low platelet values, patients should be frequently assessed for changes in level of consciousness, respiratory status, cardiovascular status, or abdominal pain.

Alterations in Laboratory Values   Thrombocytopenia is a disease of primary hemostasis reflected in the platelet count and bleeding time. PT, aPTT, and INR are of little diagnostic value in the evaluation of thrombocytopenia because they focus on secondary hemostasis.

Medical Management
Management of thrombocytopenia must address any underlying etiology. If the thrombocytopenia results from impaired production due to bone marrow suppression, a watchful waiting approach and protective measures usually are the first line of management. Exogenous thrombopoietin to stimulate platelet production currently is in investigational stages. Platelet transfusion may be administered in these populations. If the thrombocytopenia is attributable to accelerated destruction of platelets, the causative factors must be identified and addressed. Drug-induced thrombocytopenia can be addressed by cessation of the offending drug. In immune-mediated accelerated destruction, immunosuppressive treatment may be initiated to reduce antibody production. Options may include corticosteroids, splenectomy, and IV immunoglobulin. Specific treatments for immune-mediated thrombocytopenia and heparin-induced thrombocytopenia are addressed later.

Nursing Management
Nurses in a variety of clinical settings must be familiar with the risks, early signs, and management of these diseases because they can occur as a side effect of a vast array of diseases and treatments. Oftentimes, thrombocytopenia is first detected by astute nursing observation and assessment, followed up by effective collaboration. Nursing interventions implemented for the patient with thrombocytopenia focus on early detection, risk reduction, management of medical interventions, and patient education. Common bleeding precautions used to minimize risk of bleeding in high-risk patients are listed in Chart 63–17. The Nursing Process: Patient Care Plan for Thrombocytopenia and Bleeding Disorders (p. 2046) outlines appropriate care for patients with thrombocytopenia and bleeding disorders. Teaching for patients with bleeding disorders is addressed in the Patient Teaching & Discharge Priorities box (p. 2047).

Collaborative Management
Patients who have thrombocytopenia require the coordinated efforts of a multidisciplinary team to prevent exacerbation of injury and to optimize recovery. Pharmacists play a key role in the management of thrombocytopenia due to their expertise in drug side effect profiles and drug–drug interactions. Their guidance can assist the multidisciplinary team to identify drugs that might exacerbate thrombocytopenia and, moreover, to find alternative treatments with the same efficacy but with decreased deleterious side effects.

Especially in cases of bone marrow suppression, optimal nutrition plays a key role in patients' recovery from thrombocytopenia. Many patients with thrombocytopenia suffer from decreased appetite, which can result in severe nutritional deficits, or fear of oral cavity injury (and bleeding) from chewing or swallowing. Registered dietitians can develop nutrition plans that both maximize key nutrients and minimize further injury to the oral mucosa.

Immune Thrombocytopenia Purpura
Immune thrombocytopenic purpura (ITP) (previously referred to as idiopathic thrombocytopenic purpura) is an autoimmune

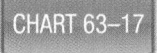 **CHART 63–17**   **Bleeding Precautions**

Although exact bleeding precautions vary among clinical sites, the following measures are widely implemented to minimize the risk of injury to patients:

- Avoid intramuscular and subcutaneous injections.
- Hold firm pressure to venipuncture sites for a minimum of 5 minutes.
- Minimize venipunctures and invasive procedures.
- Provide a soft toothbrush or tooth sponges for mouth care.
- Avoid rectal suppositories, thermometers, enemas, and other rectal/vaginal manipulation.
- Prevent constipation and straining with stools.
- Use electric razor only.
- Maintain a safe environment to avoid injury.
- Assist with ADLs and ambulation as necessary to avoid injury.
- Avoid medications with antiplatelet activity (e.g., aspirin and aspirin-containing products, NSAIDs).

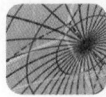

NURSING PROCESS: Patient Care Plan for Thrombocytopenia and Bleeding Disorders

Assessment of Abnormal Bleeding

Subjective Data:

Do you have any history of disease?

Do you have recent history of exposure to viruses such as measles, mumps, varicella, rubella?

Are you currently being treated with any medications? If so, which?

Do you take any OTC drugs, herbs, or street drugs?

How much alcohol do you drink on a daily basis?

Have you noticed any increased bleeding?

Objective Data:

Skin: petechiae, ecchymosis

Mucosa: color, tenderness, increased bleeding

Conjunctivae: bleeding

Urine: color

Neurological: level of consciousness (ominous sign of intracranial bleeding)

Lung sounds: crackles, diminished lung sounds

Abdominal: painful, swollen

Laboratory values: platelets less than 100,000/μL; compare to previously recorded studies

Nursing Assessment and Diagnoses	Outcomes and Evaluation Parameters	Planning and Interventions with *Rationales*
Nursing Diagnoses: *Risk for Injury* related to increased intracranial pressure, abdominal bleeding, pericardial bleeding, and/or bleeding into pleural space	**Outcome:** Free of injury due to bleeding. *Evaluation Parameters:* Laboratory: Hemoglobin values remain within normal limits. Laboratory: Platelet, APTT, PT, and INR values remain within normal limits. Vital signs: Vital signs remain within baseline normal limits for patient.	**Interventions and** *Rationales:* Frequently monitor laboratory values for signs of precipitous decrease in hemoglobin *to detect changes in level of circulating red blood cells.* Frequently monitor laboratory values for signs of increased bleeding times *to detect tendencies to bleed.* Assess vital signs especially blood pressure *as indicators of vascular space volume. In the event of bleeding, blood volume leaves vascular space.* Report critical values immediately *because health care provider may wish to initiate blood product transfusion.*
	Cerebral: Patient remains alert and well oriented. Cerebral: Pupils remain equal, round, and reactive to light. Cerebral: Gross reflex assessment remains unchanged from baseline. Abdominal: Patient denies abdominal pain. Abdominal: Bowel sounds at baseline or present in all four quadrants.	Frequently monitor neurological signs including level of Glasgow Coma Scale, papillary changes, and cranial nerves *to detect changes in level of consciousness and nerve damage.* Monitor restlessness, and confusion *as indicators of increased intracranial pressure and/or decreased oxygenation due to bleeding.* Frequently assess (inspection, auscultation, palpation, percussion) abdominal status and seek patient report of abdominal pain *to detect signs of bleeding into abdominal cavity and hypoxia in abdominal structures due to blood loss.*
	Patient denies chest pain, shortness of breath.	Assess abdomen for pain, tenderness, distention *as indicators of internal abdominal bleeding.* Assess for adventitious or diminished breath sounds. *Indicates decreased gas exchange and hypoxia.* Monitor respiratory rate and depth *to assess for respiratory distress.*
	Urine color clear. Free of blood in stool.	Frequently assess urine and stool color. *Possible early indicator of systemic internal bleeding. Detection of early signs allows for timely administration of platelet transfusion.*
Impaired Skin Integrity related to abnormal bleeding into cutaneous areas and mucosal surfaces	**Outcome:** Free of serious injury due to internal bleeding. *Evaluation Parameters:* Alert and oriented. Clear breath sounds and absence of respiratory distress. Free of reports of abdominal pain. Lab values (platelet/Hct/Hgb) within normal limits for patient. Free of petechiae, ecchymosis, hematuria. Blood pressure within normal limits. **Outcome:** Minimal or no bleeding observed. *Evaluation Parameters:* Free of petechiae, ecchymosis. Free of bleeding from gums, mucosa, and catheter sites. Urine color clear. Free of blood in stool.	**Interventions and** *Rationales:* Frequently assess skin, mucosa membrane for evidence of color change, tenderness, and bleeding. *For clinical manifestations of bleeding.* Frequently assess urine and stool color. *Possible early indicator of systemic internal bleeding. Detection of early signs allows for timely administration of platelet transfusion.* Monitor respiratory rate and depth *to assess for respiratory distress.* Assess abdomen for pain, tenderness, distention *as indicators of internal abdominal bleeding.* Assess vital signs, especially blood pressure *as indicators of vascular space volume. In the event of bleeding, blood volume leaves vascular space.*

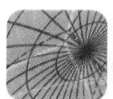

NURSING PROCESS: Patient Care Plan for Thrombocytopenia and Bleeding Disorders—*Continued*

Assessment of Patient Self-Management

Subjective Data:

What do you understand about thrombocytopenia?

Do you have any particular fears about thrombocytopenia?

What signs and symptoms might you observe that cause you concern?

Objective Data:

Skin color and condition, absence of petechiae

Mucosa membrane color

Urine and stool color

Cognition

Level of agitation and restlessness

Comprehension

Vital signs within normal values

Lab values: platelets less than 100,000/mm^3; compare to previously recorded studies

Verbalization of condition

Nursing Assessment and Diagnoses	Outcomes and Evaluation Parameters	Planning and Interventions with *Rationales*
Nursing Diagnosis: *Deficient Knowledge related to management of thrombocytopenia*	**Outcome:** Patient and family verbalize understanding of required skills and knowledge required in the management of thrombocytopenia. ***Evaluation Parameters:*** Patient verbalizes understanding of bleeding precautions including avoidance of contact sports, use of razors, oral care. Patient reports signs and symptoms that warrant immediate attention by health care provider. Patient reports understanding of medications that should be avoided including aspirin and other drugs specific to patient's history.	**Interventions and *Rationales*:** Frequently reinforce patient education regarding bleeding precautions *to minimize risk of injury.* Educate patient and family about tests and procedures *to increase understanding of disease process.* Educate patient and family concerning the disease, treatment, and potential complications *to increase understanding of disease process.* Collaborate with multidisciplinary team to *reinforce pharmaceutical, nutritional, and rehabilitation/educational interventions.*

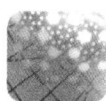

PATIENT TEACHING & DISCHARGE PRIORITIES for Generalized Bleeding Disorders

Need	Teaching Objective
Disease process	Discuss cause of disease.
Patient/family	Assist patient/family in recognition of cutaneous, GI, and genitourinary tract bleeding.
	Refer patient/family to appropriate support groups.
Pharmacologic management	Practice and discuss self-administration of blood factors or supplementation as ordered.
Patient/family	Consult with pharmacist for drug-specific teaching.
Nutrition	Discuss role of balanced nutrition emphasizing need for key elements: vitamin B$_{12}$, folate, and iron.
Patient/family	Discuss need to reduce exposure to alcohol and thiazide medications.
	Refer patient to dietitian for assistance in meal planning.
Physical exercise	Discuss and explore appropriate physical exercise options that would maintain muscle/bone/cardiovascular strength but limits risks of trauma.
Patient/family	Refer patient/family to physical, rehabilitation, and occupational therapy for outpatient consultation.
Safety	Discuss need to avoid sharp objects or sports that would cause injury.
Patient/family	Advise use of electric razors.
	Advise evaluation of home setting to eliminate sharp corners or fall hazards.
	Advise patient/family to alert dentists and other medical professionals to bleeding risks.
	Discuss signs and symptoms that require emergency intervention.

disease marked by a decrease in the number of platelets due to destruction by antibodies produced against a patient's own platelets. It is the most common of the immune-mediated thrombocytopenias. There are two distinct forms of ITP: an acute form, which affects primarily children and neonates and is usually self-limiting, and a chronic form, which lasts more than 6 months and affects primarily adults (Stasi & Provan, 2004). The following discussion will primarily address chronic forms of ITP.

Pathophysiology

Chronic forms of ITP can be subdivided into two categories: *secondary* and *primary.* Secondary immune thrombocytopenic purpura refers to the appropriate development of antibodies against invading pathogens or drugs, which then inappropriately cross-react against platelets causing their destruction. In primary ITP, antibodies against platelet surface proteins also are observed but occur in the absence of viral, bacterial, or drug exposure. The molecular mechanisms that give rise to either type of ITP are not clearly elucidated and are a focus of current research studies.

Clinical Presentation

The physical manifestations of ITP are similar to those presented earlier in the discussion about thrombocytopenia. Primary ITP can be distinguished from secondary ITP by the absence of recent infection or drug exposure. Additionally, splenomegaly usually is only observed in secondary forms. Laboratory values will reveal decreased platelet levels and perhaps anemia (due to bleeding).

Medical Management

Management of ITP has two primary goals: removal of the triggering event (if identifiable) and abatement of the immune response. In cases of secondary ITP, the underlying disease process must be treated and resolved so that the body is rid of the invading antigen responsible for antibody production. In the case of drug-induced ITP, immediate cessation of the drug is warranted.

Attention then turns to abatement of the immune response, which usually is attempted with immunosuppressive therapy. Steroids such as prednisone are the first choice in asymptomatic patients with decreased platelet counts of less than 50,000/mm³. If steroids prove ineffective, or major bleeding occurs, intravenous immunoglobulin (IVIG) is administered. IVIG has been associated with significant rates of hypersensitivity reactions and thus administration should be monitored closely. Splenectomy will be considered if patients continue to require significant doses of steroids or immunosuppressive therapy after several months (Cines & Blanchette, 2002; Stasi & Provan, 2004). The Nursing Process: Patient Care Plan for Thrombocytopenia and Bleeding Disorders (p. 2046) is appropriate for use in the patient with ITP.

Heparin-Induced Thrombocytopenia

Heparin-induced thrombocytopenia (HIT) is an example of drug-induced, immune-mediated thrombocytopenia. Although the frequency of HIT is relatively rare, 3% of patients treated with unfractionated heparin form thrombosis and 0.5% of patients exposed to diluted heparin flushes for IV therapy management experience thrombocytopenia (Rice, Nguyen, & Vann, 2002). Its incidence is steadily increasing, which is thought to be due to the ubiquitous use of heparin for DVT, pulmonary embolism, acute myocardial infarction, and IV catheter maintenance. Heparin-induced thrombocytopenia occurs most frequently in patients undergoing cardiovascular or orthopedic surgeries, because heparin is widely utilized to prevent thrombosis in these high-risk populations.

Pathophysiology

Patients on heparin therapy (including intermittent IV catheter flushes) can develop antibodies to heparin that cross-react against their own platelets. Specifically, heparin can induce the production of the antiheparin platelet factor 4 (AHPF4) antibody. This antibody causes two reactions. First, as with the autoimmune-mediated thrombocytopenia, these antibodies recognize and bind to platelets, a process that causes their accelerated destruction in the spleen. Second, and perhaps more significantly, when the AHPF4 antibody binds to platelets, it can induce platelet activation thus initiating the clotting cascade, coagulation, and, possibly, thrombosis (Lewis et al., 2003).

Clinical Presentation

A decrease in platelet count, particularly following heparin therapy often is the only indication of HIT. The onset of thrombocytopenia or a drop from baseline values typically occurs within 5 to 14 days after starting heparin therapy. Platelet counts of 80,000 to 100,000/mm³ or counts that drop by 30% or more suggest thrombocytopenia. Initially, the patient may not present with thrombotic complications such as DVT or thrombosis, despite the presence of HIT. However, thrombosis eventually does occur in approximately 35% to 75% of patients with HIT. HIT-related thrombosis leads to DVT, stroke, and cardiac events, which, in turn, carry amputation rates as high as 20% and mortality of 30% to 50% (Hirsh, Heddel, & Kelton, 2004; Warkentin & Kelton, 1996).

Medical Management

HIT can be extremely difficult to manage (1) because of its insidious presentation, (2) because heparin is normally the drug of choice for the management of thrombosis, and (3) because cessation of heparin therapy alone has proven to be an ineffective approach. Diligent observation and early intervention with appropriate drug therapies are the cornerstones of treatment for HIT. Baseline platelet levels should be measured and frequently monitored for all patients who have been recently exposed to all forms of heparin including low-molecular-weight heparin, unfractionated heparin, and heparin flushes. Patients receiving unfractionated heparin warrant even greater monitoring. Although abnormal bleeding can be observed in HIT, the absence of abnormal bleeding should not be ruled out with HIT. Clinical diagnosis of HIT is made on the basis of reduction of the platelet count, correlation with heparin administration, and when other causes (drugs, viruses, and bone marrow involvement) have been excluded (Rice et al., 2002). Laboratory tests also are available that can detect the presence of the anti-heparin platelet factor 4 (AHPF4) antibody.

Once HIT is suspected, heparin therapy (including catheter flushes and low-molecular-weight heparin) should be stopped immediately. A nonheparin anticoagulant such as direct thrombin inhibitors (lepirudin, argatroban, or bivalirudin) often is recommended as a first-line defense followed by warfarin therapy if existing thrombosis is suspected. Direct thrombin inhibitors carry similar risks to bleeding as do other anticoagulants and should be monitored using aPTT and INR.

Nursing Management

Nurses play a key role in the prevention and management of HIT. Nurses should carefully monitor the platelet counts of any patient receiving any form of heparin treatment. The rise of HIT has made the prophylactic use of heparin flushes to maintain IV catheter patency a controversial issue, especially in light of the prevalence of alternatives. Alternative options to maintain catheter patency include positive pressure valves, valved vascular access devices, use of normal saline for flushing, and specially coated central lines. Further epidemiologic research is needed in this area to develop national guidelines (Rosenthal, 2003).

If HIT is suspected, the nurse's responsibilities include the careful administration of antithrombotic therapy, monitoring of appropriate laboratory values, and assessment of bleeding risk. If bleeding also is suspected, the nurse should implement appropriate care plans to prevent anemia, hemorrhage, or injury. The Nursing Process: Patient Care Plan for Thrombocytopenia and Bleeding Disorders (p. 2046) provides details appropriate for use in this population. Other therapies for HIT are discussed in the Evidence-Based Practice box.

von Willebrand's Disease

Von Willebrand's disease (vWD), the most common inherited bleeding disorder, affects 1% to 2% of the international population. vWD results from mutations in the essential clotting factor, von Willebrand's factor (vWF), which plays key roles in both primary and secondary hemostasis. Clinical presentation of vWD depends on the extent and location of the genetic mutation (see the Genetic Considerations box, p. 2050) and varies widely, but vWD is most commonly associated with mucosal and cutaneous bleeding and prolonged bleeding times. Emerging epidemiologic studies reveal that the prevalence of the disease is underestimated and that many cases, especially in women, go widely undiagnosed with symptoms often being attributed to idiopathic menorrhagia (prolonged menstrual bleeding) (Lukes, Kadir, Peyvandi, & Kouides, 2005).

Heparin-Induced Thromboctyopenia

Clinical Problem

Intravenous therapies are a crucial component of most hospitalized patient treatments, which underscores the importance of maintaining patent IV access. Nurses have traditionally maintained IV access with a combination of regular site assessment and manual instillation of a flush solution into the IV catheter site. Without proper nursing maintenance, IV access sites can easily become occluded due to the body's natural tendency to form fibrin sheaths over any foreign object. This normally beneficial mechanism has evolved to isolate harmful pathogens; however, the fibrin sheath formation also blocks the indwelling end of the intravenous catheter. This blockage, in turn, prevents instillation of medications and blood withdrawal, thus requiring the instillation of a new IV access site, possible patient discomfort or injury related to installation, and delay in treatment.

For many years, heparinized saline flushes have been used to prevent fibrin clot formation. However, mounting evidence has revealed a growing incidence of heparin-induced thrombocytopenia (HIT). In HIT, exposure to heparin appropriately stimulates antibody formation against the heparin molecule. However, the same antibody formed against heparin has also shown efficacy activity against platelets. HIT is the depletion of platelets as a result of an autoimmune activity. Nursing practice must incorporate techniques that have shown efficacy in preserving IV access but that do not place the patient at additional risk of injury.

Research Findings

A number of studies are beginning to evaluate the efficacy of heparinized saline flushes against plain saline flushes in the maintenance of IV access. In a large study, 361 IV lock sites were assigned to either saline or heparin use exclusively. Sites were flushed every 12 hours with either 3 mL of normal saline or 3 mL of a diluted (10 units/mL) solution of heparin. At the conclusion of the study, there was no statistically significant difference in incidence of extravasation, phlebitis, clotting, or blood return between either group.

A similar study at the Mayo Clinic was conducted in the obstetric population, who are particularly prone to clotting disorders due to hematologic changes in pregnancy. In this study of 73 patients, results indicate no statistically significant differences in IV lock patency or in phlebitis between heparin or normal saline flushes. Similar results appear in arterial line maintenance. Sixty-five patients in a New Zealand intensive care unit were randomly assigned to receive either normal saline (NS) or heparinized saline (HS) (3 mL/hr as a continuous flush) to maintain their arterial lines needed for monitoring and blood sampling. Each patient's nurse was asked to score the function of the line at the end of each nursing shift. At the conclusion of the study, nursing assessment of line function revealed no difference between flush solutions.

Implications for Nursing Practice

The studies discussed here provide evidence for limiting of patient exposure to heparin in IV access flushes. The primary goal of routine flushes is to ensure patency and delivery of medications and therapies. Clearly, this goal can be achieved via the use of saline without the additional exposure to potentially life-threatening heparin-induced thrombocytopenia. For patients who do not show evidence of IV line occlusion, nurses should collaborate with their interdisciplinary team to limit flush solutions to saline only.

Critical Thinking Questions

1. Which nursing actions are most effective in preservation of intravenous line patency?

2. What are the benefits and risks of heparinized flush solutions?

Answers to Critical Thinking Questions appear in Appendix D.

References

Fujita, T., Namiki, T., Suzuki, T., Yamamoto, E. (2006). Normal saline flushing for maintenance of peripheral intravenous sites. *Journal of Clinical Nursing, 15*(1):103–104.

Niesen, K. M., Harris, D. Y., Parkin, L. S., Henn, L. T. (2003). The effects of heparin versus normal saline for maintenance of peripheral intravenous locks in pregnant women. *Journal of Obstetrics and Gynecology, 32*(4):503–508.

Whitta, R. K., Hall, K. F., Bennetts, T. M., Welman, L., & Rawlins, P. (2006). Comparison of normal or heparinised saline flushing on function of arterial lines. *Critical Care Resuscitation, 8*(3):205–208.

EVIDENCE-BASED PRACTICE

GENETIC CONSIDERATIONS for Hemophilia

Hemophilia results from inheritance of defective genes controlling the clotting system. Because hemophilia is an X-linked genetic disorder, the severity of the disease depends on whether the patient received one or two defective copies from each parent, and whether the patient is male or female. Males only bear one X chromosome, passed from the mother, implying that one copy of the mutated hemophilia gene will result in the disease. However, females, bearing two X chromosomes need to inherit two mutated versions to display the disease.

Pathophysiology

The von Willebrand's factor protein plays two roles in clot formation. In primary hemostasis, vWF acts as a binding bridge between platelets and the damaged subendothelium at the site of vascular injury. In secondary hemostasis, vWF protects Factor VIII, which is important in the contact activation (intrinsic) pathway, from degradation and delivers it to the site of injury.

vWD describes not only one distinct disease, but a heterogeneous group of disorders all involving disturbances in the vWD gene. The normal vWD gene is a very large, complex structure, usually producing a mature protein of more than 2,050 amino acids. Disturbances to this protein sequence can result in structurally abnormal vWF, too little vWF (most common), or too much vWF, accounting for more than 40 different variations of vWD. Insufficiencies in patients with vWD cause delayed platelet plug formation, prolonged bleeding times, and impaired fibrin clot formation. Alternately, excess production of vWF can lead to thrombosis.

Clinical Presentation

The severity of von Willebrand's disease varies widely depending on the extent and location of the genetic derangement. The exact genetic derangements have yet to be elucidated, but it is apparent to clinicians that patients can present with a wide variation of bleeding tendencies. In an attempt to classify vWD according to disease severity, the International Society on Thrombosis and Hemostasis proposed a simplified classification of vWD (Sadler, 1994), which has since been adopted by both researchers and clinicians worldwide. The classification system is based on the amount and characteristics of detectable vWF in the bloodstream by laboratory tests and on clinical presentation. Chart 63–18 describes the variations in clinical presentation of each classification of vWD.

As suggested in Chart 63–18, some patients may appear generally asymptomatic with only mildly increased bleeding tendencies, whereas others (type 3) with the most severe forms experience joint bleeding and hemorrhage. Fortunately, type 3 vWD requires inheritance of two copies of the mutated von Willebrand's gene, making it the rarest form of the disease. Other indicators of vWD include prolonged bleeding after minor cuts, bleeding from the gums, and mucocutaneous bleeding (petechiae, ecchymosis).

vWD will manifest as prolonged bleeding times and a reduction of vWF in the blood. The vWF quantity is directly measured by using an ELISA test that can provide a quantitative measurement. Platelet count will appear normal. PT, aPTT, and INR should also be normal.

CHART 63–18	Classifications of von Willebrand Disease
Classification	**Clinical Presentation**
Type 1	Partial quantitative deficiency of vWF Mildly decreased clotting ability
Type 2A	Qualitative defect Mildly dysfunctional ability of vWF to bind platelets Primary hemostasis defect affecting platelet plug formation
Type 2B	Qualitative defect Moderately dysfunctional ability of vWF to bind platelets Primary hemostasis defect affecting platelet plug formation
2M	Qualitative defect Severely dysfunctional or absent ability of vWF to bind to platelets Primary hemostasis defect affecting platelet plug formation
2N	Qualitative defect Mildly dysfunctional ability of vWF to bind to Factor VIII Secondary hemostasis defect affects fibrin clot formation
3	Severe or total deficiency of vWF affecting both platelet plug formation and fibrin sheath formation Patients can present with chronic mucosal and cutaneous bleeding, and/or joint bleeding Sometimes misdiagnosed as hemophilia

Source: Sadler, J. E. (1994). A revised classification of von Willebrand disease. For the Subcommittee on von Willebrand factor of the Scientific and Standardization Committee of the International Society on Thrombosis and Haemostasis. *Thrombosis and Haemostasis, 71*(4), 520–525.

Medical Management

Treatment for von Willebrand's disease is based on the current presenting symptom. In the event of problematic uncontrolled bleeding or as prophylaxis prior to invasive procedures, the patient can be treated with replacement of the deficient vWF. Desmopressin vasopressin analog (DDAVP), a synthetic hormone usually given by injection or nasal spray, induces production of vWF and subsequent increase in Factor VIII levels. DDAVP is administered at a dose of 0.3 µg/kg, with effects starting within 30 to 60 minutes and lasting for several hours. Because it is a synthetic hormone, hypersensitivity reactions including tachycardia, headache, and facial flushing are potential side effects of infusion.

Replacement therapy, the second option, is the injection of a concentrate of vWF and Factor VIII extracted either with fresh frozen plasma (FFP) or cryoprecipitate. However, very large volumes of FFP or cryoprecipitate are required to sufficiently replace vWF and Factor VIII, predisposing the patient to fluid overload and transfusion reactions. For these reasons, replacement therapy is reserved for those patients who cannot tolerate DDAVP or those with emergent bleeding in type 3 disease. Commercially prepared concentrations of vWF currently are in clinical trials as low-volume alternatives to FFP and cryoprecipitate infusions.

Nursing Management

As with other bleeding disorders, nursing responsibilities for patients with von Willebrand's disease include implementation of bleeding precautions, environmental risk reduction, and diligent assessment. Although platelet values tend to be normal in these patients, patients with severe disease can present with prolonged bleeding times (aPTT). The Nursing Process: Patient Care Plan for Thrombocytopenia and Bleeding Disorders, presented earlier in the chapter (p. 2046), is appropriate for use in these patients because it outlines physiological assessments and nursing interventions that can be applied in vWF. Because von Willebrand's disease is a chronic lifelong condition, discharge priorities for these patients emphasize education, which reinforces prevention of injury.

Disorders of Secondary Hemostasis

Disorders of secondary hemostasis refer to any disease process that disrupts the formation of the fibrin sheath via errors in the tissue factor (extrinsic) pathway or the contact activation (intrinsic) pathway. The most common cause of these disorders is deficiencies in quantity or quality of the clotting factors. Whereas disorders of primary hemostasis usually appear within minutes of injury and in superficial sites (mucosa, integumentary), bleeding associated with disorders of secondary hemostasis can occur days to weeks after injury and in the deep subcutaneous layers, the muscles, and the joints. Several disorders of secondary hemostasis have been identified; however, the most common are vitamin K deficiency and hemophilia, which is discussed next.

Hemophilia

Hemophilia is perhaps the most well-known disease of hemostasis and affected approximately 18,000 persons (primarily male) in the United States as of 2005. **Hemophilia** is a chronic condition that arises from the inheritance of mutated genes controlling Factor VIII or Factor IX. Characteristic presenting symptoms are uncontrolled bleeding particularly into large muscle groups and joints.

Pathophysiology

Patients with hemophilia inherit mutated copies of the genes controlling clotting factors VIII or clotting factor IX. Recall from the discussion on normal hemostasis above that both Factor VIII and Factor IX are required in the contact activation (intrinsic) pathway for the eventual activation of Factor X, leading to the common pathway and the conversion of fibrinogen to fibrin. Therefore, the lack of either of these factors may significantly alter formation of the fibrin sheath, clot formation, and, ultimately, clinical bleeding. Patients with hemophilia who inherit altered clotting factor VIII are considered to have hemophilia A, whereas inheritance of altered clotting factor IX is referred to as hemophilia B. Both diseases are recessive X-linked genetic disorders with implications for gender-based inheritance.

Clinical Presentation

The severity of hemophilia is related to the amount of clotting factor in the blood and is graded on a continuum from mild to severe. Mild hemophilia is characterized by insufficient clotting factor. The clinical presentation of each, hemophilia A and hemophilia B, is identical, with differentiation relying on chemical assays of blood samples.

Physical Manifestations   The hallmark clinical presentation of hemophilia is prolonged bleeding and an inability to form clots in response to injury, both of which can appear and persist for days to weeks. For patients with severe disease completely lacking any Factor VIII or Factor IX, such bleeding can have serious life-threatening consequences. Distinguished from disease of primary hemostasis, which causes increased bruising and superficial hemorrhages in the integumentary (petechiae), patients with hemophilia typically suffer from bleeding deep in the tissues. Typical bleeding sites include joints and organs. If left uncontrolled the internal bleeding can cause severe pressure on closed compartments.

Serious consequences of internal bleeding into closed spaces include increased intracranial pressure, hemiarthrosis (bleeding into the joints) leading to compartment syndrome, and oropharyngeal bleeding (into the esophagus). The eventual sequelae following each of these situations can cause lifetime disability. Increased intracranial pressure can cause ischemia and brain tissue damage. Bleeding into the joints predisposes the patient to arthritis, synovial tissue damage, and joint malformation. Oropharyngeal bleeding may occlude the airway so severely as to require intubation.

Alterations in Laboratory Values   Although the clinical presentations of hemophilia A and hemophilia B are identical, treatment options vary; thus, laboratory analysis is critical in developing an effective care plan. Patients with hemophilia have usually been diagnosed as children, prior to admission to the acute care setting. For patients known to have hemophilia, diagnostic tests such as the CBC are used to determine degree of blood loss. Bleeding and clotting studies, a platelet count, bleeding time, PT, aPTT, and INR are indicated for any patient suspected of having hemophilia. Because Factor VIII and Factor IX are disorders of the intrinsic pathway, the patient typically will have a prolonged aPTT with all other tests normal. Specific assays that detect blood levels of Factor VIII and Factor IX are used to distinguish between the two forms of hemophilia.

Medical Management

Medical management of hemophilia revolves around *factor replacement therapy*, or the administration of exogenous (donated or manufactured) Factor VIII and Factor IX. (See the Pharmacology Summary in the chapter for medications used to treat clotting disorders, p. 2054.) Previously, factor replacement therapy was achieved via fresh frozen plasma; however, possible exposure to viruses and risk of volume overload combined with the availability of commercially prepared factors has decreased the use of FFP. For mild episodes or as prophylaxis prior to procedures, DDAVP has become the treatment of choice. DDAVP stimulates the temporary production of Factor VIII.

In the event of bleeding, antifibrinolytics are sometimes used. These medications slow the fibrinolytic system, thus extending the effect of already-formed fibrin sheaths and slowing the inhibitory effects of fibrin degradation products. However, these medications have only shown significant clinical efficacy in mucosal and oral bleeding. Another principle of hemophilia treatment is the prevention of deleterious sequelae and further injury. Toward that goal, aspirin and other platelet interfering drugs are avoided.

Nursing Management

For the nurse caring for the hospitalized patient with hemophilia, cure is not the goal. Instead disease management focuses on reduction of environmental factors that increase risk and on management of the administration of the replacement factors. Bleeding precautions as shown earlier in Chart 63–17 (p. 2045) should be initiated with particular emphasis on maintaining a safe environment. Nursing problems applicable to the care of the patient with hemophilia include risk for injury (addressed with implementation of the Nursing Process: Patient Care Plan given earlier in the chapter, p. 2046), pain due to hemiarthrosis, and the need for patient education. Pain should be assessed regularly including pain level and quality. Analgesics should be administered to manage pain.

Complex Disease of the Clotting Cascade: Disseminated Intravascular Coagulation

Disseminated intravascular coagulation (DIC) is triggered by an injury or event leading to persistent activation of the clotting cascade. It manifests as widespread clot formation and thrombosis. Situations that are known to trigger DIC include sepsis, trauma (including surgery), malignancy, toxin exposure, and obstetric complications. Under normal circumstances, the clotting pathways act only transiently until vessel damage is healed. But the aforementioned situations can cause such widespread, persistent endothelial injury that the clotting pathways are required to respond with equal perseverance to seal off injured blood vessels. Eventually, this situation leads to two phenomena—the depletion of the clotting factors and the activation of the fibrinolytic system—that lead to uncontrolled bleeding. The complexity of the pathology and the simultaneous appearance of bleeding and massive thrombosis make DIC a very challenging clinical problem.

Pathophysiology

DIC is commonly associated with sepsis, trauma, cancer, or obstetric emergencies (Figure 63–14 ■). Sepsis and trauma both appear to cause DIC by widespread release of coagulation-promoting cytokines or intracellular chemical signals. In sepsis, these cytokines are released by the body in response to systemic infections with gram-negative or gram-positive bacteria and, in some cases, viruses. In severe trauma multiple mechanisms lead to DIC including endothelial damage and widespread hemolysis, which cause cytokines to be released in much the same manner as sepsis. In cancer, malignant tumors release tissue factor and other coagulation-promoting chemicals, ultimately leading to thrombosis. In obstetric emergencies, release of placental fluid or massive blood loss during childbirth is responsible for initiation of the clotting pathways.

Emerging research reveals that following initial injury by any of the mechanisms listed above, DIC appears to follow a specific sequence of molecular events (Levi, 2005). First, all of the above mechanisms cause endothelial layer damage, which in turn causes massive release of tissue factor, initiating the tissue factor (extrinsic pathway) branch of the clotting cascade. The persistence of the injury results in prolonged activation of the clotting cascade. Second, thrombin production is greatly amplified. Recall that thrombin is an extremely power-

ful promoter of coagulation. Studies show that abnormal thrombin amplification is caused by defects in the regulators that normally inhibit thrombin (antithrombin, tissue factor pathway inhibitor, and protein C). The cause and nature of theses defects are still under investigation.

These derangements cause widespread coagulation fibrin deposits and thrombosis in the microvasculature. The thrombosis occludes small vessels leading to cyanosis, tissue hypoxia, and necrosis. Eventually blood flow begins to affect the microvasculature of organs, especially the kidneys, lungs, and heart. As coagulation proceeds unchecked, the body's supply of clotting components is exhausted and eventually depleted.

Clinical Presentation

As suggested by the pathophysiology just discussed, DIC presents with paradoxical widespread thrombosis and bleeding. Laboratory values reveal prolonged clotting times and consumption of coagulation factors.

Physical Manifestations

Bleeding, although a later consequence of DIC, often is the first and most obvious sign detected. It frequently is manifested at mucocutaneous sites and as prolonged oozing from puncture

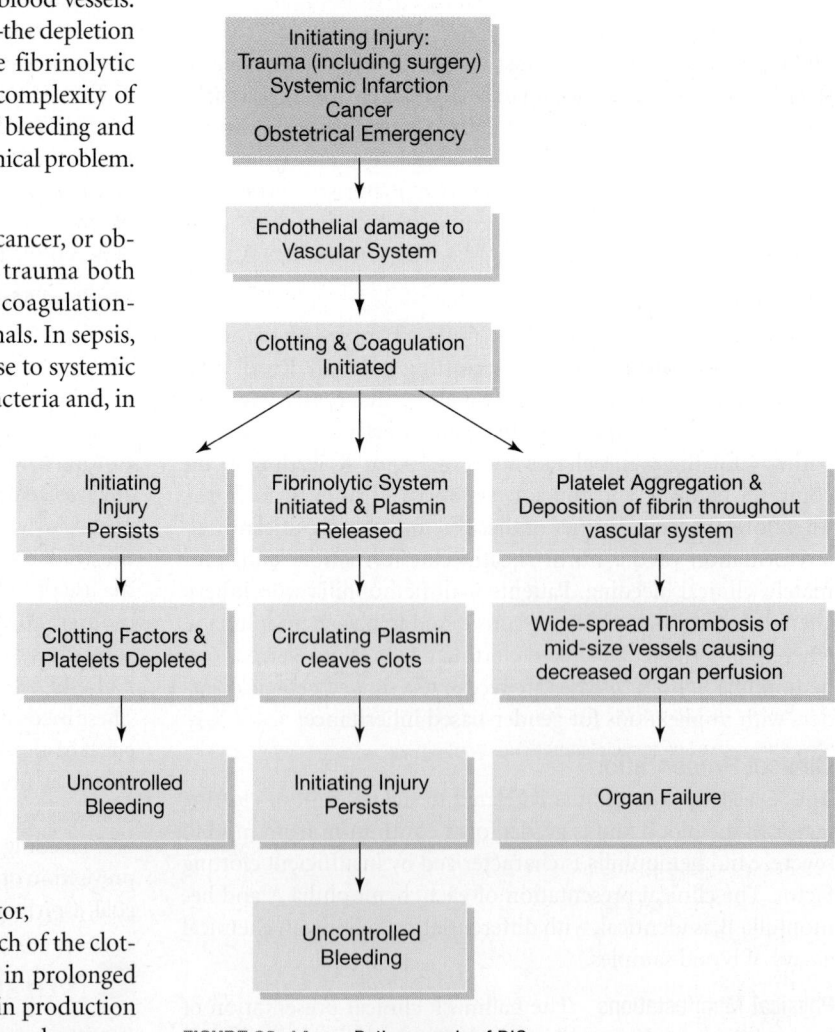

PATHOGENESIS OF DIC

FIGURE 63–14 ■ Pathogenesis of DIC.

sites. Figure 63–13 ■ (p. 2044) illustrates common bleeding sites. As DIC progresses, bleeding in gastrointestinal (GI) tract, central nervous system (CNS), heart, and genitourinary tract can occur. These are manifested as melena, a change in level of consciousness (hemorrhagic stroke), chest pain and shortness of breath, and hematuria, respectively. Extreme hypotension, tachycardia, a decreased level of consciousness, and critically low urine output (<30 mL/hr) all indicate hemodynamic shock due to blood loss.

Thrombosis can be more difficult to observe. Mild cyanosis, parasthesia (numbness), pain, and weakened pulses especially in the extremities are all indicators of microvasculature thrombosis. As the thrombi spread to affect the organs, patients can present with decreased level of consciousness (ischemic stroke), abdominal pain from GI tract occlusion, decreased urinary output (poor renal perfusion), chest pain (cardiac), and respiratory difficulty (lung). Note that many of the signs indicative of thrombosis also are indicators of bleeding. The similarity stems from the tissue hypoxia that can result from bleeding (anemia due to acute blood loss) and thrombosis (lack of circulation, hence lack of oxygenation). Clinical indicators of DIC are summarized in Chart 63–19.

Alterations in Laboratory Values

Chart 63–20 outlines the expected changes in laboratory values in the patient with DIC, which primarily reflect the consumption of clotting factors. As a result, platelet counts and fibrinogen and clotting factor titers are decreased, leading to prolonged PT, aPTT, and INR. The D-dimer test indicates excessive fibrinolysis, the end point of excessive activation of the clotting pathways.

CHART 63–19 **Clinical Indicators of Disseminated Intravascular Coagulation**

HISTORY
- Sepsis
- Trauma
- Blood transfusion
- Liver dysfunction
- Malignancy
- Recent pregnancy (retained placenta)

SIGNS
- Bleeding from mucosa
- Bleeding from catheter sights
- Petechiae, ecchymosis, and purpura
- Decreased sensation in extremities
- Extremities cool to the touch
- Altered level of consciousness
- Hemoptysis

SYMPTOMS
- Pain described as swelling, sharp
- Shortness of breath/tachypnea
- Fatigue
- Hypotension
- Tachycardia

CHART 63–20 **Expected Changes in Laboratory Values in the Patient with Disseminated Intravascular Coagulation**

Platelet Count	Decreased (<100,000 µL)
PT, aPTT	Prolonged
INR	Increased
Fibrinogen	Decreased
Clotting Factors: V, VIII, X, XIII	Decreased
Fibrin degradation products and D-dimer	Positive* (most sensitive)
Clotting inhibitors: antithrombin III and protein C	Decreased

*D-dimers and FDP can become elevated whenever the coagulation and fibrinolytic systems are activated. This occurs in a variety of conditions, and therefore the tests are not specific for any one diagnosis.

Medical Management

Complete removal of the underlying injury is required for the total resolution of DIC. All other treatments are used to mitigate the damage of thrombosis or bleeding until the sepsis, trauma, cancer, or obstetric emergency subsides. The cornerstone principle that guides treatment options is the cessation of rampant coagulation pathways. Common treatments include the following:

- **Anticoagulant therapy**—Anticoagulants such as unfractionated or low-molecular-weight heparin can prevent the formation of new thrombi. Low doses are titrated carefully and monitored to prevent exacerbation of possible bleeding in DIC. New anticoagulants that specifically target thrombin (thrombin inhibitors) currently are being studied for their potential use in DIC.
- **Replacement therapy**—Patients at risk of hemodynamic collapse from excessive bleeding may be candidates for transfusion of platelets, FFP, or concentrations of coagulation factors. The use of these treatments is reserved for patients at imminent risk due to depletion of clotting factors, because inappropriate use may exacerbate development of thrombosis (Levi, de Jonge, & van der Poll, 2006).
- **Restoration of anticoagulant (antithrombin) pathways**—Administration of antithrombin agents is a relatively new therapy approach that shows significant promise. Examples of antithromobin therapies include activated protein C and antithrombin concentrations (Levi, de Jonge, & van der Poll, 2004).

Drugs used to treat DIC and other clotting disorders are shown in the Pharmacology Summary of Medications to Treat Clotting Disorders.

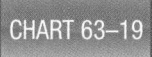 Nursing Management

DIC should be considered a medical emergency with emphasis on circulation and oxygenation, especially with respect to major organs such as heart, lungs, CNS, and kidneys. The most effective nursing intervention is anticipation of DIC in any patient with infection, trauma (including large surgeries such as GI surgeries), cancer, or obstetric emergency. Diligent assessment for

PHARMACOLOGY Summary of Medications to Treat Clotting Disorders

Medicine Category	Action	Application/Indication	Nursing Responsibility
Immune suppressive medications: Steroids Intravenous immunoglobulin	Suppression of immune response including autoimmune response.	Autoimmune thrombocytopenia (idiopathic and heparin induced) in asymptomatic patients with decreased platelet counts less than 50,000/mm³. IVIG is indicated in patients for whom steroids have proven ineffective or who have significant bleeding due to lack of platelet activity.	Assessment of laboratory values to monitor efficacy. Assessment of and patient education regarding signs and symptoms of infection since steroids will reduce immune system protection. Assessment of serum glucose levels secondary to steroid elevation. Assessment and patient education regarding mood shifts.
Clotting factor replacement therapy: Indirectly via hormone stimulation Desmopressin (DDAVP) Direct factor replacement	Induces production of deficient clotting factors (DDAVP induces production of von Willebrand's factor). Immediately replenishes deficient or depleted stores of clotting factors.	von Willebrand's disease, hemophilia, disease with uncontrolled bleeding or prophylaxis prior to invasive procedures. Direct factor replacement therapy is reserved for patients who cannot tolerate DDAVP.	DDAVP has potent antidiuretic effects, thus fluid intake should be adjusted downward to decrease the potential occurrence of water intoxication and hyponatremia. Assessment of serum electrolytes, neurological status, cardiovascular status, urinary output, and edema are to be closely monitored. Assessment of immune-mediated hypersensitivity reaction (Micromedex, 2006).

early indicators of DIC should include laboratory analysis, mucocutaneous bleeding, neurological function, and peripheral circulation. Normal findings should be documented as a baseline comparison against continual assessments. Abnormal findings should also be documented and require immediate collaboration with the health care provider.

Once DIC is suspected, attention then turns to mitigating any life-threatening sequelae. Priorities of care include implementation of bleeding precautions, maintenance of fluid balance, maintenance of acid–base balance and oxygenation, maintenance of skin integrity, and psychosocial support. Bleeding precautions were listed earlier in Chart 63–17 (p. 2045). Fluid balance derangements, which occur as a result of bleeding as well as thrombotic occlusion of the cardiovascular and renal systems, are assessed by measurement of urine output, skin turgor, and blood pressure. Oxygenation (hypoxia) problems also occur due to microvasculature occlusion and are indicated via changes in level of consciousness, cyanosis, reports of pain, and analysis of ABGs. Supplemental oxygen often is administered to prevent severe acidosis.

Attention should be paid to maintenance of skin integrity because the patient is at high risk of breakdown due to ischemia and bleeding and because additional wounds can trigger additional activation of the clotting pathways.

Emotional support also should be provided to the patient and family. DIC occurs as a serious consequence of an already existing disease process. Family and patient coping strategies may have already been exhausted by the initial injury or infection, and the addition of DIC and its treatment can cause extreme stress, especially since a diagnosis of DIC often requires transfer to an intensive care unit. Nursing assessment should always include coping ability and patients' stated fears or concerns. Nurses

should seek the collaboration of social workers, chaplains, and other professionals to assist both the patient and family.

DIC requires the application of multiple nursing skills including the administration and monitoring of transfusion therapy, oxygen therapy, and anticoagulant therapy. Monitoring of transfusion therapy should include the basic skills outlined in Chapter 22 ⬡. Oxygen therapy is used to prevent acid–base derangement and correct hypoxia due to insufficient tissue perfusion. However, oxygen therapy must be closely monitored via oxygenation saturation and ABG levels. Additionally, oxygen therapy can dry delicate mucosal tissue, thus reinforcing the need for careful skin assessment. Anticoagulant therapy is usually addressed with heparin infusions, which require careful monitoring of laboratory values (aPTT, INR) and signs and symptoms of bleeding.

Aplastic Anemia

Aplastic anemia is a relatively rare disorder characterized by severe pancytopenia (low or absent red blood cells, white blood cells, and platelets) in both the periphery and bone marrow. Incidence rates are less than 2 persons per million in the United States; however, rates are higher in patients of Asian or European descent (Mayo Clinic, 2007). The severe depletion of defensive immune cells, oxygen-carrying red blood cells, and clotting platelets is a life-threatening condition for patients requiring the urgent implementation of protective interventions.

Pathophysiology

Aplastic anemia is thought to be caused by damage to the HSCs, resulting in their inability to reproduce and differentiate. In many cases, the cause of the damage is often unknown (idiopathic); in other cases, aplastic anemia results from toxic exposure, infectious processes, or in relationship to another disease process (Sleijfer & Lugtenburg, 2003). Toxins known to cause aplastic anemia include benzene, certain insecticides, kerosene, and heavy metals. Infections associated with aplastic anemia include Epstein–Barr virus, HIV, and cytomegaloviruses. Unfortunately, some therapeutic medications also may cause the pancytopenia of aplastic anemia. These drugs include chloramphenicol, certain antiepileptics, chemotherapeutic agents, and psychotropics (especially clozapine) (Bakhshi & Abella, 2008).

The diversity of the causes implies that the underlying mechanism may be equally diverse. Molecular research has shown that in most acquired diseases, the suppression of the hematopoetic stem cell is mediated by T cells that induce apoptosis (cell death) of the HSC. However, the mechanism that causes these T cells to attack the HSC is unknown and under investigation. Drug-induced aplastic anemia has been associated with deficiency in a protein responsible for removing drug metabolites from cells; hence, affected cells may have abnormally high intracellular levels of drugs that interfere with cell function. Congenital aplastic anemia may result from chromosomal abnormalities causing early HSC death.

Clinical Presentation

Regardless of the underlying cause, the hallmark sign of aplastic anemia is pancytopenia and the absence of HSCs from the bone marrow. Patients commonly will present with evidence of mucocutaneous bleeding, easy bruising, and oozing from puncture sites due to thrombocytopenia, and hypoxia due to severe anemia. Patients may report frequent infections due to WBC depletion. Laboratory analyses will reveal correlating laboratory values such as depressed platelet, WBC, and RBC counts. Peripheral blood smears will reveal lack of reticulocytes as well. Measures of increased iron stores, increased serum ferritin, and increased serum ferritin will reveal excess iron since the vital element is not being used for RBC production. Aplastic anemia is definitively diagnosed with a bone marrow aspiration study that reveals a hypocellular marrow space that is often replaced with fatty deposits.

Medical Management

Stem cell transplant is the curative treatment for aplastic anemia. Transfusion with donated stem cells will presumably repopulate the hypocellular bone marrow with healthy hematopoietic stem cells, which will then produce fully functioning red blood cells, white blood cells, and platelets. Immunosuppressive therapy is another common approach to aplastic anemia, particularly in patients who are not candidates for stem cell transplantation. Immunosuppressive agents such as antithymocyte globulin (ATG) and cyclosporine A (CsA) depress T-cell action on the HSCs. Blood transfusions with packed RBCs and platelets are administered to replace much needed blood elements. Prophylactic antibiotics and antifungals may be ordered to protect the severely neutropenic patient. Iron chelation therapy may be administered to reduce excess iron stores.

Nursing Management

The patient with aplastic anemia benefits from nursing interventions designed for anemia, thrombocytopenia, and infection prevention. A common cause of death among these patients is death due to infection, thus prevention is a priority. Careful hand hygiene should be both stringently practiced and enforced, and also taught to the patient. All instruments and items that come in contact with the patient should be cleansed before and after each use.

The patient should be frequently assessed for signs of infection including general malaise, oozing or inflammation around puncture sites, cough, or pain. Bleeding due to thrombocytopenia and hypoxia due to anemia also are results of pancytopenia of aplastic anemia. The Nursing Process: Patient Care Plans for generalized anemia and thrombocytopenia (pp. 2013 and 2046) describe appropriate nursing interventions for use in this population.

Research

Research is essential to improve the care, quality of life, and survival of patients with hematologic disorders. The goal of research is to identify areas where practice could improve and evaluate and test methods for these improvements. The research topics related to hematologic disorders are listed in the Research Opportunities and Clinical Impact box (p. 2056). The list provides both medical and nursing research topics still under investigation. Electronic databases are a source for finding specific studies related to these topics.

Summary

Hematologic disorders comprise a broad class of diseases affecting the cells and components of the blood. The functions performed by the cells of the bloodstream include oxygen transportation, hemodynamic stability, and response to injury, all of which are necessary to adequate functioning of body systems.

Although some diseases of the hematologic system are chronic, acute illnesses including infection and surgery as well as many common medications can alter the functioning of the blood. Derangements in the hematologic system affect not only the blood system, but every system in the body including vital organ function. For these reasons, assessment of hematologic functioning is required for every patient regardless of admitting diagnosis. Nurses should include signs and symptoms of hypoxia, oxygenation, and bleeding as part of every assessment and seek consultation as necessary.

RESEARCH OPPORTUNITIES AND CLINICAL IMPACT RELATED TO BLEEDING DISORDERS

Research Area	Clinical Impact
Physiology • Manipulation of cellular signaling pathways (biotherapy) to promote normal hematopoiesis or to suppress abnormal hematopoiesis • Discovery and elucidation of the mechanisms that control clotting	Establish effective methods of treatment and ultimately cure for certain hematologic disorders that result from altered hematopoiesis. Results of molecular science are the first step in drug development for clinical trials. Development of treatment protocols to prevent thrombotic disease.
Emerging Treatment Protocols (in Clinical Trials) • Cord blood infusion for treatment of diseases of hematopoiesis • Bone marrow transplant • Novel applications of existing protocols • Manipulation of clotting factors to treat thrombotic diseases such as cardiovascular disorders, stroke, and DVT	Cord blood banking is an emerging option for parents. These studies evaluate efficacy, cost, and quality of life to determine if cord blood transfusion will become a recommended option for high-risk families. Bone marrow transplant is currently the only definitive cure for most chronic hematologic disorders. However, risks are substantial. This research develops safe and effective protocols. Drugs and treatment protocols in current clinical trials increase our understanding of both chronic and acute diseases and help establish effective treatments. The efficacy of oral vitamin B_{12} supplementation compared to parenteral. Oral supplementation is cheaper and generates much less patient anxiety. Several trials are being conducted to quantitatively and qualitatively measure efficacy.
Quality-of-Life (QOL) Research • Evaluation of QOL for adult patients with chronic hematologic disease compared to other diseases • Evaluation of QOL across the life span for aging patients with hematologic disorders	Establish domains of QOL. Benchmarks QOL in hematology against other diseases with well-understood QOL implications. As care advances, the average life span of patients with chronic hematologic disorders increases with implications for physiological, social, and medical implications.
Complementary/Alternative Approach Guided imagery and other nonpharmaceutical techniques to manage sickle cell pain	Studies impact of complementary approaches on disease management and experience.

Clinical Preparation

CRITICAL THINKING

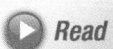 **Read**

- History of Current Illness
- Past Medical History
- Physical Exam
- Admitting Medical Orders
- Laboratory Study Results

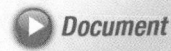 **Document**

- Summary of Hospitalization
- Pathophysiology Form
- Laboratory Values
- Laboratory Results Explanation

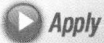 **Apply**

- List of Potential Nursing Diagnoses
- Concept Map
- Critical Thinking Questions

Log on to MyNursingKit.com to download forms you will need and to complete further steps in the Clinical Preparation assignment.

HISTORY OF PRESENT ILLNESS

Patient JS is a 60-year-old female being treated on your unit. She was admitted from the emergency department (ED) with a diagnosis of gastrointestinal bleeding in the lower GI tract. JS reports that she noticed changes in the color, odor, and consistency of her bowel movements 2 days before being seen in the emergency department. In the ED a fecal occult stool test was positive for blood. She denies any change in her diet. She denies any travel. Ms. JS has not had any major surgery or major procedures since her admission.

Medical–Surgical History

Her past medical history is unremarkable except for well-controlled non–insulin-dependent type 2 diabetes. She has no prior history of chronic GI inflammatory processes.

Social History

Ms. JS is widowed and lives by herself. She has no close relatives in the area. Ms. JS reports only drinking alcohol occasionally (defined as 1 to 2 glasses of wine per month) and a history of smoking 1 pack per day times 10 years, although she reports quitting more than 15 years ago.

Physical Exam

When you assess Ms. JS she is alert and well oriented to person, place, time, and purpose. You perform a head-to-toe physical assessment, which results in the following findings:

- Cranial nerves intact
- Small conjunctival hemorrhage in the left eye; patient reports it appeared 1 week ago
- Mild pallor noted in skin tone
- Oral mucosa clear; however, gums appear slightly pink; patient reports she noticed faint pink streaks when she brushes her teeth
- Lung sounds clear, heart sounds clear
- Vital signs: 38.2°C, BP 120/80, pulse 82 beats per minute, respirations 16
- You notice that she has shortness of breath when moving from lying to sitting and requires your assistance when moving from sitting to standing. She reports that her fatigue has been increasing during the past few weeks. She is reporting less energy throughout the day. As you continue, you notice that her peripheral pulses are intact, although you note that her extremities are cool, pale. She has small petechiae on her forearms and you notice that her IV site is oozing small amounts of blood.

Admitting Medical Orders

- Admit to general medical unit

Diagnosis: gastrointestinal bleeding in the lower GI tract; rule out anemia
Allergies: none noted
Vital signs and O_2 sats q4h
Activity: ambulate with assistance
Diet: soft diet, except when NPO prior to colonoscopy (after midnight)
Call house officer: HR < 60 or >120, systolic blood pressure < 90 or > 160, RR < 12 or > 30, temperature > 38.5°C
IVs: normal saline via IV infusion at 125 mL/hr
Intake and output q shift

Scheduled Medications

Potassium 10 mEq IV × 3 doses over 1 hour each; recheck serum potassium 1 hour following replacement
Metformin HCl tablet 500 mg 2 times daily with food

PRN Medications

None noted

Ordered Laboratory Studies

CBC, Chem 7, and reticulocytes daily
Stools for occult blood daily

Ordered Diagnostic Studies

Accu-Cheks q ac and at bedtime
Colonoscopy in a.m.

LABORATORY STUDY RESULTS

Test	On Admission	Day 1	Day 2
Hematocrit	35 g/dL	36 g/dL	38 g/dL
Hemoglobin	11%	12%	12.5%
Reticulocytes	0.45%	0.45%	0.43%
Platelets	75,000 µL	75,000 µL	70,000 µL
Sodium	135 mEq/L	140 mEq/L	140 mEq/L
Potassium	3.0 mEq/L	3.5 mEq/L	3.5 mEq/L
Chloride	95 mEq/L	100 mEq/L	100 mEq/L
CO_2	22 mEq/L	24 mEq/L	25 mEq/L
Serum glucose	110 mg/dL	114 mg/dL	115 mg/dL
Occult stool test	Positive	Positive	Positive

CRITICAL THINKING QUESTIONS

1. What syndromes do the lab values reflect?

2. Is the bone marrow attempting to compensate? Which laboratory value reflects bone marrow?

3. Which signs or symptoms correlate with and can be accounted for by the platelet count?

4. Which signs or symptoms can be correlated to the hemoglobin and hematocrit?

5. Which protective mechanisms should the nurse employ? Why would the nurse implement them?

Answers to Critical Thinking Questions appear in Appendix D.

NCLEX® REVIEW

1. A patient sustained multiple fractures to both femurs and several ribs. The nurse realizes this patient is at risk for developing:
   1. Infection.
   2. Low platelet count.
   3. Reduction in hematopoetic stem cells.
   4. Reduction in red blood cells.

2. A patient has missed receiving a vitamin B_{12} injection for two months. The nurse realizes this patient is at risk for developing:
   1. Reduced red blood cell production.
   2. Reduced white blood cell production.
   3. Reduced platelet production.
   4. Increased red blood cell destruction.

3. While conducting a physical examination, the nurse suspects a patient is experiencing iron deficiency anemia. Which of the following did the nurse assess in this patient?
   1. Fatigue
   2. Fever
   3. Tachycardia
   4. Glossitis

4. A patient with anemia due to acute blood loss has a normal hematocrit level. The nurse realizes this is due to:
   1. A compensatory mechanism.
   2. RBC mass being lost at the same rate as total blood volume.
   3. An increase in plasma volume.
   4. Diluted RBC volume.

5. The nurse is caring for a patient with thrombocytopenia. Which of the following should be included in this patient's care?
   1. Monitor volume of urine output
   2. Nutrition consult for high protein diet
   3. Encourage increased activity
   4. Frequent skin and oral mucosa assessment

6. A patient with hemophilia is in the emergency department being evaluated after being in a motor vehicle accident. The nurse realizes that this patient's injuries will be:
   1. Immediate.
   2. Minimal.
   3. Persistent and last for days or weeks.
   4. Superficial.

Answers for review questions appear in Appendix D

KEY TERMS

2,3-diphosphoglycerate (2,3-DPG) *p.2010*
absolute iron deficiency *p.2019*
anemia *p.2008*
anemic hypoxia *p.2009*
aplastic anemia *p.2054*
autoimmune hemolytic anemia *p.2038*
bioavailable *p.2020*
deoxyhemoglobin *p.2010*
desquamation *p.2018*
differentiation *p.2007*
elemental iron *p.2021*
erythropoiesis *p.2008*
erythropoietic stem cells
    (proerythroblast) *p.2007*
erythropoietin *p.2008*
ferritin *p.2018*
folate *p.2024*
functional iron deficiency *p.2019*
glucose-6-phosphate dehydrogenase (G6PD)
    deficiency *p.2037*

hematology *p.2006*
hematopoiesis *p.2006*
hematopoietic stem cell (HSC) *p.2007*
heme iron *p.2020*
hemoglobin *p.2009*
hemoglobinopathies *p.2026*
hemolytic anemia *p.2033*
hemophilia *p.2051*
hemosiderin *p.2018*
hemostasis *p.2038*
heparin-induced thrombocytopenia
    (HIT) *p.2048*
hepcidin *p.2019*
hereditary spherocytosis (HS) *p.2037*
hypochromic *p.2018*
hypoxia *p.2008*
hypoxic hypoxia *p.2009*
intrinsic factor (IF) *p.2025*

iron deficiency anemia (IDA) *p.2018*
megakaryocytic stem cells *p.2007*
megaloblast *p.2024*
megaloblastic anemia *p.2024*
melena *p.2017*
microcytic *p.2018*
myeloid progenitor cell *p.2007*
nonheme iron *p.2020*
pernicious anemia *p.2025*
progenitor cells *p.2007*
Schilling test *p.2025*
sickle cell anemia *p.2029*
thalassemia *p.2027*
thrombopoietin *p.2043*
transferrin *p.2018*
vitamin B_{12} (cobalamin) *p.2024*
von Willebrand's disease *p.2049*

EXPLORE **mynursingkit**™
PEARSON

MyNursingKit is your one stop for online chapter review materials and resources. Prepare for success with additional NCLEX®-style practice questions, interactive assignments and activities, web links, animations and videos, and more!

Register your access code from the front of your book at
www.mynursingkit.com

REFERENCES

Adamson, J. W. (2005). Iron deficiency and other hypoproliferative anemias. In D. L. Kasper, A. S. Fauci, D. L. Longo, E. Braunwald, S. L. Hauser, & J. L. Jameson (Eds.), *Harrison's principles of internal medicine* (16th ed., pp. 587–593). New York: McGraw-Hill.

Aronoff, G. (2004). Safety of intravenous iron in clinical practice: Implications for anemia management protocols. *Journal of the American Society of Nephrology, 15*, 99–106.

Armandola, E. A. (2002). Management of sickle cell anemia: New approaches. Paper presented at the *7th Congress of the European Hematology Association*, Florence, Italy.

Babior, B. M. (2000). The megaloblastic anemias. In E. Beutler, A. Lichtman, B. S. Coller, T. J. Kipps, U. Seligsohn, et al. (Eds.), *Williams' hematology* (6th ed.). New York: McGraw-Hill.

Bajaj, M., Birktoft, J., & Steer, S. (2001). Structure and biology of tissue factor pathway inhibitor. *Thrombosis and Hemostasis, 86*, 959–972.

Bakhshi, S., & Abella, E. (2008). Aplastic anemia. *Emedicine*, Retrieved October 19, 2008 from http://www.emedicine.com/MED/topic162.htm

Balducci, L (2004). Anemia, cancer, and aging, *Cancer Control, 10*(6), 478–486.

Benz, E. J. (2003). Thalassemia syndromes. In D. L. Kasper, A. S. Fauci, D. L. Longo, E. Braunwald, S. L. Hauser, & J. L. Jameson (Eds.), *Harrison's principles of internal medicine* (16th ed., pp. 594–601). New York: McGraw-Hill.

Blumenthal, M. (1999). Twenty-seven major botanicals and their uses in the United States. In D. Eskinazi, M. Blumenthal, N. Farnsworth, & C. W. Riggins (Eds.), *Botanical medicine* (pp. 18–19). Larchmont, NY: Mary Ann Liebert.

Bodhise, P. B., Dejoie, M., Brandon, Z., Simpkins, S., & Ballas, S. K. (2004). Non-pharmacologic management of sickle cell pain. *Hematology, 9*(3), 235–237.

Buchanan, I. D., Woodward, M., & Reed, G. W. (2005). Opioid selection during sickle cell pain crisis and its impact of development of acute chest syndrome. *Pediatric Blood Cancer, 45*(5), 716–724.

Bunn H. F., Rosse W. (2003). *Hemolytic anemias and acute blood loss, Harrison's Principles of Internal Medicine*, 15th edition, Japanese translation. Edited by Braunwald E. Fauci, A. S., Kasper, D. L., Hauser, S. L., Longo, D. L., Jameson, J. L.. Tokyo: Medical Sciences International, 2003, pp 704–16.

Centers for Disease Control and Prevention. (1998). Recommendations to prevent and control iron deficiency in the United States. *Morbidity and Mortality Weekly Reports, 47*, 1–29.

Cines, D. B., & Blanchette, V. S. (2002). Immune thrombocytopenia purpura. *New England Journal of Medicine, 346*(13), 995–1008.

Davoren, A., & Aster, R. H. (2006). Heparin-induced thrombocytopenia and thrombosis. *American Journal of Hematology, 81*(1), 36–44.

Dhaliwal, D. G., Cornett, P. T., & Tierney, L. M. (2004). Hemolytic anemias. *American Family Physician, 69*(11), 2599–2606.

Dharmarajan, T. S., Pais, W., & Norkus, E. P. (2005). Does anemia matter? Anemia, morbidity, and mortality in older adults: Need for greater recognition. *Geriatrics, 60*, 22–29.

Forget, B. G. (2000). Thalassemia syndromes. In R. Hoffman et al. (Eds.), *Hematology: Basic principles and practice* (3rd ed., pp. 485–510). New York: Churchill Livingstone.

Fujita, T., Namiki, T., Suzuki, T., & Yamamoto, E. (2006). Normal saline flushing for maintenance of peripheral intravenous sites. *Journal of Clinical Nursing, 15*(1), 103–104.

Gallagher, P. G. (2005). Red cell membrane disorders. *Hematology, 2005*(1), 13–18.

Gesundheit, B., Kirby, M., Lau, W., Koren, G., & Abdelhaleem, M. (2002). Thrombocytopenia and megakaryocyte dysplasia: An adverse effect of valproic acid treatment. *Journal of Pediatric Hematology and Oncology, 24*(7), 589–590.

Gillespie, T. (2003). Anemia in cancer: Therapeutic implications and interventions. *Cancer Nursing, 26*(2), 119–128.

Grinder-Pedersen, L., Bukhave, K., Jensen, M., Hojgaard, L., & Hansen, M. (2004). Calcium-fortified foods do not inhibit nonheme-iron absorption from a whole food consumed over a 4-day period. *American Journal of Clinical Nutrition, 80*(2), 404–409.

Hirsh, J., Heddel, N., & Kelton, J. G. (2004). Treatment of heparin-induced thrombocytopenia: A critical review. *Archives of Internal Medicine, 164*(4), 361–369.

Hoffbrand, V. A. (2005). Deferiprone therapy for transfusional iron overload. *Best Practice & Research: Clinical Haematology, 18*(2), 299–317.

Hoffman, M. M., & Monroe, D. M. (2005). Rethinking the coagulation cascade. *Current Hematology Reports, 4*(5), 391–396.

Hoffman, R., Benz, E., Shattil, S., Furie, B., Cohen, H., Silberstein, L., et al. (2000). Disorders of iron metabolism: Iron deficiency and overload. In R. Hoffman et al. (Eds.), *Hematology: Basic principles and practice* (3rd ed., Chap. 26). New York: Churchill Livingstone.

Hunt, J. R. (2003). Bioavailability of iron, zinc, and other trace minerals from vegetarian diets. *American Journal of Clinical Nutrition, 78*(3), 633.

Knight, K., Wade, S., & Balducci, L. (2004). Prevalence and outcomes of anemia in cancer: A systematic review of the literature. *American Journal of Medicine, 5*(116), 11S–26S.

Koury, M. J., & Ponka, P. (2004). New insights into erythropoeisis: The roles of folate, vitamin B_{12} and iron. *Annual Review of Nutrition, 24*, 105–131.

Levi, M. (2005). Disseminated intravascular coagulation: what's new? (2005). *Critical Care Clinics, 21*(3), 449–467.

Levi, M., de Jonge, E., & van der Poll, T. (2004). New treatment strategies for disseminated intravascular coagulation based on current understanding of the pathophysiology. *Annals of Medicine, 36*(1), 41–49.

Levi, M., de Jonge, E., & van der Poll, T. (2006). Plasma and plasma components in the management of disseminated intravascular coagulation. *Best Practice and Research: Clinical Haematology, 19*(1), 127–142.

Lewis, B. E., Wallis, D. E., Leya, F., Hursting, M. J., & Kelton, J. G. (2003). Argatroban anticoagulation in patients with heparin-induced thrombocytopenia. *Archives of Internal Medicine, 163*, 1849–1856.

Lipschitz, D. (2003). Medical and functional consequences of anemia in the elderly. *Journal of the American Geriatrics Society, 51*(Suppl. 3), S10–S13.

Lopez, M. A., & Martos, F. C. (2004). Iron availability: An updated review. *International Journal of Food Science and Nutrition, 55*(8), 597–606.

Lottenberg, R., & Hassell, K. L. (2005). An evidence-based approach to the treatment of adults with sickle cell disease. *ASH Education Book,* 58–65.

Lukes, A. S., Kadir, R. A., Peyvandi, F., & Kouides, P. A. (2005). Disorders of hemostasis and excessive menstrual bleeding: Prevalence and clinical impact. *Fertility and Sterility, 84*(5), 1338–1344.

Mao, T. K., Van De Water, J., & Gershwin, M. E. (2000). Effect of spirulina on the secretion of cytokines from peripheral blood mononuclear cells. *Journal of Medicinal Food, 3*(3), 135–139.

Marlowe, K. F., & Chicella, M. F. (2002). Treatment of sickle cell pain. *Pharmacotherapy, 22*(4), 484–491.

Mayo Clinic. (2007). *Myelodysplastic syndromes.* Retrieved October 20, 2008, from http://www.mayoclinic.com/print/myelodysplastic-syndromes/DS00446/DSECTION+all...

Meek, P. S., Nail, L. M., Baresvil, A., Schwartz, A. L., Stephen, S., Whitmer, K., et al. (2000). Psychometric testing of fatigue instruments for use with cancer patients. *Nursing Research, 49*(4), 181–190.

Mehta, S. R., Afenyi-Annan, A., Byrns, P. J., & Lottenberg, R. (2006). Opportunities to improve outcomes in sickle cell disease. *American Family Physician, 74*(2), 313–314.

Micromedex. (2006). University of Minnesota Libraries. Retrieved October 19, 2008 from http://www.biomed.lib.umn.edu/help/guides/micromedex

Miret, S., Simpson, R. J., & McKie, A. T. (2003). Physiology and molecular biology of dietary iron absorption. *Annual Reviews in Nutrition, 23,* 283–301.

Mock, V. (2004). Evidence-based treatment for cancer-related fatigue. *Journal of the National Cancer Institute Monographs, 32,* 112–118.

Montoya, V. L., Wink, D., & Sole, M. L. (2002). Adult anemia: Determine clinical significance. *Nurse Practitioner, 27*(3), 38–53.

Naschitz, J. E., Rozenbaum, M., Shaviv, N., Fields, M., Enis, S., Babich, J. P., et al. (2004, January 1). The feeling of fatigue: Fatigue severity by unidimensional versus composite questionnaires. *Behavioral Medicine.*

National Anemia Action Council. (2008). *Iron Deficiency Anemia.* Retrieved October 20, 2008, from http://www.anemia.org/patients/information-handouts/iron-deficiency/

National Center for Health Statistics. (2008). *National Health and Nutrition Examination Survey.* Retrieved September 30, 2008, from http://www.cdc.gov/nchs/nhanes.htm

National Comprehensive Cancer Network. (2008). Cancer and Chemotherapy-Induced Anemia, V.3.2009. Retrieved October 20, 2008, from www.nccn.org

National Institutes of Health, Office of Dietary Supplements. (2005). *Dietary supplement fact sheet: Iron.* Retrieved February 11, 2006, from http://ods.od.nih.gov/factsheets/iron.asp

National Kidney Foundation. (2001). KDOQI clinical practice guidelines for anemia of chronic kidney disease: Update 2000. *American Journal of Kidney Disease, 37,* S182–S238.

Niesen, K. M., Harris, D. Y., Parkin, L. S., & Henn, L. T. (2003). The effects of heparin versus normal saline for maintenance of peripheral intravenous locks in pregnant women. *Journal of Obstetrics and Gynecology, 32*(4), 503–508.

Nilsson, M., Norberg, B. M., Hultdin, J., Sandstrom, H., Westman, G., & Lokk, J. (2005). Medical intelligence in Sweden. Vitamin B_{12}: Oral compared with parenteral? *Journal of Postgraduate Medicine, 81*(953), 191–193.

Nyholm, E., Turpin, P., Swain, D., Cunningham, B., Daly, S., Nightingale, P. et al. (2003). Oral vitamin B_{12} can change our practice. *Journal of Postgraduate Medicine, 79*(930), 218 – 219.

Ouellette, D. R. (2005). The impact of anemia in patients with respiratory failure. *Chest 128,* 576S–582S.

Pearson, D. J. (2000). Pathophysiology and clinical effects of chronic hypoxia. *Respiratory Care, 45*(1), 39–51.

Penninx, B. J., Pahor, M., Cesari, M., Corsi, A. M., et al. (2004). Anemia is associated with disability and decreased physical performance and muscle strength in the elderly. *Journal of the American Geriatrics Society, 52*(5), 719.

Penninx, B. J., Pluijm, S. M. F., Lips, P., Woodman, M., Miedema, K., Guralnik, J. K. et al. (2005). Late-life anemia is associated with increased risk of recurrent falls. *Journal of the American Geriatrics Society, 53*(12), 2106–2111.

Ponka, P. (2001). Iron deficiency. In R. E. Rakel & E. T. Bope (Eds.), *Conn's current therapy* (pp. 369–376). London: Saunders.

Ramsey, L. T., Woods, K. F., Callahan, L. A., Mensah, G. A., Barbeau, P., & Gutin, B. (2001). Quality of life improvement for patients with sickle cell disease. *American Journal of Hematology, 66*(2), 155–156.

Rice, L., Nguyen, P. H., & Vann, A. R. (2002). Preventing complications in heparin-induced thrombocytopenias: Alternative anticoagulants are improving patient outcomes. *Postgraduate Medicine, 112*(3).

Rios, R., Sangro, B., Herrero, I., Quiroga, J., & Prieto, J. (2005). The role of thrombopoietin in the thrombocytopenia of patients with liver cirrhosis. *American Journal of Gastroenterology, 100*(6), 1311–1316.

Rosenthal, K. (2003). Consider alternative technologies to maintain vascular access devices. *Nursing Management, 34*(8), 53–56.

Sadler, J. E. (1994). A revised classification of von Willebrand disease. For the Subcommittee on von Willebrand factor of the Scientific and Standardization Committee of the International Society on Thrombosis and Haemostasis. *Thrombosis and Haemostasis, 71*(4), 520–525.

Sleijfer, S., & Lugtenburg, P. J. (2003). Aplastic anemia: a review. *Netherlands Journal of Medicine, 61*(5), 157–163.

Solovey, A. A., Solovey, A. N., Harkness, J., & Hebbel, R. P. (2001). Modulation of endothelial cell activation in sickle cell disease: A pilot study. *Blood, 97,* 1937–1941.

Stasi, R. S., & Provan, D. (2004). Management of immune thrombocytopenic purpura in adults. *Mayo Clinic Proceedings, 79,* 504–522.

Stouten, B. (2005). Identification of ambiguities in the 1994 chronic fatigue syndrome research case definition and recommendations for resolution. *BMC Health Services Research, 5,* 37.

Sturgeon, P., Itano, H. A., et al. (1955). Genetic and biochemical studies of intermediate types of Cooley's anemia. *British Journal of Haematology, 1,* 264.

Umbreit, J. (2005). Iron deficiency anemia: A concise review. *American Journal of Hematology, 78,* 225–231.

U.S. Department of Health and Human Services. (2000). *Healthy people 2010: Understanding and improving health and objectives for improving health* (2nd ed., 2 volumes). Washington, DC: Author.

U.S. Preventive Services Task Force. (2006). Screening for iron deficiency anemia, including iron supplementations for children and pregnant women: recommendation statement. *American Family Physician.* Retrieved October 17, 2008, from http://www.aafp.org/afp/20060901/us.html

Vichinsky, E. (2005). *Treating thalassemia.* Retrieved March 5, 2006, from Northern California Comprehensive Thalassemia Center website: http://www.thalassemia.com

Wang, W. C., Helms, R. W., Lynn, H. S., et al. (2002). Effect of hydroxyurea on growth in children with sickle cell anemia: Results of the HUG-KIDS study. *Journal of Pediatrics, 140*(2), 225–229.

Warkentin, T. E., & Kelton, J. G. (1996). A 14-year study of heparin-induced thrombocytopenia. *American Journal of Medicine, 101*(5), 502–507.

Weiss, G. (2002). Pathogenesis and treatment of anaemia of chronic disease. *Blood Reviews, 16,* 87–96.

Weiss, G., & Gordeuk, V. R. (2005). Benefits and risks of iron therapy for chronic anaemias. *European Journal of Clinical Investigation, 35,* 36S–45S.

Whitta, R. K., Hall, K. F., Bennetts, T. M., Welman L., & Rawlins, P. (2006). Comparison of normal or heparinised saline flushing on function of arterial lines. *Critical Care Resuscitation, 8*(3), 205–208.

Caring for the Patient with Cancer

Dawn Lambie

Outcome-Based Learning Objectives

After studying this chapter, the learner will be able to:

1. Identify the prevalence and incidence of cancer, list the common risk factors, and describe the correlation to development of malignancy.
2. Discuss the pathophysiology of cancer.
3. Compare and contrast the five common types of solid tumor cancer (prostate, breast, colorectal, lung, and brain) and cancers of the hematopoietic and lymphatic system.
4. Develop a detailed nursing plan of care for patients with cancer of the prostate, breast, colon or rectum, lung, brain, hematopoietic system, and lymphatic system.
5. Describe current treatment approaches to fatigue, nutrition, and pain and the importance of improving quality of life for patients with cancer.
6. Discuss the rationale for treatment modalities such as surgery, radiation therapy, chemotherapy, biotherapy, and transplantation.

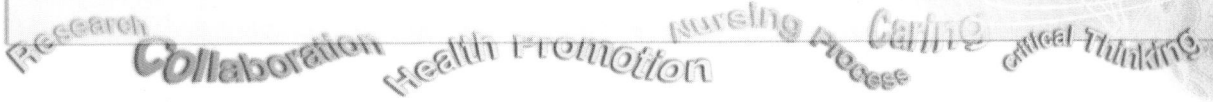

Research   Collaboration   Health Promotion   Nursing Process   Caring   Critical Thinking

FEW WORDS evoke an emotional response as dramatic as the word **cancer**. The impacts, both physiologically and psychologically, cause considerable changes in the lifestyles of both patients and families. The diagnosis of cancer in a family member will change the emotional status, finances, division of responsibility, and social activities of the entire family (Kaye, 1993). Nurses need to be aware of their own feelings and attitudes toward cancer and cancer care in order to be supportive of patients and their families.

For the past two centuries nurses have dedicated their lives to changing the experience of illness, leading to changes in nursing practice (Lynaugh, 2001). Leaders in cancer nursing have directed their efforts toward prevention, detection, education, and the creation of a specialty within nursing that embraces the whole of the human being who has cancer. Sadly, society continues to perceive malignancy as incurable with accompanied dread and hopelessness. Of critical importance is the role of nursing in the continued development of cancer screening, detection, and prevention programs. These programs have already demonstrated improved survival rates and quality of life for patients undergoing cancer treatment.

Following the first National Cancer Nursing Research Conference in 1973, oncology nurses identified the need to form a national organization to support their profession. Cancer nursing was first recognized as a subspecialty in the nursing profes-

sion in the year 1975 with the incorporation of the Oncology Nursing Society (ONS). Since its inception, ONS has grown to a membership of more than 30,000 registered nurses and other health care providers. The organization is dedicated to maintaining excellence in patient care, education, research, and administration in oncology nursing (ONS, n.d.). To be an effective oncology nurse, a nurse must possess a broad base of knowledge about the pathophysiology and psychosocial aspects of the disease and its treatment. Patients rely on nurses for support and assistance throughout all phases of their illness, from diagnosis to end-of-life care.

Epidemiology

When studying cancer, the outcome for therapeutic research is to discover a cure. In contrast, the outcome of epidemiological research is to prevent cancer (Schulmeister, 2001a). Understanding basic epidemiologic terminology will help the nurse reach a sound interpretation of literature about cancer and its causes. In addition, this knowledge will assist the nurse in identification of target population groups for education, prevention, and screening programs.

Incidence is the number of newly diagnosed cases of cancer in a specific time period in a defined population. It will be expressed as a rate per 100,000 persons, allowing for comparison between different populations. For example, when evaluating the number of estimated breast cancer cases in Minnesota for the year 2005 (3,240) and the number in California (19,790), researchers must consider the state's population or the numbers are meaningless (American Cancer Society [ACS], 2007).

Prevalence is the measurement of all cancer cases at a designated point in time. The number is divided by the total population living at the time. The prevalence rate is very useful when planning the creation of health care facilities, determining necessary manpower, and designing and implementing screening programs (Schulmeister, 2001a).

Mortality is the number of deaths from cancer in a specific period of time and within an identified population. The total number of persons dying of cancer is divided by the total population living at that time. Since 1930 the United States has been collecting mortality data. The 2007 estimated number of cancer deaths in the United States is 559,650 persons (ACS, 2007). Death certificates typically identify a single cause of death, leading to inaccuracy in the reporting of cancer deaths. Mortality figures are very useful in determining the impact of treatment, whereas incidence figures are more helpful when determining the cause of cancer.

Survival is the observation of persons with cancer over time and the likelihood of their dying over several time periods. This information is the link between incidence and mortality data, providing useful measures of the end result of treatment. In addition, survival information may provide evidence of improvement over time in the management of cancer.

Cancer Statistics

As mentioned, the ACS has estimated that approximately 559,650 Americans will die from cancer in the year 2007, resulting in 1,533 deaths per day (ACS, 2007). Refer to Chart 64–1 for details. The total number of cancer deaths continues to rise due to an aging and expanding population. Figure 64–1 ■ represents the number of cancer cases and deaths according to site and gender. This information is important for nurses to understand in order to develop and implement patient education regarding cancer prevention.

■ Etiology and Pathophysiology

Cancer is not an unruly growth of immature cells, but rather a logical, coordinated process in which normal cells undergo changes and develop special functions. An understanding of the morphology and biochemistry of the normal cell is crucial in building an appreciation of the disease itself.

Proliferative Growth Patterns

Cancer cells do not have the usual limitations on cell proliferation placed by the host. Proliferation and cancer are not always synonymous terms. Proliferation does not always insinuate the presence of

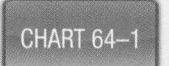 **CHART 64–1** ■ **Estimated Cancer Cases and Cancer Deaths**

Estimated Cancer Cases			Estimated Cancer Deaths*		
Total	Female	Male	Total	Female	Male
1,444,920	678,060	766,860	559,650	270,100	289,550

*Estimated number of cancer deaths expected in the United States was determined using underlying cause-of-death data from death certificates as reported to the National Center for Health Statistics.

Source: American Cancer Society. (2007). *Cancer facts and figures 2007.* Atlanta, Georgia. Retrieved from http://www.cancer.org/docroot/STT/content/STT_1x_Cancer_Facts__Figures_2007.asp.

Estimated number of new cancer cases (10 leading sites by gender), U.S. 2007

Female		Male	
Breast	26%	Prostate	29%
Lung and bronchus	15%	Lung and bronchus	15%
Colon and rectum	11%	Colon and rectum	10%
Uterine corpus	6%	Urinary bladder	7%
Non-Hodgkin's lymphoma	4%	Melanoma of the skin	4%
Melanoma of the skin	4%	Non-Hodgkin's lymphoma	4%
Thyroid	4%	Kidney/renal pelvis	4%
Ovary	3%	Oral cavity/pharynx	3%
Kidney and renal pelvis	3%	Leukemia	3%
Leukemia	3%	Pancreas	2%
Other	21%	Other	19%

Estimated number of new cancer deaths (10 leading sites by gender), U.S. 2007

Female		Male	
Lung and bronchus	26%	Lung and bronchus	31%
Breast	15%	Prostate	9%
Colon and rectum	10%	Colon and rectum	9%
Pancreas	6%	Pancreas	6%
Ovary	6%	Esophagus	4%
Leukemia	4%	Leukemia	4%
Non-Hodgkin's lymphoma	3%	Liver/intrahepatic bile duct	4%
Uterine corpus	3%	Non-Hodgkin's lymphoma	3%
Brain/CNS	2%	Urinary bladder	3%
Liver and hepatic duct	2%	Kidney and renal pelvis	3%
Other	23%	Other	24%

FIGURE 64–1 ■ Epidemiology of cancer.

CHART 64–2	Terms of Proliferative Growth Patterns	
Types of Cellular Change	**Definition**	**Example**
Hypertrophy	Increase in cell size	Increase in muscle cell size
Hyperplasia	Increase in cell number	Breast epithelium during pregnancy
Metaplasia	Replacement of one adult cell type by a different adult cell type	Replacement of columnar epithelium of respiratory tract by squamous epithelium
Anaplasia	Reverse cellular development with more primitive cell type	Irreversible changes to an accompanying cancer
Neoplasia	Abnormal cellular changes and growth of new tissue	Malignancies
Dysplasia	Abnormal growth of cells that vary in size, shape or organization of cells or tissues	Precancerous changes in cervical cells

cancer. Abnormal cellular growth is known as *nonneoplastic* and *neoplastic*. The terms are summarized in Chart 64–2.

Nonneoplastic Growth Patterns

There are four common nonneoplastic growth patterns: hypertrophy, hyperplasia, metaplasia, and dysplasia (Pfeifer, 2001). They are not neoplastic conditions, but may precede the development of cancer. Hypertrophy refers to an increase in a cell's size. Situations that create hypertrophy include increased workload, stimulation by hormones, and compensation from loss of other tissue. Hyperplasia refers to an increase in tissue mass due to a reversible increase in the number of cells of a certain tissue type. This is a normal physiological response in times of rapid growth and development such as pregnancy and adolescence. Abnormality occurs when the volume of cells produced is larger than the physiological demand. Metaplasia occurs when one mature cell type is substituted for another type not typically found in the involved tissue. A stimulus such as inflammation, vitamin deficiencies, irritation, and chemical agents can induce metaplasia. If the stimulus is removed, the process is reversible. Otherwise it will progress to dysplasia, which occurs when there are alterations in normal mature cells. These alterations can include variation from normal cell size, shape, or organization or replacement of one mature cell type with a less mature cell type. External stimuli are the usual impetus for creating dysplasia, but if removed the process may be reversible. These can include radiation, inflammation, toxic chemicals, and chronic irritation.

An irreversible change in the structure of an adult cell that deteriorates to a more immature level is known as *anaplasia*. This type of cellular change is the classic finding of cancer. Anaplastic cells no longer have the ability to implement their unique functions and overall are chaotic in their nature.

Neoplastic Growth Patterns

The term **neoplasm** means "new growth." Inherent in this definition is the understanding that there is an abnormal tissue mass that goes beyond the normal cell boundaries and results in the inability of the cell to perform its normal function. Neoplasms can be destructive to the host because they occupy space and battle for nutrients crucial to maintain its life. There are two categories of neoplasm: benign and malignant. Papillomas and warts are examples of benign neoplasms. Malignant neoplasms, referred to as cancer, have the potential to destroy the host and include solid tumors and leukemias. Refer to Chart 64–3 for a comparison between benign and malignant tumors.

CHART 64–3	Differences Between Benign and Malignant Neoplasms
Benign	**Malignant**
Usually slow growing, expansive	May proliferate rapidly or grow slowly, infiltrative patterns
Localized or encapsulated	Spread (metastasize) throughout the body invading nearby tissue
Fibrous capsule	No enclosing capsule
Rarely recur after removal	May recur even after treatment
Usually regular in shape	Irregular shape with poorly defined border
Well differentiated	Poorly differentiated
Slight vascularity	Moderate to significant vascularity

Sources: Erickson, J. (2003). Cancer. In W. Phipps, F. Monahan, J. Sands, J. Marek, & M. Neighbors (Eds.), *Medical–surgical nursing health and illness perspectives* (7th ed.). St. Louis: Mosby; Otto, S. (2001c). *Oncology nursing* (4th ed.). St. Louis: Mosby.

Characteristics of a Cancer Cell

Metabolism for normal cells is achieved through aerobic glycolysis, in which oxygen is the crucial element in maintenance of cellular activity. Malignant cells utilize higher rates of aerobic glycolysis with a resulting decrease in oxygen needed for survival. This difference in metabolism may be due to differences in intracellular enzyme structure and quantity (Volker, 1994).

Cancer cells differ according to the cell type from which they derive. It is incorrect to apply a standard definition to all cancer cells (McNance & Roberts, 2002). Some tumors may retain useful functions and closely resemble normal tissue, whereas others are chaotic enough that the tissue of origin cannot be determined. Certain cellular characteristics that are typical features of cancerous tissue include local increase in number of cells, loss of normal arrangement of cells, dissimilarity of cell shape and size, increase in nuclear size and total DNA seen by an increase in the density of staining, increase in mitotic activity, and abnormal mitoses and chromosomes.

Cancer cells are chaotic cells with significant cellular proliferation and assorted sizes and shapes. *Progression* is a term used to explain the unorganized dividing of cells and the invasion and destruction of nearby tissue. It is important to understand that progression refers to an increase of abnormal biologic properties, not always a progression in tumor size. The increase in biologic activities is related to the tumor's malignant capabilities or its lack of differentiation. Therefore, cancer can be considered an aberrant cell mass.

Tumor Growth

Malignant tumors grow in an uninhibited way and do not adhere to the normal process of cell reproduction (Volker, 1994). As the body loses cells or increases tissue function demands, there is a natural increase in the number of cells and cell replacement. Cell development approximates cell destruction (Pfeifer, 2001). Cancer cells do not reproduce faster than normal cells; in fact, many are slow growing compared to regular cells. Examples of this unique process include cells of the bone marrow and those located in the epithelial lining. All tumors contain cells that ignore the restraints typical of proliferation, but not all cancer cells proliferate indefinitely. This erratic behavior results in cell growth beyond normal margins and an increase in pressure on surrounding organs. In addition, cells may be noted to actually invade surrounding tissues and structures.

Carcinogenesis

Carcinogenesis is defined as the process of tumor development (McNance & Roberts, 2002). Normal cells are altered, resulting in the development of cancerous cells. It is a multistep process that is in constant unrest and is influenced by a variety of forces. A carcinogen (initiating agent) is a chemical, biologic, or physical agent with the potential of changing the molecular structure of the genetic component (DNA) of a cell. The transformation of the cell is due to direct contact with the carcinogen, and the result is permanent and irreversible. A co-carcinogen (promoting agent) changes the expression of the genetic information of the cell that assists in cellular transformation. Examples of co-carcinogens include hormones, drugs, and plant products. A complete carcinogen (e.g., radiation) is capable of performing functions of both an initiating agent and promoting agent. Anticarcinogens (reversing factors) are substances found in most diets, vitamins C, A, and E, and selenium. These substances may interfere with the effects of initiating agents and prevent cancerous growths.

Scientists have yet to definitively prove that the first event in carcinogenesis is a mutation, but regardless of the cause, there is an irreversible alteration in the genetic code of cells (Erickson, 2003). A number of theories have been proposed to explain the development of cancer, but no single idea has been accepted, which answers why a cause for most human cancers has yet to be determined (Pfeifer, 2001). Many of the theories of carcinogenesis discuss three common stages: initiation, promotion, and progression. In 1947 the Berenblum theory attempted to explain the first two stages, but over time the third stage of progression was proposed to further explain the complex phenomena of cancer development (Pfeifer, 2001). Figure 64–2 ■ illustrates the stages of initiation, promotion, and progression. This theory suggests that the process of changing a normal cell into a cancer cell involves three stages where all activity occurs in the cell's DNA.

In the first stage, initiation, a carcinogen alters a particular gene, resulting in damaged DNA. The three possible outcomes of this transformation include:

- Repair of the gene with no cancer development
- The occurrence of permanent changes, but there is no cancer development unless the cell is exposed to a co-carcinogen later

- Transformation into a cancer cell if the initiating agent is a complete carcinogen.

An oncogene is a slightly altered form of a normal gene that is responsible for cell growth and repair and has been associated with the development of cancer when activated (McNance & Roberts, 2002). Tumor suppressor genes hinder cellular growth, thus causing cellular death. An example of this is the p53 tumor suppressor gene on chromosome 17. This gene prohibits cells with DNA damage from multiplying. Mutations to the p53 gene have been identified in half of all human cancers (Erickson, 2003).

In promotion, the second stage, co-carcinogens produce either reversible or irreversible destruction to the proliferative mechanism of the cell (Pfeifer, 2001). Cancerous cell formation occurs with irreversible cell damage. Progression, the final stage, involves morphologic changes within cells that begin to demon-

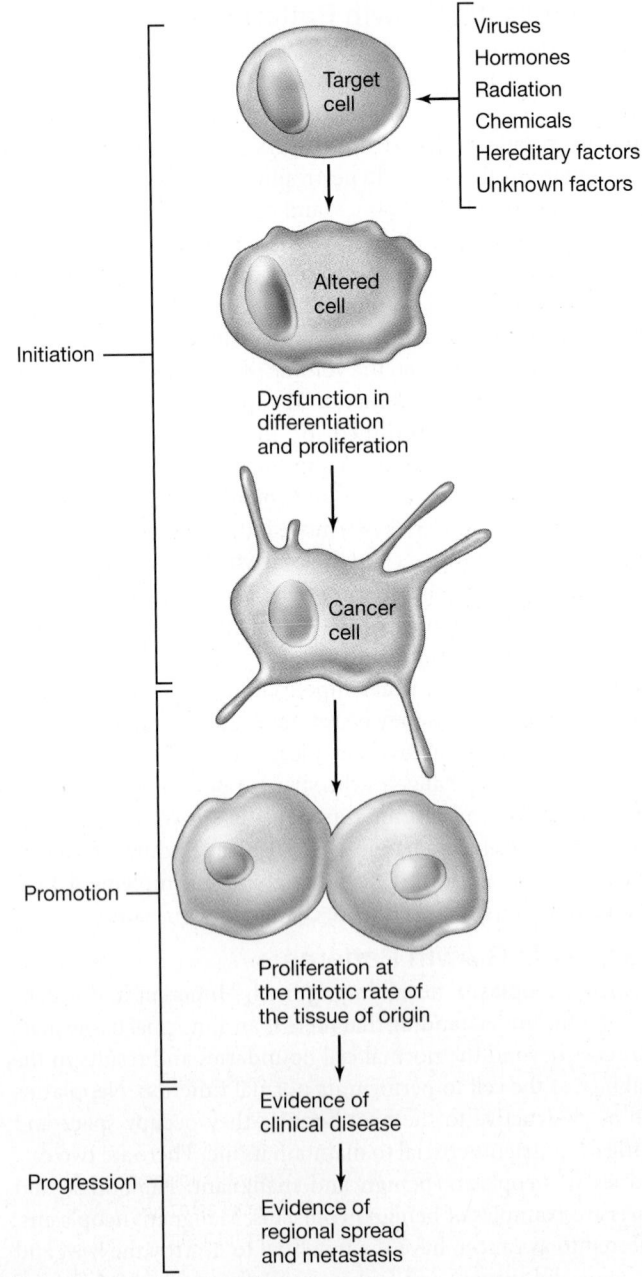

FIGURE 64–2 ■ Cellular changes with cancer.

strate malignancy and the evolution of metastatic potential. This last stage is irreversible.

In humans, the process of carcinogenesis is much more complex than any laboratory model and frequently occupies many years of an individual's life (Pfeifer, 2001). Distinguishing among the three phases is difficult because of the presence of the latent period. Occurring between the initial exposure to a carcinogen and the evidence of detectable malignancy, this period is void of specific clinical or subjective findings. Adding to the difficulty in determining the beginning and end of the stages is the absence of tests to detect latent transformed cells. This explains why it impossible to predict whether the risk of cancer exists in subsets of a population group.

Tumor Nomenclature

Tumors receive their names according to the originating tissue type as seen in Chart 64–4. The identification of the tissue is often difficult due to a variety of cell types within one malignancy.

CHART 64–4   Nomenclature and Classification of Neoplasms

Tissue of Origin	Malignant Tumor	Benign Tumor
Epithelial		
Squamous cells	Squamous cell carcinoma	Squamous cell papilloma
Basal cells	Basal cell carcinoma	No benign tumor for this type of cell
Liver cells	Hepatocellular carcinoma	Hepatocellular adenoma
Melanocytes	Malignant melanoma	Nevus
Renal epithelium	Renal cell carcinoma	Renal tubular adenoma
Glands	Adenocarcinoma	Adenoma
Endothelial/Related Tissue		
Lymphoid tissue	Lymphatic leukemia	No benign tumor for this type of cell
	Malignant lymphoma	No benign tumor for this type of cell
	Reticular cell sarcoma	No benign tumor for this type of cell
Bone marrow	Multiple myeloma	No benign tumor for this type of cell
	Leukemia	No benign tumor for this type of cell
	Ewing's sarcoma	No benign tumor for this type of cell
	Lymphosarcoma	No benign tumor for this type of cell
Lymph vessels	Lymphangiosarcoma	Lymphangioma
Mesothelium	Malignant mesothelioma	No benign tumor for this type of cell
Meninges	Malignant meningioma	Meningioma
Neural and Retinal Tissue		
Nerve fibers and sheaths	Neurofibrosarcoma	Neurilemoma, neurofibroma
	Neurogenic sarcoma	No benign tumor for this type of cell
Nerve cells	Neuroblastoma	Ganglioneuroma
	Spongioblastoma	Glioma
Muscle Tissue		
Smooth muscle	Leiomyosarcoma	Leiomyoma
Striated muscle	Rhabdomyosarcoma	Rhabdomyoma
Connective Tissue		
Fibrous tissue	Fibrosarcoma	Fibroma
Embryonic fibrous tissue	Myxosarcoma	Myxoma
Fat	Liposarcoma	Lipoma
Bone	Osteogenic sarcoma	Osteoma
Cartilage	Chondrosarcoma	Chondroma
Synovial membrane	Synovial sarcoma	Synovioma
Other		
Placenta	Chorion-epithelioma	Hydatidiform mole
	Embryonal carcinoma	Dermoid cyst
	Embryonal sarcoma	No benign tumor for this type of cell
	Teratocarcinoma	No benign tumor for this type of cell

Sources: Adapted from McNance, K., & Roberts, L. (2002). Biology of cancer. In K. McNance & S. Huether (Eds.), *Pathophysiology: The biological basis for disease in adult and children* (4th ed.). St. Louis: Mosby; Otto, S. (2001c). *Oncology nursing* (4th ed.). St. Louis: Mosby.

Within a cluster of neoplastic cells there may be benign cells as well, making identification even more difficult (Erickson, 2003). Tumors are classified according to the following: cell type, originating tissue, malignant or benign, degree of differentiation, site, and function (McNance & Roberts, 2002).

The degree of differentiation refers to the cell's maturity. Undifferentiated tumors are those that have completely lost identity with the tissue of origin. Well and moderately differentiated tumors possess cells that continue to demonstrate the tissue of origin.

Histogenetic Classification

The suffix *oma*, Greek for "tumor," is used for both benign and malignant tumors. **Benign** tumors are those whose prefix designates specific tissue, whereas **malignant** tumors use the root *carcin* (epithelial tissue) and *sarc* (connective tissue) In addition, other cancer types include lymphomas (lymphatic system), gliomas (glial cells of the central nervous system), and leukemias (blood-forming organs, usually bone marrow). Examples of benign tumors are fibromas and adenomas, which are located in fibrous and glandular tissue. The only exceptions to this are melanoma and hepatomas. Melanomas are malignancies of the melanocytes and hepatomas are malignancies of the liver. Specific connective tissue sarcomas use several different prefixes depicting the anatomic location of the tumor (Pfeifer, 2001). These include:

- *Osteo-* (bone)
- *Chondro-* (cartilage)
- *Lipo-* (fat)
- *Rhabdo-* (skeletal muscle)
- *Leiomyo-* (smooth muscle).

Preinvasive epithelial tumors with glandular or squamous cell origins are called **carcinoma *in situ***. They typically occur in the cervix, skin, oral cavity, bronchus, and esophagus. Carcinoma *in situ* neoplasms have not invaded the basement membrane of the epithelial site, thus the surrounding tissues are left untouched by malignant cells (McNance & Roberts, 2002).

Classifying Degree of Malignancy

Examination of tumor tissue under the microscope is the only way to classify, or grade, the degree of malignancy. Four grades are used as a standardized method of communicating the appearance of the cells and their potential for spread and growth. Using a standardized language allows practitioners to determine treatment options while providing prognostic information. A grade 1 tumor is small in size, more differentiated, and the least malignant. Grade 4 tumors are those with cells that appear more abnormal, are usually very aggressive in nature, and are considered to have a high degree of malignancy.

Staging is the portion of the classification system that describes the extent of the tumor and evidence of metastasis throughout the body. The TNM system is used to describe the presence and extent of local, regional, and distant disease. *T* refers to primary tumor size, *N* refers to the absence or presence of regional lymph nodes, and *M* refers to absence or presence of distant metastases. It is important to understand that not all malignancies will have similar degrees of grading and classification; ultimately, the labels will be determined by the pathologist upon

examining the tissue specimens. Details of the classification system are found in Chart 64–5.

Route of Tumor Spread

Cells that are experiencing the transformation process have abnormal or decreased anchorage. Anchorage independence is the inability of the cell to maintain cellular or extracellular matrix attachments. Cancer cells do not require a surface on which to attach and multiply. Missing this cellular characteristic that inhibits proliferation will result in cancerous cell growth in new regions, or metastases (McNance & Roberts 2002).

Cancer may invade local tissues or spread to distant areas by hematogenous or lymphatic routes. As tumors grow locally, their cells extend to and invade lymph nodes found in the same anatomic region resulting in distant metastases. Some tumors are known to metastasize to distant organs prior to or during involvement with local lymph nodes (Pfeifer, 2001).

Direct

Direct spread is the ability of a tumor to invade and eradicate adjoining tissue (Groenwald, Frogge, Goodman, & Yarbro, 1997). The following enhances this process:

- Tumor angiogenesis factor stimulates new capillary growth, which allows for continued tumor growth due to adequate nutrition and oxygen. Once a tumor reaches 2 mm^3 in size, it requires additional blood supply to grow. The new vascular growth provides not only the essential elements for growth but also a route for tumor cells to leave the primary site (Merkle & Loescher, 2005).

CHART 64–5   TNM System of Tumor Classification and Staging

Primary Tumor Size (T)

T0	No evidence of a primary tumor or lesion
Tis	Carcinoma *in situ*
T1	Lesion contained in organ of origin
T2	Localized lesion with deep growth into adjacent structures
T3	Advanced lesion limited to a region of the original organ
T4	Advanced lesion spreading into adjacent organs

Regional Lymph Nodes (N)

N0	No evidence of disease in lymph nodes
N1	Evidence of disease in regional lymph nodes but not likely metastatic
N2, 3, 4	Increasing involvement of regional lymph nodes

Anatomic Extent of Metastasis (M)

M0	No evidence of metastasis
M1, 2, 3	Worsening degrees of metastatic involvement, including distant lymph nodes and functional impairment

Sources: Erickson, J. (2003). Cancer. In W. Phipps, F. Monahan, J. Sands, J. Marek, & M. Neighbors (Eds.), *Medical–surgical nursing health and illness perspectives* (7th ed.). St. Louis: Mosby; McNance, K., & Roberts, L. (2002). Biology of cancer. In K. McNance & S. Huether (Eds.), *Pathophysiology: The biological basis for disease in adult and children* (4th ed.). St. Louis: Mosby; Pfeifer, K. A. (2001). Pathophysiology. In S. Otto (Ed.), *Oncology nursing* (4th ed.). St. Louis: Mosby.

- Mechanical pressure and increased rate of tumor growth occur when intratumor pressure causes finger-like projections to be pushed into adjacent tissue. Uncontrolled tumor growth creates expanding masses that apply pressure on local tissues.
- Cell motility and loss of cellular adhesiveness promote tumor cell distribution due to the slippery nature of the cancer cell, which enhances movement.
- Tumor-secreted enzymes may be associated with the degree to which cells have the potential to invade surrounding tissues and destroy the normal tissue barriers. An example of this is plasminogen activator.

Serosal seeding is another mechanism by which tumor cells demonstrate direct spreading (Groenwald et al. 1997). Embolization of tumor cells occurs after malignant cells invade local tissues and infiltrate body cavities. These cells then attach themselves to the serosal surface of organs within the involved cavity. The most common site for serosal seeding to occur is the lung and ovary. Penetration of the parenchyma of the organ is unlikely to occur despite the presence of tumor cells within the surface of organs in the pleural and peritoneal cavities.

Surgical instrumentation has been shown to participate in the direct spread of cancerous cells by the contamination of normal cells during surgical procedures (Volker, 1992). As needles are withdrawn during biopsies, seeding of malignant cells may occur, or manipulation of a tumor during the operative procedure may release cells into the vascular supply and into the circulation.

Metastatic

Metastasis is defined as the spread of cancerous cells from a primary site of origin to a distant site (McNance & Roberts, 2002). Of extreme importance is to recognize the effect of metastasis and that a benign tumor does not exhibit this type of behavior. The capability of malignant cells to travel to distant sites and begin invasion into adjacent tissues is very powerful and oftentimes deadly. Chart 64–6 lists the four most common cancers and their metastatic sites.

French physician Joseph Claude Recamier was the first to use the term *metastasis* in 1829 (Hawkins, 2001). Previously, researchers thought that tumors spread by direct extension and invading lymph nodes. At that time, it was thought that distant metastasis was caused by new tumor growth unrelated to the primary tumor. Recamier was the first physician to prove metastasis was caused by malignant cells separating from the primary tumor and traveling through the bloodstream and lymphatic circulation to distant anatomic locations (Liotta, 1992).

Approximately 50% to 60% of patients diagnosed with solid tumors are discovered to have metastatic disease. Some patients will have clinically detectable metastasis, whereas others will have micrometastases or clinically undetectable disease (Liotta & Kohn, 1990). Prognosis is dramatically worsened if evidence of metastasis is present at the time of diagnosis.

The metastatic process, although commonly evident clinically, is a unique, intricate series of events. A cancer cell released from a primary tumor with the mission to establish residency in a distant anatomic site has a long and difficult task in order to survive. It is believed that only 1 in 10,000 tumor cells that separate from the primary tumor are able to endure long enough to begin the metastatic process (Liotta, 1992).

Understanding the mechanism of metastasis is important to increase our appreciation of metastatic patterns; however, metastasis is known to be unpredictable in nature. Mechanisms of metastasis include (1) angiogenesis, (2) migration, (3) cell attachment, (4) cell invasion, and (5) growth factors.

Angiogenesis is the creation of new blood vessels due to migration and proliferation of endothelial cells from existing blood vessels. Although angiogenesis is a favorable occurrence in wound healing, ovulation, and embryogenesis, it is not so favorable in the development of malignancies. Vascular endothelial growth factor (VEGF) is an essential component for the growth and proliferation of cancer cells. New blood vessels provide nutrients, protein growth factors, and oxygen to the tumor mass. With the development of angiogenesis inhibitors (e.g., Avastin), this vital process for tumor growth can be slowed or stopped, affording patients better treatment options (Viele, 2005).

Because vessels created by angiogenesis tend to have permeable walls, malignant cells enter easily, allowing access to the circulatory and lymphatic systems (migration). Tumor masses produce motility factors that enable cells to move with more ease throughout the circulatory and lymphatic systems. Once in the circulation, cancer cells cluster in the first vascular bed distal to the original site. After blood circulates through the heart, the pulmonary vascular bed is the first encountered by the cancerous cells. Intestines drain their blood supply into the liver, thus exposing it to malignant cells. Understandably, the most common site of metastasis is the lung followed by the liver.

Another common vehicle for the transportation of malignant cells is the lymphatic system. Tumor emboli, which form as a result of circulating tumor cells, are trapped in lymph nodes. Not all lymph nodes will be hosts for these deadly cells; in fact, cancerous cells will bypass several lymph nodes before settling into a distant nodal site. This is known as "skip" metastasis (Hawkins, 2001).

Normally, cells adhere to one another and to the extracellular matrix (ECM). When discussing cell attachment, the nurse must understand that tumor cells form temporary attachments to ECM components and to other cells not part of their origin. Cell-to-cell adhesion is altered resulting in tumor cells attaching themselves to cells of a different origin. For example, breast cancer metastasizing to the bone occurs when a breast tissue cell relocates to the bone. This form of cell attachment is assisted by cell surface receptors such as CD44. The next type of cellular attachment is adhesion to the ECM, which promotes cellular growth and endurance. As discussed earlier, anchorage dependence is necessary for cells to attach to surfaces that nurture their proliferation.

CHART 64–6	Common Sites of Metastases of the Four Most Frequently Occurring Cancers
Origin	**Site of Metastasis**
Breast	Bone, lung, liver, brain, lymph nodes
Prostate	Bone, lung, liver, bowel, kidney, lymph nodes
Lung	Bone, liver, kidney, brain, bone marrow, lymph nodes
Colon	Lung, liver, brain, lymph nodes

Cell invasion is essential for the metastatic process. As a result, tumor cells drift from physical barriers into a vessel (intravasation) or out of a vessel (extravasation). Cancer cells are able to reach normal tissue despite numerous mechanical barriers with the assistance of tumor cell invasion. Basement membrane invasion occurs when cancer cells leave the primary tumor, penetrate into the blood or lymphatic vessels, and exit from the vasculature.

Growth factors contribute substantially to the metastatic process. Angiogenesis is potentiated or impeded by growth factors. In addition, tumor proliferation produces a decreased reliance on exogenous growth factors. The existence of growth factors at the metastatic site is imperative for continued growth of cancerous cells. Chart 64–7 illustrates various growth factors known to stimulate cancerous development.

The phenomenon of metastasis is uniquely complex as it navigates through normal body controls and regulatory functions. The process oftentimes is associated with worsened prognosis and increased mortality. Understanding the metastatic process will assist researchers in discovering and developing new and more effective treatment options.

CHART 64–7 **Correlation of Growth Factors and Cancers**

Growth Factor	Location of Cancer Cell Stimulation
Epidermal growth factor	Prostate Anal
Epidermal growth factor • Amphiregulin	Breast
Epidermal growth factor • Insulin-like growth factor	Breast Prostate Colon
Fibroblast growth factor	Breast Prostate Thyroid Bladder
Platelet-derived growth factor	Melanoma
Transforming growth factor	Colorectal

Health Promotion: Prevention, Screening, and Detection

Surviving cancer is, in part, a result of improved therapies and earlier detection. The 5-year survival rate has improved from 50% in 1975–1977 to 66% in 1996–2002 (ACS, 2007). Represented in these statistics are those people who are living 5 years after diagnosis, including those who are disease free, in remission, or under treatment with evidence of disease.

Regularly scheduled screening appointments may result in earlier detection of cancers of the breast, colon, rectum, cervix, prostate, testis, oral cavity, and skin. Earlier detection allows for diagnosis at an early stage of tumor development, which may lead to a more positive outcome for the patient (Gullatte & Otto, 2001). In 1999, the American Cancer Society set goals that would significantly lower cancer incidence and mortality rates and improve quality of life of cancer survivors by 2015 (see the National Guidelines box). One example of efforts aimed at accomplishing these goals is the collaborative work with the American Heart Association and American Diabetes Association called "Everyday Choices for a Healthier Life." These three organizations are examining tobacco use, obesity, physical inactivity, and underutilization of effective screening tests.

Nurses are becoming more involved with cancer detection and screening programs, however, assisting individuals in selecting the appropriate cancer prevention and detection options can only be done once the nurse understands the principles of each (Mahon, 2000).

Nurses play a crucial role in educating the public about cancer prevention, risk factors, and early detection. By teaching members of our society strategies to prevent cancer, how to reduce the risk of developing a malignancy, and the important tests used for early detection when the disease is easier to treat, nurses may begin to reduce the fear associated with cancer that is often portrayed in the media. It is unknown whether individuals will consider adapting behaviors and practices with ongoing health education. Influencing factors include perceived susceptibility, cost of behavior changes, and the actual health message delivered (Erickson, 2003).

Barriers exist that prevent the success of cancer screening programs. Those that are associated with health care providers

---

NATIONAL GUIDELINES 2015 American Cancer Society (ACS) Goals and Objectives for 2015

Goals

Age-adjusted mortality rates reduced by 50%.

Age-adjusted incidence rates reduced by 25%.

Measurable improvement in the quality of life from the time of diagnosis through the balance of life.

Objectives

Proportion of adults who use tobacco products reduced to 12%.

Proportion of youth who use tobacco products reduced to 10%.

Proportion of persons who follow the ACS guidelines for consumption of fruits and vegetables increased to 75%.

Proportion of adults who follow the ACS guidelines for appropriate level of physical activity increased to 90%.

Proportion of youth who follow the ACS guidelines for appropriate level of physical activity increased to 60%.

Proportion of school districts that provide school health education increased to 50%.

Proportion of all persons who use at least two or more protective measures to reduce the risk of skin cancer increased to 75%.

Proportion of women (ages 40 or older) who have ACS recommended breast screening increased to 90%.

Proportion of persons (ages 50 or older) who have ACS recommended colorectal screening increased to 75%.

Proportion of men (ages 50 or older) who follow ACS recommended guidelines for prostate cancer increased to 90%.

include the lack of time and expertise needed to integrate inclusive cancer screening programs. Those barriers experienced by patients include lack of transportation, poor financial status, or no support to access the screening programs. Our health care system struggles with the lack of resources to support a comprehensive screening program. Diverse populations are experiencing additional barriers to cancer screening programs. Access to screening programs is less common for those who are poor or less educated, those for whom English is a second language, and for certain minority groups. Creating and implementing cancer screening programs mandates the nurse to be open to a variety of issues that may impact the program's success.

The U.S. Department of Health and Human Services' *Healthy People 2010* objectives discuss goals related to increasing the quality of life, increasing the number of healthy years, and to eliminating health inequalities (see the National Guidelines box). Cancer is identified as the third area of focus out of 28. The overall goal for cancer care is to reduce the number of cases along with the disability, illness, and death associated with the disease. Suggestions for reaching these reductions include (1) smoking cessation, (2) diet modification, (3) early detection via screening programs, and (4) current cancer treatment options. To impact the morbidity and mortality associated with cancer, early diagnosis and treatment are pivotal.

Definitions

To develop sound cancer prevention and early detection programs, an understanding of the terminology used is essential. With this knowledge, nurses can assist individuals in making appropriate choices of cancer prevention and early detection strategies.

Cancer Screening

Cancer screening is the use of tests to discover cancer in someone who does not have signs or symptoms of the cancer (Mahon, 2000). An analogy would be the use of cheesecloth when straining a sauce during the preparation of a gourmet meal. The cheesecloth catches solid pieces of ingredients used to flavor the sauce but possibly undesirable to eat. These solid pieces are similar to signs of possible cancer that need to be evaluated carefully before being considered innocent or useful. A positive cancer-screening test does not indicate a definitive diagnosis of cancer; rather, it indicates that more testing needs to be done. The term *early detection* is used interchangeably with *cancer screening*.

Cancer Prevention

Cancer prevention consists of three levels. Fist, primary prevention refers to preventing diseases via immunizations and avoidance of known carcinogens. This form of prevention reduces the risk of developing cancer (e.g., educating youth regarding effects of tobacco use) with the understanding that there is no guarantee an individual will not show signs of malignancy in the future. Secondary prevention involves early detection and treatment of subclinical disease in those individuals without signs or symptoms of a malignancy. Examples include Pap smears and mammograms. Tertiary prevention is the management of a disease with the hopes to prevent progression, recurrence, or complications. Examples include monitoring for recurrence with the use of tumor markers and detecting second primary tumors early in those who are long-term survivors.

Screened Individual

Individuals who are undergoing cancer screening tests are not considered patients. Only when an abnormal screening test is discovered is the individual considered a patient. An easily understood example is that of women who routinely undergo clinical breast exams and mammography. Women with negative results are not labeled as patients. Wellness is the main focus of all cancer prevention levels.

Target Population

The target population identifies those individuals who possess characteristics that make them suitable for screening. Oncology experts believe the following characteristics are typical of a target population: (1) gender, (2) family history, (3) presence of risk factors, (4) ethnicity, and (5) age (Clark & Reintgen, 1996).

Being aware of these characteristics is important so the nurse can accurately educate the patient and family regarding the importance of recommended screening tests. Having an appreciation of the cultural beliefs and practices that influence a person's decision to be screened for cancer will give the nurse insight into how the individual approaches her health and wellness. The Cultural Considerations box (p. 2070) illustrates a few examples of how culture affects health practices.

Risk Factors

Assessing cancer risk is a common and crucial thread in all three levels of cancer prevention. Making appropriate screening

---

NATIONAL GUIDELINES *Healthy People 2010* **Cancer Goals**

GOAL: Reduce the number of new cancer cases as well as the illness, disability, and death caused by cancer.

- Overall cancer deaths
- Lung cancer deaths
- Breast cancer deaths
- Cervical cancer deaths
- Colorectal cancer deaths
- Oropharyngeal cancer deaths
- Prostate cancer deaths

- Melanoma deaths
- Sun exposure and skin cancer
- Provider counseling about cancer prevention
- Pap tests
- Colorectal cancer screening
- Mammograms
- Statewide cancer registries
- Cancer survival

Source: U.S. Department of Health and Human Services. (2000). *Healthy people 2010: Understanding and improving health.* Retrieved February 5, 2008, from http://www.healthypeople.gov.

CULTURAL CONSIDERATIONS Related to Health Practices

Temporal orientation (perceived importance of detecting health problems early) and perceptions of internal control and physical space in both African American and Caucasian women affect incidence of screening for mammograms. African American women have an increased sense of fatalism related to breast cancer. This belief about the inevitability of dying from the disease prevents them from undergoing regular mammogram screening (Russell, Perkins, Zollinger, & Champion, 2006).

The leading cause of death among Korean persons is cancer, with breast cancer being the most common cancer in Korean women (7.1% of all cancer diagnoses). The mortality rate for females has increased by 280% since 1983. Due to these staggering numbers, mammogram screening is recommended beginning at the age of 30 for Korean women, which is a decade earlier than for American women (Ham, 2006).

Greek women experience an increase in fatigue while undergoing adjuvant radiotherapy for breast cancer. Initially, the patient's fatigue is felt to be minimal but gradually increases to the point where the patient has significant changes in their health status. One known intervention to reduce the effect of fatigue is to participate in exercise activities. Because exercise is not a common behavior of many Greek women, nurses are asked to explore culturally appropriate alternatives (Lavdaniti et al., 2006).

Breast and cervical cancer screening is low among Chinese, Japanese, and Vietnamese American women. Given that Asian Americans have a high rate of liver and stomach cancer combined with infrequent screening practices for breast and cervical cancer, nurses have an opportunity to assist with health promotion and education (Lee-Lin & Menon, 2005).

Filipino women typically demonstrate avoidance when dealing with a cancer diagnosis. Several factors improve their willingness to participate in screening activities: supportive family members, suggestions from familiar health care providers, health insurance, and personal attributes (physical symptoms, family history, past diagnosis, and health literacy) (Wu & Bancroft, 2006).

RISK FACTORS for Cancer

Exogenous	Endogenous
Drugs and chemicals: Environmental and occupational factors influence the number of chemicals and drugs proven to be carcinogenic.	*Age:* Incidence increases with age.
Lifestyle behaviors: Tobacco is most deadly carcinogen.	*Genetic predisposition:* Occasional genetic link.
Nutrition: Diets low in fiber and high in fat.	*Hormones:* Influence the process of carcinogenesis.
Sexual activity: Women who engage in sex with multiple partners and begin relations early in life have increased risk of cancer.	*Immune dysfunction:* Immunocompetence is essential for identification of antigens (malignant cells).
Alcohol: Large consumptions of ethyl alcohol are linked to certain cancers of the head and neck.	
Radiation: Ionizing and ultraviolet radiation can cause cancer; the effects of EMFs, if any, are unknown.	
Viruses: Several different cancers have been linked to viruses.	
Psychosocial: Stress and the relationship to neoplasms are still being investigated.	

recommendations is extremely difficult if there has not been an accurate and complete assessment of cancer risk (Mahon, 2000). A screening program should incorporate an education portion that includes a discussion of the seven warning signs of cancer (Chart 64–8).

 **CRITICAL ALERT** *Nurses are responsible for assessing patients for the seven warning signs of cancer and alerting the health care provider or encouraging the patient to seek medical evaluation. Ongoing education about the seven warning signs of cancer is essential in order for patients and their families to understand the importance of recognizing unusual symptoms and seeking early medical attention.*

The presence of interacting cellular, genetic, immunologic, and environmental forces, potentially creating malignancy, is frequently referred to as *risk factors*. Risk factors are categorized according to whether they originate from outside the host (exogenous) or within the host (endogenous) (see the Risk Factors box). Both endogenous and exogenous risk factors cause cancer by damaging the genes that regulate normal cell growth or by perpetuating the growth of existing abnormal cells. Endogenous factors include age, genetic background (see the Genetic Considerations box), and immune competence. Exogenous factors include tobacco, radiation, diet, chemicals, and infections.

Age

As we age, the likelihood of developing a malignancy increases. Up to age 39 the probability is between 1% and 2%, and from ages 40 to 61 the chance increases to 8% to 9%. Men have demonstrated a higher incidence of cancer (33%) between the ages of 60 and 79 as compared to women (22%) (Erickson, 2003). The lifetime incidence of cancer is higher for men (43.39%) than for women (38.25%). Because of breast cancer, a woman's chance of developing cancer by the age of 60 is slightly increased (Jemail, Thomas, Murrey, & Thun, 2002).

The concept of aging as it relates to cancer development can be incorporated into the discussion of other risk factors, but to truly understand the impact of the aging process attention must be given to the theories that attempt to explain the changes. First, over time we are repeatedly exposed to a cumulative increase in the number of carcinogens, which increases the chance of a malignancy emerging. Next, cells that have aged may be less tolerant of the genetic abnormalities that occur with cancer and unable to initiate damage repair. Finally, as we age our immune system does not function as efficiently, thus opening the door for abnormal cellular growth associated with cancer formation.

Hormones

Cancer of the brain, breast, endometrium, and prostate occur in target tissues, or those that are hormone responsive. Hormones have not been proven to have a direct carcinogenic effect.

CHART 64–8	**Seven Warning Signs of Cancer**

C: hange in bowel or bladder habits

A: sore that does not heal

U: nusual bleeding or discharge from any body orifice

T: hickening or a lump in the breast or elsewhere

I: ndigestion or difficulty swallowing

O: bvious change in a wart or mole

N: agging cough or hoarseness

GENETIC CONSIDERATIONS Related to Cancer

The understanding of the link between genetics and the development of cancer is partly due to the worldwide Human Genome Project, which began in 1990. The project sought to locate, map, and sequence more than 100,000 genes that make up the human genome. Little has been linked to genetic factors (10%), but significant incidence is demonstrated among racial groups. The highest prevalence and mortality rates are seen in African Americans. Hispanics and Asian/Pacific Islanders have a 40% lower incidence, and American Indians a 50% lower incidence than African Americans.

There are three main categories of genetic cancer. First, inherited cancer syndromes typically are autosomal dominant and possess many different genes that regulate cell growth and gene repair. Diagnosis is usually done at an early age and the syndromes frequently are associated with multiple primary tumors. An example is the breast/ovarian cancer syndrome in which chromosome 17 houses a mutated tumor suppressor gene (BRCA1). The risk of developing breast and ovarian cancer is significantly increased if a female carries BRCA1. Next, a group of genetic disorders that are typically nonmalignant have been known to predispose a person to developing malignancy. For example, the presence of ataxia-telangiectasia can be correlated to the development of breast cancer and leukemia. Finally, familial "clustering" occurs when there is an increased prevalence of cancer than would be expected statistically; however, the specific genetic factors have yet to be determined. Breast cancer is the most common example of a cancer that appears to cluster in families.

Sources: American Cancer Society. (ND). *Risk factors.* Retrieved on September 22, 2008, from http://www.cancer.org/downloads/AA/CancerAtlas02.pdf; Erickson, J. (2003). Cancer. In W. Phipps, F. Monahan, J. Sands, J. Marek, & M. Neighbors (Eds.), *Medical–surgical nursing health and illness perspectives* (7th ed.). St. Louis: Mosby.

Rather, they support carcinogenesis by preparing target tissues so they are ripe for the carcinogen insult, by permitting the carcinogenesis to continue, or by modifying the growth of an established tumor. The duration in which tissue has been exposed to a hormone may influence carcinogenesis.

Immune Dysfunction

Our immune system is an intricate network of surveillance that controls the proliferation of potential cancer cells. The immune system screens the human body for these cells and activates forces to eliminate them before a tumor can be developed. Humoral factors are those that produce antibodies in the battle against cancer cells, where cellular factors include sensitized lymphocytes and macrophages. Frequently, cancer cells contain antigens that are different from the person's own antigens, which results in destruction by the immune system. The normal immune system is able to detect and destroy approximately 10 million cancer cells at one time. Tumors that replicate faster than the rate at which the normal immune system can work will continue to grow unrestrained. Today's diagnostic capabilities require a mass measuring only 1 cm in diameter for recognition. Regrettably, a tumor that is 1 cm contains at least 1 billion cells.

Most often cancers occur in individuals whose immune system is impaired due to malnutrition, chronic disease, advancing age, and stress. People with immunodeficiency states are more susceptible to developing malignancy than those whose immune system is intact. See Chapter 60 for a discussion of the immune system.

Drugs and Chemicals

Millions of chemicals have been registered with the Chemical Abstracts Service and more than 50,000 are predicted to be used regularly in business and industry. Despite acknowledging the importance of monitoring and regulating these substances, less than 1,000 chemicals or exposures have been examined to determine their role in the development of cancer (Stellman & Stellman, 1996). Great effort has been given to publishing and organizing data on cancer risk attributed to chemical carcinogens.

Chemical carcinogens are those that contain compounds or elements that alter DNA. An awareness of the relationship between chemical exposures and disease began as early as the 1700s (Pfeifer, 2001). Men employed as chimney sweeps developed an increased incidence of scrotal cancer, likely due to the continued exposure to coal burned as fuel. Although it is easy to attribute chemical carcinogens to occupational exposure, the vastness of

environmental exposures must be understood. The Occupational Safety and Health Act of 1970 authorized the Occupational Safety and Health Administration (OSHA) to impose restrictions on the amount of exposure to known carcinogens. Threshold limit values (TLVs), or the maximum allowable exposure, are difficult to determine because identification of carcinogens in the environment and workplace is very time consuming (Erickson, 2003). The U.S. Department of Health and Human Services publishes a list of known human carcinogens biannually. The *Tenth Report*, published in 2002, identifies new or changed carcinogens from previous reports. The *Tenth Report* list of carcinogens known to affect humans is shown in Chart 64–9 (p. 2072).

Drugs used for therapeutic purposes also have been known to be carcinogenic. In the 1970s the agent diethylstilbestrol (DES) was administered to prevent spontaneous abortion, but a link was discovered between its use and vaginal cancer. The relationship between cancer and drug therapy is dynamic, as can be seen in the carcinogenic history of oral contraceptives. Initially, birth control pills were identified to have a carcinogenic potential for breast cancer. Recently, it has been determined they have a protective effect against ovarian and endometrial malignancies (Erickson, 2003).

Agents used to combat cancer have also been known to increase the risk of causing secondary malignancies. Years after receiving agents such as chlorambucil and cyclophosphamide, people have experienced a notable increased likelihood of developing leukemia. Individuals who require immunosuppressive

CHART 64–9 **Known Human Carcinogens**

Aflatoxins	Estrogens
Alcohol	Ethylene oxide
4-Aminobiphenyl	Lead chromate
Analgesic mixtures with phenacetin	Melphalan
Arsenic compounds	Methoxsalen with ultraviolet A therapy
Asbestos	Mineral oils
Azathioprine	Mustard gas
Benzene	2-Naphthylamine
Benzidine	Nickel compounds
Beryllium and its compounds	Radon
1,3-Butadiene	Silica
1,4-Butanediol dimenthylsulfonate (Myleran)	Smokeless tobacco
Cadmium and its compounds	Solar radiation, exposure to sunlamps and sun beds
CCNU, methyl	Soots
Chlorambucil	Strong inorganic acid mists with sulfuric acid
Chloromethyl methyl ether	Tamoxifen
Chromium hexavalent compounds	2,3,7,8-Tetrachlorodibenzo-p-dioxin (dioxin)
Coal tar	Thiotepa
Coke over emissions	Thorium dioxide
Cyclophosphamide	Tobacco smoking
Cyclosporin A	Vinyl chloride
Diethylstilbestrol	Ultraviolet radiation, broad-spectrum UV radiation
Dyes metabolized to benzidine	Wood dust
Environmental tobacco smoke	
Erionite	

Source: Adapted from U.S. Department of Health and Human Services, Public Health Service, National Toxicology Program. (2002, December). *Report on carcinogens* (10th ed.). Washington, DC: Author.

agents to prevent transplant rejection are known to demonstrate higher incidence of the development of secondary malignancies (Antin, 2002).

Tobacco

Cigarettes are responsible for killing more Americans (440,000 predicted in 2006) than alcohol, vehicle crashes, suicide, AIDS, homicide, and illegal drugs combined (ACS, 2006a). Tobacco from pipes, cigars, cigarettes, and second-hand smoke has been reported to cause 87% of all lung cancers. Current reports indicate lung cancer as the leading cause of cancer-related deaths in both males and females and accounts for 13% of new cancer diagnoses (ACS, 2006a). Exposure to tobacco through passive means (exhaled smoke) appears to increase the risk of lung cancer in nonsmokers who live with smokers (Gullatte & Otto, 2001).

The carcinogenic effect of tobacco is demonstrated in several different agents that promote the growth of malignant cells over time. There appears to be a direct relationship between the numbers of years smoking, number of cigarettes smoked per day, and the age when smoking began. Choosing to indulge in

smokeless tobacco is not without risk. The use of chewing tobacco places a person at higher risk for developing head and neck cancer. By eliminating smoking as a lifestyle choice, a person can live longer and reduce the risk of lung cancer by approximately 50% (Erickson, 2003). Other health-related issues are positively affected by smoking cessation, such as a reduction in the risk of cardiac disease and complications from pregnancy.

Approximately one in every five Americans is addicted to tobacco products (ACS, 2006a). According to the ACS, there has been a dramatic increase in successful quit attempts in those who seek assistance with cessation. However, with inadequate health insurance coverage and the cost of treatment programs, many individuals remain addicted to tobacco products. In 2007, the Centers for Disease Control and Prevention's (CDC's) *Morbidity and Mortality Weekly Report* concluded that there continues to be a need for states to assist with funding of smoking cessation and counseling programs (CDC, 2007). Thirty-four states provide some type of coverage to assist those who wish to quit using tobacco products, including over-the-counter (OTC) products, prescription drugs, or counseling services. Seventeen states offer no tobacco treatment coverage services.

The past several years have seen a unique twist on the effect of publicity associated with tobacco use. Smoking cessation campaigns across the country have been more common in the last few years. *Healthy People 2010* objectives for tobacco use are listed in the National Guidelines box. The ACS has identified school health education as critical to the effort to assist young people in developing and maintaining health practices that reduce cancer risk. Litigation by lung cancer victims or families against tobacco companies has increased the attention paid to a behavior our society appears to be identifying as dangerous and life threatening.

Nutrition and Physical Activity

Approximately 20% of all cancer deaths are attributed to nutrition and physical activity factors (ACS, 2007). The association between food and the incidence of cancer is becoming more known and publicized. The link between high-fat foods and an increase in the development of colon, breast, and prostate cancers has been known for almost a decade (Holmes et al., 1999). The most current relationship between body weight and the development of cancer identifies an alarming rate of obesity and overweight among adolescents 12 to 19 years of age (ACS, 2007). In the past 20 years, the prevalence of obesity in African American girls has tripled. Overall, two-thirds of U.S. adults (20 years and older) are overweight or obese.

Diets high in fiber content appear to provide a protection against colon cancer. The exact mechanism of protection remains unknown, but fiber is known to reduce the concentration of fecal bile acids, dilute colon contents, and decrease colon transit time, which is helpful in decreasing the time colonic contents are exposed to carcinogens (Ziegler, Devesa, & Fravmeni, 1991). Rich sources of dietary fiber include fruits, vegetables, legumes, and whole-grain breads and cereals. Foods with vitamins C and D, beta-carotene, and selenium seem to repair cellular damage due to free radicals, which are known to destroy the genetic makeup of cells, thus creating a cellular environment that resists malignancy development.

Maintaining regular physical activity reduces the risk of deaths due to coronary heart disease and also reduces the risk of

NATIONAL GUIDELINES *Healthy People 2010* Tobacco Use Goals

Reduce coronary heart disease deaths.

Reduce lung cancer deaths.

Reduce chronic obstructive pulmonary disease (COPD) deaths.

Reduce cigarette smoking in those 18 years of age and older.

Reduce cigarette smoking in males.

Reduce cigarette smoking in females.

Reduce smoking initiation.

Increase smoking cessation attempts.

Increase smoking cessation during pregnancy.

Reduce children's exposure to smoke at home.

Reduce smokeless tobacco use in males 12 to 17 years of age.

Reduce smokeless tobacco use in males 18 to 24 years of age.

Increase number of school districts providing tobacco-free environments.

Increase number of school districts providing antismoking education in middle school.

Increase number of school districts providing antismoking education in high school.

Increase number of worksite policies banning smoking.

Increase number of states with clean indoor air laws for private workplaces, public workplaces, restaurants, public transportation, hospitals, day care centers, and grocery stores.

Increase number of states with youth tobacco laws.

Increase number of states with plans to reduce tobacco use.

Reduce oral cancer deaths in males 45 to 74 years of age.

Reduce oral cancer deaths in females 45 to 74 years of age.

Reduce stroke deaths.

Change the average age at first use of cigarettes, alcohol, and marijuana at 12 to 17 years of age.

Reduce the use of alcohol in the past month in those 12 to 20 years of age.

Reduce the use of marijuana in the past month in those 12 to 25 years of age.

Reduce the use of cocaine in the past month in those 12 to 25 years of age.

Increase high school seniors' perception of disapproval of heavy alcohol use, occasional marijuana use, cocaine use once or twice, and smoking one or more packs of cigarettes a day.

Increase high school seniors' perception of harm due to heavy alcohol use, regular marijuana use, cocaine use once or twice, smoking one or more packs of cigarettes a day, and use of smokeless tobacco regularly.

Increase tobacco excise tax for cigarettes and smokeless tobacco.

Increase number of states with preemptive clean indoor air laws.

Increase number of states with cigarette vending machine laws.

Source: Adapted from U.S. Department of Health and Human Services. (2000). *Healthy people 2010: Understanding and improving health.* Retrieved February 5, 2008, from http://www.healthypeople.gov.

---

stroke, colon cancer, breast cancer, diabetes, and hypertension (Erye et al., 2004). By keeping physically fit, people tend to control their weight better, which reduces the risk of developing cancer related to excess weight. The ACS publishes guidelines for nutrition and physical activity for cancer prevention that aims at assisting in identifying important healthy behaviors (ACS, 2004).

Sexual Activity

Never before has the correlation between sexual practices and cancer risk been more obvious and concerning. The development of genital cancer is strongly related to sexual practices. In fact, studies have identified an association between sexual activities and AIDS and cancers of the cervix, vagina, and vulva (Gullatte & Otto, 2001). Sexually transmitted infections (STIs), beginning sexual activity at a young age, multiple sexual partners, and high-risk sexual partners all have been implicated in the development of cervical cancer. Viruses, such as herpes simplex virus (HSV) and human papillomavirus (HPV), have also been known to increase the incidence of cervical cancer.

Penile cancer, although rare (1 in 100,000 men), is more common in men who are uncircumcised, infected with HPV, and use tobacco. It is speculated that males who are uncircumcised may be prone to more incidence of smegma, which leads to irritation and inflammation of the penis (ACS, 2006b). Exposure to HPV from multiple sexual partners, sexual intercourse at a young age, and unprotected sex will make a person more likely to develop malignancy. Smoking creates harmful chemicals that are absorbed into the bloodstream and disseminated throughout the body, resulting in damage to the DNA of cells. Cells of

penile tissue are not immune to this destructive process. Chapter 50 👁 presents a more detailed discussion of this rare but devastating cancer.

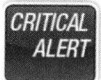 *It is important to assess patients for risky lifestyle practices that increase their chances of developing cancer. Educating patients and their families about smoking cessation, limiting the use of alcohol, and safe sexual practices as they relate to the incidence of developing cancer (and other diseases) may contribute to changing or preventing undesirable lifestyle practices.*

Alcohol

Ethyl alcohol consumption is known to cause cancers of the oral cavity, pharynx, larynx, esophagus, liver, and breast (ACS, 2008a). Men should refrain from consuming more than 2 drinks per day and women 1 drink per day. When combined with tobacco use, alcohol is the leading etiologic factor in developing squamous cell carcinoma of the oral cavity, larynx, and esophagus. It is quite possible alcohol may behave like a co-carcinogen or have a synergistic effect with tobacco (Sigler & Schuring, 1993).

Radiation

Waves and particles of energy, or **radiation**, are known to cause cancer. Radiation has the potential to be a complete carcinogen, thus possessing both initiating and promoting properties. Ionizing radiation has electromagnetic waves that are powerful enough to remove electrons from molecules, thereby weakening the cell by altering its biochemical behavior. Radiation causes mutation of the cell's DNA, which can weaken the cells' defense against a carcinogen or cause cell death. These changes take only seconds, whereas the development of a malignancy may take years. The degree of damage to the cells is related to the dose of radiation received.

Historically, radiation exposure was first recognized after the invention of the x-ray in 1895. People working with x-ray generators were noted to have skin reactions resulting in a skin sore, which led to the first radiation-caused cancer diagnosed in 1902 (ACS, 2003). In 1911, leukemia was first reported among radiation workers.

Ionizing radiation includes x-rays, gamma rays, cosmic rays, and radioactive materials such as alpha particles, beta rays, and protons. Even though each form of radiation has different energy levels, all are capable of causing cellular destruction. The three types of ionizing radiation are natural background radiation, nonmedical synthetic radiation, and medical radiation. Natural background radiation is present in cosmic rays from the solar system and radioactive elements found in the soil. This form of radiation is the major contributor to worldwide radiation exposure. Nonmedical synthetic radiation was created by aboveground nuclear weapons testing usually done prior to 1962 and some commercial and occupational sources. Medical radiation is found in diagnostic x-rays and radiation therapy. Radiation therapy is used to treat certain forms of cancer and involves the use of doses that are thousand of times higher than those of x-rays (ACS, 2003). The amount of exposure during radiographic examinations depends on the machine used and the capability of the technician. Although the amount of exposure to the average hospital nurse who may assist a patient during an x-ray is slight, nurses need to step away from the area close to the x-ray machine (Erickson, 2003).

Exposure to high-dose ionizing radiation can cause a variety of problems including leukemia, bone cancer, leukopenia, and damage to the reproductive cells. The thyroid gland and the bone marrow are most sensitive to radiation, whereas the kidney, ovaries, and bladder are least sensitive. Health care employees whose job involves exposure to radiation must wear film badges. These badges absorb radiation on a photographic film and are developed each month to determine the amount of cumulative radiation exposure. Individuals who are pregnant are usually not assigned to departments that require exposure to radiation due to the susceptibility of the fetus to the negative effects of radiation. Ultraviolet radiation is comprised of electromagnetic waves that are less powerful, but still able to produce carcinogenic effects (Erickson, 2003).

Ultraviolet radiation is present in the form of sunlight and industrial sources such as welding arcs and germicidal lights (Pfeifer, 2001). Despite the vast amount of documentation linking sunlight to the development of skin cancer, many still place the importance of tanned skin above the consequence of having cancer. Ultraviolet light is able to penetrate tissues, which results in the skin being potentially defenseless. Those at greatest risk for acquiring either basal or squamous cell cancer of the skin and melanoma are fair-skinned Caucasian individuals and outdoor workers.

Detecting skin cancers early is pivotal to decreasing mortality rates and the extent of surgical interventions. Areas such as the nose, cheek, and ears are common sites for basal and squamous cell cancers to appear. These tumors appear as waxlike, pale nodules or scaly, reddened patches. Melanomas have the appearance

of moles and erupt anywhere throughout the body. The uniqueness of melanomas is that they have the tendency to change color, shape, and size while forming localized ulcerations that may bleed. Pictures that assist the reader in better understanding how these tumors appear are found in Chapter 66 🔗. Chart 64–10 lists the warning signs of melanoma.

Radon, a colorless and odorless radioactive gas, is released when uranium decays. It is contained in soil and rocks and is located in underground mines and basements. The carcinogenic risk of radon is approximately the same as that associated with breathing second-hand smoke. According to the ACS, most radon-induced cancers are lung cancers and occur more commonly in those who smoke.

Electromagnetic fields (EMFs) are low-frequency energy fields associated with electrical power lines, household appliances, and facilities that produce electricity. Society continues to focus on the cancer risk associated with EMFs despite no scientific evidence to support the concern. Literature has identified no form of electromagnetic energy at frequency levels below that of ionizing radiation and ultraviolet radiation as a cause of cancer (Heath, 1996).

Viruses

Only recently has the relationship between viruses and cancer development in humans been established. Viruses are believed to infect the host DNA, which changes the portion that regulates normal cell proliferation and repair (proto-oncogene). In addition, cell mutation is initiated (Groenwald et al., 1997). Cancer is produced only after a prolonged incubation or latency period (usually years), which makes it very difficult for researchers to connect a viral exposure with a specific cancer (Malin, 2005). Viral carcinogens can be either slow acting or fast acting, but all are tissue specific. Slow-acting viral carcinogens include adenoviruses and herpes viruses. Human T-cell leukemia/lymphoma virus (HTLV) is an example of a fast-acting carcinogen. People are particularly vulnerable to viral carcinogens as they advance in age or their immune system begins to function inadequately.

The relationship between certain viruses and the incidence of cancer has been demonstrated in the literature. The hepatitis B virus has been linked to malignancy of the liver, and the Epstein–Barr virus (EBV) has been known to increase the incidence of developing nasopharyngeal cancer. The human papillomavirus is associated with cancer of the genitalia, especially in women. It is strongly suspected that HPV is also linked to cervical cancer. Kaposi's sarcoma is known to be caused by the presence of the cytomegaloviruses (CMVs), which are frequently seen in patients with the HIV virus.

Psychosocial

How a person's state of mind affects his immune and hormonal systems has not yet been determined, nor is it easily explained.

CHART 64–10	**Warning Signs of Melanoma: The "ABCD Rule"**	
A	is for	asymmetry
B	is for	border irregularity
C	is for	change in color or pigmentation
D	is for	diameter greater than 6 mm

It has been suggested that stressors such as death of a loved one, life changes, and personality variables may have a relationship in the development of cancer. Most reports of the link between the mind and cancer are subjective and more research needs to be done to explain how the relationship works (Erickson, 2003).

Diagnosing Cancer

Cancer treatment decisions are based on the results of accurate diagnostic findings performed by a multidisciplinary team. A person with cancer typically undergoes a battery of tests to determine the location, extent, and tumor type of the malignancy. Diagnostic modalities need to be individualized to the patient and may include a thorough history and physical, appropriate imaging tests, invasive procedures, laboratory studies, and pathology examination of tissue or blood. New diagnostic techniques have provided the opportunity for the development of sophisticated plans of treatment that positively affect patient survival. Once diagnosis is confirmed, further diagnostic studies may be necessary to stage the cancer, which will define an appropriate treatment plan.

The nurse needs to prepare the patient and family for each test and procedure. This includes explaining the rationale for the test and any preparation the patient needs to complete prior to the diagnostic procedure. Preparation examples include eliminating food and drink for a certain number of hours prior to testing (NPO) and administering bowel-cleansing agents such as enemas or oral preparations. Providing emotional support during a time when patients and families experience a tremendous amount of anxiety is crucial. Even though the term *cancer* may not have been discussed with the patient, he and family members may be experiencing an overriding fear about what the possibilities may be. During the diagnostic phase, it is critical for the nurse to offer ongoing support to patients and their families.

History and Physical

Early detection of cancer can be done through screening and is how some patients discover their diagnosis. In contrast, other patients end up in the health care provider's office after noticing unusual symptoms or after a wellness examination during which suspicious symptoms were detected (Alexander, 2001). Nurses perform a comprehensive health history and systems assessment that can be combined with the history and physical done by the health care provider. The information obtained by both disciplines provides a holistic view of the patient's health condition and needs. Listening to patients report their health history provides a perfect opportunity to identify risk factors pertinent to the individual and may elevate the suspicion of malignancy. Further diagnostic evaluation will be determined based on the assessment findings that identify potential diagnoses. The Diagnostic Tests box illustrates the tests done to evaluate for cancer, monitor treatment success and effects, and determine recurrence of disease.

DIAGNOSTIC TESTS for Cancer

Test	Expected Abnormality	Rationale for Abnormality
Serum chemistries and liver function tests	Elevated/lowered sodium, elevated potassium, elevated creatinine and BUN, elevated liver function tests.	Assess for abnormality of liver, kidney, or bone related to malignancy or treatment.
Complete blood count (CBC)	Lowered WBC, platelets, RBC, Hgb, and Hct. May have elevated WBC with leukemia.	Assess for treatment toxicity or bone marrow function.
Hemocult test	Positive (blue color) result indicates need for further diagnostic studies.	Assess for presence of blood in stool for screening purposes.
Bone marrow biopsy (aspiration)	Abnormal numbers, size, and shape of WBC, RBC, and megakaryocytes.	Assess for hematologic abnormalities.
Pap smear	Abnormal-appearing cervical cells, precancerous or malignant.	Assess for premalignant changes and cervical cancer.
Urine protein immunoelectrophoresis	Increased levels of heavy-chain M proteins (Bence-Jones proteins).	Assess urine protein and immunoglobulin levels seen in multiple myeloma.
Serum protein immunoelectrophoresis	Increased levels of heavy-chain M proteins.	Assess serum protein and immunoglobulin levels seen in multiple myeloma.
Urine catecholamines	Increased levels of epinephrine, norepinephrine, metanephrine, and vanillylmandelic.	Assess for neuroblastoma and pheochromocytoma.
CA125 (antigen, tumor marker)	Elevated in ovarian cancer and nonmalignant conditions that cause inflammation of the pleura (e.g., endometriosis, PID, pancreatitis).	Assess response to treatment in ovarian, pancreatic, breast, colon, lung, and liver cancer.
CA19-9 (tumor marker)	Elevated in colorectal, pancreatic, stomach, and bile duct cancer.	Assess response to treatment in pancreatic, colorectal, and gastric cancer.
CA27-29 (tumor marker)	Elevated in breast cancer. Occasionally elevated in cancer of the colon, stomach, kidney, lung, pancreas, ovary, uterus, and liver.	Assess response to treatment of breast cancer.

(continued)

DIAGNOSTIC TESTS for Cancer—*Continued*

Test	Expected Abnormality	Rationale for Abnormality
CA72-4 (tumor marker)	Elevated in ovarian, colorectal, and gastric cancer.	Assess response to treatment of ovarian, colorectal, and gastric cancer.
PSA (prostate-specific antigen, tumor marker)	Elevated in prostate cancer and benign prostate enlargement.	Assess response to treatment of prostate cancer. Also used for screening at-risk persons.
CEA (carcinoembryonic antigen, tumor marker)	Elevated in breast, colorectal, and lung cancer.	Assess response to treatment of breast, colorectal, and lung cancer.
HCG (human chorionic gonadotropin, tumor marker)	Elevated in germ cell cancers (ovarian and testicular) and pregnancy.	Assess response to treatment of testicular and certain ovarian cancer.
AFP (α-fetoprotein)	Elevated in liver and germ cell cancer, benign liver disease, and pregnancy.	Assess response to treatment of testicular, liver, and certain ovarian cancers.
Lactate dehydrogenase (LDH)	Elevated in most cancers.	Most helpful in monitoring treatment effect.
Neuron-specific enolase (NSE)	Elevated in lung, thyroid, kidney, testicle, and pancreatic cancer, neuroblastoma, Wilms' tumor, and melanoma.	Most helpful in small cell lung cancer (SCLC) and neuroblastoma to assess response to treatment.
IMAGING STUDIES		Least invasive diagnostic studies performed first.
Radiographic: x-ray, CT scan, mammogram, barium swallow/enema, IVP	Detects abnormal masses in abdomen, chest, pelvis, and breast.	Performed during initial diagnostic work-up and to monitor effectiveness of treatment.
Ultrasonic studies	Used to detect tumors in peritoneal space, pelvis, abdomen, prostate, and breast.	Echoes of high-frequency sound waves to visualize internal structures are helpful in distinguishing between benign cysts and malignancies. Some techniques involve inserting an ultrasound wand into a body cavity (e.g., rectum) to visualize surrounding organs (e.g., prostate).
Magnetic resonance imaging (MRI)	Detects tumors in the brain, chest, and abdomen.	Use of a magnetic field and radio-frequency waves to align hydrogen nuclei in tissues.
Nuclear medicine scans	Common organs evaluated include the brain, thyroid, and liver.	Radioactive isotopes are injected or ingested and then traced to the tissues where the isotope is attracted. Monoclonal antibodies are occasionally used to tag antigens known to be associated with malignancies. Organs with disease frequently show signs of increased or abnormal uptake of the material.
Positron emission tomography (PET)		Study glucose metabolism in body tissues and differentiate the rates of tissue metabolism. Images are obtained by detection of positron emissions from radionuclides. Tumors have more rapid rates of glycolysis compared to the tissue of origin. Gamma camera tomography maps structures and identifies malignancies.
INVASIVE DIAGNOSTIC STUDIES		
Pathology		Cells are obtained via surgical incision, biopsy, or cytologic examination techniques. These cells are examined for malignancy and, if positive, graded, which assists the health care provider in prescribing an appropriate plan of care.
Biopsy	Detects presence of abnormal tissue cells obtained from site of suspicious growth.	See above.
Endoscopy		Hollow metal tubes equipped with a light are used to visualize body cavities for diagnostic and therapeutic purposes. These tubes, known as scopes, are instruments named for the body area they visualize. Direct visualization provides the health care provider the opportunity to examine the anatomic location and obtain samples of tissue or secretions that can be used to diagnose malignancy.

Sources: Akhurst, T., & Larson, S. (1999). Position emission tomography imaging of colorectal cancer. *Seminar in Oncology, 577*(26); Alexander, J. (2001). Diagnosis and staging. In S. Otto (Ed.), *Oncology nursing* (4th ed.). St. Louis: Mosby; Erickson, J. (2003). Cancer. In W. Phipps, F. Monahan, J. Sands, J. Marek, & M. Neighbors (Eds.), *Medical–surgical nursing health and illness perspectives* (7th ed.). St. Louis: Mosby; Fischbach, F., & Dunning, M. (Eds.). (2006). *Nurses' quick reference to common laboratory and diagnostic tests.* Philadelphia: Lippincott Williams & Wilkins; Omerod, K. (2005). Diagnostic evaluation, classification, and staging. In C. H. Yarbro, M. H. Frogge, & M. Goodman (Eds.), *Cancer nursing: Principles and practice* (6th ed.). Sudbury, MA: Jones and Bartlett.

CHART 64–11	Endoscopic Instruments and Their Anatomic Use
Instrument	**Anatomic Location**
Bronchoscope	Bronchus
Gastroscope	Stomach
Colonoscope	Colon
Proctoscope	Anus and sigmoid colon
Laparoscope	Abdominal structures: • Liver • Diaphragm • Peritoneum • Gastrointestinal structures • Genitourinary structures • Gynecologic structures

Chart 64–11 explains the names of instruments and associated anatomic locations used during endoscopic procedures. In addition, the reader should review Chapter 59 ⊙, which discusses the use of monoclonal antibodies in the patient with an altered immune system, and Chapter 49 ⊙, which explains the Pap smear in more detail.

■ Commonly Occurring Cancers

Nurses who care for patients with cancer are asked to develop a knowledge base that is extensive and ever changing. Discoveries that change the diagnosis, treatment, and prognosis of this devastating disease are continuous. This fluidity demands that nurses continue to quest for more information to assist them in developing their nursing practice. Chart 64–12 (p. 2078) presents general information, clinical findings, diagnostic techniques, prognosis, and treatment modalities to assist the nurse in gaining a better understanding of the commonly occurring cancers. A more in-depth discussion of the current diagnostic studies and treatment modalities is presented later in this chapter.

Cancers of the Hematopoietic and Lymphatic Systems

Cancers of the hematopoietic and lymphatic systems are very complex and challenging disorders that are full of potentially life-threatening complications. Developing an understanding of the immune and hematologic system will assist the nurse in becoming confident when caring for patients with these disorders. Cancers occurring in the hematopoietic and lymphatic system include leukemia, lymphoma, and multiple myeloma. Due to the rare incidence of multiple myeloma, this discussion will concentrate on leukemia and lymphoma. Leukemias are classified as either acute (aggressive with severe symptoms) or chronic (slowly progressing with fewer symptoms).

The type of leukemia depends on the stem cell line affected: lymphoid or myeloid. The factors that control the organized differentiation and maturation of blood cells are absent. This disorganization results in the halting of maturation of specific cell lines, allowing for immature cells to replicate and accumulate in the bone marrow. When too many immature cells accumulate in the bone marrow, other normal cell lines are prevented from maturing and developing. Patients with leukemia will experience symptoms associated with "crowding out" of the bone marrow cells, such as platelets, red blood cells (RBCs), and white blood cells (WBCs). This will be recognized when the nurse assesses the laboratory data for a reduction in platelets, RBCs (including hemoglobin and hematocrit), and WBCs. It is important to remember that a patient with leukemia may have an abnormally high WBC count, however, the effectiveness of these cells is compromised. Nurses must be aware that patients with leukemia will have multiple laboratory abnormalities and their assessment should evaluate for signs of infection, bleeding, and anemia.

Cancers of the lymphatic system (**lymphomas**) involve organs and tissues such as the lymph nodes, spleen, thymus, bone marrow, blood, and lymph. From interstitial fluid comes lymph, which flows through lymphatic vessels and eventually into the circulatory system via the thoracic duct. Particulate is filtered through lymph nodes located in a variety of places throughout the human body. Lymphocytes originate in the bone marrow and develop into several different types of mature lymphocytes. The cells are susceptible to malignant transformation at any point during maturation and differentiation. Malignant lymphomas are grouped according to the characteristics of the lymphocyte, such as Hodgkin's disease and non-Hodgkin's disease (see Chart 64–12, p. 2078).

■ Cancer Treatment Modalities

Multiple treatment modalities are available to patients diagnosed with cancer. Each modality has certain risks, side effects, and chances for success. The nurse can assist the patient and family in obtaining information regarding treatment options so they are able to make an informed decision about their plan of care.

Surgery

Surgical approaches to cancer have existed for centuries. In 1809 Ephraim MacDowell demonstrated modern surgical approaches when he excised a 22-pound ovarian tumor from a woman who lived an additional 30 years. He performed 12 more ovarian resections which became a hallmark in the advancement of elective surgery for cancer (Hill, 1979). Surgical efforts built on the work of surgeons like MacDowell, but in the 1950s it was noted the mortality rates associated with radical procedures were not improving. The evidence was mounting to evaluate the benefit of surgery alone as treatment for all tumors.

Surgeries in patients with cancer are performed to establish a diagnosis and treat the disease. A histologic diagnosis is pivotal in establishing a definitive diagnosis of cancer along with a staging of the tumor, which determines the extent and type of the cancer. Understanding the diagnosis will allow the health care team to design a plan of care unique to each individual and his or her disease. Diagnosis is accomplished by obtaining tissue samples from an incisional biopsy, excisional biopsy, needle biopsy, or endoscopy. A **biopsy** is a procedure in which a portion of tissue is examined for the presence of abnormal cells. The technique used depends on the tumor's location, size, and growth characteristics.

| CHART 64–12 | **Commonly Occurring Cancers** | | | |

Cancer	Clinical Findings	Diagnostic Technique	Prognosis	Treatment
Breast	Noninvasive (carcinoma *in situ*): confined to the ducts and or lobules. Invasive (infiltrating): cancerous cells penetrate tissue outside of ducts (80%) or lobules (10%). Inflammatory: swelling, erythema, and invasion of dermal lymphatics.	Mass: hard, irregular, nontender. Thick breast or axilla. Nipple discharge. Nipple retraction or inversion. Dimpling or puckering of skin. Changes in size, shape, and texture of breast.	Mammogram. Self-breast exam. Biopsy, fine-needle or core needle. Pathology testing: cytologic or histologic.	Tumor size and presence of lymph node(s) have important role in predicting survival. Presence of hormone receptors has negative impact on survival. There remain percentages (20%) of those who develop recurrence.	Surgery: • Lumpectomy • Mastectomy • Breast reconstruction Radiotherapy: external beam. Chemotherapy: • Adjuvant • Hormonal High-dose chemotherapy with transplantation (for advanced cancer)
Colon and rectum	Majority are adenocarcinomas. Rectum: 40–50%. Descending sigmoid colon: 20–35%. Cecum and ascending colon: 16%. Transverse colon: 8%	Changes in bowel habits. Blood in stool. Flatulence. Indigestion. Weight loss. Fatigue	Barium enema. Colonoscopy	Distant metastases negatively impact survival. Once treatment is completed, follow-up treatment is advised (physical examination, colonoscopy, CEA levels).	Surgery: colon resection with temporary or permanent colostomy. Chemotherapy. Radiotherapy for involvement in the perineum or viscera
Prostate	Adenocarcinomas (95%). Endogenous hormones and environmental factors may be causative factors	*Early:* Painful urination. Frequency. Hematuria. *Late:* Pain (bone, joint, back). Fatigue. Weight loss	Prostate-specific antigen (PSA). Direct rectal examination (DRE). Transrectal ultrasound (TRUS). Biopsy	Transitional zone involvement is less aggressive. Metastatic disease negatively impacts survival.	Surgery: radical prostatectomy. Radiotherapy: external beam or brachytherapy. Cryotherapy. Chemotherapy. Expectant management ("watchful waiting")
Brain and CNS • Brain • Spinal cord	Intracerebral: brain, neuroglia, neurons, cells of blood vessels of connective tissue. Extracerebral: meningiomas, acoustic nerve, pituitary, and pineal gland. Classification between benign and malignant is not differentiated because surgical accessibility dictates prognosis. Astrocytoma (>50%). Glioblastoma multiforme (20%)	*Early:* Headache. Seizures. Nausea. Vomiting. *Late:* Impaired cognitive skills. Short-term memory loss. Difficulty with speech. Sensory and motor defects. Visual changes. Personality changes. Loss of sphincter control	Complete physical and neurologic examination. MRI. PET. Single-photon emission computed tomography (SPECT). Magnetic resonance spectroscopy (MRS). Biopsy	Prognosis is poor related to accessibility difficulties. Glioblastomas have poorest prognosis.	Surgery with or without placement of wafers impregnated with chemotherapy. Radiotherapy: intraoperative with radioactive seeds. Intraoperative Hyperthermia Radiosurgery. Stereotactic therapy: gamma knife, linear accelerator, and heavy beam particles. Photodynamic therapy. Chemotherapy

CHART 64–12	**Commonly Occurring Cancers—*Continued***				
Cancer	**Clinical Findings**	**Diagnostic Technique**	**Prognosis**	**Treatment**
Lung	Small cell anaplastic carcinoma Non–small cell: squamous cell carcinoma Adenocarcinomas Large cell anaplastic carcinoma Mixed cell types	Change in cough Chest pain Respiratory ailments not treated with antibiotics Dyspnea Wheezing Hemoptysis Weight loss Fatigue Dysphagia	History and physical examination Chest x-ray (anterior, posterior, lateral) CAT scan MRI CBC with differential Platelet count Chemistry panel Bronchoscopy	Prognosis for 5-year survival after surgical resection is best in patients who have carcinoma *in situ.* Prognosis for 5-year survival after surgical resection is worst for those patients who have cancer that has invaded the lymph nodes or other distant organs or structures.	Surgery Laser therapy (used for relief of complications associated with endobronchial lesions) Radiotherapy: external beam Brachytherapy Chemotherapy
Multiple myeloma	Most common in African Americans, males, age 70 Malignancy of B cell Immunodeficiency due to depressed antibody-mediated immunity	Findings are related to excess of Bence-Jones proteins. Infections: • Pneumonia • Urinary Tract Infection (UTI) • Systemic Skeletal: • Pain worse with movement • Hypercalcemia • Pathologic fractures • Vertebral collapse Renal failure: • Proteinuria • Obstructed distal and proximal tubules • Hyperuricemia Blood/bone marrow dysfunction: • Anemia • Hyperviscosity • Coagulation disorders Neurologic: • Spinal cord compression • Peripheral neuropathy	1. Serum electrophoresis to determine Bence-Jones proteins. 2. Serum immunoglobulin electrophoresis 3. Bone marrow biopsy: increase in abnormal, atypical, immature B cells. 4. Radiographic: osteolytic lesions in bones	1. Incurable, sometimes treatable 2. 1/3 patients do not respond to therapy and die within weeks of diagnosis.	Chemotherapy Corticosteroids Immunotherapy Bone marrow transplant (autologous) Radiation therapy

(continued)

| CHART 64–12 | **Commonly Occurring Cancers—*Continued*** | | | |

Cancer	Clinical Findings	Diagnostic Technique	Prognosis	Treatment
Leukemias				
Acute lymphocytic leukemia (ALL)	Most common in children *Etiology:* Radiation Chemicals Drugs Viruses	*Anemia:* Malaise Fatigue *Neutropenia:* Fever Bone pain Thrombocytopenia: Bleeding Bruising CNS involvement (10%) due to meningeal infiltrates	Peripheral blood smear: • CBC with differential • Bone marrow biopsy	Complete remission: 80–90% Cure: 30–40% Children achieve cure at rate of 60–85%	Chemotherapy: • Induction therapy to achieve remission • CNS treatment if needed • Postremission therapy Bone marrow or stem cell transplantation
Acute myeloid leukemia (AML)	*Etiology:* Radiation Chemicals Drugs Viruses Certain genetic disorders increase incidence of acquiring AML	*Anemia:* Malaise Fatigue *Neutropenia:* Fever Bone pain *Thrombocytopenia:* Bleeding Bruising Anemia is usually present when health care provider sees patient for the first time. Recurrent infections not resolved with antibiotics.	Peripheral blood smear: • CBC with differential • Bone marrow biopsy	Patients over 70 years of age are intolerant of induction therapy. WBCs > 100,000/mm^3 related to increased mortality during first week of therapy.	Chemotherapy: • Induction therapy to achieve remission • Postremission therapy Biotherapy: monoclonal antibodies Bone marrow or stem cell transplantation
Chronic lymphocytic leukemia	B-cell lymphocytes undergo a malignant transformation Few cases are of the T-cell line	25% of patients are symptom free Evidence of disease found on routine examination and laboratory work Frequent respiratory and skin infections	Peripheral blood smear: • CBC with differential • Flow cytometry to evaluate immunophenotype of cells • Bone marrow biopsy (for prognostic information)	Survival is often determined by the severity of disease when diagnosed. No pattern of predictability of disease course.	Often difficult to decide when to begin treatment. Treatment is aimed at alleviating symptoms, not cure. Treatment for complications: • Antibiotics • IV immunoglobulin Chemotherapy Splenectomy or radiotherapy (rarely done) Bone marrow or stem cell transplantation

| CHART 64–12 | **Commonly Occurring Cancers—*Continued*** | | | | |

Cancer	Clinical Findings	Diagnostic Technique	Prognosis	Treatment
Chronic myeloid leukemia	Myeloproliferative disorder Presence of Philadelphia chromosome Three stages: 1. Chronic 2. Accelerated 3. Blast crisis	*Chronic Phase:* Fatigue Pallor Dyspnea Anemia Night sweats Weight loss Sternum pain *Accelerated:* Chronic symptoms recur after treatment. *Blast crisis:* Aggressive and terminal phase that includes above symptoms with increased severity.	Peripheral blood smear: • CBC with differential • Bone marrow biopsy	Chronic phase lasts 3–4 years. Once blast crisis occurs, median survival is <6 months. 85% of patients die during blast crisis due to complications such as bleeding and infections.	Chemotherapy Biotherapy: interferon Bone marrow or stem cell transplantation
Lymphomas				
Non-Hodgkin's disease	Similar to Hodgkin's disease, but without the Reed-Sternberg cell *Etiology:* Infections Autoimmune disorders Environmental factors Typically female, Caucasian, and approximately 55 years of age	Painless lymphadenopathy (cervical or supraclavicular region) As disease worsens swelling and obstructive symptoms occur	Lymph node biopsy Chest x-ray Bone marrow biopsy Serum blood analysis: • Hepatitis B and C • CBC with differential • Chemistries	Indolent disease has most favorable prognosis. Highly aggressive disease requires high-dose therapy that increases risk of life-threatening complications.	Chemotherapy Biotherapy: monoclonal antibodies Bone marrow or stem cell transplantation
Hodgkin's disease	Presence of Reed-Sternberg cells *Etiology:* Viral exposure Epstein–Barr virus most common Woodworking Most common in young adults, age 26–31 years Occasional peak in prevalence at age 60 years	Lymphadenopathy: Cervical Supraclavicular Mediastinal Fever Night sweats Weight loss	Lymph node biopsy Staging laparotomy if receiving radiation Chest x-ray Bone marrow biopsy Serum blood analysis: • CBC with differential • Chemistries	If early stage, 20-year survival is near 80%. If receiving salvage therapy after relapse, survival is 80–95%.	Radiotherapy Chemotherapy Bone marrow or stem cell transplantation

Sources: Crane-Okada, R. (2001). Breast cancers. In S. Otto (Ed.), *Oncology nursing* (4th ed.). St. Louis: Mosby; Daniel, B. (2001). Malignant lymphoma. In S. Otto (Ed.), *Oncology nursing* (4th ed.). St. Louis: Mosby; Iovino, C., & Camacho, L. (2003). Acute myeloid leukemia: A classification and treatment update. *Clinical Journal of Oncology Nursing, 7*(5), 535–540; O'Rourke, M. (2001). Genitourinary cancers. In S. Otto (Ed.), *Oncology nursing* (4th ed.). St. Louis: Mosby; Ososki, R. (2001). Leukemia. In S. Otto (Ed.), *Oncology nursing* (4th ed.). St. Louis: Mosby.

Typically, a biopsy is done first followed by a period of approximately 2 weeks before additional surgery. This delay allows the patient and family time to adjust to the diagnosis and begin making decisions about treatment options (Pfeifer, 2001).

Primary Treatment

Primary treatment for cancer involves the removal of a malignancy and a margin of surrounding normal tissue. Reducing the amount of total body tumor burden and improving the survival rate is the goal of this surgical approach. Wide excision (en bloc dissection) approaches are used to remove the primary tumor along with regional lymph nodes, intervening lymphatic channels, and involved adjacent structures. Examples of wide excisions are radical neck dissection, radical mastectomy, and abdominal-perineal resection. Local excision is used for skin cancers and consists of the simple excision of a tumor and a small amount of surrounding tissue.

It is important for the patient to be taught the benefits and burdens of undergoing surgery for cancer. The patient and family need to be taught the potential complications, the expected length of recovery, and the degree of disfigurement associated with the procedure. In addition, the benefits of other treatment options, such as chemotherapy, radiotherapy, and conservative surgical approaches need to be presented. When given this type of information, patients can make informed decisions about the type of treatment they wish to receive.

Adjuvant Treatment

Adjuvant treatment is aimed at improving outcomes by providing additional cancer therapy. Cytoreductive therapy (debulking) is surgery used to remove a large tumor burden, which will reduce the quantity of cancer cells. Then other therapies are used on the remaining tumor burden. Occasionally, prophylactic surgery will be performed on diseased organs that have a high incidence of developing a subsequent cancer. An example of this adjuvant approach is a colectomy for a patient with ulcerative colitis because the incidence of developing colon cancer when ulcerative colitis is present is about 40% (DeVita, Hellman, & Rosenberg, 1997).

Salvage Treatment

Salvage treatment is an extensive surgical approach that is used when there has been local recurrence since prior surgery. An example of this technique would be mastectomy after breast conservation done by lumpectomy and radiation therapy (Szopa, 2005).

Palliative Treatment

Palliative surgery is a useful therapy for those patients with advanced disease. The purpose of the surgical procedure is to reduce disease or treatment-related symptoms, when a cure is not possible. Prior to recommending palliative surgery, the surgeon will consider the rate of tumor growth, the projected life expectancy, and the expected treatment outcomes. The goals of palliative surgery are to alleviate suffering and prevent the occurrence of symptoms if the patient decides to forego other treatments.

Combination Treatment

Combination treatment involves several different treatment modalities to minimize the change in the patient's appearance and functional ability. By using chemotherapy, radiation therapy, or biotherapy during the preoperative, intraoperative, or postoperative periods, tumor resectability will improve as well as the overall treatment outcomes (Pfeifer, 2001).

Reconstructive Treatment

Patients who undergo surgical procedures that leave a deficit in function or appearance may be candidates for reconstructive surgery. The goal of this treatment option is to improve function or obtain a more acceptable cosmetic effect. Discussions about possible reconstructive surgery will occur prior to the primary surgery so the patient can make a fully informed decision. Cancers of the breast, skin, and head and neck are the most commonly indicated for reconstructive surgery (Rokita, 2004).

Preoperative Care

Planning care for the surgical oncology patient should be considered comparable to the nursing care expected for any surgical patient. However, an awareness of the problems and complications exclusive to those diagnosed with cancer is essential for the nurse to provide compassionate holistic care. The health care team will assess the patient's emotional and physical status in order to predict how well she will tolerate surgery and the recovery period. The patient's functional status may be evaluated using several validated scales, such as the Karnofsky Performance Scale, Eastern Cooperative Oncology Group (ECOG) scale, and the World Health Organization scale. Chart 64–13 explains the scoring indicators included in the Karnofsky Performance Scale, which is one of the hallmark tools used in cancer treatment. These scales reflect the ability of the patient to care for self and carry out normal activities. This information will assist the health care team in developing a comprehensive plan that will maximize the patient's recovery capability (Erickson, 2003).

The presence of other medical problems, such as heart disease or lung disease, may complicate postoperative recovery. In addition, physical debilitation due to advanced disease or type of symptoms present requires special attention. Improving the patient's physical well-being includes treating symptoms such as pain, malnutrition, fatigue, insomnia, depression, and headaches. Managing a patient's symptoms in the preoperative period will affect the patient's response to surgery and recovery. The nurse needs to identify comorbidities and other symptoms prior to surgery and individualize the postoperative plan of care as needed.

During the preoperative period the nurse focuses on assessment and intervention by becoming more familiar with the patient's knowledge and adaptation of his situation. By knowing the purpose of the surgical procedure, the nurse can better understand behaviors exhibited by the patient. For instance, behaviors demonstrated by patients who recently were diagnosed with cancer are different than those by patients with metastatic disease who undergo palliative surgery for relief from spinal cord compression. The nurse must understand what kind of surgery will be performed in order to plan for appropriate preoperative preparation such as bowel preparation or nutritional support. Knowing which procedure will be performed will also alert the nurse to the location and size of the surgical incision and what type of indwelling device may be needed during the postopera-

CHART 64–13	**Karnofsky Performance Scale**
100	Normal; no complaints; no evidence of disease
90	Ability to carry on normal activity; minor signs or symptoms of disease
80	Normal activity with effort; some signs or symptoms of disease
70	Ability to care for self; inability to do normal activity or do active work
60	Occasional assistance necessary, but ability to care for most needs
50	Considerable assistance and frequent medical care necessary
40	Disabled; special care and assistance necessary
30	Severely disabled; indication for hospitalization although death not imminent
20	Very sick; hospitalization necessary; active supportive treatment necessary
10	Moribund; fatal processes progressing rapidly
0	Death

tive period. With this information the nurse can engage each patient in teaching that is customized for her or his situation.

The diagnosis of cancer has a dramatic impact on patients and their loved ones. Many feel hopeless, powerless, and depressed. Oftentimes patients will be apprehensive about the upcoming surgery, demonstrating anger, anxiety, and perhaps panic (Pfeifer, 2001). The nurse develops a therapeutic relationship with the patient and her significant others by maintaining an open, honest, and caring approach to communication. A trusting relationship can assist the patient in maintaining a realistic sense of hope.

Age and physical status play an important role in accepting the diagnosis of cancer and postoperative recovery and rehabilitation (Erickson, 2003). Those in early adulthood to middle age typically have more physical endurance; however, they may have many emotional concerns. This is the most productive time in their lives for their careers, education, child rearing, and sexual activity. Some may fear a loss of job security, financial independence, and reproductive ability, role adjustment, and disfigurement. Elderly patients may fear burdening their family, both physically and financially, and suddenly are faced with recognizing their own mortality. It is important for nurses to use a caring approach when listening to the patients' concerns and support them with information and resources appropriate for their needs.

◼ Nursing Management

Postoperative nursing care of the oncology patient varies according to the type of cancer, type of surgery performed, previous therapies, and comorbidities. A comprehensive plan of care encompasses the patient's physical and psychological needs and can be found in Chapters 25 ⊛ to 27 ⊛ where care of the surgical patient is presented. The oncology nurse knows that patients have unique medical and emotional needs that require an understanding of the overall management of the cancer patient.

Radiation Therapy

Radiation therapy is the use of ionizing rays or particles to treat cancer. More than 50% of all patients with cancer will be treated with radiation therapy during the course of their illness. The use of radiation in the treatment of disease, or radiotherapy, has been used since 1895 when radium, radioactivity, and x-rays were discovered. In 1898 the first successful radiation therapy treatment for cancer was used. Unfortunately, a host of complications occurred due to the delivery of large doses in a single treatment. During the early and mid-1900s, scientists studied the effects of radiation on tissues. Results of these studies were responsible for the inception of fractionalization, or dividing of the total dose of radiation into several small doses. During the 1950s several discoveries aided the advancement of radiotherapy including the use of vacuum tubes, which allow for higher energy to be delivered to deeper tissues, and linear accelerators, which provided deeper penetration with less scatter to normal tissues (Iwamoto, 2001).

Radiation is a localized treatment that can be used alone or in combination with other treatments such as chemotherapy and surgery. Prescribing radiation therapy in the treatment of cancer serves several purpose: to make a curative attempt to eradicate the disease; to control metastatic activity, allowing the patient relief of symptoms; to prevent microscopic disease asso-

ciated with specific primary tumors; and to improve a patient's quality of life by relieving or reducing symptoms seen with advanced cancer (Sitton, 1997). Chart 64–14 illustrates the symptoms of advancing disease targeted by radiation therapy.

Ionizing radiation destroys the ability of cancer cells to multiply and grow. This is accomplished by delivering energy potent enough to break the chemical bonds in molecules, leading to cellular damage or death. The nucleolus of a cell is penetrated by the ionizing rays or particles and interacts with its water content to form hydroxyl (free) radicals. The cells' DNA is then damaged, which results in the disruption of chromosomal strands. Cellular death depends on the ability of the chromosomal damage to repair itself (Iwamoto, 2001).

Therapeutic radiation includes electromagnetic and particulate. Electromagnetic sources are x-rays and gamma rays (energy rays without mass). Machines are the delivery mechanism for x-rays, whereas radioactive materials are responsible for emitting gamma rays. Electromagnetic sources penetrate deep into tissue layers before releasing their energy and causing cellular damage. Particulate radiation contains mass, which prohibits it from penetrating into deep tissue, but delivers energy into the cells close to the surface (Erickson, 2003).

The health care provider will determine the radiosensitivity of the cancer cells, or target tissue, prior to prescribing the course of radiation therapy. *Radiosensitivity* is the measurement of potential

CHART 64–14	Symptoms Relieved by Radiation Therapy	
Symptom	**Etiology**

Hemorrhage
  Fatigue
  Weakness
  Pallor
  Lowered blood pressure (BP),
  elevated heart rate (HR)
	Primary tumor

Pain	Bone metastasis

Vascular obstruction
  Alterations in pulses
  Cool, discolored skin
	Primary tumor

Gastrointestinal obstruction
  Abdominal pain
  Nausea and vomiting
  Absent bowel sounds
	Primary tumor

Kidney and ureter obstruction
  Flank pain
  Lower abdominal pain
  Difficulty urinating
	Primary tumor

Tracheal obstruction
  Dyspnea
  Reduced oxygen saturation
	Primary tumor

Spinal cord compression
  Numbness, tingling
  Difficulty moving
	Primary tumor

Neurological symptoms
  Headache
  Seizures
  Impaired speech
	Brain metastasis

susceptibly of cells to ionizing radiation and how rapidly destruction will occur. Rapidly dividing cells, either benign or malignant, are more sensitive (e.g., mucosa). Those cells that are slow to divide or nondividing are radioresistant (e.g., muscle or neurons) (Sitton, 2005). Because all body tissue has a degree of radiosensitivity, nurses caring for patients with cancer must understand how various tumor types will respond to radiation therapy. Chart 64–15 reviews the effect of radiotherapy on specific tumor types.

A health care provider trained in radiation oncology (radiation oncologist) will determine the maximum radiation dose possible that will not harm normal tissues surrounding the target area. Various factors are considered when calculating the dose for any given patient: patient's age, tumor size and stage, evidence of metastasis, and overall prognosis if radiation therapy is used as part of the treatment plan (Erickson, 2003). The total dose of radiation is divided into smaller doses (fractionalization) and delivered daily for several weeks. The rationale for the fractionalization is to maximize malignant cell kill, which occurs when cells enter mitosis, and to minimize damage to surrounding tissue and allow for repair to begin.

Administration of Radiation Therapy

Radiotherapy can be delivered in several ways. Teletherapy (external-beam) requires the use of a machine at a predetermined distance from the body. Brachytherapy (internal radiation) is performed using a sealed radioactive source placed in or near the malignancy. Occasionally, radioactive materials are delivered systemically via the oral or intravenous route. The most common cancer treated in this manner is that of the thyroid.

External Radiation Therapy

External radiation therapy can be used alone or with surgery to better enhance the patient's chance of survival. Typically, when radiation is used alone, it is done so with the intent of achieving cure. Cancers that are known to respond to radiation alone include cancer of the prostate, uterus, cervix, pelvis, skin, oral cavity, and early Hodgkin's disease. When radiation is used in combination with surgery, the goal is either cure or palliation of distressing symptoms. Those cancers that can be cured with both therapies include head and neck, breast, uterus, bladder, testes, and bone.

For patients who undergo both surgery and radiation and are anticipating a curative outcome, administration of radiation may be done before or after surgery. Advantages of preoperative radiation include decreasing tumor size, which increases the likelihood of successful removal of the entire mass, obliteration of cancerous cells beyond the surgical field, and elimination of lymph nodes where malignancy could form. Nurses who care for patients receiving preoperative radiation therapy will need to pay special attention to wound healing because there will be delays in normal tissue repair due to the side effects of the therapy.

The delivery of postoperative radiation therapy is intended for the elimination of residual tumor and subclinical disease. Although higher doses may be delivered, treatment is delayed until postoperative wound healing is finished.

Prior to any radiation therapy beginning, the patient will need to undergo the treatment-planning phase. The purpose of this phase of treatment is to ensure the best way to deliver the treatments needed. After a radiation oncologist examines the patient, localization of the tumor will begin. A simulator machine is used to localize the tumor, and the anatomic area that will receive radiation (port) will be marked with either ink or permanent tattoos. Figure 64–3 ■ illustrates a simulator used in the treatment-planning phase and a linear accelerator, which delivers the radiotherapy. Precise identification of the area that will receive the radiation is critical to minimize tissue damage. Other examination procedures, such as computed tomography (CT) scans, magnetic resonance imaging (MRI), intravenous pyelogram (IVP) or barium enemas, may be used depending on the area being treated (Iwamoto, 2001).

Ports, or their position, may be changed on different days to ensure the delivery of safe and optimal radiation therapy. During treatment the patient may find himself in difficult and uncomfortable positions' however, immobilization is pivotal for accurate delivery of radiation. Devices to assist with immobilization or positioning may be necessary and are made specifically for each patient. Figure 64–4 ■ shows immobilizers used to assist with positioning. Certain patient populations, such as children and the elderly, may require special molds, casts, boards, or belts to help them maintain proper positioning. The nurse educates patients that the planning phase may take several hours and encourages them to request pain medication as needed to promote comfort (Erickson, 2003).

Patients receiving external radiation therapy should expect to receive treatments daily (weekends excluded) for several weeks. The actual treatment takes approximately 5 minutes; however, more time is taken to properly position the patient. For those patients receiving palliative radiotherapy, fewer treatments will be given at higher doses. Total body irradiation is delivered to those patients who have leukemia and are preparing for bone marrow transplantation due to the multiple areas that may be harboring leukemic cells.

Several unique approaches to external radiotherapy are being used for specific cancers. Chart 64–16 (p. 2086) identifies the various approaches available.

CHART 64–15	Effect of Radiotherapy on Tumor Types	
Tumor Type	**Effect**	**Dose**
Leukemia Lymphoma Myeloma Seminoma Dysgerminoma	Highly effective	Modest
Squamous cell of oral cavity, esophagus, cervix, vagina, bladder, skin	Moderate/highly effective	High
Vasculature and connective tissue of all tumors, astrocytomas	Moderately effective	High
Tumors of bone and cartilage, renal cell, hepatomas, pancreatic cancer, salivary gland tumors, tumors of muscle, brain, and spinal cord	Fairly ineffective	High Beyond normal tissue tolerance

Sources: Erickson, J. (2003). Cancer. In W. Phipps, F. Monahan, J. Sands, J. Marek, & M. Neighbors (Eds.), *Medical–surgical nursing health and illness perspectives* (7th ed.). St. Louis: Mosby; Iwamoto, R. (2001). Radiation therapy. In S. Otto (Ed.), *Oncology nursing* (4th ed.). St. Louis: Mosby.

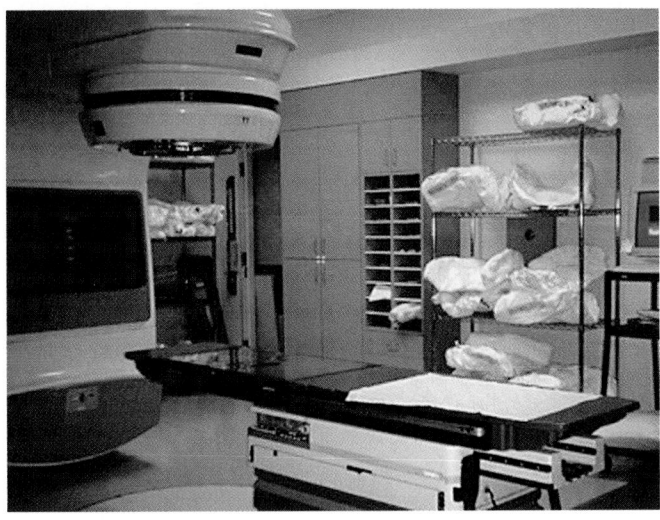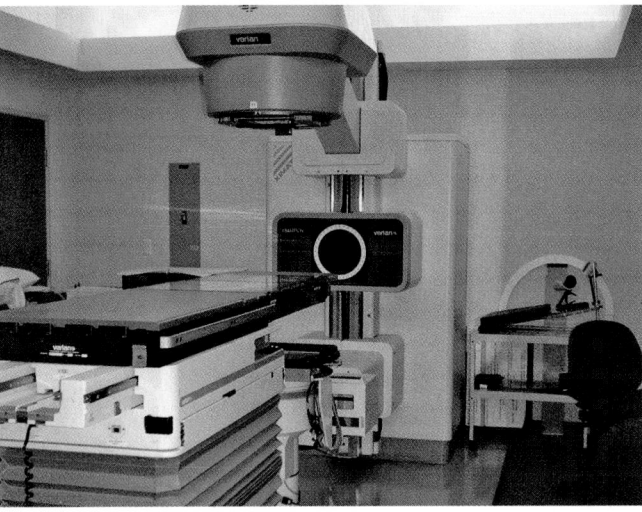

FIGURE 64–3 ■ Accelerator and simulator for radiation therapy. (Roseville Radiation Center)

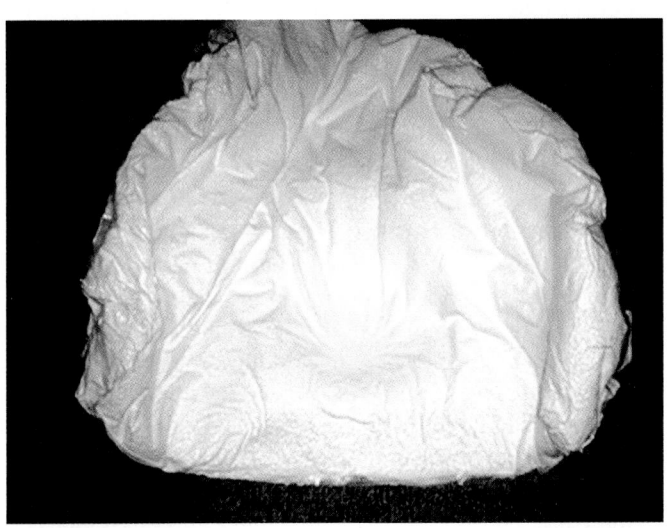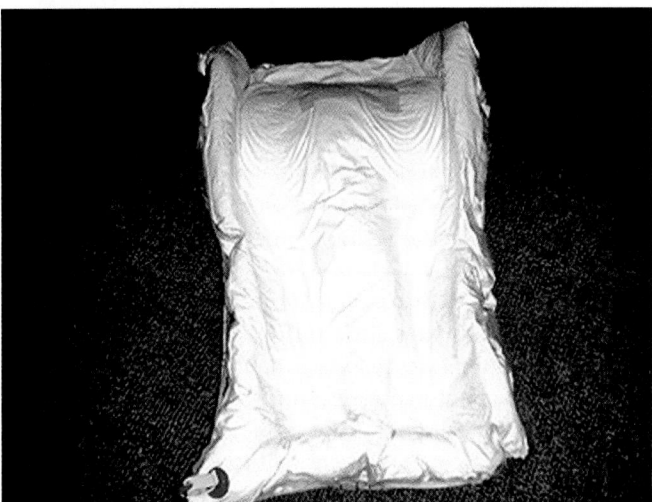

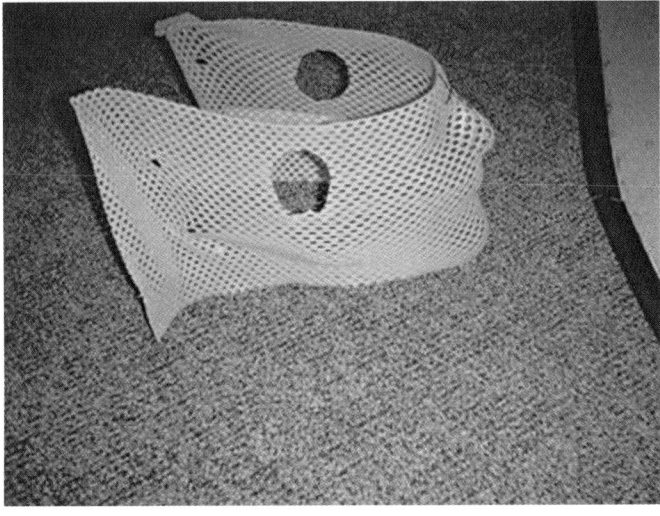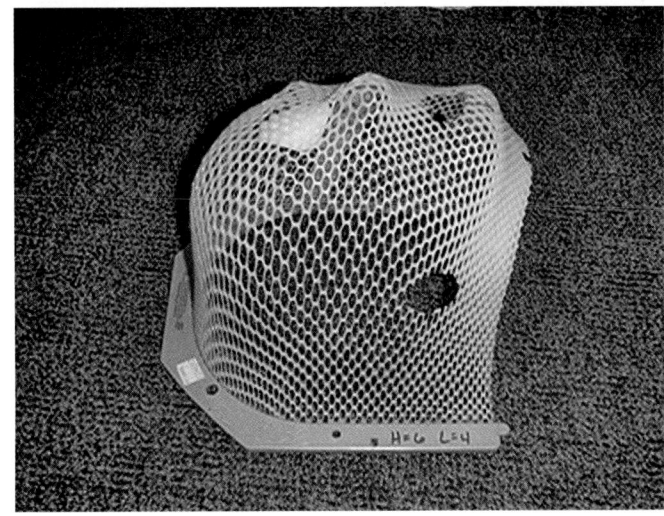

FIGURE 64–4 ■ Immobilizers for radiation therapy. (Roseville Radiation Center)

Photodynamic Therapy

An innovative approach to cancer treatment is photodynamic therapy (PDT) (Levy, 1994). Cancers of the skin, lung, esophagus, superficial bladder, and head and neck are currently the focus of this unique treatment. In addition, PDT has been used for purging bone marrow prior to autologous donor transplantation for leukemia and lymphoma (Overholt, Panjehpour, & Haydeck, 1999). PDT uses light-sensitive molecules (photosensitizers) that form oxygen radicals after exposure to light. Cellular damage or death is a

Sources: Blomgren, H., Lax, I., Goranson, H., Kraepelien, T., Nilsson, B., Naslund, I., Svanstrom, R., Tilikidis, A., et al. (1998). Radiosurgery for tumors in the body: Clinical experience using a new method. *Journal of Radiosurgery, 1*(1); Brunner, D. (1990). Report on the Radiation Oncology Nursing Subcommittee of the American College of Radiation Task Force on Standards Development. *Oncology, 4*(80); Campbell, C., & Iwamoto, R. (1992). Intraoperative radiation therapy. *Today's OR Nurse, 14*(1); Larson, D. (1998). Stereotactic external-beam irradiation. In C. Perez & L. Brady (Eds.), *Principles and practices of radiation oncology* (3rd ed.). Philadelphia: Lippincott Williams & Wilkins; Noll, L., & Riese, N. (1997). Chemical modifiers of radiation therapy. In K. Dow et al. (Eds.), *Nursing care in radiation oncology* (2nd ed.). Philadelphia: W. B. Saunders.

CHART 64–16 Unique Approaches in Radiation Therapy

Approach	Purpose
Intraoperative radiation therapy (IORT)	Control of local recurrence by directly visualizing and treating tumors.
Radiosensitizers	Medication used to enhance the effect of radiation.
Radiopharmaceuticals	Intravenous delivery of radioactive substances to treat pain from multiple osteoblastic bony metastases.
Stereotactic external-beam irradiation	Three-dimensional beam distribution, which provides high-dose treatment for small intracranial volumes. Treatment in other body areas is currently being done.

result of the radicals altering the DNA, cytoplasm, and cell membrane.

Porfimer sodium is the most commonly used photosensitizer. A laser treatment is given 48 hours after administration of the agent. Tumor masses require 48 hours to acquire a sufficient quantity of the photosensitizer. Nurses caring for those receiving PDT must be careful to educate patients and their families regarding the extreme photosensitivity and precautions necessary to prevent skin damage from sources such as examination lights and sunlight.

Internal Radiation Therapy

Brachytherapy (internal radiation therapy) uses sealed radioactive sources (implants) that are placed into or on a tumor. The term *brachytherapy* means "near treatment." This approach allows for a high concentration of radiation to be delivered to a specific site in a short period of time. The major disadvantages include the need to access the tumor by invasive procedures and the skill required of personnel administering this unique therapy (Hoskin & Coyle, 2005). Brachytherapy may also be used in combination with external radiation therapy to enhance the overall effect on the tumor. A high dose of radiation can be delivered to a small malignant mass while very little is delivered to adjacent tissues. The therapy can be received over a period of several days using a low dose rate (LDR) or over a few minutes using a high dose rate (HDR) (Flynn, 2005). Cancers of the prostate, brain, tongue, lips, lung, breast, esophagus, vagina, cervix, endometrium, rectum, and bladder may be treated with brachytherapy.

Placement of implants into the body cavity or structure is done via special applicators. Radioactive material contained in applicators such as ribbons, wires, seeds, capsules, needles, or tubes is encapsulated to prevent body fluids from becoming contaminated. Placement occurs away from the nursing unit, in the operating room, treatment room, or radiation department. After placement of the applicator, the patient returns to her hospital room and the radioactive isotope is inserted. This approach, called afterloading, is used to minimize the unnecessary risk of exposure of hospital employees to the radioactive material. The implant is left in place anywhere from a few hours to several days, during which the patient remains hospitalized.

The technique of HDR brachytherapy is another approach used to deliver radiotherapy. It involves positioning of the applicator into the cavity of a tumor, then loading the applicator with pellets or tubes with a wire by remote control. The applicator is unloaded at the end of the treatment, which lasts minutes. Figure 64–5 ■ illustrates the use of the applicator as used for prostate cancer. The HDR technique is done weekly for several weeks and does not necessitate hospitalization (Erickson, 2003).

Educating patients and their families about the implant, including the process, effects, and strategies to manage its effects, is an important role of the nurse. Prior to implantation, patients should be taught about symptom management, activity restrictions while the implant is in place, what causes current symptoms, and how the implant could change those symptoms. Once the implant is in place, patients need to be informed about when to notify the health care provider and potential side effects of the treatment along with the customary management.

Radiation Precautions

Understanding the need to protect health care providers from the risk of injury is of extreme importance when discussing patients who receive radiation therapy. Adhering to radiation safety guidelines is necessary to minimize the risk of occupational radiation exposure. Placement of internal radiation sources should be done in specially designed rooms that prevent leakage of radioactivity. Individuals working in these areas must wear a personal monitor (e.g., film badge) to measure their radiation dose. Badges contain photographic film and are worn on the person's trunk. The exchange of badges among employees should never be done because it prevents accurate determination of the amount of exposure to a specific individual. Each month badges are read for the amount of exposure and a new one is provided to the employee (Sitton, 2005).

Planning is extremely important when caring for a patient who receives radiation sources that emit gamma rays because they expose the caregivers over a varying period of time. Providers need to limit time exposed to these patients to prevent injury to themselves and others. Danger of exposure is reduced as the radioactive substance reaches its half-life or the point in time when half of the radioactivity has dissolved. Essential considerations in minimizing exposure to radiation are time, distance, and shielding. Chart 64–17 (p. 2088) explains these principles and related nursing responsibilities.

Nursing personnel also have the opportunity to educate patients and their families about the precautions needed and to alleviate fears associated with radiation therapy. Nurses need to recognize their own fears or concerns so they can develop and implement an effective plan of care for their patients. Attending in-services or educational sessions about radiation safety practices combined with a skills laboratory for practicing appropriate patient care activities will help clarify misconceptions and assist the nurse in providing comprehensive quality care. National and

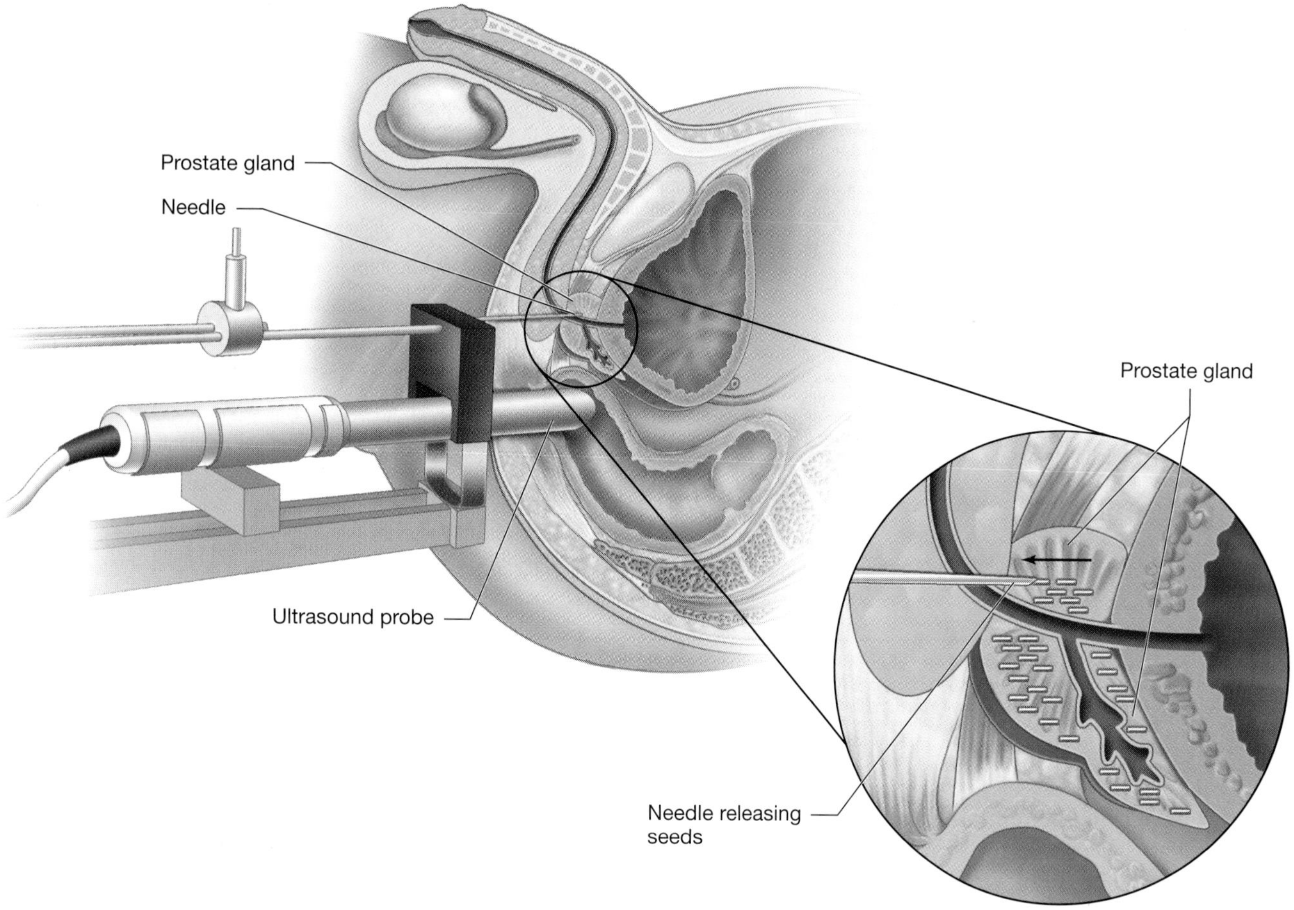

Prostate gland

Needle

Ultrasound probe

Prostate gland

Needle releasing
seeds

FIGURE 64–5 ■ Brachytherapy applicator.

state regulations mandate the monitoring of radiation levels, which provides for a safe workplace (Sedhom & Yanni, 1985).

Radiation Side Effects

Nurses play an important role in assessing, planning, implementing, and evaluating outcomes used to prevent or minimize the side effects associated with radiotherapy. Collaborating with the radiation oncology team allows for an opportunity to provide continuity and quality patient care, which will maximize efforts aimed at relief of side effects. Radiation therapy is a localized treatment that produces site-specific and general side effects that can be distressing to the patient and their loved ones.

Side effects experienced by most radiation therapy patients include skin changes, loss of appetite, fatigue, and bone marrow suppression. Radiation alters capillary blood flow leading to detectable skin changes. Skin reactions may occur within 2 weeks of beginning treatment. Erythema may be noted to range from mild, light pink to deep and dusky red (Sitton, 1997). Desquamation, first dry then moist, may occur in some patients. Moist desquamation is known to cause the epidermal layers of the skin to slough, leaving an area that is raw, painful, and draining serous exudate. Patients who have skinfolds, particularly in the axilla or groin, are more likely to develop skin reactions that progress to moist desquamation. There are ways to help minimize problems caused by skin changes associated with radiation therapy. These patients need education focused on maintaining good hygiene and when to alert their health care provider for signs of skin infection.

 **CRITICAL ALERT** *Assessing the patient's skin during the course of radiotherapy for signs of reactions (redness, erythema, and desquamation) is essential. Pay particular attention to areas with skinfolds, such as the axilla and groin. The nurse should report signs of skin breakdown to the health care provider so possible treatment can be initiated. If skin reactions are minimized, the patient will experience less suffering, fewer (if any) complications, and be more likely to continue with the therapy.*

Anorexia, or loss of appetite, can be due to the cancer or the prescribed treatment. Although it is not completely clear what causes anorexia, contributing factors include inactivity, medications, and altered ingestion and digestion of food. Another explanation for anorexia could be found in the release of tumor necrosis factor (TNF) and interleukin-1 (IL-1). These **cytokines,** which have an appetite-suppressing effect, are released from macrophages while attempting to defeat a cancer. Loss of appetite usually peaks 4 weeks into treatment and subsides shortly after treatment ends. If anorexia persists, weight loss may occur resulting in the development of fatigue (Iwamoto, 2001). Refer to the upcoming Nursing Process: Care Plan for Cancer feature (p. 2089) for detailed nursing interventions and expected outcomes related to anorexia.

Many patients who receive radiotherapy experience fatigue. The exact causative mechanism is unknown, although it is thought to be due to the result of tumor breakdown, which releases by-products into the bloodstream (Sitton, 1997). Another explanation for the development of fatigue is the increase in basal metabolic rate consuming the body's energy stores. Fatigue

| CHART 64–17 | **Principles for Minimizing Radiation Exposure** |

Principle	**Nursing Responsibilities**
Time	• Minimize time in proximity.
• Exposure directly related to time spent within specific distance of source	• Organize care activities; assemble supplies prior to entering room.
	• Prior to leaving room, place patient care items within reach.
	• Rotate staff assignments.
	• One-half hour of patient contact per shift is recommended.
	• Encourage self-care activities.
Distance	• Private room required.
• Maximize distance from source.	• Perform duties as far away from source as possible.
• Inverse square law: doubling the distance decreases exposure by one-fourth	• Never touch a source; use long-handled forceps.
	• Visit from the doorway if possible.
Shielding	• Place shield at bedside if needed.
• Type of shielding and its thickness depends on type of source	• Provide nursing care behind the shield.
	• Do not use lead aprons used in x-ray departments.

Sources: Dunne-Daly, C. (1997). Principles of brachytherapy. In K. Dow et al. (Eds.), *Nursing care in radiation oncology* (7th ed.). Philadelphia: W. B. Saunders; Erickson, J. (2003). Cancer. In W. Phipps, F. Monahan, J. Sands, J. Marek, & M. Neighbors (Eds.), *Medical–surgical nursing health and illness perspectives* (7th ed.). St. Louis: Mosby; Sitton, E. (1998). Managing side effects of skin changes and fatigue. In K. Dow et al. (Eds.), *Nursing care in radiation oncology* (7th ed.). Philadelphia: W. B. Saunders.

typically begins during the third or fourth week of treatment and will gradually wane once the treatment is over (Bender & Rosenzweig, 2004). Several other symptoms resulting from the alteration in energy production compound the effect of fatigue on cancer patients. These include pain, anorexia, infection, dyspnea, anemia, and depression.

The loss of energy and feeling of tiredness tend to be cumulative and have a significant impact on patients' quality of life. Patient education regarding the side effects of radiation begins before treatment and needs to continue once it is over. Teaching patients that side effects should be expected may decrease their fear that treatment is ineffective. Nursing care needs to be designed with energy conservation in mind. Clustering patient care activities together will allow for prolonged periods of rest for patients who are experiencing fatigue. Teaching patients and their caregivers these principles will assist the patient in coping with the tiredness experienced with fatigue while at home.

Bone marrow suppression occurs due to the prevalence of bone marrow being affected in nearly every treatment port. The common areas include pelvis, sternum, ribs, spine, metaphyses of long bones, and the skull (Iwamoto, 2001). The nursing care required is complex and challenging. Complete blood counts (CBCs) should be monitored at regular intervals during therapy or more frequently if concerning symptoms occur such as infection, bleeding, and fatigue. Providing patient and family education about precautions for neutropenia, thrombocytopenia, and anemia is essential and frequently requires reinforcement throughout the radiotherapy course.

The nurse plays a valuable role in helping the patient cope with side effects produced by radiotherapy. It also is important to recognize how the side effects will impact the patient's quality of life and how socialization may be difficult if not impossible. Many side effects are specific to the area where radiation is delivered. Site specific side effects are found in Chart 64–18.

| CHART 64–18 | **Site-Specific Side Effects of Radiation Therapy** |

Site	**Side Effects**
Head and Neck	Stomatitis (irritation of the oral mucosa):
	• *Mild:* generalized erythema, few ulcerations, and small white patches
	• *Severe:* convergent ulcerations with bleeding and white patches covering >25% of oral cavity
	Xerostomia (dryness of the mouth)
	Tooth decay and caries
	Osteoradionecrosis
	Hypopituitarism
	Taste changes
Chest	Esophagitis
	Cough
	Radiation pneumonitis
	Lung fibrosis
Abdomen	Gastritis
	Nausea and vomiting
Pelvis	Diarrhea
	Cystitis
	Erectile dysfunction
	Vaginal stenosis
	Ovarian failure
	Cessation of spermatogenesis
Brain	Cerebral edema
	Alopecia
	Changes in hair texture and color

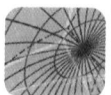

Nursing Management

A comprehensive plan of care will encompass the patient's physical and psychological needs. The Nursing Process: Care Plan for Cancer feature identifies the appropriate nursing diagnosis and pro-vides a detailed plan of care for the oncology patient. The nursing management sections for the patient receiving chemotherapy and biotherapy provide details pertinent to those patients receiving cancer-related treatments, including radiation therapy.

NURSING PROCESS: Patient Care Plan for Cancer

Assessment of Infection

Subjective Data:
Have you had fevers, chills, or body aches?
Have you noticed drainage from your skin?
Have you noticed changes in your urine odor?
Have you experienced painful urination?

Objective Data:
Signs of infection (e.g., dysuria, foul-smelling urine, elevated temperature, exudate from skin breakdown, elevated white blood count (WBC) count)

Nursing Assessment and Diagnoses	Outcomes and Evaluation Parameters	Planning and Interventions with *Rationales*
Nursing Diagnosis: *Risk for Infection* related to skin reactions, skin breakdown, multiple invasive lines, and myelosuppression	**Outcome:** No evidence of infection. *Evaluation Parameters:* Skin integrity is maintained. Urine appearance is clear, yellow, and possess no foul odor. Invasive lines are free from signs of infection. Patient demonstrates appropriate self-care behaviors.	**Interventions and *Rationales:*** Perform hand hygiene before and after working with patient. *Prevents spread of infection.* Monitor and record vital signs. *Elevated temperature and heart rate may indicate infection.* Assess for signs of infection and notify health care provider immediately: • Increased WBCs • Changes in temperature; >101°F (38.3°C) • Presence of chills, diaphoresis • Presence of myalgias • Cough, with or without sputum • Purulent drainage from site of skin reactions, intravenous site, or invasive line sites • Pain with urination, frequency with urination, foul-smelling urine • Mental status changes • Diarrhea. *Identifies need for prompt treatment.* Obtain cultures and sensitivities prior to administering antibiotic therapy. *Identifies organism responsible for infection, which directs appropriate treatment.* Administer antibiotics, antifungals, and antivirals as prescribed. Note presence of drug allergy. *Treatment of infection and prevention of drug reaction.* Initiate measures to reduce infection: • Private room if absolute neutrophil count (ANC) < 1,000/mm³ • Avoid contact with those who have known or recent infection or recent vaccination. • Hand hygiene • Avoid rectal or vaginal procedures (temperatures, examinations, medications). • Administer stool softeners to prevent straining • Meticulous hygiene • Avoid use of straight-edge razor. • Avoid raw meat and fish, fresh fruit and vegetables, fresh flowers and plants. • Provide clean liquids daily (e.g., denture cleaning solution, respiratory equipment fluid, drinking water). • Change solutions per protocol. • Avoid intramuscular injections. • Use strict aseptic technique when inserting medical devices (e.g., urinary catheters). *Infection control practice.* Instruct patient and family about infection prevention measures. *Reduces the risk of infection and encourages good infection control practices.*

(continued)

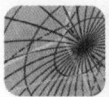

NURSING PROCESS: Patient Care Plan for Cancer—*Continued*

Assessment of Tissue Perfusion and Cardiac Output

Subjective Data:
Are you feeling breathless with minimal exertion?
Are you having chest discomfort?
Have you noticed weight gain or swelling?
Have you experienced feeling cold?

Objective Data:
Poor-quality pulses
Weight gain and edema
Increased respiratory rate
Presence of crackles in lungs

Nursing Assessment and Diagnoses	Outcomes and Evaluation Parameters	Planning and Interventions with *Rationales*
Nursing Diagnoses: *Ineffective Tissue Perfusion* and *Decreased Cardiac Output* related to chemotherapy induced cardiac toxicity and capillary leak syndrome	**Outcome:** Normal tissue perfusion and cardiac output. ***Evaluation Parameters:*** Adequate peripheral perfusion as evidenced by: • Extremity pulses present by palpation and/or ultrasound • Capillary refill < 2 seconds on distal extremities • Color and temperature normal to extremities. Adequate urinary output evidenced by 30 mL/hr. Normal neurological function. No evidence of heart failure.	**Interventions and *Rationales:*** Evaluate baseline cardiac studies (e.g., echocardiogram, ECG, MUGA scan). *Provides baseline cardiac function to allow for future comparison.* Calculate and document cumulative dose of chemotherapeutic agents, if appropriate. *Provides ongoing information regarding maximum lifetime dosage.* Assess for signs of congestive heart failure and report to health care provider: • Dyspnea • Tachycardia • Distended neck veins • Pedal edema • Crackles • Nonproductive cough • Extra heart tones (S_3) • Hepatomegaly. *Allows for prompt treatment.* Monitor vital signs for changes, and report to health care provider, such as: • Tachycardia • Tachypnea • Hypotension or hypertension. *Allows for prompt treatment.* Assess for syncope, dizziness, and weakness. *Indicates inadequate perfusion.* Monitor serum electrolytes. *Provides additional sources for alteration in cardiac function.* Administer medications to support cardiac function. (e.g., diuretics, inotropic agents, vasodilators, oxygen). *Maximizes cardiac function.* Position flat or with legs elevated. *Maximizes blood return to heart.* Encourage patient to adhere to dietary modifications (e.g., fluid restriction, sodium restriction, no alcohol, no tobacco). *Maximize cardiac function.* Instruct patient and family that cardiac effects may be irreversible. *Allows for time to consider lifestyle changes.* Collaborate with oncologist for reduced dosing of chemotherapy if ejection fraction is <55%. *Minimizes exposure to toxic effect of antineoplastic agents.* Monitor peripheral perfusion by assessing: • Capillary refill (<3.0 seconds) • Pulses present and strong throughout • Skin dry, color pink, and temperature warm. *Provides information about the quality of circulation.* Monitor urinary output for normal (> 30 mL/hr). Report abnormal findings to health care provider. *Indicates adequate renal perfusion and allows for prompt treatment if necessary.* Monitor neurological status and report abnormalities to health care provider. *Indicates possible perfusion abnormalities and need for prompt intervention.*

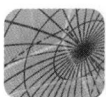

NURSING PROCESS: Patient Care Plan for Cancer—*Continued*

Assessment of Gas Exchange and Airway Clearance

Subjective Data:
Are you able to do your normal activities without breathlessness or fatigue?
Have you noticed a productive cough? If so, describe your sputum.

Objective Data:
Abnormal arterial blood gases (ABGs) and oxygen saturation
Abnormal lung sounds, rate and depth of respirations
Changes in amount and characteristics of sputum
Changes in mental status

Nursing Assessment and Diagnoses	Outcomes and Evaluation Parameters	Planning and Interventions with *Rationales*
Nursing Diagnoses: *Risk for Impaired Gas Exchange* and *Ineffective Airway Clearance* related to chemotherapy, biotherapy, and transplant-induced pulmonary toxicity	**Outcome:** Adequate gas exchange and airway clearance. *Evaluation Parameters:* Normal ABGs. No dyspnea: unlabored respirations < 24/minute. Normal neurological status. Normal breath sounds. No signs of impaired tissue oxygenation. Oxygen saturation is within normal limits.	**Interventions and *Rationales:*** Assess for adventitious or diminished breath sounds. *Indicates decreased gas exchange.* Note depth, rate, rhythm, and effort of respiration. *Assesses for respiratory distress or increased work of breathing.* Note presence of cough, amount, color, and consistency of sputum. *Assesses for development of respiratory infections or pulmonary edema.* Monitor ABGs and oxygen saturation via pulse oximetry. *Determines adequacy of gas exchange.* Monitor restlessness and confusion. *Indicators of inadequate gas exchange with resultant brain hypoxia.* Assess skin and mucous membranes for color (dusky, ashen, or cyanotic). *Indicators of tissue hypoxia and need for prompt intervention.* Instruct patient to cough and deep breathe. *Promotes gas exchange.* Administer humidified oxygen therapy as prescribed. *Promotes airway clearance.* Monitor for complaints of chest pain and report to health care provider. *May indicate acute pulmonary event such as pulmonary embolism, pleural effusion, or pneumothorax.* Instruct patient and family about symptoms of pulmonary toxicity and to report findings to health care provider. *Allows for prompt intervention.* Instruct patient and family regarding possibility of irreversible pulmonary effects. *Allows patient to consider initiating lifestyle changes consistent with pulmonary function.*

Assessment of Bleeding

Subjective Data:
Have you noticed unusual bruising?
Have you noticed any blood in your urine or stools?
Have you experienced dizziness or light-headedness?

Objective Data:
Blood studies (platelets, hemoglobin, and hematocrit) lowered
Oozing from venipunctures
Unusual amount of bruising
Bleeding gums after oral hygiene
Hematuria and guaiac-positive stools
Change in mental status or behavior
Change in vital signs

Nursing Assessment and Diagnoses	Outcomes and Evaluation Parameters	Planning and Interventions with *Rationales*
Nursing Diagnosis: *Potential for Deficient Fluid Volume* related to bone marrow suppression, hepatotoxicity, hepatic Veno Occlusive Disease (VOD), and hematologic laboratory abnormality induced by cancer treatments	**Outcome:** No evidence of bleeding. *Evaluation Parameters:* Platelet count will be within normal limits. Hemoglobin and hematocrit will be within normal limits. Hemodynamic status will be maintained. Patient will demonstrate appropriate self-care behaviors.	**Interventions and *Rationales:*** Monitor platelet counts and report a count of <50,000/mm³ to health care provider. *Identifies need for prompt treatment.* Monitor liver function tests and coagulation studies. *Identifies need for prompt treatment.*

(continued)

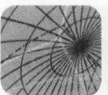

NURSING PROCESS: Patient Care Plan for Cancer—*Continued*

Nursing Assessment and Diagnoses	Outcomes and Evaluation Parameters	Planning and Interventions with *Rationales*
		Assess for bleeding and report findings to the health care provider: • Decrease in hemoglobin and hematocrit • Prolonged bleeding or oozing from invasive procedures, venipunctures, cuts, or scratches • Presence of petechiae or ecchymosis • Presence of frank or occult blood in emesis, stool, or sputum • Presence of blood from any body orifice • Change in mental status • Change in vital signs (e.g., ↑ heart rate, ↓ BP) • Skin color pale, temperature cool. *Early detection aids in early treatment.* Perform venipunctures once daily for all laboratory tests. *Minimizes the risk of bleeding.* Avoid taking rectal temperatures; avoid use of suppositories or enemas. *Minimizes the risk of bleeding.* Apply direct pressure to injection and venipuncture sites for a minimum of 5 minutes. *Minimizes bleeding.* Instruct patient regarding ways to minimize the risk of bleeding: • Perform oral hygiene with soft toothbrush or toothettes. • Avoid use of commercial mouthwashes. • Avoid straight–edge razors. • File nails with emery board. • Avoid foods that are difficult to chew. *Provides for appropriate self-care behaviors.*

Assessment of Fluid Volume Status

Subjective Data:
How frequent (if any) are your diarrhea episodes?
Are you able to consume fluids?
Do you feel dizzy or light-headed when you change positions?
Are there any remedies that have helped?
Have you noticed an increase in your weight?
Do you become breathless?

Objective Data:
Poor skin turgor, dry mucous membranes
Elevated heart rate with position changes
Output exceeds intake
Multiple diarrhea episodes
Presence of edema and weight gain
Crackles in lungs

Nursing Assessment and Diagnoses	Outcomes and Evaluation Parameters	Planning and Interventions with *Rationales*
Nursing Diagnoses: *Risk for Deficient Fluid Volume* related to nausea, vomiting, diarrhea (due to pelvic radiation & cancer), hepatic VOD, and capillary leak syndrome *Risk for Excess Fluid Volume* related to hepatic VOD	**Outcomes:** Adequate hydration. Absence of skin breakdown. Normal electrolytes. **Evaluation Parameters:** Normal serum electrolytes. Skin surrounding anus remains intact. Cessation of diarrhea episodes. No evidence of dehydration or fluid overload. Absence of skin breakdown. Normal electrolytes.	**Interventions and *Rationales:*** Assess bowel pattern. *Determines baseline.* Record frequency of diarrhea and vomiting episodes. *Indicates degree of fluid loss.* Establish and maintain IV access. *Allows for fluid volume replacement if needed.* Administer IV fluids per protocol. *Determines need for fluid administration or restriction and prevents dehydration.* Record accurate intake and output. *Determines adequacy of fluid volume replacement.* Monitor daily weights using the same scale and with the same clothing. *Indicates fluid retention or loss.* Monitor serum electrolyte values, hemoglobin and hematocrit, liver function tests, and coagulation studies and notify health care provider of critical abnormalities. *To monitor hematologic changes associated with fluid changes.* Monitor for presence of edema. *Indicates fluid retention.* Measure abdominal girth daily and apply landmark indicators to abdomen. *Indicates presence of accumulating ascites and allows for accuracy and consistency in measurements.*

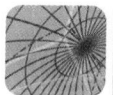

NURSING PROCESS: Patient Care Plan for Cancer—*Continued*

Nursing Assessment and Diagnoses	Outcomes and Evaluation Parameters	Planning and Interventions with *Rationales*
		Restrict sodium and water intake. *Prevents fluid retention in extracellular spaces.*
		Monitor lung sounds. *Evaluates for fluid accumulation in lung, which may require prompt treatment.*
		Place patient in semi-Fowler's position to avoid the patient lying flat. *Allows for optimal ventilation in the presence of ascites.*
		Assess for excoriation of skin surrounding anus. *Identifies need for interventions.*
		Instruct patient to cleanse area frequently. *Prevents skin breakdown.*
		Instruct patient to notify health care provider if skin breakdown occurs. *Allows for prompt treatment.*
		Administer antidiarrhea medication per protocol. *Reduces frequency of diarrhea episodes.*
		Instruct patient to use low-residue diet and limit fat content. *Reduces amount of diarrhea.*

Assessment of Skin Integrity and Oral Mucous Membranes

Subjective Data:
Have you noticed pain in your mouth?
Have you noticed sores in your mouth?
Have you noticed areas of skin breakdown?
Have you noticed hair loss?
Do you have pain, drainage, or swelling in area of skin breakdown?

Objective Data:
Presence of mouth sores
Reports of pain in mouth with citrus drinks
Poor oral intake
Presence of skin breakdown and hair loss
Presence of skin redness
Signs of pain or infection

Nursing Assessment and Diagnoses	Outcomes and Evaluation Parameters	Planning and Interventions with *Rationales*
Nursing Diagnosis: *Impaired Skin Integrity* related to alopecia, stomatitis, xerostomia, skin reactions due to radiation therapy, invasive procedures and lines, biotherapy-induced dry desquamation, rashes, and pruritus, edema, cancer diagnosis and treatment	**Outcomes:** Maintain or restore skin integrity. Cope with hair loss. Mucous membranes are intact. ***Evaluation Parameters:*** Minimal skin changes noted. Appropriate self-care behaviors are demonstrated. Skin infections are absent. Social interaction is maintained. Intact oral mucous membranes are maintained. Nutritional status is maintained. Patient is not suffering. Skin integrity is maintained or restored.	**Interventions and *Rationales:*** Inspect oral cavity daily. *Provides information needed to determine if treatment is necessary.* Instruct patient regarding proper oral care: • Brush and floss teeth as tolerated. • Use moistening gauze or toothettes instead of toothbrush if needed, for instance, if platelet count is low (<40,000/mm³). • Rinse with normal saline four times per day. • Avoid commercial mouthwashes. • Cleanse mouth before and after meals. *Prevents trauma and maintains oral hygiene.* Administer cytoprotectives as ordered (e.g., Ethyol). *Promotes comfort and reduces incidence of mucous membrane breakdown.* Provide bland and soft diet. *Allows for ease of chewing and swallowing and reduces discomfort.* Administer saliva substitutes and moisten food as needed. *Allows for ease of swallowing.* Instruct patient to report signs of stomatitis: • Burning • Pain • Areas of redness • Open lesions on the lips • Pain with swallowing • Intolerance to temperature extremes. *Identifies beginning stages of mucous membrane breakdown and facilitates prompt treatment.*

(continued)

NURSING PROCESS: Patient Care Plan for Cancer—*Continued*

Nursing Assessment and Diagnoses	Outcomes and Evaluation Parameters	Planning and Interventions with *Rationales*
		Assist in oral hygiene during mild stomatitis:
		• Normal saline rinses every 2 hours, every 6 hours during sleep.
		• Use soft toothbrush or toothette.
		• Avoid use of dentures except for meals.
		• Maintain proper fit of dentures.
		• Moisten lips with lubricating ointment.
		• Avoid eating foods that are spicy, those with temperature extremes, and those that are difficult to chew.
		Promotes hygiene, minimizes trauma, and provides for comfort.
		Assist in oral hygiene during severe stomatitis:
		• Discontinue use of dentures.
		• Rinse with prescribed agent or irrigate oral cavity with mixture of saline, anti-*Candida* agent (Mycostatin), and topical anesthetic agent.
		• Position patient properly for irrigations.
		• Provide oral suction device.
		• Use gauze or toothette with irrigation solution for cleansing.
		• Lubricate lips.
		Promotes hygiene and comfort.
		Assess patient's ability to chew, swallow, and presence of gag reflex. *Identifies risk for aspiration.*
		Encourage use of pureed diet or liquid diet. *Promotes comfort and maintains nutrition.*
		Monitor for signs of infection and notify health care provider immediately. *Facilitates prompt treatment.*
		Obtain tissue cultures as needed. *Provides evidence of infection.*
		Administer analgesics, topical and systemic, as prescribed. *Promotes comfort.*
		Discuss patterns of hair loss and regrowth with patient and family. *Provides information so preparations for loss can begin and provides an understanding of the temporary nature of alopecia.*
		Encourage expression of concerns related to hair loss. *Facilitates coping.*
		Reduce or prevent hair loss:
		• Cut long hair prior to treatment.
		• Use mild shampoo, conditioner in small amounts.
		• Gently pat hair dry.
		• Avoid electric curlers, curling irons, dryers, clips, barrettes, hair sprays, hair dyes, or other hair chemicals.
		• Avoid excessive brushing or combing; use wide-tooth comb.
		• Use scalp tourniquets or hypothermia as appropriate.
		Prevents hair loss as long as possible by decreasing the uptake of chemotherapy. Also maintains presence of hair as long as possible by reducing weight and manipulation.
		Encourage patient to avoid actions that traumatize the scalp:
		• Keep scalp lubricated to reduce itching (use vitamins A and D).
		• Use sunscreen or hat when exposed to ultraviolet rays.
		Prevents breakdown of the skin.
		Offer ways to cope with hair loss:
		• Obtain wigs or hairpieces prior to hair loss.
		• Take photograph of hair loss to wig shop to improve matching of hair color.
		• Contact American Cancer Society for available resources.
		• Wear scarf, hat, or other device as needed.
		Reduces changes in appearance.
		Assess skin integrity. *Provides baseline information.*

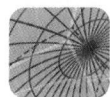

NURSING PROCESS: Patient Care Plan for Cancer—*Continued*

Nursing Assessment and Diagnoses	Outcomes and Evaluation Parameters	Planning and Interventions with *Rationales*
		Instruct patient regarding skin care of area within treatment field: • Cleanse with lukewarm water. • Avoid use of soap, powders, deodorants, and fragrances. • Avoid shaving. • Keep skinfolds dry and clean. • Use devices to protect skin from sun, heat, and cold. • Avoid use of restrictive or tight-fitting clothing. • Avoid use of tape. • Avoid massaging, vigorous rubbing, or scratching. *Minimizes skin trauma and provides protection.* Instruct patient regarding skin care if dry desquamation occurs: • Cleanse with lukewarm water. • Avoid use of soap, powders, deodorants, cosmetics, ointments, and fragrances. • Avoid shaving. • Avoid rubbing or scratching. • Avoid hyperthermia or hypothermia treatments. • Avoid use of adhesive tapes. • Avoid exposure to sunlight or cold weather conditions. • Avoid use of restrictive clothing; use of cotton materials is preferred. • Apply hydrophilic moisturizing lotion or ointment two to three times per day (e.g., vitamins A and D ointment or Aquaphor). *Prevents further skin damage and drying and aids in healing.* Instruct patient regarding skin care if moist desquamation occurs: • Notify health care provider if blistering occurs. • Keep blisters intact. • Avoid frequent cleansing of the area. • Apply saline irrigations or cold compresses three to four times per day. • Apply dressings as prescribed (e.g., Vigilon). • Apply zinc oxide or silver sulfadiazine with nonstick dressing if radiation treatments are being held. • If area is draining, apply thin layer of gauze. *Provides for healing, decreases inflammation, and prevents infection.* Administer antihistamines per protocol. *Relieves itching associated with pruritus.* Apply cold towels to affected area. *Relieves itching associated with pruritus.* Instruct patient to maintain room humidity between 30% and 40%. *Relieves itching associated with pruritus.*

Assessment of Fatigue

Subjective Data:

Do you feel unusually tired?
Do you perform your normal activities?
Do you have difficulty performing your normal activities?
How many hours per night do you sleep?
How is your appetite?
Do you have help at home?

Objective Data:

Monitor hemoglobin, hematocrit, RBCs, electrolytes
Adequate nutritional intake
Presence of pain or edema
Monitor energy expenditure

(continued)

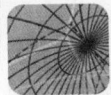

Nursing Assessment and Diagnoses	Outcomes and Evaluation Parameters	Planning and Interventions with *Rationales*
Nursing Diagnosis: *Activity Intolerance* related to fatigue, bone marrow suppression, anorexia, and hepatotoxicity	**Outcome:** Able to perform activities of daily living (ADLs). **Evaluation Parameters:** Maintain ADLs and minimize fatigue. Serum laboratory studies within normal limits. Adequate energy levels are maintained. Patient shows no evidence of suffering or discomfort. Adequate diet with recommended calorie and protein intake is maintained.	**Interventions and *Rationales:*** Encourage frequent rest periods. *Energy is conserved and replenished.* Encourage more sleep hours at night. *Restores energy levels.* Encourage patient to reorganize daily schedule of activities and seek assistance with shopping, cooking, housework, etc. *To minimize energy expenditure.* Encourage a temporary decrease in work hours. *Decreases physical and psychological stress and provides for rest.* Assess nutritional intake for adequate protein and calorie intake. *Provides source of energy.* Administer blood products per protocol. *Provides adequate oxygen availability, which will decrease fatigue.* Monitor fluid and electrolyte balance. *Provides information regarding nerve transmission and muscle function.* Assess for sources of discomfort and suffering. *Minimizes energy expenditure.*

Assessment of Nutrition

Subjective Data:
How has your appetite been?
Have you lost weight?
Have you been able to perform your normal activities?

Objective Data:
Weight loss
Decreased albumin and prealbumin levels
Poor dietary intake per calorie count and clinical nutrition consult

Nursing Assessment and Diagnoses	Outcomes and Evaluation Parameters	Planning and Interventions with *Rationales*
Nursing Diagnosis: *Imbalanced Nutrition: Less Than Body Requirements* related to chemotherapy and biotherapy-induced nausea, vomiting, hepatotoxicity, anorexia, and effects of pre- and post-transplant treatment	**Outcome:** Adequate nutritional status and maintenance of body weight. **Evaluation Parameters:** Patient experiences fewer episodes of nausea and vomiting. Adequate calorie intake maintained. Serum laboratory studies within normal limits. Adequate energy levels are maintained. Prescribed diet is tolerated.	**Interventions and *Rationales:*** Monitor accurate intake and output and record. *Indicates trends in intake pattern.* Perform nutritional assessment: • Calorie count • Ability to swallow • Food preferences • Patterns and behaviors related to eating • Ethnic and cultural preferences. *Indicates adequacy of nutrition.* Monitor serum albumin, prealbumin, glucose, magnesium, sodium, and iron. *Assesses adequacy of nutritional intake.* Assess for signs of malnutrition: • Muscle wasting • Edema • Changes in hair condition • Changes in skin. *Indicates adequacy of nutrition.* Consult nutritionist to determine appropriate needs for individual. *Assists in establishing or maintaining adequate nutrition.* Provide meticulous oral care. *Prevents infection and promotes appetite.* Administer antiemetics and appetite stimulants per orders. *Assists in improving appetite by reducing nausea and vomiting.* Encourage small frequent meals that are high in calories and protein. *Such meals are more suitable for digestion, better tolerated.* Encourage adequate fluid intake, limiting fluids during mealtime. *Prevents the development of satiety.* Increase activity level as tolerated. *Activity stimulates the appetite.* Provide environment suitable for eating: • Pain free • Relaxed environment • Presentation of food tray. *To increase appetite.* Monitor tube feedings or IV total parenteral nutrition per protocol. *Determines tolerance of nutritional delivery system.*

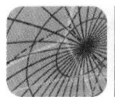

NURSING PROCESS: Patient Care Plan for Cancer—*Continued*

Nursing Assessment and Diagnoses	Outcomes and Evaluation Parameters	Planning and Interventions with *Rationales*
		Administer cytoprotectives as ordered (e.g., Ethyol). *Promotes comfort and improved nutrition by preventing dry mouth.* Provide discharge teaching to patient and family regarding nutritional needs. *Maintains nutritional status at home.*

Assessment of Pain

Subjective Data:
Are you experiencing pain?
If so, describe the quality, intensity, provoking factors, etc.
Rate pain on scale of 1–10.

Objective Data:
Unwilling to participate in care
Facial grimacing
Guarding or protecting of painful site
Using increasing doses of pain medication

Nursing Assessment and Diagnoses	Outcomes and Evaluation Parameters	Planning and Interventions with *Rationales*
Nursing Diagnosis: *Pain* related to skin reactions, cough from chest radiation, chemotherapy-induced pancreatitis, chemotherapy- and biotherapy-induced peripheral neuropathy and bone pain, mucositis, invasive procedures, and disease process	**Outcome:** Pain is controlled. ***Evaluation Parameters:*** Patient verbalizes pain level and previous interventions that were successful in alleviating pain. Pain is reduced or absent as evidenced by patient denying presence or by nonverbal behaviors: no facial grimacing, restlessness, etc. Patient reports complementary strategies of pain control are effective.	**Interventions and *Rationales:*** Assess pain using pain scale (0–10) to quantify pain level. *Provides consistency for evaluating pain.* Assess discomfort characteristics: • Location • Quality • Frequency • Duration • Alleviating therapies. *Provides baseline for assessing change.* Assess other factors contributing to pain: • Fear • Fatigue • Anger • Anxiety. *Provides data about factors that decrease the patient's tolerance to pain.* Ensure adequate fluid intake. *Minimizes frequency and intensity of cough.* Instruct patient to avoid irritants such as smoke. *Minimizes cough.* Instruct patient regarding the use of humidification in the air. *Minimizes cough.* Administer analgesics according to protocol. *Provides pain relief.* Monitor for side effects of analgesics and treat accordingly. *Ensures tolerance of analgesics.* Encourage use of pureed diet or liquid diet. *Promotes comfort and maintains nutrition.* Monitor for signs of infection and notify health care provider immediately. *Facilitates prompt treatment.* Administer analgesics prior to a procedure or treatment that may cause discomfort. *Controls increased pain level related to procedures and treatments.* Instruct patient to notify nurse when pain is not relieved or when pain begins to occur again. *Indicates need for additional pain management therapies or the administration of analgesics earlier in the pain cycle.* Collaborate with the patient and the multidisciplinary team when changes in pain management are necessary. *Increases the patient's sense of control and allows for agreement and input from all team members.* Instruct patient and family about complementary strategies to relieve pain and discomfort: • Guided imagery • Relaxation techniques • Distraction • Cutaneous stimulation. *Helps reduce anxiety and promotes relaxation.*

(continued)

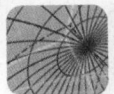

Assessment of Body Image Disturbance

Subjective Data:
What feelings do you have about the change in your appearance?
Have you been participating in your care and normal activities?
Have you been socializing?

Objective Data:
Isolating behaviors
Avoidance
Not involved with personal care

Nursing Assessment and Diagnoses	Outcomes and Evaluation Parameters	Planning and Interventions with *Rationales*
Nursing Diagnosis: *Disturbed Body Image* related to skin reactions, alopecia, long-term venous access devices, decreased sexual function, role changes, and other cancer treatments	**Outcomes:** Social integration Normal social interactions and acceptance of body image changes ***Evaluation Parameters:*** Participates in self-care activities. Demonstrates interest in appearance. Resumes or continues interactions with others in established social network. Explores alternative ways of expressing concern and affection with partner.	**Interventions and *Rationales:*** Assess patient's feelings about body image and level of self-esteem. Validate concerns. *Provides baseline for evaluating changes and determining effectiveness of interventions.* Advocate for participation in activities and decision making. *Facilitates a sense of control.* Encourage patient to verbalize concerns. *Begins coping process.* Provide personalized care. *Prevents depersonalization.* Discuss patterns of hair loss and regrowth with patient and family. *Provides information so preparations for loss can begin and provides an understanding of the temporary nature of alopecia.* Assist in self-care when fatigue, nausea, vomiting, or other distressing symptoms occur. *Improves self-esteem by ensuring physical well-being.* Help patient in selecting cosmetic devices that increase sense of attractiveness. *Promotes positive body image.* Offer ways to cope with hair loss: • Obtain wigs or hairpieces prior to hair loss. • Take photograph of hair to wig shop to improve matching of hair color. • Contact American Cancer Society for available resources. • Wear scarf, hat, or other device as needed. *Reduces changes in appearance.* Encourage dialogue between patient and partner regarding sexual function and alternatives. *Allows for affection and acceptance.*

Assessment of Urinary Elimination

Subjective Data:
Do you have difficulty urinating?
What is the color of your urine?
Do you have pain upon urination?
What is your typical fluid intake throughout the day?

Objective Data:
Presence of hematuria
Foul-smelling urine
Presence of fever
Complaints of pain with urination

Nursing Assessment and Diagnoses	Outcomes and Evaluation Parameters	Planning and Interventions with *Rationales*
Nursing Diagnosis: *Impaired Urinary Elimination* related to radiation therapy	**Outcomes:** Minimize cystitis. Able to urinate normally. ***Evaluation Parameters:*** Laboratory studies within normal limits. No evidence of discomfort or suffering. Adequate fluid intake maintained. Normal urinary patterns.	**Interventions and *Rationales:*** Assess for hematuria. *Indicates possible infection or cystitis.* Monitor fluid intake and encourage adequate intake. *Decreases incidence of cystitis.* Monitor for signs of urinary tract infection. *Promotes prompt treatment.* Obtain urine analysis and culture. *Evaluates for infection.* Assess for pain with urination. *Determines presence of symptoms needing further treatment.* Administer antibiotics, bladder analgesics, and antispasmodics as ordered. *To treat infection and pain.* Evaluate patient's understanding of cause of cystitis and measures to relieve symptoms. *Provides evidence of need for education.*

Assessment for Impaired Swallowing

Subjective Data:
Have you had difficulty swallowing?
Do you have pain with swallowing?

Objective Data:
Reports of pain with swallowing
Inability to swallow bolus of food or fluids
Refusing food or fluids

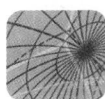

NURSING PROCESS: Patient Care Plan for Cancer—*Continued*

Nursing Assessment and Diagnoses	Outcomes and Evaluation Parameters	Planning and Interventions with *Rationales*
Nursing Diagnosis: *Risk for Impaired Swallowing* related to esophagitis or pharyngitis	**Outcome:** No difficulties with swallowing. ***Evaluation Parameters:*** Adequate nutritional status is maintained. Adequate pain management is maintained. Full course of radiation therapy is completed.	**Interventions and *Rationales:*** Instruct patient to follow a soft, bland, or liquid diet that is high in protein and calories. *Facilitates swallowing and promotes adequate nutritional intake.* Administer anesthetic and coating mouth rinses prior to eating. *Relieves discomfort associated with swallowing.* Administer analgesics per protocol. *Relieves discomfort associated with swallowing and allows for patient to continue with therapy.*

Assessment of Sexual Dysfunction

Subjective Data:
Are you satisfied with your sexual functioning?
Are you experiencing difficulty with sexual function?

Objective Data:
Minimal communication between patient and partner
Lack of touching and closeness between patient and partner

Nursing Assessment and Diagnoses	Outcomes and Evaluation Parameters	Planning and Interventions with *Rationales*
Nursing Diagnoses: *Risk for Sexual Dysfunction* related to radiation therapy of the pelvis *Altered Sexuality Patterns* related to late effects of transplantation	**Outcome:** Maintains sexual functioning as desired. ***Evaluation Parameters:*** Patient and partner understand rationale for treatment. Patient and partner maintain effective communication. Sexual functioning is improved.	**Interventions and *Rationales:*** Assess level of dysfunction via patient interview. *Determines baseline and need for interventions.* Encourage patient to discuss concerns with partner. *Facilitates effective communication.* Facilitate consultation with urologist as needed, including patient education regarding rationale. *Provides treatment and education.* Monitor for symptoms that affect libido. *Allows for treatment and understanding of changes.* Assess for fear, anxiety, diminished self-image, and depression. *Indicates need for resources for coping.* Facilitate communication about sexual issues. *Promotes open communication between patient and partner.* Instruct patient on hygiene and contraceptive measures. *Prevents infections and pregnancy.*

Assessment of Growth and Development

Subjective Data:
Parents report delayed progress in school.
Appears to be of short stature.

Objective Data:
Height and weight lower than normal
Motor abilities abnormal
Cognitive testing abnormal

Nursing Assessment and Diagnoses	Outcomes and Evaluation Parameters	Planning and Interventions with *Rationales*
Nursing Diagnosis: *Delayed Growth and Development* related to late effects of transplantation in children	**Outcome:** Normalized growth and development. ***Evaluation Parameters:*** Growth patterns are normal according to standardized charts. Educational needs are being met. Identifies need to access support systems. Actively participates in recovery.	**Interventions and *Rationales:*** Monitor patient's growth according to standard charts. *Helps determine if growth patterns are impaired.* Evaluate normal growth and development behaviors consistent with the patient's age. *Indicates need for possible treatment.* Monitor for learning disabilities. *Indicates need for special educational resources.* Administer growth hormone per protocol. *Assists in normalizing growth and development patterns.* Provide educational and emotional resources to patient and family. *Improves coping and ability to function with deficits.*

Assessment of Coping

Subjective Data:
Do you feel saddened?
Have you been withdrawing from your normal activities and routines?
Have you been sleeping well? If not, why?
Do you have a support system that comforts you?

Objective Data:
Withdrawn behavior
Unwilling to participate in care
Insomnia
Frequent episodes of crying, anger, aggressive behavior

(continued)

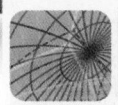

Nursing Assessment and Diagnoses	Outcomes and Evaluation Parameters	Planning and Interventions with *Rationales*
Nursing Diagnosis: *Ineffective Coping* related to alopecia, fatigue, biotherapy-induced depression, anxiety, transplant process, role changes, lifestyle changes, diagnosis of cancer	**Outcome:** Patient will demonstrate effective coping skills. ***Evaluation Parameters:*** Demonstrates effective coping strategies for living with cancer. Identifies need to access support systems. Actively participates in recovery.	**Interventions and *Rationales:*** Assess patient's and family's understanding of diagnosis, recommended treatment, and prognosis. *Provides information about need for further teaching if not consistent with actual diagnosis, treatment, or prognosis.* Encourage patient to express feelings. *Effective coping strategy.* Monitor aggressive behaviors. *May indicate ineffective coping.* Assess patient's and family's support systems. *Indicates need for recommendations.* Consult psychiatrist, psychologist, or spiritual counselor. *Provides expertise that will evaluate for effective coping and make recommendations for assistance.* Encourage family to use memory prompts with patient for orientation in regard to time, date, and location. *Allows for reorientation and participation in care.*

Assessment of Knowledge

Subjective Data:

What have you been told about your disease and treatment?

How would you manage side effects of treatment?

What symptoms would you contact your health care provider for?

Objective Data:

Assess understanding of diagnosis and recommended treatments.

Assess understanding of potential side effects and related remedies.

Nursing Assessment and Diagnoses	Outcomes and Evaluation Parameters	Planning and Interventions with *Rationales*
Nursing Diagnosis: *Deficient Knowledge* related to radiation therapy, chemotherapy, biotherapy side effects, and self-care needs	**Outcome:** Understand the use of radiation therapy for cancer and the self-care behaviors necessary to manage side effects. ***Evaluation Parameters:*** Patient verbalizes an understanding of the purpose for therapy, side effects, and measures used to minimize side effects, and protective measures. Patient demonstrates appropriate self-care behaviors. Patient understands the use of biotherapy and chemotherapy for cancer and the self-care behaviors necessary to manage side effects. Patient understands the use of transplantation for cancer and the self-care behaviors necessary to manage side effects. Patient demonstrates appropriate self-care behaviors.	**Interventions and *Rationales:*** Assess patient's expectations and concerns about therapy. *Determines baseline knowledge.* Instruct patient and family about: • The purpose of using radiation therapy to treat cancer • Routines such as consultation, simulation, treatment schedules, routine appointments, and follow-up • Expected length of each visit • Appearance of equipment and environment. *Decreases anxiety associated with treatment.* Instruct patient and family about the effects and side effects associated with radiation therapy. *Decreases anxiety associated with treatment.* Instruct patient and family about measures used to minimize side effects. *Provides for less distress associated with treatment, which maximizes chance of patient continuing with therapy.* Instruct patient and family about visiting restrictions and isolation requirements associated with internal radiation therapy. *Provides for an understanding of the need to protect others.* Instruct patient and family about: • The purpose of using chemotherapy and biotherapy, and transplantation to treat cancer • Routines such as appointments and follow-up treatments • Expected length of each visit • Appearance of infusion equipment and vascular access devices. *Decreases anxiety associated with treatment.* Assess patient's expectations and concerns about transplantation. *Determines baseline knowledge.* Instruct patient and family about the effect and side effects associated with transplantation and associated conditioning. *Decreases anxiety associated with treatment.* Instruct patient and family about measures used to minimize side effects. *Provides for less distress associated with treatment, which maximizes chance of patient continuing with therapy.*

Sources: Bender, C., & Rosenzweig, M. (2004). Cancer. In S. Lewis, M. Heitkemper, & S. Dirksen (Eds.), *Medical–surgical nursing assessment and management of clinical problems* (6th ed.). St. Louis: Mosby; Iwamoto, R. (2001). Radiation therapy. In S. Otto (Ed.), *Oncology nursing* (4th ed.). St. Louis: Mosby; Keller, C. (2001). Bone marrow and stem cell transplantation. In S. Otto (Ed.), *Oncology nursing* (4th ed.). St. Louis: Mosby; Oncology Nursing Society. (2001). *Chemotherapy and biotherapy guidelines and recommendations for practice.* Pittsburgh: Author; Rokita, S. (2004). Oncology: Nursing management in cancer care. In S. Smeltzer & B. Bare (Eds.), *Brunner & Suddarth's textbook of medical–surgical nursing* (10th ed.). Philadelphia: Lippincott Williams & Wilkins; Wikle-Shapiro, T. (1998). Nursing implications of bone marrow and stem cell transplantation. In J. K. Itano & K. N. Taoka (Eds.), *Core curriculum for oncology nursing* (3rd ed.). Philadelphia: W. B. Saunders.

Chemotherapy

Chemotherapy is defined as the systemic administration of cytotoxic drugs to treat cancer. In one form or another, this systemic therapy has been present for centuries. Current practice can be linked to the early 1900s when studies were conducted using laboratory rodents to determine the effectiveness of potential cancer chemotherapeutic agents (DeVita, 1997). During World War I and World War II soldiers were exposed to mustard gas, which was discovered to cause bone marrow and lymphoid suppression. This discovery led to the use of mustard agents in the treatment of Hodgkin's and other lymphomas for the first time in 1940. The use of chemotherapy became a standard of practice in the treatment of cancer in the 1970s (Grever & Chabner, 1997).

It was estimated that there would be 1,437,180 new cases of cancer diagnosed in 2008 (ACS, 2008b) and half of these would be treated with systemic chemotherapy. Given the prevalence of cancer, nurses need to understand the purpose of administering chemotherapy and how it is used. The primary reasons for prescribing chemotherapy are to prevent tumor cells from multiplying, spreading to adjacent tissues, or developing metastasis (Otto, 2001a). Therapy aims to provide a cure, control spread of the disease, or palliate signs of suffering. Chemotherapy may be used in several different ways, and oncologists prescribe treatment for patients with specific goals in mind. Chart 64–19 explains the five different ways of using chemotherapy and their purposes. Improvement in overall survival rate and increased periods of disease-free intervals can be attributed to the ongoing development of chemotherapy approaches to cancer treatment. The past five decades have been exciting for those caring for patients with cancer due to the dynamic state of chemotherapy research and the subsequent development of a host of new agents.

Principles of Chemotherapy

Every time a malignancy is exposed to a chemotherapeutic agent, a percentage of tumor cells are destroyed. The aim is destruction of as many cells as possible, up to 99% depending on the dose. Completely eradicating all tumor cells is virtually impossible, but the hope is to leave as few cells as possible so the body's immune system can finish the job. Chemotherapy is thought to kill a fixed percentage of the total number of cancer cells. This cell-kill hypothesis, shown in Figure 64–6 ■, suggests that if a drug has a 90% cell-kill rate and the tumor has 1,000 cells, at the end of the first treatment there would only be 100 cancerous cells remaining. The next treatment would leave the number of cells at 10, thus the reason for scheduling chemotherapy in multiple courses over a period of time.

Both cancerous cells and normal cells replicate via the various phases in the cell cycle. The cell cycle time is that time necessary for one tissue cell to divide and reproduce two identical daughter cells. The cycle for any cell has four phases each with its own important role. These include the G_1 phase, in which RNA and protein synthesis occur; the S phase, in which DNA synthesis occurs; the G_2 phase, which is the premitotic phase in which DNA synthesis is completed and mitotic spindles form; and finally mitosis (M phase) is the phase in which cell division occurs. Phase G_0, which is the resting or dormant phase, occurs after mitosis and prior to the G_1 phase (McNance & Roberts, 2002). These G_1 cells are particularly dangerous because they are not actively dividing but have the potential to replicate. Chemotherapeutic agents are meant to interrupt the cell replication at pivotal points within the cycle and are more effective when targeting cells that are actively dividing.

Because the goal of chemotherapy is to reduce the number of malignant cells present in both the primary and metastatic

The cell kill hypothesis

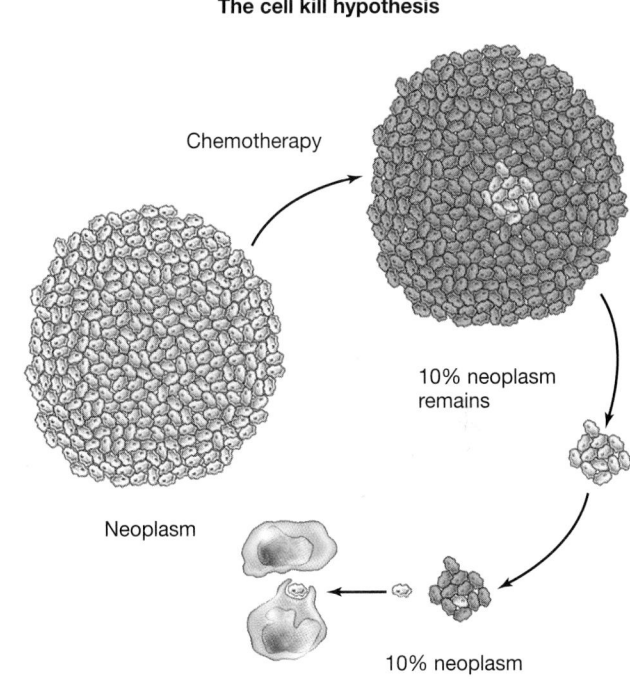

FIGURE 64–6 ■ Cell-kill hypothesis.

CHART 64–19   **Uses of Chemotherapeutic Agents in Treating Cancer**

Type of Therapy	Use	Purpose
Adjuvant	Used in combination with other cancer treatment modalities	To treat micrometastasis
Neoadjuvant	Used prior to surgical resection of tumor	To shrink tumor in order to maximize surgical resection capabilities
Primary	Used for localized cancer when other treatment options are not as effective	To maximize chance of cure or disease control
Induction	Used for cancers for which other alternatives do not exist	To maximize chance of cure or disease control
Combination	Use of two or more chemotherapeutic agents	To allow each medication to enhance the effect of the other or to act synergistically with it

tumor site, it is important to discuss the factors that determine the response of cancer cells to chemotherapy. First, the mitotic rate of the tumor affects the response of chemotherapy due to the rapid proliferation of cancerous cells. The more rapid the mitotic rate, the greater the response to chemotherapy. Tumor size affects response because the smaller number of cancer cells correlates to an improved response to treatment. In addition, when the tumor cells are young, a larger percentage of proliferating cells is more vulnerable to chemotherapy.

Certain anatomic sites offer a protected climate from the effects of chemotherapy. Few agents, such as nitrosoureas and bleomycin, cross the blood–brain barrier lending the brain protection from the effects of chemotherapy. The presence of resistant tumor cells reduces the likelihood of chemotherapy producing a positive effect. This is accomplished when mutation of cancer cells results in variant cells resistant to chemotherapy and when certain cancer cells are unable to convert the drug to an active form (Bender & Rosenzweig, 2004).

The majority of chemotherapeutic agents are most effective when working against dividing cells, not those in a resting phase as seen in G_0. As the tumor grows, more cells become inactive and convert to the resting phase. The presence of noncycling cells and drug resistance are the main difficulties encountered in the development of chemotherapeutic agents.

Classification

Chemotherapeutic drugs are classified or categorized according to their structure and mechanism of action. Similarities and differences exist between agents in the same classification. Those agents that act during a specific cell phase are classified as cell-cycle phase-specific drugs and are known to destroy cells that are actively dividing. Certain agents act on the S phase affecting DNA and RNA synthesis, whereas others act on the M phase, which terminates spindle formation. Chemotherapeutic agents that are active throughout the entire cell cycle are called cell-cycle phase-nonspecific drugs. These agents exert a longer acting effect on cells, leading to cell death or damage. Combining these two types of chemotherapeutic agents increases the number of susceptible tumor cells destroyed during a treatment period and reduces the adverse affects on normal cells, which affords the patient the possibility of achieving an improved response to treatment (Rokita, 2004). The Pharmacology Summary lists common antineoplastic (and biotherapy) agents used to treat cancer along with their common side effects and the related nursing interventions. This list is not meant to be comprehensive; rather, it gives an overview of information the nurse needs when planning care for a patient with cancer.

Administration and Safe Handling

Chemotherapeutic drugs are administered in a variety of locations and by a variety of routes. These agents can be given to patients who are in the hospital, in an outpatient infusion center, or in the home. Depending on the type of agent used, they may be given by the following routes: oral, intravenous, intramuscular, subcutaneous, arterial, intracavitary, and intrathecal. An oncology nurse knows, through experience and training, that the route is determined by the drug used, dose, type, location, and extent of tumor. Special education and training are essential in order to develop a safe practice for administering chemotherapy. The Oncology Nurses Society (ONS), together with OSHA,

has developed guidelines for the administration and handling of chemotherapy and biotherapy (Occupational Safety and Health Administration, Office of Occupational Medicine, 1995).

Safety Concerns

With the development of numerous chemotherapeutic agents in recent years came a heightened awareness of the hazards associated with those agents. Exposure to these agents can occur by inhalation, absorption, or digestion. Those handling chemotherapeutic agents need to be given training regarding the hazards and how to implement safeguards that will protect themselves and others. Hospitals and regulatory agencies recognize the risk to health care professionals and have developed precautions for those involved in the preparation, administration, and disposal of chemotherapeutic agents (Otto, 2001a). Chart 64–20 (p. 2109) lists the common precautions that should be taken by those caring for the patient receiving chemotherapy, including suggestions that would apply in home care settings. Typically nurses do not prepare chemotherapy agents, however, it is important to understand the safety precautions implemented by others to appreciate the seriousness of agents they will be asked to administer. Education of all staff is an ongoing process that should include a discussion of unique patient care situations, introduction of new equipment, and reproductive issues (Singleton & Connor, 1999).

Dose Calculations

Chemotherapeutic agents are dosed based on the body surface area (BSA) in adults and children. Pharmacists who prepare chemotherapy agents use equations to determine the appropriate dose for a patient based on his height and weight. To maintain accurate dosing, it is crucial for the nurse to monitor weight changes throughout the course of chemotherapy and communicate this information to the pharmacist. A patient's weight frequently changes throughout treatment due to drug-induced side effects such as nausea, vomiting, anorexia, and fatigue. Other factors that are considered when determining the dose of chemotherapy agents include renal function and other comorbidities (e.g., chronic obstructive pulmonary disease, heart failure, and renal failure).

Administration

The oncologist prescribing chemotherapy selects a route of administration that will deliver the optimal amount of drug to the tumor. A variety of methods are used to meet this goal. Chart 64–21 (p. 2110) explains the routes of administration along with specific nursing concerns for each. The nurse should understand the decision to use a specific delivery method and route is based on the pharmacokinetics of the drug to be used, as well as, characteristics of the patient and the cancer (Erickson, 2003).

Oral and intravenous (IV) routes are the most commonly used. All delivery methods have associated inherent risks. Intravenously administered agents pose particular concern associated with the risk of irritation to the vessel wall and extravasation (leaking of drug into tissue surrounding infusion site) causing local tissue damage. Chemotherapeutic drugs that cause severe local tissue breakdown and necrosis are called *vesicants* (Bender & Rosenzweig, 2004). Nurses need to be alert to symptoms common with extravasation such as pain, swelling, redness, and appearance of vesicles on the skin.

PHARMACOLOGY Summary of Medications for Cancer Treatment

Medication Category	Action	Application/Indications	Nursing Responsibility
Biotherapy Agents			
Interferons: • α-Interferon • β-Interferon • γ-Interferon	Antiviral and antitumor properties. Stimulate immune system or stop tumor growth. Enhance lymphocyte and antibody production. Assist with destruction of macrophages and natural killer cells. Inhibit cell replication by increasing phases of cell cycle. Mediate function of other cytokines (e.g., IL-2, TNF).	α-Interferon approved for use in hairy-cell leukemia, Kaposi's sarcoma, CML, high-grade non-Hodgkin's lymphoma, and melanoma. β-Interferon, γ-interferon approved for use in a variety of nonmalignant diseases.	Monitor for depression. Notify health care provider for possible consultation to social services and/or psychiatry. Monitor for flu-like symptoms (e.g., fevers, chills, malaise, headache, anorexia). Monitor for evidence of dehydration (e.g., concentrated urine, poor skin turgor, dry mucous membranes). Monitor electrolytes. Monitor for signs of infection (e.g., fever, increased sputum, dyspnea, urgency, and frequency). Implement neutropenic precautions as necessary. Implement safety precautions during activity. Administer antidiarrheals.
Interleukins	Produced by lymphocytes and monocytes. Known as lymphokines and monokines. Stimulate the proliferation of T lymphocytes and activation of natural killer cells. Stimulate the release of other cytokines (e.g., TNF, γ-interferon).	Most ILs are under investigation for use in the clinical setting. IL-2 is currently being used for the following conditions: • Metastatic renal cell carcinoma • Advanced metastatic melanoma • AML • Non-Hodgkin's lymphoma	Monitor for severe flu-like symptoms (e.g., fevers, chills, rigors, malaise, headache, anorexia). Monitor for capillary leak syndrome (e.g., generalized edema, decreased urine output, hypotension). Monitor for evidence of dehydration (e.g., concentrated urine, poor skin turgor, dry mucous membranes). Monitor electrolytes. Monitor for signs of infection (e.g., fever, increased sputum, dyspnea, urgency, and frequency). Implement neutropenic precautions as necessary. Implement safety precautions during activity. Administer antidiarrheals.
Granulocyte colony-stimulating factor: • Neupogen	Promote proliferation and differentiation of neutrophils. Enhance functional properties of mature neutrophils. Stimulate granulocyte and macrophage proliferation. Enhances functional properties of mature granulocytes and macrophages.	Used to treat or prevent severe thrombocytopenia and to reduce the need for platelet transfusions. Used after induction therapy in AML. Used after allogeneic and autologous bone marrow transplant (BMT).	Monitor for flu-like symptoms (e.g., fevers, chills, malaise, headache, anorexia). Monitor for bone pain and administer analgesics as needed. Monitor skin for development of rashes. Monitor for hypertension. Monitor for signs of decreased cardiac output or inadequate tissue perfusion (e.g., diaphoresis, pale color, poor-quality pulses, chest pain, edema, crackles, decreased urine output).
Granulocyte macrophage colony-stimulating factor: • Leukine	Stimulate growth and differentiation of stem cells in bone marrow to increase RBC production. Secreted by the kidney.	Used to treat chronic anemia associated with end-stage renal disease and anemia associated with cancer and HIV treatment.	
Hematopoietic growth factors: • Erythropoietin (Epogen) • Oprelvekin (Neumega)	Stimulate growth and development of platelets.	Used in acute promyelocytic leukemia, which is an extremely rare form of leukemia.	

(continued)

PHARMACOLOGY Summary of Medications for Cancer Treatment—*Continued*

Medication Category	Action	Application/Indications	Nursing Responsibility
Monoclonal Antibodies (MAbs): • Cetuximab (Erbitux) • Gemtuzumab ozogamicin (Mylotarg) • Ibritumomab tiuxetan (Zevalin) • Rituximab (Rituxan) • Trastuzumab (Herceptin) Angiogenesis inhibitor (VEGF): • Bevacizumab (Avastin)	Produced by injecting mice with tumor cells that act as antigens and obtaining antibodies from their spleens. Antibody cells are combined with cancer cells to produce more antibodies (hybridoma). Unconjugated: directly attack tumor cells; conjugated: attached to other agents (radioisotopes, toxins, chemotherapy). Aid in diagnostic evaluation by combining with a radioactive substance (radioimmunodetection).	For use in detecting and treating ovarian, breast, pancreatic, gastric, esophageal, and colorectal cancers. Used in purging tumor cells from bone marrow and peripheral blood prior to bone marrow transplantation. Treatment of cancers: • Non-Hodgkin's lymphoma • Metastatic breast cancer that overexpresses the HER2 oncogene (known to be associated with aggressive disease and decreased survival) • Leukemia (used in prevention of graft versus host disease (GVHD) after transplantation) • Metastatic colorectal cancer	Monitor CBC and differential. Monitor for signs of bleeding (e.g., bruising, bloody stool/urine, hypotension, tachycardia). Monitor for signs of infection (e.g., fever, increased sputum, dyspnea, urgency, and frequency). Implement neutropenic precautions as necessary. Monitor for signs of hypersensitivity reaction (changes in BP, rash, edema, facial flushing, dyspnea). Monitor for evidence of dehydration (e.g., concentrated urine, poor skin turgor, dry mucous membranes). Monitor electrolytes. Administer antiemetics as needed. Administer antidiarrheals as needed. Monitor for signs of decreased cardiac output or inadequate tissue perfusion (e.g., diaphoresis, pale color, poor-quality pulses, chest pain, edema, crackles, decreased urine output). Monitor renal function tests (e.g., creatinine, BUN, creatinine clearance). Encourage the use of oral saline rinses and avoiding the use of mouthwashes. Provide list of community resources for wigs, hats, caps, etc. Instruct patient about reproductive issues and provide resources as needed.
Antineoplastic Agents			
Alkylating agents: • Busulfan • Carboplatin • Chlorambucil • Cisplatin • Cyclophosphamide • Dacarbazine • Ifosfamide • Melphalan • Nitrogen mustard	Disrupt DNA replication and RNA transcription by cross-linking DNA strands. Cell cycle nonspecific.	Ovarian, breast, lung, testicular, and head and neck cancer. Multiple myeloma, leukemias, lymphoma, sarcoma.	Monitor CBC and differential. Monitor for signs of bleeding (e.g., bruising, bloody stool/urine, hypotension, tachycardia). Monitor for signs of infection (e.g., fever, increased sputum, dyspnea, urgency, and frequency). Implement neutropenic precautions as necessary. Monitor for evidence of dehydration (e.g., concentrated urine, poor skin turgor, dry mucous membranes). Monitor electrolytes. Administer antiemetics as needed. Administer antidiarrheals as needed. Encourage the use of oral saline rinses and avoiding the use of mouthwashes. Provide list of community resources for wigs, hats, caps, etc. Monitor for signs of seizures and implement seizure precautions. Monitor renal function tests (e.g., creatinine, BUN, creatinine clearance). Instruct patient to drink plenty of fluids prior to and during treatment. Administer bladder protectant as needed (Mesna). Instruct patient about reproductive issues and provide resources as needed.

PHARMACOLOGY Summary of Medications for Cancer Treatment—*Continued*

Medication Category	Action	Application/Indications	Nursing Responsibility
Nitrosoureas: • Carmustine (BCNU) • Lomustine (CCNU) • Semustine (methyl-CCNU) • Streptozocin	Block enzymes needed for synthesis of purine, resulting in immediate cell death. Similar actions to alkylating agents; cross blood–brain barrier. Cell cycle nonspecific.	Lymphomas, multiple myeloma, CNS tumors, malignant melanoma, pancreatic cancer.	Monitor CBC and differential. Monitor for signs of bleeding (e.g., bruising, bloody stool/urine, hypotension, tachycardia). Monitor for signs of infection (e.g., fever, increased sputum, dyspnea, urgency, and frequency). Implement neutropenic precautions as necessary. Monitor for evidence of dehydration (e.g., concentrated urine, poor skin turgor, dry mucous membranes). Monitor electrolytes. Administer antiemetics as needed. Instruct patient to drink plenty of fluids prior to treatment. Administer bladder protectant as needed (Mesna). Monitor renal function tests (e.g., creatinine, BUN, creatinine clearance). Monitor serum osmolarity and electrolytes. Monitor dyspnea and cough.
Antimetabolites: • Methotrexate (MTX) • Cytarabine (Ara-C) • Fluorouracil (5-FU) • Gemcitabine (Gemzar) • Hydroxyurea • Deoxycoformycin (pentostatin) • Capecitabine (Xeloda)	Hinder the synthesis of DNA by blocking the use of necessary enzymes. Cell cycle phase-specific (S phase).	Leukemias, lymphomas, myelodysplasia syndrome, breast and colon cancer.	Monitor CBC and differential. Monitor for signs of bleeding (e.g., bruising, bloody stool/urine, hypotension, tachycardia). Monitor for signs of infection (e.g., fever, increased sputum, dyspnea, urgency, and frequency). Implement neutropenic precautions as necessary. Monitor for evidence of dehydration (e.g., concentrated urine, poor skin turgor, dry mucous membranes). Monitor break in skin integrity (e.g., rashes, blistering on palms and feet). Monitor liver and renal function and electrolytes. Administer antiemetics as needed. Instruct patient to drink plenty of fluids prior to treatment. Encourage the use of saline rinses and avoiding the use of mouthwashes. Provide ice water during drug administration. Administer analgesics as needed. Provide list of community resources for wigs, hats, caps, etc. Encourage use of sunscreen year-round.

(continued)

MyNursingKit Animation: Drugs Methotrexate

PHARMACOLOGY Summary of Medications for Cancer Treatment—*Continued*

Medication Category	Action	Application/Indications	Nursing Responsibility
Antitumor antibiotics: • Bleomycin • Daunorubicin • Doxorubicin (Adriamycin) • Mitoxantrone	Interfere with function and synthesis of nucleic acids, resulting in disruption of RNA and DNA replication. Cell cycle nonspecific.	Various solid tumors. Lymphomas and acute lymphocytic leukemia.	For vesicants: IV push over 6–10 minutes, flushing with 75–100 mL solution. Monitor CBC and differential. Monitor for signs of bleeding (e.g., bruising, bloody stool/urine, hypotension, tachycardia). Monitor for signs of infection (e.g., fever, increased sputum, dyspnea, urgency, and frequency). Implement neutropenic precautions as necessary. Monitor for evidence of dehydration (e.g., concentrated urine, poor skin turgor, dry mucous membranes). Monitor electrolytes. Administer antiemetics as needed. Encourage the use of saline rinses and avoiding the use of mouthwashes. Provide ice water during drug administration. Administer analgesics as needed. Administer appetite stimulants as needed. Monitor for signs of decreased cardiac output or inadequate tissue perfusion (e.g., diaphoresis, pale color, poor-quality pulses, chest pain, edema, crackles, decreased urine output). Monitor for cough and dyspnea. Instruct patient about potential darkening of previously irradiated areas. Provide list of community resources for wigs, hats, caps, etc.
Plant alkaloids (Taxane): • Paclitaxel (Taxol) • Docetaxel (Taxotere)	Stabilize microtubule, which interferes with cell division. Cell cycle phase-specific (G_2 and M phase).	Breast, non–small cell lung, ovarian, and head and neck cancer.	For vesicants: IV push over 6–10 minutes, flushing with 75–100 mL solution. Premedicate with diphenhydramine, cimetidine, and dexamethasone. Monitor for signs of hypersensitivity reaction (changes in BP, rash, edema, facial flushing, dyspnea). Monitor neurological status (motor weakness, paresthesia). Provide list of community resources for wigs, hats, caps, etc. Monitor CBC and differential. Monitor for signs of bleeding (e.g., bruising, bloody stool/urine, hypotension, tachycardia). Monitor for signs of infection (e.g., fever, increased sputum, dyspnea, urgency, and frequency). Implement neutropenic precautions as necessary. Instruct patient to allow for frequent rest periods and to cluster activities as possible. Administer analgesics as needed. Monitor for signs of decreased cardiac output or inadequate tissue perfusion (e.g., diaphoresis, pale color, poor-quality pulses, chest pain, edema, crackles, decreased urine output).

PHARMACOLOGY Summary of Medications for Cancer Treatment—*Continued*

Medication Category	Action	Application/Indications	Nursing Responsibility
Plant alkaloids (vinca alkaloids): • Vinorelbine (Navelbine) • Vincristine • Vinblastine	Inhibit mitosis, resulting in immediate cell death (cytocidal). Cell cycle phase-specific (M phase).	Breast, testicular, small-cell lung, ovarian, and head and neck cancers. Lymphomas, acute lymphocytic leukemia (ALL), Chronic Myelogenous leukemia (CML).	For vesicants: IV push over 6–10 minutes, flushing with 75–100 mL solution. Monitor for local skin changes. Monitor CBC and differential. Monitor for signs of bleeding (e.g., bruising, bloody stool/urine, hypotension, tachycardia). Monitor for signs of infection (e.g., fever, increased sputum, dyspnea, urgency, and frequency). Implement neutropenic precautions as necessary. Monitor neurological status (motor weakness, paresthesia). Monitor liver function tests. Administer laxatives, stool softeners. Administer analgesics as needed. Provide list of community resources for wigs, hats, caps, etc.
Plant alkaloids (camptothecins): • Irinotecan • Topotecan	Alter DNA structure by inhibiting topoisomerase I. Cell cycle phase-specific (S phase).	Colorectal, non–small cell lung, and ovarian cancer. ALL.	Monitor CBC and differential. Monitor for signs of bleeding (e.g., bruising, bloody stool/urine, hypotension, tachycardia). Monitor for signs of infection (e.g., fever, increased sputum, dyspnea, urgency, and frequency). Implement neutropenic precautions as necessary. Administer atropine as needed to reduce cholinergic-induced diarrhea. Monitor for signs of dehydration (e.g., concentrated urine, poor skin turgor, dry mucous membranes). Provide list of community resources for wigs, hats, caps, etc.
Plant alkaloids (epipodophyllotoxins): • Etoposide (VP-16) • Teniposide (VM-26)	Irreversible blocking of cells during premitotic phases, resulting in destruction of DNA strands. Interferes with topoisomerase II enzyme reaction. Cell cycle phase-specific (late G_2 and S phase).	Breast, testicular, and small-cell lung cancer. Lymphomas, ALL, and multiple myeloma.	Monitor CBC and differential. Monitor for signs of bleeding (e.g., bruising, bloody stool/urine, hypotension, tachycardia). Monitor for signs of infection (e.g., fever, increased sputum, dyspnea, urgency, and frequency). Implement neutropenic precautions as necessary. Monitor for evidence of dehydration (e.g., concentrated urine, poor skin turgor, dry mucous membranes). Monitor electrolytes. Administer antiemetics as needed. Monitor blood pressure throughout infusion. Monitor for signs of anaphylaxis (changes in BP, rash, edema, facial flushing). Provide list of community resources for wigs, hats, caps, etc.

(continued)

Medication Category	Action	Application/Indications	Nursing Responsibility
Hormonal Therapy Glucocorticoids: • Prednisone • Hydrocortisone • Solu-Medrol • Dexamethasone Estrogens: • Diethylstilbestrol (DES) • Estramustine (Emcyt) • Estradiol (Estrace) Antiestrogens: • Tamoxifen Estrogen receptor antagonists: • Fulvestrant (Faslodex) Nonsteroidal aromatase inhibitors: • Anastrozole (Arimidex) Steroidal aromatase inhibitors: • Exemestane (Aromasin) Luteinizing hormone-releasing hormone (LHRH) analog • Leuprolide (Lupron) Nonsteroid antiestrogen: • Bicalutamide (Casodex) • Flutamide (Eulexin)	Interfere with proteins and hormone receptors throughout the cell cycle. Cell cycle nonspecific.	Prostate, breast, and endometrial cancers.	Monitor CBC and differential. Monitor for signs of infection (e.g., fever, increased sputum, dyspnea, urgency, and frequency). Implement neutropenic precautions as necessary. Monitor blood pressure. Instruct the patient to lower sodium intake. Instruct the patient to observe for swelling in the ankles, lower extremities, and hands. Instruct the patient to avoid discontinuing medication unless advised by health care provider. Instruct patient about signs of feminization and masculinization.
Miscellaneous: • Asparaginase (Elspar) • Bortezomib (Velcade) • Hydroxyurea • Imatinib mesylate (Gleevec)	Inhibit protein synthesis. Inhibit chymotrypsin-like activity of 25S proteasome. Act on S phase as an antimetabolite. Inhibit proliferation and induce apoptosis.	ALL. Multiple myeloma. Chronic myelogenous leukemia, melanoma, and head and neck cancer. Chronic myelogenous leukemia in blast crisis or chronic phase with failure of interferon.	Monitor CBC and differential. Monitor for signs of bleeding (e.g., bruising, bloody stool/urine, hypotension, tachycardia). Monitor for signs of infection (e.g., fever, increased sputum, dyspnea, urgency, and frequency). Implement neutropenic precautions as necessary. Monitor for evidence of dehydration (e.g., concentrated urine, poor skin turgor, dry mucous membranes). Monitor electrolytes. Monitor for signs of hypersensitivity reaction (changes in BP, rash, edema, facial flushing, dyspnea). Administer antiemetics as needed. Administer analgesics as needed (e.g., nonopioids for neuropathic pain). Administer laxatives as needed. Monitor level of sedation and implement safety measures as needed. Encourage the use of saline rinses and avoiding the use of mouthwashes. Provide ice water during drug administration.

Sources: Bender, C., & Rosenzweig, M. (2004). Cancer. In S. Lewis, M. Heitkemper, & S. Dirksen (Eds.), *Medical–surgical nursing assessment and management of clinical problems* (6th ed.). St. Louis: Mosby; Rokita, S. (2004). Oncology: Nursing management in cancer care. In S. Smeltzer & B. Bare (Eds.), *Brunner & Suddarth's textbook of medical–surgical nursing* (10th ed.). Philadelphia: Lippincott Williams & Wilkins; Viele, C. (2005). Keys to unlock cancer: Targeted therapy. *Oncology Nursing Forum, 32*(5).

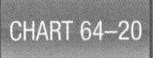

CHART 64–20   Safe Handling of Chemotherapeutic Drugs

Drug Preparation

Prepare in a biological safety cabinet (BSC):

- Vented system to outside environment
- Provide vertical laminar airflow to carry contaminated air away from BSC operator
- Blower that operates continuously
- Located in low traffic area
- Used only with trained individuals.

Handwashing prior to donning personal protective equipment (PPE).

Wear appropriate (PPE):

- Gloves that are powder free with long cuffs (change every 30 minutes)
- Gowns
- Face shields or goggles
- PPE should be replaced if torn, punctured, or soiled.

Use plastic-backed sterile absorbent pad on work surface.

Maintain sterile technique.

Use appropriate technique when opening ampules.

When reconstituting drugs in vials, use dispensing pins with venting devices to avoid aerosolization.

Use tubing and syringes with Luer-lock fittings.

Avoid overfilling of syringes.

Prime all tubing with normal saline or dextrose prior to adding cytotoxic drug.

Label each container "Cytotoxic Drug."

Place container in sealed bag before transport.

Dispose of all material that has come into contact with cytotoxic drug into appropriate receptacle.

Drug Administration

Explain to patient that protective wear minimizes the exposure of health care providers to the harmful effects of chemotherapeutic drugs.

Wear appropriate PPE.

Implement High Alert Medication Safety practice.

Administer drugs in a safe and unhurried environment, working at eye level.

Use Luer-lock fittings on all intravenous tubing, needles, and syringes used for delivery of cytotoxic drugs.

Place disposable, absorbent, plastic-backed pad under work area to collect droplets of the drug.

Implement standard precautions when handing the blood, vomitus, or excreta of a patient who has received cytotoxic drugs within the last 48 hours.

Disposal of Supplies and Drugs

Do not recap needles or break syringes.

Placed all used supplies in a leak proof, puncture proof, labeled container.

Keep containers in all areas where preparation and administration of cytotoxic drugs occur.

Environmental service personnel trained in safe handling procedures should remove containers.

Personnel should wear appropriate PPE.

Containers should be disposed of according to regulations of hazardous wastes.

In home situations:

- Place containers in an area away from children and pets until retrieved by appropriate agency.
- Check county and state regulations.

Arrange with medical supply company, health care provider's office, or private waste management company for proper disposal.

Sources: Occupational Safety and Health Administration, Office of Occupational Medicine. (1995). *Controlling occupational exposure to hazardous CPL2-2.20B CH-4.* Washington, DC: U.S. Department of Labor; Singleton, L., & Connor, T. (1999). An evaluation of the permeability of chemotherapy gloves to three cancer chemotherapy drugs. *Oncology Nursing Forum, 26*(4); The Joint Commision, (2008). *High Alert Medication: Strategies for Improving Safety,* Joint Commission Resources.

Agency policy will identify nursing actions required once symptoms of extravasation have been recognized. Oftentimes IV drugs are delivered via central vascular access devices. Refer to Chapter 22 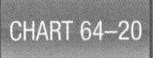 for detailed information on these types of devices along with the nursing implications.

Chemotherapy Side Effects and Toxicities

Chemotherapy produces effects on both normal cells and cancer cells. Side effects or toxic effects are the result of the destruction of normal cells that produce specific signs and symptoms and are classified as acute, delayed, or chronic. Chart 64–22 (p. 2112) lists the effects found in each category (Bender & Rosenzweig, 2004). Cells with rapid growth rates are more susceptible to damage, resulting in noticeable signs and symptoms. Examples of cells affected by this process are epithelium, bone marrow, hair follicles, and sperm. The body will respond to the products of cellular destruction by demonstrating fatigue, anorexia, and taste alterations.

Gastrointestinal System Effects

Nausea and vomiting are the most common gastrointestinal (GI) side effects. Within 1 hour of therapy commencing the patient may experience vomiting that may last up to 24 hours or more. Drugs that can reduce or eliminate nausea and vomiting are an essential part of the treatment plan for patients receiving chemotherapeutic agents and may be given prior to therapy starting and for several days after it ends. Antiemetics include serotonin blockers, which block serotonin receptors located in the GI tract and chemoreceptor trigger zone (CTZ) in the medulla, dopaminergic blockers that block dopamine receptors of the CTZ, phenothiazines, sedatives, corticosteroids, and histamines. The latter four agents are commonly used in combination with serotonin blockers when patients receive chemotherapeutic drugs that have increased emetic potential (Bremerkamp, 2000).

Nurses are responsible for being aware of the types of drugs their patients are receiving so they can anticipate what interventions may be needed to relieve suffering from nausea and vomiting. Some patients will require antiemetic therapy for several days after chemotherapy and need to be encouraged to comply with their prescribed medication regime to lessen the emetic effects of the chemotherapy. Other interventions such as relaxation techniques, guided imagery, and altering the patient's diet may also assist in reducing nausea and vomiting.

CHART 64–21   **Routes of Administration**

Route		Nursing Implications
Oral	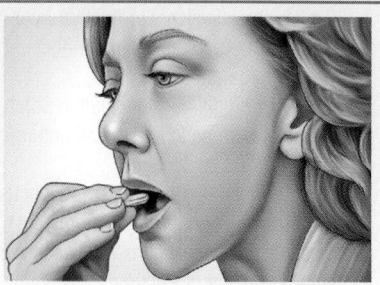	• Educate the patient about the significance of complying with prescribed schedule, optimal dosing, and patient safety. • Devise educational strategies such as individualized medication sheets to reinforce information. • Educate the patient about strategies to reduce potential for side effects (e.g., taking drugs with emetic potential with meals, taking drugs that require adequate fluid intake early in the day). • Coordinate educational sessions with oncologist and pharmacist since nurses may have minimal patient contact.
Subcutaneous	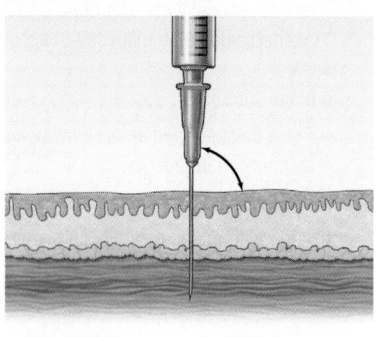	• Educate the patient and/or caregiver to give injections and allow for return demonstration. • Encourage patient to rotate injection sites and keep written log.
Intramuscular	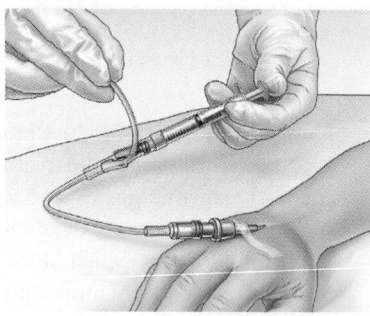	Same as subcutaneous.
Intravenous (may be given via central venous catheters or peripheral venous access) • Push • Piggyback • Side-arm • Infusion 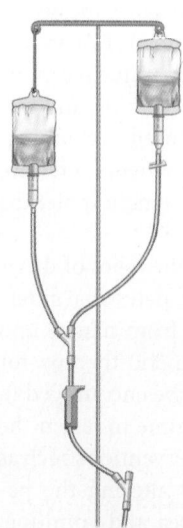	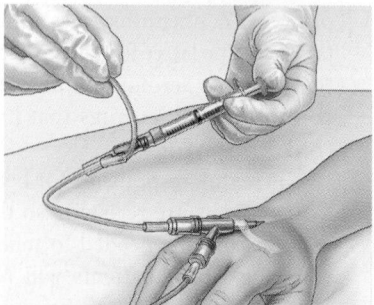 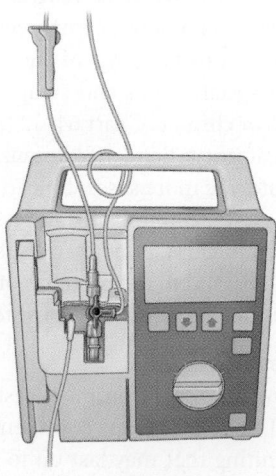	• Administered directly into vein via a syringe. • Administered using a secondary bag and tubing while primary infusion is running concurrently. • Administered into the side port of a running IV infusion. • Drug is added to appropriate size IV bag. • All medications administered via the IV route should have the blood return of the vein evaluated at regular intervals during the infusion (as determined by agency policy).

CHART 64–21 | **Routes of Administration—*Continued***

Route		Nursing Implications
Topical	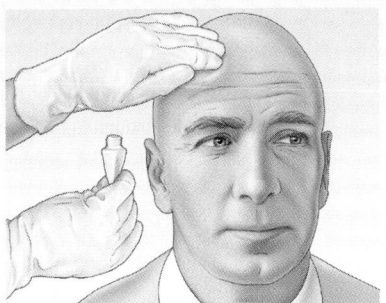	• Educate the patient to cover surface area with thin layer of medication, then wear loose-fitting clothing. • Wear gloves during application and perform hand hygiene after procedure. • Educate the patient to avoid touching the medication.
Intracavitary	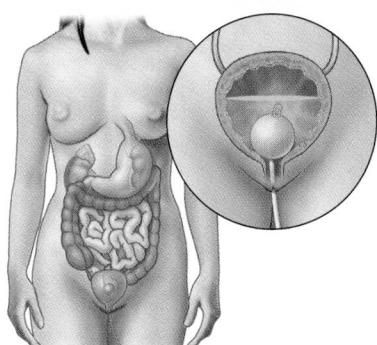	• Instill medication into either the bladder (via a catheter) or the pleural cavity (via a chest tube). • Administer premedication to reduce local irritation.
Intrathecal	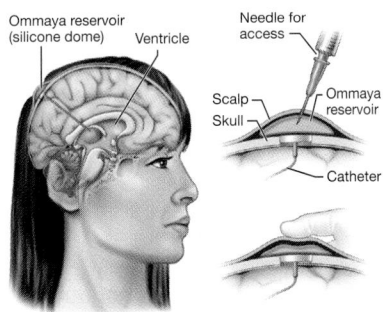	• An Ommaya reservoir, which is subcutaneously implanted, is used to gain access to ventricular cerebrospinal fluid (CSF). • Used to treat cancers that metastasize to central nervous system (CNS) (breast, lung, GI, leukemia, and lymphoma). • Does not depend on diffusion to move drug into CSF. • May last months to years without complications. • Sterile technique used throughout procedure. • Usually administered by a health care provider. • Evaluate for neurotoxicities.
Intra-arterial	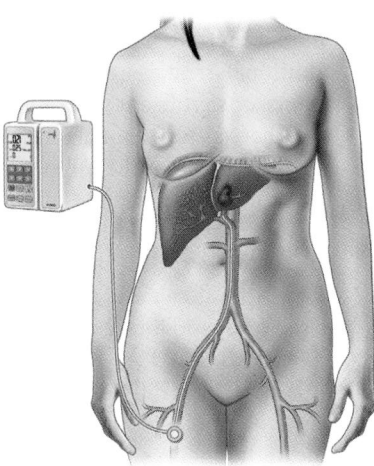	• Catheter placement into artery near inoperable tumor (liver, bladder, brain, head and neck, cervix, and bone). • Use infusion pump. • Monitor vital signs, color and temperature of extremity, and signs of local bleeding throughout therapy. • Monitor appropriate laboratory studies (e.g., liver function tests) for organ toxicity. • Educate patient about the care of the catheter and pump if to be used at home.

(continued)

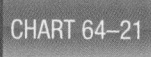

CHART 64–21	Routes of Administration—*Continued*

Route	Nursing Implications
Intraperitoneal 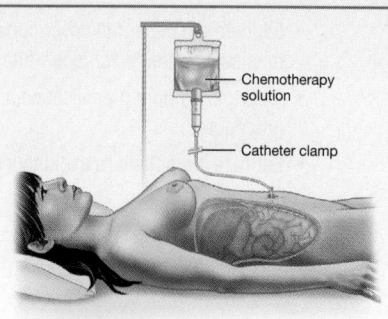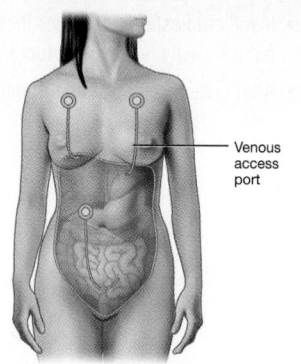	• Administration of drug via implantable port or external suprapubic catheter into the abdominal cavity. • Used typically for peritoneal metastases due to ovarian cancer. • Heat infusate solution to body temperature prior to infusing. • Infuse 1–2 liters of fluid and allow to "dwell" for 1–4 hours before draining. • Monitor for abdominal pressure, pain, fever, and electrolyte imbalance after infusing. • Measure abdominal girth.

Sources: Barber, F., & Fabugais-Nazario, L. (2003). What's old is new again: Patients receiving hepatic arterial infusion chemotherapy. *Clinical Journal of Oncology Nursing, 7*(6); Bender, C., & Rosenzweig, M. (2004). Cancer. In S. Lewis, M. Heitkemper, & S. Dirksen (Eds.), *Medical–surgical nursing assessment and management of clinical problems* (6th ed.). St. Louis: Mosby; Booker, M. (1996a). Arterial therapy. In M. Booker & D. Ignatavicius (Eds.), *Infusion therapy techniques and medications* (1st ed.). Philadelphia: W. B. Saunders; Booker, M. (1996b). Central nervous system therapy. In M. Booker & D. Ignatavicius (Eds.), *Infusion therapy techniques and medications* (1st ed.). Philadelphia: W. B. Saunders; Hartigan, K. (2003). Patient education: The cornerstone of successful oral chemotherapy treatment. *Clinical Journal of Oncology Nursing, 7*(6); Markam, M., & Walker, J. (2006). Intraperitoneal chemotherapy of ovarian cancer: A review with a focus on practical aspects of treatment. *Journal of Clinical Oncology, 24*(6).

CHART 64–22	Classification of Chemotherapy Toxicities

Classification	Toxicity
Acute	Vomiting Allergic reactions Cardiac arrhythmias
Delayed	Mucositis: • Mouth sores • Gastritis • Diarrhea Alopecia Bone marrow suppression
Chronic	Cardiac damage: • Reduced contractility Pulmonary damage: • Fibrosis and scarring Hepatic damage: • Elevated liver enzyme tests Renal damage: • Elevated creatinine and BUN

Monitoring for signs of fluid volume deficit and electrolyte imbalances should be ongoing nursing actions, and abnormal findings need to be reported to the health care provider so that additional treatment can be started in order to reduce the chance of significant weight loss and malnutrition.

Other gastrointestinal (GI) toxicities are due to the rapid rate of proliferation of the cells that line the GI tract. These include stomatitis (inflammation of the oral cavity), anorexia, mucositis (inflammation of the mucosal lining), and diarrhea. Constipation can occur in some patients receiving chemotherapeutic agents that slow motility of the large intestine and may be due to reduced food intake secondary to persistent nausea and vomiting (ONS, 2001).

Pancreatitis (inflammation of the pancreas) occurs with certain types of chemotherapeutic agents, radiotherapy to the left side of the abdomen, diabetes, tumor lysis syndrome (TLS), and the presence of intrahepatic catheters (ONS, 2001). Common signs and symptoms include abdominal pain, fever, tachycardia, and nausea and vomiting. When a patient is suspected of having pancreatitis, the nurse should review laboratory data for elevated serum amylase and lipase and hypoglycemia. Pancreatitis, if not successfully treated, can put the patient at risk for developing shock leading to possible death. Nurses administering chemotherapy agents known to cause pancreatitis should be alert to potential signs and symptoms and collaborate with the oncologist to begin prompt treatment.

Although not real common, hepatotoxicity occurs due to the direct toxic effect to the liver as a result of the metabolism of antineoplastic drugs. The likelihood of developing liver dysfunction related to chemotherapy is increased if the patient has a history of prior infections or damage (cirrhosis, hepatitis), cancer of the liver, radiotherapy to the right side of the abdomen, history of alcoholism, intrahepatic chemotherapy, and advancing age (Ludwig et al., 1999). Clinical findings associated with hepatotoxicity are those consistent with liver dysfunction, including jaundice, ascites, fatigue, malaise, anorexia, nausea and vomiting, right upper quadrant pain, dark orange urine, and bleeding tendencies. In addition, laboratory data used to determine hepatic function such as liver function tests and coagulation studies will be abnormal.

Genitourinary System Effects

A few chemotherapy agents damage kidneys due to the accumulation of end products after cell lysis and the direct effect during excretion. Chemotherapy can cause tumors to undergo rapid cell lysis, which causes an increase in uric acid production and urinary excretion resulting in kidney damage. In addition, the release of intracellular contents in the circulation causes increased levels of serum potassium and phosphates and decreased levels of serum calcium. Nurses need to be aware of the renal effect of the chemotherapy agent being administered and monitor serum blood urea nitrogen (BUN), creatinine, electrolytes, and creatinine clearance. Abnormal findings need to be reported to the health care provider so adjustments in drug dosing can be considered. Prevention of uric acid crystals can be accomplished by ensuring adequate hydration, alkalinization of the urine, and administering drugs aimed at reducing serum uric acid.

Hemorrhagic cystitis is bladder mucosal damage occurring as a result of inflammation and irritation from the metabolism of by-products of chemotherapeutic agents. The development of hemorrhagic cystitis is associated with administration of certain alkylating agents and prior radiotherapy to the pelvis or bladder. Nurses need to be alert to the few, but important, signs and symptoms that may produce suffering for most of these patients. These include dysuria, frequency, nocturia, oliguria, and hematuria.

Cardiopulmonary System Effects

Certain chemotherapeutic agents have toxic effects on the cardiopulmonary system that may produce permanent functional changes for the patient. Patients who are to receive antitumor antibiotics should have a cardiac evaluation prior to treatment to determine baseline cardiac function. During therapy the nurse needs to monitor for heart failure and signs of decreased cardiac output. A decrease in pulmonary function is a lifelong effect associated with long-term chemotherapy. Nurses need to evaluate the patient for changes in pulmonary function, including pulmonary function tests (Rokita, 2004).

Hematopoietic System Effects

The majority of chemotherapy agents cause a disruption in the normal functioning of the immune system. *Myelosuppression* is the term used to define a depression of bone marrow function. WBCs, RBCs, and platelets are susceptible to bone marrow suppression from chemotherapy. Neutropenia (reduced neu-

trophils) and thrombocytopenia (reduced platelets) along with the presence of anemia (reduced hemoglobin and hematocrit) are the main factors that limit the doses of chemotherapy given to a patient (Rokita, 2004).

Neutropenia is defined as a reduction in the number of circulating neutrophils, whereas leukopenia is defined as a reduction in the number of circulating WBCs. The importance of monitoring the neutrophils in those patients receiving chemotherapy lies in their ability to protect the host from bacterial invasion. Assessing the laboratory data includes monitoring the WBC count and calculating the **absolute neutrophil count (ANC)**. Calculation of the ANC is done by multiplying the WBC by the total percentage of neutrophils (polys and bands):

Example:

Laboratory result: WBC = 1,600 polys = 48%; bands = 5%

Calculation: Polys (48%) + bands (5%) = 53%

WBC (1,600) × polys and bands (53%) = 848.

An ANC of less than 500 is considered to put the patient at severe risk of infection (Otto, 2001a). It is important for the nurse to understand that neutropenia can occur when the total WBC is within normal range; therefore, knowing the ANC allows a correct assessment of the neutrophil status.

The term **nadir** refers to the point at which the lowest blood count is reached. Oncology nurses understand that when a patient receives chemotherapy, the nadir occurs approximately 7 to 10 days after treatment, at which point the patient is most susceptible to infection. Providing ongoing patient education regarding the signs of infection and when to report findings to the health care provider is critical. A detailed discussion of nursing management of patients experiencing side effects from chemotherapy is found in the Nursing Process: Care Plan for Cancer feature earlier in this chapter (p. 2089).

 When caring for patients receiving chemotherapy or biotherapy, the nurse should evaluate the laboratory data to determine the presence of anemia, thrombocytopenia, and neutropenia. Calculation of the ANC will provide the most accurate picture of the patient's risk for infection. The nurse should notify the health care provider immediately if the patient demonstrates signs of infection.

The availability of drugs used to stimulate the bone marrow has allowed patients to continue with chemotherapy despite the associated side effects. Granulocyte colony-stimulating factor (G-CSF) and granulocyte-macrophage colony-stimulating factor (GM-CSF) stimulate the bone marrow to produce WBCs at a more rapid pace in order to reduce the duration of neutropenia. Erythropoietin (Epogen, Procrit) is used to increase the production of RBCs, thus playing a pivotal role in preventing the anemia-induced symptoms associated with chemotherapy. The benefit of administering these agents is a reduction of the incidence of infection that allows for continuing the prescribed chemotherapeutic drug regime.

Reproductive System Effects

Both testicular and ovarian functions can be affected by antineoplastic drug therapy. Sterility and early menopause are risks a patient needs to be aware of prior to receiving chemotherapy. Males may experience an absence of spermatozoa that can be either permanent or temporary. Men should be offered the option to bank sperm prior to the start of treatment to prevent damage to sperm or sterility. Education for both patients and their partners about the potential risk to reproductive functions and appropriate protection behaviors (e.g., reliable birth control) should be provided prior to beginning therapy (Rokita, 2004).

Neurological System Effects

Neurological effects are usually reversible and disappear after completion of chemotherapy treatments. Toxicities can arise as direct or indirect damage to the central nervous system (CNS), peripheral nervous system, cranial nerves, or a combination of the three. Peripheral neuropathies, loss of reflexes, hearing loss due to damage of the acoustic nerve, and paralytic ileus are examples of the more commonly occurring effects. The nurse needs to educate the patient and family about the importance of patient safety, detection of signs and symptoms, when to notify the health care provider of evidence of toxicity, and referrals for coping strategies.

General Effects

The incidence of fatigue has been identified in research frequently enough to consider it as a major concern in cancer symptom management (Nail, 2004). Fatigue is one of the many side effects seen during cancer therapy that can affect a person's ability to function. Several factors contribute to the degree of fatigue experienced by patients receiving chemotherapy. These include immobility, malnutrition, stress, lack of sleep, anemia, hypoxia, infection or febrile states, pain, and multiple cancer therapies (e.g., biotherapy, chemotherapy, radiation therapy, and surgery). The nurse needs to encourage patients to balance activity and rest, optimize nutritional intake, and consider physical therapy consultation if necessary.

Nursing Management

Managing patients with cancer undergoing chemotherapy is complex and challenging. Nurses must be able to perform assessments that include the immune status, pain control, hemodynamic stability, and emotional coping. The ability to differentiate between toxic effects (e.g., heart failure), which can be irreversible, and expected side effects (nausea and vomiting), most of which can be managed successfully with other drugs, is one of the unique features of an oncology assessment.

The Nursing Process: Care Plan for Cancer feature earlier in this chapter (p. 2089) identifies the appropriate nursing diagnosis and provides a detailed plan of care for the oncology patient regardless of the type of treatment being given.

Collaborative Management

The use of a multidisciplinary oncology team that effectively collaborates to achieve quality patient care is essential. The diagnosis of cancer holds many emotions and experiences for both the patient and family. A plan of care needs to consider the patient's ability to tolerate diagnostic efforts, treatment recommendations, and long-term recovery. Depending on multiple variables, cancer tends to be a disease that is chronic in nature. Patients will demonstrate signs and symptoms relative to where they are in their disease trajectory and treatment plan. Each member of the team (health care providers, nurses, physical therapists, occupational therapists, speech therapists, social workers, psychiatrists/psychologists, pharmacists, and spiritual counselors) provides an expertise that will afford the patient and family the opportunity to optimize their quality of life throughout each phase of their disease.

Biotherapy

Biotherapy (biologic therapy) is known as treatment with agents whose origin, mostly mammal, is from biological sources and/or affecting biological responses (Oldham, 1991). Historically, cancer treatment has included surgery, radiotherapy, and chemotherapy, or a combination of all three therapies. Biotherapy has emerged since the 1980s as another treatment option for cancer patients receiving high-dose chemotherapy and transplantation. Nurses caring for patients receiving biotherapy need to possess an understanding of the immune system before they can begin to comprehend the rationale behind this unique treatment modality and the primary agents currently used. Refer to Chapters 59 💿 and 60 💿 for a review of the immune system. Although the mechanism of action varies with each type of biologic response modifier (BRM), the goal is the same: to destroy or halt the malignant growth of a tumor. A therapeutic effect is accomplished by altering the immunologic relationship between the tumor and the host (patient) (Rokita, 2004). Direct antitumor effects, restoration, augmentation, or modulation of host immune system mechanisms, and disrupting tumor cells' ability to metastasize or differentiate may affect host and tumor response. In addition, these agents, specifically monoclonal antibodies (MAbs), are used in diagnosing cancer by using low-dose radioisotopes tagged to MAbs that can detect tumors using special scanning equipment (Gale, 2005).

The popularity of biotherapy research has led to the development of nonspecific immunomodulating agents and new agents that include monoclonal antibodies, hematopoietic growth factors, interferons (INF), and interleukins. The latter three agents are part of a group of agents called cytokines, which are protein products from cells that function as cell regulators to enhance the production and functioning of the immune system. For example, lymphokines are products of lymphocytes and monokines are products of monocytes; interleukins are proteins that act as messengers between cells. Cytokines are described in Chapter 60 💿. Nonspecific agents surfaced when early research identified Bacille-Calmette-Guerin (BCG) and *Corynebacterium parvum*. When injected into humans these agents work as antigens that stimulate the immune response, which should destroy malignant cells. Very positive outcomes have been demonstrated with multiple trials on animal and human models. BCG is known to be effective as a treatment for localized bladder cancer and appears to have promise in the treatment for malignant melanoma.

The Pharmacology Summary chart presented earlier (p. 2103) in this chapter lists biotherapy (and chemotherapy) agents along with specific clinical indicators, administration information, and side effects. Only agents approved for use by the Food and Drug Administration (FDA) are discussed; however, it is important to realize that multiple agents are under investigation that may be determined to be beneficial for use in patients with cancer in the future.

Side effects discussed in this chapter are those generally common to all agents. When administering biotherapy agents it is the responsibility of the nurse to know the specific agent being given and become familiar with side effects specific to that drug. If side effects are not treated successfully or become too burdensome to the patient, the therapy may be dose limiting. Other concerns when administering biologic therapy include safe handling of the drugs (determined by agency policy), rate of administration, and length of time stable once reconstituted according to the manufacturer's package insert, the need for special infusion filters or equipment, and the compatibility with other medications.

Oncology nurses are becoming more familiar with administering BRMs as more agents become available for commercial use. Nurses caring for patients receiving biotherapy need to be familiar with many unique details and should be comfortable and excited with a field of cancer treatment that is rapidly changing. Nurses must have the motivation to expand their knowledge and understanding of new treatment options for cancer patients because new discoveries are frequently being made. Nurses should gain much satisfaction from being involved with developing new standards of care and mentoring new nurses in the field of cancer nursing.

■ Nursing Management

Biotherapy agents differ from chemotherapeutic agents in action and toxicity patterns, but at the same time share many of the same side effects. Nurses can use their knowledge of chemotherapy-induced side effects to assist them in planning care for those patients receiving biotherapy. A comprehensive plan of care encompasses the patient's physical and psychological needs (refer to the Nursing Process: Care Plan for Cancer, p. 2089).

Transplantation: Bone Marrow and Peripheral Blood Stem Cell

Survival rates for cancer patients have improved due to treatments such as surgery, radiotherapy, and chemotherapy. Despite this promising outcome, many cancers that initially respond to therapy tend to reappear. **Bone marrow transplantation (BMT)** offers patients the ability to receive intensive chemotherapy or radiation therapy when resistance to or failure of standard treatment occurs (Bender & Rosenzweig, 2004). BMT is the transfer of hematopoietic cells from the bone marrow of one person into another person and has been used to treat a variety of diseases. Another option, **peripheral blood stem cell (PBSC) transplantation**, is becoming more widely used in lieu of the traditional bone marrow transplantation. Long-term survival is improved with both forms of treatment, making transplantation one of the most promising cancer therapies.

Transplantation has been performed for more than a century, but only since the mid-1960s have the chances of survival really improved. In the 19th century bone marrow was fed or injected into patients with grim results; however, significant progress has been made with the discovery of human leukocyte antigen (HLA) typing (discussed in Chapter 60), antirejection medications, and antibiotics.

Indications for Transplantation
The majority of transplants are performed for malignant disorders, although success has been demonstrated for use in patients with nonmalignant diseases (Keller, 2001). Several factors determine the type of transplant that will provide the best chances for survival. These include type and stage of disease, patient's age and performance status, and donor availability.

Types of Bone Marrow Transplantation
The types of BMT are based on the where the donor cells originate (see Chart 64–23). **Autologous BMT**, which comes from the recipient, is used for disorders where the patient's bone marrow has adequate stem cells that can produce functioning erythrocytes, leukocytes, and platelets. The patient's own bone marrow or stem cells are harvested and placed into frozen storage to be reinfused into the patient when the conditioning regime (chemotherapy or radiation with chemotherapy) is completed (Keller, 2001). In the past decade more autologous BMTs have been performed, typically for hematologic malignancies. **Allogeneic bone marrow**, which is from a histocompatible donor, is used for patients with hematologic malignancies, marrow failure, severe combined immunodeficiency syndrome (SCIDS), and certain inherited metabolic disorders. The majority of allogeneic transplants are done for acute myelogenous leukemia (AML), acute lymphocytic leukemia (ALL), and chronic myelogenous leukemia (CML).

Sources of Transplantation
In 1987 the National Marrow Donor Program (NMDP) was established to allow for easier access to unrelated donors. The registry contains more than 4 million individuals who have had tissue typing and expressed a desire to donate bone marrow. In 1999 the NMDP established a central registry of cord blood banks so that transplant centers could search for these donors more easily. When a donor is chosen they do not know who will be the recipient nor does the recipient know who has made such a generous donation.

Peripheral Blood Stem Cells
Traditionally, stem cells have been harvested from within the bone marrow cavity. The use of stem cells in peripherally circulating blood was first performed in the late 1950s (Santos, 2000). It has become more common since effectiveness was demonstrated in 1986 (Voss, Armitage, & Kessinger, 1993). Currently,

CHART 64–23	**Types of Bone Marrow Transplants**

Type	Origin
Allogeneic	• Syngeneic: identical twin
	• Related: blood relative, usually sibling
	• Unrelated: located by National Bone Marrow Registry or Cord Blood Registry
Autologous	• Patient

the use of PBSC transplantation for hematopoietic support following high-dose chemotherapy is the standard of practice for several malignant and nonmalignant diseases.

Autologous PBSC collection involves two phases: mobilization and apheresis. Mobilization involves stimulating the production of PBSCs with the administration of G-CSF or GM-CSF, possibly with chemotherapy. Apheresis is the collection of PBSCs through a double-lumen central venous catheter that is placed into the patient. Blood is run through a cell separator that is programmed to collect either lymphocytes or low-density leukocytes and return other blood components to the patient. Apheresis usually takes one to three sessions each lasting 3 to 4 hours. When the collection is completed the stem cells are placed into a blood bag and cryopreserved and remain frozen at −196°C until needed for transplantation.

Allogeneic PBSC collection involves the same phases as discussed for autologous transplantation. The donor receives G-CSF for approximately 4 to 5 days, which is adequate for mobilization. Side effects that may be experienced by the donor include bone pain, headache, fatigue, nausea, and insomnia (VanBurik & Weisdorf, 1999). Apheresis is usually done via a peripheral line inserted into the antecubital veins using the cell separator. Nurses need to instruct the donor about the importance of keeping follow-up doctor appointments since the most significant side effect is a drop in platelet count of up to 50%, which places the donor at risk for bleeding.

Bone Marrow Harvesting

The process of obtaining bone marrow for transplantation is called harvesting. For an autologous donor the procedure would occur in the operating room, likely under general anesthesia. Multiple punctures are made in the posterior or anterior iliac crest to obtain the necessary amount (500 to 700 mL) of marrow needed for transplant. Once the marrow is obtained it is mixed with heparin, filtered to remove bone fragments and fat, and placed into a blood bag. At this point, the bone marrow is purged, which is the process of removing any remaining malignant cells from the marrow. Once the purging step is completed, the marrow is placed into a blood bag and frozen just like PBSCs.

Allogeneic bone marrow harvesting involves the same process as autologous harvesting, minus the purging. After the marrow is harvested from the donor, it is immediately transfused into the recipient. Nursing care of the donor includes routine postoperative care. In addition, donors need to be informed that they may expect pain at the donor sites for approximately 1 week. This pain is usually remedied by nonnarcotic analgesics. The psychological and emotional needs of donors are equally as important as their physical needs. Nurses need to encourage them to express their concerns related to the success or failure of the transplant and provide support as needed.

Umbilical Cord Blood

Collection and storage of umbilical cord blood (UCB), which is rich in stem cells, is the newest innovation in transplantation (Keller, 2001). Cord blood is obtained by withdrawing blood via the umbilical vein immediately after the umbilical cord has been clamped. The blood is then cryopreserved similar to that of PBSCs or bone marrow. Because the use of UCB is a new approach in transplantation, it is unclear how the long-term effect regarding relapse of the disease rate will be demonstrated. In addition, there are ethical issues specific to the use of UCB such as the timing of consent and identifying links between mother and baby, which may be the focus of clinical, ethical, and regulatory scrutiny.

The Transplantation Process

Selection of the appropriate donor and recipient is crucial so graft rejection and other serious complications are avoided. Criteria for the selection of a marrow or stem cell donor are few, but very important. First, histocompatibility as measured by HLA and mixed lymphocyte culture (MLC) testing must be determined. The donor's health status is evaluated to minimize the risks associated with donating and to prevent infecting the recipient with diseases such as hepatitis and HIV. Next, the donor's psychosocial profile is evaluated in an attempt to predict her attitudes and feelings toward the procedure and unknown outcomes. Finally, the donor's age is taken into consideration due to the amount of marrow needed for transplantation. Younger donors tend to be smaller in size, which limits the amount of marrow available for harvest (Keller, 2001).

A multidisciplinary approach is needed to evaluate the patient prior to receiving either bone marrow or stem cells. The pretransplant management consists of a detailed evaluation, including laboratory tests, procedures, and consultations, that is performed to determine the recipient's physical and psychosocial status (Anderson-Reitz, 2004). It is important to remember people embraced by the patient such as family and friends, all of whom may be asked to provide assistance during the transplantation process and recovery.

Once the initial evaluation is complete, the patient will undergo conditioning, which is the process of preparing the patient to receive bone marrow or stem cells. Conditioning serves three vital purposes: to eliminate malignant disease, to kill the current immunologic state, and to develop space in the marrow cavity for the transplanted stem cells as they begin reproducing. The regime will consist of high dose chemotherapy (HDCT) with or without radiotherapy and will result in severe myelosuppression. With conditioning complete, the bone marrow or stem cells may be infused. An autologous transplant is done by rapid IV push using syringes or by hanging the bag of cells and infusing over 20 to 30 minutes. During the procedure patients may experience mild dyspnea from the volume being infused and nausea and vomiting from the preservatives contained in the solution. Allogeneic marrow or stem cells are infused slowly over 1 to 5 hours. Patients may experience side effects similar to those seen in a blood transfusion, as discussed in Chapter 23 ⊖ (Keller, 2001).

Establishment of new bone marrow is referred to as **engraftment** (Rokita 2004). The time required for complete engraftment depends on the source of the stem cells. Typically, bone marrow engrafts within 3 weeks, whereas stem cells take 11 to 16 days and cord blood takes 26 to 42 days. Of utmost concern is the pancytopenia and immunosuppression experienced during the immediate period post-transplant. Nurses must be very diligent at monitoring post-transplant patients for signs of infection and bleeding.

Bone marrow transplantation nursing has evolved with the development of transplantation approaches and therapies. The complexity of this field of nursing is evident in the challenging needs of the acute care patient. Because the age of BMT patients can cross the life span, the nurse must possess skills for managing infants as well as older adults (Wingard, 2007).

Complications of Transplantation

Patients who become transplant recipients are at risk for life-threatening complications, primarily due to the effects of the conditioning regime. Complications associated with the conditioning regime are numerous and can include bleeding, infection, nausea and vomiting, diarrhea, mucositis, and graft-versus-host disease (GVHD) (Anderson-Reitz, 2004). Several months to several years after transplant, the patient may experience late effects such as chronic GVHD, avascular necrosis, osteoporosis, cataracts, gonadal dysfunction, growth failure, hypothyroidism, secondary malignancies, need for revaccinations, and changes in quality of life.

Nurses who care for those patients undergoing transplantation need to be aware of the signs of graft failure and GVHD. Graft failure (rejection) occurs very rarely, but its significance requires nurses to be astute in their ability to assess patients for signs of infection and bleeding. Graft rejection is confirmed by serial bone marrow biopsies and will require the patient to undergo another transplant or death will be the result. GVHD occurs after allogeneic transplants and is the result of an immune-mediated reaction of the new stem cells reacting to the body of the recipient.

■ Nursing Management

Transplant centers have begun to develop unique care models due to competition among health care institutions, a desire to improve outcomes, and the need to decrease costs (Schmit-Pokorny, Franco, Frappier, & Vyhlidal, 2003). Involving the patient and family members in all aspects of care has created an environment that is more personal and individualized while reducing costs and rehospitalizations. The nurse has the opportunity to assist the patient in becoming more confident and competent in self-care. Caring for patients receiving transplantation is complex and challenging, requiring a systematic approach to assessment along with the ability to remain flexible when implementing a plan of care. The patient's condition changes day to day and even hour to hour, requiring the nurse to adapt to these variations quickly and competently. A comprehensive plan of care will encompass the patient's physical and psychological needs (refer to the Nursing Process: Care Plan for Cancer earlier, p. 2089).

■ Cancer Emergencies

Oncologic emergencies occur as a result of the disease process or side effects of treatment. On occasion, patients will present to their health care provider with a variety of distressing complaints and it is determined by evaluation that the patient has a malignancy. Regardless of the cause of the emergency, catastrophic results can occur if prompt and effective interventions are not initiated (Woodard & Hogan, 1996). The two main categories of emergencies are structural and metabolic in addition to hypersensitivity (anaphylaxis) and tumor lysis syndrome (My-

ers, 2001). Chart 64–24 (p. 2118) presents the important emergencies along with a definition, clinical findings, and treatment options. Oncology nurses understand the importance of continuously monitoring their patients for both subtle and obvious changes that may indicate the development of these potential life-threatening emergencies.

■ Living with Cancer: Supportive Therapies and Symptom Management

The diagnosis of cancer does not have to be equated with miserable suffering and death. During the past 30 years a person's chance of surviving cancer has improved due to multiple factors: (1) a better understanding of the disease, (2) changes in dose-limiting treatment toxicities, (3) new targeted therapies, (4) improved screening and early detection programs, (5) evidenced-based practice, (6) improved supportive interventions, and (7) changes in sociocultural factors (Dow & Loerzel, 2004). Although these factors have given patients with cancer an improved chance of survival, patients also may need to live with a variety of symptoms or complications that have the potential to be distressing. Nurses caring for cancer patients need to be aware of the potential problems, perform accurate assessments, and determine appropriate nursing interventions to alleviate any suffering or distress.

It is not uncommon for patients to consider the use of complementary and alternative medicine (CAM) therapies throughout the course of cancer treatment (Fouladbakhsh, Stommel, Given, & Given, 2005). For example, the use of pomegranate juice by patients with cancer is discussed in the Complementary and Alternative Therapies box (p. 2119). Oftentimes patients choose not to reveal these practices to their health care providers. Of particular importance is determining the use of herbal and vitamin supplements that may interact negatively with concurrent use of traditional treatment options. Nurses need to provide education regarding the use of CAM while respecting an individual's right to make decisions.

Patients face multiple challenges throughout their cancer experience. One of the most difficult issues (for patients and nurses) is the ethics of cancer care. Ethical issues are common in oncology nursing, as evidenced by the examples listed in the Ethical Issues box (p. 2120). Nurses have opportunities to develop relationships with their patients who have cancer and their families as they go through diagnosis and treatment. This relationship provides the nurse with an understanding of the goals and values the patient possesses as they relate to their cancer experience. Collaborating with the multidisciplinary team is important to determine a plan of care that honors and respects these goals and values.

Nutrition

The nutritional status of cancer patients can be altered in a variety of ways. Emotional stress from impaired nutritional intake coupled with the metabolic demand of cancer and its treatment can have a profound effect on the patient. Nurses cannot ignore how eating can be a part of one's social presence and often is a source of enjoyment (Schulmeister, 2001b).

CHART 64–24 Oncologic Emergencies

Emergency	Findings	Treatment
Metabolic		
Disseminated intravascular coagulation (DIC) (see Chapter 63 🔗)	Signs of bleeding and clotting	• Elimination of triggering event • Supportive measures (transfusion of blood products)
Hypercalcemia: serum calcium levels >9–11 mg/dL	Lethargy Altered mental status Nausea and vomiting Anorexia Polydipsia Constipation	• Hydration • Diuresis to enhance the excretion of calcium • Pharmacology: bisphosphonates (inhibit the action of osteoclasts) • Increased mobilization
Malignant pleural effusion; accumulation of fluid in the pleural cavity	Dyspnea at rest or activity Cough (nonproductive) Chest pain Malaise Weight loss Fear of suffocation, anxiety	• Radiation or chemotherapy aimed at the primary tumor • Insertion of chest tube with drainage capability • Pleurodesis
Sepsis (see Chapter 61 🔗)	Fever Chills Changes in blood pressure Rapid respiratory rate Mental cloudiness	• Recognition of impending shock is key • Infection control practices • Private rooms • Hemodynamic monitoring while in the intensive care unit (ICU) • Antibiotic therapy
Syndrome of inappropriate antidiuretic hormone (SIADH): endocrine paraneoplastic syndrome causing water imbalance (see Chapter 52 🔗)	Hyponatremia Decreased serum osmolality Water retention Increased urine osmolality Normal skin turgor Normal blood pressure	• Treat underlying cause • Fluid restriction • Diuretic therapy
Hypersensitivity reaction (anaphylaxis): immunologic response to foreign substance or antigen; may be life threatening	Occurs within minutes of receiving certain chemotherapy agents Dyspnea Agitation Hypotension Laryngeal edema and spasm	• Prevention is the key • Careful monitoring of blood pressure, pulse, and oxygen saturation during infusion • Emergency equipment needs to be available
Tumor lysis syndrome: rapid lysis of malignant cells resulting in renal (e.g., acidosis), electrolyte (e.g., hyperuricemia, hyperkalemia), cardiac, and neurologic complications	Nausea and vomiting Edema Flank pain Hematuria Changes in blood pressure Lethargy Muscle twitching and weakness	• Prevention is the key • Pretreatment hydration • Pharmacologic therapy (diuretics, xanthine oxidase inhibitors, sodium bicarbonate) • Supportive measures for potential organ failure
Structural		
Increased intracranial pressure: volume of the brain, CSF, and cerebral blood volume increase (see Chapter 31 🔗)	Signs and symptoms of increased intracranial pressure	• Pharmacologic therapy (osmotic diuretics, corticosteroids, anticonvulsants) • Surgery to relieve pressure and evacuate fluid • Radiation and chemotherapy to shrink tumor bulk
Spinal cord compression: malignancy that invades the epidural space and cauda equina (see Chapter 32 🔗)	Signs and symptoms of cord compression are specific to the area of the cord being compressed	• Pharmacologic therapy (corticosteroids) • Radiation therapy to reduce tumor bulk • Surgery when bony instability occurs
Superior vena cava syndrome: obstruction of venous flow through the vena cava resulting in compression of intrathoracic structures, vascular congestion, and venous hypertension	Dyspnea Cough Feeling of fullness in the head Chest pain	• Pharmacologic therapy (fibrinolytic therapy) • Radiation therapy to reduce tumor bulk • Chemotherapy for specific cell types • Surgery (stents or bypass)

CHART 64–24	Oncologic Emergencies—*Continued*	

Emergency	Findings	Treatment
Cardiac tamponade: compression of the cardiac muscle by malignant fluid accumulation within the pericardial sac (see Chapter 42)	Dyspnea Chest pain Tachycardia Cough	• Pharmacologic therapy (diuretics, corticosteroids, NSAIDS) • Removal of fluid via pericardiocentesis, pericardiotomy, pericardiectomy

Sources: Bender, C., & Rosenzweig, M. (2004). Cancer. In S. Lewis, M. Heitkemper, & S. Dirksen (Eds.), *Medical–surgical nursing assessment and management of clinical problems* (6th ed.). St. Louis: Mosby; Myers, J. (2001). Oncologic complications. In S. Otto (Ed.), *Oncology nursing* (4th ed.). St. Louis: Mosby; Woodard, W., & Hogan, D. (1996). Oncologic emergencies: Implications for nurses. *Journal of Intravenous Nursing, 19*(2).

Weight loss in patients with cancer is likely to result in poor clinical and psychological outcomes (Dell, 2002). The nurse can recognize the syndrome of cancer cachexia by the presence of anorexia, weight loss, muscle and adipose tissue wasting, hyperlipidemia, and other metabolic derangements. It is present in 80% of those who die of cancer (Cunningham, 2004). Figure 64–7 ■ (p. 2120) illustrates how profoundly cachexia affects the human body. Cachexia is the result of altered absorption and changes in metabolism, such as protein, fat, and carbohydrates (National Cancer Institute, 2003). It is important for the nurse to remember that cachexia can be present in patients who have adequate caloric and protein intake but are failing to absorb the necessary nutrients.

For those patients receiving chemotherapy, inadequate nutrition is of utmost concern. One of the most dreaded side effects of chemotherapy is nausea and vomiting. Uncontrolled nausea and vomiting can eventually result in cachexia preceded by anorexia and weight loss (Finley, 2003b). Oncology nurses are vital in ensuring that the nutritional needs of these patients are being met. Recognizing the early signs of cachexia and implementing effective interventions is key in slowing or reversing the progression of cachexia syndrome.

Nutritional screening is the process of evaluating patients for the risk of developing malnutrition. The goal of screening is to identify patients at risk, prevent or treat malnutrition early, and individualize the nutritional plan of care (McMahon, 2003). Working together with a nutritionist, the nurse can perform an effective nutritional screening evaluation by determining food intake, presence of symptoms, functional status (Karnofsky Performance Scale), weight, physical assessment, and laboratory data analysis. Chart 64–25 (p. 2121) lists the signs and symptoms along with laboratory data that can be used to determine malnutrition. The nurse/nutritionist needs to use sensitivity when discussing issues associated with dietary habits because many patients are hesitant to discuss their nutritional habits.

Nutritional Support

Once the need for nutritional support has been determined, the method of delivery is the next decision to be made. For those patients with mild anorexia, nutritional counseling may be adequate, whereas those patients with severe anorexia or cachexia may require parenteral nutritional support. Oral nutrition is the preferred route, but those patients with mechanical inability to

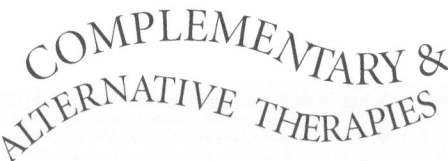 COMPLEMENTARY & ALTERNATIVE THERAPIES   Pomegranate Juice

Description:
Studies have shown that plant phytochemicals may prevent cancer due to antioxidants and nutrients (Pantuck et al., 2006). The pomegranate (*Punica granatum*) fruit has been shown to have high levels of antioxidants and other nutrients. The level of interest and research on pomegranate has surged over the last decade. The pomegranate fruit is comprised of the following components, each of which have pharmacologic activity: seed, juice, peel, leaf, flower, bark, and roots. The most notable therapeutic properties of pomegranate are antioxidant and anticancer activities, including interference with tumor cell proliferation, cell cycle, invasion, and angiogenesis (Lansky & Newman, 2007).

Research Support:
One study examined the effects of pomegranate juice on the levels of prostate-specific antigen (PSA) in men with prostate cancer and a rising PSA following conventional therapy. Patients consumed 8 oz of pomegranate juice daily. Results showed that mean PSA doubling time significantly increased with pomegranate juice consumption, from a mean of 15 months at baseline to 54 months post-treatment. Researchers concluded that the positive results from this study indicate that further testing is needed in a placebo-controlled study (Pantuck et al., 2006).

Another study examined the effect of pomegranate juice on inflammatory cell signaling proteins in patients with colon cancer. The study used pomegranate juice with a concentration of 50 mg/L. Results showed that the pomegranate juice significantly suppressed inflammatory cell signaling proteins by 79% (Adams et al., 2006).

References
Adams, L. S., Seeram, N. P., Aggarwal, B. B., Takada, Y., Sand, D., & Heber, D. (2006). Pomegranate juice, total pomegranate ellagitannins, and punicalagin suppress inflammatory cell signaling in colon cancer cells. *Journal of Agricultural and Food Chemistry, 54*(3), 980–985.
Lansky, E. P., & Newman, R. A. (2007). *Punica granatum* (pomegranate) and its potential for prevention and treatment of inflammation and cancer. *Journal of Ethnopharmacology, 109*(2), 177–206.
Pantuck, A. J., Leppert, J. T., Zomorodian, N., Aronson, W., Hong, J., Barnard, R. J., et al. (2006). Phase II study of pomegranate juice for men with rising prostate-specific antigen following surgery or radiation for prostate cancer. *Clinical Cancer Research, 12*(13), 4018–4026.

ETHICAL ISSUES Related to Cancer Treatment

1. *Informed consent and determining decision-making capacity.* Nurses reinforce and clarify information presented by health care providers. If confusion surrounding consent exists, the nurse needs to notify the health care provider for continued discussion. Documentation of the informed consent needs to be found in the medical record.

2. *Communicating bad news.* The nurse's role is one of facilitation. Nurses prepare the environment, which includes finding a meeting place and inviting the appropriate people to participate in the discussion. While the health care provider delivers the bad news, the nurse provides support, responds to the patient's and family members' feelings, and begins to plan follow-through as needed (e.g., offering spiritual support, allowing quiet private time for patient and family).

3. *Privacy and confidentiality.* Nurses are obligated to protect the patient's privacy and information related to the patient's health care situation.

4. *Clinical research trials.* Clinical research trials present multiple ethical issues for the health care team to address. These issues include poor minority involvement, patients' perspective of hope for a cure, adjustment of exclusion criteria to allow more participation, randomization that creates conflict for health care providers when they believe one intervention used in the trial is best, and cost issues.

5. *Advance directives.* Nurses educate the patient and family regarding the benefit of completing an advance directive, communicate with the health care team regarding the presence and content of the document, and refer the patient to the appropriate source for initiating.

6. *Do-not-resuscitate (DNR) orders.* Nurses' responsibilities include ensuring that the health care team and patient understand the DNR orders, advocating for independent decision making throughout the entire course of treatment while encouraging the patient to communicate openly with health care providers, ensuring proper documentation is completed and the appropriate renewal process is followed, and validating the emotional responses of patients and family members. Oftentimes forgotten, but very important, is the effect a DNR order has on the nurse and health care team. Throughout the course of an illness, oncology nurses develop a relationship with their patients and families. Although the nurse advocates for patients and their right to make decisions, a DNR order creates emotions that are important to recognize as normal.

7. *End-of-life issues.* As a patient's illness progresses, a new set of issues arises that require the patient to be given ongoing support, communication, and advocacy from the health care team. Chapter 17 💿 discusses end-of-life issues in detail.

Source: Nelson-Marten, P., & Glover, J. (2005). Selected ethical issues in cancer care. In J. K. Itano & K. N. Taoka (Eds.), *Core curriculum for oncology nursing* (4th ed.). Philadelphia: W. B. Saunders.

consume food may require enteral feedings. Parenteral nutrition is reserved for those patients whose GI tract is not functioning properly or the patient who is intolerant of enteral feedings. Chapter 14 💿 provides a detailed discussion of nutrition and the different delivery methods. Ethical questions surrounding the use of artificial nutrition and hydration with patients who have cancer are addressed in the Ethical Issues box.

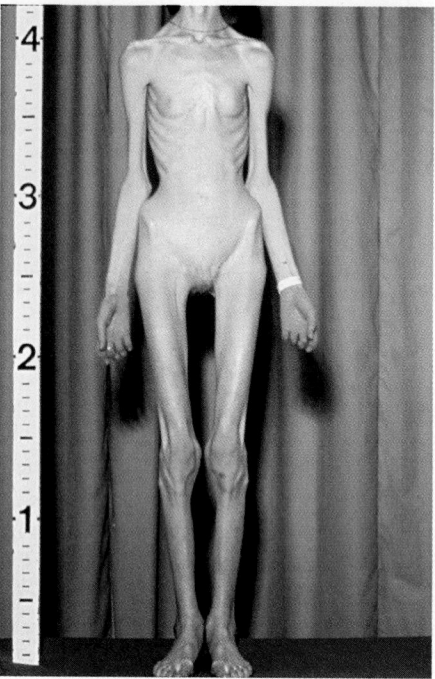

FIGURE 64–7 ■ Cancer cachexia.
Source: © Welcome Trust Images/Custom Medical Stock Photo

Fatigue

Fatigue, the most frequently experienced symptom of cancer and its therapy, has a profound effect on patients' quality of life (Barnett, 2001). Fatigue associated with cancer and cancer treatments began receiving attention from health care providers in the 1970s. A renewed interest in the topic developed in the mid-1980s when oncology nursing texts, journal articles, and research reports indicated the incidence of fatigue was more common than previously assumed (Nail, 2004). In the early 1990s, Winningham et al. (1994) described a common definition of fatigue as "a sense of tiredness." Most recently, the National Comprehensive Cancer Network (2006) expanded on this widely accepted definition to state "cancer-related fatigue is a distressing persistent subjective sense of tiredness or exhaustion related to cancer or cancer treatment that is not proportional to recent activity and interferes with usual functioning." The Evidence-Based Practice box (p. 2122) provides further discussion about fatigue related to cancer.

Influencing Factors

The cancer experience puts the patient at risk for experiencing problems that may create physical, mental, and emotional fatigue. Factors that influence fatigue include physical, functional, psychosocial, and spiritual factors, as described in Chart 64–26 (p. 2123).

Nurses caring for cancer patients are encouraged to develop a method of assessing for fatigue that can be performed quickly, but thoroughly, and can be used for patients with diseases other than cancer. Of particular importance is the timing of the nurse's assessment of fatigue. For example, if fatigue were assessed prior to receiving chemotherapy or biotherapy, the results would likely be different than if the assessment were done the day after therapies were administered. The assessment data should be used as a guide for nursing practice decisions, including reevaluation of the patient's symptoms to determine effectiveness of the nursing care plan.

CHART 64–25	Malnutrition: Signs, Symptoms, and Laboratory Data		
Signs	**Symptoms**	**Laboratory Data**	**Normal Ranges**
Weakness	Anorexia	Albumin	3.8–4.5 g/dL
Poor hair and nail condition	Alteration in mental status	Prealbumin	17–40 mg/dL
Diarrhea	Decreased immune response	Transferrin	250–450 mg/dL
Fever	Depression	Hemoglobin	Females: 12–16 g/dL Males: 14–18 g/dL
Dry mucosa	Anxiety	Hematocrit	Females: 37–47% Males: 42–52%
Edema	Fatigue	Total lymphocyte count	≥2,000/mm³
Mucositis	Pain	Nitrogen balance	Positive
Muscle atrophy		Urinary creatinine clearance	1.2 g/24 hr
Poor skin turgor		Skin test (anergy panel)	≥5 mm induration is positive

Sources: Cunningham, R. (2004). Anorexia-cachexia syndrome. In C. H. Yarbro, M. H. Frogge, & M. Goodman (Eds.), *Cancer symptom management* (3rd ed.). Sudbury, MA: Jones and Bartlett; Finley, J. (2003a). Detection and management of cachexia in cancer patients. *Advanced Studies in Nursing, 1*(1), 8–12; Finley, J. (2003b). Management of cancer cachexia and chemotherapy associated nausea and vomiting. *Advanced Studies in Nursing, 1*(1), 7; McMahon, K. (2003). Components of nutritional screening and assessment. In *Oncology Nursing Society 2003 annual congress symposium highlights* (pp. 5–6). Pittsburgh: Author.

ETHICAL ISSUES Related to Nutrition in Patients with Cancer

A declining appetite affects not only the physical well-being of patients, but also the functional, social, and psychological aspects of their quality of life. These changes are frequently noticed in patients nearing the end of their lives and should be addressed with sensitivity and compassion. One approach is to offer education, dietary modifications, and appetite stimulants; however, oftentimes these are unsuccessful and family members may begin to question if their loved one is "starving to death" (Schulmeister, 2001b).

Artificial nutrition and hydration toward the end of life are controversial therapies and have not been proven to be beneficial to the patient. In fact, administration of these therapies has been associated with complications and suffering (Ersek, 2003). It is the responsibility of the health care team to determine the patient's goals regarding end-of-life nutrition and hydration. This type of conversation may be difficult, but is paramount when trying to understand how the patient with cancer wishes to live during their final days.

Cancer Pain

Pain is a complex process that is affected by many physical and psychosocial influences. Cancer pain occurs as a result of the progression of the disease, diagnostic procedures, and/or the treatment provided. The location of the primary or metastatic lesion influences the degree of pain experienced by the patient. When there is bony involvement, such as spinal metastases, or neural involvement as is seen when tumor compresses nerve tissue, pain is intensified (Swenson, 2001). Most often it is not a problem in the early stage of the disease; however, nearly 30% of patients begin to experience pain during treatment. Advancing cancer, including metastasis, produces pain in nearly 90% of patients (Ashby & Dalton, 2000).

Up to 50% of cancer patients with pain fail to achieve adequate relief (Swenson, 2001). This statistic should compel those caring for these patients to continue to strive for more effective relief of suffering. Because cancer care produces a myriad of side effects such as fatigue, pain, infection, or bleeding, effective treatment is very challenging. It has been suggested the presence of pain and fatigue make other cancer symptoms more severe and more difficult to manage (Given, Given, Azzoouz, Kozachik, & Stommel, 2001).

In 1990, the ONS produced a position paper on cancer pain and declared "nurses are responsible and accountable for implementation and coordination of the plan for management of cancer pain" (Spross, McGuire, & Schmitt, 1990a, b, c). The National Comprehensive Cancer Network (2006) claims that cancer pain can be well controlled in most patients if the health care team uses evidenced-based guidelines, which can be individualized to each patient and involves them in decision making regarding their pain (ONS, 2006). Nurses who care for cancer patients implement frequent assessments of pain status, provide patient and family counseling or education, and participate in ongoing reevaluation and management of pain control. Chapter 15 provides detailed information on pain assessment and management that can easily be applied to patients with cancer pain.

Alternative Care Programs

Rising interest in home care and alternative settings for those patients who are facing a terminal illness such as cancer has led to the development of programs such as hospice and palliative care. Becoming familiar with the concepts of hospice and palliative care is important for the nurse who will be caring for patients with cancer. Chapter 17 discusses these programs in detail.

Quality of Life Throughout the Cancer Continuum

Although individuals with cancer have been surviving longer, they continue to search for the meaning of their illness. The search for this meaning is a process that is thought to include cognitive appraisals, reappraisals, and attributions that persons make in response to stressful experiences (Park & Folkman, 1997). Quality of life (QOL) is an important component in one's

Fatigue in Relation to Cancer

Clinical Problem

Fatigue is reported as the most prevailing symptom in patients afflicted with cancer. A common definition of fatigue is the presence of a subjective feeling of tiredness influenced by circadian rhythm (Piper et al., 1987). The incidence of developing fatigue varies throughout the disease experience: 17% to 40% in those who are disease-free cancer survivors; and 85% to 100% in those patients whose goal of care is palliative in nature (Mock, 2003). The effects of fatigue on the patient are many, including mood disturbances, poor concentration, decreased perception and capacity to work, changes in compliance with medical treatment, and decreased ability to perform ADLs. Everyone experiences fatigue throughout their daily lives; however, when it becomes constant and excessive, our ability and willingness to remain active is affected. In addition, when the effects of fatigue persist, the patient may question whether he can endure ongoing cancer treatment.

Research Findings

In the past several years, multiple research studies have looked at the effect of fatigue in patients with cancer. In 1998, Andrykowski et al. administered a fatigue questionnaire to persons with breast cancer and those with benign breast disease. The researchers were attempting to compare the presence of fatigue among these groups. Findings revealed that the breast cancer group reported greater fatigue on initial assessment and at a 4-month follow-up.

Bower et al. (2000) surveyed 1,957 breast cancer survivors and women with normal health to determine psychological factors, such as depression, known to affect fatigue. The researchers determined that the majority of survivors did not experience significant fatigue; however, of those who experienced severe fatigue, depression was a related factor.

Donovan and Ward (2005) conducted a research study that attempted to describe women's representation of fatigue and fatigue-related coping efforts by women who had received chemotherapy. Results of the study indicated that fatigue is a prevalent and severe symptom. Although it was perceived as distressing, most patients fail to report it to their health care providers.

In 2006, Sura and colleagues looked at the presence and degree of fatigue in women who received standard and dose-dense chemotherapy for breast cancer. The researchers used the revised Piper Fatigue Scale (Piper, 1998), which is designed to measure four dimensions of fatigue: physical (sensory), mental (cognitive/mood), emotional (affective), and effect on ADLs (behavioral/severity). The scale was administered prior to chemotherapy beginning, 3 days after the cycle 1 dose, and 3 days after the cycle 3 dose. Results revealed no significant difference in fatigue in all women prior to treatment, but the dose-dense group demonstrated significantly higher levels of fatigue throughout the course of treatment.

Implications for Nursing Practice

Nurses have the opportunity to positively affect the way a cancer patient experiences the effects of treatment. First, they need to be familiar with the types of patients who are likely to develop fatigue as part of their cancer experience. The studies discussed above were concerned with patients who had breast cancer; however, it is well understood that cancer treatments and severity of disease increase the risk of developing fatigue. Assessing for fatigue needs to be incorporated into routine nursing practice, specifically the presence and severity of fatigue. If patients are experiencing fatigue, the nurse can ask them to rate their distress associated with the symptom on a scale from 1 to 10. This will provide a basis of comparison for future assessments. The National Comprehensive Cancer Network (2003) has made recommendations for screening for fatigue including at the initial visit, at regular intervals, and when clinical indicators are present.

Together with the health care provider, the nurse needs to discuss treatment-related side effects and toxicities. Patients are then able to prepare and plan for the onset of fatigue. Suggesting self-care strategies to assist patients in coping helps minimize the effects of fatigue. Emphasizing energy conservation, energy restoration, exercise, good nutrition, and adequate rest should be a routine part of nursing conversation with patients who may experience fatigue.

Critical Thinking Questions

1. What components would the nurse include in an educational plan for a cancer patient (and family) who may experience fatigue?

2. Identify strategies that will facilitate coping for the patient with fatigue.

3. What nursing interventions would increase compliance with treatment for patients with fatigue?

Answers to Critical Thinking Questions appear in Appendix D.

References

Andrykowski, M., et al. (1998). Off-treatment fatigue in breast cancer survivors: A controlled comparison. *Journal of Behavior Medicine*, *21*(1).

Bower, J., et al. (2000). Fatigue in breast cancer survivors: Occurrence, correlates, and impact on quality of life. *Journal of Clinical Oncology*, *18*(4).

Donovan, H., & Ward, S. (2005). Representation of fatigue in women receiving chemotherapy for gynecologic cancers. *Oncology Nursing Forum, 32*(1).

Mock, V. (2003). Clinical excellence through evidenced-based practice: Fatigue management as a model. *Oncology Nursing Forum, 30*(4).

National Comprehensive Cancer Network. (2003). Cancer-related fatigue: Clinical practice guidelines in oncology. *Journal of the National Comprehensive Cancer Network, 1*(1).

Piper, B., Dibble, S., Dodd, M., Weiss, M., Slaughter, R., & Paul, S. (1987). The revised Piper Fatigue Scale: Psychometric evaluation in women with breast cancer. *Oncology Nursing Forum, 25*(3).

Piper, B. F., Dibble, S. L., Dodd, M. J., Weiss, M. C., Slaughter, R. E., Paul, S. M. The revised Piper Fatigue Scale: psychometric evaluation in women with breast cancer. Oncol Nurs Forum. (1998 May); *25*(4):677-84.

Sura, W., Murphy, S., & Gonzales, I. (2006). Level of fatigue in women receiving dose-dense versus standard chemotherapy for breast cancer: A pilot study. *Oncology Nursing Forum, 33*(5).

EVIDENCE-BASED PRACTICE

CHART 64–26	**Fatigue Factors**			
Physical	**Functional**	**Spiritual**	**Psychosocial**
Pain	Value/meaning given to changes in one's life	Look for value or meaning to diagnosis, treatment, suffering, recovery, and death.	Depression/isolation
Disturbed sleep–wake patterns	Ability to perform normal activities (work, home, social)	Consider the meaning and consequences of the diagnosis.	Roles/isolation
Nutrition GI difficulties Multiple medications Bone marrow suppression Performance status (Karnofsky)	Attentional fatigue: decreased capacity to concentrate	Review life to find ways to cope: • Being hopeful • Changing priorities • Learning to live with diagnosis.	Anxiety Appearance Control Relationships, affection, sexual function Finances

Sources: Barnett, M. (2001). Fatigue. In S. Otto (Ed.), *Oncology nursing* (4th ed.). St. Louis: Mosby; Blesch, K. (1991). Correlates of fatigue in people with breast and lung cancer. *Oncology Nursing Forum, 18*(1), 81; Kalman, D., & Villani, L. (1997). Nutritional aspects of cancer related fatigue. *Journal of the American Dietetic Association, 97,* 650; Miaskowski, C., & Lee, K. (1999). Pain, fatigue, and sleep disturbances in oncology outpatients receiving radiation therapy for bone metastasis: A pilot study. *Journal of Pain Symptom Management, 17*(3), 320; Nail, L., & Jones, L. (1995). Fatigue side effects and treatment and quality of life. *Quality of Life Research, 4*(1), 8.

ability to survive a major illness and the prescribed treatment. It embraces the characteristics and limitations that affect one's ability to function and obtain satisfaction in doing so. Over the years, the construct of QOL has been explored by many, but perhaps the most widely accepted description comes from Ferrell and colleagues. Their description identifies several dimensions, including physical, psychological, and social well-being, which are the hallmark components of a person's QOL (Ferrell & Dow, 1997). The health care team needs to consider both the patient and family when evaluating the effect of cancer and cancer care on QOL (Mellon, 2002). Chart 64–27 provides a list of the positive and negative aspects of cancer survivors' QOL discovered during the past decade.

Throughout all phases of cancer, it is essential for life to go on as close to normal as possible. During the diagnosis phase the patient and family are paralyzed with fear, often demonstrating behaviors consistent with denial (Shell & Kirsch, 2001). Once the diagnosis of cancer is made, others surround the patient with support in an effort to fight the disease. As the cancer advances the patient is confronted with accepting the diagnosis and possibly abandoning a hope for cure.

Nurses can support patients while they begin to adjust to the stress that accompanies the diagnosis of cancer with respectful and thoughtful communication. Although the health care provider typically delivers the news of the cancer diagnosis and prognosis to the patient, the nurse offers emotional support by providing patient and mindful listening that demonstrates compassion and concern. Patients will often express their hopes and fears when they feel someone genuinely cares. To cope with these fears cancer patients will see themselves demonstrating behaviors unfamiliar to them. These behaviors may include shock, anger, denial, bargaining, depression, helplessness, hopelessness, rationalization, acceptance, and intellectualization (Bender & Rosenzweig, 2004). A compassionate and caring nurse will reassure patients that their responses are not abnormal.

Cancer treatment is accompanied by multiple symptoms that may provoke a varying degree of suffering in the patient. The oncology nurse can positively affect QOL by prioritizing symptoms and implementing appropriate relief measures. On occa-

CHART 64–27	**Aspects of Quality of Life**	
Positive	**Negative**
Greater appreciation of life	Uncertainty and fear of the future
Improved interpersonal relationships	Lingering long-term effects of treatment
Enhanced spirituality	Changes in sexuality and self-image
Healthier lifestyles	Economic difficulties
	Family distress
	Communication difficulties with families

Sources: Dow, K., Ferrell, B., Haberman, M., & Eaton, L. (1999). The meaning of quality of life in cancer survivorship. *Oncology Nursing Forum, 26*(3), 519–528; Ersek, M., Ferrell, B., Dow, K., & Melancon, C. (1997). Quality of life in women with ovarian cancer. *Western Journal of Nursing Research, 19*(2), 334–350; Ferrell, B., Dow, K., Leigh, S., Ly, J., & Gulasekaram, P. (1995). Quality of life in long-term cancer survivors. *Oncology Nursing Forum, 22*(5), 915–922; Ferrell, B., Grant, M., Funk, B., Otis-Green, S., & Garcia, N. (1998a). Quality of life in breast cancer. Part II: Psychological and spiritual well-being. *Cancer Nursing, 21*(1), 1–9; Ferrell, B., Grant, M., Funk, B., Otis-Green, S., Garcia, N. (1998b). Quality of life in breast cancer survivors: Implications for developing support services. *Oncology Nursing Forum, 25*(4), 887–895; Ganz, P., Coscarelli, A., Fred, C., Kahn, B., Polinsky, M., & Peterson, L. (1996). Breast cancer survivors: Psychosocial concerns and quality of life. *Breast Cancer Research and Treatment, 38*(1), 183–199; Zebrack, B. (2000). Quality of life of long-term survivors of leukemia and lymphoma. *Journal of Psychosocial Oncology, 18*(4), 39–59.

sion, the patient may report distress from a symptom, such as malaise and fatigue, but with keen assessment skills the nurse may discover the presence of a more significant problem causing the patient's symptoms. This knowledge demonstrated by the nurse will be recognized by patients and will enhance their trust in those caring for them.

Key to being an effective oncology nurse is the ability to instill hope into patients and their loved ones. The meaning of hope varies depending on the status of the patient:

1. Hope that symptoms are not serious
2. Hope that treatment is curative
3. Hope for independence

4. Hope for relief of pain
5. Hope for a longer life
6. Hope for a peaceful and dignified death.

Hope allows cancer patients to maintain a sense of control over their current situation along with a positive attitude toward their disease.

Most health care organizations and cancer advocacy groups try to provide creative ways to increase cancer awareness and provide support for patients and their families. One example is the use of art as a way of explaining one's journey with cancer. Both patients and artists have begun to explain the benefit of creating art during an illness experience (Ponto et al., 2003). Patients can tell stories of their illness including initial symptoms, the diagnosing experience, hospitalizations, treatment-induced body changes, key health care providers, and recovery. Art can assist the patient in gaining a sense of control in a situation that seems uncontrollable and allows for a vehicle to communicate emotions, such as loneliness, solitude, and the need for survival (Lynn, 1994). Nurses have the unique opportunity to recognize the benefit of art in the recovery of patients afflicted with cancer.

Gerontological Considerations

Increased attention is being devoted to the care of the elderly patient with cancer. The reason for this shift in focus is dual in nature: an increased number of older people in the population, and an increased number of older people with cancer. The aging of the baby boomers (those born between 1946 and 1964) is the major cause of the increasing number of aging adults. Americans who are over the age of 65 have an 11 times more likely chance of developing cancer than people under the age of 65 years of age (Muss, 2001). Caring for the aging with cancer is quickly becoming a public health concern.

It is predicted that by the year 2030 one in five persons will be 65 years or older, compared with the current figure of one in nine persons (Kinsella & Velkoff, 2001). In addition, the number of cancer patients ages 85 and older is expected to increase more than fourfold by the year 2050. These statistics provide compelling evidence to expand the knowledge base about cancer education, screening, and management in the elderly. Of particular importance is the need for nurses to recognize the elderly's experience with cancer and to identify strategies where oncology nurses can contribute to changes in cancer care for the elderly. Understanding the 10 key facts of cancer in the elderly, as listed in Chart 64–28, will provide nurses with an appreciation of the magnitude of the problem being faced.

The future of cancer care is going to be significantly impacted by our aging population, requiring ongoing attention to the uniqueness of caring for the geriatric cancer patient. A collaborative effort by the ONS and the Geriatric Oncology Consortium (GOC) produced a position statement regarding care of the geriatric cancer patient. Within this publication, the unique attributes of older cancer patients were acknowledged, including the nature of cancer in the older adult, the specific needs found in geriatric cancer patients, and their implications for society (ONS & GOC, 2004). Nurses who are providing cancer-related care for the growing number of elderly patients need to

---

CHART 64–28 **Key Facts of Cancer in the Elderly**

Cancer is a disease of the elderly.

Most cancers are due to solid tumors.

The etiology of cancer in the elderly is controversial.

Public education of the elderly is needed.

Data regarding development of treatment toxicities are minimal.

Treatment decisions should be based on physiological (not chronological) age.

The current deficit in knowledge of the elderly with cancer is due to underrepresentation in clinical trials.

Caregiving and coping problems are important to consider.

Consider blending the specialties of oncology and gerontology.

Nursing research opportunities are endless.

---

understand the normal physiological changes associated with aging. These include impaired immune system; decreased organ function and structure; decreased skin elasticity; decreased skeletal mass, structure, and strength; changes in sensory and neurological functions; and alterations in drug absorption, distribution, metabolism, and elimination (Rokita, 2004). The Gerontological Considerations box discusses normal changes seen with aging and their impact on cancer nursing care. When administering cancer treatments to geriatric patients, the nurse must be alert to possible intolerance due to the normal changes seen with advancing age. Elderly patients with cancer frequently have comorbidities with ongoing treatments that may also limit their tolerance to prescribed cancer therapy.

Discharge Planning

Discharge planning is a process that includes assessment, identification of continuing care needs, and planning and implementation of a plan that will meet those determined needs. Typically, this process begins when the patient is admitted to the hospital, but it is reasonable to begin evaluating the patient's needs in the outpatient setting because oncology patients interface with outpatient personnel frequently for treatments and management of symptoms. A variety of health care professionals can be involved with the process, but the nurse and social worker are critical in establishing a comprehensive discharge plan. Developing a systematic approach will assist with creation of the comprehensive plan of care and provide a manner in which routine reevaluation and modification of the plan can occur.

Patients and their family need to be actively involved in the discharge planning process. Educating the patient and those caring for him or her about self-care is critical in a successful discharge plan, but first nurses must ascertain learning needs or barriers that will affect their ability to provide effective teaching. In addition, recognizing one's cultural influences needs to be recognized so the teaching can be individualized and meaningful. The Patient Teaching & Discharge Priorities box (p. 2126) describes the necessary components of the teaching plan, which includes sexuality issues and psychological adaptation.

GERONTOLOGICAL CONSIDERATIONS Related to Cancer

Changes Seen with Aging	Nursing Implications
Decreased skin elasticity, body mass, and impaired healing	Monitor for skin and mucous membrane changes. Monitor oral cavity for properly fitting prosthesis and abnormal skin condition. Provide skin care to prevent breakdown. Encourage mobility as tolerated: • Range of motion • Assist with turning. Encourage adequate nutrition. Consult with dietician as needed. Provide frequent toileting.
Impaired immune system	Monitor for signs of infection: • Fever • Chills • Exudate • Urinary symptoms • Cough • Drainage from wounds, inserted devices • Mental status changes • Laboratory data (ANC, WBC, culture and sensitivity results).
Decreased vital organ function (renal, cardiac, and pulmonary)	Monitor laboratory data as indicated: • BUN and creatinine • Oxygen saturation. Monitor for signs of decreased cardiac output and tissue perfusion. Monitor for presence of new onset of dyspnea. Collaborate with health care provider for appropriate adjustments in treatment dosages.
Decreased musculoskeletal strength	Assess for fall risk and initiate precautions as indicated.
Decreased vision, hearing, and tactile distal sensation	Modify teaching as needed for visual and hearing changes. Monitor distal extremities for skin changes and provide appropriate teaching.
Altered drug absorption, distribution, metabolism, and elimination	Collaborate with health care provider for appropriate adjustments in treatment dosages. Monitor for increased drowsiness due to medications given prior to treatment.
Changes in cognitive and emotional capacity	Assess for perceived alterations in sexuality: • Provide counseling as needed • Encourage the use of lubricants for vaginal dryness. Monitor for social concerns: • Financial burden of treatments and associated activities • Lack of transportation. Modify teaching to ensure learning.
Presence of comorbidities and treatments	Determine use of medications that may exaggerate the side effects or toxicity of cancer treatments, such as bleeding or changes in renal function. Monitor for tolerance of cancer therapy. Monitor for progression of comorbidities while receiving cancer therapy.

Sources: Iwamoto, R. (2001). Radiation therapy. In S. Otto (Ed.), *Oncology nursing* (4th ed.). St. Louis: Mosby; Otto, S. (2001a). Chemotherapy. In S. Otto (Ed.), *Oncology nursing* (4th ed.). St. Louis: Mosby. Otto, S. (2001b). Lung Cancers. In S. Otto (Ed.), *Oncology nursing* (4th ed.). St. Louis: Mosby; Rokita, S. (2004). Oncology: Nursing management in cancer care. In S. Smeltzer & B. Bare (Eds.). *Brunner & Suddarth's textbook of medical–surgical nursing* (10th ed.). Philadelphia: Lippincott Williams & Wilkins.

Research

Cancer research is crucial to improving therapy and survival along with management of symptoms associated with this devastating disease. The goal of research is to identify areas where practice could improve and then evaluate and test methods in these areas. The Research Opportunities and Clinical Impact box (p. 2127) provides a list of both medical and nursing research topics that are still under investigation. Electronic databases are a source for finding specific studies related to these topics.

Clinical Trials

Cancer treatments and symptom management have been developed and refined based on the outcome of extensive clinical trials (research). A myriad of health care professionals work collaboratively in an attempt to discover new therapies that will increase survival and improve quality of life for those individuals afflicted with cancer. Before a therapy, such as chemotherapy, is approved for clinical use, rigorous evaluations are performed to determine its beneficial effects, adverse effects, and safety

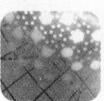

PATIENT TEACHING & DISCHARGE PRIORITIES for Cancer

Need	Teaching
Treatment side effects and toxicities: Patient/family Family/support system Setting	Instruct patient regarding proper oral care: • Brush and floss teeth as tolerated. • Use moistening gauze or toothettes instead of toothbrush if needed, for instance, if platelet count is low (<40,000/mm³). • Rinse with normal saline four times per day. • Avoid commercial mouthwashes. • Cleanse mouth before and after meals. Instruct patient to report signs of stomatitis: • Burning • Pain • Areas of redness • Open lesions on the lips • Pain with swallowing • Intolerance to temperature extremes. Take antiemetics and appetite stimulants per orders. Suggest small frequent meals that are high in calories and protein. Encourage adequate fluid intake limiting fluids during mealtime. Monitor for signs of infection and notify health care provider immediately. Avoid contact with those who have known or recent infection or recent vaccination. Avoid raw meat and fish, fresh fruit and vegetables, fresh flowers and plants. Avoid use of straight edge razor. Instruct patient regarding ways to minimize the risk of bleeding: • Perform oral hygiene with soft toothbrush or toothettes • Avoid use of commercial mouthwashes • Avoid straight-edge razors • File nails with emery board • Avoid foods that are difficult to chew Encourage frequent rest periods. Encourage more sleep hours at night. Encourage patient to reorganize daily schedule of activities and seek assistance with shopping, cooking, housework, etc. Encourage a temporary decrease in work hours. Assess availability, knowledge, and compliance with treatment regimen. Assess respite needs and resources. Assess discharge placement needs: • Home • Hospice • Extended care facility. Assess the home environment for needed assistive devices. Assess the need for professional home health. Assess the need for follow-up appointments.
In-home treatments: Patient/family Family/support system Setting	Instruct patient and family on how to operate and troubleshoot infusion equipment. Instruct patient and family on how to care for an implantable infusion device. Instruct patient and family on the proper storage of medications and solutions. Assess availability, knowledge, and compliance with treatment regimen. Assess respite needs and resources. Assess home environment for risk factors. Assess home environment for needed assistive devices. Assess the need for professional home health. Assess the need for follow-up appointments.

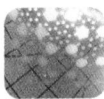

PATIENT TEACHING & DISCHARGE PRIORITIES for Cancer—*Continued*

Need	Teaching
Coping: 　Patient/family 　Family/support system 　Setting	Instruct patient to consider participating in activities and decision making. Encourage patient to verbalize concerns. Instruct about patterns of hair loss and regrowth. Encourage patient to view venous access device. Encourage patient in selecting cosmetic devices that increase sense of attractiveness. Offer ways to cope with hair loss: 　• Obtain wigs or hairpieces prior to hair loss 　• Take photograph of hair loss to wig shop to improve matching of hair color 　• Contact American Cancer Society for available resources 　• Wear scarf, hat, or other device as needed Encourage dialogue between patient and partner regarding sexual function and alternatives. Assess the need for professional home health. Assess the need for follow-up appointments.

RESEARCH OPPORTUNITIES AND CLINICAL IMPACT RELATED TO CANCER

Research Area	Clinical Impact
Physiological Research	
Photodynamic therapy for treatment of esophageal and lung cancer	Provides additional treatment options.
Effects of handling chemotherapy on the person administering the medication, offspring	Increases awareness of hazards associated with administration of chemotherapy.
Use of new interleukins as antitumor and myeloprotective agents	Provides additional treatment options and prevention of life-threatening toxicities.
Use of new interferons to treat the severity of GVHD and other cancers	Decreases incidence of metastasis.
Use of gene therapy for advanced cancers and prevention of myelosuppression	
Determining the benefit/risk ratio and efficacy of chemotherapeutic chronotherapy	
Use of drugs to prevent the development of blood vessels (antiangiogenesis therapy) in cancer treatment	
Symptom and Toxicity Management	
Evaluation of postoperative symptoms in those with lung cancer	Relieves distressing symptoms to increase healing and recovery.
Use of virtual reality interventions for chemotherapy symptoms	Relieves distressing symptoms to aid in recovery and treatment tolerance.
Innovative approaches to symptom management (cluster intervention, neutropenic protocols, fatigue guidelines, mucositis standard of care)	Increases awareness of unique symptoms and appropriate treatments to relieve suffering.
Causes of fatigue and solutions	Provides information to assist in the development of individualized nursing care plan.
Skin care for patients receiving radiotherapy	
Association between treatment and disease-related symptoms and activity	Increases awareness of need for pain control and availability of treatment modalities.
Symptoms at the end of life	
Association between patient's perceptions of treatment toxicities and ability to care for self	
Nursing pain management of inpatients and outpatients	

RESEARCH OPPORTUNITIES AND CLINICAL IMPACT RELATED TO CANCER—*Continued*

Research Area	Clinical Impact
Psychosocial and Emotional Issues	
Coping with disease and treatment	Improves psychological interventions to augment coping.
Coping of caregivers and families of patients with cancer	Provides insight into how patients make decisions regarding treatment so appropriate and effective communication can be implemented.
Decision making after cancer testing (BRCA genetic testing)	
The role of caring and the meaning of illness	Highlights importance of caring.
Quality of life	Impact of the disease and treatment.
Quality of life and influencing factors	Impact on vocation.
Employment behaviors in patients with treatment-related symptoms	Importance of family members' involvement in caregiving.
Delivery of care by family members	Importance of ascertaining patients' end-of-life choices and advocating appropriately.
Preferred versus actual location of death	
Cultural Diversity	
Symptom management in various cultural groups	Improves understanding of cultural differences in cancer management.
Participation of various cultural groups as subjects in cancer research efforts	
Use of specific treatment regimes in various cultural groups	
Decision making in various cultural groups	
Evaluating cancer risk behaviors and emotional status in various cultural groups	
End-of-life issues and ethnicity	
Prevention/Detection/Screening	
Tertiary chemoprevention to reduce the risk of cancer in those who are highly susceptible	Reduces risk of developing cancer.
Health and risk behaviors in childhood cancer survivors	Improves understanding of behaviors and allows for the development of screening programs to meet patients' needs.
Mammography decision making in women with family history of breast cancer	Allows for improved prevention and screening programs.
Disclosure of breast symptoms	
Use of telephone counseling in rural areas	
Changing health beliefs in those at risk for colon cancer	
Womens' perceptions of their risk of developing breast cancer	
Communicating breast cancer risk among family members	

(Rokita, 2004). Clinical trials can involve four phases, as described in Chart 64–29, each having a specific goal regarding research outcomes.

Oncology nurses have the unique opportunity to participate in many aspects of research efforts including obtaining informed consent, developing and implementing educational sessions for patients and their families, administering treatments under investigation, and collecting pertinent data (Gullatte & Otto, 2001). Being a patient advocate throughout all phases of clinical trials is also the role of the nurse and the health care team.

| CHART 64–29 | Phases of Clinical Trials |

Phase	Details
Phase I	Determine optimal dosing, scheduling, and toxicity.
Phase II	Further defines toxicities.
	Determines effectiveness related to specific tumor types.
	Participants usually include those who have not responded to standard treatments.
Phase III	Establish the effectiveness of new medications or procedures.
	Comparisons are made to conventional therapy.
	Nurses are involved with:
	• Identification of subjects
	• Obtaining informed consent
	• Educating subjects
	• Monitoring and assisting with compliance
	• Documenting subject responses.
Phase IV	Further investigation of new uses, dosing schedules, and toxicities.

Clinical Preparation

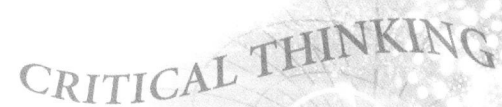

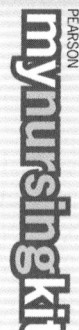

 Read

- History of Current Illness
- Past Medical History
- Physical Exam
- Admitting Medical Orders
- Laboratory Study Results

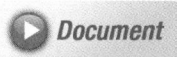 **Document**

- Summary of Hospitalization
- Pathophysiology Form
- Laboratory Values
- Laboratory Results Explanation

 **Apply**

- List of Potential Nursing Diagnoses
- Concept Map
- Critical Thinking Questions

Log on to MyNursingKit.com to download forms you will need and to complete further steps in the Clinical Preparation assignment.

HISTORY OF PRESENT ILLNESS

Mrs. S. is a 43-year-old female presenting to the Emergency Department (ED) for back pain. She was evaluated and discharged home with a prescription for a nonsteroidal anti-inflammatory drug (NSAID) and asked to follow up in the physical therapy department in 2 days. The following evening she again presented to the ED for worsening back pain along with numbness in her right buttocks. She appears well nourished, slightly pale, in obvious discomfort. While you assist her to the restroom you notice slight right foot drop and the appearance of dyspnea. Upon returning to the bed she is obviously dyspneic with a respiratory rate of 28. Oxygen saturation is 89% on room air. Lung sounds are diminished on the right side; otherwise, wheezes heard throughout. She admits to occasional productive cough. The results of a chest x-ray suggest lung cancer.

She is scheduled for a CT scan and while she is being moved from the gurney to the CT scan table, she cries out in pain while holding her right leg. The CT scan suggests a malignancy. Additional x-rays discover she has a fractured right hip. You're the nurse caring for Mrs. S. and you have received report from the nurse from surgery. Upon arrival to the floor Mrs. S. is awake, crying, groaning, and complaining of pain in her right hip area. You note on her laboratory data that her hematocrit is 22% and per order administer 2 units of packed red blood cells.

Medical–Surgical History

Allergies: none
Medical problems: hypothyroidism, depression
Medications: Prozac, Synthroid, and Motrin
Surgical history: appendectomy at the age of 13, C-section for two children

Social History

Married with two children (boys age 12 and 20)
Smokes 1.5 packs/day for 28 years
Occasional alcohol use

Physical Exam

Vital signs: BP 148/89, HR 128, RR 24, T 38.0°C
HEENT: WNL, oropharynx clear
Neck: supple, no lymphadenopathy
Lungs: diminished with wheezes throughout
Cardiovascular: JVP not elevated; normal S_1 and S_2; regular rate and tachycardic, no significant murmur, rub, or gallop; carotids 2+ without bruits
Abdomen: soft, nontender, nondistended, normoactive bowel sounds
Extremities: no edema, complaining of severe pain in her right hip
Neurological: normal, alert, and oriented × 4

Admitting Medical Orders

Ortho service
Oncology consultation
Admit to surgical floor
Diagnosis: status postrepair of fractured right hip; rule out cancer
No known allergies
Vital signs and oxygen saturation q4h
Bed rest with immobilization of right leg
Clear liquids when tolerated
I&O
Foley

Dry sterile dressing to right hip, change prn
Oxygen 1–2 L per nasal cannula as needed to maintain oxygen saturation > 90%
Call house officer: pulse < 60 and > 130/minute; BP < 90 and > 160 systolic; temperature > 38.5; urine output < 30 mL/hr for 2 hours; respiratory rate > 30/minute; oxygen saturation < 92%
Sequential compression devices (SCDs) to lower extremities
Intravenous line with 0.9% normal saline at 125 mL/hr; routine venous access device care
Neurovascular assessments to right lower extremity every 2 hours
Code status: full
Transfuse 2 units red blood cells if HCT< 24%. CBC after 2 units

Scheduled Medications

Prozac 20 mg oral every a.m.
Synthroid 0.25 mcg oral every a.m.
Duragesic patch 50 mcg; change every 72 hours

PRN Medications

Morphine sulfate PCA: 1 mg incremental dose q10min. If pain not well controlled, give morphine sulfate bolus 1–5 mg IV × 1
Tylenol 650 mg oral q4–6h as needed for pain or fever
Ativan 1–2 mg oral or IV q8h as needed for anxiety
Zofran 8 mg oral q8h as needed for nausea
Benadryl 25 mg oral q6h for itching or for sleep
Milk of Magnesia 30 mL po q4h prn constipation

Ordered Laboratory Studies

Chemistry, on admission
CBC with differential

Ordered Diagnostic Studies

Chest x-ray
12-lead ECG
CT scan of chest and spine
X-ray of right hip

LABORATORY STUDIES RESULTS

Test	Emergency Department	Postop Day 1	After Blood Transfusion
Chemistry			
Sodium	138 mEq/L		
Potassium	4.2 mEq/L		
Chloride	98 mEq/L		
Carbon dioxide	26 mEq/L		
Blood urea nitrogen (BUN)	12 mg/dL		
Creatinine	0.8 mg/dL		
Blood glucose	110 mg/dL		
Hematology			
White blood cells	11,000/mm³	12,000/mm³	20,000/mm³
Bands	4%		
Segmented neutrophils	48%		
Hemoglobin	8.6/g/dL	8.0/g/dL	9.0/g/dL
Hematocrit	26%	22%	27%
Red blood cells	4.1/mm³	3.7/mm³	3.6/mm³
Platelets	150,000/mm³	148,000/mm³	127,000/mm³

CRITICAL THINKING QUESTIONS

1. What critical assessments need to be made?

2. How can the nurse accurately determine the patient's risk for infection?

3. What nursing measures are appropriate related to infection?

4. What risk factor(s) put Mrs. S. at risk for developing lung cancer?

Answers to Critical Thinking Questions appear in Appendix D.

NCLEX® REVIEW

1. A patient tells the nurse that she doesn't want to "get cancer." Which of the following should the nurse instruct this patient?
1. There is nothing that you can do to prevent the onset of cancer.
2. Instruct in the avoidance of tobacco, excessive alcohol, and a high fat diet.
3. Avoid all types of stress.
4. The chance of developing cancer decreases with age.

2. A patient with cancer asks how a tumor can grow within an organ. The nurse explains how a blood supply is formed or the concept of:
1. Cell attachment.
2. Cell invasion.
3. Angiogenesis.
4. Migration.

3. An elderly male patient was told that he most likely has cancer and the treatment at this time will be "watch and wait." The nurse realizes this patient most likely is experiencing which type of cancer?
1. Melanoma
2. Prostate
3. Brain
4. Colon

4. The nurse is planning care for a patient with cancer. Which of the following should be included to reduce the risk of infection for this patient?
1. Measure rectal temperature every 4 hours.
2. Encourage a diet high in fresh fruit and vegetables.
3. Use strict aseptic technique when caring for venous access devices.
4. Provide intramuscular pain medications.

5. A patient receiving radiation therapy for cancer is demonstrating signs of fatigue. Which of the following can the nurse do to assist this patient?
1. Cluster care activities to increase rest periods.
2. Restrict calories.
3. Discuss activities to increase energy.
4. Review strategies to overcome fatigue over the long term.

6. A patient with cancer is scheduled to receive biotherapy. The nurse realizes the intention for this treatment is to:
1. Eliminate the need for surgery.
2. Reduce the negative impact of chemotherapy.
3. Alter the immunological relationship between the tumor and the patient.
4. Increase the patient's appetite.

Answers for review questions appear in Appendix D

KEY TERMS

absolute neutrophil count (ANC) *p.2113*
allogeneic bone marrow *p.2115*
anorexia *p.2087*
autologous BMT *p.2115*
benign *p.2066*
biopsy *p.2077*
biotherapy *p.2114*
bone marrow transplantation *p.2115*
cancer *p.2061*

carcinogenesis *p.2064*
carcinoma in situ *p.2066*
cytokines *p.2087*
engraftment *p.2116*
incidence *p.2061*
lymphoma *p.2077*
malignant *p.2066*
metastasis *p.2067*
mortality *p.2062*

nadir *p.2113*
neoplasm *p.2063*
palliative *p.2082*
peripheral blood stem cell (PBSC) transplantation *p.2115*
prevalence *p.2062*
radiation *p.2073*
staging *p.2066*
survival *p.2062*

REFERENCES

Akhurst, T., & Larson, S. (1999). Position emission tomography imaging of colorectal cancer. *Seminar in Oncology, 577*(26).

Alexander, J. (2001). Diagnosis and staging. In S. Otto (Ed.), *Oncology nursing* (4th ed.). St. Louis: Mosby.

American Cancer Society. (2001). *American Cancer Society supports closing gap between effective smoking cessation efforts and health care coverage.* Retrieved on September 22, 2008, from http://www.cancer.org/docroot/MED/content/MED_2_1x_American_Cancer_Society_Supports_Closing_Gap_Between_Effective_Smoking_Cessation_Efforts_and_Health_Care_Coverage.asp

American Cancer Society. (2003). *Radiation exposure and cancer.* Retrieved from http://www.cancer.org/docroot/PED/content/PED_1_3X_Radiation_Exposure_and_Cancer.asp?sitearea=PED

American Cancer Society. (2004). *Cancer prevention and early detection facts and figures.* Retrieved on September 22, 2008, from http://www.cancer.org/downloads/STT/CPED2004PWSecured.pdf

American Cancer Society. (2006a). *Cigarette smoking.* Retrieved from http://www.cancer.org/docroot/PED/content/PED_10_2X_Cigarette_Smoking.asp

American Cancer Society. (2006b). *Do we know what causes penile cancer?* Retrieved from http://www.cancer.org/docroot/CRI/content/CRI_2_4_2X_Do_we_know_what_causes_penile_cancer_35.asp?sitearea=

American Cancer Society. (2007). *Cancer facts and figures 2007.* Retrieved from http://www.cancer.org/docroot/STT/content/STT_1x_Cancer_Facts__Figures_2007.asp

American Cancer Society. (2008a). *Seven Steps To Reduce Your Cancer Risk.* Retrieved on September 22, 2008, from http://www.cancer.org/docroot/COM/content/div_NE/COM_1_1x_Seven_Steps_To_Take_To_Prevent_Cancer.asp?sitearea=COM

American Cancer Society. (2008b). *Cancer facts and figures 2008.* Retrieved on September 22, 2008 from http://www.cancer.org/downloads/STT/2008CAFFfinalsecured.pdf

American Cancer Society. (ND). *Risk factors.* Retrieved on September 22, 2008, from http://www.cancer.org/downloads/AA/CancerAtlas02.pdf

Anderson-Reitz, L. (2004). Supportive care of the hematopoietic stem cell transplant patient. *Oncology Supportive Care, 2*(3).

Andrykowski, M., et al. (1998). Off-treatment fatigue in breast cancer survivors: A controlled comparison. *Journal of Behavior Medicine, 21*(1).

Antin, J. (2002). Long-term care after hematopoietic cell transplantation in adults. *New England Journal of Medicine, 347*(1), 36–42.

Ashby, T., & Dalton, J. (2000). Pain assessment and management in people with cancer. In B. Nevidjon & K. Sowers (Eds.), *A nurse's guide to cancer care.* Philadelphia: Lippincott Williams & Wilkins.

Barber, F., & Fabugais-Nazario, L. (2003). What's old is new again: Patients receiving hepatic arterial infusion chemotherapy. *Clinical Journal of Oncology Nursing, 7*(6).

Barnett, M. (2001). Fatigue. In S. Otto (Ed.), *Oncology nursing* (4th ed.). St. Louis: Mosby.

Bender, C., & Rosenzweig, M. (2004). Cancer. In S. Lewis, M. Heitkemper, & S. Dirksen (Eds.), *Medical–surgical nursing assessment and management of clinical problems* (6th ed.). St. Louis: Mosby.

Blesch, K. (1991). Correlates of fatigue in people with breast and lung cancer. *Oncology Nursing Forum, 18*(1), 81.

Blomgren, H., Lax, I., Goranson, H., Kraepelien, T., Nilsson, B., Naslund, I., et al. (1998). Radiosurgery for tumors in the body: Clinical experience using a new method. *Journal of Radiosurgery, 1*(1).

Booker, M. (1996a). Arterial therapy. In M. Booker & D. Ignatavicius (Eds.), *Infusion therapy techniques and medications* (1st ed.). Philadelphia: W. B. Saunders.

Booker, M. (1996b). Central nervous system therapy. In M. Booker & D. Ignatavicius (Eds.), *Infusion therapy techniques and medications* (1st ed.). Philadelphia: W. B. Saunders.

Bower, J., et al. (2000). Fatigue in breast cancer survivors: Occurrence, correlates, and impact on quality of life. *Journal of Clinical Oncology, 18*(4).

Bremerkamp, M. (2000). Mechanisms of action of 5-HT3 receptor antagonists: Clinical overview and nursing implications. *Clinical Journal of Oncology Nursing, 4*(5).

Brunner, D. (1990). Report on the Radiation Oncology Nursing Subcommittee of the American College of Radiation Task Force on Standards Development. *Oncology, 4*(80).

Campbell, C., & Iwamoto, R. (1992). Intraoperative radiation therapy. *Today's OR Nurse, 14*(1).

Centers for Disease Control and Prevention. (2007). *State and community resources.* Retrieved on January 13, 2007, from http://www.cdc.gov/tobacco/tobacco_control_programs/stateandcommunity/index.htm

Clark, R. A., & Reintgen, D. S. (1996). Principles of cancer screening. In D. S. Reintgen & R. A. Clark (Eds.), *Cancer screening.* St. Louis: Mosby.

Crane-Okada, R. (2001). Breast cancers. In S. Otto (Ed.), *Oncology nursing* (4th ed.). St. Louis: Mosby.

Cunningham, R. (2004). Anorexia-cachexia syndrome. In C. H. Yarbro, M. H. Frogge, & M. Goodman (Eds.), *Cancer symptom management* (3rd ed.). Sudbury, MA: Jones and Bartlett.

Daniel, B. (2001). Malignant lymphoma. In S. Otto (Ed.), *Oncology nursing* (4th ed.). St. Louis: Mosby.

Dell, D. (2002). Cachexia in patients with advanced cancer. *Clinical Journal of Oncology Nursing, 6*(4), 235–238.

DeVita, V. T., Jr. (1997). Principles of cancer management: Chemotherapy. In V. T. DeVita, Jr., S. Hellman, & S. A. Rosenberg (Eds.), *Cancer: Principles and practice of oncology* (5th ed.). Philadelphia: Lippincott Williams & Wilkins.

DeVita, V. T., Jr., Hellman, S., & Rosenberg, S. A. (Eds.). (1997). *Cancer: Principles and practice of oncology* (5th ed.). Philadelphia: Lippincott Williams & Wilkins.

Donovan, H., & Ward, S. (2005). Representation of fatigue in women receiving chemotherapy for gynecologic cancers. *Oncology Nursing Forum, 32*(1).

Dow, K., Ferrell, B., Haberman, M., & Eaton, L. (1999). The meaning of quality of life in cancer survivorship. *Oncology Nursing Forum, 26*(3), 519–528.

Dow, K., & Loerzel, V. (2004). Cancer survivorship: A critical aspect of care. In C. H. Yarbro, M. H. Frogge, & M. Goodman (Eds.), *Cancer symptom management* (3rd ed.). Sudbury, MA: Jones and Bartlett.

Dunne-Daly, C. (1997). Principles of brachytherapy. In K. Dow et al. (Eds.), *Nursing care in radiation oncology* (7th ed.). Philadelphia: W. B. Saunders.

Erickson, J. (2003). Cancer. In W. Phipps, F. Monahan, J. Sands, J. Marek, & M. Neighbors (Eds.), *Medical–surgical nursing health and illness perspectives* (7th ed.). St. Louis: Mosby.

Ersek, M. (2003). Artificial nutrition and hydration. *Journal of Hospice and Palliative Care Nursing, 5*(4), 221–230.

Ersek, M., Ferrell, B., Dow, K., & Melancon, C. (1997). Quality of life in women with ovarian cancer. *Western Journal of Nursing Research, 19*(2), 334–350.

Erye, H., Kahn, R., Robertson, R., & Committee AAACW. (2004). Preventing cancer, cardiovascular disease, and diabetes: A common agenda for the American Cancer Society, the American Diabetes Association, and the American Heart Association. *CA—Cancer Journal for Clinicians, 54* (4).

Ferrell, B., & Dow, K. (1997). Quality of life among long-term cancer survivors. *Oncology, 11*(3), 565–568.

Ferrell, B., Dow, K., Leigh, S., Ly, J., & Gulasekaram, P. (1995). Quality of life in long-term cancer survivors. *Oncology Nursing Forum, 22*(5), 915–922.

Ferrell, B., Grant, M., Funk, B., Otis-Green, S., & Garcia, N. (1998a). Quality of life in breast cancer. Part II: Psychological and spiritual well-being. *Cancer Nursing, 21*(1), 1–9.

Ferrell, B., Grant, M., Funk, B., Otis-Green, S., Garcia, N. (1998b). Quality of life in breast cancer survivors: Implications for developing support services. *Oncology Nursing Forum, 25*(4), 887–895.

Finley, J. (2003a). Detection and management of cachexia in cancer patients. *Advanced Studies in Nursing, 1*(1), 8–12.

Finley, J. (2003b). Management of cancer cachexia and chemotherapy associated nausea and vomiting. *Advanced Studies in Nursing, 1*(1), 7.

Fischbach, F., & Dunning, M. (Eds.). (2006). *Nurses' quick reference to common laboratory and diagnostic tests.* Philadelphia: Lippincott Williams & Wilkins.

Flynn, A. (2005). Isotopes and delivery systems for brachytherapy. In P. Hoskin & C. Coyle (Eds.), *Radiotherapy in practice brachytherapy.* New York: Oxford University Press.

Fouladbakhsh, J., Stommel, M., Given, B., & Given, C. (2005). Predictors of use of complementary and alternative therapies among patients with cancer. *Oncology Nursing Forum, 32*(6).

Gale, C. (2005). Nursing implications of biotherapy and molecular targeted therapy. In J. Itano & K. Taoka (Eds.), *Core curriculum for oncology nursing* (4th ed.). St. Louis: W. B. Saunders.

Ganz, P., Coscarelli, A., Fred, C., Kahn, B., Polinsky, M., & Peterson, L. (1996). Breast cancer survivors: Psychosocial concerns and quality of life. *Breast Cancer Research and Treatment, 38*(1), 183–199.

Given, C., Given, B., Azzoouz, F., Kozachik, S., & Stommel, M. (2001). Predictors of pain and fatigue in the year following diagnosis among elderly cancer patients. *Journal of Pain and Symptom Management, 1*(2), 456–466.

Grever, M., & Chabner, B. (1997). Cancer drug discovery and development. In V. T. DeVita, Jr., S. Hellman, & S. A. Rosenberg (Eds.), *Cancer: Principles and practice of oncology* (5th ed.). Philadelphia: Lippincott Williams & Wilkins.

Groenwald, S., Frogge, M. H., Goodman, M., & Yarbro, C. H. (Eds.). (1997). *Cancer nursing: Principles and practice* (4th ed.). Sudbury: Jones and Bartlett.

Gullatte, M., & Otto, S. (2001). Cancer clinical trials. In S. Otto (Ed.), *Oncology nursing* (4th ed.). St. Louis: Mosby.

Ham, O. (2006). Factors affecting mammography behavior and intention among Korean women. *Oncology Nursing Forum, 33*(1).

Hartigan, K. (2003). Patient education: The cornerstone of successful oral chemotherapy treatment. *Clinical Journal of Oncology Nursing, 7*(6).

Hawkins, R. (2001). Mastering the intricate maze of metastasis. *Oncology Nursing Forum, 28*(6), 959–965.

Heath, C. W. (1996). Electromagnetic field exposure and cancer: A review of epidemiologic evidence. *CA—A Cancer Journal for Clinicians, 46*(29).

Hill, G. (1979). Historical milestones in cancer surgery. *Seminar of Oncology, 6*(409).

Holmes, M. D., Hunter, D. J., Colditz, G. A., Stampfer, M. J., Hankinson, S. E., Speizer, F. E., et al. (1999). Association of dietary intake of fat and fatty acids with the risk of breast cancer. *Journal of the American Medical Association, 281*(10).

Hoskin, P., & Coyle, C. (2005). Introduction. In P. Hoskin & C. Coyle (Eds.), *Radiotherapy in practice brachytherapy.* New York: Oxford University Press.

Iovino, C., & Camacho, L. (2003). Acute myeloid leukemia: A classification and treatment update. *Clinical Journal of Oncology Nursing, 7*(5), 535–540.

Iwamoto, R. (2001). Radiation therapy. In S. Otto (Ed.), *Oncology nursing* (4th ed.). St. Louis: Mosby.

Jemail, A., Thomas, A., Murrey, T., & Thun, M. (2002). Cancer statistics, 2002. *CA—A Cancer Journal for Clinicians, 52*(1), 23–47.

Kalman, D., & Villani, L. (1997). Nutritional aspects of cancer related fatigue. *Journal of the American Dietetic Association, 97,* 650.

Kaye, J. (1993). Psychological distress in cancer patients and their spouses. *Journal of Cancer Education, 8*(47).

Keller, C. (2001). Bone marrow and stem cell transplantation. In S. Otto (Ed.), *Oncology nursing* (4th ed.). St. Louis: Mosby.

Kinsella, K., & Velkoff, V. (2001). *An aging world: 2001* (NIH publication no. P95/01-1). Washington, DC: U.S. Government Printing Office.

Larson, D. (1998). Stereotactic external-beam irradiation. In C. Perez & L. Brady (Eds.), *Principles and practices of radiation oncology* (3rd ed.). Philadelphia: Lippincott Williams & Wilkins.

Lavdaniti, M., Patiraki, E., Dafni, U., Katapodi, M., Papathanasoglou, E., & Sotiropoulou, A. (2006). Prospective assessment of fatigue and health status in Greek patients with breast cancer undergoing adjuvant radiotherapy. *Oncology Nursing Forum, 33*(3).

Lee-Lin, F., & Menon, U. (2005). Breast and cervical cancer screening practices and interventions among Chinese, Japanese, and Vietnamese Americans. *Oncology Nursing Forum, 32*(5).

Levy, J. (1994). Photosensitizers in photodynamic therapy. *Seminars in Oncology,* (21)4.

Liotta, L. A. (1992). Cancer cell invasion and metastasis. *Scientific American, 266*(2), 54–63.

Liotta, L. A., & Kohn, E. (1990). Cancer invasion and metastasis. *Journal of the American Medical Association, 263,* 1123–1126.

Ludwig, R., Weirich, A., Abel, U., Hofmann, W., Graf, N., & Tournade, M. (1999). Hepatotoxicity in patients treated according to Nephroblastoma Trial and Study SIOP-9/GPOH. *Journal of Medical and Pediatric Oncology, 33*(5).

Lynaugh, J. (2001). Forward. In J. Johnson, S. Baird, & L. Hilderley (Eds.), *It took courage, compassion, and curiosity: Recollections and writings of leaders in cancer nursing: 1890–1970* (1st ed.). Pittsburgh: Oncology Nursing Society.

Lynn, D. (1994). *Myself resolved an artist's experience with lymphoma.* Philadelphia: Meniscus Health Care Communications.

Mahon, S. M. (2000). Principles of cancer detection and early prevention. *Clinical Journal of Oncology Nursing, 4*(4), 169–176.

Malin, A. (2005) Epidemiology. In C. H. Yarbro, M. H. Frogge, & M. Goodman (Eds.), *Cancer nursing: Principles and practice* (6th ed.). Sudbury, MA: Jones and Bartlett.

Markam, M., & Walker, J. (2006). Intraperitoneal chemotherapy of ovarian cancer: A review with a focus on practical aspects of treatment. *Journal of Clinical Oncology, 24*(6).

McMahon, K. (2003). Components of nutritional screening and assessment. In *Oncology Nursing Society 2003 annual congress symposium highlights* (pp. 5–6). Pittsburgh: Author.

McNance, K., & Roberts, L. (2002). Biology of cancer. In K. McNance & S. Huetter (Eds.), *Pathophysiology: The biological basis for disease in adult and children* (4th ed.). St. Louis: Mosby.

Mellon, S. (2002). Comparisons between cancer survivors and family members on meaning of the illness and family quality of life. *Oncology Nursing Forum, 29*(7), 1117–1125.

Merkle, C., & Loescher, L. (2005) Biology of cancer. In C. H. Yarbro, M. H. Frogge, & M. Goodman (Eds.), *Cancer nursing: Principles and practice* (6th ed.). Sudbury, MA: Jones and Bartlett.

Miaskowski, C., & Lee, K. (1999). Pain, fatigue, and sleep disturbances in oncology outpatients receiving radiation therapy for bone metastasis: A pilot study. *Journal of Pain Symptom Management, 17*(3), 320.

Mock, V. (2003). Clinical excellence through evidenced-based practice: Fatigue management as a model. *Oncology Nursing Forum, 30*(4).

Murphy, M. (2001a). Cancers of the brain and central nervous system. In S. Otto (Ed.), *Oncology nursing* (4th ed.). St. Louis: Mosby.

Murphy, M. (2001b). Colorectal cancers. In S. Otto (Ed.), *Oncology nursing* (4th ed.). St. Louis: Mosby.

Muss, H. (2001). Older age—not a barrier to cancer treatment. *New England Journal of Medicine, 345*(15), 1128–1129.

Myers, J. (2001). Oncologic complications. In S. Otto (Ed.), *Oncology nursing* (4th ed.). St. Louis: Mosby.

Nail, L. (2004). Fatigue. In C. H. Yarbro, M. H. Frogge, & M. Goodman (Eds.), *Cancer symptom management* (3rd ed.). Sudbury, MA: Jones and Bartlett.

Nail, L., & Jones, L. (1995). Fatigue side effects and treatment and quality of life. *Quality of Life Research, 4*(1), 8.

National Cancer Institute. (2003). *Nutrition.* Retrieved from http://www.cancer.gov

National Comprehensive Cancer Network. (2003). Cancer-related fatigue: Clinical practice guidelines in oncology. *Journal of the National Comprehensive Cancer Network, 1*(1).

National Comprehensive Cancer Network. (2006). *Cancer-related fatigue: Clinical practice guidelines in oncology.*

Nelson-Marten, P., & Glover, J. (2005). Selected ethical issues in cancer care. In J. K. Itano & K. N. Taoka (Eds.), *Core curriculum for oncology nursing* (4th ed.). Philadelphia: W. B. Saunders.

Noll, L., & Riese, N. (1997). Chemical modifiers of radiation therapy. In K. Dow et al. (Eds.), *Nursing care in radiation oncology* (2nd ed.). Philadelphia: W. B. Saunders.

Occupational Safety and Health Administration, Office of Occupational Medicine. (1995). *Controlling occupational exposure to hazardous CPL2-2.20B CH-4.* Washington, DC: U.S. Department of Labor.

Oldham, R. (1991). Biotherapy: General principles. In R. K. Oldham (Ed.), *Principles of cancer biotherapy* (2nd ed.). New York: Marcel Dekker.

Omerod, K. (2005). Diagnostic evaluation, classification, and staging. In C. H. Yarbro, M. H. Frogge, & M. Goodman (Eds.), *Cancer nursing: Principles and practice* (6th ed.). Sudbury, MA: Jones and Bartlett.

Oncology Nursing Society. (2001). *Chemotherapy and biotherapy guidelines and recommendations for practice.* Pittsburgh: Author.

Oncology Nursing Society (2006). *Cancer pain management position statement.* Pittsburgh: Author.

Oncology Nursing Society, Vision, Mission, Core Values (ND). Retrieved September 22, 2008 from http://www.ons.org/about/corevalues.shtml.

Oncology Nursing Society & Geriatric Oncology Consortium (2004). *Oncology Nursing Society and Geriatric Oncology Consortium joint position on cancer care in the older adult.* Pittsburgh: Oncology Nursing Society.

O'Rourke, M. (2001). Genitourinary cancers. In S. Otto (Ed.), *Oncology nursing* (4th ed.). St. Louis: Mosby.

Ososki, R. (2001). Leukemia. In S. Otto (Ed.), *Oncology nursing* (4th ed.). St. Louis: Mosby.

Otto, S. (2001a). Chemotherapy. In S. Otto (Ed.), *Oncology nursing* (4th ed.). St. Louis: Mosby.

Otto, S. (2001b). Lung Cancers. In S. Otto (Ed.), *Oncology nursing* (4th ed.). St. Louis: Mosby.

Otto, S. (2001c). *Oncology nursing* (4th ed.). St. Louis: Mosby.

Overholt, B., Panjehpour, M., & Haydeck, J. (1999). Photodynamic therapy for Barrett's esophagus: Follow-up in 100 patients. *Gastrointestinal Endoscopy, 49*(1).

Park, C., & Folkman, S. (1997). Meaning in the context of stress and coping. *Review of General Psychology, 1,* 115–144.

Pfeifer, K. A. (2001). Pathophysiology. In S. Otto (Ed.), *Oncology nursing* (4th ed.). St. Louis: Mosby.

Piper, B., Dibble, S., Dodd, M., Weiss, M., Slaughter, R., & Paul, S. (1987). The revised Piper Fatigue Scale: Psychometric evaluation in women with breast cancer. *Oncology Nursing Forum, 25*(3).

Piper, B., Dibble, S., Dodd M., Weiss, M., Slaughter, R., Paul, S. (1998) The revised Piper Fatigue Scale: psychometric evaluation in women with breast cancer. *Oncology Nursing Forum. 25*(4):677–684.

Ponto, J., Frost, M., Thompson, R., Allers, T., Will, T., Zahasky, K., et al. (2003). Stories of breast cancer through art. *Oncology Nursing Forum, 30*(6), 1007–1113.

Rokita, S. (2004). Oncology: Nursing management in cancer care. In S. Smeltzer & B. Bare (Eds.), *Brunner & Suddarth's textbook of medical–surgical nursing* (10th ed.). Philadelphia: Lippincott Williams & Wilkins.

Russell, K., Perkins, S., Zollinger, T., & Champion, V. (2006). Sociocultural context of mammogram screening. *Oncology Nursing Forum, 33*(1).

Santos, G. (2000). Historical background to hematopoietic stem cell transplantation. In K. Atkinson (Ed.), *Clinical bone marrow and blood stem transplantation.* New York: Cambridge University Press.

Schmit-Pokorny, K., Franco, T., Frappier, B., Vyhlidal, R. (2003). The cooperative care model: an innovative approach to deliver blood and marrow stem cell transplant care. *Clinical Journal of Oncology Nursing,* 7(5).

Schulmeister, L. (2001a). Epidemiology. In S. Otto (Ed.), *Oncology nursing* (4th ed.). St. Louis: Mosby.

Schulmeister, L. (2001b). Nutrition. In S. Otto (Ed.), *Oncology nursing* (4th ed.). St. Louis: Mosby.

Sedhom, L., Yanni, M. (1985). Radiation therapy and nurses' fears of radiation exposure. *Cancer Nursing, 8*(129).

Shell, J., & Kirsch, S. (2001). Psychosocial issues, outcomes, and quality of life. In S. Otto (Ed.), *Oncology nursing* (4th ed.). St. Louis: Mosby.

Sigler, B., & Schuring, L. (1993). *Ear, nose, and throat disorders* (Mosby's Clinical Nursing Series), St. Louis: Mosby.

Singleton, L., & Connor, T. (1999). An evaluation of the permeability of chemotherapy gloves to three cancer chemotherapy drugs. *Oncology Nursing Forum, 26*(4).

Sitton, E. (1997) Managing side effects of skin changes and fatigue. In K. Dow et al. (Eds.), *Nursing care in radiation oncology.* (7th ed.). Philadelphia: W. B. Saunders.

Sitton, E. (2005). Nursing implications of radiation therapy. In J. K. Itano & K. N. Taoka (Eds.), *Core curriculum for oncology nursing* (4th ed.). Philadelphia: W. B. Saunders.

Spross, J., McGuire, D., & Schmitt, R. (1990a). Oncology Nursing Society position paper on cancer pain. Part I. Scope of nursing practice regarding cancer pain, ethics, and practice. *Oncology Nursing Forum, 17*(3), 595.

Spross, J., McGuire, D., & Schmitt, R. (1990b). Oncology Nursing Society position paper on cancer pain. Part II. Education, research, and list of cancer management resources. *Oncology Nursing Forum, 17*(4), 751.

Spross, J., McGuire, D., & Schmitt, R. (1990c). Oncology Nursing Society position paper on cancer pain. Part III. Nursing administration, pediatric cancer pain and appendices. *Oncology Nursing Forum, 17*(5), 943.

Stellman, J. M., & Stellman, S. D. (1996). Cancer and the workplace. *CA—A Cancer Journal for Clinicians, 46*(2).

Sura, W., Murphy, S., & Gonzales, I. (2006). Level of fatigue in women receiving dose-dense versus standard chemotherapy for breast cancer: A pilot study. *Oncology Nursing Forum, 33*(5).

Swenson, C. (2001). Pain management. In S. Otto (Ed.), *Oncology nursing* (4th ed.). St. Louis: Mosby.

Szopa, T. (2005). Nursing implications of surgical treatment. In J. K. Itano & K. N. Taoka (Eds.), *Core curriculum for oncology nursing* (4th ed.). Philadelphia: W. B. Saunders.

U.S. Department of Health and Human Services. (2000). *Healthy people 2010: Understanding and improving health.* Washington, DC: Author.

U.S. Department of Health and Human Services, Public Health Service, National Toxicology Program. (2002, December). *Report on carcinogens* (10th ed.). Washington, DC: Author.

VanBurik, J., & Weisdorf, D. (1999). Infections in recipients of blood and marrow transplantation. *Hematology Oncology Clinics of North America, 13*(5).

Viele, C. (2005). Keys to unlock cancer: Targeted therapy. *Oncology Nursing Forum, 32*(5).

Volker, D. L. (1992). Pathophysiology of cancer. In J. C. Clark & R .F. McGee (Eds.), *Core curriculum for oncology nursing* (2nd ed.). Philadelphia: W. B. Saunders.

Volker, D. (1994). Neoplasia. In P. Beare & J. Myers (Eds.), *Principles and practice of adult health nursing* (2nd ed.). St. Louis: Mosby.

Voss, J., Armitage, J., & Kessinger, A. (1993). High dose chemotherapy and autologous transplant with peripheral blood stem cells. *Oncology, 7*(8).

Wikle-Shapiro, T. (1998). Nursing implications of bone marrow and stem cell transplantation. In J. K. Itano & K. N. Taoka (Eds.), *Core curriculum for oncology nursing* (3rd ed.). Philadelphia: W. B. Saunders.

Wingard, J. (2007). Bone marrow to blood stem cells past, present, future. In S. Ezzone and K. Schmit-Pokorny (Eds.), *Blood and bone marrow stem cell transplantation: Principles, practice, and nursing insights* (3rd ed.). Sudbury, MA: James and Bartlett.

Winningham, M., Nail, L., Burke, M., Brophy, L., Cimprich, B., & Jones, L. (1994). Fatigue and the cancer experience. *Oncology Nursing Forum, 21*(1), 23–36.

Woodard, W., & Hogan, D. (1996). Oncologic emergencies: Implications for nurses. *Journal of Intravenous Nursing, 19*(2).

Wu, T., & Bancroft, J. (2006). Filipino American women's perceptions and experiences with breast cancer screening. *Oncology Nursing Forum, 33*(4).

Zebrack, B. (2000). Quality of life of long-term survivors of leukemia and lymphoma. *Journal of Psychosocial Oncology, 18*(4), 39–59.

Ziegler, R. G., Devesa, S. S., & Fravmeni, J. F., Jr. (1991). Epidemiologic patterns of colorectal cancer. In V. T. DeVita, Jr., S. Hellman, & S. A. Rosenberg (Eds.), *Important advances in oncology.* Philadelphia: Lippincott Williams & Wilkins.

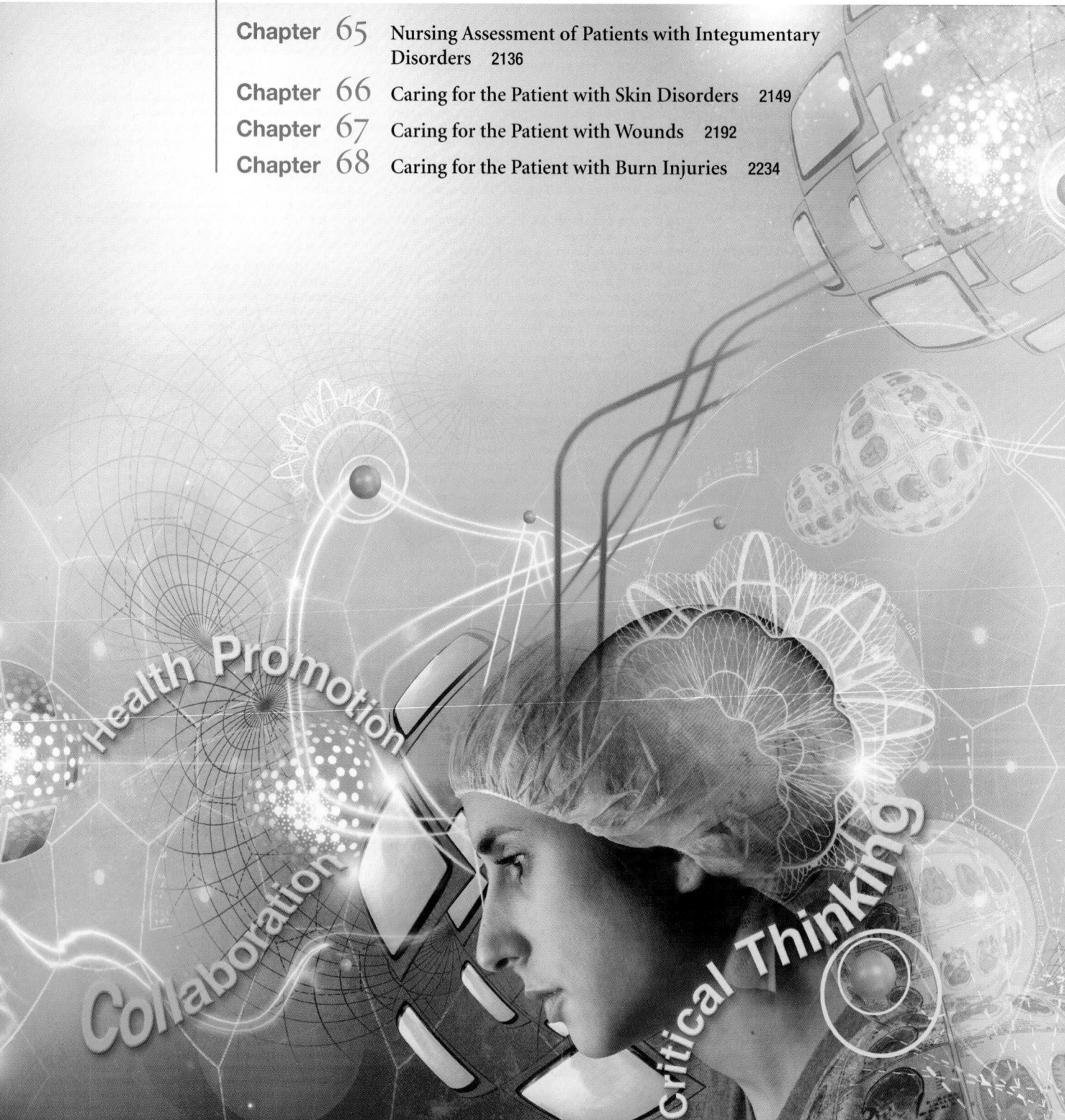

UNIT 14
Nursing Management of Patients with Integumentary Disorders

Health Promotion

Collaboration

Critical Thinking

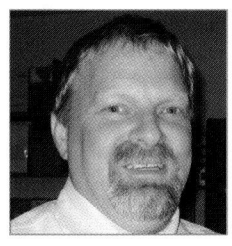

LEN My name is Len and I am the nurse manager in the Burn Intensive Care Unit (ICU) at a major teaching hospital. Although the Burn ICU specializes in the care of victims of traumatic burn injuries, we provide expert, cutting-edge care for a wide variety of other injuries and illnesses as well. Besides burn injuries, our patients are a diverse mix of people with trauma, chronic illnesses, and complex wounds.

After graduating from nursing school, I worked in a Burn Unit that also provided wound care services. I remember looking helplessly into the faces of patients with diabetes, while trying desperately to save their lower extremities from amputation. The stories they told of their cultural practices and traditions taught me valuable lessons about human compassion. I also learned that the physiological effects of their diabetes were further complicated by cultural and social gaps between native cultures and Western medicine. I developed a passion for helping those who desperately needed specialized interventions and I knew I wanted to devote my career to delivering care to a diverse population of people needing treatment for burns, complex wounds, and devastating illnesses.

The needs of burn patients and their families are even more complex than most people can possibly imagine. Teamwork and collaboration are absolutely essential for these patients to live and function. Every member of the burn team must be an expert in his or her own discipline. Health care professionals involved in the care of burn patients include burn surgeons, plastic reconstructive surgeons, pulmonologists, infectious disease experts, psychiatrists, cardiologists, ophthalmologists, respiratory therapists, physical and occupational therapists, laboratory specialists, pharmacists, dietitians, social workers, chaplains, and, of course, nurses. Burn nurses coordinate the care and implement the interventions ordered by the specialists. The role of the professional nurse does not rest with monitoring the patient's ventilator, cardiac monitor, hemodynamic status, emotional state, and pain level. We also perform daily dressing changes on large wounds and fragile skin grafts that can take up to 3 hours.

Burn patients often require very large quantities of IV fluids to prevent rapid and sudden cardiovascular collapse and hypovolemic shock. The process of infusing these large quantities of fluids is known as fluid resuscitation and is totally managed by the burn nurse. As many as three nurses, a surgeon, and a respiratory therapist may be required initially to admit and stabilize the victim of a large burn injury.

Caring about the welfare of your patients is what separates a technical nurse from a truly professional one who is committed to the profession. Due to the devastating nature of burn injuries, it is imperative for nurses to use a caring approach. A case comes to mind of a woman whose life was changed in a quick second. While getting dressed one morning, she was applying hairspray while evidently smoking a cigarette. The aerosolized hairspray ignited and she suffered full-thickness burns over a large portion of her body. After stabilization, she went to surgery to have her burns skin grafted. Our burn surgeon did such a remarkable job of placing a perfect graft over her severely damaged face. I spent 12 tedious hours with a scalpel, cotton swabs, ointment, and rolled gauze keeping serous fluid and blood from collecting under the skin graft. If fluid were allowed to collect, those portions of the graft would die due to a lack of blood supply. In spite of her injuries, I could see she was a beautiful woman whose physical appearance would now depend on me over the next few hours to make certain the skin would successfully attach. Times like these are a true test of one's commitment to others. It would have been easy to do an adequate job on this complete stranger by assessing and rolling the graft three or four times an hour. In this case, however, the fluid was collecting far too frequently. Although this woman was unknown to me, I did not see a stranger that night. I saw someone's wife and a child's mother lying in a bed on life support and placing a large portion of her future into the hands of someone she had never before met. Though I became fatigued, I stayed there never far from her face just to make sure the grafts were safe. I cannot remember whether I ate or drank much fluid that night while residing in her hot 90-degree room wrapped in a surgical gown and gloves.

Being a burn nurse is more than simply having good critical care skills, doing wound care, and managing the infusion of 30 liters of fluid into a person during a 24-hour period. It requires practicing with compassion in extreme circumstances, and accepting that the best you have to offer may not be enough. Despite the many emotionally trying circumstances I often encounter in the Burn ICU, I am more committed than ever to delivering care to a diverse population of people.

"Caring about the welfare of your patients is what separates a technical nurse from a truly professional one who is committed to the profession."

65

Nursing Assessment of Patients with Integumentary Disorders

Peggy Ellis
Teri A. Murray
Kathleen Osborn

Outcome-Based Learning Objectives

After studying this chapter, the learner will be able to:

1. Discuss the structure and function of the skin.
2. Obtain a health history relative to assessment of the skin, hair, and nails.
3. Collect subjective and objective data relative to assessment of the skin, hair, and nails.
4. Utilize correct techniques of physical exam when assessing the skin, hair, and nails.
5. Distinguish between normal and abnormal assessment findings in the skin, hair, and nails.
6. Describe skin lesions by morphologic classification.
7. Identify biologic and cultural variations in assessment of the skin.

Research   Collaboration   Health Promotion   Nursing Process   Caring   Critical Thinking

THE INTEGUMENTARY system is composed of the skin, hair, nails, and glands. The skin is the most visible organ of the body and accounts for about 7% of the body weight. It is composed of three layers: the epidermis, dermis, and subcutaneous tissue described later (Porth, 2007). The epidermal appendages of the skin include the hair, nails, sebaceous glands, and the eccrine and apocrine sweat glands. The skin is pliable, is able to withstand insults from external agents, and has a remarkable ability to heal. Additionally, through the sense of touch, it enables individuals to perceive the world around them, and its changes in color reflect emotional reactions to the environment. It is critical that the nurse be able to recognize and identify skin abnormalities. Assessment of the skin and its appendages requires a thorough understanding of the structure and function of the integumentary system and knowledge of normal and abnormal findings.

Anatomy and Physiology of the Skin

The skin is the largest organ of the body whose primary function is to provide a protective barrier to the vital organs, and it prevents harmful organisms from entering the body. It protects underlying tissues and structures from microorganisms,

chemical injury, or trauma, and it guards against excessive exposure to ultraviolet rays from the sun. Other functions of the skin include:

- Retards the loss of body heat and fluids
- Assists in the control of body temperature
- Contains the sensory receptors that allow an individual to feel heat, cold, pressure, and pain
- Contains immune systems cells
- Functions as a excretory organ (sweat glands)
- Functions as a synthesizer of vitamin D (sunlight reacts with cholesterol)
- Determines identity (race, fingerprints)
- Stores blood and fats
- Reflects emotion through color changes.

The skin also manifests diseases or injury. For example, rashes may be associated with systemic diseases such as lupus erythematosus and jaundice associated with liver disease (Porth, 2007). Redness and swelling are associated with injuries such as fractures and internal bleeding.

Skin Layers

There are three anatomical layers of the skin: the epidermis, dermis, and subcutaneous tissue (Figure 65–1 ■). Each layer is described next.

Epidermis

The epidermis is the thin, avascular outer layer that is nourished by the blood vessels from the dermis. Four distinct cell types are contained in the epidermis: keratinocytes, melanocytes, Merkel's cells, and Langerhans' cells. *Keratinocytes* are the most numerous cells of the epidermis; and as they mature they move to the surface, die, and thereby form the outermost surface of the skin (stratum corneum). These cells produce keratin, which provides the major protective barrier. The maturation and death of keratinocytes occur approximately every 4 weeks. If the process occurs too quickly, the skin appears thin and may break down more easily. If old cells have not sloughed before the formation of new cells, the skin appears thickened and scaly. *Melanocytes* are the pigment-producing cells. Pigment granules (melanin), which are black or brown, give the skin and hair its color. The more melanin an individual has, the darker the skin and hair. The primary function of melanocytes is to protect the skin from ultraviolet rays. *Merkel's cells* provide sensory information, and *Langerhans' cells* are macrophages of the immune system that arise from the bone marrow and migrate to the epidermis. These cells recognize a foreign antigen and bind it to their surface, process it, and then migrate with the antigen back to the lymphatic vessels and into the regional lymph nodes. The epidermis also contains sweat glands and sebaceous glands.

Dermis

A basement membrane connects the epidermis to the dermis. This is the layer involved in blister formation. The dermis, composed of fibrous connective tissue, contains the blood vessels, hair follicles, nerve endings, sweat glands, and sebaceous glands. It separates the epidermis from the subcutaneous tissue and provides nutrition for the epidermis. The dermis is composed of

two layers: the papillary dermis and the reticular dermis. The papillary dermis is the superficial layer, consisting of collagen fibers and ground substances (a viscid gel that is rich in mucopolysaccharides) that lie adjunct to the epidermis. This layer is densely covered by dermal papillae that contain capillary venules that nourish the epidermal layer. Lymph vessels and nerve endings are also found in this layer. The reticular dermis, the thicker layer, is composed of a complex meshwork of three-dimensional collagen bundles interconnected with large elastic fibers and ground substance. The reticular dermis also contains dermal dendrocytes, which have phagocytic properties that participate in immune function of the skin. The specific immune cells found in dermis include T cells, mast cells, and fibroblasts (Porth, 2007). The T cells provide a delayed-type hypersensitivity that is described in Chapter 60 ☉ .

Subcutaneous Tissue

Subcutaneous tissue, made up of loose connective tissue and fat cells, functions to lend support to the vascular and neural structures that supply the outer layer of skin. Because of the presence of the eccrine glands and deep hair follicles, and several skin diseases that extend into this layer, it is considered part of the skin (Porth, 2007).

Blood and Lymph Supply, Sebaceous Glands, and Innervation

The arterial vessels that nourish the skin are located between the papillary and reticular layers of the dermis and between the dermis and the subcutaneous tissue layer. Blood returns via small veins that accompany the subcutaneous vessels. The lymphatic system is located in the dermis and helps combat skin infections. The majority of the vessels are under sympathetic nervous system control. The sympathetic nervous system also controls the arrector pili muscles that cause elevation of the hair on the arms and dimpling of the skin (goose bumps). The dermis contains a rich supply of sensory neurons. The receptors for touch, pressure, heat, cold, and pain are in the dermis (Porth, 2007).

■ Gerontological Considerations

Several physiological changes occur in the skin with the aging process. Both the epidermis and the dermis thin; there is a reduction in subcutaneous tissue and collagen, and a thickening of the blood vessels. In addition, the number of melanocytes, Merkel's cells, and Langerhans' cells decreases. This results in color changes and decreased resistance to organisms. The keratinocytes actually shrink, although the amount of dead keratinized cells on the skin surface increases. These changes result in thinner skin with less padding, making it more susceptible to breakdown from trauma. There is a decrease in hormonally induced sebaceous gland activity. Therefore, older individuals have drier, more scaly skin, especially in the winter months when there is an increased need for home heating. Finally, there is less hair and nail growth, and hair permanently loses pigment with the aging process (Porth, 2007). Graying may begin as early as in the third decade of life and is caused by reduced melanin production in the hair follicles. Genetic factors tend to determine the age of the onset of graying. Chapter 66 ☉ includes an in-depth discussion of age-related skin diseases.

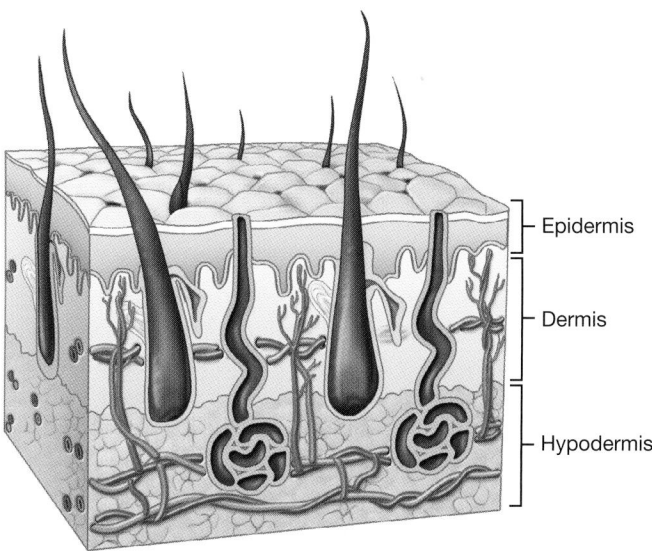

Epidermis

Dermis

Hypodermis

FIGURE 65–1 ■   Skin layers.

Physiological Impact of Ultraviolet Rays

The sun's rays are measured in wavelengths that range from 290 nanometers in the ultraviolet (UV) range to 2,500 nanometers in the infrared range. There are three types of ultraviolet rays: ultraviolet A (UVA), ultraviolet B (UVB), and ultraviolet C (UVC). The UVB rays are primarily responsible for sunburn and the cumulative damage to the skin from the sun (Porth, 2007). UVA rays produce elastic skin and actinic skin damage. Exposure to UV radiation causes sunburn and skin cancer and accelerates skin aging. A growing concern is that UV radiation can reduce the effectiveness of the human immune system, thereby enhancing the risk of infection and limiting the efficacy of immunization against disease (World Health Organization, 2001). Chapter 66 ⊕ includes an in-depth discussion of sun-related skin diseases.

 A common belief is that only fair-skinned people need to be concerned about overexposure to the sun. It is true that darker skin has more protective pigment, although the skin is still susceptible to the damaging effects of ultraviolet (UV) radiation. The incidence of skin cancers is lower in dark-skinned people; nevertheless, skin cancers occur and are often detected among them at a later, more dangerous stage. The risk of other UV-related health effects, such as eye damage, premature aging of the skin, and immunosuppression, also occurs in dark-skinned people.

(World Health Organization, 2001).

History

The health history, the major subjective source of data, provides valuable insights into the patient's past and current health status. The health history is composed of several components that provide structure for data collection and an organized record of the patient's response to skin problems. The components of the history are outlined next.

Biographic and Demographic Data

Biographic and demographic data include data such as the patient's name, address, telephone number, social security number, contact person, age, gender, race or ethnic origin, marital status, birthplace, occupation, level of education, and religious affiliation. This information is critical in identifying one patient's record from another's, and it provides a general overview of the person's communication abilities, reliability as a historian, and general personal attributes. Biographic and demographic information is needed for epidemiologic comparisons. For example, the incidence or prevalence of a particular health condition may be attributed to a certain geographic locale, a racial or ethnic group, or a specific gender. It is important to date the history so that, if the patient's condition changes, events can be correlated chronologically. Examples of biographic and demographic data that may be significant to assessment of the skin include environmental or occupational toxins, neighborhood waste, or landfills. Environmental toxins include overexposure to frost, wind, and ultraviolet rays from the sun. Neighborhood waste and landfills could involve exposure to arsenic, creosote, coal tar, and/or petroleum products. Environmental toxins, neighborhood waste, and landfills are risk factors for skin cancer. Finally the nurse also should inquire about travel to different environments such as camping or travel to rural areas of the world.

Chief Complaint

The assessment begins with identifying the patient's current issue or the reason for seeking health care, which is referred to as the chief complaint. When a patient is admitted, the nurse begins the interview by asking the patient what he considers the most current and acute health issue. It is typically best elicited by the nurse's asking "What brought you here?" It is generally a concise statement in the patient's own words indicating his rationale for seeking health care. Examples of chief complaints are "I have had a rash for 3 days"; "I've noticed discolorations on my legs and arms for 2 weeks"; "My hair has been thinning for 6 months"; "I think I have a fungal infection in my cuticle."

Presenting Symptoms

The presenting symptoms detail the chronology of each symptom, how it developed, and what events surrounded the symptoms. In the skin, the presenting symptoms may be changes in the condition of the patient's skin, such as dryness, pruritus, sores, and lumps; changes in a mole or a wart; skin lesions; or changes in skin color or texture. When obtaining information from the patient related to the presenting symptoms, the nurse should question the patient about his perception of the cause as well as what measures the patient may have already taken to remedy the condition.

Past Medical History

The past medical history can be of great value in assessing the current problem. The purpose in obtaining information about the past medical history is to identify the patient's entire past relevant health problems. Past illnesses could possibly have some effect on the patient's current health. The nurse would ask the patient about previous skin conditions, allergic reactions, unusual sensations, history of allergies, and other diseases that may affect the condition of the skin. A disease such as systemic lupus erythematosus causes a butterfly rash on the face. Use of chemotherapeutic agents to treat cancer may cause hair loss. Cancer, heart disease, liver disease, and anemia can cause changes in the nails such as grooves, ridges, and discolorations.

Childhood Illnesses

Inquire whether the patient has had any of the following childhood illnesses: measles, mumps, whooping cough, chickenpox, smallpox, scarlet fever, rheumatic fever, diphtheria, acne, and poliomyelitis. This will assist the nurse in determining the cause of any residual scarring.

Immunizations

The nurse needs to inquire about what childhood immunizations the patient had as well as adult immunizations. Ask the patient specifically about polio, diphtheria, pertussis, human papillomavirus (HPV), tetanus toxoid, influenza, last tuberculin skin test, and any skin reactions to the immunizations.

Previous Illnesses

The nursing assessment includes questions about major illnesses such as diabetes, cardiovascular disease, and infectious diseases. Patients with diabetes are prone to skin breakdown and delayed wound healing (Chapters 53 and 67 ☺). Patients with cardiovascular disease may have clubbed nail beds (Chapter 37 ☺). Infectious diseases such as cellulitis have skin manifestations, which assist with the diagnosis.

Medications

Inquire about medications taken regularly (names, dosages, frequency, reason for taking, side effects) and whether the patient complies with the medication regimen. Inquire about over-the-counter medication use; include herbal medications, vitamins, and any home remedies as well. Drugs may produce skin eruptions, decrease or increase sunlight sensitivity, and cause hyperpigmentation.

Allergies

Inquire about allergies to medications, foods, and environmental allergens. Have the patient describe what clinical skin manifestations occur when she experiences an allergic reaction as well as what makes the reaction subside.

■ Health Assessment

The current health status is the general state of health as perceived by the patient. A question to elicit this information might be "Over your lifetime, have you had ongoing skin problems?" The nurse needs to identify risk factors that impact the skin such as sun exposure and the use of cigarettes. The nurse must assess the amount of time spent in the sun as well as other risk factors associated with the development of skin cancer. These risk factors are outlined in the Risk Factors box. Other significant habits and lifestyles are assessed during the health history outlined next.

Social History

Social history includes use of alcohol or street drugs that can have adverse effects on the conditions of the patient's skin. Drugs and alcohol can have a pathologic effect on a patient's skin. This effect may result from the direct toxic effect or from personal neglect, environmental factors, and/or poor nutrition. The presence of certain cutaneous lesions in a patient should prompt an investigation into the patient's drinking and drug habits. The nurse should inquire about the patient's skin care habits and routine, use of special cleansing agents or soaps, use

---

RISK FACTORS Associated with Skin Cancer

- Age 50 or older
- Male gender
- Family history of skin cancer
- Fair complexion with light-colored hair or eyes
- Precancerous lesions
- Geographic location such as high altitude or near the equator
- Exposure to certain elements such as radium, isotopes, x-rays
- Exposure to coal, tar, creosote, and petroleum products
- Extended exposure to sunlight
- Repeated skin trauma or irritation
- Tendency to burn easily
- History of severe and/or multiple sunburns as a child.

---

of cosmetics or other dermatologic products, sun exposure patterns, use of sunscreen and sunblock, and exposure to stressors.

If suspected due to the presence of cutaneous lesion, the nurse needs to inquire about skin popping. Skin popping is a technique used by individuals to administer illicit drugs. The technique, also called "subcutaneous" or "subQ," involves injecting of the drug between skin and fat layers. Skin popping is used for several reasons including:

- Individuals not wanting to inject right into a vein
- Individuals finding it too difficult to hit the vein
- Because drugs absorb more slowly
- Less of a "rush," but the effects of the drug may last longer
- Trying to keep from getting dope sick
- To reduce the risk of drug overdose
- Individuals not having veins left to shoot the drug into. (Public Health; Seattle & King County, 2008)

Skin popping is a significant risk factor in skin and soft tissue infections, which are common among injection drug users (IDUs). There is an increased incidence of *Staphylococcus aureus* skin infections among IDUs. Additionally, outbreaks of uncommon infections including tetanus, wound botulism, and a sepsis/myonecrosis syndrome due to *Clostridium* species have been seen with IDUs (Brown & Ebright, 2002).

Occupation

This is the description of the patient's usual work. The nurse inquires about the patient's work conditions and hours, duration of employment, and any occupational exposure to irritants, pollutants, or allergens, and frequent sun exposure. Skin neoplasms do result from occupational or environmental agents. For example, individuals that work in the sun have an increased risk for the development of skin cancer.

Cultural Considerations

The nurse would inquire about any cultural habits or practices that may affect the patient's skin. This would include any culture-related dietary habits as well. For example, in Southeast Asia, there is a custom of scraping the skin when a person is sick, causing bruising and open sores. This is thought to aid in the healing process.

Environment

The nurse should inquire of the patient about environmental exposure to chemicals, toxins, animals, outdoors, paint, aerosols, petroleum products, and tar. These products can irritate the skin, causing rashes and skin breakdown.

Habits

In addition to social habits mentioned earlier the nurse should inquire about the patient's sleep patterns and whether there have been any recent changes. The nurse should ask specifically whether the patient experiences symptoms such as itching at night or night sweats. Ask the patient whether he bites or chews the nails or picks at the skin. These habits may cause a loss of skin integrity and increase the risk of a skin infection.

Exercise

The nurse should inquire about the patient's exercise habits. Does the patient exercise on a regular basis? What are the recreational activities of the patient? Do the recreational activities expose the patient to excessive weather elements, such as wind, cold, heat, or sun? Does the individual work out at community gyms? There may be a risk for contracting fungal infections or community acquired methicillin-resistant *Staphylococcus aureus* (MRSA) from the equipment or showers. Caution the patient not to share towels and to cover and protect any open areas on the skin. Ask the patient how much and how easily she perspires. Profuse, out of the ordinary perspiration may be indicative of a systemic disorder. Obesity is one cause of excessive perspiration.

Nutrition

The nurse would assess the patient's dietary pattern to see whether the patient eats well-balanced, nutritious meals. The history should focus on the patient's overall eating habits and use of chocolate, caffeine, sweets, and carbonated beverages. Inquire about recent changes in diet. Dietary changes may cause rashes and other skin reactions.

▮ Physical Examination

When conducting a physical examination of the skin, the nurse must be cognizant of age-related changes. What is normal for a young person will be changed or absent in the elderly population. Certain skin changes related to the aging process are not in and or themselves pathologic. Therefore, the nurse also must possess the knowledge of normal versus abnormal for each age group when assessing the skin. Pathologic changes are outlined in detail in Chapter 66 🔗.

Inspection

When conducting the physical assessment of the skin, the nurse must be aware of ethnic variations related to skin color and texture, mucous membrane coloring, and hair texture. The nurse must perform a thorough physical examination in a well-lit room, preferably in indirect natural daylight. To examine the skin properly, the nurse must take a brief but careful look at the patient's entire body and examine specific areas of concern in detail. A small magnifying glass and a centimeter ruler or tape are required when assessing lesions. The assessment should proceed in an orderly fashion, beginning with an examination of the most frequently exposed areas such as the face, hands, arms, legs, and feet. Along with the skin, the nurse would also examine the appendages, hair, scalp, and nails.

Inspection of the Skin

The nurse inspects the skin while the patient is in a sitting or lying position with all clothes removed except an examination or hospital gown. The nurse inspects the skin for color, temperature, thickness, moisture, texture, turgor, edema, and lesions. Special attention needs to be paid to pressure points, especially in the elderly population. If the patient has tubes and or stomas, the adjunct skin should be assessed for breakdown and rashes. The nurse needs to be aware of ethnic differences, especially in the darker skinned populations, when conducting an assessment.

 *Ethnic considerations: The best areas to assess pallor, cyanosis, and jaundice are oral mucous membranes and conjunctiva in dark-skinned people.*

Color

Skin color varies from person to person depending on the ethnicity and race of the person. Melanin, carotene, the level of oxygen in the blood, and the amount of sun exposure will all influence the color of the patient's skin. Dark skin contains more melanin than does fair skin. Asians have more carotene pigments, which gives the skin the yellow hue. In addition, skin color will vary from body part to body part. Usually, the most frequently exposed areas are noticeably different from the unexposed areas. The difference may be due to the more frequent exposure from the sun, wind, and other environmental elements on exposed skin. Normal skin color ranges from a whitish pink to a dark chocolate brown, depending on race. When evaluating skin color changes, the nurse must be cognizant of variations in skin color based on the patient's racial background, as presented in the Cultural Considerations box. When assessing for color changes, the nurse should give consideration to the room's lighting and temperature as well as the position of the patient. For example, is there a color change when the patient's leg is in a dependent position?

Palpation

Palpation is examination of the skin through the use of touch. Generally, the nurse will inspect and palpate simultaneously. When palpating the skin, the nurse assesses the skin temperature, texture, thickness, moisture, turgor, edema, and lesions. The presence or absence of a pulse needs to be determined, as it may indicate a diminished blood supply to the area.

Temperature

Using the dorsal surface of the hand, which is most sensitive to temperature, the nurse first palpates the forehead and proceeds in a systematic fashion downward, being certain to include the hands and feet. The nurse should always make side-to-side comparisons. Assess for bilateral symmetry by palpating similar areas simultaneously, using both the right and left hand. For example, are both hands the same temperature, or is one warmer or cooler than the other? Normal skin temperature ranges from slightly warm to slightly cool. This may fluctuate depending on the temperature of the patient's environment. Skin temperature will be increased with any condition that increases blood flow to the area. For example, localized skin temperature could be increased due to tissue injury, trauma, or infection. Occasionally, the temperature is slightly cooler in a person's hands and feet, but the temperature should be similar on both sides. A difference in temperature bilaterally warrants further investigation and could be indicative of vascular problems or infection.

Generalized skin temperature increases may occur in systemic infections, fever, or metabolic disorders such as hyperthyroidism. Conversely, temperature to the skin is decreased when blood flow to the skin is diminished. Conditions that may cause a decrease in local skin temperature result from diminished blood supply to the area, vasoconstriction, occlusion, or peripheral arterial insufficiency. Generalized skin temperature decreases may occur when the environment is cool and in the presence of metabolic disorders such as hypothyroidism.

CULTURAL CONSIDERATIONS for Assessing Skin Color Changes

Skin Color Variation	Description of Variation	Appearance in Light Skin	Appearance in Dark Skin
Carotenemia	A yellowish discoloration of skin that differs from jaundice because it does not involve the sclera or mucous membranes. It is often associated with a high intake of foods with carotene (sweet potatoes, squash, and carrots).	A yellowish stain in the skin.	May be difficult to assess.
Cyanosis	A bluish-gray discoloration of the skin that is often caused by decreased perfusion of the tissues with oxygenated blood.	Bluish tinge notably in skin, lower eyelid, mucous membranes, lips, earlobes, soles of the feet, and palms.	Ashen-gray discoloration of the skin, mucous membranes, lips, and tongue.
Ecchymosis	Purplish, blue, and black marks that are usually caused by trauma. Ecchymosis occurs due to the extravasation of blood. Over time the discoloration fades to greenish-brown and then yellow as the blood is reabsorbed into the vascular system.	Purplish, blue-black areas may be seen anywhere on the skin.	Purplish, blue-black areas on the skin may be difficult to see in poor lighting.
Erythema	A reddish discoloration of the skin that is caused by dilation of the capillaries. This is usually due to local irritation or inflammation, embarrassment (blushing), heat, or fever.	Redness that can be seen anywhere on the body. It may be generalized or localized.	Redness that appears on the body but is difficult to see unless in a well-lit area.
Hyperpigmentation	Hyperpigmentation can be in a specific or a general area. It results from changes in the distribution of melanin. It is often seen in pregnancy (linea nigra); persons of color are often born with dark discolorations located on the lower back and buttocks, called mongolian spots. Both linea nigra and mongolian spots disappear over time or when the pregnancy is over.	Spots or lines that appear darker than the general skin.	Spots or lines that appear darker than the general skin.
Jaundice	A yellowish discoloration of the skin, sclera, and mucous membranes that is often associated with increased amounts of bilirubin in the blood. Some newborns are born with pathologic jaundice, in which skin color changes are noted within the first 24 hours of life. Jaundice is generally caused by disorders that cause an increase in the serum bilirubin level.	A yellow staining noticeable in the skin, hard palate, sclera, palms, and soles of the feet.	Can be seen in the hard palate, sclera, palms, and soles of the feet.
Pallor	Paleness of the skin that occurs when the red-pink tones from the oxygenated hemoglobin in the blood are lost. The skin takes on the appearance of collagen (connective tissue), which is almost white.	Loss of rosy glow in the skin.	Ashen appearance. The skin will lack red tones, which normally give dark skin a luster or a glow. Pallor can best be seen in the palpebral conjunctiva, the preferred site for assessment of pallor related to anemia.
Petechiae	Pinpoint purpuric lesions of the skin.	Pinpoint purpuric lesions can be seen on the skin.	May be difficult to see except in good lighting.
Vitiligo	The absence of pigmentation in a circumscribed area.	May be difficult to see except in good lighting.	A circumscribed area or areas with loss of pigmentation.

Source: Halder, R. M. & Nootheti, P. K. (2003). Ethnic skin disorders overview. *Journal of the American Academy of Dermatology 48* (6 Supplement): S143–S148.

Texture

The texture of the skin ranges from smooth and soft to rough and hard. The nurse should use the palmar surface of the fingers and finger pads when palpating for texture. Normal skin texture is smooth, soft, and even. The texture may be rougher in exposed areas or areas of pressure, such as the elbows, palms, and soles of the feet. Conditions such as hyperthyroidism will alter the texture of the skin. Hyperthyroidism usually causes the skin to be smooth with a velvet-like texture. Hypothyroidism causes the skin to be rough and scaly. The skin of the elderly has an increased incidence of scaling as well.

Thickness

The skin should be thin and firm over most parts of the body. Normally, it is thicker on the palms, soles of the feet, elbows, and knees and thinner over the eyelids. Skin thickness varies with age or illness, as in the thin, fragile skin of the elderly or the patient who is severely emaciated. Very thin skin with a shiny appearance

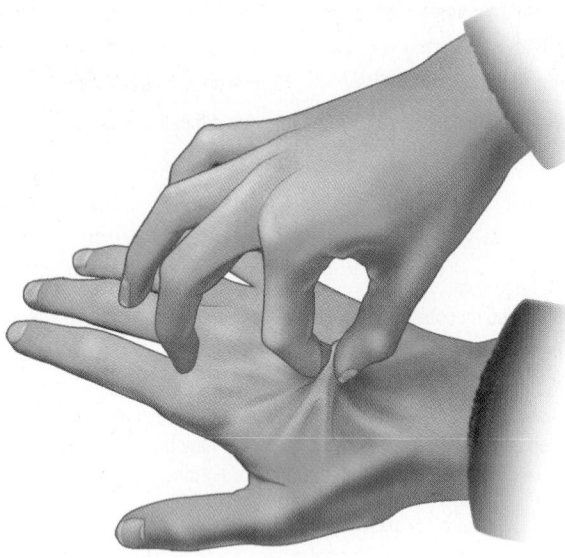

FIGURE 65–2 ■ Skin turgor.

is often indicative of impaired circulation. An individual's occupation may affect the thickness of the skin due to callous formation.

Moisture

The nurse will assess for moisture using the dorsal surface of the hand. The dorsal surface is generally drier, and using it will help to avoid confusion of the moisture on the patient's skin with that on the nurse's hand. Moisture on the skin does vary from one body part to another. The soles of the feet, the palms of the hands, and the intertriginous areas (where two surfaces are close together) contain more moisture than other parts. There should be minimal perspiration on the patient's skin unless he has just engaged in vigorous exercise, the environmental temperature is warm, or the patient has an elevated body temperature. The skin regulates body temperature by producing perspiration that evaporates, thus cooling the skin when the body temperature increases. The skin is normally drier in winter months when it is cooler and humidity is low. Dehydration will cause the skin to be drier. Medical disorders that cause dryness include myxedema and nephritis.

Turgor

Turgor refers to the elasticity and mobility of the skin. Elasticity is described as the resiliency of the skin: its ability to return to a normal position and shape. Mobility is the skin's ability to be lifted. To assess turgor, the nurse would grasp a fold of the patient's skin using the forefinger and thumb (Figure 65–2 ■). The nurse notes how rapidly the skin returns to its normal shape. Normal, healthy skin returns rapidly to its previous shape. When turgor is decreased, the skin fold holds its pinch formation before returning to its normal shape. Loss of turgor is associated with dehydration and aging. As individuals age, the skin normally loses its elasticity. The chest wall is ideal to assess turgor because it is not subject to the age-related changes associated with loss of elasticity. Increased skin turgor makes it difficult or impossible to pinch up the skin. It may be produced by conditions such as scleroderma, which causes the underlying connective tissue to become hard and immobile.

Edema

Edema is caused by the accumulation of fluid in the intercellular spaces. Edema makes the skin appear puffy and tight. Edema is often noted in dependent areas such as the hands, feet, and sacral area. To assess for edema, the nurse would palpate the patient's skin with the pads of the finger. Normally the skin surface stays smooth. If the pressure leaves an indentation in the skin, "pitting" edema is present. Pitting edema is generally evaluated on a 4-point scale, but varies among examiners:

- 1 + Mild pitting in which there is slight indentation, no obvious swelling of the leg
- 2 + Moderate pitting in which the indentation rapidly subsides
- 3 + Deep pitting in which the indentation lasts a short time
- 4 + Very deep pitting in which the indentation lasts a long time (Figure 65–3 ■).

Because measuring edema varies among examiners, some nurses prefer to record edema in terms of time duration of the

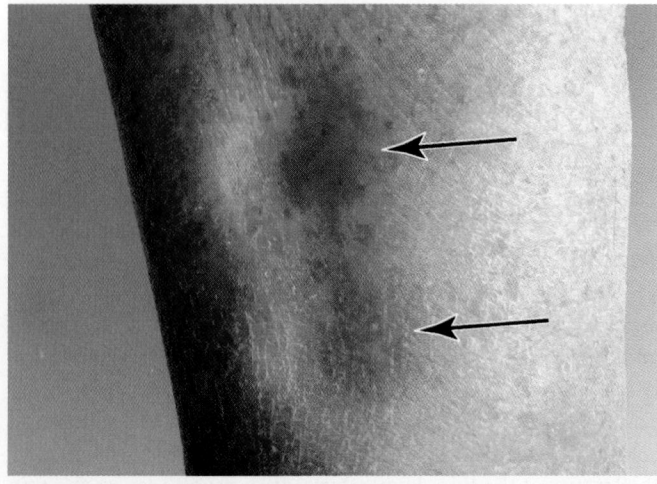

FIGURE 65–3 ■ Pitting edema.
Source: Medical-On-Line Ltd.

indentation. For example, the pitting edema lasts between 15 and 30 seconds before the skin returns to normal.

Lesions

When the nurse assesses the skin, careful attention should be paid to the presence of lesions. Lesions must be assessed using two of the techniques of examination, inspection and palpation. The nurse should use a magnification glass in order to evaluate skin lesions accurately. Lesions should be described according to distribution, location, configuration, and the presence of exudate.

Distribution and Location

Distribution of the lesions on the skin is described according to location or body region affected. Lesions may be confined to one small area (localized), confined to an entire area such as the chest (regional), or spread over the entire body (generalized). The nurse notes whether the lesions are distributed symmetrically or asymmetrically. Noting the characteristic pattern of lesions can provide additional clues in the diagnosis of a specific skin condition.

Configuration or Pattern of Arrangement

The nurse must also note the configuration of the lesions. **Configuration** refers to the pattern of arrangement or position of the lesions. The nurse should assess how lesions are patterned on the body. Are they **discrete lesions** (individual or separate), congruent (running together), grouped in a characteristic pattern, **linear lesions** (forming a line), and/or arciform lesions (arc-shaped) lesions? For example, ringworm or tinea corporis has an annular or circular configuration.

Types of Lesions

The lesion should be further examined for color, size, shape, texture, firmness, discharge, and morphologic classification. The **morphologic classification** of the skin is described in terms of type of lesion (primary, secondary, or vascular), size, shape or configuration, color, texture, elevation or depression, and pedunculation. If the lesion has drainage, the drainage is described in terms of color, odor, amount, and consistency. A **primary lesion** occurs as an initial reaction to a pathologic condition (Chart 65–1). A **secondary lesion** results from a change in the primary lesion or external trauma to the primary lesion (Chart 65–2, p. 2144). **Vascular lesions** appear as red- or purple-pigmented lesions (Chart 65–3, p. 2144). They are generally indicative of conditions that cause bleeding (petechiae and ecchymosis) or liver disease (spider angioma), or may be due to benign conditions such as telangiectasia. Determining whether the lesions blanch will help identify the type of lesion. Pectechie and ecchymosis will not blanch, whereas telangiectases will blanch.

Lesions should be measured with a small, clear, flexible ruler or tape measure. Lesion size is described in centimeters, and all dimensions should be measured (length, width, and depth). The color of individual lesions also is documented. The color of the lesion may be well circumscribed (confined to the lesion) or may be more diffuse, where the borders are not clearly defined. For example, **ecchymosis** is initially dark red or purple but gradually fades to yellowish green before it disappears.

While wearing gloves, the nurse also palpates the lesions to determine the texture or firmness. Additionally, the pattern of how the lesions appear on various areas of the body is assessed. For example, are they clustered in one area, or are they diffusely spread all over the body? It is important to ask the patient about the presence of itching and pain associated with lesions. The

CHART 65–1	**Primary Skin Lesions**		
Primary Lesion	**Description**	**Pain/Itching**	**Examples**
Abscess	A pus-filled nodule.	Localized tenderness. Typically intensity increases as size increases.	An infected wound that forms a pocket of pus under the skin surface.
Bulla	A vesicle or blister usually about 1 centimeter in diameter.	Itching and pain present.	Sunburn, poison oak, poison ivy.
Cyst	A palpable fluid-filled or solid subcutaneous sac.	Typically not painful.	Sebaceous cyst.
Furuncle	A pus-filled lesion usually greater than 0.5 centimeter.	Tender, depends on size.	Boil.
Macule	A flat, nonpalpable circumscribed area of a change in skin color.	Not painful.	Freckles, purpura.
Nodule	A well-circumscribed, firm, palpable lesion deeper within the dermis than a papule.	Not painful.	Sarcoma, subcutaneous nodules.
Papule	A solid, elevated, circumscribed mass that is generally less than 1 centimeter in diameter.	Not painful.	Wart.
Patch	A macule larger than 1 centimeter.	Not painful.	Vitiligo, port-wine stain.
Plaque	Very similar to a papule but greater than 1 centimeter in diameter.	Painful.	Psoriasis, discoid lupus erythematosus.
Pustule	A pus-filled vesicle or bulla.	May be tender.	Acne, impetigo.
Tumor	A solid mass generally larger than 1 centimeter.	Not painful.	Fibroma, lipoma.
Wheal	A circumscribed irregularly shaped elevation of the skin caused by cutaneous edema.	May or may not be tender.	Urticaria.

CHART 65–2	**Secondary Skin Lesions**		
Secondary Lesion	**Description**	**Pain/Itching**	**Examples**
Atrophy	Thinning of the skin resulting from wasting of the dermis. There is a depression in the dermis. The skin is translucent and paper-like.	Not painful.	Striae, normal aging skin.
Crust	A dried serum or blood exudate as found on the surface of an abrasion or excoriation. The size and color vary.	Crust is not tender, but wound underneath may still be tender depending on stage of healing.	Scab, healing fever blister.
Erosion	An absence of the superficial dermis. The lesion is moist and glistening.	Tender.	Syphilitic chancre.
Excoriation	The loss of superficial tissue.	Slight tenderness.	Abrasion, scratch.
Fissure	A linear crack or break from the epidermis to the dermis.	Slight tenderness depending on size and location.	Athlete's foot; chapped, cracked lips as seen in severe dehydration.
Lichenification	Rough, thickened epidermis with increased visibility of the superficial skin markings.		Chronic dermatitis.
Scale	An abundance of dry or oily keratinized cells. Color or size may vary.		Exfoliative dermatitis.
Ulcer	Destruction of the skin beneath the epidermis.	May or not be tender, depending on size, location, depth, and whether acute or chronic.	An open sore sometimes on the leg, as with peripheral vascular disease.
Scar (cicatrix)	Fibrous tissue replacing the injured dermis.	Not painful depending on stage of healing.	Healed wound or surgical wound.
Keloid	An overproduction of scar tissue that extends laterally beyond the initial wound that is usually raised and smooth in appearance. Has a high incidence of occurrence in dark-skinned races and in children.	May or may not be tender. May itch.	Healed wound or surgical wound that is larger than the original wound size.
Hypertrophy	An overproduction of scar tissue that does not extend beyond the initial wound. It has a raised thickened appearance.	May or may not be tender. May itch.	Healed wound or surgical incision that has a thickened appearance.

CHART 65–3	**Vascular Lesions**	
Lesion	**Description**	**Cause**
Cherry angioma	A distinct, benign vascular lesion 0.5–5 millimeters in diameter. A firm, deep-red papule.	Generally found on most people after age 30, and the incidence increases with age.
Ecchymosis	Red-purple nonblanchable discoloration of variable size.	Vascular wall destruction, trauma, vasculitis.
Petechiae	Red-purple nonblanchable discoloration less than 0.5 centimeter in diameter.	Intravascular defects, infection.
Purpura	Red-purple discoloration greater than 0.5 centimeter in diameter.	Intravascular defects, infection.
Spider angioma	Red central body with radiating spider-like legs that blanches with pressure to the central body.	Liver disease, vitamin B deficiency, idiopathic.
Telangiectasia	Fine, irregular red lines.	Dilation of capillaries.
Venous star	Bluish spider irregularly shaped with linear lines.	Increased pressure in superficial veins.

length of time that lesions have been present and the precipitating factors that caused them to occur, are also assessed.

If palpation is not adequate to arrive at a diagnosis, **diascopy** is used to examine superficial skin lesions with a diascope. A diascope, a high-powered spotting scope for straight or angled viewing, is often used to observe color changes of a lesion.

Inspection of the Lips

Assessment of lips includes confirming that they are symmetrical, smooth, pink, moist, and without lesions. Systemic dehydration may be manifested in dry, scaling, cracking lips. Herpes viral infections and skin cancer are disorders common to the lips. Herpes presents with vesicle on the lip that extends onto the skin. Skin cancers most commonly occur on the lower lip or the underside of the tongue (D'Amico & Barbarito, 2007). Cancer is suspected when there is an open area (sore) that does not heal. The nurse needs to inquire about a history of heavy cigarette, pipe, and cigar smoking; chewing tobacco use; and alcohol intake, as these are risk factors for the development of oral cancer.

Inspection of the Hair

Hair color is created by the production of melanin. Hair color varies from pale or platinum to dark black and is dictated by the genetic background and ethnic origin. Hair texture may be very fine to course and curly to straight. Normal hair in the absence of disease should have a vibrant appearance with a natural gloss. The normal texture of the hair may be changed due to environmental conditions and harsh treatment with colors, dyes, blowdrying, and permanent waving.

The hair should be evenly distributed on the head. **Alopecia**, loss of hair, can be a result of familial patterns of baldness, disease, medications, or a pathologic condition. Diffuse hair loss may be caused by hormonal changes, systemic infections, and reaction to chemicals or medications. Patchy hair loss can be caused by scalp infections such as ringworm, burn injuries, and trauma, and from permanent waving or other harsh chemical treatments.

The scalp should be assessed for lesions. When assessing the nurse should don gloves and separate the patient's hair into small sections and lift it. The nurse inspects the scalp for lesions, pest infestations such as lice, and dandruff.

Inspection of and Palpation of the Nails

The nurse inspects and palpates the patient's nails. The nail surface is normally slightly curved with the posterior and lateral folds smooth and rounded. The nail edges should be smooth, rounded, and clean. The normal nail bed angle is 160 degrees. The nail base is firm to palpation. A nail bed with greater than 160-degree angle suggests a clubbed nail. Clubbing of nails indicates a state of chronic hypoxia and is often seen with congenital and adult heart disease and chronic obstructive pulmonary disease.

The surface of the nail should be smooth and nonbrittle, with no splitting. Pits, transverse grooves, or lines may indicate a nutritional deficiency (Figure 65–4 ■). Patients with arterial insufficiency may have thickened, ridged nails.

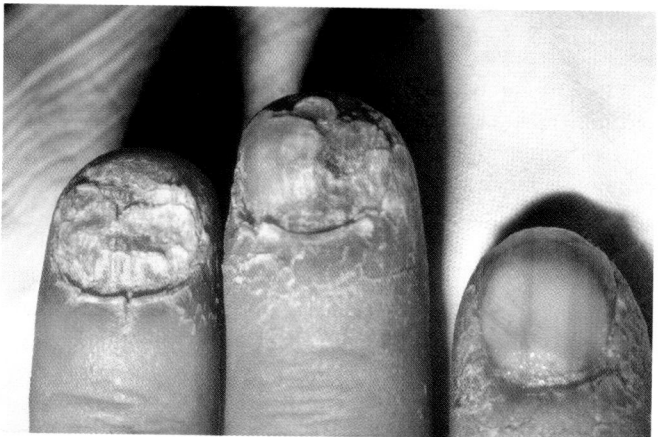

FIGURE 65–4 ■ Fingernails with pits, grooves, and lines.
Source: From Neil S. Prose, K. G. Abson, and R. K. Scher. Internat. J. Dermat. 31: 453, (1992)

The nail plate is translucent and the nurse should expect to see a pink nail bed. Dark-skinned patients may have brownish, pigmented areas or linear bands along the nail edge. The nurse palpates the nail bed to determine capillary refill. To assess capillary refill, the nurse would depress the nail edge to blanch and then release, noting the return of color. Capillary refill is usually documented as brisk, which is a normal response. However, it may have a sluggish return to color for patients with cardiovascular or respiratory disease and low hemoglobin.

Genetic Implications

The family history informs the nurse about the general health of the patient's blood relatives and spouse. This information allows the nurse to identify any illnesses that have a genetic, familial, or environmental link as well as implications for the patient's current and future health problems. The blood relatives include the maternal and paternal grandparents, parents, siblings, aunts, uncles, and children. Inquire about diseases that demonstrate genetic or familial tendencies. Familial tendencies have not been identified as genetic disorders but have been found in family clusters. Usually the information obtained about the family is documented in a genogram. The family genogram is an effective way to document a large amount of data obtained from the family history. Any family history of allergic disorders or conditions such as asthma, hay fever, skin cancer, melanoma, psoriasis, eczema, or infestations of lice or scabies should be solicited from the patient as well as familial hair loss patterns.

Critical Thinking Related to Skin Assessment

Critical thinking is essential in order to prioritize the most significant clinical manifestations that need further investigation. Skin disorders can be as benign as slight sunburn to life-threatening disorders such as necrotizing fasciitis. It is imperative that the nurse be able to distinguish normal from abnormal, benign from serious. The nurse must rely on critical thinking skills in interpreting the patient's symptoms and assessment findings to determine possible and potential patient diagnoses and to consider the appropriate actions to take. Analysis of this data allows the nurse to make a diagnosis and then follow up with an intervention. It is imperative that the nurse communicate and collaborate with other members of the health care team in developing and implementing a plan of care.

Regardless of the health problem, each symptom identified should be thoroughly described in order for the nurse to gain a full understanding. The nurse will ask the patient, "Tell me more about the problem," or "How did it start?" The patient will usually proceed with a discourse about the symptoms. The nurse uses skillful interview techniques to explore and investigate each symptom further. Any symptom analysis would be incomplete without a thorough description of symptom characteristics (Chart 65–4, p. 2146).

Symptoms related to skin conditions include itching, drainage, color changes, changes in moles or warts, or a lesion that does not heal. The nurse should inquire whether the onset was gradual or sudden and about the length of time the problem has persisted. If

MyNursingKit | Mayo Clinic: Risk Factors for Skin Cancer

CHART 65–4 **Skin Disorder Analysis Criteria**

SYMPTOM ANALYSIS

Onset

- When did it first occur?
- Did it occur gradually or suddenly?
- What are the precipitating factors?
- How long does it last?
- Is it continuous or is it intermittent?
- Is there a pattern of remission or exacerbation?

Location

- Where is it located?
- Does it radiate?

Timing

- When does it occur?
- How long does it last?
- How often does it occur?
- Is there a particular setting in which it occurs?

Quality

- How would you describe the symptom?
- How does the symptom rate on a scale of 1–10, with 10 being the most extreme?
- Is the symptom getting better or worse?

Quantity

- What is the frequency of occurrence?
- What is the extent of its occurrence?
- Does it occur in a specific setting?

Aggravating Factors

- What makes it worse?

Alleviating Factors

- What makes it go away?
- What makes it better?

Associated Phenomena

- What else happens when you experience the symptom?
- What treatments have you tried including prescription, over-the-counter, and herbal medications and remedies?

the condition were a rash, the nurse would question the patient to determine whether it is progressive and spreading. Exploring precipitating factors would provide critical clues such as whether a change in skin care products, new cologne, or a new house pet precipitated the condition. Associated symptoms would be whether the patient had a recent viral illness, had a high fever, or had exposure to increased physical or psychological stress.

■ Implications for Health Promotion

Health promotion for the skin primarily focuses on protection and early treatment. Protecting the skin will help prevent breakdown and early treatment may prevent complications. Patient teaching must include information about the risk factors that cause the various integumentary abnormalities. When assessing the patient, it is essential for the nurse to identify high-risk behaviors such as sun exposure that require education. Correct use of sunscreens and limited exposure to the sun need to be stressed. An in-depth discussion of sun protection is included in Chapter 66 .

> **CRITICAL ALERT**   *It is important for the nurse to stress that most sunscreens must be applied 15 to 30 minutes prior to sun exposure. Additionally, sunscreens need to be reapplied after swimming or excessive perspiration.*

Adequate rest balanced with a healthy exercise program has many beneficial effects. Rest is restorative to the body, and lack of it is often manifested in the color of the skin. For example, dark circles under the eyes are a common manifestation of lack of sleep. Exercise causes vasodilation, typically manifested on the skin as a "healthy glow." Increased circulation also promotes wound healing and prevents the occurrence of wound infections. Education about overexposure to heat, cold, and sun will prevent skin breakdown. The National Guidelines feature outlines safe skin care.

Hygiene

The skin and hair need to be cleansed regularly to prevent bacterial buildup, remove excess oil, and prevent odor. Education about skin hygiene needs to be tailored to match the skin type. For example, oily skin needs a cleanser that promotes drying, whereas dry skin needs a more gentle cleanser that prevents drying. The skin should be washed gently so as not to cause irritation and breakdown. If any irritation occurs, the individual must be instructed to stop using the product and try another one. Soaps tend to be more alkaline, thereby neutralizing the normal skin pH of 4.2 to 5.6. This may promote bacterial growth and increase the risk for infection. If this is occurring, the patient must be instructed to try other cleansers.

The elder population needs to use gentle, less drying cleansers and shampoos because skin and scalp dry out with age. Moisturizers are typically helpful for dry skin and scalp in preventing scaling and pruritus. Individuals may need to try different products in order to find the one that is best tailored for their skin type. Chapter 66  discusses the specific skin disorders.

Nutrition

Nutritional intake has a major impact on skin, hair, and nail health. The diet needs to be well balanced and include the daily recommended servings of each food group. The skin specifically needs vitamins A, B, C, and K. Vitamin A and C are needed to promote epithelialization and normal rate of wound healing. Lack of vitamin C is also associated with bleeding gums, petechiae, and purpura. The B complex vitamins are essential for normal metabolic processes and preventing certain dermatologic conditions such as seborrhea. Lack of vitamin K delays blood clotting and therefore can increase the risk of bruising and excessive bleeding with injuries. Protein intake is essential for normal cell growth and collagen formation, which increase wound strength, and inadequate amounts will retard wound healing. Chapter 14  contains an in-depth discussion of normal nutritional intake and the associated side effects of malnutrition.

NATIONAL GUIDELINES for Safe Skin Care

National Organization	Recommendation
American Cancer Society	Monthly skin self-examination for all adults.
	Health care provider skin examination every 3 years in persons aged 20–39 and annually in persons over 40.
	Education of patients concerning sun avoidance and use of sunscreen.
	Avoidance of artificial tanning devices.
American Academy of Family Physicians	Complete skin examination for adolescents and adults with increased recreational or occupational exposure to sunlight, a family or personal history of skin cancer, or evidence of precursor lesions.
	Skin protection from ultraviolet light for all persons with increased exposure to sunlight.
American Academy of Dermatology	Regular screening visits for skin cancer and patient education concerning periodic skin self-examination.
	Education of patients concerning sun avoidance and use of sunscreen.
	Avoidance of artificial tanning devices.
American Medical Association	Education of patients concerning sun avoidance and use of sunscreen.
	Avoidance of artificial tanning devices.
Canadian Task Force	Avoidance of sun exposure and use of protective clothing.
National Institutes of Health Consensus Panel	Regular screening visits for skin cancer and patient education concerning periodic skin self-examination.
	Avoidance of artificial tanning devices.

Source: U.S. Preventive Services Task Force. (1996). *Guide to clinical preventive services* (2nd ed.). Alexandria, VA: International Medical Publishing.

◼ Conclusion

It is essential to conduct a thorough, complete health history and an accurate assessment of the skin and the epidermal appendages to distinguish between normal and abnormal findings. As described earlier, many systemic diseases are manifested through the skin, hair, and nails. The nurse needs to possess the knowledge and skills necessary to evaluate each of these areas critically and utilize findings to help determine a nursing diagnosis. The National Guidelines box provides guidelines set forth by national organizations regarding safe skin care.

NCLEX® REVIEW

1. A patient tells the nurse that she "avoids the sun." The nurse realizes this patient could be at risk for developing:
    1. Hypothermia.
    2. Dehydration.
    3. Hypercholesterolemia.
    4. Vitamin D deficiency.

2. During an assessment, the nurse asks a patient if he has been to any foreign countries. This information would be applicable to which of the following categories of the health history?
    1. Past medical history
    2. Chief complaint
    3. Biographic and demographic data
    4. Previous illnesses

3. A 25-year-old patient is admitted with severe cutaneous skin lesions. Which area of the assessment should the nurse focus first?
    1. Culture
    2. Occupation
    3. Habits
    4. Social history

4. The nurse is preparing to examine a patient's skin. Which of the following should the nurse do when conducting this assessment?
    1. Wear sterile gloves.
    2. Assess least frequently exposed areas first.
    3. Inspect and palpate the skin at the same time.
    4. Ask the patient to stand up for the assessment.

5. The nurse assesses a patient's nails to be at a 160 degree angle with a smooth surface. These findings would be indicative of:
   1. Chronic hypoxia.
   2. COPD.
   3. A nutritional deficiency.
   4. Normal findings.

6. An African American patient has an overproduction of scar tissue along the site of a total hip replacement. The nurse realizes this scar would be considered a:
   1. Scale.
   2. Cherry angioma.
   3. Keloid.
   4. Fissure.

7. While assessing the skin of an African American patient, the nurse notes the absence of pigmentation along the right lateral thoracic region. This finding would be documented as:
   1. Jaundice.
   2. Pallor.
   3. Petechiae.
   4. Vitiligo.

Answers for review questions appear in Appendix D

KEY TERMS

alopecia *p.2145*
configuration *p.2143*
diascopy *p.2144*
discrete lesion *p.2143*
distribution *p.2143*

ecchymosis *p.2143*
edema *p.2142*
linear lesion *p.2143*
morphologic classification *p.2143*

primary lesion *p.2143*
secondary lesion *p.2143*
turgor *p.2142*
vascular lesion *p.2143*

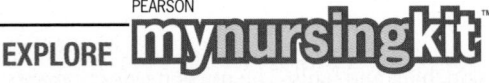

EXPLORE   PEARSON **mynursingkit**™

MyNursingKit is your one stop for online chapter review materials and resources. Prepare for success with additional NCLEX®-style practice questions, interactive assignments and activities, web links, animations and videos, and more!

Register your access code from the front of your book at
www.mynursingkit.com

REFERENCES

Brown, P. D., & Ebright, J. R. (2002). Skin and soft tissue infections in injection drug users. *Current Infectious Disease Reports, 4*(5), 415–419. Retrieved November 12, 2007, from http://opioids.com/skin-popping/index.html

D'Amico, D., & Barbarito, C. (2007). *Health and physical assessment in nursing.* Upper Saddle River, NJ: Pearson Prentice Hall.

Porth, C. (2007). *Essentials of pathophysiology.* Philadelphia: Lippincott Williams & Wilkins.

Public Health: Seattle & King County. (2008). *HIV/AIDS Program: Muscling and skin popping.* Retrieved August 29, 2008, from http://www.metrokc.gov/health/apu/harmred/muscling.htm

U.S. Preventive Services Task Force. (1996). *Guide to clinical preventive services* (2nd ed.). Alexandria, VA: International Medical Publishing.

World Health Organization. (2001). *Protecting children from ultraviolet radiation.* Retrieved November 10, 2007, from http://www.who.int/mediacentre/factsheets/fs261/en/

Caring for the Patient with Skin Disorders

Peggy Ellis
Teri A. Murray
With contributions by: John M. Osborn

Outcome-Based Learning Objectives

After studying this chapter, the learner will be able to:

1. Differentiate the etiology, pathophysiology, and interventions for infections of the skin.
2. Identify preventive measures for skin disorders.
3. Identify the impact of the environment on the skin.
4. Describe the signs and symptoms, diagnostic tests, and treatment of skin disorders.
5. Develop a nursing plan of care for a patient with a skin disorder.
6. Differentiate the psychological and physical implications for the patient with a skin disorder.
7. Describe the effects of aging on the skin.

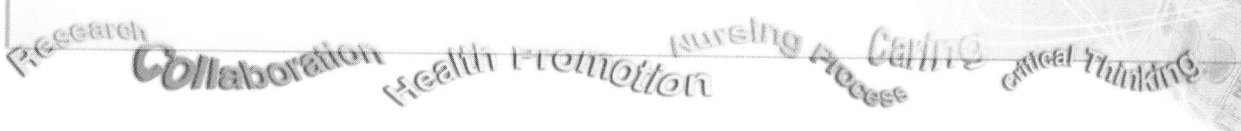

Research Collaboration Health Promotion Nursing Process Caring Critical Thinking

THE SKIN is the largest organ system of the body and serves as the protective barrier against the external environment including infectious agents. It is responsible for helping to regulate body temperature and contains receptors for sensation. The skin helps define cultural and ethnic backgrounds and helps define one's self-image. The skin also can be helpful when expressing emotion.

Disorders of the skin are a common reason for visiting the health care provider. The skin is often a mirror to the rest of the body. The patient may often complain of a rash, itching, or an unusual lesion. There can be disorders of only the skin or systemic disorders that are reflected in the skin. Certain disorders of the skin are treated with medication and/or nonpharmacologic measures, whereas others require surgical intervention.

Skin disorders are usually diagnosed by evaluating the history of onset of symptoms and precipitating factors, including systemic diseases, and performing a physical examination. Most skin disorders have distinct, recognizable lesions that assist with the diagnosis. However, if the abnormality is uncertain, it is cultured, scraped, or biopsied and microscopically examined to identify the diagnosis. The Diagnostic Tests box (p. 2150) describes the common laboratory and diagnostic tests and abnormalities associated with skin disorders.

Nails

Toenails and fingernails are considered a part of the skin and need to be assessed for abnormalities. The nails reflect nutritional status and general health as well as the presence of systemic disorders and exposure to toxic agents. Careful assessment is an important part of diagnosing both local and systemic disorders. Systemic disorders often cause changes in the shape or contour of the nail. Chart 66–1 (p. 2151) provides an overview of nail abnormalities related to systemic disease.

Brittle Nails

Brittle nails are defined as nails in which the distal plate splits, leading to peeling of the distal portion of the nail. Brittle nails are excessively ridged and dry. Usual water content of the nail is about 18%, whereas brittle nails have a water content of only about 16% (Singh, Haneef, & Uday, 2005). This is caused by prolonged immersion in water, dry skin with dryness of the nail plate, or chemical or mechanical trauma that leads to nail dehydration (Chart 66–2, p. 2151), presents other causes (Fawcett, Linford, & Stulberg, 2004). When brittle nails are noted, a thorough history and physical should be performed to help determine the cause. Note the specific nails that are involved and the changes in the nail plate.

DIAGNOSTIC TESTS for Skin Disorders

Test	Expected Abnormality	Rationale for Abnormality
Biopsy: Surgically removing all or part of the lesion for inspection under the microscope. Can be excisional, punch, shave, or immunofluorescent.	Identification of microorganisms or cell type. Can identify cancer cells, inflammatory reactions, and other types of cell abnormalities.	Enables examination of cells for identification of type, or malignant vs. benign. Helps with diagnosis and proper treatment.
Potassium hydroxide smear: A sample of the lesion is taken, wet with a solution of potassium hydroxide, and placed on a slide for examination.	Potassium hydroxide clears off debris and bacteria so that fungi can be identified.	Able to diagnose whether fungi are the cause of a skin disorder.
Tzanck smear: Scraping of lesion is taken and placed on slide. The material is stained with Giemsa, Wright's, or Sedi stain to identify multinucleated giant cells or atypical keratinocytes.	Demonstrates the presence of multinucleated giant cells, which indicates herpes simplex virus or varicella-zoster virus.	Not a very accurate test but can help to diagnose the presence of herpes simplex virus.
Culture: Sample of lesion is placed in a culture medium to allow growth of organism.	The microorganism will grow on the culture medium and can be identified.	Proper identification of the causative organism can allow for effective treatment.
Immunofluorescent studies: Tissue samples are stained for antibodies and examined under a fluorescence microscope.	Will detect immune complexes and the presence of immunoglobulins in immunologically mediated disorders.	Identifies immunologically mediated dermatitis.
Wood's lamp: "Black" light that can be shone on a rash to produce fluorescence.	Tinea will fluoresce green under a Wood's light. Other fungi may fluoresce yellow to orange.	Helps identify fungi that are the causative agent.
Polymerase chain reaction (PCR): Method of identifying the DNA in the pathogen.	Identifies mutations in DNA related to antigen–antibody reactions.	Allows the recognition of bacteria and viruses, especially those difficult to identify through a culture. Can also identify genetic disorders.
Skin scrapings: Cells can be scraped off the lesions and placed on a slide.	Allows visualization of mites, ova, and feces from infestations.	Parasites can be directly visualized and identified under the microscope.
Patch test: Suspected allergens are applied to the skin of the back or arm for 48 hours to see whether there is a reaction.	If the patient has an allergy to the substance applied to the skin, wheals and flare reactions will be evident.	Determines whether dermatitis is allergic or irritant, and identifies the allergen.

Treatment of Brittle Nails

If the hands must be immersed in water, it is important to wear gloves. The hands and nails can be massaged daily with lubricants or oils after soaking in lukewarm water for 15 minutes. Keep the nails well groomed and avoid using them as tools to scrape or pry. Systemic treatment with biotin has been found to improve the nails. Biotin is a component of the vitamin B complex that helps maintain healthy muscle, hair, and skin by stimulating keratinization. Patients who are given oral biotin at a dosage of 2.5 milligrams a day have shown improvement of nail strength over 3 to 6 months. Biotin is well tolerated with very few side effects. Therefore, it is a reasonable choice when other treatment measures fail (Scher, Fleckman, Tulumbas, McCollam, & Enfanto, 2003).

Nail Infections

The most common infection of the nail is onychomycosis, or tinea unguium, which is a chronic fungal infection under the nail. It usually occurs in the toenails but can occur in the fingernails as well. It commonly leads to deformed, cracked nails that initially become white or silvery and then turn yellow or brown. The nail beds are thickened but usually are not uncomfortable or painful. The infection can spread to other nails and is diagnosed through cultures and microscopy. This condition is difficult to treat and is typically slowly responsive to the oral and topical antifungal medications. The nail may eventually have to be surgically removed in order to clear up the infection.

Paronychia is an acute or chronic infection of the folds of tissue around the nail or the cuticle that usually begins after minor trauma. The causative organism is most frequently *Streptococcus* or *Staphylococcus*, but it can also be related to a fungus. In acute paronychia, an abscess may develop that requires surgical drainage for relief of pain. In chronic paronychia, the infection develops more slowly with progressive tenderness and swelling around the cuticle. Treatment involves the application of hot compresses and topical antibiotics.

Nail Trauma or Loss

Nail trauma can lead to disorders such as subungal hematoma and pincer nail. Trauma to the nail or nail bed may result in

CHART 66–1	**Nail Abnormalities Related to Systemic Disease**	
Nail Abnormality	**Description**	**Disease**
Beau's lines	Transverse furrows on fingernails.	Stress. Acute severe illness. Nutritional disorders. Circulation disorders. Abnormal metabolic states.
Spoon nails (koilonychia)	Nails are concave like a saucer. Nail plate is thinned.	Hypochromic anemia. Rheumatic fever. Syphilis.
Nail pitting	Thickened nail plate with small pits.	Psoriasis.
Nail clubbing	Flattened nail plate. Bulbous distal phalanx. Increased angle between nail and dorsal surface of finger.	Chronic hypoxia. Heart disease. Pulmonary disease. Cystic fibrosis. Bronchogenic carcinoma.
Mees' lines	White, transverse line.	Poisoning. Acute illness.
Lindsay's nails	Proximal portion of nail is white while distal portion is red or pink.	Chronic renal disease. Azotemia.
Terry's nails	White nail beds with distal band of reddish brown.	Cirrhosis. Hypoalbuminemia. Congestive heart failure. Diabetes type II.

CHART 66–2	**Causes of Brittle Nails**	
Occupational Causes	**Physical Causes**	
Chemicals such as acetone	Aging	
Typing	Atherosclerosis	
Playing a musical instrument	Poor nutrition with deficiencies in vitamins A, B$_6$, and C	
Grasping	Chronic renal failure	
Prying	Cardiovascular disease	
Scraping	Raynaud's disease	
Frequent hand washing	Thyroid disease	
	Psoriasis	
	Eczema	
	Onychomycosis	
	Warts	
	Squamous cell or basal cell carcinoma	

changes in the size, shape, or color of the nail. A subungal hematoma is usually related to trauma to the nail that causes bleeding and bruising under the nail. This typically leads to separation of the nail plate. The blood will cause a dark discoloration that will remain until the nail plate grows out. It may be necessary to puncture the nail to relieve the excess pressure caused by the blood building up under the nail. Pincer nail usually affects the toenail and is evidenced by the lateral edges of the nail curling in and under it, leading to a tube-like appearance of the nail. It is usually caused by pointed-toed shoes or high heels that squeeze the toes together. If the pincer nail causes pain, the nail may need to be surgically removed.

An ingrown nail occurs when the corners of the nail plate grow into the lateral nail fold and dermis. It is usually due to poorly fitting shoes, improper nail trimming, or trauma. The individual experiences pain, redness, and swelling, and an infection may develop leading to an abscess. This condition can be prevented by wearing proper fitting shoes and trimming the nails straight across. Treatment options depend on the severity of the symptoms. Soaking the nail, along with systemic and/or topical antibiotics, may be used. A cotton wick can be inserted into the lateral nail groove to allow for drainage and relief of pressure. If these strategies are unsuccessful, or if the symptoms are more severe, a wedge resection of the corner of the nail can be performed with removal of the lateral one-fourth of the nail. Removal of the lateral nail matrix may be necessary to create a new lateral nail fold and prevent the recurrence of an ingrown nail.

◼ Hair

Hair disorders include too much hair, known as hirsutism, or not enough hair, known as alopecia. **Hirsutism** is defined as the excessive growth of hair and is caused by an increased testosterone level, Cushing's syndrome, carcinoma of the adrenal gland, testicular tumors, or acromegaly. This condition occurs more commonly in women. The increase in hormones stimulates the hair follicle to grow, especially on the lip, chin, chest, areola, abdomen, lower back, buttock, inner thighs, and external genitalia. The treatment consists of diagnosing and treating the underlying cause.

Alopecia is defined as the loss of hair that can occur in men and women at any age. One of the most common forms of alopecia is **androgenetic alopecia**, also known as male pattern baldness. Androgenetic alopecia is a physiological baldness in which androgen levels are normal; however, there is a genetic predisposition to balding. In men, it usually begins with bitemporal thinning of the hair and progresses to the frontal area, whereas in women the pattern is central thinning. The degree of baldness and the age of onset are determined by the inheritance of several genes. The hair shafts gradually shrink until they become finer and thinner. It is not related to any serious health problems but can be psychologically disturbing. Certain topical medications can be applied to the scalp, but their effectiveness is variable. The two medications that have been found to be the most effective are finasteride and minoxidil. Finasteride blocks the conversion of testosterone to 5-alpha dihydrotestosterone (DHT). DHT is needed for the development of androgenetic alopecia. Minoxidil is a vasodilator applied topically that leads to enhanced hair growth due to the increased blood flow. These medications must be used for 4 to 12 months before effectiveness can be evaluated (Stough et al., 2005).

Androgenic alopecia occurs in women and is recognized as a symptom of polycystic ovary syndrome. Chapter 49 ◉ discusses polycystic ovary syndrome. It is related to excessive androgen production that causes a decrease in size of the hair follicles leading to hair loss in central and frontal areas. Hair loss also can be related to systemic medications; for example, many of the chemotherapeutic agents used for treating cancer can lead to hair loss. Systemic diseases related to hair loss include hypothyroidism, insulin resistance, and cardiovascular disease.

Alopecia also is associated with high levels of anxiety and depression, low self-esteem, poor quality of life, and poor body image. Hair is closely related to an individual's identity and attractiveness. Visits to psychologists/psychiatrists may be beneficial in helping patients deal with problems associated with alopecia (Hunt & McHale, 2005).

Skin

The skin is affected by health and healthy lifestyle choices. When teaching patients and families about how to maintain healthy skin, it is essential to discuss the importance of adequate nutrition. The skin needs protein, vitamin C, iron, and zinc to be healthy. Protein and vitamin deficiencies, along with obesity, can decrease the skin's ability to regenerate and affect the circulation to the skin, leading to skin lesions and delayed wound healing. Water is important to maintain elasticity in the skin. Approximately 64 ounces of water is needed daily to keep the skin well hydrated. Regular exercise helps maintain adequate circulation, providing oxygen and nutrients to the skin. Regular bathing keeps the excess bacteria and oils in check so that the skin can remain healthy. However, bathing more frequently than necessary should be avoided because it can cause dryness of the skin. The patient should be asked about bathing practices, including the type of cleanser used and the frequency of bathing. If the skin is dry, emollient cream or lotion should be applied immediately after bathing to maintain hydration. The skin should be inspected monthly for new growths or changes in skin lesions. (See Chapter 65 for skin assessment.) Racial differences in skin may account for changes in skin response to daily care and environmental irritants, as seen in the Cultural Considerations box.

Sunlight

The sun, along with other pollutants in the air, can irritate and damage the skin, with most of the damage occurring before the age of 18. Nearly 80% of this damage can be prevented if sunscreen is applied properly in those first 18 years of life (Samuel, Brooke, Hollis, & Griffiths, 2005). Recognizable changes occur with years of exposure to ultraviolet radiation due to repetitive tanning and sunburning. The potential for sunburn varies with skin type. Chart 66–3 lists the common descriptions of skin types and their potential for sunburn. The superficial dermis that is damaged by the sun demonstrates a breakdown of collagen and an accumulation of abnormal elastin, which lead to wrinkling and lack of resilience in the skin. When the sun damages the skin, DNA production is impaired. DNA is needed for maintenance of the genetic integrity of the skin. Therefore, impaired DNA production can lead to skin cancer and immune suppression. Sunlight also is considered a major cause of skin cancer, especially when the skin is repeatedly sunburned. Various skin cancers are discussed in this chapter. The prevention of skin cancer is an objective of *Healthy People 2010* (U.S. Department of Health and Human Services, 2000). The National Guidelines box lists the Centers for Disease Control and Prevention's guidelines related to skin cancer and protection of the skin from the sun.

Health Promotion Related to Sun Protection

The best way to avoid the damage created by the sun is to avoid the sun, wear sunscreen, or wear protective clothing when in the sun. The amount of time in the sun at midday should be limited. Sunscreens should contain avobenzne, dioxybenzone, oxybenzone, titanium dioxide, or zinc oxide for the best protection from both ultraviolet A (UVA) and ultraviolet B (UVB) rays. A sun protection factor (SPF) rates sunscreens. The higher the SPF rating the sunscreen has, the greater the protection. The current recommendation is an SPF of 15 (CDC, 2006b). Generous layers of sunscreen should be applied with special attention paid to areas often neglected such as the neck, temples, and ears. Sunscreen can be diluted or rinsed off completely by sweat, water immersion, or rubbing. Therefore, it should be applied often. The United Kingdom has begun a campaign to reduce exposure to sunlight and prevent sunburn. Part of that effort is the SunSmart program. Chart 66–4 outlines the basis of SunSmart and can be used for patient education (Affleck, 2005; Cancer Research UK, 2003).

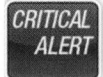 When spending time in the sun, it is important to use a sunscreen with a sun protection factor (SPF) of 15 to 30 and to reapply it often. Sunscreen should be applied 30 minutes prior to sun exposure.

CULTURAL CONSIDERATIONS for Racial Differences in Skin

Physiological skin differences among racial and ethnic groups include:

- African Americans have increased lipid content.
- African Americans have increased thickness of the stratum corneum and increased spontaneous desquamation.
- Water content of the skin is greater in Hispanics and less in Caucasians.
- An increase in melanin decreases sun damage.

The three most common disorders in darkly pigmented skin are:

- Acne
- Eczema
- Pigmentary disorders.

Source: From Halder, R. M., & Nootheti, P. K. (2003). Ethnic skin disorders overview. *Journal of the American Academy of Dermatology, 48* (Suppl. 6), S143–S148.

CHART 66–3	**Common Descriptions of Skin Types for Anticipating Sunburn**

Type	Description
Type I	Always burns, never tans
Type II	Burns easily, tans minimally
Type III	Burns moderately, tans gradually
Type IV	Burns minimally, tans well
Type V	Rarely burns, tans profusely
Type VI	Never burns, deeply pigmented

CHART 66–4   SunSmart Program

There are five points to the SunSmart program. To help remember the five points, think *SMART*:

- *S*tay in the shade 11 a.m.–3 p.m.
- *M*ake sure you never burn.
- *A*lways cover up.
- *R*emember to take extra care with children.
- *T*hen use factor 15+ sunscreen.

Sources: Affleck, P. (2005). Sun exposure and health. *Nursing Standard, 19*(47), 50–54; and Cancer Research UK. (2003). Cancer Research UK gets SunSmart with the big screen. Retrieved September 8, 2008 from http://info.cancerresearchuk.org/news/archive/pressreleases/2003/may/216205.

NATIONAL GUIDELINES for Skin Cancer Prevention

- Minimize exposure to the sun during peak hours of 10 a.m. to 4 p.m.
- Seek shade from the sun.
- Wear clothes and wide-brimmed hats that protect the skin and face.
- Wear wraparound sunglasses that block close to 100% of ultraviolet (UV) rays.
- Use a broad-spectrum sunscreen that blocks both ultraviolet A (UVA) and ultraviolet B (UVB) rays and has a sun protection factor (SPF) of at least 15 or higher. Apply generously 30 minutes before going outside, and reapply after swimming, exercising, or sweating.
- Avoid using sun lamps and tanning beds. They are also sources of UV radiation.

Source: Centers for Disease Control and Prevention (CDC). (2006b). *Health topics: Skin cancer school health guidelines.* Retrieved December 12, 2007, from http://www.cdc.gov/healthyyouth/skincancer/guidelines/summary.htm#top.

Nonmalignant Disorders Related to Sun Exposure

Exposure to the sun leads to damaged, abnormal skin cells that can be premalignant. Lesions related to these disorders are generally found on areas of the skin exposed to the sun. Photodermatitis and actinic keratosis are both skin disorders related to skin exposure to the sun.

Etiology, Epidemiology, and Pathophysiology of Photodermatitis

Photodermatitis is an inflammatory adverse reaction to sunlight. It is a common hypersensitivity to sun in which the individual sunburns more easily than usual or develops papular or vesicular lesions with exposure to the sun. It can occur in all ages and races but is more common in young women. This condition can be a true immunologic reaction that can be genetically determined. It also may occur because of the use of certain medications, in association with certain diseases, or with the use of contact agents that increase photosensitivity, such as those listed in Chart 66–5.

Clinical Manifestations of Photodermatitis

Clinically, patients develop an erythematous, papular rash that burns and itches. The rash may become vesicular with oozing and edema. It is accompanied by systemic symptoms such as

CHART 66–5   Agents Associated with Photosensitivity

Amiodarone	NSAIDs
Antipsychotic agents	Oral contraceptives
Barbiturates	Phenothiazines
Benzodiazepines	Phenylbutazone
Carbamazepine	Piroxicam
Chlorothiazide	Promethazine
Coal tar	Protriptyline
Dacarbazine	Psoralens
5-Fluorouracil	Quinidine/quinine
Furosemide	Retinoids
Griseofulvin	Simvastatin
Hypoglycemic agents	Sulfonamides
Ketoprofen	Sulfonylureas
Lomefloxacin	Sulindac
Methotrexate	Tetracyclines
Mitomycin C	Thiazides
Nalidixic acid	Tricyclics

pain, fever, malaise, chills, headache, and nausea. The rash occurs on areas exposed to the sun and persists for 7 to 10 days. Treatment consists of protection from the sun and management of the clinical manifestations.

Etiology, Epidemiology, Clinical Manifestations, and Treatment of Actinic Keratosis

Actinic keratosis lesions occur commonly after age 40 and are found on sun-exposed areas of the head, neck, arms, legs, tops of ears, and dorsal hands. **Actinic keratosis** lesions begin as hyperemic, poorly defined lesions and develop into scaly, rough, skin-colored macules with rough surfaces. Actinic keratosis is considered a premalignant lesion that may develop into squamous cell carcinoma. These lesions can be treated with topical 5-fluorouracil cream or solution, cryosurgery, or liquid nitrogen. They can also be treated with Aldara, which is thought to stimulate the immune system to remove these precancerous lesions. The patients will need instructions about sun protection measures for the remainder of their lives.

Etiology, Epidemiology, and Pathophysiology of Contact Dermatitis

Contact dermatitis is an inflammation of the skin related to exposure to an irritant or allergen in the environment. Irritant contact dermatitis is caused by a substance that is irritating to the skin but not due to an allergy. Allergic contact dermatitis is a type IV cell-mediated immune reaction that occurs after contact with an allergen. Cell-mediated immune reactions are mediated by T lymphocytes, which lead to destruction of the allergen (see Chapter 60). It may take several exposures before a reaction occurs. One of the most common types of allergic contact dermatitis is poison ivy or poison oak. It is difficult to distinguish between allergic or irritant reactions; however, an irritant reaction usually does not spread beyond the area of contact. The intensity of the skin reaction depends on the degree of sensitivity and the concentration and quantity of the exposure to the antigen. At first the dermatitis is usually confined to the area of direct exposure but may spread beyond that area.

CRITICAL ALERT *Poison ivy is a green plant with leaves arranged in threes, with one at the end and the other two opposing each other. It grows as a climbing vine on trees and poles or fences and bricks. It may have green flowers and white berries.*

Diagnosis, Clinical Manifestations, and Treatment of Contact Dermatitis

In the acute phase, the symptoms include edema, erythema (redness of the skin due to congestion of capillaries in the lower layers of the skin), vesicles, itching, and papules. If it continues into a chronic phase, the skin becomes dry, thickened, and may develop **fissures** (linear cracks or furrows in the continuity of the epidermis). The diagnosis usually requires the history of possible exposure and development of the rash, and physical examination. Patch testing can be done if necessary to determine the identity of the offending agent. Treatment includes stopping the exposure to the allergen or irritating agent. Future exposures to the causative agent should be avoided. The inflammatory process is treated using a mid- to high-potency topical corticosteroid. If the dermatitis is severe, oral steroids may be used. The itching should be treated with antihistamines. The Pharmacology Summary feature (p. 2181) presents medications used to treat skin disorders, including corticosteroids and antihistamines. Patients should be instructed not to scratch because scratching will increase the itching sensation and may cause a secondary infection.

Etiology, Epidemiology, Pathophysiology, and Clinical Manifestations of Urticaria

Urticaria, or hives, are raised, erythematous, intensely pruritic plaques or wheals that are surrounded by a white halo. These lesions vary in size and distribution and commonly occur as an allergic reaction to medications, foods, or insect bites. They also can be related to infections such as viral hepatitis, sinusitis, gingivitis, or cystitis. Aggravating factors include chemical irritants, fever, alcohol, exercise, and emotional stress. Histamine, the most common mediator of this reaction, is released by mast cells as a part of the immune response to allergens. Histamine causes an increased permeability of the microvessels of the skin, leading to a leakage of fluid into the tissues, causing edema at the site, and stimulating the itch receptors in the skin. The rash related to urticaria does not usually appear in the mucous membranes, the palms of the hands, the soles of the feet, or the axilla. Urticaria has several clinical variations outlined in Chart 66–6.

Urticaria is diagnosed by history of the exposure to possible causative agents and appearance of the lesion. Causative factors need to be identified and avoided. Most cases resolve spontaneously, but antihistamines may be given to block the action of histamine. See the Pharmacology Summary feature (p. 2181). Itching can be relieved with cold compresses or cool, colloid-type baths (Aveeno). It may be helpful to decrease stress, to avoid hot showers, and to exercise.

Etiology, Epidemiology, and Pathophysiology of Atopic Dermatitis

Atopic dermatitis, also known as eczema, is a chronic, inflammatory skin disorder characterized by dry skin related to water loss in the epidermis and decreased skin lipid levels. It can occur at any age but is more common in children. It generally cycles through periods of acute flare-ups and remissions. It can be

CHART 66–6	Urticarial Variants	
Variant	**Duration**	**Causes**
Acute	Lasts less than 6 weeks.	Food, drinks, medications, pollen, chemicals.
Chronic	Affects mostly adults. Lasts more than 2 months.	Cause is difficult to determine. May be related to underlying disease such as cancer, hepatitis, collagen disease, or Graves' disease.
Cold	Lasts 30 to 60 minutes.	Induced by exposure to cold surfaces, air, or water.
Physical urticaria	Intermittent. Lasts 1 to 2 hours.	Induced by things that increase body temperature such as showers, exercise, fever, and stress.

caused by irritants in the environment, or it can have an immunologic cause. Patients with atopic dermatitis often have a familial predisposition, including a family history of asthma or hay fever. Environmentally, it is aggravated by contact with allergens, perspiration, excessive heat, dry air, emotional stress, and rough clothing. Children often outgrow atopic dermatitis; however, it can become chronic into adulthood.

Clinical Manifestations and Diagnosis of Atopic Dermatitis

Atopic dermatitis is characterized by severe itching. The lesions are irregular, red papular patches that are weepy, shiny, or thickened. The lesions also may be plaques that are scaly and crusted. The characteristic distribution is on the face, the neck, the upper trunk, and the bends of the elbows and knees. The lesions can develop a secondary *Staphylococcus aureus* infection due to skin trauma and breakdown from scratching. It is diagnosed by history, including possible triggers for flare-ups, and physical examination to note the appearance and distribution of the lesions. Laboratory tests are not usually required; however, immunoglobin E (IgE) levels may be elevated, indicating an immune reaction. Allergy testing may be done to determine whether an allergic process is instrumental in causing the problem.

Medical Management of Atopic Dermatitis

Treatment involves controlling the aggravating factors and treating the rash. It is important to moisturize the skin to maintain the skin barrier. Bathing should be held to a minimum; however, when bathing, the patient should use tepid water and mild, unscented soap such as Cetaphil or Dove. To prevent itching and lubricate the skin, a thick, greasy moisturizer should be used at least once a day after bathing. Clothing should be soft, light, and preferably made of cotton or some natural, soft fiber. New clothes should be laundered before wearing to wash out any irritating chemicals. Any activity that causes perspiring should be avoided. Once a rash develops, the patient may be placed on a course of topical or oral corticosteroids to reduce inflammation and itching. Urea creams or nonsteroidal anti-inflammatory ointments are effective for hydrating the skin and decreasing itching. Oral antihistamines also may help decrease itching. See the Pharmacology Summary feature (p. 2181). If lesions are wet or crusted,

COMPLEMENTARY & ALTERNATIVE THERAPIES

Traditional Chinese Herbal Medicine

Description:

Atopic eczema may benefit from Chinese herbal medicines (Tse, 2003). These herbal medicines are part of an ancient medical tradition in China, otherwise known as traditional Chinese medicine (TCM). TCM is comprised of not only herbal medicines, but also acupuncture and related physical therapies, and general nutritional and life style guidelines. TCM is often performed in conjunction with conventional, or orthodox, medicine (OM) in China and other areas of Asia. In 1992, a randomized clinical trial of the use of 10 TCM herbs for atopic eczema was published and showed some benefit in treating atopic eczema. However, herbal TCM is still regarded with skepticism, as some TCM herbs provided by practitioners in the West have strayed from the standards of true TCM, and have caused liver and kidney toxicity. Some herbs have even been adulterated with pharmaceutical (OM) drugs. This has resulted in giving herbal TCM a poor reputation and recognition. These problems can be blamed on a lack of professional regulation, practitioner qualification, herbal product standards, and evidence-based clinical studies (Chan, 2005).

Research Support:

An Australian study assessed CAM use in patients with acne, psoriasis, or atopic eczema, as well as the patients' attitudes about CAM. The study involved interviewing 26 patients with acne, 29 patients with psoriasis, and 7 patients with atopic eczema. Results of these interviews showed that CAM therapy use was common, and patients had a tendency to value CAM over conventional therapies because they perceived that CAM therapies had less potential for adverse effects. Researchers concluded that, due to the extensive use of CAM therapies by patients with skin conditions, practitioners should be aware of this and alert for any implications and interactions (Magin, Adams, Heading, Pond, & Smith, 2006).

A literature review of studies was conducted in 2004 on the use of herbal TCM in treating atopic eczema. Four randomized controlled trials met the researchers' inclusion criteria. These trials showed that herbal TCM may be effective in the treatment of atopic eczema; however, researchers recommended further well-designed, larger-scale trials (Zhang et al., 2004).

References

Chan, K. (2005). Chinese medicinal materials and their interface with Western medical concepts. *Journal of Ethnopharmacology, 96*(1–2), 1–18.

Magin, P. J., Adams, J., Heading, G. S., Pond, D. C., & Smith, W. (2006). Complementary and alternative medicine therapies in acne, psoriasis, and atopic eczema: Results of a qualitative study of patients' experiences and perceptions. *Journal of Alternative and Complementary Medicine, 12*(5), 451–457.

Tse, T. W. (2003). Use of common Chinese herbs in the treatment of psoriasis. *Clinical and Experimental Dermatology, 28*(5), 469–475.

Zhang, W., Leonard, T., Bath-Hextall, F., Chambers, C. A., Lee. C., Humphreys, R., et al. (2004). Chinese herbal medicine for atopic eczema. *Cochrane Database of Systematic Reviews, 18*(4), CD002291.

---

soaking in Burrow's solution or colloidal oatmeal such as Aveeno may be helpful. Antibiotics may be needed to prevent or treat secondary skin infections. Alternative therapies such as traditional Chinese herbal medicine, as discussed in the Complementary and Alternative Therapies box, may be helpful as well.

Etiology, Epidemiology, and Pathophysiology of Skin Reaction to Medications

Skin reactions occur commonly as an allergic reaction to a medication. They can occur rapidly, as in an immediate-type hypersensitivity after exposure to the drug, or can take a few days to develop, as in a delayed hypersensitivity reaction (see Chapter 60 🔘). Allergic medication reactions are due to the function of the T cell that recognizes the medication as a foreign substance and reacts to it. This reaction usually requires a previous exposure to the medication so that the body can develop an immune response. Urticarial and maculopapular skin reactions occur most commonly with amoxicillin, trimethoprim-sulfamethoxazole, and ampicillin or penicillin. Medications such as phenolphthalein, pyrazolone derivatives, tetracyclines, nonsteroidal anti-inflammatory drugs (NSAIDs), barbiturates, and trimethoprim-sulfamethoxazole are more commonly related to fixed medication eruptions, which are rashes appearing in the same sites after each ingestion of the medication.

 **CRITICAL ALERT** *Adverse medication events in the elderly can be life threatening. Approximately 27.6% of all adverse medication events and 42.2% of life-threatening or fatal adverse medication events have been found to be preventable. These errors occurred more commonly with cardiovascular drugs and usually in the prescribing phase (60.8%) or in patient adherence (21.2%) (Gurwitz et al., 2003).*

Clinical Manifestations of Skin Reaction to Medications

The most common manifestations of an allergic skin reaction to medications are erythema, pruritus, and urticaria. The lesions are usually maculopapular occurring in a symmetrical, generalized distribution that spares the face. Fever and other systemic symptoms may accompany the rash. It is important to obtain a detailed history from the patient to identify whether a rash similar to this has occurred before and what medications the patient was taking with the prior rash as well as currently. Patients may not relate the rash to the use of a certain medication, so a specific and detailed assessment is important.

Medical Management of Skin Reaction to Medications

Treatment involves stopping the offending agent. Patients should be warned that it might take a few weeks for the rash to disappear even after stopping the medication. Antihistamines are helpful in slowing the immune response responsible for the rash and the itching, and thus promote healing. Systemic corticosteroids may be indicated if the reaction is widespread or severe. See the Pharmacology Summary feature (p. 2181). Colloidal baths are helpful to soothe extreme itching.

Skin Changes Related to Tobacco Smoking

Smoking has a negative effect on the skin, causing it to age prematurely. Smoking leads to vasoconstriction, which decreases blood supply and nutrients to the skin, and it breaks down the elastin in the skin, leading to wrinkles. There is evidence that facial wrinkling is associated with the number of pack-years smoked (Patel et al., 2006).

Skin Changes Related to Cultural Practices

Cultural practices can affect the health of the skin. For example, pomade acne is common in African Americans and Hispanics. This disorder is a form of acne caused by the use of grooming products on the scalp spreading to the forehead. These grooming agents contain substances that can lead to acne, such as lanolins and isopropyl myristate. Capsaicin-induced dermatitis is seen in Hispanic people. This condition, caused by handling hot chili peppers with bare hands, leads to erythema, burning pain, and irritation (Halder & Nootheti, 2003).

Some alternative medicine practices lead to the formation of dermatologic lesions. Coin rubbing is an Asian practice done to relieve symptoms of the flu, fever, and headaches. In this practice, a coin or a similar object is used to scrape the skin, causing ecchymotic streaks. The scraping usually occurs between the ribs, along the inner aspects of both arms, and along both sides of the spine. Cupping, another cultural practice that is done to treat pain, involves soaking a cotton ball in alcohol and igniting it. The cotton ball is then placed in a cup or jar, which is then inverted and placed on the skin. Once placed on the skin, the flame goes out and a vacuum is created. This vacuum pulls the skin into the cup or jar, leading to circular, ecchymotic, painful burns usually done symmetrically in rows of two to four cups. Moxibustion is a cultural practice that involves igniting dry weeds or incense-like material and applying the lit tip to acupuncture sites. It is used to treat a variety of disorders. It may be confused with abuse and should be considered when assessing skin disorders.

Skin Changes Related to Tattoos

Tattoos are pictures and words applied anywhere on the body, including permanent makeup applied to the eyes and lips. A tattoo is defined as a permanent mark or design made on skin by inserting ink or dye via a needle into the dermal layer of the skin with repeated punctures. The needle is connected to a small machine with tubes containing dye that apply repeated piercing to the skin, much like the action of a sewing machine. The process, which can take several hours for a large tattoo, causes a small amount of bleeding and minor to potentially significant pain. Tattooing is an increasingly popular practice; however, it is not without health risks. The skin integrity is altered, which means the individual is susceptible to skin reactions and infections. The most common infections following tattooing are caused by *Staphylococcus aureus*, which may be a result of poor hygiene on the part of either the provider or the customer, during and after the procedure. There is increased risk for potentially serious antibiotic-resistant skin infections such as community acquired methicillin-resistant *Staphylococcus aureus* with unlicensed tattoo artists who do not follow proper infection control procedures (CDC, 2006a; MayoClinic.com, 2008). Typical signs and symptoms of an infection include redness, warmth, swelling, and a pus-like drainage. Some antibiotic-resistant skin infections can lead to pneumonia, bloodstream infections, and necrotizing fasciitis.

Some degree of bleeding is inevitable during the tattooing process; therefore, the transmission of bloodborne pathogens is possible. If the equipment used to create the tattoo is contaminated with the blood of an infected person, it is possible to contract a number of serious bloodborne diseases. Bloodborne pathogen transmission is associated with the reuse of tattoo needles without proper and adequate sterilization. It is also possible that the electric equipment itself may be contaminated. Infection with hepatitis B virus is a well-documented post-tattoo complication. Other infections include hepatitis C, tetanus, tuberculosis, and the human immunodeficiency virus, the virus that causes AIDS (MayoClinic.com, 2008).

 Instructions to individuals who are planning to have either a tattoo or body piercing need to include having to question the health standards of the establishment. Many local health departments have sanitation guidelines for tattoo and body piercing establishments.

Tattoo dyes can cause allergic skin reactions, resulting in an itchy rash at the tattoo site. Red ink is most commonly associated with allergic reactions, although any color of ink may cause an allergic reaction in sensitive patients. Some allergic reactions may take years to develop; therefore, patients should be queried about old tattoos as well as newer ones during assessment. Additionally, granulomas may form around the tattoo ink, especially the red ink. Tattooing can also cause keloid scar formation if the individual is prone to them (MayoClinic.com, 2008). Tattoo ink is not regulated by the Food and Drug Administration and may contain heavy metals: alcohols, ethylene glycol (automobile antifreeze), formaldehyde, glutaraldehyde, ferrocyanides, aluminum, mercury, cadmium, cobalt, chromium, and lead. Tattoo "inks" may also be homemade and therefore may be composed of any number of potential toxins and/or allergens (County of Kern: Department of Health Services, 2007).

Due to the makeup of the dye or ink, there may be a reaction during a magnetic resonance imaging (MRI) scan. Although it happens rarely, tattoos or permanent makeup may cause swelling or burning in the affected areas during the MRI exam. In some cases, when the scan is in the immediate area of the dye such as the eye, tattoo pigments may interfere with the quality of the image (MayoClinic.com, 2008).

Care of the tattoo includes regular cleaning with soap and water and applying moisturizer. The sun should be avoided for the first few weeks after application. Tattoos may take up to several days to heal. The individual needs to be instructed not to pick at a scab, which increases the risk of infection, can damage the design, and increases the risk of scar formation.

Tattoo removal is possible, although complete removal is difficult and skin color variations and scarring are likely to remain. Methods of removal include:

- Laser surgery is the most effective way to reduce the appearance of a tattoo. Pulses of laser light pass through the top layer of skin, and the energy of the light is absorbed by the pigment in the tattoo. This process creates a very low grade of inflammation and allows the body to shed small areas of altered pigment. It requires repeated treatments over time to lighten the tattoo, and the treatment might not completely erase it.

- Dermabrasion uses a sanding process to remove the outer layer of skin and lighten the tattoo.

- Surgical removal involves cutting out the tattoo and surgically closing the open area, leaving a scar.

Skin Changes Related to Body Piercing

Body piercing involves creating a hole in a body part for the purpose of inserting jewelry. The most common body piercing areas are the lobe and other areas of the ear, nose, eyebrow, lip, tongue, and naval. Body piercing has risks similar to those of tattoos, although due to improvements in safety procedures and equipment, the popular practice of earlobe piercing is viewed as generally less risky than other body piercing. A single-use, sterilized ear piercing device or an ear piercing gun with sterilized, disposable cartridges may be safest (MayoClinic.com, 2008). Some practitioners use a reusable piercing gun for these types of piercing, which is difficult to sterilize and can more easily damage the skin. The most common infections associated with "gun"-type ear piercing are *Staphylococcus aureus* and *Pseudomonas aeruginosa* (County of Kern: Department of Health Services, 2007). In addition, any time the skin is punctured, there are risks including:

- Bloodborne diseases may occur if the equipment used to do the piercing is contaminated with the blood of an infected person. There is a risk for contracting hepatitis C, hepatitis B, tetanus, tuberculosis, and HIV.
- Allergic reactions may occur if the jewelry is made of nickel or brass.
- Oral complications that may occur with jewelry worn in tongue piercing include infection, chipped and cracked teeth, and damaged gums.
- Skin infection clinical manifestations include redness, swelling, pain, and a pus-like discharge.
- Infections from piercing in the upper ear cartilage are especially serious. Antibiotics are often ineffective. Because cartilage does not have its own blood supply, the drug cannot reach the infection site. Such infection can lead to cartilage damage and serious, permanent ear deformity.
- Body piercing can cause scarring, and if the individual is susceptible, piercing can cause keloid scar formation, discussed later.

Postprocedure care for the pierced area depends on the body part pierced. Oral piercing (tongue or lip) includes instructing the individual to rinse the mouth with an antibacterial, alcohol-free mouth rinse for 30 to 60 seconds after meals until the piercing heals. A new soft-bristled toothbrush should be used to avoid introducing bacteria into the mouth. Piercings of the nose, ears, eyebrow, and navel need to be cleaned gently with warm water and an antibiotic cleanser to remove any crusting. The jewelry should be gently turned back and forth to work the cleanser around the opening. Avoid alcohol and peroxide, as they can dry the skin; and ointments should not be applied, as they keep oxygen from reaching the piercing and can leave a sticky residue (MayoClinic.com, 2008). The piercing site will heal over without the jewelry in place.

Health Promotion Related to Tattoos and Skin Piercing

There are no licensing laws or regulations governing tattooing and piercing; therefore, individuals must protect themselves by being better informed about the entire process. Certain inherent risks, described earlier, are associated with body piercing and tattooing; however, being informed about the following will improve safety:

- Discuss the sterilization techniques by inquiring about the use of an autoclave; request to see it in operation. If none is used, go elsewhere.
- Discuss the sterilization of jewelry and instruments such as sterilization of ink pouches with intact color-change seals. If possible, ask to see the packaged sterilized instruments.
- Ask whether excess tattoo ink is being poured back into the main supply.
- Follow all after-care instructions and report complications including redness, swelling, pain, or discharge to a health care provider immediately.

Scar Formation

When patients have a full-thickness injury, healing occurs replacing the injured tissue with connective tissue forming a scar. Wounds heal in three phases: the inflammatory phase, which prepares the wound for healing; the proliferative phase during which new tissue builds to fill in the wound space; and the remodeling phase when the scar strengthens. Phases of wound healing are discussed in detail in Chapter 67 ⊙. Scars can be small and asymptomatic or large with restricted function such as occurs with a hypertrophic or keloid scar formation. Abnormal scar formation includes hypertrophic and keloid scar formation.

Hypertrophic and Keloid Scar Formation

Hypertrophic and keloid scar formation is an abnormal, excessive development of connective tissue or collagen. The cause of the development of these scars is unclear, but they seem to occur in genetically predisposed individuals. They occur more frequently when the injury occurs over the sternum, anterior chest, shoulder, upper lip, earlobe, and neck. It is believed that keloid formation arises more in African Americans, Asians, and children. Chart 66–7 compares the appearance of hypertrophic scars and keloid scars. Both scars are identified by observation and a history of trauma. If the patient has a history of keloid

CHART 66–7	Comparison of Hypertrophic and Keloid Scars	
Hypertrophic Scars	**Keloid Scars**
Begin as red, firm lesions.	Begin as pink, firm, rubbery plaque with telangiectasia.
Skin is shiny and stretched with smooth, dome-shaped surface.	Smooth, irregularly shaped, and hyperpigmented.
May be itchy and tender.	May be tender or painful, pruritic, or burning.
Usually contained within the area of injury.	Claw-like edge that extends outside the area of injury.
Resolve spontaneously without treatment in 6 to 18 months.	Resistant to therapy; may enlarge over time.

scar formation, it may be helpful to apply pressure dressings to the injury site for 8 hours a day for 4 to 6 months to decrease the scar hypertrophy and prevent decreased range of motion. Corticosteroids injected into the scar lesion may be beneficial. Surgical excision of the scar can be done but the abnormal scarring may reoccur. Referral to a plastic surgeon or dermatologist may be indicated. Chapter 68 🔗 discusses keloid scar formation with burn scars and contains graphics of the scar formation.

General Skin Lesions and Disorders

Skin disorders may result in a variety of skin lesions with multiple configurations and signs and symptoms. Skin disorders can be benign or malignant, due to infectious agents, and/or from infestations by insects. It is important for the nurse to assess these lesions, their characteristics, location, exudates, and distribution on the body. Appearance of new skin lesions occurs as a part of the aging process. Skin lesions common among the elderly are outlined in the Gerontological Considerations box.

Benign Skin Disorders

Benign skin disorders include those that are not carcinogenic. Most often these disorders are painless and asymptomatic. Any abnormal growth on the skin is of concern to a patient; therefore, it is essential that the nurse thoroughly evaluate and report skin changes. Common benign skin disorders are discussed next.

Moles or Nevi

Moles or **nevi** are common skin lesions that appear on almost everyone in almost any location but are more common in sun-exposed areas. They can be present at birth or can be acquired as an individual grows, although new ones usually do not appear after age 40. Moles are usually asymptomatic but can be irritated by clothing or trauma. The various types of moles are described in Chart 66–8. Moles are generally considered harmless but may become malignant and need to be evaluated periodically. Changes in color, diameter, or the border of the mole need to be reported to the health care provider, as these changes could indicate a premalignant or malignant change.

Skin Tags

Skin tags are common flesh-colored or brown papules that grow on a thick stalk. They are about 1 to 10 millimeters in diameter and most frequently develop on the neck, axillae, groin, eyelids, or in skin fold areas. They are usually asymptomatic unless they

GERONTOLOGICAL CONSIDERATIONS for Skin Lesions

Skin Lesion	Description
Skin tags	Soft, brown, flesh-colored papules
Keratosis	Horny or abnormal growth of keratinocytes
Lentigines	Well-bordered brown to black macules commonly called liver spots
Vascular lesions	Vascular tumors with chronically dilated blood vessels

CHART 66–8 Types of Moles or Nevi

Type of Mole or Nevus	Description
Junctional	Flat or slightly raised, brown-tan papule, less than 6 millimeters in diameter. Usually occurs at dermal–epidermal junction.
Compound	Slightly to markedly raised, pigmented papule. Symmetrical with irregular border and smooth or slightly papillary surface. Center more pigmented than border.
Intradermal	Elevated, fleshy papule. Pale or flesh colored with pigmented flecks. May have coarse, dark hairs growing from it.
Halo nevus	Mole surrounded by a ring of hypopigmentation. Usually disappears over several months with halo repigmenting.
Blue nevus	Solitary, bluish macula or papule usually located on the head, neck, or buttocks. Enlarges slowly and persists for 10 to 15 years.
Becker's nevus	Usually occurs on the shoulder, submammary area, or back. Consists of a brown macule or patch of hair. Irregular, sharply demarcated border. Varies in size but can be quite large.

are irritated by clothing or jewelry, which may cause bleeding and tenderness. Skin tags are benign and may last indefinitely without problems. They do not require treatment; however, if desired they can be removed by simple scissor excision.

Lipoma

A **lipoma** is a nodule of fat tissue that is usually benign and is identified as a soft, freely mobile growth under the skin. It is slow growing and may vary in size from 1 to several centimeters in diameter. It is most commonly located on the shoulders, legs, arms, buttocks, and back but can occur anywhere on the body. Treatment is not necessary; however, if the lesion is cosmetically bothersome to the patient, it can be surgically excised.

Epidermal Cyst

An epidermal cyst is a capsule filled with keratin that appears spontaneously in areas of friction or on hair-bearing areas, but it commonly occurs on the face, postauricular fold, posterior neck, and trunk. Occluded **pilosebaceous follicles** (sebaceous cyst containing hair follicles) probably form the wall of the cyst. A cyst is freely movable but firm and tense feeling. It is dome shaped and pale, ranging in size from 0.5 to 5 centimeters, with a central opening that drains a pasty, malodorous material made up of necrotic keratin. It generally does not cause complications but can become infected; therefore, it may need antibiotics and in some instances may require surgical removal.

Hyperpigmentation of the Skin

This category of skin disorders involves an increase in normal skin colors. It occurs because of increased or abnormally distributed melanin. It may be diffuse or limited to a specific space. Typically the major concern to the patient is the cosmetic effect.

Café-au-Lait Spots

Café-au-lait spots are asymptomatic tan macules that have smooth borders and vary in diameter from 0.5 to 20 centimeters. They are generally considered to be benign but can indicate the presence of neurofibromatosis if there are six or more spots. No treatment is necessary, but they can be eliminated with laser or bleaching agents if they are cosmetically undesirable.

Liver Spots (Solar Lentigo)

Solar lentigo, commonly referred to as an age spot or liver spot, refers to lesions that develop due to a familial tendency and chronic sun exposure in Caucasians over age 60. They are macules that are darker and larger than freckles and do not fade during winter. They occur in sun-exposed areas such as the backs of the hands, forearms, shoulders, and forehead. Their color is uniform with sharply demarcated borders. The lesions are usually asymptomatic but may be of cosmetic concern. The best treatment is prevention through the limitation of exposure to sunlight and the application of sunscreen. Bleaching creams are available that can be applied topically and will slowly fade the spots. Cosmetic resurfacing of the skin through the use of lasers or liquid nitrogen application can also decrease the pigmentation.

Hypopigmentation of the Skin

Hypopigmentation of the skin is a decrease in melanin that can be hereditary or acquired. There are diseases of the skin that lead to a loss of melanin causing a pale or gray appearance to the skin. One of the most common disorders leading to hypopigmentation is vitiligo.

Vitiligo

Vitiligo is a localized loss of melanocytes from the skin and hair creating white patches of skin (Figure 66–1 ■). The cause is unknown but may be related to an autoimmune disorder and inhibition of melanogenesis. It occurs spontaneously after emotional or physical stress or may be related to trauma. Vitiligo progresses slowly over years with new patches of hypopigmentation occurring throughout life. The white macules can occur in a symmetrical pattern or can be segmental, limited to one seg-

ment of the body. The most common sites are the backs of the hands, face, body folds, axillae, and genitalia. Vitiligo causes no discomfort and is purely of cosmetic concern. Spontaneous repigmentation can occur but is usually spotty. The white areas can be covered with dyes and cosmetics to minimize the color irregularities. Sunless self-tanning agents may also be helpful by darkening the skin through staining. If the lesions are in sun-exposed areas, sunscreens should be used because of the higher risk of sunburn. Topical corticosteroids may be used to treat inflammation associated with the areas of hypopigmentation. See the Pharmacology Summary feature (p. 2181).

Acne Vulgaris

Acne vulgaris is a skin condition that occurs most frequently during the teenage years at varying levels of severity. It is caused by obstruction of a hair follicle due to overgrowth of sebum and keratin debris, an overproduction of oil due to enlarged oil glands, and bacteria known as *P. acnes* (Gorgos, 2006). These substances provide a good medium for bacterial growth, especially *Propionibacterium acnes* (*P. acnes*). *P. acnes* contain lipases that result in the breakdown of free fatty acids. Free fatty acids irritate the skin and cause a foreign body reaction leading to inflammation. The characteristic skin lesion, known as a comedo, is typically located on the face, chest, and back (Figure 66–2 ■).

Acne is defined by type and severity. There are three types of acne: comedonal, papulopustular, and nodulocystic. Comedonal acne is defined as noninflammatory with whiteheads or closed comedos, and blackheads or open comedos. Whiteheads, or closed comedos, occur when the opening to the skin is closed, and they look like tiny flesh-colored bumps. Blackheads, or open comedos, occur when the opening to the skin is open but capped with blackened skin debris, giving them a black appearance. Papulopustular acne is inflammatory with small papules and pustules that contain a central core of purulent material. Nodulocystic acne is inflammatory with a lesion or cyst greater than 5 millimeters in diameter. These cysts can be localized or can form tracts under the skin with abscesses. Nodulocystic acne is a serious problem requiring aggressive treatment. The severity of acne is rated as mild, moderate, and severe. Mild acne is defined

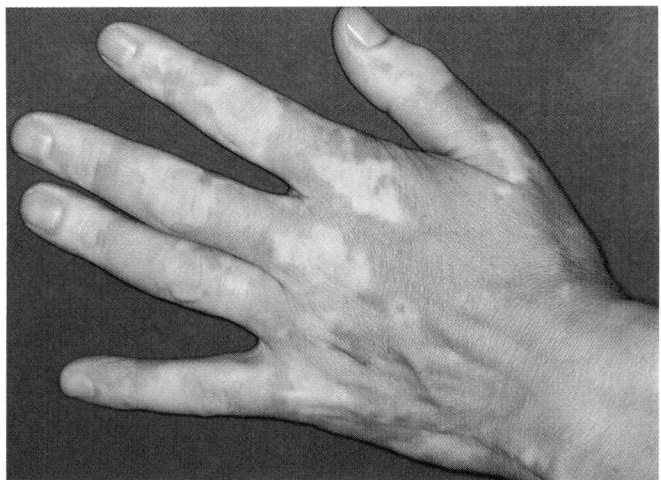

FIGURE 66–1 ■ Vitiligo.
Source: ISM/Phototake NYC

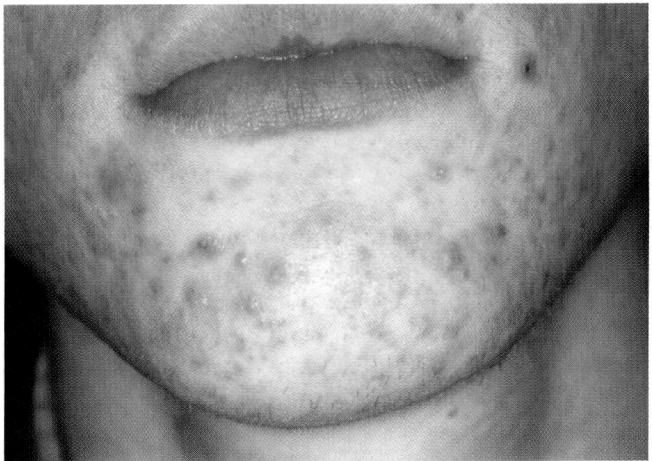

FIGURE 66–2 ■ Acne vulgaris.
Source: Dr. P. Marazzi/Photo Researchers, Inc.

as open and closed comedos and noninflamed lesions. Moderate acne is defined as open and closed comedos with some pustules and inflamed lesions. Severe acne is defined as open and closed comedos, and lesions that are inflamed and pustular. There are also nodules and significant scarring (Layton, Buchanan, & Courtenay, 2006).

Several factors have been identified as contributors to acne. Androgens play a role in the development of acne by stimulating the production of sebum, leading to obstruction of hair follicles and allowing for bacterial growth. However, estrogens can suppress the production of sebum. There is a genetic predisposition to acne as well as a link between stress and acne formation. There have, however, been no connections found between makeup use or diet and acne, which were once thought to be true. Men usually have more severe disease than women, but acne in women may persist into adulthood.

Treatment of choice for acne is based on the type and severity of the acne, the patient's skin type, and the presence or potential for scarring. Treatment will take about 6 to 8 weeks to see improvement. Nonpharmacologic approaches to therapy involve good hygiene that includes washing the face with soap and water. The patient should avoid topical exposure to oils and greases. Hats, sweatbands, and shirt collars can contribute to the collection of oil on the forehead, neck, and back and can contribute to an outbreak. Mild acne requires only topical agents such as benzoyl peroxide, salicylic acid, and azelaic acid that serve to help unblock the pores. These medications have bactericidal qualities that reduce the number of *P. acnes* and act to break down the keratin. Topical retinoids, such as Retin-A, are comedolytic agents that work as anti-inflammatory agents and normalize the abnormal growth of keratins. Oral contraceptives may be helpful for young women because they will decrease circulating androgens.

For moderate acne, a topical antibiotic should be added to the topical cleansing agent. Topical antibiotics decrease the numbers of *P. acnes* in sebaceous follicles and help to decrease inflammation. Once pustules or papules have developed, an oral antibiotic might be helpful. The antibiotic of choice is tetracycline at a dose of 500 milligrams twice daily. Erythromycin, doxycycline, and minocycline have also been shown to be effective. For severe acne, isotretinoin (Accutane) may be used. Accutane is an oral retinoid that decreases sebaceous gland activity and prevents the development of new comedos. Accutane has numerous side effects such as nosebleeds; inflammation of the lips and eyes; pain and stiffness in muscles, bones, and joints; and elevated triglyceride levels. Therefore, its use should be monitored carefully. It should never be used in pregnant women due to the major teratogenic effects. See the Pharmacology Summary feature (p. 2181). Finally, patients should be instructed not to squeeze, rub, or pick at comedos because doing so may result in scarring.

Lasers and light treatments have been used to treat acne. Lasers damage oil glands by using heat. Light treatments in the form of photodynamic therapy treat the overactive oil glands and the *P. acnes* bacteria. Both of these treatments are effective in reducing the oil production, leading to improved acne (Gorgos, 2006).

Nurses need to educate patients about the contributing factors and treatment for acne. The patient needs to understand that treatment is slow and that it will take 6 to 8 weeks to see the effects of any treatment regimen. The effects and side effects of all medications should be explained. The patient may require emotional support to deal with the psychological effects of acne because the lesions and scarring may have a negative effect on the patient's self-esteem and quality of life.

Psoriasis

Psoriasis is a chronic, noncontagious inflammatory skin disorder that affects over 4 million people in the United States (Figure 66–3 ■). Its exact cause is unknown, but there is a genetic tendency and evidence of an immune response that involves T-cell activation by an antigen stimulating the inflammatory process. The disease is chronic and incurable with exacerbations and remissions. Certain trigger factors cause an exacerbation, and these include stress, infection, medications such as beta-adrenergic blockers, smoking, and high alcohol consumption (Young, 2005). There are many types of psoriasis but chronic plaque psoriasis is the most common (Chart 66–9).

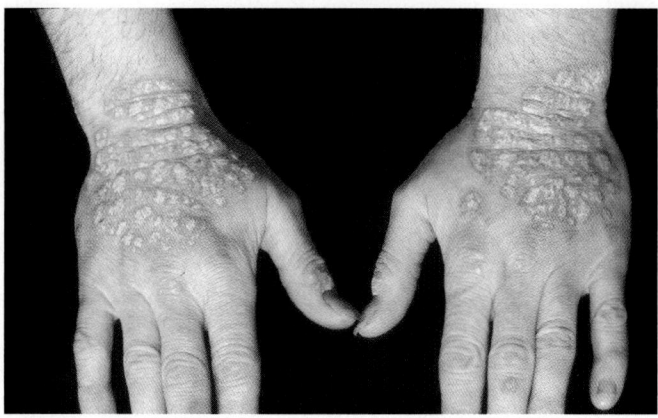

FIGURE 66–3 ■ Psoriasis.
Source: NMSB/Custom Medical Stock Photo, Inc.

CHART 66–9	Types of Psoriasis
Type	**Description**
Plaque	Red, scaly papules that coalesce. Lesions are well demarcated and symmetrical. Scale is adherent and silvery white with bleeding when removed.
Guttate	Associated with a sudden appearance of scaly papules that are "drop-like" and generally appear on the trunk.
Localized pustular	Discrete, small, sterile pustules that do not rupture but turn brown and scaly.
Generalized pustular	Erythema with sterile, generalized pustules over much of the body. Associated with systemic symptoms such as fever, chills, and leukocytosis.
Erythrodermic	Exfoliates with red skin all over body. There may be skin peeling with fluid balance problems. Very serious disease.
Nail psoriasis	Pitting of nails with separating of the nail from the nail bed. Nail plate may turn yellow.
Scalp psoriasis	Erythematous, scaly plaques that occur on the scalp or near the hairline. Usually is limited to the scalp.

The lesions of psoriasis are erythematous papules and plaques with silver-white scales that are sharply demarcated. They are the result of hyperproliferation of keratinocytes. A variety of sizes of lesions can coalesce into very large plaques. These lesions usually occur on the extensor surfaces of the knees and elbows, the scalp, the lower back, genitalia, or nails but can occur anywhere on the body. Some individuals experience pain and swelling in the joints that is associated with psoriasis called psoriatic arthritis.

Psoriasis is diagnosed by history of lesion development, trigger factors, family history, and physical examination. The appearance and distribution of the lesions can be enough to provide a diagnosis; however, skin biopsy can be done if there is question. The first line of treatment is topical agents such as emollient creams or ointments that can be used to prevent cracking and fissuring of the skin. Emollients help to moisturize the skin, easing itching and scaling. Corticosteroids are used to decrease inflammation; but the relief they provide is temporary, so they are best used in cycles for 7 to 10 days with rest periods in between. Vitamin D_3 analogue creams can be used directly on a plaque to control irritation and erythema. Coal tar preparations can be effective in resolving the lesions, although the exact mechanism of action is unknown. Phototherapy is effective when the psoriasis affects more than 30% of the body. Ultraviolet B is given three to five times weekly with exposures intense enough to cause erythema. Clearing of the lesions takes an average of 7 weeks. Phototherapy can also be used in conjunction with other medications. Most commonly used is ultraviolet A (UVA) with a photosensitizing medication such as psoralen. Psoralen is given prior to the exposure to ultraviolet light (UV). It inhibits DNA synthesis after activation with UVA, decreasing cellular proliferation. Systemic therapy is used in patients who are very uncomfortable or who have psoriasis affecting a large portion of the body. Methotrexate, a commonly used systemic medication, acts to prevent hyperkeratinization by suppressing proliferating cells or psoratic epidermal cell reproduction. Cyclosporine, an immunosuppressive drug that suppresses the growth of T cells, is used for severe inflammatory psoriasis. Etanercept is an example of biologic agents that have been used recently as a treatment for psoriasis. These medications interfere with the immunologic process, that has been found to be involved in psoriasis, with relative safety. They have been found to improve the skin lesions of psoriasis.

The psychological implications of psoriasis are great. It is a disfiguring disease that can result in low self-esteem, poor self-perception, depression, and anxiety. It can affect an individual's business, social, and sexual relationships. It may also cause problems with working due to the time off work for treatment, resulting in job loss and decreased income. Nurses need to be aware of not only the physical needs of the patient with psoriasis but also the emotional needs.

Seborrheic Keratosis

Seborrheic keratosis is a benign epidermal lesion seen predominantly in the middle-aged and elderly population. The exact cause is unknown, but it appears to be related to sun exposure. There are usually no associated symptoms, but the lesions can be irritated by clothing or jewelry. The lesions of seborrheic keratosis are warty, dirty yellow to black papules with sharp margins.

They can also be flat, and the color can vary from white to pink to black within the lesion. They have a "stuck on" appearance with a waxy feel, and they tend to occur more commonly on the back, central chest, face, and scalp. A sudden onset of numerous seborrheic keratoses, known as the Leser-Trélat sign, is often associated with the presence of an internal malignancy.

Diagnosis is made on the basis of history of sun exposure and lesion appearance, and physical examination of the lesions. The lesions will continue to grow and new lesions will continue to appear. No treatment is usually necessary, although they can be surgically removed for cosmetic or diagnostic reasons.

Dermatofibroma

Dermatofibromas are common, asymptomatic, benign, firm tan or brown papules occurring more frequently in middle-aged women. They are more commonly seen on the legs, elbows, or lateral trunk, often at the site of a previous trauma such as an insect bite. They characteristically dimple when pinched between the thumb and forefinger. Diagnosis is usually based on history of the symptoms and physical examination of the lesion. Treatment is not necessary, but dermatofibromas may be surgically removed for cosmetic reasons.

Genetic Disorder: Neurofibromatosis

Neurofibromatosis is an autosomal dominant inherited disorder; however, this condition also may arise spontaneously, without a previous family history. There are two types of neurofibromatosis. Type 1 is the most common and is known as von Recklinghausen's disease. It is characterized by multiple hyperpigmented macules; neurofibromatosis; and small, multiple, palpable, pedunculated, mobile, and pigmented nodules. These lesions become apparent after the first decade of life and are disfiguring. People with type 1 also have other associated disorders such as scoliosis and erosive bone defects. Type 2 neurofibromatosis is characterized by tumors of the eighth cranial or acoustic nerve. Symptoms associated with type 2 include headaches, hearing loss, impaired balance, facial pain, and tinnitus. This condition is often accompanied by intracranial or intraspinal tumors.

Neurofibromatosis is diagnosed by history of symptoms and physical examination. Magnetic resonance imaging may be necessary to detect tumors in the brain or spinal cord. The severity of the disease is variable. Disfigurement caused by tumors and nodules on the skin can be corrected with plastic surgery. Tumors of the spinal cord and brain can be treated surgically as well. The care of these patients is multidisciplinary, requiring visits to several specialists. Patients may need to see specialists such as an ophthalmologist for optic gliomas, a neurologist for neurofibromatosis, a dermatologist for nodules on the skin, or an orthopedist for osseous lesions. The patient must be followed closely for problems related to the formation of tumors. First-degree relatives should be screened for the presence of the disease, and genetic counseling is recommended to avoid passing the disease to future generations.

■ Malignant Conditions of the Skin

Skin cancer is the most common form of cancer occurring in the United States (CDC, 2002). Exposure to the sun's ultraviolet rays is a direct contributing factor in the development of skin cancer.

Individuals at the highest risk for skin cancer include those with fair or light skin color, those with a family history or personal history of skin cancer, individuals with chronic sun exposure, those with intermittent but intense exposure to the sun, those with sunburns early in life, and those with a large number of moles or freckles indicating sun sensitivity and sun damage. There are three types of skin cancer: The most common type is basal cell carcinoma, followed by squamous cell carcinoma, and then malignant melanoma.

Basal Cell Carcinoma

Basal cell carcinoma is more common in Caucasian people and not as common in African Americans. It is usually nonmetastasizing and occurs most frequently on the head and neck, where there is the greatest sun exposure. There are different types of basal cell carcinoma. The most common is nodular, which appears as a smooth skin-colored nodule. It is dome shaped with a rolled edge. It may have an overlying dilation of vessels seen just beneath the skin surface. The second most common type of basal cell carcinoma is superficial basal cell carcinoma. It is usually seen on the chest and back and is described as a flat, nonpalpable, erythematous plaque with distinct borders. It is often difficult to distinguish because it looks like many other skin lesions. Figure 66–4 ■ is an example of a basal cell carcinoma.

Squamous Cell Carcinoma

Squamous cell carcinoma consists of tumors of the outer epidermis that occur with frequent exposure to the sun and can be relatively aggressive when spreading. There are two types of squamous cell carcinoma: intraepidermal, which remains in the epidermis for a long time but can eventually spread to area lymph nodes and become invasive, which can be either slow or rapid growing. Squamous cell carcinoma is described as a small, red, scaling lesion sitting on an elevated base with an irregular border that may itch or be a nonhealing lesion after minor trauma. Squamous cell carcinoma develops from precancerous lesions and can metastasize through the lymphatic system to regional lymph nodes. Figure 66–5 ■ is an example of a squamous cell carcinoma.

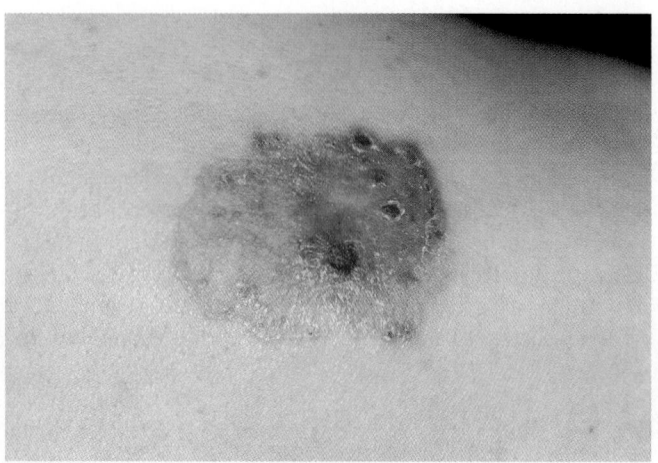

FIGURE 66–4 ■ Basal cell carcinoma.
Source: Phototake NYC

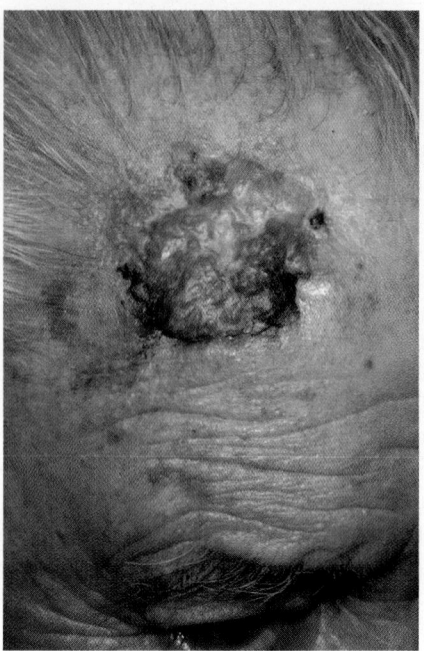

FIGURE 66–5 ■ Squamous cell carcinoma.
Source: Visuals Unlimited

Malignant Melanoma

The incidence of melanoma has more than tripled in the Caucasian population in the United States in the last 20 years. Malignant melanoma currently is the seventh most common cancer in the United States (Jemal et al., 2006; Swetter, 2008). Malignant melanoma is a skin cancer that originates from melanocytes. Early detection with early intervention is usually curative. Because of the aggressive and invasive nature of malignant melanoma, the prognosis is poor when it is diagnosed in the later stages. It is recommended that all individuals examine their skin and know the risk factors of malignant melanoma, as presented in the Risk Factors box.

Malignant melanoma is the most dangerous skin cancer because it is a rapidly growing invasive tumor that can metastasize to almost any organ in the body and result in death. It is a tumor involving melanocytes that is related to sun exposure. Fair-skinned people who sunburn easily and freckle are at the greatest risk. Severe, blistering sunburns in early childhood and intense sun exposure increase the susceptibility to melanoma. It appears as a changing or unusual mole with an irregular border, an uneven surface, and that has a varied size and shape (see the Risk Factors box). The color varies with combinations of brown, black, blue, gray, red, and white. It may be tender and will sometimes ulcerate and bleed. The four types of malignant melanoma are outlined in Chart 66–10. Because malignant melanoma is rapidly progressing, it is important to stage the disease in order to determine the best treatment option. In stage I the lesion is less than 1 millimeter thick with no evidence of tumor growth into lymph nodes. A stage II lesion is thicker than 1 millimeter with lymph nodes that are not enlarged, but there may be metastasis to other organs and lymph nodes. Stage III indicates there has been metastasis to distant organs. There is lymph node enlargement near the melanoma site, and there are

RISK FACTORS for Malignant Melanoma

Patient at high risk for malignant melanoma:

- Has a large number of typical moles.
- Has an increased number of atypical moles.
- Burns easily from exposure to the sun, freckles from sun exposure, or has difficulty tanning.
- Has a family history of malignant melanoma.
- Has previously been diagnosed with malignant melanoma.

The ABCDs of Malignant Melanoma

A *Asymmetry.*   Early melanoma is asymmetrical, as opposed to the typical mole that is symmetrical.

B *Border.*   Melanomas have irregular borders, whereas most moles have clearly delineated edges.

C *Color.*   Melanomas are usually variegated and are in shades of brown, tan, blue/black, or a combinations of colors. Typical moles tend to be uniform in color.

D *Diameter.*   Melanomas are often larger than 6 millimeters in diameter. The typical mole is generally less than 6 millimeters in diameter (the approximate size of a pencil eraser).

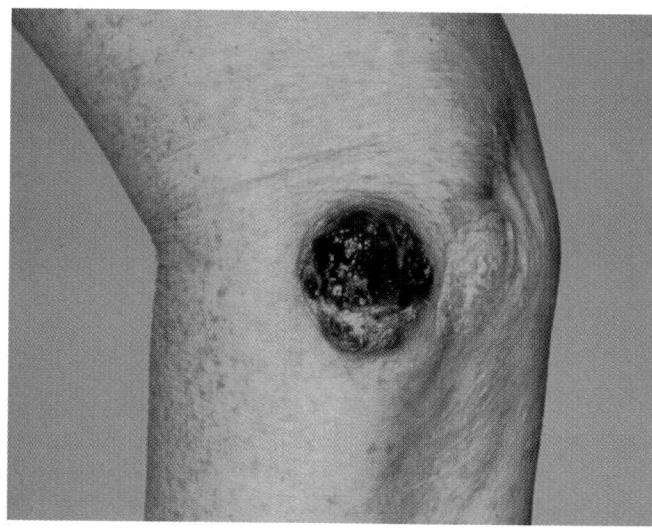

FIGURE 66–6 ■ Malignant melanoma.
Source: Biophoto Associates/Science Source

CHART 66–10   Types of Melanoma

Type	Description
Superficial spreading	Makes up 50% of the cases of melanoma. Occurs in younger adults. It looks like a nevus with a raised edge and lateral growth. It may be ulcerated and bleeding.
Nodular melanoma	Makes up 20–25% of all cases and usually occurs in young adults. Raised, dome-shaped lesion. It is usually a uniform blue-black color. It resembles blood blisters. It rapidly invades the dermis.
Lentigo melanoma	Makes up 15% of all cases and occurs in older adults. Slow-growing, flat nevus. Grows horizontally and radially.
Acral lentiginous melanoma	Least common form making up less than 10% of all cases. Occurs on the palms of the hands, soles of the feet, nail beds, and mucous membranes.

CHART 66–11   Assessing for Skin Cancer

The ABCD Method

A = Asymmetry
B = Border irregularity
C = Color variation
D = Diameter greater than the size of a pencil eraser

The Seven-Point Checklist

One or more major signs or three or four minor signs without a major sign can indicate a need to biopsy.

Major Signs

Change in size
Change in shape
Change in color

Minor Signs

Inflammation
Crusting or bleeding
Sensory changes

positive lymph nodes away from the original tumor site. Stage IV is generally widespread and incurable (Demierre, Allten, & Brown, 2005). Figure 66–6 ■ is an example of a malignant melanoma.

Assessment of Skin Cancer

Skin cancer is often asymptomatic; therefore, it is important to assess the skin frequently for changes in moles or new growths. One of the most common methods used to evaluate changes in skin lesions is the ABCD rule. Another common guideline for assessment is the seven-point checklist used for melanoma. Chart 66–11 describes both of these methods of skin evaluation. These guidelines have been found to have less than desirable di-

agnostic accuracy, especially when used for skin cancers other than melanoma; so other modalities are being evaluated for use such as total-body photography, color histogram analysis, and skin surface microscopy. The most accurate way to diagnose skin cancer is through biopsy.

Medical Management of Skin Cancer

All skin cancers should be surgically removed with the intent to cure the cancer. Basal cell and squamous cell cancer can be removed with surgical excision, chemosurgery, radiation, or curettage. Melanoma also needs surgical excision; however, it is important to go through a process of staging melanoma so that appropriate treatment can be planned. Diagnostic procedures such as chest x-ray, ultrasound, computed tomography (CT), magnetic resonance imaging (MRI), lymphoscintigraphy, and positron-emission tomography (PET) are used to detect metastasis. Melanoma is treated with deep and wide surgical excision to remove the entire tumor so that the margins are clear of melanoma cells. For stages I and II, this may be all the treatment that is necessary. For stages III and IV, when the disease has become systemic, immunotherapy, chemotherapy, or radiation therapy may be used along with regional lymph node dissection. Frequent and regular follow-up examinations should be done. An in-depth description of the diagnosis and treatment of malignant melanomas is given in Chapter 64 ☺.

Skin Infections

The skin is subject to infections caused by bacteria, viruses, or fungi. Normally the skin's flora, sebum, and immune responses help prevent infection. However, depending on the virulence of the organism and the strength of the individual's resistance, infections may occur.

Bacterial Infections

Bacteria are normally present on the skin and are not considered pathogenic. However, if they invade the skin or if the resistance of the patient is low, they can result in superficial or systemic infection. Certain organisms that are not normally on the skin also can cause infection if they invade the skin.

Cellulitis and **erysipelas** are both infections of the dermis and subcutaneous tissue layers due to a break in the skin. Cellulitis, characterized by erythema, edema, and pain, is usually caused by staphylococcus or streptococcus infections. Erysipelas is an acute, inflammatory, superficial form of cellulitis resulting from *Staphylococcus aureus* (most common) or group A beta-hemolytic streptococcus and involving the lymph system. In erysipelas, one or more well-defined lesions are bright red, tender, and warm to touch with lymphatic involvement causing a red streak along the skin leading away from the primary lesion. Associated symptoms may include fever, chills, headache, and vomiting. Due to a loss of skin integrity, patients with surgical wounds or trauma sites are susceptible to the development of these infections. The most common areas are the lower extremities, face, ears, and buttocks; however, other areas on the body can be affected as well.

Individuals with a compromised immune system have an increased susceptibility to cellulitis. In cellulitis, the skin becomes erythematous, swollen, tender, and tight over the infected area, and there is an indefinite border. There may be vesicles, blisters, or abscesses. Regional lymphadenopathy may occur in both cellulitis and erysipelas.

Diagnostic blood studies reveal mild leukocytosis with a left shift or an elevation in neutrophils, and a wound culture will identify the causative organism. Treatment involves resting the affected site with elevation if possible. Antibiotics sensitive for the causative organism are indicated. Pain medication or soaking with cool Burrow's solution can help relieve the tension and pain. Without treatment, cellulitis or erysipelas may spread to the bloodstream causing septicemia. The diagnosis, treatment, and prognosis of septicemia are described in Chapter 61 ☺.

Impetigo

Impetigo is a common skin infection caused by *Staphylococcus aureus* and/or group A beta-hemolytic streptococcus. It is a contagious, rapidly spreading infection that may occur after a minor skin injury such as an insect bite. It is usually transferred from individual to individual by direct contact and is more common in children and infants.

There are two types of impetigo: bullous and nonbullous. Bullous impetigo is characterized by a thin-roofed bulla or vesicle on an erythematous base. The bulla or vesicle collapses and drains a honey-colored crust, which dries and develops a "stuck on" appearance. Nonbullous impetigo results in vesicles or pustules on an erythematous base that also rupture, leading to a superficial honey-colored crust. Both types may develop satellite lesions. Lesions may itch or may be slightly tender.

Cultures of the lesions are not commonly done but may help in assessing antibiotic sensitivity. Treatment involves removal of crusts by soaking in warm tap water and washing with gentle antibacterial soap such as Dial or Hibiclens. Topical antibiotics such as Bactroban may be helpful, but if the infection is widespread, an oral antibiotic may be indicated. The patient should avoid contact with others and sharing towels or sheets.

Folliculitis

Folliculitis is inflammation of hair follicles that is commonly caused by *Staphylococcus* but may also be caused by trauma or *Pseudomonas aeruginosa*, which is a gram-negative organism frequently associated with nosocomial infections or infections originating in the hospital. Common causes include tight clothing, curly hair that grows back into the skin, and shaving too closely on a regular basis, leading to ingrown hairs or hairs that reenter the skin as they grow. African Americans are particularly susceptible to folliculitis due to ingrown hairs because of their curly hair. Folliculitis due to *Pseudomonas aeruginosa* is related to the use of hot tubs, whirlpools, or exposure to contaminated water. The desquamated skin cells in the water provide a good medium for bacterial growth, and free chlorine levels are decreased by the large number of people in the pool or hot tub (CDC, 2000). Folliculitis due to *Pseudomonas* is not spread from person to person but is usually due to inadequate care of the pool or tub. The *Pseudomonas* invades the hair follicle pores after superhydration of the skin by the contaminated water. Symptoms will occur 1 to 5 days after exposure to the contaminated water.

Folliculitis presents as circular papules and pustules associated with the hair follicles and surrounded by an area of erythema. They may itch and are usually located in areas of tight clothing, bathing suits, or any place where hair grows. With *Pseudomonas* folliculitis, symptoms may also include low-grade fever, sore throat, and lymphadenopathy. Folliculitis is diagnosed by history of lesion development and exposure to contaminated water, and physical exam. The lesions may be cultured to diagnose the causative organism and identify antibiotic sensitivities.

Treatment involves administration of antibiotics and other nonpharmacologic measures. If the folliculitis is limited and superficial, topical antibiotics such as Bactroban may be effective. For more involved infections, antibiotics are prescribed such as dicloxacillin when the causative agent is *Staphylococcus*, or Cipro when the causative agent is *Pseudomonas*. The affected area should be cleansed with antibacterial soap twice daily. The application of warm compresses may be helpful to soothe any itching or burning of the skin. If the folliculitis is due to ingrown hairs, the patient should be instructed to refrain from shaving until the infection is resolved. Once shaving is resumed, the patient should be instructed to shave every few days rather than daily, using a thick shaving gel to hydrate the skin. The patient should use a fresh razor blade with each shave, avoid shaving too close, and shave in the direction of hair growth. Using an electric razor instead of a straightedge blade may be helpful. Any hair tips that are beginning to grow back into the skin can be straightened out using a sterile needle or a clean soft-bristled toothbrush in a circular motion. Shaving should be followed with the use of a moisturizing lotion. Pseudomonas folliculitis is usually self-limiting.

Furuncles and Carbuncles

Furuncles and carbuncles are abscesses that develop when the infection from folliculitis becomes deeper and involves more follicles. These lesions develop when a sebaceous gland is obstructed causing a deep inflammatory reaction and infection from *Staphylococcus*. A **furuncle** is defined as a boil or a walled-off, deep, painful, firm mass that contains pus (Figure 66–7 ■). It is usually 1 to 5 centimeters in diameter. A carbuncle is a larger abscess that interconnects several hair follicles. It is about 3 to 10 centimeters in diameter and is extremely painful. A **carbuncle** will drain pus from multiple follicles, leaving crater-like nodules, and may be associated with fever and chills. Furuncles and carbuncles can occur any place where there is hair but may be more common in areas of increased friction or perspiration such as under the belt, in the groin, or in the axillae.

Furuncles and carbuncles are diagnosed by physical examination. The drainage may be cultured to help define the most effective treatment. The treatment includes incision and drainage of the abscess and warm compresses to help relieve the discomfort. Antibiotic ointments such as Bactroban or Neosporin may be used. Systemic antibiotics such as dicloxacillin or erythromycin also may be used.

Viral Infections

Viruses are intracellular pathogens that invade live cells. They contain either DNA or RNA and require host cell genetic material to replicate. They can destroy the cell during the process of entering the cell and replicating, or by causing an immune response causing cell destruction. The various types of viral infections of the skin are outlined next.

Herpes Simplex Type 1 and Type 2

Two different but similar virus types can cause herpes simplex viral infections: type 1 and type 2. Herpes simplex type 1 is found in oral lesions or cold sores, and lesions of the eye or brain that are nongenital in nature. Herpes simplex type 2 is genital and sexually transmitted. With oral–genital sexual contact, both type 1 and type 2 can present as oral. Herpes simplex is caused by a herpes virus that lives in a nerve root. It will remain asymptomatic until something triggers an outbreak. Exposure to the sun, stress, and fever are common triggers.

The lesions of herpes simplex are vesicles that are on an erythematous base and appear in groups. They are preceded by burning, stinging, or pain a few hours before the lesions erupt. The lesions may last for 2 to 6 weeks after which a second eruption may occur but be less severe. The lesions contain the live virus that can be transmitted to others through direct contact with infected lesions or genital secretions. Herpes simplex can be spread by kissing, poor hand hygiene, oral intercourse, or other sexual contact.

Diagnosis of herpes simplex is made through the evaluation of symptoms and the physical appearance of the lesions. The virus can be identified through a Tzanck smear or culture of the lesions (see the Diagnostic Tests box for skin disorders, p. 2150). The infection cannot be cured but the symptoms can be treated. Topical antiviral agents can be used to speed healing. Oral antiviral agents are available and can suppress the infection or decrease the severity if given at the onset of signs and symptoms. See the Pharmacology Summary feature (p. 2181).

Herpes Zoster

Herpes zoster is a viral infection often referred to as **shingles**. It occurs because of the reactivation of latent varicella-zoster virus, or the virus that causes chickenpox. After having the chickenpox, this virus remains dormant in the dorsal root and cranial nerve ganglia, and becomes activated usually when a person is immunocompromised due to age or some other disease process such as AIDS, Hodgkin's disease, and some cancers.

The lesions of herpes zoster are erythematous vesicles scattered over the skin surface along one or two adjacent dermatomes (Figure 66–8 ■). The vesicles occur in clusters of

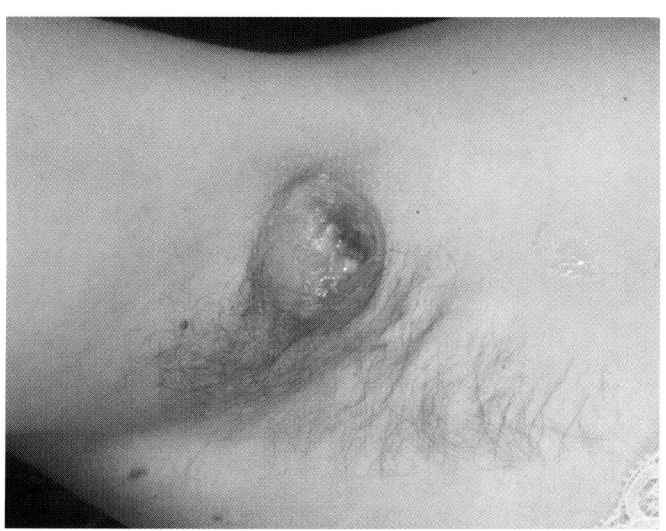

FIGURE 66–7 ■ Furuncles and carbuncles.
Source: NMSB/Custom Medical Stock Photo, Inc.

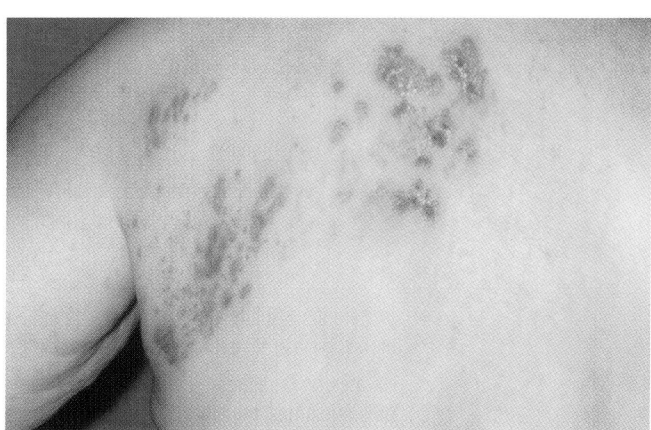

FIGURE 66–8 ■ Herpes zoster.
Source: Bart's Medical Library/Phototake NYC

various sizes and, with time, become cloudy with purulent fluid. The lesions are preceded by pain, itching, or burning in the area. The patient may also experience fever, headache, and malaise prior to the eruption of the lesions. The lesions are tender with a thoracic distribution being the most common. Lesions may also occur on the face, on the neck, and in the eye along the dermatomes of cranial nerves. A common complication is postherpetic neuralgia, which is pain for weeks, to months, and sometimes for a lifetime, after the lesions resolve. The pain is described as itching, burning, sharp, and shooting and may be severe enough to incapacitate the patient. Pain may be severe enough to cause the patient to avoid anything that touches the area, even clothing.

Herpes zoster is diagnosed by physical assessment and history. The lesions can be cultured but the virus is not easily isolated. Polymerase chain reaction (PCR), which directly identifies the virus, may be used for diagnosis. Treatment is aimed at shortening the course of herpes zoster and preventing or alleviating pain. Systemic antiviral agents are used such as acyclovir or famciclovir. See the Pharmacology Summary feature (p. 2181). Treatment can also include nerve blocks, tricyclic antidepressants, or anticonvulsants to help alleviate pain. However, there is no cure, so herpes zoster can reemerge.

Warts

Warts, or **verrucae**, are viral epidermal eruptions caused by human papillomavirus. They are benign and occur most commonly on the hands and feet. They usually are self-limiting and disappear spontaneously in months or years. However, some people prefer to be treated because the appearance of warts may be cosmetically undesirable, and warts on the sole of the foot may be painful. There are many different types of warts (Chart 66–12). The virus causing warts can be transmitted by contact when there are small breaks in the skin. Anal or genital warts are sexually transmitted. Nongenital warts are usually not precancerous; however, genital warts can increase the risk for cervical cancer (see Chapter 49).

Warts are small, hyperkeratotic flesh-colored papules that are flat or dome shaped with black dots on the surface usually seen on the extremities, especially the hands. The black dots are thrombosed capillaries. Warts can occur singly or in groups and have a rough surface. Warts are usually asymptomatic but can be tender or irritated by clothing. Plantar warts are usually tender. Plantar warts occur on weight-bearing areas where they are pushed into the skin making them appear level with the skin surface. Genital warts appear in the anogenital region and have a light-colored surface and cauliflower appearance. They are diagnosed by physical examination and history. Treatment is difficult and usually requires multiple visits to the health care provider's office. Usual treatment consists of the application of salicylic acid, use of cryotherapy or freezing of the wart, topical immunotherapy, or intralesional bleomycin. Recently, the use of duct tape to occlude the wart has been found to be effective. Duct tape is applied to the site so that the wart is completely occluded and is left in place for 2 months. The use of duct tape has been reported to be as effective as cryotherapy (Abernethy et al., 2006).

Fungal Infections

Fungi may be multicellular or monocellular but are larger than bacteria. They live on dead keratinized cells of the epidermis. Some types are considered part of the normal skin flora, but they can cause uncomfortable infections in the skin. The various fungi that affect the skin and mucus membranes are discussed next.

Candidiasis

Candidiasis is a common infection caused by the *Candida* species of fungus (Figure 66–9). This organism normally lives in the gastrointestinal tract, mouth, and vagina, and causes no harm because it is kept in control by intact skin, intact immune system, and secretions from other microorganisms that live on the skin. When the immune system is depressed, *Candida* can cause the development of opportunistic infections. It can occur with tissue damage, removal of competing organisms such as occurs with antibiotic administration, increase in glucose levels as in diabetes, or a warm, moist environment such as in skin folds. Skin candidiasis is especially prevalent in the very young, such as infants, and the very old and debilitated. The presence of predisposing factors such as wet clothing, obesity, or hyperglycemia

CHART 66–12	Types of Warts
Type	**Description**
Common wart	Flesh-toned or gray-brown, scaly papules. Usually involves the dorsal and palmar surfaces of the hands and fingers and the area around the nails.
Verruca plana (flat or juvenile wart)	Smooth, flat, or slightly elevated papule, occurring in multiples. Located on the face, backs of the hands, and shins.
Digitate or filiform warts	Lesions with multiple finger-like projections. Usually a single lesion located in the beard area, eyelids, neck, or scalp.
Plantar wart	Located on the plantar surface of the foot in pressure areas. Usually a single lesion that is tender. Often mistaken for a callus.

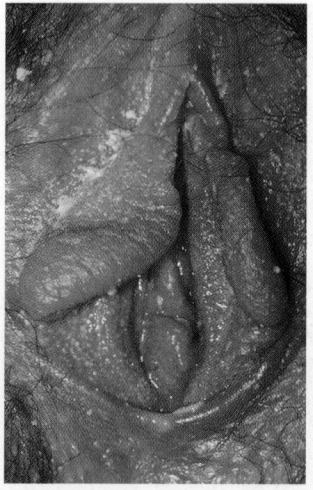

FIGURE 66–9 ■ Candidiasis.
Source: Custom Medical Stock Photo, Inc.

promotes the development of the rash. Most commonly it is seen in the perineal area, under the breasts, on the oral mucous membranes, in the vagina, and on the head of the penis. It can enter the bloodstream and infect major organs as well.

The lesions of candidiasis are pustules that peel away, leaving an erythematous, macerated patch covered by a gray-white membranous plaque with a sharply defined border. The rash appears shiny, moist, and inflamed; generally itches; and is painful. It develops satellite lesions or pustules outside the main rash area.

Candidiasis is diagnosed by history of symptoms, immunosuppression, or antibiotic use, and physical examination. A wet smear with potassium hydroxide can be used to identify the spores under the microscope (see the Diagnostic Tests box for skin disorders, p. 2150). Treatment involves the application of antifungal creams such as miconazole or ketoconazole. Cool compresses with water or Burrow's solution may help promote dryness and relief from itching and soreness. Keeping the skin dry and wearing loose, absorbent clothing help to eliminate predisposing factors. Topical agents such as Mycostatin are available in powders, vaginal suppositories, or suspensions to swish in the mouth. If the candidiasis is systemic, oral or intravenous antifungal agents can be given. See the Pharmacology Summary feature (p. 2181).

Tinea

Tinea is referred to as ringworm by the general public. However, there are many different types, and the manifestations vary with the location, duration, and pathogen involved. It commonly occurs in immunocompromised individuals but has other predisposing factors such as crowded conditions, poor hygiene, or wearing tight clothing. Tinea is diagnosed by history of signs and symptoms, and physical examination of the lesions. It is also important to do a potassium hydroxide wet mount preparation because the presence of fungal hyphae can be seen on the slide and are diagnostic (see the earlier Diagnostic Tests box on p. 2150 for skin disorders). Tinea can be treated with oral and topical antifungal agents. Usually topical agents are enough but if the infection is widespread, chronic, or the patient is immunocompromised, oral medications may be needed. See the Pharmacology Summary feature (p. 2181). The types of tinea include tinea pedis, tinea corporis, tinea capitis, and tinea cruris.

Tinea Pedis

Tinea pedis is a **dermatophyte** infection of the foot commonly referred to as "athlete's foot." It usually involves the web between the fourth and fifth toes but may occur between any of the toes and the plantar or dorsal surface of the foot. It occurs most commonly in postpubescent adolescents and adults. The infection is predisposed by the wearing of tight shoes that promote warmth and perspiration, poor hygiene, or repeated exposure to fungal organisms on locker room floors. The lesions are circular and scaly with central clearing. In the toe webs, the skin appears scaly, fissured, and macerated. The patient complains of itching and tenderness in the area.

Tinea Corporis

Tinea corporis is infection of the trunk and limbs. It occurs more commonly in warm climates and can occur at any age. The lesions are round, annular, scaly patches. They can also appear as papules, pustules, and vesicles that are inflamed and red. The lesions are multiple but uniform in appearance and are usually evident on exposed areas of the body. The lesions may be mildly pruritic but are often asymptomatic.

Tinea Cruris

Tinea cruris, also known as "jock itch," is a fungal infection of the groin and occurs almost exclusively in adult males. It is related to a warm, moist environment and obesity. The lesions are circular, beginning in the crural fold, and are erythematous or slightly brown in the center. The edge is raised, slightly scaly, and well defined. It is usually asymptomatic but may be pruritic.

Tinea Capitis

Tinea of the scalp and hair follicle is a contagious infection transmitted by personal contact. It can be spread through combs, animals, hats, blankets, telephones, and theater seats. It is more common in children and African Americans. The lesions usually appear as patchy, circular areas of hair loss. There may be visible stubs of broken off hairs within the patch of hair loss, and there may also be inflammation and scaling on the scalp. The rash may consist of fine white scales on the scalp with the appearance of dandruff or may have pustules or scabbed areas without scaling or hair loss. Tinea capitis may be associated with fever, occipital adenopathy, and leukocytosis.

▮ Infestations and Insect Bites

The skin can be invaded by insects, ticks, or parasites. Typically there is a single lesion on the skin; however, the lesion depends on the causative agent.

Bees and Wasps

The most common types of insect stings are those of honeybees followed by those of wasps. The honeybee's stinger remains embedded in the skin, whereas other species of bees and wasps leave nothing behind. Initially there is a sharp, painful sting that lasts only a few minutes. It is typically followed by mild burning and a raised white wheal with a red center that resolves in a few days.

Bee and wasp stings are dangerous only if there is a toxic systemic reaction or an allergic anaphylactic reaction. Dangerous reactions occur more commonly in adults over age 40. The symptoms of a toxic reaction include vomiting, diarrhea, headache, fever, muscle spasm, and loss of consciousness. The most severe reaction is an anaphylactic reaction, which involves itching, hives, shortness of breath, wheezing, nausea, abdominal cramps, and may lead to respiratory arrest and death. These reactions occur within minutes to hours of the sting, although allergic reactions can be delayed, occurring up to a week after the sting. Severe generalized reactions are treated with epinephrine and oral or intramuscular antihistamines, and require treatment in an emergency department. If it is a localized, nonallergic reaction, apply ice and give oral antihistamines to prevent spreading of the venom. See the Pharmacology Summary feature (p. 2181) in this chapter.

 Bee and wasp stings can result in a local reaction or a systemic anaphylactic reaction. For a local reaction, apply ice, compress the site with a tight bandage, and elevate the site. Antihistamines can be given for itching. For a systemic anaphylactic reaction, give intramuscular (IM) epinephrine; beta-2 adrenergic agonist inhalers for bronchospasm, such as albuterol; and antihistamines.

Ticks

Ticks can be bearers of diseases such as Lyme disease and Rocky Mountain spotted fever. They are very small and embed their heads in the skin to obtain blood. They can enlarge to many times their normal size while they are eating and leave toxins and microorganisms behind. Initially the tick bite leaves a local reaction involving pain, erythema, a papule, and itching. The tick should be removed totally intact if possible. If the head is left behind, a nodule may remain requiring excision. The best approach is prevention of the tick bite by wearing protective clothing, tucking the pants into the socks, and wearing closed-toed shoes.

 Ticks can be removed by grasping them as closely as possible to the skin with forceps and pulling upward. Do not squeeze the tick, or apply hot matches or nail polish. Then clean the wound with soap and water or a mild disinfectant. Instruct the patient to report any fever or unusual rash to the health care provider.

Pediculosis

Pediculosis is the infestation of the skin by lice. Lice are highly contagious parasites that survive by sucking blood. There are three types of lice: pediculosis capitis or head lice; pediculosis corporis or body lice; and pediculosis pubis or pubic lice. The female lice reproduce frequently, producing hundreds of **nits**, or eggs, that attach to the hair shaft. The nits hatch into lice that continue to reproduce. Lice secrete toxic saliva that causes trauma and releases toxins leading to itching and dermatitis. Lice are spread by personal contact through combs, brushes, sexual activity, and shared clothing and bed linens.

The major symptom of lice infestation is itching. In the scalp, the nits can be seen as yellow, oval specks attached to the hair shaft. There is extreme pruritus around the back and sides of the scalp. On the body, the lesion is a pinpoint red macule, papule, or wheal with a hemorrhagic puncture site. The center can crust and become infected. The pubic louse or "crab," as it is commonly referred to, is seen on pubic hair. Lice are diagnosed through physical examination and culture. The ova of lice will fluoresce under an ultraviolet light or Wood's lamp.

Treatment involves good hygiene and avoiding the sharing of hats, combs, or clothes. Lindane shampoo, pyrethrins, or permethrin can be used for head lice. Corticosteroid lotions or creams can be used for body lice to help relieve itching. Antihistamines are also helpful for preventing itching.

Scabies

Scabies, caused by a parasite called *Sarcoptes scabiei*, is commonly found in underdeveloped countries and areas where there is overcrowding and poor hygiene. It is contagious and transmitted by close personal contact, clothing, and bedding. The female mite tunnels into the skin, creating a burrow and depositing eggs. The eggs can sometimes be seen at the end of the burrows as tiny maculopapular dots. Intense itching that worsens at night is the primary symptom. The mite can enter the skin and travel all over the body so the itching is generalized. Lesions that are papular, vesicular, or linear occur in the wrists, web spaces of the hands, sides of the hands and feet, genital area, warm intertriginous regions, and abdomen.

Scabies is diagnosed by physical examination with identification of the mites, or burrows. Mites can be seen under a microscope after an application of mineral oil or potassium hydroxide. Treatment consists of the application of scabicide preparations such as permethrin cream or Lindane. The lotion or cream is applied to the entire skin surface including under the nails and in the umbilicus. The medication is left on for 6 hours then washed off. All contacts must be treated. Clothing and bedding should be washed and dried in a hot dryer.

■ Pressure Ulcers

Pressure ulcers are defined by the National Pressure Ulcer Advisory Panel (NPUAP) (1992) as "localized areas of tissue necrosis that develop when soft tissue is compressed between a bony prominence and an external surface for a prolonged period of time." These wounds are also referred to as decubitus ulcers or bedsores, but pressure is an important factor in their development so the term *pressure ulcer* is more appropriate. The incidence of pressure ulcer occurrence has been used to indicate quality of patient care because most are preventable. The reported incidence of pressure ulcer development in acute care settings ranges from 0.4% to 38% (Reddy, Gill, & Rochon, 2006). Pressure ulcers can occur at any age, in any socioeconomic or ethnic group, and more commonly occur on the heels and in the sacrococcygeal area. A complete description of pressure ulcer management is included in Chapter 67 🔗 .

■ Common Treatment of Skin Disorders

Common treatments for skin disorders involve creams and lotions, wet dressings, and corticosteroids. There is an old saying related to the treatment of skin disorders that "if it is dry, wet it, and if it is wet, dry it." Dry skin diseases are those that have lost water, lipids, and proteins, and they are treated with creams and lotions. Wet skin disorders are usually inflammatory disorders that are draining. When serum and exudates drain, they take lipids and proteins with them. These disorders are treated with wet compresses to suppress the inflammation and débride the wound.

Creams and lotions are used to restore the water and lipids to the skin. Creams are thicker than lotions and are more lubricating. Creams are slightly greasy in texture and best used in intertriginous areas. Ointments have a texture similar to that of petroleum jelly. They have a greater penetration in the skin than creams; therefore, they may be too occlusive for rashes with exudate or in intertriginous areas. Medications with urea or lactic acid are excellent lubricators and very effective in rehydrating the skin.

Wet dressings or compresses are used to decrease inflammation and débride draining skin lesions. Burrow's solution, acetic acid, or silver nitrate creams are often used for wet dressings. Chart 66–13 is a description of the techniques for the application of wet dressings.

Corticosteroids may be used topically or systemically. They are used because of their anti-inflammatory properties. Steroids are known to decrease the formation of several potent inflammatory mediators and to decrease vascular permeability. Topi-

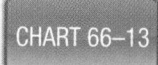

| CHART 66–13 | **Technique for Application of Wet Dressings** |

1. Use clean, soft cloth or the dressing type ordered by the health care provider. Gauze pads, wraparound gauze, cotton cloths, or clean old T-shirts may be used.

2. Fold the cloth so there are at least four to eight layers, and cut to fit an area slightly larger than the area to be treated.

3. Wet the dressings, if necessary, by immersing them in the solution, and wring them out to the point of being wet but not dripping. Solution should be room temperature.

4. Place the compresses on the affected area and smooth them out. Leave them in place for 30 minutes to 1 hour. Do not pour solution on a wet dressing to keep it wet. Remove the compress and replace it with a new one.

5. Dressings are left in place for 30 minutes. Dressings may be used two to four times a day or continuously. Discontinue use of the wet compresses when the skin becomes dry.

cal preparations are available in low, mid, and high potency. The strength needed depends on the disorder and the location on the body. Chapter 67 includes a complete description of products used to treat pressure ulcers.

Nursing Management

Nursing care for patients with skin disorders involves skills in multilevel assessment, clinical decision making, and critical thinking. Knowledge about the varied treatment strategies provides a basis for safe, quality nursing care. The nurse will need to collaborate with other members of the health care team to treat the whole patient and address the wide variety of needs the patient may have. The nursing process provides a framework for nursing management.

Assessment

The focus of nursing care is to prevent problems or recognize complications early so they can be successfully treated. The nurse must assess the patient frequently, noting changes in skin color, texture, wound size, drainage, and temperature. Analysis of the data collected during assessment will provide a basis for determining a treatment plan and assessing response to treatment. Patients with skin disorders may develop problems with hydration, fluid balance, or nutrition. Fluid loss through wounds leads to dehydration and electrolyte imbalances. The skin also provides protection against infection; so when its barrier is broken, infection becomes more likely. It is very important to assess for signs of infection both in the wound and systemically. Clinical manifestations of infection include fever, increased redness or drainage, increased pain, changes in odor or color of drainage, increased white blood cell count, and increased tissue erosion. If the infecting organism is contagious, such as occurs with *Staphylococcus,* isolation procedures may be needed (see Chapter 20).

Psychological assessment needs to be uppermost in the mind of the nurse as care is given to patients with skin disorders. The appearance of the skin affects self-esteem and body image. Skin disorders can cause the patient to withdraw from social situations. Society can be unkind to people that have scars or rashes with an unpleasant appearance. Some individuals may withdraw from the patient, fearing the disorder is contagious. Patients should be provided with an open, supportive environment in which they are comfortable voicing their concerns.

Nursing Diagnoses

The following nursing diagnoses are related to the patient with skin disorders:

- *Impaired Skin Integrity* related to epithelial skin disorder
- *Risk for Infection* related to loss of skin integrity
- *Acute Pain* related to skin disorder and exposed nerve endings
- *Fear* and *Anxiety* related to changes in health status/role functioning; situational crisis
- *Disturbed Body Image* related to disorder.

Planning

A collaborative and comprehensive approach to care will optimize the recovery process. The plan uses the assessment data to prioritize care. First, the cause must be identified and removed if possible. For example, if a rash occurs after administration of an antibiotic, the nurse must notify the health care provider and have the medication changed. Depending on the nature and extent of the skin disorder, dieticians, case managers, social workers, consultative health care providers (cardiovascular, infectious diseases, surgeons, and plastic surgeons), nursing staff, and ancillary staff should be part of the plan of care, as all play a role in the treatment.

Outcome and Evaluation Parameters

The outcome for patients with skin disorders is to heal without scarring or loss of function. The outcome goals are to promote the patient's recovery, provide support, and manage the disorder to prevent complications. The evaluation parameters include healed skin and no evidence of a systemic complication. The skin integrity will be intact and the clinical manifestations of infection will be absent. The patient will resume previous level of performing activities of daily living.

Interventions and Rationales

Interventions are based on the type of skin disorder. Once the cause has been removed the treatment begins. The involved area must have effective wound care and appropriate selection of dressing, if necessary. If the involved area is in the perineum, the nurse must make every effort to prevent urine and fecal contamination. The area needs to be kept clean and dry. Wound care, dressing, and skin barriers are described in depth in Chapter 67 .

Nutrition is essential for wound healing to occur. The nurse must assess the amount and type of food intake and intervene if lack of appetite persists. Hydration is also important for wound healing. Therefore, assessing fluid intake is essential, encouraging the patient to take in an adequate amount of fluid, and if necessary obtaining a health care provider's order for intravenous fluids.

If an infection occurs, treatment needs to be tailored to the clinical manifestations. For example, the patient may need antibiotics or antifungal medications to treat the cause. If fever is present, antipyretics and cooling measures may be necessary. Finally, if the organism is communicable, the patient will need isolation.

Evaluation

A plan for care of the patient with skin disorders should be reevaluated regularly to ensure that the plan is still effective. Any change in the patient's condition could have a negative impact on the wound healing process and the effectiveness of the plan of care. In a long-term care setting, reevaluation should be done regularly and documented. Interventions and plans of care need changing if the current treatment plan is unsuccessful. Evaluation criteria of progress would be a decrease in the size and depth of the involved area. If this healing is not occurring, then the area needs to be assessed as to why it is not, such as for infection or decreased tissue perfusion.

Collaborative Management

A collaborative approach to the management of patients with skin disorders is essential. Skin disorders have many facets that influence the patient both physically and emotionally. A multidisciplinary team that includes health care providers, nurses, psychologists/psychiatrists, occupational therapists, physical therapists, nutritionists, and pharmacists is necessary to help the patient recover. Health care provider care is discussed throughout this chapter and may include medical care as well as surgical care. In addition, psychiatric care may be needed to assist with adjustment to alterations in appearance related to the skin disorder. The occupational therapist can assist the patient to return to work or function to meet everyday needs. The physical therapist can help keep muscles strong and address the limitations of movement that may occur with scar formation. Patients with skin disorders often lose electrolytes and have increased metabolic demands that lead to weight loss and increased nutritional needs. These needs can be addressed by a nutritionist. The pharmacist will be concerned with the medications and their interactions and effectiveness. The pharmacist can assist with educating the patient about medication management and the possible side effects. The nurse's role is addressed with the specific disorders throughout this chapter. The nurse serves as the team leader to facilitate communication between members of the team and as the patient advocate.

Discharge Priorities

Most patients with dermatologic disorders are cared for at home. Discharge planning begins with the diagnosis of the condition. Patient teaching aimed at self-care is an important part of planning for discharge. The Patient Teaching & Discharge Priorities box outlines specific discharge priorities.

Life-Threatening Skin Disorders

With prompt and appropriate treatment, most skin disorders are manageable with a minimum of side effects or lifelong se-quelae. However, certain skin disorders can cause major physical disfigurement, have disfiguring sequelae, and in some instances are life threatening. These conditions begin as a skin disorder and then progress to multiple organ involvement, thereby becoming life threatening. Necrotizing fasciitis, Stevens–Johnson syndrome, and toxic epidermal necrolysis are the most common life-threatening skin disorders.

Necrotizing Fasciitis

Necrotizing fasciitis (NF), first described in 1848, is an infection of the superficial fascia or the connective tissue surrounding muscle and subcutaneous tissue, leading to fascial necrosis. It is commonly referred to as the "flesh-eating bacteria." Although relatively uncommon, it is significant because of the difficulty in recognizing it and the rapidity with which it spreads and can become fatal. This infection can occur at any age or in any location and is not specific to gender. Approximately one-half of the cases occur in young previously healthy patients (CDC, 2008). NF also occurs with a variety of conditions from simple minor injuries to complicated major surgeries or trauma. The very young and very old are at increased risk, as are those with diabetes mellitus, atherosclerosis, chronic renal failure, obesity, immunosuppression, malnutrition, illicit drug injections, alcoholism, and peripheral vascular disease. The Risk Factors box identifies those at risk for necrotizing fasciitis.

There are three types of necrotizing fasciitis (NF). Type 1 is polymicrobial and related to mixed aerobic or anaerobic bac-

---

RISK FACTORS for Necrotizing Fasciitis

Age: very young and very old

Individuals with throat or skin infections

Individuals with chronic illnesses such as:
- Cancer
- Diabetes
- Renal failure on dialysis.

People using steroids

Obesity

Poor nutrition or malnutrition

Immunosupression

Needle puncture site with illicit drug use

Frostbite

Chronic venous leg ulcers

Open bone fractures

Insect bites

Childbirth

Surgical wounds

Trauma

AIDS

Major burns

Prolonged antibiotic therapy

Alcoholics

Peripheral vascular disease

Multiple myeloma

Hypertension

Skin biopsy

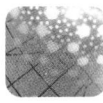

PATIENT TEACHING & DISCHARGE PRIORITIES for Skin Disorders

Need	Teaching
Wound Care	Evaluate for signs of infection such as increased redness, drainage, fever, or foul odor.
Patient/family	Perform cleaning of wounds and dressing changes as ordered by the health care provider.
	Perform hand hygiene and wear gloves while performing dressing changes.
	Avoid scratching healed areas.
	Keep unaffected skin clean and well hydrated.
	Avoid exposure to the sun.
	Wear loose-fitting, soft clothing.
Family/support system	Assess knowledge of illness: • Teach actions to decrease risk of infection. • Teach signs and symptoms that should be reported to the health care provider.
	Assess compliance with treatment: • Provide written instructions. • Assess the patient/family's abilities to provide care at home.
Setting	Assess effectiveness of available support systems.
	Assess discharge placement needs: • Home • Rehabilitation facility • Extended care facility.
	Assess home environment for need for assistive devices and safety.
	Assess need for professional home health needs.
	Assess abilities to obtain food, medications, and supplies.
Nutrition	Maintain a high-calorie, high-protein, well-balanced diet.
Patient/family	Include vitamin C, iron, and zinc in the diet.
Family/support system	Assess appetite and weight loss.
Setting	Avoid foods that cause hypersensitivity reactions.
	Teach foods to include and avoid in the diet.
	Assess financial resources.
Psychological Adjustment	Encourage verbalizations of feelings and fears.
Patient/family	Encourage positive reinforcement rather than rejection from the family.
Setting	Answer questions honestly.
	Encourage participation in support groups for the patient's specific disorder.
Pruritus	Avoid things that are irritating or intensify itching such as excessive bathing.
Patient/ family	Application of cold or emollient lotion to rehydrate the skin.
Setting	Recommend baths with cornstarch or oatmeal.
	Proper application and use of prescribed medications.
	Wear nonrestrictive, light clothing.
	Assess temperature and humidity.
Pain	Assess pain level and report increases in pain.
Patient/family	Assess effectiveness of pain medications.
Setting	Assess patient/family knowledge of pain medication and side effects.
	Assess environment for safety.

teria such as *Clostridium, Pseudomonas aeruginosa, Staphylococcus aureus, Bacteroides fragilis, Escherichia coli,* and *Klebsiella pneumoniae.* Type 2 is monomicrobial and caused by group A streptococci. Type 3 is caused by gas gangrene or clostridial myonecrosis. A variant of type 1 NF is caused by saltwater contaminated with *Vibrio* species. Sometimes group A streptococci are found in combination with *Staphylococcus aureus* or *Staphylococcus epidermidis* in type 2. Group A streptococci are normally found in the throat and on the skin. These organisms can be transmitted through coughing or sneezing, or through direct contact with secretions. Transmission can also occur through contact with infected wounds or sores on the skin. Entry through the skin can occur when there is a surgical wound or a small cut. Contaminated hands can carry the organism as well.

Pathophysiology of Necrotizing Fasciitis

Once a break in the skin occurs and is contaminated, the organisms spread from the subcutaneous tissue along the superficial and deep fascia, facilitated by bacterial enzymes and toxins, which continue to break down tissue. The infection causes:

- Tissue ischemia
- Superficial nerve damage
- Vascular thrombosis and occlusion
- Tissue liquification necrosis
- Septicemia when systemic toxicity occurs.

Certain strains of NF cause the development of streptococcal pyrogenic exotoxins A, B, and C. These exotoxins, along with streptococcal superantigen, stimulate the release of cytokines and produce hypotension (CDC, 2008). This leads to occlusion and interruption of vessels that supply the skin. The ischemia produces bullae formation, ulceration, and necrosis of the skin.

Clinical Manifestations of Necrotizing Fasciitis

Necrotizing fasciitis (NF) is difficult to diagnose because the symptoms are many and varied. One way of tracking the course of the disease is through the progression of the symptoms and laboratory findings. The symptoms usually begin about 1 week after the initiating event and can be divided into three stages: early, advanced, and critical (Chart 66–14). The early symptoms begin in the first 24 to 48 hours. The most common parts of the body affected include the extremities, the perineum, and the truncal areas, but NF can be found anywhere on the body (Hasham, Matteucci, Stanley, & Hart, 2005). The wound site looks essentially normal with wound margins not obvious, but the patient experiences flu-like symptoms, localized pain, erythema, and swelling. It is easy to misdiagnose the infection at this stage because the symptoms are vague and fit with many other problems. The hallmark sign is pain beyond what would be expected for the extent of the injury.

The second stage, known as the advanced stage, occurs within 2 to 4 days. During this phase, the early symptoms worsen. The skin becomes swollen and tight, a dusky blue color

develops, and fluid-filled blisters or bullae develop. This occurs because of ischemia and progressive thrombosis (Wong & Wang, 2005). The texture of the wound has been described as "wet wood." The skin becomes thin and hyperesthetic or anesthetic because of destruction to cutaneous nerves. This lack of sensation is a sign that the patient is not experiencing cellulitis.

The third, or critical, stage occurs within 4 to 5 days. During this stage, the bluish-colored areas become gangrenous. The skin begins to slough, and septic shock can occur leading to hypotension, high fever, delirium, loss of consciousness, pain, liver failure, renal failure, and eventually death. Without systemic complications the mortality rate for NF can be as high as 25%, although it increases to as high as 76% when sepsis and renal failure occur (Wong & Wang, 2005). Figure 66–10 ■ is an example of advanced necrotizing fasciitis.

Diagnosis of Necrotizing Fasciitis

Necrotizing fasciitis should be diagnosed early so that treatment can begin as soon as possible. The chance of the patient's surviving is better with an early diagnosis. Diagnosis is made based on

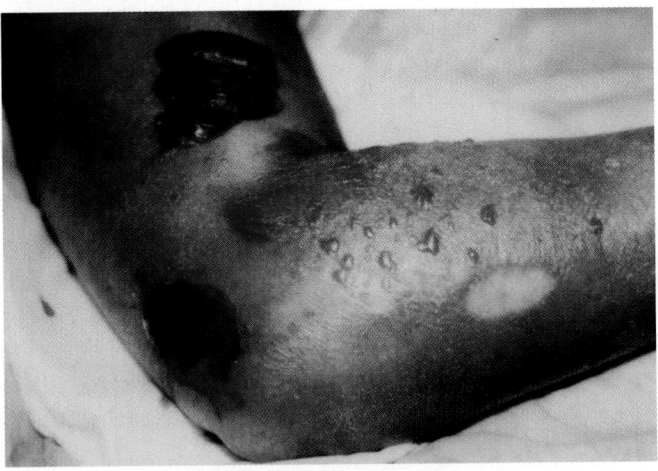

FIGURE 66–10 ■ Advanced necrotizing fasciitis.
Source: Courtesy of Donals E. Lon, B. Demers, A. E. Simor, H. Vellend, P. N. Schlievert, S. Byrne, F. Jamieson, S. Walmsely. *CID* 1:792-800, (1993)

CHART 66–14	Signs and Symptoms of Necrotizing Fasciitis

Early Stage First 24–48 hours	Advanced Stage 2nd–4th Day	Critical Stage 4th–5th Day
Flu-like symptoms such as fever, chills, myalgia, nausea, vomiting, and diarrhea. Abrupt localized pain beyond what would be expected. Patchy discoloration of skin that is violaceous to erythematous without defined borders. Nonpitting edema outside the area of discoloration. Skin is essentially normal in appearance.	Skin swollen and tight and erythema is noted. Area becomes dusky blue in color. Blisters or bullae filled with purplish, foul-smelling, thin, watery fluid. Skin has paper-like appearance. There may be palpable crepitation due to the presence of gas. Spread of the infection—increasing wound size. Increased leukocytes. Decreased sodium.	Skin sloughs. Gangrene develops. Hypotension. Delirium. Loss of consciousness. Liver failure. Renal failure. Fever. Acute respiratory distress syndrome (ARDS). Coagulopathy. Fascia appears gray to grayish green. Elevated heart rate. Tissue necrosis.

signs and symptoms and laboratory testing. The problem is that often it is difficult to make a differential diagnosis because the signs and symptoms of NF are similar to those of other conditions. It is generally believed that if the following symptoms are present, NF should be suspected:

- Rapid progression of wound size
- Poor response to therapeutic interventions
- Blistering necrosis
- Cyanosis
- Extreme local tenderness
- High temperature
- Tachycardia
- Hypotension
- Altered level of consciousness.

Laboratory findings include leukocytosis with an elevated number of neutrophils and bands. The creatine phosphokinase (CPK) levels will be elevated due to muscle damage. If there is renal damage, the blood urea nitrogen (BUN) and creatinine will be elevated. There may also be some electrolyte imbalances and anemia. However, a complete blood count, electrolyte levels, a sedimentation rate, and C-reactive protein level may look similar to those of cellulitis. Blood and wound cultures should demonstrate the presence of group A streptococcus or other organisms known to be involved in the development of necrotiz-

ing fasciitis. Computed tomography (CT) and magnetic resonance imaging (MRI) scans can help to define the extent of the fasciitis and may show gas in the subcutaneous tissues produced by the bacteria and deep fascia thickening. The Diagnostic Tests box presents the laboratory and diagnostic tests and abnormalities associated with necrotizing fasciitis. Surgeons may prefer to biopsy or may take the patient to surgery to assess the fascia directly. When directly assessed, there will be lack of bleeding in the fascia and the presence of foul-smelling pus (Wong & Wang, 2005).

Medical Management of Necrotizing Fasciitis

The best chance for survival occurs with early diagnosis and beginning treatment as soon as possible. Because of the complexity of the disease, a team approach is essential when managing the patient. Typically patients are placed in a surgical intensive care unit to monitor hemodynamic factors and provide frequent wound care. The treatment for necrotizing fasciitis is three pronged: antibiotics, surgical débridement, and supportive care. Treatment begins with the early administration of broad-spectrum antibiotics and intensive surgical débridement. Broad-spectrum antibiotics are started initially; however, once the culture results have returned, an antibiotic that targets the organism is preferred. The most common antibiotic is benzylpenicillin, given intravenously in large doses. Penicillin by itself may not be successful, so the addition of clinidamycin is helpful in producing a favorable outcome. Metronidazole and third-generation cephalosporin

DIAGNOSTIC TESTS for Necrotizing Fasciitis

Test	Expected Abnormality	Rationale for Abnormality
White blood count (WBC) with differential	Elevated with an elevated number of bands signifying left shift.	Due to acute infectious process.
Creatine phosphokinase (CPK)	Elevated.	Released from muscle cells when damaged.
Blood urea nitrogen (BUN) and creatinine	Elevated.	Will occur if there is renal damage. Also some antibiotics can affect renal function.
Red blood count (RBC), hemoglobin, hematocrit	Decreased.	Demonstrates anemia due to bleeding and possibly renal failure.
Blood and wound cultures	Growth of causative organism: usually group A streptococcus.	Demonstrates organisms involved.
Serum sodium	Decreased.	Due to wound infection and leakage.
Computed tomography (CT) and magnetic resonance imaging (MRI)	Demonstrates extent of fasciitis and gas in subcutaneous tissues.	Can show breakdown of tissue. Organisms responsible produce gas. Will assist in directing rapid surgical débridement.
T2-weighted MRI	Shows well-defined regions of high signal intensity in the deep tissues.	Will assist in directing rapid surgical débridement.
Excisional deep skin biopsy / Cultures of the affected tissue / Gram staining of the exudates	Helpful in diagnosing and identifying the causative organisms. May provide a clue as to whether a type 1 or type 2 infection is present.	The type influences the antibiotic therapy.
Histologic findings	A dense infiltration of neutrophils may be observed in deeper parts of the subcutaneous tissue and fascia. Subcutaneous fat necrosis and vasculitis are also evident. Eccrine glands and ducts may be necrotic. Alcian blue or periodic acid-Schiff (PAS) staining with diastase may show clusters of bacteria and fungi.	Sections show superficial fascial necrosis with blood vessels occluded by thrombi.

antibiotics have also been useful. Some health care providers may opt to use intravenous immunoglobulin (IVIG) with severe streptococcal infections associated with NF. The use of intravenous immunoglobulin may be a useful adjunct treatment to increase the immune response.

Early surgical débridement is necessary to remove all necrotic tissue and prevent the spread of the infection. Initially the patient is taken to surgery as often as every 12 to 24 hours, where débridement is done until clear margins are obtained. This regimen is continued until tissue necrosis stops and fresh viable tissue begins to grow. It may be necessary surgically to excise organs and amputate involved limbs to remove irreversible necrosis and gangrene or because of overwhelming toxicity. Prompt surgery increases the likelihood of survival.

Skin grafting is typically required to close the full-thickness injuries. Chapter 68 🔗 has a complete description of the various skin grafting techniques.

Supportive therapies may include high-calorie diet, hyperbaric oxygen therapy, and the application of a vacuum assisted closure device. Because patients with necrotizing fasciitis are breaking down tissue and have a high metabolic state, extra calories are required. A description of hypermetabolic state is included in Chapter 68 🔗.

A vacuum assisted closure device (wound VAC) is typically applied to the wound after débridement when clear edges have been obtained. This device does three things to improve wound healing:

- It creates a negative pressure in the wound by applying suction. The suction drains interstitial edema fluid, thus decreasing pressure on capillaries and improving perfusion.
- The negative pressure also provides a mechanical stretch/distortion of the cells in the wound bed, which stimulates production of granulation tissue.
- The suction removes stagnant fluid in the wound, thus decreasing the bacterial burden in the healing wound bed.

Vacuum assisted closure is discussed in detail in Chapter 67 🔗.

Streptococcal toxic shock syndrome, which is characterized by hypotension and multiorgan failure, can lead to death. Therefore, fluid resuscitation and hemodynamic monitoring are required. The management of shock is discussed in detail in Chapter 61 🔗.

▪ Nursing Management

Nursing care for patients with necrotizing fasciitis requires excellent assessment, clinical decision making, and critical thinking skills. Nurses need to be aware of the possibility of necrotizing fasciitis, even with the smallest of traumatic injuries. It is important to recognize those patients at risk (see the Risk Factors box for necrotizing fasciitis, p. 2170) and to alert the health care provider when warranted.

The usual infection control precautions are important, such as hand hygiene to prevent the chances of spreading the bacteria. The patient should be in a private room and under contact isolation (see Chapter 20 🔗). It is important to assess the patient's status regularly. The nurse should check vital signs, oxy-

gen saturations, intake and output, and laboratory values frequently and report abnormalities to the health care provider. The possibility of septic shock or fluid imbalances should be monitored. The wound is assessed for expansion of the erythema, changes in edema, changes in color, and drainage.

Pain is an important issue in the patient with necrotizing fasciitis. Pain may be difficult to monitor because it often seems out of proportion to the patient's injury. It is important to assess the pain because it is an indication of the pathologic process. Therefore, changes in pain need to be reported to the health care provider, and pain should be treated accordingly. The dressing changes are long, complex, and very painful, requiring premedication. The usual pain medication is morphine sulfate; however, alternative therapies such as imagery and music therapy may be helpful as well. The nurse is responsible for monitoring the administration of medications and assessing for side effects or signs of toxicity. Chapter 15 🔗 provides a complete description of the pain management protocol.

 **CRITICAL ALERT** *Remember that pain is a subjective experience and may be more or less than is typical for other patients with a similar diagnosis. Assess pain carefully using a pain scale.*

Nutritional needs of the patient are a concern to promote wound healing. Because of the infection, pain, and wound healing, the patient's calorie needs are increased. The patient with necrotizing fasciitis requires two to three times the normal amounts of calories and protein for healing. Supplements may also be required for wound healing such as vitamin C, vitamin E, and iron. The nutritionist should be consulted, and if the patient can eat, frequent, high-calorie meals are indicated. To increase compliance with nutritional intake, the patient's likes, dislikes, and cultural needs must be considered. If the patient is not able to eat, total parenteral nutrition (TPN) or enteral feeding may be indicated. The nurse also must monitor the administration of parenteral or enteral nutrition.

A fluid balance chart is needed to keep track of urine output and intravenous and oral intake. The patient should be assessed for signs of fluid imbalance such as crackles in the lungs, edema in dependent areas, or decreased urine output. Any abnormalities should be reported to the health care provider.

Wound care of the affected skin is important. The patient's wounds are assessed frequently for any changes such as in drainage, color, odor, or increasing size. Unaffected skin is assessed as well. Evaluation of pressure areas and maintenance of skin integrity in unaffected skin are essential parts of the assessment. The patient is repositioned at least every 2 hours and assessed for signs of skin breakdown. Wound care and dressing changes are complicated procedures requiring planning and the support of the patient. Strict sterile technique is used.

The patient with necrotizing fasciitis has many psychological needs. There is frequently a long hospital stay followed by months of rehabilitation. The interruption in skin integrity leads to an altered body image, threatens the patient's self-esteem, and may lead to extreme anxiety and grief. The physical appearance, along with the fact that the patient is often in isolation, may affect the number of visitors, leading to depression and social isolation. The prolonged illness may have a financial impact, especially if the patient is the main wage earner of the family. Additionally, disabilities after recovery may keep the patient from returning to work. The patient should be encouraged to voice concerns and feelings, and a mental health specialist should be consulted.

Application of the nursing process will facilitate a comprehensive, holistic approach to the patient. The assessment data, which include sample questions specific to skin disorders, are found in the Nursing Process: Patient Care Plan feature. This care plan applies the nursing process to the relevant nursing diagnoses and provides a comprehensive care plan for the patient with necrotizing fasciitis.

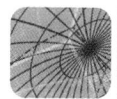 **NURSING PROCESS: Patient Care Plan for Necrotizing Fasciitis**

Assessment of Skin Integrity

Subjective Data:
Where are the lesions located?
Are there any associated symptoms?
How long have the lesions been present?
Is there any drainage? If so, what color and consistency?
Do you have any chronic health problems?
Has there been any recent exposure to drugs, environmental or occupational toxins, or people with similar skin conditions?

Objective Data:
Skin color
Presence of drainage: color, consistency, odor
Pattern of the lesions
Skin temperature around the lesions

Nursing Assessment and Diagnoses	Outcomes and Evaluation Parameters	Planning and Interventions with *Rationales*
Nursing Diagnosis: *Impaired Skin Integrity* related to skin lesions	**Outcomes:** No signs of infection or worsening of infection. *Evaluation Parameters:* Skin will not have drainage, or drainage will not be yellow or green with a foul odor. Skin color will be pink; no blue or gray. Wound will show signs of healing.	**Interventions and *Rationales:*** Assess skin for drainage, warmth, and redness. *Indicates presence of infection.* Assess skin lesions for changes. *Indicates progression or healing of skin disorder.* Implement an individualized treatment plan for site of skin impairment. Use aseptic technique. *Treatment should be implemented according to patient needs and to prevent infection.* Remove or control impediments to wound healing. Reposition every 2 hours, and assess for signs of skin breakdown. *Wound healing can be delayed if impediments are not relieved.* Teach patient care of skin wounds. *It is important for the patient to understand and comply with care.* Patient should be placed in a private room with contact isolation. *To decrease the chance of infection.*

Assessment of Fluid Status

Subjective Data:
Are you having any difficulty breathing?
Do you have edema?
Do you have any chronic health problems?

Objective Data:
Lung sounds
Presence of edema in ankles, in dependent areas, or around lesions
Vital signs

Nursing Assessment and Diagnoses	Outcomes and Evaluation Parameters	Planning and Interventions with *Rationales*
Nursing Diagnosis: *Risk for Imbalanced Fluid Volume* related to fluid loss	**Outcome:** Adequate fluid balance. *Evaluation Parameters:* Lung sounds will be clear with a normal respiratory rate. Urine output will be within 1,000 milliliters of intake. Extremities and wounds will not be edematous. Laboratory values, such as electrolytes, will be within normal range.	**Interventions and *Rationales:*** Assess the patient's preoperative status. *Awareness of preexisting fluid overload or dehydration can prevent fluid problems postoperatively.* Monitor vital signs. *Vital signs, such as increased pulse or respiration, can indicate fluid volume overload or dehydration.* Monitor intake and output of fluids. *Can help monitor fluid status. Intake should be within 1,000 milliliters of output for 24 hours.* Assess for signs of edema in dependent areas or around lesions. Weigh patient at least weekly. Monitor fluid status. *Can indicate fluid retention.* Assess electrolyte levels. *Electrolytes can be altered with fluid overload or dehydration and can cause problems.*

(continued)

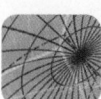

NURSING PROCESS: Patient Care Plan for Necrotizing Fasciitis—*Continued*

Assessment of Physical Mobility

Subjective Data:
How active are you physically?
Has your activity level changed with your skin problems? How?
What limits your activity?

Objective Data:
Assess range of motion of all extremities.
Assess patient's strength.
Assess oxygen saturation levels.

Nursing Assessment and Diagnoses	Outcomes and Evaluation Parameters	Planning and Interventions with *Rationales*
Nursing Diagnosis: *Impaired Physical Mobility* related to discomfort	**Outcome:** Patient is mobile and independent. ***Evaluation Parameters:*** Physical activity is increased as the patient's condition allows. Patient verbalizes a feeling of increased strength and ability to move. Patient is able to perform activities of daily living.	**Interventions and *Rationales:*** Assess mobility skills. *Provides a baseline and makes nurse aware of opportunities for improvement.* Monitor patient's ability to tolerate activity. *Provides information about problems that might inhibit activity.* Treat pain before activity. *Pain limits mobility.* If patient is immobile, perform passive range of motion or any activity that is not contraindicated. *Helps to maintain joint mobility and increase circulation.* Help patient to achieve mobility and independence as soon as possible. *Early mobilization can help prevent complications related to immobility.*

Assessment of Pain

Subjective Data:
Using a scale of 1–10, with 1 being very little pain and 10 being the worst imaginable pain, what is your pain level?
What is your experience with pain?
Do you routinely take pain medication at home? If so, how much and what kind? What kind of pain do you experience at home?
Are you allergic to any pain medication?
Do you have any cultural or religious beliefs that impact your pain control?
Where is your pain located?
Can you describe what type of pain you are having?
Does your pain radiate or stay in one place?
Is your pain constant or intermittent?
What brings your pain on or relieves it?

Objective Data:
Grimacing with movement
Restlessness and irritability
Taut facial expression
Watch how the patient moves
Vital signs
Check skin for diaphoresis and pallor
Clenched teeth

Nursing Assessment and Diagnoses	Outcomes and Evaluation Parameters	Planning and Interventions with *Rationales*
Nursing Diagnosis: *Acute Pain* related to exposed nerve endings	**Outcome:** Adequate pain control. ***Evaluation Parameters:*** Patient reports pain before it becomes unbearable. Patient reports pain relief. Pain decreases, requiring less medication. Patient is able to perform activities without pain.	**Interventions and *Rationales:*** Assess severity and quality of pain frequently. *Helps to determine cause and presence of pain so it can be relieved.* Explore need for medications to relieve pain. *Pharmacologic interventions should be used when needed to relieve pain.* Discuss patient's fears of unrelieved pain, overdose, or addiction. *The patient's concerns may prevent reporting of pain.* Review patient records to determine effectiveness of medications for pain relief. *Systematic tracking of pain relief will help identify and improve problems with pain management.* Support the patient's use of nonpharmacologic interventions for pain relief. *Nonpharmacologic interventions can be effective as a supplement to pharmacologic interventions.* Plan care and activities around periods of pain. *Pain diminishes ability to be active.*

Assessment of Body Image Disturbance

Subjective Data:
How has your lifestyle changed since the skin disorder started?
Do you have negative feelings about your body or your appearance?
Do you fear rejection by others?

Objective Data:
Is there an actual change in the appearance of the patient?
Is the patient hiding from or avoiding others?

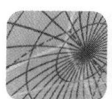

NURSING PROCESS: Patient Care Plan for Necrotizing Fasciitis—*Continued*

Nursing Assessment and Diagnoses	Outcomes and Evaluation Parameters	Planning and Interventions with *Rationales*
Nursing Diagnosis: *Disturbed Body Image* related to illness	**Outcome:** Patient accepts or is satisfied with body image. ***Evaluation Parameters:*** Patient states acceptance of body changes. Patient returns to previous social involvement.	**Interventions and *Rationales:*** Acknowledge the patient's feelings related to changes in body image. *Changes in body image may lead to a variety of reactions. Patients should feel supported and able to express their feelings.* Allow the patient to explore the changes gradually. *Patient should be able to explore the changes when ready.* Encourage the patient to be involved in the decision making and accept inadequacies and strengths. *When patients have a say in their care, they are more likely to adapt to changes.* Assess the influence of cultural beliefs, norms, and perceptions on body image. *The patient's body image is influenced by culture and the norms of that social context.*

Assessment of Sleep Pattern

Subjective Data:
How are you sleeping?
Do you have trouble falling asleep?
Do you wake up in the middle of the night?
What keeps you from sleeping?
What are your bedtime rituals?

Objective Data:
Observe patient sleeping.
Assess environment for noises, temperature, lighting, or disturbances.

Nursing Assessment and Diagnoses	Outcomes and Evaluation Parameters	Planning and Interventions with *Rationales*
Nursing Diagnosis: *Readiness for Enhanced Sleep* related to pain and anxiety	**Outcomes:** Patient falls asleep and sleeps without interruption. ***Evaluation Parameters:*** Patient sleeps throughout night. Patient verbalizes a feeling of not being fatigued.	**Interventions and *Rationales:*** Assess patient's sleep patterns and bedtime rituals. Sleep patterns are individual. *Sleep can be enhanced by adhering to usual rituals when possible.* Determine current level of anxiety or pain. *Anxiety and pain prevent sleep.* Provide measures before bedtime to assist with sleep. *Simple interventions such as warm milk or a back massage can help induce sleep.* Keep environment quiet and interruptions at a minimum. *Noise can interfere with sleep.* Plan for long periods of uninterrupted sleep. Discourage long naps during the day. *Can interfere with prolonged good sleep.*

Assessment of Ineffective Protection

Subjective Data:
Is there pain in the lesions or skin, and has it changed?
Has the appearance of the skin lesions changed?
How have you been caring for the skin lesions?
What has your diet been like?
Have you been sleeping well?
Have you been following the prescribed treatment such as medications and wound care?

Objective Data:
Inspect skin lesions for redness, warmth, and drainage
Vital signs
Signs of infections other than on the skin
Age

Nursing Assessment and Diagnoses	Outcomes and Evaluation Parameters	Planning and Interventions with *Rationales*
Nursing Diagnosis: *Ineffective Protection* related to interrupted skin integrity	**Outcome:** Patient is free of any new signs of infection. ***Evaluation Parameters:*** Patient verbalizes precautions to prevent infection. Patient eats a well-balanced diet. Patient performs proper wound care.	**Interventions and *Rationales:*** Monitor vital signs. *Vital signs can demonstrate signs of infection.* Assess nutritional status. *Nutrition is important for supporting the immune system.* Assess for signs of new or worsening infection. *Infection should be identified early, and treatment initiated to decrease the chances of mortality or complications.* Implement interventions to prevent the spread of infection. *Infection is easily spread from one patient to another or one site to another if infection control measures are not observed.* Teach the patient and family about precautions to take to avoid infection. *Reduce the risk of infection from visitors.*

(continued)

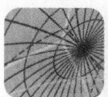

NURSING PROCESS: Patient Care Plan for Necrotizing Fasciitis—*Continued*

Assessment of Nutrition

Subjective Data:
How is your appetite?
Do you have sores in your mouth?
What kinds of foods are you eating?
What kinds of foods do you like or dislike?
Are there any cultural practices that would influence your diet?

Objective Data:
Assess nutritional status.
Assess 24-hour food intake.
Assess for sores in the mouth.

Nursing Assessment and Diagnoses	Outcomes and Evaluation Parameters	Planning and Interventions with *Rationales*
Nursing Diagnosis: *Imbalanced Nutrition: Less than Body Requirements*	**Outcome:** Patient will have an adequate intake to meet the body's needs for repair. **Evaluation Parameters:** Patient eats most of the food served. Weight will be improved or maintained at a healthy level.	**Interventions and *Rationales:*** Monitor food intake. *Food intake needs to be adequate for healing.* Serve small amounts of high-calorie, high-protein food every 2 hours. *Patient is more likely to eat small amounts more frequently than large amounts less often.* Provide a well-balanced diet with foods the patient likes. *Patient will be more likely to eat.* Consult with a dietician. Assess the need for parenteral or enteral feedings. *If the patient is unable to eat enough food orally to keep up with the body's demands, other avenues may need to be explored and utilized.*

Assessment of Social Isolation

Subjective Data:
Is there anyone depending on you for care at home?
Are you the breadwinner for the family?
Can your loved ones visit you?

Objective Data:
Loved ones are visiting.

Nursing Assessment and Diagnoses	Outcomes and Evaluation Parameters	Planning and Interventions with *Rationales*
Nursing Diagnosis: *Social Isolation* due to prolonged illness	**Outcomes:** Patient will have a plan for care of others who are dependent. Patient will have plan for care of self at home. **Evaluation Parameter:** Patient returns to previous life roles.	**Intervention and *Rationale:*** Consult social worker or case manager. *Allows for plans to be made for needed care and decreased anxiety in patient.*

Collaborative Management

The care for a patient with necrotizing fasciitis is multidimensional and multidisciplinary, requiring the nurse to serve as the team coordinator and patient advocate. The goals are to assure that the patient receives high-quality care and has an understanding about the disease process and treatment. These patients require intensive nursing and medical management, along with the expertise of the physical and occupational therapists, psychologists/psychiatrists, pharmacists, and nutritionists. To ensure complete closure and prevention of infection, wound care is managed by both the nurses and the health care providers. The initial medical team needs to include a surgeon, an infectious disease specialist, a pathologist, and a microbiologist. The remainder of the team members depends on the severity and location of the wound and may include an urologist; a specialist in plastic surgery; or an ear, nose, and throat (ENT) surgeon in cases of infections of the cervical area. The members of the nursing team depend on the severity of the wound and the hemodynamic stability of the patient. Nurses knowledgeable in wound care are essential, and critical care nurses may be needed to monitor and maintain the hemodynamic parameters.

As the wound heals, the scar formation causes contracture formation, which, depending on the site of the wound, may decrease joint range of motion. Physical therapy is initiated as soon as possible and continues after hospital discharge to maintain and increase range of motion in the joints. When contracture formation is severe, the surgeon needs to release the contractures surgically.

The pharmacist assists the medical team with pain and infection control management. The infection must be controlled to prevent further tissue and organ loss. The antibiotics are monitored by the nurses, health care providers, and pharmacists to ensure sensitivity to the organisms. Pain management is a major concern for this patient. During dressing changes, the use of conscious sedation is frequently required due to the severity of the pain. Additionally, ongoing pain management between the dressing changes is necessary to ensure patient comfort. Because of the longevity of the hospitalization, the pain management protocols require frequent adjustment. The pharmacist is an essential part of this process.

The disabilities experienced by the patient may lead to changes in lifestyle and occupation. Often the patient is unable to return to the previous profession due to physical limitations. Family dynamics and role function often change at least temporarily and perhaps permanently depending on the degree of disability. The occupational therapist, social worker, and psychologist/psychiatrist all assist the patient with physical and psychological adjustments after discharge.

Finally, the nutritionist must develop a comprehensive plan for nutrition for enhancing wound healing, regaining strength, and preventing complications. The dietician works with the health care team from the time of admission through discharge to ensure proper nutritional support.

Health Promotion

Because necrotizing fasciitis can occur at any age or location and is not specific to gender, it is imperative to educate patients, families, and the general public about the risk factors (see the earlier Risk Factors box for necrotizing fasciitis, p. 2170) and how to avoid them. As stated earlier, about one-half of the cases occur in young previously healthy patients; therefore, avoiding behaviors such as skin popping (Chapter 65 😊) will decrease the risk. If the individual has already contracted the disease once, education needs to include avoiding being reexposed. Patients need to be told to seek medical help for wounds that are not healing or appear infected.

Stevens–Johnson Syndrome

Stevens–Johnson syndrome (SJS) is a severe, acute, self-limiting skin reaction to infection or certain medications. It affects the epidermal layer of the skin and mucous membranes. SJS usually begins with flu-like symptoms or symptoms of an upper respiratory infection and progresses to mucosal erosions and erythematous skin macules that blister and cause denudation or skin detachment. The incidence is approximately 4 to 7 cases per million inhabitants per year, and SJS occurs most commonly in children and young adults (Khalili & Bahna, 2006).

Etiology of Stevens–Johnson Syndrome

The cause of Stevens–Johnson syndrome (SJS) is most commonly an adverse reaction to medication or an infection. In children the cause is usually infection, whereas in adults the cause is typically drugs or malignancy (Hockett, 2004). The most common medications leading to SJS are sulfonamides, beta-lactam antibiotics, penicillin, anticonvulsants, some nonsteroidal anti-inflammatory medications, and allopurinol. The most common infections implicated as a cause include herpes simplex virus and *Mycoplasma pneumoniae*. HIV infection, cancer, or the presence of an autoimmune disorder increases the risk of developing SJS. Symptoms generally appear within 14 days of exposure to the causative agent (Hockett, 2004).

The triggering mechanism for SJS is unclear, but the pathophysiology is immunologic with a cell-mediated cytotoxic reaction against epidermal cells. Cell destruction is thought to be caused by a cytokine such as tumor necrosis factor (Hockett, 2004; Khalili & Bahna, 2006). Immune complexes made up of the drug metabolites and antibodies develop and become trapped in the microvasculature of the skin (Letko et al., 2005). They are attacked by lymphocytes and macrophages, leading to destruction and necrosis of the epidermis (Tsang, Tsang, & Wong, 2004).

Diagnosis and Clinical Manifestations of Stevens–Johnson Syndrome

The diagnostic criteria of SJS are defined differently by different authors. There is no universally accepted definition. However, SJS generally begins with flu-like symptoms such as headache, rhinorrhea, cough, and body aches. Target skin lesions are present and are described as having a bright-pink or red inner ring, a ring of lighter pink, and then a ring of dark pink. These lesions are concentric macular exanthemas that focus on the face, neck, and extremities, which then become blisters that grow together and break open such as might be seen in burns (Hockett, 2004). The lesions are found on less than 20% of body surface area in the first 48 hours and result in skin detachment (Letko et al., 2005). SJS is diagnosed by skin biopsy and immunofluorescent studies that demonstrate the presence of immunoglobulin M (IgM) and C3 deposits in the vascular walls. Letko et al. (2005) defined SJS by the following: (1) involvement of at least two mucous membranes, (2) presence of target lesions with sudden epidermal detachment, (3) fever, (4) skin biopsy compatible with erythema multiforme and Stevens–Johnson syndrome, (5) positive Nikolsky's sign, and (6) involvement of less than 20% of the total body surface area. Nikolsky's sign can be assessed by applying slight thumb pressure that leads to separation of the epidermis from the dermis when the thumb slides laterally on the skin (Hockett, 2004). At least 61% of patients with SJS have mucous membrane involvement with the mouth, eyes, skin, genitalia, esophagus, and respiratory tract affected. Ocular involvement occurs in 39% of all patients with SJS (Forman, Koren, & Shear, 2002). The mucosal lesions are painful and have a crusted surface. They may lead to blindness or impaired nutrition.

SJS is often misdiagnosed because the first symptoms can be attributed to the flu or an upper respiratory infection and are vague, such as fever, cough, headache, fatigue, sore throat, and malaise. Approximately 1 to 3 days after these symptoms, the target lesions appear and are concentric, quickly becoming confluent blisters. Within hours the skin becomes painful and Nikolsky's sign may be positive.

Medical Management of Stevens–Johnson Syndrome

Mortality rates for SJS are 1% to 5% (Khalili & Bahna, 2006). Early diagnosis and withdrawal of the causative agent are essential to decrease morbidity and mortality. There is no universally accepted treatment other than supportive care. Treatment with glucocorticoids is controversial. Some studies have suggested that glucocorticoids lead to increased morbidity and mortality, whereas others report that short-term use of glucocorticoids in high doses improves outcomes (Letko et al., 2005). The use of intravenous immunoglobulin (IVIG) has shown some success and improved outcomes; however, more research is needed (Khalili & Bahna, 2006). Intravenous fluid replacement similar to that initiated with the treatment of burns must be started to prevent dehydration and treat electrolyte loss through skin lesions (see Chapter 68 😊). Often these patients are taken to burn units for care. Total parenteral nutrition (TPN) is necessary to treat protein loss that occurs with skin detachment and to help prevent stress ulcers. Prevention of infection is important. Prophylactic antibiotics are generally unnecessary but careful aseptic technique is needed.

Skin cultures may be taken every 48 hours to aid in the decision to start antibiotics if necessary. Dressings are used to protect the epidermis but tape should be avoided. Dressings consist of gauze with petrolatum or silver nitrate. Biologic skin covers such as cadaveric allografts may also be used. Topical anesthetics and systemic pain medication may be needed to decrease pain related to dressing changes. Emotional and psychiatric support is essential.

Toxic Epidermal Necrolysis

Toxic epidermal necrolysis (TEN) is a part of the same syndrome of diseases as is Stevens–Johnson syndrome, described earlier. It is a more severe form of the disorder and is life threatening with more extensive skin detachment. Although the disorder is rare, occurring in only 1 person per million, it can have mortality rates of 40% (Klein, 2006). It generally occurs in people between the ages of 46 and 63 but can occur at any age. It more commonly affects women. The causes are the same as those for Stevens–Johnson syndrome with the most common being an adverse reaction to drugs such as sulfonamide antibiotics, anticonvulsant agents, and allopurinol. The pathophysiology is unknown; however, it is thought to be related to an immune response that is cell mediated by the T lymphocytes. Skin lesions have been found to have macrophage infiltration of the dermis and epidermis with tumor necrosis factor in the epidermis (Letko et al., 2005).

Diagnosis and Clinical Manifestations of Toxic Epidermal Necrolysis

TEN is diagnosed by skin biopsy and immunofluorescent studies. The criteria for defining TEN include the following: (1) involvement of at least two mucous membranes, (2) loss of confluent sheets of epidermis leaving an exposed dermis, (3) fever, (4) erosions of more than 30% of the total body surface area, and (5) skin biopsy compatible with TEN. There is also a positive Nikolsky's sign. Like SJS, TEN begins with symptoms of an upper respiratory infection. Approximately 2 to 3 days after the respiratory symptoms, the epidermis blisters and begins splitting and sloughing from the dermis. There are no target lesions, but there are large areas of epidermal sloughing with a dark-red, oozing dermis. These areas are painful and tender. Mucous membranes are also affected. Once diagnosed, patients with TEN can be assessed to predict mortality. The SCORTEN scoring system is used for that purpose. It gives points to 7 parameters, which are added to result in a score between 0 and 7. A score of 0 to 1 is related to a mortality of 3.2%, whereas a score of 5 or more predicts a mortality of at least 90%. The SCORTEN should be performed during the first 24 hours after hospital admission and again on day 3 of hospitalization. The ability to predict mortality can be useful in discussing the patient's condition with family members and in evaluating the effectiveness of new treatments (Guegan, Bastuji-Garin, Poszepczynska-Guigne, Roujeau, & Revuz, 2006).

Medical Management of Toxic Epidermal Necrolysis

Early diagnosis and withdrawal of offending agents are important in decreasing mortality. To achieve the best outcomes, treatment should occur in a burn unit or intensive care unit for patients with TEN. There is no definitive treatment, so the care provided is mostly supportive and symptomatic. The development of an in-

fection or sepsis increases the risk of mortality. Treatment goals are the same as for SJS. Intravenous fluid replacement is needed to prevent dehydration and treat electrolyte losses. TPN is needed to supply badly needed nutrients for growth and repair and to address the protein loss that occurs with the hypermetabolic state. The hypermetabolic state is described in Chapter 68 ⊛. Wounds are generally débrided in the operating room, and biologic dressings, such as homografts and xenografts, are used to decrease the chance of infection, reduce pain, prevent fluid loss, and control body temperature. Reepithelialization begins about 18 days after the development of the first symptoms. As with SJS, treatment with corticosteroids is controversial.

■ Nursing Management for Stevens–Johnson Syndrome and Toxic Epidermal Necrolysis

Like necrotizing fasciitis, nursing care for Stevens–Johnson syndrome and toxic epidermal necrolysis requires knowledgeable assessment skills and critical thinking. Nurses need to be cognizant of the possible development of these conditions. At the first signs of a drug reaction, the health care provider must be alerted and the offending agent stopped immediately. Once either of these conditions develops, it is best managed in a burn unit using a multidisciplinary approach with the nurse as the gatekeeper. The nursing process provides the framework to manage these patients.

Assessment

The extent of total body surface area involvement determines the systemic impact for both Stevens–Johnson syndrome and toxic epidermal necrolysis. The nurse needs to assess the amount of skin involved by using a standard measurement such as the rule of nines described in Chapter 68 ⊛. Fluid loss is not as severe as that seen in burn patients but can be significant, especially if the mucous membranes are involved in areas that cannot be observed, such as the lungs and gastrointestinal tract. Fluid status needs ongoing assessment by monitoring vital signs, urine output, central venous pressure, and cardiac output if a Swan-Ganz catheter is in place. The hemoglobin (Hgb) and hematocrit (HCT) also need to be assessed frequently because they both increase with the loss of intravascular volume; and in the presence of inadequate fluid resuscitation, the Hgb and HCT become abnormally elevated. Chapter 68 ⊛ includes a complete description of fluid management. The patient should be assessed for involvement of mucous membranes. The eyes should be assessed daily for involvement and daily eyedrops may be needed.

Nursing Diagnoses

The nursing diagnoses for patients with Stevens–Johnson syndrome or toxic epidermal necrolysis include:

- *Deficient Fluid Volume* related to increased capillary permeability, increased intravascular hydrostatic pressure, and increased evaporative loss
- *Risk for Imbalanced Fluid Volume* related to excessive IV fluid administration and diminished organ capacity for excessive volume load

PHARMACOLOGY Summary of Medications Used to Treat Skin Disorders

Medication Category	Action	Application/Indication	Nursing Responsibility
Topical corticosteroids: • Betamethasone (Diprolene) • Fluocinonide (Lidex) • Mometasone (Elocon)	Inhibits inflammatory process leading to vasoconstriction of dilated vessels.	Used for inflammatory and pruritic conditions, and hyperplastic and infiltrative disorders. This includes conditions such as atopic and allergic dermatitis, hypertrophic scars, and psoriasis.	Should be applied in a thin layer and rubbed in thoroughly on wet skin. Areas of the body with thin skin, such as the face, or intertriginous areas are more susceptible to side effects. Some infections may be made worse by corticosteroids.
Antiacne medications: • Benzoyl peroxide (Benoxyl 10)	Broad-spectrum bacteriostatic activity against *P. acnes* with anti-inflammatory actions as well.	Decreases inflammation and is keratolytic. It is rubbed into the acne lesions once or twice daily.	Patients should be taught how to use it and the side effects. May irritate the skin. Use should start slow and be gradually increased. Can be irritating to the skin. Produces phototoxicity. May aggravate acne during the first 2–4 weeks of therapy until the skin becomes acclimated.
• Retinoic acid/tretinoin	Keratolytic agent used to increase cell turnover and prevent comedos. Reduces inflammation.	Used as a cream, gel, or solution, and applied topically. Applied sparingly at bedtime. Avoid using around nose, eyes, or mouth.	
• Antibacterial agents such as erythromycin and tetracycline	Antibacterial agents effective against *P. acnes*. Reduces inflammation.	Taken orally or topically. Is used orally for deep acne.	There is no toxicity with topical use. Monitor for allergic reactions with oral use.
Antifungal agents: • Miconazole (Lotrimin) • Nystatin (Mycostatin) • Ketoconazole (Nizoral)	Kills or inhibits the growth of fungi.	Applied topically. Each drug is specific to a particular organism. Applied sparingly once or twice daily.	Monitor for side effects or allergies. Thoroughly rub the drug into the skin. Do not use with occlusive coverings unless prescribed by the health care provider. Keep areas clean and dry.
Antihistamines: • Diphenhydramine (Benadryl) • Loratadine (Claritin) • Fexofenadine (Allegra)	Blocks histamine leading to vasoconstriction and decreased capillary permeability. Decreased itching and edema.	Decreases itching and signs of urticaria. Taken orally.	May cause drowsiness and dryness of the mouth. Some are nonsedating.
Antiviral: Acyclovir (Zorivax)	Inhibits the growth of herpes virus.	Effective against herpes simplex 1 and 2, varicella-zoster, herpes zoster, Epstein–Barr virus, and cytomegalovirus. Given topically or orally.	Monitor for effectiveness of the drug. Monitor for side effects. Prevent spread of infection. Encourage adequate fluid intake. Inform patient that this drug is not a cure for herpes.

- *Ineffective Tissue Perfusion* related to constricting edema formation and circumferential wounds
- *Impaired Gas Exchange* related to lung involvement and fatigue
- *Impaired Skin Integrity* related to epithelial skin loss
- *Risk for Infection* related to loss of skin integrity and impaired nonspecific and specific immunity
- *Acute Pain* related to burn injury and exposed nerve endings
- *Imbalanced Nutrition: Less than Body Requirements* related to hypermetabolic demands of disorder, decreased appetite, immobility, pain, nausea/vomiting, and depression
- *Fear* and *Anxiety* related to changes in health status/role functioning; situational crisis
- *Ineffective Thermoregulation* related to epithelial skin loss

- *Disturbed Body Image* related to loss of skin and potential loss of function.

Planning

A collaborative and comprehensive approach to care will optimize the recovery process. The plan uses the assessment data to prioritize care. First, the cause must be identified and removed if possible. Depending on the nature and extent of the disorder, dieticians, case managers, social workers, consultative health care providers (cardiovascular, infectious diseases, surgeons, and plastic surgeons), nursing staff, and ancillary staff should be part of the plan of care, as all play a role in the prevention and treatment. Stevens–Johnson syndrome and toxic epidermal necrolysis disorders can be life threatening; therefore, it is essential that the plan be correctly prioritized. As always, protection of airway and maintenance of normal oxygen levels are the first priority. Due to fluid shifts, it also is essential to monitor the patient's hemodynamic status and electrolyte levels. Infection prevention is another critical priority for these patients due to loss of skin integrity.

Outcomes and Evaluation Parameters

The immediate outcome is to stabilize the patient's airway, hemodynamic status, fluids and electrolytes, and pain control. Until the skin can be replaced, another critical outcome is infection prevention, which is manifested by absence of fever, increased white blood count, and clinical manifestations of wound infection, discussed earlier. The long-term outcome for patients with Stevens–Johnson syndrome and toxic epidermal necrolysis is to heal without scarring or loss of function, as manifested by a return to previous level of functioning.

Interventions and Rationales

Initial nursing interventions include managing the patient's airway, and monitoring and intervening to maintain a normal hemodynamic status. Ventilator support may be necessary, especially if the mucous membranes of the lung are involved. Pneumonia may occur related to mucus retention and sloughing of the tracheobronchial mucosa. Adequate oxygenation should be maintained through frequent respiratory assessment and delivery of oxygen when necessary (Hockett, 2004). A complete description of nursing management of the ventilated patient can be found in Chapter 36 ⊕.

The fluid shifts out of the intravascular space into the interstitial space with these types of disorders, thereby decreasing the circulating blood volume. Fluid replacement and monitoring of urine output and electrolyte balance are critical to survival. As described earlier, the nurse must closely assess the patient's individual response to fluid replacement to maintain hemodynamic stability. A complete description of fluid replacement for patients who have loss of skin integrity is included in Chapter 68 ⊕. Hemodynamic monitoring is found in Chapter 24 ⊕.

Due to exposed nerve endings, these disorders are very painful. Pain management is an ongoing issue that requires frequent reassessment. Augmenting pain medications during dressing changes and any other painful procedures is essential and will promote healing. Dressing changes can be long and involved, as well as painful. Patients are given continuous morphine infusions by patient-controlled analgesia (PCA) pumps. Nurses need to monitor for breakthrough pain and give medication as needed.

The patient needs to be protected from infection until skin integrity has occurred. Skin and mucous membrane care should be meticulous to avoid infection. Strict aseptic technique is mandatory when performing skin assessment and dressing changes. The patient should be placed in a private room and closely monitored for the presence of infection by daily blood and wound cultures. Oral lesions can be treated with mouthwashes and topical anesthetics. Gastrointestinal involvement may be mild or severe requiring nasogastric intubation or parenteral nutrition. If the eyes are affected, medication to prevent infection may be necessary, and direct light and brightly lit rooms should be avoided because of photophobia.

Typically there is no scarring or contractures. However, physical therapy and range-of-motion exercises are essential to pre-

serve joint function. Psychological support is very important in the nursing care of patients experiencing Stevens–Johnson syndrome or toxic epidermal necrolysis. These diseases are severe, life threatening, and progress rapidly. The patient can become almost unrecognizable overnight. Counseling and spiritual support should be made available to the patient and family members.

Due to the hypermetabolic state and the increased need for calories for wound healing, nutrition also is a priority. Early consultation with a dietician to establish calorie, protein, carbohydrate, and nutrient needs will help prevent a malnourished state. Nursing care includes recording accurate intake and output, and a calorie count every shift. Maintain oral hygiene and monitor the gastrointestinal tract for bowel sounds and distention. If enteral feeding is being done, tube placement and function are monitored as well as the patient's tolerance of the prescribed diet. Daily weight measurement and laboratory values such as total protein levels, complete blood count, glucose, iron, and prealbumin, as well as wound healing, are also measures of adequate nutrition.

Evaluation

A plan for care of the patient with Stevens–Johnson syndrome or toxic epidermal necrolysis must be reevaluated regularly to ensure that the plan is still effective. Any change in the patient's condition could have a negative impact on the wound healing process and the effectiveness of the plan of care. Evaluation criteria of progress would be a decrease in the size and depth of the involved area. If this healing is not occurring, then the area needs to be assessed as to why it is not, such as for infection or decreased tissue perfusion.

■ Cosmetic Surgical Procedures

Cosmetic surgery is done to enhance the attractiveness of certain normal features related to the skin and its underlying structures. This surgery includes reshaping of the nose, body contouring, breast surgery, and facial rejuvenation for the aging process such as resurfacing or tightening of the skin. Reconstructive surgery is performed in those who may have deformities related to cancer, congenital abnormalities, disease, and structural and/or traumatic injuries that result in functional disabilities or abnormal appearance. Congenital deformities include prominent ears, cleft lip and palate deformities, and congenital nevi.

Cosmetic surgery is individualized depending on one's race or ethnicity. For example, darker skinned non-Caucasian individuals present a unique set of needs separate from those of Caucasians. The Cultural Considerations box outlines concerns related to ethnic skin and cosmetic surgery. Today, many surgical procedures can be done to correct skin-related problems for all ethnic groups, and a number of them are discussed next.

Blepharoplasty

Blepharoplasty is a surgical procedure performed to remove the excess skin and fat and occasionally a portion of the orbicularis oculi muscle around the eye. With aging, the relocation of fat, loss of skin elasticity, and excess muscle around the eye can interfere with vision or cause an unwanted appearance. A blepharoplasty can be done alone or along with a face-lift or brow lift (Figure 66–12 ■, p. 2184). Local anesthetic and conscious se-

CULTURAL CONSIDERATIONS for Cosmetic Surgery

Darker skinned individuals are less prone to the signs of aging due to the photoprotective nature of the melanin in darker skin. However, sometimes people of different cultures elect to undergo cosmetic surgery. It is important to understand that the ethnic characteristics of the facial features need to be maintained. Darker skin types are more prone to changes in pigmentation of the skin and scarring; therefore, those concerns also need to be considered when planning the surgery.

dation is usually enough to allow the procedure to be performed. There is some swelling and bruising at the site that will subside in about 10 to 14 days. Complications are unusual but include bleeding, hematoma formation, epidermal inclusion cysts of the incisions, ectropion, infection, and asymmetry.

Rhinoplasty

Rhinoplasty is the surgical alteration of nasal structures, which usually includes the bone and cartilage. It is performed for cosmetic reasons and is often done at the same time as surgical procedures to correct functional problems associated with the obstruction of the nasal passages. Rhinoplasty also is performed for reconstructive conditions such as abnormalities associated with cleft lip and palate deformities or nasal trauma. Rhinoplasty is considered one of the most difficult surgical procedures a plastic surgeon performs. It requires consideration of a myriad of anatomic factors as well as psychological and ethnic factors.

Rhinoplasty can be performed under local or general anesthesia. Topical and injectable vasoconstrictors and anesthetic agents are used. The patient may or may not be hospitalized. The nose will be packed postoperatively for a few days to prevent bleeding and support the nasal structures, and an exterior nasal splint is applied for about a week to a week and a half. There is swelling and periorbital bruising that takes about 2 weeks to subside. However, it takes up to a year for all swelling and sensation to stabilize and to appreciate the final result. This procedure has an increased incidence of needing a secondary procedure to achieve the best result, which is usually done after a year. Figure 66–11 ■ is an example of before and after a rhinoplasty.

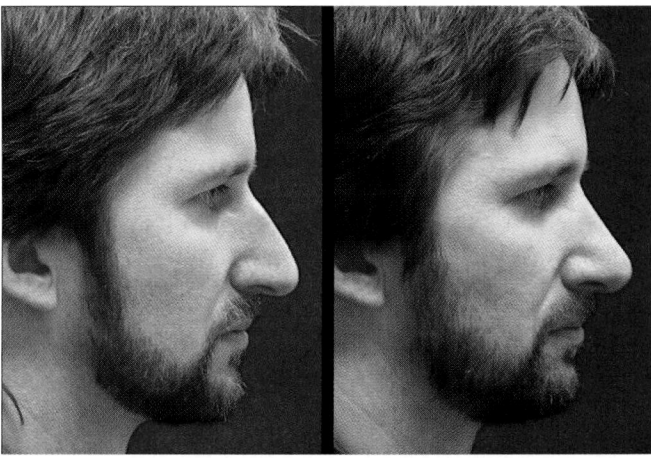

FIGURE 66–11 ■ Before and after a rhinoplasty.
Source: Michael Bermant, MD, Board Certified, American Board of Plastic Surgery/ http://www.plasticsurgery4u.com

Preoperatively, it is important to assess the patient's motivation and desires. An assessment should be made of what the patient's expectations are for the procedure and whether these can be met considering the patient's unique anatomy. Some surgeons perform computer imaging to allow the patient to visualize the results of the surgery preoperatively (Tysome & Sharp, 2006). It is also important to note anything in the patient's history that could affect the outcomes of the surgery. Prior nasal trauma or surgery, sinus or allergy disease, systemic illnesses, medication abuse, respiratory impairments, and emotional stability are examples of factors that need to be evaluated. The surgeon also should consider the ethnicity of the patient. The noses of many African American, Hispanic, and Asian patients may look different from the noses of other nationalities and will require individualized approaches and goals for surgery.

Postoperative complications from rhinoplasty are rare but may include epistaxis, infection, prolonged edema, nasal airway obstruction, and an unsatisfactory cosmetic result. Rhinoplasty is commonly performed and is considered safe and effective.

Rhytidectomy

Rhytidectomy is surgery on the skin to eliminate wrinkles and improve the appearance of the face. It is also referred to as "facial rejuvenation" or "face-lift." The purpose of a rhytidectomy is to set back the signs of aging by approximately 10 years or more. The patient will continue to look younger by approximately 10 years for the rest of her life, even as aging progresses. The Gerontological Considerations box outlines the normal facial changes caused by aging. The rhytidectomy is becoming more common with people wanting natural-looking results because physical appearance is important in how individuals are perceived by others. Appearance also is linked to body image, self-esteem, and confidence. The lines on the face help communicate feelings that occur when interacting with others. Therefore, a youthful appearance may affect an individual in social and professional arenas. Surgery cannot reverse all the effects of aging, but it can reposition tissues and redistribute volume to create a more youthful and rested appearance.

Several anatomic areas can be improved as a part of the rhytidectomy, including the forehead and eyebrows, nasolabial

GERONTOLOGICAL CONSIDERATIONS for the Effects of Aging on the Face

Many anatomic changes occur during the aging process:
- Skin loses elasticity and water content.
- The texture and turgor of the skin change.
- The retaining ligaments of the soft tissue of the face weaken.
- Face loses volume from decreased subcutaneous adipose stores and muscle mass.
- Facial bones undergo resorption.
- The eye orbit changes shape, allowing for positional changes of the eye globe.
- Face becomes elongated and flattened.
- Smoking, genetics, and sun exposure contribute to the loss of skin elasticity and wrinkle formation.

folds, jowls, skin and the platyoma muscle of the neck, and malar fat pads. It is important for the surgeon to identify what the patient's expectations are and to discuss what can and cannot be accomplished, so that the expectations are realistic.

Rhytidectomy can be performed with either local anesthesia and conscious sedation, or general anesthesia. The incisions are made at or within the hairlines, behind the ears, or in natural skin creases so that the scars are less noticeable. Typically this procedure is done on an outpatient basis, although in some instances a surgeon may opt to keep a patient hospitalized the first night. There may be drains and padded dressings to protect the face, and swelling of the face and eyelids is present postoperatively, being the most severe at about the second postoperative day. Complications are rare but may include hematoma, infection, asymmetry, skin necrosis, transient facial weakness, and permanent loss of sensation. With makeup, patients are usually presentable in about 1 to 2 weeks. Figure 66–12 ■ demonstrates before and after pictures.

Dermabrasion

Dermabrasion is the process of removing the epidermis and the outer portion of the dermis, creating a partial thickness skin loss. The purpose of this procedure is to allow new skin to regenerate into a smoother surface. See Chapter 68 🔗 for a complete description of a partial thickness injury. Dermabrasion is used to improve scars, fine wrinkles, sun spots, and areas of hyperpigmentation. A diamond fraise cylinder that has abrasive properties is used to perform the procedure, thus allowing for regrowth of new skin over the abraded area. This procedure is generally limited to use on the face, and either local or general anesthesia is necessary. An open wound is created, which eventually heals in about 7 to 14 days depending on the depth of the abrasion. The patient may need to apply an emollient during this time. Complications include infection, changes in skin color, and scarring. Patients have generally reported being very satisfied with the outcome of the procedure when it has been realistically presented preoperatively.

Microdermabrasion

Microdermabrasion is a skin-freshening technique that helps repair skin that has been damaged by the sun and the effects of aging. The purpose of the procedure is much the same as dermabrasion, just not as deep, and is used to improve scars, fine wrinkles, and hyperpigmentation. The back of the hands and the face are the common areas that benefit from this procedure. A plastic surgeon or esthetician uses a device like a fine sandblaster to spray tiny crystals across the skin, mixing gentle abrasion with suction to remove the dead outer layer of skin. More than one treatment may be needed to reduce or remove fine wrinkles and unwanted pigmentation. No anesthesia is necessary, although the patient may describe a feeling of warmth and throbbing afterward. The skin remains reddened and dry for approximately 4 to 5 days. The patient is instructed to use moisturizers, and long-term use of sunscreens is necessary because the abraded area is more sensitive to burning. If performed properly, complications from this procedure are extremely rare.

Laser

The laser has been used for treating wrinkles, acne, nevi, seborrheic keratosis, actinic keratosis, hemangiomas, tattoos, scars, and unwanted hair. There are many different types of lasers, but the basic principle is that a laser light generates heat that is absorbed into the skin. Different types of tissue will absorb only specific laser wavelengths; thus, the choice of the laser depends on the type of tissue being treated and the problem. The laser beam focused on the skin quickly heats and leads to resurfacing of only the area being treated. Most lasers are used in private offices and small surgical suites under no anesthesia or only local anesthesia. However, the deeper procedures involving greater surface areas may need general anesthesia.

Preoperative preparation of the patient involves detailed teaching about what is involved and what can be expected from the treatments. Depending on the type of laser used, the condition being treated, and the depth of the treatment, treatments may include up to 3 to 5 sessions occurring biweekly or monthly.

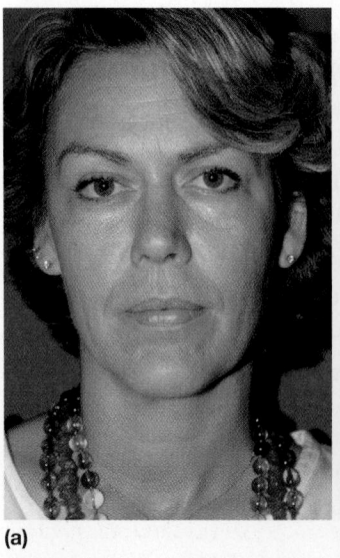 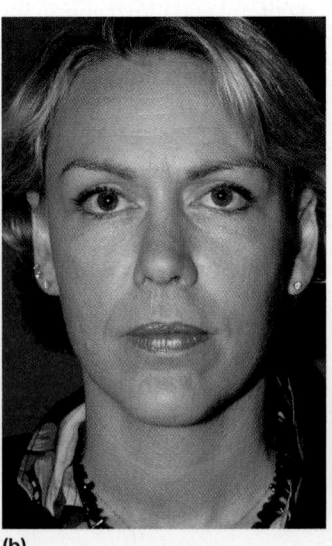 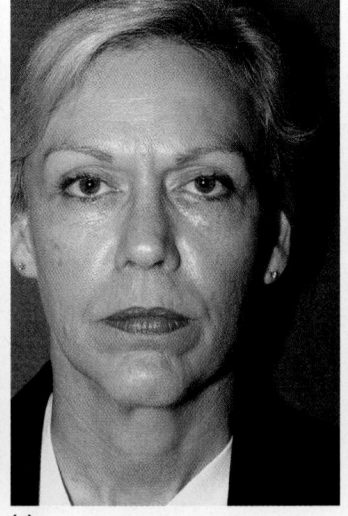 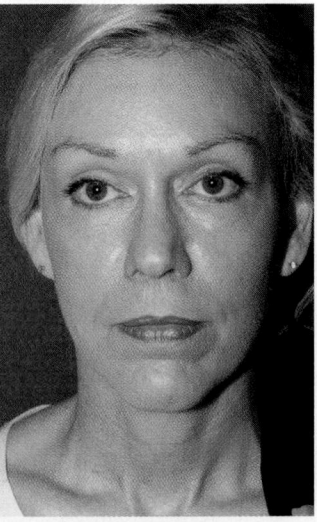

(a)   (b)   (c)   (d)

FIGURE 66–12 ■ Same patient, different ages. A and B: Age 40 years, before and after rhytidectomy and blepharoplasty: C and D: Age 54 years, before and afer rhytidectomy and brow lift.
Source: Courtesy of John M. Osborn MD, FACS, Plastic Surgery Center, Sacramento, CA

Improvement occurs on a continuous basis for up to 6 months after the treatments have been completed. After the procedure, there will be mild to severe localized erythema and swelling at the site of the treatment. Again, depending on the depth of the treatment area, there may be mild to moderate discomfort with the skin feeling dry and tingly for up to a few months. Complications postoperatively are rare but include permanent erythema, edema, acne formation, contact dermatitis, pruritus, infections, and pigmentary alterations.

Injectable Tissue Fillers

As a result of the aging process, a loss of facial fullness and the development of wrinkles occur. A nonsurgical treatment to soften these facial lines and help restore volume and facial contours is injectable fillers. These fillers also are used to treat scars, sun-damaged skin, and thin lips. Outlined here are the different types of tissue fillers on the market:

- Collagen is a natural protein that supports the skin. The two sources are human and bovine collagen. Bovine collagen requires prior allergy testing. The results may last 2 to 4 months.
- Hyaluronic acid is a natural substance found in human bodies. It is used to enhance lips and fill facial creases such as nasolabial folds. It may also be appropriate for some surface wrinkles and concave scars. The results may last 6 months or longer.
- Hydroxyapatite is a mineral-like compound found naturally in human bones, suspended in a gel-like formulation. It is the heaviest of facial fillers and is recommended to fill deeper creases such as nasolabial folds, marionette lines, and frown lines, as well as to enhance fullness of the cheeks and other facial contours.
- Human fat, harvested from the patient's own body, can be injected to enhance facial fullness, fill deep creases, and build up shallow contours. Fat injection requires a more extensive procedure than injection of other fillers because it uses liposuction techniques to extract the fat used for injection. Treatment can last up to a year or more in some cases, and results are highly variable. Fat can be stored for future treatment, although the results from the use of preserved fat are not as favorable.

All tissue fillers except fat are injected by either the health care provider or a specially trained nurse. Fat injections are done solely by the health care provider because the fat needs to be harvested by liposuction. Prior to the injection, the site is cleaned by an antibacterial agent, and icing or a topical numbing agent may be offered to make patients more comfortable. Some tissue fillers contain an anesthetic agent. In other cases, local anesthetic may be administered to the treatment site.

Complications from fillers are uncommon, and the risks vary depending on the specific filler used and the relative permanence of the filler substance. Complications outlined by the American Society of Plastic Surgeons (ASPS) (2007) include:

- Infection at the injection site
- Development of nodules that may require surgical excision
- Acne-like skin eruptions
- Antibody reaction to filler material that may reduce the effectiveness of future injections

- Facial asymmetry
- Bleeding, bruising, and swelling
- Temporary paralysis of other muscle groups or other unintended effects due to migration of the filler material from the original site
- Skin necrosis
- Skin rash, itching, and swelling
- Skin redness
- Skin sensitivity
- Under- or overcorrection of defects

Botulinum Injections

Botulinum toxin type A (Botox) is purified protein complex derived from bacterium *Clostridium botulinum*. Once injected into the muscle, it blocks the release of chemical acetylcholine, thereby temporarily paralyzing the muscles (ASPS, 2007). It is currently being used as a safe and effective cosmetic agent to temporarily improve frown lines between the eyebrows (glabellar lines), forehead creases, laugh-line wrinkles near the eyes, and thick bands in the neck. Botox also can be used to combat migraine headaches and to treat hyperhidrosis (excessive perspiration). A new and still evolving role for Botox is that of a pain reliever for mastectomy patients. Women injected with Botox in the pectoral muscles following the surgical removal of their breast experienced significantly less pain and shorter hospital stays (ASPS, 2007).

Liposuction

Liposuction, is a form of body sculpting or body contouring. It is one of the most common cosmetic surgeries performed. Depending on the elasticity of the skin, it can be performed on anyone after the age of 16. Older patients with less elasticity are not as good candidates as younger patients and need to be realistic about their expectations. The purpose of liposuction is to remove subcutaneous fat in diet-resistant areas of the body that are out of proportion. Liposuction is not viewed as a treatment for obesity but can help contour the body of someone with normal body weight and good skin tone but localized areas of fat accumulation. Patients need to be evaluated and instructed so that unrealistic expectations will not be an issue.

Tumescent liposuction involves infiltrating diluted lidocaine and epinephrine into the subcutaneous tissue to provide anesthesia prior to the actual liposuction. Therefore, general anesthesia is not required but may be used along with the infiltrate at the discretion of the patient or the health care provider (Kucera et al., 2006). Tumescent liposuction allows for the aspiration of a higher amount of fat and a smaller amount of blood (Coldiron et al., 2006). Prior to the procedure, the areas to be removed are marked while the patient is in an upright position, because fat tends to shift when the patient is horizontal and sedated. The diluted mixture of lidocaine and epinephrine is injected into the site to provide anesthesia, cause vasoconstriction, and allow for greater volumes of fat to be aspirated. A small cannula is then inserted through a 2- to 10-millimeter incision and advanced throughout the fat using back-and-forth movements. The fat is mechanically broken up, and tunnels are created. The loosened fat is then removed using suction. The average amount suctioned is between

2 and 3 liters, although any amount up to 10 liters may be aspirated. Any patient who has over 5 liters aspirated should remain in an overnight care facility for observation of vascular complications and hemodynamic compromise. The risk of complications from this procedure is relatively small. The most common complications include contour irregularities, the development of a hematoma or seroma, transient numbness, asymmetry, and persistent postoperative edema (Coldiron et al., 2006).

Postoperatively, patients are usually discharged home once they are stable. Compression dressings are worn over the areas treated to compress the tunnels created by the cannula, to ensure a more even result, to prevent fluid from collecting in the tunnels, and to increase patient comfort. Recovery is rapid with most discomfort resolved within 5 days, although the compression dressings are used from 1 to 6 weeks postoperatively.

Patients are generally satisfied with the results and are able to maintain the fat loss. With weight gain, some fat buildup in the treated areas will occur, but the gain will be in the same proportion as the gain in the rest of the body. Fat cells enlarge with weight gain and do not multiply.

Abdominoplasty

An abdominoplasty is performed to remove excess skin and fat from the lower abdomen and to tighten the muscles of the abdominal cavity. Usually as a result of pregnancy, but also as a result of obesity and the accumulation of intra-abdominal fat, the rectus abdominis muscles separate in the midline, causing a weakness in the muscular support of the abdominal contents. The surgery consists of making an incision across the lower abdomen just above the symphysis pubis out to and sometimes beyond the anterior iliac crest. The skin and adipose tissue are undermined over the abdominal muscles to the level of the lower sternum and the medial ribs, creating a skin and fat flap. The umbilical stalk is left intact but separated from the surrounding skin during the dissection. The muscles are then plicated (sewn together) in the midline to tighten the abdominal musculature and support the abdominal contents. The overlying skin and fat are then redraped inferiorly, and the excess skin and fat are excised. The umbilicus is then reattached through a new hole created in the skin above it, and the skin inferiorly is closed, leaving a scar across the lower abdomen and around the umbilicus.

Panniculectomy

A panniculectomy is the surgical excision of just excess skin and fat that hang over the pubic area as a skin apron, most commonly following excessive weight loss. With this procedure there is no undermining of the skin and fat and no plication of the muscles, as described for the abdominoplasty. It is usually performed to reduce strain on the back and to prevent intertrigo rashes that form under the apron between the skin layers. With the increasing popularity of bariatric surgical procedures, this procedure is becoming more common; and because it is usually performed for functional versus cosmetic reasons, it is usually covered financially by insurance carriers. Bariatric surgery is described in detail in Chapter 14 ☜.

Nursing Management

Dermatologic surgery is generally an elective procedure that may be done in the outpatient setting or as an inpatient, depending on the patient and the procedure. The patient has generally had several discussions with the health care provider about the procedure, its possible complications, and the patient's expectations. The needs of the patient, however, are very much like the needs of any patient undergoing surgery. Chapters 25, 26, and 27 ☜ discuss the preoperative, intraoperative, and postoperative needs of the patient.

Immediately after surgery, the patient will be monitored in a postanesthesia care unit (PACU) for complications related to the surgery and anesthesia. Chapters 26 and 27 ☜ discuss patient care in the PACU. Depending on the type of surgery, there may be a pressure dressing to prevent bleeding and decrease edema. The nurse will need to check the dressings frequently for bleeding and to monitor the patient for signs of hemorrhage, such as increased pulse rate, decreased blood pressure, or changes in level of consciousness. The patient also may have drains in place that the nurse will need to monitor for amount and color of drainage. The patient needs to be kept comfortable. This may require special positioning and pain medication.

The patient should be instructed not to remove scabs, and the incisions should be kept clean and dry. Any redness, increased warmth, or drainage should be reported to the surgeon. The patient will need teaching about treatments or care of the incision at home.

Postoperative care for the abdominoplasty or panniculectomy includes instructing the patient to minimize tension on the suture line by sleeping in a semi-Fowler's position, not lifting heavy objects, and avoiding strenuous exercise. Instruct the patient not to smoke tobacco, as it constricts blood vessels, which diminishes the blood supply needed for wound healing. It is essential to teach pain management techniques such as splinting the wound when coughing, walking in a hunched over position, and consistent use of pain medications. It also is important to discuss the clinical manifestations of wound infection, which include wound separation, drainage, redness, increased pain, and fever. The nurse must stress to the patient what signs and symptoms need to be reported to the surgeon.

Health Promotion

The patient undergoing cosmetic surgery and the patient's family will need teaching related to the type and extent of surgery. Specific instructions should be given related to the type of incision, length of surgery, length of recovery, and possible complications. Although the surgeon will generally provide the patient with this information, is it important that the nurse reinforce and clarify that the patient understands the information. The patient needs to be aware of any postoperative limitations or special care needs.

There may be special preoperative preparations. For example, rhytidectomy patients need to be instructed to wash their hair and face with antibacterial soap several times to decrease the bacterial count. The patient should be instructed not to ingest aspirin, ibuprofen, or other platelet coating drugs for at least 2 weeks before and after surgery because of the increased risk of bleeding. The patient will need a physical examination and routine diagnostic laboratory tests prior to surgery to assess physical readiness for anesthesia. Chapter 25 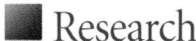 discusses preoperative instructions in detail. The patient should be prepared psychologically for postoperative edema and discoloration. Due to this bruising and edema, the true effects of the surgery cannot be evaluated for several weeks.

Research

Research opportunities exist related to skin disorders and cosmetic surgery. The goals of research are to identify effective means of caring for patients with skin problems and to support patients psychologically who have experienced changes in appearance. The research topics related to skin disorders are identified in the Research Opportunities and Clinical Impact box.

RESEARCH OPPORTUNITIES AND CLINICAL IMPACT RELATED TO SKIN DISORDERS AND COSMETIC SURGERY

Research Area	Clinical Impact
Effects of various moisturizers on the skin.	Keeping the skin intact and avoiding dryness.
Mechanisms to diagnose skin cancer accurately.	Early detection and treatment.
Treatment for common skin conditions.	Many skin conditions do not have adequate treatment available for cure or control.
Lifestyle outcomes of cosmetic surgery. Social and psychological implications of cosmetic surgery.	There is a need to determine whether cosmetic surgery makes a difference in lifestyle and body image.
Risk factors for herpes zoster.	More information is needed about who might be at risk other than those who are immunocompromised.
The effects of cosmetic surgery on the ethnic population.	Most research related to cosmetic surgery has been done with the Caucasian population. How does ethnic skin respond?
Define epidemiology with necrotizing fasciitis using population-based studies. Factors that help predict who might develop necrotizing fasciitis.	Identify those with the greatest risk for acquiring necrotizing fasciitis.
Testing of computer health care provider's orders. Interventions to improve patient understanding of and compliance with medication dosage and administration.	There is a need to decrease medication errors.
The role of nonsteroidal anti-inflammatory drugs (NSAIDs) in the development of necrotizing fasciitis.	Clarifies whether NSAIDs aggravate or initiate the development of necrotizing fasciitis.

Clinical Preparation

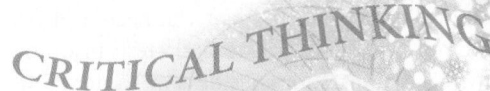
CRITICAL THINKING

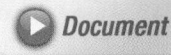 **Read**

- History of Current Illness
- Past Medical History
- Physical Exam
- Admitting Medical Orders
- Laboratory Study Results

 **Document**

- Summary of Hospitalization
- Pathophysiology Form
- Laboratory Values
- Laboratory Results Explanation

Apply

- List of Potential Nursing Diagnoses
- Concept Map
- Critical Thinking Questions

Log on to MyNursingKit.com to download forms you will need and to complete further steps in the Clinical Preparation assignment.

HISTORY OF PRESENT ILLNESS

Mr. Tatum is a 47-year-old white male who was admitted to the hospital with necrotizing fasciitis located in a wound in his right lower leg. He reports being hit on the lower leg with a log while he was chopping wood about 7 days ago. At the time of the injury, he removed several splinters. Following the injury the pain increased to the point that it became difficult for him to walk. He noted that there was increased swelling and a mottled appearance where the splinters were, and that the wound had doubled in size in the last 2 days. He brought himself to the emergency department for an evaluation of the leg and to rule out a fracture. No fracture was found, however the assessment revealed a cellulitis with a hard "woody" texture to the wound. He was admitted for further wound evaluation.

Upon admission Mr. Tatum was taken to surgery for a debridement and culture of his wound. The culture showed group A streptococcus. He is scheduled for a second debridement in 12 hours. The surgical debridement will continue until clear borders are obtained. Application of a vacuum-assisted closure device was done in surgery.

Medical–Surgical History

Mr. Tatum has been in relatively good health. Lately he has had some problems with tendonitis in the left elbow and was on Naprosyn. No other chronic health problems. He was on no medications prior to admission other than Naprosyn.

Social History

Mr. Tatum lives in the country but works as a mechanic at the local steel plant.

He reports that he drinks approximately 6 beers per week, mostly on the weekend. He does not use illicit drugs. He smokes about 1 pack of cigarettes per day.

Physical Exam
Vital signs; BP 120/76; P 96; RR 16; T 99.4°F
Oxygen sat 93% on room air
HEENT: normal but poor dentition
Heart: regular rate and rhythm; normal S_1, S_2
Lungs: clear to auscultation in all fields
Abdomen: obese, soft, nontender
Normal neuro exam
No rash
Chest x-ray: clear
ECG: WNL
Weight: 210 lbs (95.4 kg); height: 6'1"
Extremities: left leg appears normal with good color, no edema, dorsalis pedis and posterior tibial pulses 2+ bilaterally
Anterior right lower leg has wound approximately 5 inches in diameter about mid-shin. The area around the wound is erythremic with bluish patches and bullae draining clear watery liquid. The wound is surrounded by nonpitting edema from the knee to the ankle. Area around wound is very tender to touch.

Admitting Medical Orders
Plastic Surgery Service
Surgical floor

Diagnosis: necrotizing fasciitis of right leg
Allergic to codeine
Oxygen at 2–3 liters nasal cannula, keep oxygen saturation ≥ 92%
Bed rest with bathroom privileges
Vital signs and O_2 saturation levels q2h
Call house officer: pulse < 60 and > 110/minute; BP < 90 and > 130 systolic; temperature > 38.5°C; urine output < 30 mL/hr for 2 hours; respiratory rate > 30/minute; oxygen saturation < 92%
Sequential compression device (SCD) to lower left extremity
Incentive spirometer every 2 hours while awake
Foley
I&O
NPO after midnight for OR
Calorie count
IV: D5 lactated Ringer's at 100 mL/hr
Contact isolation
Wound VAC to right lower leg with 125 mmHg of continuous suction

Scheduled Medications
Clindamycin 900 mg IV q8h
Ampicillin 1.0 gm IV q6h

Gentamicin 90 mg IV three times per day
Famotidine 20 mg IV twice daily
Naprosyn 500 mg po twice/day (when taking po)

PRN Medications

Morphine sulfate via patient-controlled analgesia: concentration:
  1 mg/mL Basal rate 1 mg/hr; incremental: 1 mg;
  6-minute lock-out
Phenergan 25 mg IV q6h prn nausea
Triazolam 0.125–0.25 mg po q noc, prn sleep (when taking po)
Ativan 0.5–2 mg IV q6–8h prn anxiety

Milk of Magnesia 30 mL po daily prn constipation (when taking po)
Tylenol 650 mg po/PR prn q4h for fever > 38.5°C

Ordered Laboratory Studies

STAT wound culture (done in OR)
CBC, Chem 20 panel, CK now
Daily: CBC, PT-INR/PTT, Ca, Mg, phosphorus, Chem 7 panel
Blood culture every 24 hours prn temp > 38.5°C

Ordered Diagnostic Studies

ECG
CT scan of right leg

LABORATORY STUDY RESULTS

Test	Day 1	Day 2	Day 3
White blood cells (WBCs)	18,000/mm^3	22,000/mm^3	28,000/mm^3
Neutrophils	80%	88%	96%
Hemoglobin	12 g/dL	11 g/dL	10 g/dL
Hematocrit	36%	33%	30%
Red blood cells (RBCs)	4.5/mm^3	4.1/mm^3	3.8/mm^3
Platelets	250,000/mm^3	400,000/mm^3	540,000/mm^3
Sodium	136 mEq/L	138 mEq/L	139 mEq/L
Potassium	4.0 mEq/L	4.8 mEq/L	5.0 mEq/L
Chloride	96 mEq/L	97 mEq/L	101 mEq/L
Carbon dioxide	30		
Magnesium	1.8 mEq/L		
Phosphorus	4 mg/dL		
Blood urea nitrogen (BUN)	22 mg/dL	34 mg/dL	49 mg/dL
Creatinine	1 mg/dL	1.3 mg/dL	1.7 mg/dL
Glucose	198 mg/dL	192 mg/dL	160 mg/dL
Calcium	9.2 mg/dL		
Total protein	5.2 g/dL		
Albumin	3.6 g/dL		
Alkaline phosphatase	105 units/L		
Aspartate aminotransferase (AST)	38 units/L		
Total bilirubin	1.1 mg/dL		
Creatine kinase	280 units/L		
PTT	32 seconds		
PT	9.6 seconds		
INR	1.2		
Wound culture	Group A beta-hemolytic streptococcus		
CT scan	Asymmetric fascial thickening with gas tracking along the fascial planes		

CRITICAL THINKING QUESTIONS

1. What complications should you assess for in Mr. Tatum and why?

2. How is Mr. Tatum's necrotizing fasciitis transmitted and how can you protect the other patients you are caring for?

3. Mr. Tatum is concerned about his leg and asks you whether it will ever be back to normal. How should you respond?

Answers to Critical Thinking Questions appear in Appendix D.

NCLEX® REVIEW

1. The nurse is instructing a patient to reduce bathing and use a mild unscented soap. These interventions are appropriate for which of the following skin disorders?
   1. Atopic dermatitis
   2. Poison ivy
   3. Urticaria
   4. Contact dermatitis

2. The nurse is instructing a patient with a skin disorder on nutrition. Which of the following should be included in this instruction?
   1. Restrict calories.
   2. Eat foods high in vitamin C, iron, and zinc.
   3. Limit high-water content foods.
   4. Limit fatty foods.

3. A patient asks what she could do to make sure her teenage daughter doesn't develop skin cancer. Which of the following should the nurse instruct this patient?
   1. Eat a well-balanced diet.
   2. Maintain a normal weight for height.
   3. Take a daily multivitamin.
   4. Instruct in the use of sunscreen.

4. A patient with a skin disorder is prescribed a topical corticosteroid. Which of the following should the nurse instruct this patient about the use of this medication?
   1. Rub the medication into wet skin thoroughly.
   2. Apply a thick layer of the medication and allow it to air dry.
   3. Stay out of the sun when you use this medication.
   4. It may cause drowsiness.

5. A patient has been admitted to the hospital with a skin disorder. Which of the following should the nurse include in the assessment of this patient?
   1. Signs of infection
   2. Employment history
   3. Social activities
   4. Neurological status

6. A patient tells the nurse that she "doesn't socialize much in the summer" because she needs to wear long sleeves to cover the psoriasis on her arms. Which of the following should the nurse respond to this patient?
   1. That's too bad.
   2. You probably like the winter much better.
   3. There are light materials that you could wear to protect your arms while still enjoying the summer activities.
   4. I would go out anyway.

7. A patient tells the nurse that as she gets older, it seems like her face is getting longer. Which of the following should the nurse respond to this patient?
   1. It is a sign of disease.
   2. This is a normal part of aging.
   3. It happens because of exposure to smoke.
   4. It happens because of sun exposure.

Answers for review questions appear in Appendix D

KEY TERMS

acne vulgaris *p.2159*
actinic keratosis *p.2153*
androgenetic alopecia *p.2151*
androgenic alopecia *p.2151*
atopic dermatitis *p.2154*
blepharoplasty *p.2182*
café-au-lait spot *p.2159*
candidiasis *p.2166*
carbuncle *p.2165*
cellulitis *p.2164*
contact dermatitis *p.2153*
dermabrasion *p.2184*
dermatofibromas *p.2161*
dermatophyte *p.2167*

erysipelas *p.2164*
fissure *p.2154*
folliculitis *p.2164*
furuncle *p.2165*
hirsutism *p.2151*
impetigo *p.2164*
lipoma *p.2158*
liposuction *p.2185*
necrotizing fasciitis (NF) *p.2170*
neurofibromatosis *p.2161*
nevi *p.2158*
nits *p.2168*
paronychia *p.2150*
pediculosis *p.2168*

photodermatitis *p.2153*
pilosebaceous follicles *p.2158*
psoriasis *p.2160*
rhinoplasty *p.2183*
rhytidectomy *p.2183*
scabies *p.2168*
seborrheic keratosis *p.2161*
shingles *p.2165*
solar lentigo *p.2159*
Stevens-Johnson syndrome (SJS) *p.2179*
toxic epidermal necrolysis (TEN) *p.2180*
urticaria *p.2154*
verrucae *p.2166*
vitiligo *p.2159*

REFERENCES

Abernethy, H., Cho, C., DeLanoy, A., Khan, O., Kerns, J. W., & Knight, K. (2006). What nonpharmacological treatments are effective against common nongenital warts? *Journal of Family Practice, 55*(9), 801–802.

Affleck, P. (2005). Sun exposure and health. *Nursing Standard, 19*(47), 50–54.

American Society of Plastic Surgeons (ASPS). (2007). *Injectable fillers.* Retrieved January 5, 2008, from http://plasticsurgery.org/patients_consumers/procedures/InjectableFillers.cfm?gclid=CKPEo4_V35ACFRdPagodPzDOWQ

Cancer Research UK. (2003). *Cancer Research UK gets SunSmart with the big screen.* Retrieved September 8, 2008, from http://info.cancerresearchuk.org/news/archive/pressreleases/2003/may/216205

Centers for Disease Control and Prevention (CDC). (2000). *Pseudomonas dermatitis/folliculitis associated with pools and hot tubs—Colorado and Maine, 1999–2000. Morbidity and Mortality Weekly Report, 49*(48), 1087–1091. Retrieved September 3, 2008, from http://www.cdc.gov/mmwr/preview/mmwrhtml/mm4948a2.htm

Centers for Disease Control and Prevention (CDC). (2002). *Skin cancer: Preventing America's most common cancer, fact sheet 2002.* Retrieved February 18, 2004, from http://www.cdc.gov/HealthyYouth/skincancer/pdf/facts.pdf

Centers for Disease Control and Prevention (CDC). (2006a). *Methicillin-resistant* Staphylococcus aureus *skin infections among tattoo recipients—Ohio, Kentucky, and Vermont, 2004–2005.* Retrieved December 12, 2007, from http://www.cdc.gov/mmwr/preview/mmwrhtml/mm5524a3.htm

Centers for Disease Control and Prevention (CDC). (2006b). *Health topics: Skin cancer school health guidelines.* Retrieved December 12, 2007, from http://www.cdc.gov/healthyyouth/skincancer/guidelines/summary.htm#top

Centers for Disease Control and Prevention (CDC). (2008). *Division of bacterial and mycotic diseases. Group A streptococcal (GAS) disease.* Retrieved August 30, 2008, from http://www.cdc.gov/ncidod/dbmd/diseaseinfo/groupastreptococcal_g.htm

Coldiron, B., Coleman, W. P., Cox, S. E., Jacob, C., Lawrence, N., Kaminer, M., et al. (2006). ASDS guidelines of care for tumescent liposuction. *Dermatologic Surgery, 32,* 709–716.

County of Kern: Department of Health Services. (2007). *Complications associated with body piercing and tattooing.* Retrieved December 12, 2007, from http://www.co.kern.ca.us/health/tattooing513.asp

Demierre, M., Allten, S., & Brown, R. (2005). New treatments for melanoma. *Dermatology Nursing, 17*(4), 287–295.

Fawcett, R. S., Linford, S., & Stulberg, D. L. (2004). Nail abnormalities: Clues to systemic disease. *American Family Physician, 69,* 1417–1424.

Forman, R., Koren, G., & Shear, N. H. (2002). Erythema multiforme, Stevens–Johnson syndrome and toxic epidermal necrolysis in children: A review of 10 years' experience. *Drug Safety, 25*(13), 965–972.

Gorgos, D. (2006). Dermatology nursing news: Skin update. *Dermatology Nursing, 18*(1): 89–92, 95–98, 107.

Guegan, S., Bastuji-Garin, S., Poszepczynska-Guigne, E., Roujeau, J., & Revuz, J. (2006). Performance of the SCORTEN during the first five days of hospitalization to predict the prognosis of epidermal necrolysis. *Journal of Investigative Dermatology, 126*(2), 272–276.

Gurwitz, J. H., Field, T. S., Harrold, L. R., Rothschild, J., Debellis, K., Seger, A. C., et al. (2003). Incidence and preventability of adverse drug events among older persons in the ambulatory setting. *JAMA, 289,* 1107–1116.

Halder, R. M., & Nootheti, P. K. (2003). Ethnic skin disorders overview. *Journal of the American Academy of Dermatology, 48*(Suppl. 6), S143–S148.

Hasham S., Matteucci, P., Stanley, P. R., & Hart, N. B. (2005). Necrotizing fasciitis. *British Medical Journal, 330*(9), 830–833.

Hockett, K. C. (2004). Stevens–Johnson syndrome and toxic epidermal necrolysis: Oncologic considerations. *Clinical Journal of Oncology Nursing, 8*(1), 27–30.

Hunt, N., & McHale, S. (2005). The psychological impact of alopecia. *British Medical Journal, 331*(7522), 951–953.

Jemal, A., Siegel, R., Ward, E., Murray, T., Xu, J., Smigal, C., et al. (2006). Cancer statistics, 2006. *CA: A Cancer Journal for Clinicians, 56*(2), 106–130. Retrieved September 4, 2008, from http://caonline.amcancersoc.org/cgi/content/full/56/2/106

Khalili, B., & Bahna, S. L. (2006). Pathogenesis and recent therapeutic trends in Stevens–Johnson syndrome and toxic epidermal necrolysis. *Annals of Allergy, Asthma, & Immunology, 97,* 272–281.

Klein, P. A. (2006). Stevens-Johnson Syndrome and Toxic Epidermal Necrolysis. *eMedicine.* Retrieved September 8, 2008 from http://www.emedicine.com/derm/TOPIC405.HTM

Kucera, I. J., Lambert, T. J., Klein, J. A., Watkins, R. G., Hoover, J. M., & Kaye, A. D. (2006). Liposuction: Contemporary issues for the anesthesiologist. *Journal of Clinical Anesthesia, 18*(5), 379–387.

Layton, A., Buchanan, P., & Courtenay, M. (2006). Continuing professional development. Treatment of acne vulgaris. *Primary Health Care, 16*(4), 41–49.

Letko, E., Papliodis, E. N., Papliodis, G. N., Daoud, Y. J., Ahmed, A. R., & Foster, C. S. (2005). Stevens–Johnson syndrome and toxic epidermal necrolysis: A review of the literature. *Annals of Allergy, Asthma, & Immunology, 94*(4), 419–436.

MayoClinic.com. (2008). *Tattoos: Risks and precautions to know first.* Retrieved August 30, 2008, from http://www.mayoclinic.com/health/tattoos-and-piercings/MC00020

National Pressure Ulcer Advisory Panel (NPUAP). (1992). *Statement on pressure ulcer prevention.* Retrieved September 8, 2008, from http://www.npuap.org/positn1.htm

Patel, B. D., Loo, W. J., Tasker, A. D., Screaton, N. J., Burrows, N. P., Silverman, E. K., et al. (2006). Smoking related COPD and facial wrinkling: Is there a common susceptibility? *Thorax, 61*(7), 568–671.

Reddy, M., Gill, S. S., & Rochon, P. A. (2006). Preventing pressure ulcers: A systematic review. *Journal of the American Medical Association, 296*(8), 974–984.

Samuel, M., Brooke, R. C. C., Hollis, S., & Griffiths, C. E. M. (2005). Interventions for photodamaged skin. *The Cochrane Database of Systematic Reviews,* Issue 1. Retrieved August 30, 2008, from http://www.cochrane.org/reviews/en/ab001782.html

Scher, R. K., Fleckman, P., Tulumbas, B., McCollam, L., & Enfanto, P. (2003). Brittle nail syndrome: Treatment options and the role of the nurse. *Dermatology Nursing, 15*(1), 15–24.

Singh, G., Haneef, N. A., & Uday, A. (2005). Nail changes and disorders among the elderly. *Indian Journal of Dermatology, Venereology, and Leprology, 71*(6), 386–392.

Stough, D., Stenn, K., Haber, R., Parsley, W. M., Vogel, J. E., Whiting, D. A., et al. (2005). Psychological effect, pathophysiology, and management of androgenetic alopecia in men. *Mayo Clinic Proceedings, 80*(10), 1316–1322.

Swetter, S. (2008). Malignant melanoma. *eMedicine from Web MD.* Retrieved August 30, 2008, from http://www.emedicine.com/derm/topic257.htm

Tsang, M. O., Tsang, K. Y., & Wong, W. (2004). The use of recombinant human epidermal growth factor (rhEGF) in a gentleman with drug-induced Steven Johnson syndrome. *Dermatology Online Journal, 10*(1), 25. Retrieved September 4, 2008, from http://dermatology.cdlib.org/101/correspondence/TEN/tsang.html

Tysome, J. R., & Sharp, H. R. (2006). Current trends in photographic imaging for rhinoplasty surgery. *The Internet Journal of Otorhinolaryngology, 5*(2). Retrieved August 30, 2008, from http://www.ispub.com/ostia/index.php?xmlFilePath=journals/ijorl/vol5n2/imaging.xml

U.S. Department of Health and Human Services (DHHS). (2000). *Healthy People 2010 understanding and improving health.* Washington, DC: Author.

Wong, C., & Wang, Y. (2005). The diagnosis of necrotizing fasciitis. *Current Opinion in Infectious Disease, 18*(2), 101–106.

Young, M. (2005). The psychological and social burdens of psoriasis. *Dermatology Nursing, 17*(1), 15–19.

Zhang, W., Leonard, R., Bath-Hextall, F., Chambers, C. A., Lee, C., Humphreys, R., et al. (2004). Chinese herbal medicine for atopic eczema. *The Cochrane Database of Systematic Reviews.* Issue 4. Retrieved August 30, 2008, from http://www.cochrane.org/reviews/en/ab002291.html

Caring for the Patient with Wounds

Harold Engle
Kathleen Osborn

With contributions by:
Jan Clark

Outcome-Based Learning Objectives

After studying this chapter, the learner will be able to:

1. Compare and contrast the clinical manifestations of the three phases of wound healing.
2. Describe wound characteristics and nursing documentation that are required in a periodic wound assessment.
3. Describe key factors that are relative to the prevention of pressure ulcers.
4. Compare and contrast wound classifications and respective treatments.
5. Evaluate therapies and their benefits with respect to wound healing.
6. Understand the psychosocial and liability factors pertaining to wound care.
7. Describe how research in wound care will lead to better efficiency and outcomes with evidence-based practice.

Research Collaboration Health Promotion Nursing Process Caring Critical Thinking

WHAT IS the largest organ of the human body? The skin is the largest organ of the human body and functions to protect internal organs from insults such as infection and injury. These insults may be as minor as a bump or bruise or as major as a life-threatening infection or trauma. Whether the injury is caused by a surgeon's scalpel, trauma from a bullet or stab wound, or tissue damage from a myocardial infarction, the repair process is similar. The primary objective of the wound healing process is to restore skin integrity and structural continuity of the injured area (Porth, 2007).

Skin is an organ of the integumentary system that is comprised of three layers of tissue: epidermis, dermis, and subcutaneous tissue. Each layer has a different composition and function. The outermost layer of skin is the epidermis. It contains melanocytes for pigmentation, Langerhans' cells as part of the immune system, sensory nerves, and keratinocytes. The main function of the epidermis is protection and sensation. The dermis, the thickest layer of the skin, contains the microvascular system along with hair follicles, sweat glands, lymph vessels, sebaceous (oil) glands, and nerve endings. It is constructed of collagen, a protein made from fibroblasts. It is also comprised of elastin, which makes the skin flexible and elastic. The main functions of the dermis are thermoregulation and blood supply to the epidermis. The last layer of the skin, the subcutaneous fat layer (also known as hypodermis), is comprised of stored fat cells. It is an avascular layer as well. Its main function is insulation and protection of the underlying organs (Porth, 2007). Chapter 65 🖙 discusses the anatomy of the skin in detail.

Physiology of Wound Healing

What happens when the skin is compromised by an injury? Once tissue injury has occurred, the primary objective is to restore tissue integrity through the healing process. There are three phases of wound healing: homeostasis/inflammation, proliferation, and remodeling (Figure 67–1 ■). These phases represent a cascade of events that overlap and are dependent on one another. Each phase contributes to the desired result of healing the wound. Any disruption or absence of a phase can result in a delayed or prolonged healing. Each phase is discussed next.

Phase One: Homeostasis/Inflammatory Phase

Homeostasis is the tendency of the human body to maintain stability, and maintaining stability is the first reaction when a wound occurs. Injury to the epidermis, dermis, and subcutaneous tissue causes blood cells to spill into the wound, and the first step toward homeostasis is to get the bleeding stopped. A vasoconstric-

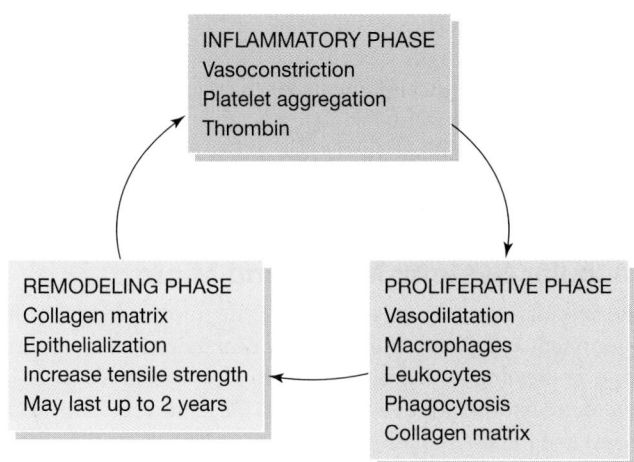

INFLAMMATORY PHASE
Vasoconstriction
Platelet aggregation
Thrombin

PROLIFERATIVE PHASE
Vasodilatation
Macrophages
Leukocytes
Phagocytosis
Collagen matrix

REMODELING PHASE
Collagen matrix
Epithelialization
Increase tensile strength
May last up to 2 years

FIGURE 67–1 ■ Phases of wound healing.

tive substance is released by the platelets that assist in this process. Coagulation factors, which promote platelet aggregation in the endothelium of the injured vessel at the site of injury, are also released. The bleeding is usually stopped by a thrombus formation. Thrombus formation is discussed in detail in Chapter 62 🔘 .

The next step in regaining homeostasis is the secretion of **growth factors**, which are a group of extracellular polypeptides (secreted by platelets and macrophages) that affect cell growth, reproduction, movement, and function. Growth factors recruit the necessary cells to synthesize and regulate the wound repair. Scientists have identified several of these growth factors and their effects on the wound repair process: for example, platelet-activating factor (PAF), which induces platelet aggregation (Porth, 2007), and epidermal growth factor (EGF), which may have an important part in wound healing by stimulating keratinocyte proliferation and migration of cells (Gibbs et al., 2000). The keratinocyte growth factor impacts the remodeling process by stabilizing epidermal turnover and barrier function (Gibbs et al., 2000).

The **inflammatory phase** of wound healing begins at the time of the injury or surgery. The purpose of this critical phase is to prepare the site for growth of new tissue. This phase of wound healing cleans the wound in preparation for closure. In a clean acute wound, the inflammatory phase lasts approximately 3 to 5 days, but in a wound complicated by infection or necrosis, the inflammatory phase is prolonged and wound healing is delayed (Waldrop & Doughty, 2000). Within hours after injury, histamines are released from mast cells, causing local vasodilation and increased capillary permeability. This allows leakage of serous fluid into the injured site, which results in erythema, edema, and the production of exudates.

Prostaglandin, which is released during the inflammatory phase, is a long-chain fatty acid that regulates platelet aggregation and controls inflammation and vascular permeability. The inflammatory phase is characterized by the presence of granulocytes, macrophages, and lymphocytes, which are attracted to the injured site by the complement factors and antigens. These cells, called **phagocytes**, perform **phagocytosis**, the process of absorbing and enzymatically degrading foreign matter and devitalized tissue, thus preparing the wound for closure. The by-product of phagocytosis is exudate. Exudate, or drainage

from the wound, is usually at its peak during the inflammatory phase. Note that the drainage from the wound during the inflammatory phase does not indicate infection in the wound; it is the body's normal response to injury.

Suppression of the inflammatory phase can contribute to a delay in wound healing. Radiation therapy can suppress the inflammatory phase by causing depletion of the neutrophils and macrophages, which release the growth factors. Malnutrition, dehydration, and chronic steroid use also can suppress the inflammatory phase. Chronic use of steroids specifically results in decreased production of histamines, suppressing the inflammatory response.

Phase Two: Proliferation

The proliferative phase is the next phase in the healing process. Reconstruction occurs at this phase. It can last up to 3 weeks after the inflammatory phase in a normal, healthy person. Growth factors described earlier originating from injured vessels stimulate the formation of vascular buds and regrowth of vascular loops. Stimulated endothelial cells multiply and form tubular structures differentiating into arterioles or venules, a process referred to as **angiogenesis**. These new blood vessels can begin to form in a wound within 3 days of injury, provided there is sufficient blood circulation to the wound bed.

Simultaneously, in the process of revascularization, connective tissue begins to form at the wound margins. **Fibroblasts** are the small cells that migrate along the fibrin network to produce the connective tissue and collagen fibers. **Collagen synthesis** is the multistep process in which fibrin proteins form a matrix to support the newly forming tissue. Collagen synthesis is dependent on adequate amounts of vitamin C, iron, and copper in the diet. The newly formed collagen fibers are not organized in the same tension contours as in healthy tissue, thus decreasing the tensile strength and elasticity in a repaired wound. Collagen fibers in scar tissue actually have a disorganized appearance (Christian, Talavera, Stadelmann, Slenkovich, & Downey, 2006). The end result is that scar tissue never has the same tensile strength as normal tissue.

Due to angiogenesis, granulation tissue develops. **Granulation tissue**, aptly named for the recognizable tiny, round, granule-like nodules, is a highly vascular connective tissue that contains newly formed capillaries, proliferating fibroblasts, and residual inflammatory cells (Porth, 2007). Granulation tissue appears beefy red and moist because of the dense revascularization process. Granulation tissue gradually fills the defect of the wound. If granulation tissue is slow to form, one can presume that there is an insufficient blood supply, there is a wound infection, or one of the growth factors necessary for revascularization is deficient, all of which interrupt the normal rate of wound healing. This part of the proliferative phase begins about 3 days after initial injury and may overlap with the inflammatory phase.

Epithelialization is the process by which the wound closes from its margins, covering the defect with a layer of new skin. This is accomplished by cell migration from the wound edges over granulation tissue. The wound bed must be moist and well perfused with blood in order for epithelialization to occur. Epithelialization, usually first seen at the wound margins, appears as a small pink or pearl-like area. Islands of epithelial cells can

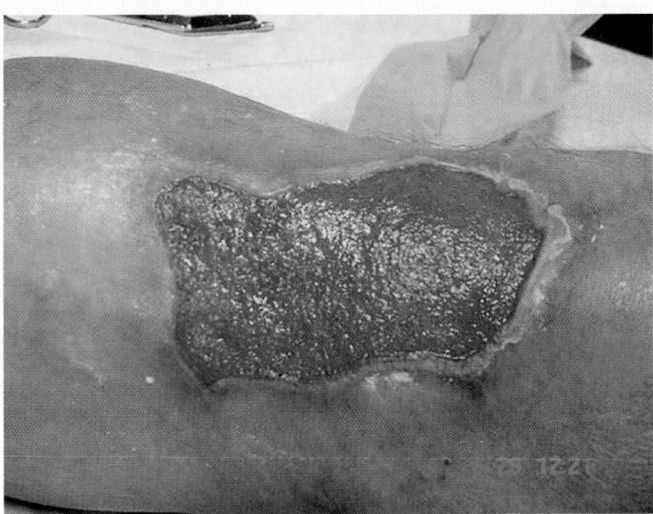

FIGURE 67–2 ■ Granulation and epithelialization tissue.
Source: Courtesy of Harold Engle

appear within the wound defect on the surface of the granulation. This new skin is quite fragile and must be protected from injury. A moist environment encourages the migration of these cells across the wound surface from all directions. Granulation and epithelialization, if not interrupted, continue to develop for up to about 14 to 21 days (Figure 67–2 ■).

Partial thickness wounds (e.g., skin tears, abrasions) do not require granulation to heal because epithelial cells are able to migrate across the wound, rebuilding dermis.
Full-thickness wounds require granulation to fill the defect caused by the wound. This is not regenerated tissue but scar tissue.

Phase Three: Remodeling

Remodeling, the third and final phase of wound healing, occurs after the wound is closed. It begins about 3 weeks after the injury and can still be in progress from 6 months to 2 years later. During this phase the scar changes and matures. The bulk decreases and the color changes from pink to pearly white. The incisional strength builds, and by the end of 8 weeks it is about 70% of its original strength. During remodeling collagen fibers are partially broken down by enzymes and reconfigured. Contraction due to the myofibroblasts can cause collagen fibers to become taut; scar tissue shrinks and cutaneous tissue becomes smaller. Tension lines are frequently visible on the cutaneous surface (outer skin) of scar tissue. Healed wounds achieve only part of the original tensile strength and therefore are at a greater risk of future breakdown. The remodeling phase leaves the affected area with only 65% to 80% of its original tissue strength, and the affected area will be more prone to reinjury in the future. The remodeling phase may last up to 2 years.

The nurse needs to teach the patient that the scar tissue will never reach its preinjury strength. Therefore, it is essential to protect it from trauma and overexposure to the sun to prevent future skin breakdown.

■ Wound Healing Assessment

There are many factors that influence the wound healing process or lack thereof. A wound develops as a result of some type of insult or injury. The body has a normal process for wound heal-

ing, as described earlier in the phases of healing. Many factors play a role in the progression or lack thereof in wound healing. These factors are critical elements for the phases of wound healing to proceed. Any factors that are not adequate will delay healing until they are sufficiently corrected. The nurse must be aware of the risk factors that may impact the rate of wound healing when assessing patients.

Vascular System: Macro and Micro

The vascular component to healing is the most essential of all components; without it, no phase of healing can begin and no hope of healing can occur. The vascular system consists of macrocirculation (large vessels such as the femoral or carotid arteries) and microcirculation (small vessels such as capillary beds or superficial artery systems). The vascular system is essential to deliver the clotting factors, oxygen, leukocytes, macrophages, prostaglandins, and growth factors that contribute to the healing process. Without adequate circulation, a wound will not heal. There are multiple tests that can determine circulation. Macrocirculation of the lower extremities can be tested by performing an ankle-brachial index (ABI). The measurement is a ratio of ankle systolic pressure to brachial systolic pressure. Normally, the ankle systolic pressure is at or slightly higher than the brachial systolic pressure. A ratio of less than 0.9 is indicative of circulatory disease in the lower extremities. The ABI is a noninvasive, inexpensive tool to determine whether additional testing for circulatory disease is warranted. Chapter 43 ⬢ further describes the ABI.

Other noninvasive tools to test circulation are Doppler studies that utilize ultrasound to test arterial blood flow and estimate arterial circumference and/or occlusion. An invasive study for circulatory evaluation is a femoral angiogram, whereby a catheter is inserted into the femoral artery and pictures are taken with enhancement by a dye that reveals actual blood flow and determines a percentage of blockages, if any. A procedure to restore circulatory flow to the lower extremities can be performed that utilizes a blade that cuts through the plaque and a vacuum suction to remove the plaque.

Microcirculation can be evaluated as well. Microcirculation involves the capillary beds that actually "feed" the wound area itself. A test, best known as a transcutaneous oxygen measurement (TCOM), can evaluate the tissue at a depth of one-fourth inch. The test utilizes an electrode that is heated to vasodilate the capillary bed. A solution is used as the medium for the diffusion of gases, including oxygen, and a measurement of the partial pressure of oxygen is recorded. Chart 67–1 notes the areas and partial pressures one expects to see for adequate circulation to heal.

Venous System

The venous system is also a component of and a factor in the wound healing process. The venous system returns the deoxygenated blood to the heart. The dilation of the venous system due to incompetent valves causes edema. The edema compresses the tissue and thus compresses the capillary beds and decreases circulation. Due to changes in capillary permeability in the edematous areas, fluid leaks into the local tissues. Infection then can set in as bacteria on the skin invade the area and are attracted to the fluid-filled medium.

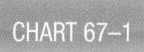

CHART 67–1   **Transcutaneous Oxygen Measurement (TCOM)**

PO$_2$

Chest 60–80 mmHg (reference lead).

Extremity 30–40 mmHg (desired).

If extremity < 30 mmHg, apply 100% O$_2$ and measure response.

If response increases PO$_2$ in mmHg, patient is possible candidate for hyperbaric oxygen therapy.

CHART 67–2   **Systemic and Situational Factors Impacting Wound Healing**

Smoking	Incontinence
Age 75 or over	Diaphoresis
Inadequate nutrition	Paralysis
Low albumin/protein	Neurological disease
Anemia	Immunosuppression
Dehydration	Infection
Immobility	Dementia
Edema	Cancer
Spasticity	Kidney disease
Contractures	Lung disease
Emphysema	Dermatologic conditions
Heart disease	Impaired circulation
Emaciation/cachexia	Obesity
Diminished sensation	Diabetes
Steroid use	Present pressure ulcers
Stress	Uncontrolled pain

A simple and noninvasive clue that there is venous insufficiency besides edema is the presence of hemosiderin staining (Figure 67–3 ■). Hemosiderin staining is a direct result of red blood cells that are "trapped" in the interstitial tissues and the breakdown of heme, or iron, into the tissue itself. Venous Doppler tests using ultrasound measure venous congestion and regurgitation (a direct result of incompetent valves) and can accurately detect venous insufficiency. Chapter 43 ☺ discusses peripheral vascular disease.

■ Risk Factors That Impact Wound Healing

Many important factors can cause a delay in wound healing. Some are directly controlled by the patient, whereas others have an effect that is less easily controlled by the patient. The following factors will be discussed: nutrition and hydration, infection, comorbid conditions, medications, stress, glucose control and diabetic management, smoking, and gerontological considerations. Chart 67–2 outlines systemic and situational factors impacting wound healing.

Nutrition and Hydration

Nutrition is one of the most understated and undervalued components of and factors in wound healing. Nutrients are essential for normal healing because malnutrition interrupts the rate of normal tissue repair. The diet must be high in protein and calories with vitamin and nutritional supplements. Proteins are the

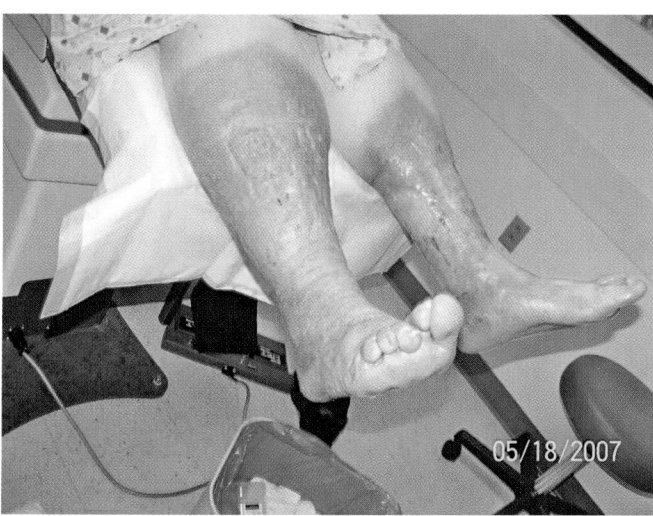

FIGURE 67–3 ■ Hemosiderin stain.
Source: Courtesy of Harold Engle

building blocks of collagen, a cellular matrix that forms the basis of tissue granulation. Micronutrients, those that are needed in small amounts, include the fat soluble vitamins A, D, E, and K and the water soluble vitamins C and the B family. Vitamins such as A, D, E, and K play a role in the wound healing process as cofactors, antioxidants, antiplatelet properties, cell membrane stability, and in other vital functions. Supplemental vitamins and nutritional supplements should be monitored.

Supplements that are high in proteins and vitamins can assist in replacing low levels of albumin and aid in the formation of collagen to "fill" the wound to a level depth. Supplemental amino acids include arginine, glutamine, and hydroxy-methyl butyrate (HMB). A therapeutic nutrition drink is available that contains all three amino acids; it is called Juven (Ross Products, Abbott Laboratories).

The need for nutrients continues throughout the healing process. Using every opportunity to get patients to take in nutrients can be a nursing challenge. A comprehensive nutritional assessment should be done for nonhealing and chronic wounds. Chart 67–3 (p. 2196) outlines the specific vitamins and nutrients and their roles in the wound healing process. Diagnostic tests to check protein levels are albumin and more recently prealbumin tests. Prealbumin helps to determine whether the decrease in albumin is due to dietary intake or some organic issue independent of dietary intake. Chapter 14 ☺ includes a discussion of albumin and prealbumin.

CRITICAL ALERT   *If prescribed diet allows, offer medications with one of the canned nourishment supplements or Instant Breakfast mixes. The opportunity to offer calorie-laden fluids can be helpful to those patients who have difficulty consuming enough calories.*

Maintaining adequate hydration assists in healing and decreases the risk of development of additional wounds. Proper hydration is often overlooked after intravenous fluids are discontinued. Offering patients fluids on a regular basis assists in

| CHART 67–3 | Essential Vitamins and Nutrients for Wound Healing |

Vitamin and Nutrients	Function in Wound Healing
Vitamin A	Stimulant for onset of wound healing process. Stimulant of epithelialization and fibroblast deposition of collagen.
B vitamins (B$_6$, B$_{12}$)	Critical to metabolism and to synthesis of protein, fat, and carbohydrate, but no reported benefits of vitamin B specific to wound healing.
Vitamin C	Collagen synthesis, capillary wall integrity, fibroblast function, and immunologic function.
Vitamin E	By fighting oxidative damage, it can be effective in reducing infection risk, but daily levels in excess of 100 international units retard healing.
Vitamin K	Essential for blood clotting (coagulation).
Iron	Excessive consumption could result in bacterial proliferation.
Zinc	Essential for protein synthesis and collagen formation. Necessary for formation of T lymphocytes, supporting immunity. Deficiency leads to decreased epithelialization and fibroblast proliferation.
Copper	Cofactor for connective tissue production. Collagen cross-linking.
Arginine (amino acid)	Produces nitric oxide, which is essential for collagen accumulation and angiogenesis, and enhances immunity.
Glutamine (amino acid)	Critical role in preserving nitrogen balance, protein synthesis, cellular structure, and metabolism. Source for cellular respiration.

maintaining hydration. Intake and output must be documented in order to monitor hydration status. Fluid intake should be measured every 24 hours if inadequate hydration is suspected. Chapter 14 ☺ includes a complete description of nutritional requirements.

Infection

Infection, the process of organisms invading and destroying cells, can also determine the rate of wound healing or lack thereof. Wounds can be contaminated, colonized, and infected. Contamination is the presence of bacteria on the wound surface with no multiplication of the bacteria. Colonization is the presence of bacteria that are multiplying on the wound surface but are not invading tissue. Infection means the bacteria are invading viable tissue. The presence of bacteria in pus, slough, or necrotic tissue does not mean the tissue is infected (McGuckin, Goldman, Bolton, & Salcido, 2003). Three basic elements must exist for a clinical definition of infection (Gardner & Frantz, 2004):

- Microorganisms must be present in viable tissue.
- Microorganisms must multiply enough to impair healing or cause injury.
- Invading microorganisms must produce a host response or tissue injury.

It is generally accepted that clinical infection in acute wounds has been correlated with tissue levels greater than 10^5 organisms per gram. To diagnose infection, laboratory microbiologic results must be evaluated in conjunction with local clinical findings. It is important to recognize the classic signs and symptoms of infection: erythema, heat, edema, pain, and purulent exudate. These symptoms are the host's response to invading organisms. These symptoms are reliable indicators of infection in acute wounds.

Infection requires the body to "fight" infection with white blood cells, macrophages, and leukocytes, and the attention to healing becomes secondary as the body focuses on the immediate problem of the infection at hand. Infection also leaves *bioburden*, or waste, that must then be disposed of before collagen synthesis and granulation can occur. Microorganisms such as methicillin-resistant *Staphylococcus aureus* (MRSA) and *Klebsiella pneumoniae* with a resistant erythromycin sensitive beta lactamase (ESBL) strain are now invading wounds. These multidrug-resistant strains require multiple antibiotics with long durations.

The tissue injury produced by microorganisms is more likely found in chronic wounds. These symptoms include delayed healing, friable granulation tissue that bleeds easily, discoloration, unexpected pain/tenderness, wound breakdown, and abnormal smell (Cutting & White, 2005; Gardner & Frantz, 2004). Nursing management includes obtaining a culture when ordered by the health care provider. It is important to know the proper procedure: Cleanse the wound thoroughly with saline; and then with the sterile culturette swab, apply pressure and roll the swab over and over a 1 centimeter square. The portion of the wound to be cultured can be anywhere within the wound bed; choose a spot where tissue fluid can be expressed by pressing with the swab. The purpose is to take a culture of the tissue fluid, not of the exudate on top of the wound. Tissue biopsy is the gold standard to determine infection, but this is not done by nurses and is not readily available in all institutions. The Diagnostic Tests box outlines laboratory and diagnostic findings related to wound healing.

Comorbidities

Comorbidities, which are concurrent disease processes, also affect the wound healing process. For example, diabetes, a disorder characterized by the inability to store glucose and thus the

DIAGNOSTIC TESTS Related to Wound Healing

Test and *Normal Values*	Expected Abnormality	Treatment
White blood cells (WBC): *4,500–11,000/mm³*	Increased with inflammation and acute infection. Decreased with thrombocytopenia, cancers, anemias, or liver disease.	Diagnose and track infection. WBC alone does not tell health care providers anything without differential.
Platelets: *150,000–400,000/mm³*	Increased with inflammation and infection. Indication of concealed bleeding (i.e., gastrointestinal [GI]).	Basic element of coagulation. Decreased count can drive treatment.
Red blood cells (RBC): *Female: 4–5.5 million/mm³* *Male: 4.5–6.2 million/mm³*	May be decreased due to bleeding from the wound. Menses in women. Renal disease. Decrease might indicate depleted blood volume. Chronic infections.	Monitor for need for medications or blood administration to increase value.
Hemoglobin (Hgb): *Female: 12–15 g/dL* *Male: 14–16.5 g/dL*	May be decreased due to bleeding from the wound, hypoxia, anemias, or overhydration. Some prescription medications can decrease count.	Monitor with hematocrit for need for medications or blood administration to increase value.
Hematocrit (HCT): *Female: 35–47%* *Male: 42–52%*	May be decreased due to bleeding from the wound.	Monitor for need for medications or blood administration to increase value.
Total proteins: *6.3–8.3 g/dL*	May be decreased with malnutrition. Decrease indicates immunosuppression.	Monitor need for nutritional supplements.
Serum albumin: *3.5–5.5 g/dL*	May be decreased with malnutrition injury because albumin catabolism increases as a result of injury.	Monitor need for nutritional supplements. Half-life is 21 days; easily influenced by medications and fluid status.
Serum prealbumin: *16–40 mg/dL*	Reflects immune and inflammatory status.	Current protein status.
Wound culture and sensitivity: *Negative*	Will be positive if there is contamination, colonization, or infection.	Assess for wound infection and which antibiotic will be effective in treating it.

Source: Adapted from Corbett, J. V. (2004). *Laboratory tests and diagnostic procedures with nursing diagnoses* (6th ed.). Upper Saddle River, NJ: Pearson Prentice Hall.

occurrence of elevated blood glucose levels, is the single most prevalent comorbidity in patients requiring chronic wound care. Diabetes causes neuropathy, or decreased sensation. (See the discussion on wound healing and diabetes later in this chapter.) Diabetes also interferes with the immune system and circulation by the hardening of the vessels and capillary beds. This hardening is the process whereby the vessel and capillary beds are infiltrated by fatty deposits that accumulate, cause localized damage to the endothelial lining of the vessel, and cause it to scar over repeated damage and healing.

Hypertension and atherosclerotic disease also cause problems with circulation and edema that compromise wound healing. Autoimmune disorders such as lupus or scleroderma decrease the body's ability to fight off infection; and when a wound is found in patients with these disorders, the delayed healing due to decreased immunity is evident.

Medications

Some medications can affect the wound healing process. Steroids decrease the immune system by delaying white blood cell migration and fibroblasts, thus impacting the inflammatory phase of wound healing. The ground matrix, collagen synthesis, regeneration of blood vessels, and epithelialization are also significantly delayed due to steroid use. One area of research now

in progress is in the use of retinoids, vitamin A, to combat these effects. Retinoids have been shown in some trials to combat the ill effects of steroids directly and potentially reverse some of their adverse effects (Wicke et al., 2000). Chemotherapy drugs, specifically methotrexate, can delay the wound healing process by decreasing the immune system as well as by bone marrow suppression and anemia. Communication with patients is crucial to develop a realistic plan of care. The medications they take are a necessity; therefore, the plan of care must include educating the patient that the process of wound healing will be delayed. Realistic timelines should be provided, as these will help decrease anxiety.

Stress

Stress causes a release of hormones, including glucocorticoids, which reduces the production of cytokines, an essential component of the inflammatory process. The glucocorticoids also alter leukocyte movement. Reduction in these two factors causes immunosuppression. Because wound healing begins with inflammation, if this phase becomes suppressed, there is a delay in wound healing. Previous research has demonstrated that stress was associated with a 25% to 40% delay in wound closure across the models tested (Marucha, 2005). Stress also causes catecholamine release, which in turn causes vasoconstriction that will reduce perfusion and oxygenation to subcutaneous tissue and wounds.

Minimizing the patient's level of stress will promote the progression of wound healing. Pain and noise are common stressors for hospitalized patients. When pain is present, energy is spent in enduring the pain and not in healing the wound. Control of pain with analgesics and diversional activities will help decrease stress.

Manipulation of the patient's environment will reduce external stressors. Nurses are in a unique position to control the patient's environment. The nurse needs to be sensitive to the environmental noise and mitigate it when possible. Chapter 12 🔗 provides an in-depth discussion of the impact of stress on the human body. The impact of stress on the immune system is discussed in Chapters 59 and 60 🔗.

Glucose Control and Diabetic Management

Glucose control is essential for normal healing. High levels of glucose impair wound healing, and it is important to control the blood sugar very early in wound care to maximize wound healing potential. For example, high glucose levels result in altered leukocyte functioning and increased risk of infection. Monitoring the daily blood glucose levels and HgA1c values is important and helps to educate the patient about the need for glucose control. Recommended HgA1c value is 6.5% (Frykberg, 2002). This roughly estimates a blood glucose level of 120 mg/dL. Optimal glucose control is currently 70 to 110 mg/dL. Assess the patient's knowledge of diabetes and glucose control, and reinforce areas where it is lacking. If necessary, a consultation with a diabetes educator can refresh the patient's knowledge and address knowledge deficits about the disease. Diabetes education classes provide a foundation for the beginning of a lifetime of disease management. High levels of glucose impair wound healing, and it is important to control the blood sugar very early in wound care management. Careful monitoring and blood sugar should extend beyond wound healing and into the remodeling phase.

Smoking

The association between cigarette smoking and delayed wound healing is a common phenomenon in the clinical setting. The effects of nicotine, carbon monoxide, and hydrogen cyanide contained in cigarettes are the culprits that impact the normal rate of wound healing. Nicotine has the following effects on the tissues, which result in delayed wound healing:

- It is a vasoconstrictor that reduces blood flow to the skin, resulting in a loss of oxygen and nutrients, ischemia, and impaired healing of injured tissue.
- It increases platelet aggregation, thereby increasing the risk of thrombotic microvascular occlusion and tissue ischemia.
- It reduces the proliferation of red blood cells, fibroblasts, and macrophages.

Carbon monoxide decreases oxygen transport and slows metabolism. Finally, hydrogen cyanide inhibits the enzyme systems necessary for oxidative metabolism and oxygen transport at the cellular level. The overall effect of smoking on wound healing is a slower healing process. Open wounds are at an increased risk for wound infection and increased scar formation. Patients should be advised to stop smoking prior to elective surgery or when recovering from wounds resulting from trauma, disease, or emergent surgery. The nurse needs to assess the patient for the clinical manifestations of delayed wound healing and report them to the health care provider.

Gerontological Considerations and Comorbidities

Age-related changes in skin occur normally. **Rete pegs** (or epidermal ridges) are protrusions in the fifth layer of the epidermis that extend down into the dermis to help anchor the epidermis to the dermis. In the elderly (as in neonates), the ridges are flatter, failing to anchor the epidermis and making it easier for the epidermis to slide away from the dermis, resulting in skin tears (Figure 67–8 ■, p. 2203). Additionally, sweat glands decrease production, which results in drier skin. The increased incidence of **xerosis** (a skin condition characterized dry, pruritic, cracked, or fissured skin with scaling and flaking) in persons over the age of 60 can be attributed to (1) a decrease in the lipid component of skin, (2) a loss in water retention, and (3) frequent fragranced baths and showering (Norman, 2003). There is decreased dermal thickness causing thinning of the skin, especially along lower legs and forearms, as evidenced by the prominence of skin tears on extremities. Fewer collagen and elastin fibers cause less elasticity (recoil) in the skin. The skin is less effective as a barrier against water loss and bruising. There is a natural loss of thermal regulation, tactile sensitivity, and pain perception. **Senile purpura**, another age-related change, is a type of hemorrhaging under the skin due to thinner, more fragile blood vessels. Senile purpura often occurs at the site of skin tears. All of these factors place an elderly person at higher risk of dehydration, skin tears, burns, and traumatic injury. In addition, wound healing is prolonged in older adults for the following reasons:

- Re-epithelialization takes almost twice as long.
- The rate of wound dehiscence is greater in older adults and thought to be due to the decreased tensile strength of the wound.
- A greater number of comorbidities results in prolonged wound healing. Healing may be prolonged by conditions that result in poor cardiac output or low oxygen-carrying capacity such as heart failure. Diabetes, peripheral vascular disease, and poor nutrition all result in longer healing times in any age population.

Careful attention to aged skin is good prevention. Emollient skin care products help the skin retain moisture. Protect arms and legs from sun and trauma with clothing. Consistent use of sunscreen also is beneficial to prevent skin breakdown. A review of medications that may affect skin is in order. Gentle cleansing and physical assistance are essential.

Preinjury Status

All of the factors described earlier impact the wound healing process. When a patient is admitted, it is essential to assess the physical and emotional status. Lifestyles and habits that will impact healing such as smoking and poor nutrition must be identified. Both physiological and psychological factors alter the rate of wound healing as well as morbidity and mortality. The longer the illness existed before surgery or trauma, and preinjury nutritional status both contribute to rate of wound healing and risk of infection.

■ Classification of Wounds and Treatment

Several classifications for wounds exist. This chapter covers the most common types of wounds: diabetic, venous, arterial, vasculitic, traumatic, cancer, and pressure wounds. They all come from different origins, and their plans of treatment vary based on wound type. Wound classifications are helpful when documenting wound assessment and care because they tell a history of the wound. For example, identifying a wound as chronic or acute provides an immediate awareness of the direction that wound care should follow and expectations of the healing process. **Chronic wounds** are defined as wounds that do not follow the expected sequence of repair in a timely and uncomplicated manner. **Acute wounds** are recent wounds that are either traumatic or iatrogenic in etiology. Examples of **traumatic wounds** are abrasions, blisters, cuts, bites, stab wounds, gunshot wounds, and burn injuries. **Iatrogenic wounds** include intravenous (IV) puncture sites, incisions, radiation-induced skin damage, and grafts. Acute wounds progress through the stages of wound healing normally.

Chronic wounds generally occur due to inadequate blood supply in the tissue, repeated prolonged insults to the tissue, and disruptive underlying pathologic processes. The wound healing cascade is interrupted at some point by systemic deficiencies or extrinsic insults. Examples of chronic wounds are pressure ulcers, diabetic ulcers, vascular ulcers, and fungating tumors. Wounds that do not respond to appropriate treatment within 6 weeks are considered chronic in nature and should be referred to a wound specialist.

The type of wound determines the basic plan of care and treatment for that wound, but keep in mind that everyone responds differently to treatment and that the plan must be individualized. Wound care is not just a science but an art, and "thinking outside the box" has led to a great many strides in aggressive wound care therapy. Described next are classifications to describe further the extent of damage and current phase of healing, including diabetic, venous, arterial, vasculitic, traumatic, pressure, pyoderma gangrenosum, cancer, pressure, fungal, partial thickness and full-thickness wounds, and skin tears.

Diabetic Wounds

Diabetic ulcers are the most common form of chronic ulcer seen in outpatient and inpatient settings (Frykberg, 2002). The most frequent areas to find a diabetic ulcer are on the plantar surface of the foot or toe/metatarsal head (Figure 67–4 ■). The mitigating factors that promote development of a wound in a patient with diabetes are neuropathy, macro/microvascular changes, and a slow, decreased immune response. Neuropathy is decreased or absent sensation in an area due to elevated blood glucose levels that over time affect the myelin sheath surrounding the nerves and degrade the sheath, exposing the nerves. The nerves then die over time without the

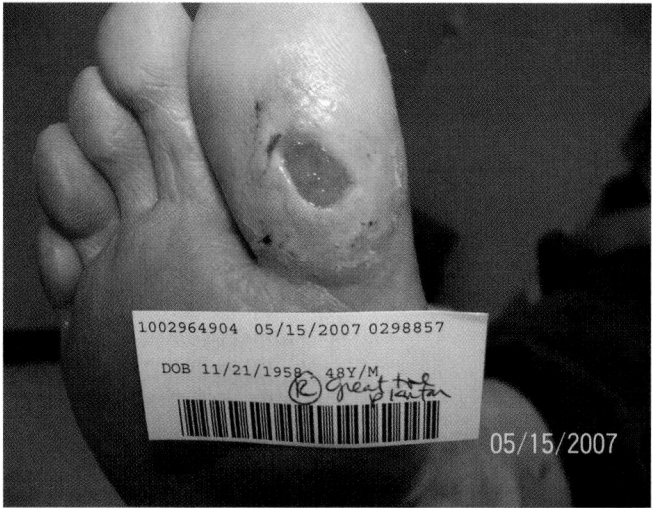

FIGURE 67–4 ■ Diabetic plantar ulcer.
Source: Courtesy of Harold Engle

myelin sheath to protect them from the body's own immune response.

Macro- and microvascular changes are due to elevated blood glucose levels that over time cause fatty deposits to stick to the endothelial lining of vessels and cause narrowing and then blockage of circulation (Porth, 2007). The immune response is also delayed in a patient with diabetes. Although the exact cause is unknown, it has been well documented that a slow response to a wound or infection, and thus slow-to-develop outward signs of a problem, causes a delay in the wound healing process and a delay in alerting the patient with diabetes that a problem is occurring. Delay in seeking care causes a delay in treatment (Shah & Hux, 2003).

Diabetic wounds usually appear on the feet but also may occur in other places on the body. These wounds are typically caused by traumatic injury to the foot because the patient with diabetes suffers from neuropathy, which may result in little or no sensation in the feet. Not being aware of the injury, the patient may continue to traumatize the wound by walking. Two reliable methods of classifying diabetic wounds exist. The original Wagner Ulcer Grade Classification System has been modified to take into account ischemia and infection along with depth of penetration (Chart 67–4). In this system ulcers graded with low scores are less complex. Higher scores indicate more complex ulcers that may require surgical intervention. Wagner's classification system is the

---

CHART 67–4   Wagner Ulcer Grade Classifications

A. Grade 1: Superficial diabetic ulcer

B. Grade 2: Ulcer extension
   1. Involves ligament, tendon, joint capsule, or fascia
   2. No abscess or osteomyelitis

C. Grade 3: Deep ulcer with abscess or osteomyelitis

D. Grade 4: Gangrene to portion of forefoot

E. Grade 5: Extensive gangrene of foot

most widely used to describe the natural history of the dysvascular foot, even though evidence of its validity and reliability are lacking (Smith, 2002). Smith (2002) proposes that the University of Texas Wound Classification System—known as the Size (Area and Depth), Sepsis, Arteriopathy, and Denervation (S[AD]SAD) classification system—will become the standard with a detailed breakdown regarding vascularity and infection. The University of Texas classification system for diabetic wounds is in Chart 67–5. New wound care products such as tissue engineered grafts and ointment containing platelet-derived growth factors (Regranex) have been effective treatments. Offloading (relieving the pressure from a specific site) still remains the most likely method of ensuring a plantar or heel ulcer will heal (Steinberg, 2004).

Medical Management

After reviewing the factors affecting a diabetic wound, a plan of care is developed that involves diagnostic studies to evaluate the extent of those factors. A test to check for neuropathy is called the loss of protective sensation (LOPS) test. LOPS uses a monofilament called 5.07 Semmes-Weinstein nylon monofilament, which measures sensation in eight areas in order to determine the extent of neuropathy (Wood et al., 2005). LOPS, arterial Doppler studies to check circulation, cultures of the wound, and basic chemistry and differentials are evaluated to correct any of those factors if possible. Differentials show the various types of immune cells that are present in the body. The main focus is on the percent of neutrophils, because the percentage goes up when an acute reaction occurs in response to infection. Neutrophils, also called PMNs or polymorphonuclear leukocytes, respond to inflammation and have phagocytic (microorganism-killing) properties. The other types of immune cells are eosinophils, which respond to parasitic infections and allergic reactions, and basophils, which respond to leukemia and myelo diseases of the muscle (Porth, 2007). One serious result of a diabetic wound is bone infection, or osteomyelitis. A diagnostic test such as magnetic resonance imaging (MRI), computed tomography (CT), bone scan, or indium scan (tagged white blood cells with indium, a radioactive material) can determine the presence of a bone infection. A biopsy of the bone can be performed as well. A biopsy can be read by a pathologist, and the shape or morphology of the tissue can be determined to be present with infection or not. If aggressive therapy and advance treatment modalities such as hyperbarics (100% oxygen under pressure) are not successful, an amputation may be necessary to protect the patient from an infection that spreads throughout the entire limb, body, and bloodstream. Offloading, the process of relieving pressure, should be accomplished, particularly in the plantar areas, so that compression of the microcirculation due to pressure does not occur. (See the discussion on offloading in the Wound Management section later in this chapter.)

Venous Ulcers

Venous ulcers are another type of chronic wound. Most venous ulcers are on the lower extremities and the pretibial area but can occur almost anywhere on the leg. One recent contributor to the number of venous ulcers that are now observed relates to the vein harvesting for coronary artery bypass grafting. Pregnancy and occupation can also lead to venous congestion and the development of venous ulcers. Venous ulcers are not well defined in their margins from an assessment standpoint. They are accompanied by edema and often hemosiderin staining. **Hemosiderin staining** occurs when the heme part of the red blood cell is deposited in the tissues as red blood cells get trapped and accumulate due to venous congestion (Figure 67–3 ■, p. 2195). As the red blood cell dies, the heme is deposited, and the staining color of brownish hue results. When venous congestion occurs in the lower extremities, the veins are stretched like a rubber band. Over time, the constant stretching of the veins decreases their elasticity (the ability for a rubber band to retract to its original position and shape). There are valves in the veins that open and close and allow venous return to the heart. If the veins become inelastic over time, the valves become incompetent or "leaky" and regurgitate the fluid, allowing pooling of the fluid in the lower extremities. The venous congestion, or edema, now compresses the capillary beds and constricts the fluid's flow in the dermis to feed the skin. If an injury occurs or the fluid accumulates so much that it leaks through the skin pores, bacteria can set in and an ulcer develops.

CHART 67–5	University of Texas Classification System for Diabetic Wounds			
Stage	**Grade 0**	**Grade I**	**Grade II**	**Grade III**
A	Preulcerative or postulcerative lesion completely epithelialized	Superficial wound not involving tendon, capsule, or bone	Wound penetrating to tendon or capsule	Wound penetrating to bone or joint
B	Preulcerative or postulcerative lesion completely epithelialized with infection	Superficial wound not involving tendon, capsule, or bone with presence of infection	Wound penetrating to tendon or capsule with presence of infection	Wound penetrating to bone or joint with presence of infection
C	Preulcerative or postulcerative lesion completely epithelialized with ischemia	Superficial wound not involving tendon, capsule, or bone with presence of ischemia	Wound penetrating to tendon or capsule with presence of ischemia	Wound penetrating to bone or joint with presence of ischemia
D	Preulcerative or postulcerative lesion completely epithelialized with infection and ischemia	Superficial wound not involving tendon, capsule, or bone with presence of infection and ischemia	Wound penetrating to tendon or capsule with presence of infection and ischemia	Wound penetrating to bone or joint with presence of infection and ischemia

Source: From Lavery, L. A., Armstrong, D. G., & Harkless, L. B. (1996). Classification of diabetic foot ulcerations. *Journal of Foot and Ankle Surgery, 35*(6), 528.

The decreased circulation does not allow the normal healing process to occur, as the platelets, growth factors, and leukocytes can no longer reach the area of insult and the ulcer becomes worse.

Medical Management

The treatment for the patient is to decrease the edema by compression. Compression therapy will allow pressure to be increased to the lower extremity to promote venous return and decrease venous congestion, allowing the capillary beds at the level of the wound to open and the healing process to occur. The patient should be instructed that the venous congestion is chronic and that, most often, the patient will have to undergo compression therapy of some type for the rest of his life to prevent further ulcers and associated complications. Compression can be achieved by the use of compression stockings, wraps, or a compression pump. One caution before using compression as treatment is to make sure the patient has adequate arterial circulation and no deep venous thrombosis. Performing venous and arterial Doppler ultrasounds can determine flow and presence or lack thereof of a deep venous thrombosis. Another caution is that compression therapy can lead to an increase in the patient's preload volume, and those patients with concurrent cardiac maladies such as heart failure and low ejection fractions may not tolerate the additional volume. These patients must see their cardiologist, and an adjustment on their diuretic therapy may need to occur. In addition to compression therapy, the wound may need to be débrided to allow the healing phases to begin.

Arterial Ulcers

Arterial wounds may perhaps take the longest to heal. They are often located on the malleolar area of the lower extremity (Figure 67–5 ■). They present with a "punched out" appearance with well-defined margins, unlike the venous ulcer. Associated assessment reveals poor palpable pulses and a Doppler may be needed to auscultate the pulse. The lower extremity is cool to the touch, discolored, and hair loss may be evident. Chart 67–6 presents a comparison of arterial and venous ulcers.

Medical Management

An arterial ulcer requires surgical intervention to restore the blood flow. A débridement of the wound should not occur until circulation is restored, because the wound cannot heal at all and a débridement, especially of protective dead skin, can actu-

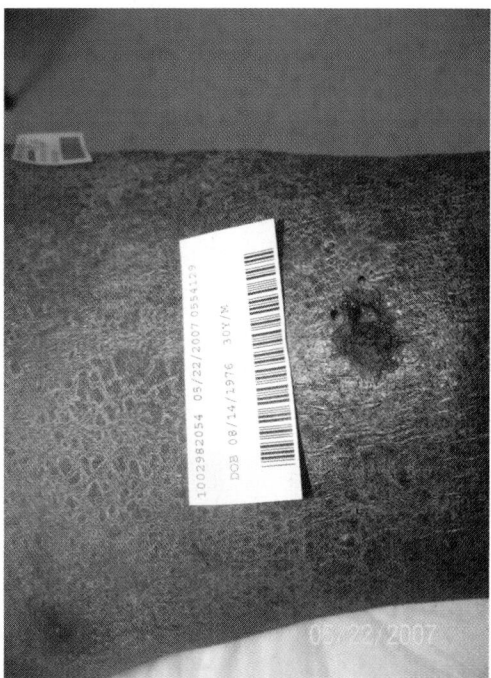

FIGURE 67–5 ■ Arterial ulcer.
Source: Courtesy of Harold Engle

ally worsen the ulcer. With arterial circulation restored, the process of débridement and wound healing can occur, over time.

Vasculitic Ulcers

Vasculitis is the inflammation of the vascular bed system at the micro and possibly macro level that is extremely painful (Figure 67–6 ■, p. 2202). Vasculitic ulcers are associated with collagen vascular disorders such as systemic lupus erythematosus (SLE) or rheumatoid arthritis. They can also occur in patients with other associated vasculitic conditions such as polyarteritis, livedo vasculitis, and Takayasu's disease. Vasculitic ulcers usually present as a small ulcer noted on the leg that appears at first to be benign and inconsequential but takes a long time to make any progress in healing. (Hiok, 1997). These ulcers are more prevalent in females. Vasculitic ulcers are some of the most painful ulcers that a patient can develop.

CHART 67–6   Differing Characteristics of Arterial and Venous Ulcers

Characteristic	Arterial Insufficiency Ulcer	Venous Stasis Ulcer
Location	Distal aspect of extremity (toe tips), pressure points on foot	Medial malleolus Distal and lateral aspects
Size and shape	Deep, small craters with well-defined margins	Normally limited to dermis; shallow subcutaneous tissue with irregular margins Can be "pinholes" through which serous fluid leaks
Wound bed	Pale or necrotic	Red or yellow slough, adhering or loose
Volume of exudate	Minimal	Normally large amount
Periwound skin appearance	Pale in color and faint erythema can be seen	Macerated, crusted, or scaling
Pain	Cramping or constant deep-aching pain	Variable; dull, aching, intermittent burning, etc.

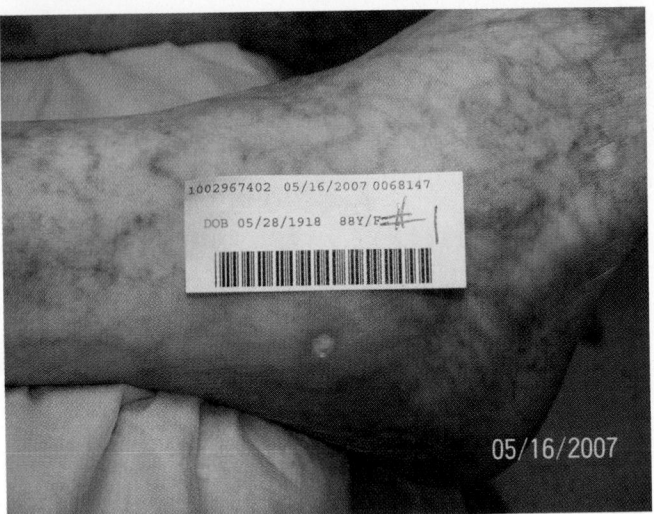

FIGURE 67–6 ■ Vasculitis.
Source: Courtesy of Harold Engle

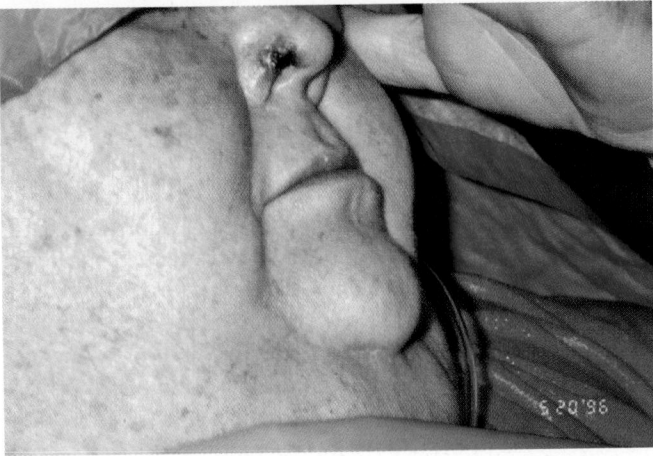

FIGURE 67–7 ■ Cancer lesion.
Source: Jan Clark

Medical Management

A biopsy can be taken to confirm the diagnosis of a vasculitic ulcer because the pathogenesis of the process is not fully known. Medications such as pentoxifylline, dapsone, calcium channel blockers, and corticosteroids have been used in the treatment of the ulcer.

Traumatic Wounds

Traumatic wounds develop from some type of blunt or sharp trauma. Adequate cleaning and removal of foreign debris are the most important steps in the healing of these wounds because infection causes a delay in the healing process. Comorbidities such as diabetes, heart failure, and autoimmune disorders may contribute to the severity and response to the healing process of these wounds.

Medical Management

Prophylactic antibiotic therapy can assist in the progress of healing. If an affected area is down to exposed bone, osteomyelitis is a risk. Skin grafts and flaps may be required to cover any areas of missing tissue that cannot be replaced. The patient and family must be educated on signs and symptoms of infection, dehiscence, or evisceration, discussed later in the chapter.

Pyoderma Gangrenosum

Pyoderma gangrenosum is an uncommon dermatosis that can be diagnosed with a biopsy of the affected skin. It presents as small red bumps that may look like an insect bite. The reddened areas open up over time as sores and have a reddish-purple hue around the margins. They most often occur on the legs but may affect other areas of the body as well. Pyoderma gangrenosum is rare and treatable but also may return in the future. Treatment may include a combination of corticosteroids and immunosuppressants in addition to good general wound care (MayoClinic.com, 2006).

Cancer

Wounds that have been identified as unable to heal over an extended period of time (months to years) and not classified as another type of wound may be suspected as cancerous (Figure 67–7 ■). A biopsy of the wound can confirm this suspicion. Usually, the wound has irregular margins, irregular hues of color, and the skin in the affected area may be friable and unhealthy in general appearance.

Medical Management

Removal of the affected cancerous lesions via surgery is the treatment of choice along with possibly immunosuppressants or radiation therapy, depending on severity. The patient should be instructed to inspect her skin vigilantly on a routine basis, have a caregiver inspect the hard-to-visualize areas of the body, and report any suspicious-looking areas to her primary health care provider or dermatologist.

Partial Thickness or Full-Thickness Wound Depths

The current discussion among wound care experts is that staging pressure ulcers should give way to a simpler method of describing injury that is appropriate for all wounds, including pressure ulcers: A wound is either a partial thickness or a full-thickness injury. Partial thickness wounds involve only the skin layers of the epidermis and/or part of the dermis. These wounds are shallow and appear bright pink to red. When they involve the dermis, the wounds may be pale pink with islets of red basement membrane. The **basement membrane** is a thin, acellular layer between the dermis and epidermis. It acts as scaffolding for the epidermis. Blood supply and nutrients reach the epidermis by passing through the basement membrane. Wound healing with partial thickness injuries occurs primarily by epithelialization, which is the migration of epithelial cells from the edges of the wound and from the base of hair follicles, sweat glands, and sebaceous glands. This process continues until the wound is healed.

Full-thickness wounds involve both the epidermis and the dermis and may extend into the subcutaneous tissue, fascia, muscle, and bone. Repair of full-thickness injuries occurs by granulation and wound contraction or with sutures or skin grafts. Chapter 68 ⊙ includes a diagram of partial versus full-thickness wound depth.

Medical Management

Partial thickness and full-thickness wounds require an assessment of all factors of wound healing for any deficiencies. Débridement is essential to stimulate the phases of healing and to keep the wound acute so that the body responds to those chemical signals. Prevention of infection and decreasing bioburden will also speed up the healing process. Finally, the proper choice of dressing to maintain an optimal healing environment will facilitate healing as well.

With proper wound management, partial thickness injuries involving only the superficial dermis heal spontaneously in about 2 weeks, and they usually cause no cosmetic or functional impairment. Partial thickness wounds involving the deep dermis heal spontaneously, but may require a prolonged period (greater than 21 days) to do so. These wounds may result in some scar or contracture formation. Closure of full-thickness injuries occurs by granulation, epithelial migration, contracture, and/or surgical intervention.

Skin Tear Classifications

Skin tears (Figure 67–8 ■) are common in elderly patients whose skin has become fragile and thin. Payne-Martin Classification for Skin Tears provides health care providers with a means to enhance

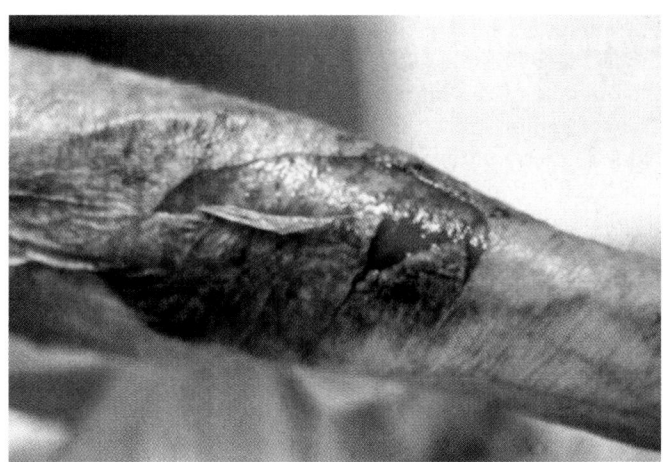

FIGURE 67–8 ■ Skin tear.
Source: Jan Clark

documentation and track outcomes of care. It improves assessment, prevention, and treatment of skin tears. The system uses three categories based on the amount of tissue lost (Chart 67–7).

Nurses should recognize patients at risk for skin tears. Some factors to be considered are age, condition of skin, use of steroids, unsteady balance and gait, easy bruising, and vision impairment. Prevention of skin tears includes avoiding use of harsh soaps and alcohol-based cleansers; using a patting motion to clean and dry skin; avoiding scrubbing skin; applying moisturizers; and adding padding to wheelchair arms, bed rails, and other objects that can do harm. Consider long sleeve clothing, long socks with the toes cut out, or commercial arm protectors to protect upper extremities. Educate staff, family, and caregivers to use caution in repositioning those patients at risk.

 CRITICAL ALERT *Nurses need to take special care when removing tape from patients' skin that is at high risk for skin tears. Hold the skin down as the tape is being pulled off. Best of all, do not use tape on the skin, but bandage and put the tape on the bandage.*

Medical Management

Treatment of skin tears should include irrigating the tear with saline and trying to reposition any skin flap back in place. Skin flaps that are kept moist are more likely to adhere and heal. Use of adhesive tapes or transparent films can result in additional skin tears. Steri-Strips stay in place but become crusted with dry blood and can harbor pathogens. Preferred dressings should be nonadherent such as foam, hydrogel sheets, and alginates that are absorbent and become gel like. Some health care providers handling wound care have had success with zinc-impregnated gauze wraps secured with an elastic-like tape, such as Coban, on the zinc wrap itself and not stretched tight. These dressings can be left for several days without being changed if the wound drainage is minimal.

Telfa dressings are also widely utilized for skin tears. Telfa is a nonstick application that protects the wound from outside injury or infection, has some absorptive properties, and allows the dressing to be removed without further damage to the skin.

CHART 67–7 **Payne-Martin Classification and Treatment for Skin Tears**

Category	Description
Category I:	Skin tear without tissue loss. A. Linear type: epidermis and dermis pulled apart as if an incision has been made. B. Flap type: epidermal flap completely covers the dermis to within 1 millimeter of the wound margin.
Category II:	Skin tear with partial tissue loss. A. Scant tissue loss: a loss of 25% or less of the epidermal flap. B. Moderate to large tissue loss: loss of more than 25% of the epidermal flap.
Category III:	Skin tear with complete tissue loss. No epidermal flap: black (necrosis), yellow drainage, pink or red granulation tissue completely exposed.
Treatment	
Appropriate skin tear treatment Little or no bleeding	Adhesive dressings or tapes should never be used to secure dressings onto fragile skin. A moisture barrier applied to periwound skin will help protect it and prevent further trauma. A gauze bandage wrapped around the extremity should be secured with tape onto the bandage, not the skin. Hydrogel sheet dressings or foam. Foam dressings.
Moderate bleeding	Zinc-impregnated gauze and cotton Webril wrapped around extremity, secured with Coban on bandage; none of it should be wrapped tightly.

Pressure Ulcers

Pressure ulcers develop when pressure causes decreased circulation to an area. The compression interferes with the tissue blood supply, leading to vascular insufficiency, tissue anoxia, and cell death, resulting in tissue necrosis. According to the National Pressure Ulcer Advisory Panel (NPUAP) (2007b), "A **pressure ulcer** is localized injury to the skin and/or underlying tissue usually over a bony prominence, as a result of pressure, or pressure in combination with shear and/or friction." Pressure ulcers are often related to the elderly, but that is not the only at-risk population for the disease. Patients with paraplegia, those with quadriplegia, those who have had strokes, patients with depression, and anyone who is not moving or will not move to relieve pressure off an affected area can develop a pressure ulcer. The most common areas of where pressure develops are those areas when lying in a bed or sitting in a chair or wheelchair that come in contact with the surface. Heels, sacral areas, ischial areas, and the lower back are the most common areas. Other areas include the elbows, the occiput of the head, the spine, and even the ears. The ears can develop pressure ulcers as a result of long-term oxygen use with a nasal cannula. The nasal cannula is held in position behind the ears, and time can cause that area to develop a pressure ulcer.

Etiology of Pressure Ulcers

Pressure ulcers occur when pressure, due to the compression of the skin between bone and another surface over time, impedes blood flow causing tissue ischemia leading to necrosis and ulcer formation. There can be deep internal pressure causing deep internal tissue damage with no evident epidermal damage, or the pressure can be evident first in the epidermal tissue. Pressure ulcers are caused by intrinsic and extrinsic factors. Intrinsic factors are defined as the internal conditions that exist related to the patient's physical or mental health such as nutritional status, mobility, incontinence, age, and skin condition. Extrinsic factors are derived from the environment such as skin hygiene, medication, shear, and friction. Shear occurs as the skeleton moves against the muscles and other internal structures, causing the tissues to be pulled in opposite directions. This causes the bone to rub against the internal structures and distorts the shape of the capillaries, causing them to be occluded and contributing to the formation of a pressure ulcer. Friction occurs when the body moves against an unyielding surface causing the epidermis to be stripped away and ulcers to form (Baranoski, 2006). Common sites for pressure ulcers are seen in Chart 67–8.

CHART 67–8	Common Sites for Pressure Ulcers

Patient Position	Pressure Ulcer Sites
Supine	Scapula, occiput, sacrum, heels
Lateral	Ear, shoulder, trochanter, medial knee, malleolus, foot edge
Prone	Nose, forehead, chest, iliac crests, foot edge, toes

Risk Factors for Pressure Ulcer Development

Risk factors have been identified that make a patient more prone to the development of a pressure ulcer. Risk assessment requires the evaluation of the presence of those factors. Patients who have restricted activity, as would occur with quadriplegia, strokes, and fractured hips, are at risk. Not only are these patients inactive, but they also may have decreased sensation preventing them from feeling the pain associated with the development of a pressure ulcer. Patients with poor nutrition are more susceptible. Patients who are very thin or have decreased protein in the diet have skin that is more likely to ulcerate. Patients who have urinary or fecal incontinence or are exposed to other types of moisture such as perspiration, wound drainage, or emesis are more prone to ulcers. Moisture causes a weakening of the cell wall of skin cells and changes the protective pH of the skin, making the skin more susceptible to skin breakdown (Arnold, 2003). The existence of a comorbid condition such as diabetes mellitus, hypertension, respiratory disease, or vascular disease also increases the risk for pressure ulcers.

Pressure Ulcer Staging

Pressure ulcers are staged according to depth of injury. In 1994 the National Pressure Ulcer Advisory Panel (NPUAP) followed the example of the International Association of Enterostomal Therapists (now known as the Wound, Ostomy and Continence Nurses Society) and adopted Shea's descriptions of pressure sores as a classification system of staging pressure ulcers according to the depth of tissue involved. A staging classification system was developed to allow for consistency in the assessment and description of these wounds; however, it should be noted that a wound that is necrotic and covered with eschar cannot be staged because the depth cannot be measured. The National Guidelines box outlines the NPUAP's four stages of pressure ulcers (2007b). In 1992 these stages were incorporated into the clinical practice guidelines for prevention and treatment of pressure ulcers by the Agency for Health Care Policy and Research (AHCPR) (which is now the Agency for Healthcare Research and Quality, or AHRQ). Stage I pressure ulcers were redefined in 1997 to reflect the new knowledge of accumulated clinical experience. The new definition included more subtle skin changes detected by skilled wound/skin assessments, such as skin temperature, tissue consistency, and color inconsistencies of dark skin tones. In 2002, NPAUP proposed a new description, *deep tissue injury* (DTI) to describe the purple ecchymotic injury seen in intact skin that indicates pressure-related injury to subcutaneous tissues, which may develop into a Stage III or IV pressure ulcer even with optimal treatment. Staging describes the tissue involved in a pressure ulcer, but it alone does not provide a basis for determining topical treatment of wounds. Only pressure ulcers can be staged with this classification system (Figure 67–9 ■, p. 2206). Skin tears, diabetic ulcers, surgical wounds, and burn injuries each have their own classification system. Once the ulcer begins to heal, it is not appropriate to use the staging in a reverse order to describe healing. Once an ulcer has reached a certain stage, such as Stage IV, it is always considered a Stage IV ulcer.

Scales for Predicting Pressure Score Risk

Several risk assessment tools exist to determine the probability of pressure ulcer development. They include the Gosnell, Nor-

NATIONAL GUIDELINES for Pressure Ulcer Staging from the National Pressure Ulcer Advisory Panel

Stage of Wound	Guideline
Deep tissue injury (DTI)	Deep tissue injury is a new stage that is characterized by purple or maroon tissue over bony prominence areas from pressure or shear with intact skin. It often feels "boggy" (soft) or indurated (hard). It should be classified as a DTI, and close monitoring for further deterioration should be performed.
Stage I	Intact skin with nonblanchable area of redness. A keynote for other clues, especially for those with darker skin tones, is any change in color, warmth, edema, or pain over a bony prominence area of pressure.
Stage II	Classified most often as an open or fluid-filled blister. Partial thickness avulsion of skin into dermis layer and may present as a shallow open ulcer.
Stage III	Involves full-thickness loss in which the hypodermis or subcutaneous fat layer may be exposed. It may be shallow or deep, depending on the amount of hypodermis tissue.
Stage IV	Full-thickness wound with exposed tendon, muscle, and/or bone. Most often has slough (dead cells) or eschar (dead tissue). Assessment for undermining and tunneling is prudent as they most often accompany this stage of wound. Again, one cannot use depth to determine the stage because certain anatomic locations may have less depth to tendon, muscle, and/or bone.
Unstageable	Eschar and/or slough that covers the wound area cannot be staged because the underlying tissue cannot be assessed. It is therefore classified as unstageable until the eschar is removed, and then the wound should be documented related to its defining characteristics.

Source: National Pressure Ulcer Advisory Panel (NPUAP). (2007b). Updated staging system. Pressure ulcers stages revised by NPUAP. Retrieved September 1, 2007, from http://www.npuap.org/pr2. htm. "Reproduction of the National Pressure Ulcer Advisory Panel (NPUAP) materials in this document does not imply endorsement by the NPUAP of any products, organizations, companies, or any statements made by any organization or company."

ton, Braden Scale, and other versions developed for specific institutions or populations or for items considered such as concurrent pressure ulcer, comorbidities, age, and continence issues. The Braden Scale for Predicting Pressure Sore Risk is the most widely used and most clinically validated tool that allows nurses and other health care providers to score a patient's level of risk for developing pressure ulcers reliably (Figure 67–10 ■, p. 2207). There are institutional variations of the Braden scale to serve special populations such as in pediatric and intensive care units. The scale consists of six categories with subscales: sensory perception, moisture, activity, mobility, nutrition, and friction and shear. Each category and subscale condition needs to have a score assigned to it for an individual patient. The first category is sensory perception. The patient can be awake and alert with no impairment, partially paralyzed or in a coma and totally unresponsive, and anywhere in between. The nurse decides where on that range the patient is closest. The moisture score pertains to perspiration as well urinary and fecal incontinence. Activity refers to bed rest, up to chair, ambulate, and up ad lib. The subscales of nutrition are given very specific parameters. Some institutions have substituted prealbumin values in some of the ranges. Each category is assigned a score of 1 to 4 with the exception of friction and shear. The scores are assigned and added up. Lower scores indicate higher risk of pressure ulcer development. The highest score is 23 and the lowest is 6. A score of 18 or lower indicates a risk for pressure ulcer development. The nurse can look at the subscales and identify specific risks and implement prevention interventions.

A second widely used scale to predict the risk for pressure ulcer development is the Norton Scale (Figure 67–11 ■, p. 2208). It was originally developed in 1960, was subsequently modified, and is still being used (Halek & Mayer, 2002). The modified Norton Scale uses a point system to assess the patient's physical condition, mental condition, activity, mobility, and incontinence. Points are assigned to each area based on the nurse's assessment. Higher points are assigned to higher function. Therefore, a score of 25 or less places a patient at risk for pressure ulcers. The lower the score, the higher the risk for the development of a pressure ulcer. The risk is identified as: low (25–24 points); medium (23–19 points); high (18–14 points); and very high (13–9 points).

Pressure ulcer prevention interventions should be outlined in the institution's policy and procedure manual and be based on the recommendations of the nationally accepted standards of care for pressure ulcers: the Agency for Health Care Policy and Research (AHCPR) Publication No. 92-0047, *Pressure Ulcers in Adults: Prediction and Prevention* (1992), and Publication No. 95-0652, *Treatment of Pressure Ulcers in Adults* (1994). The subsequently published Wound, Ostomy and Continence Nurses Society's (WOCN) *Guideline for Prevention and Management of Pressure Ulcers* (2003) is a secondary review of the literature and an establishment of a level of evidence rating. It supports the findings and recommendations of the original AHCPR guidelines, with the agency now known as the Agency for Healthcare Research and Quality (AHRQ).

Medical Management

Prevention is the key to pressure ulcers, and education of the patient and family/caregiver can provide the patient with the ability to prevent or at least minimize the development in the future. Once a pressure ulcer develops, the goals of treatment are to maintain or improve oxygenation to the area, prevent infection, and promote healing. Many products may be used to treat pressure ulcers. Some work by absorbing exudate and keeping the skin dry; some products débride the wound, whereas others are used for protection and insulation of the wound. Treatment decisions are generally guided by the stage of the ulcer. For Stage I

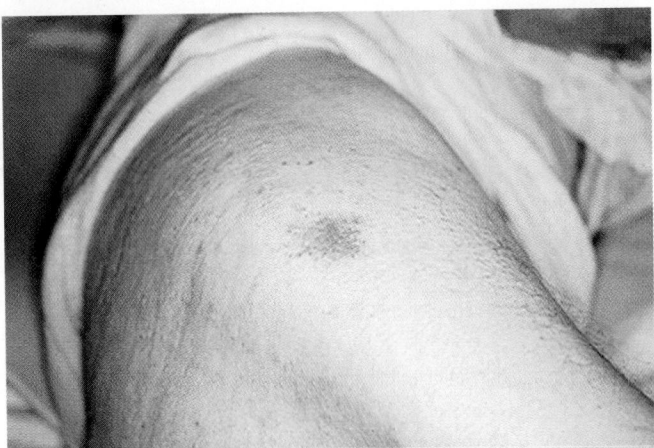

1.

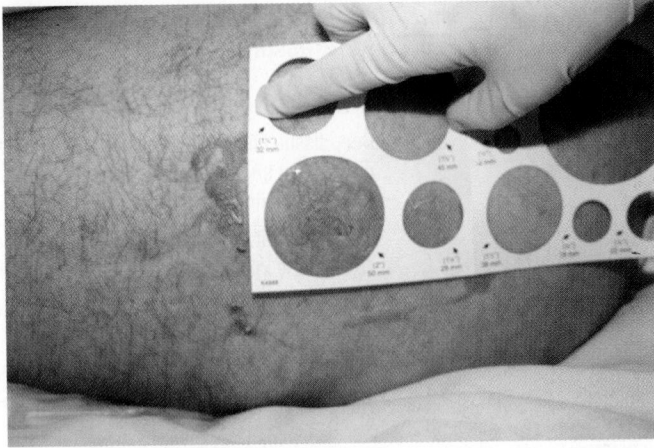

2.

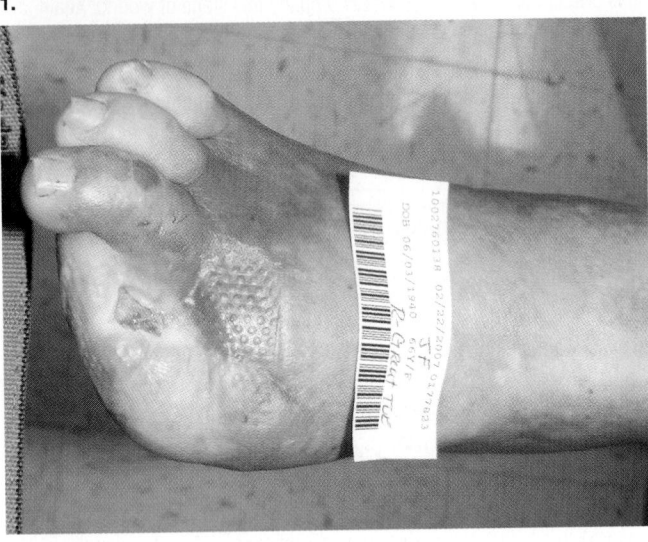

3.

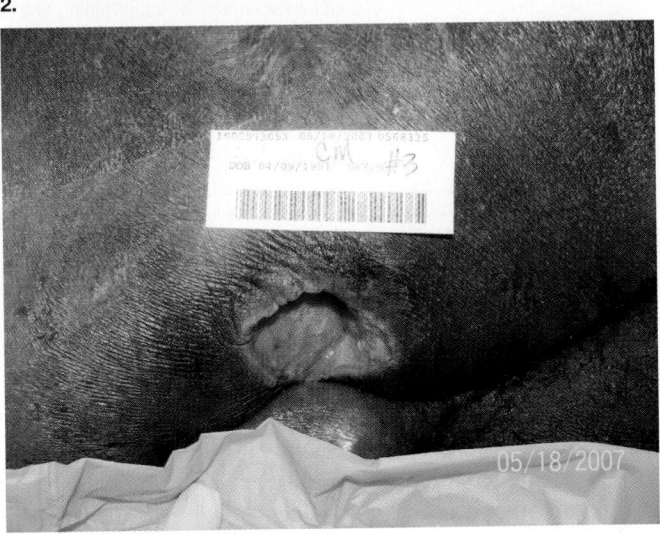

05/18/2007

4.

FIGURE 67–9 ■ Four stages of pressure ulcers.
Source: 1, 3, 4: Courtesy of Harold Engle; 2: Jan Clark

ulcers, frequent turning and removal of pressure should be done to prevent progression of the ulcer. Stage II and Stage III ulcers need a moist healing environment. Stage IV wounds maybe require débridement either surgically or mechanically through dressings or enzymes. Normal saline, hydrogen peroxide, or other commercial cleansers can be used to clean the ulcer. Minimal pressure should be used during cleaning to avoid trauma to the tissues in the wound bed. Topical dressings may be used to protect the wound and keep it moist and insulated. It may be necessary to pack the wound to fill dead space and tunnels. Adjunct therapies such as hyperbaric oxygen, application of growth factor, biosynthetic agents, and negative pressure therapy may be used, which are discussed later in this chapter.

Nursing Management

Once a pressure ulcer develops, the nurse is responsible for assessing the wound at periodic intervals for improvement and response to treatment. The nursing process provides a framework for the management of patients with pressure ulcers. An assessment of pressure ulcers starts with accurate documentation. The Centers for Medicare & Medicaid Services (CMS) is changing how one codes a pressure ulcer. A pressure ulcer will now be coded as community acquired (outside of the area one is working) or hospital acquired (developed in the area in which one is working). CMS will not reimburse for hospital acquired pressure ulcers, and documentation is the key on admission of the patient.

Assessment

An in-depth assessment can identify patients at risk, and actions can be taken to prevent the development of a pressure ulcer. The National Institute for Health and Clinical Excellence (NICE, 2005) supports that the skin should be inspected daily to observe for any changes in skin condition. The nurse must assess and document the location of the wound because that can provide clues about the cause of the ulcer. A wound on the ischial tuberosity would suggest pressure during sitting, whereas a wound over the sacrococcygeal area indicates shear along with pressure (Arnold, 2003). The size of the wound should be assessed and documented with the patient in the same position each time. The wound's greatest length, greatest width, and depth at the deepest point should be noted. It is important to identify any sinus tracts or undermining, and the presence of any foreign bodies in the wound. The "red, yellow, black" system (see the Wound Assessment section later in this

Braden Risk Assessment Scale

NOTE: Bed and chairbound individuals or those with impaired ability to reposition should be assessed upon admission for their risk of developing pressure ulcers. Patients with established pressure ulcers should be reassessed periodically.

Patient Name: _____ Room Number: _____ Date: _____

Sensory Perception	1. Completely Limited	2. Very Limited	3. Slightly Limited	4. No Impairment	Indicate Appropriate Numbers Below
Ability to respond meaningfully to pressure-related discomfort	Unresponsive (does not moan, flinch or grasp) to painful stimuli, due to diminished level of consciousness or sedation. OR limited ability to feel pain over most of body surface.	Responds only to painful stimuli. Cannot communicate discomfort except by moaning or restlessness. OR has a sensory impairment which limits the ability to feel pain or discomfort over 1/2 of body.	Responds to verbal commands, but cannot always communicate discomfort or need to be turned. OR has some sensory impairment which limits ability to feel pain or discomfort in 1 or 2 extremities.	Responds to verbal commands. Has no sensory deficit which would limit ability to feel or voice pain or discomfort.	
Moisture	**1. Constantly Moist**	**2. Very Moist**	**3. Occasionally Moist**	**4. Rarely Moist**	
Degree to which skin is exposed to moisture	Skin is kept moist almost constantly by perspiration, urine, etc. Dampness is detected every time patient is moved or turned.	Skin is often, but not always, moist. Linen must be changed at least once a shift.	Skin is occasionally moist, requiring an extra linen change approximately once a day.	Skin is usually dry. Linen only requires changing at routine intervals.	
Activity	**1. Bedfast**	**2. Chairfast**	**3. Walks Occasionally**	**4. Walks Frequently**	
Degree of physical activity	Confined to bed.	Ability to walk severely limited or non-existent. Cannot bear own weight and/or must be assisted into chair or wheelchair.	Walks occasionally during day, but for very short distances, with or without assistance. Spends majority of each shift in bed or chair.	Walks outside the room at least twice a day and inside room at least once every 2 hours during waking hours.	
Mobility	**1. Completely Immobile**	**2. Very Limited**	**3. Slightly Limited**	**4. No Limitations**	
Ability to change and control body position	Does not make even slight changes in body or extremity position without assistance.	Makes occasional slight changes in body or extremity position but unable to make frequent or significant changes independently.	Makes frequent though slight changes in body or extremity position independently.	Makes major and frequent changes in position without assistance.	
Nutrition	**1. Very Poor**	**2. Probably Inadequate**	**3. Adequate**	**4. Excellent**	
Usual food intake pattern	Never eats a complete meal. Rarely eats more than 1/3 of any food offered. Eats 2 servings or less of protein (meat or dairy products) per day. Takes fluids poorly. Does not take a liquid dietary supplement. OR is NPO and/or maintained on clear liquids or I.V.'s for more than 5 days.	Rarely eats a complete meal and generally eats only about 1/2 of any food offered. Protein intake includes only 3 servings of meat or dairy products per day. Occasionally will take a dietary supplement. OR receives less than optimum amount of liquid diet or tube feeding.	Eats over half of most meals. Eats a total of 4 servings of protein (meat, dairy products) each day. Occasionally will refuse a meal, but will usually take a supplement if offered. OR is on a tube feeding or TPN regimen which probably meets most of nutritional needs.	Eats most of every meal. Never refuses a meal. Usually eats a total of 4 or more servings of meat and dairy products. Occasionally eats between meals. Does not require supplementation.	
Friction and Shear	**1. Problem**	**2. Potential Problem**	**3. No Apparent Problem**		
	Requires moderate to maximum assistance in moving. Complete lifting without sliding against sheets is impossible. Frequently slides down in bed or chair, requiring frequent repositioning with maximum assistance. Spasticity, contractures or agitation lead to almost constant friction.	Moves feebly or requires minimum assistance. During a move, skin probably slides to some extent against sheets, chair restraints, or other devices. Maintains relatively good position in chair or bed most of the time, but occasionally slides down.	Moves in bed and in chair independently and has sufficient muscle strength to lift up completely during move. Maintains good position in bed or chair at all times.		

NOTE: Patients with a total score of 16 or less are considered to be at risk of developing pressure ulcers.
(15 or 16 = low risk; 13 or 14 = moderate risk; 12 or less = high risk)

Total Score: _____

© Copyright Barbara Braden and Nancy Bergstrom, 1988

FIGURE 67–10 ■ Braden Risk Assessment Scale.

Source: Barbara Braden and Nancy Bergstrom.

The Norton Scale

NOTE: Scores of 14 or less rate the patient as 'at risk'

	Physical Condition		Mental Condition		Activity		Mobility		Incontinence		Total Score
	Good	1	Alert	1	Ambulant	1	Full	1	Not	1	
	Fair	2	Apathetic	2	Walk/help	2	Slightly	2	Occasional	2	
	Poor	3	Confused	3	Chairbound	3	Limited	3	Usually-urine	3	
	Very bad	4	Stupor	4	Bedridden	4	Very limited, Immobile	4	Doubly	4	
Name: Date:											
Name: Date:											
Name: Date:											
Name: Date:											
Name: Date:											
Name: Date:											
Name: Date:											
Name: Date:											

FIGURE 67–11 ■ Norton Scale.

Source: Doreen Norton, Rhoda McLaren, and A. N. Exton-Smith, *An Investigation of Geriatric Nursing Problems in Hospital,* copyright National Corporation for the Care of Old People (now Centre for Policy on Ageing), London, 1962.

chapter) is often used to describe the wound bed with black indicating eschar, yellow indicating subcutaneous tissue or devitalizing necrotic tissue, and red indicating the presence of muscle or granulation tissue (Arnold, 2003). The color of the wound bed can provide information about the vascular supply, presence of infection, nutritional status, and presence of healthy versus necrotic tissue. The presence of exudates should be noted, paying particular attention to the amount, color, consistency, and odor. The characteristics of the exudates can provide clues to the presence and type of infection. The presence of pain both during dressing changes and separate from dressing changes should be noted. Periwound description, drainage, presence of infection, and tissue type (eschar, slough, and granulation) are also to be recorded. Record a concise history with comorbidities, past treatments, pain scale, and any psychosocial aspects that impact the plan of care. Risk scales such as the Braden scale or Norton Scale should be performed to identify those at risk. Interventions will be derived from the risk score.

Newer technology includes pressure mapping, which is a form of computerized technology that allows for the assessment of areas of increased pressure. A thin mattress or sensor pad is placed under the patient and is connected to a computer screen. The screen then shows the patient's pressure points (Hanson,

Langemo, Anderson, Hunter, & Thompson, 2006). This allows the nurse to identify patient positions that may increase the risk of the development of pressure ulcers and to evaluate the use of a variety of support surfaces.

Nursing Diagnoses

The following nursing diagnoses are related to pressure ulcers:

- *Risk for Infection*
- *Impaired Tissue Integrity*
- *Ineffective Tissue Perfusion*
- *Disturbed Body Image.*

Planning

A collaborative and comprehensive approach to wound care is essential. Many hospitals have wound care protocols, and others have wound care nurses or teams designed specifically to accomplish the task of leading the plan of care. Dieticians, case managers, social workers, consultative health care providers (cardiovascular, infectious diseases, surgeons, and plastic surgeons), nursing staff, and ancillary staff should be part of the plan of care, as all play a role in the prevention and treatment of pressure ulcers. The plan must focus on alleviating pressure, treatment of existing ulcer with sound wound care, education, nutrition, rehydration, mobility, and bed support surfaces (if applicable). Here are some examples of interventions as they relate to the Braden scale scores:

Low Risk (15–18)

1. Keep skin clean and dry.
2. Use moisturizer on dry skin.
3. Do not massage bony prominences.
4. Protect skin from moisture; use underpads and briefs.
5. Use skin-protecting ointments (Aloe Vesta or equivalent) to protect skin exposed to urine, stool, or wound drainage.
6. Decrease friction and shear.
7. Increase mobility and activity as tolerated.
8. Assess skin daily.

Moderate Risk (13–14)

1. ALL OF THE ABOVE+
2. Wound care coordinator evaluation.
3. Use lift pads/trapeze (trapeze requires health care provider's order) to minimize friction and shear.
4. Consider a pressure reduction device on the beds and chair.
5. Consider utilizing a turning schedule.
6. Encourage proper dietary intake, and consider a dietician consult.
7. If bed- or chair-bound, reposition the patient every 1 to 2 hours.
8. Protect heels and elbows; elevate heels off the bed surface, and use pillows between knees.
9. Increase mobility and activity in patients that are bed- or chair-bound.

High Risk (10–12)

1. ALL OF THE ABOVE +
2. Consult dietitian and wound care coordinator evaluation (must enter as consult evaluations in computer).
3. Elevate head of bed only as necessary for meals, treatments, and as medically necessary.
4. Obtain order from health care provider for pressure reduction/relief therapeutic bed.

Note: Low air loss beds do not substitute for turning.

Very High Risk (9 or below)

1. ALL OF THE ABOVE+
2. Obtain order from health care provider for pressure relief therapeutic bed.

A head-to-toe assessment can determine areas where pressure ulcers are already developed or at-risk areas. Bed support services can reduce or relieve pressure as can gel cushions for wheelchairs. Pressure mapping, as described earlier, can determine a patient's "hot areas" where pressure in a wheelchair is the most intense, and a special wheelchair pad can be customized to redistribute the pressure to other areas of less concern.

Outcomes and Evaluation Parameters

In an acute care setting in which an average length of stay is 4 to 5 days, one will not see great improvement of a pressure ulcer in regard to dimensions. However, changes in the amount of drainage, the size and appearance of the periwound area, and the clinical manifestations of infection are noticeable in this time frame. At a minimum, one should not see regression of the pressure ulcer.

The National Pressure Ulcer Advisory Panel (NPUAP) developed a tool to document healing of the pressure ulcer. This tool, known as the Pressure Ulcer Scale for Healing (or PUSH) tool, requires assessing and scoring of the ulcer based on three elements: length times width, exudate amount, and tissue type. The scores are summed and graphed over time so that changes in the ulcer can be monitored. If the score goes down, the wound is healing; and if the score goes up. the wound is deteriorating (NPUAP, 1998). Other methods for evaluation may be similar to the PUSH tool in looking at other factors in healing. An example of the PUSH tool is shown in Chart 67–9 (p. 2210) (NPUAP, 2007a).

Interventions and Rationales

The first intervention is to relieve the pressure. It may be as easily accomplished as using pillows to offload, turning at least every 2 hours or less, or as concrete as pressure reduction or relief devices such as the bed support surfaces. It may require an offloading device such as a shoe or sometimes a total contact cast. The rationale for this first intervention is obvious, as the source of the ulcer was the pressure. Next the existing pressure ulcer must be treated with good wound care and an appropriate selection of dressings. An appropriate dressing promotes the optimum wound environment and serves as protection from outside insult. Dressings are described in detail in the Wound Management section later in this chapter.

The nurse must also assess for incontinence with regard to the specific area around the perineum. Incontinence causes the skin to break down. Acids from the urine and/or stool, along with a warm, moist environment, can be an enhancement for fungal and yeast growth. Moisture barrier and antifungal/antiyeast creams protect and promote good healthy skin in an environment where incontinence occurs. One may also consider an indwelling catheter or a diverting colostomy to remove the incontinence from an existing pressure ulcer.

Nutrition supplementation is an essential intervention. Protein is the building block for collagen synthesis, interstitial fluid balance, granulation, and epithelialization. Vitamins and minerals support the chemical agents of healing as cofactors. Vitamins also have antioxidant properties to prevent free radical formation and ensure healthy skin reproduction. ProMod or other supplements can be added to gastrostomy feedings or as dietary supplements on trays. The patient should have an intake of sufficient calories and protein to prevent weight loss and maintain normal prealbumin levels.

Baths should be given only when needed to avoid drying out the skin. When bathing, use gentle cleansers with warm, not hot,

CHART 67–9	**NPUAP PUSH Tool**

Observe and measure the pressure ulcer. Categorize the ulcer with respect to surface area, exudate, and type of wound tissue. Record a sub-score for each of these ulcer characteristics. Add the sub-scores to obtain the total score. A comparison of total scores measured over time provides an indication of the improvement or deterioration in pressure ulcer healing.

Length × Width	0	1	2	3	4	5	Sub-score
	0 cm²	<0.3 cm²	0.3–0.6 cm²	0.7–1.0 cm²	1.1–2.0 cm²	2.1–3.0 cm²	
		6	7	8	9	10	
		3.1–4.0 cm²	4.1–8.0 cm²	8.1–12.0 cm²	12.1–24.0 cm²	>24.0 cm²	
Exudate Amount	0	1 Light	2 Moderate	3 Heavy			Sub-score
	None						
Tissue Type	0	1	2	3	4		Sub-score
	Closed	Epithelial Tissue	Granulation Tissue	Slough	Necrotic Tissue		
							Total Score

Source: National Pressure Ulcer Advisory Panel (NPUAP). (2007a). Updated staging system. Retrieved October 1, 2007, from http://www.npuap.org/push3-0.htm. "Reproduction of the National Pressure Ulcer Advisory Panel (NPUAP) materials in this document does not imply endorsement by the NPUAP of any products, organizations, companies, or any statements made by any organization or company.

water. The skin should be kept well hydrated with nonalcohol moisturizers used for dry skin. Friction during bathing and massage over bony prominences should be avoided because it can cause additional tissue damage. It is important to use proper positioning and to use techniques to avoid friction when moving the patient. Friction can also be avoided by using cornstarch. If incontinence occurs, the skin should be cleansed at the time of soiling, a topical moisture barrier should be applied, and absorbent underpads or briefs should be used to provide a quick drying surface.

Positioning is important in the prevention of pressure ulcers. The goal is to get the patient mobile and active as soon as possible; however, when mobility is physically impossible, the patient's position should be changed a minimum of every 2 hours. A sufficient number of people should be available to move the patient so that shearing and friction during movement can be avoided. Assistive devices such as transfer boards or mechanical lifts may be helpful to minimize tissue injury during movement. The "rule of 30" is used for positioning. This rule states that the head of the bed should be elevated 30 degrees or less and the body placed in a 30-degree laterally inclined position when placed on either side. These positions avoid pressure directly over the trochanter and promote improved circulation to the skin over the sacrum and ischial tuberosities (Black et al., 2007). Pillows or foam wedges may be used to keep the patient properly positioned. The prone position may also be used if the patient is able to tolerate it. Attention should be focused on maintaining proper alignment so that functional ability can be maintained.

Education is the main key to keeping the plan of treatment on the right track postdischarge. The next level of care must be communicated too as far as the plan of care and past failures and successes. The family must be active participants if the patient is being discharged home. Home health help may be needed to continue support and evaluation as well as continued education. The patient and family must know how to prevent further pressure ulcers from developing as well as early intervention and the

resources available to them. Education is essential for the future success of the patient with pressure ulcers, as most often the conditions are chronic and the environment for continued deterioration still exists.

Evaluation

A plan for care of pressure ulcers should be reevaluated regularly to make sure the plan is still effective. Any change in the patient's condition could have a negative impact on the wound healing process, and reevaluation of effectiveness of the plan of care should occur. In a long-term care setting, reevaluation should be done weekly and documented, and interventions and plans of care changed if the current treatment plan is unsuccessful. An evaluation criterion of progress would be a decrease in the size and depth of the wound. If this is not occurring, then the wound needs to be assessed as to why the healing is not occurring, such as the presence of infection or decreased tissue perfusion.

Collaborative Management

Collaborative management involves the use of an interdisciplinary team to assist in correcting or optimizing the influential factors involved in wound healing. A health care provider may consult a wound care center and wound care specialist to collaborate. A general or plastic surgeon may be needed for an incision and drainage (I&D), débridement, flap, or other surgical procedure. A registered dietician (RD) may be required to evaluate nutritional status and offer suggestions. A physical therapist may be needed to increase mobility and alleviate pressure from immobility. A pedorthist may be needed to develop specialized footwear and offloading devices to alleviate pressure to wound area. A vascular specialist may be needed to restore circulation to the wound area. An infectious disease health care provider may be needed to follow the patient with an infected wound and provide antibiotic coverage that is appropriate. A social worker or case manager may be needed to ensure that proper wound care follow-up at home is performed and that the patient has that necessary social support system to be at home. Home health care may be needed for advanced wound care and continued evaluation. There could be many disciplines involved in a patient's care to heal a wound, and communication and a good plan of care are necessary to coordinate all the aspects of healing.

Health Promotion

Pressure ulcers occur in 10% to 17% of all hospitalized patients and 20% to 40% of all nursing home patients (Pressure Ulcers, 2005). These figures are important because they forecast the anticipated number of persons needed in health care jobs to take care of the patients with these wounds. The figures also forecast the expense of treating and healing the pressure ulcers. In 2010 the National Pressure Ulcer Advisory Panel (NPUAP) will publish new findings about the rate of pressure ulcer development in conjunction with *Healthy People 2010*, the U.S. Department of Health and Human Services (2000) blueprint for national health goals. One of the many objectives of this federal initiative is to reduce the incidence of pressure ulcers by 50% by the year 2010. With the increased attention of regulatory agencies, pressure ulcer prevention should be of great concern to the nurse.

The goals of the nurse are to identify and teach other caregivers to identify those at risk of developing pressure ulcers and implement prevention. If pressure ulcers should develop, then treatment should reflect good healing rates and efficient expenditures. The institution or agency is expected to achieve implementation of prevention and treatment through the education of its staff. Nursing is actually graded in a report card by the American Nurses Association (ANA) on how successfully pressure ulcers are being prevented and treated. Nurse-sensitive outcome indicators have been established by the ANA to help demonstrate nursing's unique contributions to health care. ANA instituted the Nursing Care Report Card for Acute Care in which 10 specific quality indicators of nursing were developed and defined. One of these indicators is the maintenance of skin integrity. The ANA Safety and Quality Indicator Project national database is growing through participating acute care institutions and is beginning to show evidence that nursing does indeed impact health outcomes (Duffy & Korniewicz, 2000).

Interventions are where the nurse can make a difference with attentive care, expert skills, and critical judgment. Above all things, it is essential that pressure is relieved from the pressure ulcer in order to have healing begin. The cause of the ulcer must be removed to see improvement.

■ Wound Assessment

Wound assessment requires the use of four of the five senses. Palpation can determine softness (maceration), hardness (induration), or edema. Olfaction can determine infection and dead/slough tissue. Inspection can determine periwound condition, size, and drainage. Auditory sense requires active listening to the patient with regard to pertinent history, past failures/successes for healing, and pain.

Measurement

A wound must be objectively assessed to determine a baseline and effectiveness of a plan of care. Measurements can be made from a head-to-toe reference or longest length and perpendicular width. Either way, the main function of measurements is consistency from a reference standpoint. A wound should be measured for length, width, and depth. The wound is usually measured in centimeters. The depth measurement should be directly perpendicular to the patient's skin and down into the wound and not a measurement parallel to the patient's body. Again, subsequent measurements should use the same point of reference to denote progress or regression adequately. The surface area of the wound is the length multiplied by the width in centimeters squared (cm^2). The volume is the length multiplied by the width and the depth in centimeters cubed (cm^3). A wound routinely heals by decreasing depth first and then contraction by decreasing length and width. That being said, a combination of changes can occur in any dimension, and the volume changes most accurately capture and note wound progression/ regression.

Additional measurements refer to how the wound is shaped underneath the skin surface. A sinus tract is an area, sometimes referred to as a tunnel, where there is nonhealed detached tissue under intact skin. These areas tend to become infected and may develop abscesses if the opening is sealed, blocking drainage. Sinus tracts are measured in centimeters. Referring to location, the area of tunneling is defined on a clock face with 12 o'clock being the head of the body. For example, if a wound located on the anterior aspect of the leg has tunneling on the medial side of the left leg, the measurement would be x amount of centimeters at the 9 o'clock position. There is also a measurement for undermining. Undermining is like a cliff without tissue below and more broad, and is measured from each point or side using the clock-face method (Figure 67–12 ■).

Location

The correct assessment and documentation of the location of the wound is necessary for consistency and accuracy in follow-up of the wound care. There may also be some additional areas of breakdown, and there should be no confusion as to the number

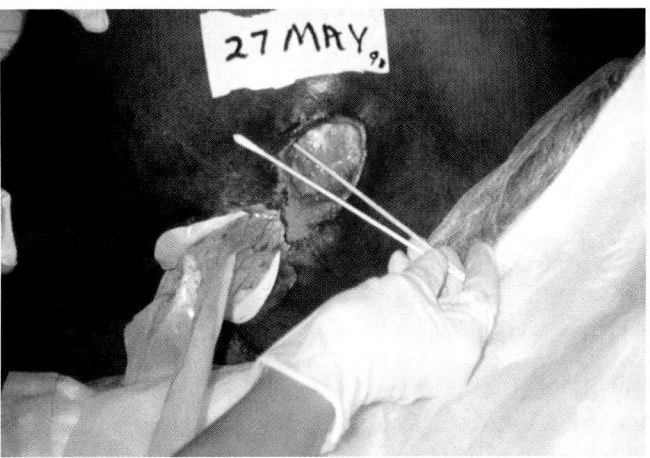

FIGURE 67–12 ■ Undermining.
Source: Jan Clark

and locations of the wounds so that consistent and accurate documentation can occur. Using words such as *medial, lateral, proximal, distal,* and other anatomic location definitions will give clear and concise information.

Wound Drainage

A wound may have many different types of drainage. The drainage may be sanguineous (bloody), serosanguineous (bloody with plasma fluid), serous (plasma only), or purulent (infected). Sanguineous drainage occurs when there is acute trauma to the vascular bed. It may be a result of further insult either due to environmental causes such as hitting the wound area on a foreign object, or from insult due to intentional causes such as a sharps débridement. Serosanguineous drainage is more related to overall edema leading to capillary weakness and leakage. Serous drainage may occur when edema has forced fluid to move from the intravascular department into the tissue and then leakage through the wound bed. Purulent drainage is a sign of infection and indicates the need for antibiotic therapy and/or silver dressing treatment. The amount and type of drainage are documented in the patient's record at regular intervals.

Bioburden

Bioburden is when foreign material, collagen debris, and other biofilms and breakdown from bacterial load and injury cause a delay in the wound healing process and a decrease in biochemical response to healing. Bioburden may be controlled with a combination of irrigation with a syringe, anti-infective agents, or surfactant cleansers.

Periwound Assessment

The periwound area is defined as the area surrounding the wound base circumferentially. The periwound area is a very important indicator of how severe the wound is and of progression or regression of wound closure. The periwound area may be reddened around the wound base. The reddened area indicates that an acute inflammatory process is occurring that may be due to further injury underlying the skin around the wound or infection. If the periwound area is "boggy" or soft, it indicates that there is maceration. Maceration is when excessive moisture destroys the skin's integrity and leaves the skin layers suboptimal. A hardened area referred to as induration indicates tissue that is edematous, infected, injured, or dead. Typically the induration area is opened to relieve the pressure and remove any dead tissue that may exist. The periwound area may also have a yeast or fungal infection due to use of intravenous, oral, or local antibiotic use.

Effective wound management requires one to pay particular attention to the periwound area. Creams that contain dimethicone can protect the periwound area from drainage with a moisture-barrier effect. A moisture product may be required for dry and flaky periwound skin that may be under an occlusive dressing. Antifungal and yeast creams may be applied to the periwound areas to prevent these conditions that commonly occur after chronic antibiotic use and in dark, moist areas. Some lotions can contain lidocaine, an anesthetic to control pain, or hyaluronic acid to control redness and inflammation.

Wound Descriptions

Describing the appearance of the wound helps determine prognosis and treatment plan. One system of wound description is the red, yellow, black system. Red identifies a beefy-red to pink granular bed and identifies the most common treatment for the wound stage based on that wound bed. The yellow stage identifies a wound with fibrin or slough and a plan of treatment designed for that stage of the wound bed. The black stage is when the wound bed has eschar, and a plan of treatment is designed for that stage as well. It is simple to use because the color system is easily identifiable and easily treatable with a set of guidelines to follow for treatment as described in the next section.

■ Wound Management

It is essential that the health care team remember that dressings assist in the body's overall ability to heal itself. They are not intended to be a substitute to identifying and treating the underlying causes of a wound. They simply promote an optimal environment for wound healing progression to occur.

Healing can occur by three methods: primary, secondary, or tertiary intention. **Primary intention** is a closure by sutures, stitches, Steri-Strips, or staples. It is utilized when healing is expected within 10 days and new tissue formation is minimally required. **Secondary intention** is a wound that is allowed to remain open to granulate in and contract. Many traumatic and postsurgical wounds are treated in this manner. **Tertiary or third intention** is a delayed closure to allow for drainage of fluid, contamination control, and/or a plan for surgical intervention at a later date (Smith & Nephew Clinical Staff, 2001).

Physiological local wound environment means that through appropriate topical therapies a wound will ultimately return to the characteristics of healthy or normal functioning (Rolstad, Ovington, & Harris, 2000). Principles of topical therapy are derived from scientific studies of the wound healing process and evidence-based practice. These principles are described in this section.

Offloading

Offloading is a very important factor that influences the wound healing process. Offloading is the process of relieving pressure on a bony prominence, callus, or wound. Standing places 50% of one's body weight on each leg. Walking, dependent on the speed, can equal one to one and one-half times the body weight on an affected area. Offloading devices such as boots, wheelchair cushions, splints, and total contact casting can redistribute pressure or relieve pressure entirely, depending on the device. Turning a patient every 2 hours and floating a patient's heels off the bed on pillows are also forms of offloading. The object is to relieve the pressure that causes a decrease in circulation by compression of the capillary beds and localized tissue destruction. The affected area will form a hardened area called a callus to protect the area from further damage (Martin, Oldani, & Claxton, 2005).

Remove Necrotic Tissue and Foreign Bodies or Particles

Foreign bodies or particles in a wound may be there because of trauma (splinters, glass, and grass). When the wound is cleaned, efforts are made to flush out any loose debris. Hydrogen peroxide may be helpful to clean the initial trauma-induced wound; but after its initial use, refrain from cleansing the wound with hydrogen peroxide because when used in full strength it is toxic to the new fibroblasts that are trying to rebuild the wound. The foreign body may be a suture or staple in a wound that has healed over, and now the wound is reopening because the suture or staple may be working its way to the surface of the skin.

Necrotic tissue is devitalized tissue that ranges from the yellow fibrinous slough to a thick, leathery-like dark brown or black scab-like wound, referred to as eschar. Chapter 68 🖭 discusses burn eschar. Débridement of necrotic tissue is very important because it harbors bacteria. One exception to the rule is eschar covering ischemic wounds, such as dry gangrenous toes. The eschar in an ischemic wound serves as protection against infection, and there is little chance of adequate microcirculation being able to help heal the wound if débrided. The consensus for treatment is painting the ischemic wound with an antiseptic solution such as povidone-iodine and covering it with dry dressings (Drosou, Falabella, & Kirsner, 2003).

Four methods of débridement are sharp, mechanical, enzymatic, and autolytic (Chart 67–10). Sharp débridement is done with scalpel, scissors, or nippers. Anesthetics or the operating room may be required depending on wound size and depth. Mechanical débridement is the dislodging of necrotic tissue, which is accomplished in several ways, including:

- Wet-to-dry dressings are used for mechanical débridement: The slough adheres to the dressing as it dries and is pulled off when the dressing is removed.
- The whirlpool method of débridement also is a mechanical débridement method. It is currently out of favor because of the increased risk of infection and has been replaced with pulse lavage (Vaughn, 2002).
- Pulse lavage is an electrically powered device that emits a regular, automatic interruption of fluid flow with a handheld device. The most common irrigant is saline.

Enzymatic débridement is chemically induced by prescriptive ointments that contain papain urea or collegenase, which penetrates the slough and eschar causing them to soften and "melt down." Once softened, the slough and eschar are mechanically débrided.

Autolytic débridement is allowing the body to utilize the phagocytes to destroy the necrotic tissue. This is often a preferred method of débridement for those persons for whom daily (or more frequent) dressing changes would be a hardship; that is, patients who are critically ill that cannot be turned. Autolytic débridement is a slow and nonaggressive treatment. Occlusive dressings are often used to soften eschar before sharp débridement to avoid débridement of viable tissue. Occlusive dressings are contraindicated on infected wounds.

CHART 67–10 Débridement Methods

Method	Advantages	Disadvantages
Sharp Necrotic tissue removed with scalpel, nippers, or scissors.	Can be used on wound with any amount of slough or eschar. Treatment is swift.	Performed by only skilled nurses or health care providers. Patient may experience pain. May require local anesthetic. May require surgical time procedure (known as incision and drainage).
Autolytic Example: Occlusive dressings, such as transparent film, or hydrocolloids cause physiological "melting" of the necrotic tissue by phagocytes.	Pain free. Can be used on any wounds with slough or eschar. Often preferred for patients who are in the intensive care unit (ICU) and may not be able to tolerate the multiple dressing changes necessary after sharp débridement. Transparent films and wound gel are easy methods to use to achieve autolytic débridement.	Requires more time than sharp or enzymatic methods. Cannot use for infected wounds.
Enzymatic Examples: Accuzyme (papain). Panifil. Xenoderm. Urea active ingredient causing disintegration of slough and eschar.	Faster than autolytic, normally. Usually pain free. Can use for infected wounds. Tissue specific.	Patient may be sensitive to active ingredient. Educate patient that method will increase exudate production. Exudate management.
Mechanical Examples: Wet-to-dry dressing is classic example: the pulling away of tissue that has adhered to the dry dressing. Pulse lavage using high-pressure water streams to dislodge necrotic tissue.	Can be used for infected wounds. Removes loose devitalized tissue.	May be painful. Not tissue specific (removes good granulation tissue with necrotic tissue).

MyNursingKit | Video: Infection Control: Wound Irrigation—Wet to Dry Dress

Obliterate Dead Space

Dead space refers to tissue destruction under intact surface tissue, such as tunneling or sinus tract formation. Dead space areas provide a fluid medium and a desirable environment for pathogen growth. The nurse needs to probe margins of the wound to identify any tracts, undermining, or tunneling. These areas need to be packed with a retrievable material to prevent the tract from closing prematurely and forming an abscess. Pack these areas with one piece of dressing to obliterate the dead space, always leaving a tail of the packing material to prevent granulation tissue closing over the wound that has packing in it. Always document the size and shape, and direction of the sinus tract or tunnel and how much dressing it took to pack the wound. There is always the possibility of packing material being left in the wound.

 Always use a continuous piece of dressing for packing the wound rather than several small pieces because they might get inadvertently left in the track—especially deep wounds with sinus tracts.

Absorb Excess Exudate

Large amounts of exudates may macerate wound margins. Bacterial toxins in the exudate may inhibit the wound healing process (White & Cutting, 2006). A highly exudating wound also may be infected. Measures to protect the intact periwound skin include using liquid skin barriers, moisture barriers, and absorbent dressings. Dressings past their absorbent capacity should be changed promptly.

Provide Thermal Insulation and Protection

Wounds need to be kept at the body's core temperature. When the temperature of the wound is lowered, leukocyte mobility is impaired, and phagocytic efficiency and affinity of hemoglobin for oxygen are reduced (Enoch & Harding, 2003). These conditions slow wound healing. Therefore, dressing changes need to be done quickly because leaving wounds open without dressings can slow blood flow to the wound and delay epidermal migration due to reduced temperatures. Cleansing a wound can reduce the local tissue temperatures for up to 40 minutes. Mitosis and leukocyte activity can be delayed for up to 3 hours after cleansing. If a dressing change is interrupted, cover the wound with sterile gauze to help slow down temperature reduction in the wound and to protect it from airborne organisms. Protect the healing wound from trauma such as wheelchair legs, furniture, pets, and or other objects that may harm the wound. New trauma disrupts newly formed vessels, connective tissue, and epidermis.

Maintain a Moist Wound Surface

Keeping the wound bed moist prevents desiccation and cell death. It facilitates epithelial migration promotes angiogenesis, and connective tissue synthesis. Additionally, moist wound beds are less painful. Three investigations in the mid-20th century showed that "moist wound healing" was achieved by covering the experimental wounds with an occlusive membrane consisting of thin plastic film. Starting in 1958 with Odland observing that a blister healed faster if it were left unbroken, the idea that dressings were pharmacologic agents was taken

seriously (Odland, 1958). In 1962 Winter showed that occlusion of wounds with a polyethylene film more than doubled the wound healing rate in domestic pigs (Winter, 1962). Hinman and Maiback established the beneficial effect of occlusion on resurfacing of experimental wounds in normal human subjects (Hinman & Maibach, 1963). These principles still hold true today.

A moist wound environment created by occlusive dressings facilitates granulation tissue development through increased gel-matrix secretion, new blood vessel growth, collagen secretion, fibroblast proliferation, and epidermal migration (Smith, 2002). Benefits of moist wound healing are faster epidermal resurfacing and fewer infections.

Protection from maceration of the periwound skin is part of the delicate balance of moist wound healing (Clark, 2002). A variety of products described later support this concept. Products that add moisture, protect from moisture, absorb moisture, and maintain moisture are all available to the health care provider for promotion of optimal wound healing. Moist wound healing is not a new concept, but has been slow to become the automatic choice of health care providers. Moist wound healing has, however, become the mantra of specialists trained in wound care management. These specialists recognize the benefits of occlusive dressings that facilitate moist wound healing. Chart 67–11 outlines dressing categories, characteristics, and uses.

Wound Cleansers

Wound cleansing is a controversial topic within the ranks of wound care experts. Antiseptics such as hydrogen peroxide, povidone-iodine, acetic acid, and Dakin's solution, which can kill bacteria, can also be cytotoxic to white blood cells and fibroblasts. Removing bacteria from the wound bed can be done with normal saline at pressure between 4 and 15 pounds per square inch (psi). Above 15 pounds per square inch the pressure tends to drive bacteria into the tissue. Many commercial cleansers may inhibit the viability and phagocytic activity of leukocytes unless they are diluted due to toxic ingredients. Commercial wound cleansers contain surfactants and preservatives, and many come with a built-in sprayer achieving a desirable pounds per square inch pressure. An accepted rule of using saline as a cleanser is that after sterile saline is opened, it is good for only 24 hours; then it should be discarded. Saline kept refrigerated may be safe longer than 24 hours, but it is always a good idea to check labels or ask the manufacturer. Water is acceptable as a wound cleanser as long as it is free from contaminants. Some wound cleansers that are promoted as killing bacteria are not toxic to tissues; for example, Techni-Care Surgical Scrub (Care-Tech Laboratories, Inc.).

 *Skin cleansers should never be used on wounds. Skin cleansers are formulated to break chemical bonds that bind fecal matter to the skin; they are not suitable for the delicate tissue of a wound bed.*

Wound Care Products

Nurses may choose from several different types of dressings for wound management. The factors in making a decision on a

CHART 67–11 **Dressing Categories, Characteristics, and Uses**

Dressing Category and Description	Brand Names	Indications for Use	Advantages	Disadvantages
Transparent Films Primary or secondary dressings. Polyurethane with a porous adhesive layer that allows oxygen to pass through the membrane and moisture vapor to escape.	Opsite Bioclusive CarraFilm Polyskin Tegaderm UniFlex	Partial thickness wounds. Stages I and II pressure ulcers. Donor sites. Superficial burns.	Wound visible. Promotes autolytic débridement. Reduces friction. Pain reduction. Waterproof. Conformable.	Nonabsorptive. Fluid retention properties may lead to maceration or increased risk of fungal infection. May be difficult to apply for some persons. Contraindicated for infected wounds and sensitive or fragile skin.
Hydrogels Primary or secondary dressings. Amorphous or sheet design. Nonadherent, water or glycerin based.	Sheets: ClearSite Vigilon Elasto-Gel XCell Gels: DuoDerm gel Carrasyn Curasol gel Hypergel	Painful wounds. Skin tears. Radiation burns. Donor sites. Necrotic wounds. Partial or full-thickness wounds. Stages II–IV pressure ulcers. Wound edges. Neuropathic (diabetic) ulcers.	Nonadherent. Moisture retentive. Encourages autolytic débridement. Keeps wound edges supple. Pain reduction. Easy to apply and remove.	May macerate. Little absorption. Sheet dressing can dehydrate. Gels require secondary dressing. Sheets require tape or bandage to keep in place or may come with adhesive border. (Do not use the adhesive border on fragile skin; cut it away and secure with bandage.)
Hydrocolloids Primary dressings. Hydrophilic colloid particles bound to polyurethane foam; impermeable to bacteria.	DuoDerm CGF DuoDerm, thin Restore SignaDress Tegasorb Nu-Derm Cutinova Hydro	Partial thickness wounds. Stages II and III pressure ulcers.	Enhances autolytic débridement. Self-adherent, but not to wound. Pain reduction. Good for 2–5 days. Waterproof. Moisture retentive. Thermal insulation.	Minimal absorption. Some with aggressive adhesive. Contraindicated for infected wounds. Characteristic odor may be confused with infection.
Foams Primary dressings. Hydrophilic polyurethane.	3M Allevyn PolyMem Tielle Hydrasorb Lyofoam Mepilex	Venous stasis ulcers (can use under compression wraps). Tracheostomy. Draining wounds. Dermal wounds. Surgical incisions. Skin tears. Neuropathic (diabetic) ulcers.	Absorptive. Cushioning. Thermal insulation. Easy to apply and remove. Nonocclusive. Nonadherent.	May require secondary dressing or tape to secure. May macerate periwound skin if not changed appropriately. Not for dry, nondraining wounds.
Alginates Highly absorptive dressing of brown seaweed fibers; forms a soft gel when mixed with wound fluid. Available in ropes or sheets.	Kaltostat Sorbsan Algiderm Carrasorb Comfeel Seasorb	Highly exudative, draining wounds. Incisions. Venous stasis ulcers. Dermal wounds. Stages III and IV pressure ulcers. Tunneling or undermined areas. Split-thickness skin grafts.	Nonadherent. Can be used on infected wounds. Hemostatic properties for minor bleeding. Reduced frequency of dressing changes.	Requires secondary dressing. Contraindicated for wounds with exposed tendons, bone due to possible desiccation.
Composite Combination of products that provide multiple functions (i.e., bacterial barrier, absorption layer, and adhesive border). It can be any combination of dressings.	Primapore Versiva Viasorb Alldress	Surgical incisions. Stages II–IV pressure ulcers. Partial or full-thickness wounds.	Multiple sizes and shapes. Easy to apply. Usually absorbent. Check insert instructions for each brand dressing.	Adhesive borders may limit use due to fragile skin. Does not necessarily provide moist wound healing. Check insert instructions for each brand dressing.

(continued)

CHART 67-11	Dressing Categories, Characteristics, and Uses—*Continued*			
Dressing Category and Description	**Brand Names**	**Indications for Use**	**Advantages**	**Disadvantages**
Silver dressings	Aquacel Ag Acticoat Biostep Ag Silverlon Prisma Silversorb Maxsorb Ag Silverfoam (for wound VAC)	Silver is used as an antimicrobial in its ionic form, Ag^+. It may be used in a gel form to provide moisture, an absorbent form like a foam or alginate, or with a collagen product. The wound VAC has a foam with silver in it as well now.	Can be used in multiple different types of dressings. Bacteriocidal to methicillin-resistant *Staphylococcus aureus* (MRSA) and vancomycin-resistant enterococcus (VRE) infections. Useful for prophylaxis as well.	Some studies show that too much silver may be inhibitory to healthy epithelialization. Further studies are underway.
Collagens	Biostep Collagenase Puracol Fibracol, SkinTemp Promogran	Collagens are used to provide collagen to the wound bed after the body denatures the initial injured collagen. Collagen is the protein matrix that is the major part of the extracellular matrix (ECM) and provides stability and tensile strength.	It is used to speed up the healing process by filling in the wound bed faster than the body could on its own. Some forms now also control the amount of matrix metalloproteinases (MMPs) and therefore prevent the body from breaking down the new collagen bed.	Timing, initially, the wound bed will have MMPs that denature the injured collagen, so it can be replaced with healthy collagen. In acute wounds, collagen may not be indicated. In chronic wounds, the amound of MMPs should be controlled to allow the dressing to be assimilated into the wound bed without denaturing by MMPs.

particular product are protection, degree of drainage or lack thereof, antimicrobial activity, biochemical needs, collagen requirements, and pain relief. As the wound treatment plan continues, it may be necessary to switch dressing types based on the needs for that wound bed at the time of assessment. The same dressing will most often not be required the entire treatment of the wound. It is very important to understand that despite algorithms and protocols, what drives choices for dressings is a skilled assessment of the wound on which to base decisions about dressings. The wound is viable and changing; flexibility regarding the type of dressings used is necessary to continue to show improvement in the wound. Moist wound healing is a delicate balance of moisture—keeping the wound bed moist and the periwound skin dry and intact. Basic, good wound care is pretty simple: If a wound is dry, add moisture; if a wound is wet, use an absorbent dressing; and always protect the periwound skin.

The most common type of dressings are presented next with the understanding that there are many different variations in size, brand, and combinations to provide a highly individualized plan of treatment that is cost effective, convenient, and outcome driven. See Chart 67–11 for a summary of common dressing categories, characteristics, and uses.

Moisture Retentive Dressings

The goals of moisture retentive dressings, occlusive dressings, or semiocclusive dressings are all the same: maintaining a moist wound environment. There are hydrogels, calcium alginates, silver dressings, collagens, foams, polyurethane films, hydrocolloids, contact layers, composites, and combinations, all of which are described here. Generally these dressings are painless, reduce the need for multiple dressing changes daily, and result in faster heal-

ing rates. On the cellular level, cells desiccate without moisture and cannot do their job of building tissue to fill in and cover a wound. Moist wound healing is facilitated by moisture retentive dressings.

 *To the patient who tells the nurse that he leaves the dressing off at night so the wound can get air, the nurse needs to explain that the wound gets oxygen from the blood supply, not from the ambient air. Do not let the wound dry out.*

Hydrogels

Hydrogels are made of a saline base. They provide moisture to the wound bed that is required for epithelialization to occur as the cells migrate across the wound bed. Hydrogels can come in a tube of gel, in sheets, or impregnated in a gauze pad. Hydrogels are used for wounds that are dry and require moisture. They are not intended for wounds with excess drainage. A caution with this dressing is that maceration, the tendency for the periwound area of good skin to get wet and soft and potentially break down, can occur. Close supervision of the wound's progress and astute assessment are required.

Alginates

Alginates are composed of algae or seaweed. These dressing can absorb at least about five to ten times their surface area of drainage. In chronic wounds, the chemical's matrix metalloproteinases, or MMPs, are out of ratio for wound healing to occur. MMPs degrade collagen and denature it. As a reminder, collagen is the scaffold whereby tissue growth occurs. A certain amount of MMPs are necessary to control other biochemical signals and degrade collagen that is injured. Alginates absorb the excess wound drainage to inactivate some MMPs as well as prevent against maceration, as described earlier.

Silver Dressings

Silver in its ionic form is a natural bactericidal agent, even against the most resistant bacterial strains such as MRSA (methicillin-resistant *Staphylococcus aureus*) and VRE (vancomycin-resistant enterococcus). Silver, when in contact with the bacteria, interferes with bacterial cell DNA, bacterial enzymes, and proteins in the cell wall to create its bactericidal effect. Silver has been used since the late 1800s for its antimicrobial activity. It can be found in gels, alginates, saturated gauze, metallic nylon, and other media to deliver the silver cation Ag^+. Some silver dressings require saline to be activated and some do not. There is a debate as to how much silver is effective and whether larger than required amounts of silver can be harmful and destructive. The main focus, however, should be the rate at which the silver is deposited into the wound bed and the wound bed's characteristics. Silver will kill only the surface bacteria it comes in contact with, and oral antibiotic therapy should continue.

Collagens

Collagen dressings are also utilized for wound care treatment. Native collagen that is stable and can resist early degradation by MMPs can provide an extracellular matrix (ECM) that allows wound healing to continue. Extracellular matrix is the matrix of native collagen, connective tissue, and basement membrane that forms the foundation or scaffold on which the epithelial tissue is embedded. There are many different types of collagen dressings. Characteristics such as size, depth, shape, drainage, or lack thereof, infection, and bioburden, all factor into selecting the right type of collagen medium to utilize (Nataraj et al., 2007).

Foams

A foam dressing is made of a spongy material that is highly absorptive as compared to its surface area. It is also soft and pliable so that it can conform to any environment. Foams can be used in two ways. One use is for absorption. They can be used alone or in combination with an alginate to "wick" away excess moisture and prevent maceration. They can also be utilized for protection as a barrier against foreign insult. For example, a patient in a wheelchair with a lower leg wound is prone to further trauma due to hitting the wound on the wheelchair with transfers. The foam then provides a cushion for the insult and protects the already compromised wound bed from further damage. It can also be utilized to protect from friction and shear forces from surfaces and contact with other body parts.

Transparent Films

Transparent films are made of a clear sticky wrap much like the plastic wrap used for storage of food with glue on one side. Transparent films can be used to visualize a wound bed and for an occlusive dressing. It should be noted however, that on elderly patients with frail skin, another option should be considered. This film tends to stick and protect so well that when it is time to remove it, it can cause further damage by clinging to and separating the skin during its removal. Transparent films are excellent, however, for protection from incontinence and foreign contact getting to the wound bed and can allow the wound dressing to remain intact for a greater duration.

Gauze

Gauze is the most widely used dressing and may be wrongly alluded to as a standard of care (Ovington, 2002). Research has shown that wet-to-dry dressings and gauze are commonly ordered for wounds in which there is scant evidence to support their use, such as with open surgical wounds healing by secondary intention (Armstrong & Price, 2004). Wet-to-dry dressings consist of saline-moistened gauze placed inside or on a wound bed, covered with dry gauze, and secured. When the moistened gauze dries, it adheres to the wound. When it is removed, it pulls away good tissue along with the necrotic tissue and debris. This is nonselective débridement, and there is a high risk for reinjury of the wound bed. Plus, it is usually painful.

Wet-to-moist or moist gauze dressings are saline-moistened gauze placed in the wound and kept moist until removed. This may require rewetting the gauze, but generally it means that the dressing is changed before it dries out, which in reality may or may not happen. More frequent dressing changes may mean more pain for the patient, more work for an elderly caregiver spouse, and more expense for a home health nurse or hospital staff nurse.

Negative Pressure Therapy

Negative pressure therapy is a dressing that uses a vacuum or negative pressure to assist in drainage collection and promotion of granulation and angiogenesis. Wound vacuum assisted closure (VAC) is a system that uses controlled negative pressure (vacuum) to help promote wound healing (Figure 67–13 ■, p. 2218). This therapy helps remove infectious materials and other fluids from the wound. The wound VAC system consists of a computer-controlled therapy unit, canister, sterile plastic tubing, foam dressing, and a clear VAC drape dressing. The foam dressing is gently packed into the open wound bed, taking care not to leave any on normal skin. A tube is then connected to the foam at one end and the VAC control unit at the other end. Once the foam is in place, it is sealed with a clear drape that is similar to a large bandage. Suction is applied and infectious materials and other fluids from the wound are pulled through the tube and into the canister. The wound VAC works best in a clean, granular bed; and débridement and infection control should be accomplished first before a wound VAC is applied. It is changed every 2 to 3 days.

Wound VAC negative pressure wound therapy (NPWT) can be prescribed for many chronic and traumatic wound patients in the hospital, in the extended care facility, and in the home. The negative pressure and drainage system (1) promotes granulation tissue formation through the promotion of wound healing (Argenta & Morykwas, 1997; Joseph et al., 2000); (2) uniformly draws wounds closed by applying controlled, localized negative pressure; (3) removes interstitial fluid allowing tissue decompression; (4) removes infectious materials; and (5) provides a closed, moist wound healing environment. Wound VAC is used in the hospital setting, in the extended care facility, and at home for the following conditions:

- Chronic open wounds (diabetic and pressure ulcers)
- Acute and traumatic wounds
- Meshed grafts
- Subacute wounds (i.e., dehisced incisions)
- Skin grafts and flaps. (MedTech1.com, 2005)

Nursing care includes maintaining and documenting the negative pressure level, changing the foam per the health care provider's order, and assessing wound healing.

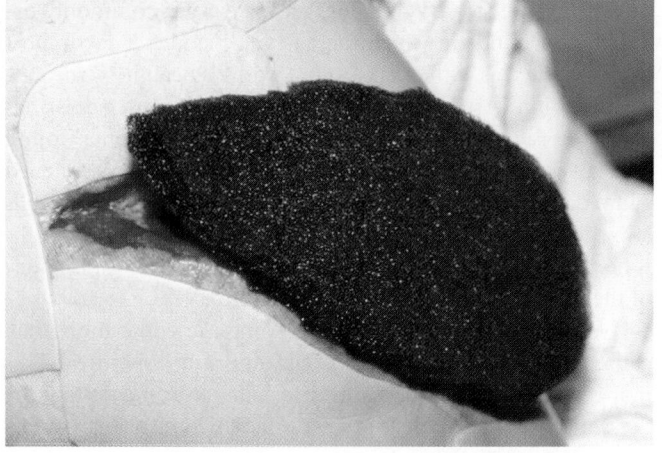

1.

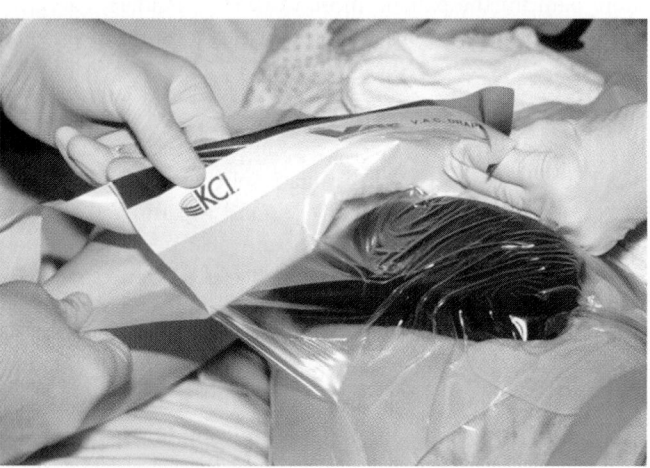

2.

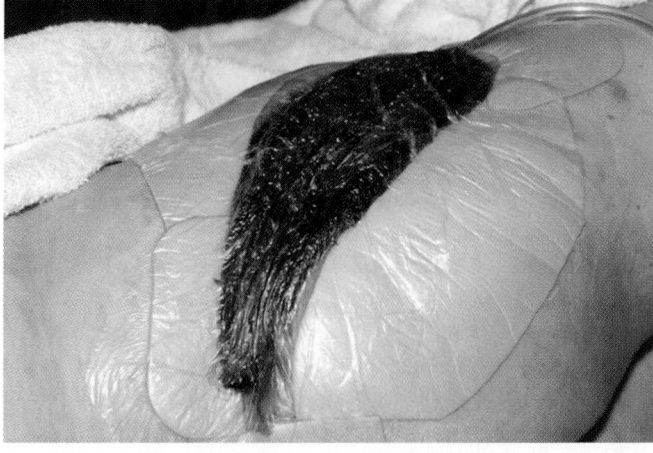

3.

4.

FIGURE 67–13 ■ Wound vacuum assisted closure (VAC).
Source: 1, 2: Jan Clark; 3, 4: Cheryl Wraa

▌Adjuvant Therapy

There are adjuvant treatments one could consider in a plan of care to promote the healing process. These treatments are used in conjunction with good wound care and identification of the causative factors that relate to wound healing or lack thereof. One such treatment is the use of skin grafts or flaps to close or fill in a wound. A skin graft requires an area of the patient's healthy skin on the body (usually from the lower extremity thigh area) to be excised and placed over the wound area and sutured or stapled in to affix the graft. Of note, the wound should be a clean (free of infection and debris), granulating wound that is ready to accept the graft. One must also consider the patient's vascular and nutritional status to ensure graft survival and take. Pressure must not be applied to the affected area, and that may require a pressure relief device like a "sand bed," which is made of silicone beads that are heated and effectively move under the patient so that no pressure is applied to the affected area. Skin grafting is described in detail in Chapter 68 ☺ .

Tissue Grafts

Another adjuvant treatment is the use of tissue grafts. These grafts can be derived from human tissue or from animal tissue.

They contain collagen and/or fibroblasts and keratinocytes, the major components of the dermal and epidermal layers of skin. These applications are placed directly to the wound bed and affixed or anchored so that the graft stays in place. The benefit of this graft over a skin graft is that there is no donor site required to heal, no requirement of anesthesia or invasive surgery, and it is minimally invasive. Tissue grafts can also be performed repetitively to get the intended result.

Whirlpool Therapy

Whirlpool therapy is another adjuvant treatment. A whirlpool is a tub that has circulating water to remove debris and bioburden in the wound to promote wound healing. It is often performed daily and can be found in many inpatient and outpatient physical therapy departments. One side effect of whirlpool use is infection (Vaughn, 2002).

Hyperbaric Oxygen Therapy

Hyperbaric oxygen therapy is also an adjuvant treatment. **Hyperbaric oxygen therapy (HBOT)** refers to intermittent treatment of the entire body with 100% oxygen at 20 times greater than normal atmospheric pressures. HBOT has been used to improve wound healing in patients with compromised oxygenation and/or perfusion because it stimulates the growth of new blood vessels in areas with reduced circulation and arterial blockage (Cranton, 2005). Patients are placed in either chambers that can be individual or large, room-like chambers that can accommodate several people at one time. The patient breathes in this oxygen under pressure in a chamber. The oxygen under pressure forces the oxygen into the plasma surrounding the red blood cells to "supersaturate" the patient with oxygen. Its benefits are increased tissue oxygen levels, angiogenesis (new blood vessel formation), antibacterial activity (oxygen kills anaerobic bacteria and its toxins), enhanced leukocyte killing (T-cell formation), and prevention of reperfusion injury. There are about 14 approved diagnoses accepted by the Centers for Medicare & Medicaid Services (CMS) for hyperbaric oxygen therapy. One example is that patients who have diabetic wounds at a depth of Wagner Grade 3, failed conventional wound therapy for 30 days, and had vascular and glucose optimization can receive hyperbaric therapy. Patients with osteomyelitis and patients at risk of failing a surgical flap can receive hyperbaric oxygen therapy as well. HBOT also is used to treat extensive wounds such as burn injuries, infected wounds, and wounds in patients who are at high risk for delayed healing. Wherever blood flow and oxygen delivery to vital organs are reduced, function and healing can potentially be aided with HBOT. Recently HBOT has been used for treatment of chronic degenerative health problems related to atherosclerosis, stroke, peripheral vascular disease, diabetic ulcers, wound healing, cerebral palsy, brain injury, multiple sclerosis, macular degeneration, and many other disorders (Cranton, 2005).

There must be a trained hyperbaric technician and health care provider that supervise the hyperbaric treatment as well. Special precautions muse be taken with regard to fire hazards when considering oxygen under pressure. The treatment lasts about 2 hours and is given daily for anywhere from 20 to 60 treatments. There are rare side effects of hyperbaric oxygen therapy, such as oxygen toxicity seizures, eardrum rupture, pneumothorax, hypoglycemia in patients with diabetes, and temporary visual changes; but because these effects can be potentially serious, constant supervision is required, as stated earlier (Undersea & Hyperbaric Medical Society, 2007).

Electrical Stimulation

Electrical stimulation (ES) is the use of electrical current to stimulate cellular processes. The literature remains unclear as to the exact "dosage" (Sussman, 1998). Benefits are reported to be an antibacterial effect, increased blood flow, cell proliferation, edema reduction, and autolytic débridement facilitation.

Normothermia (Radiant Heat)

Radiant heat is believed to increase blood flow through vasodilation, thereby promoting cell proliferation. New methods of delivering the radiant heat have been developed. The system consists of a power supply, control unit, warming insert, and dressing that supports the warming insert and protects the wound. The system maintains appropriate levels of temperature and moisture in and around the wound.

Specialty Support Surfaces

Specialty support surfaces are mattresses or overlays that provide pressure reduction or pressure relief. Pressure reduction and pressure relief are based on the principle of decreasing interface pressure. The pressure between a bony prominence and surface such as a hospital bed or seating surface is **interface pressure**. Decreasing interface pressure decreases pressure on capillaries. Ischemia results when capillaries are occluded, shutting down oxygen and nutrients necessary for cellular viability. Cellular death results in tissue necrosis—pressure ulcers. On admission to the hospital, nursing assessment of the patient includes pressure ulcer risk. Ideally a primary part of the care plan is selection of an appropriate surface (Coats-Bennett, 2002). To be able to make decisions about which specialty support surface will most benefit the patient requires an in-depth understanding not only of the specialty support surface performance but also of the patient's condition. An assessment of the patient should include risk for skin breakdown, location of present ulcers or wounds, sensory perception, mobility status, chronic illness, nutritional status, moisture and continence issues, and the patient's ability to be repositioned due to procedures, surgeries, hardware (e.g., fixators), and hemodynamic stability.

A "gatekeeper" is essential to provide the patient with the correct support surface and to control costs. Frequently that position is filled by the wound ostomy continence nurse or someone else who has had extensive education about specialty support surfaces and an understanding of the Centers for Medicare & Medicaid Services (CMS) categories for reimbursement purposes. Detailed descriptions of a patient's wound, activity level, and state of health are important documentation in obtaining reimbursement for specialty support surface. Evidence-based decision tools to select appropriate specialty surfaces are helpful and can be formulated specific to institutions and the products they use (Warren, Yoder, Young-McCaughan, 1999). In addition to the specialty support surfaces, institutions and home health services can utilize overlays of gel, foam, or air for pressure reduction. Other specialty support surfaces facilitate pulmonary rescue of patients and support bariatric patients.

Pressure Reduction and Pressure Relief

Standard hospital mattresses have interface pressures of approximately 100 mmHg. Without frequent repositioning, healthy individuals can experience occluded capillaries. Pressure reduction surfaces can lower interface pressure, but will not consistently lower interface pressure below 32 mmHg, which is capillary closing pressure (Coats-Bennett, 2002). Pressure relief products vary in interface pressure. Many are dynamic, so that the interface pressure is constantly changing to ensure that pressure load is distributed.

Therapeutic Mattress Replacements

Therapeutic mattress replacements (TMR) are called so because they replace the standard hospital mattress. They are made of various layers, usually with a 4- to 6-inch layer of high-density foam. TMRs can include layers of air or gel. They are covered by waterproof covers, which help reduce pressure, friction, and shear.

CHART 67–12	**Skin Breakdown Protection Overlays**	
Overlay	**Description**	**Use**
Foam	Construction of a foam overlay's height, density, and indention load deflection (ILD) produces the characteristics to evaluate for effective pressure reduction. Base height should be measured from the base of the overlay to the lowest point of convolution in an "egg-crate" foam construction. To provide pressure relief, 4 inches or more of height is necessary.	At risk for pressure ulcers Stages I and II pressure ulcers
Gel	Gel overlays are filled with silicon elastomer, silicon, polyvinyl chloride, or similar gel materials. They help reduce friction. The gel is displaced by the patient's body weight and provides flotation.	At-risk patients Stages I and II pressure ulcers
Air	Powered air overlays are considered dynamic (air is in motion). Air overlays consist of air cells that are inflated and produce consistent pressure reduction. Alternating air overlays consist of air cells constantly deflated and inflated, effectively reducing the effects of pressure duration by changing pressure distribution. Some of these are designed so the airflow moves quickly into small chambers so the effect is pulsating. Nonpowered air overlays are static (no air motion). Static air overlays have connecting air cells that conform to body weight to displace pressure load.	At-risk patients Stages I, II, III, and IV pressure ulcers Burns Surgical flaps
Water	Water-filled overlays are vinyl mattresses filled with water. The patient should displace the water without bottoming out, effectively floating the patient.	At-risk patients Stages I, II, and III pressure ulcers

Overlays are to be placed on top of a TMR or standard hospital mattress. Overlays can be powered or nonpowered. Nonpowered overlays are static air, foam, water, or gel filled. Powered overlays may provide alternating pressure or low air loss. They differ widely in pressure reduction: the ability to support the patient and redistribute pressure load. Chart 67–12 summarizes the various overlays available.

Pressure Relief

Two types of pressure relief are low air loss therapy and air fluidized therapy.

In *low air loss therapy*, low air loss overlays sit on top of the standard or therapeutic mattress replacement, or as a mattress that replaces the mattress on the frame. A pump is connected to the mattress or overlay, attached to the foot of the bed, and plugged in to electricity. Some models feature a short-term battery to keep the mattress from deflating. Low air loss mattresses arriving within a special frame are considered "air support systems." A series of pillows are inflated with air in continuous motion, to specific patient measurements of weight and height. Therapy provided by low air loss beds includes maintaining capillary blood flow, eliminating shear and friction, and reducing moisture. NEVER place a patient with spinal injury on a low air loss mattress until the injury has been radiologically cleared or the neurosurgeon or orthopedic surgeon orders it. (Each institution needs to have a specific policy.) The potential for further injury exists because the "air bed" does not support the spine.

 *Do not diminish the pressure-relieving effects of the low air loss surface by using extra layers of sheets or pads. Extra padding increases pressure. Use only the pads recommended by the bed manufacturer.*

Air fluidized therapy utilizes a high rate of airflow to fluidize fine particulate material to produce a support medium that has characteristics similar to liquid. The support system does not utilize a mattress; the fluidized particulate matter is contained within a sheet that conforms around the patient's body. One-third of the body is floating and the rest is enveloped within the sheet of constantly moving matter. Indications for these beds are

surgical flaps and grafts and in some cases intractable pain. Pain relief occurs because the fluidized air relieves pressure on painful areas as well as bony prominences or surgical flaps/grafts.

Bariatric Systems

Patients weighing more than 500 pounds or having a body mass index above 40 should be considered for placement on a bariatric system for safety reasons. Bariatric systems utilize a reinforced frame to support body mass. Most can be converted to a chair position. Some systems provide a wider area to help support and facilitate the repositioning of patients. Low air loss mattresses are available on bariatric systems. Newer models can make full-body lateral rotation turns with the low air loss surface.

Kinetic or Oscillation Therapy

Pulmonary rescue is another function of a specialty support surface. These special frames actually turn patients to mobilize the secretions in their lungs. Overlays can systematically deflate and inflate on opposite sides to create a shift in the patient's chest, although the turn is not as significant as that of a turning frame. The frames now come with controls to turn patients in incremental degrees, and to select turning positions and time involved in each turn. Certain models have incorporated a low air loss support surface into the frame. They also usually come with scales for weighing patients. In addition, options for percussion and or/gentle pulsation modes to aid in pulmonary toilet and enhance circulation are available. Long periods of the turning mechanism being turned off require reevaluation of the bed's impact on the patient, and other options should be considered (Coats-Bennett, 2002). Most importantly, it must be understood that these "turning" beds do not replace the need for repositioning patients or protecting heels to prevent pressure ulcers.

Summary

Pressure reduction surfaces include therapeutic mattress replacements, 4-inch foam overlays, static air, gel, water, and dynamic air overlays. Pressure relief surfaces include low air loss and air fluidized surfaces. Kinetic or "turning beds" are used for pulmonary rescue. Bariatric beds are for patients who are obese. These must be considered therapy and documented as such with

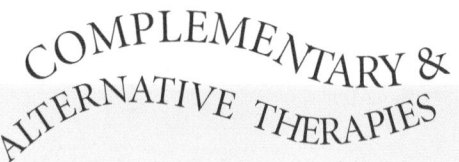

Horse Chestnut Seed Extract

Description:

The horse chestnut is the fruit of the horse chestnut tree (*Aesculus hippocastanum L.*). A medicinal extract, horse chestnut seed extract (HCSE), is prepared from the seed of the fruit. HCSE is commonly used in Europe for chronic venous insufficiency (CVI). CVI is a condition that includes symptoms such as leg swelling, varicose veins, leg pain, itching, and skin ulcers.

Research Support:

A literature review was conducted to evaluate the efficacy and safety of oral HCSE for the treatment of CVI. Researchers sought randomized controlled trials that compared use of oral HCSE single preparations with placebo in people with CVI. Researchers excluded trials if the HCSE was one of several active components in a combination preparation, or as a part of a combination treatment. Study results showed that HCSE treatment improved CVI-related signs and symptoms compared to placebo, and that there were only mild and infrequent adverse effects associated with HCSE treatment. Although researchers concluded that HCSE may be effective as a safe short-term treatment for CVI, they felt that more rigorous trials are needed to confirm its efficacy (Pittler & Ernst, 2006).

In an Australian prospective triple–blind randomized placebo-controlled trial, 54 patients with venous leg ulcers from a large South Australian community nursing service were randomly allocated to receive horse chestnut seed extract (n=27) or placebo (n=27) for 12 weeks. Ulcers were assessed at weeks 0, 4, 8 and 12 utilizing a wound assessment tool and the Alfred/Medseed Wound Imaging System. The difference between groups in the number of healed leg ulcers and change in wound surface area, depth, volume, pain and exudate was not statistically significant. However, horse chestnut seed extract did have a significant effect on the percentage of wound slough over time and on the number of dressing changes at week 12. Even though horse chestnut seed extract is likely to attenuate the pathogenesis of venous insufficiency and, in turn, facilitate venous ulcer

healing, the current study did not statistically support such a claim. However, taking into account the small sample and insufficient power of the trial, and the significant improvement in wound slough and visit frequency, it appears that it may be useful in the management of venous leg ulcers (Leach, Pinocombe, & Foster, 2006a).

Another study assessed the cost-effectiveness of using HCSE for venous ulcer treatment versus conventional therapy, which involves dressings and compression, alone. The randomized, placebo-controlled study, which was conducted for 12 weeks in South Australia, involved 54 patients with venous ulcers. Researchers compiled the cost of HCSE in addition to dressing materials, travel, staff salaries, and infrastructure for each patient when comparing HCSE treatment to conventional treatment. Results showed that HCSE therapy combined with conventional therapy was more cost effective than conventional therapy alone considering only dressing materials costs per patient. Researchers pointed out that the total cost of wound care is significantly impacted by dressing change frequency. They concluded that the use of HCSE in venous ulcer treatment may enhance clinical efficiency due to less frequent nursing visits (Leach, Pinocombe, & Foster, 2006a).

References

Leach, M. J., Pincombe, J., & Foster, G. (2006a). Clinical efficacy of horse chestnut seed extract in the treatment of venous ulceration. *Journal of Wound Care, 15*(4), 159–167.

Leach, M. J., Pincombe, J., & Foster, G. (2006b). Using horse chestnut seed extract in the treatment of venous leg ulcers: A cost–benefit analysis. *Ostomy Wound Management, 52*(4), 68–70, 72–74, 76–78.

Pittler, M. H., & Ernst, E. (2006). Horse chestnut seed extract for chronic venous insufficiency. *Cochrane Database of Systematic Reviews, 25*(1), CD003230.

---

observed outcomes and achieved goals. They should be used in conjunction with optimal nutrition, appropriate positioning, optimal transferring and turning techniques, and routine skilled nursing care and assessments. Support surfaces should be changed to reflect the goals and objectives of the patient's current plan of care (Coats-Bennett, 2002).

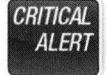 *It is essential to debunk the myth that once a patient is on a specialty support surface she does not need to be repositioned. Manufacturers of specialty beds and wound care experts agree that nurses need to reposition patients on specialty beds frequently.*

Complementary and Alternative Therapies

The use of complementary and/or alternative therapies may be attractive to patients for wound healing, especially of nonhealing chronic wounds. Alternative medicine products may include honey, aloe, chamomile, calendula, and tea tree oil. A number of over-the-counter topical and ingestible agents promote wound healing, decrease scar formation, and prevent bruising. These agents are frequently less costly and more accessible than prescription pharmaceutical agents and dressings. One example of a topical agent is ordinary honey. It has successfully healed

chronic wounds in patients who have failed to get closure with other methods. The Complementary and Alternative Therapies feature outlines the use of horse chestnut seed extract for the treatment of chronic venous insufficiency.

Management of Drains

Care of surgical drains and tubes in postoperative patients is important in order to avoid complications. Nurses in home health and in long-term acute care facilities must learn to manage drains and tubes because of shorter lengths of stay in acute care facilities. To care for the postoperative patient with drains, the nurse must know the type, purpose, and location of the surgical drain, proper management strategies, potential problems, and how to troubleshoot complications. The nurse also must ensure that the system is securely stabilized and assess patency on a regular basis. Because drains are removed when they are no longer needed, monitoring the amount of drainage is important in order to determine the length of time the drain needs to stay in place. If the tube or drain is not draining fluid, there may be a problem with the system. The nurse should make a systematic check from where the drain leaves the patient's body to the collection device to check for kinks, blood clots, or mucous or tissue shreds. Milking the tube away from the patient can be done to sustain patency of the tube. Any significant change in amount or character of drainage must be reported to the health care provider.

Nurses need to protect the skin from any drainage or leakage to prevent irritation. Dry gauze dressings can be used to help lift the drainage tube away from the skin and help stabilize the device. Stabilizers such as the Hollister Drain Tube Attachment Device keep drains and tubes from migrating in and out of the exit site. Constant friction due to migration of the tube causes the space around the tube to enlarge, allowing more movement of the tube and more leakage around the tube. With more moisture and friction, hypergranulation can occur. **Hypergranulation** is the formation of soft, pink, fleshy projections in the open area, which is the body's attempt to heal the enlarged track. Silver nitrate sticks are often used to burn down this tissue because it creates more moisture and causes pain in some instances. Moisture barriers can be used to protect the skin from breakdown if there is leakage from in or around the drain insertion site.

Preventing complications should be the goal of drain/tube management. Therefore, the nurse should consistently use hand hygiene before and after patient care, use aseptic techniques when cleaning and dressing surgical drains/tubes, and dispose properly of drainage containers and drains when removed. Skin around the drain needs to be kept clean and dry.

Surgical drains are often indicated for decompression in areas with a significant amount of fluid accumulation, fistulas, infected tissue, and potential dead space. Two types of drains are used: active or passive.

Active Drains

Active drains are low-pressure suction devices that are constantly removing fluids via a closed drainage system. The drain is attached to a collapsible reservoir that exerts negative pressure to pull fluids from the wound bed. Active drain advantages include minimal tissue trauma, accurate drainage measurements, and the closed system decreases infection risk. Examples of common active drains are Jackson–Pratt and Hemovac (Figures 67–14A, 67–15 and 67–16 ■).

Nursing interventions for active drains include:

- Keep the drain tubing straight without kinks.
- Keep the reservoir compressed (a collapsed position) to maintain the negative pressure.

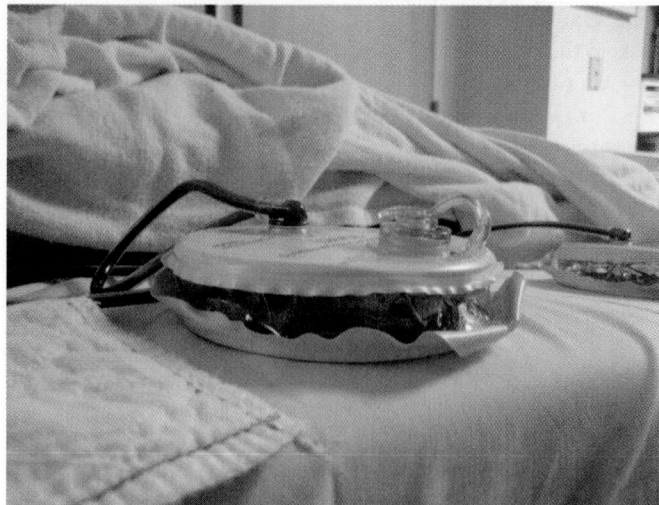
FIGURE 67–15 ■ Hemovac drain.
Source: Cheryl Wraa

- For optimal function, the reservoir should be emptied before it is half full.
- Unclog blood or tissue shreds from the drain tubing by milking or stripping toward the reservoir.
- Document amount and color of drainage.

Wounds initially have sanguineous or serosanguineous drainage. As the wound heals, there is less amount of drainage, and it becomes more serous.

Passive Drains

Passive drains are made of soft, flat, flexible material and are usually placed in a stab wound near an incision site. Pus, blood, necrotic debris, and fluids interfere with wound healing and can provide a milieu for pathogens. Passive drains provide a conduit that functions by gravity for the removal of this drainage, which may be too viscous for the active drains. An example of a common passive drain is a Penrose drain (Figure 67–14B ■).

The drain is typically sutured to secure it and keep it from migrating in or out of the wound. Flat gauze sponges or fenestrated sponges are used at the end of the drain to absorb the exudates. They are removed and new ones applied when the dressing be-

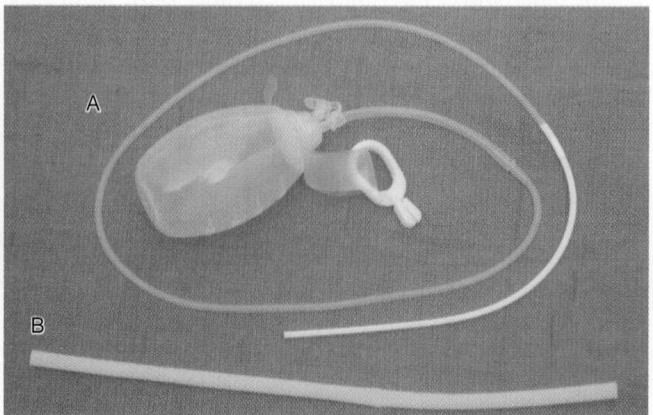
FIGURE 67–14 ■ A Jackson–Pratt and B Penrose drain.
Source: Courtesy of John M. Osborn, M. D., FACS, Sacramento, CA Plastic Surgery Center

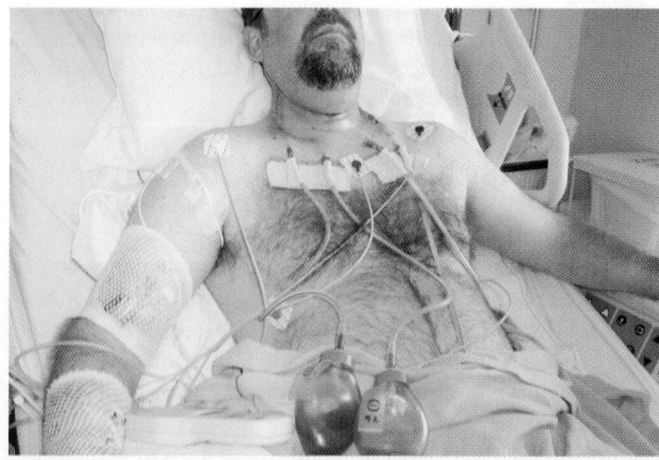
FIGURE 67–16 ■ Jackson-Pratt drain with serosanguineous drainage.
Source: Ann E. F. Sievers, RN

comes saturated, as these dressings may become wet with irritants to the skin. Care must be taken not to pull the drain out of the wound inadvertently during the dressing change. The nurse must protect the skin with a moisture barrier and frequently check the dressing to assess need for replacement.

Percutaneous Drainage Catheters

Interventional radiologists implant a percutaneous drainage catheter to allow drainage from sites where fluid collection may be infected, or to collect the fluid for laboratory studies to determine the nature of the fluid. The catheter is connected to a dependent drainage system such as a urinary leg bag. Placement sites include the biliary, peritoneal cavity, groin, breast, or anywhere infection is suspected.

Nursing care includes assessment for patency and irrigation of the catheter to maintain patency. Aseptic technique is used, and a health care provider's order is needed for the irrigation procedure, which includes the frequency and volume of irrigating solution to be used. Forceful instillation of fluid and forceful aspiration are never used. Accurate documentation is required regarding the color, amount, and consistency of fluid and the patient's tolerance of the procedure. Sterile dressings are used to cover the percutaneous site.

Impaired Wound Healing

Impaired wound healing is defined as the disruption of the normal biochemical repair or regeneration process. Abnormalities may be manifested in a number of ways, described next. If healing is occurring at a normal rate, the wound edges of an incision should not separate after the first 24 hours. Assessing the wound edges will give the nurse information about the healing process. If the edges are separated or there is serous or serosanguineous drainage, the nurse needs to assess the wound frequently for signs of impaired wound healing.

Dehiscence

Wound dehiscence is the separation of sutures or staples along the incision in a previously closed wound (Figure 67–17 ■). Dehiscence can be caused by infection or tension on the skin pulled together tightly with sutures or staples. Patients that are obese and patients on steroids are at a higher risk for the development of dehiscence. A sign of impending dehiscence is the leakage of serous or serosanguineous fluid from the incision for several days after injury or surgery. This indicates that collagen is not being properly formed and the tensile strength of the wound is impaired. If there is serosanguineous drainage, it should be absorbed by a sterile cover dressing. The characteristics of wound dehiscence drainage (amount, color, and odor), along with the length of the separation, should be reported to the surgeon emergently. The patient may need to return to surgery for wound closure, or the wound may need to be packed with dressings. To prevent maceration or irritation of the normal skin adjacent to the wound edges, liquid skin barriers or moisture barriers should be applied to the periwound skin with each dressing change.

Evisceration

Wound evisceration is defined as the protrusion of organs from a wound site (Figure 67–18 ■). It typically occurs following a wound dehiscence. The nurse needs to cover the organs with a sterile saline-moistened dressing and call the surgeon emergently. The patient will need to return to surgery for repair of the evisceration.

Hematoma and Seroma Formation

Hematoma is defined as an area of swelling or a mass of blood confined to an organ, tissue, or space due to a broken blood vessel. Due to the abnormal collection of blood in the tissues, hematomas are typically painful. It is the increased pain in the area when it should be decreasing that often leads to the diagnosis of hematoma. A hematoma can become infected and large enough to split the skin open and cause drainage. The treatment consists of cold compresses for the first 24 hours to decrease bleeding, elevation of the affected area, and, if large enough, aspiration is necessary. Antibiotics may be necessary if the hematoma becomes infected. The nurse needs to report the presence of a hematoma to the health care provider and do serial assessments to assess changes in the size. The wound will not completely heal until the hematoma has dissolved.

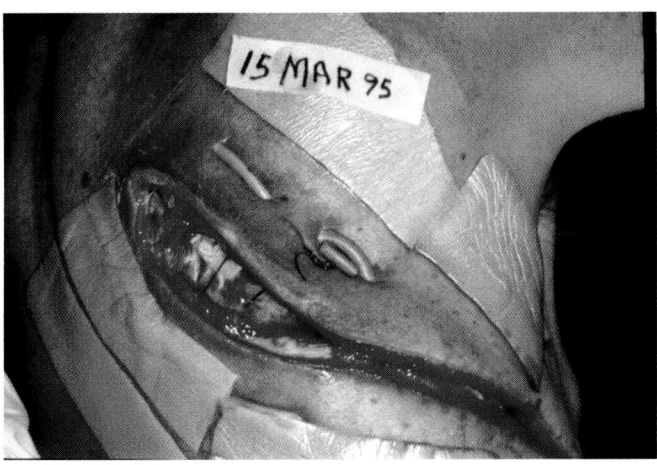

FIGURE 67–17 ■ Wound dehiscence.
Source: Jan Clark

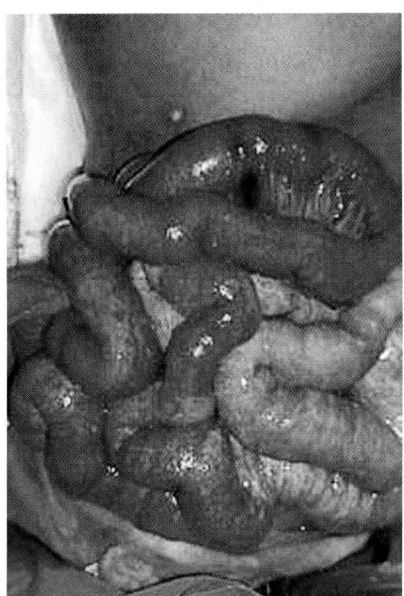

FIGURE 67–18 ■ Wound evisceration.
Source: Jan Clark

A **seroma** is the same as a hematoma except that instead of a collection of blood it is a collection of serous fluid. Its presence impacts wound healing; therefore, the typical treatment is aspiration or incision, and drainage procedure with postprocedure packing and secondary intention closure.

Literature suggests that patients that are obese are more prone to hematoma and seroma formation. Donor-site infections, donor-site seromas, and hernias also occur more frequently in patients that are obese. The large pannus predisposes patients to fluid accumulation, creating an environment conducive to seroma formation, infection, and wound edge separation or dehiscence (Wilson & Clark, 2004).

Nursing Management

Use of the nursing process guides the management of wounds. Beginning with a thorough nursing assessment of the wound is important in making decisions about treatment and goals because of the viable and changing nature of a wound. The treatment plan may need to be changed to facilitate these changes in the wound (Ovington, 2002). Typically guided by the health care provider's orders, the nurse is responsible for daily management of the wound. Therefore, the nurse is in a unique position to detect changes in the wound environment that indicate complications. Reporting these changes could prevent problems that may become life threatening. The nurse is in a pivotal position as a patient advocate to facilitate management by all the members of the health care team.

Assessment

Nurses are required to do routine scheduled and interventional assessments of their patients in all settings: acute and long-term acute care, home health, and nurse-managed clinic visits. The assessment becomes a written record of subjective and objective data. A systematic approach ensures a continuity of documentation and an accurate history of interventions and results. Assessment tools such as the Braden scale (p. 2207) are a reliable resource for the nursing documentation because of the succinct terminology. For example, assessment tools provide scores, numbers, and categories or indications of the acuity of a condition and specifically identify areas for intervention.

Skin Assessments

Skin assessments are different from wound assessments. Basic skin assessment should include observation of the entire body, checking temperature, color, moisture, turgor, and integrity. Chart 67–13 combines the elements of basic and comprehensive skin assessments as developed by Baranoski and Ayello (2004). Maintaining skin integrity in special populations—that is, the aged with frail skin, who have chronic diseases, or those who are immunosuppressed—can be a challenge. Routine assessments,

CHART 67–13 **Basic and Comprehensive Skin Assessment Elements**

Basic Skin Assessment	Characteristics	Comprehensive Skin Assessment	Characteristics
Temperature	Normally warm to touch. Warmer than normal could signal inflammation. Cooler than normal could signal poor vascularization.	Inspection	Normally smooth, slightly moist, and same general tone throughout. Tone: Melanocytes provide ranges from light ivory, light to deep brown, black, yellow to olive, light pink to dark ruddy pink or red.
Color	Intensity: paleness. Normal color tones. Hyperpigmentation or hypopigmentation reflecting blood flow or melanin deposits.	Palpation	Moisture: perspiration. Edema: eyes, extremities, sacrum. Tenderness. Turgor, elasticity. Texture.
Moisture	Dry or moist to touch. Hyperkeratosis (flaking, scales). Eczema. Dermatitis, psoriasis, rashes. Edema.	Olfaction	Normal body odor. Absence of pungent odor. Poor hygiene. Odor may indicate presence of bacteria or infection.
Turgor	Normally returns quickly to its original state. Slow return to original shape: dehydration or effect of aging.	Hair and Nails	Hair: • Hirsutism: excessive body hair • Alopecia: hair loss. Nails: • Color, shape, contour • Clubbing, texture thickness.
Integrity	No breakdown. Type of skin injury (record appropriate classification system to identify injury).	Skin Alterations	Previous scars. Graft sites. Healed ulcer sites. Piercings.

Source: Baranoski, S., & Ayello, E. (Eds.). (2004). *Wound care essentials: Practice principles.* Philadelphia: Lippincott Williams & Wilkins.

preventive interventions, and maintenance hydration are key elements of maintaining skin integrity.

Wound Assessments

Fresh postoperative wounds do not require the intense scrutiny of historical data like a chronic wound does because these data are available in the chart, but a systematic approach to assess wound characteristics is still useful. Initial chronic wound assessments should include the patient's immune status, allergies, blood glucose levels, hydration, nutrition, latest blood albumin levels, oxygen and vascular supply, social history, habits (e.g., smoking), a review of current medications, and if possible the patient's history of wound (etiology, age of wound, treatments thus far). These factors give the health care provider clues about why a chronic wound is not healing.

Measuring and tracking wound size is an outcomes approach to intervention. Special products are available to assist in proper measurement techniques. Length, width, and depth of the wound are standard measurements. Special measuring instruments, such as Puritan DM Stick (Puritan Medical Products Co., LLC), a sterile foam-tipped plastic swab marked in millimeters, safely and comfortably give accurate, consistent measurements. Tracing graphs of transparent film, such as E-Z Graph System of wound assessment (E.S. Graph of Victoria, Inc.), enable health care providers to outline the shape of the wound and show progress of the wound surface contracture. These tracings offer a great psychological boost to patients whose wounds are healing by millimeters, when they can see progress as compared to original wound size. Several measurement tools are available that graph or assign scores to the progress of the wound. Many institutions and agencies have protocols to include these tracking tools (Chart 67–14, p. 2226).

Nursing Diagnoses

The following nursing diagnoses are related to wound healing:

- *Risk for Infection*
- *Impaired Tissue Integrity*
- *Ineffective Tissue Perfusion, peripheral*
- *Disturbed Body Image.*

Planning

A plan for care is identified by the type of wound and the factors that coexist to impede the healing process. The plan of care should be individualized, and the patient and family should be involved in the planning process. The patient and family must agree to the plan of care and the interventions because they are responsible for the accurate and complete implementation of the plan overall. The plan will include diagnostic studies to follow up on factors that may or may not impede progress. All the information must be gleaned so that a correct and meaningful treatment plan is pursued.

Outcomes and Evaluation Parameters

The outcomes of interventions provide a basis for performance evaluation. By combining assessment skills and reviewing collected data, nurses are prepared to do an evaluation of the patient's overall condition. Connecting the specialized pieces such as wound assessment, respiratory assessment, and vascular assessment with integrated interventional data can result in an evaluation that is specific; for example, poor perfusion is contributing to slow wound healing and subsequent increased risk for infection.

The outcome or goal for the patient must be identified after all the diagnostic data are considered. The outcome may be driven by the goal of healing, the goal of preventing further damage, or even amputation. The outcome is directly related to how the plan of care impacts the factors that impede healing and the interventions to promote the most optimal environment. A good wound care plan addresses all the factors in wound healing to allow the body to heal itself. The wound will heal if all the factors that affect wound healing are addressed.

Evaluation parameters would include the clinical manifestations of effective wound healing. The wound is getting smaller in diameter as well as in depth. There is an absence of drainage, odor, and normal white blood count. The patient would be experiencing less pain and tenderness. Complete wound closure is the final evaluation parameter.

Interventions and Rationales

Nursing interventions are aimed at prevention of wound complications and promotion of healing. Interventions are developed based on assessment and diagnostic results. Wound management needs to follow the four principles of wound management. Débridement (see Chart 67–10, p. 2213) by any method will cause the body to respond to its signals through the phases of wound healing. For example, débridement will send signals that trigger platelet aggregation, MMP (matrix metalloproteinases) to denature harmed collagen, leukocytosis and phagocytosis to clean up the environment, and growth factors to heal the wound with new collagen synthesis. Dressings can be applied to provide moisture for epithelial migration in a dry wound or moisture retention and absorption to prevent maceration and further collagen damage in a wet wound. Silver can be applied as an antimicrobial agent. Offloading devices such as specialized shoes, splints, wheelchair cushions, or bed surfaces will alleviate pressure and restore circulation for healing. Nutrition should be addressed and supplements given to assist in correcting any deficiencies. Vascular status should be addressed and corrected if possible. Bioburden and infection must be controlled. Perineal care of the incontinent patient will help prevent skin breakdown. Keeping skin dry decreases friction and prevents breakdown from abrasive force. With microabrasions the skin has reduced barrier capability, allowing permeability to irritating substances and proliferation of bacteria and fungal infections. Protect the skin from wetness and fecal irritants by using moisture barriers on a regular basis on anyone who cannot get up and go to the bathroom on his own. Most soap leaves a difficult-to-rinse residue and has high pH levels that interfere with the skin's protective acid mantle. Soap can be irritating and strip the natural lubricant from skin. Skin cleansers should have nonionic surfactants that do not strip natural body oil. Skin cleansers can be any combination of products: antibacterial; 3-in-1 products for cleansing, moisturizing, and protecting; and pH balanced. Moisture barriers protect the skin from too much moisture (incontinence, perspiration). Many types and brands

CHART 67–14 Wound Assessment Guidelines

Wound Characteristic	Descriptors	Assessment Verbiage
Location	Upper/lower extremities Lateral/medial Left/right Midline Central Dorsal/plantar	Use anatomic location, such as malleolar or occipital. Describe proximity to other wounds consistently. Number wounds if more than one. Identify wound by classification and/or location. Example: "#1 skin tear, right upper extremity."
Size	length, width, and depth in centimeters	Always measure in centimeters; never estimate size by comparison; i.e., a quarter, the size of an orange.
Tracks	Centimeters and direction	Use a clock face as a frame of reference with 12 o'clock being toward the head. Example: "3-centimeter track at 2 o'clock."
Undermining	Centimeters and location	Example: "Undermining from 11 to 2 o'clock, from 1 to 1.5 centimeters."
Color	Red, yellow, black	Use percentages and shades of color. Example: "Pale red 60%, yellow 25%, black 15%."
Tissue	Granulation Epithelialization Necrotic Slough Eschar	Use descriptors: "Thick black eschar with 0.3-centimeter rim of pink tissue." "Beefy red granulation." "Pink epithelial tissue migrating toward center from 3 to 5 o'clock."
Exudate/drainage	Serous Sanguineous Serosanguineous Purulent	Use color and amount in descriptions: "Moderate serosanguineous, pink-tinged." "Minimal sanguineous, dark red." "Foam dressing saturated to edges of dressing and accumulation of exudates under dressing." (This might indicate increased drainage [infection?] or just a need for a more absorbent dressing.)
Odor	Subjective and difficult to quantify Indicate presence or not, foul	Remember that moisture retentive dressings also retain wound odor. When trying to control odor, description of presence of odor can measure outcomes: "Odor in room." "Odor at bedside." "Odor when dressing removed."
Wound margins	Rolled With epithelial tissue Defined, well demarcated Nondefined or nondemarcated	Describe margin appearance.
Periwound		
Erythema	Presence or not Intensity (color)	Use a marker pen on the skin to outline presence of suspicious erythema that might indicate infection/cellulitis.
Induration	Presence or not	May describe as increasing or resolving.
Maceration	Presence or not Extent in centimeters	Tissue maceration occurs when wound drainage or dressing moisture drowns cells. When the offending reason is contained or removed, the condition is repaired autolytically: The macerated tissue sloughs off and new skin has been generated.
Intervention and Tolerance		
Pain	Scale of 0–10	Clarify pain: "Tender when probed." "Premedicated with. . . ." "Pain subsided after packing completed."
Tolerance of procedure	Cleaning Packing Débridement	May overlap with pain assessment. A record here determines whether the patient needs premedication. Or does pain occur only during probing and packing and then subside?

of moisture barriers, body cleansers, and moisturizers are available. Emollients help keep moisture in the skin. Moisturizers add moisture to skin.

When a patient has a factor that impedes healing that cannot be corrected, the patient may be placed in conservative care and treated to prevent any further deterioration. Sometimes an amputation may be required to save the patient's life. It is not an easy decision, and the patient, family, and health care providers should come to an agreement that preservation of life overrides preservation of limb.

Evaluation

A wound and its environment and contributing factors determine the plan of care. The plan and treatment are altered in response to the assessment results of the wound, the periwound area, and any factors impeding its progress in healing. For instance, a wound may initially be draining a large amount of fluid and require an alginate. Once the drainage has decreased to a minimum, the wound bed may become dry and then require a moisture dressing such as a hydrogel to facilitate epidermal cell migration. Daily wound evaluation and documentation are indicated until there is complete wound closure. At this point the patient may also have returned to activities of daily living and so requires an offloading device. Education about protecting the newly healed wound until it matures is essential, or wound breakdown will occur.

Nursing Documentation

Nursing documentation in the patient's record must be accurate and complete in documenting the assessment, interventions, and outcomes, as well as the patient's responses to treatment. For example, wound characteristics noted after an assessment must be descriptive enough for someone who has not seen the wound to get a good mental picture. Note whether there has been a measurable outcome; that is, decrease in size, decreased drainage, increased epithelial tissue. The documentation needs to include what was used to clean the wound (saline or wound cleanser), type of dressing used and amount, and how the dressing was secured if necessary. Note significant changes that might indicate infection, and report them to the health care provider. Wound documentation also should include a patient's emotional response toward the wound and participation in wound care management. Specific to documentation of wound care, the following items should be part of the record:

- Be specific with date and time.
- Was the wound present on admission? This can be ascertained only if a head-to-toe inspection of the skin is done by the nurse.
- Record the name and score of any risk assessment tool that is used.
- How long has the patient had the wound?
- What is the specific location of the wound?
- What are the wound's surface dimensions and depth?
- What types of dressings were used and how much?
- Note changes in quantity and odor of exudates/drainage.
- What is the condition of skin surrounding the wound?
- What support surface is the patient on? Remember that specialty support surfaces are therapeutic treatment and

should be acknowledged in interventions/assessment and documentation.
- Is there progress or deterioration of the wound?
- What are the patient's and family/caregiver's reactions to the wound? Do they participate in wound care? Are their expectations reasonable?

It is necessary for the records to reflect the health care provider's orders requiring specific dressing type, frequency of dressing changes, dressing amounts used, and expected length of need. The record must reflect a diagnosis with wound description and classification if applicable. Each wound should be described separately and evaluation of wound is required monthly. Documentation can make the difference in whether treatment and/or supplies are reimbursed.

■ Collaborative Management

The primary aim of clinical management for wound healing is expedient closure of the wound with no complications. The interdisciplinary team members including the primary health care provider, certified wound care specialist nurse, nutritionist, hospitalist, vascular surgeon and/or oncologist, pharmacist, and the nurse should be included in the wound care plan. Typically wounds are not an isolated problem for most patients. The patient's comorbidities must continue to be treated. In the acute setting, the wound is often not the admitting diagnosis. Traumatic wound treatment is begun on admission in the emergency department. Frequently the certified wound care nurse is called for these wounds by surgeons to provide continuing care of the wound. If the patient is admitted with a chronic wound, the certified wound care nurse should be notified; an assessment of wound will be made; the admitting or referring health care provider will be notified of recommended treatment; orders will be obtained; and staff nurses will institute them. Staff nurses doing admission assessments need to remove existing dressings and assess, document, and report the presence of wounds. Most hospitals ensure that a nutritionist sees a patient within 24 hours of admission. Nutritionists will make recommendations for dietary considerations such as calorie intake, supplements, and vitamins, and place them in the chart. Nurses are expected to monitor intake. Plastic or vascular surgeons may be consulted for nonhealing chronic wounds as well as traumatic injuries. They may be called to perform sharp débridement. Dermatologists may be consulted for other skin issues such as rashes. Podiatrists may be consulted for foot and diabetic wounds. Endocrinologists may be consulted to control diabetes. Pharmacists may be depended on to advise about medications that will slow down wound healing and the timing for tests for antibiotic efficacy with peaks and troughs. Blood samples are drawn at specific intervals before and after antibiotic administration and sent to the laboratory to determine the amount of antibiotic in the system. This can determine whether the amount of antibiotic should be adjusted for efficacy. Respiratory therapists ensure that the patient's oxygenation is optimal. Physical therapists may do wound care in some settings. Physical therapists need to be informed about wounds so dressings and drains are free of tension. Some treatment/therapies may be covered by different services in different settings such as Unna's boot (Chapter 43) for venous stasis ulcers or application of plaster casts to take the pressure off of diabetic wounds. A growing trend is the service of the hospitalist, a health care provider that specializes in coordinating and communicating the care of patients while in the hospital with the primary care health care provider and all other services consulted. A collaborative team approach ensures that all aspects of the wound healing process are being guided by people that are knowledgeable in each aspect of care.

> **CRITICAL ALERT** *Most chronic wounds are not emergencies (unless sepsis is present). Remember that saline and gauze are the safe universal dressing and that pressure relief is essential in preventing ulcer formation.*

All these individuals may or may not actually meet to discuss a patient's care. Charting by all of the individuals is ideally read as each comes to assess and treat the patient. Nurses have an obligation to read the notes to become informed of patient status. In home health, communication of patient status to the health care provider is of paramount importance, because the home health nurse may be the only one doing a physical assessment for long periods of time. Accurate descriptions of existing wounds are valuable to the health care providers making decisions regarding patient care.

Health Promotion

Education of the patient or caregiver regarding decisions and goals of treatment has been found to be an important factor in successful wound healing. Tenets of an effective teaching plan include:

- Wound care
- Infection prevention/assessment
- Nutrition
- Lifestyles and habits that prevent or slow wound healing
- Prevention of wound breakdown
- Follow-up care.

Each of these factors must be taught to the patient and family/caregivers in a logical, understandable fashion. For example, a written plan and return demonstrations from the patient/family help facilitate teaching.

Identifying the patient's needs for discharge begins on admission to the health care setting. The process includes assessment, identification of continuing care needs, planning, and implementing a plan that will meet those determined needs. Today it is a common practice to send patients home before wounds have completely healed and to have their care continued at home and in the outpatient clinic setting. A variety of health care professionals can be involved with the process, as described earlier, but the nurse is the pivotal figure in establishing a comprehensive discharge plan. Developing a complete plan of care and providing a manner in which routine reevaluation and modification of the plan can occur will facilitate the process until wound closure has occurred. Nurses must educate patients and family/caregivers about all aspects of the wound care. Concise written instructions beginning with a statement about hand hygiene should be given to the patient or caregiver. Return demonstration ensures that the patient and caregiver understand the procedures. If the patient is

to be discharged with a drain in place, the patient should know the purpose of the drain, expected output, drain care and emptying, how to troubleshoot, whom to contact for questions, and whom to contact for an emergency.

Discharge Planning

Patients and their family need to be actively involved in the discharge planning process. The nurse must evaluate the knowledge and willingness to participate in the wound care and then develop instructions and guidelines for the patient and caregiver. If barriers exist that will affect their ability to provide effective care, an alternative plan must be instituted. For example, recognizing cultural influences and family roles is essential, so the teaching can be individualized and meaningful. An assessment of resources and transportation also is an essential component of the plan. The nurse needs to evaluate the patient and family's ability to afford and obtain the necessary supplies for the wound care. State and federal resources may need to be sought to provide the necessary equipment and supplies. The Patient Teaching & Discharge Priorities box describes the necessary components of the discharge teaching plan.

■ Psychological Considerations

Acute and chronic wounds affect quality of life. Patients often experience depression, isolation, and financial burdens caused by wounds. Cultural issues may create misunderstanding or "compliance" issues. Nurses are often first aware and most aware of these conditions. Assessing the meaning and significance of the wound to the patient and family or caregiver is often overlooked. Frequently pain is associated with wounds and body image may be disturbed. Pain occurs due to the nerve endings being exposed, and some of the interventions utilized to heal the wound can cause varying degrees of pain. As with all assessment of pain, it is what the patient states it is as far as severity, character, duration, and tolerance level. Medications can be prescribed to alleviate the pain. Nonnarcotic medications such as nonsteroidal anti-inflammatories (NSAIDs) can alleviate pain and decrease inflammation. Narcotic medications such as opioid or opioid derivatives can be given. One should consider adequate pain coverage before dressing changes, changes in position, or mobility. Controlling pain can help patients to be more compliant with the treatment plan and willing to investigate other treatment modalities if their pain is sufficiently controlled to a tolerance level that they can withstand. Pain can be assessed on a number scale, facial scale, vital sign assessment, or combinations of such scales. Chapter 15 ☺ includes an in-depth discussion of pain management.

Depression can occur when a patient has a wound. It may affect the way she sees herself or the way she perceives that others see her, especially if the wound is easily visible. Not only does the patient have an emotional response to her wound, but almost everyone the patient encounters has an emotional response to her wound. Wounds are perceived as unpleasant, disgusting, scary, and a nuisance. Depression may affect the patient's ability to perform the daily activities he desires to do, and it may limit patient independence. It can be very costly for the treatments and medications. The patient may have to wear some special type of shoe or device that makes her self-conscious.

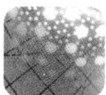

PATIENT TEACHING & DISCHARGE PRIORITIES for the Management of Wounds

Need	Teaching
WOUND CARE Patient/family Family/support system Setting	Perform daily cleansing and dressing changes: • How often to change the dressing • Type of dressing and solutions. Elevate areas where edema formation occurs. Avoid sunlight, as it can cause, among other things, healed wounds to discolor or darken permanently: • Avoid overexposure to sun. • Use sunscreen products when exposed to sunlight. • Use clothing and hats for added protection. Avoid exposure to extreme temperatures and harsh chemicals. Wear loose-fitting, soft clothing. Assess availability of, knowledge of, and compliance with treatment regimen. Have family perform return demonstration. Assess discharge placement needs: • Home • Rehabilitation facility • Extended care facility. Assess need for professional home health needs. Assess need for follow-up appointments.
WOUND INFECTION Patient/family Family/support system Setting	Assess for infection of open wounds and healed wound breakdown with each dressing change, and report as necessary. Signs and symptoms include: • Odor and exudate • Fever • Increased drainage • Swelling • Lack of wound closure • Increased pain. Teach minimization of risk factors for infection: • Hand hygiene • Clean technique with dressing changes. Explain signs and symptoms that require medical attention. Assess environment for risk factors that increase the risk of infection.
NUTRITION Patient/family Setting	Maintain a high-calorie, high-protein diet. Continue taking vitamins and mineral supplements as ordered. Observe for appetite and weight loss, and food intolerance. Assess financial resources. Home. Rehabilitation center.
PAIN MANAGEMENT Patient/family Setting	Assess pain level and report any increase in pain. Assess effectiveness of pharmacologic interventions. Wean patient off pain medication when pain lessens. Report a sudden increase in pain. Assess environment for safety and promotion of therapeutic needs.

MyNursingKit | Video: Infection Control: Dressing Change—Clean Technique

The nurse needs to assess the patient for her feelings about her wound and associated treatment. Empathize with the patient, and try to devise a plan that is least intrusive and yet realistic. A nurse can address the concerns by providing privacy during dressing changes; factual explanation of the wound to patient and family or caregiver; frank discussions with the patient and caregiver about how the wound is affecting them; scheduling wound care at the best time for the patient; and applying appro-priate dressings and performing timely dressing changes. Instruct the patient on what can or will happen if treatment is not followed according to the individualized plan. Patients want to be informed and want honest feedback but need some compassion with the delivery of their care. Educational sites on the Internet for them to visit as well as support groups may be helpful. The wound affects one's daily lifestyle and thus cannot help but be a nuisance and a factor in the way that the patient feels about himself and how others perceive him to be. An individual who has had a recent amputation, has a whole new set of restrictions and adaptations to overcome. The patient will need education to prevent further insults from occurring to preserve the best way of life he can expect. Document the patient's response to the wound. Chapter 13 🔗 includes an in-depth discussion of the psychosocial aspects of nursing.

Ethical Issues

Treatment of wounds can also lead to a discussion about aggressive versus conservative care. For example, what is the appropriate care for a nursing home resident patient who has previously had multiple strokes and is now aphasic and bedbound? A sacral pressure ulcer develops and eschar is observable. The patient is debilitated and has failure to thrive. Is aggressive treatment of the wound with surgical intervention appropriate? Does the patient have the ability to heal if surgical intervention is performed? Can the patient even be cleared for surgery safely? These are all questions that must be asked and considered before developing a treatment plan. The patient may not be a candidate for aggressive care, and a conservative approach may be the ethical and prudent action. The goal may be to prevent the further deterioration of the wound. Obviously, a collaborative approach among the health care team, patient, and family must occur to make a decision on what ultimate goal or outcome is desired. As hard as it is at times as health care professionals, sometimes the best plan is not the most aggressive but the most realistic plan that requires acceptance. Decisions for care and the degree of aggressiveness or lack thereof, must be consistent with the patient's overall physiological status and well as the patient's and family's goals. Those goals may be complete restoration, ability to function, or provision of comfort. Caregivers experience a myriad range of emotions. Balancing the needs of the patient with that of the caregiver can be a difficult role. As the nurse it is important to understand that the health-related quality of life is the patient's perception of well-being and not an evaluation of clinical status.

▊ Research

Research is essential in order to continue improving wound care, complication rates, healing time, and scar formation. The goal of research is to identify areas in which practice needs to be improved and then to evaluate and test methods in these areas. The Research Opportunities and Clinical Impact box related to wound healing provides a list of both medical and nursing research topics still under investigation. Electronic databases are a source for finding specific studies related to these topics.

▊ Liability

It is essential that the nurse understands how the regulatory and accrediting bodies such as the Joint Commission assess individual wound interventions and their effectiveness. These regulatory bodies monitor what nurses do as individuals and what they accomplish aggregately within an institution. Hospitals must have quality assurance records regarding pressure ulcer incidence and measures for reduction.

The development of wounds, in particular pressure ulcers, has led to a lot of controversy over quality of care and thus liability. Pressure ulcers, for the most part, are preventable. Prevention requires a plan of action that is individualized and vigilant. As a result of so many preventable ulcers that have developed over the years, the U.S. government has taken steps to try to ensure that all necessary action be taken to prevent pressure ulcers from developing due to negligence. A federal tag, called F-tag 314, requires long-term care facilities (nursing homes) to comply with certain regulations concerning prevention and treatment of pressure ulcers in the long-term care setting. The long-term care facility must assess those at risk for development of a pressure ulcer, follow certain preventative guidelines, demonstrate compliance with those guidelines, and, if the patient still develops a pressure ulcer, show appropriate intervention. The patient must then be monitored for progress and the plan of care altered if the plan fails to achieve the desired result of healing. The Centers for

---

RESEARCH OPPORTUNITIES AND CLINICAL IMPACT RELATED TO WOUND HEALING

Research Area	Clinical Impact
Wound healing dressings that promote faster healing.	Prevent infection.
Wound healing cleansers.	Prevent infection.
Topical hyperbaric oxygen treatment.	Increase healing rates.
Dietary factors that impact wound healing.	Increase healing rates.
The nature of pain induced by direct tissue injury.	Patient comfort and increased wound healing.
Nursing pain management.	
Pain and anxiety measurement and management during procedures.	
Mechanisms to prevent scar formation.	Improve wound appearance and prevent contracture formation.
Prevention of hypertrophic and keloid scar formation.	Improve wound appearance and prevent contracture formation.
Techniques to increase tensile strength and reduce wound breakdown.	Improve techniques to increase wound healing and prevent scarring.
Role of growth factors in wound healing.	Improve techniques to increase wound healing.

Silver as an Antimicrobial Agent

Clinical Problem

Infection is a common complication for a patient with a wound, especially a chronic wound. Prophylactic antibiotic use has allowed more resistant bacterial organisms to proliferate. Because wounds that are chronic may now be colonized with bacteria, deciding when and how to treat can be a complicated decision. Silver is a product that has come into wide use as a local antimicrobial agent, and the evidence surrounding its effectiveness, how much to use, and in what medium has been the subject of great debate in wound care.

Research Findings

Ip, Lui, Poon, Lung, and Burd (2006) performed a study that utilized an agar medium and various types of microorganisms such as methicillin-resistant *Staphylococcus aureus* (MRSA) and vancomycin-resistant enterococcus (VRE), as well as other microbes. Different silver dressings were applied. The result revealed that those with a higher concentration of ionic silver had a quicker and broader bactericidal effect. It was noted, however, that too much silver could potentially damage tissue and kill keratinocytes and fibroblasts. The most important factors relative to antimicrobial effectiveness are the bioavailability concentration and rate of delivery to the tissue. Indeed, different concentrations of silver ions could be used depending on intended desire. Prophylactic treatment could contain fewer silver ions than treatment of an active infection. The goal is to deliver the minimum amount of silver ions to perform the intended outcome.

Implications for Nursing Practice

It appears that silver is an important part of antimicrobial activity for a wound to prevent infection or treat an active infection. Silver should be treated as any other drug and utilized appropriately to the individual situation and only for its intended use. Silver is relatively cheap, abundant, and highly effective against resistant microorganisms. Its success has been repeatedly demonstrated and makes it a useful tool in wound care.

Critical Thinking Questions

1. What are some goals for the use of silver as it relates to wound care?

2. Ionic silver (Ag+) is the effective chemical against bacteria. What would happen if it were to meet the chloride ion (Cl−) *in situ* (in its environment in the wound)?

3. Identify other nursing measures to prevent infection in a wound.

Answers to Critical Thinking Questions appear in Appendix D.

Reference

Ip, M., Lui, S., Poon, V., Lung, I., & Burd, A. (2006). Antimicrobial activities of silver dressings: An *in vitro* comparison. *Journal of Medical Microbiology, 55,* 59–63.

EVIDENCE-BASED PRACTICE

Medicare & Medicaid Services (CMS) guidelines for October 2008 will not pay for treatment of a pressure ulcer that develops during the hospital stay. A hospital acquired pressure ulcer will have its own diagnosis-related group (DRG) code, and it will be differentiated from a community acquired DRG code. The statistics of the hospitals will be available to the public in the near future. CMS ultimately will not pay for the continuation of care for the patient with a hospital acquired pressure or decubitus ulcer, and the hospital will be responsible for all care of that patient related to that ulcer going forward. The hospital will bear the financial responsibility for the care of that patient's pressure ulcer even if the patient is no longer physically in that hospital. Documentation by health care providers and nursing staff will be pivotal in establishing whether the pressure ulcer was present on admission (POA).

◼ Summary

Many recent advancements have been made with regard to wound care treatment. For example, living tissue dressing applications such as Apligraf have decreased the recovery time of healing effectively. Other xenografts (from a nonhuman animal source) such as Primatrix and Oasis have been developed as rich collagen sources to "fill in" a wound and again speed up the healing process. Ultraviolet light therapy and ultrasound therapy are being utilized to control bioburden and promote the healing process as well. The future may hold many significant advances with gene therapy and alteration/replication. Research and advancements will occur in wound therapy and healing; but the factors required for a wound to heal will not change, and the body will "heal thyself" as long as those factors required are present.

NCLEX® REVIEW

1. A patient with poor circulation has a leg wound. The nurse realizes that which phase of the wound healing process could be compromised in this patient?
   1. Homeostasis
   2. Inflammatory
   3. Proliferation
   4. Remodeling

2. A patient has been diagnosed with a tunneling wound. The nurse would document the size of the wound:
   1. In inches.
   2. In centimeters squared.
   3. Using the clock face method.
   4. In centimeters cubed.

3. A patient, prone to pressure ulcer development, is unable to move independently in bed. Which of the following should the nurse to do assist this patient?

   1. Move the patient's limbs every hour.
   2. Use the rule of 30 to reposition the patient every two hours.
   3. Minimize the use of assistive devices to move the patient.
   4. Avoid the use of foam wedges.

4. A patient has a category II skin tear on her forearm. Which of the following would be appropriate to care for this wound?

   1. Use compression therapy.
   2. Plan for surgical intervention.
   3. Apply a moisture barrier and secure with gauze.
   4. Plan for debridement of the wound.

5. A critically ill patient needs to have a leg wound debrided. The nurse realizes that the best approach to use for this patient wound be:

   1. Autolytic debridement.
   2. Sharp debridement.
   3. Mechanical debridement.
   4. Enzymatic debridement.

6. A patient with a leg wound tells the nurse that she's ugly and is not really sure if she wants to take care of the wound when she goes home. Which of the following should the nurse say in response to this patient?

   1. It's not that bad.
   2. Tell me why you think the wound is ugly.
   3. I have to agree with you.
   4. Maybe you can stay in the hospital until it's healed.

7. A patient with a wound has a poor appetite. The nurse realizes this will impact the patient's:

   1. Risk of infection.
   2. Healing rate.
   3. Wound appearance.
   4. Comfort level.

Answers for review questions appear in Appendix D

KEY TERMS

acute wounds *p.2199*
angiogenesis *p.2193*
basement membrane *p.2202*
chronic wounds *p.2199*
collagen synthesis *p.2193*
epithelialization *p.2193*
fibroblasts *p.2193*
granulation tissue *p.2193*
growth factors *p.2193*
hematoma *p.2223*
hemosiderin staining *p.2200*

homeostasis *p.2192*
hyperbaric oxygen therapy (HBOT) *p.2218*
hypergranulation *p.2222*
iatrogenic wounds *p.2199*
impaired wound healing *p.2223*
inflammatory phase *p.2193*
interface pressure *p.2219*
phagocytes *p.2193*
phagocytosis *p.2193*
pressure ulcer *p.2204*
primary intention *p.2212*

prostaglandin *p.2193*
remodeling *p.2194*
rete pegs *p.2198*
secondary intention *p.2212*
senile purpura *p.2198*
seroma *p.2224*
tertiary or third intention *p.2212*
traumatic wounds *p.2199*
wound dehiscence *p.2223*
wound evisceration *p.2223*
xerosis *p.2198*

PEARSON

EXPLORE   mynursingkit™

MyNursingKit is your one stop for online chapter review materials and resources. Prepare for success with additional NCLEX®-style practice questions, interactive assignments and activities, web links, animations and videos, and more!

Register your access code from the front of your book at
www.mynursingkit.com

REFERENCES

Agency for Health Care Policy and Research (AHCPR). (1992). *Pressure ulcers in adults: Prediction and prevention* (Publication No. 92-0047). Rockville, MD: Author. Retrieved September 11, 2008, from http://www.ncbi.nlm.nih.gov/books/bv.fcgi?rid=hstat2.chapter.4409

Agency for Health Care Policy and Research (AHCPR). (1994). *Treatment of pressure ulcers in adults* (Publication No. 95-0652). Rockville, MD: Author. Retrieved September 11, 2008, from http://www.ncbi.nlm.nih.gov/books/bv.fcgi?rid=hstat2.chapter.5124

Argenta, L. C., & Morykwas, M. J. (1997). Vacuum assisted closure: A new method for wound control and treatment: Clinical experience. *Annals of Plastic Surgery, 38*(6), 563–577.

Armstrong, M. H., & Price, P. (2004). Wet-to-dry gauze dressings: Fact and fiction. *Wounds, 16*(2), 56–62.

Arnold, M. C. (2003). Pressure ulcer prevention and management: The current evidence for care. *AANC Clinical Issues: Advanced Practice in Acute Critical Care, 14*(4), 411–428.

Baranoski, S. (2006). Raising awareness of pressure ulcer prevention and treatment. *Advances in Skin and Wound Care, 19*(7), 398–405.

Baranoski, S., & Ayello, E. (Eds.). (2004). *Wound care essentials: Practice principles.* Philadelphia: Lippincott Williams & Wilkins.

Black, P. et al., (2007). National pressure ulcer advisory panel's updated pressure ulcer staging system. Medscape Nurses from web MD.

Retrieved on September 13, 2008, from http://www.medscape.com/viewarticle/563159

Christian, P., Talavera, F., Stadelmann, W., Slenkovich, N., & Downey, S. (2006). Wound healing, growth factors. *eMedicine.* Retrieved September 7, 2008, from http://www.emedicine.com/plastic/topic457.htm

Clark, J. J. (2002). Wound repair and factors influencing healing. *Critical Care Nursing Quarterly, 25*(1), 1–12.

Coats-Bennett, U. (2002). Use of support surfaces in the ICU. *Critical Care Nursing Quarterly, 25*(1), 22–32.

Corbett, J. V. (2004). *Laboratory tests and diagnostic procedures with nursing diagnoses* (6th ed.). Upper Saddle River, NJ: Pearson Prentice Hall.

Cranton, E. M. (2005). *Hyperbaric oxygen therapy.* Retrieved September 13, 2008, from http://drcranton.com/hbo.htm

Cutting, K. F., & White, R. J. (2005). Criteria for identifying wound infection—Revisited. *Ostomy Wound Management, 51*(1), 28–34.

Drosou, A., Falabella, A., & Kirsner, R. (2003). Antiseptics on wounds: An area of controversy (Part one). *Wounds.* Retrieved October 29, 2007, from http://www.woundsresearch.com/article/1586

Duffy, J., & Korniewicz, D. (2000). Outcomes measurement using the ANA safety and quality indicators. *Nursing World.* Retrieved October 29, 2007, from http://nursingworld.org/mods/archive/mod72/ceomfull.htm

Enoch, S., & Harding, K. (2003). Wound bed preparation: The science behind the removal of barriers to healing (Part two). *Wounds.* Retrieved October 29, 2007, from http://www.woundsresearch.com/article/1798

Frykberg, R. G. (2002). Diabetic foot ulcers: Pathogenesis and management. *American Family Physician, 66*(9), 1655–1662.

Gardner, S. E., & Frantz, R. A. (2004). Wound bioburden. In S. Baranoski & E. A. Ayello (Eds.), *Wound care essentials: Practice principles* (pp. 91–116). Philadelphia: Lippincott Williams & Wilkins.

Gibbs, S., Silva Pinto, A. N., Murli, S., Huber, M., Hohl, D., & Ponec, M. (2000). Epidermal growth factor and keratinocyte grow factor differentially regulate epidermal migration, growth and differentiation. *Wound Repair Regeneration, 8*(3), 192–203.

Halek, M., & Mayer, H. (2002). Predictive validity of the original and expanded Norton Scale in geriatric nursing. *Pflege, 15*(6), 309–317.

Hanson, D., Langemo, D., Anderson, J., Hunter, S., & Thompson, P. (2006). Pressure mapping: Seeing the invisible. *Advances in Skin and Wound Care, 19*(8), 432–434.

Hinman, C. D., & Maibach, H. (1963). Effect of air exposure and occlusion on experimental human skin wounds. *Nature, 200,* 377–378.

Hiok, T. L. (1997). *Leg ulcers: A multidisciplinary approach.* Retrieved September 1, 2007, from http://www.nsc.gov.sg/cgi-bin/WB_ContentGen.pl?id=242&gid=49

Ip, M., Lui, S., Poon, V., Lung, I., & Burd, A. (2006). Antimicrobial activities of silver dressings: An *in vitro* comparison. *Journal of Medical Microbiology, 55,* 59–63.

Joseph, E., Hamori, C. A., Bergman, S., Roaf, E., Swann, N. F., & Anastasi, G. W. (2000). A prospective randomized trial of vacuum assisted closure versus standard therapy of chronic nonhealing wounds. *Wounds, 12*(3), 60–67.

Lavery, L. A., Armstrong, D. G., & Harkless, L. B. (1996). Classification of diabetic foot ulcerations. *Journal of Foot and Ankle Surgery, 35*(6), 528.

Leach, M. J., et al. (2006a). Clinical efficacy of horse chestnut seed extract in the treatment of venous ulceration. *Journal of Wound Care, 15*(4), 159–167.

Leach, M. J., et al. (2006b). Using horse chestnut seed extract in the treatment of venous leg ulcers: A cost–benefit analysis. *Ostomy Wound Management, 52*(4), 68–70, 72–74, 76–78.

Martin, N., Oldani, T., & Claxton, M. (2005). A guide to offloading the diabetic foot. *Podiatry Today, 9*(18), 67–74.

Marucha, P. T. (2005). *Modulation of inflammation by stress and psychosocial factors.* Retrieved August 6, 2005, from http://medicine.osu.edu/mindbody/project_2.html

MayoClinic.com. (2006). *Pyoderma gangrenosum.* Retrieved September 1, 2007, from http://www.mayoclinic.com/health/pyoderma-gangrenosum/DS00723

McGuckin, M., Goldman, R., Bolton, L., & Salcido, R. (2003). The clinical relevance of microbiology in acute and chronic wounds. *Advances in Skin & Wound Care, 16,* 12–25.

MedTech1.com. (2005). *What is V.A.C.® therapy?* Retrieved December 14, 2006, from http://www.medtech1.com/companies/kci.cfm

Nataraj, C., Ritter, G., Dumas, S., Helfer, F., Brunelle, J., & Sander, T. W. (2007). Extracellular wound matrices: Novel stabilization and sterilization method for collagen-based biologic wound dressings. *Wounds.* Retrieved September 1, 2007, from http://www.woundsresearch.com/article/7374

National Institute for Health and Clinical Excellence (NICE). (2005). *Pressure ulcer management.* Retrieved September 11, 2008, from http://www.nice.org.uk/CG029

National Pressure Ulcer Advisory Panel (NPUAP). (1998). *Instructions for using the PUSH tool.* Retrieved September 13, 2008 from http://www.npuap.org/pushinstr.htm

National Pressure Ulcer Advisory Panel (NPUAP). (2007a). *Updated staging system.* Retrieved October 1, 2007, from http://www.npuap.org/push3-0.htm

National Pressure Ulcer Advisory Panel (NPUAP). (2007b). *Updated staging system. Pressure ulcer stages revised by NPUAP.* Retrieved September 1, 2007, from http://www.npuap.org/pr2.htm

Norman, D. (2003). The effects of stress on wound healing and leg ulceration. *British Journal of Nursing, 12*(21), 1256–1263.

Odland, G. (1958). The fine structure of the interrelationship of cells in the human epidermis. *Journal of Biophysical, Biochemistry and Cytology, 4,* 529–535.

Ovington, L. (2002). General principles of wound care. In P. J. Sheffield, A. P. S. Smith, & C. E. Fife (Eds.), *Wound care practice* (pp. 159–187). Flagstaff, AZ: Best Publishing.

Pittler, M. H., & Ernst, E. (2006). Horse chestnut seed extract for chronic venous insufficiency. *Cochrane Database of Systematic Reviews, 25*(1), CD003230.

Porth, C. (2007). *Essentials of pathophysiology* (2nd ed.). Philadelphia: Lippincott Williams & Wilkins.

Pressure ulcers. (2005). *Professional guide to diseases* (8th ed.). Retrieved October 24, 2007, from http://www.wrongdiagnosis.com/b/bedsores/book-diseases-7a.htm

Rolstad, B. S., Ovington, L. G., & Harris, A. (2000). Principles of wound management. In R. A. Bryant (Ed.), *Acute and chronic wounds: Nursing management* (2nd ed., pp. 85–124). St. Louis: Mosby.

Shah, B. R., & Hux, J. E. (2003). Quantifying the risk of infectious diseases for people with diabetes. *Diabetes Care.* Retrieved September 1, 2007, from http://care.diabetesjournals.org/cgi/content/abstract/26/2/510

Smith, A. P. S. (2002). Etiology of the problem wound. In P. J. Sheffield, A. P. S. Smith, & C. E. Fife (Eds.), *Wound care practice* (pp. 3–48). Flagstaff, AZ: Best Publishing.

Smith & Nephew Clinical Staff. (2001). *Treatment options for surgical wounds.* Retrieved September 13, 2008, from http://wound.smith-nephew.com/au/node.asp?NodeId=3746

Steinberg, J. S. (2004). Understanding growth factors and matrix metalloproteinases in the diabetic foot wound. *Wounds, 16*(Suppl. B), 13S–24S.

Sussman, C. (1998). *Electrical stimulation.* Retrieved October 1, 2007, from http://www.medicaledu.com/estim.htm

Undersea & Hyperbaric Medical Society. (2007). *Indications for hyperbaric oxygen therapy.* Retrieved October 1, 2007, from http://www.uhms.org/Default.aspx?tabid=270

U.S. Department of Health and Human Services (DHHS). (2000). *Healthy People 2010 understanding and improving health.* Washington, DC: Author.

Vaughn, M. (2002). Physical therapeutic modalities in wound healing. In P. J. Sheffield, A. P. S. Smith, & C. E. Fife (Eds.), *Wound care practice* (pp. 159–187). Flagstaff, AZ: Best Publishing.

Waldrop, J., & Doughty, D. (2000). Wound-healing physiology. In R. A. Bryant (Ed.), *Acute and chronic wounds: Nursing management* (2nd ed., pp. 17–40). St. Louis: Mosby.

Warren, J. B., Yoder, L. H., & Young-McCaughan, S. (1999). Development of a decision tree for support surfaces: A tool for nursing. *MEDSURG Nursing, 8*(4), 239–248.

White, R., & Cutting, K. (2006). *Modern exudate management: A review of wound treatments.* Retrieved October 1, 2007, from http://www.worldwidewounds.com/2006/september/White/Modern-Exudate-Mgt.html

Wicke, C., Halliday, B., Allen, D., Roche, N. S., Scheuenstuhl, H., Spencer, M., et al. (2000). Effects of steroids and retinoids on wound healing. *Archives of Surgery, 135,* 1265–1270.

Wilson, J. A., & Clark, J. J. (2004). Obesity: Impediment to postsurgical wound healing. *Advances in Skin & Wound Care, 17*(8), 426–435.

Winter, G. D. (1962). Formation of scab and the rate of epithelialization of superficial wounds in the skin of the young domestic pig. *Nature, 193,* 293–294.

Wood, W. A., et al. (2005). Testing for loss of protective sensation in patients with foot ulceration: A cross-sectional study. *Journal of the American Podiatric Medical Association, 95,* 469–474.

Wound, Ostomy, and Continence Nurses Society (WOCN). (2003). *Guideline for prevention and management of pressure ulcers.* Glenview, IL: Author. Retrieved September 11, 2008, from http://www.guideline.gov/summary/summary.aspx?doc_id=3860

68

Caring for the Patient with Burn Injuries

Kathleen Osborn

Outcome-Based Learning Objectives

After studying this chapter, the learner will be able to:

1. Differentiate between the three classifications of burn injury: mild, moderate, and major.

2. Compare and contrast the causes, incidence, prevalence, types, and prevention of burn injuries.

3. Describe the pathophysiological response of burn injury at the tissue and organ level.

4. Compare and contrast the three periods of burn care.

5. Describe the significance and components of burn severity assessment including size and depth of injury, impact of patient's age on injury, part of the body burned, and past medical history.

6. Describe the components of a comprehensive burn treatment plan for each of the three periods of burn care including fluid resuscitation, pain management, wound care, surgical management, contracture prevention, nutritional needs, and emotional adjustment.

7. Describe the discharge teaching needed to facilitate an optimal recovery and return to society.

8. Identify the potential complications associated with each period of burn injury.

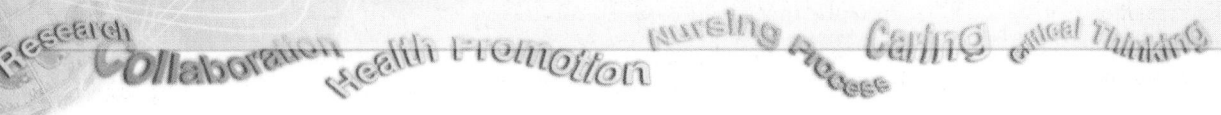

BURN INJURIES are a traumatic, dehumanizing injury that can be fatal, disfiguring, and incapacitating. Burns cause a loss of skin integrity that ranges from a minor superficial injury to a deep full-thickness injury that extends into the underlying structures and organs. As noted in National Guidelines box, according to the American Burn Association (ABA), burns are classified as minor, moderate, or major. All three categories of injury may cause a systemic response; but the deeper and more extensive the injuries are, the greater and more serious the systemic reaction becomes.

Epidemiology

The incidence of burn injuries has been declining in the last 50 years, although the United States (U. S.) remains one of the leading countries in the developed world in the number of fire- and burn-related fatalities. Burn injuries are second only to motor vehicle crashes as the leading cause of accidental death in the U. S. (Burn Survivor Resource Center, 2002b). According to the American Burn Association, each year in the U. S., 1.1 million burn injuries require medical attention, and approximately 45,000 of these require hospitalization (National Institutes of General Medical Sciences, 2006). Approximately 4,500 people die each year from burn injuries, and up to 10,000 people in the U. S. die every year of burn-related infections. Pneumonia is the

most common infection among hospitalized patients with burns (Murray, 2008). Fire departments respond to fires every 15 seconds, and residential fires occur every 60 seconds (Burn-surgery.org, 2004).

For fire-related injuries, the home is the most common site, accounting for the majority of all fire-related deaths. Cigarettes are a leading cause of fatal homes fires. Annually between 900 and 1,000 people die from fires started by cigarettes, and an additional 2,500 to 3,000 are injured. The cost of human life and property damage is in the billions of dollars each year from cigarette-related fires.

The decline in the death rate from burn injuries is mostly attributed to early excision and closure of the burn wound. Additional reasons for improved survival rates are improved resuscitation, control of infection, and support of the hypermetabolic response. The mortality rate for burns is highest in the very young and in the elderly population. (Reasons for this are discussed later in this chapter.)

Etiology

Burn injuries occur when there is direct or indirect contact with a heat source. No matter what the causative factor, burn injury results in a loss of skin integrity. Depending on the cause and extent of the injury, there can be both localized and systemic

NATIONAL GUIDELINES for the Classification of Burn Injury

Minor Burn Injury	Moderate Burn Injury	Major Burn Injury
Excludes:	Excludes:	Includes:
Electrical injury	Electrical injury	All electrical injuries
Complicated injuries (multiple trauma)	Inhalation injury	Inhalation injury
High-risk patients such as older adults and those with chronic illnesses.	Complicated injuries (multiple trauma)	Complicated injuries (multiple trauma)
Includes:	High-risk patients such as older adults and those with chronic illnesses.	High-risk patients such as older adults and those with chronic illnesses
Partial-thickness injuries < 15% of total body surface area (TBSA) in adults	Includes:	All burns involving ears, eyes, face, hands, feet, and perineum
Full-thickness injuries < 2% of TBSA not involving ears, eyes, face, hands, feet, and perineum.	Partial-thickness injuries 15–25% of total body surface area in adults	Partial-thickness injuries > 25% of total body surface area in adults
	Full-thickness injuries 10% of TBSA not involving ears, eyes, face, hands, feet, and perineum.	Full-thickness injuries 10% or greater of TBSA.

Source: American Burn Association. http://www.ameriburn.org/

tissue damage. Inhaling smoke causes injury to the lungs, referred to as **inhalation injury**. Management of burns is standard regardless of the cause except for inhalation and electrical burns. The unique aspects of inhalation and electrical burn injuries are outlined later, as they involve more than just trauma to the skin.

Types of Burn Injury

Burns occur as a result of exposure to fire (thermal); direct contact with electricity, radiation, or chemicals; and scalds. It is important to know how the patient was burned because each type of burn injury has unique treatments, morbidity and mortality statistics, and sequelae. Chart 68–1 outlines the various types of injury and the associated causes.

Thermal Burns

Thermal burns from flames are the most common type of burn injury. These injuries occur when heat is transferred to the body from an external source; for example, flames from a fire. The depth of the injury is related to the length of exposure and the temperature of the heat source.

Scald Burns

Scald burns are a type of thermal injury that occurs from contact with hot foods or liquids, including steam. The severity of the burn is related to the temperature of the hot liquid and the length of time it is in contact with the body. At 120°F (48°C), skin requires 5 minutes for a full-thickness burn to occur. When the temperature of the liquid is 140°F (60°C), it takes only 5 seconds or less for the a serious burn. Coffee, tea, and other hot drinks are usually served at 160° to 180°F (71° to 82°C).

Electrical Burns

Electrical burns tend to be deeper than most burn injuries. The depth and severity of the injury depends on the amount of voltage, the length of exposure, the type of current, the pathway of flow, and the local tissue resistance. It is difficult to assess the extent of damage accurately for two reasons. First, much of the damage occurs internally due to the electrical current traversing along the tendons and vessels as it flows through the body, creating deep wounds that often extend into the subcutaneous tissue and muscle fascia (Cancio et al., 2005). Second, the destructive process initiated at the time of injury continues for weeks afterward. At the time of contact, the electrical flow follows the path of least resistance through the body, which is typically along muscles, long bones, blood vessels, and nerves. The entry and exit sites give a clue as to how much damage has been sustained. For example, if the entry wound is the hand and the exit is the bottom of the foot, the current traveled through most of the major organs. If the entry/exit was hand to shoulder, then just the arm sustained injury. Figure 68–1 ■ (p. 2236) is an example of tissue damage from an electrical injury. The damage to the skin appears deceptively small as compared to the damage that is sustained by internal muscle, fat, and fascia along the path of electrical flow. When deep muscle injury has occurred, myoglobin is released into the circulation from the muscle tissue. It is transported to the kidneys where it can block the renal tubules due to its large size, causing acute tubular necrosis.

CHART 68–1	Causes of Burn Injuries

Type of Injury	Cause
Thermal	Flame, flash injuries (explosion), contact with hot metal and hot, sticky tar
Electrical	Contact with electrical current, sparks or electrical arcing, alternating current, direct current, high-voltage lines, and lightning
Radiation	Overexposure to sunlight, radiation treatment for cancer
Chemical	Contact with strong acids, alkalis, or an organic compound
Scalds	Steam, hot liquids
Inhalation	Exposure of upper airway to intense heat, flames, and smoke Exposure of lung parenchyma to chemicals, steam, or aspiration of hot liquids
Nuclear	Nuclear power plant accidents

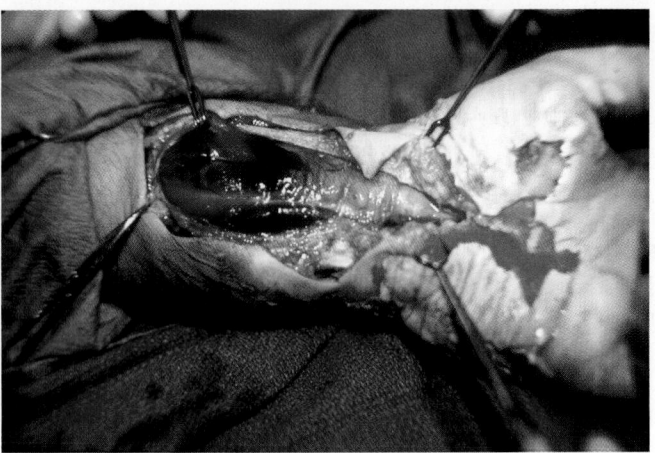

FIGURE 68–1 ■ Black muscle from electrical injury.
Source: Courtesy of: John M. Osborn, M.D., FACS, Sacramento, CA Plastic Surgery Center

Additionally, at the time of the injury, contact with the electrical current can cause tetanic muscle contractions that can be strong enough to cause fractures of long bones and vertebrae. These tetanic contractions also can occur in the respiratory muscles and cardiac muscles, causing suffocation and disruption of the cardiac conduction system resulting in dysrhythmias and cardiac arrest. Delayed neurological changes and cataract formation also may occur (Benson, Sidor, Schwartz, Desposito, & Hostetler, 2006).

Radiation Burns

Radiation burns are usually a result of overexposure to the sun or are associated with radiation treatment for cancer. Radiation injury also may occur from industrial accidents such as at nuclear power plants. Tissue damage occurs from the transfer of radiant energy to the body, which stimulates reactions with body chemicals resulting in cell death. The cells most susceptible to injury are those that divide rapidly such as bone marrow, skin, and the gastrointestinal tract. The depth of the injury depends on how close the individual was to the source as well as the length of time to exposure. Typically radiation injuries involve only the epithelial layer of skin (Wolf & Herndon, 2000).

Chemical Burns

Chemical burns occur when the skin is in contact with caustic chemical compounds such as strong acids, alkalis, or organic compounds. There are common household chemicals that cause burns such as bleach, boric acid, creosote, paint thinner, and plumbing pipe decloggers such as Drano or Liquid-Plumr. In the workplace occupational agents such as liquid concrete in the road construction and paving industry are also the source of chemical burns (Burn Survivor Resource Center, 2002a). The depth of the injury from a chemical is directly related to the length of exposure. Liberal washing of the skin and removing clothing and jewelry as quickly as possible will limit the depth of the injury (Surgical-tutor.org.uk, 2006). Emergency treatment of chemical burns is discussed later in this chapter.

Inhalation Injury

Inhalation injuries occur in 20% to 30% of patients admitted to burn centers (Lucile Packard Children's Hospital at Stanford, 2008). These injuries resulting from inhalation of heated air and smoke present a unique set of problems, one of which is difficulty in diagnosing the full extent of the injury. There is a set of criteria used to evaluate for the presence of an inhalation injury, which includes that the injury occurred in an enclosed area; there are burns of the face and neck; and there are singed nasal hairs, a hoarse, dry cough, bloody/sooty sputum, and labored respirations. Additionally, there may be edema, blisters, and ulcerations along the mucosal lining of the oropharynx and larynx. The edema continues to increase for 24 to 48 hours after the injury; thus, close monitoring for pulmonary complications, including acute respiratory distress syndrome (Chapter 36), is essential. Smoke inhalation in addition to cutaneous external burn injuries results in increased morbidity and mortality as compared to external injuries alone (Demling, 2005). The majority of deaths from burn injuries are due to smoke inhalation rather than to surface burns. Associated smoke inhalation injuries increase mortality rate by 77% when combined with cutaneous injuries (Mandel & Hales, 2008).

Nursing care includes vigorous pulmonary toilet, continuous monitoring of oxygen saturation levels, daily chest radiographs, and an early assessment of the need for intubation and mechanical ventilation. Respiratory distress may or may not develop, but evidence of it needs to be part of an ongoing assessment. Due to the edema from the injury, ongoing assessment for airway obstruction is essential. Signs of airway obstruction include:

- Stridor
- Use of accessory muscles
- Respiratory distress
- Hypoxia
- Deep burns of the face and neck
- Blister or edema of the oropharynx. (Mandel & Hales, 2008)

Continuous monitoring of arterial blood gases (ABGs) is necessary to assess the need for intubation and ventilatory support. Have necessary supplies ready for emergent intubation with inhalation injuries.

Health Promotion

The decline in burn injuries in the U. S. is due in part to the focus on injury prevention. High-risk populations have been identified, as listed in the Risk Factors box, and prevention programs have been established to increase knowledge of burn prevention. Firefighters and health care workers teach burn prevention to various populations in multiple settings. These education programs include information about teaching children and adults caring for them that if clothing catches fire, the person needs to "stop, drop, and roll," as this will assist in putting the flames out. Wrapping the victim in a blanket, coat, or sheet also will help extinguish the flames because the oxygen needed to sustain the flame is cut off. Applying copious cool water immediately after the injury helps decrease the severity of the burn. The older adult population is the most susceptible to burns caused by clothing catching fire while cooking or smoking; therefore, education programs about burn prevention also need to target this population.

The nurse is in a pivotal position to collaborate with other disciplines to develop prevention programs in local communities. The majority of fires are started in the home through igno-

RISK FACTORS for Burn Injuries

Population	Risk
Older adults	Clothing catching fire while cooking or smoking Living in apartments above the first floor
Infants and children	Matches and cigarette lighters Sun exposure Electrical outlets Clothing Scald injuries Microwave ovens Kitchen stoves Fireplaces Chemicals Fireworks
Young adults	Motor vehicle crashes Stun guns Sun exposure Methamphetamine laboratories Fireworks Taser
Firefighters	Exposure to all types of fires while in the line of duty

rance and carelessness. Children playing with matches and cigarette lighters account for approximately 35% of all burn injuries (Lucile Packard Children's Hospital at Stanford, 2008). Prevention education focuses on keeping children safe by keeping matches and lighters out of reach. Parents also need to be taught that uncovered electrical outlets in homes pose a threat to small children. Plastic plugs need to be inserted in every plug within reach of a child.

Scald burns from hot tap water are totally preventable. The ABA recommends the following simple safety tips to decrease the risk of scald burns:

- Set home water heaters no higher than 120°F.
- Provide constant adult supervision of young children or those who may have difficulty removing themselves from hot water on their own.
- Fill the bathtub to the desired level before getting in. Run cold water first, then hot.
- Mix tub water thoroughly and check the temperature with one's elbow before getting in the water.
- Install antiscald temperature devices that stop or interrupt the flow of water when the temperature reaches a predetermined level.
- Cook on back burners when children are present.
- Keep children out of cooking areas when hot food or liquids are being transported.
- Place hot items in the center of the table during mealtime.
- Never drink or carry hot liquids while carrying a child.

The focus of chemical burn prevention is, first, keeping chemicals in a safe place and, second, knowing how to neutral-

ize them when they occur. All home chemicals need to be locked away from children. If contact occurs, copious amounts of water irrigation will decrease the severity of the burn.

Radiation burns typically are not deep injuries, but repeated exposure increases the risk of skin cancer. The goal for the prevention of radiation burns is to educate the public to limit exposure to sun, wear protective clothing and sunscreen when exposed to the sun, and avoid the use of artificial sources of ultraviolet light (tanning booths, sunlamps, and tanning beds). The amount of protection offered by a sunscreen is referred to as the sun protection factor (SPF). The higher the SPF number, the greater the protection. Protection from the sun offered by sunscreens may be classified as follows:

- Minimal: SPF 2 to 11
- Moderate: SPF 12 through 29
- High: SPF 30+. (Some sunscreens claim SPFs higher than 30, although the added protection at such higher levels is insignificant.) (Centers for Disease Control and Prevention, 2006).

In the industrial setting, the most effective means of preventing exposure to radiation is proper maintenance of equipment, education of employees who work near equipment, and regularly scheduled safety checks.

Approximately three-fifths of burn injuries occur in homes where there are no smoke detectors or the smoke detectors are nonfunctioning; thus, the education focus has centered on installation and periodic checking of smoke detectors. The Centers for Disease Control and Prevention (CDC) gives funding to state health departments to provide the Smoke Alarm Installation and Fire Safety Education (SAIFE) program in high-risk homes in 16 states. The programs use local fire department contractors to canvass neighborhoods, installing long-lasting lithium-battery-powered smoke alarms and providing general fire safety education and a 6-month battery checkup (Ballesteros, Jackson, & Martin, 2005). Additionally, most cities in the United States have fire departments that will install smoke detectors free of charge for older adults.

One goal of the Federal Emergency Management Agency (FEMA) focuses on decreasing residential fire deaths by increasing awareness of hazards in the home and the need for smoke detectors and a fire extinguisher. The National Guidelines box (p. 2238) outlines the national guidelines for fire prevention set forth by FEMA.

Lawmakers' role in fire prevention is multifaceted. First, laws requiring public buildings to have protective measures in place such as fire-retardant fabrics, proper egress routes, smoke detectors, and sprinkler systems must be enforced. Second, the government must enforce laws requiring proper labeling of not only flammable products but also toxic chemicals and their associated antidotes.

On a national level, the ABA has succeeded in getting key pieces of legislation passed. Additional funding for burn centers was approved as part of bioterrorism legislation in the event of a bioterrorist act against the United States (ABA, 2002). Representatives of the ABA testified before a congressional committee and were successful in passing a law to increase the flammability standards for clothing worn by children up to age 7 (HR 4896 and S 2188). Legislation on "safe cigarettes" is another issue that

NATIONAL GUIDELINES for Fire Prevention

Guideline	Prevention Measures
Smoke alarms	Working smoke alarms can double the chances of survival.
	Every home needs at least one smoke alarm.
	Test it monthly, keep it free of dust, and replace the battery at least once a year.
	Smoke alarms themselves should be replaced after 10 years of service, or as recommended by the manufacturer.
Electrical fires	Never overload circuits or extension cords. Do not place cords and wires under rugs, over nails, or in high-traffic areas.
	Immediately shut off and unplug appliances that sputter, spark, or emit an unusual smell.
	Have appliances professionally repaired or replaced.
Appliances	When using appliances, follow the manufacturer's safety precautions.
	Overheating, unusual smells, shorts, and sparks are all warning signs that appliances need to be shut off and then repaired or replaced.
	Unplug appliances when not in use.
	Use safety caps to cover all unused outlets, especially if there are small children in the home.
Alternate heaters	Portable heaters need their space.
	Keep anything combustible at least 3 feet away.
	Keep fire in the fireplace.
	Use fire screens and have chimneys cleaned annually. The creosote buildup can ignite a chimney fire that could easily spread.
	Kerosene heaters should be used only where approved by authorities.
	Never use gasoline or camp stove fuel.
	Refuel outside and only after the heater has cooled.
Affordable home fire safety sprinklers	When home fire sprinklers are used with working smoke alarms, the chances of surviving a fire are greatly increased.
	Sprinklers are affordable; they can increase property value and lower insurance rates.
Escape plan	Practice an escape plan from every room in the house.
	Caution everyone to stay low to the floor when escaping from fire and never to open doors that are hot.
	Select a location where everyone can meet after escaping the house.
	Keep window escape ladders on any floor above the main level.
	Get out and then call for help.
Caring for children	Children under age 5 are naturally curious about fire.
	Many play with matches and lighters.
	Children set over 20,000 house fires every year.
	Take the mystery out of fire play by teaching children that fire is a tool, not a toy.
	Check labels on clothing for young children to ensure that the fabrics are fire retardant.
Caring for older people	Every year more than 1,200 senior citizens die in fires.
	Many of these fire deaths could have been prevented.
	Seniors are especially vulnerable because many live alone and cannot respond quickly.
Smoking precautions	Careless smoking is the leading cause of fire deaths and the second leading cause of injuries among people age 65 and older.
	Cigarettes continue to burn when they are not properly extinguished.
	When a resting cigarette is accidentally knocked over, it can smolder for hours before a flare-up occurs.
	Put cigarette or cigar out at the first sign of feeling drowsy while watching television or reading.
	Use deep ashtrays and put cigarette all the way out.
	Never smoke in bed.
	Do not walk away from lit cigarettes and other smoking materials.
	Do not put ashtrays on the arms of sofas or chairs.

Source: U.S. Fire Administration. (2006). *Working together for home fire safety.* Retrieved October 5, 2006, from http://www.usfa.fema.gov/downloads/pdf/fswy11.pdf

the ABA has actively lobbied for changes. A fire-safe cigarette, which would require manufactures to institute small design changes, has significantly less propensity to ignite furniture and mattresses. The ABA supports legislation that would require manufacturers to institute these changes (HR 4607 and S 2317).

Pathophysiology of Tissue Injury

As discussed earlier, burn injuries are caused when tissue is exposed to thermal, electrical, radiation, or chemical energy. The tissue injury resulting from these agents causes coagulation of cellular protein. The amount of tissue damage is related to the length of exposure and the temperature of the offending agent. As the temperature increases, cellular functions become impaired. Cell membranes are disrupted when exposed to temperatures between 40° and 44°C (104° and 110°F). Exposure of tissue to 60°C (140°F) for longer than 1 second will cause a **partial-thickness injury** (epidermis and part of the dermis). A **full-thickness injury** (epidermis and dermis) will occur with temperatures greater than 70°C (158°F) (Flynn, 2002). Full-thickness versus partial-thickness injury is described later in this chapter.

Tissue Injury

When thermal damage occurs on the skin surface, three distinct zones of injury are created. These zones relate to the level of damage in a given area. The center of the wound, referred to as the **zone of coagulation**, is the area where there is the greatest amount of injury to the tissue. If all the layers of the skin have been destroyed, this area contains denatured protein and coagulated nonfunctioning blood vessels. The appearance of the tissue is white or pearly gray and has a leather-like texture. Nerve endings have been destroyed; therefore, there is no sensation in this area. If all the layers of the skin are not destroyed, the zone of coagulation appears red and is very painful. With both types of injury, there is edema formation in the surrounding area because of the release of vasoactive mediators such as histamines, serotonin, interleukin-1, and prostaglandins from the injured cells (Demling, 2005). An in-depth discussion of the effect of vasoactive mediators is covered in Chapter 61 🔗.

Surrounding the zone of coagulation is an area of potentially viable but injured cells referred to as the **zone of stasis**. The microvasculature in this area is clogged with heat-injured erythrocytes. Vasoactive mediators from these injured cells cause edema formation, further impairing blood flow to the area. This decrease in blood flow to the area continues for approximately 16 to 24 hours after the injury. Survival and recovery of the cells in the zone of stasis depend on prompt and appropriate wound care, edema control, and systemic fluid resuscitation. These interventions decrease the incidence of cellular dehydration, ischemia, and infection. If prompt measures are not instituted, these extremely vulnerable cells die, becoming part of the zone of coagulation. The tissue in this area initially appears moist, red, and blanches with pressure because of the presence of viable capillaries.

In the outermost portion of the injured area, there is minor cell damage; this area is referred to as the **zone of hyperemia**. Once again, due to the vasoactive mediators, there is prominent blood flow to this area. This blood contains the nutrients needed to support the zone of stasis, and it contains the necessary mediators to continue the inflammatory process within the zones of stasis and coagulation. Like the zone of stasis, the zone of hyperemia has viable capillaries and, therefore, will blanch with pressure (Oliver, Spain, & Stadelmann, 2005). Tissue in this area appears pink and moist. Complete healing of this area is expected, unless there is additional insult such as infection or profound tissue inflammation (Figure 68–2 ■).

Systemic Injury

Burn injuries, depending on the size and depth, potentially could impact every organ system in the body. Immediately after a burn injury, fluid begins to shift from the intracellular and intravascular compartment into the interstitial space. This is

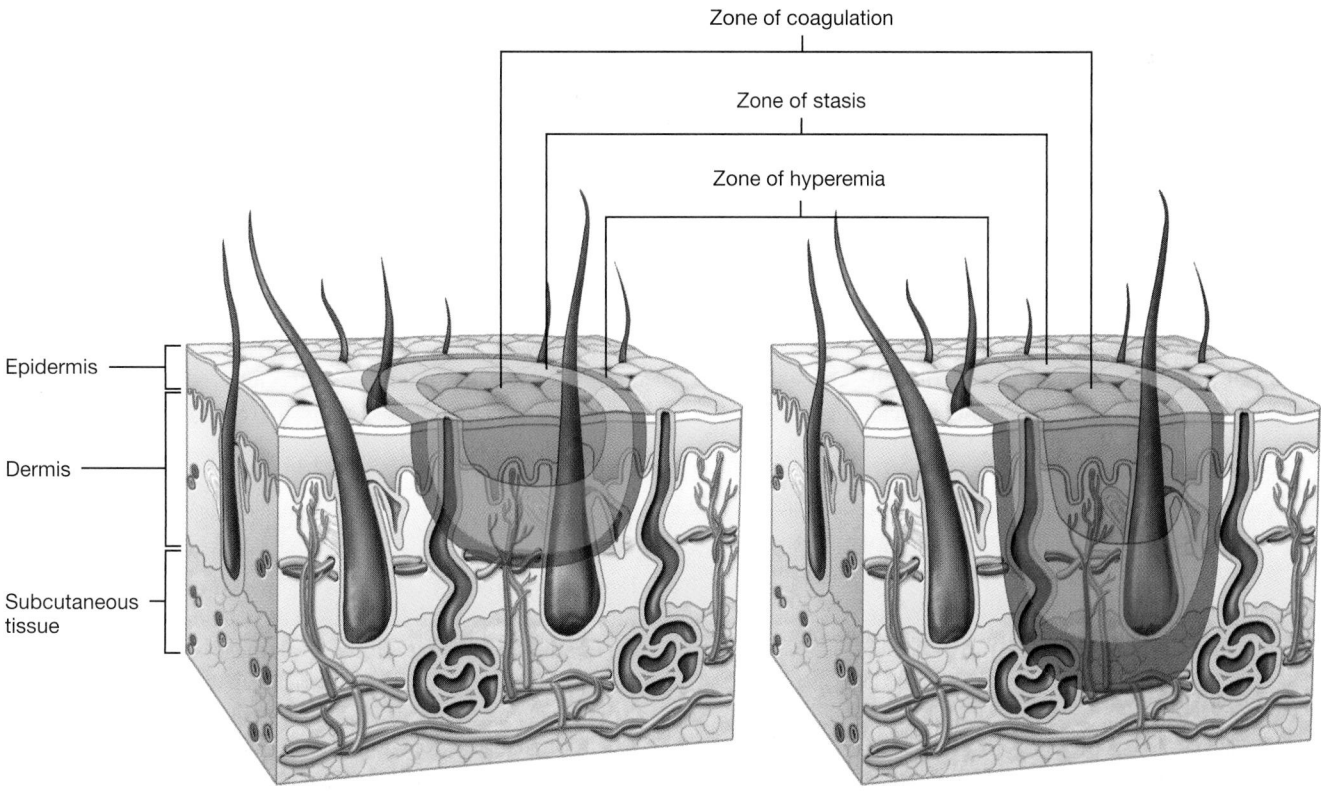

FIGURE 68–2 ■ Three zones of injury.

commonly referred to as "third spacing" of fluid and, if left untreated, will lead to burn shock. Additionally, edema develops in unburned tissues and organs distant from the site of injury when the burn size exceeds 20% total body surface area (Ahrns, 2004). Burn shock is the pathophysiological mechanism that underlies most of the systemic effects of a burn injury on the tissues and organs of the body. Burn shock occurs because of a loss of intravascular fluid and, thus, circulating blood volume. This loss of fluid occurs for two reasons; First, fluid is lost to the environment through the wound (insensible loss), and second, fluid is lost due to movement from the intravascular space into the interstitial space (Oliver et al., 2005).

Pathophysiologically, what is occurring is that at the time of the injury there is a release of an excessive amount of the Hageman factor (factor XII), which initiates and activates the inflammatory cascade (Porth, 2007). Proinflammatory mediators such as histamines, arachidonic acid metabolites, prostaglandins, bradykinin, and catecholamines are released from the injured tissue (Porth, 2007; Wolf & Herndon, 2000). These mediators cause arteriolar and venular dilation, which results in increased capillary permeability and, thus, leaking of fluid, electrolytes, and protein out of the intravascular space into the interstitial space causing interstitial edema. This leaking is due to changes in the osmotic pressure within the injured tissue. Because of oncotic changes, fluid moves with the protein that is leaving the vascular space, further increasing the edema formation in the wound. The outcome is a dramatic outpouring of fluids, electrolytes, and proteins into the third space, resulting in the decrease in circulating blood volume and consequently a decreased cardiac output. The development of shock is due to loss of the circulating blood volume, causing an intravascular hypovolemic state. The end result is decreased oxygen and nutrients to the tissues. Both localized and systemic edema occur because of the fluid shifts. This process of fluid movement begins at the time of injury, peaks in 12 to 24 hours after the injury, but will continue for 48 to 72 hours until the vascular permeability is at least partially reestablished and the leaking ceases.

The edema formation occurring during burn shock impairs peripheral circulation and results in tissue necrosis of the underlying tissues. Therefore, treatment during this initial period of fluid shifting focuses on aggressive fluid resuscitation for the hypovolemia, maintaining normal oxygen levels, and blocking the mediators to decrease the edema formation. These treatments will help prevent the conversion of the zone of stasis to the zone of coagulation. Because fluid continues to leak even after capillary integrity is restored, fluid resuscitation continues to be monitored closely.

What is unique to the patient with burns is that very little fluid leaves the body. Therefore, when the fluid stops leaking and begins to return to the vascular space, a marked increase in the intravascular volume occurs. When this process begins, fluid resuscitation needs to be adjusted so as not to cause fluid overload. Fluid resuscitation and monitoring are discussed later in this chapter.

Organ Injury

Virtually all systems in the body are affected in a major burn injury because the mediators leave the confines of the local tissue injury through the circulation and travel to remote organs causing injury (Oliver et al., 2005). Under normal conditions these medi-

ators are efficient and immune protective, but in the case of major trauma such as burn injury, they become poorly regulated, causing overwhelming inflammation and coagulation, and fibrinolysis can ensue, which can constantly be reactivated (Porth, 2007).

Cardiac Response

The initial hypovolemic state of burn shock significantly alters cardiovascular function with burns of greater than 40% total body surface area. One reason for this alteration is the loss of circulating blood volume, which decreases cardiac output and results in a loss of nutrients and oxygen delivered to the tissues. The second mechanism that impacts cardiac output is stimulation of the sympathetic nervous system (flight or fight), which causes the release of catecholamines (epinephrine and norepinephrine). These catecholamines cause vasoconstriction and an increase in systemic vascular resistance, which increases cardiac workload. Release of tumor necrosis factor, an inflammatory mediator, has a significant negative inotropic effect causing myocardial depression. The effect of this mediator goes on even after adequate fluid resuscitation (Porth, 2005). Due to these combined effects, heart failure is a major risk factor when attempting to achieve homeostasis in the early phase of burn care. This is especially true in the elderly population.

The cardiac conduction system also may be affected by increased serum potassium levels. Cell damage causes the release of intracellular potassium, which may cause hyperkalemia. Increased levels of potassium cause changes in the myocardial action potential, resulting in abnormalities in the cardiac conduction system. These abnormalities increase the risk of ventricular dysrhythmias and cardiac arrest. The Diagnostic Tests box describes the laboratory and diagnostic tests and the initial and later abnormalities associated with burn injuries.

Pulmonary Response

Increased pulmonary vascular resistance created by the release of the mediators such as serotonin, impacts pulmonary function, even in the absence of inhalation injury. This increased resistance also is compounded by the increase in systemic vascular resistance. Pulmonary edema, therefore, occurs because of increased capillary pressure combined with the vasoconstriction of the microcirculation. If left-sided heart failure also is present, this further increases capillary pressure and impacts oxygen exchange.

In summary, both the heart and lungs are affected by the proinflammatory mediators on a microvascular level. These changes are marked by a loss of fluid volume, increased vascular resistance, and finally a decreased cardiac output (Wolf & Herndon, 2000).

Gastrointestinal Response

With activation of the sympathetic nervous system, there is an increase in circulating catecholamines, which causes blood to be shunted away from the gastrointestinal (GI) organs. This results in decreased gut motility and absorption of nutrients. When a burn injury occurs, there is a subsequent increase in metabolism, which can rapidly deplete body stores. With the loss of motility, which is referred to as a *paralytic ileus,* nutrients may not progress through the GI tract and be absorbed. This lack of motility leads to gastric distention, nausea, and vomiting. A paralytic ileus is an indication to withhold administration of enteral feedings, further compromising the nutritional state. There is some evidence that early administration of enteral feedings actually decreases the incidence of

DIAGNOSTIC TESTS for Burn Injuries

Test	Initial Expected Abnormality	Later Expected Abnormality	Rationale for Abnormality
Potassium level	Increased.	Decreased after burn shock; fluid shifts back to intracellular and intravascular spaces.	Increased due to cell lysis and fluid shifts to extracellular spaces. Decreases with fluid resuscitation.
Sodium level	Increased.	Normalizes with fluid replacement. Will decrease with repeated Hubbard tank treatments.	Due to dehydration and then decreased with fluid shifts.
Hematocrit (HCT)	For the first 12–48 hours after the burn injury, there is an increase in the hematocrit due to hemoconcentration related to intravascular fluid volume loss.	Decreased with adequate hydration due to cell destruction from injury. Once fluid balance has been reestablished, a lower and more accurate hematocrit reading occurs.	Red blood cells are lost both directly in the burn and as a result of increased fragility. Circulating red blood cell mass becomes trapped and destroyed within the burn wound at the time of injury. Erythrocyte losses continue to occur for several days after the injury.
Hemoglobin (Hgb)	Increased due to hemoconcentration.	Decreased with adequate hydration due to cell destruction from injury.	Red blood cells are lost both directly in the burn and as a result of increased fragility. Circulating red blood cell mass becomes trapped and destroyed within the burn wound at the time of injury. Erythrocyte losses continue to occur for several days after the injury.
Platelets	Decreased due to dilution and consumption.	Normal if bone marrow manufactures enough. May be increased in the presence of infection.	Dilution and consumption immediately after a burn injury cause an abnormal decrease both in the platelet count and in clotting factors. It is believed that a large number of platelets are utilized to stabilize the vasculature in and around the burned area.
White blood cells (WBC)	Granulocytes continue to increase for the first 24 hours after the injury, and then the count begins to fall.	Increased with infection and decreased in immunodeficient states.	This increase is due to mobilization of preexisting stores. The decrease in the granulocyte level is due in part to the dilutional effects of fluid replacement therapy, and due to concentration in the injured areas.
Creatinine/blood urea nitrogen (BUN)	Normal to increased depending on fluid replacement.	Low if malnourished. Increased in presence of renal insufficiency.	Increases seen with electrical burns where extensive tissue damage is suspected.
Blood glucose; nondiabetic	Increased.	Increased or decreased depending on nutritional replacement.	Due to stress response and changes that occur with fluid resuscitation and type of nutritional replacement.
Total protein	Decreased.	Increased or decreased depending on nutritional status.	Fluid shifts cause a decrease, and nutritional replacement will increase it.
Prealbumin	Decreased.	Increased or decreased depending on nutritional status.	Massive inflammation causes a decrease, and nutritional replacement will increase it.
Creatine kinase (CK) level	Elevated.	Returns to normal after 48 hours.	Electrical burns due to extensive tissue damage.
Urine specific gravity	Elevated.	Decreased to normal levels with rehydration.	Dehydration.

paralytic ileus and helps maintain mucosal integrity (Chen, Xie, & Jiang, 2001). This issue of whether or not to administer enteral feedings remains a topic of research.

Blood flow to the GI tract immediately after burn injury also is affected by the release of angiotension II, a potent vasoconstrictor. This substance, which is released in response to low systemic fluid volume, has a direct vasoconstrictive effect on the splanchnic vasculature smooth muscle, causing ischemia to the gut (Tadros, Traber, Heggers, & Herndon, 2000, 2003). This ischemia causes intestinal mucosal atrophy and an increased permeability of the mucosa molecules (Yamamoto et al., 2001). Bacteria that are normal in the GI tract are held there by the mucosa. In burn injuries and burn wound sepsis, GI mucosal atrophy causes movement of intraluminal bacteria to extraluminal sites, referred to as *bacterial translocation* (Yamamoto et al., 2001). Bacterial translocation is thought to be one of the mechanisms that cause systemic sepsis and multisystem organ failure (Menchaca-Diaz et al., 2003). Research continues to investigate how to decrease the rate of bacterial translocation. Glutamine, a dietary supplement, has demonstrated to partially reverse gut atrophy and integrity. Glutamine administration decreases the incidence of gram-negative bacteremia and improves mortality rates (Tadros et al., 2003; Wischmeyer et al., 2001). Early enteral feedings appear to prevent or at least slow down mucosal atrophy (Chen et al., 2001).

Patients with severe burn injuries experience stress gastritis within 72 hours. Gastrointestinal (GI) erosions can occur within 5 hours of injury in 80% of all patients with severe burns. These erosions cause only minor upper bleeding, but within 72 hours this minor bleeding may progress to frank GI ulcerations (Curling's ulcer), resulting in major hemorrhage. This sequence of events was frequently seen in the patients when no ulcer prophylaxis (either antacids or H_2-receptor antagonists) was used (Fadaak, 2000).

Renal Response

The hypovolemia that occurs as a result of fluid shifts causes a decrease in renal blood flow and filtration rates. Therefore, abnormal increases in renal function studies (blood urea nitrogen [BUN] and creatinine), coupled with a marked decrease in or no urine output, may be seen during the early resuscitation phase (see the earlier Diagnostic Tests box, p. 2241). The kidney is able to recover if fluid resuscitation is initiated quickly and adequately.

After a major burn injury, the dead or damaged erythrocytes release large amounts of hemoglobin. If the burn extends deep enough to cause muscle injury, myoglobin also may be released into the bloodstream, such as seen with electrical injuries. Under normal circumstances, both of these substances are conjugated by haptoglobin and transferred to the liver. But if large amounts are released at once, the liver is unable to handle the increased load, and these substances are excreted in the urine. Myoglobin and hemoglobin will damage the renal tubules and promote renal failure. There is a higher risk for renal failure when any of the following is also present: dehydration, acidosis, massive presence of necrotic tissues after third- and fourth-degree electrical and chemical burns, hypercatabolic state, and/or shock.

Immune Response

The three major functions of the normal mature immune system are defense, homeostasis, and surveillance. The defense function provides the body with the ability to fight infection, while the homeostatic function controls the activities of the defense system. Finally, the surveillance function recognizes foreign materials.

The body's first line of defense, the skin, is destroyed with a burn injury. As discussed earlier, these injuries trigger the inflammatory response, causing the release of proinflammatory mediators, which induce localized vasodilation and increased capillary permeability. As a result, venous stasis and microthrombi occur at the injury site. The hypovolemia that occurs immediately after a burn injury causes an increase in blood viscosity, which results in sluggish blood flow to the wound bed. This results in a decreased delivery of oxygen, antibodies, and nutrients, which retards wound healing and increases the risk of

infection. A second manifestation of mediators, such as tumor necrosis factor and interleukin, is impairment of the function of lymphocytes, macrophages, and neutrophils, causing a decreased ability to fight infection. See Chapter 59 ⊕ for a complete description of the immune system.

The protein that is lost due to third spacing from capillary leaking impairs both the cell-mediated and humoral immune systems. The humoral immune response needs B cells to produce antibodies and immunoglobulins. In the patient with burns, the serum levels of immunoglobulins are decreased, therefore diminishing the normal immune response. A decrease in the production of T cells negatively impacts cell-mediated cytotoxic activity. The decreased function of both cell-mediated and humoral immune responses creates a state of immunodeficiency and increases the risk of the development of opportunistic infections and death despite aggressive antimicrobial therapy.

A final insult to the immune system may occur because of the relationship between nutrition and immunocompetence. When the burn injury occurs, a hypermetabolic state is created, which places the victim at high risk for malnutrition (Pereira, Murphy, & Herndon, 2005). Without adequate calories, proteins, and trace elements, there is a decrease in the function of the immune system and, therefore, susceptibility to infection increases.

Integumentary Response

The skin protects against infection, prevents loss of body heat, helps control body temperature, functions as an excretory organ (sweat glands), is a sensory organ, and produces vitamin D when sunlight reacts with cholesterol. Finally, it determines identity; that is, race and fingerprints. Burn injuries cause a transient and, in some cases, permanent loss of many of these functions. With partial-thickness injuries, enough of the substructures of the skin remain intact to regenerate function. However, with full-thickness injuries, many functions such as hair growth, perspiration, and sensory functions are permanently lost.

The overall thickness of the skin varies depending on the part of the body it covers. For example, the skin on the back tends to be thicker than the skin on the inner aspect of the arms. Therefore, similar temperatures produce different depths of injury depending on the part of the body burned.

Multisystem Dysfunction

In major burn injuries, proinflammatory mediators, such as cytokines, are released in a chaotic, repeatedly reactivated fashion. This causes a continual reactivation of the inflammatory response, which in turn causes distant and multiorgan involvement leading to dysfunction and death (Gosian & Gamilli, 2005; Porth, 2007). Chapter 61 ⊕ discusses in detail the sequence of events that causes multiorgan involvement and dysfunction.

■ Periods of Burn Injury Management

Three distinct periods of care for the acute burn injury have been identified: the emergency or resuscitative period, the acute period, and finally the rehabilitative phase. Each phase has different goals and priorities, even though these stages tend to overlap. In order for the patient to have optimal physical as well as emotional healing, each stage of care requires a multidisciplinary team of health care providers with specialized training. The goals and treatments of each phase or period are described next.

Emergency Phase

The emergency period of burn care begins at the time of the injury and lasts for the first 2 to 3 days. The goal during this phase is to resolve the immediate insult by certain means, which include maintaining an airway and oxygen levels, treating concurrent injuries, correcting the fluid imbalance, preventing wound infection, conserving body heat, relieving pain, and providing emotional support.

Prehospital Care and Transport

The focus of treatment at the scene of the injury is first to ensure the safety of the rescuers and then to remove the victim from the burn source. An initial assessment is required to determine vital signs and the severity of the burn and other injuries. This assessment follows the ABCDEF format: A = airway, B = breathing, C = circulation, D = disability, neurological deficit, E = exposure and evaluation, and F = fluid resuscitation. Any smoldering clothing and restrictive jewelry must be removed to decrease the depth of the injury. Burn victims are unlikely to develop shock in the first 30 minutes; therefore, after airway stabilization the patient can be transported to a local emergency department or directly to a burn center. If the patient is less than 60 minutes away from a hospital, the American Burn Association teaches that intravenous line insertion is not necessary at the scene of the accident.

Application of clean normal saline-soaked towels helps with cooling the burned skin, often is effective for pain relief, and may limit the extent of burn damage. These cold soaks must be used cautiously; limit them to 5% to 10% of the body surface at any one time, and limit them in time to prevent systemic hypothermia. Ice is not used because it may cause further injury to the skin and exacerbate hypothermia. The burning process generally stops after 5 minutes of water cooling, and any further cooling only contributes to hypothermia. For patient comfort the burn should be covered with clean, dry blankets.

Chemical burns require copious irrigation with water for at least 20 minutes to reduce the concentration of chemicals and, thus, the depth of the injury. If the chemical is in the eyes, contact lenses must be removed, and the eyes are irrigated with copious amounts of water. A minimum of 2 liters of fluid is used for each eye, and irrigation may be needed for several hours after the injury (EmedicineHealth, 2006).

No oils or salves should be applied to any type of burn injury. If the patient has not had tetanus toxoid in the last 5 years, it is administered early, often in the field. If the patient has never received tetanus or has not had a booster in the last 10 years, tetanus immunoglobulin is given. Due to a loss of skin integrity, body temperature drops; therefore, the patient should be covered with clean blankets before transfer.

Emergency Department Care

Once the patient reaches the emergency department (ED), a rapid and thorough initial assessment is done, beginning with the respiratory and cardiovascular systems. As always, the first priority is to assess the patency of the patient's airway and the adequacy of gas exchange. If the burns occurred on the face and neck, massive airway edema can cause airway obstruction and death. An assessment for heat or smoke inhalation is done emergently, as these agents can cause damage to the airways and lung parenchyma. The nasal passages and oral airway are assessed for

soot. If respiratory distress is present and/or there are burns of the face and neck, nasotracheal or endotracheal intubation is indicated within 1 to 2 hours after the injury, before swelling further compromises the airway (McCall & Cahill, 2005). After intubation, the need for oxygen and ventilatory support is assessed and instituted. Ongoing monitoring of arterial blood gases and oxygen saturation levels determines the effectiveness of the interventions. The nurse is responsible for monitoring the patient's airway and assessing the adequacy of gas exchange. An in-depth discussion of respiratory assessment, intubation, and mechanical ventilation is in Chapters 33 and 36.

An assessment of the cardiovascular system is essential because it provides information regarding fluid volume status and the potential for the development of shock. A 12-lead electrocardiogram (ECG) is necessary to detect myocardial ischemic changes and cardiac dysrhythmias, especially with electrical injuries. The carotid and peripheral pulses are assessed for rate and quality. The skin is inspected for color, sensation, and capillary refill. Finally, the blood pressure and apical pulse are assessed. Due to the progressive nature of fluid volume loss, these assessments must be performed on a frequent and ongoing basis.

Concurrent with airway management and cardiovascular assessment, it is essential to place large-bore intravenous (IV) catheters. Most health care providers believe that shortening the time from injury to IV insertion and beginning of fluid resuscitation will decrease the mortality rate. The best insertion site is through nonburned tissue, if possible. If there is no nonburned area for intravenous access, then placement through burned tissue is necessary and justifiable, given the risk for the development of hypovolemic shock. This is done as early as possible while the nonviable tissue (**eschar**) is still sterile (Figure 68–3 ■). Placement of an indwelling urinary catheter also is necessary, as urine output is considered the most reliable indicator of fluid status.

In burn injuries greater than 20% of total body surface area (TBSA), the patient is prone to nausea and vomiting because of a loss of blood flow to the gastrointestinal tract, as discussed earlier in this chapter. Due to the risk of aspiration, oral fluids are withheld, and a nasogastric tube may be inserted to prevent abdominal distention and vomiting. The next priority during the emergency period is to assess for any concurrent injuries. Life-threatening injuries such as pneumothorax, spinal cord, or acute

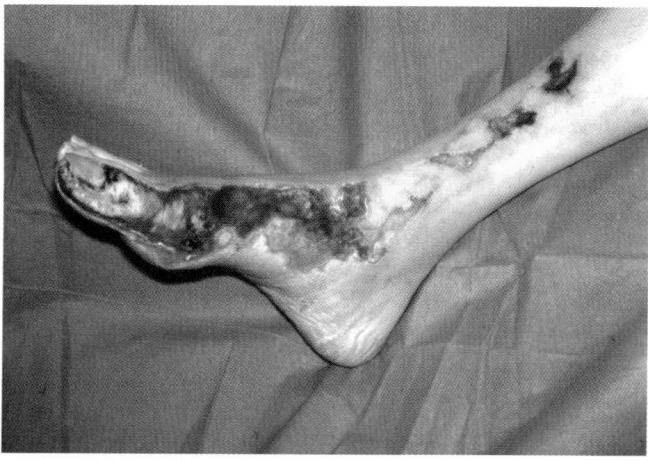

FIGURE 68–3 ■ Eschar.
Source: Courtesy of: John M. Osborn, M.D., FACS, Sacramento, CA Plastic Surgery Center

brain injuries need to be stabilized and treated. Final treatment of concurrent injuries, such as surgery, is typically delayed if possible until the patient is hemodynamically stable.

The loss of skin integrity decreases the patient's ability to retain and maintain body heat. When body temperature decreases, shivering occurs as a compensatory mechanism to increase body heat. This shivering increases oxygen and metabolic needs, and must be avoided. Burn wounds are covered with dressings, blankets are applied, and the room temperature is elevated to increase and maintain body temperature.

Blood studies are obtained to provide baseline data and to assist in identifying preexisting conditions. For patients with 30% or greater TBSA, the blood studies should include a complete blood count, serum electrolytes, blood glucose, blood urea nitrogen (BUN), serum creatinine, and coagulation studies. If substance abuse is suspected or if there is an altered level of consciousness in the absence of a head injury, a toxicology screen is indicated. If inhalation injury is suspected or the patient is in respiratory distress, arterial blood gases and a chest x-ray are necessary. In the case of electrical burns where extensive tissue damage is suspected, serum creatine kinase (CK), blood urea nitrogen, and creatinine levels should be evaluated, typically on an ongoing basis (see the Diagnostic Tests box, p. 2241). To diagnose any concurrent injuries, x-rays and scans need be completed where indicated.

Burns are a life-threatening, disfiguring injury that has a major emotional impact on both the patient and family. Thus, emotional support is essential in all stages of burn recovery and must begin in the emergency period.

Prevention of wound infection is a critical concern from the time of injury to final wound closure. Therefore, once the patient has been stabilized, the focus of care shifts to the assessment of burn size and depth. Burns are categorized as minor, moderate, or major (see the National Guidelines box for the ABA's classification of burn injury, p. 2235), and a determination is made as to whether the patient requires hospitalization. If hospitalization is indicated, then the decision needs to be made as to whether to admit the patient to a medical–surgical floor or to a specialized burn center.

Burn Center Criteria

In order to qualify as a burn center, the unit must be capable of delivering all therapy required, including rehabilitation. Additionally, the center must provide training and conduct research. Typically burn centers are associated with university hospitals and/or hospitals with 500 or more beds. Burn centers provide treatment for minor, moderate, and major burn injuries. A burn center must contain a minimum of six beds and have a designated medical director who is board certified in general or plastic surgery, with one additional year of specialized training in burn care. Besides specially trained nurses, the center must also employ licensed physical therapists, occupational therapists, and licensed dieticians with previous experience in burn care (Demling, DeSanti, & Orgill, 2004). Most major burn centers also have social workers, clergy, child life specialists, and psychologists. Each member of the team must understand the critical aspects of wound care, infection control, and the psychological and rehabilitative needs of the patient with burns. Transfer of any patient, whether it is from the field or the ED,

must be coordinated with the burn center health care provider. All pertinent information regarding injuries, hemodynamic status, fluid resuscitation, and treatments must be reported to the burn center staff.

The American Burn Association and the American College of Surgeons have established these criteria for admission to a burn center:

1. Partial-thickness and full-thickness burns greater than 10% body surface area (BSA) in patients under 10 years or over 50 years of age.
2. Partial-thickness and full-thickness burns greater than 20% BSA in other age groups.
3. Partial-thickness and full-thickness burns involving the face, hands, eyes, ears, feet, genitalia, perineum, or those that involve skin overlying major joints.
4. Full-thickness burns greater than 5% TBSA in any age group.
5. Electrical burns, including lightning injury (significant volumes of tissue beneath the surface may be injured and result in acute renal failure and other complications).
6. Significant chemical burns.
7. Inhalation injury.
8. Burn injury in patients with preexisting illness that could complicate management, prolong recovery, or affect mortality.
9. Any patient with burns in whom concomitant trauma poses an increased risk of morbidity or mortality may be treated initially at a trauma center until stable before being transferred to a burn center.
10. Children with burns seen in hospitals without qualified personnel or equipment for their care should be transferred to a burn center with these capabilities.
11. Burn injury in patients who will require special social and emotional or long-term rehabilitative support, including cases involving suspected child abuse and neglect. (Demling & DeSanti, 2006b)

Admission to a Burn Center

If the patient meets the criteria listed, admission to a burn center is indicated. During the admission process, both the local and systemic effects of the burn injury are quickly assessed and treated. The admission process begins with airway management, hemodynamic stabilization, and an assessment of the burn size and depth. After an in-depth assessment, a comprehensive treatment plan is instituted that provides the care needed to ensure an optimal recovery. The nurse is pivotal in coordinating the admission process and the treatment plan.

Admission Assessment

The admission assessment of a patient following a burn injury needs to include the history of the event that caused the injury, the time the injury occurred, the causative agent and the duration of exposure, where the injury occurred (e.g., enclosed space), any concurrent injuries, and any on-the-scene first aid treatments.

This assessment is vital because portions of the treatment plan depend on this information. For example, fluid resuscitation calculations are based on the time of the injury as opposed to the time of admission to the hospital. The causative agent is especially important with chemical burns such as from strong acids or alkaline agents, which may require neutralization to stop the ongoing burning effect. If the injury occurred in an enclosed area, such as a house, there also may be inhalation injuries that require special consideration and treatment. Concurrent injuries, such as fractures, often are associated with burns and require a treatment plan for stabilization. Finally, first aid treatments and home remedies applied prior to arrival at the hospital need to be documented and reported to the health care team.

Clinical Manifestations and Determinants of Burn Wound Severity

In order to treat a burn injury adequately, its severity must be evaluated using the following five factors: the size of the injury, the depth of injury, the age of the patient, past medical history, and the part of the body burned. Each of these factors impacts the treatment plan as well as the morbidity and mortality for a given patient.

Burn Size

When estimating burn size, it is expressed as a percent of total body surface area. Two common formulas are used to estimate percent of body burned. The first formula is the **rule of nines** that divides the body into seven areas, which each represent 9% or multiples of 9% of the body surface area. For an adult, the head and neck are 9%, the arms are 9% each, the lower extremities are 18% each, the trunk is a total of 36% (18% anterior, 18% posterior), and the perineum is 1%. Thus, the total = 100%. Age and growth and development are factors in determining the distribution of the body surface area. Figure 68–4 ■ outlines the rule of nines for both adults and children. The rule of nines is an easy-to-remember general estimate of body surface area and is considered adequate for the prehospital and emergency care periods.

The second formula is the **Lund-Browder formula** (Figure 68–5 ■, p. 2246). This formula divides the body into smaller percentage areas and is considered more accurate, especially for chil-

dren and infants. The formula determines surface area measurements for each body part according to the age of the patient.

When a patient is admitted, the affected areas are shaded in on a chart using either the rule of nines or the Lund-Browder formula. The total body surface area (TBSA) involved in the burn injury is then calculated. Most burn centers total the partial-thickness and full-thickness injuries separately. The totaled sum of body surface burned is used when calculating fluid resuscitation needs, as well as metabolic and immunologic responses. The TBSA also is a critical determinant of overall morbidity and mortality (Osborn, 2003).

Burn Depth

The depth of a burn injury is an important predictor of morbidity and mortality as well as of surgical management and functional and cosmetic outcomes (Osborn, 2003). There are a number of accepted terms used to refer to the depth of the injury. Burn depth is expressed in terms of full-thickness and partial-thickness, and/or first, second, third, and fourth degrees. First- and second-degree burns are partial-thickness injuries, which result in partial destruction of the skin layers. Enough epithelial cells, hair follicles, and sweat glands remain intact to provide a new epidermis.

Partial-thickness injuries involving only the superficial dermis (first degree), heal spontaneously in about 2 weeks and usually cause no cosmetic or functional impairment. Partial-thickness wounds involving the deep dermis (second degree), heal spontaneously, but may require a prolonged period (greater than 21 days) to do so, and may result in some scar or contracture formation (Figure 68–6 ■, p. 2246). Infection, trauma, and a decreased blood supply increase the risk of a partial-thickness injury converting to a full-thickness injury.

Full-thickness injuries (third degree) result in the destruction of all skin layers, and there may be destruction of subcutaneous tissue, muscles, and bones (Figure 68–7 ■, p. 2247). Some health care providers refer to burns that involve muscles and bones as fourth-degree injuries. Full-thickness burns have no sensation to pain on light touch due to the destruction of the pain and touch receptors. Closure of the wound occurs by granulation, epithelial migration, contracture, and/or surgical intervention. (See the discussion of wound management later in this chapter.) Figure 68–8 ■ (p. 2247) demonstrates the difference in skin depth between a partial-thickness and a full-thickness injury.

The differential diagnosis of burn depth is based on the cause of the injury, the appearance of the wound, and the presence or absence of sensation in the area. Chart 68–2 (p. 2248) provides guidelines for helping make the determination between partial-thickness and full-thickness injury.

An assessment of the pattern of the burn injury during the emergency period also is essential. If the injury is circumferential (involving the entire circumference of an area), there is an increased risk for diminished blood supply to the area distal to the injury. (See the treatment of circumferential injuries later in this chapter.)

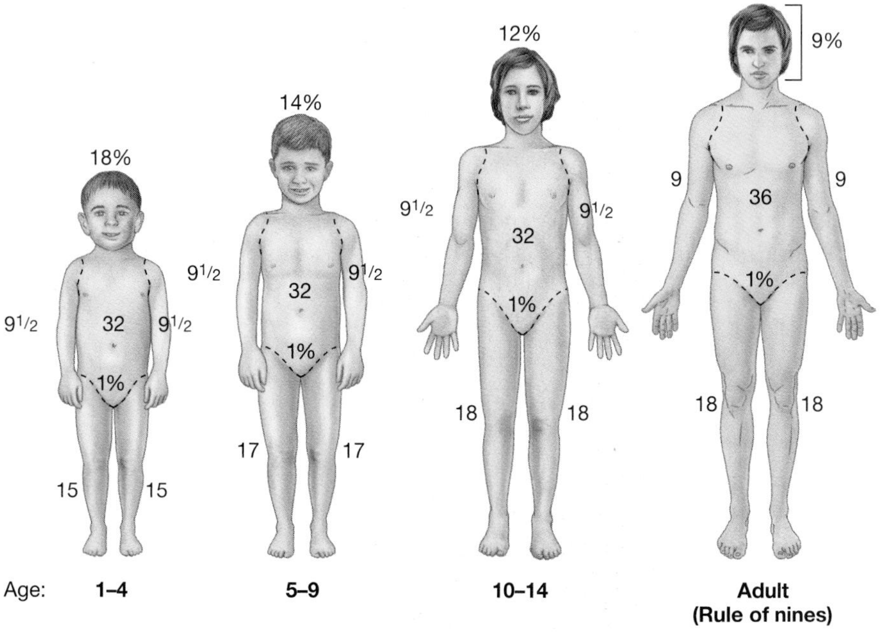

FIGURE 68–4 ■ Rule of nines.

Area	Age (years)					% 1°	% 2°	% 3°	% Total
	0–1	1–4	5–9	10–15	Adult				
Head	19	17	13	10	7				
Neck	2	2	2	2	2				
Ant. trunk	13	13	13	13	13				
Post. trunk	13	13	13	13	13				
R. buttock	2½	2½	2½	2½	2½				
L. buttock	2½	2½	2½	2½	2½				
Genitalia	1	1	1	1	1				
R.U. arm	4	4	4	4	4				
L.U. arm	4	4	4	4	4				
R.L. arm	3	3	3	3	3				
L.L. arm	3	3	3	3	3				
R. hand	2½	2½	2½	2½	2½				
L. hand	2½	2½	2½	2½	2½				
R. thigh	5½	6½	8½	8½	9½				
L. thigh	5½	6½	8½	8½	9½				
R. leg	5	5	5½	6	7				
L. leg	5	5	5½	6	7				
R. foot	3½	3½	3½	3½	3½				
L. foot	3½	3½	3½	3½	3½				
					Total				

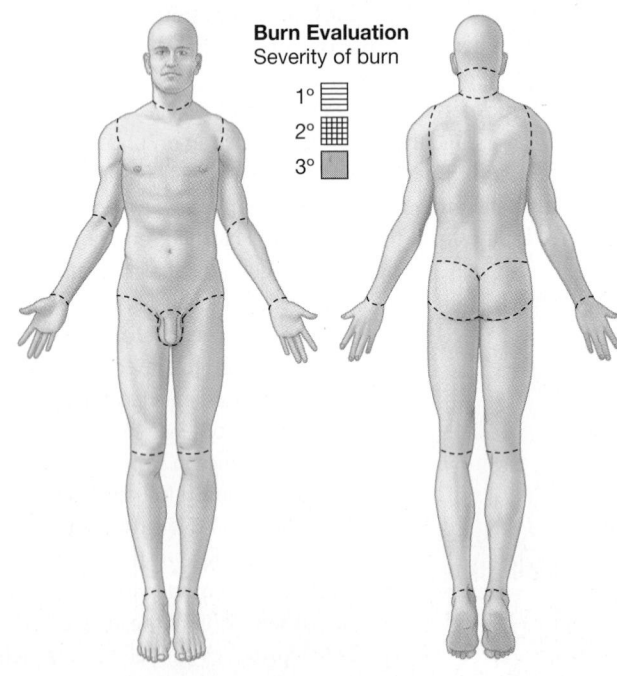

Burn Evaluation
Severity of burn

1° ▤
2° ▦
3° ▨

FIGURE 68–5 ■ Lund-Browder formula.

Age

The very young and the elderly have higher mortality rates than a young adult with the same percentage of burn injury. In the younger population (usually under 2 years of age), there are two specific reasons for increased mortality. First, infants and young children have an immature immune system with a weak antibody response to infection and tend to die of septicemia. Second, the very young have a greater proportion of body surface area per amount of body mass. As a result, there is a higher risk for fluid volume loss, requiring greater fluid resuscitation for total percent burn as compared to adults. Therefore, there is an increased risk for the development of hypovolemic shock.

In the older population (over 60 years of age), burns tend to exacerbate previous medical problems such as cardiovascular disease, renal insufficiency, diabetes, and chronic obstructive pulmonary disease. This population tends to have decreased physiological reserves, which are needed to respond to the stress of a burn injury; therefore, older adults are at a higher risk for shock and multisystem organ failure. Additionally, the older population tends to heal more slowly, resulting in a greater risk for the development of infection and pneumonia.

Past Medical History

Cardiac, respiratory, renal, and endocrine diseases and/or a history of substance abuse decreases the rate of survival of a major burn injury at any age. The added insult of a burn injury exacerbates these preexisting conditions and increases morbidity and mortality.

Part of Body Burned

The area of the body affected by burns is significant due to the associated side effects and the potential for cosmetic and functional deformities. For example, burns of the head, neck, and chest tend to have pulmonary complications and are considered more serious than a burn of the same size on the lower leg. Burn injuries occurring in the perineum and upper thighs are more prone to infections due to local contamination. For cosmetic as well as functional reasons, burns of the face, neck, and hands require special treatment for both physical as well as psychological reasons.

In summary, many health care providers believe as a general rule of prognosis that if the age of the patient and the percentage of burn add up to more than 100, there is little chance of survival. Adding any prior chronic medical problems to this situation decreases the chances of survival even further. The single most powerful factor in predicting mortality from fire is smoke inhalation, which is covered in this chapter.

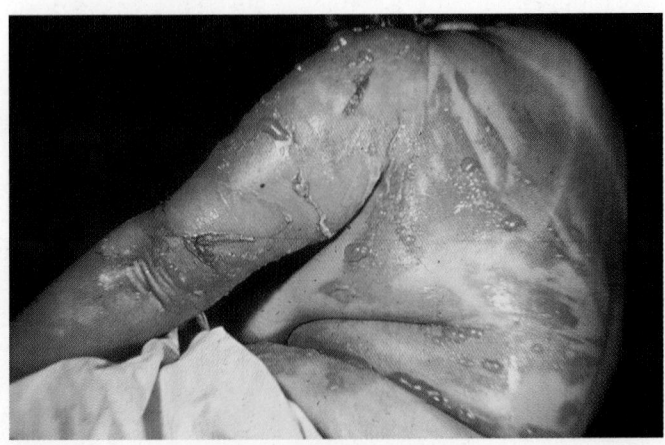

FIGURE 68–6 ■ Partial-thickness injury.
Source: Courtesy of: John M. Osborn, M.D., FACS, Sacramento, CA Plastic Surgery Center

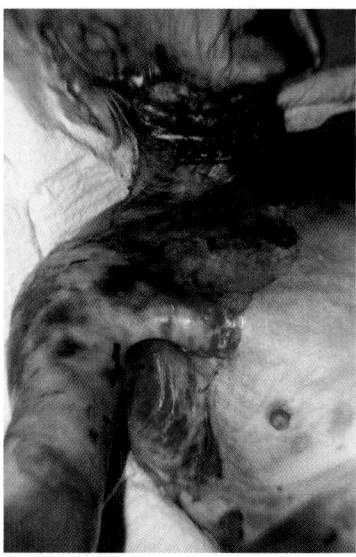

FIGURE 68–7 ■ Full-thickness injury.
Source: Courtesy of: John M. Osborn, M.D., FACS, Sacramento, CA Plastic Surgery Center

Laboratory and Diagnostic Evaluation

Tissue and cell destruction, and fluid and electrolyte shifts, cause many hematologic changes following a burn injury. The most radical changes occur in the first 24 to 48 hours after the injury. Therefore, careful monitoring of laboratory values is critical during this hemodynamic stabilization period, although careful monitoring of laboratory data must continue throughout all phases of burn recovery. Hematologic response to burn injury is discussed next and outlined in the earlier Diagnostic Tests box (p. 2241).

Red Blood Cells

Red blood cells are lost both directly in the burn and as a result of increased fragility. Circulating red blood cell mass becomes

trapped and destroyed within the burn wound at the time of injury. The cell loss is not only due to direct heat damage because erythrocyte losses continue to occur for several days after the injury. What is somewhat misleading is that in the first 12 to 48 hours after the burn injury there is an increase in the hematocrit. This increase is not due to an increase in erythrocytes but instead is the result of hemoconcentration related to intravascular fluid volume loss. Once fluid balance has been reestablished, a lower and more accurate hematocrit reading occurs. Red blood cell production is dependent on adequate iron stores and normal metabolism. Circulating levels of iron are depressed after burn injury, which may explain why erythrocyte production is decreased despite normal production of erythropoietin from the kidney.

Leukocytes

Immediately after the burn injury there is an increase in granulocytes, which constitute 60% to 80% of the total number of normal blood leukocytes (white blood cells). This increase is not due to an increased production but rather is from mobilization of preexisting stores. The granulocytes continue to increase for the first 24 hours after the injury, and then the count begins to fall. The decrease in the granulocyte level is due in part to the dilutional effects of fluid replacement therapy and because the granulocytes have concentrated in the injured areas. Within 48 hours after the injury, stores of granulocytes are depleted, and the patient is dependent on the bone marrow for the production of new cells. Infection and septicemia are factors that stimulate the production of granulocytes.

Platelets

Dilution and consumption of platelets immediately after a burn injury cause an abnormal decrease both in the platelet count and in clotting factors. In addition, it is believed that a large

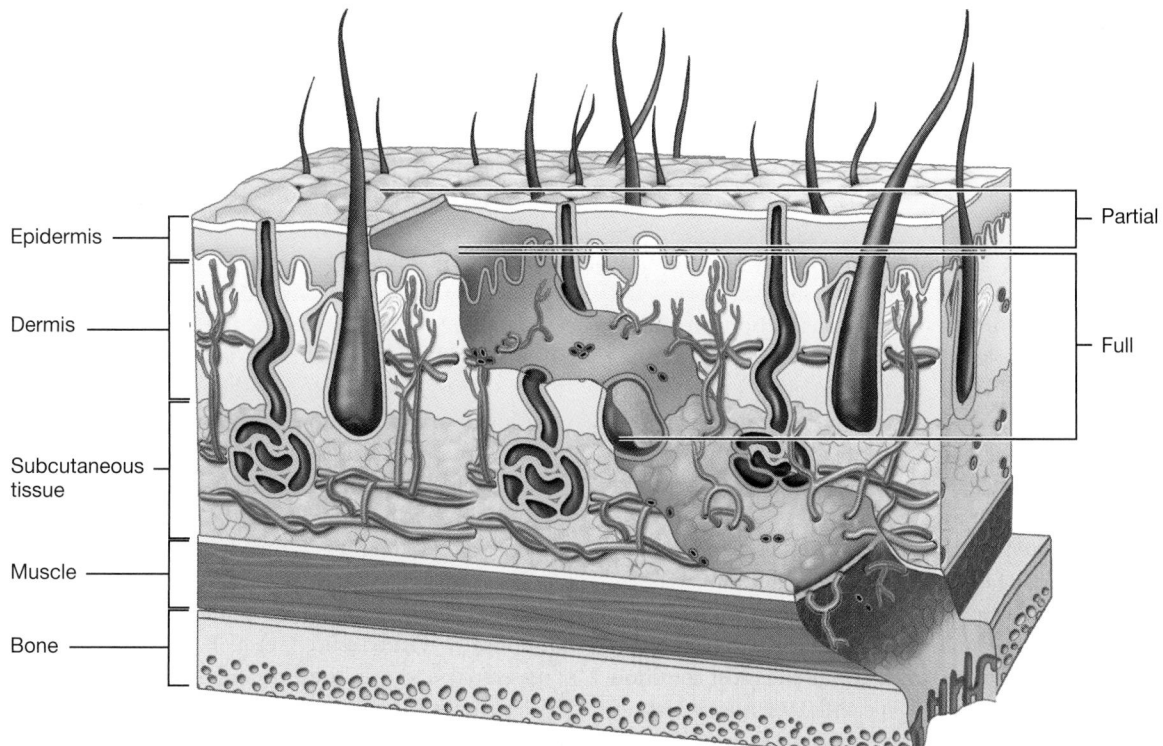

Epidermis

Dermis

Subcutaneous tissue

Muscle

Bone

Partial

Full

FIGURE 68–8 ■ Skin layers of partial-thickness versus full-thickness injury.

CHART 68–2	**Determination of Burn Depth**		
	Superficial Injury	**Partial-thickness Injury**	**Full-Thickness Injury**
Skin Depth	Epidermis	Epidermis and most of the dermis Base structures of sebaceous and sweat glands intact	Epidermis, dermis, and may include subcutaneous tissue, muscle, and bones
Skin Appearance	Red, may have local edema Blanches with pressure	Pink or dark-pink May appear dull, white, tan, or cherry Blanches with pressure	Dark red, white, charred black, gray Pearl, dark tan, waxy No blanching Charred blood vessels visible
Pain	Increased sensitivity	Increased sensitivity	Absent: nerve endings destroyed
Blister Formation	None	Large, thick walled, and will increase in size	Usually none or, if present, thin walled and will not increase in size
Texture	Slightly firm if edema present	Firm due to edema	Dry and leather like
Possible Causes	Sun Ultraviolet light Flash flame	Hot liquids or solids Flash or direct flame to clothing Chemicals Ultraviolet light	Hot liquids or solids Flame Chemicals Electrical contact
Healing Time	2–5 days No scarring	5–35 days No grafting unless converts to full-thickness injury	Little to no healing potential Requires grafting

number of platelets are utilized to stabilize the vasculature in and around the burned area. The bone marrow does not store platelets, and therefore, increased production is necessary to meet the needs of the body. It is not uncommon to replace platelets during the first 36 hours after the injury.

Medical Management

Survival following a burn injury is dependent on an in-depth, timely assessment and the development of a treatment plan. The health care provider will supply the orders for patient management, and the nurse coordinates the plan with the members of the health care team. After airway stabilization, it is critical to begin fluid resuscitation in order to prevent the development and progression of hypovolemic shock. Specific orders are outlined next.

Fluid Resuscitation

As described earlier, large amounts of fluid are lost in the first 24 to 48 hours after injury due to increased capillary permeability. Therefore, fluid replacement is critical to survival during the emergency period. The purpose of fluid resuscitation is to maintain circulating blood volume and cardiac output, which become compromised due to fluid shifting out of the intravascular space into the interstitial space. The goal is to prevent hypovolemic shock, tissue ischemia, and death. The amount of fluid needed for replacement depends on the size of injury, depth of burn, patient's age, and past medical history.

A number of different formulas have been devised in an attempt to standardize the amount and type of fluid for replacement. All of the formulas use either crystalloids or colloids or a combination of both. A crystalloid is an electrolyte solution that may be either isotonic or hypertonic. Two of the most common isotonic solutions are lactated Ringer's and 0.9% normal saline. Lactated Ringer's is most commonly the solution of choice because it most closely mimics the body's extracellular fluid. Crystalloid solutions typically are used in the first 12 hours until

capillary permeability begins to stabilize. Once the capillary leaking has slowed, some formulas give colloid products such as fresh frozen plasma, dextran, and albumin. These hypertonic solutions not only provide volume but also generate an osmotic pressure, which pulls fluid back from the interstitial space into the intravascular space. Fresh frozen plasma also restores lost clotting factors, and red blood cell replacement is indicated if a significant change has occurred in the hemoglobin and hematocrit levels. Some formulas also give 5% dextrose solution for maintenance and replacement of insensible losses.

The guidelines of the Advanced Trauma Life Support course and the Advanced Burn Life Support course recommend the use of a simple formula that is readily available at the hospital. The most common formulas are listed in Chart 68–3. Generally, health care providers use the Parkland/Baxter formula, which administers 4 milliliters of lactated Ringer's (LR) solution per kilogram of body weight multiplied by percent of TBSA of burn (4 mL/kg of weight × % burn). Because most of the fluid loss occurs in the first hours after the injury, 50% of the fluid is given in the first 8 hours, 25% in the second 8 hours, and 25% in the third 8 hours. Over the second 24 hours, the LR generally is discontinued and a hypotonic solution such as 5% dextrose and water with potassium is titrated to maintain an adequate urine output (Demling & DeSanti, 2006a). Plasma and albumin are administered in boluses during the second 24 hours to maintain hemodynamic stability (Flynn, 2002).

These formulas were designed as a guideline for fluid administration. Each patient has to be monitored individually for his response to fluid resuscitation. For example, due to the increased risk of diminished organ function in the elderly, fluid resuscitation will be less aggressive than with the very young who are more susceptible to dehydration. Therefore, all patients with burn injuries require close monitoring for adequacy of fluid replacement and organ perfusion.

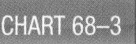

CHART 68-3   Fluid Replacement Formulas for Burn Injuries

Parkland/Baxter Formula

First 24 hours:

4 mL/kg × % total body surface area (TBSA) of lactated Ringer's

1/2 given in first 8 hours, 1/4 in second 8 hours, 1/4 in third 8 hours

Second 24 hours:

Dextrose and water, plus potassium

Colloid: 20–60% of calculated plasma volume (0.35–0.5 mL/kg × % TBSA)

Consensus Formula

First 24 hours:

2–4 mL/kg × % TBSA of lactated Ringer's

1/2 given in first 8 hours, 1/4 in second 8 hours, 1/4 in third 8 hours

Second 24 hours:

0.3–0.5 mL/kg × % TBSA of colloid solution

Electrolyte-free solution to maintain urine output

Brooke Army Formula

First 24 hours:

1.5 mL/kg × % TBSA of lactated Ringer's

0.5 mL/kg × % TBSA of colloid solution

1/2 given in first 8 hours, 1/4 in second 8 hours, 1/4 in third 8 hours

Second 24 hours:

0.5–0.75 mL/kg × % TBSA of lactated Ringer's

2,000 mL of dextrose and water

Evans Formula

First 24 hours:

1 mL/kg × % TBSA of 0.9 normal saline

1 mL/kg × % TBSA of colloid solution

1/2 given in first 8 hours, 1/4 in second 8 hours, 1/4 in third 8 hours

Second 24 hours:

0.5 mL/kg × % TBSA of 0.9 normal saline

2,000 mL of dextrose and water

Fluid Resuscitation Assessment   End points are objective criteria that define a measured outcome or goal of treatment. If end points are not achieved, resuscitation measures must be adjusted and reassessed. End points are important with burn resuscitation because then fluids are titrated using objective data instead of being only formula driven (Ahrns, 2004). Therefore, assessing normal organ function provides a means of monitoring fluid replacement. Fluid resuscitation end points include:

- **Mentation**—Orientation and level of consciousness are sensitive to changes in oxygen delivery because the brain needs constant blood for normal function. Deficient fluid resuscitation resulting in inadequate oxygen delivery to the brain can cause agitation, restlessness, confusion, and even stupor. In the absence of head trauma, a well-hydrated patient should be alert and oriented.
- **Skin color and temperature**—Vasoconstriction caused by intravascular depletion is manifested by cool, pale, and clammy skin or mottled skin with advanced shock. Additionally, due to loss of skin and subsequent temperature regulation, core body temperature may be decreased.
- **Heart rate**—Tachycardia, a heart rate greater than 100 beats per minute, is a better indicator of hypovolemia and with hydration will return to the upper limits of normal for the age range.
- **Blood pressure**—The blood pressure (BP) tends to be a poor indicator of perfusion in the very early stage because pronounced catecholamine release results in an increased systemic vascular resistance (SVR), causing normal BP to be maintained even in the presence of hypovolemia.
- **Urine output**—Most health care providers agree that the urine output is the best gauge of adequate hydration and in an adult it should be 0.5 to 1 mL/kg of body weight per hour (Demling & DeSanti, 2006a). Typically, a minimum urine output of 30 mL/hr is the gauge.

- **Specific gravity**—Specific gravity, which is also monitored on an hourly basis, becomes elevated (>1.025) with dehydration and decreases as fluid is replaced.
- **Central venous pressure (CVP)**—A CVP of between 4 and 12 indicates adequate fluid volume (Ahrns, 2004).
- **Hemoconcentration factors**—Hemoglobin (Hgb) and hematocrit (HCT) increase with the loss of intravascular volume; and in the presence of inadequate fluid resuscitation, the Hgb and HCT become abnormally elevated. The level of these values is proportional to the level of fluid volume. As fluid returns to the intravascular space, the Hgb and HCT levels will return to normal and typically become abnormally low due to cell destruction (see the Diagnostic Tests box, p. 2241). Overhydration will give false low readings.
- **Gastrointestinal function**—Normal gastrointestinal function is inferred by the return of bowel sounds.

 A hemoglobin (Hgb) of > 20 g/dL and/or a hematocrit (HCT) of > 60% is an indication that fluid resuscitation is inadequate and needs to be increased. The Hgb and HCT are not the best indicators of fluid balance because many blood cells are destroyed with the initial tissue injury. Use other indicators of fluid balance, such as heart rate, central venous pressure (CVP), and blood pressure (BP), because they are more reflective of the adequacy of hydration.

Pain Management

Pain management is a complex issue for a burn victim in that pain varies in character and intensity throughout all phases of burn treatment. Pain is related to tissue injury and the healing process and is complicated by fear, anxiety, depression, and the chronicity of the injury. The goal of pain management is to provide maximal comfort on an ongoing basis. To accomplish this, it is necessary to establish a partnership with the patient regarding how to manage pain relief.

Once fluid resuscitation has begun, narcotic analgesics are administered intravenously to help control pain. For effective pain management, interventions must be evaluated and modified on an ongoing basis. Pain causes an activation of the sympathetic nervous system, causing vasoconstriction, which decreases blood flow to the wound and delays healing.

If pain is not managed appropriately at the outset of the injury, then long-term pain management issues may ensue. The main tenets of pain management for patients with burns are:

- Analgesics are more effective if given on a scheduled basis rather than only as requested by the patient.
- Intramuscular (IM) injections are not used during the emergency period because of poor absorption.
- IM injections are avoided in children, because they fear the injection as much as the pain.
- Bowel management begins with narcotic pain management.
- Doses of medication should be modified as the clinical situation dictates (e.g., dressing changes).
- Anxiety needs to be treated for effective pain management.
- Pain management must be individualized to the patient with consideration being given to the time since the injury, patient's age, percentage burn, or burn depth.

A comprehensive approach to pain management includes assessing the pain level, anticipating prophylactic analgesic needs, and administering narcotics as ordered. In the event that the patient cannot verbalize or assist in the assessment of pain relief, there are physiological responses that must be assessed on a regular basis. These include increased heart rate, diaphoresis, increased agitation, grimacing, and rhythmic movement or lack of movement (Flynn, 2002).

In the beginning acute stages of burn injury, the most commonly used agents are opioids such as morphine sulfate, fentanyl, and codeine. Small, frequent doses on a non–pain-contingent schedule are indicated for the continuous pain or background pain that is associated with loss of skin integrity. Procedural pain such as dressing changes are best managed by additional intravenous opioids. Patients typically report excruciating pain with dressing changes, especially with partial-thickness injuries. As the burn injury heals, less potent drugs are indicated such as nonsteroidal analgesics. The length of time required to treat burn injuries necessitates a comprehensive interdisciplinary team approach that is essential for maximizing a patient's functional outcome while minimizing psychological distress. Adequate management of pain requires that the plan be reevaluated frequently. Chapter 15 provides an in-depth discussion of pain management principles.

Alternative Therapies for Pain Management It is essential to allow the patient to verbalize the pain experience and explore alternative therapies for pain relief. These therapies include guided imagery, hypnosis, and music and are used as an adjunct to medication. The Complementary and Alternative Therapies box details music therapy's use in the management of pain.

> **CRITICAL ALERT** *Assess adequacy of pain management for dressing changes daily. Secure health care provider's orders for more medication, and have these orders available as backup if needed. Be sensitive to cultural diversity in response to pain and medicate accordingly.*

COMPLEMENTARY & ALTERNATIVE THERAPIES   Music

Description:

Pain management is a vital issue in burn care. Research has shown that the experience of pain affects both the body and the mind. Therefore, nurses must use a holistic view of pain management and healing when caring for patients with burns. In addition to the use of cognitive, behavioral, and pharmacologic interventions for pain management, nurses should consider the use of music as an intervention. Research has shown that music is helpful for pain management. Music provides a simple, inexpensive intervention that the nurse can easily adapt to the individual needs of patients with burns (Prensner, Yowler, Smith, Steele, & Fratianne, 2001).

Research Support:

A Korean study assessed whether music therapy could affect anxiety and pain for patients undergoing burn dressing changes. The study involved 32 adult patients with burns, 15 of whom received the routine burn dressing changes (the control group) and 17 of whom listened to self-selected music through headphones during burn dressing changes for 3 days (the experimental group). Participants in the experimental (music) group completed the State Anxiety Inventory and a self-report of pain scores before and after burn dressing changes. Results showed that the participants who received music therapy reported significant reductions in both anxiety and pain before and after burn dressing changes as compared to participants who did not receive music therapy. Researchers concluded that music therapy with self-selected music is a valuable intervention for the treatment of pain and anxiety in patients undergoing burn dressing changes (Son & Kim, 2006).

Another study assessed the effect of music therapy on 14 randomly selected pediatric burn patients. The experimental group listened to live music and the control group received verbal interaction only. Psychological, behavioral, and physiological outcomes were reported using the Wong Baker FACES Pain Rating Scale, the Fear Thermometer, the Nursing Assessment of Pain Index, heart rate, and respiration rate. Although the results of the study were mixed and inconclusive, researchers recorded improved pain and anxiety through anecdotal reports from the experimental group. Based on these results, researchers stated that further study is needed in order to recommend use of music therapy for patients with burns (Whitehead-Pleaux, Baryza, & Sheridan, 2006).

References

Prensner, J. D., Yowler, C. J., Smith, L. F., Steele, A. L., & Fratianne, R. B. (2001, January-February). Music therapy for assistance with pain and anxiety management in burn treatment. *Journal of Burn Care and Rehabilitation, 22*(1), 82–88.

Son, J. T., & Kim, S. H. (2006). The effects of self-selected music on anxiety and pain during burn dressing changes. *Taehan Kanho Hakhoe Chi, 36*(1), 159–168.

Whitehead-Pleaux, A. M., Baryza, M. J., & Sheridan, R. L. (2006). The effects of music therapy on pediatric patients' pain and anxiety during donor site dressing change. *Journal of Music Therapy, 43*(2), 136–153.

Nursing Management

The nursing care needs of the newly admitted patient with burns are complex and multifaceted. Use of the nursing process will facilitate a comprehensive approach to patient assessment and care. The Nursing Process: Patient Care Plan feature applies the nursing process to the applicable nursing diagnoses and provides a comprehensive care plan for a patient with burns during the emergency period.

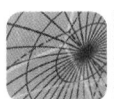

NURSING PROCESS: Patient Care Plan for the Emergency Period

Assessment of Fluid Volume Loss

Subjective Data:
Do you know where you are?   Are you feeling light-headed or dizzy?
Tell me your name.   Are you feeling thirsty?

Objective Data:
Blood pressure   Urine output
Cardiac output   Hemoglobin and hematocrit

Nursing Assessment and Diagnoses	Outcomes and Evaluation Parameters	Planning and Interventions with *Rationales*
Nursing Diagnosis: *Deficient Fluid Volume* related to increased capillary permeability, increased intravascular hydrostatic pressure, and increased evaporative loss	**Outcomes:** Adequate intravascular volume. Fluid and electrolytes within normal limits. No signs and symptoms of hypovolemic shock. Mental alertness and cognitive orientation. ***Evaluation Parameters:*** Normal vital signs. Normal serum electrolytes, hemoglobin, and hematocrit. Urine specific gravity between 1.010 and 1.020. Urine output at 0.5 mL/kg per hour.	**Interventions and *Rationales:*** Insert large-bore intravenous (IV) catheter through nonburned tissue per order. *To facilitate fluid replacement.* Administer and titrate IV fluids per ordered formulas and parameters. *To replace lost volume.* Record amount of IV fluid infused. *To monitor fluid replacement.* Assess vital signs and urine output at least hourly until stable and then per health care provider's order/unit policy. *To assess adequacy of fluid replacement.* Monitor central venous pressure (CVP) and pulmonary artery wedge pressure (PAWP) if possible. *To assess adequacy of fluid replacement and cardiac output.* Monitor arterial blood gases (ABGs). *To assess acid–base balance and presence of shock.* Obtain baseline weight if possible and monitor regularly. *To monitor adequacy of nutritional replacement.* Test all stools and emesis for blood. *To monitor for blood loss from stress ulcers.* Maintain a heated environment. *To prevent loss of body heat due to loss of skin integrity.* Monitor serum electrolytes, hemoglobin, and hematocrit, and report critical abnormalities to the health care provider. *To monitor hematologic changes associated with fluid loss and tissue destruction.* Monitor for blood loss from burns or other injuries. *To assess need for blood replacement therapy.* Assess orientation frequently and regularly. *Monitor adequacy of fluid replacement and presence of associated head injury.* Provide oral fluids, if patient is able to drink. *Encourage fluid intake to replace lost fluid.*

Assessment of Excess Fluid

Subjective Data:
Do you feel short of breath?
Do you have a cough?

Objective Data:
Congested lungs   Increased PAWP
Increased heart rate   Increased rate and depth of
Increased blood pressure   respirations
Increased CVP   Increased weight

Nursing Assessment and Diagnoses	Outcomes and Evaluation Parameters	Planning and Interventions with *Rationales*
Nursing Diagnosis: *Risk for Imbalanced Fluid Volume* related to excessive IV fluid administration and diminished organ capacity for excessive volume load	**Outcome:** Adequate hydration with no evidence of fluid overload. ***Evaluation Parameters:*** Normal vital signs. Normal CVP, PAWP. Normal ABGs, electrolytes. Vesicular lung sounds clear. No dyspnea. No increase in body weight. Normal urine output and specific gravity.	**Interventions and *Rationales:*** Assess body weight if possible. *Monitor for excess fluid buildup.* Assess urine output and specific gravity. *Monitor hydration status.* Assess arterial blood gases (ABGs) and electrolytes. *To assess acid–base balance, severity of shock state, and electrolyte changes due to fluid shifts.* Monitor intake and output hourly. *To assess rate of fluid replacement.* Monitor lung sound. *To assess for fluid build-up.*

(continued)

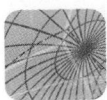

NURSING PROCESS: Patient Care Plan for the Emergency Period—*Continued*

Assessment of Tissue Perfusion

Subjective Data:
Can you feel me touch your fingers and toes?
Can you move your fingers and toes?
Where are you having pain?

Objective Data:
Nail bed color and capillary refill
Temperature of fingers and toes
Peripheral pulses

Nursing Assessment and Diagnoses	Outcomes and Evaluation Parameters	Planning and Interventions with *Rationales*
Nursing Diagnosis: *Ineffective Peripheral Tissue Perfusion* related to constricting edema formation and circumferential burns	**Outcome:** Adequate peripheral tissue perfusion. ***Evaluation Parameters:*** Extremity pulses present by palpation and/or ultrasound. Capillary refill < 3 seconds on distal extremities. Absence of numbness or tingling. Absence of increased pain.	**Interventions and *Rationales:*** Remove constricting clothing, jewelry, and dressings. *To promote tissue perfusion.* Elevate affected extremities above the heart. *To reduce edema formation.* Monitor arterial pulses by palpation and/or ultrasound every hour during the first 24–48 hours. *To assess perfusion status during edema formation.* Assess pain and capillary permeability on both burned and unburned areas. *To assess the impact of edema formation.* Assess for numbness or tingling. *To assess perfusion status during edema formation.* If pulses diminish or become absent, if pain increases, or if capillary refill slows, notify the health care provider immediately. *These are indications of a loss of perfusion and need medical intervention to prevent necrosis formation.* If indicated, prepare patient for escharotomy. *To prevent loss of affected extremity or prevent respiratory depression.*

Assessment of Airway and Gas Exchange

Subjective Data:
How did you get burned?
Did the injury occur in an enclosed space?
Do you have any preexisting health problems such as heart, lung, or kidney disease?

Objective Data:
Lung sounds
Oxygen saturation
Work of breathing; e.g., gasping, increased rate, loudness
Vital signs
Skin and nail bed color

Nursing Assessment and Diagnoses	Outcomes and Evaluation Parameters	Planning and Interventions with *Rationales*
Nursing Diagnoses: *Impaired Gas Exchange* related to inhalation injury and fatigue *Ineffective Airway Clearance* related to tracheal edema	**Outcome:** Adequate gas exchange. ***Evaluation Parameters:*** Normal arterial blood gases. Free of dyspnea: unlabored respirations < 24/minute. Alert and oriented. Clear breath sounds. No restlessness, cyanosis, or fatigue. Oxygen saturation is within normal limits.	**Interventions and *Rationales:*** Assess for adventitious or diminished breath sounds. *Indicates decreased gas exchange.* Note presence of cough, and amount, color, and consistency of sputum. *Assessing for inhalation injury.* Monitor ABGs and oxygen saturation. *To assess adequacy of gas exchange and level of shock state.* Monitor respiratory rate and depth. *To assess for respiratory distress.* Monitor restlessness and confusion. *Indicators of inadequate gas exchange with resultant brain hypoxia.* Observe for cyanosis, especially in the mucous membranes. *Indicators of inadequate gas exchange with resultant tissue hypoxia.* Turn, cough, deep breathe, elevate head of bed, and instruct on use of incentive spirometry. *Measures to promote gas exchange.* Administer humidified oxygen as prescribed. *To loosen secretions and promote airway clearance.* Report respiratory distress to the health care provider. *Medical intervention may be indicated to prevent respiratory failure.* Assess need for suctioning and/or endotracheal intubation. *To maintain adequate gas exchange.*

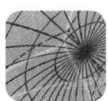

NURSING PROCESS: Patient Care Plan for the Emergency Period—*Continued*

Assessment of Skin Integrity

Subjective Data:
Where are you having pain?

Objective Data:
Percent total body surface area burn using standardized measurement scales
Depth of injury

Nursing Assessment and Diagnoses	Outcomes and Evaluation Parameters	Planning and Interventions with *Rationales*
Nursing Diagnosis: *Impaired Skin Integrity* related to epithelial skin loss	**Outcome:** Normal wound healing to reestablish skin integrity. ***Evaluation Parameters:*** Burn wounds will heal spontaneously or by surgical closure as evidenced by no open wound, no drainage, and no odor. Absence of clinical manifestations of wound infection.	**Interventions and *Rationales:*** Assess extent of total body surface area (TBSA) of burn. Cleanse and débride wound. *Determines treatment and prognosis.* Assess wound for depth, location, and dimensions. *Determines treatment and prognosis.* Elevate affected areas. *To decrease edema.* Position therapeutically. *To prevent contracture formation.* Apply antibiotic cream and/or dressing per health care provider's order. *To prevent infection.* Clean, débride wounds daily, and assess for separation of eschar and evidence of granulation tissue. *Preparation for skin grafting.* Assess for presence or absence of granulation tissue and necrotic tissue. *Assess wound status for grafting.* Assess for infection (see *Risk for Infection* nursing diagnosis). *To prevent occurrence and spread of infection.* Establish a skin breakdown prevention plan. Monitor blood glucose. White blood count (WBC) daily. *Infection assessment.* Monitor donor sites for infection. *May convert site to a full-thickness injury.* Administer vitamins and minerals per order. *To promote wound healing.*

Assessment for Infection

Subjective Data:
Is your pain increasing?
Do you feel weaker?

Objective Data:
Previously healed wounds are breaking down
Open wounds not healing
Partial-thickness injuries/donor sites converting to full-thickness injuries
Increased odor and drainage from wound sites
Wound cultures positive for organisms
Fever
Increased WBC

Nursing Assessment and Diagnoses	Outcomes and Evaluation Parameters	Planning and Interventions with *Rationales*
Nursing Diagnosis: *Risk for Infection* related to loss of skin integrity and impaired nonspecific and specific immunity	**Outcome:** Effective infection prevention. ***Evaluation Parameters:*** Burn will not be colonized by organisms. Healing and re-epithelialization as noted by wound closure. Skin integrity will be restored.	**Interventions and *Rationales:*** Cleanse and shave wound per protocol. *To prevent contamination from surrounding tissue and hair.* Assess for infection and document with each dressing change. *To prevent spread of infection.* Assess for drainage: exudate, color, odor, and amount. *Factors that indicate infection.* Assess for undermining or sinus tract formation. *Indicates infection.* Use strict aseptic technique. *To prevent infection.* Notify health care provider of presence of infection or wound enlargement. *To facilitate medical intervention.* Monitor serum WBC daily. *Increased WBC indicates presence of infection.* Maintain nutritional therapies. *Malnutrition increases the risk of infection.* Monitor and record temperature hourly. *Indicates infection.* Culture wounds and body secretions per protocol. *To assess for infection.*

(continued)

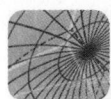

NURSING PROCESS: Patient Care Plan for the Emergency Period—*Continued*

Assessment of Nutritional Status

Subjective Data:
How is your appetite?
What can be done to help improve it?
Do you understand the importance of maintaining adequate nutrition?
Do you feel nauseated?
What kinds of food do you enjoy?

Objective Data:
Presence of bowel sounds
Calorie count
Prealbumin level
Weight changes

Nursing Assessment and Diagnoses	Outcomes and Evaluation Parameters	Planning and Interventions with *Rationales*
Nursing Diagnosis: *Imbalanced Nutrition: Less than Body Requirements* related to hypermetabolic demands of burn injury, decreased appetite, immobility, pain, nausea/vomiting, and depression	**Outcome:** Adequate nutrition maintained. **Evaluation Parameters:** Adequate calorie and nutrient intake maintained. Tolerates prescribed diet. Nutritional laboratory values within normal limits. Regular bowel pattern. Maintains preinjury body weight (+ or − 10%). Gastric pH > 5. Stool and gastric aspirate are negative for blood. Fluid and electrolyte balance is normal. Progressive wound healing. Free of complications. Adequate energy levels.	**Interventions and *Rationales:*** Record accurate intake and output, and calorie count every shift. *Indicates adequacy of nutrition.* Maintain oral hygiene. *Helps promote appetite and prevents infection.* Monitor gastrointestinal tract for bowel sounds and distention. *Assesses normal digestive process.* Monitor feeding tube placement and function. *To prevent complications such as aspiration.* Administer enteral tube feedings at prescribed rate and concentration. *To maintain nutrition.* Monitor for residual formula by aspiration per health care provider's order. *To assess tolerance and absorption of feedings.* Monitor weight daily. *Indicates adequacy of nutrition.* Consult nutritionist to establish calorie, protein, carbohydrate, and nutrient needs. *To maintain nutrition.* Allow patient to select desired foods. *To promote appetite.* Involve family in meal planning. *To assess patient's likes and dislikes.* Provide high-calorie, high-protein, high-carbohydrate diet, including snacks. *To augment between meal calorie intake.* Avoid painful procedures near mealtime and make the environment pleasant for eating. *To increase appetite.* Monitor laboratory values; i.e., total protein levels, complete blood count, glucose, iron, and prealbumin. *To ensure adequacy of nutrition.* Monitor elimination patterns. *To assess gastrointestinal (GI) function.* Monitor wound healing progress. *Wound healing progress is impacted by nutritional status.* Monitor pH and guaiac tests on gastric aspirate and stools. *To assess for GI bleeding.* Administer antacids, stool softeners, laxatives, and antiulcer agents per health care provider orders. *To prevent GI bleeding.* Assess dietary patterns in culturally diverse populations. *To tailor diet to foods of a particular culture.*

Assessment of Pain

Subjective Data:
What is your pain level using the 0–10 scale? A 1 is very little pain and a 10 is the worst imaginable pain.
What is your experience with pain?
Do you routinely take pain medications at home; if so, what for and what kind?
Are you allergic to any pain medication?
Do you have any cultural or religious beliefs that impact your pain control?

Objective Data:
Grimacing on movement
Restlessness and irritability
Taut facial expression

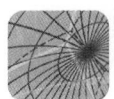

NURSING PROCESS: Patient Care Plan for the Emergency Period—*Continued*

Nursing Assessment and Diagnoses	Outcomes and Evaluation Parameters	Planning and Interventions with *Rationales*
Nursing Diagnosis: *Acute Pain* related to burn injury and exposed nerve endings	**Outcome:** Comfort level maintained. ***Evaluation Parameters:*** Able to communicate pain level and therapies that help alleviate it. Pain reduced and/or absent as evidenced by patient report and no pain behaviors: grimacing. Nonpharmacologic method of control is effective as evidenced by patient report and no pain behaviors. Reports satisfaction with pain management program.	**Interventions and *Rationales:*** Use pain scale (0–10) to quantify pain level. *Quantifying pain increases consistency.* Instruct patient to inform nurse if pain is not relieved. *Indicates need to change pain management plan.* Assess cultural and religious impact on patient's responses. *Different cultures and religions respond differently to pain.* Correct misconceptions about risk of addiction and overdose. *To decrease anxiety related to medication addiction.* Explain, prepare, and medicate patient for painful procedures (dressing change) and anticipated discomforts. *To control increased pain level related to procedure.* Provide a supportive environment wherein patient is able to express pain level. *Opens communication and facilitates pain management.* Use pain control measures before pain becomes severe. *This increases comfort and decreases need for medication.* Teach nonpharmacologic method of control; i.e., guided imagery and massage, and breathing exercises. *These measures augment pain relief.* Cover wounds. *Covering areas where there is no skin decreases the pain.* Elevate affected areas. *Elevation decreases edema formation, which can be painful.* Provide rest periods between procedures to assist with coping with ongoing pain. *Decreases the fatigue related to long-term pain.* Revise pain management plan as wounds heal and pain decreases. *To prevent overmedication.* Plan diversional activities. *To augment pain-relief measures.*

Assessment of Fear and Anxiety

Subjective Data:

Tell me what you are feeling about your injuries.

Who are the people in your life that are your support system?

How have you handled fearful situations in the past?

Objective Data:

Facial expressions

Mood

Verbalization of fear regarding injury, impact on family, and future

Nursing Assessment and Diagnoses	Outcomes and Evaluation Parameters	Planning and Interventions with *Rationales*
Nursing Diagnoses: *Fear* and *Anxiety* related to changes in health status/role functioning; situational crisis	**Outcome:** Anxiety level minimized. ***Evaluation Parameters:*** Verbalizes anxious feelings. Verbalizes what relieves anxiety. Anxiety relieved by consistently demonstrating aggression and anxiety control, coping, impulse control, self-mutilation restraint, and substantially effective social interaction skills. Verbalizes absence of sensory perceptual disorders. Verbalizes absence of physical manifestations of anxiety. Behavioral manifestations of anxiety absent.	**Interventions and *Rationales:*** Assess and document level of anxiety. *To track trends in anxiety levels.* Explore with the patient/family techniques to reduce anxiety. *This gives the patient a sense of control and opens communication about the subject.* Provide factual information concerning diagnosis, treatment, disfigurement, disabilities, and prognosis. *Truthful explanations increase trust and potentially decrease anxiety.* Explain all procedures and allow time for mental preparation. *This decreases fear and anxiety of the unknown.* Explore with patient effective ways to minimize anxiety. *This gives the patient a sense of control.* Instruct patient on use of relaxation techniques. *To relieve anxiety.* Assess need for and administer antianxiety and pain medication. *If alternative measures are not effective, may need antianxiety agents.* Assist patient/family in setting realistic goals for progress. *Indicates effectiveness of emotional adjustment.* Consider psychiatric counseling for patients/families who exhibit inability to accept situation. *Provide an ongoing plan and interventions to promote long-term relief from anxiety.*

(continued)

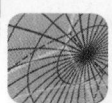

Assessment for Temperature Regulation

Subjective Data:
Do you feel cold/too warm?

Objective Data:

Body temperature   Shivering   Dusky nail beds

Nursing Assessment and Diagnoses	Outcomes and Evaluation Parameters	Planning and Interventions with *Rationales*
Nursing Diagnosis: *Ineffective Thermoregulation* related to epithelial skin loss	**Outcome:** Normal thermoregulation maintained. ***Evaluation Parameter:*** Body temperature maintained between 37.5° and 38.7°C (99.5°–101.5°F).	**Interventions and *Rationales:*** Minimize heat loss by covering patient with dressing and blankets. *To decrease heat loss due to a lack of skin integrity.* Apply heat lamps and radiant heat shields. *To decrease heat loss due to a lack of skin integrity.* Keep room temperature elevated, especially during dressing changes. *To decrease heat loss due to a lack of skin integrity.* Monitor rectal and core temperatures as per orders and report changes. *To assess effectiveness of interventions.*

Assessment of Patient Perception of Environment and Injury

Subjective Data:
What questions do you have about your injury and the necessary therapy for healing?
Have you been in situations in your life in which you feel you have very little control?
How do you typically cope with situations in which you are not in control?

Objective Data:
Compliance with treatments

Nursing Assessment and Diagnoses	Outcomes and Evaluation Parameters	Planning and Interventions with *Rationales*
Nursing Diagnosis: *Powerlessness* related to foreign environment and critical injury	**Outcome:** Realistic perception of control. ***Evaluation Parameters:*** Verbalizes realistic perception of abilities to perform. Identifies health outcome priorities. Verbalizes powerlessness. Identifies actions that are within his control. Verbalizes ability to perform necessary actions. Reports adequate support from staff and family.	**Interventions and *Rationales:*** Determine knowledge of health and injury. *Determines where to begin teaching.* Discuss realistic options for self-care. *Gives patient hope and realistic view of limitations.* Reinforce personal strengths. *Decreases sense of powerlessness.* Encourage verbalization of feeling of powerlessness. *Opens communication.* Assist patient to increase independence when realistic. *Decreases powerlessness.* Allow control over surroundings and schedule when possible. *Decreases powerlessness.* Keep items within reach. *Decreases powerlessness.* Set short-term realistic goals. *Decreases powerlessness.* Explore patient's support mechanisms: family, church, and friends. *Needed as a source of support.*

Assessment of Patient and Family Knowledge of Injury

Subjective Data:
What do you understand about your injury?
Do you have questions about the injury/treatment program?
What would you like me to tell you about your injury?

Objective Data:
Patient/family verbalizes knowledge of seriousness of injury and prognosis.

Nursing Assessment and Diagnoses	Outcomes and Evaluation Parameters	Planning and Interventions with *Rationales*
Nursing Diagnosis: *Deficient Knowledge* regarding burn resuscitation	**Outcome:** Adequate knowledge of treatment regimen. ***Evaluation Parameter:*** Patient and family will verbalize understanding of treatments and care.	**Interventions and *Rationales:*** Assess patient/family's readiness and ability to learn, and individual learning needs. *The person must be psychologically ready to learn.* Determine level of existing knowledge. *Begin the teaching where existing knowledge ends.* Provide factual information about diagnosis, treatments, and prognosis. *To increase knowledge and understanding.* Explain all procedures in simple, concise language—allowing for questions. *Increases understanding.* Encourage questions. *Keeps open communication and augments understanding.* Ongoing education of treatment plan and rationale. *Ongoing education is necessary as situation and condition change.* Document response to teaching. *Assists health care team when implementing a teaching plan.*

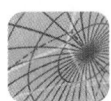

NURSING PROCESS: Patient Care Plan for the Emergency Period—*Continued*

Assessment of Psychological Adjustment to Scarring and Contractures

Subjective Data:
What impact does the change in your physical appearance have on your life?
How do you plan to cope with these changes?

Objective Data:
Does patient look at burn wounds?
Does patient ask questions about the wounds?
Is patient's perception realistic regarding body image changes?
Are the patient/family willing to learn and participate in the required care after hospital discharge?

Nursing Assessment and Diagnoses	Outcomes and Evaluation Parameters	Planning and Interventions with *Rationales*
Nursing Diagnoses: *Disturbed Body Image* related to scar formation and functional loss *Risk for Complicated Grieving* related to body image change, risk of family role change, and possible occupational change	**Outcome:** Acceptance of body image changes. ***Evaluation Parameters:*** Patient verbalizes understanding of body changes. Patient verbalizes acceptance of self.	**Interventions and *Rationales:*** Assess patient's level of anxiety and knowledge related to body image changes. *Body image changes occur as healing progresses.* Encourage discussion of meaning of loss. *Increases adjustment.* Observe interaction with significant people. *Indication of adjustment.* Assess for signs of grieving. *Indication of adjustment.* Establish therapeutic environment with an atmosphere of acceptance. *Increases adjustment.* Explain expected appearance. *Increases adjustment.* Offer mirror for viewing of facial burns. *Assesses adjustment.* Be realistic and positive during explanations. *Increases adjustment.* Plan family involvement during teaching. *Increases adjustment.* Set realistic goals for future. *Increases trust and is reality based.*

Source: Wilkinson, J. M. (2009). *Nursing diagnosis handbook; with interventions and outcomes* (8th ed.). Upper Saddle River, NJ: Prentice Hall.

Collaborative Management

To achieve optimal recovery and return to society, patients with burns need a multidisciplinary team approach, including health care providers, nurses, physical and occupational therapists, social workers, psychologists/psychiatrists, and dieticians. To ensure complete closure and prevention of infection, wound care is managed by both the nurses and the health care providers. As the burn scar heals, it continues to contract, thereby decreasing range of motion in the surrounding area. Physical therapy is begun within a few days after admission and continues for at least a year after hospital discharge. Ongoing physical therapy will help increase range of motion in the joints. When contracture formation is severe, the surgeon needs to release the contractures surgically. Due to the scarring and contractures, it may not be possible for the patient to return to her previous profession. The occupational therapist assists the patient with exercises that will enhance fine motor movements, while the social worker and a psychologist/psychiatrist are used to help the patient adjust to body image changes and perhaps loss of profession. Family dynamics often are impacted by the prolonged hospitalization and change in role function within the family structure. The psychologist/psychiatrist also assists the patient with the adjustments of these changes. Finally, a comprehensive plan for nutrition is important for enhancing wound healing, regaining strength, and preventing complications. The dietician works with the health care team from the time of admission through discharge to ensure proper nutritional support.

Acute Phase

The acute period of burn management begins when the patient is hemodynamically stable and ends with closure of the burn wounds. The goals of treatment during this period include wound cleansing and healing; pain relief; preserving body heat; preventing infection; promoting nutrition; and splinting, positioning, and exercising affected joints.

Wound Care

After airway and hemodynamic stabilization, wound care is the next priority. Infection is the most serious threat to further tissue injury and the development of sepsis; therefore, survival may be dependent on preventing wound contamination. Nurses generally coordinate and perform wound care; thus, nursing assessment and interventions are critical. Care of the wound includes cleansing, débridement, shaving, culturing, assessment for infection and adequate circulation, and applying topical antibiotics. These aspects of wound care are discussed next.

Cleansing

Cleansing of the burn wound at the time of admission may be accomplished by a number of methods depending on the preference of the health care provider, available equipment, and the stability of the patient. The purpose of the cleansing is to remove debris from the wound, eliminate dead tissue, and prevent further destruction of viable tissue by infection. For the cleansing process, the patient may be submerged in a Hubbard tank, hosed over a spray table, placed in a shower, or washed at the bedside. The advantage of using a Hubbard tank is that the patient can be totally submerged in the water, which helps remove topical antibiotics and dead tissue (eschar), and facilitates range-of-motion exercises. Submersion in a Hubbard tank is typically limited to 30 minutes or less because submersion in water leaches sodium from the open wound, causes heat loss, and is very painful. Whichever method is used, the wound is washed with gauze and a mild bacteriostatic soap such as chlorhexidine gluconate (Hibiclens) or any noncytotoxic cleansing agent. Removal of blisters is controversial; most health care providers believe that if blisters are intact they should be left in place, but if they are open the loose tissue should be removed. Washing of open wounds is a painful process; therefore, it is imperative that the patient be premedicated prior to dressing changes. Heat shields, warm blankets, and increased room temperature are methods used to help maintain body temperature during dressing changes.

Wound Débridement

The purpose of wound débridement is to remove loose tissue, wound debris, and eschar (nonviable tissue) in order to prepare the wound for closure. In Figure 68–9 ■ the white tissue is dead eschar, which needs to be débrided before the wound is ready for grafting. Débridement of a burn wound can be accomplished by three methods: mechanically, chemically, and surgically. Mechanical débridement is accomplished by using wet-to-dry dressings. Mechanical débridement is done by manually cutting the dead tissue with scissors and forceps, as well as with hydrotherapy. During daily dressing changes, nurses use scissors and forceps to remove and cut away the dead tissue. Use of the Hubbard tank, a spray table, and/or the shower gradually softens the dead tissue, which facilitates easier removal. Chemical removal of eschar is accomplished by the use of commercially prepared enzymatic or fibrinolytic agents that digest necrotic tissue, such as Elase (Parke-Davis Division of Warner-Lambert Co., Morris Plains, New Jersey). This agent is a combination of two lytic enzymes in a petroleum base. Enzymatic débridement agents must be applied only within the open wound and must be discontinued once the eschar is gone and granulation tissue is present. More extensive wound débridement is done in surgery by excising the burn wound. The techniques used to remove eschar are discussed in the Surgical Management section later in this chapter.

Shaving, Culturing, and Photographs

With the exception of the eyebrows, body hair is shaved within the wound itself and up to 2.5 centimeters from the periphery of the wound. This is done to avoid wound contamination because hair attracts and shelters bacteria. Wound culturing is typically done on admission to obtain baseline information and is repeated approximately every 7 days unless the wounds become symptomatic with exudate and odor. Culturing protocols are specific to site and health care provider. Photographs are taken on admission to provide baseline data and then repeated periodically throughout the healing process.

Escharotomies

During the initial phase of management, a surgical intervention may be required to maintain adequate circulation to the underlying tissues. Burn-induced changes in capillary permeability and the infusion of large volumes of crystalloid solutions to maintain vascular volume, cause edema to form beneath the inelastic eschar. If a full-thickness injury involves an entire circumferential area, the edema creates a tourniquet-like effect and diminishes or completely cuts off circulation distal to the injury site. If left untreated, there is a high risk for tissue necrosis and in some instances total loss of the tissue including limbs. Doppler ultrasound signals are often used to assess perfusion in the involved areas. Loss of ultrasound signals is an indication for an escharotomy. Incisions or **escharotomies** are made through the burn tissue to relieve the constricting effects of the edema. These incisions should extend the entire length of a full-thickness injury, including joints, to ensure release of neural and vascular compression (Figure 68–10 ■). The incisions penetrate the eschar and immediate subadjacent connective tissue to permit expansion of the edematous underlying tissue. Frequent monitoring of the circulation distal to the escharotomy site is part of the ongoing nursing assessment and includes pulses, tissue color including paleness and cyanosis, sensation, increased pain, capillary refill, and decreased temperature. Often it is necessary to monitor circulation every 15 to 20 minutes. If distal blood flow does not improve, a second escharotomy is needed.

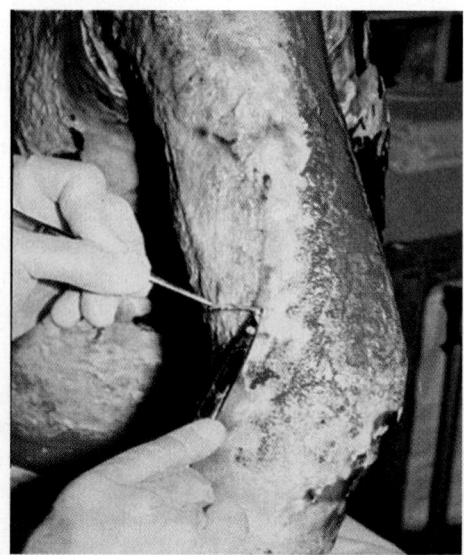

FIGURE 68–9 ■ Débridement of eschar.
Source: Courtesy of: Robert M. Faggella, Jr. M.D., FACS Sacramento, CA

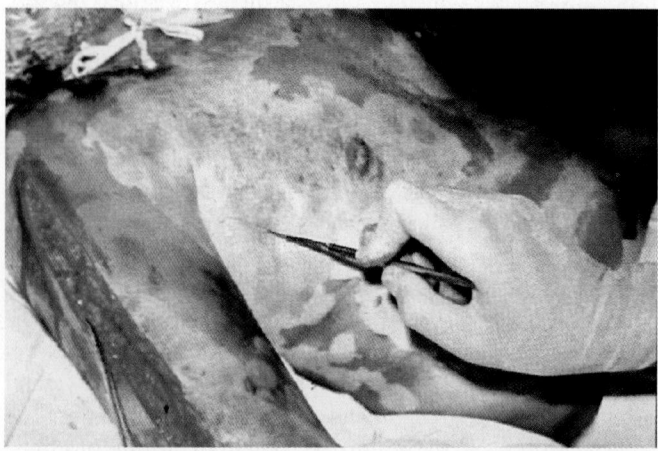

FIGURE 68–10 ■ Escharotomy.
Source: Courtesy of: Robert M. Faggella, Jr. M.D., FACS Sacramento, CA

Typically, no anesthesia is required because full-thickness injuries have limited or no sensation, and generally blood loss is minimal and is readily controlled with pressure.

Circumferential burns of the neck and chest may occlude the airway and decrease chest expansion and pulmonary function, resulting in respiratory distress. A chest escharotomy may be needed to restore a patent airway and effective ventilation. Monitoring respiratory effort is a critical part of the initial nursing assessment and includes respiratory rate, oxygen saturations, arterial blood gases, cyanosis, lung sounds, and shortness of breath (see Chapter 33 for complete respiratory assessment). Mechanical ventilation may be necessary due to low tidal volumes.

In Figure 68–11, the broken lines are the preferred sites for escharotomy incisions. The solid segments emphasize the importance of extending the incisions across joints with a full-thickness injury.

Fasciotomy

On rare occasions an incision of the muscle fascia beneath the burned tissue is required to restore circulation in a burned limb. This procedure is required for very deep burns involving the fas-

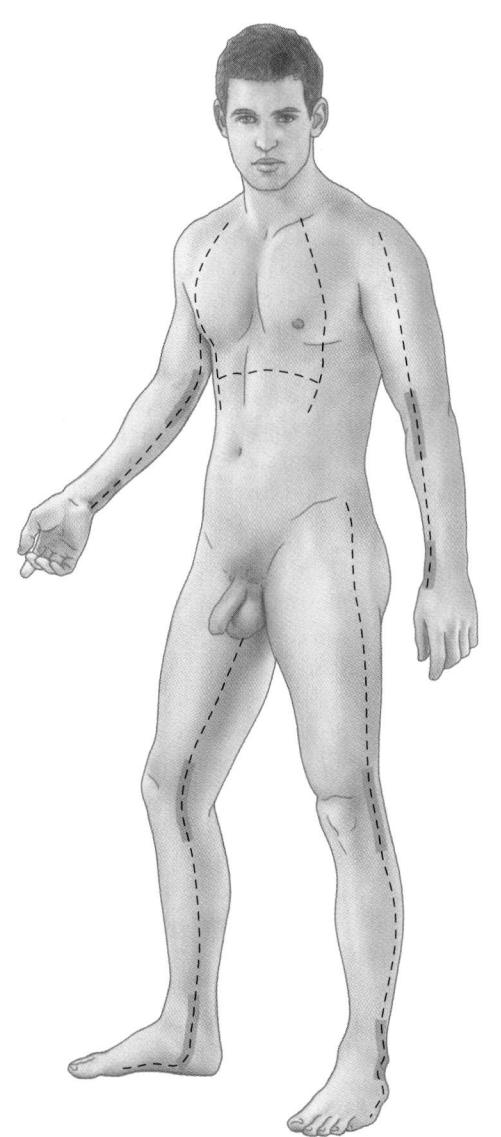

FIGURE 68–11 ■ Common escharotomy sites.

cia and muscle, for associated traumatic limb injuries, and for high-voltage electrical injury. Stony, hard edema of the muscle compartments and absence of peripheral pulses distal to the site of the electrical contact should prompt immediate fasciotomy and exploration of the muscle compartments. The circulation can be assessed with a Doppler ultrasound.

 Assessment of pulses, capillary refill, and color of the area distal to the escharotomy is critical. Any changes in the circulatory status need to be reported to the health care provider immediately. If an escharotomy is done in the chest area, close monitoring of lung sounds is essential to assess gas exchange. Until the swelling subsides, the need for repeated escharotomies continues.

Application of Topical Antibiotics/Dressing

The use of topical antibiotics started in the late 1940s when infection was the leading cause of death in patients with burns. The overall objective for the use of these agents is to prevent infection and to penetrate the burn wound. The penetrating action helps the burn tissue (eschar) separate from the deep viable tissue, and the antimicrobial action of the topical agents assists in preventing infection. These agents are usually applied once or twice daily after the wound has been cleaned and débrided. The Pharmacology Summary feature (p. 2260) outlines the most commonly used agents. Silver sulfadiazine appears to be the most frequently used medication in the United States, although a number of health care providers use a combination of drugs to maximize antimicrobial protection and minimize the associated side effects (Murphy, Lee, & Herndon, 2003).

Two techniques are commonly used for antibiotic application. First, with the open method, the antibiotic cream is applied directly to the wound with a gloved hand, and the wound is left open to air. Ointment is reapplied as necessary to ensure constant coverage. This method is used most frequently for the face and ears. The advantages are better visualization of the wound, easier mobility and joint range of motion (ROM), cost, and simplicity of wound care.

Disadvantages include an increased risk of hypothermia with extensive injuries and easy removal of the ointment with patient activity. The second method is referred to as the closed method, whereby either the antibiotic cream is applied directly to the wound with a gloved hand and then covered with a dry gauze dressing, or the dressing itself is impregnated with the cream and then applied to the wound. Even though there is less mobility with the closed method, the advantage is less heat and fluid loss from the wound surface.

Special Care Sites

For burns in and around the eye, special care must be taken because the skin is very thin and delicate. When cleansing and applying topical antibiotics to this area, care must be taken to keep the cleanser as well as the antibiotic cream out of the eye itself to help prevent conjunctivitis. The nose is another area where special consideration is needed because full-thickness burns of the nose could lead to a loss of tissue and cartilage. Débridement and cleansing must be gentle, and any nasal tubes should be monitored for placement to prevent erosion of nasal tissue. Burns of the ears also require special attention because the skin overlying the external ear, the auricle, is thin and prone to infection. This area must be cleaned gently and inspected frequently for infection. Pillows and gauze dressing beneath the head are contraindicated for burns

PHARMACOLOGY Summary of Topical Medications for Burns

Medication Category	Action	Application/Indication	Nursing Responsibility
Silver sulfadiazine (Silvadene)	Broad-spectrum antimicrobial with limited penetration ability.	Deep partial- to full-thickness burns. Wound infection.	Apply 1/4 inch thick using either open or closed dressing method, 2–3 times daily. Discontinue when eschar is gone. Not painful—soothing.
Silver nitrate	Broad-spectrum antimicrobial; poorly penetrates eschar.	Deep partial- to full-thickness burns. Wound infection.	Apply using either open or closed dressing method. Will turn wound black and is painful.
Mafenide Acetate (Sulfamylon)	Bacteriostatic for gram-positive and gram-negative organisms; penetrates thick eschar and cartilage.	Deep partial- to full-thickness burns. Wound infection.	Apply 1/4 inch thick using either open or closed dressing method, 2–3 times daily. Painful.
Petroleum- and mineral-based antimicrobials (Neosporin, Bacitracin)	Mild bactericidal for gram-positive and gram-negative organisms; poor penetration.	Partial-thickness burns.	Maintain adequate layer to prevent wound drying.

of the ear because the external pressure could decrease circulation and lead to pressure necrosis. Burns of the fingers and toes require individual dressing to each digit to help prevent web space contracture formation. Finally, deep burns where bone and tendons are exposed, must be kept moist until complete wound coverage is achieved. This requires the use of moist dressings that must be changed every 4 to 8 hours.

Temporary Dressings

Biologic, biosynthetic, synthetic, and composite dressings are useful as temporary coverings for burn wounds. The agent selected for use is determined by the condition of the wound, the inherent properties of each agent, and the goals of treatment. Chart 68–4 outlines the common agents, their indications for use, and the associated nursing care.

Biologic Dressings Biologic dressings include **heterografts** such as pigskin or allografts obtained from living or deceased humans. Heterografts are usually impregnated with silver nitrate to retard bacterial infection. Both of these dressings mimic human skin and are used for several purposes, including (1) covering clean superficial or partial-thickness wounds, (2) protecting granulation tissue or excised ungrafted wounds, (3) preventing fluid and temperature losses, and (4) testing the receptivity of the wound for **autografting** (patient's own skin). As seen in Figure 68–12 ■, pigskin (black) is being used when there is not enough of the patient's own skin to cover the wound. **Allografts,** skin harvested from human cadavers, are stored in skin banks located throughout the United States. Typically an allograft is rejected within 14 to 21 days following application. During the dressing, the nurse assesses, trims, and removes the biologic dressings where healing has occurred.

Biosynthetic Dressings **Biosynthetic dressings** are a combination of biologic and synthetic materials and are effective as temporary covering for a variety wounds. One of the more common biosynthetic dressings is Biobrane (Dow B. Hickman Pharmaceuticals, Inc., Sugar Land, Texas), which has been effective in the treatment of superficial partial-thickness burns such as scalds and as a donor-site dressing. A **donor site** is the

area on the body where the skin is surgically harvested to use for covering burn wounds. Biobrane (Figure 68–13 ■) is a semi-transparent dressing that is typically soaked in 0.9 normal saline and stretched over the wound and secured with staples, tape, and/or Steri-Strips. Once applied the patient is able to use the involved area such as hands for performing activities of daily living. As the wound heals, the Biobrane loosens and is trimmed away.

A second biosynthetic dressing that is more commonly used in the United Kingdom is calcium alginate. This product is manufactured from seaweed and contains calcium, which reacts with the sodium in the wound and creates a protective gel. This dressing is able to absorb as much as 20 times its own weight in wound fluid while creating a warm, moist environment for healing. Calcium alginate typically is used for exudative wounds and for split-thickness donor sites. After the wound is irrigated, calcium alginate is applied and covered with a dressing. The dressing is changed when it is saturated.

Synthetic Dressings There are three general categories of synthetic dressings: thin filmed, composite, and nonadherent. The thin-filmed dressings are composed of polyethylene and, when applied, provide a transparent, moisture-retentive, waterproof environment that promotes wound healing. These dressings are useful only for the treatment of superficial, clean partial-thickness burns and to cover donor sites. Commonly used products are Op-Site, Tegaderm (3M, Medical Division, St. Paul, Minnesota), and Bioclusive (Johnson & Johnson, Arlington, Texas).

Composite dressings (Lyofoam) are foam dressings used in the treatment of exudative burn wounds and graft sites. One layer of the dressing wicks away exudate while another layer maintains a moist environment that facilitates wound healing. The third type of commonly used synthetic dressing is nonadherent fine mesh gauze. Examples of nonadherent dressing include Xero-form gauze (Kendall Inc., Mansfield, Massachusetts) and Scarlet Red ointment dressing (Sherwood Medical, St. Louis, Missouri). These products are to cover clean partial-thickness wounds, new split-thickness skin grafts, and donor sites. The dressings are applied directly over the wound and then changed if they fall off. If

CHART 68-4 Temporary Coverings for Burn Wounds

Covering	Description	Indications/Uses	Nursing Care
Biologic Dressings			
Xenograft (heterograft)	Porcine (pigskin).	Clean partial-thickness injuries. Débrided full-thickness injuries.	Left covered with gauze dressings may be used for the first 24 hours.
Allograft (homograft)	Human cadaver skin harvested within 24 hours of death and preserved by refrigeration and cryopreservation.	Protect excised wounds and test for receptivity of wound bed for autograft.	Left covered with gauze dressings are used to protect site and absorb drainage.
Biosynthetic Dressings			
Biobrane	Collagen-embedded nylon fabric partially bonded to a silicone film.	Partial-thickness injuries. Secured to wound with staples, Steri-Strips, or gauze. Will adhere to wound.	Remove dressing once Biobrane has adhered to wound—left open to air. Trimmed away as wound healing occurs.
Calcium alginate	From alginates found in brown seaweed.	Exudative wounds. Split-thickness donor sites.	Applied to wound after irrigation and covered with absorbent dressing. Changed when cover dressing is saturated.
Synthetic Dressings			
Thin-filmed dressings: OpSite Tegaderm Bioclusive	Semipermeable, adherent polyurethane film dressings.	Protect and facilitate healing in small, clean partial-thickness burns. Cover partial-thickness donor sites.	Dressing needs to have intact skin margins to adhere to the dressing. Does not need dressing over the top unless draining exudate. Remove when wound healed.
Composite dressings: Lyofoam	Polymeric dressings designed to provide moisture-retentive, absorbent, insulating environment.	Cover moderate to highly exudative wounds.	Placed directly over exudative wounds and covered with absorbent dressing. Dressing change frequency depends on amount of exudate.
Nonadherent dressings: Xeroform	Fine mesh gauze impregnated with 3% bismuth tribromophenate. Mild antimicrobial.	Clean partial-thickness wounds. Provides protective barrier, and promotes epithelial growth.	Monitor for and maintain adherence to wounds: Change if nonadherent. Monitor for infection.
Scarlet Red	Fine mesh gauze impregnated with lanolin, olive oil, petrolatum, and red dye.	Promotes epithelial development and protects wound.	Applied to clean partial-thickness injury. Applied in surgery to donor sites.

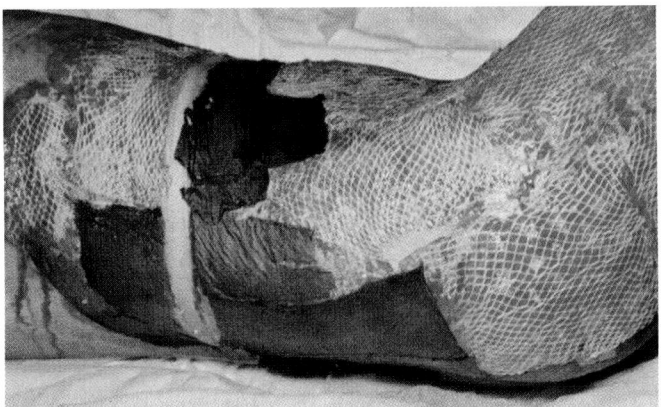

FIGURE 68–12 ■ Black pigskin and meshed skin grafts.
Source: Courtesy of: Robert M. Faggella, Jr. M.D., FACS Sacramento, CA

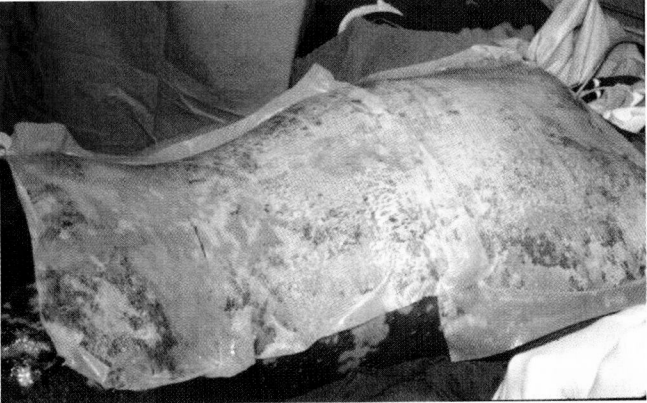

FIGURE 68–13 ■ Application of Biobrane.
Source: Courtesy of: UC Davis, University of California

used for donor-site covering, they are covered with an outer dressing, which typically remains in place for 24 hours. Once the outer dressing is removed, the fine mesh gauze remains in place for 5 to 7 days and is allowed to dry out and loosen as healing oc-

curs. If used for skin grafting, a single layer is applied over the graft site and then reinforced with several layers of coarse mesh gauze and left in place for 5 to 7 days. See Chart 68–4 for a summary of the temporary coverings for burn wounds.

Infection Assessment

Early recognition of a wound infection is critical in limiting morbidity and mortality. Due to immunosuppression and open wounds, the patient with burns is at a high risk for the development of an infection. Wound infection is defined as the presence of bacteria, fungi, or viruses in or around the open wound. The nursing management plan to prevent infection includes (1) vigilant monitoring for signs and symptoms of infection and sepsis, (2) maintaining a hygienic environment to reduce the presence of microorganisms, (3) use of aseptic technique for wound care and invasive procedures, and (4) timely administration of both systemic and topical antibiotics. Daily assessment of the wound is primarily a nursing responsibility. When dressings are removed, the wound is assessed for changes in wound exudate (color, odor, and amount), signs of cellulitis (inflammation/erythema of surrounding tissue), increased wound pain, and loss of previously healed skin.

If infection goes undetected or untreated, it can progress to a deeper wound infection leading to sepsis. Infection also can convert a partial-thickness injury to a full-thickness injury. Characteristics of an invasive infection include focal, dark, red, brown, or black discoloration in the eschar; rapid conversion (necrosis) of an area of partial-thickness injury to full-thickness injury; early, rapid separation of the eschar (fungal infection characteristic); and hemorrhagic fat necrosis.

The prevention of the introduction of exogenous organisms, which cause infection, requires strict adherence to standard precautions and adherence to strict aseptic technique. The nurse must assess all personnel and visitors entering the patient's room for the presence of infection. A sign should be placed on the patient's door indicating the need not to enter if the visitor is sick.

Hyperbaric Oxygen Therapy

Hyperbaric oxygen therapy (HBO) is a means of providing additional oxygen to the body tissues by placing the patient's entire body under increased atmospheric pressure in a closely monitored airtight chamber. During HBO therapy, the patient breathes 100% oxygen for a predetermined period of time. Hyperbaric oxygen therapy has been used for split-thickness skin graft acceptance, flap survival and salvage, wound reepithelialization, and acute thermal burns. Research continues on the impact of HBO on wound healing to try to take advantage of the angiogenic properties of increasing oxygen gradients resulting from hyperbaric therapy (Neumeister, 2005).

Surgical Management

The surgical management of burn injuries is a complex process involving a sequence of carefully planned surgical stages. The process begins with surgical débridement of damaged tissue, followed by wound closure using a number of techniques described next.

Burn Wound Excision

Historically, treatment for full-thickness injuries involved waiting for the eschar to separate over time with cleansing and débridement. Then the patient was taken to surgery for grafting to close the open wound. This method of treatment was associated with frequent wound infections, prolonged, painful daily débridement and dressing changes, and lengthened hospital stays. Since the late 1970s surgical techniques have been developed to excise eschar, allowing early closure of the burn wound. Early surgical débridement and grafting have decreased the length of hospital stay, decreased the number of septic episodes, and improved survival rates.

Two types of excision are used for burn wounds: tangential excision and fascial excision. Tangential excision, the most frequently used procedure, involves sequential removal of thin layers of eschar until viable dermis or subcutaneous fat is exposed. The depth of the excision is determined by the appearance of healthy tissue and bleeding from dermal or subcutaneous beds. The goal is to create a clean living wound bed with circulation to support graft adherence. The advantage of the tangential excision is decreased risk of infection due to early closure and better preservation of surrounding tissues and body contours, thus, resulting in a better cosmetic result. The disadvantage is that blood loss may be considerable if large surface areas are tangentially excised.

Fascial excision involves removal of eschar and the underlying subcutaneous tissue to the level of the muscle fascia. This technique is usually reserved for patients with very deep, life-threatening burns, typically from electrical injury. The advantages of this technique are that there is less blood loss, it provides a viable graft bed, and less time is required for surgery. The disadvantages include an unsightly cosmetic deformity, loss of superficial nerves, near complete cutaneous denervation, and a high incidence of distal edema when the excision is superficial.

Burn Wound Closure

Burn wounds are usually closed with cutaneous autografts (patient's own skin). Split-thickness skin grafts and occasionally full-thickness skin grafts can be used to accomplish closure. The skin grafts are harvested from the patient's healthy tissue (donor site) and applied to the burn wound.

Harvesting of Skin   Harvesting of skin is accomplished by two methods, and the choice of which to use depends on the desired depth of graft. **Full-thickness skin grafts** are removed surgically by excising the entire thickness of the donor skin to the level of the subcutaneous tissue, typically 0.025 to 0.3 inch thick. Donor sites need to be closed by either sutures or split-thickness skin grafts, and therefore, full-thickness grafts are limited to the repair of small wounds or defects. The advantage of this technique is that it permits the transfer of the entire dermal layer, resulting in greater durability and less wound contracture than the split-thickness grafts. Full-thickness skin grafts are used most frequently for areas that require thicker skin to prevent breakdown, such as the palm of the hand, the bottom of the foot, and over joints. Full-thickness grafts also are used for facial defects because there is less contracture formation and a better cosmetic result.

The more common method used for covering a burn wound is a **split-thickness skin graft**, which is a partial layer of skin, including the epidermis and part of the dermis. The skin is harvested from the patient's donor site with a surgical instrument called a dermatome. The dermatome is guarded, making it easier to control the thickness of the harvested skin, which is usually 0.008 to 0.0012 inch thick (Figure 68–14 ■).

When the skin has been harvested, it can be used as either a sheet skin graft or a **meshed skin graft**. Meshing a graft means cutting holes in the harvested skin, which allows it to be stretched over a greater surface area. To mesh the graft, the harvested skin is placed on a plastic template and guided through a

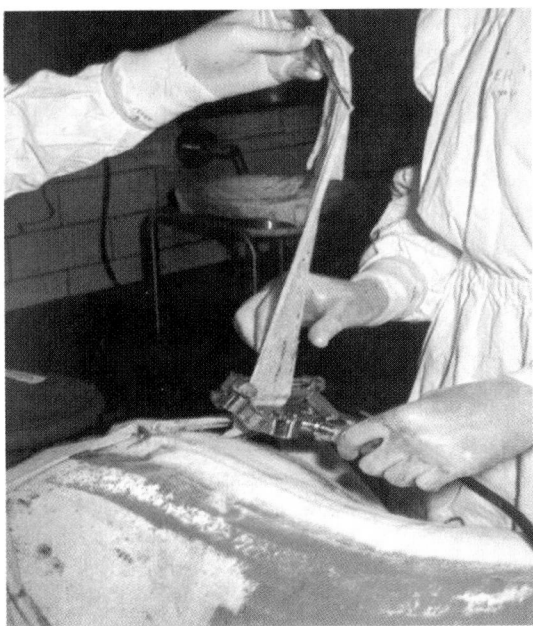

FIGURE 68–14 ■ Dermatome harvesting skin.
Source: Courtesy of: Robert M. Faggella, Jr. M.D., FACS Sacramento, CA

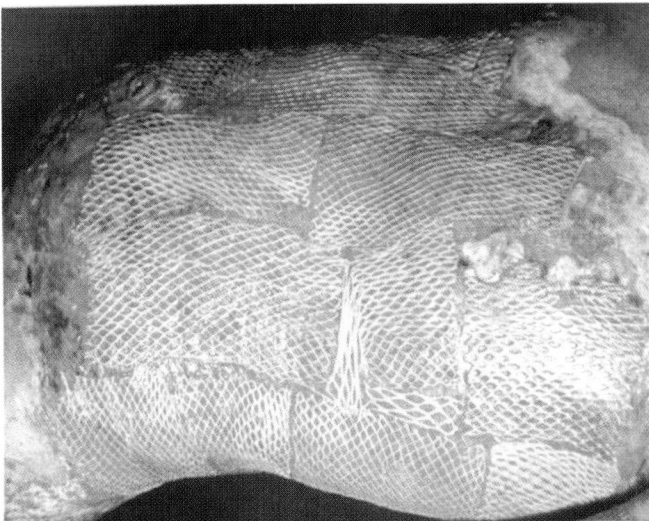

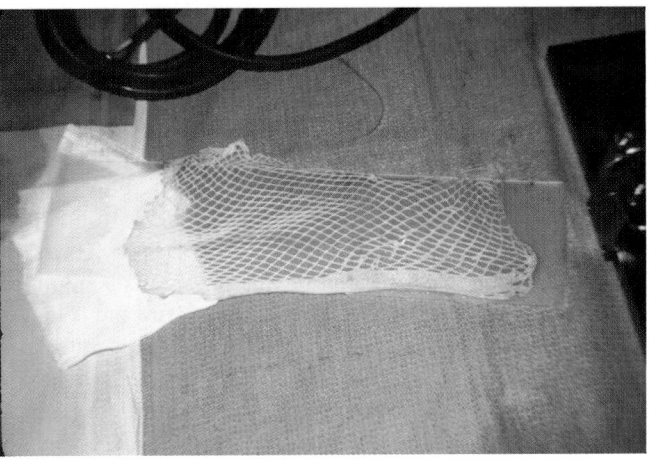

FIGURE 68–15 ■ 3:1 meshed skin graft.
Source: (top): Courtesy of: Robert M. Faggella, Jr. M.D., FACS Sacramento, CA; (bottom): Courtesy of: John M. Osborn, M.D., FACS, Sacramento, CA Plastic Surgery Center

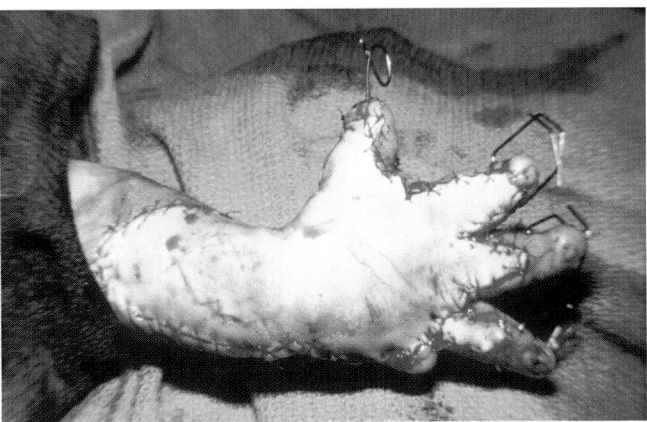

FIGURE 68–16 ■ Sheet skin grafts.
Source: Courtesy of: John M. Osborn, M.D., FACS, Sacramento, CA Plastic Surgery Center

mechanical meshing apparatus, thereby cutting the diamond-shaped pattern of holes (Figure 68–15 ■). The meshed skin graft can be increased from two to nine times its original size, depending on the size of the holes. Skin grafts expanded beyond four times, referred to as 4:1, their original size require longer healing time, have a greater propensity for scar formation, and are usually used only for patients with massive injuries and limited donor sites. The holes in the graft will close over time by epithelialization from the skin edge. With meshed split-thickness skin grafts, there is less of a concern of blood and serous fluid collecting under the grafted area, increasing the percentage of graft adherence. The disadvantage of this method is that the epithelial scar formation from these meshed grafts is in the shape of a diamond, producing a characteristic checkerboard appearance.

Split-thickness grafts that have not been meshed are referred to as **sheet skin grafts** (Figure 68–16 ■). Sheet grafts provide a better cosmetic and functional result and should be used when adequate donor sites are available. Priority areas for using sheet grafts, if the burn is small, include the head, face, hands, neck, upper torso in women, and joint surfaces for growing children. A disadvantage of sheet grafts as compared to meshed grafts is that when blood, bacteria, and serous drainage collect under the graft, the graft has difficulty adhering to the wound surface. Both sheet and meshed skin grafts initially adhere to the wound by means of surface tension and later because of fibrin formation. Within 48 hours, circulation begins to occur, as evidenced by an increasing pink or red color on the graft surface. Depending on the preference of the surgeon, grafts may be sutured or stapled in place. Loss of the skin graft may occur for several reasons. First, hematoma or seroma formation beneath the graft will prevent it from adhering to the wound surface. During the first few days following surgery, the sheet grafts must be examined frequently so that subgraft hematoma or seroma formation can be removed either by needle aspiration, incising the graft to express blood and fluid, or by physically pulling a hematoma through an incision with forceps. Fluid collecting under the graft can be rolled to the side with cotton-tipped applicators.

Second, persistent motion of the grafts will prevent vascular connections and graft adherence; therefore, the grafted area must remain immobilized. Splinting of the grafted area ensures immobilization of the graft for the first few days. Normal movement may be resumed at approximately 5 days, depending on the area involved and the health care provider's preference. Finally, an infection in the grafted area will create exudate under the graft and prevent graft adherence. The wound surface should be meticulously clean and free of infection at the time of graft application. All health care personnel must use strict aseptic technique when caring for the skin grafts.

Cultured epithelial autografting (CEA) is a method to obtain the patient's own skin when there is limited donor-site availability. Once a patient has been identified as a candidate, skin biopsies (usually 2 to 3 centimeters long by 1 centimeter wide) are taken from nonburned tissue and sent to a commercial site where they are cultivated in a medium of epidermal growth factor. This tissue is grown for 18 to 25 days to where it expands to 10,000 times its original size. The cultured grafts are returned to the burn center and applied surgically using the same procedure as for split-thickness skin grafts. Enough CEA to cover an entire body can be grown in 24 days; however, there continue to be limitations to its use. The skin has no dermal layer; therefore, it is thin and friable, resulting in breakdown and contracture formation (Supp, Neely, Supp, Warden, & Boyce, 2005).

Donor-Site Care

When skin is harvested from a donor site, a superficial partial-thickness wound is created (Figure 68–17 ■). Healing occurs by epithelial migration in about 10 to 14 days. Donor sites can be reused approximately three to four times with a 10- to 14-day healing period between each use. As much as the size of the injury permits, the donor-site skin should be selected to match the recipient-site skin in texture and color.

The focus of care for the donor sites in the postoperative period is preventing infection. If the site becomes infected, it may convert from a partial-thickness to a full-thickness injury, which then must be grafted. Several dressing options are available for donor sites in the postoperative period. Currently, Vaseline gauze with bismuth; antibacterial polyurethane film; and silver-impregnated mesh are common donor-site dressings. A more traditional approach to donor-site care has been to use a dry fine mesh gauze or gauze impregnated with petrolatum or antimicrobial agents (i.e., Xeroform) to cover the donor site. The choice of donor-site dressing is made by the health care provider. See Chart 68–4 (p. 2261) for a description of the agents

used to cover donor sites. As the donor site heals, it dries out (scab formation) and the dressing separates from the wound. The healing process takes about 10 to 14 days. The primary nursing goals are to allow airflow around the donor site to assist in the drying process and prevention of infection.

Donor sites may have a tendency to form hypertrophic scarring, especially in dark-skinned or very fair people. A single harvest from an individual area usually does not cause scarring; however, repeated harvesting from the same site increases the risk of scarring. After the donor site has healed, it requires the same long-term care as do burn wounds, such as avoiding the sun and use of moisturizing creams. Some health care providers use pressure garments to reduce donor-site hypertrophy.

 *Nurses are primarily responsible for prevention of infection in a donor site. Early detection and reporting will help prevent conversion of a donor site from a partial-thickness to a full-thickness injury.*

Alternative Skin Covering

In patients with large burn injuries, there is a limited amount of unburned skin suitable as a donor site; therefore, available donor sites need to be used repeatedly. Several products that are currently available provide a deep dermal layer covering of the burn wound, which then can be covered with an ultra-thin split-thickness skin graft. Ultra-thin donor sites heal faster, complications are minimized, and they are ready for reuse sooner where repeated autograft harvesting is necessary. AlloDerm and Integra (Integra Life Sciences Corporation, Plainsboro, New Jersey) are two products currently in use. AlloDerm is an acellular, nonimmunogenic dermal substitute derived from human cadaver skin (Livesey et al., 1995). This product is meshed and applied to a full-thickness injury after it has been excised of dead tissue. A thin split-thickness skin graft is placed over the AlloDerm during the same surgical procedure. AlloDerm is useful for wounds extending over joints where a thicker layer of skin will help prevent contractures, thereby increasing range of motion. Integra is a two-layered skin substitute composed of an internal layer of collagen net and an external layer of silicone. After wound débridement, Integra is placed into the wound. It takes the dermal layer 2 to 3 weeks to become vascularized; then the outer layer is removed and an ultra-thin split-thickness skin graft is applied (Figure 68–18 ■).

If replacement of normal functioning skin is the goal for skin substitutes, then there is no perfect skin substitute. Each of these products has limitations and all are expensive to use. Further

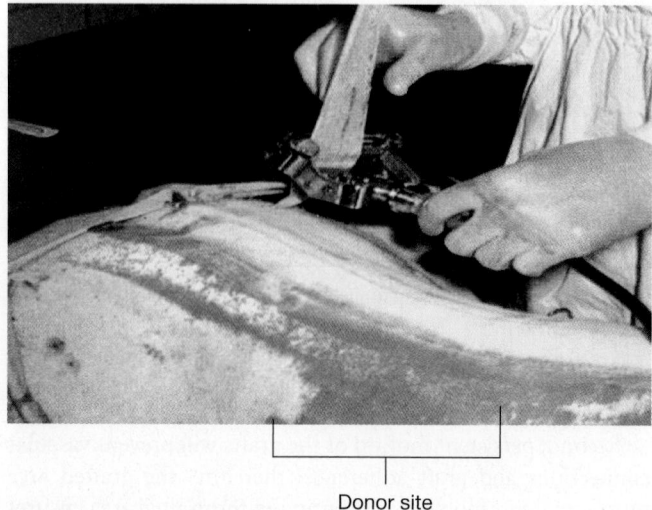

FIGURE 68–17 ■ Donor site.
Source: Courtesy of: Robert Fagella, Jr. MD FACS, Sacramento, CA

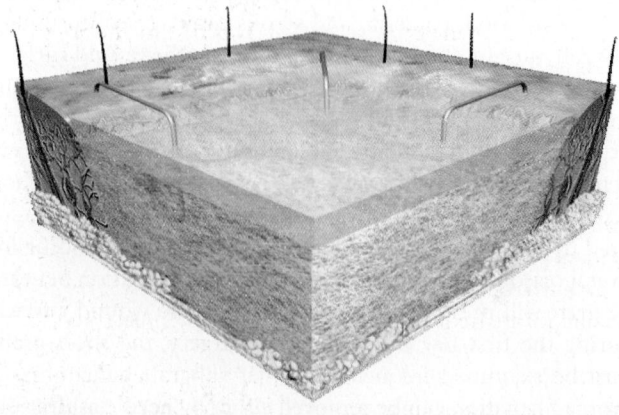

FIGURE 68–18 ■ Integra.
Source: Courtesy of: Johnson and Johnson Wound Management a Division of Ethicon, Inc.

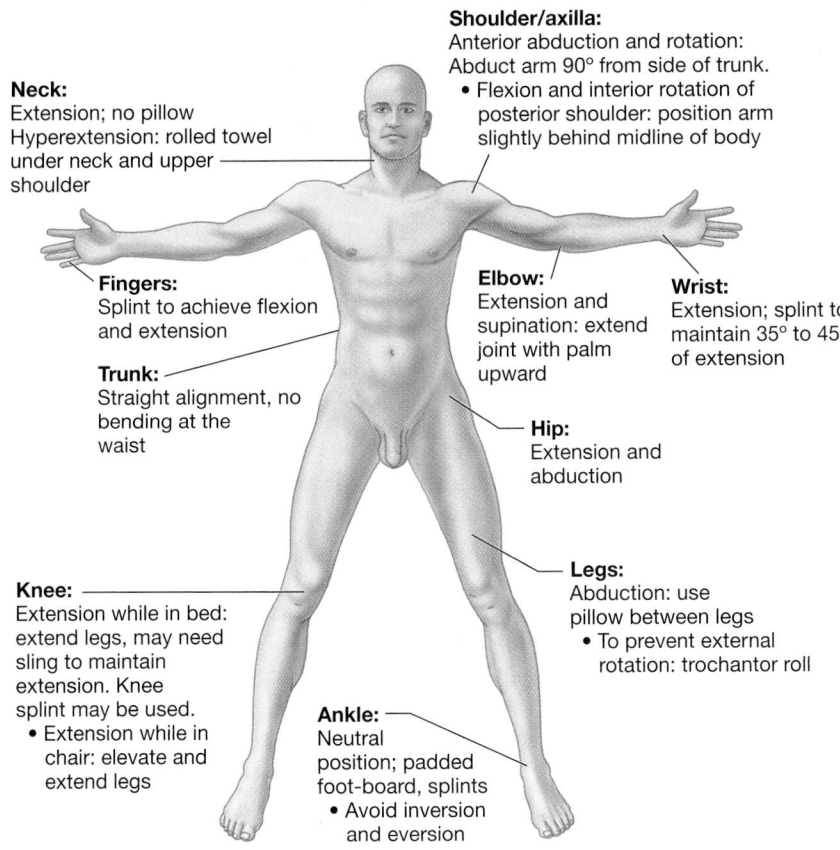

Neck:
Extension; no pillow
Hyperextension: rolled towel
under neck and upper
shoulder

Shoulder/axilla:
Anterior abduction and rotation:
Abduct arm 90° from side of trunk.
• Flexion and interior rotation of
posterior shoulder: position arm
slightly behind midline of body

Fingers:
Splint to achieve flexion
and extension

Trunk:
Straight alignment, no
bending at the
waist

Elbow:
Extension and
supination: extend
joint with palm
upward

Wrist:
Extension; splint to
maintain 35° to 45°
of extension

Hip:
Extension and
abduction

Knee:
Extension while in bed:
extend legs, may need
sling to maintain
extension. Knee
splint may be used.
• Extension while in
chair: elevate and
extend legs

Legs:
Abduction: use
pillow between legs
• To prevent external
rotation: trochantor roll

Ankle:
Neutral
position; padded
foot-board, splints
• Avoid inversion
and eversion

FIGURE 68–19 ■ Common anticontracture positions.

evaluation and testing are needed to improve efficacy and bring down the cost of the products.

Promoting and Maintaining Normal Mobility

As wound healing progresses, the need for promoting and maintaining mobility increases and changes. The goal of therapy is to regain strength, endurance, and joint mobility in order to achieve optimal functioning. Therapeutic positioning, splinting, and range-of-motion exercises are essential in meeting this goal and cannot be overemphasized. It is essential that the family be actively involved because the program needs to continue after discharge for at least a year.

Positioning

From the day of admission, therapeutic positioning is used to protect the patient's wounds, decrease edema, and counteract scar contraction. The anatomic sites where contracture formation is a risk must be identified in the early stages and anticontracture measures instituted to counter scar contraction. Involved extremities are placed in a functional position, and joints are typically placed in extension. Figure 68–19 ■ demonstrates the correct therapeutic anticontracture positions. Pillows, ropes, gauze rolls, linen, and pulleys are used to accomplish these positions. Finally, frequent position change is necessary to prevent skin pressure and breakdown. Beds with special mattresses and pressure-reducing capabilities are frequently used to prevent skin breakdown.

Splinting

Splinting begins as soon as possible after the injury for several reasons, including protection of joints and skin grafts, anatomic positioning to prevent contracture formation, and maintenance and

elongation of scar length. Ideally, splints should be made of a material that allows them to be reshaped as edema decreases and the burn scar changes and heals (Figure 68–20 ■). If the patient experiences pain, sensory impairments, or wound breakdown, the splint is removed and redesigned to prevent these complications. Padding of the splints decreases the occurrence of skin breakdown. Simple everyday items such as high-top shoes can be used for splinting purposes, and serial casting (e.g., removed and replaced as contour extremity changes) also can serve to maintain normal positioning of affected areas.

Exercise Program

An active, progressive exercise program is essential to prevent permanent burn scars from forming contractures and to maintain normal range of motion (ROM) in affected joints. Exercise increases circulation and pulmonary function, decreases edema formation, offsets some of the manifestations of immobilization, and allows for the preservation of functional motor skills. The exercise program begins on the day of admission and continues until the scars have matured. Exercise is very difficult in the beginning due to pain, edema, and loss of tissue elasticity. The health care team must assist the patient in understanding the importance of exercise despite painful limitations imposed by the injury.

Varying levels of physical assistance are required depending on the extent of the injury and the motivation of the patient. If, for example, weakness prevents true ROM, assistance is provided to help the patient complete the motion. This is referred to as active–assistive exercise and is frequently used with patients that are burn injured. The active component provides the same benefits as active ROM exercises, and the assistive component facilitates complete, properly directed motion. Passive ROM exercises are used for patients who are unable to move on their own. They also may be used to assess motion, maintain and mobilize joints and soft tissue, and minimize contracture formation.

The patient's ability to ambulate is affected by strength, endurance, pain, edema, and contracture formation. A progressive ambulation program is essential to prevent contracture formation

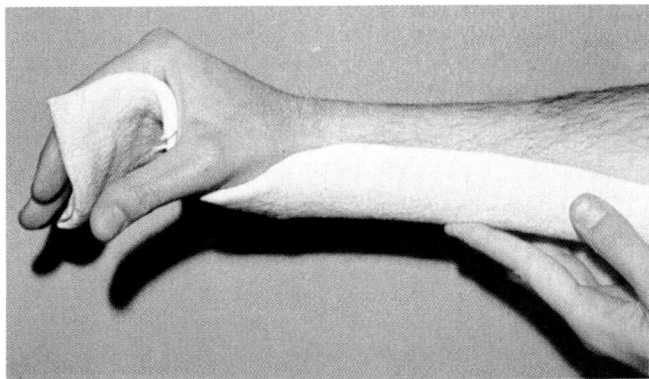

FIGURE 68–20 ■ Arm splint.
Source: Courtesy of: Robert M. Faggella, Jr. M.D., FACS Sacramento, CA

and needs to begin as soon as the patient is able to tolerate it. Initially the program begins with sitting, followed by standing and pivoting, and gradually ambulating. Prior to getting the patient out of bed, some type of elastic dressing or pressure garment is applied to prevent orthostatic hypotension, venous stasis, and edema formation.

Nutritional Requirements

Nutrients are essential for normal healing, and inadequate nutrition has a negative impact on the immune response, wound healing, metabolic function, and survival. The key cause of ineffective wound healing is malnutrition (Greenhalgh, 2005). At the time of the burn injury, patients experience extreme metabolic stress that is proportional to the size of the injury. After a burn injury, the resting energy expenditure (REE) increases by as much as 50% to 150% higher than that of the average trauma patient (Demling et al., 2004). This hypermetabolic response and the mobilization of glucose are necessary for wound healing. Without adequate glucose, excessive protein catabolism occurs (Demling et al., 2004; Pereira et al., 2005). Thus, early and adequate nutritional interventions are critical to the survival of the patient with burns. The hypermetabolic state tends to decrease in the weeks following the injury, but the metabolic rate does not return to normal until the wound is completely healed.

The goal of a nutritional replacement program during the acute phase is to provide adequate calories to promote wound healing (Greenhalgh, 2005). A number of formulas are used to estimate amount of calories needed to accomplish this goal. One generally accepted formula is (25 kilocalories X kilograms of body weight) + (40 kilocalories × % TBSA burn). It is not unusual for caloric needs to exceed 5,000 calories per day. The goal is to have the patient not lose more than 10% of his preburn weight. Calorie requirements need to be recalculated frequently because nutritional needs change with the healing process and changes in the hypermetabolic state. Specific nutrients needed for tissue repair include proteins, carbohydrates, lipids, and vitamins and trace minerals.

1. Proteins are needed for collagen synthesis, for wound remodeling, and for normal immune response. Protein loss, the stress of the injury, and tissue destruction all contribute negative nitrogen. There are differing opinions on the exact amount of protein needed to prevent proteolysis of lean body mass. The formulas used to calculate protein replacement generally estimate up to 2 grams of protein per kilogram per day (Greenhalgh, 2005).

2. Carbohydrates supply most of the energy needed for cell function and the immune response. Most practitioners believe that nonprotein energy intake should be primarily carbohydrates, with exogenous insulin added as clinically indicated to prevent hyperglycemia (Hart et al., 2001).

3. Lipids are essential in all nutritional regimens, but due to the impact on the immune system, many burn centers use no lipids at all (Borde, Bernier, & Garrel, 2002).

4. Vitamins and trace minerals are an integral part of the immune response, protein synthesis, and cell repair. They stimulate epithelialization, capillary budding and strength, and collagen formation, and are cofactors in enzymatic reactions (Greenhalgh, 2005). The exact vitamin and mineral requirements for optimal healing differ between patients,

although there are general guidelines for replacement. Patients with major burn injuries typically receive a multivitamin, 10,000 units of vitamin A, and 200 milligrams of zinc once per day, and 500 milligrams of ascorbic acid twice per day, depending on the health care provider's preference.

Whenever possible, patients with burns are encouraged to use the oral route for nutritional replacement. It is not uncommon, however, for patients to have difficulty consuming sufficient calories and protein by mouth. When this occurs it is essential to meet the metabolic demand with additional supplements. Meals are supplemented with high-calorie (1 to 1.5 calorie/mL) snacks. The enteral route is preferred because it maintains the structural and functional integrity of the gastrointestinal tract (Andel, Kamolz, Horauf, & Zimpfer, 2003). Many burn centers institute early enteral feedings within 24 hours of admission for any burn greater than 40% total body surface area. Early feeding is believed to improve the gastrointestinal, immunologic, nutritional, and metabolic responses to the burn injury. Enteral feedings instituted before 18 hours after the injury have shown a significantly decreased mortality rate (Gottschlich et al., 2002). Typically the enteral feedings are trickled very slowly via a feeding tube, and patients are monitored closely for aspiration.

Regular monitoring of laboratory values related to adequacy of intake is essential. Total protein levels, complete blood count (CBC), glucose, iron, and prealbumin all indicate adequacy of nutrition. There is a complete discussion of nutritional replacement and monitoring provided in Chapter 14 ⊙.

■ Nursing Management

The aim of nursing care during the acute phase is to ensure optimal healing and prevent complications. Use of the nursing process will facilitate a comprehensive approach to patient assessment and care. The Nursing Process: Patient Care Plan feature applies the pertinent nursing diagnoses and provides a comprehensive care plan for a patient with burns during the acute period.

■ Collaborative Management

A collaborative care approach is optimal for management of patients with burn injuries. Utilizing a multidisciplinary team approach that includes health care providers, nurses, physical and occupational therapists, psychologists/psychiatrists, and a pharmacist will facilitate the best possible quality of life for the patient and the family. The occupational therapist helps facilitate realistic occupational goals, while the physical therapist assists in the rehabilitation of affected areas to prevent contracture formation. In addition to the nursing care described earlier (p. 2251) and in the Nursing Process: Patient Care Plan for the Acute Phase feature, the nurse plays a pivotal role in coordinating the efforts of the health care team.

Rehabilitative Phase

The rehabilitative phase typically begins when there is less than 20% open wound and the patient is functioning at the highest possible level since admission. Depending on the size of the injury, the rehabilitative phase may begin as early as 2 weeks or as

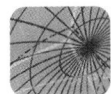

Assessment of Fatigue and Ability to Perform Activities

Subjective Data:
Do you feel fatigued after physical activities?
Do you feel like you are gaining or losing strength as your burns heal?

Objective Data:
Heart rate, blood pressure, and respiratory rate increase with activity.
Strength and endurance change as burn wounds heal.
Ability to perform activities of daily living.

Nursing Assessment and Diagnoses	Outcomes and Evaluation Parameters	Planning and Interventions with *Rationales*
Nursing Diagnosis: *Activity Intolerance* related to severity of injury	**Outcomes:** Increased endurance and energy conservation. ***Evaluation Parameters:*** Patient reports improvement in fatigue levels. Patient demonstrates more daytime wakefulness. Patient demonstrates ability to pace activities to conserve energy. Tolerates usual activities. Recognizes energy limitations. Balances activity with rest. Endurance level adequate for activity.	**Interventions and *Rationales:*** Discuss with patient/family the relationship of burn injury to fatigue. *As wounds heal and nutritional state stabilizes, energy will increase.* Assess emotional, spiritual, and physical responses to activity. *To institute changes to plan if necessary.* Evaluate patient's motivation and desire to increase activity. *To institute changes to plan if necessary.* Determine causes of fatigue. *To modify plan if necessary.* Monitor cardiorespiratory response to activity. *To assess appropriateness of activity level.* Monitor oxygen saturation response to activity. *To assess appropriateness of activity level.* Pace daily activities to conserve energy. *Prevent overexertion.* Ensure adequate nutritional support. *To increase strength and endurance.* Ensure sleep and rest period, record hours of sleep on record. *To increase strength and endurance.* Consult with physical therapist and occupational therapist to develop exercise program. *A progressive program to sustain progress.* Establish a conditioning program with patient-centered goals. *To increase compliance.*

Assessment of Mobility

Subjective Data:
How far are you able to ambulate?
Do you feel any change in the range of motion in the affected areas with exercise?
What is your understanding of the need for and importance of daily exercise?

Objective Data:
Range of motion in affected areas
Ability to perform active exercises
Wound healing progress
Patient/family's knowledge of need for continued exercise and splinting of affected areas

Nursing Assessment and Diagnoses	Outcomes and Evaluation Parameters	Planning and Interventions with *Rationales*
Nursing Diagnosis: *Impaired Physical Mobility* related to burn wounds and contracture formation	**Outcome:** Joint movement normal for injury level. ***Evaluation Parameters:*** Patient verbalizes understanding of restricted activity. Patient maintains strength and position of function in all affected areas. No contracture formation.	**Interventions and *Rationales:*** Consult with physical therapist and occupational therapist to formulate a plan for maintaining and increasing mobility. *A progressive program is necessary to sustain progress and prevent contracture formation.* Perform active and passive range-of-motion (ROM) exercises every 2 hours. *To prevent contracture formation.* Apply splints as prescribed. Maintain antideformity positions and reposition hourly (Figure 68–19 ■, p. 2265). *To prevent contracture formation.* Elevate affected extremities. *To decrease edema.* Maintain limbs in functional alignment. *To prevent contracture formation.* Anticipate need for analgesia. *To increase mobility.* Ambulate when stable. *Essential to begin activity program to increase endurance and decrease contracture formation.* Assess for loss of ROM and muscle atrophy related to immobility. *High risk for contracture formation.* Educate patient/family regarding rationale for imposed activity restrictions; i.e., recent skin grafting. *To prevent loss of skin graft.* Provide diversional activities to increase compliance with immobility. *To prevent loss of skin graft.*

(continued)

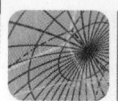

Assessment of Ability to Perform Activities of Daily Living

Subjective Data:
To what extent are you able to take care of your physical needs?
Is this ability increasing as your wounds heal?
Do you have people that can help you after you are discharged?

Objective Data:
Ability to perform activities of daily living
Psychological motivation to function independently

Nursing Assessment and Diagnoses	Outcomes and Evaluation Parameters	Planning and Interventions with *Rationales*
Nursing Diagnosis: *Readiness for Enhanced Self-Care* related to wounds and activity intolerance	**Outcome:** Increasing ability to perform activities of daily living. **Evaluation Parameters:** Verbalizes increased sense of control. Demonstrates self-care activities within limits of functional ability. Accepts assistance when needed. Progressively increases mobility.	**Interventions and *Rationales:*** Consult with occupational therapist regarding need for assistive devices. *These will increase self-care ability.* Ensure patient has adequate time to perform tasks at own pace. *Patients are slow and tentative in the beginning.* Increase self-care activities as soon as possible. Ensure patient participation in planning care. *To decrease powerlessness and increase self-confidence.* Monitor for changes in functional abilities. *To monitor progress.* Instruct patient/family on alternative ways to perform activities of daily living. *To increase patient/family involvement.*

Assessment of Patient and Family Coping Skills

Subjective Data:
What skills have you used in the past to cope with stressful situations?
What people in your life do you use for emotional support?
Tell me your perception of your injuries.
Tell me your perception of your limitations.

Objective Data:
Willingness to be compliant with therapy.
Determine patient's level of independence.
Assess effectiveness of support systems.

Nursing Assessment and Diagnoses	Outcomes and Evaluation Parameters	Planning and Interventions with *Rationales*
Nursing Diagnoses: *Readiness for Enhanced Individual Coping* related to situational crisis, inadequate support systems, and unrealistic perceptions of recovery	**Outcome:** Effective coping. **Evaluation Parameters:** Patient/family: Verbalize feelings. Identify and utilize effective coping strategies, appropriate for injury status. Identify ineffective coping strategies and patterns. Seek information about injury, treatment, and prognosis. Employ behaviors to reduce stress. Report decrease in negative feelings. Demonstrate impulse control. Demonstrate normal information processing. Recognize support systems. Employ behaviors to reduce stress. Report decrease in negative feelings.	**Interventions and *Rationales:*** Assess and determine degree of impairment. *To assist in the development of a plan to promote coping.* Determine past coping skills. *To assist in the development of a plan to promote coping.* Assess current coping skills. *To assist in the development of a plan to promote coping.* Explore with patient feelings about injury, and explore previous methods of dealing with life problems. *Assessment will assist in augmenting patient's ability to cope, or it will determine need for intervention.* Identify patient's view of injury and its congruence to view of health care team. *To assess patient's perception of reality.* Monitor aggressive behaviors. *A sign of ineffective coping and that intervention is needed.* Identify patient/family's view of condition and how it relates to actual condition. *Assessment of how realistic their perceptions are. Determines where intervention is needed.* Assess patient/family's support systems. *May be used as a source of support.* Evaluate impact on patient/family's life situation. *Loss of previous life function impacts coping.* Determine risk for self-harm. *Severe alterations in body image and functional level place the patient at a high risk for self-harm.* Provide factual information about diagnosis, treatments, and prognosis. *Realistic, factual information is essential to augment adjustment.* Encourage verbalization of fears and let patient know these reactions are normal. *To enhance open, factual communication.* Explain procedures. *To increase knowledge and decrease fear of unknown.* Assist patient in dealing with changes in body image, and appraise adjustment. *To enhance adjustment.* Discuss future treatment options for changes in body image. *To increase knowledge and decrease fear of unknown.* Encourage family and friends to participate in care. *Enhances adjustment of significant others.* Consult psychologist if necessary. *To enhance adjustment.*

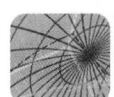

NURSING PROCESS: Patient Care Plan for the Acute Period—*Continued*

Nursing Assessment and Diagnoses	Outcomes and Evaluation Parameters	Planning and Interventions with *Rationales*
Deficient Fluid Volume due to evaporative loss *Impaired Skin Integrity* related to burn wounds *Risk for Infection* related to loss of skin integrity and impaired nonspecific and specific immunity *Ineffective Thermoregulation* related to loss of skin integrity *Acute Pain* related to burn injury and exposed nerve endings *Imbalanced Nutrition: Less than Body Requirements* related to hypermetabolic demands of burn injury *Fear* and *Anxiety* related to changes in health status/role functioning; situational crisis *Deficient Knowledge* related to burn wound care and treatment, disfigurement, and functional loss *Disturbed Body Image* related to scar formation and functional loss *Risk for Complicated Grieving* related to body image change, risk of family role change, and possible occupational change	See the earlier Nursing Process: Patient Care Plan for the emergency period of care for the information pertinent to each of the nursing diagnoses in the left column (p. 2251).	

Source: Wilkinson, J. M. (2009). *Nursing diagnosis handbook; with interventions and outcomes* (8th ed.). Upper Saddle River, NJ: Prentice Hall.

long as several years after the burn injury. During the rehabilitative phase, the patient with burns has stabilized physically and frequently is more aware of the long-term ramifications of her injury. Emphasis is placed on physical and psychological restorative therapy. Treatment aims include physical therapy to increase strength, endurance, function, and ROM; ongoing functional and cosmetic reconstruction; and psychological preparation for the patient's return to society. Pain management and nutrition are still concerns during the rehabilitative phase. Discharge planning and occupational preparation also are addressed during the rehabilitative phase.

Scar and Contracture Formation

With newly healed skin of partial-thickness wounds, there is minimal scar formation because the epidermis does not thicken. Frequently patients complain of dryness and itching in the newly healed areas, which are treated with frequent application of lotions and in more severe cases oral medication such as diphenhydramine hydrochloride (Benadryl). With a full-thickness injury, the dermal layer of skin has been affected, and the skin is repaired through scar formation. During the healing process, hypertrophic scars and contractures can form. **Hypertrophic scar** (Figure 68–21 ■) formation is defined as an overgrowth of dermal tissue that remains within the boundaries of the wound. There is a higher risk of hypertrophic scar formation in areas of stress and movement such as the hands, chest, and legs. If the hypertrophic scar extends beyond the wound

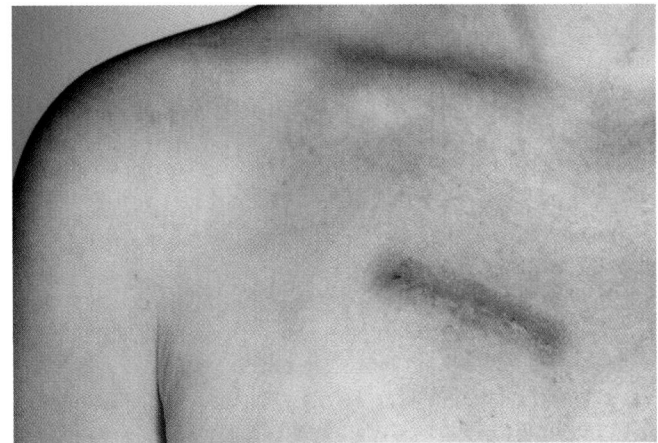

FIGURE 68–21 ■ Hypertrophic scar.
Source: Bart's Medical Library/Phototake NYC

edges, it is referred to as a **keloid scar** (Figure 68–22 ■, p. 2270). Certain areas of the body that are more prone to keloid formation include the chest, the presternal area, and the shoulders and deltoid region. Once keloid scars have formed, there is limited treatment available. Current treatments that have experienced some success are injecting steroids into the scar and laser therapy. There is a genetic predisposition for the development of keloid scarring, which is discussed in the Genetic Considerations box (p. 2270).

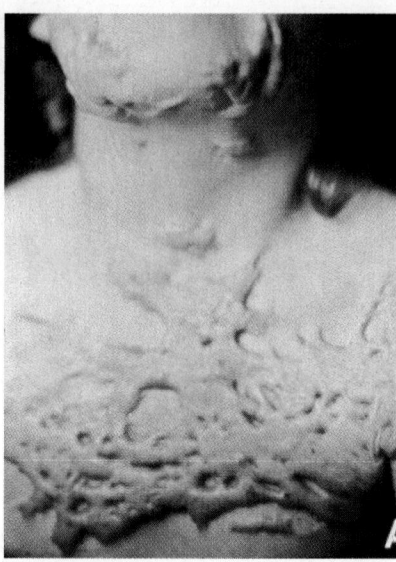

FIGURE 68–22 ■ Keloid scar.
Source: Courtesy of: Robert M. Faggella, Jr. M.D., FACS Sacramento, CA

GENETIC CONSIDERATIONS for Keloid Scar Formation

There is a genetic predisposition for the development of keloid scar formation in the African American race. African Americans have approximately a 15 times greater incidence of keloid formation.

Source: Tuan, T., et al. (2003). Increased plasminogen activator inhibitor-1 in keloid fibroblasts may account for their elevated collagen accumulation in fibrin gel cultures. *American Journal of Pathology, 162*(5), 1579–1589.

During the healing process of full-thickness injuries, the burn scar shrinks and becomes inelastic, resulting in contracture of the wound. A contracture (Figure 68–23 ■) is defined as a permanent shortening of connective tissue. Once formed, contractures resist stretching, limiting body motion and flexibility. Splinting, exercise, and constant pressure help prevent the formation and progression of contractures.

Exercise Program

As the burn wound heals, continual contraction of the scar creates the majority of the chronic problems. This contraction process causes a decrease in function in the involved area. Beginning rehabilitation on admission to a treatment center helps prevent contractures and diminishes the need for reconstructive surgery. Several therapies are used by the health care team to assist in preventing contracture formation, described earlier. The exercise program includes promotion of functional skills, stretching exercises, and scar massage.

Functional Skills

Functional skills are defined as the specific motor abilities necessary to perform activities of daily living (ADL) in order to function independently. In the beginning, exercises should focus on basic activities including ambulating, hygiene, and self-feeding. During the rehabilitative phase, exercise programs need to be expanded to include the specific skills needed for functioning in the home and the job environment.

All exercise programs are progressive in order to increase the patient's strength and endurance. Protein catabolism associated

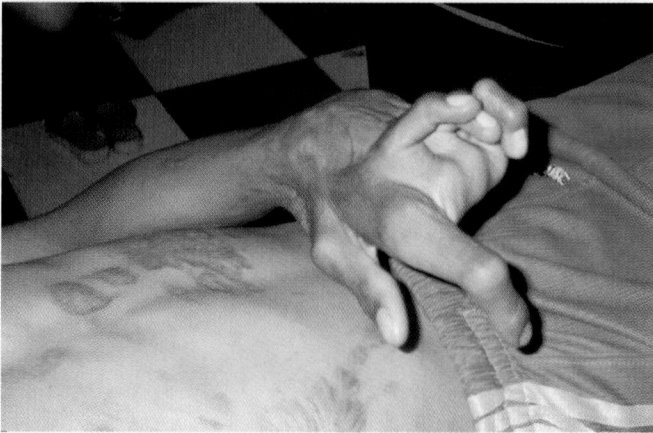

FIGURE 68–23 ■ Contracture formation.
Source: Courtesy of Kathleen Osborn

with the burn injuries as well as days of immobility lead to a decrease in muscle mass and strength. It is important to remember that endurance and conditioning underlie the success of any exercise program. Exercise programs need to be at regular intervals throughout the day and followed by periods of rest. It is the repetitive nature of the programs that builds strength and endurance and prevents contracture formation. Range-of-motion exercises are omitted for 3 to 7 days after skin grafting.

Stretching Exercises

Stretching exercises are used to elongate shortened soft tissue. The fundamental goal of a stretching program is to increase ROM. Stretching can be a passive or an active activity, although patients must learn to perform self-stretching exercises as they prepare for discharge. Stretching is done primarily after wound closure during the rehabilitative phase. The stretch should be gentle, slow, and sustained. Blanching of the scar represents appropriate stretch. Immediately after a stretching session, positioning and splinting are used effectively to maintain the elongation of the tissue.

Scar Massage

Completely healed burn wounds are massaged with oil or lotion to break down hardened areas, increase circulation, decrease hypertrophy, possibly increase range of motion, and improve appearance. Massage is performed one to four times daily. Patients and families are taught to continue scar massage after discharge.

Pressure Dressing and Garments

The use of pressure dressings and garments to decrease hypertrophic scar formation and increase wound pliability is a widely accepted practice (Figure 68–24 ■) (O'Brien, Weinstock-Zlotnick, Sanchez, Gorga, & Yurt, 2005). It is believed that the pressure from the garments causes ischemia, thereby decreasing collagen production, which thickens scars. In general, wounds that require more than 14 days to heal will scar and therefore should be placed in pressure garments. Elastic bandages are used initially for wound compression and edema formation. During the rehabilitative phase before hypertrophy begins, patients are measured for custom-fit elastic garments that provide three-dimensional pressure on all affected areas (Burn Survivors Throughout the World, 2006). In order to be effective, the pressure exerted by the garment must exceed capillary pressure (25 mmHg). Pressure garments are worn continuously (23 hours per day) for several months and/or years, depending on the hy-

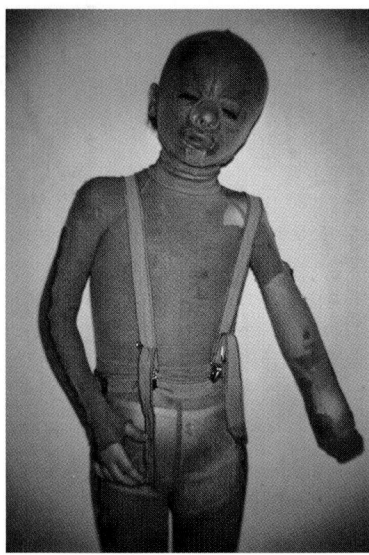

FIGURE 68–24 ■ Compression garment.
Source: Courtesy of: John M. Osborn, M.D., FACS, Sacramento, CA Plastic Surgery Center

pertrophic scarring. Even though the garments reduce scar formation, patient compliance—especially in the hot weather—has long been an issue. Patient teaching needs to stress the benefits of the garments in an effort to increase compliance. Periodic refitting is necessary to ensure proper fit and pressure.

Functional and Cosmetic Reconstruction

Once burn scars have healed, certain surgical options are available to improve function and cosmetic appearance. Typically, reconstruction begins after the scar has matured, which takes about a year. However, surgery may be indicated earlier if there is a serious functional impairment. Surgical intervention includes both scar excision and/or scar realignment. Small hypertrophic scars can be completely excised in one surgery. Larger hypertrophic areas need serial surgeries to remove the scar segmentally, one portion at a time.

Scar realignment is a technique used when the scar develops in a different direction than the normal tissue. Abnormal scar alignment causes excessive wound contracture and decreased ROM in the area. Scars can be surgically reoriented to increase ROM and decrease the visibility of the scar. A Z-plasty is a common method utilized for scar realignment (Figure 68–25 ■).

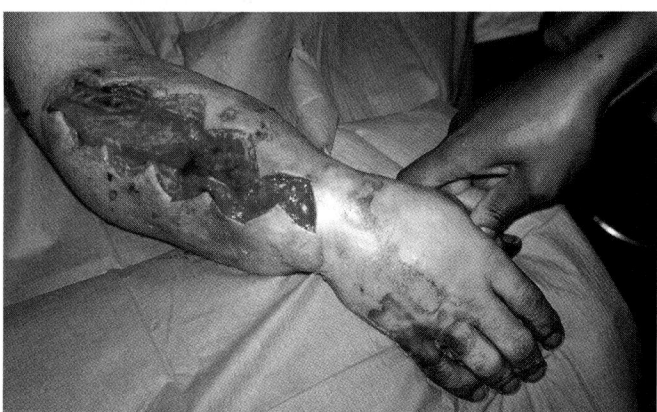

FIGURE 68–25 ■ Z-plasty.
Source: Courtesy of: John M. Osborn, M.D., FACS, Sacramento, CA Plastic Surgery Center

Psychological Recovery

Burn injuries that cause scarring, regardless of size, alter patients' perceptions of body image. The preinjury coping mechanisms have a major impact on how a patient copes following a burn injury. Some of the most common preinjury disorders found in people that are burn injured include depression, antisocial behavior, personality disorder, organic brain syndrome, and alcohol and drug abuse. Patients with preexisting psychiatric issues are at a higher risk for self-inflicted burns either as attempted suicide or self-mutilation (Erzurum & Varcellotti, 1999; Mabrouk, Mahmod, Massoud, Magdy, & Sayed, 1999). Research supports that there is a higher incidence of psychological maladjustment among people who sustain burn trauma than in people who sustain other types of trauma (Fauerbach, Lawrence, Munster, Palombo, & Richter, 1999).

During the healing process, a number of psychological reactions occur. In the beginning stages of treatment during the emergency period, patients often use withdrawal and denial as coping mechanisms. These patients tend to keep their eyes closed, remain immobile, and have little interaction with family and staff. Regression also is a common reaction in the patient that is burn injured, manifested by child-like behaviors such as dependence and temper tantrums. Other psychological reactions during the healing process include anger, hostility, depression, and anxiety. These reactions are manifested in a number of ways including restlessness, agitation, sleep disturbances, hostility toward staff and family, and self-degradation. Recently, post-traumatic stress disorder is being diagnosed with increasing frequency in patients with burns after discharge from the acute care setting (Van Loey & Van Son, 2003; Yu & Dimsdale, 1999). The Ethical Issues box (p. 2272) discusses some of the dilemmas that burn victims and their families, as well as the health care team grapple with while recovering from the burn injuries.

Grief is a natural and frequent reaction to burn injuries. Besides the change in body image, other contributing factors to the grief reaction include loss of physical functioning, potential changes in vocation, and separation from home and family. The patient that is burn injured must be given an opportunity to express concerns and feelings about the body image change and be reassured that this grieving process is normal and will eventually dissipate. The nurse's role is to be an active, nonjudgmental listener, allowing the patient time to express feelings and grieve the loss of former self. The nurse must answer questions honestly, acknowledge the patient's difficulty with coping, and encourage positive behaviors. Patients typically cope better if they are kept informed of planned treatments and surgeries. It is anxiety producing to be faced with unexpected events, especially when the patient has had to give up most of his independence. As wounds heal, the patient must resume control of as many activities and functions as is possible.

Measures to assist the patient in coping with grief and loss include resuming activities of daily living and socializing with family and friends. These activities enhance self-efficacy and worth, and give the patient more control. Additionally, a combination of psychotherapy and pharmacologic treatments often are effective in promoting adjustment. Burn support groups have also been effective in promoting adjustment to the disfigurement and reentrance into society.

ETHICAL ISSUES In the Treatment of Burn Injuries

There are a multitude of ethical issues related to the resuscitation, care, and rehabilitation of burn victims and their families. A comprehensive team approach is needed to achieve the most effective outcome. Initially burn injuries may be life threatening. Therefore, decisions must be made about the extent of resuscitation, especially with a massive injury; when to withhold or withdraw care; quality of life, both immediate and long term; and achieving a dignified and comfortable death in the case of futility. These issues are evaluated by the team and presented to the patient and family for their decision. The nursing role is to advocate for the patient, be supportive of the decision, and provide the family with factual, realistic data about the patient's condition and medical interventions.

Ethical dilemmas may arise for the nurse when it is difficult to support the decision for personal and/or professional reasons. One example would be an elderly patient who has sustained an injury that is not survivable due to age and past medical history. The family has made the decision that it wants everything done for this patient. The nurse is aware that this decision is going to cause a great deal of suffering for this patient with little hope of survival. In this case the nurse is obliged to treat this patient with the hope of survival. The dilemma for the nurse may be the conflict between being a patient advocate, supporting the family's decision, and dealing with one's own personal belief system. This is typically a very difficult ethical dilemma for the health care team. Team conferences typically occur to discuss a team approach to care and a plan to provide consistency in the approach to patient care.

Specific ethical issues for patients that are burn injured and their families include:

- Quality of life after the injury, both immediate and long term
- Extent of resuscitation after a massive injury
- When to withhold or withdraw care
- Body image adjustment
- Dignified and comfortable death
- Psychological adjustment
- Considerations of futility
- Nonmaleficence
- Financial costs.

Sensitivity to the patient's spiritual beliefs also is an essential part of the psychological recovery. A person's faith often will help guide her in life especially when a crisis has occurred, such as burn injury. The health care team needs to evaluate the need for spiritual guidance and support with each individual patient and then follow through with providing a spiritual guidance counselor of the patient's choice (priest, minister, rabbi, etc.).

Pain Management

Pain is markedly decreased with closure of the wound. Small areas of open wound may still need dressing changes that are painful, and newly healed skin is sensitive. In addition, the exercise therapies are often painful due to stiff, noncompliant skin in the affected areas. Therefore, pain management is still an issue and needs to be evaluated individually and on an ongoing basis. Along with diversional activities and relaxation techniques, oral analgesics typically relieve the pain experienced in the rehabilitative phase. Patient report of the absence of symptoms and/or an assessment of lack of pain behaviors, such as guarding, is necessary to assess when tailoring pain management therapies.

Nutritional Requirements

During the rehabilitative phase, the negative nitrogen balance and anorexia have resolved. Because the wound is still healing, high-calorie and high-protein diets are necessary. A nutritionist can assist with a nutrition plan to ensure adequate daily caloric intake. Promotion of independent eating also is important. If it is functionally difficult for the patient to eat due to involvement of hands, occupational therapy is needed to obtain devices that will facilitate self-feeding. Finally, in preparation for discharge, the patient and family need instructions about meal planning and the reporting of difficulties such as cachexia, weight loss, and food intolerance.

Discharge Priorities

Discharge planning is a complex process that begins when the patient is admitted to the hospital. An organized comprehensive plan of care with both short-term and long-term goals will ensure the highest level of recovery. As healing progresses, the patient and family need to be prepared for discharge. The ultimate goal is to return the patient to as close as is reasonably possible to the preinjury state.

Discharge planning requires a team approach with each member contributing from his or her area of expertise. In order to institute a realistic plan and ensure compliance, the patient and family have to be active, participating members of the team. Teaching is essential in order to prepare the patient and family for self care. Nurses play a key role in the implementation of the teaching plan because they coordinate and evaluate patient needs on an ongoing basis.

Health Promotion

To augment understanding, an organized, comprehensive teaching plan is necessary. The Patient Teaching & Discharge Priorities box outlines the necessary components of the discharge teaching plan, which includes wound care, infection assessment, nutrition, pain management, sexuality issues, scar and contracture prevention, psychological adaptation, and vocational rehabilitation.

Major burn wounds take 12 to 18 months to heal completely. Discharge instructions include care of both the open and healed wounds. Normal manifestations of newly healed wounds include dryness, itching, and an increased sensitivity to sunlight. Specific instructions need to stress how to assess the wound for complications such as newly formed open areas, blister formation, and signs and symptoms of infection. The instructions also need to include when and why it is necessary to notify the health care provider of complications. Discharge teaching plays a major role in preventing excessive scar and contracture formation. Teaching regarding ongoing pain management, sexuality issues, and emotional adaptation are all critical to ensure an optimal recovery. Comprehensive instructions are outlined in the Patient Teaching & Discharge Priorities box.

Occupational Recovery

Vocational adjustment is a common problem during the first year after discharge from the hospital. Often the patient has an extended recovery time after hospitalization before he is physically

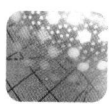

PATIENT TEACHING & DISCHARGE PRIORITIES for Burn Management

Need	Teaching
WOUND CARE	Perform daily cleansing and dressing changes for open areas.
	Elevate areas where edema formation occurs.
Patient/family/support system	Avoid scratching the healed areas, as this could cause breakdown:
	• Encourage liberal use of emollient lotions for dryness and flaking.
	• Use diphenhydramine hydrochloride (Benadryl) for pruritus (itching).
	• Keep fingernails short and use gloves when sleeping.
	Avoid sunlight, as it can cause, among other things, healed wounds to discolor or darken permanently:
	• Avoid overexposure to sun.
	• Use sunscreen products when exposed to sunlight.
	• Use clothing and hats for added protection.
	Avoid exposure to extreme temperatures and harsh chemicals.
	Wear loose-fitting, soft clothing.
Setting	Assess availability of, knowledge of, and compliance with treatment regimen.
	Assess respite needs and resources.
	Assess discharge placement needs:
	• Home
	• Rehabilitation facility
	• Extended care facility.
	Assess home environment for need for assistive devices.
	Assess for professional home health needs.
	Assess need for follow-up appointments.
WOUND INFECTION	Assess for infection of open wounds and healed wound breakdown with each dressing change, and report as necessary.
Patient/family/support system	Signs and symptoms include:
	• Odor and exudate
	• Fever
	• Increased drainage
	• Swelling
	• Lack of wound closure.
	Apply antibiotic ointments as prescribed.
	Teach minimization of risk factors for infection.
Setting	Explain signs and symptoms that require medical attention.
	Assess environment for risk factors.
NUTRITION	Maintain a high-calorie, high-protein diet.
Patient/family/support system	Continue taking vitamins and mineral supplements as ordered.
Setting	Observe for appetite and weight loss, and food intolerance.
	Taper calorie intake once preinjury or ideal weight has been achieved to prevent excessive weight gain.
	With professional guidance, institute an exercise program; i.e., physical therapist.
	Assess financial resources.
PAIN MANAGEMENT	Assess pain level and report any increase in pain.
Patient/family/support system	Assess effectiveness of pharmacologic interventions.
Setting	Wean patient off pain medication when pain lessens.
	Assess environment for safety and promotion of therapeutic needs.
SEXUALITY	Answer questions about sexual potential.
Patient/partner	Encourage both partners to express fears and concerns.
Setting	Encourage privacy and a familiar environment.

(continued)

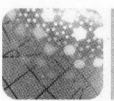

Need	Teaching
SCAR FORMATION PREVENTION AND EXERCISE PROGRAM Patient/family/support system Setting	Stress and assess compliance with wearing of pressure garments 23 hours a day. • If pressure garment is too loose, it is ineffective; discontinue use and will need new garment. • If it is too tight, it can cause numbness, tingling, and skin breakdown; discontinue use and will need new garment. • Need two sets. Ace wraps need to be worn per health care provider's order, usually when out of bed. Progressive passive and active range-of-motion (ROM) exercises. Progressive stretching and ambulation. Progressive exercise program to increase overall stamina (walking). Referral to physical therapy for development of an exercise program.
EMOTIONAL ADJUSTMENT Patient/family/support system Setting	Answer questions honestly. Encourage verbalization of frustrations and anger. Encourage positive reinforcement from the family. Encourage independent functioning as soon as possible. Stress that it is not uncommon to feel a letdown after discharge. Encourage participation in a burn support group.
OCCUPATIONAL RECOVERY Patient/family/support system Setting	Referral to the local office of the state labor and industry board for vocational counseling. Referral to vocational interest, aptitude, and psychological testing to determine areas of interest. Provide realistic plan, patient and family education, and engage an employer in the process.

and emotionally ready to return to work. Additionally, due to disfigurement and functional limitations, the patient may be unable to resume his previous job/profession. Therefore, the patient may need a referral to the local office of the state labor and industry board for information on job retraining programs. For many patients, vocational interest, aptitude, and psychological testing may be necessary to determine areas of occupational interest. Successful reentry into the work environment depends on a realistic plan, patient and family education, and engaging an employer in the process.

Nursing Management

The aim of nursing care during the rehabilitative phase is to prepare the patient both physically and psychologically to return home and to work. Use of the nursing process will provide a comprehensive approach to achieve these goals.

Nursing Diagnoses

A number of nursing diagnoses may be applicable in the rehabilitative phase. The most significant diagnoses for the patient that is burn injured include:

- *Acute Pain*
- *Impaired Skin Integrity*
- *Impaired Physical Mobility*
- *Activity Intolerance*
- *Deficient Knowledge related to injuries and limitations*
- *Disturbed Body Image*
- *Fear and Anxiety*

- *Readiness for Enhanced Self-Care*
- *Readiness for Enhanced Nutrition.*

These diagnoses depend on the degree of disfigurement and loss of functional capacity, as well as the home environment and support systems. The patient's personal coping skills and ability to adapt to the change in body image also impact applicable nursing diagnoses. Additional diagnoses related to the rehabilitative phase include:

- *Social Isolation* related to disfigurement and loss of function
- *Readiness for Enhanced Family Processes* related to risk of role change and loss of earning capacity
- *Readiness for Enhanced Individual Coping* related to ongoing maladjustment to burn injury
- *Risk for Complicated Grieving* related to ongoing realization of extent of injury
- *Noncompliance* related to wearing the elastic garments and continued need for physical therapy
- *Disturbed Sensory Perception* related to sensory overload/deprivation and sleep pattern disturbance
- *Impaired Home Maintenance* related to unavailable support system.

Collaborative Management

In the rehabilitative phase, the need to collaborate with all of the health care specialties continues. As the patient is prepared for discharge, each aspect of the physical and psychological needs is evaluated, and a plan is put in place to address them all. As is consistent with the entire hospital stay, the nurses coordinate the health care team to ensure that all aspects of care are addressed. The length of time that physical therapy and occupational therapy continue on an outpatient basis depends of the size and area of injury. The psychosocial needs of returning to society, family, and hopefully occupation are addressed by psychologists/psychiatrists prior to discharge as well as on an ongoing basis after discharge. Because the hypermetabolic state continues until all the wounds are healed, the need for dietary consultation continues. Finally, the surgeons begin the reconstructive process that may continue for months or years, depending on the extent of the injury.

Complications of Burn Injuries

It is a generally believed that complications are a "rule" rather than an exception for patients that are burn injured. Burn injuries should never be viewed in isolation because of their profound effect on multiorgan systems. The most common complications that lead to increased mortality include wound infection, nosocomial pneumonia, sepsis, acute renal failure, gastrointestinal ulcers, and respiratory failure. Certain complications occur more frequently in a given period or phase of burn treatment. Chart 68–5 outlines the complications specific to each period of burn management.

Gerontological Considerations

The incidence of burn injuries is less in the adult population under age 60, but the mortality rates continue to be higher than in the younger population (U.S. Library of Medicine and the National Institutes of Health, 2006). One-third of all persons who die in home fires are adults older than age 65. There is a greater incidence of inhalation injury in the elder adults because of their inability to escape the fire. Elderly patients with burns suffer from greater morbidity and mortality than do younger patients with similar burn extents (Redlick et al., 2002). In addition, the elderly often delay seeking medical care for burn injuries, which predisposes them to complications such as cellulitis and infec-

tion. With the onset of early wound excision and grafting, the mortality rates have declined in the last three decades. It is a general belief that the elderly survivors of burn injuries have decreased functional recovery. In addition elderly people tend to have other conditions that impact their recovery. See Evidence-Based Practice box on page 2277.

Each period of burn recovery is prolonged in the elderly. This is due in part to diminished reserve capacity of organ systems. For example, wound healing is delayed because of diminished host resistance and impaired cell-mediated and humoral immunity. Therefore, older adults have a decreased ability to fight infections and are more prone to sepsis. Once wounds are healed, there is a decreased tensile strength; thus, they break down and reopen easily.

Special nursing care considerations for the elderly include a careful assessment of the cardiovascular and pulmonary systems during early fluid resuscitation. This population is more prone to the development of pulmonary edema and heart failure. Monitoring of heart rate, blood pressure, and breath sounds on a frequent and ongoing basis is critical during rapid fluid administration to detect early signs and symptoms of heart failure. Mobilizing the patient as early as possible to maintain pulmonary function and promote independence also is an important aspect of care. Strict asepsis is critical because of the diminished immune response and increased susceptibility to infection. Finally, consistent attention to the nutritional intake of an elderly person is essential in that it impacts wound healing and survival.

Research

Research is essential to improve the care, quality of life, and survival of patients with burn injuries. The goal of research is to identify areas where practice could improve and evaluate and test methods for these improvements. The research topics related to burn injuries are included in the Research Opportunities and Clinical Impact box (p. 2276). The list provides both medical and nursing research topics still under investigation. Electronic databases are a source for finding specific studies related to these topics.

CHART 68–5 **Complications of Burn Injuries**

Emergency Phase	Acute Phase	Rehabilitative Phase
Immunosuppression: both humoral and cell mediated. Sepsis: highest incidence in burns greater than 40%. Bacterial translocation from the gut. Pneumonia and acute respiratory distress syndrome (ARDS), especially if an inhalation injury has occurred. Renal and heart failure from shock. Stress ulcers: rare due to medications and early tube feedings. Psychological problems. Normal grieving begins: denial.	Wound infection. Psychological problems; grieving process; patients fear both death and survival.	Scarring and contracture formation. Psychological problems. Loss of function and deformities. Normal grieving process switches to a focus on what are realistic future goals in terms of function and interpersonal issues.

RESEARCH OPPORTUNITIES AND CLINICAL IMPACT RELATED TO BURN INJURY MANAGEMENT

Research Area	Clinical Impact
Physiological Research	Mediating the shock state and potentially decreasing the mortality rate.
Drugs to reverse the release of natural dilators to prevent the shunting of blood from the vascular system.	
Fluid resuscitation techniques: high-concentration salt mixtures and high molecular weight salt mixtures instead of balanced salt mixtures for larger burn injury resuscitation.	
Hyperdynamic resuscitation and role of serum lactate in severely burned patients.	
Complex multiorgan response to burn injuries.	
High-frequency percussive ventilation for the treatment of inhalation injuries.	Prevent respiratory failure.
Direct instillation of combined aerosolized medications and hormones into the lungs of inhalation injury patients to decrease airway damage.	
Selective decontamination of the gastrointestinal (GI) tract to decrease wound infections and pneumonia.	Prevent systemic infection.
Early feeding of patients with burns to prevent translocation of bacteria to the bloodstream, causing sepsis.	
Use of glutamine supplements and the hypermetabolic response.	Augment wound healing.
Pain Management	Patient comfort and increased wound healing.
The nature of pain induced by direct tissue injury.	
Nursing pain management.	
Brief cognitive interventions for burn pain.	
Rapid induction analgesia for the alleviation of procedural pain during burn care.	
Relationship of itch to pain.	
Factors predicting hypnotic analgesia in patients with clinical burns.	
Pain and anxiety measurement and management during procedures.	
Emotional and Psychological Research	Assess factors that influence compliance and acceptance of burn injury and permanent scarring.
Predictors of post-traumatic stress syndrome and distress following acute burn injuries.	
Anxiety: current practices in assessment and treatment of anxiety in patients with burns.	Impact on vocation.
Chronic sorrow.	
Self-blame, compliance, and distress among patients with burns.	Impact on long-term adjustments to changes in body image.
Return to vocational stability.	
Massage therapy to reduce anxiety and cortisol levels.	Improve psychological interventions to augment coping.
Music influencing postprocedural recall.	
Factors that enhance positive long-term psychological adaptation.	
Family characteristics that augment psychological adaptation.	
Sexuality after burn injury.	
Burn Wound Research	Improve techniques to increase wound healing and prevent scarring.
The nature of fabric flammability and its effect on human skin.	
Living skin grafts (cultured autografts) used with Integra, for permanent burn wound closure.	
Treatment of pruritus and burn wounds.	
Hypnosis and burn wound healing.	
Massage therapy and itching.	
Comparative study of burn wound cellulitis treatments.	
Use of Integra artificial skin in preventing skin contractures to joints of burn wounds.	
Burn size estimation using direct template drawings.	
Use of music during wound débridement.	
Direct measurement of cutaneous pressures generated by pressure garments.	
Techniques to increase tensile strength and reduce wound breakdown.	
Regulation and secretion of human growth factors used to modulate the hypermetabolic response to burn, and augment wound and donor-site healing.	

Diabetes and Burns

Clinical Problem

Treating patients with diabetes for any other disease or disorder is associated with an increased risk for complications. For example, peripheral neurological impairments associated with diabetes result in a decrease in protective sensation and tissue vascularity. The lack of vascularity results in slowing the rate of wound closure, thereby increasing the risk for infection. Nurses need to understand and apply evidence-based findings when caring for patients with diabetes that are burn injured in order to prevent infection and promote wound healing.

Research Findings

Kowal-Vern & Latenser (2004) conducted a research study to determine the demographic characteristics of patients with diabetes that sustain burns and their rate of community-acquired and nosocomial infections. A 46-month retrospective chart and patient registry review was completed comparing patients with diabetes that have sustained burn injuries with patients without diabetes that have had such injuries. The infection rate, patient's age, mechanism of injury, time of year injuries occurred, time from injury to treatment, and complications were all evaluated. Adult patients with diabetes had a significant increase in community-acquired burn wound cellulitis and sepsis as compared to the population that was nondiabetic. The most common organisms in diabetic burn infections were *Streptococcus, Proteus, Pseudomonas, Candida* species, and methicillin-resistant *Staphylococcus aureus* (MRSA). Only 38% of the patients with burns presented for treatment promptly. Based on the study's findings, the researchers concluded that peripheral neuropathy may have precipitated the injury and delayed medical treatment in lower extremity burns of patients with diabetes. The researchers also concluded that there was an increased risk of nosocomial infections, which prolong hospitalization.

Implications for Nursing Practice

This study clearly indicates a need for nurses to educate patients with diabetes about the potential for burn injuries, the need for immediate medical treatment, and the possible complications of burn injuries. Additionally, nurses need to understand that when caring for patients with burns there is a significantly increased risk for wound infection and sepsis. Ongoing nursing assessment of the burn wound for infection needs to be rigorous with the understanding of the risk for patients that have diabetes. The nurse needs to understand the importance of reporting the first signs of infection so that treatment can be instituted as soon as possible.

Critical Thinking Questions

1. In order of priority, what are the most important points that would be included in an education plan for patients with diabetes and their families?

2. Compile a list of high-risk environmental and patient factors that would increase the risk of burn injuries.

3. Identify nursing measures that would decrease the risk of infection for patients with diabetes.

Answers to Critical Thinking Questions appear in Appendix D

Reference

Kowal-Vern, A., & Latenser, B. A. (2004). Infections in diabetic burn patients. *Diabetes Care, 27*(10), 229–233.

EVIDENCE-BASED PRACTICE

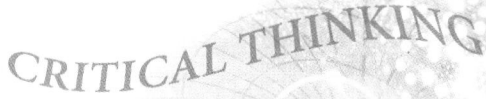

Clinical Preparation

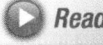 **Read**

- History of Current Illness
- Past Medical History
- Physical Exam
- Admitting Medical Orders
- Laboratory Study Results

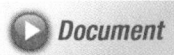 **Document**

- Summary of Hospitalization
- Pathophysiology Form
- Laboratory Values
- Laboratory Results Explanation

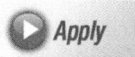 **Apply**

- List of Potential Nursing Diagnoses
- Concept Map
- Critical Thinking Questions

Log on to MyNursingKit.com to download forms you will need and to complete further steps in the Clinical Preparation assignment.

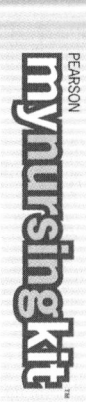

HISTORY OF PRESENT ILLNESS

As the on-coming nurse in a major burn center, you are receiving report about Mrs. X, a 60-year-old housewife who was admitted to the hospital following a fire that occurred in her home. A neighbor noted the smoke coming from the house and called 911 for emergency assistance. The firefighters had to carry Mrs. X from the burning house because she was unconscious. Despite resuscitative efforts, Mrs. X's husband was declared dead at the scene of the fire. Mrs. X's two grown children have been notified of the accident and are currently in the waiting room. This is the patient's hospital day 2. A large-bore triple lumen subclavian catheter was placed, and lactated Ringer's solution is infusing using the Brooke Army Formula guidelines. A Foley catheter was inserted, and her urine output is being monitored hourly and has been at least 30 mL/hr. A femoral arterial line was placed and has a good wave form. She is being medicated for pain with moderate relief.

Her last vital signs were temperature: 39°C, pulse: 126 beats per minute, respiratory rate: 16/minute, and BP: 104/80. A nasogastric (NG) tube was placed in order to decompress the stomach if nausea and vomiting should occur and for medication instillation. The patient denies nausea and she is tolerating NG medications. Her abdomen is soft with hypoactive bowel sounds noted in all four quadrants. She has not had a bowel movement since admission.

Medical–Surgical History

No known allergies
Hypertension
Myocardial infarction 2 years ago
Non–insulin-dependent diabetes
Atrial fibrillation
Depression
Two live births via vaginal delivery
Medications: Digoxin, Captopril, Paxil, and Glipizide

Social History

Was living independently with husband up to time of the fire
Two grown children
One son lives in local area
No tobacco use

Physical Exam

27% total body surface area burned
Approximately 12% is full-thickness injury, primarily on left arm and leg
Left arm and leg: circumferential injuries that required escharotomies
Remainder of burn wounds are on face and chest
Following escharotomies, pulses present in both left arm and leg, and patient able to wiggle toes on command
Restless, anxious, and complaining of severe pain
Moving all four extremities equally, on command
Pupils respond to light equally at 4 millimeters
Apical pulse: can be heard at the apex; peripheral pulses: +4 (0–4 scale) and slightly irregular, no extra heart sounds
Cardiac monitor: sinus tachycardia with occasional premature ventricular contractions
Capillary refill < 3 seconds in all extremities
Inhalation injury: currently intubated on ventilatory support with 50% oxygen
Lungs: wheezes and diminished breath sounds in bilateral bases; suctioned every hour for carbon-stained thick mucus
Oxygen sat 94–96%

Admitting Medical Orders

Burn service
Admit to burn intensive care unit
No known allergies

Diagnosis

27% burn injury

Orders

Vital signs, oxygen saturation, and urine output every hour
Foley

AccuCheck before meals and at bedtime
IV lactated Ringer's solution 180 mL/hr
Hubbard tank and dressing change with Silvadene daily
Bed rest
Strict I&O
Elevate left arm and left leg on 2 pillows each
HOB 30 degrees
PT/OT daily
NG feeding: replete at 5 mL/hr
Check residual q4h, stop feeding for 1 hour if > 100 milliliters
Ventilator: FIO$_2$ at 50%, TV: 700, Rate: 10, Peep: 5, PS/PC: 18/22
Suction prn
Daily weight
Call house officer: Pulse < 60 & > 110/minute; BP < 90 & > 130 systolic; temperature > 38.5; urine output < 30 mL/hr for 2 hours; respiratory rate > 30/minute; oxygen saturation < 92%

Scheduled Medications

MVI 1 NG daily
Folic acid 1 mg NG daily
Vitamin A 20,000 units NG daily
Zinc 220 mg NG daily
Thiamine 100 mg NG daily
Pepcid 20 mg IV q12h
Cefataxime 1 g IV q8h
Digoxin 0.25 mg IV daily
Captopril 25 mg NG 3 × daily, hold for SBP < 100
Paxil 30 mg NG daily
Glipizide SR 10 mg NG daily
Tobramycin 5 mg/kg on call to OR

PRN Medications

Tylenol 650 mg q6h NG/PR prn pain and temp > 101.5
Benadryl 50 mg IV/NG q6h prn itching and insomnia
Fentanyl 50–150 mcg IV prn dressing change
Phenergan 25 mg IV q6h prn nausea and vomiting
Versed 2–4 mg IV prn dressing change
Morphine sulfate drip 1 mg/mL at 1–7 mg/hr titrate to effect
Versed drip 0.5 mg/mL at 0.5–3 mg/hr titrate to effect for agitation/anxiety

Laboratory Studies

ABG, CBC, Chemistry 7 daily
Type and cross for 4 units of packed red blood cells
Blood, sputum, and urine culture

Diagnostic Studies

Chest x-ray daily

LABORATORY STUDY RESULTS

Test	Day 1	Day 2	Day 3
Sodium	138 mEq/L	148 mEq/L	135 mEq/L
Potassium	4.8 mEq/L	5.8 mEq/L	5 mEq/L
Chloride	103 mEq/L	110 mEq/L	108 mEq/L
Carbon dioxide (CO_2)	28 mg/dL	31 mg/dL	25 mg/dL
Blood urea nitrogen (BUN)	10 mg/dL	10 mg/dL	9 mg/dL
Creatinine	1.1 mg/dL	1.3 mg/dL	1.8 mg/dL
Blood glucose	141 mg/dL	135 mg/dL	132 mg/dL
Calcium	8.6 mg/dL	9 mg/dL	9 mg/dL
Magnesium	1.9 mg/dL	1.9 mg/dL	2 mg/dL
Phosphorus	2.2 mg/dL	3.4 mg/dL	3.8 mg/dL
Albumin	2.7 g/dL	2.27 g/dL	1.97 g/dL
White blood cells (WBC)	15,800/mm³	9,900/mm³	4,600/mm³
Red blood cells (RBC)	6.9/mm³	5.88/mm³	4.73/mm³
Hemoglobin (Hgb)	19.3/mm³	18.2/mm³	14.7/mm³
Hematocrit (HCT)	56.6%	54.1%	43.5%
Platelets	188,000/mm³	180,000/mm³	149,000/mm³
International normalized ratio (INR)	0.8		
Arterial blood gases (ABGs)			
PO_2	135 mmHg	96 mmHg	94 mmHg
Oxygen saturation	98%	99%	97%
pH	7.31	7.37	7.39
PCO_2	52 mmHg	49 mmHg	44 mmHg
HCO_3	26 mEq/L	28 mEq/L	26 mEq/L

CRITICAL THINKING QUESTIONS

1. Besides burn wound assessment and fluid resuscitation needs, what other priorities would be essential to assess Mrs. X for?

2. What is the rationale for performing an escharotomy, and what clinical manifestations would result if an escharotomy were not done?

3. What impact does diabetes have on Mrs. X's prognosis?

4. What impact does fluid resuscitation have on Mrs. X's sodium, chloride, hemoglobin, and hematocrit levels?

Answers to Critical Thinking Questions appear in Appendix D.

NCLEX® REVIEW

1. The nurse is assessing the patient with an electrical burn. It is noted that the patient has a 1% partial-thickness burn to the left foot and a 2% full-thickness burn to the right shoulder, where they contacted the electrical source. The patient is awake, alert and oriented. Vital signs are HR 97 with frequent ectopy, BP 136/75, RR 22, SpO₂ 94% on room air. The nurse knows that this patient's injuries should be classified as a:
   1. Minor burn injury.
   2. Moderate burn injury.
   3. Major burn injury.
   4. Medium burn injury.

2. A nurse is teaching a class on injury prevention to a group of new mothers. Which of the following statements made by one of the participants indicates the need for further instruction regarding burn injury prevention?
   1. "Every house should have at least one clean working smoke detector."
   2. "SPF 30+ can help reduce the likelihood of getting a radiation burn."
   3. "Make sure all children's sleepwear is made from fire retardant fabrics."
   4. "Liquid at 140° F requires five minutes to cause a full-thickness burn."

3. It is important to understand the pathophysiological changes that occur in the severely burned patient. When the student nurse inquires about these changes, the most appropriate response by the nurse would be:

1. "With bacterial translocation the gastrointestinal mucosal atrophy that occurs causes intraluminal bacteria to migrate to extraluminal sites."

2. "Decreased cardiac output can occur early after a burn because stimulation of the parasympathetic nervous system causes vasoconstriction."

3. "Hepatic failure ensues when damaged erythrocytes and muscle tissue cause the excess release of hemoglobin and myoglobin, respectively."

4. "It is not uncommon to transfuse leukocytes within the first two days because granulocyte stores and circulating iron stores are depleted."

4. Upon admission to the burn unit the patient with a 35% TBSA thermal burn begins to undergo intensive wound care and physical therapy. Pain control and topical antimicrobial medications are also important. The nurse understands the patient is in which period of burn care?

1. The resuscitative period
2. The acute care period
3. The emergency period
4. The rehabilitative period

5. Four victims of a house fire arrive in the emergency department. Based on what you know about burn severity assessment, which of the following patients should the nurse see first?

1. A 35-year-old with a history of migraines and 40% TBSA full-thickness thermal burns to the neck, left upper extremity and circumferentially around the chest. Vital signs are HR 116, BP 90/68, RR 26 and shallow, SpO_2 90%.

2. A 70-year-old with a history of diabetes and 14% TBSA partial-thickness thermal burns to the back and right shoulder and 1% TBSA full-thickness burn to the right arm. Vital signs are HR 88, BP 130/75, RR 22 and regular, SpO_2 98%.

3. A 12-year-old with a history of astigmatism and 20% TBSA partial-thickness thermal burns to the anterior left lower extremity, left foot and abdomen. Vital signs are HR 80, BP 110/65, RR 24 and regular, SpO_2 100%.

4. A 44-year-old with a history of hypertension and 8% TBSA full-thickness thermal burns to the right upper extremity and 15% TBSA partial-thickness burns to the abdomen and anterior chest. Vital signs are HR 98, BP 148/92, RR 22 and regular, SpO_2 98%.

6. Which of the following nursing diagnoses is most important during the emergency period of burn care?

1. Altered skin integrity related to epithelial skin loss
2. Fluid volume deficit related to increased capillary permeability
3. Increased risk for infection related to loss of skin integrity
4. Acute pain related to burn injury and exposed nerve endings

7. The nurse is preparing the previously burned patient for discharge home. Which of the following statements by the patient would indicate the need for further teaching?

1. "I know I should maintain a progressive exercise program to help increase my strength and endurance."

2. "The hardened areas in my healed scars can be broken down if I massage them daily with lotion or oil."

3. "I can tell that my stretching exercises are being done appropriately when my burn scars start to blanch."

4. "My pressure garments should be removed one to four times a day to allow for adequate circulation."

8. There are many complications associated with burn injuries. Which of the following would be the best indicator of an early complication during the emergency phase of burn care?

1. Blood pressure 118/66
2. Central venous pressure 6
3. Heart rate 114
4. Urine output 30 mL/hr

Answers for review questions appear in Appendix D

KEY TERMS

allograft *p.2260*
autografting *p.2260*
biologic dressing *p.2260*
biosynthetic dressing *p.2260*
chemical burns *p.2236*
donor site *p.2260*
eschar *p.2243*
escharotomies *p.2258*
full-thickness injury *p.2239*

full-thickness skin graft *p.2262*
heterografts *p.2260*
hypertrophic scar *p.2269*
inhalation injury *p.2235*
keloid scar *p.2269*
Lund-Browder formula *p.2245*
meshed skin graft *p.2262*
partial-thickness injury *p.2239*
radiation burns *p.2236*

rule of nines *p.2245*
scald burns *p.2235*
sheet skin grafts *p.2263*
split-thickness skin graft *p.2262*
thermal burns *p.2235*
zone of coagulation *p.2239*
zone of hyperemia *p.2239*
zone of stasis *p.2239*

REFERENCES

Ahrns, K. (2004). Trends in burn resuscitation: Shifting the focus from fluids to adequate end point monitoring, edema control, and adjuvant therapies. *Critical Care Nursing Clinics of North America, 16*(1), 1–25.

American Burn Association. (2002). *Burn care resources: Burn facts.* Retrieved on October 4, 2006, from http://www.ameriburn.org/advocacy/firesafety.html

Andel, H., Kamolz, L., Horauf, K., & Zimpfer, M. (2003). Nutrition and anabolic agents in burned patients. *Burns, 29,* 592–595.

Ballesteros, M. F., Jackson, M. L., & Martin, M. W. (2005). Working towards the elimination of residential fire deaths: The Centers for Disease Control and Prevention Smoke Alarm Installation and Fire Safety Education (SAIFE) program. *Journal of Burn Care & Rehabilitation, 26*(5), 434–439 (11 ref.).

Benson, B. E., Sidor, M. I., Schwartz, R. A., Desposito, F., & Hostetler, M. A. (2006). Burns, electrical. *eMedicine.com.* Retrieved September 9, 2008, from http://www.emedicine.com/ped/topic2734.htm

Borde, V. D., Bernier, J., & Garrel, D. R. (2002). Effects of dietary fatty acids on burn-induced immunosuppression. *Cell Immunology, 220*(2), 116–124.

Burnsurgery.org. (2004). *Burn center transfer criteria.* Retrieved September 18, 2008, from http://www.burnsurgery.org/Modules/initial_mgmt/sec_4.htm

Burn Survivor Resource Center. (2002a). *Chemical burns.* Retrieved October 4, 2006, from http://www.burnsurvivor.com/injury_examples_chemicalburns.html

Burn Survivor Resource Center. (2002b). *Medical care guide: Burn statistics.* Retrieved October 5, 2006, from http://www.burnsurvivor.com/burn_statistics.html

Burn Survivors Throughout the World. (2006). *Rehabilitation of burn scars.* Retrieved October 5, 2006, from http://www.burnsurvivorsttw.org/burns/burnrehab.html

Cancio, L. C., Jimenez-Reyna, J. F., Barbillo, D. J., Walker, S. C., McManus, A. T., & Vaughan, G. M. (2005). One hundred ninety-five cases of high-voltage electrical injury. *Journal of Burn Care & Rehabilitation, 26*(4), 331–340.

Centers for Disease Control and Prevention. (2006). *Skin Cancer: School Health Guidelines.* Retrieved September 18, 2008, from http://www.cdc.gov/healthyyouth/skincancer/guidelines/questions.htm

Chen, G., Xie, W., & Jiang, H. (2001). Clinical observation of the protective effect of oral feeding of glutamine on intestinal mucosal membrane. *Chinese Journal of Burns, 17*(4), 210–211. Retrieved May 1, 2002, from http://firstsearch.oclo.com/WebZ/FSFETCH

Demling, R. H. (2005). The burn edema process: Current concepts. *Journal of Burn Care & Rehabilitation, 26*(3), 200–206.

Demling, R. H., DeSanti, L., Orgill, D. R. (2006a). *Initial management of burn patient.* Retrieved May 11, 2006, from http://www.burnsurgery.org/modules/initial/part_two/sec9. html

Demling, R. H., & DeSanti, L. (2004). Initial management of the burn patient. *Burnsurgery.org.* Retrieved September 18, 2008 from http://www.burnsurgery.org/Modules/initial_mgmt/index_mgmt.htm

Demling, R. H., & DeSanti, L. (2006b). *Transfer criteria for referral to a burn facility.* Retrieved October 5, 2006, from http://www.burnsurgery.org/modules/initial/part_two/sec9.htm

Demling R. H., DeSanti, L., & Orgill, D. R. (2004). The metabolic response to burn injury and the role of nutritional support. *Burnsurgery.org.* Retrieved October 4, 2005, from http://www.burnsurgery.org/Modules/burnmetabolism/index_metabolism.htm

emedicine Health. (2006). *Chemical burns.* eMedicineHealth.com Retrieved October 5, 2006, from http://www.eMedicineHealth.com/chemical_burns/page6_em.html

Erzurum, V. Z., & Varcellotti, J. (1999). Self-inflicted burn injuries. *Journal of Burn Care & Rehabilitation, 20*(1), 22–24.

Fadaak, H. A. (2000). Gastrointestinal haemorrhage in burn patients: The experience of a burn unit in Saudi Arabia. *Annals of Burns and Fire Disasters, 13*(2).

Fauerbach, J. A., Lawrence, J. W., Munster, A. M., Palombo, D. A., & Richter, D. (1999). Prolonged adjustment difficulties among those with acute post-trauma distress following burn injury. *Journal of Behavioral Medicine, 22*(4), 359–378.

Flynn, M. B. (2002). Burn injuries. In K. McQuillan, K. Von Rueden, R. Hartsock, M. Flynn, & E. Whalen (Eds.), *Trauma nursing: From resuscitation through rehabilitation* (3rd ed., pp. 788–809). Philadelphia: W. B. Saunders.

Gosian, A., & Gamilli, R. L. (2005). A primer in cytokines. *Journal of Burn Care & Rehabilitation, 26*(1), 7–12.

Gottschlich, M., Jenkins, M., Mayes, T., Khoury, R. T., Kagan, R. J., & Warden, G. D. (2002). The 2002 research award. An evaluation of the safety of early vs. delayed enteral support and the effects on clinical, nutrition, and endocrine outcomes after severe burns. *Journal of Burn Care & Rehabilitation, 23*(6), 401–415.

Greenhalgh, D. (2005). Models of wound healing. *Journal of Burn Care & Rehabilitation, 26*(4), 293–305.

Hart, D. W., Wolf, S. E., Zhang, X. J., Chinkes, D. L., Buffalo, M. C., Matin, S. I., et al. (2001). Efficacy of a high-carbohydrate diet in catabolic illness. *Critical Care Medicine, 29*(7), 1321–1324.

Lucile Packard Children's Hospital at Stanford. (2008). *Safety and injury prevention: Fire safety and burns—Injury statistics and incidence rates.* Retrieved September 9, 2008, from http://www.lpch.org/DiseaseHealthInfo/HealthLibrary/safety/firestat.html

Lvsey, S. A., Herndor, D. N., and Hollyoak, M. A. (1995). Transplanted acollular allograft dermal matrix: Potential as a template for the reconstruction of viable dermis. *Transplantation 60*(1), 1–9.

Mabrouk, A. R., Mahmod, O. A., Massoud, K., Magdy, S. M., & Sayed, N. (1999). Suicide by burns: A tragic end. *Burns: Journal of International Society for Burn Injuries, 25*(4), 337–339.

Mandel, J., & Hales, C. A. (2008). *Smoke inhalation.* Retrieved September 9, 2008, from http://www.uptodate.com/patients/content/topic.do?topicKey=~9DITT3s_pPmii9&selectedTitle=1~147&source=search_result

McCall, J. E., & Cahill, T. J. (2005). Respiratory care of the burn patient. *Journal of Burn Care & Rehabilitation, 26*(3), 200–206.

Menchaca-Diaz, J. L., Silva, R. M., Figueiredo, L. F. P., Bugni, G. M., Watanabe, A. Y., Silva, F. J. P., et al. (2003). Bacterial translocation consequential to intestinal bacterial overgrowth provokes aggravation of mortality by sepsis. *Critical Care, 7*(Suppl. 3), P28. Retrieved October 12, 2005, from http://ccforum.com/content/7/S3/P28

Murphy, K. D., Lee, J. O., & Herndon, D. N. (2003). Expert opinion on pharmacotherapy. *Expert Opinion, 4*(3), 369–384.

Murray, C. (2008). *Burn wound infections.* eMedicine from Web MD. Retrieved on September 18, 2008, from suapple@verizon.net.

National Institutes of General Medical Sciences. (2006). *Fact sheet: Trauma, shock, burn, and injury: Facts and figures.* National Institutes of Health. Retrieved October 5, 2006, from http://www.publications.nigms.nig.gov/factsheets/trauma_burn_facts.html

National Institutes of Health. (2006). *Fact sheet: Burns and traumatic injury.* Retrieved October 5, 2006, from http://www.nih.gov/about/researchresultsforthepublic/BurnsandTraumaticInjury.pdf

Neumeister, M. (2005). Hyperbaric oxygen therapy. *Emedicine.com.* Retrieved October 5, 2006, from http://www.emedicine.com/plastic/topic526.htm

O'Brien, K. A., Weinstock-Zlotnick, G., Sanchez, J., Gorga, D., & Yurt, R. Y. W. (2005). Comparison of positive pressure gloves on hand use in uninjured persons. *Journal of Burn Care & Rehabilitation, 26*(4), 363–370.

Oliver, R. I., Spain, D., & Stadelmann, W. (2005). Burns, resuscitation and early management. *eMedicine.com.* Retrieved August 29, 2005, from http://www.emedicine.com/plastic/topic159.htm

Osborn, K. (2003, May). Nursing burn injuries. *Nursing Management,* 49–56.

Pereira, C. T., Murphy, K. D., & Herndon, D. N. (2005). Altering metabolism. *Journal of Burn Care & Rehabilitation, 26*(3), 197–199.

Porth, C. M. (2007). *Pathophysiology: Concepts of altered health states* (7th ed., pp. 391–397). Philadelphia: Lippincott Williams & Wilkins.

Prensner, J. D., Yowler, C. J., Smith, L. F., Steele, A. L., & Fratianne, R. B. (2001). Music therapy for assistance with pain and anxiety management in burn treatment. *Journal of Burn Care & Rehabilitation, 22*(1), 83–88; discussion 82–83.

Redlick, F., Cooke, A., Gomez, M., Banfield, J., Cartotto, R. C., & Fish, J. S. (2002). A survey of risk factors for burns in the elderly and prevention strategies. *Journal of Burn Care & Rehabilitation, 23*(5), 351–356.

Son, J. T., & Kim, S. H. (2006). The effects of self-selected music on anxiety and pain during burn dressing changes. *Taehan Kanho Hakhoe Chi, 36*(1), 159–168.

Supp, A. P., Neely, A. N., Supp, D. M., Warden, G. D., & Boyce, S. T. (2005). Evaluation of cytotoxicity and antimicrobial activity of Articoat® Burn Dressing for management of microbial contamination of cultured skin substitutes grafted to athymic mice. *Journal of Burn Care & Rehabilitation, 26*(3), 238–246.

Surgical-tutor.org.uk. (2006). *Burns.* Retrieved October 5, 2006, from http://www.surgical-tutor.org.uk/default-home.htm?core/trauma/burns.htm~right

Tadros, T., Traber, D. L., Heggers, J. P., & Herndon, D. N. (2000). Angiotensin II inhibitor DuP753 attenuates burn-and-endotoxin-induced gut ischemia, lipid peroxidation, mucosal permeability, and bacterial translocation. *Annals of Surgery, 231*(4), 566–576.

Tadros, T., Traber, D. L., Heggers, J. P., & Herndon, D. N. (2003). Effects of interleukin-1alpha administration on intestinal permeability and bacterial translocation in burn sepsis. *Annals of Surgery, 237*(1), 101–109.

Tuan, T., et al. (2003). Increased plasminogen activator inhibitor-1 in keloid fibroblasts may account for their elevated collagen accumulation in fibrin gel cultures. *American Journal of Pathology, 162*(5), 1579–1589.

U.S. Fire Administration. (2006). *Working together for home fire safety.* Retrieved October 5, 2006, from http://www.usfa.fema.gov/downloads/pdf/fswy11.pdf

U.S. Library of Medicine and the National Institutes of Health. (2006). *Dementia.* Retrieved March 9, 2005, from http://www.nlm.nih.gov/medlineplus/ency/article/000739.htm

Van Loey, N., & Van Son, M. (2003). Psychology and psychological problems in patients with burn scars. *American Journal of Clinical Dermatology, 4*(4), 245–272.

Whitehead-Pleaux, A. M., Baryza, M. J., & Sheridan, R. L. (2006). The effects of music therapy on pediatric patients' pain and anxiety during donor site dressing change. *Journal of Music Therapy, 43*(2), 136–153.

Wilkinson, J. M. (2009). *Nursing diagnosis handbook; with interventions and outcomes* (8th ed.). Upper Saddle River, NJ: Prentice Hall Health.

Wischmeyer, P. E., Lynch, J., Liedel, J., Wolfson, R., Riehm, J., Gottlieb, L., et al. (2001). Glutamine administration reduces gram-negative bacteremia in severely burned patients: A prospective, randomized, double-blind trial versus isonitrogenous control. *Critical Care Medicine, 29*(11), 2075–2080.

Wolf, S. E., & Herndon, D. N. (2000). Burns and radiation injuries. In K. L. Mattox, D. V. Feliciano, & E. E. Moore (Eds.), *Trauma* (4th ed., pp. 1137–1151). New York: McGraw-Hill.

Yamamoto, S., Tanabe, M., Wakabayashi, G., Shimazu, M., Matsumoto, K., & Kitajima, M. (2001). The role of tumor necrosis factor-alpha and interleukin-1 beta in ischemia-reperfusion injury of rat small intestine. *Journal of Surgical Residents, 99*(1), 134–141.

Yu, B. H., & Dimsdale, J. E. (1999). Posttraumatic stress disorder in patients with burn injuries. *Journal of Burn Care & Rehabilitation, 20*(5), 426–433; discussion 422–450.

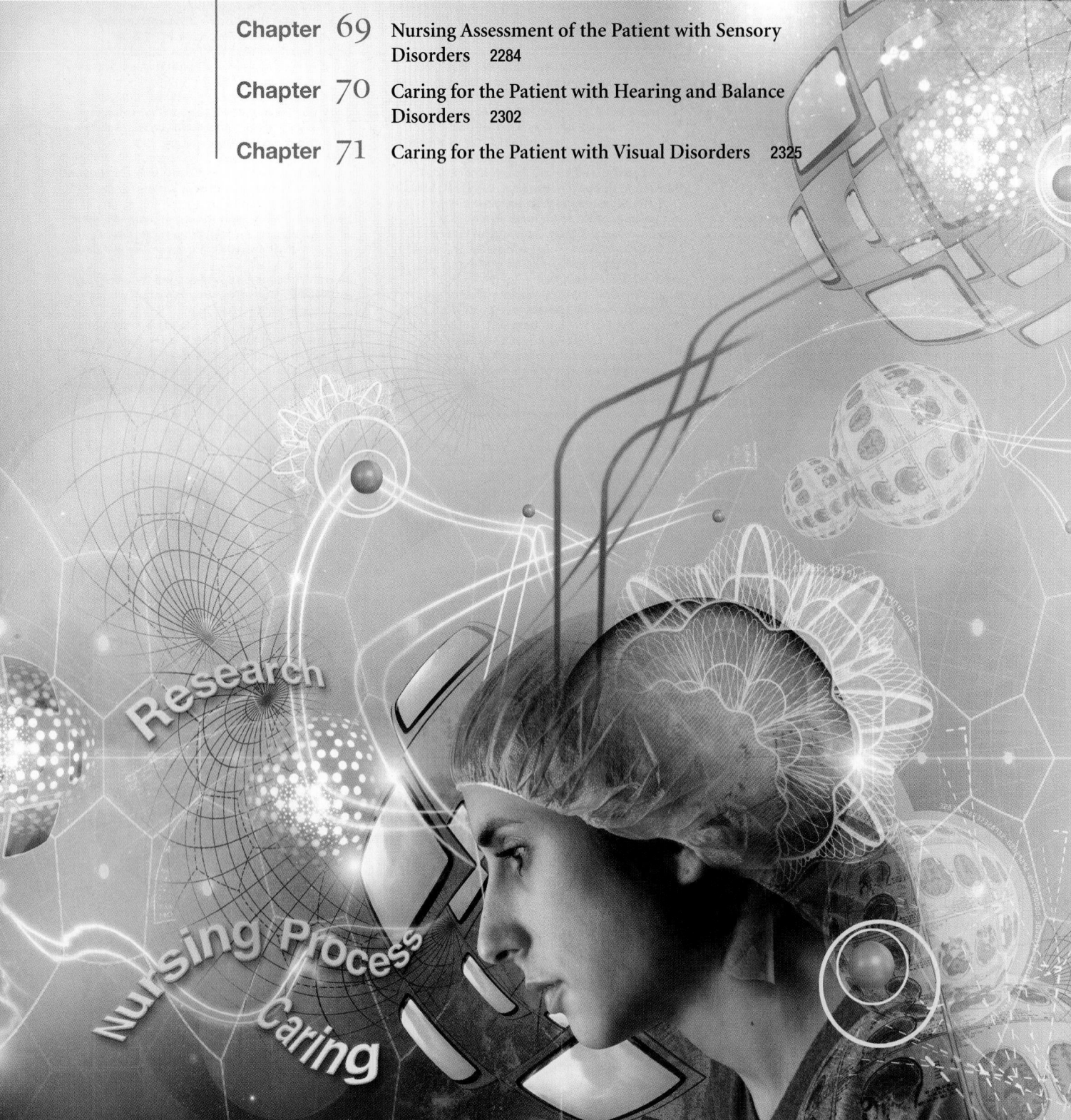

UNIT 15

Nursing Management of Patients with Sensory Disorders

Research

Nursing Process

Caring

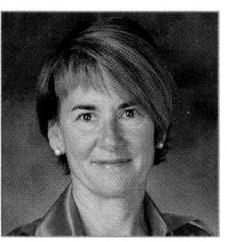

JOYCE My name is Joyce I have been a nurse practitioner specializing in family practice for more than 20 years. After graduating from the University of San Francisco, I worked as a public health nurse for VISTA (Volunteers in Service to America) at a migrant and seasonal farm workers' clinic in Toppenish, Washington. My practice included visiting migrant camps, providing immunizations and antibiotics, checking conditions regarding hygiene, and evaluating the general condition of the camps. During this experience I discovered the existence of nurse practitioners, their role, and their independence—that was what I wanted to become.

As a practicing family nurse practitioner (FNP), I am fortunate to have found a role in the delivery of health care that is completely fulfilling, that allows me to practice independently and utilize the holistic nursing model when providing care. As an FNP I want to know more about patients than just their chief complaints; I want to know about their lives. By delving more deeply into patients lives, I have often found an underlying condition, physical or emotional, that contributes to either the disease state or potential effectiveness of treatment.

In 1992 I received my master's in nursing at Sacramento State University. I received a doctor of education in leadership from St. Mary's College in 2007. While completing my doctorate, I accepted a faculty position at Sacramento Stare University. I am able to continue my practice as an FNP while teaching, pursuing research, and publishing.

It is impossible for me to think of a typical day—they are all so different. As an FNP I care for a wide range of patients, from infants to the elderly, with all systems affected from ENT to GI/GY. I counsel those who have had acute heart attacks and provide reassurance to new mothers that their babies will let them know when they are hungry. Over the years I have seen and cared for hundreds of ENT problems, some very simple, others much more complicated, including multiple sore throats, conjunctivitis, corneal abrasions, tonsillar abscesses, acute otitis media, sinusitis, and the common cold. This can be rather mundane, but then there are conditions that are complicated and frightening due to their potentially troubling lifelong consequences, such as abscessed sinusitis, temporary loss of vision secondary to a corneal burn or significant trauma, and hearing loss due to a medication or trauma. Some ENT complaints are aspects of a larger problem such as a brain mass, an acoustic neuroma, or other neurological condition. Recently, I cared for a deaf couple about to be married, one of whom was receiving a cochlear implant, the other was not. Many implications surrounded this decision—medically, surgically, psychologically, and personally. It was complicated and frightening to them and what this might mean for their marriage.

Navigating through these clinical situations takes **conscientious** patience, **competence, compassion,** and a total **commitment** to the complete health and well-being of each person. One of the most troubling situations I dealt with was the case of JM, a 72-year-old male with a history of upper respiratory complaints and progressively poor generalized health. Over a 2-year period, he was diagnosed with acute and chronic sinusitis, asthma, and GERD (reflux), He was treated with multiple antibiotics, Protein Pump Inhibitors, and nasal and respiratory inhalers. Still the problems persisted. Then his granddaughter noticed his aberrant behavior of swearing and using foul language. Upon reflection, his wife noted other abnormal behavior, such as the inability to remember simple equations or the passwords to his bank accounts. JM was referred to an ENT specialist who found that he had chronic sinusitis that had abscessed into his frontal lobe, causing his confusion and other neurological/cognitive problems. Neurosurgery was performed, but JM experienced a massive cerebral hemorrhage during the procedure and died 4 days later. Recognizing how long the situation was left unaddressed and allowed to progress with a failure of appropriate interventions and referrals that could have possibly changed the clinical outcome or improved the quality of JM's life was frustrating and frightening. It caused me to review my own practice—not just treating symptoms but looking at the person as a whole, the big picture.

Have I listened to the patient? Am I paying attention to what he is worried about? Does she understand the diagnosis and treatment plan? Have I **collaborated** with my patients or have I simply told them what to do? Even after many years of practice, I continue to review my clinical knowledge and my approach to patients and their care. It is my obligation, my **commitment,** to bring to patients the belief that they are in control of their situations. It is not about me—it is about the patient. I must be sure that I am **competent** and **confident** when dealing with health problems, **conscientious** in seeking out consultation if not, and **compassionate** about recognizing the person behind the diagnosis. It is essential that I *always* remember there is a human being at the center and all treatment and care focuses on that center.

"As a practicing family nurse practitioner (FNP), I am fortunate to have found a role in the delivery of health care that is completely fulfilling, that allows me to practice independently and utilize the holistic nursing model when providing care."

69 | Nursing Assessment of the Patient with Sensory Disorders

Arlene McGrory

Outcome-Based Learning Objectives

After studying this chapter, the learner will be able to:

1. Differentiate normal from abnormal findings of a physical assessment of the ear, nose, and throat.
2. Identify the subjective and objective history data related to ear, nose, and throat disorders that needs to be obtained.
3. Identify the risk factors for ear, nose, and throat disorders.
4. Describe the psychosocial impact of disorders of the ear, nose, and throat and how it impacts nursing care.
5. Describe the purpose, nursing responsibility, and significance of results of diagnostic exams of the ear, nose, and throat.

Research   Collaboration   Health Promotion   Nursing Process   Caring   Critical Thinking

THE SPECIALTY of otorhinolaryngology focuses on ear, nose, and throat (ENT) disorders. These disorders are common, may occur at any age, and often require immediate attention. Disorders of the ear, nose, and throat may affect the ability to perceive sound, speak, and breathe. Additionally, some of these disorders can be cosmetically disfiguring and affect body image and ultimately may be socially isolating. Early diagnosis and treatment can help keep people active and get involved in the world normally.

Nurses have numerous opportunities to identify risk factors and encourage healthy behaviors in patients. The modifiable risk factors related to ear, nose, and throat illnesses are primarily environmental, social, and occupational. These risk factors are discussed in the various chapter sections related to ear, nose, and throat conditions. Nurses need to assess patients for these risk factors and educate the patient and family to promote healthy behaviors. Nursing assessment using inspection, palpation, auscultation, and percussion, as well as a review of patients' social and occupational histories and laboratory results, provides information that can help identify conditions.

■ Anatomy and Physiology of the Ear, Nose, and Throat

The ear, nose, and throat encompass several organs and multiple systems including the integumentary, respiratory, gastroin-

testinal, neurological, endocrine, lymphatic, and circulatory systems. The following sections describe the anatomy and physiology of the ear, nose, and throat.

Ear

The external ear contains the cartilaginous auricle, or pinna. The external ear canal or meatus connects the auricle to the tympanic membrane (Figures 69–1 and 69–2 ■). **Cerumen**, or earwax, lubricates the external ear canal. Fine hair protects the canal from foreign objects. The canal protects the tympanic membrane.

The middle ear includes the tympanic membrane or eardrum, which conducts sound to the ossicles. In the tympanic cavity a small air-filled space in the temporal bone contains the ossicles and oval and round windows. The eustachian tube, the auditory tube from the middle ear to the nasopharynx, maintains equal pressure on both sides of the tympanic membrane.

The malleus, incus, and stapes are the auditory ossicles, which transmit sound waves to the inner ear. The inner ear consists of the bony labyrinth, which includes the vestibule and the utricle and saccule, which are filled with endolymph and are sensory receptors. Semicircular canals contain christa ampullaris receptors. The utricle, saccule, and semicircular canal help equilibrium. The shell-like cochlea is filled with perilymph and endolymph, which transmit sound vibrations. The organ of Corti contains supporting cells and hair cells that transmit

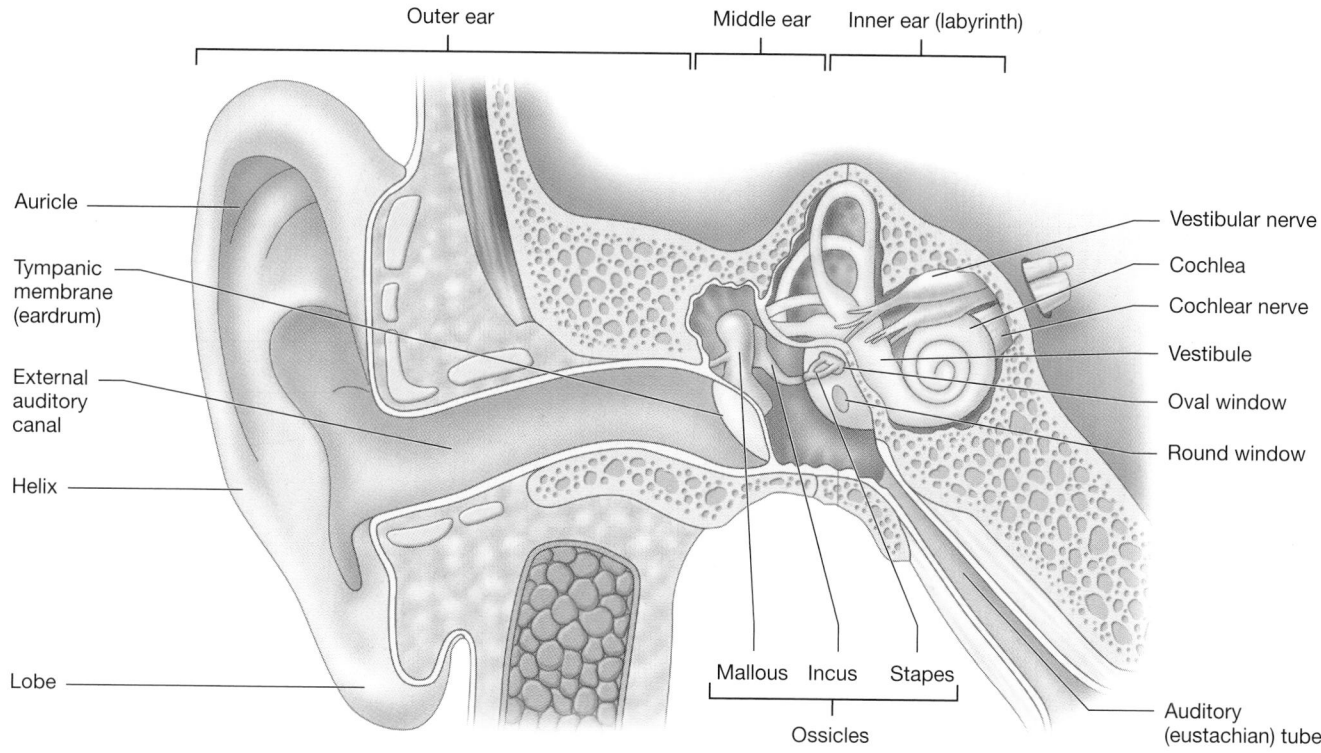

FIGURE 69–1 ■ Outer, middle, and inner ear.
From Lemone, P., and Burke, K. (2003). *Medical–Surgical Nursing: Critical Thinking in Client Care*, 3/e.

Right auricle

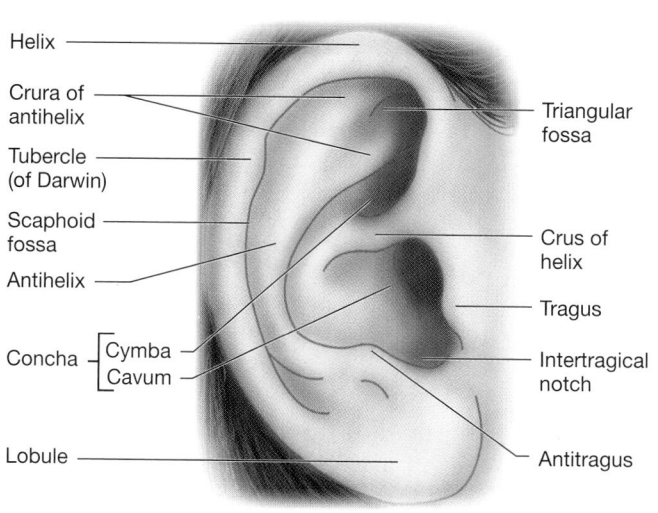

FIGURE 69–2 ■ External ear.

sound to the vestibulocochlear nerve (cranial nerve [CN] VIII). Hearing occurs as a result of sound waves vibrating the eardrum, malleus, incus, stapes, and oval window of the inner ear, the perilymph and endolymph of the cochlea, and the hair cells of the organ of Corti. The eighth cranial nerve carries the impulses to the auditory area in the temporal lobes.

Nose

The external nose has a bridge, which includes the nasal septum, tip, and nares or nasal opening (Figure 69–3 ■, p. 2286). Inter-

nally the nose is surrounded superiorly by the olfactory bulb and nerves and frontal sinus, and inferiorly by the hard palate. The interior is open to air and the posterior is surrounded by the sphenoid sinus, pharyngeal tonsil, eustachian tube, nasopharynx, soft palate, oropharynx, and palatine tonsil. The nares are lined with cilia, are highly vascular, and contain mucous membranes with ciliated goblet cells that produce mucus. The olfactory nerve (CN I) in the upper part of the nasal cavities controls the sense of smell. The paranasal sinuses, which include frontal, ethmoid, and sphenoid sinuses, are air cavities that surround the nasal cavity (Figure 69–4 ■, p. 2286). They add resonance to the voice and drain mucus through the nares.

Oral Cavity

The oral cavity includes, from superior to inferior surfaces, the upper lip, gingiva, hard and soft palate, glossopalatine arch, pharyngopalatine arch, palatine tonsil, posterior pharyngeal wall, uvula, and tongue (Figure 69–5 ■, p. 2286). Centermost inside the upper and lower lips, the superior and inferior labial frenulum connects the lips to the gingiva. The gingiva secure the teeth in the mouth. Thirty-two permanent and 20 deciduous teeth, needed for chewing food, are anchored by the gingiva, which is part of the oral mucosa and covers alveolar bone. The tongue is controlled by hypoglossal (CN XII) speech, chewing, and swallowing. The sensory function of the tongue is innervated by the facial nerve (cranial nerve VII) and glossopharyngeal nerve (CN IX). Oral mucosa is pink, moist, and without sores or bleeding.

The pharynx is the tube that extends from the nasopharynx behind the nasal cavity, to the oropharynx part of the oral cavity, to the laryngopharynx. The anterior portion of the laryngopharynx

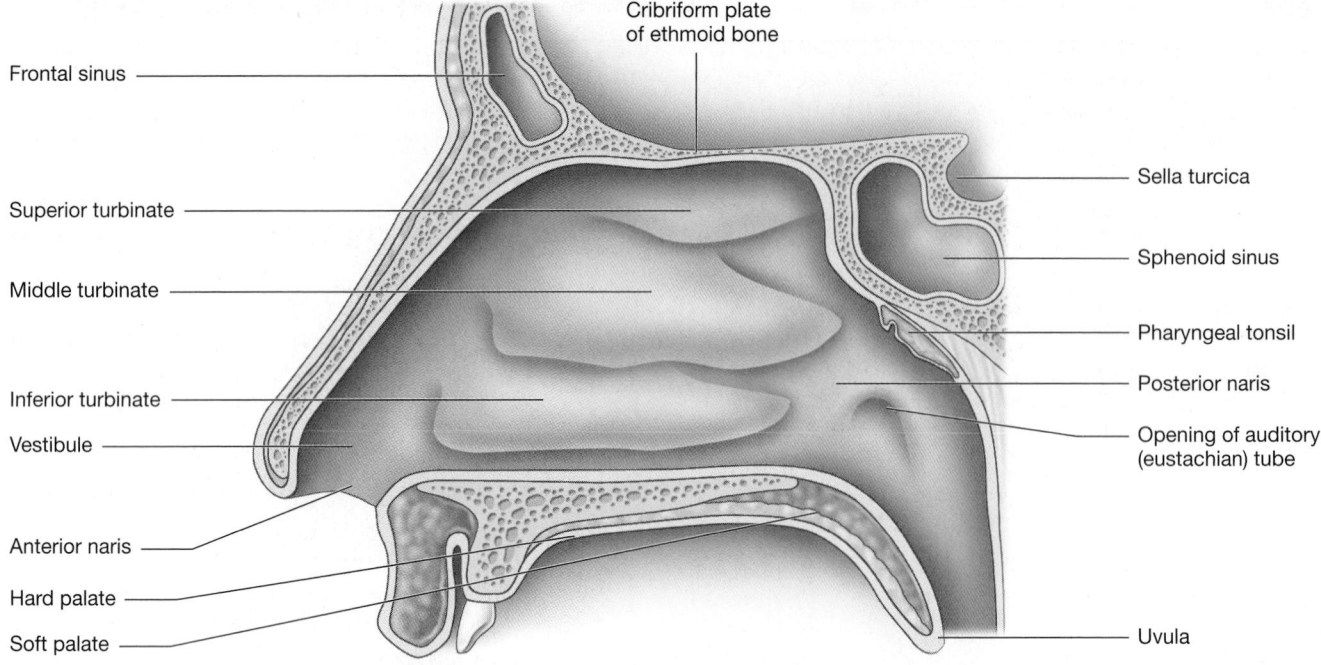

FIGURE 69–3 ■ The nose.

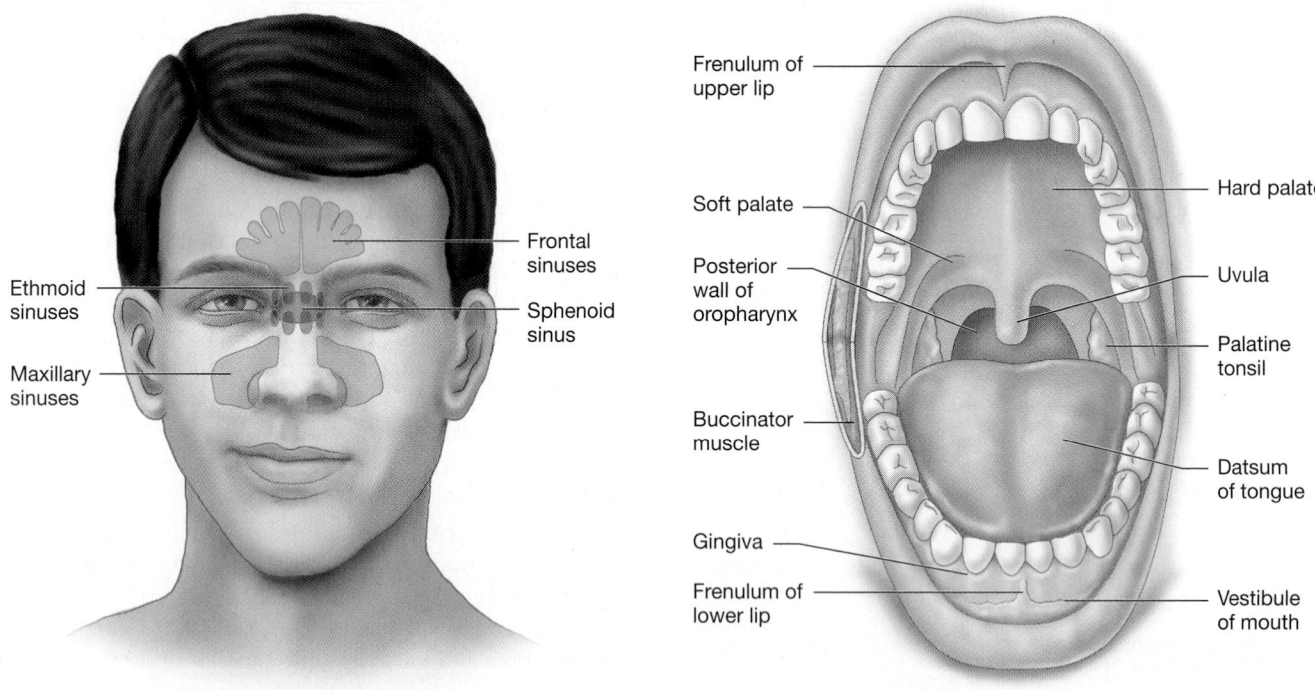

FIGURE 69–4 ■ The sinuses.
From Thompson, J. M. (1993). *Mosby's clinical nursing.* St. Louis: Mosby.

FIGURE 69–5 ■ Structures of the mouth.
From Seidel, H. M., et al. (1991). *Mosby's guide to physical examination,* 2/e, St. Louis: Mosby.

opens onto the larynx, and the posterior portion opens into the esophagus. Both the oropharynx and the laryngopharynx participate in swallowing.

The palatine tonsils are visible on either side of the soft palate. The lingual tonsils are on the base of the tongue. The pharyngeal tonsils or adenoids are behind the nose. The tonsils are lymphatic tissue that helps fight infections. The hard palate is the floor of the nasal cavity. Posterior to the hard palate is the soft palate, which helps prevent aspiration by elevating when swallowing. The uvula is a conelike structure centered on the soft palate that prevents food from entering the nasal passage. Several glands—the salivary, parotid, submandibular, and sublingual glands—and Wharton's duct surround the mouth and drain saliva.

Neck

The neck contains the thyroid gland, which produces thyroid hormone to control metabolism; thyroxine (T_4) and triiodothyronine (T_3); and calcitonin, which decreases calcium and phosphate levels (Figure 69–6 ■). Four parathyroid glands are attached to the thyroid gland posteriorly and serve to increase serum calcium levels. Cervical lymph nodes drain the structures of the head and neck.

The nurse must have a sound working knowledge of the anatomy and physiology of the ear, nose, and throat to be able to understand when the patient has problems with these structures. Along with the nurse's physical assessment skills, diagnostic tests and the patient's current functional abilities will help the interdisciplinary health care team choose interventions.

History

In order for the nurse to make an accurate assessment of the patient with an ENT problem, the patient's history needs to be explored. The personal, family, and social aspects of a person's life provide clues to the causes of health problems and the patient's receptivity to the care offered by health care professionals. Chart 69–1 (p. 2288) provides an assessment format that will help keep the nurse focused on the patient's complaint and allow the nurse to systematically assess the patient. Within this framework the patient's functional abilities are also assessed.

Biographic and Demographic History

The biographic information obtained is important in assessing risk for and identifying the presenting problem of patients with ENT problems. Medical, family, and social issues particular to the patient need to be explored. Specific questions are discussed under each organ.

Chief Complaint and Presenting Symptoms

The patient's primary complaint or the reason the person sought health care assistance is the presenting symptom. Examples of primary complaints include pain, breathing difficulties, and pruritus. The nurse's knowledge of the occurrence of diseases and conditions in certain population groups helps to focus the subsequent history.

Common ear problems include conductive deafness, sensorineural hearing loss, and tinnitus. **Conductive hearing loss** results from a lesion between the external auditory canal and the cochlea. **Sensorineural hearing loss** involves defects in the sensory end organ of the cochlea or in nerve transmission to the central nervous system (CNS). Patients can have hearing problems at any age. Knowledge of gender differences also is important. For example, otosclerosis is a familial disorder in which irregular ossification occurs in the stapes of the middle ear causing conductive deafness, sensorineural hearing loss, and tinnitus. It is more common in women than men (Mosby, 2002). Otosclerosis also can be triggered by pregnancy (Sigler, 2002).

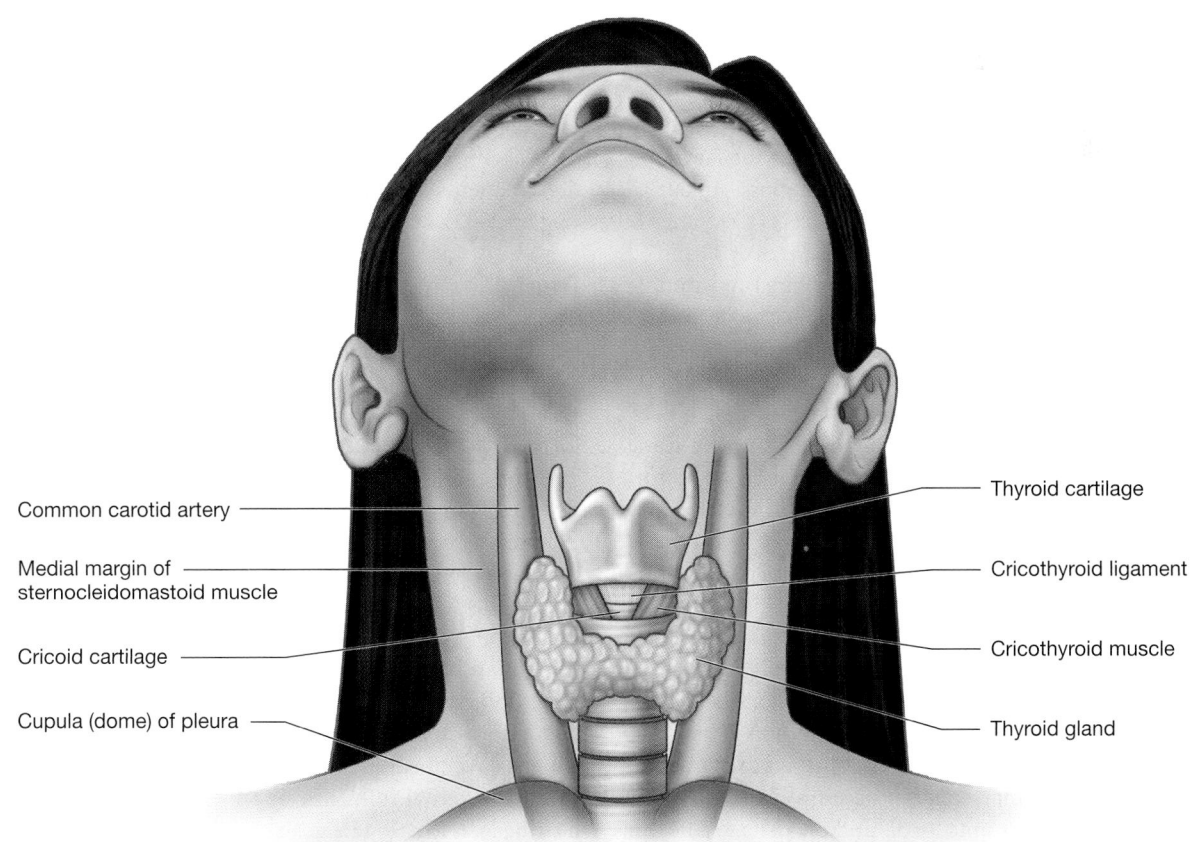

Common carotid artery

Medial margin of sternocleidomastoid muscle

Cricoid cartilage

Cupula (dome) of pleura

Thyroid cartilage

Cricothyroid ligament

Cricothyroid muscle

Thyroid gland

FIGURE 69–6 ■ The neck.

CHART 69–1	Ear, Nose, and Throat Assessment Format			
	Inspection	**Palpation**	**Auscultation**	**Percussion**
Subjective presenting symptom				
History (family, occupational, allergy)				
Current medications				
Ear				
Hearing test results				
Nose and paranasal sinuses				
Mouth				
Lips				
Gingiva and teeth				
Buccal mucosa				
Pharynx and larynx				
Nursing diagnosis				

Age impacts hearing ability. For example, *presbycusis*, hearing loss in the high-frequency range, is the most common sensorineural hearing loss in older people (Heron & Wharrad, 2000; Rabinowitz, 2000). The patient experiencing the gradual hearing loss of aging may limit social interactions as it becomes so difficult to understand the spoken word. During the assessment the nurse should inquire about functional ability and social interactions. Loss of hearing also can be perceived as mental status changes. Nurses need to be more aware of the impact of hearing loss on the elderly (Heron & Wharrad, 2000).

The nurse also should be aware of specific problems with at-risk populations. Acoustic neuromas, which are benign tumors of the Schwann cell sheath, are more common in women ages 40 to 50 years. Ménière's disease is a dysfunction of the labyrinth with symptoms of vertigo (dizziness), hearing loss, unilateral aural fullness, and **tinnitus**, or ringing in the ears (Crummer & Hassan, 2004). It is most common between the ages of 30 and 60 years. Any patient with obstruction of the ear canal, any middle ear disorders, or trauma to the ears or those receiving certain medications can develop tinnitus (Sigler, 2002). Ototoxic drugs are outlined in Chapter 70 🔗 .

Race is also an important consideration when assessing ENT problems, because some ethnic groups are more prone to some medical conditions. Otosclerosis is more common in the southern Indian population and much less common in Asians and blacks (Sigler, 2002).

Epistaxis, nasal bleeding, can occur at any age but is most common in children and in adults over 50 years old. Ten percent of the population experiences epistaxis at least once. It is more prevalent in the winter from inhaling dry air and is of particular concern in patients who have a history of hypertension, hemophilia, or leukemia. In adults nasal fractures are more common in men and are usually from sports injuries, assaults, or other kinds of trauma.

Sinusitis is of particular concern because it occurs at all ages and both sexes. It accounts for 32 million visits to a health care provider each year (National Institutes of Health [NIH], 2006). Smokers have more problems with sinusitis than nonsmokers.

Mouth and pharyngeal and laryngeal conditions occur from infections, tumors, or trauma. These conditions affect a person's ability to breathe and eat. Peritonsillar abscess occurs most often in young adults. Retropharyngeal abscesses are most common in children under 6 years old but are becoming more common in adults (Sigler, 2002). Ludwig's angina, severe cellulitis of the floor of the mouth, occurs as a result of dental disease. Laryngitis can occur from viruses or bacteria, inhaling noxious fumes, excessive use of the voice, or gastric reflux. Patients with head and neck cancer have problems with dysphasia and obstructive sleep apnea (Bailey, 2004; Koliha, 2003).

Vocal cord paralysis occurs more frequently in men than women and is usually the result of thyroid surgery, anterior cervical fusion, carotid endarterectomy, or cancer of the larynx. Elderly patients sometimes have presbylaryngeus, or dysphonia (Sigler, 2002).

Past Medical History

The patient's past medical history provides information about past health-related problems and, in particular, gives clues to the residual problems that may impact current treatment.

Childhood Diseases and Immunizations

The nurse should consider that any adult presenting with an ear, nose, and throat problem may have had a history of problems as a child. The frequency, clinical manifestations, and treatment of ENT disorders are essential information that must be obtained during the assessment. Inquire about any childhood history of ENT problems. Many children are prone to ear infections, sore throats, and tonsillitis. Complications of otitis media, which is either inflammation or infection of the middle ear, include frequent upper respiratory infections and sinus infections. Did the patient have tonsils and adenoids removed? Intrauterine exposure to maternal influenza or rubella can result in congenital hearing loss. Hearing loss can be very isolating and be perceived as mental status change.

Inquire about the presence of genetic diseases, especially those affecting the ear, nose, and throat. Hearing loss in children can occur from infections and genetics. Did the patient have all the childhood illnesses or immunizations? The nurse should inquire about childhood and adult immunizations, including the immunization dates and reactions.

Genetic conditions that affect otolaryngology can be divided into minor and major problems. Major genetic malfunctions include cleft lip and palate, sensorineural hearing impairment, absent or abnormal ears, eye abnormalities, blindness, and microcephaly. Minor genetic problems include high-arched palate, cleft uvula, wide-set eyes, abnormal slant of palpebral fissures, large auricles, and short neck (Jafek & Murrow, 2001).

Previous Illnesses and Hospitalizations

Past illnesses and hospitalizations can give the nurse clues to residual problems and how the patient coped with previous illnesses. In terms of diagnosing problems, the nurse needs to inquire about what has been done thus far. Has the patient had audiologic tests to determine the degree of hearing loss? Has the patient had surgery to correct hearing loss? Sinusitis is a very common condition and many patients have endoscopic sinus surgery for relief of the infection and pain. Has the patient had any cosmetic surgery? The nurse should ask about injuries and accidents, particularly foreign objects lodged in the ear, nose, or throat area. Has the person had any harmful ingestions or falls or been involved in a motor vehicle crash?

Head and neck cancer patients may have had various kinds of surgery, for example, a glossectomy or laryngectomy. Patients with head and neck cancer who have had surgery will need to have a barium swallow to ascertain whether or not the patient can resume normal eating.

Medications

List all current medications including prescribed, over-the-counter (OTC) medications, vitamins, and especially decongestants and sleeping medications. It is important to include systemic medications that may have an effect on the ENT assessment. Many medications are ototoxic and cause permanent bilateral hearing loss with eighth cranial nerve damage and some cause tinnitus (refer to Chapter 70 ☺). In particular, patients with compromised renal function are at risk for developing deafness and tinnitus from medications. To minimize this damage, while patients are taking these drugs serum drug levels and serial hearing evaluations should be done. Patients receiving long-term antibiotics can also develop vertigo because of damage to the eighth cranial nerve (Jafek & Murrow, 2001). Medications and chemicals that cause vertigo are outlined in the Risk Factor box in Chapter 70 (p. 2309) ☺. Also ask the patient about the use of herbal and home remedies for ENT problems. Patients who take herbal remedies and OTC products may experience unwanted side effects.

Allergies

All allergies, including medication, food, environmental, chemical sensitivities, and latex allergies should be documented. What are the patient's symptoms when exposed to these allergens? Some common symptoms of allergy experienced by the patient include headache; fatigue; sore mouth or tongue; edema; fluctuating hearing loss; tinnitus; dry, cracking skin; and muscle and joint pain. Conditions that are frequently associated with allergies include chronic sinus disease, recurrent tonsillitis, or ear infections (Jafek & Murrow, 2001).

Cough and Sputum Production

Patients with upper respiratory and sinusitis conditions frequently have copious sputum production and cough from postnasal drip. Any patient with oropharyngeal dysphagia is at risk of aspiration. This kind of patient would cough on attempted swallowing and needs to be referred to a speech therapist (National Guideline Clearinghouse, 2006).

Family Health History

Some ear, nose, and throat conditions are genetically transmitted. Damage to hearing can occur *in utero* from genetic or infectious conditions (influenza or rubella) (Dillon, 2003). Half of the incidence of severe hearing loss occurring in 1 in 1,000 live births comes from genetic causes. It is typically noticed because of impaired speech development. Half the people who have otosclerosis have a family history of the condition (Sigler, 2002). The nurse needs to investigate whether any family members were hard of hearing before 50 years old and, if so, what caused the hearing loss. Have any family members had ear surgery? Do other family members have any type of ear problems?

It may be helpful to draw a genogram of living and dead family members to trace the incidence of any genetically linked conditions. Inquire about illnesses of other family members, including allergies, asthma, diabetes mellitus, and alcohol or other drug abuse.

Social History

Social history and habits include occupational and recreational pursuits, cultural considerations, and environmental exposures. Each of these areas has the potential to impact normal ear, nose, and throat functioning. Each is discussed next.

Occupational and Recreational

Occupational and recreational related ear problems can occur for a variety of reasons. Anyone who experiences high levels of noise occupationally or recreationally without wearing hearing protection risks hearing impairment and potential deafness. The major sources of high levels of noise (90 to 170 dB) include chain saws and other power tools, rock concerts, gunshots, jets, diesel locomotives, motorcycles, and lawn mower engines. One-third of all hearing loss can be attributed to occupational noise exposure (American Academy of Audiology, 2003). Experiencing recreational and occupational noise on an acute or chronic basis can cause bilateral sensorineural hearing loss at higher frequencies (3,000 to 6,000 Hz).

For patients who present with symptoms of sinusitis, the nurse must inquire about occupational exposure and the onset or worsening of symptoms. If the symptoms continue or become intolerable, the patient may need a referral to a career counselor to investigate a job change.

Sinus congestion occurs frequently with airline pilots, flight attendants, swimmers, and divers because the changes in barometric pressure may inhibit the clearance of sinus secretions. Smoking cigars or cigarettes or chewing tobacco increases the chance of precancerous and cancerous lesions on the nose, throat, mouth, pharynx, and larynx. A history of alcohol use is strongly associated with head and neck cancer. Exposure to noxious fumes or chemicals can lead to tumor development. Recreational activities also may increase the risk. For example, swimming can cause bacterial otitis externa, also called swimmer's ear (Smith & Osborne, 2003).

Cultural Considerations

Culture can impact how receptive the patient is to the prescribed medical treatment. Many people in the deaf community refuse genetic services because of a history of stigmatization. For example, at one time in the United States, deaf people were sterilized and prohibited from marrying, and programs were developed to extinguish their language.

Some Native American and Alaskan Indians prefer to use the traditional methods of healing, such as the medicine man, before resorting to Western methods of health care. People of other cultures, such as Asian Americans, Pacific Islanders, and Hispanics, may also prefer to use traditional methods of healing. Chinese patients rarely complain verbally but nonverbal communication, such as leaving uneaten food on a plate, may be used to express their dislike. Chinese people are particularly reluctant to accept surgical procedures (Spector, 2004). This may be seen by practitioners of Western methods of treatment as noncompliance.

In relation to the assessment of the ear, nose, and throat, during history taking the nurse needs to be sensitive to cultural norms. For example, for American Indian and Alaska Native populations note taking during the interview is taboo (Spector, 2004). In this case the nurse needs to directly address the issue with the patient or devise a culturally sensitive method of recording the information.

Environmental Exposures

Patients can be exposed to many allergens such as seasonal pollen in the environment. Environmental chemicals, both those occurring naturally (seasonal pollen) and those produced by industry, can create acute and chronic health hazards. Since the 1970s U.S. industry has produced an excess of 70,000 chemicals that potentially cause ill health (Chalupka, 2001). Nurses need to be more aware of the pervasiveness of these chemicals, their toxic effects, and the symptoms these chemicals produce particularly as they relate to the ear, nose, and throat examination. The *NIOSH Pocket Guide to Chemical Hazards* (U.S. Department of Health and Human Services 1997) can help identify chemical health hazards and symptoms.

In assessing the ear, nose, and throat several chemicals are common irritants. Adult exposure to environmental smoke may cause rhinitis, pharyngitis, and nasal congestion. Volatile organic compounds and formaldehyde can cause tingling in the ears, nose, and throat, rhinitis, epistaxis, and nasal congestion and may exacerbate childhood asthma. Combustion from poorly vented wood stoves and fireplaces, kerosene lamps, and garage exhaust may cause rhinitis, cough, and asthma. Sulfur dioxide gas causes nose and throat irritation (Chalupka, 2001).

Habits

Evaluating the patient's health habits can be an opportunity for health teaching. The nurse should inquire about the use and amount of tobacco products and alcohol ingestion. Does the patient use sunscreen? The nurse should inquire about the use of recreational drugs. A history of recreational drug use, such as cocaine, which is inhaled through the nasal passages, can cause perforation of the septum, bleeding, crusting, and a whistling sound with respiration. The nurse should teach the patient that

using cotton tip applicators, hairpins, paper clips, or other such objects in the ear can damage the tympanic membrane and cause possible acute bacterial otitis externa (Smith & Osborne, 2003).

Travel

Changes in air pressure during airplane travel can cause ear discomfort. Common measures used to prevent this discomfort are to swallow more frequently and/or yawn. Another technique is to pinch the nostrils shut, take a mouthful of air, and force it into the back of your nose and try to blow your thumb and fingers off your nostrils. Subsequently the ears should be cleared and hearing returned. If none of these techniques is successful, the individual may try to use a decongestant or nose spray. Feeding a baby with a bottle or putting a pacifier in the baby's mouth will help the baby's ear pop. Because a cold, sinus infection, or allergy commonly blocks the eustachian tube, postponing the trip until the symptoms are less bothersome may be helpful. Any patient who has undergone ear surgery should consult with their health care provider about a safe time to travel by air (American Academy of Otolaryngology-Head and Neck Surgery, 1993).

Ear

The ears are sensory organs that, in conjunction with the nervous system, provide rich aural stimuli that enhance the quality of our lives. The ability to hear is essential for the normal development and maintenance of speech. The external and middle ear captures, transmits, and amplifies sound. The inner ear's vestibular structures are stimulated by sound waves to assist in balance.

Current Health and Risk Factors

The nurse needs to understand the current health of the patient and any risk factors, that might impact on possible problems of the ear, nose, and throat. Disorders of the external ear occur from obstruction or inflammation. Disorders of the middle ear occur because of abnormal patency, functional or mechanical obstruction, and infection (refer back to Figure 69–1 ■, p. 2285).

Disorders of the middle ear impair hearing, and can cause tinnitus or ringing in the ears. Conductive hearing loss occurs from loss of transmission of sound to the inner ear from diseases such as external ear infections, cerumen impaction, and middle ear effusion or obstruction (Crummer & Hassan, 2004; Marzo, 2003). Sensorineural hearing loss occurs when there is damage to the eighth cranial nerve or the end organ of hearing. This hearing loss can occur in a variety of ways. Presbycusis followed by noise exposure is the primary cause of sensorineural hearing loss followed by noise exposure. Congenital factors such as birth trauma and prenatal infections or exposure to toxic substances also cause sensorineural hearing loss. In addition, neoplastic conditions, acoustic neuromas, Ménière's disease, **ototoxicity** from drugs or other chemicals, infections, and systemic diseases can cause sensorineural hearing loss (Rabinowitz, 2000) (see Chapter 70 ☺).

Disorders of the ear also can be associated with neurological problems. The nurse needs to inquire about a history of meningitis, double vision, numbness in hands or feet, weakness in arms or legs, tingling in the mouth or face, loss of consciousness, fainting, or seizures. When noise-induced hearing loss occurs, the hair cells of the basilar membrane of the cochlea have been damaged.

In any patient with sudden hearing loss, the nurse must investigate the possibility of trauma and ask the patient what medications are being taken and for how long.

Hearing loss can be exacerbated by concurrent exposure to ototoxic solvents or heavy metals (Rabinowitz, 2000). The nurse should be aware of this important modifiable health risk, screen for risk factors, and teach the proper use of hearing protection. Is the patient's workplace very noisy? Does the patient wear any personal protective ear protection? How often does the patient wear earplugs?

Current Issue

What is the patient's current ear problem? The focus of the interview and assessment should be on identifying hearing loss, **otalgia** (ear pain), tinnitus, vertigo, and infection. A risk factor analysis should be done and any acute injury should be assessed.

Hearing Loss

Each year 60,000 people are diagnosed with unilateral hearing loss (Kim & Toriumi, 2003). About 28 million Americans have some hearing loss (Marzo, 2003). The nurse needs to inquire about difficulty hearing high- or low-pitched sounds, or both. Questions included in this assessment include the following:

- Does the patient have difficulty discriminating sounds in a group setting?
- Has the change in hearing been sudden or gradual?
- Do family members complain that the patient cannot hear them?
- What were the events leading to the perception of hearing loss?
- Does the patient perceive distortion in hearing, differences in pitch or sound, fullness or pressure in the ear?
- Has the patient ever had a hearing examination and, if so, why?
- What were the results of the hearing examination?
- Does the patient work in a profession where there is chronic loud noise and, if so, is ear protection worn?

Some occupational pursuits require the use of hearing protection, for example, people working with jet engines. A standard set of hearing tests can be performed depending on the symptoms, as outlined in Chapter 70 ☺ Diagnostic Tests for Hearing Loss box (p. 2312).

Is the patient wearing a hearing aid and, if so, in one or both ears? Are they turned on? Do the hearing aids help hearing? How old are the batteries? How recently did the patient change batteries? Does the hearing aid cause any irritation of the ear canal? Does the patient have an implantable hearing device? The nurse needs to observe any behavioral cues that may indicate possible hearing loss:

- Irritability
- Difficulty hearing higher frequency consonants (e.g., *sl* or *sh*)
- Complaints about people mumbling or giving inappropriate answers
- Use of a high volume on the television or radio
- Frequently asking for words to be repeated
- Leaning forward or turning head to hear better
- Avoiding group situations or anyplace with increased background noise

- Appearing aloof
- Using a very soft or loud voice.

Otalgia

The nurse needs to inquire about the presence, duration, and intensity of otalgia (ear pain). Is it unilateral or bilateral, constant or intermittent, and where is the location of the pain? Does the patient have a sense of fullness in the ears? Is it worse when moving and relieved by staying still? Does the application of warmth help? Use a pain scale to determine the intensity of pain. Ask about a history of trauma to the ears. What measures have been used to relieve it and have they been successful? Ask if the patient uses a cotton applicator or other implement to clean the ears.

Tinnitus

Tinnitus (ringing in the ears) affects approximately 50 million Americans (Sigler, 2002). It is usually an unwanted, primarily localized, internal auditory perception usually not heard by others. Objective tinnitus can be heard by others and is caused by vascular problems of the carotid arteries or jugular veins. Subjective tinnitus can only be heard by the patient and can be caused by metabolic, pharmacologic, psychogenic, and/or neurological abnormalities (Crummer & Hassan, 2004). The nurse needs to assess when the patient first noticed ringing in the ears and/or any kind of head noise. What is the intensity or frequency? Is the noise high or low pitched, buzzing, humming, or hissing or is it loud and persistent? Is it intermittent or constant, unilateral or bilateral, and what, if anything, relieves the symptoms? Has the patient been taking medications such as aspirin? A thorough history, head and neck exam, and audiometric exams are warranted (Crummer & Hassan, 2004).

Vertigo

Vertigo is the illusion of rotational movement, tilting, or swaying with feelings of imbalance during standing and walking. More than 90 million Americans over the age of 17 years report vertigo to their health care providers (Sandhaus, 2002). It can be a symptom of serious central cerebral dysfunction (acoustic neuroma, brain tumor, or trauma) or a benign peripheral problem (semicircular canals, peripheral nerve). It is a cardinal symptom of vestibular dysfunction.

With objective vertigo the patient perceives moving surroundings and the body stays still. Subjective vertigo is just the reverse, with the perception that the body is moving and the surroundings are still. Nausea and vomiting may persist but loss of consciousness is not usually a problem. Other symptoms that the patient may experience include presyncope, disequilibrium, and light-headedness. Presyncope is a feeling of faintness. Disequilibrium is the feeling of falling. Light-headedness may be psychogenic or idiopathic. Peripheral causes are usually intensely vertiginous, whereas central causes are mildly vertiginous with nystagmus (Sandhaus, 2002). To rule out the possibility of other system involvement, all cranial nerves should be tested. Cardiac rate, rhythm, and orthostatic blood pressure, which can mimic positional vertigo, also should be checked.

The nurse needs to ask the patient to describe the physical sensation of vertigo. Has the patient fallen or been injured because of the vertigo? Does this vertigo happen when changing positions? Is it intermittent or constant? Is there any unsteadiness of gait? It is also important for the nurse to inquire about

MyNursingKit | Video: Eyes, Ears, Nose, Throat

current medications that may cause vertigo (Chapter 70). The assessment must include an evaluation of both prescription and OTC medications that may cause ototoxicity, which is hearing loss resulting from eighth cranial nerve (vestibulocochlear) damage, and sometimes loss of balance or vertigo. The patient needs to be referred to a health care provider for further testing for causes, such as brain tumors.

Hearing Loss, Tinnitus, Vertigo, and Medications

The combination of vertigo, tinnitus, and hearing loss can be very disabling for a person. Eighty-five percent of patients with tinnitus also have hearing loss. Ototoxic tinnitus can be caused by ACE inhibitors; some anesthetics, such as bupivacaine and lidocaine; and antibiotics, specifically gentamicin, sulfisoxazole, trimethoprim-sulfamethoxazole, and vancomycin (Jafek & Murrow, 2001).

Many patients who take medications, specifically salicylates, erythromycin, and loop diuretics, can develop bilateral and permanent ototoxic hearing loss. Loop diuretics damage stria vascularis in the organ of Corti. Aminoglycosides damage the cochlear hair cells, causing bilateral hearing loss and dizziness. Vancomycin's toxic effect results in high-frequency hearing loss, which may lead to permanent deafness. This occurs due to damage to the auditory receptor cells (Jafek & Murrow, 2001). Note that benign positional vertigo is usually not associated with hearing loss or tinnitus.

Infection or Drainage

The nurse needs to inquire about any spontaneous purulent, clear (cerebrospinal fluid), or bloody drainage. What is the consistency and amount of drainage? Is it unilateral or bilateral, acute or chronic? Does the patient have a fever, recent upper respiratory infection, cough, earache, or other symptoms that would indicate an infection? These questions all help diagnose infection. If present the patient needs referral to a health care provider for further evaluation and treatment.

Barotrauma

Barotrauma, which is physical injury or rupture of the tympanic membrane, results from changing air pressure (Mosby, 2002). The nurse should inquire about any problems with the ears subsequent to diving or an airplane flight. Has the patient had any sports injuries or been involved in a car crash? Air bags deploying in an enclosed space (car windows closed) can cause ear barotrauma.

Physical Examination

Ear conditions do not occur in isolation from the other body systems. For instance, checking the temperature of a patient with complaints of otalgia is important when assessing for infection. Checking the blood pressure and pulse of a patient who has symptoms of possible vestibular dysfunction such as vertigo is important to rule out cardiovascular conditions. All cranial nerves should be checked because their proper functioning or impairment in relation to ear, nose, and throat problems is integral to understanding the other body systems. For example, an abnormality of the facial nerve (CN VII) with asymmetric facial movements can suggest Bell's palsy or a cerebrovascular accident. Chapter 28 describes the assessment of the cranial nerves.

Inspection and Monitoring

External structures of the ear are inspected visually. The top of the ears should cross a line from the outer canthus of the eye. An auricle below this line or at a posterior angle greater than 10 degrees may indicate chromosomal aberrations. Inspect for size, symmetry, shape, skin color, redness, drainage, scaling or nodules (may be cancer or gout). If drainage is present, is it sanguineous, serous, mixed, purulent, or odiferous? Inspect the mastoid bone for size or color of skin. Note any tenderness.

The inside of the ear is inspected with an otoscope. An otoscopic examination includes inspection of the auditory canal and tympanic membrane. Look for inflammation, exudates, lesions, and foreign bodies. Check for narrowing of the ear canal, nodules, redness, scales, edema, and drainage. Normally the eardrum is slightly conical, shiny, smooth, and pearl gray. Cerumen should be moist and may vary in color from brown to white, but hardened, dry, or foul-smelling cerumen may indicate infection. In a majority of Asians and Native Americans, cerumen is dry, white, and flaky. In African Americans and Caucasians, cerumen is brown, wet, and sticky. Look for the structures of the tympanic membrane, for landmarks indicating the border of the annulus, the light reflex, umbo, the short process, and the long handle of the malleus. Note the color and presence of perforations, bulging, or retraction of the tympanic membrane, dilation of the vessels, bubbles, or fluid. Normal middle ear fluid is thin and amber (Anderson et al., 1998). To test the mobility of the tympanic membrane, a pneumatoscope is used. A **pneumatoscope** is an otoscope with a bulb attachment in which the nurse introduces air in to the ear canal and middle ear. A ruptured tympanic membrane will not move.

Palpation

During the physical assessment gently palpate the auricle (refer back to Figure 69–1 ■, p. 2285), which is the external ear or pinna, with the thumb and forefinger to check for tenderness, pain, or nodules. Palpate the mastoid behind the auricle. It should be smooth, hard, and nontender. Abnormalities of the auricle include Darwin's tubercle (a benign protrusion on the upper part of the helix). Keloid scar formation from ear piercing or trauma is common in African Americans. Sebaceous cysts in the meatus or in back of the auricle can become painful, as well as at nodules along the rim of auricle. Exostoses are benign bony lumps arising from the ear canal near the tympanic membrane. They are more frequent in men than women and originate from irritated periosteum from swimming in cold water (Sigler, 2002). The nurse should palpate the preauricular and postauricular lymph nodes (Jafek & Murrow, 2001).

Hearing Tests

During the nursing assessment the nurse observes for any obvious clues to hearing loss like asking for words to be repeated. If any hearing test abnormalities are found, the patient should be referred to an audiologist for further testing. Hearing acuity is tested to determine the presence of hearing loss and, if present, whether it is conductive or sensorineural. The **Weber test** screens hearing acuity and helps distinguish whether hearing loss is conductive or sensorineural. A tuning fork tapped at the base will emit a vibratory frequency range of 512 to 1,024 Hz, which corresponds to normal speech. When conducting the Weber test, place an activated tuning fork midline on top of the patient's head, bridge of the nose, or the chin. A negative or normal Weber test occurs when the patient perceives sound equally in both ears or "in the middle." Sound that lateralizes to the affected ear is conducted through bone and is a conductive hearing loss from external or middle ear disorders. Sound that lateralizes to the unaffected ear indicates nerve damage or sensorineural hearing loss from inner ear or auditory or brain pathology.

The **Rinne test** is used to measure the conduction of sound by bone. In this text an activated tuning fork is placed on the right and left mastoid bone sequentially. The patient should indicate when the sound is no longer heard. The tuning fork is then placed in front of the auditory canal. Normally air conduction through the external auditory canal is twice as long as with mastoid bone conduction. With a conductive hearing loss, bone conduction is greater than air conduction (Crummer & Hassan, 2004). With the **Schwabach test** the nurse places an activated tuning fork on the mastoid process of the patient and alternately tests for both air and bone conduction. With the **voice whisper test** the examiner stands approximately 1 to 2 feet in back of the patient and whispers several words near each ear. The patient should be able to hear bilaterally and equally.

Vestibular hearing function tests the receptors for the vestibular system, which are located in the semicircular ducts of the inner ear. The vestibular nerve fibers travel in the vestibulocochlear (VIII) cranial nerve to the vestibular nuclei of the oculomotor (III), trochlear (IV), and abducens (VI) cranial nerves. Disorders of the vestibular function can be peripheral, involving the labyrinth, or central, involving the vestibular connections. Abnormal nystagmus, tinnitus, or hearing loss are other common manifestations of vestibular dysfunction. Vestibular function tests are outlined in the Diagnostic Tests for Vestibular Function box in Chapter 70 ⊙ (p. 2310).

The **caloric test** is used to assess the abnormal nystagmus, tinnitus, or hearing loss that is a result of vestibular dysfunction. This test can differentiate peripheral lesions from eight cranial nerve lesions (Sandhaus, 2002). Warm or cold water is introduced into the ear. The normal response is vertigo and nystagmus within 30 to 60 seconds. When cold water is introduced into the left ear, the normal response is a right beating nystagmus. When warm water is introduced into the left ear, a left beating nystagmus is elicited (Jafek & Murrow, 2001). This test is only done on a person with an intact eardrum and no visible blood or fluid behind the tympanic membrane. A caloric test is done on an unconscious patient to test for severe brainstem injury. A patient with a brain injury does not have nystagmus.

The **Romberg test** assesses the patient's ability to maintain an upright posture when arms are out in front, with eyes open and closed. This is used to test for inner ear balance and the proprioceptive ability of the visual and cerebellar system.

Auscultation

When assessing for objective tinnitus, the nurse can auscultate over the head and neck, periauricular area, orbits, and mastoid and verify for audible sounds (Crummer & Hassan, 2004). If noted this indicates objective tinnitus is present and helps differentiate between subjective and objective tinnitus.

Ear Monitoring Equipment

In addition to the tests and monitoring equipment described earlier, the otoscope also is used to inspect the ear canal and tympanic membrane. Hearing aids remain the most common and effective interventional devices to correct hearing impairments.

Hearing aids should be checked for cleanliness. The audiologist can provide the patient with a small wire brush to remove built-up cerumen. In addition, patients should keep an extra supply of batteries on hand. Indications and types of hearing aids are discussed in detail in Chapter 70 ⊙ .

Health Promotion

To prevent hearing loss, individuals should avoid exposure to continuous, very loud noises as well as sudden, sharp loud noises. It is important for persons who are exposed to very noisy environments to wear hearing protection to prevent hearing loss. Swimmers may be at risk for frequent ear infections and should be encouraged to wear earplugs when in the water. Patients should be advised not to dry their ears after bathing with an applicator or any other small object. Gently use the end of a towel to remove excess water or use a cotton ball to wick the water out. Some people develop excess cerumen, which can cause temporary hearing loss, and need periodically to have the nurse remove the cerumen by irrigation.

▨ Nose and Paranasal Sinuses

The nose is the external opening of the respiratory system (refer back to Figure 69–3 ■, p. 2286). It warms, moistens, filters air, and provides a sense of smell. The nasal cavity is surrounded by paranasal sinuses, which lighten the skull, help speaking, and produce mucus (refer back to Figure 69–4 ■, p. 2286). Obstruction of the nasal passages due to inflammation, infection, or neoplasms can occur.

Current Health and Risk Factors

Proper functioning of the nose and paranasal sinuses is essential for an adequate airway. The nurse assesses these areas both subjectively and objectively, as discussed later. The external disorders of the nose are related to the skin. Chapter 66 ⊙ discusses skin disorders that occur on the face and nose.

Current Issue

Medical conditions that impair proper nasal airway functioning need immediate attention and include pain, headache, difficulty breathing, bleeding and drainage, trauma, sense of smell, sneezing, and sleep patterns/obstructive sleep apnea. It is important to assess when the symptoms began, what brings them on, whether they are intermittent or constant, and what relieves them.

Pain

The source of pain in the nose or paranasal sinuses may be infection, trauma, or tumor. Poor preventive care of teeth and gums can be a source of infections that can spread to the sinuses and cause pain. Sinusitis or rhinosinusitis is the most common health problem in the United States (Smith & Osborne, 2003). Human immunodeficiency virus (HIV) can cause severe sinusitis from gram-negative and opportunistic infections. Chapter 60 ⊙ includes a complete description of HIV.

Headache

When the source of the headache is the nose and paranasal sinuses, the nurse should inquire about the frequency, intensity, and duration of the headache that localizes to the sinuses. Inquire if the headache is accompanied by nasal congestion, maxilla or dental pain, fetid breath, fever, or lethargy (Smith & Osborne,

2003). If headaches persist or become worse, the patient needs to be referred for diagnostic testing of the sinus tracks.

Difficulty Breathing

Inquire about the circumstances that occur when the patient has difficulty breathing. In addition to investigating cardiac and respiratory causes, difficulty breathing due to nasal problems can be caused by obstruction, infection, or inflammation. Inquire about a history of allergies, and upper respiratory infections and self or medical treatment. Inflammation and edema from eustachian tubes extending to the nasal mucosa may obstruct airflow between the middle ear and nose. An assessment of the lungs would assist in ruling out pulmonary versus upper airway causes of the shortness of breath.

Bleeding or Drainage

Bleeding or other drainage from the nose needs to be investigated in relation to a primary or secondary cause. Epistaxis, or blood draining from the nose, occurs in approximately 10% of the population at any age (Sigler, 2002). It can be caused by hypertension, malignancy, coagulation defects, or trauma or its causes may be idiopathic. Inquire about clear drainage from the nose, especially if the patient has had recent head trauma, because this might indicate cerebrospinal fluid leak. The nurse needs to evaluate the type, amount, and frequency of nasal drainage as well as any associated symptoms.

Trauma

A history of trauma to the nose such as a fracture may cause a deviated septum, which can obstruct breathing. A deviated septum also may be congenital. The obstruction is typically unilateral, and can be surgically corrected to reopen the nasal passage. Other trauma to the nose includes burns, abrasions, and lacerations. Each of these situations needs to be assessed and appropriate referrals made for treatment.

Sense of Smell

The sense of smell can be partially or completely impaired due to obstruction from trauma, polyps, sinus infections, hormonal disorders, and dental problems. Patients who receive radiation therapy for head and neck cancer also can have diminished sense of smell (National Institute on Deafness and Other Communication Disorders, 2002a). Under normal circumstances, the sense of smell diminishes slightly with age. **Anosmia** is the complete loss of smell. It can be associated with the presence of nasal polyps (Sigler, 2002). To test the sense of smell, use a variety of pungent substances such as cloves and vanilla to assess the olfactory nerve (CN I).

Sneezing

The nurse needs to inquire about a history of upper respiratory infection. Sneezing, particularly at specific times of the year or under specific environmental circumstances, should be investigated for the possibility of allergies or respiratory infection. **Allergic rhinitis** is an inflammation of the nasal mucosa caused by an allergic substance, for example, hay fever or pollen (Tierney, McPhee, & Papadakis, 2001). The nurse needs to inquire if the allergies are related to a specific time of year. Does the patient regularly take medications for allergic rhinitis, sinus infections, stuffy nose, or frequent respiratory infections? Some nasal sprays and decongestants may cause rebound nasal swelling. OTC oral decongestants may have an adverse effect on patients with diabetes, hypertension, hyperthyroidism, and cardiac illnesses.

Sleep Patterns/Obstructive Sleep Apnea

Sleep patterns need to be assessed by the nurse. Disorders of sleep related to the nasal passage range from habitual snoring to **obstructive sleep apnea (OSA)** (Gupta & Reiter, 2004). OSA is defined as brief periods of breathing cessation or a marked reduction in tidal volume with a minimum of five episodes of apnea per hour during sleep accompanied by excessive daytime somnolence (Flemmons, 2002). Patients with severe obesity, cardiac conditions, hypertension, increased neck circumference, craniofacial abnormalities, hypothyroidism, and acromegaly are at increased risk of OSA (Flemmons, 2002; Gupta & Reiter, 2004). The usual treatments include continuous positive airway pressure (CPAP) at night or oral appliances. Additionally, a variety of surgical procedures can be used to relieve OSA, including palatoplasty, septoplasty, tonsillectomy, tracheostomy, and turbinate reduction. Newer innovative technologies include genioglossus or hyoid advancement, tongue-base reduction, and laser palatoplasty (Gupta & Reiter, 2004).

Physical Examination

The nose should be examined for external and internal problems. The sinuses need to be assessed by palpation, inspection with transillumination, and percussion of the frontal and maxillary sinuses. The absence of transillumination reveals mucosal thickening or sinus fullness. Tenderness with gentle percussion reveals fullness in the sinus cavity. These assessments are described later.

Inspection

During the physical exam the nurse inspects the nose for contour, symmetry, and color, and its relationship to other facial structures (Anderson et al., 1998). The face is assessed for the presence of edema around the nose and eyes. The external nose is inspected for deformities, tumors or masses, dryness or ulcerations, and signs of trauma or bleeding. Nostrils should be symmetrical and without nasal flaring, which indicates increased respiratory effort.

To inspect the internal nasal passages, use a penlight, a nasal speculum, or a nasopharyngeal mirror to assess for color abnormalities, lesions, swelling, drainage, and bleeding. The nasal membrane is normally redder than the mouth, but can be pale, edematous, and bluish gray in patients who have allergic rhinitis. Inspect the nasal mucosa for bleeding and the nasal septum for perforation or deviation. To check for patency and airflow, ask the patient to occlude one nare at a time and breathe. Air movement may be impeded if the patient has a deviated septum, polyps, foreign body obstruction, allergies, or an upper respiratory infection. Observe any drainage and note the consistency and any postnasal drip, bleeding, or blood-tinged mucus.

Palpation

The nose and frontal and maxillary paranasal (frontal and maxillary) sinuses are palpated to detect fullness, tenderness, displacement, movement, crepitus, or edema. In a darkened room use a penlight against the patient's cheek to transilluminate through the roof of the mouth. Normally a faint glow can be seen through the bones of the sinuses, but with sinusitis there is absent or diminished light transmission. The nurse also needs to palpate the submaxillary and submental lymph nodes for swelling.

Percussion

The nurse percusses the periorbital and nasal sinuses for tenderness. Under normal circumstances these areas should not be painful. Tenderness or pain may indicate an allergic sinusitis, trauma, or an infectious process (Dillon, 2003). Discuss the pain with the patient, identifying specific areas of discomfort, and inquire about any recent injury to the area.

Nose and Paranasal Sinuses Monitoring Equipment

The equipment needed to monitor the nose and paranasal sinuses includes a flashlight to transilluminate the sinuses, an otoscope with a nasal speculum, and an oxygen saturation monitor. The nurse should monitor oxygenation routinely for any patient with a nasal or sinus problem. Oxygen saturation should be maintained between 93% and 100% for individuals with normal lung function. It is important to assess the range within which a particular patient stays. If the oxygen level is not adequate, supplementary oxygen should be provided. In addition, the nose and paranasal sinuses should be monitored for the amount, type, and color of mucous production. Frequently nose and sinus congestion causes pain, and a valid and reliable pain scale should be used on admission and throughout the hospital stay to assess the results of the treatment.

Health Promotion

Sinus pain is a common reason patients self-medicate and visit the doctor. It is important to caution the patient to not self-medicate and to instead consult a health care provider or nurse practitioner regarding appropriate remedies. It may helpful for the patient with chronic sinus congestion to address the possible allergic basis of the sinusitis and try to eliminate or minimize allergen exposure in daily life.

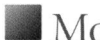 Mouth

The mouth is an integral part of the respiratory and alimentary tract. The mouth is used for eating, speaking, and breathing. The mouth includes the lips, gingiva, buccal mucosa, and tongue.

Current Health and Risk Factors

Good health of the mouth allows people to function at the most basic levels: breathing and eating. A systematic assessment of the mouth can reveal local and systemic problems that need to be addressed. When assessing the mouth the nurse can promote health when observing dental and gingival disease or poorly fitting dentures. In addition, health promotion activities regarding hydration and nutrition can be incorporated into the assessment. The nurse can also assess the patient's self-care abilities. Inquire about how frequently the patient visits the dentist, brushes, and flosses teeth. Refer back to Figure 69–5 ■, p. 2286, which displays the structures of the mouth.

Current Issue

The disorders of the mouth include fetid breath, change in taste, poor dentition, pain, change in voice, infection and inflammation, and trismus. During the assessment the nurse must inquire about the occurrence of any of these problems, how often they occur, and what treatment has been sought.

Fetid Breath

Fetid breath, or halitosis, may be a symptom of tooth decay, poor oral hygiene, gum, and tonsil or sinus disease. Fruity breath commonly occurs with patients who are malnourished or in diabetic ketoacidosis. A musty smell to the breath, or fetor hepaticus, is the result of liver failure and nitrogenous breakdown. The odor of ammonia is caused by end-stage renal disease.

Poor Dentition

The dental assessment includes evaluating the patient for any difficulty with chewing or swallowing. Poorly fitting dentures or orthotic appliances and inadequate dentition can cause difficulty chewing, nutritional problems, and mouth sores. Ask the patient if partial or full dentures are worn. Tooth loss resulting from oral disease may affect normal closure of mouth and jaw alignment. Inquire about dental habits such as flossing of teeth, frequency of brushing, how often the teeth are professionally cleaned, and occurrence of dental caries.

Infection and Inflammation

An infection or inflammation of the pharynx or tonsil can be detected easily by observing the condition of the mucosa, presence of drainage, and pain. A yellow or green streaked posterior pharynx indicates postnasal drainage. A gray membrane is indicative of diphtheria. White exudative patches with a reddened mucosa (exudative pharyngitis) are the result of streptococcal, chlamydial, or gonorrheal bacteria or a virus. Tonsillitis and peritonsillar abscess with erythema and exudates are also visible upon inspection (Dillon, 2003).

Trismus

Trismus is restricted jaw movement from shrinkage of connective tissue in the posterior mandibular or temporomandibular region. It is usually due to radiation treatment for head and neck cancer, trauma, infection, surgery (MedicineNet, 2007) or structural abnormalities, or it may be a symptom of temporomandibular joint syndrome.

Physical Examination

The physical examination of the mouth is essential to understand the systemic problems of the patient as well as local conditions. The mouth reveals much about the overall nutritional state. The National Guidelines box (p. 2296) lists oral assessment guidelines.

Inspection

Inspect the mouth for color, moisture, and lesions and the overall condition of teeth, gingiva, tonsils, uvula, and hard and soft palate. Normally the mouth is pink and moist with intact mucous membranes, no lesions, and no alteration in taste. Inquire whether the patient has experienced a change in taste. Fluid intake and output need to be assessed because signs of dehydration can be observed in the dry mucosa.

 A healthy oral cavity can reflect general good health. Poor nutrition and hydration are revealed in problems with the gingiva, lips, and tongue.

Inspect the hard and soft palate for ulcerations or lesions (Chart 69–2, p. 2296). Normally the hard and soft palates are concave and pink. The hard palate has many ridges and the soft

MyNursingKit Video: Health and Physical Assessment: Mouth/Throat—Oral Examination

NATIONAL GUIDELINES for Oral Assessment

Area to Be Observed	Rating 1 Normal	Rating 2 Mild Abnormality	Rating 3 Severe Abnormality
Voice	Normal	Deep, rasp, hoarse	Difficulty talking, pain
Swallow reflex	Normal	Some pain on swallowing	Unable to swallow
Lips	Smooth, pink, moist	Dry, cracked	Ulcerated or bleeding
Tongue	Pink, moist, papillae present	Coated or loss of papillae with a shiny appearance, with or without redness	Blistered or cracked
Saliva	Watery	Thick	Absent
Mucous membrane	Pink and moist	Reddened or coated, without ulceration	Ulcerated with or without bleeding
Gingiva	Pink, stippled, and firm	Edematous with or without redness	Spontaneous bleeding or bleeding with pressure
Teeth or denture-bearing area	Clean with no debris	Plaque or debris in localized area if teeth are present	Plaque or debris generalized along gum line or denture-bearing area

Source: National Guideline Clearinghouse. (2004). *Nursing management of oral hygiene.* Retrieved February 17, 2007, from http://www.guideline.gov/summary/summary.aspx?doc_id=7153&nbr= 004285&string=ear+AND+nose+AND+throat.

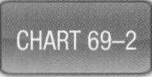

CHART 69–2 Signs and Symptoms of Oral and Pharyngeal Cancer

Sore that bleeds easily and does not heal

Lump or thickening

Red or white patch that persists

Difficulties chewing, swallowing, or moving tongue or jaw—late symptoms

Source: American Cancer Society. (2006). *Cancer facts and figures 2006.* Atlanta, GA: Author.

palate is smooth. White patches in the mouth could be *Candida albicans*, streptococcal infection, leukoplakia, or a precancerous condition. Note the color, pigmentation, ulcers, or nodules.

To assess for trismus, ask the patient to open the mouth widely. There should be no restricted jaw movement or pain. Palpate the temporomandibular joint (TMJ) just below the earlobe where the mandible and maxilla join. Assess for sounds or clicks or friction sounds. Assess for pain and restricted jaw movement when opening the mouth. Gently palpate the trachea for deviation, mobility, tenderness, and consistency. Avoid firm palpation, because it will cause gagging. With a folded gauze pad and a tongue blade, inspect the mucosa around the tongue.

Health Promotion

To maintain good oral health, the patient should see the dentist at regular intervals and use good oral hygiene measures. Because the use of tobacco in any form and the excessive use of alcoholic beverages are the primary risk factors in the development of oral cancer, it is important for the nurse to encourage the cessation of tobacco and excessive alcohol use (American Cancer Society, 2006; National Guideline Clearinghouse, 2004).

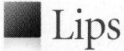

Lips

The lips function to keep food and saliva in the mouth during chewing, and they help form words and facial expressions. The proper functioning of the lips reflects the patient's state of health. The lips are a sphincter muscle, the orbicularis oris covered by skin externally and internally by mucous membrane. The sensory receptors in lips help judge the temperature and texture of food.

Current Health and Risk Factors

The lips are an important part of the physical examination of the oral cavity. The lips can develop local problems and can reflect systemic problems. The chief complaint is most frequently related to hydration, ulcerations, lesions, bleeding, and infections.

Hydration

When a person is hydrated their lips are moist and pink to brown in color. Dehydration produces cheilitis or dry and cracked lips. Dehydration can develop from poor intake of fluids, diuretics, sun exposure, or fever.

Color

Lip color may be an indicator of more systemic problems. Cyanosis can indicate hypoxia or vasoconstriction. A cold body temperature also will cause the lips to become cyanotic. Pale lips may be a clinical manifestation of anemia. Reddened lips reveal an infectious or inflammatory disorder.

Ulcerations, Lesions, or Bleeding

Lesions can reveal a generalized inflammatory disorder. Any local lesion on the lip needs to be evaluated for the possibility of basal cell or squamous cell cancer, infections, or nutritional deficiencies. Cheilosis, manifested by increased moisture in the corners of the mouth, reflects a riboflavin deficiency, poorly fitting dentures, or immune deficiencies. Bleeding from the lips can occur as a result of certain drugs that cause a deficiency in clotting mechanisms or from some congenitally acquired conditions that manifest as generalized bleeding disorders.

Infections

Local and systemic infections commonly appear on the lips. A local viral infection called herpes simplex, or a cold sore, can commonly appear on the lips. A chancre on the lips is a painless ulcer of primary syphilis.

Physical Inspection

During the physical exam the color, moisture, swelling, lesions, or other signs of inflammation in and around the lips are assessed. Lips should be moist, pink or darker and have no lesions, bleeding, dryness, or swelling. Local problems that can easily be inspected are asymmetrical lips resulting from a congenital deformity, for example, a cleft lip, or from trauma, paralysis, or surgical intervention. Many systemic problems can be revealed by inspecting the lips. Fissures at the corners of the lips or cheilosis reveals a vitamin B deficiency. Swollen, inflamed lips are a sign of an allergic response called angioedema. Drying and cracking lips or cheilitis (inflammation of the lips) can occur from allergies and lip licking.

Palpation

When palpating the lips for tenderness and consistency, use the gloved thumb and forefinger to gently pull down on the lower lip and pull up on the upper lip. Palpating the lips should reveal soft tissue and the lips should be nontender and have no masses. Abnormal masses or lesions should be noted and followed up.

Health Promotion

Implications for health promotion as it relates to lips should focus on encouraging the patient to use lip gloss with sunscreen protection. Use of any type of tobacco should be avoided because it can cause lip cancer. A patient with cheilosis needs nutritional counseling to improve dietary intake. The use of a daily multivitamin might be helpful. A patient with cyanotic lips may need to be referred to cardiac rehabilitation to maximize cardiac efficiency. A patient with pale lips may need to have a complete physical examination to assess the reason for the anemia.

Gingiva and Teeth

Gingiva (gums) is a dense, strong oral mucosa that provides the support for and surrounds the teeth. Adults normally have 28 to 32 teeth if the third and fourth molars have erupted. The teeth function to cut, grind, and chew food. The muscles of mastication are innervated by the trigeminal (CN V) and facial (CN VII) cranial nerves.

Current Health and Risk Factors

The condition of the gingiva and teeth reflects the patient's health habits and nutrition and can reflect the side effects of treatment for some conditions. With the aging process bone resorption and receding and pale gingiva can make the teeth appear larger. The teeth and gingiva can have problems with inflammation and drainage; teeth become loose, broken, or fall out, and gingiva is subject to gingival hypertrophy.

Purulent drainage from the gingiva can occur from an infectious process such as upper respiratory infections or a local abscess. Other inflammations can occur from poorly fitting dentures, leukemia, and HIV. *Candida albicans* can occur with white patches overlying reddened inflamed gingiva (Dillon, 2003). Periodontitis is inflammation of the area around the teeth. Brownish colored gums may reflect Addison's disease. Loose, broken, or missing teeth may result from general poor oral care, poor nutrition, or trauma. Gingival hypertrophy is a painless hyperplasia that can occur with pregnancy and some medications including phenytoin and calcium channel blockers (Dillon, 2003).

Physical Examination

The teeth and gingiva are integral to the eating and drinking of fluids. Their poor health can have an impact on overall health. The essential nursing physical assessment of the teeth and gingiva is described next. Referral to dental specialists is appropriate for routine care and treatment.

Inspection

Ask the patient to open his mouth. Does the patient have his own teeth, full dentures, partial dentures, or orthodontic appliances? Count the upper and lower teeth. The 32 teeth (or 28 if the third molars have been extracted) should be white and firmly set in the gingiva, with good occlusion. Are the teeth in good condition or do they have caries? Ask the patient when he last visited the dentist and how often he receives preventive care for his teeth. Observe for exposed root of the tooth from receding gums. If the patient wears dentures, do they fit well? A patient with loose teeth, dental decay, and discolored teeth should be referred to a dentist. The patient's breath should smell fresh.

Observe for redness, tenderness, edema, retraction, discoloration, or easy bleeding of the gingiva. This can represent gingivitis, scurvy, or poorly fitting dentures. Pale mucous membranes can be an indication that the patient is anemic. Oral cancer lesions usually associated with smoking and alcohol use can present on gums. Any lesion should be investigated by the health care provider.

Health Promotion

Dental visits should occur at regular intervals. Patients should be taught to floss their teeth to remove plaque and help with gingival health. A patient with gingival hypertrophy should visit the dentist more frequently and use a soft toothbrush to avoid irritation.

Buccal Mucosa

The buccal mucosa consists of the gingiva and the hard and soft palate. The palate forms the roof of the mouth and separates the mouth from the oropharynx. It is divided into the anterior hard palate and the posterior soft palate. The soft palate is flexible with chewing and swallowing and is covered with a thin mucosa membrane that extends to the uvula.

Current Health and Risk Factors

The oral mucosa is easy to assess for local and systemic problems. General nutritional status, infections, tumors, mouth sores, and pain can be easily identified. Normal oral mucosa is pink, moist, and intact and has no lesions. Poor nutritional status is seen in swollen, dry, and red mucosa. Mouth infections can occur especially when there is poor nutrition and inadequate dental care. Patients who use antibiotics or have HIV are susceptible to oral candidiasis, which manifests as white patches on an inflamed mucosa (Dillon, 2003).

Cancer of the mouth can occur on any part of the oral mucosa. The chance of developing oral cancer increases with habitual drinking of alcohol and the use of smoking and chewing tobacco. The symptoms of oral cancer are nonhealing lip or mouth sores, a mass in the mouth or throat, leukoplakia, bleeding, pain or numbness, chronic sore throat, foreign body sensation in the mouth or throat, dysphasia, a voice change, or ear pain (American Cancer Society, 2006).

Leukoplakia is a white adherent mucosal coating, which may lead to cancer. Stomatitis, also called mucositis, can occur as a secondary problem with patients who have decreased immune status, and as a consequence of radiation therapy or chemotherapy from cancer treatment. Canker sores, or herpes simplex, can occur with some frequency in some people.

It is important for the nurse to inquire about the location, duration, and intensity of mouth pain. Does the patient have a sore throat, and dental, jaw, or mouth pain, or any pain opening the jaw? The nurse needs to assess whether or not the patient has trismus which is restricted jaw movement and pain (Dillon, 2003).

Physical Examination

The normal buccal mucosa is moist, color consistent with that of gingiva, intact, and without bleeding or sores. When assessing the mouth the following areas should be evaluated: voice, swallow reflex, lips, tongue, saliva, mucous membrane, gingiva, teeth, or denture-bearing area.

Inspection

Prior to inspecting the mouth the nurse needs to request that the patient remove her dentures or other mouth prosthesis. The palate, dentures, and gingiva were discussed earlier. Inspect the tonsils for the presence or absence of edema, spots, exudates, lesions, or drainage. Tonsils are graded from 1+ (visible), 2+ (between pillars and uvula), 3+ (touching the uvula), to 4+ (one or both tonsils extend to the midline of the oropharynx).

Approximately 1,500 mL of saliva is produced daily by the Wharton's ducts, Stenson's ducts, parotid (beneath each ear), submandibular, sublingual (on the floor of the mouth), and buccal glands (the lips and cheeks). Wharton's ducts contain about 20 papillae and are located at the openings for the submandibular glands at the base of the tongue on either side of the frenulum. They should be patent, be secreting saliva, and be without lesions or inflammation.

Palpation

Palpate the oral mucosa with a gloved hand. Stenson's ducts, the openings for the parotid glands, are found at the second molars. Palpate with a gloved hand the floor of the mouth for swelling or tenderness of the tonsillar and submental lymph nodes. Note any palpable nodules, which may indicate cancer. Palpating the back of the oral cavity with a tongue blade will make the patient gag. This tests the sensory function of the hypoglossal nerve (CN IX) and the motor function of the vagus nerve (CN X).

Health Promotion

The National Guidelines box (p. 2296) recommends best practices for oral health include tooth brushing with fluoridated toothpaste twice a day. Avoid using hydrogen peroxide unless prescribed by a dentist or a health care provider.

■ Tongue

The tongue is a muscular organ essential to speaking and chewing food. The anterior two-thirds of the tongue is covered with papillae, which contain approximately 10,000 taste buds. People identify five different tastes: sweet, bitter, salty, and umami (glutamate found in chicken broth, meat extracts, and some cheeses) (National Institute on Deafness and Other Communication Disorders, 2002b). The intrinsic and extrinsic muscles of the tongue help move food during mastication. The extrinsic muscles are used during swallowing and speech.

Current Health and Risk Factors

The tongue can reflect the general health and local problems. Abnormalities of the tongue include inflammatory or infectious lesions, enlargement, allergic reactions, limited movement, and loss of sense of taste. Glossitis, an inflammation of the tongue, can be caused by chemotherapy or a vitamin B_{12}, iron, or niacin deficiency. *Candida albicans*, or thrush, can cause a thick white coating or redness on the tongue. Thrush can be caused by changes in normal flora from chemotherapy or radiation therapy, AIDS, antibiotic therapy, or alcohol, tobacco, or cocaine use (Dillon, 2003).

An enlarged tongue can occur with myxedema, acromegaly, Down's syndrome, or amyloidosis. Infectious processes such as glossitis can cause enlargement of the tongue. An allergic reaction can cause an enlarged tongue and subsequently compromise the airway.

A tongue that cannot move normally or a tongue paralyzed from trauma to CN XII or syringobulbia will cause difficulty with speaking and eating. A patient who has had a cerebrovascular accident may have limited movements of the tongue.

Sense of Taste

About 200,000 people each year visit health care providers with complaints of problems with their sense of taste. It frequently is associated with problems with their sense of smell. Loss of a sense of taste can be temporary or permanent. A diminished sense of taste is called hypogeusia. A complete loss of a sense of taste is called ageusia. Diminished sense of taste can be congenital, but it usually occurs from a head injury or an illness such as upper respiratory disorder. Exposure to chemicals such as insecticides and some medicines can cause a diminished sense of taste (National Institute on Deafness and Other Communication Disorders, 2002b). Patients who have received radiation therapy for head and neck cancer may have a diminished sense of taste. In addition, taste disorders can occur concurrently with obesity, diabetes, hypertension, malnutrition, Parkinson's disease, Alzheimer's disease, smoking, and Korsakoff's psychosis. The elderly experience changes in taste with less distinct perception of sweetness, reduced saliva, and thinner mucosa (National Institute on Deafness and Other Communication Disorders, 2002b).

Physical Examination

The tongue has multiple functions, each of which needs to be assessed during a physical examination. Changes or abnormalities of the tongue may indicate both a local and systemic disorder. The nurse must document and report changes to the health care provider.

Inspection

The tongue should be midline; the dorsum should be pink, moist, and rough (taste buds) and have no lesions. It should move freely and have symmetrical strength. The ventral surface should have large blood vessels visible, no lesions and no inflammation.

During the assessment the nurse evaluates the patient's ability to speak and swallow. The patient may need referral to a speech therapist who will evaluate and treat the speech deficit. Referral for a swallow study may be necessary if paralysis is present. The risk of aspiration increases with tongue paralysis.

To assess for proper functioning of the hypoglossal nerve (CN XII), ask the patient to stick out her tongue. Observe the dorsal surface for color, hydration, texture, symmetry, fasciculation, atrophy, position in the mouth, and the presence of lesions. There should be no pain, ulcerations, or lesions. The tongue should be pink, moist, symmetrical, and midline. The patient should be able to move the tongue up and down and side to side. Ask the patient to press the tongue against the cheek on each side. Also ask the patient to touch the tip of the tongue to the roof of the mouth. Ask the patient to taste and identify several different kinds of flavors. The ventral surface should be moist, rough from taste buds, have prominent blood vessels, and have no lesions.

Palpation

Palpate the submandibular glands in front of the ear. Use your gloved finger on the outside of the cheek to press against the tongue to assess bilateral tongue strength.

Tongue Monitoring Equipment

The nurse should use a gloved hand and a tongue blade to look carefully at all areas of the tongue. In addition, asking a patient to swallow a small sip of water will help assess swallowing. Listening to the patient speak will help assess speech and tongue movements. Test the patient's taste with sweet, bitter, salty, and many other flavors.

Health Promotion

To prevent allergic reactions to environmental allergens and medications that might cause edema of the tongue, the patient should wear a medic alert bracelet. Patient's who have allergies to bee stings should carry and be given instructions about how to use an EpiPen. A patient who has trouble swallowing because of limited tongue movement needs to be referred to a speech and swallowing therapist to learn techniques to swallow without choking or pocketing food. Any patient with a lesion on the tongue needs to see a health care provider who can diagnose and treat it.

■ Pharynx and Larynx

The pharynx and larynx integrate components of the respiratory, neurological, lymphatic, endocrine, vascular, and musculoskeletal systems. The larynx includes the supraglottis, glottis, and subglottis, the thyroid cartilage, and vocal cords. The trachea is a flexible cylindrical tube, 2.5 cm by 11 cm, extending in front of the esophagus from the cricoid cartilage to right and left bronchi. The trachea has C-shaped hyaline cartilage rings that protect the airway. The trachea is a passageway for air, and the esophagus is a passageway for food. Thyroid cartilage, cricoid cartilage, and epiglottis surround the larynx.

Current Health and Risk Factors

The patient may present with problems originating in the pharynx or larynx with difficulty speaking, breathing, or having a sense of a lump in his throat. These symptoms can be the result of tumor, infection or inflammation, foreign body, or trauma to

the neck and may be very painful. The patient should be encouraged to seek immediate treatment to preserve the airway. The patient's habits are also important to assess, including smoking and/or alcohol intake, because it is frequently associated with cancer of the vocal cord or larynx. A smoking history is expressed as packs per day for a number of years. Alcohol history is expressed as the number of drinks per day, kind of alcohol, and the number of years of drinking. Has the patient had any change in voice recently? Has the patient had any episodes of respiratory distress?

Tumors of the head and neck particularly occur with slow-growing basal cell carcinoma and rapidly invasive squamous cell carcinoma. Inquire about the patient's use of tobacco and ingesting alcohol. Diagnosis and treatment of head and neck cancer are discussed in Chapter 34 ⊚. A partial or total laryngectomy is the permanent removal of the voice box. From then on the patient breathes through the neck and will have to learn alternative methods of communication such as esophageal speech.

Neck and throat infections may be life threatening because of the potential to cause airway compromise. Epiglottitis, for example, is an infection of the supraglottic larynx usually caused by *Haemophilus influenzae* type B. Pharyngitis, which may include the tonsils, palate, and uvula, may be caused by bacteria, viruses, and fungi. An infection of the tonsils, tonsillitis, can be caused by bacteria or viruses. Inadequate treatment of tonsillitis may cause a peritonsillar abscess or quinsy sore throat.

A foreign body in the trachea requires emergency treatment. The Heimlich maneuver can be useful in dislodging the foreign body. If unsuccessful, take the patient to the emergency department immediately.

Trauma to the neck can occur from a sports injury or violence or may be work related and it can cause airway compromise and vocal change. Trauma damage requires immobilization, an x-ray, and immediate treatment to preserve the damaged airway.

Change in Voice

Change in the sound of the voice can occur from an infectious process, such as epiglottitis, or from neoplasms and chronic smoking. It also may occur from vocal cord paralysis, which is more common in elderly men than women. Thyroid surgery, anterior cervical fusion or carotid endarterectomy, and cancer of larynx and lung are the most common causes of vocal cord paralysis (Sigler, 2002). Vocal cord paralysis is a particularly important issue because of the potential for dyspnea and stridor to accompany it (Sigler, 2002). Inquire about how long the voice change has been present, whether it is getting worse, and whether there any other associated symptoms. Does the patient have difficulty swallowing food and saliva, which would indicate the presence of a mass? Chart 69–2 (p. 2296) in the chapter outlines the signs and symptoms of oral cancer. The patient's voice should be normal without any hoarseness, be clear and spontaneous, and not have a nasal intonation.

 *The nurse must investigate any changes in voice because they could relate to airway obstruction. The first priority is to assess oxygenation, so begin by checking the oxygen saturation and vital signs. Assess for shortness of breath. Report abnormal assessment findings to the health care provider.*

Physical Examination

The physical examination should address whether the patient has any of the above problems. Knowledge of normal anatomy of the structures of the neck is essential. It takes time and practice to learn how to inspect and palpate the thyroid, carotid artery, and lymph nodes.

Inspection

Observe the trachea for inflammation, pain, excessive salivation or dryness, drainage, masses, and lymphoid tissue in the throat. Inspect the neck in a neutral position and when hyperextended. It should be erect and midline and have no tracheal deviation or visible lumps, bulges, or masses. Involuntary contraction of the neck so that the neck tips to the side is acquired or congenital torticollis. Inspect the lower third of the neck for enlargement of the thyroid. Normally the thyroid is not visible and has no masses, swelling, or hypertrophy. Any enlargements may indicate malignant or benign disorders or infectious processes. Are lymph nodes visible or is the jugular vein distended? Is the patient in any respiratory distress? Does the patient have full range of motion of the neck?

Swallow and gag reflexes are tested with a tongue blade touching the back of the mouth, which causes gagging to occur. To test the glossopharyngeal nerve (CN IX) and vagus nerve (CN X), use a tongue depressor to press down on the tongue when the patient says "aaah." Note the rise and fall of the uvula and check for symmetry, edema, or discharge.

Palpation

Palpate the preauricular, postauricular, tonsillar, submandibular, and submental lymph nodes along the mandible between two fingers to determine the dimension, texture, and consistency. Palpable lymph nodes should be described according to shape, dimension, size, consistency, masses, crepitus, mobility, and tenderness. Palpable lymph nodes should be soft to rubbery, freely mobile, distinct, round, and nontender. Because the thyroid gland moves as a person swallows, ask the patient to swallow while palpating the thyroid gland from the anterior or posterior. An enlarged thyroid gland indicates thyroid disease, and further laboratory tests are warranted. Palpate the trachea for normal midline position and the absence of crepitus. Does the patient complain of any pain during palpation?

Auscultation

If a mass is palpated, auscultate the thyroid gland with the bell of the stethoscope over each lobe to identify a possible bruit. Normally there should be no thyroid sounds. Sounds are sometimes associated with hyperthyroidism (Dillon, 2003). Auscultate the larynx and trachea for breath sounds.

Pharynx and Larynx Monitoring Equipment

Patients who have pharyngeal or laryngeal problems may need to be assessed with a tongue blade and flashlight to inspect for pharyngeal tumors or drainage, and/or to test the gag reflex. Some patients need to have their oxygen saturation monitored. Some patients are dependent on alternative methods of breathing, for example, a patient with a tracheostomy, laryngectomy, or endotracheal or nasopharyngeal tube.

Health Promotion

The most important implication for health promotion measures that patients can take is to avoid the use of any tobacco products and minimize the use of alcohol. Patients who are on antibiotics need to be reminded to complete the cycle of medications. Families need to be taught the Heimlich maneuver.

■ Summary

Diseases of the ear, nose, and throat are some of the most common health problems that bring a patient to seek health care. The nurse has an important role in assessing the potential and actual problems associated with these disorders. Promoting healthy behaviors in relation to the ears, nose, and throat can help reduce the cost of health care. Early treatment can prevent increasing disability.

NCLEX® REVIEW

1. A patient's ear canal is shiny with brown sticky cerumen. The nurse would consider these findings as being:
   1. An infection.
   2. Normal.
   3. Evidence of a foreign body.
   4. Abnormal exudate.

2. A patient begins to sneeze soon after entering an examination room. Which of the following should the nurse ask this patient?
   1. How long have you had a head cold?
   2. How long have you been using nasal sprays?
   3. Has anyone ever told you that you snore when asleep?
   4. Do you think that there is something in the room causing you to sneeze?

3. An elderly patient has several sores on his gums and tells the nurse that he hasn't been to a dentist since he received his dentures. Which of the following should the nurse respond to this patient?
   1. Maybe you should stop wearing the dentures.
   2. Even though you have dentures, seeing a dentist regularly is necessary for good oral health.
   3. I'm sure that you don't miss going to the dentist.
   4. Those sores will heal; just give it some time.

4. An elderly patient sits quietly and does not engage in conversation with those seated nearby. The nurse realizes this patient might be experiencing:
   1. Mental status changes.
   2. Dementia.
   3. Social isolation because of hearing loss.
   4. Antisocial behavior disorder.

5. A patient is unable to hear words that the nurse whispers to the health care provider who is standing about two feet away from the patient. The nurse would interpret this finding as being:

   1. Normal.

   2. Evidence of hearing loss in the ear closest to the examiner.

   3. Evidence of acoustic nerve damage.

   4. Evidence of a blocked ear canal.

Answers for review questions appear in Appendix D

KEY TERMS

allergic rhinitis *p.2294*
anosmia *p.2294*
barotrauma *p.2292*
caloric test *p.2293*
cerumen *p.2284*
conductive hearing loss *p.2287*
epistaxis *p.2288*

fetid breath *p.2295*
obstructive sleep apnea (OSA) *p.2294*
otalgia *p.2291*
ototoxicity *p.2290*
pneumatoscope *p.2292*
Rinne test *p.2293*
Romberg test *p.2293*

Schwabach test *p.2293*
sensorineural hearing loss *p.2287*
tinnitus *p.2288*
trismus *p.2295*
vertigo *p.2291*
voice whisper test *p.2293*
Weber test *p.2292*

EXPLORE   **PEARSON**   **mynursingkit**™

MyNursingKit is your one stop for online chapter review materials and resources. Prepare for success with additional NCLEX®-style practice questions, interactive assignments and activities, web links, animations and videos, and more!

Register your access code from the front of your book at
www.mynursingkit.com

REFERENCES

American Academy of Audiology. (2003). *Position statement: Preventing noise-induced occupational hearing loss.* Retrieved February 1, 2004, from http://www.audiology.org/layouts/aaa/login. aspx?ReturnURL=%2fresources% 2fdocumentibray%2fPages%2fHearingConservation.apx

American Academy of Otolaryngology-Head and Neck Surgery. (1993). *Ear, altitude and airplane travel.* Alexandria, VA: Author.

American Cancer Society. (2006). *Cancer facts and figures 2006.* Atlanta, GA: Author.

Anderson, H. G., Cyr, M. M., Guadagnini, J. P., Hickey, M. M., Higgins, T. S., Harris, L. L., et al. (Eds.). (1998). *General history, risk factors, and normal physical assessment.* Huntoon, M. B. (Eds.) (1998) *Core curriculum for otorhinolaryngology and head and neck nursing.*

Bailey, K. (2004). Management of dysphagia in patients with advanced esophageal cancer. *Gastrointestinal Nursing, 2*(2), 18–22.

Chalupka, S. (2001). Essentials of environmental health, enhancing your occupational health nursing practice (part 1), *AAOHN Journal, 49*(3), 137–154.

Crummer, R. W., & Hassan, G. A. (2004). Diagnostic approach to tinnitus. *American Family Physician, 69*(1), 120–127.

Dillon, P. (2003). *Nursing health assessment.* Philadelphia: F. A. Davis.

Flemmons, W. (2002). Obstructive sleep apnea. *New England Journal of Medicine, 347*(7), 498–504.

Gupta, V., & Reiter, E. (2004). Current treatment practices in obstructive sleep apnea and snoring. *American Journal of Otolaryngology, 25*(1), 18–25.

Heron, R., & Wharrad, H. (2000). Prevalence and nursing staff awareness of hearing impairment in older hospital patients. *Journal of Clinical Nursing, 9*(6), 834–841.

Jafek, B. W., & Murrow, B. W. (2001). *ENT secrets* (2nd ed.). Philadelphia: Hanley & Belfus.

Kim, D., & Toriumi, D. (2003) What's new in otolaryngology–head and neck surgery? *Journal of American College of Surgeons, 297*(1), 97–114.

Koliha, C. A. (2003). Obstructive sleep apnea in head and neck cancer patients post treatment . . . something to consider. *ORL-Head and Neck Nursing, 21*(1), 10–14.

Marzo, S. (2003). Implantable hearing devices. *ORL-Head and Neck Nursing, 21*(4), 22–25.

MedicineNet. (2007). *Definition of trismus.* Retrieved on July 22, 2007, from http://www.medterms.com/script/main/art.asp?articlekey= 40739

Mosby *(2002) Mosby's medical, nursing, and allied health dictionary* (5th ed.). (2002). St. Louis: Mosby.

National Guideline Clearinghouse. (2004). *Nursing management of oral hygiene.* Retrieved from http://www.guideline.gov/summary/ summary.aspx?doc_id=7153&nbr=004285&string=ear+AND+ nose+AND+throat

National Guideline Clearinghouse. (2006). *Cough and aspiration of food and liquids due to oral-pharyngeal dysphagia: ACCP evidence-based clinical practice guidelines.* Retrieved February 17, 2007, from http://www.guideline.gov/summary/summary. aspx?ss= 15&doc.id=8664&string=ear+AND+nose+AND+throat

National Institute on Deafness and Other Communication Disorders. (2002a). *Smell and smell disorders fact sheet.* Bethesda, MD: Author.

National Institute on Deafness and Other Communication Disorders. (2002b). *Taste and taste disorders fact sheet.* Bethesda, MD: Author.

National Institutes of Health. (2006). *NIAID fact sheet: Sinusitis.* Retrieved March 24, 2007, from http://www.niaid.nih.gov/factsheets/ sinusitis.htm

Rabinowitz, P. (2000). Noise-induced hearing loss. *American Family Physician, 6*(5), 2749–2756, 2759–2760.

Sandhaus, S. (2002). Stop the spinning: Diagnosing and managing vertigo. *Nurse Practitioner, American Journal of Primary Health Care, 27*(8), 19–25.

Sigler, B. A. (2002). *Ear, nose and throat.* In J. M. Thompson, G. K. McFarland, J. E. Hirsch, & S. Tucker (Eds.), *Mosby's clinical nursing.* St. Louis: Mosby.

Smith, L., & Osborne, R. (2003). Infections of the head and neck. *Topics in Emergency Medicine, 25*(2), 106–116.

Spector, R. (2004). *Cultural diversity in health and illness* (6th ed.). Upper Saddle River, NJ: Pearson Prentice Hall.

Tierney, L. M., McPhee, S. J., & Papadakis, M. A. (Eds.). (2001). *Current medical diagnosis and treatment.* Stamford, CT: Appleton & Lange.

U.S. Department of Health and Human Services. (1997). *NIOSH pocket guide to chemical hazards.* Washington, DC: Author.

70 Caring for the Patient with Hearing and Balance Disorders

Barbara Moyer
Kathleen Osborn

With contributions by:
Dawna Martich

Outcome-Based Learning Objectives

After studying this chapter, the learner will be able to:

1. Identify and define the major structures included in the sense of hearing.
2. Compare and contrast the two mechanisms of hearing.
3. Distinguish the three types of hearing loss.
4. Apply health promotion strategies to prevent hearing loss in all age groups.
5. Compare and contrast the three different pathologic causes for a hearing disorder.
6. Discuss discharge priorities for a patient with a hearing disorder.
7. Explain specific aspects of the nursing management for a geriatric patient with a hearing disorder.
8. Apply the nursing process to a patient with a hearing disorder.

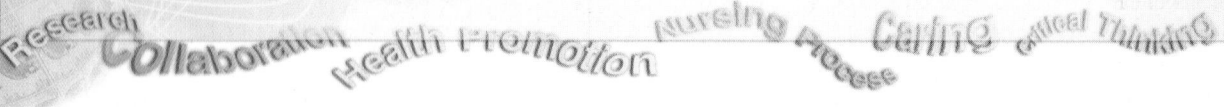

Research Collaboration Health Promotion Nursing Process Caring Critical Thinking

AN INTACT SENSE OF HEARING AND BALANCE is essential to health and daily function. Damage to the ears and accompanying structures will have a negative impact on individuals in all age groups. Identified as being one of the five major senses, hearing is often taken for granted. Many times an alteration in the sense of hearing is not detected until the person is questioned about her voice volume or atypical responses to environmental and verbal stimuli. Loss of hearing may lead to problems in both an individual's professional and personal life, and it also can impact safety. To function in society, one must be able to give and receive information accurately.

Balance also is partially controlled by the ear. A normal functioning inner ear is necessary to maintain body balance. Along with the ear, the joints, the muscles, and the eyes send messages to the cerebellar portion of the brain for coordination and perception. Problems with balance increase the risk for accidental falls, thereby impacting safety.

Anatomy and Physiology of the Ear

The complexities of hearing are best understood when each part of the ear is analyzed (Figure 70–1 ■). The ear is divided into three parts: external/outer, middle, and inner. The external or outer ear

is comprised of some structures visible to the naked eye and others that are not. The pinna, or the most visible portion of the ear, is made up of cartilaginous tissue. The pinna is the portion of the ear that is most easily seen. The pinna collects and directs sound waves into the external auditory ear canal. The ear canal is also made up of cartilaginous material and is relatively short at approximately 1 inch in length. Within this structure sits ceruminous and sebaceous glands that produce cerumen, which is commonly referred to as earwax. The bony portion of the ear canal, which covers the mastoid process, is also considered a structure of the external/outer ear. The tympanic membrane (eardrum), comprised of tissue that makes up the ear canal, is the final structure within this portion of the outer ear anatomy. It is this structure that transmits sounds from the outer to the middle ear.

The middle ear begins from the inner side of the tympanic membrane and extends to the eustachian tube. Within this portion of the ear sit the three auditory bones: the malleus, the incus, and the stapes (Figure 70–1 ■). The malleus is attached to the inner portion of the tympanic membrane. When the tympanic membrane vibrates with sound, so does the malleus. The incus is attached to the malleus and also vibrates in response to sound. The stapes is the structure that separates the middle from the inner ear. The base of the stapes, the footplate, fills the oval

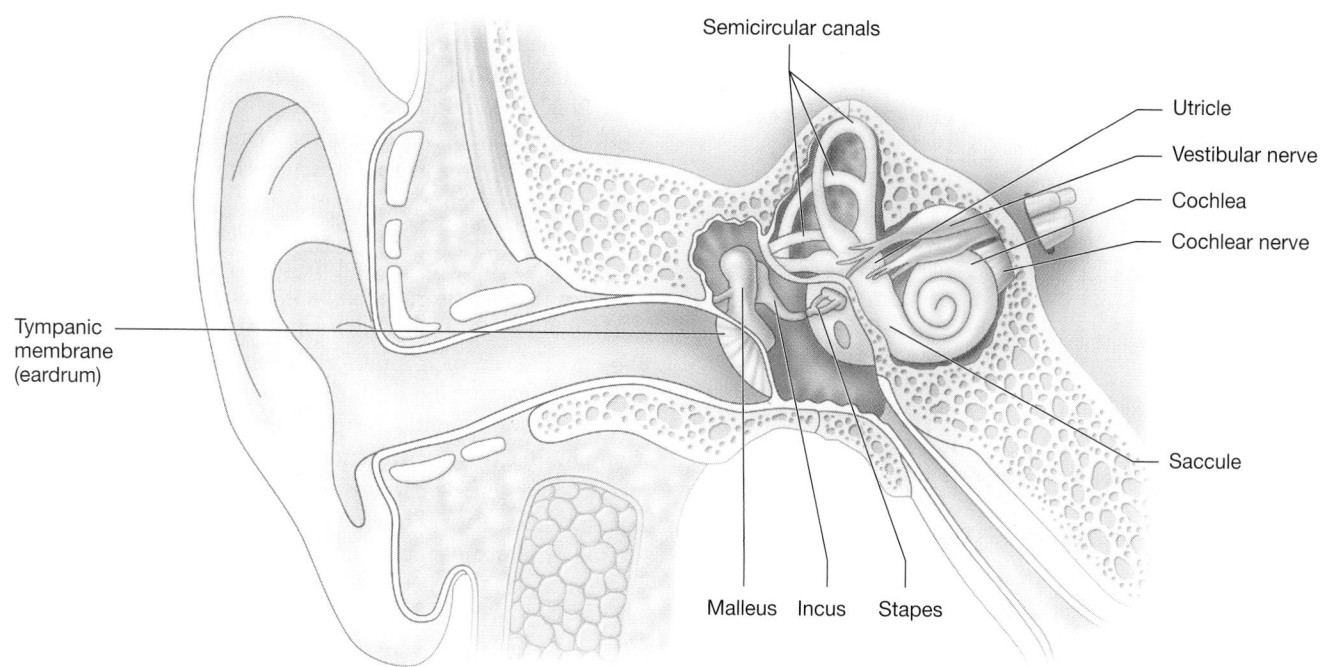

FIGURE 70–1 ■ Anatomical structures of the ear.
Source: AMA's Current Procedural Terminology, Revised 1998 Edition.

window, which leads to the inner ear. The footplate of the stapes fits tightly into a tiny oval window of the bony cochlea that opens into the inner ear. The stapes vibrates and makes the fluid in the inner ear vibrate.

The inner ear includes the cochlea, the vestibular system that contains the bony labyrinth and the semicircular canals, and the acoustic nerve. The cochlea is responsible for hearing, whereas the vestibular system is responsible for balance. The cochlea, shaped like a snail, contains a structure termed the organ of Corti. The small hairs within this organ change sound vibrations into neural signals that are transmitted to the brain via the acoustic nerve. The bony labyrinth consists of the saccule and utricle, organs that provide position sense. Within the inner ear are found the semicircular canals, specifically the horizontal, anterior, and posterior canals, which help with balance and movement. The acoustic nerve consists of two separate parts, the vestibular and cochlear branches. This eighth cranial nerve (CN) controls hearing and equilibrium.

Mechanism of Hearing

There are actually two mechanisms involved with hearing: bone conduction and air conduction. **Bone conduction** is the conduction of sound to the inner ear through the bones of the skull. **Air conduction** begins the process when noise enters the external ear and travels to the middle ear. Once inside the middle ear, the sound is transmitted through the three auditory bones, the malleus, incus, and stapes. Once the sound or noise reaches the stapes, it is then transmitted to the inner ear where it reaches the acoustic nerve and is transmitted to the brain for interpretation. Hearing disorders can be caused by an alteration anywhere within the auditory structures.

■ Etiology and Epidemiology of Hearing Impairment

The most prevalent disorder associated with the structures of the ear is hearing loss. This disorder is estimated to affect approximately 30 million Americans and is considered a chronic health condition seen in all types of people in all age groups, although the percentage of those affected accelerates with age. Also, men are twice as likely as women to have hearing loss (Isaacson, 2005). The degree of hearing loss can range from mild to complete. Causes of this disorder are varied and have distinct types: conductive, sensorineural, or mixed. In **conductive hearing loss**, sound waves cannot reach the inner ear for processing and interpretation. With **sensorineural hearing loss**, the cause is damage to the auditory nerve or possibly damage to the small hair cells within the inner ear. **Mixed hearing loss** refers to both conductive and sensorineural hearing loss caused by a dysfunction of both air and bone conduction processes.

In the case of sensorineural hearing loss caused by noise, the culprit is prolonged exposure to sounds with an elevated decibel level. Typically, exposure to decibel levels of 85 or greater can lead to sensorineural hearing loss (American Academy of Otolaryngology–Head and Neck Surgery [AAO-HNS], 2002). Higher decibel levels cause death of nerve endings in the ear structures. Over time, and if enough of the nerve endings are damaged or destroyed, hearing loss will occur. Nerve endings will not regenerate therefore this type of hearing loss is permanent. Chart 70–1 (p. 2304) describes causes of conductive and sensorineural hearing loss in more detail.

Sounds create vibrations measured in frequencies. A sound with a low frequency vibrates slower than a sound with a high

CHART 70–1 **Causes of Conductive and Sensorineural Hearing Loss**

Conductive Hearing Loss	Sensorineural Hearing Loss
Buildup of cerumen (earwax) in the auditory canal	Aging
Infection of the external or middle ear (otitis media)	Head injury
	Infection
	Ototoxic medications
Fluid in the middle ear	Genetics
A punctured eardrum	Prolonged noise exposure
Edema	Myxedema
Tumors	Labyrinthitis
Foreign body	Diabetes mellitus
Otosclerosis	Acoustic neuroma
Perforation of the tympanic membrane	Ménière's disease
	Presbycusis

frequency. With a loss or change in the nerve endings in the ear structures, the brain is unable to pick up or interpret these frequencies. The first change seen in individuals with sensorineural hearing loss is a loss of high-frequency sounds. This manifests as the inability to interpret or understand the words spoken by females or children in addition to losing the ability to discern the spoken sounds of *s, f, sh, ch, h,* or a soft *c.* The last type of hearing loss, mixed, is caused by both conductive and sensorineural factors.

Pathophysiology and Treatment of Hearing Impairment or Loss

The causes of hearing impairment or loss can be categorized as mechanical, inflammatory, or an obstructive disorder. Causes of mechanical hearing loss include external otitis, exostosis, foreign bodies, trauma, and otosclerosis. **Otitis externa,** or swimmer's ear, is an infection of the skin covering the outer ear canal. External otitis is commonly a bacterial infection caused by *Streptococcus, Staphylococcus,* or pseudomonal types of bacteria. Swimmer's ear is usually caused by excessive water exposure. When water pools in the ear canal (frequently trapped by earwax), the skin becomes soggy, diluting the acidity that normally prevents infection. A cut in the lining of the ear canal also can allow bacteria to penetrate the skin. When this happens bacteria and fungi (from contaminated water or objects placed in the ear) continue to grow and the ear canal gets red and swollen. Diffuse external otitis can lead to irreversible skin conditions, canal stenosis, and deafness.

Exostosis, or surfer's ear, is a condition of the ear canal in which the bony lining under the skin develops a number of lumps that grow into the tube. Exostosis is found among salt-water enthusiasts, usually males 20 to 39 years of age (UCSD Student Health Service, 2007). Possibly due to cold water, the bony portion of the external canal becomes thickened and eventually creates a knoblike projection. Over time, several of these bony growths may close the ear canal causing hearing loss. The condition is painless and may go unnoticed for a number of years until hearing loss becomes obvious. Surgical removal of the outgrowths is necessary to restore hearing.

The lodging of a foreign body within the ear canal also causes a reduction in hearing and possible blockage of cerumen. Treatment in this case is to remove the foreign body and instruct the individual to avoid placing objects within the ear. This occurs most frequently in small children. The nurse should provide parents or caregivers with instructions on what is the appropriate size toy for each age group of young children.

Traumatic injury to the ear can also lead to a mechanical loss of hearing caused by a rupture of the tympanic membrane (eardrum). This disorder can be the result of a sudden trauma such as a head injury or skull fracture, explosive injury, or severe blow to the ear, or from a foreign object pushed into the ear canal. Most tympanic membrane ruptures heal spontaneously within weeks to months. Surgical intervention in the form of a **tympanoplasty,** reconstruction of the tympanic membrane, is needed to restore damage to the membrane and possible middle ear structures. Patient teaching includes ways to reduce the likelihood of tympanic membrane rupture such as protect the ears in blast areas (construction workers), avoid instrumentation such as cotton-tipped applicators, and avoid water sports until cleared by the health care provider.

Another mechanical cause of hearing loss is due to otosclerosis or a primary bone dyscrasia that leads to conductive hearing loss. **Otosclerosis** is a condition in which the structures of the ear begin to harden. Symptoms of this disorder are hearing loss, tinnitus, and dizziness and other sensations of motion. Otosclerosis affects both ears in 80% of patients (Kim, Chang, & Lim, 2000). Also, hearing might appear to be better in noisy environments. Seen as a common cause of conductive hearing loss, treatment options are limited to a **stapedectomy.** A stapedectomy is a surgical procedure in which the innermost bone (stapes) is removed and replaced with a small plastic tube of stainless steel wire (prosthesis) to improve the movement of the sound to the inner ear. Under local or general anesthesia, the surgeon opens the ear canal and uses an operating microscope to separate the stapes from the incus. Next a laser vaporizes the tendon and arch of the stapes bone, which helps remove it from the middle ear. The surgeon opens the window that joins the middle ear to the inner ear and acts as a platform for the stapes bone. Finally, the laser makes a tiny opening and gently clips the prosthesis to the incus bone. This prosthesis bridges the gap between the incus and the inner ear providing sound conduction.

Hearing loss due to an inflammatory process is seen in conditions that cause the accumulation of drainage in the ear canal (otitis external, acute/chronic otitis media), and chronic mastoiditis. When exposed to pathogens, as in otitis externa or media, the individual can usually recall a recent infective process such as the flu or a cold. Possibly the individual might have recently participated in water-related activities. In both diagnoses the patient experiences fullness in the ears with varying degrees of hearing impairment and pain. Depending on the cause, treatment could be with local or systemic antibiotics and instruction to protect the ears. Should the offending organism be isolated to the middle ear area and if the infections reoccur frequently, further treatment may include tube placement or other surgical interventions. The insertion of tubes in the ears, or a **myringotomy,** can be done on an outpatient basis. After creating an incision in the tympanic membrane (eardrum), a small plastic or metal tube is placed through the opening. The purpose of the tube is to ventilate the middle ear and equalize the pressure within the ear and the outside environment. The tubes typically stay in place for 6 to 12 months or until they spontaneously fall out. Anyone with tubes in the ears should avoid getting water inside them. After removal, if the symptoms return, the tubes might need to be reinserted.

An acute or chronic infection of the mastoid process can also lead to changes in hearing and balance referred to as **mastoiditis**. Most often the cause of mastoiditis is a bacterial infection. The individual will experience signs of a systemic infection along with drainage from the ear and subsequent changes in hearing and position sense. Systemic antibiotics are usually the first treatment. However, if chronic mastoiditis occurs, a **mastoidectomy** (removal of the mastoid process) is indicated. This procedure can either be done through the ear or externally through an incision to the occipital bone. Postoperative care depends on the approach used in addition to prevention of infection, maximizing safety, and promoting healing.

An obstruction might be the cause of the change in a person's ability to hear. Examples of such obstructions may include a malignancy within any of the ear structures or a benign acoustic neuroma, described in Chart 70–2 (p. 2306). In the case of a malignancy, surgical intervention and subsequent chemotherapeutic agents may be required. This depends on the type of malignancy following identification of the cause of hearing change. With an acoustic neuroma, treatment begins with surgical removal of the neuroma followed by medications and therapy as prescribed.

Hearing Loss in the Newborn

Hearing loss can have a variety of causes. In the newborn, it can be linked to birth trauma, toxicity, infection, fetal anoxia during delivery, premature or low birth weight, genetics, or an elevated serum bilirubin level. In addition, deafness upon birth has been seen in those women who have been exposed to highly communicable diseases such as rubella and syphilis or who have ingested known **ototoxic** (impairs hearing and balance) medications while pregnant. Ototoxic medications are outlined in Chart 70–3 (p. 2307).

The presence of hearing can be assessed as early as 2 to 3 days of life. Hearing loss is one of the most common developmental abnormalities present at birth. Approximately 1 to 3 infants per 1,000 are born with significant hearing loss. If left undiagnosed, it will impede speech, language, and cognitive developments. Currently 27 states and the District of Columbia have mandatory early hearing screening programs (National Conference of State Legislators, 2007). Individuals with hearing impairment at this early age will face a lifetime of challenges. Learning how to communicate with sign language and lip reading are just two ways to aid the person born without the sense of hearing.

 CRITICAL ALERT *Sudden hearing loss is considered a medical emergency. Individuals who suddenly lose their hearing should seek immediate medical attention.*

Hearing Loss in Children

Otitis media, an inflammation of the middle ear, is the most frequently diagnosed disease in infants and children. The eustachian tube, a passage between the middle ear and the back of the throat, is smaller and more nearly horizontal in children than adults. Thus it is more easily blocked by conditions such as large adenoids and infections. Until this tube changes in size and angle as the child grows, children are more susceptible to otitis media. As mentioned, the three tiny bones in the middle ear carry sound vibrations from the eardrum to the inner ear. When fluid is present, the vibrations are not transmitted. This results in mild or even moderate hearing loss. Generally this type of hearing loss is conductive and temporary. Repeated episodes of otitis media, however, may lead to permanent sensorineural hearing loss. Genetic factors are thought to cause more than 50% of all incidents of congenital hearing loss in children (Smith & Camp, 2007). Some genetic syndromes such as Down syndrome may lead to hearing loss. Finally, there are a variety of conditions that may cause acquired hearing loss (loss after birth). Some examples are ear infections, meningitis, measles, encephalitis, chickenpox, influenza, mumps, head injury, use of ototoxic drugs, and noise exposure.

Hearing Loss in Adults

Hearing loss in adults affects all portions of the ear. Some causes of outer and middle ear sound wave interference are malformation, skull fractures, infections, impacted earwax or foreign objects, a punctured eardrum, or a cyst or tumor. The most common causes of hearing loss in adults are damage to the structures of the inner ear and damage to the auditory nerve that sends those impulses to the brain (University of Iowa Hospital & Clinics, 2006). Other causes are injury, exposure to noise, infection or disease, use of ototoxic drugs (salicylates, aminoglycosides, antibiotics, loop diuretics), tumors, trauma (including acoustic neuroma), and the aging process. Other conditions are otosclerosis and Ménière's disease.

Hearing Loss in Older Adults

Hearing loss is one of the three most common chronic conditions among older adults after high blood pressure and arthritis. Approximately 25% to 40% of adults older than 65 years have some degree of hearing loss, and it is estimated that 40% to 60% of people ages 75 years or older have hearing loss commonly caused by gradual changes in the inner ear (Parmet, Lynm, & Glass, 2003). **Presbycusis** is the loss of hearing that gradually occurs in most individuals as they grow older. Presbycusis is usually a sensorineural hearing disorder. It is most commonly caused by gradual changes in the inner ear as a result of loss of hair cells in the organ of Corti within the ear. The individual might first experience the symptom of **tinnitus**, a constant ringing or roaring within their ears, and then over time the degree of hearing loss will vary. Some individuals might have loss of the middle ranges of hearing. Others might be unable to hear normal conversation in a noisy room. Treatment of this type of loss usually involves a hearing aid.

Hearing loss can also be caused by a virus or bacteria, changes in blood supply to the ear because of heart conditions or stroke, head injuries, tumors, and certain medications previously mentioned. Sometimes presbycusis is a conductive hearing disorder, meaning the loss of sound sensitivity caused by abnormalities of the outer and/or middle ear. Such abnormalities may include reduced function of the tympanic membrane or reduced function of the three tiny bones in the middle ear that carry sound waves from the tympanic membrane to the inner ear.

CHART 70–2 **Common Disorders of the Ear**

Disorder	Cause	Clinical Manifestations	Treatment
External Ear			
Otitis externa (swimmers' ear)	Hot humid environment Water sports Sharp objects that cause open lesions Headphones	Open lesions Itching Pain with movement of tragus Plugged ear Pressure Hearing loss Exudate	Reduce local inflammation and pain Moist heat Topical antibiotics Topical steroids Pain medications Instruct patient not to use cotton-tipped applicators Instruct patient to use earplugs when swimming
Cerumen or foreign body	Cerumen buildup Small objects placed in ear	Pressure Pain Hearing loss	Irrigation Mineral oil
Middle Ear			
Otitis media Acute Chronic Serous	Infectious agent in middle ear causes swelling of mucosa and ossicles If untreated may cause rupture of tympanic membrane	Pressure Pain Hearing is diminished Headache Malaise Fever Nausea Vomiting	Systemic antibiotics Rest Quiet environment Analgesics Antipyretics Antihistamines Myringotomy
Mastoiditis	Complication of otitis media	Swelling behind the ear Pain with movement of tragus, pinna, or head Localized cellulitis	Systemic antibiotics Surgical removal (mastoidectomy) of involved tissue, if no response to antibiotics
Trauma to the tympanic membrane	Complication of infection Rapid changes in middle ear cavity pressure Direct damage with a foreign body (pencil) Slapping of external ear Excessive nose blowing	Hearing loss (transient or permanent) Pain	Avoid inserting objects into the ear Hearing aid Surgical reconstruction of the ossicles and tympanic membrane
Inner Ear			
Tinnitus	Medications Trauma Ménière's disease	Mild ringing to loud roaring that may disturb thought and attention span	Stop medications. No cure if cause cannot be found. Mask sound with noise, music, and background sound during sleep. Ear molds and hearing aids can amplify sounds to drown out tinnitus. Contact American Tinnitus Association for further therapy.
Labyrinthitis	Infection of the labyrinth from a complication of otitis media	Hearing loss on affected side Tinnitus Spontaneous nystagmus to the affected side Vertigo with associated nausea and vomiting	Systemic antibiotics Stay in darkened room Antiemetics Antivertiginous medications
Ménière's disease	Either overproduction or decreased reabsorption of endolymphatic fluid causing a distortion in the inner canal system	Tinnitus Unilateral sensorineural hearing loss Vertigo Clinical manifestations occur in attacks that can last for several days	Instruct to move head slowly to prevent worsening of vertigo Salt and fluid restrictions Stop smoking Antivertiginous medications Antiemetics Mild diuretics Antihistamines Antianxiety medications Labyrinthectomy Endolymphatic decompression
Acoustic neuroma	Benign tumor of CN VIII	Mild vertigo Tinnitus Gradual sensorineural hearing loss	Surgical removal with resultant permanent hearing loss

CHART 70–3	Ototoxic Medications

Chemotherapeutic Agents That Can Cause Ototoxicity

Actinomycin	Methchlorethamine
Bleomycin	Methotrexate
Carboplatin	Nitrogen mustard
Cisplatin	Procarbazine
DCM	Vincristine
Fluorouracil	

Antibiotics with a High Potential for Ototoxicity

Amikacin	Lincomycin
Ampicillin	Metronidazole
Capreomycin	Minocycline
Chloramphenicol	Neomycin
Clindamycin	Netilmicin
Colistin	Polymyxin B
Dihydrostreptomycin	Streptomycin
Erythromycin	Tobramycin
Etiomycin	Vancomycin
Gentamicin	Viomycin
Kanamycin	

Antibiotics with a Suspicion for Ototoxicity

Floxins

Diuretics with a High Degree of Ototoxicity

Bumetanide	Furosemide
Diamox	Mannitol
Ethacrynate acid	Torsemide
Ethacrynate sodium	Piretanide

Medications with Quinidine Known to Produce Ototoxicity

Atabrine	Plaquenil
Chloroquine	Quinidex
Lariam (mefloquine)	Quinine sulfate

Ototoxicity Associated with Aspirin and NSAIDs

Advil	Lodine
Aleve	Naprosyn
Anaprox (Naproxen)	Nuprin
Dolobid	Relafen
Feldene	Toradol
Ibuprofen (Motrin)	Voltaren
Indocin	

Ototoxicity Associated with Aspirin

Ascriptin	Empirin
Bufferin	Excedrin
Disalcid	Fiorinal
Ecotrin	Trilisate

Ototoxicity Associated with Analgesics

Hydrocodone with acetaminophen

Exposure to Environmental Chemicals

Butyl nitrite	Mercury
Carbon disulfide	Styrene
Carbon monoxide	Tin
Hexane	Toluene
Lead	Trichloroethylene
Manganese	Xylene

Chemicals

Alcohol	Metals
Aniline dyes	Nicotine
Caffeine	Potassium bromide
Carbon monoxide	Povidone–iodine

Sources: Gale encyclopedia of medicine (3rd ed.). (2006). Farmington Hills, MI: Gale Cengage; http://www.dizziness-and-balance.com; http://www.healthatoz.com; Vestibular Disorders Association (2004, February 16), http://www.vestibular.org.

Noise-Induced Hearing Loss

Noise-induced hearing loss (NIHL) is seen most frequently after an individual has had a prolonged exposure to noise or sound at the level of 85 to 90 dB or a sudden exposure to sound/noise at greater than 90 dB. Often viewed as an occupational hazard, NIHL can occur in anyone who has been exposed to loud noises or sounds. Treatment of NIHL begins with overnight rest. Removing the source of the noise or sound with rest typically restores hearing function. Continuous exposure may cause permanent damage. Individuals who have repeated exposure, such as factory/construction workers, rock musicians, and other individuals exposed to loud sounds on a regular basis, should be counseled to use protective devices. For research about NIHL, see the Evidence-Based Practice box (p. 2308).

Acoustic Neuroma

Acoustic neuroma is a benign tumor of the eighth cranial nerve (Chart 70–2). As the tumor grows it extends from the internal auditory canal to the cerebellopontine angle, the angle between the cerebellum and pons, a common site for the growth of acoustic neuromas, and eventually presses on the brainstem. Clinical manifestations include tinnitus and unilateral sensorineural hearing loss, which may progress to mild vertigo. As the tumor enlarges other cranial nerves are impacted.

After the unilateral hearing loss has been confirmed, definitive diagnosis is made by computed tomography (CT) and magnetic resonance imaging (MRI). Surgical removal via a craniotomy is necessary, with permanent loss of hearing on the affected side.

Balance and Equilibrium

Balance of the body is maintained by the interactions between the eyes, the joints and muscles (proprioceptive system), the brain, and the labyrinth (vestibular apparatus). These structures all function together to maintain position sense and equilibrium.

Noise-Induced Hearing Loss

Clinical Problem

Exposure to excessive loud sounds causes damage to sensitive hair cells in the inner ear and to the nerve of hearing. Every day, people experience sound in the environment such as sounds from television and radio, traffic, and equipment. Normally these sounds are at safe levels that do not affect hearing. When exposed to excessive loud and repetitive loud sounds, the pure force of these vibrations can cause damage to hair cells leading to noise-induced hearing loss (NIHL).

Research Findings

The National Institutes of Health is conducting several research studies on NIHL. One is looking at the effects of noise on hair cells within the ear. Findings thus far support that noise damages these hair cells, leading to a hearing loss. Another study is trying to determine if noise causes a disruption in the blood flow to the cochlea within the ear. Researchers are studying the effects of peripheral vascular disease medication to maintain blood flow to the cochlea while exposed to noise that would otherwise lead to NIHL. Both of these studies are still under investigation.

Implications for Nursing Practice

Nurses should serve as advocates in the prevention, education, identification, and interventions for individuals with NIHL. They also should promote healthy lifestyle practices for all individuals who are at risk for NIHL.

Critical Thinking Questions

1. Identify ways to prevent NIHL.
2. Who is affected by NIHL?
3. What types of activities predispose individuals to the development of NIHL?

Answers to Critical Thinking Questions appear in Appendix D.

Reference

Dangerous decibels. (2007). Retrieved September 26, 2008, from http://www.dangerousdecibels.org.

An alternation or change in any one of their functioning will lead to a disorder with balance (Figure 70–2 ■).

Balance Disorders

The primary symptom of a balance disorder is the development of vertigo. Defined as an attack of dizziness, **vertigo** is often described as a "spinning" sensation. This sensation can last from 10 minutes up to several hours or days. Oftentimes, the most comfortable position for a patient experiencing vertigo is lying flat, immobilizing the head. Sudden head movements can precipitate nausea and vomiting. In addition to irritability, the patient might complain of tinnitus and reduced hearing on the involved side. The Risk Factors box outlines the risk factors associated with balance disorders.

The term *motion sickness* is often used to describe the symptoms associated with vertigo. In motion sickness, vertigo is present with nausea and possible vomiting. Motion causes

nystagmus, an oscillation of the eyes that is linked to the body's ability to maintain balance with motion or movement. Treatment includes reducing the motion and possibly using antiemetic (Droperidol) and antivertiginous (Dramamine) medications until the sensation passes.

Labyrinthitis

One of the pathophysiological causes of vertigo is **labyrinthitis** (Chart 70–2, p. 2306). Labyrinthitis, an inflammation of the inner ear, affects both the cochlear and/or vestibular portion of the labyrinth. A recent infection within the sinuses or upper respiratory tract might be the cause. Infection can enter from the meninges, the middle ear, or from the bloodstream. The individual experiences a sudden onset of dizziness and vertigo that might last briefly, such as 3 to 6 days. Seen as self-limiting, the dizziness and vertigo might take up to 6 weeks to resolve. Tinnitus, nausea and vomiting, hearing loss, and spontaneous nystagmus also occur. Meningitis, or infection in the brain, is a complication of labyrinthitis.

If chronic, the individual might need surgical intervention in the form of a labyrinthectomy or **vestibular nerve dissection** to reduce the impulses and remove the subjective sensation of dizziness/vertigo. A **labyrinthectomy** (removal of the labyrinth) will cause total deafness of the affected ear. In the case of a vestibular nerve dissection, the patient will need a craniotomy to access the vestibular nerve. The surgeon will partially sever the nerve. The outcome will be a reduction or removal of the vertigo and hearing loss. Diagnostic tests for vestibular function are outlined in the Diagnostic Tests for Vestibular Function box (p. 2310). Treatments are outlined on Chart 70–2 (p. 2306).

Other infectious causes of balance disorders include the common cold, childhood diseases such as measles and mumps, and more complex diseases such as meningitis, encephalitis, and syphilis. The common cold is discussed in Chapter 34 ⚙, and meningitis and encephalitis are discussed in Chapter 29 ⚙.

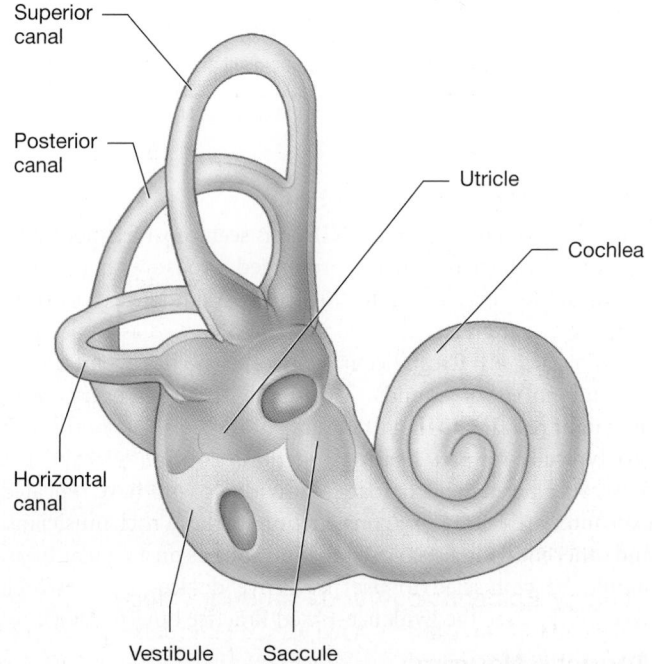

FIGURE 70–2 ■ Anatomical structures of balance.
Source: Balance Disorders (NIH Publication No. 00-4374).

RISK FACTORS Associated with Balance Disorders or Problems

Things to Avoid	Things to Encourage
Driving vehicles if dizzy or unsteady	Change positions slowly
Operating hazardous machinery	Move from lying to upright position in stages
Prolonged periods of standing	Remove throw rugs, litter, and avoid highly polished floors
Exposure to excessive heat or sunlight	Use assistive devices for picking things up from floor
Climbing step ladders	Replace fluids if excess fluid loss
Stooping to pick things up from floor	Take antihypertensive medications after meals
Using over-the-counter medications	Apply nonslip surfaces in bathtub or shower
Using alcohol or drugs that cause vertigo	Provide hand grips in bathroom
Smoking in bed or near oxygen	Provide railings in hallways and stairs
Prolonged bed rest, which causes skeletal muscle weakness and tone	Remove protruding objects (hooks, shelves) from stairway walls
Unsafe conditions while cooking	Wear shoes or slippers with nonskid soles
Increased susceptibility to glare	Install good lighting in hallways or stairs
High heels or unsafe footwear	
Things that cause increased dizziness	
Medications and chemicals that cause vertigo:	Avoid when possible
Alcohol	
Aminoglycosides	
Anticonvulsants	
Antihypertensives	
Cocaine	
Cytotoxic agents	
Furosemide	
Nitroglycerin	
NSAIDs (indomethacin)	
Salicylates	
Tranquilizers	

Ménière's Disease

A second pathologic cause of vertigo, **Ménière's disease**, is defined as a metabolic alteration in the labyrinthine fluid. Individuals with this diagnosis experience a sudden onset of dizziness, nausea, vomiting, giddiness, and hearing loss that can range from several minutes to hours or days in length. Treatment includes medications (Chart 70–3, p. 2307 and in the Pharmacology Summary on p. 2313) and avoidance of tobacco, alcohol, and caffeine. If extremely limiting, surgical intervention includes surgical destruction of the labyrinth with resulting irreversible hearing loss. Another procedure that is done early in the disease is endolymphatic decompression. A small tube is placed in the endolymphatic sac to allow for drainage to reduce vertigo. Treatments are outlined in Chart 70–2 (p. 2306).

Benign Paroxysmal Positional Vertigo

In benign paroxysmal positional vertigo (BPPV) the symptom of dizziness is thought to be due to the formation of otoconia, which are small crystals of calcium carbonate derived from the utricle (Figure 70–1 ■, p. 2303).

Etiology, Epidemiology, and Pathophysiology

The formation occurs due to the utricle being damaged by head injury, infection, or other disorder of the inner ear, or it may have degenerated because of advanced age. Viruses affecting the ear causing vestibular neuritis, minor strokes involving the an-

terior inferior cerebellar artery, and Ménière's disease are significant but unusual causes. BPPV is also common in persons who have been treated with ototoxic medications such as gentamicin (Black, Pesznecker, Homer, & Stallings, 2004). In about 50% of the cases, the cause is idiopathic. BPPV accounts for approximately 20% of all occurrences of dizziness in the general population and about 50% in the older population (Hain, 2007).

Clinical Manifestations

The symptoms of BPPV include dizziness or vertigo, lightheadedness, imbalance, and nausea. Activities that bring on the symptoms of BPPV vary among individuals, although a change in position most commonly precipitates them. It is the change in the position of the head with respect to gravity that causes the vertigo. Getting out of bed and/or rolling over in bed are triggers. As the name implies, BPPV may be present for a few weeks, then stop, then come back again (Hain, 2007).

Diagnostic Procedures

A variety of diagnostic tests are used to help in the diagnosis of hearing and balance disorders. The diagnosis is made based on the patient's medical history, findings on physical examination, and the results of vestibular and auditory tests. The medical history must evaluate the use of ototoxic medications and a review of what triggers the symptoms. It is significant if the dizziness is triggered by lying down or by rolling over in bed.

DIAGNOSTIC TESTS for Vestibular Function

Test	Normal	Expected Abnormality	Hearing Loss
Caloric test (assesses the degree of vestibular and brainstem function, differentiating peripheral lesions from CN VIII lesions) (Sandhaus, 2002) Perform only if tympanic membrane is intact. Irrigate the ear canal with a few drops of cold water.	Nausea, horizontal nystagmus, vertigo toward unirrigated side.	No eye movement (nystagmus) in unconscious patient	Impaired brainstem function
Romberg test (assesses ability to maintain an upright posture when arms are out in front, with eyes open and closed) Stand with feet close together without swaying with eyes open and eyes closed.	Slight swaying is normal. If patient maintains balance, the Romberg test is negative.	Swaying and inability to maintain balance	Impairment in inner ear balance (vestibular nerve [CN VIII] functions), proprioceptive ability, visual, and cerebellar

The Dix-Hallpike test is used to aid the diagnosis. The patient is brought from sitting to a supine position, with the head turned 45 degrees to one side and extended about 20 degrees backward. If the test is positive, the patient will experience a burst of nystagmus (jumping of the eyes). The eyes jump upward as well as twist so that the top part of the eye jumps toward the down side. Electronystagmography (ENG) testing may be needed to look for the characteristic nystagmus (jumping of the eyes) induced by the Dix-Hallpike test and an MRI scan is done if a stroke or brain tumor is suspected (Hain, 2007).

When evaluating a person's ability to hear, three characteristics are assessed: frequency, pitch, and intensity. **Frequency** is the number of sound waves emanating per second and is measured in Hertz (Hz). The ability to hear frequencies from 500 to

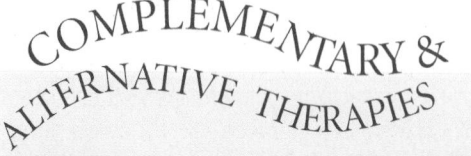

COMPLEMENTARY & ALTERNATIVE THERAPIES   T'ai Chi

Description:

T'ai chi chun (TCC), often called just t'ai chi, is an Asian form of exercise that dates back to the 12th century. It is comprised of a series of flowing, graceful movements designed to circulate the body's vital energy, or chi. Those who practice t'ai chi do so to increase their balance, circulation, and overall health. T'ai chi has become a popular method of exercising to maintain good health.

Research Support:

Studies on t'ai chi published from 1996 and 2004 show that it may have the following benefits:

- better balance
- less fear of falling
- greater strength
- greater functional mobility
- increased flexibility
- improved psychological well-being
- better sleep for elderly individuals who are sleep disturbed
- improved cardiovascular functioning

One study examined whether t'ai chi improves balance, muscular strength and endurance, and flexibility in older adults with at least one cardiovascular disease (CVD) risk factor. The study involved 39 older Chinese adults who engaged in a 60-minute t'ai chi class three times per week for 12 weeks. Researchers found that t'ai chi created statistically significant improvements in all balance, muscular strength and endurance, and flexibility measures after 6 weeks. Those improvements also increased further after 12 weeks. Researchers concluded that t'ai chi is a valid intervention for improving balance, upper- and lower-body muscular strength, endurance, and flexibility in older adults (Taylor-Piliae, Haskell, Stotts, & Froelicher, 2006).

The impact of t'ai chi on balance and fear of falling was assessed in another study that used a novel way of involving them in exercise: videoconferencing. A group tele-exercise program was designed so that participants could participate in t'ai chi exercise classes in their own homes through a videoconferencing system. These classes were structured, interactive, and supervised, and were conducted three times per week for 15 weeks. At the completion of the 15-week study, results showed significant improvement in fear of falling and balance (Wu & Keyes, 2006).

References

Kuramoto, A. M. (2006). Therapeutic benefits of t'ai chi exercise: Research review. *Wisconsin Medical Journal, 105*(7), 42–46.

Taylor-Piliae, R. E., Haskell, W. L., Stotts, N. A., & Froelicher, E. S. (2006). Improvement in balance, strength, and flexibility after 12 weeks of t'ai chi exercise in ethnic Chinese adults with cardiovascular disease risk factors. *Alternative Therapies in Health and Medicine, 12*(2), 50–58.

Wu, G., & Keyes, L. M. (2006). Group tele-exercise for improving balance in elders. *Telemedicine Journal and E–Health, 12*(5), 561–570.

Source: Kuramoto, 2006.

2,000 Hz is needed to understand everyday speech. The term **pitch** describes frequency; low pitch is 100 Hz and high pitch is 10,000 Hz.

The **decibel (dB)** is a measurement of loudness or the intensity of sound. Sounds typically range from 0 to 140 dB or greater, with a critical level for hearing being 30 dB. Zero decibel is the sound measurement of slight whispering, whereas the blast of a gun approaches 140 dB.

The various tests used to determine these three components of hearing are outlined in the Diagnostic Tests box (p. 2312). These tests also assist in determining the reason for hearing loss (i.e., conductive versus sensorineural) and the degree of loss.

Medical Management

BPPV is not life threatening and is frequently self-limiting because symptoms often subside or disappear within 2 months of onset (Imai et al., 2005). Therefore, patients can opt to just wait it out. Certain modifications in daily activities may be necessary to cope with the dizziness. For example, instruct the patient to:

- Use two or more pillows at night.
- Avoid sleeping on the "bad" side.
- In the morning get up slowly and sit on the edge of the bed for a minute.
- Avoid bending down to pick up things and extending the head.
- Be careful when lying back such as in the dentist's chair or at a hair salon sink.

Motion sickness medications are sometimes helpful in controlling the nausea associated with BPPV but do not prevent the dizziness.

Some maneuvers will help move the otoconia out of the sensitive part of the ear (posterior canal) to a less sensitive location. The health care provider sequentially moves the head into four positions, staying in each position for roughly 30 seconds. The recurrence rate for BPPV after these maneuvers is about 30% at 1 year; in some instances a second treatment may be necessary. Use of an antiemetic medication prior to the maneuver may be helpful if nausea is anticipated (Hain, 2007). The patient should continue with the daily modifications described above for at least 1 week to avoid provoking head positions that might bring BPPV on again.

If the exercises are ineffective in controlling symptoms, and the symptoms have persisted for a year or longer, a surgical procedure called *posterior canal plugging* may be recommended. This procedure blocks most of the posterior canal's function without affecting the functions of the other canals or parts of the ear. The surgery poses a small risk to hearing—about 3%—but is effective in about 85% to 90% of individuals who have had no response to any other treatment (Shaia et al., 2006). See Complementary & Alternative Therapies box for additional treatment for balance disorders.

Other Causes of Balance Disorders

Other causes for a balance disorder include an intracranial neoplasm (brain tumor) or a cerebrovascular accident (stroke). With a brain tumor, a balance disorder might be one of the first presenting symptoms. The mass will be found while the patient is undergoing a thorough diagnostic evaluation to determine the cause of the balance disorder. In the case of a stroke, a change in balance might also be one of the first presenting symptoms. A stroke can be caused by either an intracranial hemorrhage or a cerebral embolism. Depending on the location of the bleeding or blood clot, the structure of the cerebrum is affected, tissue displaced, and pressure placed on other brain structures. A change in balance oftentimes will be the first indication of a pending or actual stroke. The causes and treatment of strokes are discussed in detail in Chapter 30 ⊕.

Interventions for Hearing Loss

Treatment of a hearing loss will depend on the underlying cause. This could range from simply removing the cause, as with noise-induced hearing loss or ear canal obstruction, to a surgical procedure. In the case of an infection, antibiotics or a myringotomy might be indicated to treat the infection and drain any fluid and pressure within the middle ear. (The Pharmacology Summary feature, p. 2313 discusses antibiotics and other medications used to treat hearing as well as balance disorders.) Should the cause of hearing loss be due to otosclerosis, a stapedectomy may be the treatment of choice.

Removal of Foreign Body

Foreign bodies of the ear are relatively common in emergency medicine. They are seen most often but not exclusively in children. Various objects may be found, including toys, beads, stones, folded paper, and biologic materials such as insects or seeds. Patients in extreme distress secondary to an insect in the ear require prompt attention. The insect should be killed prior to removal, using mineral oil or 2% lidocaine. Methods of removal consist of irrigation, suction, and instrumentation. Irrigation with water is contraindicated if the tympanic membrane is perforated. Irrigation is also contraindicated for soft objects, organic matter, or seeds, which may swell if exposed to water. Suction is sometimes a useful way to remove foreign bodies. Suction the ear with a small catheter held in contact with the object. Grasp the object with alligator forceps. Place a right-angled hook behind the object and pull it out. Form a hook with a 25-gauge needle to snag and remove a large soft object such as a pencil eraser. It is imperative to avoid any intervention that pushes the object deeper into the ear. After the foreign body is removed, inspect the external ear canal. For most foreign bodies, no medications are needed. However, if infection or abrasion is evident, fill the ear canal several times a day for 5 to 7 days with a combination antibiotic and steroid otic suspension (e.g., Cortisporin).

Removal of Impacted Cerumen

In the event of impacted cerumen, the treatment of choice is removal of the impaction. A health care provider or trained nurse should remove the impaction. Typically this is accomplished by flushing the ear canal with a syringe filled with water that is at or near body temperature. Some health care providers prefer a mixture of hydrogen peroxide and water. The flushing action loosens the impaction from the walls of the canal, and the warm water facilitates drainage from the ear. If the impaction does not clear, the patient is instructed to place mineral oil in the ear three times per day for 2 days. This will soften the dry impacted cerumen, and then the irrigation may be repeated. After removal of the impaction, the patient should be instructed not to insert any objects into the ear canal and to have frequent ear examinations.

DIAGNOSTIC TESTS for Hearing and Balance

Test	Expected Abnormality	Rationale for Abnormality
Voice and watch tick Used to test high-frequency hearing loss The examiner stands 1–2 feet behind and to the side of the patient, while the patient occludes each ear sequentially and the examiner whispers four unrelated words near each ear.	With a hearing abnormality, the patient will not be able to hear words whispered.	If the patient is unable to hear whispering, there is then some degree of hearing loss. The loss of the ability to hear a watch ticking is considered to be a loss of high-frequency sounds.
Weber test (tuning fork test) Used to test sensorineural hearing loss Place an activated tuning fork midline on top of the patient's head, bridge of nose, or chin.	Hear sound in the damaged ear. Hear no sound in the damaged ear.	If the patient has conductive hearing loss, the sound will lateralize to the ear with the loss because the sound is being conducted directly through the bone to the ear. It the patient has sensorineural hearing loss, the sound will lateralize to the hearing ear because nerve damage in the nonhearing ear prevents hearing.
Rinne test (tuning fork test) Used to test conductive hearing loss Place activated tuning fork on the right and left mastoid bone sequentially and in front of each ear.	Hear sound longer through bone. Hear sound longer through air.	This test compares bone conduction with air conduction. If the patient hears sounds longer through bone, then the patient has a conductive hearing loss. If the patient hears sounds longer through the air, then the patient has a sensorineural hearing loss.
Schwabach test (compares the patient's perception of bone conduction to the examiner's) Place an activated tuning fork on the mastoid process of the patient and alternately test for both air and bone conduction.	Diminished—the examiner hears the sound longer than the patient does. Prolonged—the patient hears the sound longer than the examiner does.	Sensorineural loss Conductive loss
ACOUSTIC IMMITTANCE TESTS		
Tympanometry Used to test the flexibility of the tympanic membrane	Tympanic membrane does not move.	Tests for mobility and if there is anything impeding movement of the tympanic membrane and ossicles of the middle ear.
Acoustic reflexes Used to test the flexibility of the stapedius muscle	Stapedius muscle will not contract.	Measures the change in admittance produced by contraction of the stapedius muscle as it responds to an intense sound; stimulation of one ear causes reaction in both ears.
Pure tone audiometry Used to determine type and degree of hearing loss	Unable to hear certain decibel levels.	Provides a record of which decibel levels the patient is unable to hear. This test will not provide the cause of the hearing loss.
Auditory brainstem response Used to test decibel levels of hearing	Cannot hear clicks.	This test measures hearing by measuring the decibel levels the patient hears and if there is anything in the way of nerve pathways.
Electronystagmography Used to test for Ménière's disease	There will be changes in the electrical potentials (waveforms) created by eye movements during spontaneous, positional, or calorically evoked nystagmus.	This test is used to assess the oculomotor and vestibular systems. It is helpful when trying to confirm the diagnosis of Ménière's disease.
Platform posturography Used to test for balance disorders	The patient will not be able to maintain balance or position sense.	Checks for impairments with position sense and balance.
Sinusoidal harmonic acceleration Used to test balance disorders	Eye movements will be uncoordinated.	Another test for balance disorders, this test uses a rotary chair. Through the movements of the chair, the vestibulo-ocular system can be assessed.
Middle ear endoscopy Used to test new-onset hearing loss	Some disorder exists within the middle ear, seen by direct visualization of these structures.	Office procedure to evaluate cause of new-onset hearing loss and to diagnose vertigo.

PHARMACOLOGY Summary of Medications to Treat Select Hearing and Balance Disorders

Medication Category	Action	Application/Indication	Nursing Responsibility
• Isopropyl alcohol drops (dries moisture) • Acetic acid (VoSoL) solution • Antiseptic	Restores acidity and helps keep ear canals dry. Has an antibacterial and antifungal action.	Reduces infection of otitis externa	Dry ears post swimming. Place 1 to 2 drops into each ear after swimming.
• Polymyxin, neomycin, hydrocortisone (Cortisporin, Pediotic) ciprofloxacin (Cipro HC Otic) and ofloxacin (Floxin Otic) • Otic antibiotics	Disrupts cell wall synthesis of susceptible bacteria.	Reduces infection of otitis externa	Note any allergies prior to starting antibiotics. Stop treatment if irritation occurs when using medication. Report any unusual symptoms related to ears or hearing (tinnitus, roaring sounds, loss of hearing acuity, or dizziness).
Amoxicillin (Amoxil) • Cephalosporins, macrolides, trimethoprim-sulfamethoxazole (Bactrim) • Amoxicillin/clavulanic acid (Augmentin) Antibiotic	Disrupts cell wall synthesis of susceptible bacteria.	Acute otitis media	Check for previous allergies to penicillin (amoxicillin) or sulfa (Bactrim). Report any unusual symptoms such as rash, irritation, itching.
Antibiotics • Neomycin, Garamycin, tobramycin, quinolones (Cipro) • IV antibiotics: ampicillin, Unasyn, Ceftin Antibiotic	Disrupts cell wall synthesis of susceptible bacteria.	Chronic otitis media	Note any allergies to specific medications. Report unusual symptoms related to ears or hearing (tinnitus, roaring sounds, loss of hearing acuity, or dizziness).
Steroid eardrops	Has an anti-inflammatory effect on ear canals.	Chronic otitis media	Assess for new onset of ear drainage, earache, erythema, pain, or vertigo. Assess that the ear canal is clear and not impacted with cerumen before medication administration. Consider giving in combination with antibiotics to treat infections. Be aware that steroids may mask infections.
Meclizine (Antivert, Bonine) Antihistamine Antivertigo agent	Long-lasting piperazine antihistamine, structurally and pharmacologically related to cyclizine.	Ménière's disease	Advise caution while driving or engaging in hazardous activities until response to drug is known. Be aware that sedative action may add to that of other central nervous systems (CNS) depressants.
Diphenhydramine (Benadryl) Antihistamine	H_1-receptor antagonist and antihistamine with significant anticholinergic activity.	Ménière's disease	Advise caution while driving or engaging in hazardous activities until response to drug is known. Be aware of additive CNS depressant effects with concurrent use. May cause a drying effect, thus it is important to increase fluid intake if not contraindicated.
Streptomycin IM or gentamicin (transtympanic injection) Aminoglycoside antibiotic Anti-infective	Disrupts cell wall synthesis of susceptible bacteria.	Ménière's disease (selectively destroys vestibular apparatus if vertigo uncontrollable)	Note allergies. Monitor for ototoxicity and hearing problems. Report tinnitus, roaring noises, impaired hearing, sense of fullness in ears. Monitor intake and output to be on alert for nephrotoxicity.

(continued)

PHARMACOLOGY Summary of Medications to Treat Select Hearing and Balance Disorders—*Continued*

Medication Category	Action	Application/Indication	Nursing Responsibility
Diazepam (Valium) Antianxiety CNS agent	Psychotherapeutic agent related to chlordiazepoxide.	Ménière's disease	Monitor for CNS effects such as hypotension, muscular weakness, tachycardia and respiratory depression. Use safety precautions because drowsiness and ataxia may occur. Avoid CNS depressants because of additive effects.
Phenergan (antiemetic)	Long-lasting derivative of phenothiazine with marked antihistamine activity.	Ménière's disease (may be needed to reduce nausea)	Supervise ambulation because sedation and dizziness may occur. Take initial dose 30–60 minutes before anticipated travel. Avoid sunlamps or prolonged exposure to sunlight. Do not take OTC medications without health care provider approval. Avoid CNS depressants because of additive effects. Relieve dry mouth by increasing fluid intake, chewing sugarless gum, or sucking on hard candy.

Assistive Devices

Assistive devices are available for individuals who have partial or total hearing loss. These include phone amplifiers, which allow the caller to speak in a normal tone while amplifying the sound for the person with the hearing impairment. Small portable amplifiers also are available and are carried by those with hearing impairments to assist with communication. Additionally, special apparatus can be connected to doorbells and telephones that cause lights to flash when activated.

The two main types of assistive devices for individuals who have partial or total hearing loss are assistive listening devices (ALDs) and alerting devices (ADs). ALDs help with listening, whereas ADs signal the presence of a sound. Basic ALD systems are devices that amplify the sound, which allow the caller to speak in a normal tone while amplifying the sound for the person with the hearing impairment, or enhancement systems that produce higher frequencies (pitches), which are important for understanding speech through microphones or transmitters. Alerting devices may be modified so that one is alerted when sound devices (telephones, alarm clocks, doorbells) ring. Lamps throughout the house can be made to "flash" when someone rings the doorbell or a small "vibrator" can be placed under a pillow to wake one up in the morning when the alarm goes off.

Hearing Dogs

Hearing guide dogs are specially trained to alert the deaf person or a person with a hearing impairment to ringing doorbells, potential dangers, and other sounds that require a response. The dog alerts the person by physical contact. In public, the dog positions itself between the person with the hearing impairment and possible danger, such as oncoming traffic. Information about qualifying for a dog is obtained through International Hearing Dog Inc., which is a nonprofit organization fully funded by donations. Its mission is to train and place hearing dogs with persons who are deaf or hard of hearing with or without multiple disabilities at no charge to the recipient.

Hearing Aid

A hearing aid is a small electronic sound amplifier that fits either into the external ear canal or just behind the ear. The purpose of the hearing aid is to improve hearing, thereby preventing social isolation and anxiety. The aid can be worn in one or both ears. The patient should be fitted for the hearing aid based on type and degree of hearing loss as determined by a certified licensed audiologist. For sensorineural hearing loss there are aids that will depress the low-frequency sound and enhance the high-frequency sound. The hearing aid will only make sounds louder; it will not help with discriminating words or understanding speech. Hearing aids amplify all sounds including background noise, so the person needs to learn to filter out background noise. Initially, patients are typically encouraged to use the hearing aid for only part of the day and use television/radio to get used to the change in volume. The patient needs to learn to adjust the tone or volume on the aid to achieve the best sound. The newer digital/programmable hearing aids are programmed by the audiologist with a computer, so the sound quality and response time can be adjusted on an individual basis (National Institute on Deafness and Other Communication Disorders [NIDCD], 2002a). These hearing aids are better able to compensate for background noise because they allow amplification at certain programmed frequencies, rather than all of them.

Hearing aids are delicate devices that need careful handling and care in order to work properly. The nurse needs to instruct the patient on care and cleaning requirements for the hearing aid. The following items are typical maintenance tasks for hearing aids:

- Clean the ear mold with mild soap and water.
- Check the battery regularly.

- Clean the hole in the middle of the device.
- Always have an extra battery on hand.
- Avoid spraying hairspray or other beauty products on the hearing aid.
- Turn off the hearing aid when not in use.

The patient also will need instructions about side effects or complications. The patient should contact the health care provider if skin irritation or accelerated cerumen accumulation occurs. If the hearing aid does not improve hearing, the patient may need to try another brand. Chart 70–4 lists the different types of hearing aids.

Cochlear Implants

A cochlear implant is a small, complex electronic device that can help to provide a sense of sound to a person who is profoundly deaf or severely hard of hearing. The intention was for this implant to aid individuals with neurofibromatosis, one of the hereditary forms of deafness, to hear. An implant does not restore or create normal hearing, although it can give a deaf person a useful auditory understanding of the environment and help him or her to understand speech. With a cochlear implant, electrodes are placed in the cochlea and attached to a microphone and signal processor, which are surgically placed under the skin behind the ear. The microphone and signal processor transmit electrical stimuli to the 22 implanted electrodes. The electrical signals stimulate the auditory nerve fibers and then the brain where the sounds are interpreted. Once implanted the patient undergoes extensive cochlear rehabilitation. Several months of training with an audiologist and speech pathologist are needed to learn to interpret the sounds.

Cochlear implants are beginning to be used in children with promising results. A longitudinal study was conducted on 107 children with hearing impairments who received cochlear implants before the age of 7. The findings showed that these children developed communication skills within a few months (NIDCD, 2002b).

Speech Reading and Sign Language

Speech reading, also known as lip reading, uses the eyes to assist with understanding what is being said to the deaf person. There are formal speech reading classes where the deaf person is taught special clues and how to understand body language. The deaf person or someone with a hearing impairment typically understands only a portion of the words, but communication is enhanced.

Sign language is another means of enhancing communication for the deaf person or person with a hearing impairment. American Sign Language is one example of a complex visuospatial language that is used by the deaf community. Sign language is a linguistically complete, natural language that is native to many deaf men and women, as well as some hearing children born into deaf families.

A program designed to test the self-efficacy for health-related behaviors among deaf adults is discussed in the Evidence-Based Practice box.

◼ Nursing Management

Preparing to provide care to a patient with a hearing or balance disorder should begin with an assessment of the patient's current status. From this information, the nurse can then determine

---

On Efficacy of Deaf Heart Health Intervention

Clinical Problem

Performing activities of daily living (ADLs) or working in society produces self-perception or task-related problems for culturally deaf individuals.

Research Findings

A quasiexperimental pre/post-test study was performed to test the effectiveness of the Deaf Heart Health Intervention (DHHI) in increasing self-efficacy for health-related behaviors among culturally deaf adults. The DHHI targets modifiable risk factors for cardiovascular disease. A sample of 84 participants completed a time 1 and time 2 data collection process. The sign language version of the Self-Rated Abilities Scale for Health Practice (SRAHP) was used to measure self-efficacy for nutrition, psychological well-being/stress management, physical activity/exercise, and responsible health practices. Total self-efficacy scores were significantly higher in the intervention group than in the comparison group at time 2, controlling for scores at baseline ($F < 1, 81 > = 26.02$, $p < 0.001$). Results support the development of interventions specifically tailored for culturally deaf adults to increase their self-efficacy for health behaviors.

Implications for Nursing Practice

Nurses need to be aware of health and mental behaviors that cause problems with self-efficacy among culturally deaf individuals and promote intervention strategies that help improve these individuals.

Critical Thinking Questions

1. What are some health-related behaviors that may increase self-efficacy for culturally deaf adults?

2. Identify ways in which culturally deaf adults can adjust to their environment.

3. What role might school nurses play in helping to identify culturally deaf adolescents?

Answers to Critical Thinking Questions appear in Appendix D.

Reference

Jones, E. G., Renger, R., & Kang, Y. (2007). Research in nursing and health: Self-efficacy for health related behaviors among deaf adults. *Research in Nursing and Health 30*(2), 185–192.

CHART 70–4	**Basic Types of Hearing Aids for Sensorineural Hearing Loss**

Type	Description
In-the-ear	Fit in outer ear; used for mild to severe hearing loss.
Behind-the-ear	Worn behind the ear and connected to a plastic earmold that fits inside the outer ear; used for mild to profound hearing loss.
Canal aids	Fit into the ear canal and used for mild to moderately severe hearing loss.
Body aids	Aid attaches to a belt or pocket and is connected to the ear by a wire; used for profound hearing loss.

Source: Extracted from National Institute on Deafness and Other Communication Disorders at http://www.nidcd.nih.gov/health/hearing/hearingaid.asp.

diagnoses appropriate to address these findings. Examples of nursing diagnoses may include the following:

- *Disturbed Sensory Perception: Auditory*
- *Impaired Social Interaction*
- *Social Isolation*
- *Risk for Loneliness*
- *Ineffective Coping*
- *Impaired Walking*

- *Deficient Knowledge*
- *Anticipatory Grieving*
- *Risk for Situational Low Self-Esteem*
- *Risk for Injury*

From the diagnoses, the nurse can then plan interventions to aid in the care of a patient with special needs. Refer to the Nursing Process: Patient Care Plan for a Hearing or Balance Disorder feature for more information on nursing care for these disorders.

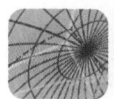

NURSING PROCESS: Patient Care Plan for a Hearing or Balance Disorder

Assessment of Hearing

Subjective Data:
When did you first notice that you had a change in your ability to hear?
Did you have a recent exposure to a loud noise or infection?

Objective Data:
Results of hearing tests.
Test ability to hear at normal voice range.
Test lower and higher pitch.
Speak into both ears to test unilateral verses bilateral hearing loss.

Nursing Assessment and Diagnoses	Outcomes and Evaluation Parameters	Planning and Interventions with *Rationales*
Nursing Diagnoses: *Disturbed Sensory Perception: Auditory* and *Impaired Verbal Communication*	**Outcomes:** Patient/family understand that the disease causes progressive hearing loss. Patient/family understand what treatments will help. ***Evaluation Parameters:*** Patient can communicate. Assistive devices are helping with hearing and communication.	**Interventions and *Rationales*:** Assess degree of hearing loss. *Helps determine best approach to communicate.* Teach about disease process. *Helps reduce anxiety and stress related to the change or loss in hearing.* Speak clearly and slowly in a normal to deep voice; face the patient when speaking; use touch to gain the patient's attention. *Aids in verbal and nonverbal communication with the patient.* Respond to call light as soon as possible; answer questions; teach about medications/treatments *to decrease fear and anxiety.* Provide emotional support to the member having difficulty coping with the new sensory deficit *to decrease fear and anxiety.* Instruct or reinforce instruction on use of hearing aid. *Aids in retention of training and reinforces the need for using the assistive device for hearing.* Provide sensory stimulation; encourage expressing feelings of concern and loss for hearing deficit; teach to watch for visual cues. *Provides additional support for the patient.*

Assessment of Balance

Subjective Data:
How long have you been experiencing dizziness/vertigo?
Have you fallen?
How long have you been dizzy with walking?
Are you using any hazardous machinery such as a car or equipment at work?
Are you nauseated with the dizziness/vertigo?
Do you drive an automobile?

Objective Data:
Observation of ataxia while ambulating
Observation of bumping into things while ambulating

Nursing Assessment and Diagnoses	Outcome and Evaluation Parameters	Planning and Interventions with *Rationales*
Nursing Diagnoses: *Risk for Falls, Risk for injury,* and *Impaired Walking*	**Outcomes:** Patient will understand that balance disorder is temporary. Patient will participate in rehabilitative activities to maximize position sense. Patient will adhere to medication regime prescribed for balance disorder. ***Evaluation Parameters:*** Dizziness and vertigo subside. Patient is able to resume normal activities of daily living (ADLs) and lifestyle.	**Interventions and *Rationales*:** Explain the cause for dizziness and vertigo. *Helps the patient understand the reason for the symptoms.* Assist the patient with ambulation and other ADLs *to ensure the patient does not experience any injuries while dizzy.* Utilize safety measures such as keeping bedside rails in elevated position and call light within reach. *Safety precautions.* Teach family how to assist patient with ambulation and ADLs upon discharge *to ensure ongoing safety measures until the dizziness and vertigo subside.*

Discharge Priorities

When planning for discharge from an acute care facility for treatment of a hearing or balance disorder, the nurse is in the best position to help the patient and family with physical, psychological, and future occupational needs. Helping the patient and family deal with the cause of the hearing or balance deficit and identify choices to avoid future problems associated with hearing and balance are the approaches of choice. The Deaf Mental Health Charter (2007) commissioned by the Sign and Mental Health Foundation, London, England, has identified a variety of areas that need implementation to address the types of choices that the deaf community may make. These areas are outlined in the Patient Teaching and Discharge Priorities box.

If discharging a patient from an acute care facility, physical teaching needs might include postoperative wound care, medication therapy, coping, and a return-to-work plan. In the outpatient setting, teaching needs might be focused on adherence to a prescribed medication regime, avoidance of behaviors that caused the hearing/balance disorders, protective devices for the workplace, and other health promotional activities.

Should the hearing or balance disorder lead to a long-term change in the ability to hear, other instructions would include communication instruction such as sign language, use of a hearing aid, suggestions to family for communicating with the family member who has the hearing impairment, and learning to avoid the same exposure that caused the hearing impairment in their loved one.

Health Promotion

The Deaf Community has limited access to health promotion information and care. Health care providers, educators, and policy makers could improve medical care to the Deaf Community by (1) better understanding its culture and language, (2) creating more health education programs specifically for the Deaf Community, (3) developing opportunities for more deaf people and American Sign Language (ASL) users to enter the health professions, and (4) creating incentives for hearing health care professions to become ASL proficient (Sadler, Huang, & Padden et al., 2001).

Neonate/Baby/Childhood

The instructions on how to protect hearing can begin when the mother brings her newborn child to the pediatrician for routine checkups. The infant should be tested for hearing prior to reaching 1 month of age. Children of all ages should be examined immediately if exhibiting symptoms of an ear infection. If left untreated, hearing loss might ensue.

Mothers should be instructed on the risk of using cotton swabs to clean the ears of their children. Alternative methods to clean the ear should be provided such as using a wick to absorb fluid in the

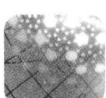

PATIENT TEACHING & DISCHARGE PRIORITIES for the Hearing and Balance Disorders

Need	Teaching
Usable information techniques	Provide access to easily understood information in appropriate formats, such as plain language, visual representation in subtitled DVDs and videos.
	Assist with location of classes for American Sign Language, if applicable.
	Provide for health information or programs (including mental health promotion) that are accessible to the Deaf community. Design these programs in close cooperation with organizations that serve the Deaf community.
Safe environment	The inpatient, outpatient, day services, or work settings need to have services that make the environment safer; for instance, visual fire safety provisions and access to alerting and telephone services, TVs with teletext ability, pagers, and inclusive ways to operate remote door-entry systems.
Communication support	Deaf people who use BSL as their first and preferred form of communication have the right to qualified interpreter support. Deaf people who use English and hearing aids have the right to use lipspeaker-cued speech or speech to text transcription.
Health promotion	Provide access to health information or programs (including mental health promotion) to the deaf community. These programs should be designed in close cooperation with organizations that serve the deaf community. Different means of promotion, such as face-to-face delivery in BSL, may be more effective to reach deaf people.
Assessment, care, and treatment	Deaf people have the right to be assessed by a trained worker who has deaf/deaf blind awareness and skills. Deaf-specific advisory services should be considered. Using these services aims to ensure that deaf persons can fully participate in any assessment and discussion of services.
Placement	Any placement decision should take into account the deaf person's preferred communication method and language.
Advocacy	Deaf people have the right to independent advocacy in health, mental health service, education, employment, and social care. This is to ensure that the deaf person can fully participate in any assessment and discussion of services to make informed choices.
Physical teaching needs	In the outpatient setting, teaching needs might be focused on adherence to prescribed medication regime, avoidance of behaviors that caused the hearing/balance disorders, protective devices for the workplace, and other health promotional activities. If the patient had surgery, include teaching on postoperative wound care, medication therapy, coping, and a return to work plan.

Source: Deaf Mental Health Charter. (2007). *Mental Health Foundation.* Retrieved June 21, 2007, from http://www.mhf.org.uk/our-work/service-development/all-age-groups/deaf-charter. Commissioned by Sign and Mental Health Foundation, London, England.

ear canal. Children should not have small objects as toys for play since these small objects can become lodged within the ear canal. Children also should have their ears protected with earplugs while participating in water activities and with muffs prior to being exposed to loud noises. Even though most, if not all, children experience head colds, if not treated properly, head colds can lead to infections that settle in the ears. Children who experience repeated colds should have an examination of their ears and associated structures to make sure the ears are not becoming affected or damaged from ongoing nasal and sinus inflammation and infection.

Adolescence

Teenagers who frequently listen to loud music can experience a temporary loss of hearing. Over time, this hearing loss can become more permanent. Parents should caution their teenagers to reduce the volume of music to avoid this damaging effect.

Adults

Adults also are at risk for hearing and balance disorders. Causes might include the indiscriminate use of cotton swabs to clean the ear canal and loud noise from factory work, jack hammers, music, explosive devices, automobile engines, and the like. Engaging in water activities or sports also can lead to infections within the ear structures. If not treated, these infections also can lead to hearing loss similar to that which is seen more frequently in children.

Because balance and position sense are intimately related to the structures of the inner ear, changes in balance should not be ignored. Individuals who find they struggle to maintain a sense of balance should seek medical attention. The examination will most likely include a thorough study of the ear structures in efforts to determine the cause of dizziness or vertigo.

Individuals of all ages should learn to protect their ears and hearing by having earplugs for water activities/showers, earmuffs to reduce exposure to loud noises, and common sense to reduce the volume of music or entertainment activities such as television.

Patient, Family, and Community Perspectives

Having a loss of hearing creates unique challenges for the individual. Environmental noise cannot be discerned, leaving the person prone to hazards such as an oncoming automobile or even the warning buzz of a bee. Communities need to provide street warning signs for motorists driving in areas where residents with hearing impairments live. Schools should provide educational programs for students to learn the hazards of hearing impairment and loss. Adults should be encouraged to seek advice for hearing loss and be supported when needing to purchase and care for hearing aids. Those who cannot have their hearing restored through surgery or devices need to be supported with training and education to learn sign language or provided with a telephonic device to aid with communication.

Rehabilitative programs exist for these individuals to help them regain position sense and balance. Individuals with a known balance disorder should be advised to avoid operating motor vehicles or machinery. The Risk Factors box (p. 2309) lists those needs to be included in the rehabilitative programs. The patient's health care provider may need to contact the Department of Motor Vehicles to report the patient's balance disorder. The patient's driver's license could be suspended until the disorder passes and the patient passes a medical clearance prior to resuming the use of a motor vehicle.

Collaborative Care

The patient with a hearing or balance disorder may need the aid of additional caregivers. These caregivers include therapists in occupational and physical medicine and speech and hearing. Learning to care for a hearing aid might first be reviewed with an audiologist and then turned over to the nurse for instructional reinforcement. If the patient is experiencing a balance disorder and being treated with rehabilitative services, the nurse's role is to reinforce the instructions provided by the therapist.

National Guidelines for Hearing Loss Prevention

A program led by the U.S. Department of Health and Human Services (DHHS), termed *Healthy People 2010,* has identified specific objectives to help with the problem of hearing loss, as outline in the National Guidelines box. The *Healthy People 2010* focus area on vision and hearing stresses the importance of early intervention to protect and conserve the vision and hearing of young children and to mitigate the severity of vision and hearing impairments that can heavily degrade the quality of life of older Americans. The vision and hearing section of the *Healthy People 2010* document (U.S. Department of Health and Human Services, 2000)) stresses the following:

- Increase the proportion of persons who have a hearing examination on schedule.
- Increase the number of persons who are referred by their primary care health care provider for hearing evaluation and treatment.
- Increase the use of appropriate ear protective devices, equipment, and practices.
- Decrease noise-induced hearing loss in children and adolescents ages 17 years and younger.
- Decrease adult hearing loss in the noise-exposed public.

**NATIONAL GUIDELINES for *Healthy People 2010*
Objectives for Reducing Hearing Loss**

1. Increase the number of newborns having a first hearing examination by 1 month of age. Babies with a hearing loss should have additional testing by 3 months of age. If hearing loss continues, enrollment in a rehabilitative program by 6 months of age.

2. Decrease the number of ear infections in children.

3. Increase the number of Deaf/hard-of-hearing individuals who use adaptive devices such as hearing aids or cochlear implants.

4. Increase the number of individuals who have routine hearing examinations.

5. Increase the number of individuals who are referred by their primary health care provider for a hearing evaluation and treatment.

6. Increase the use of protective devices, such as earplugs or earmuffs, in people of all ages.

7. Reduce the number of individuals of all ages who suffer from noise-induced hearing loss.

Source: U.S. Department of Health and Human Services. (2000). *Healthy people 2010: Understanding and improving health.* Retrieved February 5, 2008, from http://www.healthypeople.gov.

A radiologist-funded group of health care providers has written a set of guidelines to aid in the diagnosis of hearing and balance disorders. These guidelines, entitled the *American College of Radiology Appropriateness Criteria for Vertigo and Hearing Loss* (2008), recommend specific diagnostic tests as a precursor to prescribing treatment for a balance or hearing disorder (see the National Guidelines box). Commonly referred to as national guidelines, this list names specific hearing/balance disorders then states the ideal diagnostic tests that should be used to diagnose the disorder. Tests frequently recommended include an MRI, with and without contrast, a CT scan, with and without contrast, skull films, and tomography. The intention of these diagnostic tests is to first determine or possibly rule out the presence of cerebral pathology as the cause for the change in hearing or balance.

Cultural Considerations

Very few cultural differences are seen in hearing and balance disorders. One interesting difference is with the Vietnamese. These individuals have dry earwax, which is gray in color and brittle to the touch. In a majority of Asians and Native Americans cerumen is dry, white, and flaky. In African Americans and Caucasians cerumen is brown, wet, and sticky (Hunter, 1996; Mitchell, 1997).

Genetic Implications

Congenital hearing loss occurs when a trait found within the chromosomes of both parents passes to the infant. The trait can be dominant, recessive, or sex linked. Congenital conditions that include some degree of hearing impairment are outlined in the Genetic Considerations box.

GENETIC CONSIDERATIONS Related to Hearing and Balance Disorders

Disorder	Results	Ear Structure
Usher syndrome	Balance problems	Inner ear
Treacher Collins syndrome	Bone development	Middle ear
Nonsyndromic deafness	Conductive problems	Inner ear
ESPN	Changes in hairlike projections	Inner ear
Pendred syndrome	Hearing loss and goiter	Inner ear
Neurofibromatosis	Tumor (acoustic neuroma)	Inner ear
Diastrophic dysplasia	Cartilage and bone	External ear
Von Hippel Lindau syndrome	Endolymphatic sac tumors	Inner ear
Jervell and Lange-Nielsen syndrome	Flow of potassium ions	Inner ear
Alport syndrome	Organ of Corti	Inner ear
Crouzon syndrome	Ear canals	Middle and inner
Chromosome 18	Low-set ears	Outer and middle

Source: *Genetics Home Reference* website: http://ghr.nlm.nih.gov. A Service of U.S. National Library of Medicine.

The risk of giving birth to a child with a hearing deficit depends on the health of the parents and their respective health backgrounds. Histories of known deafness in families should cause those of childbearing years to seek genetic testing and counseling prior to conception. To proceed with the understanding that a child could be born deaf will undoubtedly cause prospective parents much anxiety around the decision to reproduce at all.

Treatment of congenital deafness will vary depending on the underlying congenital cause. As more research is conducted on the different congenital disorders, treatment options will likely expand.

Gerontological Considerations

More often than not, deafness is associated with aging. It is estimated that one-third of adults over the age of 60 have some degree of hearing loss. This percentage increases to approximately 50% of all adults over the age of 85 experiencing an alteration in their ability to hear (NIDCD, 2001).

The causes of hearing loss and balance disorders in the elderly can be from a metabolic disorder, such as type II diabetes mellitus, or from the aging process. In diabetes, the disorder can go undetected for many years. By the time of diagnosis, the patient might already have long-term complications to the nervous system. Included in these complications could be damage to the auditory nerve leading to a change in the ability to hear. The impact of unstable blood glucose levels can also lead to a balance disorder.

Exposure to known ototoxic medications (see Chart 70–3, p. 2307) throughout life could finally manifest in later years. A patient might have ingested a medication that was not known to

---

NATIONAL GUIDELINES for Vertigo and Hearing Loss

The *American College of Radiology Appropriateness Criteria for Vertigo and Hearing Loss* (2008) provides the radiologic diagnostic tests used to aid in the diagnosis of vertigo and hearing loss. This document addresses the hearing and balance disorders based on presenting symptoms, categorized as variants from normal. With the clinical condition of hearing loss/vertigo the variants are:

1. Sensorineural hearing loss, acute vertigo
2. Sensorineural hearing loss, intermittent vertigo
3. Sensorineural hearing loss, no vertigo
4. Conductive hearing loss, rule out petrous bone abnormality
5. Episodic vertigo, new onset (hours to days)
6. Vertigo, no hearing loss, normal neurological exam
7. Total deafness, cochlear implant candidate, surgical planning
8. Fluctuating hearing loss, history of meningitis or to rule out congenital anomaly.

Based on the patient's presenting hearing or balance disorder, these guidelines are consulted to determine which diagnostic test to perform to aid in the diagnosis of the disorder.

American College of Radiology (2008). Guideline title: Vertigo and hearing loss. Retrieved on September 29, 2008 from http://www.guideline.gov/summary/summary.aspx?ss=15&doc_id=9602&nbr=5123.

be ototoxic until after years of pharmacologic study. Older individuals might be experiencing presbycusis. Because the onset of hearing loss associated with presbycusis is slow and gradual, individuals might not even recognize that their hearing is changing until a significant amount of deterioration has occurred. Oftentimes, the individual finds he can no longer hear high-pitched sounds or voices, particularly with loud or noisy background sounds. The individual might also identify tinnitus, because this symptom is common in those diagnosed with presbycusis as the cause for their hearing deficit/change.

Nursing Assessment of the Elderly

When providing care to an elderly patient with a hearing deficit or balance disorder, the nurse needs to include specific items in the assessment process. First the method of communication must be determined. A loud voice does not ensure successful hearing or comprehension. Depending on the cause and degree of hearing loss, the nurse might simply drop the tone of the voice to be successful with vocal communication with an elderly patient who has a hearing impairment because the loss of high-frequency sounds occurs first.

The review of systems or head-to-toe assessment should include any known cardiac disorders, blood pressure history or known hypertension, and any metabolic disorders such as diabetes. Conditions that involve the arteries and veins such as peripheral vascular disease or atherosclerosis could provide answers for any cause of hearing or balance disorders linked to an alteration in blood flow to the brain.

The reason for the current hospitalization or visit to the health care provider's office should include a reference to any change in hearing or balance. The current blood pressure and pulse should be assessed for possible association with the patient's current cardiovascular status. In addition, assess whether the patient is able to ambulate without assistance or appears wobbly or unbalanced when attempting to walk. This could be linked to a disorder within the ears or balance-related structures.

Questions to the patient about her health should include any history of a cardiovascular accident or transient ischemic attacks. Additionally, ask if the patient has a history of cerebral brain tumors or other diagnosed pathologic conditions that could be linked to the current symptoms of the hearing/balance disorder.

Finally, an assessment of the past medical history of the elderly patient presenting with a hearing or balance disorder should include any and all exposure to communicable diseases that might have been treated with antibiotics that have known ototoxic side effects. An example might be pulmonary tuberculosis that was treated with streptomycin.

Psychosocial and Economic Needs

The elderly patient experiencing a change in hearing or balance might be embarrassed to admit the change. Oftentimes, elderly patients might not have adequate finances to purchase a hearing aid or they might feel that needing such a device is a sign of weakness or aging. Patients who are unstable with ambulation caused by a balance disorder might find they stay close to home to avoid falling. This can lead to social isolation, which in turn can lead to depression. Couple a balance disorder with a hearing

loss and an elderly person might become a social recluse, lost in a world of increasing silence. Previous joys found in living might diminish as elderly patients realize that they might be approaching the end of their life.

Medications and Compliance

The medications used to treat hearing and balance disorders can be a hindrance as well as beneficial. Medications to treat other diseases or conditions can have the side effects of hearing disturbance or tinnitus (antibiotics, aspirin) or dizziness (beta blockers, ACE inhibitors). Taking medications to aid with a balance disorder might adversely interact with other prescribed medications (opioids, central nervous system depressants). Depending on the medications and results of combining medications, patients might choose to stop taking some medications in favor of others that have less of an impact on their general sense of well-being.

Laboratory Test Alterations

The elderly patient being evaluated for a hearing or balance disorder will most likely have a complete battery of serum laboratory tests done. The purpose of the findings might be to indicate whether the patient has an electrolyte or blood glucose disorder. An electrolyte disturbance, such as low sodium or low potassium levels, can be associated with light-headedness. A low blood glucose level also can present with light-headedness and lack of coordination. Diagnostic tests to determine the degree of presbycusis (see the Diagnostics Tests box, p. 2312) would undoubtedly reveal the condition and offer the patient treatment choices including a referral for a hearing aid or surgery to replace the stapes.

Prognosis and Complications

Depending on the diagnosis, the prognosis would vary. Should the patient need surgery, such as a stapedectomy, some degree of hearing might be restored. Should the course of treatment include medications and hearing aids, other issues might interfere with the prognosis. If the patient were unable to afford the medications or hearing aid, the situation would continue to exist and possibly worsen in time. Care should be taken to address the needs of the elderly should they hesitate to commit to a referral for a hearing aid.

Caregiver Needs

Needs for those providing care to an elderly individual with a hearing or balance disorder vary. If the elderly person were independent, the caregiver would most likely be able to adjust his own lifestyle and activities to those of the individual to whom he is providing the care. If a balance disorder is added to the mix of other health issues, the caregiver might need additional support. The caregiver might not be able to leave the elderly individual alone due to the risk of falling or injury. Each situation needs to be assessed to determine the best options for both the elderly patient and caregivers alike.

■ End-of-life Issues

It is often believed that the sense of hearing is the last sense "to go" when an individual is facing an inevitable death. Should this be the case, conversations need to be adjusted accordingly. The nurse's responsibility is to control the environment as much as possible to ensure that no inappropriate conversations occur near the patient.

Research

Research opportunities focus on the causes and treatment of hearing and balance disorders. The Research Opportunities and Clinical Impact box identifies just a few of these opportunities.

Summary

Most nurses will care for an individual with a hearing and balance disorder during the course of their careers. The nurse must be knowledgeable and sensitive to the needs of people with hearing impairments to ensure safety and decrease anxiety. These unique challenges will provide extreme rewards especially when the prescribed therapy restores hearing to someone who might otherwise live the rest of their years in progressive silence.

RESEARCH OPPORTUNITIES AND CLINICAL IMPACT RELATED TO HEARING AND BALANCE DISORDERS

Research Area	Clinical Impact
Hearing aids for sensorineural hearing loss	Improved hearing.
	Three new types of hearing aids designed to help individuals with a sensorineural hearing loss are under investigation: linear peak clipper (PC), compression limiter (CL), and wide dynamic range compressor (WDRC).
	Researchers have found that all three new hearing aids have increased hearing between 10% and 30% in individuals with sensorineural hearing loss.
Occupational hazard	Research ways to decrease hearing loss due to continuous exposure to loud noise.
Prevent genetic deafness	Normal hearing

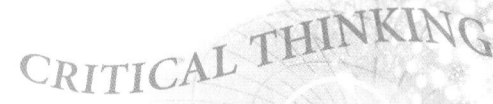

Clinical Preparation

 Read

- History of Current Illness
- Past Medical History
- Physical Exam
- Admitting Medical Orders
- Laboratory Study Results

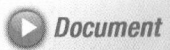 **Document**

- Summary of Hospitalization
- Pathophysiology Form
- Laboratory Values
- Laboratory Results Explanation

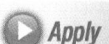 **Apply**

- List of Potential Nursing Diagnoses
- Concept Map
- Critical Thinking Questions

*Log on to MyNursingKit.com to download forms you will need and to complete further steps in the Clinical Preparation assignment.

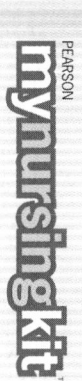

HISTORY OF PRESENT ILLNESS

Mrs. M. is a 78-year-old Caucasian female admitted through the emergency department for substernal chest pain. Even though Mrs. M. was admitted to the hospital with rule-out myocardial infarction, one health issue of concern was her inability to hear or follow simple commands. On closer evaluation it was determined that Mrs. M. had a definite hearing problem, one worthy of more investigation.

Once Mrs. M.'s cardiac status was stabilized, the concern turned to her hearing problem. Mrs. M. stated that she has noticed a progressive decline in her ability to hear, so much so that she has asked her family to provide a telephone with an amplifier so that she can hear conversations better. After an audiology examination conducted several years ago, she was diagnosed with presbycusis in addition to some degree of sensorineural hearing loss, probably due to ototoxic medications.

Medical–Surgical History

Allergies: naproxen sodium, hives

Medications: Lanoxin 0.125 mg po q a.m., aspirin 85 mg po q a.m., Toprox XL 100 mg po daily, Altace 2.5 mg po bid

Previous illnesses: pulmonary tuberculosis, 1944, treated with repeated pneumothorax treatments; history of taking streptomycin in 1955 prophylactically for tuberculosis; diagnosed with type II diabetes mellitus in 1993, diet controlled; progressive alteration in hearing

Surgeries: bilateral knee replacements, 1994

Social History

Family history: parents deceased; husband, two daughters alive/well

Social history: married, lives with husband split-level home

Physical Exam

Elderly white female

Height: 5 ft 3 inches; weight: 154 lbs

Temperature: 98.0°F

Pulse: 64 and regular

Respirations: 18 and regular

Blood pressure: 138/88 right arm

O_2 saturation: 93% on room air

HEENT: uses reading glasses; own teeth/no dentures

Neck: no JVD; carotid pulses present bilaterally

Heart: NSR, rate/rhythm regular

Lungs: present right lobes, reduced left upper lobe

Abdomen: soft, nontender, mildly obese

Extremities: no edema; pedal pulses strong; bilateral scars present over both knees

Neuro: Alert and oriented × 3

CXR: mild cardiomegaly

ECG: changes consistent with mild ischemia

Admitting Medical Orders

Admit to telemetry unit

Cardiology

Condition: stable

Allergies: naproxen sodium, hives

Diagnosis: R/O pending MI; status postcardiac catheterization; 80% blockage of LAD coronary artery; stent placed

Audiology consult

IV: saline lock; flush q8h

Diet: NAS

Oxygen: 2 L NC

Daily weight

I&O

Accu-Chek ac and at bedtime

Sequential compression devices (SCDs) to lower extremities

Bed rest with bathroom privileges

Vital signs and oxygen saturation q4h

Incentive spirometer q2h while awake

Call house officer if: pulse < 60 & > 110/minute; BP < 90 & > 160 systolic; temperature > 38.5; urine output < 30 mL/hr for 2 hours; respiratory rate > 30/minute; oxygen saturation <92%; Accu-Chek < 70 and > 130

Scheduled Medications

Lanoxin 0.125 mg po q a.m.

Aspirin 81 mg po q a.m.

Toprox XL 100 mg po daily

Altace 2.5 mg po bid

Postcatheterization: Plavix 75 mg po q a.m.

Glipizide SR 10 mg po daily

PRN Medications

Nitroglycerin 0.4 mg sublingual prn chest pain q5min × 3

Morphine 0.3–5 mg IV q3–5min; maximum dose 15 mg q3hr prn pain

Phenergan 25 mg IV q6h prn nausea

Mylanta 30 mL q4–6h po prn dyspepsia

Triazolam 0.125–0.25 mg po q noc, prn sleep

Ativan 0.5–2 mg IV q6–8h prn anxiety

Milk of Magnesia 30 mL po daily, prn constipation

Tylenol 650 mg po/PR q4h for pain

Ordered Laboratory Studies

Fasting blood sugar

Hemoglobin A1c

Troponin I q8h × 3

CPK-MB q8h × 3

Basic chemistry panel, CBC, magnesium q a.m.

Lipid panel in a.m.

Ordered Diagnostic Studies

Chest x-ray on admission

12-lead ECG

Echocardiogram

Cardiac catheterization

LABORATORY STUDY RESULTS

Test	Before Heart Catheterization	After Heart Catheterization	Day 2
Sodium	140 mEq/L	138 mEq/L	139 mEq/L
Potassium	4 mEq/L	4.2 mEq/L	4.2 mEq/L
Chloride	101 mEq/L	99 mEq/L	103 mEq/L
Carbon dioxide (CO_2)	22 mEq/L	24 mEq/L	25 mEq/L
Blood urea nitrogen (BUN)	19 mg/dL	18 mg/dL	18 mg/dL
Creatinine	1.2 mg/dL	1.0 mg/dL	1.1 mg/dL
Fasting blood sugar	160 mg/dL		
Hemoglobin A1c	7.0%		
Phosphorus	2.1 mg/dL	3.2 mg/dL	3.7 mg/dL
Calcium	8.1 mg/dL	8.2 mg/dL	8.6 mg/dL
Magnesium	2.0 mEq/L	1.9 mEq/L	2.0 mEq/L
Creatine kinase	4,018 units/L	3,612 units/L	2,000 units/L

Test	Before Heart Catheterization	After Heart Catheterization	Day 2
Relative index	>5.9%	>10.1%	>9.2%
CK–MB	>300.00%	>300.00%	259.7%
Troponin I	>100 ng/mL	80.91 ng/mL	51.00 ng/mL
WBC	11.5/mm³	11.0/mm³	9.3/mm³
RBC	4.21/mm³	4.89/mm³	4.92/mm³
Hemoglobin	12.9 g/dL	11.5 g/dL	12.7 g/dL
Hematocrit	37.5%	36.8%	37.6%
Platelets	262,000/mm³	280,000/mm³	300,000/mm³
Cholesterol	256 mg/dL		
High-density lipoproteins (HDL)	30 mg/dL		
Low-density lipoproteins (LDL)	158 mg/dL		
Very low-density lipoproteins (VLDL)	60%		
Apolipoproteins	152 mg/dL		
Triglycerides	201 mg/dL		

CRITICAL THINKING QUESTIONS

1. Mrs. M. needs to have the television on extremely loud and her roommate is complaining. What can you do to help the situation?

2. Knowing the type of hearing loss Mrs. M. is experiencing, what would be the best treatment for her?

3. Is Mrs. M. a candidate for a hearing aid or cochlear implant? Why?

4. Identify four specific discharge instructions to help the family work with Mrs. M.'s hearing disorder until further treatment is prescribed.

Answers to Critical Thinking Questions appear in Appendix D.

NCLEX® REVIEW

1. A patient tells the nurse that she's had her right eardrum punctured many times when she was a child. The nurse realizes this patient might have difficulty with:
   1. Balance.
   2. Movement.
   3. Sound transmission.
   4. Equilibrium.

2. A patient tells the nurse that she hears better when she isn't wearing a scarf over her head. The nurse realizes this patient is describing which mechanism of hearing?
   1. Bone conduction
   2. Air conduction
   3. Middle ear conduction
   4. Acoustic nerve conduction

3. A young male was brought into the emergency department because he suddenly couldn't hear. Upon examination, it was determined that a small object was lodged deeply into his ear canal. Which type of hearing loss did this patient experience?
   1. Mixed
   2. Acoustic
   3. Conductive
   4. Sensorineural

4. A young mother with a 2-week-old infant tells the nurse that she hopes her baby has good hearing since deafness "runs in her family." Which of the following should the nurse instruct this patient?
   1. The baby can't be tested for hearing until at least the age of 1.
   2. Even if tested, the baby's hearing will change as he grows.
   3. The baby should be tested now.
   4. The baby's sense of hearing hasn't developed yet.

5. A patient is scheduled for a stapedectomy. The nurse realizes this procedure is used to most likely treat which of the following causes of a hearing disorder?
   1. Mechanical
   2. Inflammatory
   3. Obstructive
   4. Mixed

6. The nurse is caring for a patient with a hearing deficit. Which of the following should be included in this patient's discharge planning for environmental safety?
   1. Assist with location for American Sign Language classes
   2. Removal of scatter rugs throughout the home
   3. Mechanism to ensure a visual alert in the event of a home fire
   4. Instruction on electrical cord safety

7. An elderly patient tells the nurse that she has a difficult time hearing. Which of the following should the nurse do to assist this patient's hearing deficit?

1. Shout directly into the patient's ear.

2. Drop the tone of the voice when talking.

3. Clap hands directly into the patient's face to gain the patient's attention.

4. Write everything down for the patient to read.

8. A patient with a new onset of a hearing loss becomes anxious when the nurse begins to leave the room. Which of the following should the nurse do to help this patient?

1. Assure the patient that the call light will be answered as soon as possible.

2. Tell the patient that there are other patients who have more important needs at this time.

3. Suggest that the patient walk in the hall to see other people.

4. Turn on the television for the patient.

Answers for review questions appear in Appendix D

KEY TERMS

acoustic neuroma *p.2307*
air conduction *p.2303*
bone conduction *p.2303*
conductive hearing loss *p.2303*
decibel (dB) *p.2311*
exostosis *p.2304*
frequency *p.2310*
labyrinthectomy *p.2308*
labyrinthitis *p.2308*

mastoidectomy *p.2305*
mastoiditis *p.2305*
Ménière's disease *p.2309*
mixed hearing loss *p.2303*
myringotomy *p.2304*
noise-induced hearing loss (NIHL) *p.2307*
otitis externa *p.2304*
otitis media *p.2305*
otosclerosis *p.2304*

ototoxic *p.2305*
pitch *p.2311*
presbycusis *p.2305*
sensorineural hearing loss *p.2303*
stapedectomy *p.2304*
tinnitus *p.2305*
tympanoplasty *p.2304*
vertigo *p.2308*
vestibular nerve dissection *p.2308*

EXPLORE PEARSON **mynursingkit**

MyNursingKit is your one stop for online chapter review materials and resources. Prepare for success with additional NCLEX®-style practice questions, interactive assignments and activities, web links, animations and videos, and more!

Register your access code from the front of your book at
www.mynursingkit.com

REFERENCES

American Academy of Otolaryngology–Head and Neck Surgery. (2002). *Noise and hearing protection.* Retrieved June 25, 2007, from http://www.entnet.org/healthinfo/hearing/noise_hearing.cfm

American College of Radiology. (2008). Guideline title: *Vertigo and hearing loss.* Retrieved on September 29, 2008 from http://www.guideline.gov/summary/summary.aspx?ss=15&doc_id=9602&nbr=5123

Black, F. O., Pesznecker, S. C., Homer, L., & Stallings, V. (2004). Benign paroxysmal positional nystagmus in hospitalized subjects receiving ototoxic medications. *Otol. Neurotol., 25*(3), 353–358.

Deaf Mental Health Charter. (2007). *Mental Health Foundation.* Retrieved June 21, 2007, from http://www.mhf.org.uk/our-work/service-development/all-age-groups/deaf-charter

Hain, T. C. (2007). *Benign paroxysmal positional vertigo.* Retrieved on August 21, 2007, from http://www.dizziness-and-balance.com/disorders/bppv/bppv.html

Holloway, N. M. (2004). *Medical-surgical care planning* (4th ed.). Philadelphia: Lippincott Williams & Wilkins.

Hunter, J. (1996). *Genetics and inheritance.* Retrieved July 2007 from Dartmouth University website: http://www.dartmouth.edu/~cbbc/courses/bio4/bio4-1997/01-Genetics.html

Imai, T., et al. (2005). Natural course of the remission of vertigo in patients with benign paroxysmal positional vertigo. *Neurology, 64,* 920–923.

Isaacson, J. E. (2005). In C. M. Porth (Ed.), *Pathophysiology: Concepts of altered health* (7th ed.). Philadelphia: Lippincott Williams & Wilkins.

Jones, E. G., Renger, R. and Kang, Y. (2007). Self efficacy for health related behaviors among deaf adults. *Research in Nursing and Health. 30*(2), 185–192.

Kim, C. S., Chang, S. O., & Lim, D. (Eds.). (2000). Updates in cochlear implantation. *Advances in Otorhinolaryngology, 57,* 22–27.

Mitchell, R. (1997). *Genetics and inheritance.* Retrieved July 2007 from Dartmouth University website: http://www.dartmouth.edu/~cbbc/courses/bio4/bio4-1997/01-Genetics.html

Kuramoto AM. (2006). Therapeutic benefits of t'ai chi exercise: research review. WMJ. 105(7):42-6.

Murray, R. B. and Zentner, J. P. (2001). *Health promotion strategies through the life span* (7th ed.). New Jersey: Prentice Hall, pages 765–767, 782–783.

National Conference of State Legislators. (2007, May). *50 State summary of newborn hearing screening laws.* Retrieved June 21, 2007, from http://www.ncsl.org/programs/health/hear50.htm

National Institutes on Deafness and Other Communication Disorders. (2001, January). *Hearing loss and older adults* (NIH Publication No. 01-4913). Retrieved June 25, 2007, from http://www.nidcd.nih.gov

National Guidelines Clearinghouse. (1999). ACR Appropriateness Criteria for vertigo and hearing loss. www.guideline.gov

National Health and Nutrition Exam Survey (2004). Retrieved on June 25, 2007 from www.cdc.gov/nchs/nhanes.htm

National Institute of Health. (2000). Clinical advisory: NIDCD/VA clinical trial finding can benefit millions with hearing loss. Retrieved from www.nlm.nih.gov. on June 25, 2007. October 2000.

National Institutes on Deafness and Other Communication Disorders. (2002a, November). *Cochlear implants* (NIH Publication No. 00-4798). Retrieved June 25, 2007, from http://www.nidcd.nih.gov

National Institutes on Deafness and Other Communication Disorders. (2002b, February). *Hearing aids* (NIH Publication No. 99-4340). Retrieved June 25, 2007, from http://www.nidcd.nih.gov

Parmet, S., Lynm, C., & Glass, R. (2003). Adult hearing loss. *Journal of the American Medical Association, 289,* 2020.

Sadler, G. R., Huang, J. T., Padden, C. A., et al. (2001). Accommodating Deaf Patients in Non-Hospital Settings. *Journal of Cancer Education, 16*(2) 105-8.

Sandhaus, S. (2002). Stop the spinning: Diagnosing and managing vertigo. *Nurse Practitioner, American Journal of Primary Health Care, 27*(8), 19–25.

Shaia, W. T., Zappia, J. J., Bojrab, D. I., LaRouere, M. L., Sargent, E. W., & Diaz, R. C. (2006). Success of posterior semicircular canal occlusion and application of the dizziness handicap inventory. *Otolaryngology–Head Neck Surgery, 134*(3), 424–430.

Smith, R. J. H., & Camp, G. V. (2007). *Deafness & hereditary hearing loss: Overview.* Seattle: University of Washington.

UCSD Student Health Service. (2007). Retrieved July 2007 from http://studenthealth.UCSD.edu

University of Iowa Hospital & Clinics. (2006). *Hearing loss in adults.* Retrieved July 2007 from http://www.uihealthcare.com/topics/hearing/hear4685.html

United States Department of Health and Human Services. (2000). *Healthy people 2010: Understanding and improving health.* Retrieved February 5, 2008, from http://www.healthypeople.gov

Caring for the Patient with Visual Disorders

Lucie S. Elfervig

Outcome-Based Learning Objectives

After studying this chapter, the learner will be able to:

1. Identify the normal basic anatomy and physiology of the eye.

2. Perform basic assessment, tests, and examination of the eye in obtaining meaningful data for management and treatment.

3. Describe different types of visual and ocular conditions and problems.

4. Apply nursing diagnoses, nursing process, and patient teaching associated with the visual and ocular problems of adults.

5. Discuss and provide meaningful resources for patients with visual and ocular problems.

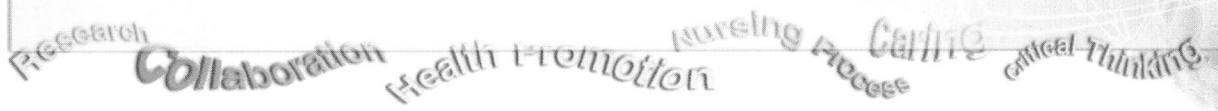

THE SENSE of sight is one of the primary means of being active and taking joy in the visual world, being that the other senses seem to direct one toward seeing what is heard, what is touched, what is smelled, and what is tasted. So, truly sight guides most of one's daily activities. The eyes also provide a window or insight into the body's functions. Systemic problems or conditions that have visual or ocular manifestations can be discovered for the first time on an ocular examination. Chart 71–1 (p. 2326) outlines the more common systemic problems that may be manifested through ocular conditions. Often, ocular impairment can be preventable with early recognition and treatment that will save vision and prevent blindness. Visual disorders, depending on the degree of vision loss, can be very disturbing, with a sense of hopelessness, loss, powerlessness, and bereavement for the patient as well as the patient's family. Vision loss may be as minor as a refractive error that can be corrected with glasses, contact lenses, or laser or as severe as ocular trauma with functional vision loss, no light perception, or enucleation. Visual impairment creates both a physical and a psychological adjustment that can limit a patient's activities of daily living (ADL).

Visual assessment is a vital part of the nurse's function in caring for the whole patient and giving reassurance to patients that the nurse is there for their total well-being. Nurses play a key role in assisting, planning, implementing, evaluating, and educating patients and their families in adapting to new cop-

ing skills for everyday changes that can come with visual disorders. This chapter provides an overview of visual disorders for the adult through the aged, clarifying in greater detail the ocular disorders that appear more often today, and how best to evaluate and manage eye and ocular conditions. Many eye professionals perform specific roles in the evaluation, assessment, and treatment of medical and surgical ocular diseases and conditions. Typically health care providers adhere to the vision objectives set forth for the first time in *Healthy People 2010.* These objectives, commonly referred to as *Healthy Vision 2010,* provide a framework to assessment and promotion of ocular health through the chapter. These are detailed in the National Guidelines feature entitled Healthy Vision 2010 for Eye Evaluation (p. 2327).

■ Anatomy and Physiology Overview

The eyeball and its structures can be examined externally and internally. The orbit and ocular adnexa structures include the orbital contents and walls, eyebrows, eyelashes, eyelids, lacrimal puncta, lacrimal system, and extraocular muscles (Figure 71–1 ■, p. 2326). The eye structures include the canthus, conjunctiva, limbus, sclera, cornea, anterior and posterior chambers, trabecular meshwork, choroid, ciliary body, iris, pupil, lens, vitreous body, and retina.

CHART 71–1	**Ocular Conditions Resulting from Systemic Problems**
Systemic Problem	**Ocular Condition**
Atopic dermatitis	Keratoconus
	Trichiasis
Cerebrovascular accident (stroke)	Vascular occlusion
	Hemianopia, blindness
Cirrhosis	Xanthelasma
Diabetes mellitus	Rubeosis iridis
	Dot/blot hemorrhages
	Exudates
	Vitreous hemorrhage
Giant cell arteritis	Anterior ischemic optic neuropathy (AION)
	Amaurosis fugax
	Cilioretinal artery occlusion (CAO)
	Cotton-wool spots (CWS)
Gout	Asteroid hyalosis
	Bilateral conjunctival hyperemia
Herpes zoster (shingles)	Disciform keratitis
	Unilateral facial lesions
	Trigeminal dermatomes
Histoplasmosis	Choroiditis
	Peripheral hypopigmented spots
	Choroidal neovascular membrane (CNV)
Hypertension	Hard exudates, edema
	Narrow arterioles
	Cotton-wool spots
Hyperthyroidism (Graves' disease)	Exophthalmos
	Eyelid retraction
	Braley's sign*
Immunosuppressive disease (AIDS)	Cytomegalovirus retinitis
Inflammatory bowel disease	Frequent subconjunctival hemorrhages
	Limbal infiltrates
	Episcleritis
Leukemia	Roth's spots**
	Papilledema
Multiple sclerosis (MS)	Optic nerve edema
	Nystagmus
	Diplopia
Rheumatoid arthritis	Anterior scleritis
	Episcleritis
	Filamentary keratitis
Systemic Lupus Erythematosis (SLE)	Keratoconjunctivitis sicca (KCS)***
	Cotton-wool spots
	Central serous retinopathy (CSR)
Third nerve palsy	Ptosis
	Ophthalmoplegia
Toxoplasmosis	Retinochoroiditis
	Cystoid macular edema (CME)
Usher's syndrome	Posterior subcapsular cataract (PSC)
	Pigmentary retinopathy
	Bull's-eye retinal lesions
	(Other key symptom: deafness)

*Braley's sign: Intraocular pressure increases in an upward gaze, as compared to looking in a normal position.
**Roth's spot: retinal hemorrhage that has a white center.
***Keratoconjunctivitis sicca (KCS): dry eye syndrome.

Sources: Gold, D. H., & Weingeist, T. A. (2001). *Color atlas of the eye in systemic disease.* Philadelphia: Lippincott Williams & Wilkins; Kanski, J. J. (2001). *Systemic diseases and the eye: Signs and differential diagnosis.* London: Mosby International Limited; and Watson, P. G., Hazleman, B. L., Pavesio, C. E., & Green, W. R. (2004). *The sclera & systemic disorders* (2nd ed.). Philadelphia: Butterworth-Heinemann.

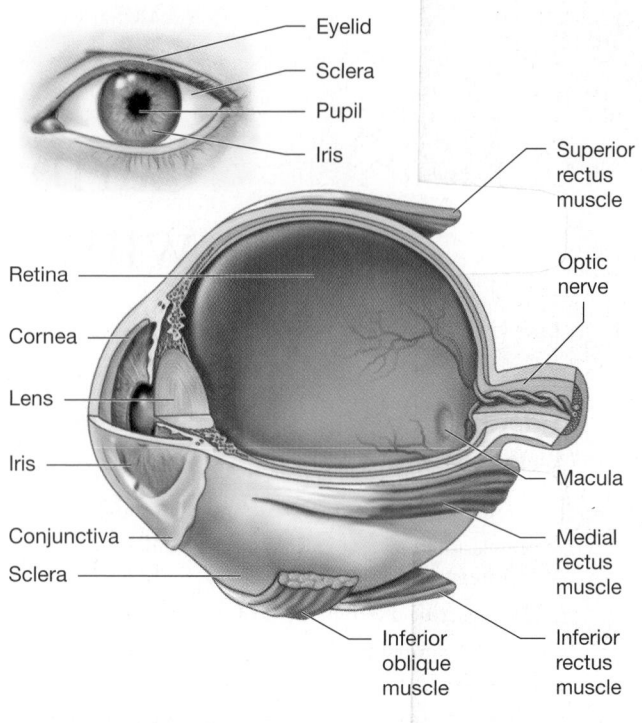

FIGURE 71–1 ■ The human eye.

Orbit and Ocular Adnexa

The eyeball is encased on three sides by the bony cavity called the orbit, which protects the eyeball from injury. The orbit is lined with muscles, connective, and adipose or fat tissue. It is approximately 40 millimeters in all three dimensions (height, width, and depth), like a pear lying on its side. The orbital walls are made up of seven bones that include the frontal, zygomatic, sphenoid, ethmoid, lacrimal, palatine, and maxillary bones. The eyebrow lies over the bony prominence (superior orbital ridge) above the eyelids that acts as a protective ridge from falling debris or foreign objects getting into the eye. The upper and lower eyelashes are the ciliary hairs of the eyelids that help keep debris from falling into the eye. The eyelids contain the ocular glands, which include oil glands (meibomian and glands of Zeis), mucous glands (goblet cells), sweat glands (Moll), and aqueous glands (lacrimal and accessory lacrimal glands of Krause and Wolfring).

The space or exposed area between the upper and lower eyelids is called the interpalpebral fissure. The eyelids have a blink mechanism that operates by the levator palpebrae superioris muscle to protect the anterior portion of the eye and the spreading of tears across the cornea. This blink mechanism is very important to the health of the cornea. Upper and lower lacrimal puncta are the small openings at the nasal end of the upper and lower eyelid margins for the drainage of tears produced by the lacrimal system. The lacrimal gland lies under the upper eyelid skin between the lateral eyebrow edge and outer canthus.

The eyeball is able to move in all cardinal fields of gaze by the six extraocular muscles, which are the four rectus muscles (superior, medial, inferior, and lateral) and two oblique muscles (superior and inferior). The extraocular muscles are innervated by the third, fourth, and sixth cranial nerves, which coordinate the vision of both eyes with the occipital lobe of the brain to view a single image.

HEALTHY VISION NATIONAL GUIDELINES for Eye Evaluation

Healthy Vision 2010 (DHHS, 2000b), objectives provide a way to identify vision and eye problems and an opportunity to improve the vision of all Americans with prevention measures established by the following organizations: the American Academy of Ophthalmology, National Eye Institute, Centers for Disease Control and Prevention's Vision Health Initiative, Glaucoma Foundation, and American Academy of Optometry. The focus of *Healthy Vision 2010* is to make Americans aware of eye diseases that can result in loss of vision and the necessary measures for prevention of eye disease and injury. The promotion of vision health and quality of life for all people, at all stages of life, addresses issues that affect cost, disability, and diseases in vision loss. To achieve its overall prevention goals, *Healthy People 2010* supports comprehensive community-based eye screenings and regular vision checkups—these vary between age and disease entity—with an eye health care provider. Regular eye examinations are a means of prevention, diagnosing eye problems early, as well as treatment for people diagnosed with diabetic retinopathy, cataracts, glaucoma, macular degeneration, and any vision problems that might lead to blindness. *Healthy People 2010* recommends comprehensive programs that must be applied universally to the general population and in a more intensive fashion to selected and indicated persons known to be at high risk for vision impairment; for example, those with diabetes (DHHS, 2000a). *Healthy People 2010* recognizes vision as the primary cue for conducting everyday activities. Vision is instrumental in development, learning, communicating, working, health, and quality of life. Vision loss creates many environmental, social, and psychological challenges for individuals and their families.

Healthy Vision 2010 has 10 main objectives related to vision assessment:

1. *Dilated eye examination.* To detect early diseases and disorders of the eye, because many eye conditions have no signs or symptoms, or warning. This should be done at least every 2 years for adults.

2. *Vision screening for children (under 5 years).* To detect vision problems before beginning school, in an effort to save sight.

3. *Impairment due to refractive errors.* Over 60% of Americans have refractive defects that could benefit from corrective lenses.

4. *Impairment in children and adolescents (under 18 years).* Reduce blindness and visual impairment, especially nearsightedness (myopia), which affects about 25% of schoolchildren.

5. *Diabetic eye disease.* Reduce vision loss and impairment due to diabetic retinopathy. Early diagnosis and treatment can prevent about 90% of vision loss with an annual dilated eye examination. About 50% of patients with diabetes are diagnosed too late for effective treatment.

6. *Reduce visual impairment due to glaucoma.* Optic nerve damage is a major health problem, and left untreated it will lead to blindness. Up to 3 million Americans have glaucoma and as many as 120,000 are blind. Glaucoma is the number-one cause of vision loss in African Americans. Half of the people with glaucoma are not being treated because they are unaware they have this condition; it is known as the silent blinder.

7. *Cataracts.* Reduce vision loss due to cataracts. They can occur in children, but are mostly a problem for adults age 50 and older. Treatment is readily available with surgery and intraocular lens implantation.

8. *Occupational injury.* Reduce vision loss from occupational injury and lost workdays. It is reported that 3 out of every 5 occupational eye injuries are due to not wearing safety goggles or protective eyewear. The Occupational Safety and Health Administration requires that employees be provided with protective eyewear, which can prevent 90% of eye-related accidents.

9. *Protective eyewear.* Increased use of personal protective eyewear for recreation, for hazardous projects at home, and for sports (hockey, racquetball, tennis, baseball, basketball, and paintball), which all bring some risk of eye injury.

10. *Vision rehabilitation.* Increase in the use of services for the visually impaired and the use of adaptive devices in aiding vision.

Nurses need to be knowledgeable of these objectives and guidelines in educating patients and families in the prevention of vision loss, in providing educational materials on eye health, and in promoting early detection and treatment of eye diseases.

Sources: U.S. Department of Health and Human Services (DHHS). (2000a). *Healthy People 2010: Vision and hearing.* Retrieved April 26, 2007, from http://www.healthypeople.gov/document/HTML/Volume2/28Vision.htm; and U.S. Department of Health and Human Services (DHHS). (2000b). *Healthy Vision 2010.* Retrieved April 26, 2007, from http://www.healthyvision.2010.org

Eye Structures

It is necessary to understand the anatomic structure of the eye as a whole in order to identify pathophysiological conditions and their impact on the individual. The basic anatomic structures are explained next.

The temporal and nasal canthi are the outer and inner tissue edges where the upper and lower eyelids meet. The palpebral and bulbar conjunctivas are the mucous membrane lining of the undersurface of the eyelids and eyeball itself, up to the limbal margin, respectively. The fornix or cul-de-sac is the junction where the palpebral and bulbar conjunctivas meet. The limbus or the corneoscleral junction is the margin between the sclera and the cornea. The sclera, which is the white part and the outer protective layer of the eyeball, helps maintain its shape. The cornea, which is the transparent, avascular center at the anterior surface of the eyeball, is the major refractive surface of the eye. The refractive media of the cornea bend light rays to a single focus on the retina. The epithelium is the outermost layer of the cornea that is protected by the tear film layers that also gives the cornea its smooth surface. The tear film is composed of three layers, and if any of the layers is defective, the health of the eye can be compromised. The tears are formed by a natural reflex response or emotional stimulus.

The anterior chamber is the space between the back of the cornea and the front of the iris. The posterior chamber is the space between the back of the iris and the front of the lens. Both these chambers contain aqueous humor, which is a clear fluid that provides nutrients for the eye. The aqueous humor is produced by the ciliary body, which also helps regulate intraocular pressure. The trabecular meshwork is a mesh-like filtering structure located at the iris–scleral junction (limbal region) at the angle in the anterior chamber. The meshwork assists in the regulation of the intraocular pressure of the eye with the filtering and flow of aqueous humor as it drains into the canal of Schlemm at the angle.

Uveal Tract

The uveal tract is composed of the choroid, ciliary body, and iris. The choroid is the middle layer of the eyeball between the retina and the sclera. The choroid contains the major vascular system of the eye that nourishes the outer retina. The ciliary body makes up the ciliary processes and ciliary muscles. The processes produce the aqueous humor that flows through the chambers and can affect the intraocular pressure of the eye. The ciliary muscles control the accommodative ability of the lens by the attachment of the zonular fibers between the lens and ciliary muscles. The ciliary muscle contractions can change the configuration of the trabecular meshwork or canal of Schlemm by increasing aqueous outflow and, in turn, can affect the intraocular pressure of the eye. The iris is a vascular and pigmented fiber that forms the colored portion of the eye that encompasses the pupil. The iris (iris diaphragm) is the division between the anterior and posterior chambers. The pupil is the black middle space of the iris, which constricts and dilates by the sphincter and the dilator muscles, respectively. This allows the refraction of light to enter the eye for vision. The pupils normally react to bright light by constricting, and they are usually equal, round, and accommodative.

Lens

The lens divides the aqueous humor from the vitreous humor or gel. It is the focusing structure of **accommodation** that allows seeing objects at close and at far range. The lens is supported by the zonular fibers that are attached to the ciliary body. It is the one ocular structure that continues to grow with aging.

Vitreous Body

The vitreous body is the largest chamber (roughly two-thirds) of the eye that maintains the shape of the eyeball. The vitreous gel is made up mainly of water with a collagen framework, which includes collagen (structure), hyaluronic acid (which gives the vitreous its viscosity), proteins, and solutes. The collagen network can be aggregated by vitreous collapse due to aging that forms vitreous opacities, which cast shadows on the retina. These shadows are referred to as **floaters**. The posterior and peripheral vitreous interfaces with the retina.

Retina

The retina is composed of 10 thin layers. Two of the major retina layers are the photoreceptor layer and the retinal pigment epithelium. The photoreceptor layer is composed of cones and rods for photopic (day) and scotopic (night) vision. The center of the retina, called the macula, is where the greatest number of cone receptors is located for central and color vision. The rod receptors mainly are in the peripheral retina for side or field vision. The very center of the macula is called the fovea or fovea centralis, where the greatest concentrations of cones are located for the sharpest visual acuity. The two main functions of the retinal pigment epithelium are the metabolism of vitamin A and the absorption of light, which aid in visual acuity by providing nutrients to the photoreceptors.

Other major structures in the retina are the optic disc and vessels. The optic disc is oval or circular, pinkish orange in color, with distinct margins; has a central depression or cup; and is the physiological blind spot on a visual field. The central cup of the disc is where the retinal vessels (arteries and veins) enter and branch out to form the superior and inferior arcades that are the outer borders of the macula. The optic nerve is an extension of the central nervous system that forms a visual pathway behind the eyes. The pathway crosses at the chiasm where the optic nerve of each eye meets and crosses nasally and uncrosses temporally to form the optic tracts. The optic tracts continue to the lateral geniculate bodies, to the optic radiations, and then to the visual cortex of the occipital lobe of the brain.

Visual Assessment

Visual assessment should follow a thorough health history. Chart 71–2 outlines the categories and assessment of a health and ocular history. The categories include the general medical history, the visual history, and the history of clinical manifestations. It is important to ask the patient specifically about any inherited conditions such as diabetes, hypertension, macular degeneration, glaucoma, or unexplained vision loss. And if an injury has occurred, the nurse needs to make certain to question whether the trauma involved any metal-on-metal contact, as this tends to cause intraocular penetration.

Initial Examination

The initial examination should include the following procedures: visual acuity (VA) at far range (Figure 71–2 ■) and at near range (Figure 71–3 ■), external eye examination, the direct ophthalmoscope examination, and an intraocular pressure reading. For patients that cannot read, use a picture chart to obtain acuity. Chart 71–3 (p. 2330) outlines the steps for visual acuity testing.

The external evaluation can be done with the use of a penlight and visual observation. The components for completing

CHART 71–2	Health and Ocular History Assessment
Category	**Assessment**
General history	Any known allergies (drugs, foods, environment)? Using any prescription or over-the-counter medications? Any recent illnesses or surgeries? Any known medical history (especially diabetes, ulcers, strokes, hypertension, and pulmonary)?
Visual history	Wears glasses, contact lenses, or no correction? Are one or both eyes involved? Using any topical eyedrops or oral eye medications? Vision prior to problem, injury, or trauma (if applicable)? Any vision or eye test already obtained previously? Any prior eye surgery or laser?
History of clinical manifestations	Any signs and symptoms? Duration of signs and symptoms? Time and place of signs and symptoms, problem or injury/what happened? Any penetrating or perforating injury? Any metal?

Eye test chart for 10 feet

Actual size   20 ft. equivalent

$\frac{10}{100}$	K V D	$\frac{20}{160}$
$\frac{10}{60}$	Z S H C	$\frac{20}{125}$
$\frac{10}{50}$	H S K R N	$\frac{20}{100}$
$\frac{10}{40}$	C H K R V D	$\frac{20}{80}$
$\frac{10}{30}$	H O N S D C V	$\frac{20}{60}$
$\frac{10}{25}$	O K H D N R C S	$\frac{20}{50}$
$\frac{10}{20}$	V H D N K U O S R C	$\frac{20}{40}$
$\frac{10}{15}$	B D C L K Z V H S R O A	$\frac{20}{30}$
$\frac{10}{12}$	H K G B C A N O M P V E S R	$\frac{20}{25}$
$\frac{10}{10}$	P K U E O B T V X R M J H C A Z D I	$\frac{20}{20}$
$\frac{10}{8}$	D K N T W U L J S P X V M R A H C F O Y Z G	$\frac{20}{15}$

FIGURE 71–2 ■ Visual acuity chart for far.

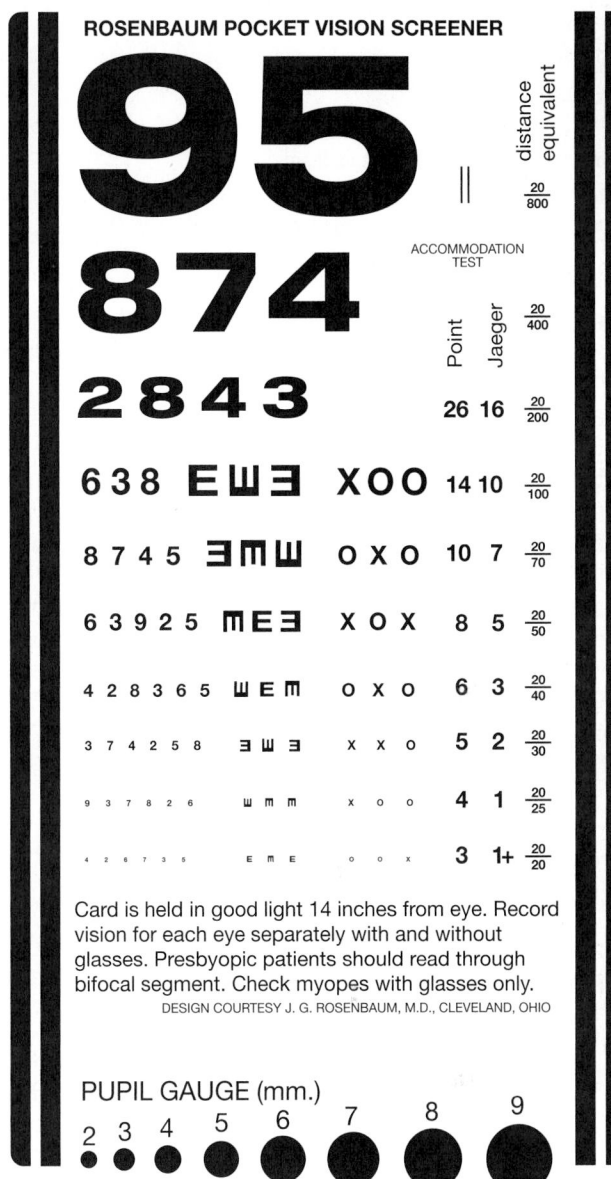

FIGURE 71–3 ■ Visual acuity chart for near.

the external examination and procedures are listed in Chart 71–4 (p. 2330) and Chart 71–5 (p. 2331).

Direct ophthalmoscope examination is used to check the fundus of the eye by viewing through the pupil. During the process, the nurse needs to view the cornea, anterior chamber, lens, and vitreous for clarity; check for any opacity in the visual pathway; and check the optic nerve (disc) for color, shape, and vessels (Figure 71–4 ■, p. 2332). Most medical offices, clinics, ambulatory centers, outpatient facilities, and emergency departments will be equipped with a direct ophthalmoscope.

It also is important to check intraocular pressure (IOP) if one has a tonometer (Figure 71–5 ■, p. 2332), or the nurse may need to gently palpate over the eyelid to indicate whether the eyeball is hard or soft (Figure 71–6 ■, p. 2332).

Diagnostic eye tests are essential for a complete ocular and visual evaluation to decide on the most definitive diagnosis and treatment regimen. Many of the diagnostic tests require anesthetic or dilating eyedrops. These drops are described in the

Pharmacology Summary feature (p. 2346). The tests can include preoperative evaluations for cataract surgery for proper lenses implant, assessment of corneal health, visualization for possible retinal opacities and breaks, advancement of glaucoma, and genetic anomalies. Some of these diagnostic tests may include baseline fundus photography, fluorescein angiography, or ultrasonography. Other tests may be necessary to order for a more systemic assessment, such as x-rays, computed tomography (CT) scan, magnetic resonance imaging (MRI), and carotid ultrasound, in addition to specific blood tests and cultural sensitivities. Diagnostic tests that are used to assess ocular and visual health are outlined in the Diagnostic Tests box (p. 2333).

■ Visual Impairment

Visual impairment can be anything from correctable refractive errors, inherited anomalies, acquired visual changes, nutritional deficiencies, to aging changes. Refractive errors are the most

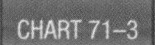

CHART 71–3	Visual Acuity Testing		

Types		Distances	Charts
Take Visual Acuity (VA)*			
Far VA (right eye, left eye, and both eyes): with glasses or contact lenses if the patient wears them.		20 feet (6 meters)	Snellen acuity or equivalent distance chart
Near VA (right eye, left eye, and both eyes): with glasses or contact lenses if the patient wears them.		14–16 inches (38–40 centimeters)	Near reading chart

*Test vision with each eye separately: right eye, then left eye (covering the eye not being tested); once vision is obtained with each eye, then test vision with both eyes open.

- **Record VA**—20/20, 20/30, etc. whatever line the patient reads, and document each eye separately and together (e.g., 20/30 right eye, 20/50 left eye, 20/40 both eyes) for far and near acuity. If the patient cannot see the chart at the standard distance, then walk up to the patient with the chart until he can read the largest letter (this is usually the 200 letter).

- **Record Count Fingers (CF)***—If the patient cannot see the nurse's fingers, then the nurse moves her hand and sees whether the patient can detect the motion; the nurse moves increasingly closer to the patient until he sees the nurse's hand moving. For example, the recording might read: CF at 5 feet with right eye, left eye, and both eyes.

- **Record Hand Motion (HM)****—If the patient cannot see the nurse's hand move, then shine a light in the patient's eyes (best to dim the room lights) and see whether he can detect the light; the nurse moves increasingly closer to the patient until the light is perceived. For example the recording might read: HM at 2 feet with right eye, left eye, and both eyes.

- **Record Light Perception (LP) or Record No Light Perception (NLP)*****—If the patient cannot see the nurse's light, then the visual acuity is no light perception (NLP), with right eye or left eye. When doing LPs, make sure the light is bright, room lights are dimmed, and the opposite eye is covered well. For example the recording might read: LP at 3 inches with right eye, left eye, and both eyes.

* At the distance seen (e.g., CF at 5 feet), with right eye, left eye, and both eyes.
** At the distance seen (e.g., HM at 2 feet), with right eye, left eye, and both eyes.
*** At the distance seen (e.g., LP at 3 inches), with right eye, left eye, and both eyes.

CHART 71–4	Ocular and Vision Evaluation Tests	

Test	Procedure
Extraocular muscle movement (cardinal fields of gaze)	The patient is seated directly opposite the tester, facing each other about 1 foot apart. The patient is instructed to look at a pen or target that is held in the tester's hand at a distance of 16 inches (40 centimeters). The patient is asked to follow the pen when the tester moves it in the primary position (looking straight ahead) to eight cardinal fields of gaze: from the primary position to look right upward, straight up, left upward, left temporal, left downward, straight down, right downward, and right temporal. The tester is to observe the patient and note whether her eyes move equally together in all fields of gaze, note whether both eyes are symmetrical, and record either as normal or, if any deviation from normal, as minimal (−1), moderate (−2), severe (−3), or total (−4) loss of eye movement.
Cover–uncover test for tropia	The patient is to wear his own corrective lenses, if he has them. Have the patient fixate on a target about 20 feet (6 meters) away for far and 16 inches (40 centimeters) for near; it can be a visual acuity chart, picture chart, E chart, or toy, the smallest line of clear acuity. The tester is to sit in front of the patient, but does not block target view. Note the eye that is fixating, cover that eye with an occluder, and note what the fellow eye does. If the uncovered eye moves to pick up fixation, note the direction it moves— toward the nose, then it was fixated outward, so it is exo; or toward the ear, then it was fixated inward, so it is eso. If the uncovered eye does not move and has steady fixation, no strabismus exists. The eye would move up and down to indicate vertical tropia.
Alternating cover test for phoria	The patient is to wear her own corrective lenses, if she has them. Have the patient fixate on a target about 20 feet (6 meters) away for far and 16 inches (40 centimeters) for near; it can be a visual acuity chart, picture chart, E chart, or toy, the smallest line of clear acuity. The tester is to sit in front of the patient, but does not block target view. Place the occluder in front of the right eye, hold it for about a second or so, and then move it swiftly over the left eye. This alternating cover test is repeated many times. Repeat with the occluder in front of the left eye for a second or so, then move it swiftly over the right eye, and repeat. The tester observes the eye that is just being uncovered to see whether it deviates. If the just uncovered eye moves inward, then it was fixed outward, so it is exo; and if the just uncovered eye moves outward, then it was fixed inward, so it is eso. If the just uncovered eye does not move and has steady fixation, no strabismus exist. The eye would move up and down to indicate vertical phoria.
Confrontation fields (visual field testing)	The tester is comparing the range of the patient's visual field in relation to the tester's visual field, which is assumed normal. The light source should be behind the patient, and the background behind the tester should be dark and uniform. The patient is seated, and the tester sits or stands directly opposite and facing the patient about 2 feet away. The patient's right eye is open and left eye is closed or occluded, while the tester's left eye is open and right eye is closed, and each fixes on the other's open eye. The tester will move her fingers or bright test object from the far periphery and note when it comes into the field of view; the tester and patient should see it at the same time. This is done for the four major quadrants (superior, nasal, inferior, and temporal) and repeated for the patient's left eye. The approximate normal degrees of angle recognition of the test object are 60° superior, 60° nasal, 70° inferior, and 80° temporal. Record results, and if any visual field defects are noted, the patient should be sent in for sophisticated visual field testing.

CHART 71–5	Ocular and Visual Evaluation and Assessment

Examination	Assessment
Initial Examination	
Central visual acuity	Take visual acuity (VA) of each eye separately and together at far and at near, with patient glasses if he wears them: with Snellen acuity chart or reading card; or use a newspaper, read a wall clock, or recognize faces at the bedside or at the doorway. Make some record of visual acuity.
Peripheral visual acuity	Take side vision; see whether the patient can see movement and objects coming in from the periphery. Confrontations can be done here; a visual field (VF) screening test.
Intraocular pressure (IOP)	Check IOP, if one has a tonometer, or may need to gently palpate over the eyelid to indicate whether the eyeball is hard or soft.
External Examination (Observations and Penlight Test)	Observe face and all structure surrounding the eye for any asymmetry or color, size, shape, or expression differences; and overall general appearance.
Eyelids	Does the eyelid close automatically (blink reflex)? Does the eyelid cover the cornea completely when closed? Does the eyelid lag or droop (ptosis)?
Eyelashes	Do the eyelashes curve inward (entropion) or outward (ectropion)? Are there any misaligned or missing lashes (trichiasis)?
Eyeball	Observe for obvious laceration, trauma, bruises, or black eye (ecchymosis). Does the eyeball appear sunken (enophthalmos) or protruding (proptosis)?
Conjunctiva	Observe and check for tearing, itching (pruritus), drainage, injection (hyperemia), swelling (edema), discoloration, lesions, scaling, or irregularities.
Sclera	Observe color (white) and vascular (red).
Cornea	Observe for clarity.
Anterior chamber	Check anterior chamber for whether it is clear and deep, meaning without discharge, deposits, or opaques; pus (hypopyon); or blood (hyphema). Sclera white and conjunctiva clear.
Pupils	Check pupils for size (in millimeters), shape, and whether pupils are equal, round, reactive to light and accommodation (PERRLA).
Iris	Observe color, shape, and size.
Muscles	Check eye mobility by checking the primary and eight cardinal fields of gaze for extraocular muscle function. Check for cross-eyes (exo = out, eso = in) by doing cover eye tests. Draw pictures of what is seen if indicated for documentation.
Direct Ophthalmoscope Examination*	Check for a red reflex, and note whether present or whether a different reflex is noted between the eyes (e.g., leukocoria-white reflex). View for media clarity (cornea, anterior chamber, lens, and vitreous), checking for any opacities or foreign bodies in the visual pathway. Check the optic nerve (disc) for color, shape, vessels, and cup/disc (C/D) ratio. View fovea (central vision area of the macula) for edema, color abnormalities, and foveal reflex (yellowish-orange reflex) to determine whether present or not, and whether there is asymmetry or atrophy.

*See Figures 71–2, 71–3, and 71–4 (pp. 2329 and 2332).

common vision problem in the general population. Four of the leading causes of visual impairment are macular degeneration, diabetic retinopathy, glaucoma, and cataracts. Measuring refractive error is referred to as a manifested refraction (MR) that is performed on a phoropter, a refractive device used to measure the degree of optical correction needed for one's best-corrected visual acuity (BVA) with the use of spherical, cylindrical, and prismatic lenses.

Refraction

Refraction refers to refractive errors or the bending of light rays through different media (cornea, anterior humor, lens, and vitreous humor) as the rays enter the eyes (Miller & Scott, 2004).

Refractive errors now are being referred to as first-order aberrations, with the new wavefront technology able to measure more precisely each layer of the eye and eye structures for more meticulously customized correction (Thall, Thammano, & Miller, 2004). **Aberration** is more ideally defined as any deviation from perfect behavior; in other words, the lower the aberration, the sharper the image (Thall et al., 2004).

Emmetropia

The term for no refractive error or normal vision without any corrective optical devices is **emmetropia**, meaning the eye is able to focus light rays on the retina to form a clear and sharp image on its own. *Surgically induced emmetropia* is a term used to describe

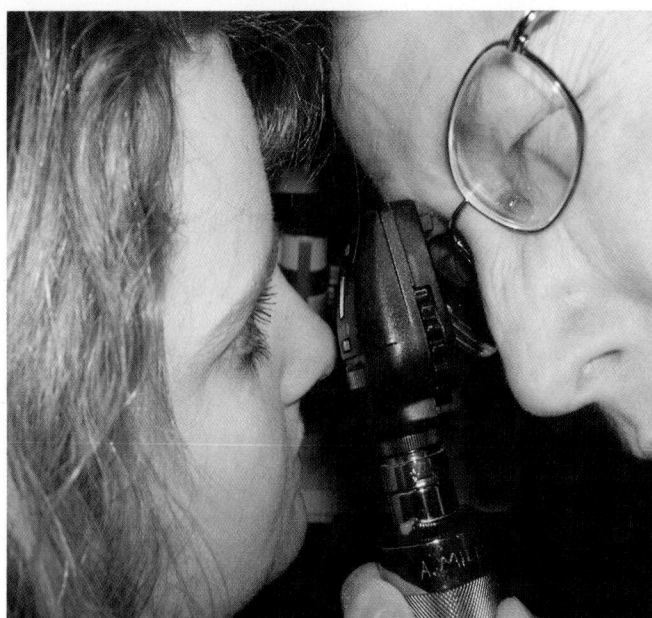

FIGURE 71–4 ■ Direct ophthalmoscope examination.
Source: Lucie S. Elfervig

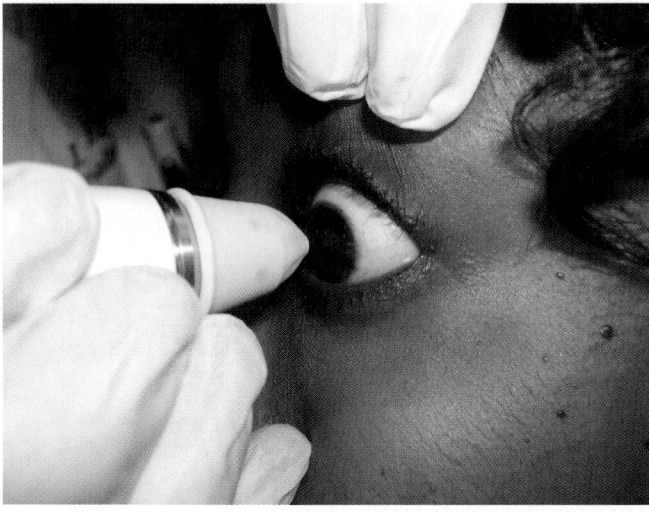

FIGURE 71–5 ■ Application of Tono-Pen for intraocular pressure.
Source: Lucie S. Elfervig

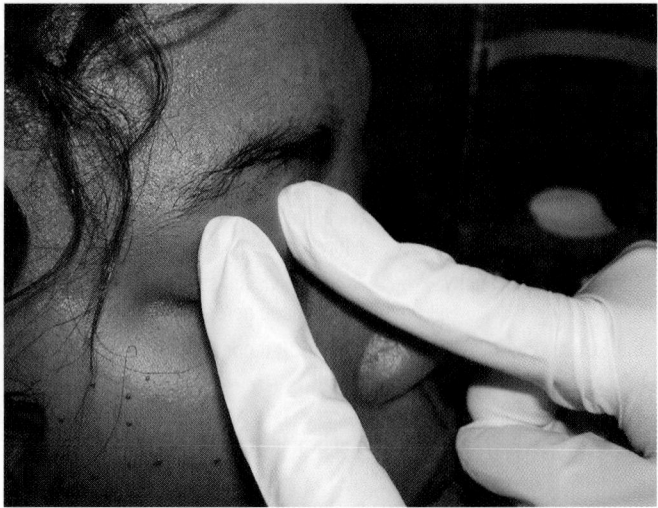

FIGURE 71–6 ■ Palpation of intraocular pressure.
Source: Lucie S. Elfervig

patients who have had previous refractive surgical correction to create 20/20 visual acuity without any corrective optical devices such as glasses or contact lenses. Refractive surgery is the use of a laser to reshape the corneal curvature to eliminate or to reduce refractive errors. Refractive surgery gradually is becoming the norm, instead of the exception, with the advent of decreased cost, increased advertisement, and social pressure to keep looking youthful. Contact lenses and glasses are becoming less "in vogue," even though they are an alternative to refractive surgery. Potential contraindications that negate refractive surgery may be unrealistic expectations, too high of a refractive or astigmatic error, cornea that is too thin (< 560 micrograms), pupil natural dilation that is too large (> 6.5 to 9 millimeters), severely dry corneas, previous eye surgery, and lack of understanding of the procedure and its risks and benefits (Abad & Azar, 2004). The preoperative refractive laser surgery evaluation may include an extensive interview and

visual/ocular measurements. A number of refractive laser surgical correction procedures are available, depending on the patient and/or surgeon preference and the particular presenting problem.

Ametropia

Ametropia is a general term used to indicate a refractive error that is present, which usually can be corrected with glasses, contact lenses, or possibly refractive surgery. The four most common forms of ametropia are myopia, hyperopia, astigmatism, and presbyopia.

Myopia

Myopia, nearsightedness, is the condition in which distance objects are unclear. The parallel light rays fall in front of the retina, because of a longer axial length of the eyeball, which requires a minus (concave) corrective lens to focus the image on the fovea for sharp vision. Other myopic shifts can be created when a patient with diabetes has elevated blood sugar, which makes the natural crystalline lens swell, or there are nuclear sclerosis cataracts in the elderly. Myopia is the most common ametropia, making up over 80% of the refractive errors in the general population (Abad & Azar, 2004).

Hyperopia

Hyperopia or hypermetropia, farsightedness, is the condition in which near objects are unclear. The parallel light rays fall behind the retina, because of a shorter axial length of the eyeball, which requires a plus (convex) corrective lens to focus the image on the fovea for normal or correct vision.

Astigmatism

Astigmatism, irregular corneal surface or asphericity, means that the refractive power is not homogeneous in all meridians, which prevents light rays from focusing on a single point (AAO-3, 2008–2009). Astigmatism usually can be corrected with the required lens or contact lens correction at a specific optical axis.

Presbyopia

Presbyopia is lack of accommodation, the ability to focus from distance to near images, because of aging. Presbyopia usually requires a plus lens correction, bifocals, or trifocals, depending on

DIAGNOSTIC TESTS for Visual Disorders

Test	Definition
Exophthalmometry	The measuring of the degree the eyeball extends from the edge of the eyelids or protrudes from the orbit (e.g., a sign of hyperthyroidism).
Schirmer's test	The measuring of tear production; to treat variations of dry eye syndrome.
Glare test	The measuring of artificial sunlight's effect at various degrees of bright light intensity (usually three: low, medium, and high); for cataract surgery readiness determination.
Potential acuity meter (PAM)	The measuring of potential visual acuity returns after cataract surgery.
Gonioscopy	Using a microscopic instrument to view and to examine the anterior chamber angle structures for patency or any obstructions.
Visual field (VF) perimetry	The measuring of peripheral or side vision with standard machines or manual screenings for vision loss or blind spots (scotoma).
Glaucoma diagnostic test (GDx)	The measuring of the optic nerve health and glaucomatous changes.
Pachymetry (PACH)	The measuring the thickness of the cornea; used in the treatment of glaucoma and refractive surgery.
Keratometry readings (K-readings)	The measuring of the corneal curvature for detecting astigmatism; used in refractions, refractive surgery, and cataract surgery.
Corneal topography (topo)	The measuring of the corneal layers for use in refractive surgery and treating keratoconus and other corneal anomalies.
Ultrasonography:	The use of high-frequency sound waves to detect and outline intraocular and orbital structures by measuring the distance between them. Changes and opacities can be easily recognized by this method.
• A-scan	Measuring axial length for cataract surgery: distinguish between benign and malignant eye tumors.
• B-scan	Two-dimensional image for viewing intravitreal opacities, detachments, tumors, muscles, and inflammation.
Fundus photography (FP)	The photographs of the posterior pole of the retina.
Fluorescein angiography (FA) or indocyanine green (ICG) angiography	The intravenous injection of a dye into the bloodstream to measure the retinal vascular perfusion, infarcts, stenosis, ischemia, leakages, neovascularizations, avascular obstructions, microaneurysms, and retina defects for the evaluating, diagnosing, monitoring, and treating of ocular diseases.
Optical coherence tomography (OCT)	The viewing and measuring of the retinal layers for edema, holes, degeneration, and other anomalies.
Ophthalmodynamometry (ODN)	The measuring of the blood pressure of the ophthalmic artery by increasing intraocular pressure; and it induces pulsations in the central retinal artery at the optic nerve, to determine carotid artery insufficiency or poor disc perfusion.
Color vision tests	The measuring of color vision for any deficiency, such as the lack of red-green discrimination or blue-yellow discrimination.
Electrophysiology:	The measuring of the visual pathways from the retinal photoreceptors to the visual cortex of the brain.
• Visual evoked potential (VEP)	The measuring of vision potential of seeing (occipital cortex); in diagnosing visual function, unexplained vision loss, retinal vascular diseases, ocular traumatic problems, visual pathway lesions, toxic or nutritional eye diseases, glaucoma, and optic nerve diseases.
• Electro-oculogram (EOG)	The measuring (from cornea to retinal layers) of retinal pigment epithelium functions; in diagnosing ocular melanoma, opacification, retinal toxicities, retinal disorders (especially in macular dystrophies), and inherited retinal diseases (especially Best's disease).
• Electroretinogram (ERG)	The measuring of cone/rod functions (diffuse electrical response generated by the neural to nonneural cells of the retina); in diagnosing intracranial lesions, inherited retinal diseases (e.g., retinitis pigmentosa), retinal vascular diseases, visual opacities/traumatic problems, toxic or nutritional diseases, glaucoma, and unexplained vision loss.
Ophthalmic radiography: • Plain x-ray	Right oblique, left oblique, and lateral views of the affected side for the diagnoses of orbital fractures and tumors are usually sufficient.
• Computed tomography (CT) scan, with and without contrast	For serial section views of the orbit and eye; especially in diagnosing tumors, intraocular masses, orbital disease, intracranial diseases, and bone structure.
• Magnetic resonance imaging (MRI)	For high magnetic field to evaluate the brain, orbit, and eye; giving better definition of tissue and fluid locations, especially edema that involves the orbital area and surrounding tissue.

(continued)

Test	Definition
• Carotid ultrasound	Used to determine blockage of the carotid arteries, uses high frequency sound waves to create images of the insides of the carotids to determine whether plaque has formed in the arteries. May also be used with a Doppler to show blood flow through the arteries.
Laboratory tests: • Elevated erythrocyte sedimentation rate (ESR) in temporal arteritis • Normal ESR in anterior ischemic optic neuropathy	Laboratory tests are usually not very significant in the diagnoses of ocular or vision problems. The erythrocyte sedimentation rate (ESR or sed rate) would be one significant blood test used for diagnoses in ophthalmology in relation to temporal arteritis versus anterior ischemic optic neuropathy.

the patient's needs or preferences. As one ages, the nucleus fibers become compressed with additive cortical fibers, resulting in decreasing accommodation (AAO-11, 2008–2009) or a more rigid lens. It generally is during the fourth decade of life that one experiences the loss of elasticity of the natural crystalline lens, which causes the loss of the ability to focus up close, resulting in presbyopia.

Strabismus

Strabismus is a functional misalignment of the extraocular muscles that causes the eyes not to focus together or to a single point. The eye can misdirect in any of the following positions; *eso* meaning toward the nose or medial, *exo* meaning toward the ear or temporal, *hyper* meaning upward or superior, and *hypo* meaning downward or inferior. This is normally a childhood condition, but it can affect one's vision throughout life.

Adult Strabismus

Adult strabismus refers to adults with cross-eyes, those that have lost their ability to fuse. Adult onset of strabismus is usually the result of head trauma and insult to the brain, especially if one is unconscious for a long period of time (AAO-6, 2008–2009). Adults with strabismus will see double (diplopia), because they do not suppress vision. Asthenopia may be another common symptom, which includes eye discomfort on use, such as headache, eyestrain, and brow ache (Pratt-Johnson & Tillson, 2001).

Adult strabismus may be treated with eye muscle exercises, eyeglasses containing prisms, botulinum toxin (Botox) injections, and eye surgery. Eye muscle exercise usually is used when treating a form of adult strabismus, called convergence insufficiency, in which eyes cannot align themselves for close work or reading. These exercises can retrain eyes to focus inward together. Prism eyeglasses can be used to correct mild double vision associated with adult strabismus. Botox injections are an effective treatment when overactive eye muscles are causing strabismus. Eye muscle surgery is the most common treatment; it is used to loosen or tighten the muscles around the eye in order to correct the misalignment.

Diplopia

Diplopia describes double vision, the phenomenon when one object appears as two. Diplopia can be binocular or monocular (AAO-5, 2008–2009). Binocular diplopia can be functional or real. Monocular diplopia usually is an optical or refractive error, and glasses or contact lens correction will solve the problem

(Pratt-Johnson & Tillson, 2001). With functional diplopia, the person is not moving eyes properly for single focus vision (Pratt-Johnson & Tillson, 2001).

Amblyopia

Amblyopia, or more commonly called "lazy eye," is when a person has an eye with decreased or impaired vision with no obvious anatomic explanation. It is usually due to the lack of proper maturation during the growth and development stages, or just to not having the proper refractive correction, meaning no glasses, or the lack of use of correction by patients.

Other possible causes of amblyopia could be toxins, such as poison, alcohol, or tobacco; psychological (hysterical) problems; nutritional (e.g., vitamin B) insufficiency; cataracts (physical occlusion); and strabismic (cross-eyed or wall-eyed) phenomenon (AAO-6, 2008–2009). For all of these reasons and possibly others, the microscopic connections between the brain and visual receptors are not making the necessary links for good visual outcome. Amblyopia usually occurs about age 7 from not using the affected eye, and if not corrected by then, it may become irreversible. One treatment for amblyopia may be occlusion of the normal vision eye, attempting to force the poor vision eye to function properly (Guttman, 2004). Amblyopia does not develop in adulthood from not using an eye for vision.

Phoria

Phoria is a tendency toward a function deviation or defect that results from a break in visual fusion by covering an eye. **Esophoria** is a tendency of the eye to turn inward toward the nose or nasal canthus when that eye is covered or when the eye becomes tired. Exophoria is a tendency of the eye to turn outward toward the ear or temporal canthus when that eye is covered or possibly when the eye becomes tired.

Tropia

Tropia is a definite functional defect that results from a break in visual fusion due to an imbalance or misalignment of the extraocular muscles when both eyes are not covered. Esotropia is misalignment of one eye when it crosses inward toward the nasal canthus and the other eye is in normal alignment whether covered or not (Figure 71–7 ■). Exotropia is misalignment of one eye when it crosses outward toward the temporal canthus and the other eye is in normal alignment whether covered or not. When a tropia is mild, it is difficult at times to distinguish from a phoria; cover tests are very useful in making a distinction.

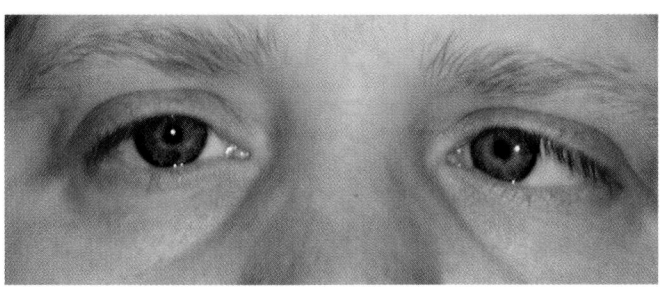

FIGURE 71–7 ■ Esotropia.
Source: Lucie S. Elfervig

Nystagmus

Nystagmus is an involuntary tremor, oscillation, or jerky movement of the eyeball. Nystagmus usually is divided into two types: sensory and motor. Sensory nystagmus is the result of loss of foveal fixation due to the pathology of the macula, retina, or optic nerve (Pratt-Johnson & Tillson, 2001). This condition or symptom often is seen in albinism due to foveal hypoplasia. Other causes may be congenital cataracts; aniridia (no iris); macular anomalies, optic nerve defect or abnormal rod photoreceptor function; and achromatopsia (color blindness) (Pratt-Johnson & Tillson, 2001). Motor nystagmus is the result of not finding a sensory cause of dysfunction and no obvious foveal organic pathology; it is usually less severe than sensory nystagmus (Pratt-Johnson & Tillson, 2001).

The assessment should include a screening cover eye test to rule out any strabismic tendencies or poor visual acuity. During a cover test, the health care provider directs the patient to focus on a small object both at a distance and close up. Each eye is covered alternately; as the cover paddle is moved from one eye to the other, the health care provider notes how much each eye has to move when uncovered to pick up the fixation target. If the alignment of the eyes is outside normal limits or the patient is experiencing symptoms, the health care provider may recommend treatment.

Easy tests with the use of a direct ophthalmoscope can be performed to gain meaningful information. These include checking the foveal reflexes to see whether they are equally bright in color and checking corneal reflexes to determine whether they are equally aligned. Unequal foveal reflexes may indicate a deviating eyeball, which would be the one with the brighter reflex (Brueckner test). Unequal alignment of corneal reflexes (Hirschberg test) also may indicate a deviation in the visual gaze, meaning the eyes have different fixation points (Pratt-Johnson & Tillson, 2001).

Macular Degeneration

Macular degeneration (**MD**) is defined as deterioration of the macula, the area of central vision in the posterior pole or retina, causing central acuity loss. Age-related macular degeneration (ARMD or AMD) is the most common cause of vision loss in those over age 60. Vision loss due to aging is a major health problem today, especially with the advent of the baby boomer generation. Vision loss may affect one's cognitive ability with aging; vision and cognition may share a similar nervous system cell loss, as indicated in recent research (Age-Related Eye Disease Study [AREDS] Research Group, 2006; Wong et al., 2002). The Evidence-Based Practice feature (p. 2336) examines the possible link between age-related macular degeneration and cognitive function.

Age-related macular degeneration is progressive, causing atrophic or deteriorating changes of the macula and retinal pigment epithelial (RPE) layer (Elfervig, 1998). The more common risk factors associated with macular degeneration include aging, hypertension, atherosclerosis and cardiovascular disease, smoking, lung conditions, diabetes, hyperlipidemia, hyperopia, light-colored iris, ultraviolet light exposure, and heredity (Rosenfeld & Gorin, 1999). Age-related macular degeneration is classified into two major types, dry and wet, discussed later. The degeneration of the macula occurs with time and can eventually lead to legal blindness. **Legal blindness** is defined as the best-corrected visual acuity of 20/200 of both eyes or worse, or 20 degrees or more of peripheral field loss.

Drusen

Drusen usually is the earliest fundus sign of age-related macular degeneration. **Drusen** (Figure 71–8 ■, p. 2337) is yellowish, round, slightly elevated, different-sized subretinal pigment epithelial deposits in the macula (Maguire, 1999). However, not all drusen are diagnostic of macular degeneration. Over half the population over age 70 has drusen; however, usually only when vision loss is associated with it, is it referred to as a sign of early age-related macular degeneration.

Patients with macular degeneration may notice at first that it is a little more difficult to see with the affected eye while doing close-up work, or that they have trouble seeing at a distance, especially with driving. A frequent symptom is **metamorphopsia**, a condition characterized by vision distortion; that is, when straight lines such as door frames or posts look crooked or irregular. Other symptoms also may include a difference in the sizes and colors of objects between eyes, meaning the loss of **contrast sensitivity** (**CS**). The individual may find she is having trouble with daily activities, such as sewing, gardening, reading, watching television, and almost any activity that requires looking directly at some object to accomplish a task or skill. The Amsler grid, as shown in Figure 71–9 ■, (p. 2337) is a self-testing tool for daily use, highly recommended for this population, to notice early macular changes from macular degeneration.

Dry Age-Related Macular Degeneration

Dry age-related macular degeneration (AMD) is referred to as nonexudative, geographic, or atrophic changes in the macula (see Figure 71–8 ■, p. 2337). Dry AMD occurs when the light-sensitive cells in the macula slowly break down, gradually blurring central vision in the affected eye. As it gets worse, an individual may see a blurred spot in the center of vision. Over time, as less of the macula functions, central vision is gradually lost in the affected eye. The most common symptom of dry AMD is slightly blurred vision. One may have difficulty recognizing faces or need more light for reading and other tasks. Dry AMD generally affects both eyes, but vision can be lost in one eye while the other eye seems unaffected. One of the most common early signs of dry AMD is drusen (see Figure 71–8 ■, p. 2337) (National Eye Institute, 2006).

Wet Age-Related Macular Degeneration

Wet age-related macular degeneration is exudative, serous, or neovascular changes in the macula (Figure 71–10 ■, p. 2337). Wet AMD occurs when abnormal blood vessels behind the retina start to grow under the macula. These new blood vessels

Age-Related Macular Degeneration and Cognitive Function

Clinical Problem

Vision loss due to aging is a major health problem today, especially with the aging of those of the baby boomer generation, who are now over 50 years of age. Vision loss may affect one's cognitive ability with aging; vision and cognition may share a similar nervous system cell loss, indicated in other studies (AREDS Research Group, 2006; Wong et al., 2002). Vision loss from age-related macular degeneration (AMD) is the leading cause of visual impairment among people age 60 and older (Singerman et al., 2005). According to the United States Census Bureau (2000), 35 million Americans are age 60 and older; and among these, approximately 14% have some sensory impairment (vision and hearing loss), and about 11% have some mental decline. Evidence has shown that when one cannot visually focus clearly, one cannot think clearly either. Early detection of visual impairment and employing the best current means of prevention, treatment, and stabilization may make the difference between chronicity and quality of life for aging adults both visually and mentally. Nurses must understand how to apply evidence-based findings when managing patients with vision loss, especially older citizens with AMD.

Research Findings

The AREDS Research Group (2006) conducted an investigation into the association between cognitive ability and visual impairment from AMD. These investigators hypothesized that aging of mind and vision are related in functional ability. Participants numbered about 2,900 in taking the AREDS Cognitive Function Battery to identify differences of macular abnormalities from AMD and severity of visual acuity loss. The findings suggested a possible association of advanced AMD with visual acuity loss with decreased cognitive function in older people with vision loss worse than 20/40.

Implications for Nursing Practice

This study clearly indicates a need for nurses to educate patients with AMD to keep regular follow-ups with their vision health care provider in order to maintain good visual acuity and health as long as possible. They should be advised to avoid smoking, to limit exposure to air pollution and ultraviolet rays, and to maintain good general health (stabilize any hypertension and hyperlipidemia) in order to age well. Treatments for AMD may include the use of antioxidants, intravitreal injections, or laser as applicable. Patients that are visually impaired need to be informed about the importance of maintaining cognitive stimulating activity, through regular activity, large print books, and special visual systems. Auto reading books or tapes also may prove to be beneficial in keeping one cognitively active. The relationship between decreased vision and cognitive function may also be based on the fact that visual impairment can affect the quality of interactive experiences of older adults in developing meaningful relationships. The nurse needs to understand the relationship of cognitive functions with decreases in visual function gained from this study (AREDS Research Group, 2006) in order to counsel the patient significantly. Keeping active on a regular basis may enrich mental, physical, and psychosocial well-being.

Critical Thinking Questions

1. In order of priority, what are the most important points to include in an education plan for the patient with visual impairment from AMD?

2. What methods would be effective in increasing compliance with the stabilization of vision loss from AMD?

3. Identify nursing measures that would decrease the risk of vision loss from AMD.

Answers to Critical Thinking Questions appear in Appendix D.

References

Age-Related Eye Disease Study (AREDS) Research Group. (2006). Cognitive impairment in the Age-Related Eye Disease Study. AREDS Report No. 16. *Archives of Ophthalmology, 124*(4), 537–543.

Singerman, L. J., Brucker, A. J., Jampol, L. M., Lim, J. I., Rosenfeld, P., Schachat, A. P., et al. (2005). Neovascular age-related macular degeneration: Roundtable. *Retina, 25*(Suppl. 7), S1–S22.

United States Census Bureau. (2000). Demographic Summary. Retrieved February 2, 2007, from http://www.census.gov/main/www/cen2000.html.

Wong, T., Klein, R., Nieto, F., Moraes, S., Mosley, T., Couper, D., et al. (2002). Is early age-related maculopathy related to cognitive function? The atherosclerosis risk in communities study. *American Journal of Ophthalmology, 134*(12), 828–835.

---

tend to be very fragile and often leak blood and fluid, which raise the macula from its normal place at the back of the eye. Damage to the macula occurs rapidly, and loss of central vision can develop quickly. An early symptom of wet AMD is that straight lines appear wavy. Wet AMD is also known as advanced AMD (National Eye Institute, 2006).

Disciform Scar

Disciform scar is a chronic sign of age-related macular degeneration formation. Disciform scar is associated with hemorrhage and serous fluid in and beneath the retinal pigment epithelial layer causing retinal pigment epithelium and photoreceptor damage (Martidis & Tennant, 2004). If this goes untreated, the fibrocytes (scar tissue) from the choroid will accumulate between and within the retinal pigment epithelium and photoreceptors. This will develop finally into a disc-shaped scar that results in severe vision loss; it is referred to as the end stage of macular degeneration.

Laboratory and Diagnostic Procedures and Medical Management

Medical management options for dry macular degeneration can include the possibility of doing nothing and letting aging take its course. Management also may include a recommendation of taking antioxidant eye vitamins (Age-Related Eye Disease Study [AREDS] Research Group, 2003) or supplementing one's diet with the consumption of dark-green leafy vegetables, orange/yellow vegetables, and fruits to try to revitalize the aging retina. Of note, antioxidants also are contraindicated for patients on anticoagulants. Chapter 14 🔗 discusses antioxidants.

 *Patients on blood thinners should not take antioxidant eye vitamins, because antioxidants can improve clotting. Check with the health care provider first before taking.*

Medical management options for wet macular degeneration are nonsteroidal anti-inflammatory medications (D'Amato,

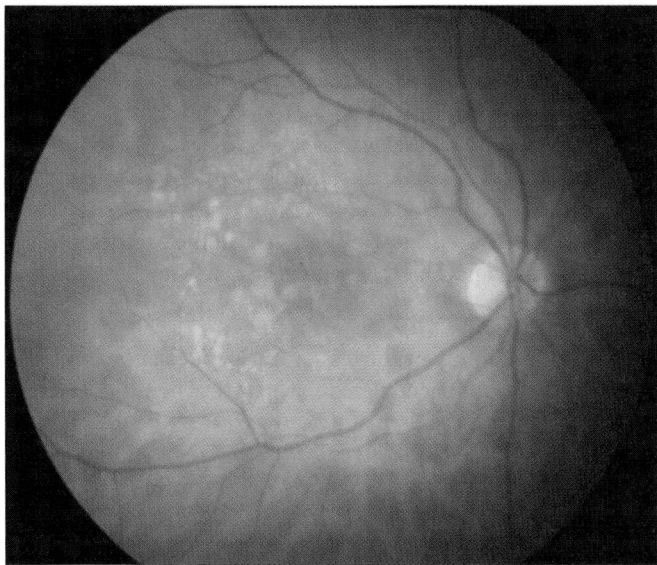

FIGURE 71–8 ■ Dry age-related macular degeneration with drusen.
Source: Lucie S. Elfervig

Amsler grid testing

- Hold card about 16 inches away (normal reading distance)
- Use good lighting
- Wearing best corrected glasses for near
- Cover or close left eye
- Look at the center black spot with right eye
- Notice if any irregularities or distortions in the grid lines, such as, missing, crooked or bent, doubled, light gray in color, blotch or gray shaded area
- Cover or close right eye
- Look at the center black spot with left eye
- Repeat: noticing any irregularities or distortions in the grid lines

FIGURE 71–9 ■ Amsler grid.

1999), laser photocoagulation, photodynamic therapy, vitrectomy with choroidal neovascularization removal (Elfervig, 2000b), and intravitreal injection of anti–vascular endothelial growth factor (anti-VEGF) antigen binding drugs (Ferrara,

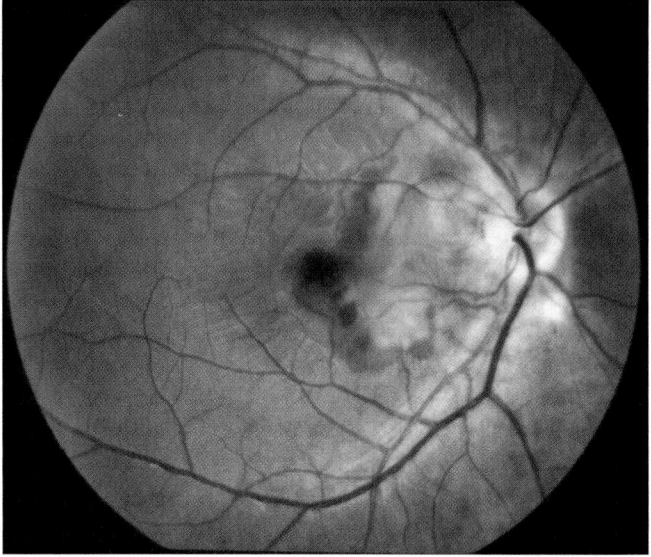

FIGURE 71–10 ■ Wet age-related macular degeneration (choroidal neovascularization).
Source: Lucie S. Elfervig

Damico, Shams, Lowman, & Kim, 2006). The fluorescein angiogram and optical coherence tomography are required diagnostic tests (see the Diagnostic Tests box, p. 2333) to be evaluated for photodynamic therapy and are used to determine who is a good candidate for the procedure.

Photodynamic therapy laser is a clinical procedure that requires an intravenous injection of a special verteporfin dye that is photosensitive, so that the laser beam treats only the leaking blood vessels and not the surrounding retinal tissue. The therapy can be repeated on a 3-month cycle, and it usually takes at least two laser procedures to obtain therapeutic results. After patients have had photodynamic therapy, their eyes and skin are very sensitive to sunlight and they must avoid direct sunlight exposure for 3 to 5 days. Photodynamic therapy (PDT) was once the treatment of choice for wet age-related macular degeneration. Now, it is also being used in combination therapy with anti-VEGF treatments (Dhalla et al., 2006). The day of the laser procedure, patients must wear sunglasses, a long-sleeve shirt, pants, gloves, socks, shoes, and a wide-brimmed hat, so they are protected from direct sunlight. Patients will be monitored by the health care provider every 3 months until the neovascularization is arrested.

CRITICAL ALERT *Verteporfin dye is a light-activated medication or photosensitive dye used in photodynamic therapy (PDT) with a nonthermal laser. Injection of the dye into the vein makes the eyes and skin photosensitive. On the day of laser surgery, the patient should wear or bring to wear the following after the surgery for the trip home: dark sunglasses, wide-brimmed hat, gloves, long-sleeve shirt, pants, socks, and shoes (no sandals).*

Direct sunlight exposure can result in third-degree burns or severe skin irritation. Avoid sunlight and bright light exposure for 4 to 5 days postsurgery. During daylight, close curtains and window shades; avoid skylights, tanning beds, halogen lights, and dental or surgical appointments or procedures. One can use regular indoor lights, watch television, go to the movies, but must wait until after sundown to go outside to do any chores.

Intravitreal injection of anti-VEGF drugs is becoming the treatment of choice for wet age-related macular degeneration. An injection of the anti-VEGF drug is administered into the vitreous cavity (Eye Tech Study Group [ETSG], 2003; Ferrara et al., 2006). The frequency of the injections is determined by the leakage regression response to the drug found on fluorescein angiography (FA) or optical coherence tomography (OCT). Injections can be as frequent as every 4 to 6 weeks for stabilizing vision and consistent visual acuity improvements (Dhalla et al., 2006; Ruiz-Moreno, Montero, Barile, & Zarbin, 2006).

Nursing Management

The quality of life with central vision loss can significantly affect one's perception with communicating and just getting about on a daily basis. Nursing management of patients with age-related macular degeneration can be complex and multifaceted. Application of the nursing process will facilitate a comprehensive approach to patients' assessment and care. The nursing assessment and management data, which include specific questions to patients that are visually impaired with wet macular degeneration, are found in the Nursing Process: Patient Care Plan for Macular Degeneration feature. This care plan applies the nursing process to the relevant nursing diagnoses and provides a comprehensive care plan for patients that are visually impaired during the early stages of wet macular degeneration.

Collaborative Management

To achieve potential vision restoration and return to society as before, patients with wet macular degeneration need a multidisciplinary team approach, including the ophthalmologist, ophthalmic advance nurse practitioner, nurse, social worker, and optometrist or low vision rehabilitation specialist. To ensure maximum vision potential, vision care is managed by both

nurses and the health care provider. As the wet macular degeneration starts to dry and stop leaking, some macular scarring may develop, leaving a degree of visual impairment or possibly legal blindness. The optometrist and low vision rehabilitation specialist will provide the necessary glasses or low vison aids to enhance patients' visual acuity, hopefully to a functional level. Patients will need instructions as well as practice in the best use of vision aids. The social worker is accustomed to helping patients adjust to a new lifestyle with vision deficit.

Health Promotion

Due to the possibility of the loss of independence as a result of legal blindness from age-related macular degeneration (AMD), it is important for the patient to know whether he has a family history of AMD, because this directly affects the patient's quality of life. Regular eye examinations are a means to detect early changes of AMD and to assess the use of eye vitamins and any new investigative findings in the treatment of AMD. Nutritional supplements for age-related macular degeneration are presented in the Complementary & Alternative Therapies box.

Diabetic Retinopathy

Retinopathy generally refers to degenerative changes in the retina. The most common causes of retinopathy result from diabetes mellitus (DM) or diabetes, thus causing weak and leaking blood vessels in the retina. The various stages of diabetic retinopathy include nonproliferative, preproliferative, and proliferative (Bhavsar & Drouilhet, 2006; Elfervig & Elfervig, 2001; Eliott, Lee, & Abrams, 2001; Porth, 2007) (Figure 71–11 ■, p. 2342).

Epidemiology, Etiology, and Risk Factors

Diabetic retinopathy (DR) is the leading cause of legal blindness among young adults and working-age Americans—those

COMPLEMENTARY & ALTERNATIVE THERAPIES — Nutritional Supplements for Age-Related Macular Degeneration

Description:
Age-related macular degeneration (ARMD) is the third most common cause of blindness in the world. ARMD creates partial or complete blindness in thousands of people. Its prevalence is expected to increase as the population ages. A small number of patients experience slowed disease progression from laser therapy and surgery, but these treatments are unlikely to restore lost vision. However, there are many CAM therapies that can improve this condition; the two most common therapies are antioxidants and omega-3 fatty acids ("Nutritional Supplements," 2006).

Research Support:
Studies have shown that dietary intake of omega-3 fatty acids benefits visual development. In addition, several other studies show that omega-3 fatty acids may be useful for conditions of the retina and lens. A Canadian literature review assessed and analyzed the evidence for whether omega-3 fatty acids prevent the development or progression of retinitis pigmentosa. Researchers found six studies published between 1995 and 2004 that met their eligibility criteria. These studies showed that omega-3 fatty acids improved some retinitis pigmentosa outcomes (Hodge et al., 2006).

Another review of published studies examined the role of nutritional and herbal medicines in treating ARMD, cataracts, diabetic retinopathy, and

glaucoma. Although the evidence did support the use of certain vitamins and minerals in patients with certain forms of ARMD, it did not support use of these supplements to prevent or treat cataracts, diabetic retinopathy, or glaucoma (West, Oren, & Moroi, 2006).

Another review of literature included eight trials and found one major U. S. trial that showed that antioxidant (beta-carotene, vitamin C, and vitamin E) and zinc supplementation prevented progression to advanced ARMD and loss of visual acuity (Evans, 2006).

References
Evans, J. R. (2006). Antioxidant vitamin and mineral supplements for slowing the progression of age-related macular degeneration. *Cochrane Database of Systematic Reviews, 19*(2), CD000254.
Hodge, W. G., Barnes, D., Schachter, H. M., Pan, Y. I., Lowcock, E. C., Zhang, L., et al. (2006). The evidence for efficacy of omega-3 fatty acids in preventing or slowing the progression of retinitis pigmentosa: A systematic review. *Canadian Journal of Ophthalmology, 41*(4), 481–490.
"Nutritional supplements for macular degeneration." (2006). *Drug Therapy Bulletin, 44*(2), 9–11.
West, A. L., Oren, G. A., & Moroi, S. E. (2006). Evidence for the use of nutritional supplements and herbal medicines in common eye diseases. *American Journal of Ophthalmology, 141*(1), 157–166.

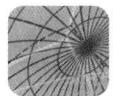

NURSING PROCESS: Patient Care Plan for Macular Degeneration

Assessment of Patient/Family Understanding of Vision Loss

Subjective Data:
Are you taking any eye systemic medications or antioxidant eye vitamins?
Are you on any blood thinners?
Do you smoke?
Do you wear glasses, contact lenses, or use any low vision aids?
Have you had any eye problems or vision problems in the past?
Are you seeing black spots or wavy lines in your vision?
Have you had any eye treatments, surgeries, lasers, or photodynamic therapy?
Do you spend a lot of time outdoors, and do you wear ultraviolet protective glasses or sunglasses?
Does anyone else in the family have macular degeneration?
What is your occupation?
Does it involve one or both eyes?
Have you had any vision or eye tests done?
Has treatment already been started for this problem?
What has your health care provider told you about this disease?

Objective Data:
Distance visual acuity
Near visual acuity
Intraocular pressure
Central blind spot
Eye examination
Vital signs
Interview behavior

Nursing Assessment and Diagnoses	Outcomes and Evaluation Parameters	Planning and Interventions with *Rationales*
Nursing Diagnosis: *Deficient Knowledge* related to macular degeneration	**Outcomes:** Patient/family able to verbalize visual limitations and the necessary lifestyle changes. ***Evaluation Parameters:*** Verbalizes understanding of reason for visual loss. Identifies vision loss. Identifies alternative devices of assistance. Demonstrates ability of skills to use alternative devices.	**Interventions and *Rationales:*** Provide education and resources about vision loss, means of treatment and management, and role in self-care and alternative devices in assisting. *To assess understanding of vision loss by means of care, management, and follow-up.* Encourage self-care in keeping compliant with and proactive in maintaining vision health. *To assess self-care compliance and management.* Educate about and promote normalization with enhancement of skills in self-esteem and socialization, and means to access support systems. *To monitor knowledge of social interaction deficits by assessing means of improvement. To use skills that enhance social interactions.* Provide presence, good listening, and skills in socialization, anxiety reduction, relationship building, and accessing support resources. *To monitor active social encounters.* Provide the necessary means to maintain functional activities as long as possible for a better quality of life. Assess needs in maintaining everyday functional activities. *To mark appliances with Velcro or material that is recognizable to touch for identification.* Assess needs in limiting frustrations. *To provide access to auto reading or large television screens for entertainment enjoyment. To provide magnifier or bright lights for enhancing vision when applicable.* Provide continued independence. *To monitor everyday activities in assessing continued independence.*

Assessment of Patient/Family Coping

Subjective Data:
How are you handling your vision problems?
How long have you had this eye problem?
Do you have any other health or medical problems?
How would you describe your ocular or vision problems, signs, and symptoms?
Who are your support systems?

Objective Data:
Body language
Family support systems
Ability to adjust lifestyle

(continued)

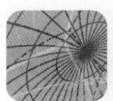

NURSING PROCESS: Patient Care Plan for Macular Degeneration—*Continued*

Nursing Assessment and Diagnoses	Outcomes and Evaluation Parameters	Planning and Interventions with *Rationales*
Nursing Diagnoses: *Anxiety* related to altered self-concept secondary to vision loss, especially centrally, and the fear of becoming legally or totally blind *Ineffective Coping* due to the inability to ask for help related to low self-esteem secondary to vision loss *Interrupted Family Processes* related to the shock of patient's vision loss	**Outcomes:** Experience a reasonable level of anxiety and fear. Evidence of effective family coping. *Evaluation Parameters:* Explains levels of anxiety and fear and coping patterns to overcome them. Relates less anxiety and fear after teaching. Expresses an improved level of psychological and physical comfort. Exhibits useful coping mechanisms in managing anxiety and fear. Assertive in asking for assistance when vision is not adequate to perform a given task. Expresses a need for assistance. Obtains the help needed to get the task done. Enjoys family support and meaningful family functions. Identifies altered family processes and reasons why. Exhibits effective family functioning. Comfortable in communicating without the means of observing facial expressions. Expresses self well in communicating with others. Engages sociably. Demonstrates a positive self-image with lifestyle adaptations and the resources of support to assist in keeping a positive attitude. Identifies changes in one's self-esteem. Identifies self in a realistic light with current circumstances. Expresses positive feelings about oneself. Exhibits healthy coping and adaptive skills.	**Interventions and *Rationales:*** Monitor level of anxiety and fear from mild to panic. *To assess for lower levels of anxiety and fear.* Provide reassurance and comfort with presence and active listening. *To observe improved levels of comfort.* Teaching disease process. *To assess less anxiety and fear with understanding.* Educate patient that peripheral vision is not lost with macular degeneration. *To assess improved self-concept with acceptance of vision loss.* Assist and teach patient in using other senses of hearing and touching more effectively to enhance communication skills. *To observe communicating with others well to increase sociability.* Assist patient in not feeling embarrassed or less of a person by teaching effective means of asking for assistance when necessary. *To observe obtaining help when needed with a sense of self-satisfaction of obtained task.* Provide presence, active listening, and emotional support. Teach and provide skills for coping; body image, self-role, self-awareness, and self-concept enhancements; and cognitive rethinking, value clarifications, and support resources. *To monitor positive lifestyle adaptations.*

Assessment of Home Environment

Subjective Data:
What kind of work do you do?
Are you able to perform your activities of daily living (ADL)?

Objective Data:
Home environment
Need for assistance
Financial stability

Nursing Assessment and Diagnoses	Outcomes and Evaluation Parameters	Planning and Interventions with *Rationales*
Nursing Diagnosis: *Impaired Home Maintenance* related to functional ability secondary to vision loss	**Outcomes:** Manage and maintain a clean and safe environment to live. *Evaluation Parameters:* Identifies obstacles in home management. Exhibits means to use support system. Exhibits ability to use alternative and adaptive devices that are safe.	**Interventions and *Rationales:*** Assist in family integrity promotion, involvement, mobilization, process, maintenance, and support. *To observe engaging in usual family functions, with acceptance of family support and love.* Assist in providing resources for home cleaning assistance and support system enhancement. *To report factors that are obstacles in home maintenance and management.* *To assess the use of resources for home help by using the necessary devices for a clean and safe home environment.*

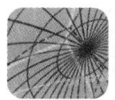

NURSING PROCESS: Patient Care Plan for Macular Degeneration—*Continued*

Assessment of Patient Response to Illness

Subjective Data:
Tell me about your perceptions of your disease.
What impact has this had on your life?
How has it impacted family dynamics and your role in the family?

Objective Data:
Facial expressions
Family relationships
Evidence of making necessary adjustments

Nursing Assessment and Diagnoses	Outcomes and Evaluation Parameters	Planning and Interventions with *Rationales*
Nursing Diagnoses: *Hopelessness* related to vision loss *Powerlessness* related to loss of controls in one's lifestyle secondary to vision loss	**Outcomes:** Express a sense of hope and feelings of hopefulness. Express a sense of power and express control over one's life situations. ***Evaluation Parameters:*** Verbalizes feelings and expresses hope. Identifies the future and sets realistic goals. Exhibits a positive feeling for now and later. Expresses self-confidence and trust of others. Demonstrates self-direction in decision making and problem solving. Identifies factors that can be controlled. Identifies the needs for care, treatment, and future situations in one's life.	**Interventions and *Rationales:*** Instill and provide presence, active listening, emotional and spiritual support, and hope. *To open communications and to facilitate feeling of hopefulness.* Teach and provide skills for behavior modification, coping skills, and crisis intervention. *To assist in setting future realistic goals and the ability to achieve set goals. To observe trust in making informed decisions and using effective problem solving.* Provide presence, and emotional and spiritual support. Teach and provide skills for coping, crisis intervention, decision making, and support system enhancement. *To assess factors of control and power by decision making concerning future care and treatment. To provide the resources of support and assistance, when indicated.*

Assessment of Safety Measures

Subjective Data:
Describe the physical layout of your residence.
How much are you able to get around independently?
What are your support systems?

Objective Data:
Ability to perform ADL
Use of aids such as a cane
Caregiver presence and ability to assist

Nursing Assessment and Diagnoses	Outcomes and Evaluation Parameters	Planning and Interventions with *Rationales*
Nursing Diagnoses: *Risk for Injury* or *Risk for Falls* related to vision loss *Readiness for Enhanced Self-Care* related to vision loss	**Outcomes:** Remain free from injury and falls related to vision loss. Perform self-care adequately in performing all the necessary activities of daily living. ***Evaluation Parameters:*** Identifies potential areas of injury and places of risk. Demonstrates appropriate measures to provide and to maintain safety. Identifies self-care deficits. Exhibits ability to use support systems. Exhibits ability to use necessary adaptive devices. Verbalizes knowledge of the options of antioxidant eye vitamins, when indicated.	**Interventions and *Rationales:*** Educate on visual defects and provide the necessary safety skills and management to prevent injury or falls. *To assess understanding of visual deficits with seeking the means to provide a safe environment to prevent injury or falls.* Provide resources for normal daily activities, self-care needs and tools, and support system information. *To observe self-care using the necessary information for support and resources to perform activities of daily living in maintaining a normal life with known self-care deficits. To provide means to keep an adequate supply of antioxidant eye vitamins, when indicated (contraindicated for smokers and patients on anticoagulants).*

persons under the age of 60—typically affecting individuals in their most productive years (Bhavsar & Drouilhet, 2006). It is the leading cause of blindness for all ages in the United States (Porth, 2007). From the initial diagnosis of diabetes, if occurring during adulthood or at a prepubertal age, patients may have a 5-year so-called "grace period" during which retinopathy usually is not visually detectable. This is referred to as diabetes without ophthalmic complications.

Approximately 16 million Americans have diabetes, with 50% of them not even aware that they have it. Of those that know, only one-half receive appropriate eye care. Thus, it is not surprising that diabetic retinopathy is the leading cause of new blindness in persons aged 25 to 74 in the United States and is responsible for more than 8,000 cases of new blindness each year (Fong et al., 2003). This means that diabetes is responsible for 12% of blindness, and the rate is even higher among certain ethnic groups. An

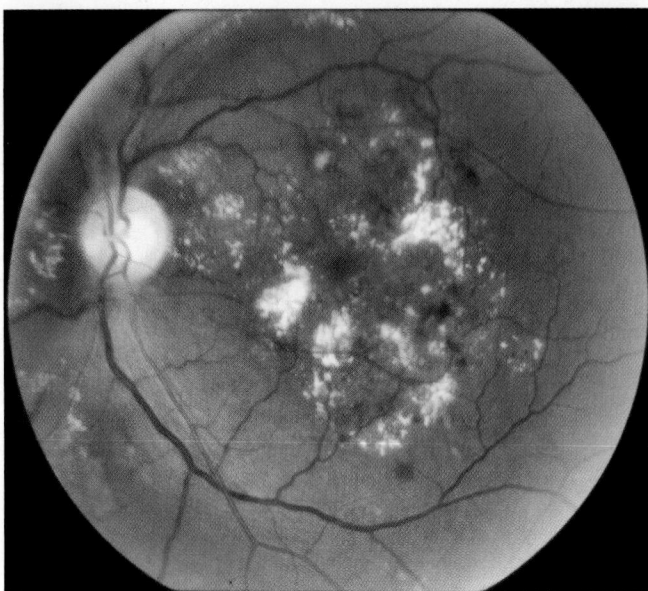

FIGURE 71–11 ■ Diabetic retinopathy.
Source: Lucie S. Elfervig

increased risk of diabetic retinopathy appears to exist in patients with Native American, Hispanic, and African American heritage (Bhavsar & Drouilhet, 2006). The major risk factors for diabetic retinopathy are years of being diabetic, family history, hyperglycemia, hypertension, hyperlipidemia, smoking, anemia, and renal disease.

Pathophysiology and Clinical Manifestations

Diabetic retinopathy results in edema from leaking capillaries that hemorrhage. Other signs are **cotton-wool spots (CWS)** from ischemic tissue that can advance to neovascularization (Elfervig & Elfervig, 2001). Diabetic retinopathy progresses in stages: from nonproliferative diabetic retinopathy, to preproliferative diabetic retinopathy, proliferative retinopathy, neovascularization of the disc or elsewhere in the retina, vitreous hemorrhage, gliotic (scar) tissue or traction retinal detachment, retinal detachment, or neovascular glaucoma of the iris. Nonproliferative diabetic retinopathy is manifested by cotton-wool spots or soft exudates caused by lack of blood supply to the tissue, **flame-shaped hemorrhages** from the nerve fiber layer of the retina, and dot/blot hemorrhages from the outer plexiform layer of the retina (Rosenblatt & Benson, 2004). Once a person is diagnosed with diabetes mellitus, she should have a baseline dilated eye examination and evaluation. Patients with diabetes usually are followed annually if no signs or symptoms of diabetic retinopathy are present and are seen more often if active diabetic retinopathy is in progress. Sometimes just by getting blood sugar and blood pressure under control, the vessel leakage from diabetes will clear on its own. Thus, it is very important to emphasize good blood sugar and blood pressure controls, and to educate patients about not smoking or giving up smoking. Diabetic retinopathy signs and symptoms can range from none to floating spots, streaks, lines, scattered lights, distortion, hazy and cloudy view, darkness, and poor color vision, depending on the location of the retinopathy in the retina (Elfervig & Elfervig, 2001; Porth, 2007).

Laboratory and Diagnostic Procedures

Fasting glucose and hemoglobin A_{1c} (Hb A_{1c}) are laboratory tests that are performed to help diagnose diabetes. The Hb A_{1c} level also is important in the long-term follow-up care of patients with diabetes and diabetic retinopathy. Controlling diabetes and maintaining the Hb A_{1c} level in the 6% to 7% range are the goals in the optimal management of diabetes and diabetic retinopathy. If these levels are maintained, the progression of diabetic retinopathy is reduced substantially. Fluorescein angiography also is used in the diagnosis and management of diabetic retinopathy (see the Diagnostic Tests box, p. 2333). These scans reveal microaneurysms, blot and dot hemorrhages, areas of nonperfusion, and evidence of collateral vessels that do not leak (Bhavsar & Drouilhet, 2006).

Medical Management

Preventing diabetic retinopathy from developing or progressing is considered the best approach to protecting vision. Therefore, glucose control may retard the progression of retinopathy. Management of hypertension and hyperlipidemia also is important, as these conditions also may contribute to the risk of developing or furthering diabetic retinopathy.

Laser photocoagulation provides the major direct treatment modality for diabetic retinopathy (Bhavsar & Drouilhet, 2006). This laser treatment is applied directly to leaking microaneurysms, and grid photocoagulation with a checkerboard pattern of laser burns is applied to diffuse areas of leakage and thickening. It is not recommended near the disc. Vitrectomy has proved effective in removing vitreous hemorrhage and severing vitroretinal membranes that develop (Porth, 2007).

■ Nursing Management

The nurse has many opportunities for education and intervention with patients and family in preserving vision function and promoting eye health to prevent the advancement of diabetic retinopathy. Nursing management of patients with diabetic retinopathy can be complex and multifaceted. Application of the nursing process facilitates a comprehensive approach to patients' assessment and care.

Assessment and Nursing Diagnoses

Assessment data includes specific questions related to blood sugar and blood pressure controls and vision fluctuation. It also establishes the background of the patient by determining how long the patient has been a diabetic and other contributing factors to the diagnosis of retinopathy. Specific questions might be asked of the patient:

- What type of medication are you on for diabetic control?
- How is your blood glucose and your blood pressure?
- Are you taking any other systemic medications?
- Do you smoke?
- Do you wear glasses, contact lenses, or have you had any eye problems in the past?

From an objective perspective, the nurse should assess the patient for visual acuity, blood sugar, and blood pressure values. An eye examination also is in order as is an assessment of behavioral manifestations.

Nursing diagnoses are developed from the assessment data, and a patient care plan depicts the nursing process used in caring for patients with diabetic retinopathy. In determining diagnoses the nurse must recognize that the patient is undergoing changes in self-perception and in the ability to maintain familiar and constant roles in caring for self and for participating as a member of a social group, e.g., family, friends. Typical diagnoses to be considered are those related to anxiety, ineffective coping, infection potential related to surgery, altered family processes, and impaired home maintenance and self-care deficits along with impaired social interaction.

Outcomes and Evaluation Parameters

Outcomes and evaluation parameters should be focused on the desired response of the patient in adapting to the overall diagnosis of diabetic retinopathy: reduced anxiety and coping patterns. They are demonstrated patient behaviors, both subjective and objective, that indicate the patient is adjusting to the overall diagnosis of diabetic retinopathy.

Planning and Interventions

Planning and nursing interventions focus on communication and education and monitoring the patient's verbal and nonverbal behaviors. For instance, the nurse is responsible for instructing the patient on the relevance of blood sugar to the diagnosis and how to control it. Information on the reduction of risk factors also is shared as is education regarding available resources for maintaining self-care and a safe environment to those with visual defects. Anxiety and comfort levels also are monitored in order to determine on-going patient needs and provide assistance as appropriate.

◼ Collaborative Management

A multidisciplinary team approach consists of the health care provider, internist or endocrinologist, ophthalmologist, ophthalmic advance nurse practitioner, nurses, nutritionist, and optometrist. They all serve to provide comprehensive care to patients with diabetic retinopathy. Management of diabetic retinopathy may include medical controls or surgical intervention, such as laser photocoagulation or surgical vitrectomy (Rosenblatt & Benson, 2004) (Figure 71–12 ◼) by the ophthalmologist. Sometimes just by having the internists adjust patients' medications to stabilize blood sugar and/or blood pressure will negate any need for laser. Severe hypertension or hyperglycemia also can prevent laser treatment, especially if the diastolic blood pressure is above 100 mmHg or the blood sugar is over 300 mg/dL, because the laser is less effective under these conditions. Laser also can be a means to stabilize the fundus for impending vitrectomy, to improve the surgical outcome. It is not uncommon for patients with diabetes who have diabetic retinopathy to have anywhere from three to six laser sessions per eye over their lifetime. The nurse practitioner or nurse can provide the necessary education and follow-up monitoring of patients' progress to assist them in complying with a diabetic regimen. The nutritionist assists with establishing a diet regimen to enhance health and control diabetes. The optometrist provides

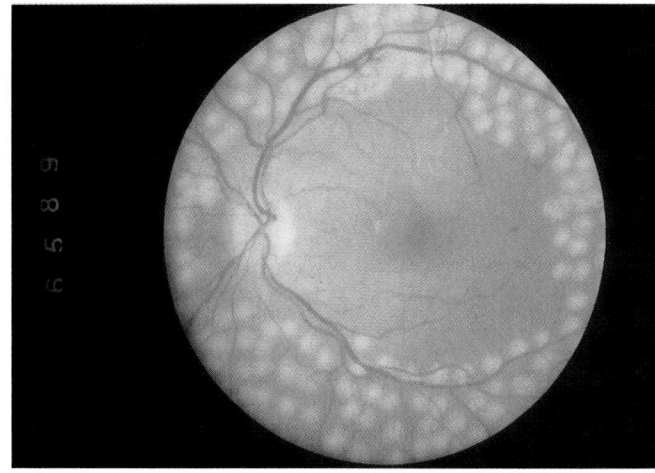

FIGURE 71–12 ◼   Laser photocoagulation.
Source: Lucie S. Elfervig

visual evaluations between regular health care provider visits and makes the necessary refractive corrections when indicated.

Because blood sugar fluctuation can cause changes in vision, it is recommended that periodic blood sugar checks be established. Hyperglycemia may cause the natural crystalline lens to swell, creating myopic shift and a temporary change in refractive error. Hypoglycemia may cause a cerebral response creating temporary blurred vision, diplopia, drowsiness, faintness, confusion, anxiety, headache, slurred speech, sweating, tremor, seizures, and even coma. It is recommended that the blood sugar be gotten under control and stabilized for at least 6 to 9 weeks before changing glasses or contact lenses. A possible cure for diabetes is islets of Langerhans transplant or pancreatic transplant, which will consequently stop the progression of diabetic retinopathy, but retinopathy damage that is already present, does not reverse. See Chapter 53 ⊘ for more information on diabetes.

Health Promotion

Due to the progressive nature of diabetic retinopathy, especially after the 5-year grace period, health promotion begins as soon as the patient is diagnosed with diabetes. Patient/family education focuses on controlling the blood sugar and risk factors that aggravate the disease progression, such as hypertension, hyperlipidemia, smoking, overeating, and lack of exercise. Education includes all of the latter and possible lifestyle changes and preventive care. It is important for patients to have regular eye examinations annually if no diabetic retinopathy is present and more frequently if diabetic retinopathy is already in progress.

Glaucoma

Glaucoma includes a group of conditions that feature an optic neuropathy accompanied by optic disc cupping and visual field loss. It generally is associated with an increase in intraocular pressure; however, some people with normal intraocular pressure may develop characteristic optic nerve and visual field changes. Glaucoma is a very significant health condition, especially with aging Americans, because its incidence increases with age.

Epidemiology and Etiology

Glaucoma is the second most common form of legal blindness in the United States, and the third most common in the world

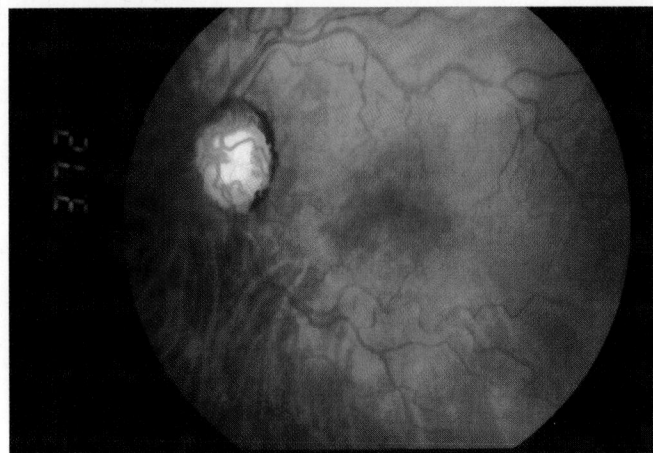

FIGURE 71–13 ■ Glaucoma with collaterals on the disc.
Source: Lucie S. Elfervig

(Elfervig, 2002a), but with treatment loss of sight can be prevented (Figure 71–13 ■). An estimated 60 million people worldwide have glaucoma. About 6 million people worldwide are blind from glaucoma, including 100,000 Americans, making it the leading cause of blindness in the United States (Porth, 2007). Normal range of intraocular pressure is between 10 and 21 mmHg, but not all persons with elevated intraocular pressure (greater than 22 mmHg) have glaucoma or optic nerve damage (ocular hypertension), and not all persons with normal intraocular pressure are glaucoma free (low- or normal-tension glaucoma) (Elfervig, 2002a).

Pathophysiology

Generally glaucoma is described as open angle or closed angle, depending on its outflow mechanism, and primary or secondary, depending on its etiology. Primary glaucoma infers that it has no relation to other ocular conditions, and secondary glaucoma is the result of another preexisting ocular condition. Aqueous humor, which is produced by the ciliary body and secreted by ciliary processes, flows from the posterior chamber through the pupillary space and is deposited into the anterior chamber. Aqueous humor exits from the anterior chamber in the anterior angle into the trabecular meshwork, Schlemm's canal, intrascleral channels, and through episcleral and conjunctival veins, into venous circulation (AAO-10, 2008–2009). This continuous production and dissemination of aqueous fluid is responsible for maintaining normal intraocular pressure. Glaucoma is the condition that develops when any sequence of the production of aqueous humor or the drainage of aqueous humor does not function properly. This causes aqueous fluid to build up intraocularly, which causes the intraocular pressure to increase in the eye, thus putting pressure on the optic nerve and causing it to atrophy. This can lead to permanent blindness if left untreated (AAO-10, 2008–2009). Ocular changes may include optic nerve neuropathy, retinal ganglion cell dropout, poor optic nerve perfusion, and nerve fiber layer destruction. The retinal ganglion cell layer of the sensory retina is composed of the neurons that project to the vision center of the brain, and the axons converge to form the optic nerve. The ganglion cell normally dies with aging (apoptosis), but glaucoma accelerates this process; and when over half the ganglion cells die, visual acuity loss becomes more apparent (Stewart, 2004).

More recent studies (Walker & Piltz-Seymour, 2004) have illustrated that central corneal thickness, measured with pachometry, can alter intraocular pressure readings. Diurnal intraocular pressure is intraocular pressure that can vary at different times of the day (PDR, 2004a). Intraocular pressure elevation puts pressure on the optic nerve, which can cause destruction of the nerve fiber layer of the retina, possibly causing a permanent vision loss. Hallmark signs of glaucoma are elevated intraocular pressure, visual field defects, optic nerve cupping or notching, and nerve fiber layer hemorrhages.

Open-Angle Glaucoma

Open-angle glaucoma (OAG) is the condition that exists when a patient has an open angle, meaning there is adequate anterior chamber space for proper drainage of aqueous fluid, but elevated intraocular pressure is present. The elevated pressure is due to the increase in aqueous production or the decrease in aqueous drainage due to trabecular meshwork obstruction, canal of Schlemm obstruction, or degenerative changes of the drainage tissue (AAO-10, 2008–2009). Open-angle glaucoma is sometimes referred to as the "silent blinder" or "thief in the night," because patients experience no symptoms in the early stages, and possibly it is first recognized due to noticeable vision loss. Side vision loss usually comes later in the course of the disease. Standard terms for open-angle glaucoma (OAG) are chronic (COAG), primary (POAG), or pigmentary. Pigmentary occurs when pigment pieces of the iris are blocking the drainage canal. Primary open-angle glaucoma, the most common form of glaucoma, occurs when the mechanical blockage may be caused from the iris being too near the Schemm's canal, thus bulging forward and blocking the trabecular meshwork (Zimmerman, Sakiyalak, Krupin, & Rosenberg, 2004). Chronic open-angle glaucoma is long-standing glaucoma.

Ocular Hypertension

Ocular hypertension refers to elevated intraocular pressure with no other signs or symptoms, no damage to the optic nerve, and no visual field loss. Ocular hypertension can be a precursor to impending glaucoma. Treatment includes observation only, unless intraocular pressure becomes unstable, there is a strong family history of glaucoma, or the intraocular pressure starts to elevate. Then medical treatment would indicate the starting of antiglaucoma drops (Walker & Piltz-Seymour, 2004). See the later Pharmacology Summary feature (p. 2346).

Low-Tension Glaucoma

Low-tension glaucoma (LTG), or normal-tension glaucoma (NTG), refers to normal intraocular pressure readings, but even though the pressure is within normal parameters, it is still too high for patients if optic nerve atrophy or visual field loss occurs. This usually results from inadequate blood perfusion to the optic nerve, possibly due to vasospastic etiology, such as in patients that suffer with frequent migraine headaches (Hitchings, 2004).

Secondary Glaucoma

Secondary glaucoma refers to elevated intraocular pressure due to a secondary cause, such as congenital anomalies, hyphema, inflammation (uveitis, iridocyclitis), tumors, drugs (topical steroids), hypermature cataract, or choroidal neovascularization (Choplin & Lundy, 1998). Conditions that interrupt the aqueous fluid drainage system, such as trauma, exophthalmos, or advanced diabetes, can cause structural changes that give rise to elevated intraocular pressure (Choplin & Lundy, 1998).

Acute Angle-Closure Glaucoma

Acute angle-closure glaucoma (AACG) is when the angle in the anterior chamber closes suddenly due to a shallow or narrow anterior angle (which is between the iris and cornea) by iris blockage, thereby preventing aqueous flow through the trabecular meshwork (Elfervig & Elfervig, 2007; Trobe, 2006) and into the canal of Schlemm (Traverso, Bagnis, & Bricola, 2004). This causes the intraocular pressure to rise very high, creating extreme eye pain and pressure with blurry vision, fixed mid-dilated pupil, corneal edema, hyperemia, photophobia, light halos, epiphora, and frontal headaches (Trobe, 2006) that can be accompanied by nausea, vomiting, and abdominal ache (Elfervig & Elfervig, 2007; PDR, 2004a). Typically, the ocular pain alone will motivate patients to seek immediate eye care in the clinic or emergency department.

CRITICAL ALERT   *With acute angle-closure glaucoma:*
Do not dilate the pupils!
Assess for pupils, hazy cornea, eye pain, and vision loss.
Assess for any systemic symptoms of headache, nausea, or vomiting.

Obtain intraocular pressure frequently, by the nurse, every 20 to 30 minutes until the intraocular pressure is lower, below 30 mmHg, with a health care provider's standing order for proper eye medication and systemic medications for emergency use.

The treatment goal of acute angle-closure glaucoma is to lower intraocular pressure, as quickly as possible, with systemic medications orally or intravenously, as well as topical ophthalmic drops that are ordered by the health care provider. The application of topical ophthalmic antiglaucoma drops, systemic or intravenous carbonic anhydrase inhibitors, or osmotic agents is common treatment, in addition to the administration of topical ophthalmic steroid drops every 10 to 15 minutes for the first hour, then hourly until intraocular pressure is stable (Netland & Allen, 1999). See the later Pharmacology Summary feature (p. 2346). Peripheral iridectomy (PI) or laser iridotomy is the standard immediate surgical procedure to ease high intraocular pressure and relieve blockage (Traverso et al., 2004). Measures are continued and the pressure is checked every 30 to 40 minutes, until it is lowered enough to clear corneal swelling and quiet the anterior chamber. Once the eye is quiet and comfortable, a more extensive ocular examination can be conducted. One means for angle closure to occur is when pupils normally dilate in the dark or at night. This can be intermittent at first, and then suddenly permanent closure may take place (Campbell & Netland, 1998). Other predispositions to angle closure are hyperopia, increased iris thickness with drug dilation, a large natural crystalline lens (cataracts), and a pupillary block that traps aqueous fluid. Sometimes acute angle-closure glaucoma subsides without intervention, but usually medical and surgical intervention is indicated to prevent ocular damage and keep open angle patency.

Clinical Manifestations

The usual onset of glaucoma is asymptomatic, slow, silent, and painless. Some symptoms may be blurred vision or eye ache; but usually by the time these symptoms develop, some permanent

optic nerve damage has occurred along with vision loss or insidious visual field defects. The aged, males, and African Americans seem to be at greater risk for open-angle glaucoma (PDR, 2004a). Open-angle glaucoma is one of the major causes of vision loss or legal blindness in the aged, second only to age-related macular degeneration. It usually is bilateral and has a hereditary predisposition, but pressure can vary in each eye. Family history, diabetes, and being very farsighted can put one at greater risk for developing glaucoma.

Laboratory and Diagnostic Procedures

Pachometry is a new device to measure central corneal thickness. It is now used as one of the standard devices in determining accurate intraocular pressure. (See the Diagnostic Tests box, p. 2333.) Average central corneal thickness is about 545 ± 20 micrometers, which has a bearing on the final intraocular pressure recorded for a diagnosis of open-angle glaucoma. If the cornea is too thick, the intraocular pressure reading can be falsely read as too high; or if the cornea is too thin, the intraocular pressure reading can be falsely read as too low (PDR, 2004a; Walker & Piltz-Seymour, 2004). The intraocular pressure is obtained by tonometry reading; that number reading is adjusted according to corneal thickness.

Medical Management

There is no known cure for glaucoma, but it can be well controlled with early diagnosis and treatment. Without treatment glaucoma eventually will cause blindness. Chronic untreated glaucoma can result in a rigid eyeball, sightlessness, and eye pain, and may even require enucleation for a very painful blind eye. The eye health care provider determines the best target pressure as a goal to be reached in conjunction with the extent of optic nerve damage and type of glaucoma. Treatment may include antiglaucoma eyedrops, oral medications, and laser or surgery intervention, depending on the type of glaucoma, the stage of the disease process, and the number of risk factors present. The different types of antiglaucoma eyedrops, categorized in the Pharmacology Summary feature (p. 2346), are usually the first line of therapy. When medical treatment is unsuccessful, intolerable, or patients are noncompliant, surgical options are considered. Surgical and laser options for glaucoma treatment are YAG laser (neodymium: yttrium-aluminum-garnet) for peripheral iridectomy or iridoplasty, laser trabeculoplasty (LTP), laser trabeculectomy, viscocanalostomy, ciliodestructive procedure, or trabeculotomy and trabeculectomy filtering procedure (AAO-10, 2008–2009).

■ Nursing Management

The nurse plays a major role in educating patients about glaucoma and proper management to prevent the advancement of glaucoma. Nursing management of patients with glaucoma can be complex and multifaceted. Application of the nursing process facilitates a comprehensive approach to patients' assessment and care.

Assessment and Nursing Diagnoses

The assessment data includes specific questions related to intraocular pressure controls and vision fluctuation. Subjective data which the nurse needs to gather include: family history of glaucoma, status of eye exam, any current medications being

PHARMACOLOGY Summary of the Topical Ophthalmic Drops for Diagnostic Procedures and Treatment of Glaucoma

Medication Category	Action	Application/Indication	Nursing Responsibility
Anesthetics			
Proparacaine Tetracaine	Anesthetizes corneal nerves and surrounding tissue (conjunctiva); partial or complete loss of sensation.	*Numbing of the cornea:* Applanation tonometry to check intraocular pressure (IOP) or gonioscopy for glaucoma. Removal of a superficial corneal foreign body or sutures. Perform minor corneal or conjunctival procedures. Schirmer's diagnostic test. Contact lenses fitting. Lacrimal canalicular manipulation. Preop preparation, especially in laser therapy. Trauma evaluation. Dosage: 1 to 2 drops over cornea. Onset: within 12 seconds. Duration: about 10–20 minutes. Reapply as needed.	Assessment of clinical signs of allergic reaction, especially to "caines." Explain that the patient's eye is being numbed. Temporary elimination of blink reflex. May need to patch eye following a procedure for protection. Caution: The patient is not to rub or touch eye for several minutes, until numbing sensation dissipates. Never give a patient numbing drops for self-administration; they can cause serious corneal damage, opacity, and vision loss. Monitor for adverse ocular reactions: corneal edema, redness, burning, stinging, keratitis, and delayed epithelial wound healing.
Fluorescein sodium with topical anesthetic		*Numbing and staining of the cornea:* Applanation tonometry or gonioscopy to check IOP for glaucoma. Access corneal abrasion/injury, herpetic lesions, or foreign body. Access tear flow in lacrimal drainage tests. Assist in contact lenses fitting. Evaluate postop closure of sclerocorneal wound in delayed anterior chamber reformation. Removal of superficial corneal foreign body or sutures. Perform minor corneal or conjunctival procedures.	Explain to patient that her tears and edges of eyelids and lashes will be yellow temporarily; the color washes out with her tears. Make sure the drops are current and have not been contaminated by touching the patient's eyelashes or lids with tip of bottle; fluorescein drops can grow *Pseudomonas* if contaminated. Caution: Topical use only and not to be used for long periods (can delay wound healing if overused). Patients with cardiac disease or hyperthyroidism. Observe for adverse ocular reactions: stinging, burning, redness, keratitis, corneal opacity, decreased vision, and iritis. Observe for adverse systemic reactions: dermatitis and depression (rare).
Mydriatics			
Phenylephrine (Neo-Synephrine)	Contends for binding site on muscarinic receptors with activation of α-adrenoceptors on sympathetically innervated iris dilator muscle, arterioles, and Muller's muscle. Produces pupillary dilation by this stimulation of iris dilator muscle and paralyzes iris sphincter and ciliary muscle.	*Pupillary dilation required:* Diagnostic procedures, fundus examination, uveitis (posterior synechiae), preoperatively for laser therapy, etc. Dosage: 1 to 2 drops 20–30 minutes prior to examination or procedure. Onset: 20–60 minutes. Duration: 3–5 hours.	Assess for clinical signs of allergic reaction. Contraindicated in patients with narrow-angle glaucoma. Caution: topical use only. May cause an exaggerated adrenergic effect if used with monoamine oxidase inhibitor (MAOI) agents (up to 21 days after). Instruct patient to wear sunglasses to block ultraviolet (UV) light exposure. Advise patient that driving with eyes dilated may cause difficulty, especially on a sunny day. Practice good hand hygiene to avoid iatrogenic dilation. Advise of possible additive effect if patient is on tricyclic antidepressants. Observe for adverse ocular reactions: stinging and burning. Observe for adverse systemic reactions: collapse, tremor, palpitation, perspiration, and pallor.

Sources: Elfervig, L. S. (2002b). Pharmacology. In K. Goldblum & P. Lamb (Eds.), *Core curriculum for ophthalmic nursing* (2nd ed.). Dubuque, IA: Kendall/Hunt; PDR. (2004a). *Glaucoma: Disease management guide* (1st ed.). San Francisco: Allergan; and PDR. (2004b). *Physicians' desk reference for ophthalmic medicines* (32nd ed.). Montvale, NJ: Thomson.

Medication Category	Action	Application/Indication	Nursing Responsibility
Cycloplegics Atropine (Atropine Care 1%) Cyclopentolate (Cyclogyl) Homatropine (Equipin) Scopolamine Tropicamide	Blocks postganglionic innervation of ciliary body, longitudinal muscle, and iris sphincter, to produce paralysis of ciliary muscle (blocking accommodation) and iris sphincter (blocking constriction).	*Pupillary dilation required:* Refraction requiring mydriasis and cycloplegia, especially in children, who have a large accommodative ability. Acute inflammation of the anterior uveal tract (relieve iris spasm). Preop or postop mydriasis for iridocyclitis. Optical aid in axial lens opacity. Diagnosis procedures. *Atropine:* Dosage: 1 to 2 drops bid, qid. Onset: 45–120 minutes. Duration: 7–14 days. *Cyclopentolate:* Dosage: 1 to 2 drops. Onset: 30–60 minutes. Duration: 6–24 hours. *Homatropine:* Dosage: 1 to 2 drops. Onset: 30–60 minutes. Duration: 3 days. *Scopolamine:* Dosage: 1 to 2 drops 1 hour before refraction. Onset: 30–60 minutes. Duration: 4–7 days. *Tropicamide:* Dosage: 1 to 2 drops; repeat in 5 minutes as necessary. Onset: 20–40 minutes. Duration: 4–6 hours.	Assess for clinical signs of allergic reaction. Contraindicated in patients with narrow-angle glaucoma. Caution use in Down syndrome patients and the elderly. The darker the iris pigmentation, the greater the dosage for effect. Pressure placed with fingers at the bridge of the nose (lacrimal sac compression) may prevent excess systemic absorption. Instruct patient to wear sunglasses to block UV light exposure. Driving with eyes dilated may cause difficulty, especially on a sunny day. Perform good hand hygiene to avoid iatrogenic dilation. Topical use only. Observe for adverse ocular reactions: redness, conjunctivitis, lid inflammation, dry eyes, edema, and follicles. Observe for adverse systemic reactions: fever, dermatitis, flushing, dry mouth and skin, irritability, tachycardia, urinary retention, loss of coordination, hallucinations, coma, death, progressive respiratory depression, and stroke symptoms (which stop in 7 hours when drop is discontinued).
Miotics Carbachol Pilocarpine	Constricts pupils for ocular hypotension. Cholinergic agonist agents–induce, muscarinic receptor contraction of ciliary muscle in facilitating aqueous outflow, and increases trabecular meshwork outflow to decrease intraocular pressure (IOP).	*Open-angle glaucoma, good second- and third-line therapy.* *Preop and postop IOP controls.* *Acute glaucoma attack prevention in noneffected eye or antidote for mydriasis.* Dosage: 1 to 2 drops tid, qid, or 5–6 times a day, depending on eyedrop selection to the affected eye.	Promote compliance with eyedrops. Assess for relief of elevated intraocular pressure, drug effectiveness. Review patient history, due to contraindications of patients with iritis, conjunctivitis, or keratitis, and post–cataract surgery to prevent posterior synechiae. Inform patient that he may have difficulty with dark adaptation with field of vision reduced. Caution with night driving and working with hazardous equipment in dim light. Instruct to stop use prior to general anesthesia. Assess for clinical manifestation of allergic reaction. Observe for adverse ocular reactions: blurred vision, stinging, red eye, ciliary spasm, and induced myopia. Observe for adverse systemic reactions: sweating, headache, syncope, salivation, arrhythmias, hypotension, asthma, pulmonary distress, cramping, vomiting, diarrhea, and urinary frequency. Observe for systemic toxicity with overdose; antidote atropine.

(continued)

PHARMACOLOGY Summary of the Topical Ophthalmic Drops for Diagnostic Procedures and Treatment of Glaucoma—*Continued*

Medication Category	Action	Application/Indication	Nursing Responsibility
Beta Blockers			
Nonselective ß-adrenergic antagonist: Carteolol (Cartrol) Levobunolol (AKBeta) Metipranolol (Toprol) Timolol (Apo-timol) *Selective ß-adrenergic antagonist:* Betaxolol (Betoptic) Levobetaxolol (Betaxon)	Antagonist agents inhibit agonist actions (blockers). ß-Adrenergic antagonist affects ocular function by competing with agonist for ß-adrenergic receptor binding sites, thereby blocking the effects of sympathetic stimulation. This results in decreased aqueous production and may increase aqueous outflow to decrease IOP.	*Primary open-angle glaucoma (POAG), ocular hypertension, aphakic glaucoma, or secondary glaucoma.* Dosage: 1 drop daily, bid, or tid, depending on eyedrop selection to the affected eye.	Promote compliance with eyedrops. Assess for relief of elevated intraocular pressure, drug effectiveness. Review patient history, due to contraindications of patients with chronic obstructive pulmonary disease (COPD), asthma, sinus bradycardia, overt cardiovascular failure, cardiogenic shock, greater than 1° atrioventricular (AV) block, and patients on catecholamine (reserpine). Selective β-adrenergic antagonist poses less risk of pulmonary adverse effects. May mask hypoglycemia in insulin-dependent diabetes mellitus (IDDM) and clinical signs of hyperthyroidism. Can elevate triglycerides. Protect drops from light. Instruct patient of possible additive effects if on systemic beta-blockers. Assess for clinical manifestation of allergic reaction. Observe for adverse ocular reactions: blurred vision, foreign body sensation, photophobia, ptosis, diplopia, and decreased corneal sensitivity. Observe for adverse systemic reactions: insomnia, arrhythmias, pulmonary distress, and bronchospasm (can cause death).
Alpha₂ Agonists			
Apraclonidine (Iopidine) Brimonidine (Alphagan P)	Mimics endogenous adrenergic compounds. Affects ocular function by select binding to α_2 receptors with sympathetic nervous system influence on aqueous formation, pupil width, and ocular blood flow to decrease IOP from glaucoma by decreasing aqueous production and increasing uveoscleral outflow.	*POAG, ocular hypertension, or preop IOP controls for laser therapy.* Dosage: 1 drop bid, tid, or 1 drop preop and postop laser therapy.	Instruct regarding need for compliance with eyedrops. Assess for relief of elevated intraocular pressure, drug effectiveness. Review patient history, due to contraindications of patients on clonidine and monamine oxidase inhibitors (MAOI) therapy. Can develop a vasovagal response during laser surgery and overreduction in IOP. Caution in patients with cardiovascular disease, renal dysfunctions, hepatic dysfunctions, depression, cerebral insufficiency, or Raynaud's disease. Assess for history of drug allergies prior to administration. Assess for adverse ocular reactions: red eye, mydriasis, upper lid elevation, burning stinging, blurriness, follicles, and itching. Observe for adverse systemic reactions: drowsiness, fatigue, headaches, blood pressure changes, dry mouth, nasal congestion, respiratory, or gastrointestinal (GI) discomforts.

PHARMACOLOGY **Summary of the Topical Ophthalmic Drops for Diagnostic Procedures and Treatment of Glaucoma—*Continued***

Medication Category	Action	Application/Indication	Nursing Responsibility
Prostaglandins Bimatoprost (Lumigan) Latanoprost (Xalatan) Travoprost (Travatan)	Increases uveoscleral outflow, increasing aqueous outflow.	*POAG, ocular hypertension, or elevated IOP lowering.* Dosage: 1 drop daily at bedtime.	Encourage compliance with eyedrops. Assess for relief of elevated intraocular pressure, drug effectiveness. Review patient history, due to contraindications. Inform patient of possible red eye (usually goes away within 8–12 weeks), increased eyelash growth, and discoloration of iris and tissue around the eye. Do not drop over contact lenses. Caution: Patients with pulmonary compromise, renal or liver dysfunctions, uveitis, or iritis; aphakic, pseudophakic, or macular edema; do not use Latanoprost with thimerosal. Assess for clinical manifestation of allergic reaction. Observe for adverse ocular reactions: persistent red eye, hyperpigment of iris and adnexa, increased growth of eyelashes, blurriness, stinging, itching, foreign body sensation, conjunctivitis, and macular edema. Observe for adverse systemic reactions: chest pain, angina, respiratory infection, colds, rash, back pain, and joint pain.
Carbonic Anhydrase Inhibitors (CAIs) Brinzolamide (Azopt) Dorzolamide (Trusopt)	Decreases the pressure in the eyes by reducing how much fluid (aqueous humor) is produced in the eye.	*Glaucoma treatment for IOP lowering.* Dosage: 1 drop bid or tid, depending on eyedrop selection.	Encourage compliance with eyedrops. Assess for relief of elevated intraocular pressure, drug effectiveness. Review patient history, due to contraindications if on sulfa drugs; patients with severe renal failure and hepatic insufficiency may have low levels of electrolytes (sodium [Na] and potassium [K]), hyperchloremic acidosis (especially po CAI medication). Caution: May mask hypoglycemia in IDDM, patients with pulmonary or cardiac disease, and patients on high dose of aspirin. Evaluate for clinical manifestation of allergic reaction. Observe for adverse ocular reactions: blurred vision, foreign body sensation, photophobia, ptosis, diplopia, and decreased corneal sensitivity. Observe for adverse systemic reactions: arrhythmias, pulmonary distress, drowsiness, Na and K imbalance, GI upset, and paresthesia.

taken, and past and present eye problems. The nurse also should assess the patient to determine how one is adapting to the visual problems and what anxieties or fears the patient might be experiencing. Is the patient experiencing feelings of loss of control? From an objective perspective the nurse will assess actual visual acuity, body language for distress, family support systems, and the patient's ability to adjust to lifestyle behaviors.

Nursing diagnoses are developed from the assessment data, and a patient care plan applies the nursing process to the relevant nursing diagnoses and provides a comprehensive approach for caring for patients with glaucoma. Diagnoses may include anxiety and fear based on altered self-concept, potential ineffective coping, pain related to intraocular pressure, and health maintenance issues. The nurse also must consider impaired home maintenance issues, risks for injury or falls, self-care deficits related to vision loss, and feelings of powerlessness related to loss of control.

Outcomes and Evaluation Parameters

Evaluation of the patient's response to treatment and nursing interventions is measured through outcome parameters. The focus of evaluation is the ability of the patient to keep intraocular pressure under control, to maintain a level of anxiety and fear at a reasonable level, and to prevent eye pain. Also noteworthy is the patient's ability to maintain and manage a clean and safe environment in which to live.

Planning and Interventions

Planning and implementation of nursing interventions focus on ways to help the patient achieve desired outcomes. Emphasis should be placed on helping the patient find resources and assistance to manage at home and to resume normal activities. Emotional and spiritual support should be provided as should education and specific instructions on how to care for self. Identification of risk factors and instructions on self-care and community resources also is very important.

▮ Collaborative Management

The best results for patients with glaucoma are achieved through a multidisciplinary team approach, including the ophthalmologist, ophthalmic advance nurse practitioner, nurse, and optometrist. Management of glaucoma may include medical controls with the continuous use of eyedrops or surgical intervention by the ophthalmologist. The nurse practitioner or nurse can provide the necessary education and follow-up monitoring of patients' progress to ensure compliance with the glaucoma regimen. Nursing assessment and education include patients' compliance with regular use of eyedrops and follow-up, which is one of the main goals in treating glaucoma. The major reason for the cause of blindness from glaucoma, besides not knowing one has glaucoma, is noncompliance in using eyedrops and not taking glaucoma as a disease seriously. It is imperative that patients understand that the long-term goal of treatment is to lower intraocular pressure to prevent optic nerve damage, and only with continued use of drops can this goal be reached. The new generation of glaucoma eyedrops can lower intraocular pressure with once or twice a day dosage, which eliminates confusion, saves

time, and makes compliance feasible. It is essential to inform patients of potential side effects of the drops and let patients know that some side effects may be only temporary for a couple of months and then dissipate. Patients may need to change eyedrops if side effects are persistent. Eyedrops must be administered properly to gain the full benefit of the medication and prevent waste. Having patients give a return demonstration with artificial tears will allow the nurse to determine patients' ability for self-medication. If multiple drops are prescribed, it is helpful to give patients an index card with the list of drops and when to use them. This will assist patients in preventing drug errors and promoting compliance. The optometrist can provide visual evaluations between regular health care provider visits and make necessary refractive corrections when indicated, thereby, contributing to patients' compliance with eye medications.

Discharge Priorities and Health Promotion

Patient education includes information on risk factors for glaucoma such as family history, myopia, previous eye trauma, low blood pressure, African ancestry, diabetes, longtime exposure to steroids, and aging. On early detection of glaucoma and subsequent treatment to prevent permanent vision loss, health care providers need to focus on patient compliance with glaucoma eyedrops, as outlined in the Pharmacology Summary feature (p. 2346), and regular follow-ups. The patient is taught how to instill eyedrops properly for the full benefit of treatment. Regular eye examination is imperative to know whether treatment prescribed for glaucoma is effective; because no symptoms will occur until vision becomes blurry or lost, and this may not be reversible.

Cataracts

Cataracts are opacity (loss of transparency) of the natural crystalline lens, usually as a result of natural aging, that causes oxidative damage to the lens solubility and increasing cloudiness. The term *phakic* refers to the mature crystalline lens. The crystalline lens is one of the anatomic body structures that continue to grow with the passage of time. Sometimes the lens is compared to an onion with its additive layers; therefore, increased compression and density result in opacity. Cataracts can normally be recognized in adults as early as in the late 20s or early 30s, as the beginning of cataract formation is classified as lenticular changes. Risk factors that may accelerate cataract growth are ultraviolet light, x-ray exposure, smoking, poor diet, diabetes, and corticosteroid therapy. Congenital or traumatic cataracts are the exception to the normal growth phase of cataract formation and may need immediate treatment with surgical removal. Cataracts can be the leading cause of blindness, especially in remote areas of the world, where cataract surgery is not accessible. Cataracts are curable, and if people live long enough, most will experience them at some point in their lifetime.

The onset of the signs and symptoms of cataracts are usually gradual. Patients start to notice that headlights from automobiles look like starbursts. They are bothered with glare, have difficulty reading street signs at night, and experience progressive reading difficulty even with glasses or bifocals. The refractive index changes and the power increases possibly may make patients more nearsighted. This is called a myopic shift and temporarily provides better vision without glasses for the hyperopic or farsighted person.

This is referred to as "second sight" (AAO-11, 2008–2009). Usually cataracts are a painless, progressive loss of vision with aging.

Cataracts are classified according to the opacity formation location in the crystalline lens. The four most basic types of cataract are nuclear, cortical, posterior, and anterior. The other classifications of cataract formations that may be used pertain to specific conditions or inheritance. Chart 71–6 is inclusive of the types of cataract types.

Immature Cataracts

The immature cataract is still in the earlier stages of maturation or ripening, beginning with sectors of opacity and intervening clear areas (AAO-11, 2008–2009) (Figure 71–14 ■). Mature cataracts are easily recognizable with an ophthalmoscope and more definitively with a slit-lamp biomicroscopy. Sometimes the cataract is so dense and noticeable, a penlight will do. *Senile* or *mature cataract* is a term used in describing the later stages of formation and most commonly is reached by the time one reaches 70 to 80 years of age.

Diagnosis is made by a vision test with best-corrected visual acuity of about 20/50 or worse, and a glare test, which mimics sunlight for 20/200 or worse vision, to be considered for cataract surgery. A potential acuity meter (PAM) test also is performed to gauge the approximate visual acuity return after cataract surgery. (See the Diagnostic Tests box, p. 2333.) This may vary depending on whether any other vision problems existed preoperatively; for example, if patients have age-related macular degeneration, diabetic retinopathy, or had previous eye surgery.

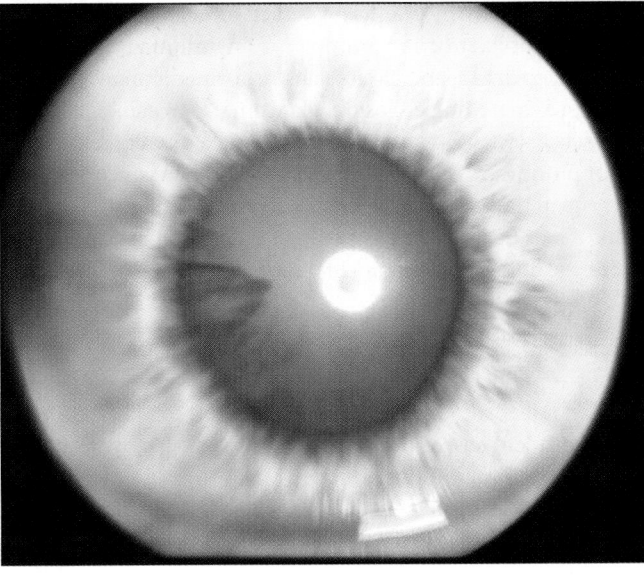

FIGURE 71–14 ■ Nuclear sclerotic with spokes (cortical cataract).
Source: Lucie S. Elfervig

Cataract Surgical Implications

The decision to operate is ultimately determined by the patient when the individual is no longer able to perform activities of daily living, work, drive a motor vehicle, watch television, read, or use a computer. Cataract removal, with few exceptions, usually is recommended by the time one is past 85 years of age.

CHART 71–6 **Categories of Cataract Types**

Type	Description
Nuclear sclerotic (NS) cataract	The nuclear cataract refers to the thickening or hardening (opacity) of the nucleus or central location of the natural crystalline lens (AAO-11, 2008–2009).
Senile, mature, or brunescent cataract	The advanced stage of cataract formation, when it turns brown in color, is most commonly reached by the time the patient is in his 70s or 80s.
Hypermature or Morgagni's cataract	The nuclear sclerosis has gone past maturity into a liquid state.
Cortical or spokes cataract	The cataract thickening is in the peripheral cortex of the natural lens. The radial opacities look like spokes on a wagon wheel, and visual acuity disturbances come on later, if the nucleus is still clear.
Anterior subcapsular cataract (ASC)	The thickening of the natural lens at the anterior or front capsular surface. This more commonly develops from ocular trauma or uveitis conditions (Streeten, 2000).
Posterior subcapsular (PSC) or cupuliform cataract	The thickening of the crystalline lens at the posterior or back capsular surface. This type of cataract is seen more commonly after long systemic steroid usage or a long period of intraocular inflammation. This can cause more difficulty with reading, and bright lights and glare compound this difficulty (AAO-11, 2008–2009).
Hereditary cataract	The lens opacity that has a genetic precondition that usually develops in the third to fifth decade of life. A precondition may be an autosomal dominant inherited disorder or genetic abnormalities, such as Down syndrome or Marfan's syndrome (AAO-6, 2008–2009).
Traumatic cataract	The opaque lens formation due to trauma to or about the eye. This type of cataract usually develops within a brief period (only months) and affects only the involved eye. Manifested symptoms may be blurry vision, glare, photophobia, pain, and iritis (AAO-11, 2008–2009).
Surgically induced or oil-droplet cataract	The cataract that mimics a tear droplet in the nucleus of the lens, which more commonly develops after a vitrectomy surgery (Eliott, Lee, & Abrams, 2001), especially in younger adults ages 30 to 50. The vision is usually blurry enough to interfere with work performance or activities of daily living. Common complaints are unexplained vision loss, the need for frequent glasses changes, and increasing myopia. Oil droplet describes the appearance of a type of opacity that results.

Sources: American Academy of Ophthalmology (AAO-6). (2008–2009). *Basic and clinical science course: Pediatric ophthalmology and strabismus* (Section 6). San Francisco: Author; American Academy of Ophthalmology (AAO-11). (2008–2009). *Basic and clinical science course: Lens and cataract* (Section 11). San Francisco: Author; Eliott, D., Lee, M. S., & Abrams, G. W. (2001). Proliferative diabetic retinopathy: Principles and techniques of surgical treatment. In S. J. Ryan (Ed.), *Retina* (3rd ed., Vol. 2). St. Louis: Mosby; and Streeten, B. W. (2000). Pathology of the lens. In D. M. Albert & F. A. Jakobiec (Eds.), *Principles & practice of ophthalmology* (2nd ed., Vol. 4). Philadelphia: W. B. Saunders.

Sometimes when one has cataract surgery, it can possibly solve two problems; for example, if an intumescent cataract (swollen, enlarged, and cloudy lens) is formed, it may be a precursor to acute angle-closure glaucoma (Streeten, 2000). As cataracts grow and mature, the crystalline lens enlarges, crowding or putting pressure on the anterior chamber, which results in narrowing the angle. Cataract surgery can solve both the problems of lens opacity and of opening the anterior chamber angle, thus restoring vision and normal intraocular pressure.

Cataract Surgery

Cataract surgery is 98% successful (Streeten, 2000). The surgery usually is performed one eye at a time, and if the fellow eye also needs cataract surgery, it is performed about 6 to 8 weeks later. This is prudent to see how the patient recovers postoperatively. If unforeseen complications do arise from the first cataract surgery, they can be taken into consideration when the fellow eye has cataract surgery. Some conditions that may predispose patients to less than ideal results are age-related macular degeneration, diabetes, Marfan's syndrome, or previous retinal detachment. Before cataract surgery is done, a good dilated eye examination is done, to make sure there are no existing problems. If any problems are present, they will need to be addressed before the surgery is performed; for example, active diabetic retinopathy.

Cataract surgery usually is done in an ambulatory surgery center (ASC) under topical or local anesthesia. The anesthesia may vary depending on the surgeon and patient's preference. Preoperative ophthalmic antibiotic/anti-inflammatory drops for surgical preparation and dilation are administered. Preparation for surgery usually includes lid scrubs, and the facial area around the eyes is cleaned with antiseptic solution and well rinsed prior to surgery. Cataracts usually are removed by phacoemulsification with the use of ultrasonic power to fragment (break up) the lens, and the lens fragments are then aspirated with vacuum and flow irrigation. Extracapsular cataract extraction (ECCE) usually is done with a single small surgical incision near the sclerolimbal margin, called no stitch surgery. Extracapsular cataract extraction is the removal of the entire lens (nucleus and cortex) and the central portion of the anterior capsule, leaving the posterior capsule fully intact. The lens implanted is placed in the lens sulcus. On rare occasions an intracapsular cataract extraction (ICCE) may be the best option. This is when the entire lens with capsule is removed. An artificial lens is surgically implanted, called an intraocular lens (IOL) implant. A posterior chamber intraocular lens (PCIOL) is the most commonly used intraocular lens. An anterior chamber intraocular lens (ACIOL) or sutured intraocular lens is used when a posterior chamber intraocular lens cannot be stabilized due to surgical or ocular complications, such as broken zonules, or other systemic problems, such as Marfan's syndrome. New custom IOL implantations that are now available for patients having cataract removals can correct for accommodation or astigmatism. *Pseudophakic* is the term used after cataract surgery when patients have an intraocular lens implant and no longer have a natural crystalline lens. Aphakic refers to no lens implant or without lens implant after cataract surgery of the natural lens removal. These patients will need to wear thick glasses or contact lenses for best-corrected visual acuity. The goal of the lens implant is to restore best-corrected vision for patients so that pa-

tients do not have to wear glasses or contact lenses. However, unless a multifocal lens implant is used (a combination lens for near and distance vision), patients most often will still need reading glasses for seeing up close.

Secondary intraocular lens implant implies that an intraocular lens is implanted after the primary cataract surgery was performed at an earlier date (AAO-11, 2008–2009). For whatever reason, a primary intraocular lens was never implanted at the time of the original cataract surgery. The secondary intraocular lens implant is placed in the aphakic eye (that without a lens).

On completion of the surgery, eyedrops are put in the surgical eye, followed by the application of an eye patch and shield, and postoperative topical ocular medications are prescribed. See the Pharmacology Summary feature (p. 2346). Patients usually are given a postoperative take-home pack, which may include eye patches, sterile eyewash, sunglasses, topical eye medications or prescriptions, and an analgesic prescription for minor operative discomfort. Patients need to know how to care for the postsurgical eye properly with appropriate cleaning and wearing an eye patch or shield as directed.

Postoperative Cataract Care

Postoperative treatment and follow-up care on postoperative day 1 include removal of the eye patch and shield and assessment of visual acuity and intraocular pressure, followed by slit-lamp biomicroscopy and ophthalmoscopy to check the wound stability and any potential postoperative problems (Oetting, 2001). Depth perception may be temporarily impaired following cataract surgery due to the eye patch, being the first eye done, or being aphakic. Patients that are aphakic will need glasses or contact lenses for corrective vision. It often is recommended to postpone getting new corrective lenses for about 6 to 12 weeks after cataract surgery, thus giving the eyes the needed time to heal completely, and sparing patients the expense of more than one pair of glasses. Patients should be instructed to take it easy for a few days and to use topical ophthalmic antibiotic/anti-inflammatory drops as prescribed, for approximately 4 weeks.

Possible cataract surgery complications may include a dropped natural crystalline lens or intraocular lens implant, surgical astigmatism, and decentered or tilted intraocular lens. These and other complications are outlined in Chart 71–7 (AAO-11, 2008–2009).

■ Nursing Management

Nursing management for cataract surgery focuses on preparing patients for the procedure by explaining that it is typically an outpatient procedure performed under local or topical anesthesia. Preoperatively, patients are informed by the ophthalmologist and confirmed by the nurse about what a cataract is, the surgical procedure, and the benefits and risks of cataract surgical removal. The nurse should assess understanding, answer misconceptions or questions, and relieve anxieties. Postoperative instructions should be discussed with patients and significant others prior to surgery for understanding. Instruction should include a demonstration of proper eyedrop instillation, with a return demonstration from the person who will be instilling postoperative eyedrops. Assessment of the operative and nonoperative eye prior to surgery should be completed and documented. It is essential to record all current medications, prescription and over

CHART 71–7	Potential Complications Post-Cataract Surgery

Complication	Description
Decentered/tilted intraocular lens	The intraocular lens falls out of central position or tilts in any direction, causing aberrations or less than clear vision. If not a problem, leave well enough alone. If a problem, surgeon may need to go back in to straighten the intraocular lens, suture it in place, or remove it.
Surgical astigmatism	Abnormal curvature of the cornea is induced with sutures; once healed, the sutures can be cut and refractive adjustments made.
Bullous keratopathy	Corneal edema from surgical manipulation and vitreocorneal adherence; complaining of blurry vision, epiphora, and photophobia; treated with topical eye medication (antibiotics).
Hyphema	Blood in the anterior chamber; complaining of blurry vision and pain; treated with topical eye medication and patching, and quiet; check intraocular pressure often.
Glaucoma	Elevated intraocular pressure; complaining of nothing, but noted on intraocular pressure check; may have pain and blurry vision; treated with topical antiglaucoma eye medication, and occasionally oral medication is indicated if intraocular pressure is > 50 mmHg.
Dropped natural lens Dropped intraocular lens	The natural crystalline lens or the intraocular lens implant is dropped in the vitreous; this requires a pars plana vitrectomy with air–fluid–gas exchange to retrieve the lens, usually immediately at the time of surgery or shortly afterward.
Cystoid macular edema	Edema of the choroidal layer in the macula (central vision); treated with topical eye medication and possibly vitrectomy with air–fluid–gas exchange.
Retained crystalline lens material	Lens material in the capsule is an irritant that can become infectious and cause inflammation; complaining of blurred vision and pain. Treat the problem it is causing, or Elschnig's pearls, lens remnants, can be polished.
Vitreous prolapse	If the rupture of the posterior capsule results, this allows vitreous into the anterior chamber, which may cause pupillary block, poor healing, infection, retinal breaks, or retinal detachments; usually this is corrected at the time of surgery with an anterior vitrectomy to remove vitreous from the anterior chamber.
Retinal detachment	Retinal layers detach or separate from their base; complaining of a curtain, a veil, floaters, or light flashes in vision; treated with endolaser or a vitrectomy with air–fluid–gas exchange.
Vitreous hemorrhage	Blood in the vitreous chamber; complaining of blurry vision and floaters; treated with head elevated during rest or sleep, and let the blood settle inferiorly, or may need a vitrectomy with air–fluid–gas exchange.
Uveitis	Inflammation of the uveal tract (iris, ciliary body, and choroid) from surgical trauma or allergy to intraocular lens; complaining of photophobia, epiphora, and pain; treated with topical eye medication (possible mydriatics, antibiotics/anti-inflammatories, or steroids) or intraocular lens removal.
Endophthalmitis	Intraocular infection and inflammation of the eyeball and tissue; complaining of pain, blurred vision, purulent discharge, hypopyon, and corneal edema; treated with intravitreal, fortified topical, topical, and/or oral antibiotics, and may also require a vitrectomy with air–fluid–gas exchange.
Posterior capsular opacity	This is the most common complaint after cataract surgery, because the posterior capsule is left intact. This capsule prevents other potential major complications that could occur if the capsule were opened. Opacity or haziness of the posterior capsule membrane may take place within several weeks to years or may never develop; complaining of hazy or blurry vision and cataract coming back; cannot read or drive; treated with Nd:YAG laser to open the capsule.

Source: Adapted from American Academy of Ophthalmology (AAO-11). (2008–2009). *Basic and clinical science course: Lens and cataract* (Section 11). San Francisco: AAO.

the counter (OTC), with dosage and frequency, especially any anticoagulants, because they may need to be stopped temporarily before and immediately following surgery.

Infections and Inflammation

All structures of the adnexa and eyeball are subject to infection and inflammation. This section covers some of the most common and serious inflammatory conditions. Inflammatory eye conditions usually are very responsive to treatment, and in most cases the eye is restored to normal with little or no treatment. However, some severe eye infections can mean hospitalization and result in the loss of vision and possibly the eye.

Dry Eye Syndrome

Keratoconjunctivitis sicca, or dry eye syndrome (DES), is the result of poor tear production and formation, or excessive evaporation (AAO-8, 2008–2009). With aging, especially with menopausal women, dry eyes can become a chronic problem, with less tear surface tension. This results in tears running down the face instead of adhering to the cornea epithelial surface. Dry eyes also can be a side effect of some systemic medications (e.g., propranolol) or systemic disease (e.g., Sjögren's syndrome) (AAO-8, 2008–2009). Dry eyes give the sensation of a sandpaper or "gritty" feeling in the eye, blurred vision, and difficulty focusing up close. Treatment usually includes frequent use of artificial tear supplements and/or puncta plugs. Patients are instructed on frequent instillation of artificial tears and being consistent with application. If patients find that using the tears once, twice, or a number of times a day provides relief, they are instructed to use the tears the same number of times each day, so as to prevent the eye from drying out completely between applications. Puncta plugs are plastic or collagen devices that are inserted by an eye health care provider into the puncta to obstruct tears from leaving the eye. If dry eyes become so chronic that they result in corneal defects and scarring, surgical intervention may be indicated with various degrees of tarsorrhaphy, which is the suturing of the upper and lower eyelids together, to lessen corneal exposure (AAO-8, 2008–2009). Artificial tears usually are over-the-counter medication, but a new artificial tear by prescription (cyclosporine ophthalmic emulsion) is available that may keep the eye moist for a longer period of time and help increase tear production.

Blepharitis

Blepharitis, or meibomitis, is inflammation of the eyelids, with redness and crustiness (dry flaky dermis). The use of warm compresses and lid scrubs often is adequate treatment. If the condition is more chronic and becomes ulcerative, the addition of antibiotic ointment may be indicated. This is a very common condition in the aged population, in which the meibomian glands build up with a waxy deposit, the tears do not function properly, and dry eyes develop (Lamb, 2002; Rougé, 2004). Patients complain of **foreign body sensation (FBS)**, nasal canthus deposits, itching, tearing, burning, and irritation. This can be difficult to eliminate and usually requires continuous weekly or daily lid scrubs and warm compresses, which are described in Chart 71–8.

Conjunctivitis

Conjunctivitis is inflammation of the conjunctiva, the clear mucous membrane that covers the sclera of the eye (bulbar conjunctiva), the underlining of the eyelids (palpebral conjunctiva), and the space between the lid and globe (forniceal conjunctiva, fornix, or cul-de-sac) (AAO-2, 2008–2009). On an initial evaluation, it is important to try to obtain a culture or cytologic/serologic study on the type of discharge (especially if mucopurulent). The three most common types of conjunctivitis—viral, allergic, and bacterial—are outlined in Chart 71–9.

CHART 71–8	Eyelid Cleaning and Comfort Measure
Warm Compresses	This is the use of a facecloth or washcloth placed in lukewarm water. Fold it in half and place gently over eyelids for 3 to 8 minutes, especially trying to feel the warmth at the margin of the eyelids to dissolve or melt the waxy discharge that collects at the base of the eyelashes.
Eyelid Scrubs	This is the use of baby shampoo or no tears shampoo diluted in warm water (3 drops of shampoo to 125 milliliters of water). Use a Q-tip applicator or the soft edge of a facecloth to scrub eyelid margins gently. Commercial lid scrubs are also available in local pharmacies.

CHART 71–9 — Three Most Common Forms of Conjunctivitis

Form	Discharge	Eyelid Edema	Lymph Node	Pruritus
Viral conjunctivitis	Clear, sticky	Minimal	Usually	None
Allergic conjunctivitis	Clear, runny	Moderate to severe	None	Intense
Bacterial conjunctivitis	Purulent	Moderate	None	None

Viral Conjunctivitis

Viral conjunctivitis, commonly referred to as "classic pinkeye," is inflammation caused by an adenovirus. This also is referred to as an epidemic keratoconjunctivitis (EKC) when the inflammation encompasses both the cornea and the conjunctiva (AAO-8, 2008–2009). Initially the inflammation starts unilaterally and quickly spreads bilaterally. After about a week of incubation time, such signs and symptoms as clear mucous sticky discharge, excessive tearing (epiphora), hyperemia, small white conjunctival elevations (follicles), light sensitivity (photophobia), foreign body sensation, conjunctival inflammation and irritation, and tissue edema to the point of a transparent bluish hue (chemosis) develop. Preauricular lymph node enlargement and soreness also can be symptoms of viral conjunctivitis (Elfervig & Elfervig, 2007; Trobe, 2006). Causative agents may include adenovirus, herpes simplex, herpes zoster, or influenza virus (Rubenstein & Jick, 2004). Treatment includes good hand hygiene, which is imperative, plus not sharing washcloths, towels, and pillows due to this condition's extremely contagious nature. Viral conjunctivitis usually will take its course and clear on its own.

Patients can use artificial tears, topical ophthalmic antibiotic/steroid, or decongestant eyedrops for 7 to 10 days. Cold compresses for eye comfort also may help increase the healing time and shorten the disease course. Patients should not return to school or to work if in the active stages for at least 4 days, and possibly a week to 10 days, due to the severity and the epidemic nature of viral conjunctivitis.

 *Viral conjunctivitis is highly contagious. The nurse should use effective hand hygiene frequently, before and after putting in medicated eyedrops. The examination area should be sanitized with antibacterial solutions after examination.*
The patient should be instructed in effective hand hygiene technique and advised not to touch eyes or faces of others, and to keep a distance from others. The patient also should be instructed to use clean sheets and towels and not to share them with others.

Allergic Conjunctivitis

Allergic conjunctivitis, sometimes referred to as hay fever conjunctivitis, is caused by environmental changes and contaminants. This also is referred to as a vernal keratoconjunctivitis when the inflammation involves both the cornea and the conjunctiva during seasonal changes, and appears to be most common in young males (Lamb, 2002; Wu & Ariyasu, 1999). It usually is bilateral, with whitish discharge, hyperemia, swelling, burning, stinging, epiphora, and pruritus (Elfervig & Elfervig, 2007; Trobe,

MyNursingKit | Video: Eyes, Ears, Nose, Throat: Conjunctivitis: Etiology and Pathophysiology

2006). This commonly is a seasonal occurrence, especially in the spring and fall, and usually reoccurs annually. Symptoms seem to lessen after sleeping and with less environmental exposure by staying indoors. Causative agents may include animal dander, dust, wind, smoke, feathers, ingested foods, makeup, creams, systemic medications, and anything that can cause an allergic response. Medical management includes topical decongestant eyedrops for 7 to 10 days, good hand hygiene, cold compresses, and oral antihistamines. These measures usually will bring the allergies under control. If this is a seasonal episode, using preventive measures such as taking oral antihistamines a couple of weeks prior to the season may abate clinical manifestations. It may be necessary for patients to seek medical evaluation and treatment.

Bacterial Conjunctivitis

Bacterial conjunctivitis usually is unilateral in the early stages, but often becomes bilateral, with mucopurulent discharge, hyperemia, chemosis, eyelid inflammation and irritation (blepharitis), lid crusting, eyelid edema, and eyelids sticking and matting together, especially on awakening in the morning (Elfervig & Elfervig, 2007; Trobe, 2006). The preauricular nodes usually are not enlarged (Trobe, 2006). Causative agents may include *Staphylococcus aureus, Neisseria gonorrhoeae, Streptococcus pneumoniae, Corynebacterium diphtheriae, Haemophilus influenzae, Listeria,* and *Moraxella* (Rubenstein & Jick, 2004). Medical management includes topical ophthalmic antibiotic drops or ointment for 7 to 10 days, warm compresses, and good hand hygiene technique.

Other common infections and inflammations of the eye are outlined in Chart 71–10 (p. 2356) by description, signs, causes, and management. The conditions include subconjunctival hemorrhage, sty, chalazion, pinguecula, pterygium, dendritic keratitis, herpes zoster ophthalmicus, episcleritis, and scleritis.

Uveitis

Uveitis is inflammation of the uvea or uveal tract, which includes inflammation of the iris, the ciliary body, and the choroid. An in-depth medical history is prudent if uveitis is suspected because of endogenous uveitis, meaning the cause originated from systemic conditions, such as arthritis, oncologic causes, infections, or lupus (Nussenblatt & Whitcup, 2004). Other definitive locations are iritis (includes the iris), cyclitis (includes the ciliary body), anterior uveitis or iridocyclitis (includes the iris and ciliary body), or posterior uveitis or choroiditis (includes the choroid) (Elfervig, 2002a). Clinical manifestations may include blurry vision, tearing, floaters, erythema, hyperemia, edema, or photophobia. Eye pain is usually described as dull with an ache inside the eye. Dark glasses do not seem to help the photophobia.

Noticeable ciliary infection signs when observing the eye may include a small, irregular pupil and dilated or engorged episcleral vessels on the sclera (Nussenblatt & Whitcup, 2004). A slit-lamp examination could reveal cells and flare in the anterior chamber. Cells are white blood cells, and flare is protein deposits floating in the aqueous humor (Harper, Chorich, & Foster, 2002). If patients complain of floaters and blurry vision, the adjacent connecting structures may be inflamed: the vitreous (vitritis), the retina (retinitis), or the retina and choroid (retinochoroiditis) (AAO-9, 2008–2009; Elfervig, 2002a).

Medical management usually includes topical antibiotics to treat the infection, topical or periocular injected steroids to treat the inflammation, and topical mydriatic and cycloplegic drops for temporary dilation and paralysis of the ciliary muscle for comfort (Foster & Vitale, 2002). See the Pharmacology Summary feature (p. 2346). The cycloplegic drops will affect accommodation, so if patients do not have reading glasses or bifocals, they may have temporary difficulty reading small print while on these drops (Foster & Vitale, 2002).

Bullous Keratopathy

Bullous keratopathy or Fuchs' dystrophy is edema and degeneration of the corneal epithelium causing scarring and reduced vision that result from membrane endothelial outgrowths into Descemet's corneal layer (Beers & Berkow, 1999). The severity of the condition can result in corneal ulcer from an epithelial infection and may require a corneal graft later. Initially, it may present with guttata, petite whitish hyaline deposits in Descemet's membrane (Wu & Ariyasu, 1999). This also can be a result of surgical trauma. Medical management includes corneal contact lens bandage, hypertonic saline drops, and intraocular pressure–lowering drops, as indicated (Wu & Ariyasu, 1999).

Corneal Ulcer

Cornea ulcers are local necroses of the corneal tissue due to incursion by bacteria, fungi, or viral infections. These invasions can be the result of contact lens overwear, foreign body penetration, wound or trauma, ocular surgical trauma, chronic conjunctivitis or blepharitis, nutritional vitamin A deficiency, entropion, exophthalmos, exposure keratitis, and chronic, severe dry eyes. All of these conditions allow infectious organisms to penetrate the cornea, resulting in degeneration of corneal tissue (Wu & Ariyasu, 1999). The most common invading organisms are *Pseudomonas, Staphylococcus, Streptococcus,* herpesvirus, and *Acanthamoeba* (AAO-8, 2008–2009). Patients may complain of foreign body sensation, epiphora, and blurry vision initially.

On examination with the biomicroscope, a small dull-grayish deposit can be noted in the epithelium, which progresses to a whitish circumscribed opacity in the cornea that necroses into an ulcer. Other ocular signs may be chronic hyperemic eye, **hypopyon** (pus in anterior portion of eye) or corneal neovascularization with later progression (AAO-8, 2008–2009; Elfervig & Elfervig, 2007). A dendritic infiltrate is very diagnostic of a fungal infection (McLeod, 2004). The deeper the ulcer is in the corneal layers, the more severe the disease and complications, and it is considered an urgent condition to be treated aggressively by an ophthalmologist. Medical management options can vary from fortified eyedrops to corneal transplant (penetrating keratoplasty).

Trachoma

Trachoma is chronic inflammation of the conjunctiva that ranges from mild to severe, even scarring. It is caused by repeated invasion of *Chlamydia trachomatis*, which causes chronic infection and inflammation (Rubenstein & Jick, 2004). Ocular manifestations can be follicles, hyperemia, entropion, and trichiasis, and can result in blindness from corneal opacification. This ocular disease is more common in Third World

CHART 71–10 **Infections and Inflammations of the Eye**

Condition	Description/Sign	Cause/Management
Non-traumatized eye (subconjunctival hemorrhage)	Dilated blood capillaries or small capillary leakage on the sclera or conjunctiva.	Coughing, sneezing, sudden motion, or straining, especially if a patient is on a blood thinner; usually resolves spontaneously.
Hordeolum (sty or stye)	Infection of the eyelid glands. Internal hordeolum is located within the eyelid itself, a pustular infection of the meibomian gland; and external hordeolum is located at the eyelid margin, a pustular infection of the oil glands of Zeis.	Can resolve spontaneously, when warm compresses are applied two to four times a day to the infected area to aid in localization and rupture of the pustule; topical ophthalmic antibiotic ointment and incision and drainage of the pustule also may be indicated if it does not resolve spontaneously.
Chalazion	Inflammation in the meibomian gland of the eyelid; referred to as an internal hordeolum or meibomian cyst. Appears as a raised, round, inflamed (erythematic), and tender area near the lid margin.	Blockage of the sebaceous material in the meibomian gland. Treat with warm compresses and ophthalmic antibiotic ointment. If this becomes a nuisance or interferes with vision, it can be surgically excised.
Pinguecula	Small, yellowish conjunctival elevation at the 3 and 9 o'clock positions on the scleroconjunctival area, which results from prolonged ultraviolet, sunlight, or environmental exposure.	Usually does not cause any symptoms and does not require treatment. If it becomes irritating, use artificial tears.
Pterygium	Yellowish-white triangular growth of conjunctival tissue at the 3 and 9 o'clock positions close to the limbus that results from prolonged ultraviolet exposure and can spread onto the cornea.	If it continues to grow across the cornea, passing the central visual axis causing vision loss, then laser or surgical intervention is indicated. Otherwise, it is just observed, with no treatment, or treated with artificial tears if it becomes irritating.
Herpetic keratitis (dendritic keratitis)	Inflammation of the cornea. Staining of the corneal epithelium reveals a bare branch-like configuration on the cornea (dendrite). Signs and symptoms are photopia, epiphora, foreign body sensation, and hyperemia.	Caused by the herpes simplex virus. Treatment with antiviral drops usually is sufficient, but systemic drugs may be indicated if drops are not effective in clearing the inflammation. Epithelial débridement around the dendrite of loose tissue with a cotton-tip applicator may aid in accelerating the healing process. Atropine Care 1% drops also may help in healing and comfort (AAO-8, 2008–2009).
Herpes zoster ophthalmicus	Varicella-zoster virus (shingles or chickenpox) involves the globe of the eye. Nose lesion (nasociliary nerve affected) can be diagnostic (McLeod, 2004). Signs are eyelid edema, hyperemia, corneal edema, keratitis, and elevated intraocular pressure.	Forehead dermatitis. Infection treated with antiviral oral medications, topical steroid drops, and atropine drops. The intraocular pressure is monitored often until it returns to normal and remains stable. Patients over age 60 may need a short course of oral corticosteroids to prevent acute postherpetic neuralgia or persistent pain (McLeod, 2004).
Episcleritis	Inflammation of the episclera (outermost layer of the sclera); appears with single, large, dilated vessels in the episcleral layer at about the 3 and 9 o'clock positions on the sclera (Goldstein & Tessler, 2004). The patient complains of hyperemia, photophobia, local tenderness, and epiphora.	Treatment may range from nothing and observation; to topical vasoconstrictor, topical steroid drops, or oral nonsteroidal anti-inflammatory drugs to shorten the course of discomfort. It usually is self-limiting and rarely becomes serious (Daly, 2002).
Scleritis	Inflammation of the sclera and deep episclera. This can be serious and vision threatening and is found more commonly in women between 45 and 65 years of age (Daly, 2002). Complaints may be localized eye pain, tenderness, photophobia, epiphora, and hyperemia. The irritated area appears bluish (meaning deep vessel involvement); this can range from being diffuse, nodular, or necrotizing tissue. About 15% of patients develop vision loss within the first year (Beers & Berkow, 1999).	Treatment may include cytotoxic immunosuppression, but usually systemic corticosteroid is the initial treatment of choice. Patients should be closely monitored for hematopoietic, renal, and other organ involvement.

Sources: American Academy of Ophthalmology (AAO-8). (2008–2009). *Basic and clinical science course: External disease and cornea* (Section 8). San Francisco: Author; Beers, M. H., & Berkow, R. (1999). *The Merck manual of diagnosis and therapy* (17th ed.). Whitehouse Station, NJ: Merck Research Laboratories; Daly, S. W. (2002). Scleral disorders. In K. Goldblum & P. Lamb (Eds.), *Core curriculum for ophthalmic nursing* (2nd ed.). Dubuque, IA: Kendall/Hunt; Goldstein, D. A., & Tessler, H. H. (2004). Episcleritis, scleritis, and other scleral disorders. In M. Yanoff & J. S. Duker (Eds.), *Ophthalmology* (2nd ed.). St. Louis: Mosby; and McLeod, S. D. (2004). Infectious keratitis. In M. Yanoff & J. S. Duker (Eds.), *Ophthalmology* (2nd ed.). St. Louis: Mosby.

countries and is the second leading cause of preventable blindness in the world, second only to cataracts (Mayo Clinic, 2006).

Preseptal Cellulitis

Preseptal cellulitis is inflammation of the eyelid tissue in front of the orbital septum and does not involve the eyeball (Elfervig & Elfervig, 2007; Trobe, 2006). It can exhibit the following signs and symptoms of the eyelid: warmth, tenderness, swelling, redness, and chemosis. It usually does not involve problems with eye movement or pain. Patients also may be febrile and irritable from the inflammation and discomfort. Systemic antibiotics and warm compresses for 10 days is the recommended medical treatment.

Orbital Cellulitis

Orbital cellulitis is inflammation of the postseptal orbital tissue from the spread of bacteria from elsewhere (endogenous), usually from the nasal and sinus system, or the traumatic induction of bacteria into the orbit (AAO-7, 2008–2009) (Figure 71–15 ■). The most common causative organisms in adults are staphylococci and streptococci from bacterial sinusitis (Dutton, 2004). Clinical manifestations may include fever, red and edematous eyelids, periocular pain, hypopyon, proptosis, impaired ocular motility, afferent pupillary defect, optic nerve swelling, corneal abscess, decreased vision (can be a rapid onset), hyperemia, and erythema (Elfervig & Elfervig, 2007; Trobe, 2006). Patients should be referred immediately to a health care provider, so that the primary locus of the infection can be identified with thorough examination and history of any trauma, flu or upper respiratory infection, sinusitis, or toothaches. Test requirements may be x-rays, computed tomography (CT) scan, and Gram stain and culture of any discharges from the eye, nose, mouth, or skin. Medical management may involve hospitalization with aggressive intravenous and systemic broad-spectrum antibiotics, topical fortified antibiotic eyedrops and subconjunctival antibiotics, surgical

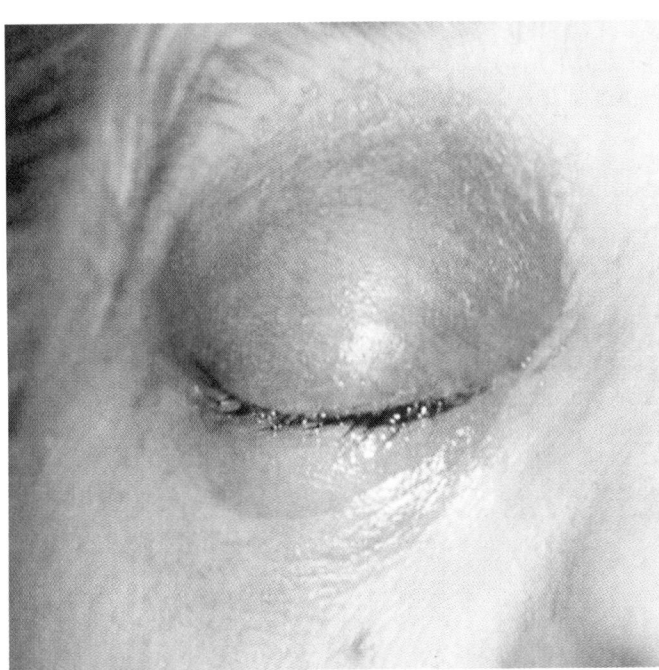

FIGURE 71–15 ■ Orbital cellulitis.
Source: Courtesy of Lucie S. Elfervig

débridement/drainage or vitrectomy, whatever is indicated pending culture result. Vision and pupil functions should be checked every 5 to 6 hours. Orbital cellulitis can lead to intracranial abscess and cavernous sinus thrombosis, which when involved has the added symptoms of nausea, vomiting, headache, and possible loss of consciousness, a life-threatening complication. When patients are ready to be discharged, it is very important for them to follow the discharge regimen, or recurrent infection and loss of the eye may develop, which could be life threatening.

Discharge Priorities and Health Promotion

Discharge planning starts with admission to the hospital and is continuous throughout the hospitalization. An organized plan of care with set goals will ensure the highest level of recovery. The ultimate goal is to return patients home with no complications or added problems.

To assist and to augment understanding, an organized and comprehensive instructional plan is necessary with patient brochures and information. The Patient Teaching & Discharge Priorities box (p. 2358) outlines the necessary components of the teaching plan for orbital cellulitis, which includes the healing regimen, risks of recurrent infection and other potential complications, pain management, emotional adjustment, and sensory deprivation or recovery. Discharge instructions include continuous use of systemic antibiotics and topical antibiotic eyedrops or ointment, use of good hygiene technique to prevent reinfection, ways to achieve altered comfort, monitoring the healing process of the eye, health care provider notification of complications, and compliance with follow-up care. Care specialists may include an ophthalmologist, an otolaryngologist, a health care provider, and a nurse consultant.

Endophthalmitis

Endophthalmitis is a mucopurulent intraocular inflammation that occurs most often after intraocular surgery, such as for cataract, glaucoma, strabismus, or penetrating keratoplasty. The incidence of endophthalmitis is approximately 1 in 1,000 population. The exogenous pathogens harbored on the lids and in the conjunctival fornix invade the eye and inflammation results (Elfervig & Elfervig, 1999). Endophthalmitis also can be a consequence following incisive eye trauma, especially by a contaminated foreign body (Elfervig & Elfervig, 1999). It is an infection of the vitreous in combination with the retinal and the uveal layers of the eye. Endophthalmitis is classified as endogenous as the result of hematogenous dissemination of infection from elsewhere in the body, or exogenous as a result of surgery infectivity (more frequent) or acute ocular injury (Campochiaro, 1999). Causes of endophthalmitis can be bacterial (more frequent) or fungal infection (Elfervig & Elfervig, 1999). *Staphylococcus epidermidis* is the most widespread exogenous infecting organism of the eye (Campochiaro, 1999). Fungal endophthalmitis can be the result of *Candida* species and *Aspergillus* species organisms (Seal, Bron, & Hay, 1998). Fungal infections are less common and more endogenous (Hamza, Loewenstein, & Haller, 1999). Endogenous infection is tainted organisms in the blood that settle in the choroid or retina, resulting in retinitis, choroiditis, or chorioretinitis that invades the vitreous chamber, causing an inflammatory reaction and acute endophthalmitis (Hamza et al., 1999).

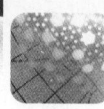

PATIENT TEACHING & DISCHARGE PRIORITIES for Orbital Cellulitis

Need	Teaching

HEALING REGIMEN

Patient/family

Follow antibiotic regimen, as prescribed:
- Daily application of fortified topical antibiotic ointment and drops
- Daily administration of systemic antibiotics
- Daily monitor for signs of improvement.

Perform daily eye patch changes, as indicated by amount of purulent discharge and healing; or the eye may need no patching as healing takes place and there is no discharge or drainage.

Eye shield as a protection and safety measure if eye is not too proptotic.

Monitor visual acuity changes frequently:
- Increased blurriness
- Diplopia
- Any improvements.

Monitor for increase in infection:
- Proptosis (eye bulging out more)
- Corneal dullness and loss of sensitivity
- Increase in swelling
- Appears cross-eyed
- Eye movement impaired
- Pupil size changes
- Increase in erythema or discoloration
- Increase in warmth to touch or pain/soreness.

Observe for any central nerve system involvement:
- Nausea or vomiting
- Febrile
- Level of consciousness decreased
- Headaches.

Maintain quiet and rest at home:
- No going out
- No strenuous activity
- No heavy lifting.

Follow-up appointments:
- Daily to weekly visits to the ophthalmologist
- Follow-up with otolaryngologist if sinus infection involvement.

Family/support system

Assess availability of, knowledge of, and compliance with treatment regimen.

Assess respite needs and resources.

Setting

Assess discharge placement needs.

Assess home environment for need for assistive devices.

Assess for need for professional home health needs.

Assess for a healing environment.

Assess need for follow-up appointments.

RISK OF INFECTION

Patient/family

Assess for clean techniques:
- Use good hand hygiene before changing any dressings or applying topical medications.
- Soiled linens are changed.
- Keep hands clean and fingernails short; do not scratch or rub swollen eyelid, as may introduce germs or break down tender tissue.
- Use protective eye shield or wear gloves when sleeping, if the healing process creates itching and the stimulus to touch eyelid.

Assess for any signs or symptoms of infection increase, and report as needed.

Signs and symptoms include:
- Proptosis (eye bulging out more), increase in swelling of eyelid
- Appears cross-eyed; eye movement impaired; pupil size changes
- Increase in redness or discoloration to eyelid
- Increase in warmth to touch or soreness to eyelid
- Increase in vision blurriness or eye pain
- Nausea or vomiting
- Febrile
- Level of consciousness, if decreased.

Teach clean techniques to minimize the risk of infection.

Describe signs and symptoms that need immediate medical attention.

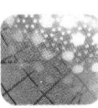
Need	Teaching
Setting	Assess environment for risk factors.
PAIN MANAGEMENT	Assess for altered comfort.
Patient/family	Assess for pain: • Increase in redness (hyperemia or injection) • Swelling • Increase in blurriness of vision • Increase in discharge • Proptosis does not subside. Reduce or relieve discomfort with healing promotion by using warm compresses to eyelid. Promote the use of analgesic medication as prescribed for discomfort. Encourage the patient that with each day of healing, increased comfort should follow.
Setting	Assess environment for safety and endorsement of therapeutic needs.
EMOTIONAL ADJUSTMENT	Anxiety and fear of going totally blind or of condition being life threatening.
Patient/family	Assist with anxiety coping. Answer any questions or concerns truthfully. Encourage expression of frustrations and fear of vision loss. Encourage frequent family contact and positive support. Encourage self-care and individual recovery to normal activity as soon as applicable and safe. Express that it is normal to feel some fear and discouragement after discharge.
Setting	Encourage the patient to seek information if there is a lack of understanding. Incorporate family and friends for support and interaction. Seek spiritual guidance and understanding.
SENSORY DEPRIVATION OR RECOVERY	Monitor whether visual acuity is getting worse or improving. Monitor whether mental acuity is declining.
Patient/family	Monitor visual acuity and whether eyelid appears to be healing. Monitor mental status: • Level of consciousness or awareness. Report changes in visual acuity or mental awareness. Seek medical attention if visual acuity or mental acuity becomes worse. Vision loss may make patient feel isolated and alone. Mental awareness or the lack thereof may require further assistance, reevaluation, and immediate follow-up and examination. Encourage family interaction frequently.
Setting	Assess environment for injury prevention and needs if vision or mental awareness is impaired.
RISK OF COMPLICATIONS	Potential complications: • Blindness, intracranial abscess, cranial nerve palsies, cavernous sinus thrombosis, or meningitis can be fatal.
Patient/family	Should be suspicious of complications if daily improvement is not observed, increased bulging of the eye, or increased globe misalignment. Assess for any reinfection of orbit, and report as needed any reoccurring signs and symptoms, or if eye does not appear to be improving. Monitor visual acuity changes: increase in blurriness, pain. Monitor for increase in infection and clinical deterioration: • Progressive proptosis (eye bulging out) • Globe displacement • Increase in swelling • Appears cross-eyed • Eye movement impaired • Pupil size larger • Increase in redness or discoloration • Increase in warmth to touch. Observe for any central nervous system involvement: • Nausea or vomiting • Febrile • Level of consciousness. If unusual signs or symptoms observed, even if not sure what they are, question any problems and notify the health care provider.

(continued)

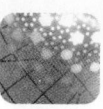

PATIENT TEACHING & DISCHARGE PRIORITIES for Orbital Cellulitis—*Continued*

Need	Teaching
Setting	Hospital.
	Readmission if orbital infection does not start to improve in 24–48 hours.
	Very aggressive treatment with intravenous antibiotics.
	Orbital abscess surgical incision and drainage if indicated.
	Culture and sensitivity, Gram stain, computed tomography (CT) scan, x-rays, magnetic resonance imaging (MRI), or lumbar puncture.

Risk factors for the development of endophthalmitis include a possible complication following cataract surgery; which can be related to the patient's history, aseptic technique, or intraocular lens implant (Falk, Beer, & Peters, 2006; Seal et al., 1998). Patients on immunosuppressive therapy also may be at a higher risk for endophthalmitis due to poor wound healing (Seal et al., 1998). Additional risk factors for endophthalmitis include diabetes, torn posterior capsule, iris manipulation, lens fragments in the vitreous, and prolonged surgery time (Montan et al., 1998). The incidence of fungal endophthalmitis increases with immunocompromised persons and intravenous drug abusers, especially by contaminated needles (Montan et al., 1998).

Clinical Manifestations

Clinical manifestations of endophthalmitis usually are blurred vision (the most general symptom), which can occur rapidly, eye pain, hypopyon (most familiar sign), cells and flare in the anterior chamber, corneal edema, photophobia, conjunctival injection, and chemosis (Elfervig & Elfervig, 2007; Trobe, 2006). Fungal involvement causes a vitreous clouding (poor media clarity) and light perception visual acuity (Hamza et al., 1999).

Diagnostic and Laboratory Procedures and Medical Management

Diagnostic tests may include fluorescein angiography and ultrasonography (B-scan), which is useful for cloudy media. (See the Diagnostic Tests box, p. 2333.) Anterior chamber and vitreous tap or vitreous biopsy is recommended if a specimen is indicated (Seal et al., 1998). Vitreous and aqueous Gram stain and semiquantitative cultures are essential (Campochiaro, 1999). Certain gram-positive organisms seem to have a better visual prognosis (Campochiaro, 1999).

Aggressive treatment is crucial to avoid a severe and enduring vision loss, thus improving the chances of the visual acuity outcome (Seal et al., 1998). Evisceration often is the treatment of choice for advanced endophthalmitis with severe recurrent mucopurulent infection and no light perception vision. The outcome of surgical management of endophthalmitis has a good prognosis for vision restoration, possibly as high as 20/50 in about half the cases (Falk et al., 2006; Seal et al., 1998). Being aware of early changes in patients' vision or recognizing suspicious complaints, with immediate intervention, especially if endophthalmitis is suspected, can save sight.

■ Eye Trauma and Injury

Eye injury is a significant and disabling health problem. Injuries to the eye from traumatic events are a common occurrence that should be treated as emergencies requiring immediate attention. In the United States approximately 2.5 million individuals experience an eye injury requiring treatment in an emergency department, inpatient or outpatient facility, or private health care provider's office (Mulrooney, 2006). In persons under 25 years of age, ocular trauma is the number-one cause of vision loss. Fortunately, advances in microsurgical techniques over the past decade have allowed vision to be saved in some of these injured eyes. Common and frequent injuries to the eyes and eyelids are discussed next.

Epidemiology and Etiology

Eye emergencies include cuts, scratches, foreign objects in the eye, burns, chemical exposure, and blunt injuries to the eye or eyelid. Because the eye is easily damaged, any of these conditions can lead to vision loss if left untreated. A recent study estimated that from 2002 to 2003 there were 27,152 injuries in the United States related to the wearing of eyeglasses. The same study concluded that sports-related injuries due to eyeglasses wear were more common in those under the age of 18, and that fall-related injuries due to eyeglasses wear were common in those aged 65 and over (Sinclair, Smith, & Xiang, 2006). On the other hand, eyeglasses have been found to offer protection, resulting in a lower incidence of severe eye injuries to those wearing them (May et al., 2000).

A chemical injury to the eye can be caused by a work-related accident or by common household products, such as cleaning solutions, garden chemicals, solvents, or many other types of chemicals. Fumes and aerosols can also cause chemical burns. With acid burns, the haze on the cornea often clears with a good chance of recovery. However, alkaline substances—such as lime, lye, commercial drain cleaners, and sodium hydroxide found in refrigeration equipment—may cause permanent damage to the cornea. Ongoing damage may occur in spite of prompt treatment. It is important to flush the eye with clean water or saline while seeking urgent medical care. Dust, sand, and other debris can easily enter the eye. Persistent pain and redness indicate that professional treatment is needed. A foreign body may threaten vision if the object enters the eye itself or damages the cornea or lens. Foreign bodies propelled at high speed by machining, grinding, or hammering metal on metal present the highest risk.

Trauma from sports is very common. Some of the more recurrent injuries occur during the following activities: hockey, archery, darts, BB guns, bicycling, sports that involve rackets, baseball, boxing, and basketball. Trauma also may be caused by flying pieces of wood, metal, glass, stone, and other materials. Blunt injury by fist also should be considered, as should road traffic accidents with head and facial trauma. Other causes of intraocular trauma may arise from workplace tools or even common household implements.

A black eye usually is caused by direct trauma to the eye or face. Certain types of skull fractures can result in bruising around the eyes, even without direct trauma to the eye. The bruise is caused by bleeding under the skin. The tissue surrounding the eye turns black and blue, and gradually becomes purple, green, and yellow over several days. The abnormal coloring disappears within 2 weeks. Usually, swelling of the eyelid and tissue around the eye also occurs. Occasionally, serious damage to the eye itself occurs from the pressure of the swollen tissue. Bleeding inside the eye can reduce vision, cause glaucoma, or damage the cornea. Accidents, occupational injuries, sports injuries, and fights are some of the risk factors associated with black eyes.

Pathophysiology with Clinical Manifestations and Medical Management

The actual pathophysiology resulting from an eye injury is dependent on the type of injury. Clinical manifestations, laboratory and diagnostic procedures, and specific medical management also are contingent on the type of injury. The most common types of eye trauma or injury are discussed next.

Chemical Burns

Chemical burns require immediate irrigation by washing the eye continuously for 15 to 25 minutes. If suspicious or aware that the chemical is an *alkali*, the eye should be irrigated for a good 35 plus minutes or more, especially over the cornea. The most common alkaline agents are lye, lime, potash, ammonia, drain cleaners, chemical cleaners and detergents, fertilizers, and industrial solvents (Elfervig & Elfervig, 2007; Trobe, 2006). If litmus paper is available, use it as an indicator, and do not stop irrigating until litmus paper illustrates neutral, pH of 7 to 7.3. It is important to keep in mind that chemical agents can come in many forms: liquid, gas, or solid. Alkali (pH > 7) burns usually are more serious than acid (pH < 7) burns, because an alkali (hydroxyl ions) continues to burn or damage tissue after contact if it is not completely removed or neutralized. The most common offensive acid agents are battery acid and laundry bleach.

In checking for foreign bodies, never remove a penetrating foreign body, and refer the patient immediately to an ophthalmologist. Signs and symptoms might be painful loss of vision with a burning sensation, corneal swelling, excessive tearing, hyperemia, chemosis, photophobia, and blepharospasm. Emergency treatment involves copious irritation that may require flipping the upper lid (Figures 71–16, 71–17, and 71–18 ■) and pulling down the lower lid (fornix), using a lid speculum, or instilling topical ophthalmic anesthetic drops to allow the eye to be open well enough to complete a more effective irrigation. Evaluation of the eye should be done using the format stated in the Visual Assessment section earlier in this chapter. Treatment indications may include topical ophthalmic cycloplegics for comfort, topical ophthalmic antibiotic eyedrops and ointment for infection, topical ophthalmic steroid drops for inflammation, and a sterile eye patch and/or shield, pending the health care provider's orders. Refer back to Charts 71–4 and 71–5 (pp. 2330 and 2331) for ocular and vision evaluation tests and assessment.

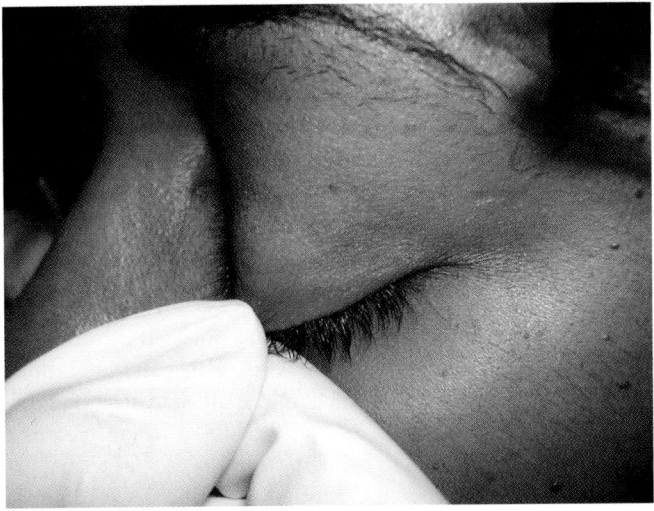

FIGURE 71–16 ■ Demonstration of flipping the upper eyelid. First step, placing finger on eyelid.
Source: Courtesy of Lucie S. Elfervig

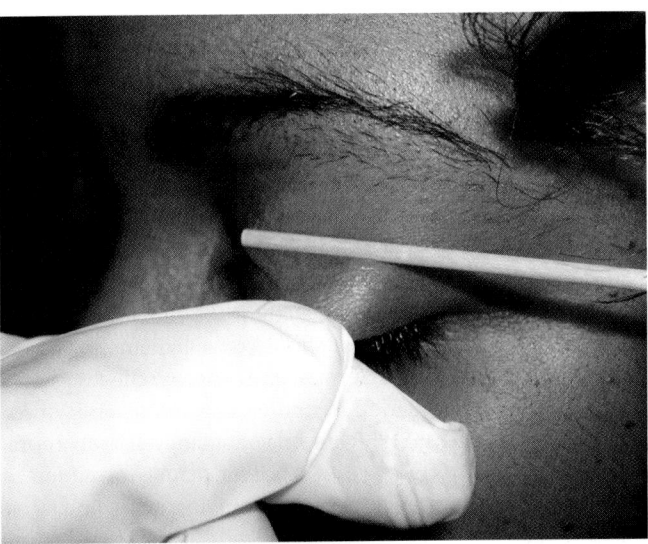

FIGURE 71–17 ■ Demonstration of flipping the upper eyelid. Placing wooden dowel to roll eyelid.
Source: Lucie S. Elfervig

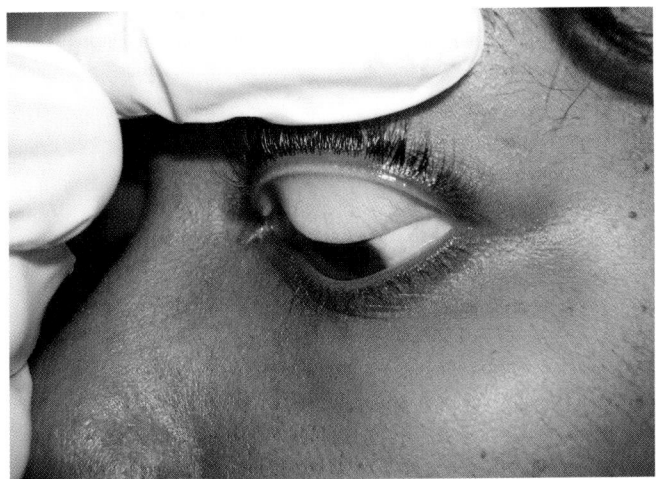

FIGURE 71–18 ■ Demonstration of flipping the upper eyelid. Lid back exposing conjuctivitis.
Source: Lucie S. Elfervig

It is important to keep in mind that chemical agents that may cause burns come in many forms; that is, liquid, gas, or solid. When a chemical burn to an eye occurs, seconds count! The affected eye should be irrigated with copious amounts of water or normal saline for no less than 20 to 35 minutes or until litmus paper pH is neutral. The eyelid may be inverted for better irrigation.

Central Retinal Artery Occlusion

Central retinal artery occlusion (CRAO) is a vascular infarction to the central retinal artery wherein blockage by an embolus results in acute unilateral vision loss, afferent pupillary defect, and decreased carotid pulse with associated carotid bruit (Elfervig & Elfervig, 2007; Trobe, 2006). Other manifestations may include narrowed retinal arterioles, pale optic disc, and diffused pale posterior retina, except in the fovea where there is a classic "cherry-red spot," a hallmark sign for central retinal artery occlusion that generally vanishes in about 2 weeks (Sharma & Brown, 2001b) with the return of normal color. Emergency measures are taken to decrease intraocular pressure with topical antiglaucoma drops, oral carbonic anhydrase inhibitors, and an anterior chamber tap (paracentesis). Other desperate attempts to restore perfusion to the central retinal artery, but which have not been proven effective, may include trying to restore vasodilation by rebreathing CO_2 (breathing inside a paper bag), using hyperbaric chamber treatment, and performing intermittent digital massage of the globe with the eyelid closed, as soon as possible and best within less than 24 hours (Elfervig & Elfervig, 2007; Trobe, 2006). Once stability is established and the nurse or ophthalmologist is able to take a medical history, it is imperative that the nurse ask about vascular diseases that cause hardening of the arteries and listen with a stethoscope for carotid bruits. The ophthalmologist or nurse should refer patients to the internist or family health care provider for appropriate tests and a complete physical evaluation. Tests often ordered are an erythrocyte sedimentation rate (ESR) to rule out giant cell or temporal arteritis, a carotid ultrasound to check for plaque formation or carotid insufficiency, an echocardiogram for heart and valve malfunctions, a blood pressure check, and a diabetic evaluation (Sharma & Brown, 2001b). Typically, most patients seek medical attention after 24 hours; so for patients with cardiovascular anomalies, instruct them to seek emergency eye care immediately if any of the earlier ocular signs or symptoms occur.

CRITICAL ALERT *Immediate actions to be taken in the event of central retinal artery occlusion include:*

Have patient breathe inside a paper bag for vasodilation, if it is within minutes of the occlusion taking place.

Do an intermittent gentle digital massage of the globe to aid perfusion, if it is within the first 24 hours of occlusion taking place.

Check intraocular pressure, by the nurse.

Assess eye for pain and vision loss.

Access standing orders to obtain an erythrocyte sedimentation rate.

Open Globe

Open globe or ruptured globe refers to an open eyeball with a laceration, penetrating injury, or intraocular foreign body. These ruptures usually are from a blunt trauma, motor vehicle crash, sporting event, fistfight, or high-velocity object creating an open, jagged-edged wound (Elfervig & Elfervig, 2007; Robson, Behrman, & Abbuhl, 2007; Trobe, 2006). Ruptured globe commonly is associated with a dislocated lens, retinal detachment, vitreous hemorrhage, and a wide area of tissue damage. Patients can present with the following ocular signs: **hyphema** (bleeding in the eye), edema, chemosis, acute diffuse subconjunctival hemorrhage, corneal laceration, irregular pupil, and lens cloudiness. Open globes often can have orbital fractures, so it is important to observe for facial hypoesthesia (insensitivity to touch) over the cheek, to palpate gently along the orbital rim for a step-off notch area, and to note whether diplopia is present (Elfervig & Elfervig, 2007; Trobe, 2006). Once the confirmation of ruptured globe is made, immediate surgical priority is instituted. The prognosis is guarded toward expected final visual outcome.

CRITICAL ALERT *Immediate actions to be taken in the event of an open globe injury include:*

Assess open wounds, intraocular foreign body or protrusion, and support appropriately; and refer immediately to the emergency department.

Obtain visual acuity and assess for other ocular symptoms; if this is not possible, an immediate referral to the emergency department is indicated.

Observe for facial hypoesthesia (loss of sensation).

Obtain a history surrounding the circumstances.

Laboratory and Diagnostic Procedures

Visual acuity is a must and usually is the first test done following an eye injury, using standard visual acuity charts for near and distance acuity, unless other urgent matters preclude doing this test first (see Chart 71–3, p. 2330, for proper testing). It is a good idea to keep a couple of pairs of standard reading glasses (e.g., +2.00 and +3.00) on hand at the clinic or workplace, because often patients forget or lose their glasses. Using a pinhole is one way to take a distance visual acuity without corrective lenses. When standard testing charts are not available, use the best means available to obtain some measure of vision; often a newspaper or book (standard print read at 14 to 16 inches is ~ 20/40 acuity) is used for near vision, and looking out a window at a license plate may work for distance vision. Sometimes one has to be a little inventive when testing for visual acuity. When recording vision results, it is necessary to document devices and materials used for obtaining distance and near vision, especially if one is not using standard equipment (e.g., patient was able to read a license plate appropriately 10 feet away without corrective lenses with each eye separately and together). Any type of acuity should be recorded, whether it is count fingers, hand motion, light perception, or no light perception. Pupil check should be done to see whether pupils are equal, round, and reactive to light and accommodation (PERRLA); and the nurse should be alert to afferent pupillary defect. Normal eyes constrict when light is shined in one of them; if they dilate it may indicate optic nerve injury. If a patient is complaining of minor eye irritation and not a true eye emergency, and if a foreign body is found on evaluation to be an eyelash, dust, or lint that is easily removable with a tissue or irrigation, this can be done by the nurse. It is essential to document the type of foreign body and how it was removed.

■ Nursing Management

Time is crucial in true eye emergencies, where minutes count. When first assessing eye injuries, it is imperative to provide timely and appropriate triage, treatment, and referral, as this can affect the final visual outcome. When a patient presents with a chemical burn to the eye, copious irrigation of the eyeball, fornix, and facial area with water for the first 15 to 25 minutes is crucial in possibly saving the cornea, and therefore vision, before doing anything else. After the rinsing, an initial evaluation can be made. If the evaluation indicates that it is not a true emergency situation or that an immediate referral is not necessary, and the patient's condition is stable, it is appropriate to take a detailed history to identify the offending chemical and determine whether a neutralizing agent is available. The nurse should record the necessary information, take the visual acuity of both eyes, check pupil responses, and assess how much ocular involvement seems to have taken place. See Charts 71–2, and 71–5 (pp. 2328 and 2331) for assessment protocols. After initial assessment of an eye emergency and initial treatment is instituted, and if no intraocular foreign body is present, the nurse should place a protective shield over the eye, if indicated.

When an intraocular foreign body is present, it is critical to leave the object in place and stabilize it, especially if it is protruding from the eye. The object should not be removed, and the nurse should be very careful not to put pressure on the intraocular foreign body. This provides safety in transportation. It usually is best to keep patients in a sitting position, because lying down or reclining may advance the intraocular foreign body deeper into the eye with the natural force of gravity. The nurse should instruct patients not to eat or drink anything from that time forward, because emergency surgery may be done promptly. Time and contents of the last meal consumed should be documented for the record. Patients' activity should be restricted and patients should be kept comfortable and quiet at all times. The ophthalmologist will perform further evaluation with a complete ocular examination. Be aware that any type of ocular emergency, trauma, injury, intraocular foreign body, or laceration may need tetanus prophylaxis, as indicated. If ordering magnetic resonance imaging (MRI) of patients, there are two things to keep in mind. It should not be done if a metal intraocular foreign body is suspected, because the MRI could move or dislodge the intraocular foreign body, thereby causing more ocular damage. Second, if previous retinal repair surgery was done, it is necessary to check with the patients' ophthalmologist to determine whether an encircling band or scleral buckle was used in the retinal surgical repair; in the past (over 5 years ago), metal clips or staples were used to secure the encircling band or scleral buckle on the retina, and the MRI magnification could remove or dislodge these clips. These metal clips have not been used in retinal repair more recently.

CRITICAL ALERT *Precautions related to magnetic resonance imaging (MRI) of the eye include:*

In the past, an encircling band or scleral buckle in retinal repair surgery was secured with metal clips or clasps.

Patients with a history of retinal repair surgery should check their past medical history or with their surgical ophthalmologist to find out whether they had an encircling band or scleral buckle used in their retinal repair surgery and whether it was secured with metal clips or clasps.

Magnets pull on metal and can pull metal out of position.

MRI magnification can pull out metal intraocular foreign bodies, and surgical metal clips or clasps, thus causing damage to eye tissue.

Eye Urgencies

Some eye injuries are described as urgencies, meaning that treatment is imperative. These conditions include penetrating and perforating trauma, blunt trauma, neovascular glaucoma, **flashes** and floaters, retinal vascular occlusions, and sudden vision loss, when response time could be several minutes, several hours, or even several days. Sudden vision loss can be divided into acute macular hole, retinal occlusions, anterior ischemic optic neuropathy, temporal arteritis, amaurosis fugax, and ocular migraines. A comprehensive discussion of each of these eye urgencies follows.

Penetrating or Perforating Trauma

Penetrating trauma refers to an injury that penetrates or enters the eye, but does not exit the eye. Perforating trauma refers to an injury that goes through the eye completely and exits the eye. Common weapons of injury are knives, scissors, guns, branches/sticks, wood, arrows, darts, and nails. Depending on the seriousness of the trauma, ocular manifestations will vary. Some of the signs and symptoms are epiphora, hyperemia, subconjunctival hemorrhage, hyphema, proptosis, ecchymosis, edema, iris defects, laceration, abnormal intraocular pressure, blurry vision, diplopia, eye pain, and foreign body sensation or actually seeing the intraocular foreign body in the eye. Once the type of wound is confirmed, appropriate management is instituted, and if a penetrating intraocular foreign body is present, surgery probably will be recommended. Treatment also will include topical ophthalmic antibiotics, systemic antibiotics and anti-inflammatory medications, plus a topical ophthalmic mydriatic for comfort (AAO-8, 2008–2009). See the Pharmacology Summary feature (p. 2346).

Blunt Trauma

Blunt trauma refers to an eye injury from a blunt object, such as fists, projectile objects (tennis balls, paintballs), or a motor vehicle crash, which can present with hyphema, chemosis, ecchymosis, edema, subconjunctival hemorrhage, epiphora, decreased vision, photophobia, and any degree of discomfort. Nursing management includes using the same measures as if patients have a ruptured globe. Re-bleeding after an initial hyphema occurs in about 10% of the cases, usually within about 7 to 10 days. Treatment varies with the level of seriousness (AAO-7, 2008–2009). There are many other eye injuries that commonly are seen, such as corneal abrasions, contact lens overwear, and corneal foreign body. These injuries are outlined in Chart 71–11 (p. 2364).

Neovascular Glaucoma

Neovascular glaucoma (NVG) is intraocular pressure elevation due to a new blood vessel growth network within the iris and the trabecular meshwork causing angle closure (Fanous, 2004). Neovascular glaucoma can be an end stage to severe diabetic retinopathy, when blood glucose is uncontrolled, resulting in retinal hypoxia and capillary nonperfusion (AAO-10, 2008–2009). Treatment for neovascular glaucoma has a low success rate, so prevention is the best means of therapy. Laser photocoagulation is one surgical recommendation.

Ocular Flashes and Floaters

Flashes (photopsias) and floaters are symptoms that can occur from many intraocular conditions, but more commonly from posterior vitreous detachment (PVD), vitreous hemorrhage,

CHART 71–11   **Common Ocular Eye Injuries**

Injury	Description	Signs/Symptoms	Assessment
Corneal abrasion	Scratched area of the cornea causing corneal defect.	Foreign body sensation, eye pain, epiphora, photophobia, blurry vision.	Take a good history, evaluate with topical ophthalmic anesthetic drop and fluorescein stains (strips), and examine with a blue (cobalt) light; the abrasion appears yellowish-green in color. Draw a picture of the corneal defect, and invert the upper eyelid to evaluate further for debris or foreign body, if indicated. Seek medical treatment if further evaluation and ophthalmic medications are indicated (Visto, 2000).
Contact lens overwear (superficial punctuate keratitis [SPK] or giant papillary conjunctivitis [GPC])	Result of contact lens abuse, because of sleeping in them too long, poor hygiene of maintaining contact lenses, or wearing damaged or infected lenses.	Above, plus: injection, pruritus, halos, mucous discharge.	Contact lenses need to be removed or—if contaminated with an infection or deposits, or if damaged—thrown away. Stay out of contact lenses for 1 to 2 weeks, or until all eye irritation is cleared. Take a good history; evaluate the eye with topical anesthetic drop and fluorescein stain, and use blue light check for corneal abrasions. Record contact lens type, age, length of time worn, type of cleaning and storage solutions, and last time cleaned. All contact lens wearers should have a pair of backup glasses for such occasions. Depending on the severity and stage of overwear, the patient may need to seek medical treatment (Dabezies et al., 1998).
Corneal foreign body	Small, superficial corneal lesions that give the sensation of having sand or grit in the eye.	Above, plus corneal edema.	Mineral matter can be less irritating, as metal, vegetation, and insects usually cause an inflammatory response, which can result in swelling and infection. Take a good history, and note whether the patient was wearing safety glasses or goggles. Evaluate the eye with topical anesthetic ophthalmic drop and staining; and upper eyelid inverted to check for foreign bodies (if indicated). Management may require irrigation only to remove a minor irritant. If a corneal defect is present, seek medical treatment (Parrish & Chandler, 1998).

Sources: Dabezies, O., Klyce, S., Morgan, J., Hartstein, J., Donshik, P., Boswall, G., et al. (1998). Corneal changes from contact lenses. In H. Kaufman, B. Barron, & M. McDonald (Eds.), *The cornea* (2nd ed.). Boston: Butterworth-Heinemann; Parrish, C. M., & Chandler, J. W. (1998). Corneal trauma. In H. Kaufman, B. Barron, & M. McDonald (Eds.), *The cornea* (2nd ed.). Boston: Butterworth-Heinemann; and Visto, D. A. (2000). Corneal abrasion: To patch or not to patch. *Insight, 25*(1), 4–6.

and retinal breaks or detachments (AAO-12, 2008–2009). (See the Retinal Detachment section later in this chapter.) Photopsias (flashes) are when a person notices a light flashing in the eye, something like a lightbulb when it blows out. Floaters are described as gnats or grayish filament floating in one's line of sight. Photopsias and floaters can be the first warning signs for more serious eye problems and need to be distinguished by a comprehensive dilated eye examination with slit-lamp biomicroscopy and indirect ophthalmoscopy. An ultrasonogram (B-scan) is performed when the fundus cannot be viewed adequately with an indirect ophthalmoscope due to some opacity. Treatment measures are indicated by cause, from observation to surgery.

Retinal Vascular Occlusions

Retinal vascular occlusions include central retinal artery occlusion (CRAO) (see the discussion in the Eye Trauma and Injury section earlier in this chapter). Central retinal vein occlusion (CRVO) is a compression of the central retinal vein that causes a tumultuous blood flow giving rise to thrombosis (AAO-4, 2008–2009). Branch artery occlusion (BAO) refers to an occlusion of the branch artery off the central retinal artery (Sharma & Brown, 2001b). Branch vein occlusion (BVO) is an occlusion of the branch vein off the central retinal vein, commonly the superior temporal vein (Fekrat & Finkelstein, 2001). Occlusion is a stroke to the eye that can cause a sudden loss of vision by ocular vascular infarction to the arterial or venous circulation of the optic nerve, either centrally or peripherally (branch vessels). The blood flow is blocked by an acute vascular plaque or embolus, which creates an ischemic retinal defect. The signs may include a pale or swollen optic disc, nerve fiber layer (NFL) infarctions, retinal apoplexy, cotton-wool spots, or soft exudates, which can cause vision loss and visual field defects (Schachat, 2001). Other signs for a central retinal vein occlusion can be peripapillary flame-shaped hemorrhages or intraretinal hemorrhages; a branch vein occlusion can be flame-shaped or intraretinal hemorrhages and distended vessels off the disc near the superior or inferior arcades. Arterial occlusions will cause white retina, areas of nonperfusion, and arterial attenuation (Schachat, 2001). The longer the occlusion is present, the greater the vision loss. Arteriole occlusions seem to cause more of a permanent or greater vision deficiency. With venous occlusions some vision seems to return with early treatment. One of the most severe complications of central retinal vein occlusion is developing neovascular glaucoma (Clarkson, 2001).

A complete medical evaluation should be done by a health care provider to evaluate for vascular insufficiency, hyperlipidemia, hypertension, or diabetes. It is important to educate known patients with cardiovascular anomalies or arteriosclerosis about seeking eye care immediately if any of the earlier ocular signs or symptoms are manifested. Many patients that have had retinal occlusions state that they experienced a sharp pain or severe headache to the temporal area of the face on the side of the involved eye just minutes to hours before the stroke to the eye and loss of vision occurred. Nursing management includes obtaining a good history and making proper referrals. The oph-

thalmologist or ophthalmic nurse specialist will do an ocular examination and order a fluorescein angiogram and visual field test. (See the Diagnostic Tests box, p. 2333.) The treatment may include systemic anticoagulants, such as an aspirin or pentoxifylline, antiglaucoma ophthalmic drops, laser photocoagulation, or radial optic nerve neurotomy.

Sudden Vision Loss

Sudden loss of visual acuity is a very frightening experience that usually is unexplainable at first to patients. This leaves patients wondering what happened. Some of the ocular problems that can cause a sudden loss of vision are acute macular hole, retinal occlusions, anterior ischemic optic neuropathy, temporal arteritis, amaurosis fugax, and ocular migraines. These ocular conditions are outlined in Chart 71–12 with descriptions and management.

Eyelid Laceration

Eyelid laceration refers to any cut or open wound to the eyelid that has many possible causes such as from an open globe, penetrating trauma, blunt trauma, falls, or motor vehicle crash

---

CHART 71–12 **Sudden Vision Loss Eye Problems**

Problem	Description/Management
Acute macular hole	A hole in the central area of the retina, where one's 20/20 vision is located, called the fovea. Signs and symptoms include unilateral, painless, and substantial loss in central vision that appears as a round orangish-red spot in the macula. There is a grayish area surrounding the hole, which usually indicates edema and drusen (yellow deposits) may be present. Medical management for a true macular hole probably will mean a vitrectomy with air–fluid–gas exchange and intraocular steroids.
Anterior ischemic optic neuropathy (nonarteritic ischemic optic neuropathy)	An ischemic attack to the optic nerve (ON). Signs and symptoms include unilateral, painless decrease in vision; afferent pupillary defect; disc edema; and normal erythrocyte sedimentation rate (ESR) (which distinguishes this from arteritic ischemic optic neuropathy). No effective management is known at this time. The degree of vision loss depends on the extent of ischemia.
Temporal arteritis (giant cell arteritis or arteritic ischemic optic neuropathy)	A unilateral loss of vision. Signs and symptoms may include altitudinal visual field loss and decreased color vision, afferent pupillary defect, optic nerve swelling, forehead and scalp tenderness, arthritis-type discomfort, painful chewing, loss of weight, and elevated erythrocyte sedimentation rate. This usually occurs in patients around the age of 65. The patient needs a comprehensive medical work-up, a temporal artery biopsy for diagnosis confirmation, erythrocyte sedimentation rate, plus a complete ocular examination with visual field. Medical management with systemic steroid is of an urgent nature to prevent vasculitis and contralateral eye disease, to prevent the possibility of rendering the patient legally blind.
Amaurosis fugax	A transient, sudden, and painless decrease in vision unilaterally is caused by Hollenhorst plaques, which obstruct arterial blood flow to the ophthalmic artery. The temporary or fleeting loss of vision can last from about 30 minutes to hours, and usually gives the patient a panic attack of possibly going blind. On complete ocular examination, the plaques might be visualized in the retinal vasculature coupled with retinal edema, and very rarely for ophthalmic artery stenosis. The eye exam also will include fluorescein angiography and fundus photography. A complete medical and neurological evaluation is indicated to rule out transient ischemic attack (TIA) and carotid stenosis. Medical management may include systemic anticoagulants and hypolipidemic agents, or endarterectomy.
Ocular migraine (occipital lobe ischemia)	A mirage-like image, shimmering edge, heat waves, or smoke-like screen that appears in one's vision, something like an aura. Usually no headache is involved; however, the patient may experience mild discomfort and sudden peripheral vision loss or transient visual obscuration. This visual impairment occurs mainly in the temporal quadrant. The peripheral vision disappears for about 10 to 20 minutes, and vision returns to normal after the episode. No treatment is required if this is a true ocular migraine. Aspirin or acetaminophen may help to prevent the reoccurrence if one is going through a period of ocular migraine episodes and can possibly remove the cause, such as particularly stressful circumstances.

Sources: Arnold, A. C. (2004). Ischemic optic neuropathy, diabetic papillopathy, and papillophlebitis. In M. Yanoff & J. S. Duker (Eds.), *Ophthalmology* (2nd ed.). St. Louis: Mosby; Jabs, D. A. (2001). Rheumatic diseases. In S. J. Ryan (Ed.), *Retina* (3rd ed., Vol. 2). St. Louis: Mosby; Lee, A. G., & Brazis, P. W. (2003). *Clinical pathways in neuro-ophthalmology: An evidence-based approach* (2nd ed.). New York: Thieme; Sharma, S., & Brown, G. C. (2001a). Ocular ischemic syndrome. In S. J. Ryan (Ed.), *Retina* (3rd ed., Vol. 2). St. Louis: Mosby; and Sjaarda, R. N., & Thompson, J. T. (2001). Macular hole. In S. J. Ryan (Ed.), *Retina* (3rd ed., Vol. 3). St. Louis: Mosby.

(AAO-7, 2008–2009). Lid laceration injuries are divided into six levels of severity, which are shown in Chart 71–13 (Elfervig & Elfervig, 2007). Patients should be made aware of the signs and symptoms of a possible infection, such as hyperemia, inflammation, edema, discharge, or pain. The use of ice packs to control hemorrhaging and reduce swelling will offer some comfort. Medical treatment can be as minor as an adhesive butterfly strip, topical antibiotic/anti-inflammatory drops or ointments, and a sterile patch. A patch is contraindicated if an intraocular foreign body is present. Surgical treatment may be the best option when greater tissue is involved with the injury, which may include surgical repair or reconstruction, as indicated according to the level of severity (AAO-7, 2008–2009).

Nurses should educate patients on good hand hygiene before applying eyedrops or ointment to prevent the risk of infection. The nurse should assist in pain management for *Readiness for Enhanced Comfort* and psychological support for *Ineffective Coping* for patients with severe vision losses, those who commonly express *Anxiety* and *Fear*. Patient education is a must to prevent the risk of noncompliance. Education about the prescribed treatment regimen and regular follow-up care should be reinforced by the nurse to promote healing for the best possible visual outcome and patient's hopefulness.

Retinal Detachment

Retinal detachment is the separation of the sensory retinal layers from the retinal pigment epithelium, where subretinal fluid collects in the potential space (AAO-12, 2008–2009). This condition usually requires immediate surgical repair, especially if the macula is still on or intact. If the macula is off or detached and there is choroidal edema, there is time to place patients on steroids for a few of days before surgery. This allows time to decrease the edema and give the retinal tissue time to heal, thus, providing more surgical manipulability and possibly a better surgical outcome.

Clinical manifestations of a retinal detachment vary and are outlined in Chart 71–14. There literally may be no clinical manifestations, or patients may have blurry vision, a shower of floaters, light flashes, and a curtain or veil in the line of vision. It is most likely that patients will not experience pain, but they may experience a panic attack (Steidl & Hartnett, 2003). Primary high-risk factors may include trauma, high myopia, lattice degeneration, retinoschisis, retinopathy, tumors, and post-cataract surgery. Secondary risk factors may include vitreous hemorrhage, diabetic retinopathy, severe uveitis, severe hypertension, Marfan's syndrome, and toxemia from pregnancy. Retinal detachment that involves the macula may be recognizable through a direct ophthalmoscope without dilation and can have a whitish retinal reflex (Figure 71–19 ■). If the macula is still intact and the retinal detachment is in the periphery, then a dilated eye examination is necessary to view the retinal detachment. An ultrasonogram (B-scan) is indicated for any detachment to view the extent of the detachment, tissue involvement, and location. (See the Diagnostic Tests box, p. 2333.)

CHART 71–13 **Lid Laceration Categories**

Category	Involvement
Superficial	Usually can be treated by a nonophthalmologist with Steri-Strips, butterflies, or Band-Aids.
Full thickness	Lid margin and lid function, and ocular abnormality; be cautious.
Medial one-third of upper and lower lids	May involve the canalicular (tear) system; be cautious.
Deep laceration of upper lid	Ptosis; indicates levator muscle may be involved; be very cautious.
Fat prolapse	Globe penetration, foreign body, and impaired lid function; be cautious.
Loss of tissue	Grafting of the skin or reconstructive surgery may be necessary.

Sources: Elfervig, L. S., & Elfervig J. L. (2007). Recognition and triage of ocular emergencies. *Refinements: Clinical Education Modules for Today's Ophthalmic Team, 2*(1), 1–14. Manuscript updated and submitted for republication; and Green, J. P., Charonis, G. C., & Goldberg, R. A. (2004). Eyelid trauma and reconstruction techniques. In M. Yanoff & J. S. Duker (Eds.), *Ophthalmology* (2nd ed.). St. Louis: Mosby.

CHART 71–14 **Clinical Manifestations of a Retinal Detachment**

Sign	Description
Absence (none)	The patient does not realize anything is wrong when the retinal detachment is so far in the periphery near the ora.
Blurry vision	The patient will notice her central vision is blurry or cloudy; this is because the retinal detachment involves the central macula and edema.
Shower of floaters	The patient will notice black/gray spots or clear ameba-type spots in his vision, which are more noticeable against a light background or blue skies; these are clumps of vitreous proteins or clumps of red blood cells from a hemorrhage.
Flashes of light	The patient will notice flashing lights (like a lightbulb breaking) in her peripheral vision; more common when getting up from a lying position or entering a dark environment. This is usually caused by the vitreous pulling on the retinal sensory layer.
Curtain or veil	The patient will notice a curtain- or a veil-like shape come across his central vision; this is usually the detached retinal flap or retinal layers' separation moving around in the vitreous crossing in the central line of sight. The superior temporal quadrant is the most common location for a retinal detachment, so the patient will notice an inferior nasal flap or vision loss.
No pain	The patient does not experience any pain with a spontaneous retinal detachment, but may panic when noticing vision changes or loss.
Loss of tissue	Grafting of the skin or reconstructive surgery may be necessary.

Source: Adapted from Steidl, S. M., & Hartnett, M. E. (2003). *Clinical pathways in vitreoretinal disease.* New York: Thieme.

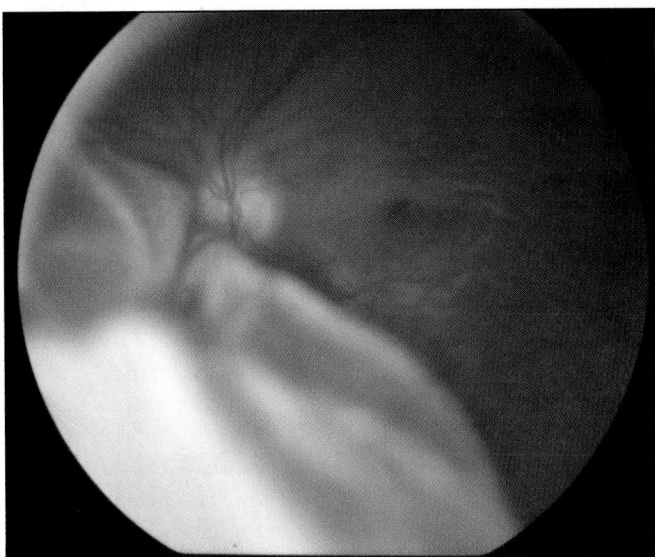

FIGURE 71–19 ■ Retinal detachment with macula off.
Source: Lucie S. Elfervig

Posterior Vitreous Detachment

Posterior vitreous detachment (PVD) occurs when the vitreous separates from the retinal surface and liquefies (syneresis), usually due to aging and increased axial length of the eye. This occurrence typically starts unilaterally and the fellow eye usually starts later (Hikichi & Yoshida, 2004). Symptoms of only occasional flashes and floaters usually are the most common signs and can be annoying. If the diagnosis proves to be the latter, bilateral PVD, and there are no tears, holes, or detachments located, time would allow the ophthalmologist an opportunity to observe the condition and have patients return to the office in 2 to 3 weeks for a reevaluation. If symptoms increase or become more obvious, patients should be instructed to return to the ophthalmologist's office sooner. Posterior vitreous detachment can also be a procurer of retinal detachments. The vitreous is firmly attached at the vitreous base (near ora serrata), the disc margins, the macula, and large vessel margins; retinal breaks can occur more easily in these areas with a spontaneous or traumatic posterior vitreous detachment (AAO-12, 2008–2009).

Retinal Breaks

Retinal breaks are retinal tears or holes. They can give the same warning signs as a retinal detachment. These patients need to be seen by an ophthalmologist to be evaluated by a dilated fundus examination. If a retinal detachment is highly probable, the patient should be instructed to stay quiet and refrain from straining, lifting heavy objects, or participating in activities. If it is only a small retinal break, it can usually be treated with cryopexy or laser photocoagulation.

Vitreous Hemorrhage

Vitreous hemorrhage is the presence of blood or red blood cells in the vitreous humor or cavity that commonly is caused by diabetic retinopathy, retinal detachment, or trauma. Vision is usually blurry to very poor depending on the degree of blood present, resulting in painless, unilateral vision loss. Vitreous hemorrhages often are observed over time to see whether the blood will reabsorb spontaneously. If it does not reabsorb, surgery may be indicated.

Nonrhegmatogenous and Rhegmatogenous Detachment

The two major types of retinal detachment are nonrhegmatogenous and rhegmatogenous. Nonrhegmatogenous may include serous and traction retinal detachment. Serous detachment occurs from serous leakage (clear fluid) that separates retinal intraocular layers between the retina and retinal pigment epithelium, or separates choroidal intraocular layers between the choroid and sclera, which pulls the retina off as a result of inflammation (Elfervig & Elfervig, 1998). Traction detachment occurs from scar tissue, fibrovascular formation of the vitreous that detaches the retina. This type of detachment is more common in long-standing diabetes with inflammation and with patients that have had previous ocular trauma (Elfervig & Elfervig, 1998). Rhegmatogenous detachment occurs from a break or a tear in the retina. The break or tear can occur when the vitreous degenerates and tugs the retina off by separating its sensory layers (Elfervig & Elfervig, 1998).

Retinal Detachment Surgical Implications

Retinal detachment surgical repairs usually are outpatient procedures that do not require hospitalization. The surgical procedures can be as simple as a cold (cryopexy) or hot laser (photocoagulation), or can be more invasive with pneumatic retinopexy or vitrectomy.

Cryopexy

Cryopexy (cryo) or cryotherapy means basically to fix by freezing, with the use of nitrous oxide (N_2O). Cryopexy is a type of cold laser that seals a retinal hole or retinal tear in the peripheral retina, usually present in an anterior position, meaning between the equator and the ora of the peripheral retina (Williams & Aaberg, 2001). Laser photocoagulation means to seal with light energy that converts to thermal heat. When a retinal hole or retinal tear is too posterior, meaning behind the equator, fundus photocoagulation laser usually is the treatment of choice (Williams & Aaberg, 2001). The photocoagulation laser uses argon or dye to seal the retinal hole or retinal tear. Cryopexy and thermal laser scars are both permanent, leaving a micropigmented or white scarred area in the retina tissue.

Vitrectomy

Vitrectomy is the surgical removal of the vitreous by a pars plana incision and air, gas, or fluid exchange (Charles, 2001). The air, gas, or fluid exchange is to realign and reattach the retina, to keep the retina in its proper anatomic position. A scleral buckle or encircling band sometimes is used during vitrectomy to enforce and stabilize the weak area of the retina, to lessen the chance of a re-detachment (Charles, 2001). A scleral buckle and encircling band are usually permanent and can make the eyeball more myopic, thus changing the refractive error of vision and possibly requiring a change in glasses or the addition of glasses. Once patients have a retinal detachment, they are considered to be at high risk for future retinal detachments, because they are now known to be more prone to them.

■ Eye Tumors or Neoplasms

Tumors of the eye can be life threatening, but many are not and are said to be benign. Medical and surgical treatment should include a good eye examination and observation; and suspicious-looking

CHART71–15	Signs of Ocular Tumors
Sign	**Ocular Change**
Vision change	The vision becomes less clear or distorted.
Strabismus	An eye being crossed; may complain of diplopia.
Changed moles, freckles, or wart-like lesions	A pigmented area in and around the eye that appears to grow larger and darker.
Periorbital ecchymosis	A dark circle discoloration of the eyelids, around the eyes; the child appears somewhat like a raccoon.
Proptosis	An eye appears to "bug out"; or globe displacement.
Ptosis	An eyelid that droops; look for misalignments.
Subcutaneous mass	A notable growth or elevation noted on the face, adnexa, or eyeball; or palpable nodule.

Sources: American Academy of Ophthalmology (AAO-6). (2008–2009). *Basic and clinical science course: Pediatric ophthalmology and strabismus* (Section 6). San Francisco: Author; Shields, J. A., & Shields, C. L. (1999a). *Atlas of eyelid and conjunctival tumors.* Philadelphia: Lippincott Williams & Wilkins; Shields, J. A., & Shields, C. L. (1999b). *Atlas of intraocular tumors.* Philadelphia: Lippincott Williams & Wilkins; and Shields, J. A., & Shields, C. L. (1999c). *Atlas of orbital tumors.* Philadelphia: Lippincott Williams & Wilkins.

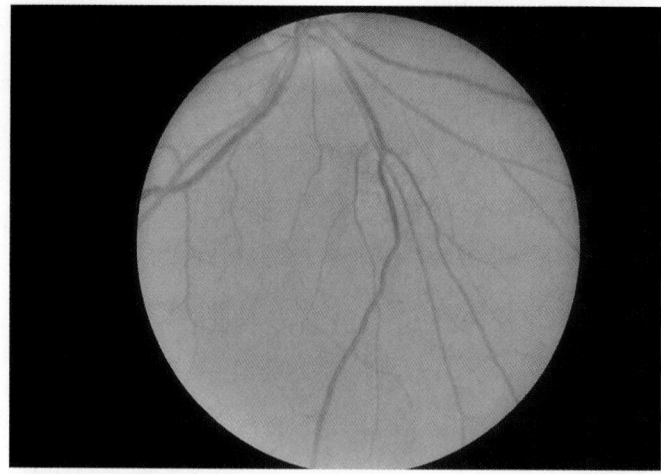

FIGURE 71–20 ■ Choroidal nevus.
Source: Lucie S. Elfervig

tumors should be biopsied by an ophthalmologist or neuro-ophthalmologist. The eyes and surrounding tissue are subject to both benign and cancerous lesions, but due to the limitations of this chapter they will not be discussed in their entirety. This section covers some of the more common eye neoplasms, which will be divided into benign eye lesions, precancerous eye lesions, and malignant eye lesions. Some signs of an ocular tumor may seem like ordinary ocular changes, but if certain signs are manifested without a reasonable explanation, a neoplasm may be awakening. Chart 71–15 outlines possible signs of ocular tumors.

Benign Eye Tumors

Benign eye lesions are tumors in or around the eyeball that are not cancerous or are nonmalignant and not life threatening. These lesions are sometimes called a nevus, hyperplasia, pigmented hypertrophy, or freckle. Most of the time benign eye tumors just need watching or close observation, but they can be excised if they impair vision or cause significant cosmetic alterations.

Nevus

Nevus, sometimes called a freckle, is a brownish pigmented area of eye tissue that usually is flat or slightly elevated, varies in size and shape, varies in pigment intensity, and can be amelanotic, meaning without pigment or whitish. Nevi often are located near the corneoseral limbus on the iris, conjunctiva, and eyelid, and on the choroidal retina (Figure 71–20 ■). Nevi rarely have malignant potential (Shields & Shields, 1999a). They usually are just observed unless they change in color or continue to grow, and then further evaluation is warranted with possible treatment.

Hypertrophy of Retinal Pigment Epithelium

Hyperplasia or pigmented hypertrophy of retinal pigment epithelium is a black pigment area or dot in the retina or on the eyelid where pigmented cells have accumulated. This condition

usually is benign and needs only periodic observation, every 1 or 2 years. No treatment is necessary, unless the dot enlarges or changes color, which usually is uncommon.

Lymphoid Hyperplasia

Lymphoid hyperplasia is the proliferation of lymphoid infiltrates with benign lymphocytes and plasma cells that can invade the iris, ciliary body, and choroid, and also can involve conjunctiva and orbit. It is unilateral and occurs largely in adults, and it is manifested in the choroid as circumscribed or diffused yellow thickening, usually accompanied with a secondary retinal detachment (Shields & Shields, 1999a). Treatment is surgical excision, irradiation, and chemotherapy; it is difficult to distinguish benign lymphoid tumors from malignant lymphoid lesions, even on the basis of histological appearance (Green, 2002). Laboratory analysis was done using microscopy, immunophenotyping, and gene rearrangement using the Southern blot technique, necessary for differentiation. DNA-rearrangement analysis allows a very precise determination of the benign and malignant lymphoid infiltrates of the ocular region. These tumors can also generally be distinguished by their signal intensity on T2-weighted images (Abe et. al., 2005).

Papilloma

Papilloma is a frequent benign epithelial growth or lesion (looks like a wart) that usually grows on or near the upper or lower eyelid margins of older adults (Green, 2002). Treatment is observation or cosmetic excision. It generally is the same color as the adjacent skin, and it is formed from small projections of fibrovascular connective tissue lined by hyperkeratotic epidermis (Shields & Shields, 1999a). Papillomatous configurations can be pedunculated (granular and whitish or pigmented), sessile (smooth surface and pinkish), and consist of solitary or multiple benign lesions (Shields & Shields, 1999a).

Seborrheic Keratosis

Seborrheic keratosis is a common benign basal cell papilloma or seborrheic wart cutaneous lesion that is usually a focal, periocular, light-brownish pigmented, discrete, slightly elevated, and placoid lesion (Shields & Shields, 1999a). In African Americans, it is characterized as dermatosis papulosa nigra. Other characteristics are acanthotic (basal cell proliferation) or adenoid (keratin cysts) types (Shields & Shields, 1999a). Treatment is observation or cosmetic excision. Inverted follicular keratosis seen in middle-aged males is a discrete, benign cutaneous nodule that is usually on an eyelid margin as papillomatous (wart like) or pigmented; usually surgical excision is warranted (Shields & Shields, 1999a). *Basosquamous cell acanthoma* may be a more accurate term, because it is not related to hair follicles (Shields & Shields, 1999a).

Xanthelasma

Xanthelasma is a bilateral benign deposit of yellowish-white, slighted elevated lipid plaques in the subcutaneous dermis of the upper and lower eyelids (Green, 2002). Normolipemia or an indication of secondary hyperlipidemia (e.g., such as in patients with diabetes) may be diagnostic of Erdheim-Chester disease (Shields & Shields, 1999a). Xanthelasma is referred to as xanthoma or tuberous xanthoma when the deposits become quite enlarged, which are more indicative of hypercholesterolemia (Shields & Shields, 1999a). These growths are removed only if unattractive and bothersome to patients. Blood cholesterol levels should be checked, because hyperlipidemia may be symptomatic of increasing lipid deposits.

Telangiectasis

Telangiectasis is a small focal red lesion associated with dilated conjunctival capillaries. Small dilated vessels are differentiated from systemic vascular hematoma in Louis-Bar syndrome or Rendu-Osler-Weber syndrome. Parafoveal telangiectasis shows central endothelial degeneration with lipid accumulation within the vessel walls, and advanced degeneration of the pericytes (AAO-4, 2008–2009). Pericytes are the protective basement membrane (mural cells) around ocular and kidney vessels that gives strength and vascular endurance to keep cells from degenerating (AAO-2, 2008–2009). This is why patients with diabetes have increasing vessel leakage (endothelial damage), because the pericyte membrane is absent, which protects the capillary lumen (AAO-12, 2008–2009).

Precancerous Eye Tumors

Precancerous eye lesions are premalignant tumors. The lesions not only can be stable benign tumors but also can continue to grow and develop into cancer or malignant tissue.

Actinic Keratosis

Actinic keratosis (senile or solar keratosis) is a familiar precancerous cutaneous lesion, is caused by repeated exposure to sunlight, and can develop into cutaneous squamous cell carcinoma (Shields & Shields, 1999a). Characteristics may include multiple erythematous, excoriated (scab-like), sessile plaques, or papillary dermis buds (Shields & Shields, 1999a). This commonly is seen in older Caucasians with prolonged sun exposure; for example farmers, fishermen, and carpenters. Treatment is observation, but excision is recommended if it is at all suspicious. Other treatment options are chemotherapy or cryotherapy, especially if keratosis has multiple characteristics.

Melanocytic Nevus

Melanocytic nevus, which can be congenital or acquired, is a benign cutaneous nevus of the eyelid or peripunctal conjunctiva. It can be pigmented or amelanotic, usually does not cause a loss of eyelashes if on the eyelid, and can be a precancerous state to malignant melanoma (Shields & Shields, 1999a). Treatment is

observation, but if it is suspicious, excision is suggested. This can be problematic if much of the eyelid is involved; and a possible radical removal with cosmetic surgery may be indicated, especially if metastasis is suspected (Shields & Shields, 1999a).

Malignant Eye Tumors

Malignant eye lesions are cancerous tumors. They are in or around the eyeball, are local and definite, or can be diffused and life threatening through metastasis.

Basal Cell Carcinoma

Basal cell carcinoma is most commonly eyelid cancer, usually in light-skinned adults in their fifth decade of life or older, most often located in the nasal canthus of the upper cheek (Vaughn, Dortzbach, & Gayre, 2004). Diagnosis is confirmed with a biopsy and surgical excision or radiation. The two most principal types are the noduloulcerative (firm, round nodule with fine dilated capillaries and ulcerated center) and the diffuse morpheaform (hard, pale, flat with undefined margins); but presentations can vary from cystic, pigmented, and other forms (Vaughn et al., 2004). Treatment may include wide excision with frozen section. Surgery may be multiple procedures for a large lesion, which also might include reconstruction and skin grafts. Radiation and cryotherapy may be used if surgical resection is not a good option.

Squamous Cell Carcinoma

Squamous cell carcinoma or Bowen's disease of the eyelid and the conjunctival and lacrimal sacs is clinically presented as an erythematous, crusted, keratotic (horny growth) local lesion (Vaughn et al., 2004). This is common in adults with a history of chronic sun exposure. Treatment of choice is complete surgical excision and eyelid reconstruction, if indicated. Small tissue biopsy may be warranted before extensive surgery for reconfiguration. Management also may include radiotherapy or cryotherapy for nonresectable cases. Metastasis is more common with squamous cell carcinoma compared to basal cell carcinoma.

Intraocular Lymphoid

Intraocular lymphoid is infiltration of malignant lymphocytes of the uveal tract, vitreous, optic nerve, or retina that can be unilateral or bilateral. The most common lymphoid is reticulum cell sarcoma or non-Hodgkin's B-cell lymphoma (Shields & Shields, 1999b). Treatment usually follows along with the systemic course (e.g., leukemia) of management combined with ocular irradiation.

Intraocular Choroidal Metastasis Tumor

Intraocular choroidal metastasis tumor is a secondary cancer arising from another systemic cancer, such as lung or breast carcinoma (Figure 71–21 ■, p. 2370). Typically, it can appear like "leopard skin" over the choroidal retina, which causes changes in the retinal pigment epithelium, secondary retinal detachment, or choroidal detachment (AAO-4, 2008–2009). Treatment of choice usually is chemotherapy or radiation external beam, or plaque. Secondary complications are treated as indicated, such as vitrectomy for a retinal detachment.

Merkel Cell Carcinoma

Merkel cell carcinoma is a primary cutaneous neuroendocrine tumor, which is aggressive and can involve the eyelid and eyebrow as a painless red nodule (Vaughn et al., 2004). Management

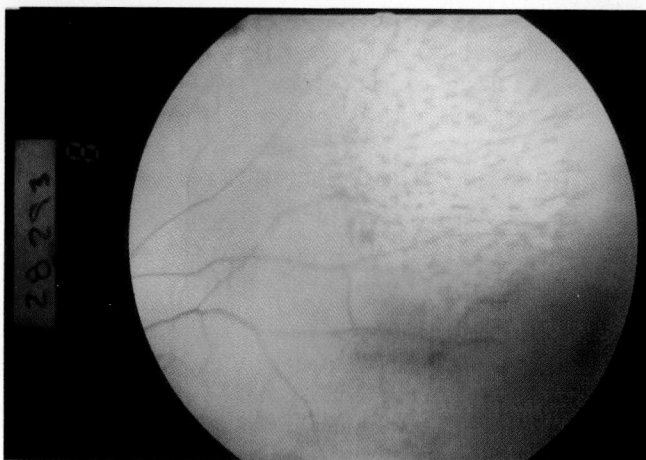

FIGURE 71–21 ■ Metastatic tumor of the choroid.
Source: Lucie S. Elfervig

requires a wide surgical excision, because this tumor can reoccur and metastasize.

Kaposi's Sarcoma

Kaposi's sarcoma is a malignant vascular tumor seen more commonly in young adults with AIDS (Vaughn et al., 2004). It is a smooth, bluish, subcutaneous eyelid tumor that is commonly associated with immunosuppression and in conjunction with many other cutaneous lesions. Medical management is chemotherapy and radiation.

Orbital Tumors

Orbital tumors are malignant metastatic lesions that have spread to the orbit from the bloodstream. One of the first signs may be proptosis or eye displacement. Other manifestations are pain, diplopia, or edema of the eyelid or conjunctiva. Orbital tumors are diagnostic of carcinomas in adults, in which lesions originate from epithelial structures of the breast, prostate, lung, or other anatomy (Dutton, 2004). Often when an orbital tumor is metastatic in females, they have a history of breast cancer or in males, prostate cancer. Lung cancer also can be the primary site of an orbital metastatic tumor. Findings that will influence treatment options are whether the tumor is benign or malignant, whether it has metastasized, the size and location of the tumor, and whether the tumor is vision threatening or life threatening. Treatment options may include observation, radiation, plaque, or excision, depending on the type of tumor.

Nursing Management and Health Promotion

The nurse should instruct patients about risk factors, detection, self-examination, regular follow-up care, and possible treatment options concerning ocular neoplasms. It can be very difficult to distinguish between benign and malignant neoplasms. It always is wise to refer to a health care provider for extensive evaluation if a discoloration, growth, or lesion is noticed on a patient, especially if it is changing in size or color, appears to be growing, has a discharge, or will not heal.

Gerontological Considerations

Many ocular and visual changes can occur with aging, and most are normal with passage of time. Descriptions of some of the ocular and visual changes that occur due to aging, and that can affect one's lifestyle significantly, are presented in the Gerontological Considerations box.

Cultural Considerations

Culture and geographic locations also can have a significant impact on the types of visual impairment people may manifest or experience. The Cultural Considerations box (p. 2372) outlines some visual disorders that are more common in specific cultures and certain geographic locations due to climate and environmental conditions.

Genetic Considerations

Genetics is the study of the gene matrix that makes each person unique and provides the molecules and cellular processes for anatomic description of visual development and outcome. Understanding some of the inherited mutations can assist in the treatment and prognosis of specific visual defects. Descriptions of some of the hereditary conditions that might be factors in visual impairment of adults are presented in the Genetic Considerations box (p. 2372).

Ethical Issues

The decision to donate a cornea is a difficult one, fraught with ethical considerations. It is based on the wish to donate an organ in order to benefit another in the restoration of vision. Some are eligible to make this decision; others are not. The ethical issues to be considered are discussed in the Ethical Issues box (p. 2374). The national guidelines that identify donor contraindications for corneal transplants are shown in the National Guidelines box (p. 2374).

Research

Research is another mechanism by which to explore and find answers for those that are visually impaired as new devices and clinical outcomes are developed. Vision researchers are striving to meet population needs as well as individual needs. Research topics related to vision research aimed at discovering cures and solutions to visual disorders are outlined in the Research Opportunities and Clinical Impact box (p. 2374).

Summary

This chapter has focused on the most common eye disorders, including eye emergencies. The majority of these disorders are treated in an outpatient setting. However, should the need arise or the setting change to inpatient due to geographical circumstances the principles and guidelines set in this chapter are applicable. The clinical preparation vignette is written to assist the learner in caring for a patient with an ocular disorder, but one who also suffers from diabetes, and comprises a very typical situation found by nurses in many settings.

GERONTOLOGICAL CONSIDERATIONS for the Aging Eye

Aging Eye Change	Explanation
Facial Features, Eyebrows, Eyelids, and Eyelashes	
Eyebrow and eyelash pigmentation loss	The eyebrows and eyelashes turn gray to white.
Senile enophthalmos	The recession or sinking of the eyeball into the orbit as a result of the loss of subcutaneous fat, decreased elastic tissue, and decreased muscle tone, but does not affect vision. No intervention necessary.
Ptosis senilis	A pseudoparalytic drooping of the upper eyelid; if it causes a problem by crossing the visual axis, it can be surgically corrected.
Blepharochalasis or dermatochalasis	An atrophy of elastic tissue of the eyelids resulting in the upper eyelid hanging over the eyelid margin or lashes. Redundant eyelid tissue creates wrinkles and folds. If it causes a problem with vision or cosmetically, it can be surgically corrected.
Senile entropion or blepharelosis	The inward turning (inversion) of the eyelid margin; if it causes a problem with irritation or foreign body sensation to the cornea, it can be surgically corrected.
Senile ectropion	The outward turning (eversion) of the eyelid margin; if it causes a problem with dry eye syndrome with the loss of tears and cannot be corrected with artificial tear use, it can be surgically corrected.
Conjunctiva	
Conjunctivochalasis	The loss of transparency and more laxity of the conjunctiva, wherein the bulbar conjunctiva wrinkles into the lower eyelid margin.
Sclera	
Sclera rigidity	The sclera becomes harder or rigid with loss of elasticity. This can also affect accurate intraocular pressure reading with indentation tonometry.
Senile scleral translucency	The sclera thins and becomes more transparent, exhibiting dark-grayish oval areas of the sclera, anterior to muscle insertion.
Scleral lipid deposition	The anterior sclera will appear yellowish due to lipid depositions in the deeper scleral tissue.
Pupil and Iris	
Pupil sclerosis	The pupil size decreases with age (senile miosis) because of pupil sphincter sclerosis, which narrows the visual field and affects peripheral vision to a mild degree. No intervention is usually necessary.
Cornea	
Keratoconjunctivitis sicca or dry eye syndrome	A deficiency of tear production, especially in postmenopausal women, can make the cornea feel gritty or have a foreign body sensation. This is usually relieved with frequent use of artificial tear drops or ointments.
Arcus senilis or gerontoxon	A grayish-white ring that develops at the peripheral edge of the cornea (limbus) from lipoid deposits into the corneal stroma, and does not affect vision; no intervention is required.
Guttata or corneal dystrophy	The thickening of Descemet's membrane (fourth layer of the cornea) with hyaline deposits from the loss of endothelial cells. These cells help maintain the health of the cornea and vision clarity.
Lens	
Cataract	The yellowing or opacity of the natural crystalline lens that is corrected surgically when a cataract is mature. In the meantime, corrective lenses can help; may also notice an alteration in color perception, especially for blues, violets, and greens.
Optic Nerve, Retinal, Vitreous	
Glaucoma	An elevated intraocular pressure due to aging, whereby trabecular meshwork is sluggish due to the loss of elasticity.
Age-related macular degeneration	The degeneration of the macula due to aging; the loss of retinal pigment epithelium and visual function.
Senile circumpapillary choroidal atrophy or peripapillary halo	The degeneration of arterioles in the choriocapillaris causing sclerosis, especially around the optic nerve; usually does not affect vision. No intervention is necessary.
Senile retinoschisis or schisis	A primary, acquired, gradual splitting of the retina into two distinct layers. SR develops from the coalescence of intraretinal microcysts located in an area of peripheral cystoid degeneration near the ora serrata and extends posteriorly and circumferentially. This process leads to the splitting of the retina at the outer plexiform layer or, less commonly, at the inner nuclear layer
Syneresis	Degeneration of the vitreous humor with loss of gel consistency, acts as a precursor to posterior vitreous detachment of gel, which is commonly called floaters. This occurs during the aging process and seldom calls for an intervention unless secondary complications result, such as retinal detachment.

(continued)

GERONTOLOGICAL CONSIDERATIONS for the Aging Eye—*Continued*

Aging Eye Change	Explanation
Vision	
Presbyopia	The loss of accommodation about the fourth decade of life is the loss of the ability to focus up close and necessitates the need for reading glasses or bifocals.
Astigmatism	The cornea can flatten more with age; this changes the corneal curvature and may result in new astigmatism or changes in astigmatism. This can be corrected with lenses.
Stereopsis loss	The loss of depth perception due to light scatter or glare that affects vision performance, causing difficulty with night vision, especially driving and judging heights properly. This can possibly be helped with brighter, nonglare lights and brighter colors, such as reds, oranges, and yellows.

CULTURAL CONSIDERATIONS for Visual Disorders

Culture	Ocular Condition
African Americans	Glaucoma
African Caribbeans	Sickle hemoglobinopathies
Africans, Central Americans, and South Americans	River blindness
Africans, Middle Easterners, Indians, and Southeast Asians	Trachoma
Caucasians	Age-related macular degeneration
Hispanic Americans and African Americans	Diabetic retinopathy
Japanese and Spaniards	Progressive myopia

Source: Yanoff, M., & Duker J. S. (Eds.). (2004). *Ophthalmology* (2nd ed.). St. Louis, MO: Mosby.

GENETIC CONSIDERATIONS in Adults with Visual Impairments

Consideration	Definition
Color blindness:	A hereditary condition that disables vision to distinguish colors.
• Protanomaly	Mild red-green discrimination, deficient red photoreceptors.
• Deuteranomaly	Red-green discrimination; most common form of color blindness (X linked).
• Tritanomaly	Mild blue-green discrimination.
• Protanopia	Severe red discrimination, appearing very dark; no red photoreceptors.
• Deuteranopia	More severe red-green discrimination.
• Tritanopia	Only two cone pigments and no blue photoreceptors.
Refractive errors	The inheritance of hyperopia, myopia, and/or astigmatic refractive errors.
Keratoconus	A hereditary central thinning of the cornea, making it a cone-shaped elevation of the central cornea that is usually progressive and more noticeable in those 20 years or older.
Corneal dystrophy (or Fuchs' dystrophy)	It can be hereditary deterioration of the cornea due to loss of endothelial cells from Descemet's membrane (fourth corneal layer) thickening, and possibly progressing to poor vision and cornea transplant.
Cataracts	A hereditary cataract usually matures faster, and cataract surgery can be necessary as early as in the second to fourth decade of life, instead of the usual sixth to eighth decade of life.
Glaucoma (Mendelian inheritance)	It can be hereditary, causing intraocular pressure elevation, optic nerve atrophy, and poor perfusion of the optic nerve.
Uveitis	It can be hereditary with inflammation of the uveal tract, which includes the iris, ciliary body, and choroid.
Leber's hereditary optic atrophy	A hereditary, rapidly developing bilateral optic nerve degeneration; vision loss usually stabilizes and occurs in males in their 20s and 30s.

GENETIC CONSIDERATIONS in Adults with Visual Impairments—*Continued*

Consideration	Definition
Disorder	
Marfan's syndrome	A hereditary condition whereby the bone structure is very long and thin, especially arms, legs, fingers, and toes. Weak ligaments, bone deformities, and heart disease are prevalent. Those with Marfan's syndrome often are myopic, with large corneas, early cataracts, dislocated lenses, ptosis, strabismus, and choroidal malformations.
Usher's syndrome	A hereditary combination of bilateral deafness and night blindness.
Alport's syndrome	A hereditary combination of kidney disease, deafness, and lens abnormality; such as small and round lenses, early cataracts, and anterior lenticonus (cone-shaped protrusion of the lens).
Joubert syndrome	A hereditary central nerve system defect with severe psychomotor deficiencies, breathing problems, and nystagmus.
Wagner's disease	A hereditary vitreoretinal degeneration syndrome that makes one more prone to retinal tears and detachments. Other ocular signs are myopia, lattice degeneration, strabismus, and cataracts in the teen years.
Stickler syndrome	A hereditary progressive connective tissue disease that causes enlarged and degenerative joints, arthritis, flattened midface, cleft palate, and deafness. Ocular signs are vitreoretinal degeneration, high myopia, and early cataracts.
Grönblad-Strandberg syndrome (pseudoxanthoma elasticum)	A hereditary elastic connective disorder that gives skin a leathery appearance, something like a plucked chicken's skin, with major artery defects. The retinal symptoms are angioid streaks, which are subretinal pigmented lines from cracks in Bruch's membrane that form macular hemorrhages and scars.
Age-related macular degeneration	A deterioration of the macula causing central vision loss and distortion. It is often hereditary, developing as early as in one's 50s.
Kandori's syndrome	A hereditary form of nonprogressive night blindness with numerous irregular and large gray-yellowish flecks in the retina.
Refsum's disease	A hereditary disease that is characterized by footdrop, inability to sleep, increased cerebrospinal fluid, accumulation of fatty acids, and electrocardiogram changes. Ocular signs are poor dark adaptation, constricted visual field, nystagmus, ptosis, and small pupil (miosis).
Retinitis pigmentosa (night blindness)	A hereditary bilateral rod/cone dysfunction with diminished or loss of side vision that can slowly progress to central vision loss and blindness.
Retinoblastoma	A hereditary malignant retinal tumor (most common in childhood); this may be the reason for an adult to have an eye removed or be blind in both eyes. If untreated, it can metastasize to the brain and cause death.
Nursing Assessment	Assess family history for glaucoma, cataracts, night blindness, color blindness, or other visual anomalies. Assess family history for other systemic disorders, such as deafness and cutaneous, metabolic, and connective tissue disorders. Assess physically for body asymmetry, deafness, and cutaneous, metabolic, and connective tissue disorders.
Management Issues	Question about DNA testing or other genetic testing that has been done in this family. Refer family for genetic counseling and evaluation to discuss inheritance, family risk factors, and gene-based intervention. Provide genetic information, materials, and resources. Provide assessment and understanding of genetic information and inherited conditions. Provide support and coping with new genetic findings. Be a patient advocate in management of care with genetic conditions and others that are predisposed to genetic problems. Being a counselor for the whole family may be indicated, so that the family members understand what genetic traits may be transmitted to the following generations.
Genetic Resources	Genetic Alliance[a] Gene Clinic[b] National Organization of Rare Diseases[c] Online Mendelian Inheritance in Man (OMIM)[d] "Genetic Testing for Inherited Eye Disease"[e] *Archives of Ophthalmology:* January and February 2007 issues devoted to ophthalmic genetics for in-depth details on inherited eye diseases and conditions

[a] http://www.geneticalliance.org

[b] http://www.geneclinics.org

[c] http://www.rarediseases.org

[d] http://www.ncbi.nlm.nih.gov/Literature/index.html or http://www.ncbi.nlm.nih.gov/genome/guide/human/

[e] Stone, E. M. (2007). Genetic testing for inherited eye disease. *Archives of Ophthalmology, 125*(2), 205–212.

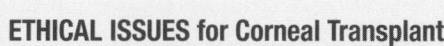

ETHICAL ISSUES for Corneal Transplants

Approximately 40,000 corneal transplants are done in the United States each year (Rabinowitz, 2005). The decision to donate corneal tissue for transplantation can have ethical considerations. It is important for the family that is being asked to donate a cornea for the benefit of someone else's vision, that the decision be a well-informed one, one that is freely chosen, and one that is compatible with the ethical beliefs of the individuals concerned. It is important for the family members to know that whatever decision they make, to donate or not to donate, they have freedom of choice. Under the circumstances of facing the loss of a loved one, any decision they make is the right decision for them. Usually the decision is one of three choices: Donate all organs, donate only the cornea, or do not donate at all. The two most common reasons not to donate are (1) the fear of something being done before the person is dead, and (2) the fear that the health care provider may hasten the death to benefit another.

Thoughts for Consideration

- Donation is an ethical decision to benefit another person.
- With treatment of the body after death, respect is the greatest issue, especially for psychological, religious, spiritual, moral, and cultural reasons.
- Donation is the last giving act the person donor does to reflect his life.
- The family knows that the loved one still lives on in another person. (NHMRC, 1997)

Sources: American Academy of Ophthalmology (AAO-8). (2008–2009). *Basic and clinical science course: External disease and cornea* (Section 8). San Francisco: Author; National Health and Medical Research Council (NHMRC). (1997). *Donating organs after death: Ethical issues.* Canberra, Australia: Australian Government Publishing Service; and Rabinowitz, Y. (2005, August 29). *Corneal transplants.* Retrieved April 26, 2007, from http://www.laser-prk.com/corneal.htm.

NATIONAL GUIDELINES for Criteria for Donor Contraindications of the Cornea

Acquired or congenital eye disorders that would prevent successful surgical outcome include:

- Active disseminated lymphoma or leukemia
- Active fungal or bacterial endocarditis
- Active intraocular or ocular inflammation
- Active septicemia
- Immunosuppressant diseases (HIV, syphilis, or hepatitis)
- Intrinsic malignancies
- Prior intraocular surgery of donor
- Prior refractive corneal surgery
- Unknown cause of death
- Unknown central nervous system (CNS) disease or CNS infection. (AAO-8, 2008–2009)

Sources: Eye Bank Association of America. (2001). *Frequently asked questions.* Retrieved October 4, 2008, from http://www.rsotresight.org/general/faqs.htm; Main, S. (2005). Regulation of eye banking and uses of ocular tissue for transplantation. *Clinical Laboratory Medicine, 24*(3), 607–624.

RESEARCH OPPORTUNITIES AND CLINICAL IMPACT RELATED TO VISUAL DISORDERS

Research Area	Clinical Impact
Vision Research	
Bradyopsia, light blindness, a new eye disease discovery caused by bright light exposure limiting function visual acuity with 20/20 acuity on Snellen vision chart due to phototransduction failure (Nishiguchi & Dryja, 2004).	Identification of patients that cannot see when moving from the indoors to the outside in bright sunlight or vice versa. They are blind for at least 5–10 seconds and are stopped in their tracks before vision starts to return, but vision is never comfortable. Contrast and swift-moving objects are difficult to track or see.
Diabetic Retinopathy Research	
Anti-VEGF therapy: Lack of oxygen to retinal tissue produces the release of vascular endothelial growth factor (VEGF), which causes blood vessels in the retina to leak, resulting in edema, tissue thickening, and growth of new vessels (Campochiaro, 2004).	Repair the progress of edema and scarring from diabetic retinopathy; to restore and preserve vision.
Oxygen therapy may improve decreased vision from diabetic retinopathy (Nguyen et al., 2004).	Supplement oxygen to prevent the growth of new vessels due to ischemic tissue for long-term vision restoration.
New anti-VEGF therapy: for the treatment of proliferative diabetic retinopathy (PDR) complicated with vitreous hemorrhage (Spaide & Fisher, 2006).	Treat the progress of PDR and vitreous hemorrhage in advanced diabetic retinopathy; to preserve vision.

RESEARCH OPPORTUNITIES AND CLINICAL IMPACT RELATED TO VISUAL DISORDERS—*Continued*

Research Area	Clinical Impact
Cornea Research	
Keratoprostheses, artificial cornea, and polymethymethacrylate (PMMA) device for implantation on the cornea (Alfonso, 2004).	Yield long-term vision restoration and lessen the rejection of donor tissue.
Melanoma Research	
Quality-of-life issues following choroidal melanoma treatment (Collaborative Ocular Melanoma Study—Quality of Life Study Group, 2006; Marr, 2006).	Anxiety of enucleation vs. brachytherapy in the treatment of eye melanoma; enucleation treatment anxiety was less in the long run.
Macular Degeneration Research	
Sunlight exposure and the incidence of macular degeneration that takes away central visual acuity with aging (Tomany, Cruickshanks, Klein, Klein, & Knudtson, 2004).	Prevent damage of the macula by wearing protective eyewear to block ultraviolet light, such as wearing sunglasses and hats to prevent long periods of sunlight exposure to central vision.
Age-related macular degeneration is a potential public health crisis: Antioxidant dietary supplements are a possible means to regress this threat to low vision (AREDS Research Group, 2003).	Supplement of antioxidants or vitamins to diet may slow down or improve macular tissue from breaking down, to restore some degree of healthy tissue function for increased vision.
Macular degeneration being the leading cause of legal blindness in older adults, especially the wet form. Patients may have hope with statin and aspirin therapy to lower the risk of going legally blind (Wilson, Schwartz, Bhatt, McCulloch, & Duncan, 2004).	Taking statin and aspirin could lessen the chances of going legally blind from wet macular degeneration.
Independence and the quality of life with vision loss from age-related macular degeneration and other health morbidity for older adults. The study to address all these areas of impact on one's life (Elfervig, 1997).	With increased vision loss, older adults have more difficulty carrying out activities of daily living, especially shopping, laundry, and handling finances. The more systemic illnesses a person has along with vision loss, the more difficulty with housekeeping, handling finances, and just doing daily chores. Married persons with vision loss and other health problems had greater satisfaction with life than did single persons with the same problems. Patients with macular degeneration can keep active and maintain a good degree of independence, with varying degrees of vision deficiency, if they have proper equipment and home setup, with new learned skills.
Evidence impact of vision-related quality of life (QOL) in patients with age-related macular degeneration (Berdeaux, Nordmann, Colin, & Arnould, 2005; Ferris, 2005).	Preserving minimal visual acuity in the worse eye may contribute to vision-related QOL for the better.

Sources: Age-Related Eye Disease Study (AREDS) Research Group. (2003). Potential public health impact of age-related eye disease study results. *Archives of Ophthalmology, 121*(11), 1621–1624; Alfonso, E. C. (2004). Keratoprostheses: Artificial corneas yield long-term vision. *Ophthalmology Times, 29*(12), 1, 60; Berdeaux, G. H., Nordmann, J. P., Colin, E., & Arnould, B. (2005). Vision-related quality of life in patients suffering from age-related macular degeneration. *American Journal of Ophthalmology, 139*(2), 271–279; Campochiaro, P. A. (2004). Reduction of diabetic macular edema by oral administration of kinase inhibitor. *Investigative Ophthalmology & Visual Science, 45*(3), 922–931; Collaborative Ocular Melanoma Study—Quality of Life Study Group (COMS QOLSG). (2006). Quality of life after iodine 125 brachytherapy vs. enucleation for choroidal melanoma. *Archives of Ophthalmology, 124*(2), 226–238; Elfervig, L. S. (1997). *Functional independence and life satisfaction with vision loss from age-related macular degeneration: A study of older adults.* Doctoral dissertation, Louisiana State University Medical Center, UMI No. 9717113; Ferris, F. L. (2005). Vision-related quality of life in patients suffering from age-related macular degeneration. *Evidence-Based Ophthalmology, 6*(3), 163–164; Marr, B. (2006). Quality of life after iodine 125 brachytherapy versus enucleation for choroidal melanoma five-year results from the collaborative ocular melanoma study: COMS QOLS Reports No. 3. *Evidence-Based Ophthalmology, 7*(3), 154–156; Nguyen, Q., et al. (2004). Supplemental oxygen improves diabetic macular edema: A pilot study. *Investigative Ophthalmology & Visual Science, 45*(2), 617–624; Nishiguchi, K. M., & Dryja, L. (2004, March). New eye disease: Light blindness. *EyeNet,* 13–14; Spaide, R. F., & Fisher, Y. L. (2006). Intravitreal bevacizumab (avastin) treatment of proliferative diabetic retinopathy complicated by vitreous hemorrhage. *Retina, 26*(3), 275–278; Tomany, S. C., Cruickshanks, K. J., Klein, R., Klein, B. E., & Knudtson, M. D. (2004). Sunlight and the 10-year incidence of age-related maculopathy. *Archives of Ophthalmology, 122*(5), 750–757; and Wilson, H. L., Schwartz, D. M., Bhatt, H. R., McCulloch, C. E., & Duncan, J. L. (2004). Statin and aspirin therapy are associated with decreased rates of choroidal neovascularization among patients with age-related macular degeneration. *American Journal of Ophthalmology, 137*(4), 615–624.

Clinical Preparation

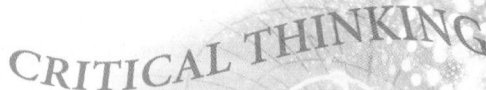 CRITICAL THINKING

PEARSON **mynursingkit**™

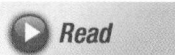 **Read**

- History of Current Illness
- Past Medical History
- Physical Exam
- Admitting Medical Orders
- Laboratory Study Results

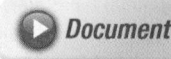 **Document**

- Summary of Hospitalization
- Pathophysiology Form
- Laboratory Values
- Laboratory Results Explanation

 **Apply**

- List of Potential Nursing Diagnoses
- Concept Map
- Critical Thinking Questions

Log on to MyNursingKit.com to download forms you will need and to complete further steps in the Clinical Preparation assignment.

HISTORY OF PRESENT ILLNESS

As the on-coming nurse to a clinic facility, you are presented with the following patient in the examination room as your first patient of the morning. Mrs. M is a 55-year-old executive at a local bank, who presented at the clinic with sudden vision loss in her left eye, seeing darkness with some floaters when she awakened this morning. She arrived at the clinic with her husband, who did the driving, along with her grown daughter.

Medical–Surgical History

Mrs. M's past medical history includes hypertension, hyperlipidemia, and non–insulin-dependent diabetic mellitus for the past 10 years. She is currently taking aspirin, Avapro, Zocor, and Glucotrol; is on a low-salt diabetic diet; and does not smoke. Her only surgery was an appendectomy as a child. She has a family history of diabetes and hypertension, no known vision problems, no known allergies, and she is not on any eyedrops. When asked when she had her last professional eye examination, Mrs. M states she has never had one. Mrs. M states her vision was good until this morning.

Physical Examination

In your findings Mrs. M is 5'2" tall, weighing 175 pounds. She states she did not hit her head or her eye; she just awakened this morning with blurry vision in the left eye. When you shine a penlight in her right eye, you get a bright, clear reflex, and in her left eye you get a dull, flat reflex. Her pupils are equal at 3.5 millimeters, are round, and react to light and accommodation. Her facial features, ocular adnexa, and eyes appear symmetrical: There are no discolorations, no discharges, no pain, no growths, no size difference, and no misalignments; the only asymmetry is that the left eyelid droops slightly. The visual acuity is 20/30 right eye and 20/200 left eye with glasses for both near and far vision. Her blood glucose is checked and found to be 300 mg/dL, and urinalysis showed a trace of protein. Her vital signs are temperature 98°F, pulse 75 beats per minute, respiratory rate 17/minute, and blood pressure 160/100. Mrs. M is referred to a local vitreoretinal ophthalmologist for further evaluation, examination, and treatment.

CRITICAL THINKING QUESTIONS

1. What might be the cause of a sudden vision loss in a patient with diabetes?

2. Besides blood sugar and vital signs checks, what else might you test Mrs. M for; what test might be most diagnostic?

3. What possible treatments may clear Mrs. M's vision?

4. What changes might her health care provider make in Mrs. M's treatment for diabetes?

5. What measures will Mrs. M have to take at home to improve her vision?

Answers to Critical Thinking Questions appear in Appendix D.

NCLEX® REVIEW

1. A patient tells the nurse that she thinks there's something wrong with her vision because she sometimes sees black things "moving" in her vision. The nurse realizes this patient is describing:
   1. Glaucoma.
   2. Cataracts.
   3. Floaters.
   4. Detached retina.

2. While conducting a cover-uncover test for tropia, the nurse notes that a patient's uncovered eye moves toward the nose. This finding would indicate:
   1. The uncovered eye is fixated inward.
   2. The uncovered eye is fixated outward.
   3. The uncovered eye has steady fixation.
   4. Vertical tropia.

3. A patient with a history of head trauma is in need of treatment for adult strabismus. Which of the following would be considered as appropriate for this patient?
   1. Contact lenses
   2. Occlusion of the normal vision eye
   3. Bifocal lenses
   4. Eye muscle surgery

4. The nurse is planning care for a patient with glaucoma. Which of the following should be included in this plan of care?
   1. Diet
   2. The correct use of eyedrops
   3. Control of heart disease
   4. Use of corrective lenses

5. A patient has been diagnosed as being brain dead and the family is not sure if the patient's corneas should be donated. Which of the following can the nurse provide to this patient's family?
   1. Explain that since there is an organ shortage, the family really should donate the patient's corneas.
   2. Explain that whatever decision they make, they have freedom of choice.
   3. Explain to the family that time is of the essence and they need to decide before the patient dies.
   4. They can always visit the person who received the donated corneas.

Answers for review questions appear in Appendix D

KEY TERMS

aberration *p.2331*
accommodation *p.2328*
acute angle-closure glaucoma
  (AACG) *p.2345*
amblyopia *p.2334*
ametropia *p.2332*
astigmatism *p.2332*
cataracts *p.2350*
central retinal artery occlusion
  (CRAO) *p.2362*
contrast sensitivity (CS) *p.2335*
cotton-wool spots (CWS) *p.2342*
diabetic retinopathy (DR) *p.2338*

diplopia *p.2334*
drusen *p.2335*
emmetropia *p.2331*
esophoria *p.2334*
flame-shaped hemorrhages *p.2342*
flashes *p.2363*
floaters *p.2328*
foreign body sensation (FBS) *p.2354*
glaucoma *p.2343*
hyperopia *p.2332*
hyphema *p.2362*
hypopyon *p.2355*

legal blindness *p.2335*
macular degeneration (MD) *p.2335*
metamorphopsia *p.2335*
myopia *p.2332*
nystagmus *p.2335*
open globe *p.2362*
phoria *p.2334*
presbyopia *p.2332*
retinal detachment *p.2366*
retinopathy *p.2338*
strabismus *p.2334*
tropia *p.2334*

PEARSON
EXPLORE mynursingkit™

MyNursingKit is your one stop for online chapter review materials and resources. Prepare for success with additional NCLEX®-style practice questions, interactive assignments and activities, web links, animations and videos, and more!

Register your access code from the front of your book at
www.mynursingkit.com

REFERENCES

Abad, J. C., & Azar, D. T. (2004). Current concepts, classification, and history of refractive surgery. In M. Yanoff & J. S. Duker (Eds.), *Ophthalmology* (2nd ed.). St. Louis: Mosby.

Abe, S., Tamakawa, M., Andoh, M., Kohda, K., Teranishi, C., & Ohta, I. (2005). Lymphoid tumor in the orbit: malignant or benign? MRI, histomorphological and molecular genetic analysis of eight cases. *European Journal of Plastic Surgery, 27*(8), 378–382.

Age-Related Eye Disease Study (AREDS) Research Group. (2003). Potential public health impact of Age-Related Eye Disease Study results. AREDS Report No. 11. *Archives of Ophthalmology, 121*(11), 1621–1624.

Age-Related Eye Disease Study (AREDS) Research Group. (2006). Cognitive impairment in the Age-Related Eye Disease Study. AREDS Report No. 16. *Archives of Ophthalmology, 124*(4), 537–543.

Alfonso, E. C. (2004). Keratoprostheses: Artificial corneas yield long-term vision. *Ophthalmology Times, 29*(12), 1, 60.

American Academy of Ophthalmology (AAO-2). (2008–2009). *Basic and clinical science course: Fundamentals and principles of ophthalmology* (Section 2). San Francisco: Author.

American Academy of Ophthalmology (AAO-3). (2008–2009). *Basic and clinical science course: Optics, refraction, and contact lenses* (Section 3). San Francisco: Author.

American Academy of Ophthalmology (AAO-4). (2008–2009). *Basic and clinical science course: Ophthalmic pathology and intraocular tumors* (Section 4). San Francisco: Author.

American Academy of Ophthalmology (AAO-5). (2008–2009). *Basic and clinical science course: Neuro-ophthalmology* (Section 5). San Francisco: Author.

American Academy of Ophthalmology (AAO-6). (2008–2009). *Basic and clinical science course: Pediatric ophthalmology and strabismus* (Section 6). San Francisco: Author.

American Academy of Ophthalmology (AAO-7). (2008–2009). *Basic and clinical science course: Orbit, eyelids, and lacrimal system* (Section 7). San Francisco: Author.

American Academy of Ophthalmology (AAO-8). (2008–2009). *Basic and clinical science course: External disease and cornea* (Section 8). San Francisco: Author.

American Academy of Ophthalmology (AAO-9). (2008–2009). *Basic and clinical science course: Intraocular inflammation and uveitis* (Section 9). San Francisco: Author.

American Academy of Ophthalmology (AAO-10). (2008–2009). *Basic and clinical science course: Glaucoma* (Section 10). San Francisco: Author.

American Academy of Ophthalmology (AAO-11). (2008–2009). *Basic and clinical science course: Lens and cataract* (Section 11). San Francisco: Author.

American Academy of Ophthalmology (AAO-12). (2008–2009). *Basic and clinical science course: Retina and vitreous* (Section 12). San Francisco: Author.

Arnold, A. C. (2004). Ischemic optic neuropathy, diabetic papillopathy, and papillophlebitis. In M. Yanoff & J. S. Duker (Eds.), *Ophthalmology* (2nd ed.). St. Louis: Mosby.

Beers, M. H., & Berkow, R. (1999). *The Merck manual of diagnosis and therapy* (17th ed.). Whitehouse Station, NJ: Merck Research Laboratories.

Berdeaux, G. H., Nordmann, J. P., Colin, E., & Arnould, B. (2005). Vision-related quality of life in patients suffering from age-related macular degeneration. *American Journal of Ophthalmology, 139*(2), 271–279.

Bhavsar, A. R., & Drouilhet, J. H. (2006). Retinopathy, diabetic, background. *Emedicine.* Retrieved June 16, 2008, from http://www.emedicine.com/oph/topic414.htm

Campbell, D. G., & Netland, P. A. (1998). *Stereo atlas of glaucoma.* St. Louis: Mosby–Year Book.

Campochiaro, P. A. (1999). Acute posterior bacterial endophthalmitis. *Ophthalmology Clinics of North America, 12,* 83–88.

Campochiaro, P. A. (2004). Reduction of diabetic macular edema by oral administration of kinase inhibitor. *Investigative Ophthalmology & Visual Science, 45*(3), 922–931.

Charles, S. (2001). Principles and techniques of vitreous surgery. In S. J. Ryan (Ed.), *Retina* (3rd ed., Vol. 3). St. Louis: Mosby.

Choplin, N. T., & Lundy, D. C. (1998). *Atlas of glaucoma.* London: Martin Dunitz Ltd.

Clarkson, J. G. (2001). Central retinal vein occlusion. In S. J. Ryan (Ed.), *Retina* (3rd ed., Vol. 2). St. Louis: Mosby.

Collaborative Ocular Melanoma Study—Quality of Life Study Group (COMS QOLSG). (2006). Quality of life after iodine 125 brachytherapy vs. enucleation for choroidal melanoma. *Archives of Ophthalmology, 124*(2), 226–238.

Dabezies, O., Klyce, S., Morgan, J., Hartstein, J., Donshik, P., Boswall, G., et al. (1998). Corneal changes from contact lenses. In H. Kaufman, B. Barron, & M. McDonald (Eds.), *The cornea* (2nd ed.). Boston: Butterworth-Heinemann.

Daly, S. W. (2002). Scleral disorders. In K. Goldblum & P. Lamb (Eds.), *Core curriculum for ophthalmic nursing* (2nd ed.). Dubuque, IA: Kendall/Hunt.

D'Amato, R. J. (1999). Pharmacologic therapy: Angiogenesis inhibition. In J. W. Berger, S. L. Fine, & M. G. Maguire (Eds.), *Age-related macular degeneration.* St. Louis: Mosby.

Dhalla, M. S., Shah, G. K., Blinder, K. J., Ryan, E. H., Mittra, R. A., & Tewari, A. (2006). Combined photodynamic therapy with verteporfin and intravitreal bevacizumab for choroidal neovascularization in age-related macular degeneration. *Retina, 26*(9), 988–993.

Dutton, J. J. (2004). Orbital diseases. In M. Yanoff & J. S. Duker (Eds.), *Ophthalmology* (2nd ed.). St. Louis: Mosby.

Elfervig, L. S. (1997). *Functional independence and life satisfaction with vision loss from age-related macular degeneration: A study of older adults.* Doctoral dissertation, Louisiana State University Medical Center, UMI No. 9717113.

Elfervig, L. S. (1998). Age-related macular degeneration. *Nurse Practitioner Forum, 9*(1), 4–6.

Elfervig, L. S. (2000). Photodynamic therapy (PDT). *TNA District 1 Dispatcher, 2*(1), 5.

Elfervig, L. S. (2002a). Uveal disorders (glaucoma). In K. Goldblum & P. Lamb (Eds.), *Core curriculum for ophthalmic nursing* (2nd ed.). Dubuque, IA: Kendall/Hunt.

Elfervig, L. S. (2002b). Pharmacology. In K. Goldblum & P. Lamb (Eds.), *Core curriculum for ophthalmic nursing* (2nd ed.). Dubuque, IA: Kendall/Hunt.

Elfervig, L. S., & Elfervig, J. L. (1998). Retinal detachment. *Insight, 23*(2), 66–70.

Elfervig, L. S., & Elfervig, J. L. (1999). Endophthalmitis. *Insight, 24*(3), 99–103.

Elfervig, L. S., & Elfervig, J. L. (2001). Proliferative diabetic retinopathy. *Insight, 26*(3), 88–93.

Elfervig, L. S., & Elfervig J. L. (2007). Recognition and triage of ocular emergencies. *Refinements: Clinical Education Modules for Today's Ophthalmic Team, 2*(1), 1–14. Manuscript updated and submitted for republication.

Eliott, D., Lee, M. S., & Abrams, G. W. (2001). Proliferative diabetic retinopathy: Principles and techniques of surgical treatment. In S. J. Ryan (Ed.), *Retina* (3rd ed., Vol. 2). St. Louis: Mosby.

Eye Bank Association. (2001). *Frequently asked questions.* Retrieved October 4, 2008, from http://www.restoresight.org/general/faqs.htm

Eye Tech Study Group (ETSG). (2003). Anti-vascular endothelial growth factor therapy for subfoveal choroidal neovascularization secondary to age-related macular degeneration. *American Journal of Ophthalmology, 110*(5), 979–986.

Falk, N. S., Beer, P. M., & Peters, G. B. (2006). Role of intravitreal triamcinolone acetonide in the treatment of postoperative endophthalmitis. *Retina, 26*(5), 545–548.

Fanous, M. M. (2004). Neovascular glaucoma. In M. Yanoff & J. S. Duker (Eds.), *Ophthalmology* (2nd ed.). St. Louis: Mosby.

Fekrat, S., & Finkelstein, D. (2001). Branch retinal vein occlusion. In S. J. Ryan (Ed.), *Retina* (3rd ed., Vol. 2). St. Louis: Mosby.

Ferrara, N., Damico, L., Shams, N., Lowman, H., & Kim, R. (2006). Development of ranibizumab, an anti-vascular endothelial growth factor antigen binding fragment, as therapy for neovascular age-related macular degeneration. *Retina, 26*(8), 859–870.

Ferris, F. L. (2005). Vision-related quality of life in patients suffering from age-related macular degeneration. *Evidence-Based Ophthalmology, 6*(3), 163–164.

Fong, D. S., Aiello, L., Gardner, T. W., et al. (2003). Diabetic retinopathy. *Diabetes Care, 26,* 226–229.

Foster, C. S., & Vitale, A. T. (Eds.). (2002). *Diagnosis and treatment of uveitis.* Philadelphia: W. B. Saunders.

Gold, D. H., & Weingeist, T. A. (2001). *Color atlas of the eye in systemic disease.* Philadelphia: Lippincott Williams & Wilkins.

Goldstein, D. A., & Tessler, H. H. (2004). Episcleritis, scleritis, and other scleral disorders. In M. Yanoff & J. S. Duker (Eds.), *Ophthalmology* (2nd ed.). St. Louis: Mosby.

Green, D. (2002). Neoplastic disorders. In K. Goldblum & P. Lamb (Eds.), *Core curriculum for ophthalmic nursing* (2nd ed.). Dubuque, IA: Kendall/Hunt.

Green, J. P., Charonis, G. C., & Goldberg, R. A. (2004). Eyelid trauma and reconstruction techniques. In M. Yanoff & J. S. Duker (Eds.), *Ophthalmology* (2nd ed.). St. Louis: Mosby.

Guttman, C. (2004). Experience underlines efficacy of full-time occlusion for amblyopia. *Ophthalmology Times, 29*(4), 1, 20.

Hamza, H. S., Loewenstein, A., & Haller, J. A. (1999). Fungal retinitis and endophthalmitis. *Ophthalmology Clinics of North America, 12,* 89–108.

Harper, S. L., Chorich, L. J., & Foster, C. S. (2002). Diagnosis of uveitis. In C. S. Foster & A. T. Vitale (Eds.), *Diagnosis and treatment of uveitis.* Philadelphia: W. B. Saunders.

Hikichi, T., & Yoshida, A. (2004). Time course of development of posterior vitreous detachment in the fellow eye after development in the first eye. *American Journal of Ophthalmology, 111*(9), 1705–1707.

Hitchings, R. (2004). Normal-tension glaucoma. In M. Yanoff & J. S. Duker (Eds.), *Ophthalmology* (2nd ed.). St. Louis: Mosby.

Jabs, D. A. (2001). Rheumatic diseases. In S. J. Ryan (Ed.), *Retina* (3rd ed., Vol. 2). St. Louis: Mosby.

Kanski, J. J. (2001). *Systemic diseases and the eye: Signs and differential diagnosis.* London: Mosby International Limited.

Lamb, P. A. (2002). Conjunctival disorders. In K. Goldblum & P. Lamb (Eds.), *Core curriculum for ophthalmic nursing* (2nd ed.). Dubuque, IA: Kendall/Hunt.

Lee, A. G., & Brazis, P. W. (2003). *Clinical pathways in neuro-ophthalmology: An evidence-based approach* (2nd ed.). New York: Thieme.

Maguire, M. G. (1999). Natural history. In J. W. Berger, S. L. Fine, & M. G. Maguire (Eds.), *Age-related macular degeneration.* St. Louis: Mosby.

Marr, B. (2006). Quality of life after iodine 125 brachytherapy versus enucleation for choroidal melanoma five-year results from the collaborative ocular melanoma study: COMS QOLS Reports No. 3. *Evidence-Based Ophthalmology, 7*(3), 154–156.

Martidis, A., & Tennant, M. T. (2004). Age-related macular degeneration. In M. Yanoff & J. S. Duker (Eds.), *Ophthalmology* (2nd ed.). St. Louis: Mosby.

May, D. R., Kuhn, F. P., Morris, R. E., Witherspoon, C. D., Danis, R. P., Matthews, G. P., et al. (2000). The epidemiology of serious eye injuries from the United States Eye Injury Registry. *Graefe's Archive for Clinical and Experimental Ophthalmology, 238*(2). Retrieved September 24, 2008, from http://www.springerlink.com/content/u0pxmaf7p4hd5vh6/

Mayo Clinic. (2006). Trachoma overview. *Revolution Health.* Retrieved October 5, 2008, from http://www.revolutionhealth.com/condidions/ eye/trachoma/understand-overview?section=s,,,

McLeod, S. D. (2004). Infectious keratitis. In M. Yanoff & J. S. Duker (Eds.), *Ophthalmology* (2nd ed.). St. Louis: Mosby.

Miller, D., & Scott, C. A. (2004). Epidemiology of refractive errors. In M. Yanoff & J. S. Duker (Eds.), *Ophthalmology* (2nd ed.). St. Louis: Mosby.

Montan, P., Koranyi, G., Setterquist, H., Stridh, A., Philipson, B., & Wiklund, K. (1998). Endophthalmitis after cataract surgery: Risk factors relating to technique and events of operation and patient history. *Ophthalmology, 105,* 2171–2175.

Mulrooney, B. C. (2006). Cataract, traumatic. *Emedicine.* Retreived October 2, 2008 from http://www.emedicine.com/oph/TOPIC52.HTM

National Eye Institute. (2006). *Age-related macular degeneration.* Retrieved June 3, 2008, from http://www.nei.nih.gov/health/maculardegen/armd_facts.asp

National Health and Medical Research Council (NHMRC). (1997). *Donating organs after death: Ethical issues.* Canberra, Australia: Australian Government Publishing Service.

Netland, P. A., & Allen, R. C. (Eds.). (1999). *Glaucoma medical therapy: Principles and management.* San Francisco: The Foundation of the American Academy of Ophthalmology.

Nguyen, Q. et al. (2004). Supplemental oxygen improves diabetic macular edema: A pilot study. *Investigative Ophthalmology & Visual Science, 45*(2), 617–624.

Nishiguchi, K. M., & Dryja, L. (2004, March). New eye disease: Light blindness. *EyeNet,* 13–14.

Nussenblatt, R. B., & Whitcup, S. M. (2004). *Uveitis: Fundamentals and clinical practice* (3rd ed.). Philadelphia: Mosby.

Oetting, T. A. (2001). A paradigm shift in cataract surgery: Less for the surgeon to do—More for the nurses and technicians to do. *Insight, 26*(1), 23–30.

Parrish, C. M., & Chandler, J. W. (1998). Corneal trauma. In H. Kaufman, B. Barron, & M. McDonald (Eds.), *The cornea* (2nd ed.). Boston: Butterworth-Heinemann.

PDR. (2004a). *Glaucoma: Disease management guide* (1st ed.). San Francisco: Allergan.

PDR. (2004b). *Physicians' desk reference for ophthalmic medicines* (32nd ed.). Montvale, NJ: Thomson.

Porth, C. M. (2007). *Essentials of pathophysiology: Concepts of altered health states.* Philadelphia: Lippincott Williams & Wilkins.

Pratt-Johnson, J. A., & Tillson, G. (2001). *Management of strabismus and amblyopia: A practice guide* (2nd ed.). New York: Thieme.

Rabinowitz, Y. (2005, August 29). *Corneal transplants.* Retrieved April 26, 2007, from http://www.laser-prk.com/corneal.htm

Robson, J., Behrman, A. J., & Abbuhl, S. (2007). Globe rupture. *Emedicine.* Retrieved June 18, 2008, from http://www.emedicine.com/emerg/TOPIC218.HTM

Rosenblatt, B. J., & Benson, W. E. (2004). Diabetic retinopathy. In M. Yanoff & J. S. Duker (Eds.), *Ophthalmology* (2nd ed.). St. Louis: Mosby.

Rosenfeld, P. J., & Gorin, M. B. (1999). Genetics. In J. W. Berger, S. L. Fine, & M. G. Maguire (Eds.), *Age-related macular degeneration*. St. Louis: Mosby.

Rougé, L. J. (2004, April). Breaking the blepharitis cycle. *EyeNet*, 25–26.

Rubenstein, J. B., & Jick, S. L. (2004). Disorders of the conjunctiva and limbus. In M. Yanoff & J. S. Duker (Eds.), *Ophthalmology* (2nd ed.). St. Louis: Mosby.

Ruiz-Moreno, J. M., Montero, J. A., Barile, S., & Zarbin, M. A. (2006). Photodynamic therapy and high-dose intravitreal triamcinolone to treat exudative age-related macular degeneration: 1-year outcome. *Retina, 26*(6), 602–612.

Schachat, A. P. (2001). Medical retina. In S. J. Ryan (Ed.), *Retina* (3rd ed., Vol. 2). St. Louis: Mosby.

Seal, D. V., Bron, A. J., & Hay, J. (1998). *Ocular infection: Investigation and treatment in practice*. St. Louis: Mosby.

Sharma, S., & Brown, G. C. (2001a). Ocular ischemic syndrome. In S. J. Ryan (Ed.), *Retina* (3rd ed., Vol. 2). St. Louis: Mosby.

Sharma, S., & Brown, G. C. (2001b). Retinal artery obstruction. In S. J. Ryan (Ed.), *Retina* (3rd ed., Vol. 2). St. Louis: Mosby.

Shields, J. A., & Shields, C. L. (1999a). *Atlas of eyelid and conjunctival tumors*. Philadelphia: Lippincott Williams & Wilkins.

Shields, J. A., & Shields, C. L. (1999b). *Atlas of intraocular tumors*. Philadelphia: Lippincott Williams & Wilkins.

Shields, J. A., & Shields, C. L. (1999c). *Atlas of orbital tumors*. Philadelphia: Lippincott Williams & Wilkins.

Sinclair, S. A., Smith, G. A., & Xiang, H. (2006). Eyeglasses-related injuries treated in U.S. emergency departments in 2002–2003. *Ophthalmic Epidemiology, 13*(1), 23–30.

Singerman, L. J., Brucker, A. J., Jampol, L. M., Lim, J. I., Rosenfeld, P., Schachat, A. P., et al. (2005). Neovascular age-related macular degeneration: Roundtable. *Retina, 25*(Suppl. 7), S1–S22.

Sjaarda, R. N., & Thompson, J. T. (2001). Macular hole. In S. J. Ryan (Ed.), *Retina* (3rd ed., Vol. 3). St. Louis: Mosby.

Spaide, R. F., & Fisher, Y. L. (2006). Intravitreal bevacizumab (avastin) treatment of proliferative diabetic retinopathy complicated by vitreous hemorrhage. *Retina, 26*(3), 275–278.

Steidl, S. M., & Hartnett, M. E. (2003). *Clinical pathways in vitreoretinal disease*. New York: Thieme.

Stewart, W. C. (2004). New (pending) glaucoma medical therapy. In M. Yanoff & J. S. Duker (Eds.), *Ophthalmology* (2nd ed.). St. Louis: Mosby.

Stone, E. M. (2007). Genetic testing for inherited eye disease. *Archives of Ophthalmology, 125*(2), 205–212.

Streeten, B. W. (2000). Pathology of the lens. In D. M. Albert & F. A. Jakobiec (Eds.), *Principles & practice of ophthalmology* (2nd ed., Vol. 4). Philadelphia: W. B. Saunders.

Thall, E. H., Thammano, P., & Miller, R. (2004). Perspectives in aberrations of the eye. In M. Yanoff & J. S. Duker (Eds.), *Ophthalmology* (2nd ed.). St. Louis: Mosby.

Tomany, S. C., Cruickshanks, K. J., Klein, R., Klein, B. E., & Knudtson, M. D. (2004). Sunlight and the 10-year incidence of age-related maculopathy. *Archives of Ophthalmology, 122*(5), 750–757.

Traverso, C. E., Bagnis, A., & Bricola, G. (2004). Angle-closure glaucoma. In M. Yanoff & J. S. Duker (Eds.), *Ophthalmology* (2nd ed.). St. Louis: Mosby.

Trobe, J. D. (2006). *The physician's guide to eye care* (3rd ed.). San Francisco: American Academy of Ophthalmology.

U.S. Census Bureau. (2000). Demographic profiles. Retrieved February 2, 2007, from http://www.census.gov/main/www/cen2000.html

U.S. Department of Health and Human Services (DHHS). (2000a). *Healthy People 2010: Vision and hearing*. Retrieved April 26, 2007, from http://www.healthypeople.gov/document/HTML/Volume2/28Vision.htm

U.S. Department of Health and Human Services (DHHS). (2000b). *Healthy Vision 2010*. Retrieved April 26, 2007, from http://www.healthyvision.2010.org

Vaughn, G. J., Dortzbach, R. K., & Gayre, G. S. (2004). Eyelid malignancies. In M. Yanoff & J. S. Duker (Eds.), *Ophthalmology* (2nd ed.). St. Louis: Mosby.

Visto, D. A. (2000). Corneal abrasion: To patch or not to patch. *Insight, 25*(1), 4–6.

Walker, R. S., & Piltz-Seymour, J. R. (2004). When to treat glaucoma. In M. Yanoff & J. S. Duker (Eds.), *Ophthalmology* (2nd ed.). St. Louis: Mosby.

Watson, P. G., Hazleman, B. L., Pavesio, C. E., & Green, W. R. (2004). *The sclera & systemic disorders* (2nd ed.). Philadelphia: Butterworth-Heinemann.

Williams, G. A., & Aaberg, T. (2001). Techniques of scleral buckling. In S. J. Ryan (Ed.), *Retina* (3rd ed., Vol. 3). St. Louis: Mosby.

Wilson, H. L., Schwartz, D. M., Bhatt, H. R., McCulloch, C. E., & Duncan, J. L. (2004). Statin and aspirin therapy are associated with decreased rates of choroidal neovascularization among patients with age-related macular degeneration. *American Journal of Ophthalmology, 137*(4), 615–624.

Wong, T., Klein, R., Nieto, F., Moraes, S., Mosley, T., Couper, D., et al. (2002). Is early age-related maculopathy related to cognitive function? The atherosclerosis risk in communities study. *American Journal of Ophthalmology, 134*(12), 828–835.

Wu, W., & Ariyasu, R. G. (1999). Cornea and external disease. In D. A. Lee & E. J. Higginbotham (Eds.), *Clinical guide to comprehensive ophthalmology*. New York: Thieme.

Yanoff, M., & Duker, J. S. (Eds.). (2004). *Ophthalmology* (2nd ed.). St. Louis: Mosby.

Zimmerman, R., Sakiyalak, D., Krupin, T., & Rosenberg, L. F. (2004). Primary open-angle glaucoma. In M. Yanoff & J. S. Duker (Eds.), *Ophthalmology* (2nd ed.). St. Louis: Mosby.

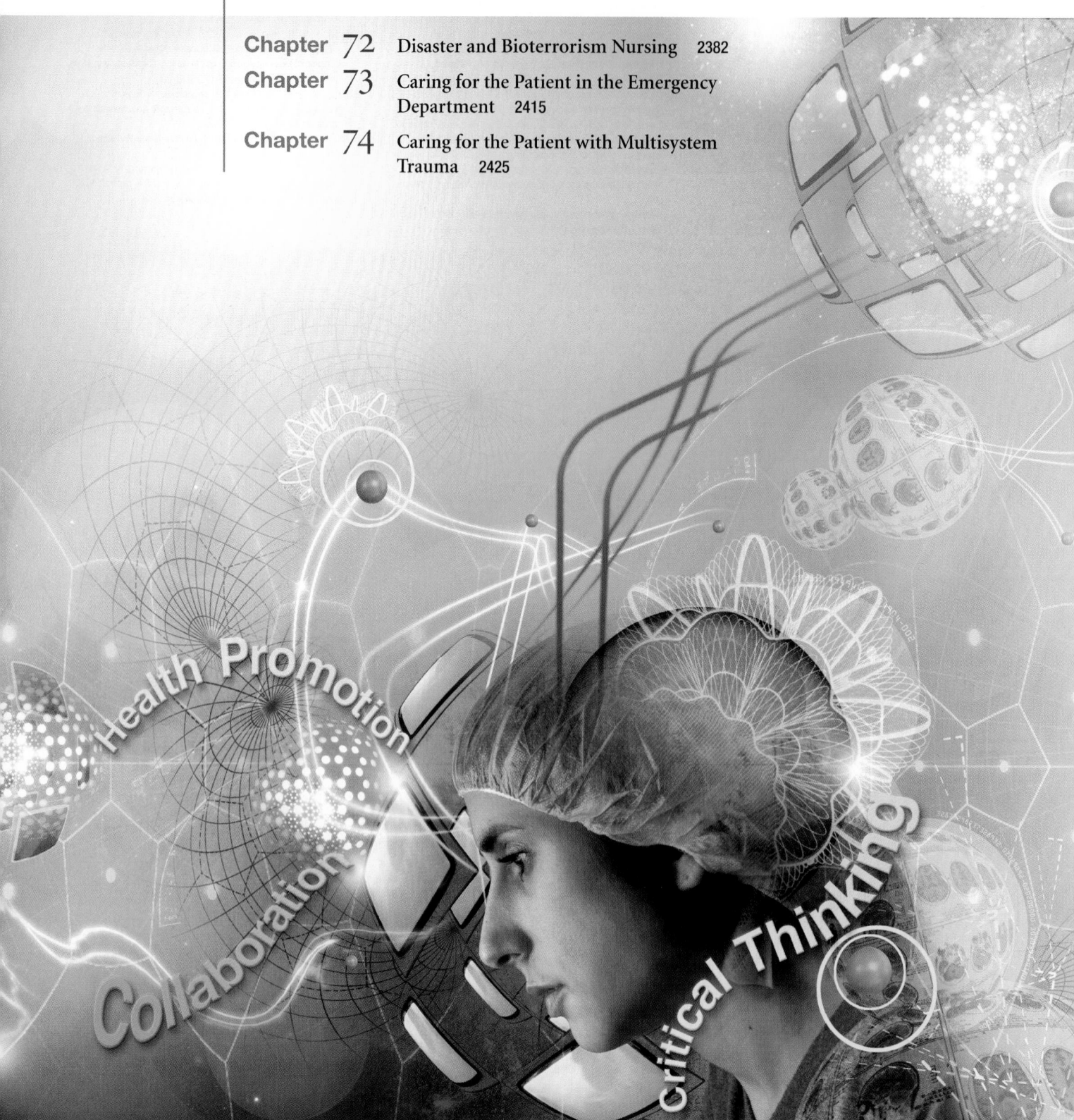

UNIT 16

Disaster, Emergency, and Trauma Nursing

Health Promotion

Collaboration

Critical Thinking

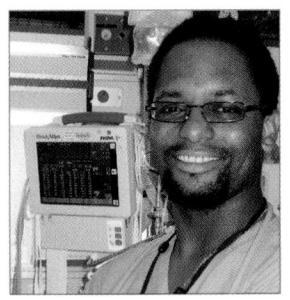

CHRISTOPHER My name is Christopher and I am a registered nurse and part of the specialized and unique staff that make up the Emergency Department (ED) in a large hospital. ED nurses specialize in variety and diversity because our patient population is everybody and everyone. The institution where I work is a Level I trauma teaching hospital in a midsize urban city serving hundreds of patients daily. We never close and offer all specialties of medical care for 24 hours out of every day. We see and do things during our typical workday that cannot be imagined. I function with my peers (physicians, pharmacists, nurses, technicians, respiratory therapists, etc.) in a collaborative effort with the goal of a better outcome for all those we encounter during our day.

Life is unpredictable as is the vast population of patients who visit the ED. With that being said, it is vital as an ED RN that I respond in a predictable, competent, and conscientious way. I have a commitment to those who come to the ED to respond with compassion and competence, doing all that I can to end my patients' "emergencies." As an RN, I am driven by the how and the why: How did this happen? Why did this happen?—two questions that are essentially behind what I and my colleagues do as medical professionals. A patient presents to the department with a chief complaint (CC) and as a collaborative team we attempt to answer the how/why questions. Sometimes the answers are straightforward, sometimes they are incomplete, but we are committed to finding the answer. Regardless of the seriousness of the complaint, the nurses in the ED treat all patients with the same level of comportment and caring.

Consider this example shift report: Today's assignment is the resuscitation room (RR), also known as the Trauma Bay. The RR is usually where patients who are severely ill or injured start for stabilization. It is important for ED nurses to have excellent assessment skills and a strong knowledge base about injury and illness so they can anticipate events that might occur.

The start of the shift is uneventful. One patient is in the RR; a restrained driver of a rollover motor vehicle crash (MVC). The patient is stable: three stable hematocrits, no fractures and some bumps and bruises, soon to be discharged home alive because "seat belts save lives!" I start to check the supplies in the room because it is important to be prepared at all times. The triage nurse tells me that a report has been received from the prehospital providers that they are bringing in a 19-year-old male who was found down at a party and could not be awakened. His level of consciousness is 9 out of 15 on the Glasgow Coma Scale (eyes, 2; verbal, 2; motor, 5) and decreasing. Fundamental to life are the ABCs: A = airway (EMS came in manually ventilating the patient, who is moved from stretcher to bed and the team moves quickly to secure an airway); B = breathing (something the patient is not doing effectively on his own, so he will need to be supported by a ventilator); and C = circulation (the patient's heart rate and blood pressure were within normal limits and not an immediate concern).

Having confidence in your coworkers and your own abilities allows many things to happen at once: The physicians prepare to intubate the patient as intravenous lines are established by the nurses and labs sent. The patient is stabilized with a safe effective airway, and within 25 minutes the patient is back from the CT scanner (no head injury) and moved to another area of the ED to "metabolize to freedom" (the patient's blood alcohol level was over four times the legal limit.)

I work 12-hour shifts. During that time I see and do too many things to begin to list. There are also those days where you feel that despite all of your efforts, something more could have been done. Every day there are emergencies, some are more subjective than others, but it is not my place to judge but to have compassion as I work with the patients. The patient who comes in after an MVC and succumbs to injuries, the patient with an active GI bleed who is stabilized and sent to the ICU, or the patient with just a burning sensation upon urination all receive the same attention and my total commitment.

"I have a commitment to those who come to the ED to respond with compassion and competence, doing all that I can to end my patients' "emergencies.""

CHAPTER 72

Disaster and Bioterrorism Nursing

Karen Silady

Outcome-Based Learning Objectives

After studying this chapter, the learner will be able to:

1. Define terrorism.
2. Describe the historical use of various agents.
3. Discuss various chemical agents, signs and symptoms, and treatment.
4. Compare and contrast biologic agents, signs and symptoms, and treatment.
5. Delineate the signs and symptoms of radiation illness.
6. Apply the principles of an incident command system in the hospital setting during a WMD event.
7. Describe the role of DMAT, DMORT, and the Strategic National Stockpile.
8. Apply critical incident stress principles to WMD events.

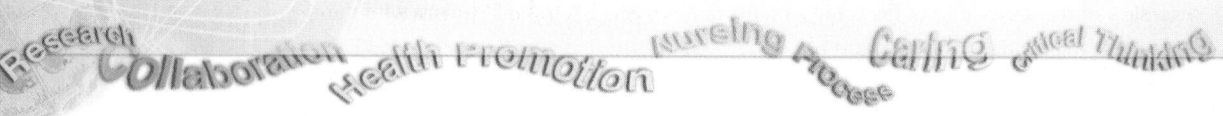

Research   Collaboration   Health Promotion   Nursing Process   Caring   Critical Thinking

Terrorism is an act, the purpose of which is to disrupt daily life and/or to cause terror and panic. Terrorism is defined by the Federal Bureau of Investigation (FBI) as "the unlawful use of force or violence against persons or property to intimidate or coerce a Government, the civilian population, or any segment thereof, in furtherance of political or social objectives" (FBI, 2006).

The FBI further describes terrorism as "international" when the use of force or violence is committed by a group or individual that is foreign based and/or has some connection to a foreign power, or whose activities cross international boundaries. This can include groups such as al Qaeda in the Middle East, the Irish Republican Army (IRA) in Ireland, the Freedom for the Basque Homeland (Euskadi Ta Askatasuna: ETA) in Spain, and the individual suicide bombers in Israel (FBI, 2006).

Terrorism

Terrorism is defined as "domestic" when the group or individuals operate out of the United States or Puerto Rico without foreign direction and their activities are directed at the U.S. government or the U.S. population This includes such groups as the Ku Klux Klan, Greenpeace, white supremacist groups, the Black Panthers, and lone individuals such as Timothy McVeigh (FBI, 2006).

It is often said that one man's terrorist is another man's freedom fighter. Politics aside, the problem with terrorism for nursing is that it creates large numbers of dead and injured that will require physical as well as psychosocial care. In addition, those who have witnessed the event will also need psychosocial care to deal with what was witnessed.

Targets

Ideal targets for terrorists would be anything and anywhere that large-scale disruption would ensue and are often based on the idealism behind the terrorist group. This includes large gatherings of people; nuclear power plants; chemical plants; federal buildings and other governmental institutions; infrastructure systems such as public utilities; military installations; religious buildings such as churches, synagogues, and mosques; controversial businesses such as abortion clinics; and world headquarters of companies. The point of terrorist events is to attract media attention, increase support for the cause, undermine the government or the agency attacked, influence policy, and create a sense of vulnerability. Occasionally the purpose is solely revenge (Sidell, Patrick, Dashiell, Alibel, & Layne, 2002).

Historical Use of Various Agents

Terrorism is not a new phenomenon, and different agents have been used throughout history.

Chemical Agents

In war and in terrorist events, there are numerous accounts of the use of chemical weapons. The Chinese in 1000 B.C. used arsenic smoke as a weapon (Lee, 2003). During World War I, on April 15, 1915, the Germans released 150 tons of chlorine gas near Ypres, Belgium. Because chlorine is heavier than air, it hugged the ground and settled into the trenches of the allied forces. This characteristic gives chlorine its nickname "the dragon." There were approximately 800 deaths, but psychologically the event was devastating to the 15,000 troops, resulting in a complete retreat. Because the allies had gas masks, chlorine came to be more of a tactical weapon. On June 12, 1917, at a site near Ypres, sulfur mustard was released; sulfur affects the eyes, lungs, and skin. This caused 20,000 casualties and forced the troops to don hot, bulky protective clothing along with the gas masks (Christopher et al., 1997). Mustard was also used by Iraq against Iran from 1980 to 1988 and against Kurdish citizens in Halahja, Iraq, in 1988, resulting in 5,000 deaths (Durham, 2002; U.S. Army Medical Research Institute of Chemical Defense [USAMRICD], 2000).

In 1994 and again in 1995, the Aum Shinrikyo cult released sarin gas into the Tokyo subway system. This was accomplished by carrying dilute sarin in plastic bags and then puncturing the bags with the tip of an umbrella. Sarin is a very potent nerve gas that can cause death in minutes. It was first invented as an insecticide by the Germans in 1937. This incident in Tokyo is the largest disaster caused by a nerve gas during a time of peace (Lee, 2003).

Accidents with respect to chemical agents abound. In Bhopal, India, in 1984 there was the accidental release of 50,000 pounds of methyl isocyanate (composed of phosgene, methylamine, and isocyanate) from a Union Carbide plant, which killed thousands in the initial exposure, with ultimately over 150,000 casualties (Durham, 2002).

Biologic Agents

As long ago as the 6th century B.C., there is documented use of **biologic agents**, bacteria, viruses and toxins, in warfare. The Assyrians poisoned enemy water wells with rye ergot, a fungus that grows on rye. This causes hallucinations and cardiac problems.

During the French and Indian War (1754–1763), Jeffrey Amherst, commander of the British forces in North America, authorized blankets and handkerchiefs used by smallpox victims to be distributed to the Indians who were sympathetic to the French (Christopher, Cieslak, Pavlin, & Eitzen, 1997; Durham, 2002; Kortepeter, 2001). During World War I (1914–1918), there is credible evidence that German agents infected horses and cattle in the United States with glanders (*Burkholderia* [*Pseudomonas*] *mallei*) before the animals were shipped to France. There are multiple allegations of many other biologic agents having been used in a similar fashion during that war (Christopher et al., 1997; Durham, 2002; Kortepeter, 2001).

During World War II (1939–1945), the Japanese had an extensive biologic experimentation program. The program was centered near Pingfang with other sites in Mukden, Changchun, and Nanjing. Agents used included *Yersinia pestis*, *Vibrio cholerae*, *Shigella*, *Neisseria meningitidis*, and *Bacillus anthracis*. It is said that 10,000 prisoners died from infection or execution following infection experimentation. The United States was accused by North Korea, China, and the Soviet Union of using biologic weapons during the Korean War. During the Cold War, there were numerous allegations on all sides regarding the use of and experimentation with biologic agents. Then-President Richard Nixon by executive order terminated the United States offensive biologic weapons program in 1970 (toxins) and 1971 (microorganisms).

During the Vietnam War, pungi sticks were routinely used by the Vietcong. These were sharpened bamboo sticks placed in rice paddies that had been rubbed with human waste to create great infected sores. The famous "yellow rain" from that war caused people and animals to become disoriented and ill, including some fatalities. Although still controversial, it is believed that some of these were clouds of trichothecene toxins (T-2 mycotoxin). Others believe that these were simply large clouds of tropical bee feces (Christopher et al., 1997; Kortepeter, 2001).

In April 1979 in Sverdlovsk (now Yekaterinburg), Russia, there was an accidental release of anthrax from a military microbiology facility secondary to a significant problem with the air filters. At least 77 cases, with 66 deaths, due to inhalation of anthrax were reported in relation to this incident (Christopher et al., 1997; Kortepeter, 2001). In the fall of 1984, there was a large salmonella outbreak in the city of The Dalles, Oregon. It was traced back to a religious commune, the Rajneeshees, who had intentionally contaminated a local salad bar with *Salmonella typhimurium*. This resulted in 751 cases of enteritis and 45 hospitalizations (Christopher et al., 1997; Torok et al., 1997).

The Bulgarian defector Georgi Markov lived in London. He was assassinated in 1978 by Bulgarian agents who had shot him in the leg with a pellet using a spring-loaded weaponized umbrella. The pellet had been hollowed out and filled with ricin, then sealed with wax that melts at body temperature. It is believed that similar weapons have been used in 60 known assassinations (Christopher et al., 1997).

Radiologic Agents

The only known wartime use of nuclear devices was the bombing of Nagasaki and Hiroshima by the United States during World War II (Jacocks, 2003; Udeani & Aguilera, 2002). This is widely accredited with assisting in ending the war.

In 1979 there was a small accidental leak of radiation at the Three Mile Island nuclear power plant in the Unites States from an overheated reactor coil. Over 2,000 lawsuits were filed, although no effects on physical health were ever documented. All the lawsuits were eventually dismissed (Raso, 1999).

On April 26, 1986, the Chernobyl Nuclear Reactor Unit 4 accidentally released a large cloud of radioactivity 80 miles northwest of Kiev in the Ukraine. This cloud was known to have gone over Belorussia, the Baltic republics, and headed toward Scandinavia. Due to many political factors at the time, acknowledgment of the incident by the then–Soviet Union took over 7 days. There are 56 official victims recorded, but virtually no data are available regarding numbers of casualties from this incident (World Nuclear Association, 2008; Jacocks, 2003). Much of what is known regarding radiation injuries comes from the Japanese incidents in World War II, Chernobyl, and Soviet weapons workers who had little to no safety procedures for protection (Jacocks, 2003).

Alexander Litvinenko, a former Russian spy, was poisoned with polonium-210 in the autumn of 2006. It is suspected that he was poisoned while dining in a restaurant in London. He ultimately died of acute radiation sickness (BBC, 2007).

Explosive Agents

The chronicles of war over the centuries are filled with the use of explosive devices since the invention of gunpowder. In the United States, recent incidents include 168 deaths and 759 injured from the bombing of the Alfred P. Murrah Federal Building in Oklahoma City April 19, 1995, by Timothy McVeigh. He made a bomb using items commonly found in home improvement stores (WashingtonPost.com, 1998).

The World Trade Center, which ultimately collapsed when struck by airplanes in the September 11, 2001, terrorist incident, was also bombed in 1993 with 6 deaths and 1,000 injured (Durham, 2002). The September 11, 2001, attack by al Qaeda of flying hijacked planes into the World Trade Center, the Pentagon, and then crashing one plane in Pennsylvania resulted in approximately 3,000 deaths. The 1996 Summer Olympics in Atlanta, Georgia, were rocked by an explosion in Centennial Park killing 1 person and injuring at least 100 (Cable News Network [CNN], 1996).

Worldwide, the recent frequent suicide bombings in Israel have given health care professionals extensive experience in caring for the victims of blast injuries. Frequent worldwide and local threats are defused prior to explosion or injury. A recent event involved police defusing an 8-pound bomb planted at the Pamplona Running of the Bulls festival in Spain in July 2003 by Freedom for the Basque Homeland (Euskadi Ta Askatasuna: ETA) (BBC, 2003).

Planning for Disasters

Dr. Eric Auf der Heide, from the U.S. Department of Health and Human Services, reviewed the literature regarding "lessons learned" from actual disasters and wrote:

> Disaster planning is only as good as the assumptions on which it is based. However, some of these assumptions are derived from a conventional wisdom that is at variance with empirical field disaster research studies. Knowledge of disaster research findings might help planners avoid common disaster management pitfalls, thereby improving disaster response planning. (Auf der Heide, 2006)

He then compared common assumptions about disasters and compared them with research findings, and discussed the implications for planning. Chart 72–1 presents these findings.

National Standards of Nursing Education

There was a time when nursing education regarding terrorism in the United States was considered unnecessary. Because of the events surrounding the September 11, 2001, World Trade Center disaster in New York, this education is now considered core information for all nurses. Since August 29, 2005, the events surrounding Hurricanes Katrina and Rita have forced the nation to focus on disaster response. Although this chapter focuses on terrorism and the issues involved, it is recognized that an all-hazards approach to planning and response is necessary.

In the aftermath of Hurricane Katrina, President George W. Bush, in a speech from Jackson Square in New Orleans in 2005, announced his order to the Department of Homeland Security

to review all emergency plans in every major city in America. The final results of that study were published June 16, 2006, entitled *Nationwide Plan Review Phase 2 Report* (Chertoff, 2006). In this report, 15 major areas of deficiency for state and urban areas were identified, including such things as a clear command structure, care of special needs populations, patient tracking, communication, and the ability to provide care for large numbers of casualties. Regardless of the cause of the catastrophe, whether terrorism or hurricane, the nurse needs to be prepared to work within an alternate structure and care for numerous patients, often with fewer resources.

Gebbie and Qureshi (2002) published a simple set of competencies for working nurses in regard to emergency and disaster preparedness based on previous work done for public health workers in the American Journal of Nursing (Chart 72–2, p. 2386). This has become something of a classic work and is frequently quoted.

The International Nursing Coalition for Mass Casualty Education (**INCMCE**), now called the Nursing Emergency Preparedness Education Coalition (NEPEC), coordinated by Vanderbilt University, consists of representatives from nursing education, nursing organizations, accrediting bodies, and governmental agencies. This coalition has a stated purpose to "assure a competent nurse workforce to respond to mass casualty incidents" (INCMCE, 2003). The INCMCE has published a lengthy document "Educational Competencies for Registered Nurses Responding to Mass Casualty Incidents." This document defines core competencies in the areas of critical thinking, assessment, technical skills, and communication. It describes core knowledge in the areas of health promotion, risk reduction, and disease prevention; health care systems and policies; illness and disease management; information and health care technologies; ethics; and human diversity. It also defines professional role development.

In the post–September 11th environment, multiple agencies and groups have developed educational programs regarding terrorism and health care with varying levels of complexity and varying focus. A recent Google.com search with key words "terrorism education" delivered almost 27 million sites. The vast majority of these programs are still grossly based on a handful of core government/military documents considered by experts to be the most solid sources of information available today about biologic, chemical, and radiologic agents (Chart 72–3, p. 2387).

Types of Events

Because of the massive damage and injury caused, the agents used by many terrorists are termed *weapons of mass destruction* (**WMD**). Although there are numerous acronyms for these agents, the acronym suggested for common use by the Department of Justice is **CBRNE**, which stands for chemical, biologic, radiologic, nuclear, and explosive devices, with incendiary (fire-causing) devices being included under explosive devices. Depending on the agent used and the target, many vectors, or means, of spreading the agent are available. These include spraying devices, letters and packages, contaminated water or food, insects and animals, and the wind. The various agents enter the body in basically one of four ways: ingestion, inhalation, injection, or dermal exposure.

Effective dissemination can be difficult. Many agents must be finely aerosolized and some clump in humid weather. The device

| CHART 72–1 | Common Disaster Planning Assumptions versus Research Observations | | |

Assumption	Research Observation	Planning Implications	Potential Interventions
Dispatchers will hear of the disaster and send emergency response units to the scene.	Emergency response units, both local and distant, will often self-dispatch.	Effective disaster planning requires planning not only for the jurisdiction but also at the intercommunity level. Plans should anticipate the likelihood that more help than needed will arrive, whether requested or not.	Expect unsolicited responders, and develop a plan for coordinating them. Establish intercommunity or statewide mutual aid plans and training. Use staging or check-in areas outside of rapidly established security perimeters.
Trained emergency personnel will carry out field search and rescue.	Most initial search and rescue is carried out by the survivors themselves.	Planners may incorrectly assume that they will have control over disaster emergency medical service (EMS) responses. Disaster search and rescue is often ad hoc and uncoordinated. Even if they are not part of the planned response, law enforcement officers often become involved in search and rescue. Survivors involved in search and rescue may have the best information on the location of the missing.	Train first responders how to coordinate with survivors carrying out search and rescue. Designate personnel to obtain information from survivors about the location of the missing.
Trained EMS personnel will carry out triage, provide first aid, or stabilize medical care, and if necessary decontaminate casualties before patient transport.	Casualties are likely to bypass on-site triage, first aid, and decontamination stations and go directly to hospitals.	Hospitals should not assume that casualties will be triaged, decontaminated, or given first aid in the field. Patients arriving in private cars may need to be extricated carefully so that injuries are not aggravated.	Develop real-time instructions that can be given to survivors (by commercial radio) on how to protect themselves; give first aid; and deal with contaminated casualties. Provide courses on first aid, search and rescue, and disaster care for the public. Send first responders to hospitals to extricate casualties from private vehicles.
Casualties will be transported to hospitals by ambulance.	Most casualties are not transported by ambulance. Rather, they arrive at hospitals by a variety of nonambulance vehicles (private cars, police vehicles, buses, or on foot).	EMS authorities often have little control over time of transport or hospital destination for disaster casualties. Transport outside of the EMS system also poses challenges for patient tracking.	Educate the public about precautions to take when transporting casualties and about which should not be moved. Establish procedures for collecting information after the fact from hospitals about what casualties they have received.
Casualties will be transported to hospitals appropriate for their needs and in such a manner that no hospital receives a disproportionate number.	Most casualties are transported to the closest or most familiar hospitals.	Although specific hospitals may be designated to receive contaminated casualties, it is the patients who will often choose their destination. Thus, all hospitals must be prepared to do decontamination. Although it may not be possible to prevent inefficient casualty distribution, it may be possible to influence or plan around it.	Consider having ambulances bypass hospitals closest to the disaster. Establish area and intercommunity EMS/hospital mutual aid plans and radio systems so that ambulances can be directed to hospitals best able to treat their patients. Use a "first-wave" protocol to divide initial casualties among area hospitals.

(continued)

CHART 72–1 Common Disaster Planning Assumptions versus Research Observations—*Continued*

Assumption	Research Observation	Planning Implications	Potential Interventions
Authorities in the field will ensure that area hospitals are promptly notified of the disaster and the numbers, types, and severities of casualties to be transported to them.	Hospital notification of a disaster may be from the first arriving victims or the news media rather than from the authorities in the field. Often, information and updates about incoming casualties are insufficient or lacking.	Initial hospital response may have to depend on the resources in house. Hospital procedures that require time-consuming activities before casualty arrival (donning chemical-resistant suits, etc.) may not be practical.	Base initial hospital response plans on in-house rather than on-call resources. Provide in-house staff with authority to activate and modify the plan. Develop plans for the expedient decontamination of unannounced casualties, which might include the use of fire hoses supplied with warm water, until more sophisticated decontamination equipment can be set up.
The most serious casualties will be the first to be transported to hospitals.	The least serious casualties often arrive first.	Because accurate and timely information from the field is often lacking, emergency departments (EDs) may not know of the more serious patients yet to come. As a result, when these patients arrive, they may find all beds occupied.	Assign field responders to communicate casualty information to hospitals. Hold beds open at hospitals for the possibility of later arriving, more serious casualties.

CHART 72–2 Emergency and Disaster Preparedness Core Competencies for Nurses

1. Describe the agency's role in responding to a range of emergencies that might arise.
2. Describe the chain of command in emergency response.
3. Identify and locate the agency's emergency response plan (or the pertinent portion of it).
4. Describe emergency response functions or roles, and demonstrate them in regularly performed drills.
5. Demonstrate the use of equipment (including personal protective equipment) and the skills required in emergency response during regular drills.
6. Demonstrate the correct operation of all equipment used for emergency communication.
7. Describe communication roles in emergency response.
8. Identify the limits of one's own knowledge, skills, and authority, and identify key system resources for referring matters that exceed these limits.
9. Apply creative problem-solving skills and flexible thinking to the situation, within the confines of one's role, and evaluate the effectiveness of all actions taken.
10. Recognize deviations from the norm that might indicate an emergency and describe appropriate action.
11. Participate in continuing education to maintain up-to-date knowledge in relevant areas.
12. Participate in evaluating every drill or response and identify necessary changes to the plan.

ADDITIONAL CORE COMPETENCIES FOR MANAGERS

13. Ensure that there is a written plan for major categories of emergencies.
14. Ensure that all parts of the plan are practiced regularly.
15. Ensure that gaps in knowledge or skills are filled.

Source: Gebbie, K. M., & Qureshi, K. (2002). Emergency and disaster preparedness: Core competencies for nurses. *American Journal of Nursing, 1*(102), 46–51. With permission.

may be technically difficult to use. The so-called "shoe bomber" was caught because he could not get the bomb fuse to light with repeated strikes of his lighter. The agent can potentially be hazardous to the terrorist, requiring extensive protective gear such as with some of the biologic agents.

Identification of an incident can be difficult, especially if the agent is one in which the symptoms have a delayed onset from the time of exposure. Patients will self-present to a variety of health care facilities, so there often is a delay before the event is recognized. It is important to maintain a high index of suspicion.

The key is in recognizing clusters. In chemical events, this would include the symptoms suggestive of the agent (Agency for Toxic Substances and Disease Registry [ATSDR], 2001a, 2001b; Community Research Associates [CRA], 2003: USAMRICD, 2000).

In biologic agents, it is harder to discern initially without a direct clue such as a threatening note or direct identification of munitions or tampering. Biologic clusters are found using usual public health epidemiologic methodology. Clues would include a large epidemic of a particular set of symptoms, more severe symptoms than are usually seen for a particular pathogen, an

CHART 72–3 Core Sources of Information Regarding Terrorism Response

Agency for Toxic Substances and Disease Registry (ATSDR). (2001). *Managing hazardous materials incidents.* Atlanta, GA: U.S. Department of Health and Human Services.
Three-volume set from the U.S. Public Health Service.

Jacocks, J. (Ed.). (2003). *Medical management of radiological casualties* (2nd ed.). Bethesda, MD: Armed Forces Radiobiology Research Institute.
The armed forces' handbook for nuclear and radiologic agents.

Kortepeter, M. (Ed.). (2001). *USAMRIID's medical management of biological casualties handbook* (4th ed.). Fort Detrick, MD: U.S. Army Medical Research Institute of Infectious Diseases.
The armed forces' handbook for biologic agents.

Sidell, F. R., Patrick, W. C., Dashiell, T. R., Alibel, K., & Layne, S. (Eds.). (2002). *Jane's chem-bio book* (2nd ed.). Alexandria, VA: Jane's Information Group.
A handbook developed by a think tank regarding chemical and biologic agents.

U.S. Army Medical Research Institute of Chemical Defense (USAMRICD). (2000). *Medical management of chemical casualties handbook* (3rd ed.). Aberdeen Proving Ground, MD: Author.
The armed forces' handbook regarding chemical agents.

U.S. Department of Transportation (DOT). (2008). *2008 Emergency response guidebook.** Washington, DC: U.S. Government Printing Office.
The core hazardous materials book used in the United States, Mexico, and Canada.

Websites

http://www.bt.cdc.gov
The Centers for Disease Control and Prevention's website. Is a center of information pertaining to all aspects of terrorism and health care.

http://www.emsa.ca.gov
The California Emergency Medical Services Authority (EMSA) website. Has the entire hospital incident command system (HICS) and training available; free downloading.

*Also available at http://hazmat.dot.gov/pubs/erg/guidebook.htm

unusual disease or a disease unusual for the region, unusual strains, and a large number of cases of unexplained disease or death. The onset of a biologic agent event would depend on the agent used, especially the incubation period (Kortepeter, 2001). Illness in the animal population often will act as a herald that a significant event is occurring.

Symptoms, clustering, and onset in radiologic incidents depend greatly on the type of radiation involved and the delivery method. A radiological dispersion device (**RDD**), or so-called "dirty bomb," would have a different presentation than a fission device (atomic bomb) (CRA, 2003; Jacocks, 2003). Note that the likelihood of the use of a fission device in a terrorist event is considered very low. Explosions are fairly easy to identify because they create patients with traumatic injuries.

Personal Protective Equipment

Personal protective equipment (**PPE**) is the clothing and equipment that are protective to the person from whatever agent to which one is exposed, be it chemical, biologic, or radiologic. PPE is classified according to the degree of protection it delivers: Level A, Level B, Level C, and Level D (Chart 72–4, and Figures 72–1 and 72–2 ■, p. 2388). Many daily exposures to hazardous materials that are not even related to terrorist events will require personal protection and perhaps even decontamination.

No one suit is protective for all agents. Factors to determine the level of PPE to use include not only the agent but also other practical matters such as the temperature, humidity, body size,

CHART 72–4 Personal Protective Equipment Levels

LEVEL A
Highest level of respiratory, skin, and eye
Fully encapsulated chemical-resistant suit
Full face piece and supplied air (self-contained breathing apparatus, or SCBA)
Inner chemical-resistant gloves
Chemical-resistant safety boots
"Moon suit"

LEVEL B
Same respiratory as Level A but less skin
Full face piece and supplied air (SCBA)
Chemical-resistant clothing
Inner and outer chemical-resistant gloves
Chemical-resistant safety boots
Hard hat

LEVEL C
Full face piece with air purifying canister–equipped respirator
Chemical-resistant clothing
Hard hat

LEVEL D
Regular work clothing
Safety shoes
Safety goggles/splash shield

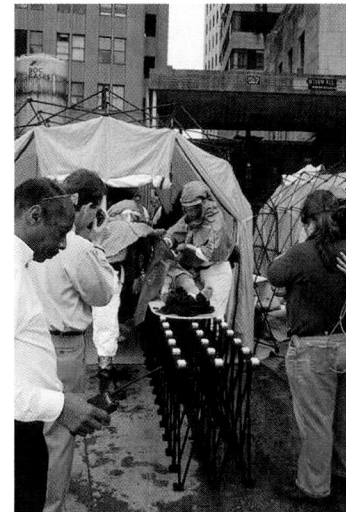

FIGURE 72–1 ■ Decontamination drill in PPE suit.
Source: Photo courtesy of Robert J. McBride RN, New Orleans

MyNursingKit | Center for Disease Control and Prevention

MyNursingKit | The California Emergency Medical Services Authority

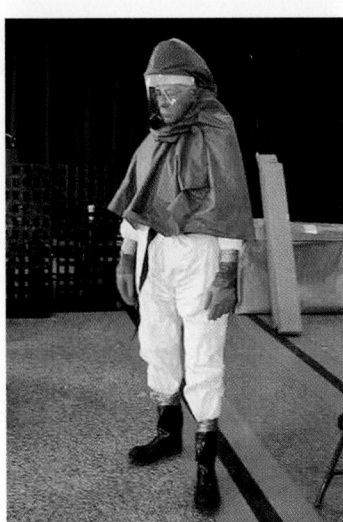

FIGURE 72-2 ■ PPE suit.
Source: Photo courtesy of Robert J. McBride RN, New Orleans

facial hair, and strenuousness of the expected activity. There are many problems with PPE for the user, including hyperthermia, dehydration, and claustrophobia. In addition, there are limited vision, limited dexterity, limited movement, and communication problems. During operations, there need to be preset hand signals indicating distress that can be used by the person in the gear.

Proper donning and doffing of PPE are essential to prevent contamination. Extensive training and practice are required. Proper donning includes such things as correct use of all gear, taping all openings, and checking for breaches in gear before entering contaminated area; there need to be specific checklists for removing protective clothing at the end of an incident or end of a tour of duty. The person in the PPE will require decontamination before being allowed into noncontaminated areas.

While wearing the PPE, there is constant concern about possible breach of protection as well as whether the level of protection is appropriate for the situation. In general, the greater the level of protection, the greater the risk of an adverse effect. There are very specific medical criteria regarding who is allowed to don higher level PPE. Once in the PPE, the safety officer and medical management personnel must monitor the wearer for problems (ATSDR, 2001a, 2001b; Hick et al., 2003; Lehmann, 2002; Sidell et al., 2002; USAMRICD, 2000). The United States Department of Labor, Occupational Safety and Health Administration (OSHA) published the final draft of *OSHA Best Practices for Hospital-Based First Receivers of Victims from Mass Casualty Incidents Involving the Release of Hazardous Substances* in January 2005 (OSHA, 2005). This document contains recommendations for PPE purchasing and training based on a hospital's hazard analysis. Safety concerns for the personnel wearing the PPE are also discussed.

Level A

Level A protection is the highest level of protection for the skin, eyes, mucous membranes, and respiratory system. This is what is commonly referred to as the "moon suit." Level A has a fully encapsulated, vapor-tight, chemical-resistant suit; chemical-resistant boots/shoes with steel toe and shank; chemical-resistant inner

and outer gloves; coveralls; hard hat; two-way communications system; and completely self-contained breathing apparatus (SCBA). There are cooling units available to extend the time a person can tolerate being in these suits as well as lower level suits.

SCBA has a full face piece connected to a compressed air source. Some are closed circuit. This system uses a small tank of supplemental oxygen, and recycled exhaled gases are rebreathed ("rebreather"). The open circuit SCBA has a tank of air, and the exhaled air is released into the atmosphere. SCBAs give the person freedom to travel within the time limit of the air bottle. Supplied air respirators (SARs) have a long hose that attaches the person to a more distant air supply. This system limits the person to an area the length of the air supply hose, but the person has no time limit on air supply. SCBAs and SARs require individual fit testing (ATSDR, 2001a, 2001b; Hick et al., 2003; Sidell et al., 2002; USAMRICD, 2000).

Level B

Level B is similar to Level A except that chemical protective clothing (CPC) is used instead of the fully encapsulating suit. This provides splash protection but is not vapor proof. Chemical protective clothing includes two-piece chemical splash suits, disposable chemical-resistant overalls, and other chemical-resistant clothing. Inner and outer resistant gloves and resistant steel toe and shank boots are used. SCBA is used with a full face shield. Level B is the minimum level recommended for initial entry into sites until the hazard has been identified.

Chemical protective clothing can be affected by chemical degradation of the suit, whereby through aging or contact with a chemical the suit's structural integrity is damaged. Level B does use the self-contained breathing apparatus. Chemicals can eventually permeate protective clothing depending on the exact chemical. Manufacturer's literature will include permeation "breakthrough" times for various chemicals. Penetration of the suit occurs when the integrity is breached; there may be an opening in the suit (such as an untaped zipper), the suit tears, or the suit has a defect (ATSDR, 2001a, 2001b; Hick et al., 2003; Sidell et al., 2002; USAMRICD, 2000).

Level C

By the time patients arrive to a hospital or other health care facility, they will have had a prolonged exposure to the agent and yet are still alive. Many hospitals and health care facilities therefore use a Level B suit with Level C respiratory protection. Level C consists of full face piece with an air purifying canister–equipped respirator and chemical-resistant clothing. This level is used when skin and eye exposures are unlikely, the agent is known, and the criteria for the exact respiratory equipment being used are met.

Air purifying respirators (APRs) and powered air purifying respirators (PAPRs) purify ambient air based on the type of canister and filter connected to the system. PAPRs use a battery-operated blower that delivers essentially decontaminated air at slight positive pressure into a face piece. Both APRs and PAPRs can protect against particulates, some gases, and vapors, depending on the filters, absorbents, and canisters used. When used with high efficiency particulate air filtration (HEPA filters) in combination with organic vapor cartridges, a level of biologic protection can be achieved. Radiologically contaminated particles can also be trapped (ATSDR, 2001a, 2001b; Hick et al., 2003; Sidell et al., 2002; 3M, 2002; USAMRICD, 2000).

Level D

Level D PPE is regular clothing. It affords simple protection, but no respiratory or skin protection. Safety goggles, splash shields, and regular latex-type gloves can be considered part of Level D protection (ATSDR, 2001a, 2001b; Hick et al., 2003; Sidell et al., 2002; USAMRICD, 2000).

Decontamination

Decontamination is the reduction or removal of contaminating agents. In instances of radiologic contamination, the point is to remove the radioactive contaminants. In these cases, the runoff needs to be contained. Decontamination in the hospital or health care setting can involve persons who received "gross" decontamination at the scene prior to arrival and persons who presented to the facility outside of the emergency medical services route without any prior treatment. It is important to recognize that contaminated persons must be fully decontaminated before being admitted to the facility to prevent the facility from being contaminated. The axiom is "there are no patients until they are decontaminated." Victims, first responders from the scene, equipment, and personnel assisting with the process all will undergo decontamination.

Gross decontamination, or field decontamination, is a process whereby the greater part of the agent is removed or washed away. This is usually done by some type of high-volume rinse system such as systems created using fire hoses. It is estimated that 80% of the agent can be removed by simply removing the clothing (ATSDR, 2001a, 2001b; Jacocks, 2003; Medical Center of Louisiana at New Orleans (MCLNO), 2003; Sidell et al., 2002; Texas Engineering Extension Service, National Emergency Response and Rescue Training Center [TEEX], 2003; USAMRICD, 2000).

The area set up for decontamination is outside. In setting up this area, there are three zones: the hot zone, warm zone, and cold zone. It is best if the hospital is upwind of the decontamination area. The **hot zone**, also called the exclusion or red zone, is the area of highest contamination. This is where persons waiting to be decontaminated are staged. There is usually

a triage area set up here to sort those requiring quicker treatment (see the START Triage section later in this chapter), and each person receives a numbered tag. A brief registration is done to collect basic information such as name, date of birth, and social security number. This is logged with the triage number. Many hospitals have prenumbered sets of triage kits with tags, registration sheets, and belongings bags on the disaster cart.

The **warm zone,** or yellow zone, is also referred to as the contamination reduction corridor (Figure 72–3 ■). This is where the actual decontamination process takes place. The **cold zone,** or green zone, is also known as the support zone. The hospital is in the cold zone. No one is allowed into the cold zone without being decontaminated (ATSDR 2001a, 2001b; MCLNO, 2003; Sidell et al., 2002; TEEX, 2003; USAMRICD, 2000). Chart 72–5 outlines the three zones of decontamination.

The decontamination lines are usually divided into male and females, and also into those who are ambulatory and the nonambulatory. The first step is to disrobe completely. Clothing is generally collected in red bags and labeled. Personal belongings, such as watches, wallets, jewelry, and eyeglasses, are usually collected in clear plastic bags and labeled. In the shower area, the person will fully lather up, including in all body creases, the hair, and the genital area. Attention should be directed toward contaminated wounds first, as agents are more rapidly absorbed by broken skin. There has been controversy regarding the best agents for decontamination. Common current consensus is some type of liquid soap or baby shampoo. A 0.5% bleach is still used for some equipment decontamination. For those who are ambulatory, only guidance will be needed in the process of being cleaned. The nonambulatory patients will require physical washing by specially trained personnel in full personal protective gear. Once washing is complete, they will dry off, are given some type of hospital gown or clothing, and are admitted into the cold zone disposition area from where they are sent into the hospital system (ATSDR, 2001a, 2001b; MCLNO, 2003; Sidell et al., 2002; TEEX, 2003; USAMRICD, 2000).

In suspected terrorist events, all of the clothing and personal belongings collected are considered evidence from a crime scene. The Federal Bureau of Investigation (FBI) will confiscate these items as evidence. It is important that these items be handled using usual chain-of-custody procedures. If the personal items can be decontaminated, after the FBI is finished with these items, an effort is made to return them to the correct owner (ATSDR, 2001a, 2001b; MCLNO, 2003; Sidell et al., 2002; TEEX, 2003; USAMRICD, 2000).

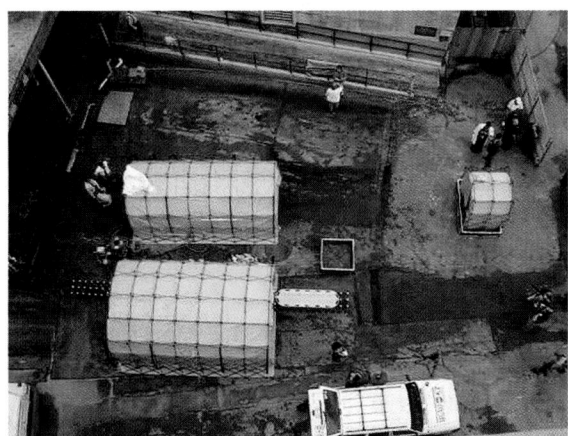

FIGURE 72–3 ■ Decontamination setup.
Source: Photo courtesy of Robert J. McBride RN, New Orleans

CHART 72–5	Zones of Decontamination	
Hot Zone	**Warm Zone**	**Cold Zone**
Red	Yellow	Green
Patient entry	Decontamination	Clean treatment area
EMS access	Ambulatory	Clean evacuation
Triage	Nonambulatory	Staging area for personnel
Initial disrobing		
Emergency first aid		

Chemical Agents

Chemical agents are generally considered either industrial or military depending on their use. From here they are further divided based on the military's original view on how these chemicals affect the body. Chemical agents include nerve agents and vesicants, or blistering agents, which are generally considered to be military agents only. Blood agents, choking agents, and irritants are the other categories, and they are mostly toxic industrial chemicals (Chart 72–6).

Spread

Most dissemination of chemical agents is by aerosol. The spread of chemical agents by this method depends on the agent's vapor pressure, how fast it goes from a liquid to a gas at room temperature, and its vapor density, its weight relative to air. High vapor pressure agents evaporate quickly, such as acetone (fingernail polish remover). High vapor density agents, such as chlorine, tend to sink and hug the ground. Low vapor pressure agents and high vapor density agents are said to be **persistent**, that is, they stay around for a long time, creating a hazardous environment for a longer period and thus a longer exposure time. An agent is considered persistent if it lasts longer than 24 hours as a liquid on surfaces. Persistent agents such as mustard and VX become useful in denying access to an area or to materials. Nonpersistent agents, such as sarin (used in the Tokyo attacks) and cyanide, are more useful as tactical agents within a population (ATSDR, 2001a, 2001b; CRA, 2003; Sidell et al., 2002; USAMRICD, 2000).

Nursing Management of the Patient Exposed to Chemical Agents

Nursing management of the patient exposed to chemical agents depends greatly on the agent and the severity of the exposure. Application of the nursing process will facilitate a comprehensive approach to patient assessment and care. Nursing diagnoses depend on the agent and symptoms seen. For all chemical agents, *Risk for Injury* related to gross contamination with chemical will apply. Patient assessment parameters will follow the signs and symptoms expected, based on the class of agent. (A sample Nursing Process: Patient Care Plan for nerve agents is in the Nerve Agents section, p. 2392.)

Collaborative Management

The main categories of nerve agents, vesicants, blood agents, choking agents, and irritants are presented with common signs and symptoms and basic treatment. Much of the care is symptomatic. All patients with chemical exposure require comprehensive care from a health care team including nurses, health care providers, toxicologists, and specialists from all fields, depending on the nature and severity of the injury. Psychological and emotional care of these patients needs to be included while providing physical care.

Routes of Entry

There are several means for chemical agents to be spread. It is important to attempt to identify the route of entry in order to identify other potential patients.

Ingestion

Chemicals can be put in food, medicines, and water or other liquids. Ingestion through the public water supply is a less likely scenario due to dilution and the treatment water receives at the plants. Water wells and individual buildings are considered more likely targets. An example of the oral route was the 1982 episode of product tampering whereby bottles of Tylenol were contaminated with cyanide and seven people died. Although the casualty count was low, it created tremendous terror in the population (ATSDR, 2001a, 2001b; CRA, 2003; USAMRICD, 2000).

Inhalation

Inhalation is considered the most common route for chemicals, as most episodes of chemical agent release will be by aerosol. Many devices can be used for dissemination including mosquito trucks, aerial sprayers such as crop dusters, and various industrial spray equipment pieces including pesticide sprayers, wind dispersion, and using buildings' heating and cooling systems. The new term for this activity is *aerobiology* (ATSDR, 2001a, 2001b; CRA, 2003; USAMRICD, 2000).

Injection

Injection can be by needle or dart or any other sharp object such as broken glass. The number of casualties is low by this method. Other injection methods include the shrapnel from a chemical dispersion devise. The shrapnel containing the chemical in the device would enter the body and be absorbed into the tissue (ATSDR, 2001b; CRA, 2003; USAMRICD, 2000).

Dermal Exposure

Dermal exposure would cause external damage to the skin and eyes. It could then be absorbed through the skin and into the body. This would occur through either an aerosol release or an intention spill. With an aerosol release, the agent would have to have a high vapor density so that it would fall on the intended population. With an intentional spill, the agent would most likely be persistent in nature (ATSDR, 2001b; CRA, 2003; USAMRICD, 2000).

CHART 72–6	**Chemical Agents by Class**

NERVE AGENTS	CHOKING AGENTS (ASPHYXIATES)
Sarin (GB)	Ammonia
Soman (GD)	Chlorine
Tabun (GA)	Phosgene
V agent (VX)	
	IRRITANTS
VESICANTS	Mace (CN)
Mustard	Tear gas (CS)
Lewisite	Pepper spray (OC)
Phosgene oxime	
BLOOD AGENTS	
Hydrogen cyanide	
Cyanogen chloride	

Nerve Agents

Nerve agents are the most toxic of the known chemical agents. During World War II, Germany developed many nerve agents but for unknown reasons never used them. The only known use of nerve agents was in the Iran–Iraq War and by terrorists. Nerve agents work in a manner similar to organophosphate insecticides in that they inactivate acetylcholinesterase, thereby increasing the acetylcholine at the receptor site. This process results in an overstimulation at the synapse. The effect on the patient is dose related. The most common routes of exposure are inhaled and topical. The agents are readily absorbed from the skin and eyes.

The signs and symptoms seen, which are the same as with organophosphate poisoning, are remembered by the mnemonic SLUDGEM: salivation, lacrimation, urination, defecation, gastric upset, emesis, and miosis. Often there is a complaint of dim vision. The nerve agents also cause cardiac dysrhythmias, confusion, fasciculations and convulsions, along with unconsciousness. Almost all people affected by a nerve agent will have miosis, and most will have a runny nose and shortness of breath. The combination of pinpoint pupils and muscle fasciculations is the most reliable sign of nerve poisoning (Abramowicz, 2002; Dang, Kare, Schneiderman, & Dang, 2002; McKee et al., 2000; Sidell et al., 2002; USAMRICD, 2000).

The attachment of the nerve agent to the enzyme is permanent unless removed by therapy. Atropine assists with symptomatic relief and is the most common drug used in the treatment of nerve gas exposure. Atropine will help with the muscarinic effects such as rhinorrhea, salivation, sweating, bronchoconstriction, bronchorrhea, nausea, vomiting, and diarrhea. The most common reversal agents are the oximes such as Protopam chloride (2-PAM chloride). Protopam helps with muscle twitching and respirations. Atropine and Protopam are packaged together into what is called a MARK I kit. The MARK I kit is administered intramuscularly via an auto injector. The reversal agents must be used early in the course, because, once aging has occurred, the reversal agent is of no effect. Diazepam can help with the convulsions. With all nerve agents, those who survive need full decontamination. Their clothing must be double sealed in plastic and handled as little as possible to avoid secondary exposure to others (Abramowicz, 2002; ATSDR, 2008; Dang et al., 2002; McKee et al., 2000; Sidell et al., 2002; USAMRICD, 2000).

The remainder of the care is outlined in the Nursing Process: Patient Care Plan for Known Nerve Agent Exposure feature (p. 2392).

Sarin (GB)

Sarin is a clear, colorless, and tasteless liquid that has no odor in its pure form. Sarin easily evaporates into a gas, as occurred in the Tokyo event. Sarin mixes easily with water so it can be used to poison food and water. It is heavier than air, so it tends to sink. Once a person is exposed, sarin will continue to release from a person's clothing for about 30 minutes, causing secondary exposures. Low-dose exposure would produce symptoms within seconds to hours. Even a small drop of sarin can cause sweating and muscle twitching at the site of exposure (Centers for Disease Control and Prevention [CDC], 2006e; Sidell et al., 2002; USAMRICD, 2000).

Soman (GD)

Soman is a clear, colorless, and tasteless liquid. It does have a slightly fruity camphor odor, but this cannot be relied on to provide warning against toxic exposure. It can discolor with aging to a dark brown. Soman is highly volatile and so poses a short-lived threat when released. However, soman is heavier than air and so sinks when released. Soman mixes readily with water, so it also can be used to poison food and water. Soman breaks down slowly in the body; therefore, it has a cumulative effect with repeated exposures (ATSDR, 2001c; CDC, 2006f; Sidell et al., 2002; USAMRICD, 2000).

Tabun (GA)

Tabun is a clear, colorless, and tasteless liquid. It has a slightly fruity odor that cannot be relied on to give warning of exposure. Tabun can become a vapor when heated. It also mixes easily with water and is heavier than air. Compared to sarin, tabun is less volatile and therefore will last longer on surfaces than sarin does (ATSDR, 2001c; CDC, 2006h; Sidell et al., 2002; USAMRICD, 2000).

V Agent (VX)

V agent, more commonly called VX, is the most toxic substance known to man. Less than one drop on the skin can be fatal. It is believed by some that any skin exposure to VX is lethal unless washed off immediately on contamination. VX is an amber-colored, odorless, and tasteless oily liquid and is very persistent. It evaporates at about the same rate as motor oil. VX is primarily a liquid exposure hazard, but when exposed to high heat can become a gas. Although it cannot be mixed as readily into water as the other nerve agents, VX can be used to contaminate water and food sources. VX is heavier than air, so it will sink to low-lying areas. Its persistence and toxicity make it the worst of the nerve agents (ATSDR, 2001c; CDC, 2006i; Sidell et al., 2002; USAMRICD, 2000).

Vesicants

Vesicants are **blister agents** that cause redness and irritation to skin that progresses to partial thickness and often full-thickness blisters. In the eyes, the vesicants can cause irritation and conjunctivitis to corneal burns and blindness. With inhalation, vesicants can cause mucosal sloughing and airway obstruction. In high doses, bone marrow suppression can be seen in 3 to 5 days. Especially after oral ingestion, nausea, vomiting, and diarrhea can occur. Emesis and feces may be blood stained. Systemic absorption from any route can cause symptoms such as headache, nausea and vomiting, leukopenia, and anemia.

With most agents except lewisite, there is an asymptomatic period of hours following exposure. The damage is being done to the tissue; it is the overt signs that are delayed. Complete decontamination is required with clothing being double bagged for protection. If eye exposure is suspected, eye irrigation is recommended. There are numerous reports of apathy, lethargy, and sluggishness in people exposed to mustard after exposure and for a period of time afterward. This phenomenon has not been well studied. There is no specific therapy for vesicant exposure. All treatment is supportive (Abramowicz, 2002; ATSDR, 2001c; CDC, 2006a; McKee et al., 2000; Sidell et al., 2002; USAMRICD, 2000).

Mustard

Mustard has been used as a chemical weapon many times in recent history. Mustard is an oily liquid ranging in color from light yellow to brown. It has an odor like garlic, horseradish, onion, or mustard, from which it derives its name. Odor should not be relied on for detection of exposure. Mustard freezes at 57°F, so it is primarily a liquid hazard, but it is a definite vapor hazard at

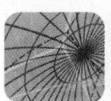

NURSING PROCESS: Patient Care Plan for Known Nerve Agent Exposure

Assessment of Exposure

Subjective Data:
Determine from information sources the agent suspected.
Ask assessment questions of the patient regarding nerve agent symptoms, including dim vision and abdominal discomfort, circumstances of exposure and previous decontamination, and past medical history.

Objective Data:
Assess readiness for decontamination, including equipment and personnel.
Perform pre–personal protective equipment (PPE) assessments of personnel including vital signs and weight.
Perform full patient assessment for nerve agent exposure. (See the Nerve Agents section in this chapter.)

Nursing Assessment and Diagnoses	Outcomes and Evaluation Parameters	Planning and Interventions with *Rationales*
Nursing Diagnosis: *Injury, Risk for* related to gross contamination with chemical	**Outcomes:** The patient is fully decontaminated. No exposures to health care workers or facility. No injury to the health care providers. ***Evaluation Parameters:*** Patient has no chemical left on body as measured with chemical strips or other devices. No increase in symptomatology following decontamination. Health care workers and decontamination workers have no exposure to chemical and no symptoms of chemical exposure or exhaustion. Clean areas maintained. No contamination of the facility.	**Interventions and *Rationales:*** Decontamination area set up into hot, warm, and cold zones, with a triage area in the hot zone as well as re-triage in the cold zone. Areas monitored to maintain zones. Health care workers and other decontamination personnel don full and appropriate PPE prior to contact with contaminated patients. Monitor personnel during decontamination process for signs of agent exposure and heat exhaustion. *To prevent contamination of and injury to personnel.* Fully undress patients and place belongings in clear bags, double bagged, with identification easily seen through bag. *To preserve evidence and prevent secondary exposure.* Fully scrub patients, including creases and hair, using warm soapy water, and rinse. *To remove remaining chemical.* Assess patient prior to decontamination and reassess patient in the cold zone for symptoms of exposure. *To determine severity of symptoms and care needed.*

Assessment of Airway

Subjective Data:
Does the patient complain of shortness of breath (SOB), difficulty breathing, drowning sensation, or weakness?

Objective Data:
Assess for amount of salivation, lacrimation, emesis, rhinorrhea, and bronchorrhea in airways. Assess for fasciculations, level of consciousness and degree of confusion, seizures, respiratory rate, degree of work of breathing, breath sounds, cough effort, vital signs, and skin and nail bed color.

Nursing Assessment and Diagnoses	Outcomes and Evaluation Parameters	Planning and Interventions with *Rationales*
Nursing Diagnosis: *Airway Clearance, Ineffective* related to copious secretions, weakness, depressed level of consciousness, and ineffective cough	**Outcomes:** The patient will maintain a patent airway and adequate gas exchange. ***Evaluation Parameters:*** Clear breath sounds. Clear airways. Pulse oximeter above 95%. Skin warm, dry, and pink with brisk capillary refill.	**Interventions and *Rationales:*** Assess patient for amount and type of secretions. Full respiratory assessment including vital signs, breath sounds, work of breathing, cough effort, skin vital signs, and pulse oximeter. *To determine degree of distress.* Observe for cyanosis, increased confusion, and restlessness. *These are signs of increased hypoxia.* Allow patient to sit in high Fowler's position. *To facilitate respiratory effort and airway clearance.* Suction airways as needed for ineffective/inadequate cough. Endotracheal intubation as indicated. *To maintain clear airway.* Administer oxygen as needed. *To maintain adequate gas exchange.* Administer atropine and Protopam as ordered. *To dry secretions and assist with shortness of breath.* Teach effective coughing techniques such as huff cough. *To improve airway clearance and reduce fatigue from constant coughing.*

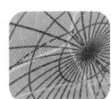

NURSING PROCESS: Patient Care Plan for Known Nerve Agent Exposure—*Continued*

Assessment of Cardiac Status

Subjective Data:
Sensation of palpitations, racing heart, skipping beats.

Objective Data:
Cardiac monitor.
Radial and apical pulse. Blood pressure.
Level of consciousness.

Nursing Assessment and Diagnoses	Outcomes and Evaluation Parameters	Planning and Interventions with *Rationales*
Nursing Diagnosis: *Cardiac Output, Decreased* related to dysrhythmias	**Outcomes:** The patient will have a normal sinus rhythm with adequate cardiac output. **Evaluation Parameters:** Sinus rhythm without ectopy on cardiac monitor. Awake, alert, and oriented level of consciousness.	**Interventions and *Rationales:*** Measure apical and radial pulses and blood pressure, and level of consciousness. *To determine relative perfusion.* Place on cardiac monitor. Monitor with at least 2 leads. *To determine dysrhythmias and need for treatment.* Monitor electrolytes. *Altered electrolytes can affect the cardiac rhythm.*

Assessment of Fluid Status

Subjective Data:
Degree of thirst, headache, amount of cramping, and nausea.
Previous amounts of fluid lost.

Objective Data:
Assess degree of dehydration.
Monitor electrolytes and serum osmolality, physical signs of dehydration, vital signs, and level of consciousness.

Nursing Assessment and Diagnoses	Outcomes and Evaluation Parameters	Planning and Interventions with *Rationales*
Nursing Diagnosis: *Fluid Balance, Readiness for Enhanced* related to copious secretions, high urinary output, vomiting, and diarrhea	**Outcome:** The patient will attain fluid and electrolyte balance. **Evaluation Parameters:** Diarrhea and emesis halted. Intake and output equal. Secretions controlled. Serum osmolality and electrolytes within normal limits. Vital signs within normal limits.	**Interventions and *Rationales:*** Assess hydration status such as oral mucous membrane moisture, intake and output, sunken eyes, skin tenting, thirst, and headache. *To determine degree of dehydration and any improvement in or deterioration of condition.* Strictly monitor intake and output. *To determine fluid balance and any improvement in or deterioration of condition.* Assess vital signs, orthostatic vital signs, cardiac rhythm, and level of consciousness. *To identify signs of hypovolemic shock, perfusion, and electrolyte imbalances.* Monitor serum osmolality and electrolytes when ordered. *To determine replacement needs.* Assess for nausea and administer antiemetics as ordered. *To decrease nausea and vomiting.* Administer atropine and Protopam. *To decrease secretion production and decrease diarrhea and emesis.* Administer normotonic intravenous solutions and oral replacement when tolerating oral fluids. *To replace lost fluids and restore fluid balance.* Administer electrolyte replacement intravenously or orally when tolerated. *To replace lost electrolytes and restore balance.*

Assessment of Coping

Subjective Data:
Assess for feelings of apprehension, fear, uneasiness, palpitations, loss of concentration, degree of sense of threat, feelings of helplessness, powerlessness, increased tension, and worry.

Objective Data:
Assess for decreased concentration, narrow focus.
Signs of tension-reducing behaviors such as biting fingernails, cursing, and rocking.
Altered pitch and tone of voice.
Other typical signs and symptoms—such as increased heart rate, increased respiratory rate, tremor, dry mouth, and increased gastrointestinal symptoms—are not reliable signs due to the nerve agent exposure.

(continued)

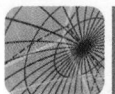

NURSING PROCESS: Patient Care Plan for Known Nerve Agent Exposure—*Continued*

Nursing Assessment and Diagnoses	Outcomes and Evaluation Parameters	Planning and Interventions with *Rationales*
Nursing Diagnosis: *Coping, Ineffective* related to perceived and actual threat from situation, unknown outcome, and possible further danger	**Outcome:** There will be a decrease in the patient's anxiety. **Evaluation Parameters:** The patient will report no sensation of palpitations. Will answer simple questions clearly without lag. Will report a subjective decrease in sensation of anxiety and helplessness and an increased sense of control. Anxiety-reducing behaviors will be greatly decreased or absent, such as no rocking and no nail biting.	**Interventions and *Rationales:*** Use calm, reassuring approach. *To increase confidence in caregiver and reduce anxiety of unknown.* Reassure patient that appropriate medical care is being rendered for condition. Explain procedures and purpose of medications and interventions in simple terms. Explain in simple terms the effects of the nerve agent. *Reduce anxiety by decreasing the fear of the unknown and learning what to expect.* Identify for patient the safety of the facility/situation, if true. *To reassure of current safety.* Stay with patient. If the nurse must leave the patient, the nurse should tell the patient when he will return and do so. *To build a trusting relationship and provide sense of security in care.* Acknowledge patient's fears and anxiety. *To identify feelings as a normal reaction, provide insight into situation, and decrease anxiety.* Teach simple stress reduction exercises such as imagery. *To allow for self-comforting and assist with relaxation.* Administer antianxiety agents if ordered and indicated. *To decrease anxiety and promote rest.*

100°F, which is common in the more arid regions of the world. Because of its chemical properties, mustard is often mixed with other chemicals to keep it liquid at lower temperatures. The effects from mustard are seen anywhere from 2 to 48 hours postexposure. Mustard also has some mild cholinergic properties, which may be responsible for the early gastrointestinal symptoms and the miosis seen (Abramowicz, 2002; ATSDR, 2001c; McKee et al., 2000; CDC, 2006g; Sidell et al., 2002; USAMRICD, 2000).

On the skin, the erythema starts with itching. As the erythema fades, areas of increased pigmentation are left. The erythema usually starts in warm, moist thin-skinned locations such as the axillae, perineum, antecubital fossae, and neck. The blisters usually start 4 to 24 hours postexposure. The vesicles start small and then coalesce to form bullae. These large blisters are usually dome shaped with thin walls, yellowish in color, and surrounded by erythema. The fluid is clear, thin, and straw colored at first. Later, the fluid turns more yellow and tends to coagulate. The fluid does not contain mustard and is not harmful to those exposed. In high-dose exposures, the lesions may develop central necrotic areas, which are extremely slow to heal. These blistered areas are extremely painful, and it takes large doses of narcotics to control the pain. These burns cause less fluid loss than thermal burns, and care must be given to avoid overhydration in fluid resuscitation (ATSDR, 2001c; CDC, 2006g; Sidell et al., 2002; USAMRICD, 2000).

The early respiratory effects are usually irritation or burning of the nares, sinus pain or irritation, nosebleeds, and irritation of the pharynx. Laryngitis with voice changes can occur with a nonproductive cough. Damage to the trachea and upper airways can lead to a productive cough. With the lower airways involved, there is increasing dyspnea and increased sputum production. Signs of a

chemical pneumonitis can appear 2 to 3 days postexposure. Pseudomembranes can form from necrosis of the airway mucosa. Death in mustard exposure is usually from respiratory failure (ATSDR, 2001c; CDC, 2006g; Sidell et al., 2002; USAMRICD, 2000).

The eyes are the most sensitive to mustard. Blisters do not form. Usually the symptoms are in a range from conjunctivitis, to photophobia, blepharospasm, pain, and then corneal damage. Severe corneal damage, perforation of the cornea, and scarring can occur, including blindness (ATSDR, 2001c; CDC, 2006g; Sidell et al., 2002; USAMRICD, 2000).

Lewisite

Lewisite is an oily and colorless liquid with the odor of geraniums. It is more volatile than mustard. Lewisite causes stinging and burning on contact in such severity that the person will take immediate steps to remove it. Lewisite also causes more immediate blistering. The blisters tend to be smaller and in clusters, as opposed to large bullae with mustard. There is almost no human data from lewisite; most data are from animal investigations. (ATSDR, 2001c; CDC, 2006b; Sidell et al., 2002; Truab & Hoffman, 2002; USAMRICD, 2000).

Within 5 minutes of exposure, lewisite will cause a grayish area of dead epithelium. Redness and blistering follow rapidly, but do not reach their height for 12 to 18 hours. The lesions have more necrosis and tissue sloughing than those of mustard. With eye exposure, pain and blepharospasm occur on contact. The eyes are often swollen shut within an hour. Because of the extreme irritancy to the respiratory system, the person usually self-limits exposure by masking or exiting the area. There is evidence that third spacing of fluid occurs after a massive exposure causing a hypotensive state called "lewisite shock." British anti-lewisite agent was created to use topically to limit toxicity of this agent. Although no longer formulated for this use, it is still used in heavy metal poisoning (ATSDR, 2001c; CDC, 2006b; Sidell et al., 2002; USAMRICD, 2000).

Phosgene Oxime

Phosgene oxime is a different chemical from the choking agent phosgene discussed later. Phosgene oxime is solid below 95°F. It is colorless as a solid, but yellow to brown as a liquid, and it can have a peppery or pungent odor. It can be released into food and water. It is not a true vesicant, as it does not cause blisters. Phosgene oxime is known as an urticant or nettle agent, as it causes intense itching and a hive-like rash on contact. There is very little experience with this agent (ATSDR, 2001c; CDC, 2006d; Sidell et al., 2002; Truab & Hoffman, 2002; USAMRICD, 2000).

The liquid or vapor of phosgene oxime causes pain on contact, followed by blanching with an erythematous ring, then wheals within 30 minutes, with later necrosis. The pain can persist for several days. It can cause extreme pain in the eyes. It is very irritating to the airways, causing pulmonary edema after both skin exposure and inhalation (ATSDR, 2001c; CDC, 2006d; Sidell et al., 2002; Truab & Hoffman, 2002; USAMRICD, 2000).

Blood Agents

Blood agents include the gases such as hydrogen cyanide and cyanogen chloride and crystals such as sodium cyanide and potassium cyanide. Although it has a bitter almond odor, only about 50% of the population has the genetic ability to detect it. Cyanide is naturally present in some fruit pits and lima beans. It is used extensively in industry such as in ore extraction and the manufacturing of paper and plastics. It is present when many common household items burn in fires and thus represents a frequent threat to many in the course of daily work, as well as a possible terrorist agent. The primary route of exposure is through inhalation, although liquid is absorbed through the skin, eyes, and oral mucosa. If the exposure was with a liquid, then decontamination is needed. Cyanide acts by blocking the mitochondrial enzyme cytochrome oxidase, which leads to reduced aerobic metabolism. Glucose breakdown continues, resulting in a buildup of pyruvate, which is converted to lactic acid resulting in lactic acidosis and intracellular shortage of adenosine triphosphate (ATP) (ATSDR, 2001c; CDC, 2004; Dang et al., 2002; Martin, 2002; Sidell et al., 2002; USAMRICD, 2000).

In higher concentration exposures to cyanide, death is usually within 3 to 8 minutes. In lower exposures or with ingestion, the onset of symptoms is slower. The initial transient rapid respiratory rate may be followed by apprehension, anxiety, agitation, and vertigo. There can be a feeling of general weakness, nausea with or without vomiting, and muscular trembling. Later respirations slow, with loss of consciousness, convulsions, and apnea with cardiac standstill. Because of the slow onset of symptoms, treatment is possible (ATSDR, 2001c; CDC, 2004; Dang et al., 2002; Sidell et al., 2002; USAMRICD, 2000).

Medical management of cyanide poisoning starts with administration of 100% oxygen. Amyl nitrate by inhalation or sodium nitrate by intravenous injection is used to create methemoglobin,

as cyanide has a higher affinity for methemoglobin. Sodium thiosulfate is administered to convert the cyanide to thiocyanate, which is excreted in the urine. Hyperbaric oxygen treatment has been shown to be efficacious, especially when the patient is cyanotic. Supportive therapy includes intravenous bicarbonate for severe acidosis, vasopressors to support blood pressure, and valium to treat seizures. Long-term disorders of the basal ganglia are often seen after cyanide poisoning (ATSDR, 2001c; CDC, 2004; Dang et al., 2002; Sidell et al., 2002; USAMRICD, 2000).

Choking Agents (Asphyxiates)

Choking agents are also called **asphyxiates** or lung-damaging agents. Inhalation is the usual route of exposure. Initially, irritation of the nasopharynx causes sneezing, pain, and erythema, which are difficult to distinguish from exposure to a riot control agent. Dysphagia, a choking sensation, and a cough often follow. Central airway damage is characterized by signs and symptoms such as hoarseness, stridor, and coarse crackles. Within 2 to 24 hours, signs of pulmonary edema begin, starting with shortness of breath on exertion, wheezes, fine crackles, and large amounts of white to pink frothy sputum. It is important to note that the pulmonary edema is not of cardiac origin, so diuretics are contraindicated. Pulmonary edema within 4 hours of exposure indicates a poor prognosis. Treatment is largely supportive, with oxygen, ventilatory support if indicated, and bronchodilators. Bed rest with absolute minimal activity is a must, as physical activity exacerbates the symptoms. Steroids and ibuprofen have been used for phosgene exposure to decrease inflammation, but their use in other choking agent exposure is unknown. Decontamination is indicated if liquid or solid materials are present (Abramowicz, 2002; Dang et al., 2002; Sidell et al., 2002; USAMRICD, 2000).

Ammonia

At room temperature, anhydrous ammonia is a colorless, highly irritating gas with a strongly pungent odor. It is a common agent in household cleaners and found in fertilizers. In higher concentrations, it is used extensively in industrial settings. It is also a key ingredient in the manufacture of crystal methamphetamine. Anhydrous ammonia is highly irritating to the eyes and respiratory tract, causing lacrimation and rhinorrhea, swelling of the throat and bronchi, coughing, and pulmonary edema. In higher concentrations, it causes chemical pneumonitis and can cause lung hemorrhage. Skin exposure in higher concentrations can cause pain and corrosive injury. For survivors of severe inhalation injuries, residual chronic lung disease is common. Three clinical patterns of presentation are described for phosgene and chlorine depending on the exposure. In the first 3 to 5 days postexposure, there can be a chemical bronchitis and pneumonitis with fever and a high white blood cell count (ATSDR, 2001c, 2004; Sidell et al., 2002; Truab & Hoffman, 2002; USAMRICD, 2000).

Chlorine

Chlorine is a widely recognized odor as it is common in household bleach and swimming pool chemicals. As a gas, it has a yellow-green color and tends to settle on the ground. In mild exposure to chlorine, there is a choking sensation, eye and nose irritation, a cough, and exertional dyspnea. In moderate exposure, there is hoarseness, stridor, and pulmonary edema within 2 to 4 hours. In a severe exposure, respiratory distress at rest and pulmonary edema can occur within 30 to 60 minutes. Copious upper respiratory secretions are present. Sudden death from laryngeal edema, laryngospasm, or bronchospasm can occur. Sodium bicarbonate is sometimes used for the metabolic acidosis seen in massive exposures (ATSDR, 2001c; CDC, 2006a; Sidell et al., 2002; Truab & Hoffman, 2002; USAMRICD, 2000).

Phosgene

Phosgene is a colorless gas that has the odor of newly mown hay, freshly cut grass, or corn but forms a white cloud that hugs the ground. Although highly volatile, phosgene is twice as potent as chlorine. Phosgene is distinguished by its odor and its generalized mucous membrane irritation in high concentrations including causing laryngospasm. With phosgene there is dyspnea, and the onset of pulmonary edema is delayed. In mild exposure, cough, dyspnea, and or chest tightness first occurs. Eye irritation and lacrimation are indicative of moderate phosgene exposure. In severe exposure, the pulmonary edema occurs in about 4 hours with respiratory distress at rest. With phosgene, sudden death may also occur from the laryngeal edema, laryngospasm, or bronchospasm (ATSDR, 2001c; CDC, 2006c; Sidell et al., 2002; Traub & Hoffman, 2002; USAMRICD, 2000).

Irritants

Irritants, commonly known as **riot control agents**, produce transient discomfort and eye closure so that the recipient is temporarily unable to fight or resist. They generally cause pain, burning, lacrimation, or discomfort on exposure to mucous membranes within seconds of exposure, but these effects rarely persist for more than a few minutes. Fresh air is the treatment, but showering will be helpful in alleviating symptoms. Clothing should be double bagged in plastic and handled as little as possible. Large and prolonged doses in contained areas can cause eye injury and respiratory failure (McKee et al., 2000; USAMRICD, 2000).

Tear Gas (CS)

Tear gas is colorless to gray with a sharp, irritating odor some describe as that of hair spray. With exposure to tear gas, there is usually a burning sensation in the nose, rhinorrhea, and sneezing and increased salivation when it contacts the mouth. With inhalation into the airways, there is bronchorrhea, coughing, and a sensation of chest tightness. If there is damaged skin, such as abrasions, there will be a tingling or burning sensation, and sometimes an erythematous reaction. With sustained exposure (hours) in hot and humid conditions, a second-degree–type burn can occur. Nausea and vomiting can also occur (USAMRICD, 2000). Although normally the signs and symptoms are of short duration and severity, there are reports of young, healthy nonsmoking subjects requiring intensive care treatment following exposure for hypoxia, hemoptysis, and pulmonary infiltrates when combined with strenuous exercise (Thomas, 2002).

Mace (CN) is available commercially for self-protection but is otherwise not used. Its effects are similar to those of tear gas (USAMRICD, 2000).

Pepper Spray (OC)

Pepper spray, also known as "oleoresin capsicum," is a suspension of red pepper initially used by the U.S. Postal Service against aggressive dogs. Police use it in riot control situations and to assist in difficult apprehensions. Although there have been many accusations of deaths from pepper spray, the April 2003 report by the Department of Justice, *The Effectiveness and Safety of Pepper Spray*, concluded that no deaths have been caused directly by pepper spray, although there are indications that it has contributed to two deaths (National Institute of Justice, 2003).

Other Agents

It is worth mentioning that the military does have other agents that will most likely never be encountered by the civilian population. Incapacitating agents include BZ from the family benzilates. **Incapacitating agents** cause symptoms that are the opposite of nerve agents, as they decrease the effective acetylcholine at receptor sites. Central nervous system signs and symptoms can include stupor, confusion, and confabulation. Other signs and symptoms include mydriasis, blurred vision, dry mouth, and an initial rapid heart rate followed by a normal or slow heart rate. **Vomiting agents** include diphenylchloroarsine (DA) and diphenylcyanoarsine (DC). They cause a strong pepper-like irritation in the upper respiratory tract, leading to irritation of the eyes, lacrimation, sneezing, cough, nausea, and vomiting. These would most often be used in combination with another agent so as to cause persons to unmask (McKee et al., 2000; Sidell et al., 2002; USAMRICD, 2000).

■ Biologic Agents

Biologic agents include bacteria, viruses, and toxins. Biologic agents are usually in a liquid or dry form. Most agents tend to be off white to amber, brown, or red. This color can easily be changed with the addition of simple food dyes so as to blend these agents into the background of the area of dispersion. Unlike chemical agents, biologic agents are not detectable with the usual five human senses. Because the period of illness is longer than with chemical agents, the impact on health care is much longer and larger than with chemicals. If such an agent were dispersed, there would be waves of patients depending on the incubation and population affected, as opposed to a single influx (Franz et al., 1997; Kortepeter, 2001; Sidell et al., 2002). Chart 72–7 outlines the biologic agents by class: bacteria, viruses, and toxins.

CHART 72–7	Biologic Agents by Class
BACTERIA	**VIRUSES**
Anthrax	Dengue fever
Brucellosis	Ebola
Cholera	Rift Valley fever
Glanders	Smallpox
Plague	Venezuelan equine encephalitis (VEE) virus
Q fever	Viral hemorrhagic fever (VHF)
Rickettsia	**TOXINS**
Tularemia	Botulinum
Typhus	Ricin
	Saxitoxin
	Staphylococcal enterotoxin B (SEB)
	Trichothecene mycotoxins

Biologic agents are categorized as Category A, B, or C. Category A agents are those that pose the highest risk to national security because they (1) cause high mortality with the potential for major public health effects including special actions for public health preparedness, (2) are easily disseminated or easily spread person to person, and (3) may cause public panic and public disruption. Category A agents include smallpox, anthrax, plague, botulism, tularemia, and viral hemorrhagic fever. Category B agents are moderately easy to disseminate, can cause moderate morbidity and low mortality, and require specific actions and enhancements by the Centers for Disease Control and Prevention (CDC). Category B agents include brucellosis, glanders, ricin, staphylococcal enterotoxin B, and some of the food- and water-borne illnesses such as salmonella, *Shigella*, and *Vibrio*. Category C agents are emerging pathogens that could be engineered in the future because they are readily available, are easily produced and disseminated, and have the potential for high morbidity and mortality. The Category C agents include Hantaviruses, tick-borne encephalitis virus, and yellow fever (CDC, 2006a, 2006j, 2008; House, Graber, & Scheckel, 2003).

Nursing Management of WMD Infection

Nursing management of the patient with an infection from a WMD event is the same as that of any other patient with the same infection. Refer to Chapter 20 🔗 for the care of the patient with infectious disease. Application of the nursing process will identify an assessment data cluster that will assist in identifying the agent involved.

Collaborative Management

As with other infectious agents, weaponized biologic agents require aggressive infectious disease management. A health care team that includes nurses, health care providers, public health personnel, and infectious disease specialists will be required. When large numbers of patients are involved, public health's role becomes key in managing the spread of the disease. As with chemical agents, psychological and emotional care needs must be included in the comprehensive approach.

Spread

There are multiple routes in which biologic agents can be dispersed.

Aerosol Route

The spread of biologic agents would usually be by an aerosol method. Most biologic agents can be aerosolized to a size of 1 to 10 microns. Particles larger than 15 microns will not stay suspended in the air but will fall out to the ground. Secondary aerosolization occurs when the particles that have fallen to the ground are stirred by currents created by passing people or objects such as cars. Breathing in through the nose filters out only those particles larger than 10 microns (Hagler, 2004). Most aerosolized biologic agents will be taken deeply into the lungs by those exposed (Franz et al., 1997). The aerosols can be created using simple sprayers such as a garden or paint sprayer, crop duster planes, mosquito trucks, fire extinguishers, all the way to a dispersion bomb, much as with chemical agents. These all take a high level of knowledge and sophistication to create (Franz et al., 1997; Kortepeter, 2001; Sidell et al., 2002).

Oral Route

Foods and fruits can be contaminated either during distribution or in the manufacturing process. Outbreaks of food poisoning at various restaurants or at family picnics are examples of accidental contamination of foods. The oral route was used in the Oregon salad bar incident mentioned earlier (Torok et al., 1997). The accidental contamination of food usually produces few casualties.

Most public-type water supplies are at very low risk for significant contamination due to the chlorination treatment process. Reverse osmosis systems have been shown to be effective against the toxins of ricin, microcystin, T-2 mycotoxin, and saxitoxin. Contamination of a personal water well or single building's water supply at the intake would be a more likely scenario (Sidell et al., 2002).

Injection

The injection route for biologic agents is not a common terrorist method. It is more commonly used in specific assassination attempts, such as that of Georgi Markov (Christopher et al., 1997). It would be possible to contaminate hospital equipment and thus have injection be the vector, but this is unlikely.

Dermal Exposure

Intact skin affords an excellent barrier for most biologic agents, so dermal exposure is not an effective means of transmission for most bacteria and viruses. Open wounds such as paper cuts or other small abrasions will provide a portal of entry. Cutaneous anthrax is commonly acquired this way. Some of the toxins such as T-2 mycotoxin ("yellow rain") are believed to be able to penetrate skin (Sidell et al., 2002).

Vector Transmission

Biologic agents can intentionally be spread with fleas, ticks, and mosquitoes, just as they are in nature. This is a complicated process but is known to have been accomplished. This route is not considered as a likely scenario because other methods are easier and less expensive (Sidell et al., 2002).

Bacteria

Bacteria generally cause disease by invading host organisms and or producing toxins. *Rickettsia* is unique in that these bacteria rarely can grow without a living host cell and yet are most susceptible to antibiotics. Some bacteria form spores that are resistant to heat, cold, drying, chemicals, and radiation and can therefore germinate under favorable conditions (Kortepeter, 2001).

Anthrax

Anthrax, which is spore forming, is caused by *Bacillus anthracis*. The spores are very stable and may remain for years in soil and water. There are three clinical forms of anthrax: cutaneous, inhalation, and gastrointestinal. Anthrax typically has an incubation period of 1 to 5 days. Those with known exposure can receive ciprofloxacin or doxycycline prophylactically. There is a vaccine available used primarily in the active duty military. Treatment is with ciprofloxacin, doxycycline, or penicillin with streptomycin, along with symptomatic treatment (Franz et al., 1997; Hardin, 2002; Inglesby et al., 2002; Kortepeter, 2001; Sidell et al., 2002).

A terrorist attack using anthrax would most likely be with aerosol, resulting in inhalation anthrax, as in the 2001 U.S. Postal Service incidents on the East Coast ("Follow-Up of Deaths," 2003). Following the primary aerosolization, the spores settle onto surfaces and can be resuspended when disturbed. This occurrence is uncertain and depends on many factors. Anthrax is also known as "woolsorter's disease" because it is known to occur in workers handling contaminated wool, hair, and hides. Standard (universal) isolation precautions are adequate for anthrax. There is no indication that health care workers caring for these patients need any type of prophylaxis (Franz et al., 1997; Hardin, 2002; Inglesby et al., 2002; Kortepeter, 2001; Sidell et al., 2002).

Cutaneous Anthrax

Cutaneous anthrax, also known as malignant pustule anthrax, occurs most frequently on the arms and hands of those working with infected livestock. Spores enter through broken skin. The lesions can occur up to 12 days postexposure. The lesion initially appears as a pruritic macule or papule that enlarges to a round ulcer by the second day. Vesicles may appear. The central lesion develops into eschar, which dries and loosens, falling off in 1 to 2 weeks. Painful lymphadenopathy and lymphangitis can occur with some systemic symptoms. Antibiotics do not change the course of the lesion but do help with the systemic symptoms. Especially when treated, death from cutaneous anthrax is rare (Franz et al., 1997; Hardin, 2002; Inglesby et al., 2002; Kortepeter, 2001; Sidell et al., 2002).

Inhalation Anthrax

The initial symptoms of inhalation anthrax are nonspecific and last for a few days or less: cough, dyspnea, fever, headache, chills, diaphoresis, chest pain, weakness, and sometimes abdominal pain. There is usually a short period of improvement followed by the abrupt development of the second phase. The second phase is more severe with fever, more severe dyspnea, shock, and a classic widening mediastinum and pleural effusions. Up to half of the patients develop hemorrhagic meningitis. Inhalational anthrax has a high mortality rate (Franz et al., 1997; Hardin, 2002; Inglesby et al., 2002; Kortepeter, 2001; Sidell et al., 2002).

Gastrointestinal Anthrax

Gastrointestinal anthrax is rare in humans and occurs most frequently by eating the undercooked meat of infected animals. A large amount of anthrax must be ingested to cause the disease. In the oral pharyngeal form, an oral or esophageal ulcer forms along with sepsis, regional lymphadenopathy, and edema. In the lower gastrointestinal tract, the lesions tend to occur in the end of the ileum or in the cecum. It usually presents with nausea and vomiting, and progresses rapidly to bloody diarrhea, acute abdomen, and sepsis. Massive ascites has been known to occur (Franz et al., 1997; Hardin, 2002; Inglesby et al., 2002; Kortepeter, 2001; Sidell et al., 2002).

Brucellosis

Brucellosis, also called "undulant fever," was the first disease weaponized by the United States in 1954. Undulant fever is caused by one of six species of *Brucellae*. Undulant fever has a variable incubation, from 5 to 60 days, but it is believed that the incubation would be shorter if this agent were weaponized for

inhalation. Brucellosis typically presents as a nonspecific flu-like illness, with fever, headache, myalgias, arthralgias, back pain, diaphoresis, chills, and general malaise and weakness. Vertebral osteomyelitis, intervertebral disk space infection, paravertebral abscess, and sacroiliac infections are rare but severe complications. Gastrointestinal symptoms occur in 70% of adults. No human vaccine is available. Treatment is with doxycycline plus rifampin or ofloxacin with rifampin. For those with known exposure, prophylaxis is with doxycycline plus rifampin. Trimethoprim-sulfamethoxazole can be substituted for rifampin; however, the relapse rate may reach 30% (Franz et al., 1997; Kortepeter, 2001; Sidell et al., 2002).

Plague

Plague, caused by *Yersinia pestis*, occurs in three forms: bubonic, septicemic, and pneumonic. Plague is spread from rodents to humans by the bite of infected fleas. Incubation is generally 2 to 10 days. As it can be spread person to person, droplet precautions are indicated with pneumonic plague. Bubonic plague requires standard (universal) precautions. Those exposed to plague can receive doxycycline, ciprofloxacin, or tetracycline prophylactically. Plague is usually treated with streptomycin, gentamicin, ciprofloxacin, or doxycycline. Plague meningitis is treated with chloramphenicol. Untreated plague has a high mortality rate (Franz et al., 1997; Inglesby et al., 2000; Kortepeter, 2001; Sidell et al., 2002).

A vaccine did exist at one time. The CDC references a 1982 article from the *Morbidity and Mortality Weekly Report (MMWR)* regarding recommendations for the administration of this vaccine ("Plague Vaccine," 1982). The Computer Sciences Corporation is in clinical trials for a plague vaccine that uses recombinant technology. This vaccine was originally developed by USAMRICD. No results of the clinical trials are yet available (Computer Sciences Corporation, 2008).

Bubonic Plague

The onset of disease is abrupt with fever, chills, weakness, myalgias, headache, and an acutely swollen and painful lymph node near the site of the flea bite. This is called a **bubo** and is normally seen in the lower leg or groin, because the legs are the most common site of flea bites in humans. The bubo is so painful that it usually prevents motion in the affected area. The bubos recede with antibiotic therapy. Incision and drainage of these lesions is contraindicated as that would present an exposure risk to the health care worker. Diagnostic sampling can be done by needle aspiration, which may provide short-term symptomatic relief (Franz et al., 1997; Inglesby et al., 2000; Kortepeter, 2001; Sidell et al., 2002).

Septicemic Plague

Septicemic plague can present primarily or secondary to bubonic plague. Septicemic plague presents similarly to other gram-negative septicemias with high fever, chills, malaise, hypotension, nausea, vomiting, and diarrhea. With plague, purpuric lesions, necrosis of small vessels, gangrene of the nose and fingertips, and disseminated intravascular coagulopathy can occur, from whence it is believed the name the "black death" originated (Franz et al., 1997; Inglesby et al., 2000; Kortepeter, 2001; Sidell et al., 2002).

Pneumonic Plague

Pneumonic plague usually occurs secondary to bubonic or septicemic plague; however, it is expected to be the primary event in a weaponized plague attack that would be in an aerosolized form. The incubation period is usually 1 to 6 days. The onset is acute and fulminant with high fever, chills, headache, malaise, and myalgias followed within 24 hours by a productive cough. Although the sputum is usually bloody, it can be watery or purulent. Abdominal pain, nausea, vomiting, and diarrhea can also be present. The pneumonia progresses rapidly to dyspnea, stridor, and cyanosis with respiratory failure and circulatory collapse (Franz et al., 1997; Inglesby et al., 2000; Kortepeter, 2001; Sidell et al., 2002).

Tularemia

Tularemia is caused by *Francisella tularensis*. It is considered to be one of the more likely biologic choices for weaponization. It is found in a variety of small mammals. Tularemia is known to be spread by ticks, flies, and mosquitoes as well as by contact with or ingestion of infected soil, food, or water. It can be spread in aerosol, as seen in laboratory workers, but no person-to-person spread has been documented. Tularemia has an incubation period of about 3 to 5 days. Prophylaxis for known exposure is with doxycycline, tetracycline, or ciprofloxacin. Treatment of the disease is with streptomycin, gentamicin, or ciprofloxacin. A vaccine has been used in laboratory workers but is not in general release. Standard (universal) isolation precautions are indicated for tularemia (Barrueto & Hoffman, 2002; Dennis et al., 2001; Franz et al., 1997; Kortepeter, 2001; Sidell et al., 2002).

Typhoidal Tularemia

Typhoidal tularemia is seen with inhalation exposure. It has an abrupt onset of fever, body aches (especially the lower back), shaking chills, and sore throat, along with chest pain or tightness and a cough that may or may not be productive. A true and extremely severe pneumonia can develop. Symptoms can be progressive and include nausea, vomiting, diarrhea, and weight loss (Barrueto & Hoffman, 2002; Dennis et al., 2001; Franz et al., 1997; Kortepeter, 2001; Sidell et al., 2002).

Ulceroglandular Tularemia

Ulceroglandular tularemia is characterized by a cutaneous papule, which becomes ulcerative, with regional lymphadenopathy at the inoculation site. The lesion appears at the same time as the general symptoms of fever, chills, headache, and malaise (Barrueto & Hoffman, 2002; Dennis et al., 2001; Franz et al., 1997; Kortepeter, 2001; Sidell et al., 2002).

Oropharyngeal Tularemia

Oropharyngeal tularemia is from drinking contaminated water or eating contaminated food. Occasionally, it can be from inhalation. A stomatitis can develop, but most commonly there is an exudative tonsillitis or pharyngitis, sometimes with ulceration. There is usually pronounced cervical lymphadenopathy (Barrueto & Hoffman, 2002; Dennis et al., 2001; Franz et al., 1997; Kortepeter, 2001; Sidell et al., 2002).

Q Fever

Q fever was first called "query fever" because the cause was unknown. Q fever is caused by the *rickettsia Coxiella burnetii*, which is highly infectious by the aerosol route. The common vectors are cattle, sheep, goats, dogs, cats, and birds. Q fever has an incubation of 2 days to 2 weeks, most commonly 10 to 14 days. Symptoms can be slow or abrupt in onset and usually consist of fever, chills, myalgias, and headache, with fatigue, anorexia, and weight loss less commonly. It can develop into pneumonia. About one-third of the patients with Q fever will develop abnormal liver function tests. Those patients with pre-existing valvular heart disease can occasionally develop endocarditis. A vaccine is under development. Q fever is generally treated with tetracycline or doxycycline. For known exposure to Q fever, prophylaxis is tetracycline or doxycycline (Franz et al., 1997; Kortepeter, 2001; Sidell et al., 2002).

Viruses

Viruses have either DNA or RNA as genetic material. Viruses are intracellular parasites and lack a system for their own metabolism. They require a host for replication (Kortepeter, 2001).

Smallpox

Smallpox is caused by the variola virus. There are two forms: variola major: and the less severe variola minor. In 1980 the World Health Organization declared that smallpox had been eradicated. It is estimated that 80% to 90% of adults and 100% of children are highly susceptible to the disease. Monkeypox, cowpox, and vaccinia are of the same genus, but only smallpox is spread person to person, primarily by droplet or aerosol. Smallpox is thought to be the most likely biologic agent to be used in a terrorist attack. Because it is supposed to have been eradicated, a single case of smallpox should be considered suspect and treated as an international emergency, beginning with notification of local health authorities (Franz et al., 1997; Hardin, 2002; Henderson et al., 1999; Kortepeter, 2001; Sidell et al., 2002).

Following exposure, the incubation period varies from 7 to 19 days, with an average of 12 days. Symptoms usually begin abruptly with fever, vomiting, headache, backache, rigors, and malaise. About 15% of patients develop delirium. Two to three days later, oral lesions appear at the same time as a red rash appears on the face, hands, and forearms. It spreads next to the legs and then the trunk. This centrifugal distribution is an important diagnostic feature. The rash begins as macules and progresses quickly to papules and then pustular vesicles. In contrast to varicella (chickenpox), which has multiple crops, smallpox has one crop of lesions. This single crop of lesions remains in roughly the same stage of progression. In the second week after onset, the pustules form scabs that leave depressed, depigmented scars after healing. The virus can be recovered from scabs, so the patient needs to remain isolated and considered infectious until all the scabs separate.

In the event of an outbreak of smallpox, vaccination of all persons is recommended. Even 4 days after true exposure, the vaccine can prevent or decrease the severity of the symptoms. Smallpox vaccine is not without its problems. The smallpox vaccine is actually vaccinia, a related virus. There are side effects including fever and axillary lymphadenopathy all the way to a postvaccine encephalitis. There are 1 to 2 deaths per million vaccinated along with cases of vaccinia and eczema vaccinatum. In the absence of known true exposure, vaccination is contraindicated in the immunosuppressed (including HIV infection), those with a history of or current eczema, or those in current close contact with persons with one of these conditions (Franz et al., 1997; Hardin, 2002; Henderson et al., 1999; Kortepeter, 2001; Neff, Lane, Fulginiti, & Henderson, 2002; Sidell et al., 2002).

As soon as the diagnosis of smallpox is made, droplet isolation of the patient should be instituted (preferably at home), and all household and face-to-face contacts should be vaccinated and placed under surveillance. If there is a large number of cases, cohorting is indicated, including consideration of a cohort health care facility if indicated (Franz et al., 1997; Hardin, 2002; Henderson et al., 1999; Kortepeter, 2001; Sidell et al., 2002).

Venezuelan Equine Encephalitis

Venezuelan equine encephalitis (VEE) virus is a complex group of eight alpha viruses that are mosquito borne. VEE was tested by the United States in the 1950s and 1960s as a biologic weapon. It can be spread in weaponized form as an aerosol or by deliberately infected mosquitoes. It has an incubation of 1 to 6 days followed by sudden onset of symptoms. Symptoms are severe and include spiking high fevers, shaking chills, severe headache, photophobia, and aching in the lumbar region and legs. Nausea, vomiting, diarrhea, cough, and sore throat may follow. The acute phase lasts approximately 24 to 72 hours, with recovery in 1 to 2 weeks. Neurological involvement is rare (0.5% to 4%). There are a variety of investigational vaccines, each specific to one virus but not to all. Treatment for those with uncomplicated VEE includes analgesia for the headache and myalgias. Those with encephalitis may need anticonvulsants and intensive care–level supportive therapy. Universal precautions are used for VEE, except that the patient should be treated in a screened-in area, with residual insecticides, as the patient is an infection reservoir for mosquitoes for at least 5 days after onset of symptoms (Franz et al., 1997; Kortepeter, 2001; Sidell et al., 2002).

Viral Hemorrhagic Fevers

Viral hemorrhagic fevers (VHFs) encompass a large number of RNA viruses. The syndrome is an acute febrile illness characterized by prostration, myalgias, and evidence of vascular involvement such as easy bleeding, petechiae, and postural hypotension. These symptoms can progress to include all organ systems. The mortality rate ranges widely, depending on the disease, with Ebola being approximately 90%, and the rates for yellow fever and Dengue fever being lower. Lassa, Congo-Crimean, Hantaan, Ebola, and Marburg viruses can be spread by aerosol; so full respiratory isolation, including hair, face, eye, and shoe protection, with negative airflow is indicated. Full respiratory protection with high efficiency particulate air (HEPA) filtered respirators, battery-powered air purifying respirators, or a positive pressure–supplied air respirator is indicated when the patient has a prominent cough, vomiting, diarrhea, or hemorrhage. Downstream personnel, such as linen handlers and environmental service workers, must also use full precautions. Prompt burial or cremation with minimal handling of the remains is recommended. Routine (universal) isolation with special attention to proper disposal of sharps is satisfactory for most of the others, as these patients have a large amount of the virus in their blood and secretions. A vaccine is available for yellow fever. There are other vaccines in various stages of testing and development. Ribavirin has been shown to be of some use in Lassa virus, Rift Valley fever, and Congo-Crimean fever (Borio et al., 2002; Franz et al., 1997; Kortepeter, 2001; Sidell et al., 2002).

Toxins

Toxins are produced by living organisms. Except for the mycotoxins, they are generally not active on the skin. Toxins have a variety of chemical properties in that some are easily denatured by heat or light. For some, such as ricin and mycotoxins, very large quantities would be needed for an effective open air attack. The bacterial toxins, such as Botulinum, are the most toxic substances by weight (Kortepeter, 2001).

Botulinum

Botulinum toxin is derived from *Clostridium botulinum* and two other clostridia species. There are seven recognized forms: A, B, C, D, E, F, and G, all of which produce similar symptoms. This is significant in that different antitoxins are available based on species. Botulinum, which causes botulism, is the most potent toxin known to humans, being 15,000 times more toxic than the nerve agent VX. When untreated, there is an approximate 60% mortality rate. Food-borne botulinum is common in improperly prepared canned foods. The mechanism of action is that the botulinum toxin acts to prevent release of acetylcholine presynaptically, thus, interrupting nerve transmission, the opposite of what occurs in chemical nerve agents. Botulinum is best spread through foods, but it can be aerosolized as well. There is no vaccine (Arnon et al., 2001; Franz et al., 1997; Kortepeter, 2001; Sidell et al., 2002).

Botulinum presents 12 to 72 hours postexposure with symptoms of an afebrile, symmetric, and descending paralysis. Ptosis, diplopia, blurred vision, photophobia, and dilated pupils, with trouble talking, swallowing, and an altered voice, are early signs. Mucous membranes are often dry and the patient may complain of a dry mouth and sore throat. The gag reflex may be absent. Paralysis of the respiratory muscles requires intubation and ventilation. There is generalized weakness followed by the descending flaccid paralysis. Sensory symptoms usually do not occur. Intensive nursing care is required for up to 3 months with full recovery taking up to 1 year. The antitoxin must be administered early, as it can neutralize the circulating toxin only in patients with symptoms that are progressing (CDC, 2006k; Franz et al., 1997; Kortepeter, 2001; Sidell et al., 2002).

Staphylococcal Enterotoxin B

Staphylococcal enterotoxin B (SEB) is one of the exotoxins produced by *Staphylococcus aureus*. It is generally spread through food, but it can be weaponized as an aerosol. SEB is one of the most common causes of food poisoning. Exotoxins are actually excreted from the organism. Because SEB's primary site of action is in the intestine, it is called an enterotoxin. Related toxins include toxic shock syndrome toxin-1. When ingested, SEB can cause extremely high fevers, nausea, vomiting, and diarrhea with profound fluid loss. After oral ingestion, onset of symptoms is 1 to 12 hours, usually 3 to 4 hours. With inhalation, onset of symptoms is 3 to 12 hours. When inhaled, SEB causes a sudden onset of high fever, headache, myalgias, chills, a nonproductive cough, dyspnea, and retrosternal chest pain. Severe cases can lead to pulmonary edema, respiratory failure, and death. The fever lasts up to 5 days in the range of 103° to 106° to 108°F. The cough may last 4 weeks. Vaccines are currently under development (Franz et al., 1997; Kortepeter, 2001; Sidell et al., 2002).

Ricin

Ricin is a toxin made from the mash left over when castor beans are processed to make castor oil. It is fairly easy to extract and can be spread in food or aerosolized. It is less potent than many other agents, so it would take large amounts of product to cover a significant area. When injected, as in the Georgi Markov incident in London in 1978 (Christopher et al., 1997), ricin causes severe necrosis of muscles and lymph nodes near the site of injection, with moderate organ failure following. After ingestion of ricin, symptoms would occur in less than 6 hours.

Expected symptoms in ricin poisoning include nausea, vomiting, necrosis of the gastrointestinal epithelium with resultant upper and lower gastrointestinal bleeding, and renal, hepatic, and splenic necrosis and failure. Dehydration, hypotension, hallucinations, and convulsions can occur. Depending on the dose inhaled, symptoms may occur 4 to 8 hours postexposure. With inhalation, the symptoms may include coughing, fever, chest tightness, dyspnea, nausea, and myalgias and arthralgias. The onset of profuse sweating is often the sign of the symptomatology ending. Humans would be expected to develop severe lung inflammation, with progressive respiratory symptoms including cyanosis and pulmonary edema. Management is primarily supportive, although if it is a known ingestion, vigorous gastric lavage and cathartics are recommended. Vaccines are under development (CDC, 2008; Kortepeter, 2001; Sidell et al., 2002).

Trichothecene Mycotoxins

The trichothecene (T-2) mycotoxins are a group of about 40 compounds produced by the mold (fungi) of *Fusarium, Myrothecium, Trichoderma*, and *Stachybotrys* genus and others. They are extremely stable to heat and ultraviolet light, requiring autoclaving at 1500°F for 30 minutes to be inactivated. When one of these molds is baked into bread and ingested, some individuals developed a lethal illness called alimentary toxic aleukia characterized by initial signs of abdominal pain, nausea and vomiting, and diarrhea with prostration. Within days, chills, fever, myalgias, with bone marrow suppression and secondary sepsis occurred. Those that survived to this point then developed painful throat and laryngeal ulcers with petechiae and ecchymosis, bloody diarrhea, hematemesis, hematuria, epistaxis, and vaginal bleeding (Kortepeter, 2001; Sidell et al., 2002).

Mycotoxins can be released by aerosol, commonly called yellow rain. In an air release, the toxins can be inhaled, absorbed through the skin, and ingested. Within minutes of exposure, burning skin, redness, tenderness, and blistering with progression to skin necrosis with leathery blackening and sloughing of large areas of skin occurs. From eye exposure, symptoms of eye pain, redness, lacrimation, blurred vision, and foreign body sensation occur. Nasal contact results in nasal itching and pain, sneezing, epistaxis, and rhinorrhea. Mouth and throat exposure causes pain and blood-tinged saliva and sputum. Tracheobronchial and pulmonary exposure is characterized by dyspnea, wheezing, and coughing. With ingestion, and thus gastrointestinal exposure, nausea, vomiting, and cramping abdominal pain with watery or bloody diarrhea occur. Systemic findings include weakness, prostration, dizziness, ataxia, and loss of coordination. Tachycardia with hypothermia and hypotension follows in fatal

cases. Death may occur in minutes to hours or days. The only treatment is supportive (Kortepeter, 2001; Sidell et al., 2002).

Radiologic Agents

The environment holds many sources of radiation. People are exposed to diagnostic x-rays, the sun, luminous paints, ceramics, and cosmetics daily. Radiologic accidents and terrorist incidents are on a much different scale in terms of the amount of radiation received and the type of radiation involved (Jacocks, 2003). **Radiologic agents** include any agent that is a source of alpha, beta, or gamma radiation that can be used as a weapon.

Nursing Management of the Patient Exposed to Radiologic Agents

Nursing management of the patient exposed to radiologic agents depends greatly on the dose and severity of the exposure. Application of the nursing process will facilitate a comprehensive approach to patient assessment and care. This again is a situation in which psychological, emotional, and spiritual care are important.

Collaborative Management

All patients exposed to radiologic agents require comprehensive care from a health team including nurses, health care providers, various specialists, and radiologists, depending on the systems involved and the severity of the injury.

Devices

Of all the WMD scenarios, according to experts, the least likely is a nuclear blast because of the materials and technology required, as well as the uncontrolled results. This would be an event such as the atomic bombs dropped in Nagasaki and Hiroshima. For radiologic events, a radiological dispersion device (RDD), the so-called dirty bomb, or a simple radiologic device is considered to be more probable. A simple radiologic device is the spread of radioactive material without an explosion. An example is placing a container on a street corner to expose passersby. A radiological dispersion device does not cause a nuclear reaction. It is an explosive device that releases radioactive material into the environment. This type of device mostly creates trauma patients from the explosion, but complicates medical evacuation of the area and care of the victims because of the contamination. The radiologic contamination from an RDD also causes widespread fear, panic, and terror even if it is too low level to cause actual bodily harm (Jacocks, 2003; Udeani & Aguilera, 2002).

In a nuclear explosion there is the blast, an intense shock wave, thermal radiation manifested as heat and light, followed by nuclear radiation. Nuclear blasts create injury just as blasts from conventional weapons do. The heat and light will create thermal burns. The nuclear radiation will cause acute radiation syndrome (Udeani & Aguilera, 2002). The care of these burns and traumatic injuries would be no different than that of those sustained by other means. Burn injuries are covered in Chapter 68 ⊚, and traumatic injuries are covered in Chapter 74 ⊚.

Types of Radiation

Nonionizing radiation is low energy and nonharmful, such as from classroom lights. Ionizing radiation produces charged ions in the material it strikes. The three most common ionizing particles are alpha, beta, and gamma. The radiation absorbed dose (rad) is a measure of energy deposited in matter by the ionizing radiation. This term is being replaced by the international system *gray* (Gy). One gray equals 100 rad. A roentgen-equivalent-man (rem) is a unit that describes the biologic effect of one rad (Jacocks, 2003; Veenema & Karam, 2003).

Exposure

To describe severity of exposure, the measure of a lethal dose is used. An exposure of 350 rad, or 3.5 gray, will cause death in half the people exposed, if no medical care is received, within 60 days. This is referred to as a lethal dose of 50/60 (LD 50/60). With medical treatment the lethal dose can be increased to between 600 and 800 rads. Unlike chemicals, radiation cannot be detected with the five senses. Geiger counters, dosimeters, and various other detection equipment are employed when radiation is suspected (CRA, 2003; Jacocks, 2003; Udeani & Aguilera, 2002).

Ionizing Radiation

Alpha particles are very big and heavy. They penetrate poorly, traveling only 1 to 2 inches. They are easily stopped by a piece of paper or clothing and do not penetrate the dead skin layer. External alpha radiation rarely causes a health risk, although decontamination is necessary. If introduced through broken skin, inhaled, or ingested causing internal contamination, alpha particles can cause extensive damage especially to the kidneys, lungs, liver, and skeletal system (Fell-Carlson, 2003; Jacocks, 2003; Udeani & Aguilera, 2002; Veenema & Karam, 2003). This is the radiation particle in polonium-210, the material found in the former Russian spy Alexander Litvinenko at his death (BBC, 2007).

Beta particles are smaller than alpha particles. Beta particles can travel about 10 feet through the air and can penetrate skin a short distance causing severe burns ("beta burns"). Damage to the eyes can occur from beta particles, and when ingested or inhaled internal injuries can occur. Shielding with heavy clothing, walls, or thin metals is effective protection against penetration of beta particles (Fell-Carlson, 2003; Jacocks, 2003; Udeani & Aguilera, 2002; Veenema & Karam, 2003).

Gamma rays are emitted during nuclear detonation and are present in fallout. Gamma rays can travel several hundred feet in air and travel through tissue to the deep organs. Gamma radiation is also referred to as "penetrating radiation." Because of this penetration, gamma rays are an external and internal hazard. Dense materials such as lead, concrete, and steel can block penetration of gamma rays. Neutrons are also released in nuclear detonations, and they can penetrate thick concrete (CRA, 2003; Fell-Carlson, 2003; Jacocks, 2003; Udeani & Aguilera, 2002; Veenema & Karam, 2003).

Routes of Entry

Gamma radiation can enter the body by penetration, and this is termed irradiation. In this type of exposure, the victim is not radioactive. This is the same process by which diagnostic x-rays are performed.

Radiologic contamination occurs when particulate matter that is radioactive is released. People become contaminated when the material is deposited on the skin, ingested, inhaled, or absorbed in some manner. Internal contamination can lead to incorporation, whereby the radioactive material is assimilated into body tissue. This can cause both immediate and delayed problems.

Alpha and beta particles can be inhaled if they are airborne. Radiation can be injected and ingested. With dermal exposure, radiation can cause an external burn and or be absorbed into the body if the skin is broken.

Radiation exposure depends on the three principles of time, distance, and shielding. The shorter the time of exposure, the less absorption by the tissue. Radiologic exposure follows the inverse square law in relationship to distance, so that if the distance from the source is doubled, the dose rate of exposure is decreased by a factor of 4. If a source has a radiation level of 100 radiation absorbed dose (R/hr) at 1 foot, at 2 feet the radiation would be 25 R/hr, and at 8 feet it would be 1.56 R/hr. Shielding refers to the materials between the person and the source of radiation. The more dense the material, such as lead, the more protection is afforded (CRA, 2003; Jacocks, 2003).

Radiation Exposure

In most hospitals, one of the radiologists is usually the designated radiation safety officer in charge of determining exposure and risk. Most hospitals have Geiger counters readily available to determine the simple presence or absence of a certain level of radiation in the environment. Personnel involved in the care of radiation victims will need dosimeters to determine their exposure. These personnel will more than likely need decontamination. Depending on the severity of the exposure, many different effects can be seen. Those exposed to low-level external contamination may have skin burns that will heal, to no sequelae. These are *not* considered to be at higher risk later for cancer. Many of those with internal contamination will need follow-up monitoring to measure clearance of the radionuclides from the body. These individuals are also not considered to be at higher risk for cancers later in life. Those exposed to higher levels of radiation that have caused symptoms are considered to be at elevated risk for cancer later (Veenema & Karam, 2003).

In lower level radiation exposure, early treatment can be the key to decrease incorporation (the uptake of radiation into the cells of the body) and decrease symptoms and sequelae. Potassium iodide can have a protective effect on the thyroid if taken before, or within 3 to 4 hours after, exposure to a radioactive cloud. It comes in capsules as well as in liquid. It protects the thyroid gland by filling the receptor sites so that radioactive iodines cannot bind (CDC, 2006n).

Prussian blue is a blue dye first produced in 1704 for use in Prussian military uniforms. Prussian blue can be taken to help remove certain ingested radioactive substances. It works by binding to cesium and thallium in the gut, which are then excreted in the stool. Prussian blue reduces cesium's half-life from approximately 110 days to approximately 30 days. It reduces thallium's half-life from approximately 8 days to approximately 3 days. Prussian blue is still commonly available as a dye and as a paint in art stores (CDC, 2006l; Seed, 2002).

Acute Radiation Syndrome

Acute radiation syndrome (ARS) is an acute illness caused by irradiation of the whole body, or at least a significant part of the body. Radiation generates highly reactive free radicals and directly damages proteins, messenger RNA (mRNA), and DNA. In smaller doses, it interferes with cell proliferation whereas in higher doses it causes cell death. Those body tissues with a higher turnover rate are more susceptible to the effects of radiation, such as the bone marrow (Merck Manuals, 2005). Acute radiation syndrome varies in severity based on dose and the age and relative state of wellness of the person exposed. The severity and extent of the symptoms increase and the duration of each phase shortens as the radiation dose goes up. There are four phases to ARS (Jacocks, 2003).

Prodromal Phase

The prodromal phase has an onset of minutes to hours, and lasts from hours to days, depending on the dose of radiation. It is characterized by the relatively rapid onset of nausea, vomiting, and malaise. At higher levels, fever, hypotension, and diarrhea can also be present. Onset of symptoms within 30 minutes of exposure is most likely indicative of a lethal dose. The gastrointestinal symptoms usually resolve within 2 days, but the fatigue and malaise often continue. At higher doses, 200 rads and above, lymphocyte counts will decrease and cognitive impairment can occur (Jacocks, 2003; Udeani & Aguilera, 2002; Veenema & Karam, 2003).

Latent Phase

Following the prodromal phase, there is a transition phase in which the individual will be relatively symptom free. This latent phase varies from no time to 2 weeks, depending on the dose received (Jacocks, 2003).

Illness Phase

In the illness phase, also called the manifest stage, there is overt illness. This phase presents as a hematopoietic (blood-forming) system, gastrointestinal system, central nervous system, or skin syndrome, or a combination of any of these, based on the system injured.

The hematopoietic system shows the earliest indications of the severity of the radiation exposure. There will be a drop in all cell counts due to death of the bone marrow. A depressed immune system, fever, sepsis, and hemorrhage are common. Those with lower level exposure can recover if they receive medical support and their bone marrow regenerates. Medical support includes blood transfusions, protection from infection, and antibiotic therapy. Occasionally, stem cell transplantation is needed (Jacocks, 2003; Udeani & Aguilera, 2002; Veenema & Karam, 2003).

Gastrointestinal symptoms, nausea, vomiting, and diarrhea are usually seen in doses greater than 600 rad and are a result of damage to the epithelial cells lining the small intestine. The symptoms lead to fluid and electrolyte imbalances and opportunistic infections, which can lead to septicemia. Symptomatic care is prescribed including antiemetics, sedatives, fluid replacement, and a bland diet. Persistent high fevers and bloody diarrhea are ominous signs (Jacocks, 2003; Udeani & Aguilera, 2002; Veenema & Karam, 2003).

The central nervous system is one of the most radiation-resistant tissues in the body. Central nervous system symptoms are seen with doses in excess of 1,000 rads. With this level of radiation, there is usually almost immediate nausea, vomiting, disorientation, and seizures from the loss of fluid, electrolytes, edema, and increased intracranial pressure. Death follows within hours to days. Care involves administering sedatives and analgesics to control seizures and anxiety, as this syndrome is fatal (Jacocks, 2003; Udeani & Aguilera, 2002; Veenema & Karam, 2003).

Recovery or Death

Mortality from ARS is directly related to the amount of radiation exposure. Those with a large exposure will usually die within several months of the exposure. The deaths are most commonly related to opportunistic infections as a result of bone marrow destruction. Survivors' recovery phase may last for several months up to two years.

◼ Explosions

Injuries from explosions run the gamut of traumatic injuries from extremely minor ones, not needing medical attention, to complete crush and incineration. Blasts cause injuries that are not always described in basic trauma chapters. Although the mechanism of injury for these problems is a blast force, these injuries are treated in the usual manner (CDC, 2006m; Riley, Clark, & Wong, 2002; Udeani & Aguilera, 2002).

Blast Injuries

There are a few injuries specific to blasts. Blasts are divided into high order explosives (HE) and low order explosives (LE), based on the strength of the ordinance (Chart 72–8, p. 2404). The injuries are divided into primary, secondary, and tertiary. Primary blast injuries are usually caused by high order explosives. Primary blast injuries result from the direct effect of increases in atmospheric pressure causing barotrauma. Ruptured eardrums are the most common injury. The most severe injuries are to the lung and include pneumothoraces, contusions, hemorrhage, bronchopleural fistulas, thrombosis, disseminated intravascular coagulation (DIC), and adult respiratory distress syndrome (ARDS). High order explosives can also cause bowel perforation, gastrointestinal bleeding, shearing injuries to the mesentery, rupture of the testicles, and other solid organ damage. Concussion and traumatic brain injury may also result (CDC, 2006m) (Chart 72–9, p. 2404).

Secondary blast injuries are from flying debris. These include minor lacerations, contusions, and abrasions; dust and smoke inhalation; all the way to impaled large foreign objects and being trapped by large pieces of debris. Tertiary blast injuries occur when the person is thrown by the blast through the air and the person strikes another object. Any variety of injuries can be expected (CDC, 2006m; Riley et al., 2002; Udeani & Aguilera, 2002).

◼ How These Events Affect the Health Care System

In the after action reports of the Tokyo sarin gas attack, numerous problems with the hospital disaster plan were identified. Although over 4,000 presented for treatment, less than 1,000 were found to have any symptoms. There was no plan for moving casualties, family, and media through the hospital system. People came into the hospital from all three entrances, causing mass chaos. The entire hospital was contaminated, as the agent was not

CHART 72–8 Blast Injury from High Order Explosives

Category	Mechanism	Body Part Affected	Types of Injuries
Primary	Impact of the overpressurization wave with body surfaces	Gas-filled structures the most susceptible: lungs, gastrointestinal (GI) tract, and middle ear	Blast lung Tympanic membrane (TM) rupture and middle ear damage Abdominal hemorrhage and perforation Eye rupture Concussion and traumatic brain injury (TBI)
Secondary	Flying debris and bomb fragments	Any body part	Penetrating ballistic (fragmentation) or blunt injuries Eye penetration (can be occult)
Tertiary	Individual thrown by the blast wind	Any body part	Fracture and traumatic amputation Any blunt traumatic injury Closed and open brain injuries
Quaternary	All explosion-related injuries, illnesses, or diseases not due to primary, secondary, or tertiary mechanisms Includes exacerbation or complications of existing conditions	Any body part	Burns (flash, partial, and full thickness) Crush injuries Closed and open brain injuries Asthma, chronic obstructive pulmonary disease (COPD), or other breathing problems from dust, smoke, or toxic fumes Angina Hyperglycemia, hypertension

Source: Adapted from Centers for Disease Control and Prevention (CDC). (2006, June 14). *Explosions and blast injuries: A primer for clinicians.* Table 1, Mechanisms of blast injury. Retrieved December 12, 2006, from http://www.bt.cdc.gov/masscasualties/explosions.asp.

CHART 72–9 Blast Injuries by System

System	Injury or Condition
Auditory	Tympanic membrane (TM) rupture, ossicular disruption, cochlear damage, foreign body
Eye, orbit, face	Perforated globe, foreign body, air embolism, fractures
Respiratory	Blast lung, hemothorax, pneumothorax, pulmonary contusion and hemorrhage, arteriovenous (AV) fistulas (air embolism), airway epithelial damage, aspiration pneumonitis, sepsis
Digestive	Bowel perforation, hemorrhage, ruptured liver or spleen, sepsis, mesenteric ischemia from air embolism
Circulatory	Cardiac contusion, myocardial infarction from air embolism, shock, vasovagal hypotension, peripheral vascular injury, air embolism–induced injury
Central nervous system (CNS)	Concussion, closed and open brain injury, stroke, spinal cord injury, air embolism–induced injury
Renal	Renal contusion, laceration, acute renal failure due to rhabdomyolysis, hypotension, and hypovolemia
Extremity	Traumatic amputation, fractures, crush injuries, compartment syndrome, burns, cuts, lacerations, acute arterial occlusion, air embolism–induced injury

Source: Adapted from Centers for Disease Control and Prevention (CDC). (2006, June 14). *Explosions and blast injuries: A primer for clinicians.* Table 2, Overview of explosive-related injuries. Retrieved December 12, 2006, from http://www.bt.cdc.gov/masscasualties/explosions.asp.

identified until 3 hours after the event. Although gowns, gloves, and simple masks were available, chemical-resistant personal protective equipment was not accessible. Many hospital workers suffered secondary exposure. The hospital used 700 ampoules of pralidoximine and 2,800 ampoules of atropine. Additional supplies had to be flown in to meet the demand (Lee, 2003).

WMD as Medical Disasters

Routine life in a hospital currently revolves around overcrowding and understaffing with shortages of needed supplies. The addition of a WMD event is expected to break most already overstretched health care systems. WMD events are the ultimate mass casualty incident and are medical disasters. These events overwhelm the hospital's ability to allocate resources because the high number of casualties affects the infrastructure of the health care delivery system. About 80% of victims walk in for health care, and hospitals provide the majority of that care; and yet most disaster plans still rely on field triage to assess and spread out the people needing care. Personal protective equipment (PPE) is a must in all situations. All disaster plans must address mass casualty incidents and WMD, with a structured plan in which there are clear lines of command and communication, and clearly delineated roles; and the media need to be included in the plan. The media can be used to decrease the mass hysteria and get vital information to the public (Compton, Stewart-Craig, & Doak, 1999; Scharoun, Van Caulil, & Liberman, 2002; U.S. General Accounting Office, 2003). President Bush (2002), in the *National Strategy to Combat Weapons of Mass Destruction*, states, ". . . appropriate civilian agencies must possess the full range of operational capabilities to counter the threat and use of WMD by states, and terrorists against the United States, our military forces, and friends and allies." This is a call for action and preparation, including for the health care team.

Specific Problems

According to the August 2003 U.S. General Accounting Office (GAO; in 2004 it became the U.S. Government Accountability Office) report on hospital preparedness, most urban hospitals have plans, or are working on plans, but most do not have the capacity to handle a large increase in patient load. This includes staffing, supplies, equipment, and space. Of particular note were few ventilators, few isolation beds, few PPE suits, and the inability to handle more than 6 patients for decontamination per hour. (The GAO report indicates that 2,700 ventilators are being added to the Strategic National Stockpile.) The tremendous expense for rarely, if ever, used resources was cited as a concern regarding preparation.

In the initial response, quick identification of the agent, isolation, decontamination, and care needed must be identified. The verification and appropriate use of volunteers must be addressed. Health care workers may be reluctant to go to work because of family care issues and fear of exposure to the agent. Identification of the patients present and family and friends searching for loved ones needs an action plan (Compton et al., 1999; Scharoun et al., 2002; U.S. General Accounting Office, 2003). Telephone lines, including cell phones, are usually quickly overwhelmed. Especially because of outside calls, the hospital telephone system is usually unusable. Two-way radios, ham radios, e-mail, and cable television can all be used to facilitate communications (Lenzer, 2003). Initiating the disaster plan, decontamination concerns and protecting personnel, having adequate initial supplies and personnel, and initiating care to the patients, while preserving the crime scene and evidence, presents a daunting task. For adequate preparation, drilling of the disaster plan must be routinely done.

Problems After the Initial Response

Problems after the initial response include continuing with identifying the patients that are present, including full demographic information. Family and friends will be looking for missing loved ones, and there needs to be a communications system for this information. The need for good communication and a functioning communications system cannot be overemphasized. In a WMD event, a large number of patients admitted to the hospital will need ongoing care. Many of the patients will have similar symptoms and require similar care. This will overtax the pharmacy, hospital equipment, and supplies for some time to come. In addition, decontamination of the hospital or parts of the hospital may be necessary (Compton et al., 1999; Scharoun et al., 2002; U.S. General Accounting Office, 2003).

There will be bigger issues of obtaining supplies and adequate staff for the long term. A sample suggestion regarding supplies is that hospitals keep atropine in the dry form, as the usual stock will be almost immediately depleted due to the amounts used. Staff will face long hours, poor work conditions, and tremendous stress and pressure. Along with nurses and health care providers, food service workers, secretaries, maintenance, environmental services, laundry, central supply technicians, and a host of other personnel will be needed. Special attention needs to be paid to the psychological and emotional health of the worker. The stress on the patients, families, and community will all also be factors (Compton et al., 1999; Scharoun et al., 2002; U.S. General Accounting Office, 2003).

National Incident Command System

Managing a terrorist event requires the cooperation of multiple agencies working together. To this end, President George W. Bush wrote the February 28, 2003, *Homeland Security Presidential Directive Five (HSPD-5)*, which directs the secretary of the Department of Homeland Security to establish a comprehensive national incident management system (Bush, 2003). Appropriately called the National Incident Management System (NIMS), NIMS provides a framework for all levels of government and local agencies to work together in preparing for, responding to, and recovering from domestic incidents. NIMS is housed in the Federal Emergency Management Agency (FEMA) Emergency Management Institute (EMI). EMI's main goal is emergency management training (Ridge, 2004).

NIMS is based on the **incident command system (ICS)**, initially designed for use at California wildfire sites by its fire departments. NIMS creates a standard but flexible all-hazards organizational structure whereby the various agencies involved can interact and communicate in an organized manner. It is designed to be used in all phases of disaster management: prevention, preparedness, response, recovery, and mitigation (Ridge, 2004). NIMS has an incident commander (IC), one person in charge of the entire operation. The operation itself is broken into four main areas: operations, planning, logistics, and finance, with a "chief" over each division. Those four chiefs report directly to the incident commander. Also reporting directly to the commander are a safety officer, public information officer, and liaison officer. Room is made in the structure for an expert position who would answer directly to the incident commander (Ridge, 2004). Extensive training on the NIMS system is available from FEMA; its website is kept up to date with new training sessions as they are developed.

The incident command system was adapted to the hospital environment initially by the state of California and evolved into what is now called the hospital incident command system (HICS). The new version of HICS was released in October 2006.

Hospital Incident Command System

HICS uses this same structure adapted to a hospital environment. The HICS manual and supporting documents, available free online, contain the structure with all job descriptions, sample policies and procedures, as well as sample documents/tracking sheets, which can be copied and/or adapted for use as needed (CRA, 2003; California Emergency Medical Services Authority [EMSA], 2006). The hospital incident command system naturally fits into the National Incident Command System, which allows the hospital to speak the same language and use the same divisions as all other agencies.

Organization

The hospital incident command system would be used in the hospital any time there is an incident with the potential to overwhelm resources (Figure 72–4 ■, p. 2406). This could include large accidents with multiple victims all the way to massive WMD events. With HICS, the plan is flexible to the situation. Only those positions and functions that are required by the incident need to be

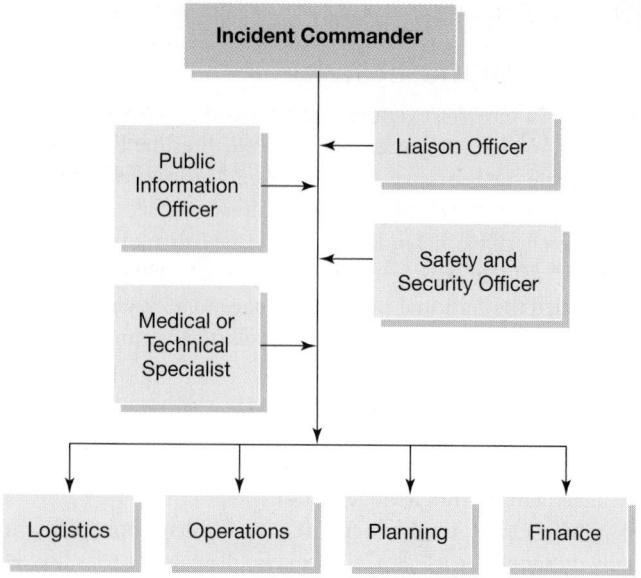

FIGURE 72-4 ■ Hospital incident command system.

activated. Many of the positions can be combined and filled by one person. The plan gives a clear chain of command and clear responsibilities, has a common language and common mission, prioritizes duties, and ensures thorough documentation of actions. The comprehensive documentation allows for a more complete evaluation of the event in the after action sessions. It also improves recovery of expenses while decreasing liability (EMSA, 2006).

HICS uses the same basic structure as NIMS. There is an incident commander (IC) to whom the public information officer, the safety and security officer, the liaison officer, and the section chiefs answer. The incident commander organizes and directs the emergency operations center and gives overall direction for the hospital operations. The public information officer provides information to the media, releases other information as indicated, and assists with communication. The safety and security officer monitors and has authority over the safety of rescue operations and hazardous conditions. This position organizes and enforces scene, facility, and traffic protection and security. The liaison officer functions as the contact person for representatives of other agencies such as the fire department and police departments. As with NIMS, there is room made in the administrative structure for a medical or technical specialist if needed. An example of a needed specialist might be a radiation specialist in the event of a dirty bomb (EMSA, 2006).

Sections

There are four sections: planning, logistics, finance, and operations. The head of each section is a chief. Each section can be further divided if needed. This subdivides the work and allows for a manageable span of management responsibility for each individual (EMSA, 2006).

The planning section ensures the formulation and documentation of an overall response plan and helps to set objectives. It gathers data and status reports from various areas within the hospital to aid in decision making. The planning section is responsible for duties such as providing a situation status report to the hospital and hospital workers every 4 to 6 hours. Planning

also interacts with other sections such as assisting in establishing a plan for medical staff rotation in cooperation with personnel from the operations section.

The logistics section provides the hospital environment and materials to meet all objectives. This includes organizing and directing all operations associated with maintaining the physical environment; adequate food for patients, visitors, and personnel; shelter; and adequate medical and pharmaceutical supplies. This includes such duties as transportation, assessing damaged areas for use or evacuation, communications, and materials supply.

The finance section provides the funding for operations and ensures hospital-wide documentation of activities and expenses to assist with recovery of costs. Large events typically cost millions of dollars in salaries, materials, equipment, and other costs. A single incident can bankrupt a facility without reimbursement. Even federal relief dollars require documentation of expenses for receipt of reimbursement.

The operations section covers much of the day-to-day work of delivering medical care. This includes matching staff to patient needs, organizing inpatient care, and managing the treatment areas such as triage, the emergency department, operating rooms, discharging of patients, and morgue operations (EMSA, 2006).

START Triage

To sort through the massive influx of people during mass casualty incidents, there needs to be a method of identifying those most in need of decontamination and care. The Simple Triage and Rapid Treatment (START) system was designed by Hoag Hospital and the Newport Beach, California, Fire Department for use in multicasualty incidents. It has become the standard method of triage in mass casualty. This method is effective both in the field at the scene of an incident and for sorting at the door of the hospital. START is not designed for use in the pediatric population. A corollary system called "Jump START" has criteria for children based on the same categories (Disaster Management Systems, 2005; Romig, 2008).

The START triage system uses four categories: Red means immediate care needed, with usually two or more systems affected. Yellow means delayed care needed, with usually one system involved. Green means minor care is needed; and black means deceased or that death is expected, with no life-extending care to be delivered (Figure 72-5 ■).

To determine the appropriate category, respirations, perfusion, and neurological status are checked. The first step is to identify the "walking wounded." An announcement is made that all who can walk go to a designated area. These persons are all automatically assigned to the green or minor category. For those left, the airway is opened and respirations are ranked as a red if greater that 30 and the person receives a tag; if respirations are less than 30, no tag is given; and a black tag is given if respirations are zero. Next, major hemorrhage is controlled and perfusion is assessed by checking for a radial pulse, as one must have a blood pressure of at least 80 mmHg to have a radial pulse. If there is no radial pulse, the legs are elevated and a red immediate tag is applied; if there is a pulse, no tag is applied. The last step is to check the neurological status. If the person can answer a simple yes–no question, the tag applied is a yellow delayed tag. If unable to answer, the person receives a red immediate tag.

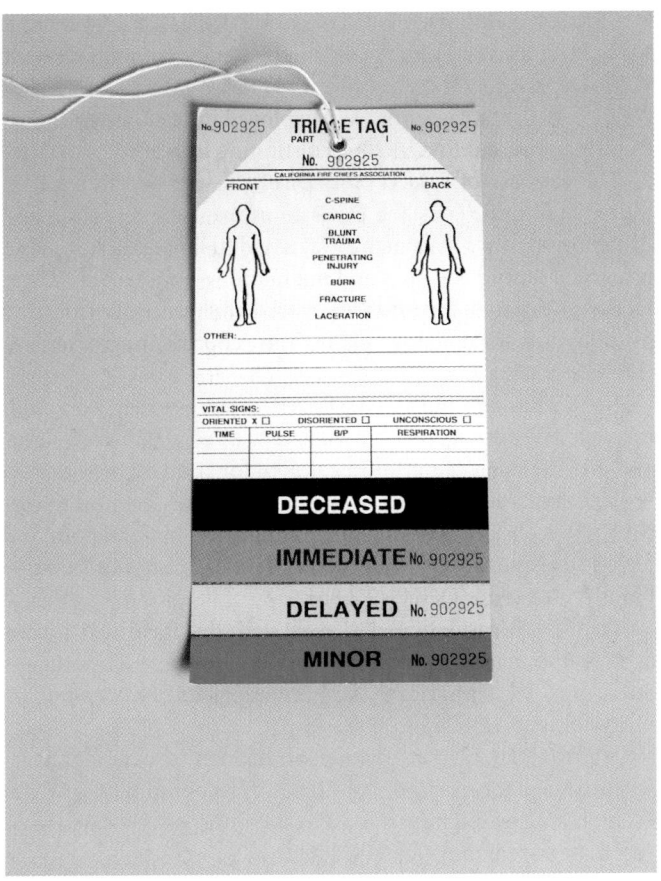

FIGURE 72–5 ■ Triage tag.

For a red tag, the immediate care needed category, classic assessment findings include that respirations are present only after repositioning the airway, respiratory rate is less than 8 or greater than 30, capillary refill is delayed more than 2 seconds, and there may be a significant decrease in level of consciousness. For a yellow tag, the delayed care needed category, the injuries can be controlled or treated for a limited time in the field. Green, the minor care designation, includes those who are ambulatory, with or without minor injuries, that do not require immediate or significant treatment. The black, the deceased or expectant category, is for those with no spontaneous effective respiration after the airway is repositioned (Community Emergency Response Team–Los Angeles [CERT-LA], 2003; Disaster Management Systems, 2005; MCLNO, 2003).

As with any methodology, the START triage system requires practice for proficiency. Some hospitals use START tags on designated days throughout the month during routine operations as a drill for personnel to remain familiar with the tags and system.

■ National Resources

In addition to regional and state supplies, there are national resources available to assist in a disaster situation.

Strategic National Stockpile

The National Pharmaceutical Stockpile program was created in 1999 during the Clinton administration under the auspices of Centers for Disease Control and Prevention (CDC). Its original funding was only $5.2 million per year. The National Pharmaceutical Stockpile program was renamed the **Strategic National Stockpile (SNS)** program and was moved into the new Department of Homeland Security on March 1, 2003. The purpose of the stockpile is to maintain a national repository of pharmaceutical agents, vaccines, medical supplies, and equipment that will be delivered to the site of a large-scale disaster to augment local and state resources in order to decrease morbidity and mortality in the civilian population (Esbitt, 2003; Williams, 2002).

Organization

The Strategic National Stockpile is organized using a five-tiered approach. These are the 12-hour push packs, vendor managed inventory, storage and rapid deployment of vaccines, buying power with surge capacity, and technical assistance. To obtain Strategic National Stockpile assets, the affected state's governor must request the SNS from the CDC. The CDC director will evaluate the request and release the supplies if deemed necessary (CDC, 2005; Esbitt, 2003).

Although the SNS delivers material and technical assistance, the state and local agencies must provide the manpower to use and distribute the materials to the population. There is no charge for the supplies themselves. The state will need nurses, pharmacists, and health care providers for the dispensing sites, but can use nonmedical volunteers to assist with crowd control, move materials, and operate machinery such as forklifts (Esbitt, 2003; Williams, 2002).

Push Packs

Although the 12-hour push pack is less than 4% of the stockpile, it is what is most commonly considered in terms of the SNS. The push packs are so named because they can be shipped within 12 hours of the decision to deploy the assets (Chart 72–10). There are 12 of these located around the United States. Each set consists of 100 containers weighing approximately 50 tons total. Each container is on wheels and is easily moved by one or two people. The containers are designed to fill a 747 cargo jet completely. The receiving site must have about 12,000 square feet of space for storage, repackaging bulk supplies, performing inventory control, and distributing the supplies (Esbitt, 2003; Williams, 2002).

The contents of the push packs are reviewed by content experts frequently and changed based on the current perceived threats. The contents of the push packs include bulk oral antibiotic agents, intravenous and intramuscular medications, analgesics, and other emergency medications. They also include equipment such as pill-counting equipment and an automatic packaging machine. Other supplies include intravenous supplies, airway supplies, and

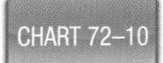 **Contents of 12-Hour Push Pack**

Antibiotics and other pharmaceuticals

IV supplies

Airway supplies

Bandage supplies

Pill counting and packaging equipment

Through vendor managed inventory (VMI): vaccines, antivirals/antitoxins bandaging supplies. It costs about $9 million per month to store and maintain the push packs (Esbitt, 2003; Williams, 2002).

The SNS delivered a team of technical advisers to New York on September 11, 2001, and a 12-hour push pack. The technical advisers arrived 5 hours after deployment and the push pack arrived 7 hours after deployment (Esbitt, 2003). The SNS was most recently deployed to the Gulf Coast region following Hurricanes Katrina and Rita in 2005.

Vendor Managed Inventory

Vendor managed inventory (VMI) is federally owned inventory that is stored by the vendor until needed. Vendor managed inventory is designed to be used to provide specific pharmaceuticals and supplies when the WMD agent is known or for smaller scale events when an entire push pack is not needed. It can also be used to resupply at the scene when a push pack has been deployed. When needed as part of the initial response, the goal is to deliver the VMI within 12 hours. During the anthrax events of 2001, more than 50 requests for antibiotics were filled and shipped to 11 states and the District of Columbia. Each shipment delivery time was less than 5 hours (Esbitt, 2003).

Vaccine and antitoxins are stockpiled using VMI. When shipped, special cooler containers are used to maintain the products at the correct temperature. For smallpox, only the vaccine, diluent, bifurcated needles, and transfer needles are sent. The location must supply items such as gloves, gauze, Band-Aids, sharps containers, and waste bags (Williams, 2002).

The federal government has special prearranged contracts that allow for the purchase of large amounts of supplies and pharmaceuticals should the need arise. In this surge capacity contracting, there are over 97 lines of inventory (Williams, 2002).

Technical Support

A team of advisers, called the Technical Advisory Response Unit (TARU), is 5 to 7 experts in logistics, public health, communications, operations, and emergency response. The TARU can help state and local authorities with receiving, managing, distributing, dispensing, and replenishing the SNS. These units can provide technical assistance with operation of the machinery such as the repackaging unit. They can assist in recovering the support equipment and cargo containers, and in recovering unused SNS assets and materials (Esbitt, 2003).

National Disaster Medical System

Housed in the Department of Health and Human Services, the Office of Preparedness and Response directs and manages the National Disaster Medical System (NDMS), which ensures resources are available after a disaster that overwhelms the local health care resources. Under the National Response Plan, NDMS is responsible for coordinating and managing the federal response to federally declared disasters and major emergencies including natural disasters, technologic disasters, major transportation incidents, and acts of terrorism. Within NDMS are six major divisions: Disaster Medical Assistance Teams (DMATs), Disaster Mortuary Operational Response Teams (DMORTs), National Veterinary Response Teams (NVRTs), National Pharmacy Response Teams (NPRTs), National Nurse Response Teams (NNRTs), and Federal Coordinating Centers (FCCs). All of these teams are made up of volunteers who, when deployed, become federal employees for the duration of their tour. There

is a modest reimbursement. For most of these teams, there is special training and online continuing education requirements (U.S. Department of Health and Human Services [DHHS], 2008a). All of the divisions were deployed in response to Hurricanes Katrina and Rita in 2005 continuing into 2006.

The services of DMAT and DMORT will be discussed in more detail next. First, the FCCs coordinate the reception and distribution of patients being evacuated to an area. They play a role in recruiting hospitals and maintaining non–federal hospital participation in NDMS. They work with local authorities and hospitals in developing plans and coordinating exercises (DHHS, 2008b).

NVRTs are very much like DMAT teams, but they work with animals. The purpose of these teams is to assess the medical needs and provide stabilization and treatment for animals; provide surveillance regarding animal disease, biologic and chemical terrorism, public health assessments, animal decontamination, and technical assistance regarding food and water quality; and provide hazard mitigation (DHHS, 2008b).

The NPRT was designed to assist with the chemical prophylaxis or vaccination if needed for a biologic event. These teams are comprised of pharmacists, pharmacy technicians, and pharmacy students (DHHS, 2008b).

The NNRT will be used when an incident occurs that overwhelms the nation's supply of nurses in responding to a WMD event. It is also designed to assist in chemoprophylaxis or a mass vaccination program (DHHS, 2008b).

Disaster Medical Assistance Teams

The Disaster Medical Assistance Team (DMAT) is part of NDMS (DHHS, 2008b; Dayton DMAT, 2008; Riley, 2003). A **DMAT** is a group of volunteer health care providers, nurses, emergency medical technicians, technical staff, and other health care professionals and support staff designed to provide emergency medical services. They can provide care at a temporary site such as a tent, or at a fixed site such as a hospital. In mass casualty situations, the team can provide triage, medical care, and prepare patients for evacuation. The DMAT may assist overloaded local staff at local health care facilities and/or provide primary health care. When deployed, the team arrives with enough supplies and equipment to sustain itself for 72 hours (Dayton DMAT, 2008; Riley, 2003). Following Hurricanes Katrina and Rita, multiple DMAT teams were deployed to the entire Gulf region. They performed duties ranging from vaccination clinics, to relieving local hospital staff in the hospital, to providing the primary source of medical care in a decimated area.

Types of DMAT Teams

A level 1 DMAT travels with all of its own supplies and equipment, including tents (Figure 72–6 ■). It is fully self-contained for 72 hours. A level 2 DMAT is deployed with another team, or it relieves a level 1 team. It is not considered self-sufficient, as it does not carry its own supplies. A level 3 team has local responsibilities only. There are about 55 DMAT teams. Other specialty teams include burn teams, pediatric teams, veterinary teams, and mortuary teams (Dayton DMAT, 2008; Riley, 2003).

Deployment

DMATs are completely voluntary and used only within the United States. Once activated for deployment, the team member becomes a temporary federal employee. As a federal em-

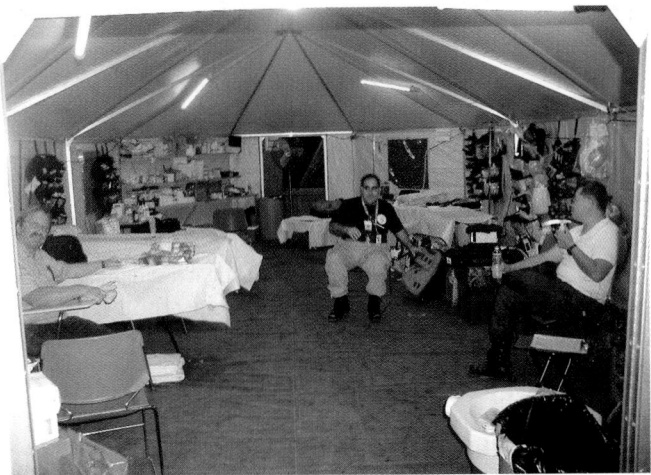

FIGURE 72–6 ■ DMAT tent and team members.
Source: Kathleen Osborn

ployee, any license or certification is automatically recognized in all 50 states. Team members are paid wages, travel is reimbursed, and there is a food stipend. There are meetings and training to attend including such things as setting up the tents, familiarization with the equipment, and learning how to work within the team. Each member is required to provide certain personal gear needed for deployment such as eye and ear protection, leather work gloves, canteen, sleeping bag, camping knife, hand cleanser gel, and toilet paper. Further information on becoming part of a DMAT team is available online (Dayton DMAT, 2008; Riley, 2003).

Disaster Mortuary Operational Response Teams

In large-scale events, along with large numbers of ill or injured people, there will be large numbers of the dead. Management of the dead requires special training and resources. Disaster Mortuary Operational Response Teams (**DMORTs**) are designed to assist with this task. The DMORTs are under the NDMS through OEP in the Department of Health and Human Services in the same manner as the DMAT. DMORTs can provide comprehensive mass fatality management for incidents that overwhelm local resources. As with DMATs, these are volunteers who become temporary federal employees when deployed. As people in the United States expect full identification, federal level assistance is needed in large events due to the tremendous drain on resources and finances (DHHS, 2008b).

Services

DMORT extensive services include mobile morgue operations, forensic exam assistance, DNA acquisition, remains identification, search and recovery, scene documentation, medical and psychological support, embalming and casketing, a family assistance center, antemortem and postmortem data collection, record keeping, processing of personal effects, coordination of release of remains, communication, and safety officers and specialists (Chart 72–11). DMORT teams can identify those requiring decontamination prior to release or autopsy. In identifying remains, they have extensive data gathering, which has helped in identifying even minute remains allowing the family to have closure. Recent missions have included the Space Shuttle *Columbia* disaster and the World Trade Center disaster (DHHS, 2008b; Smith, 2003).

CHART 72–11   What Can DMORT Do to Help?

- Mobile morgue operations
- Forensic examination
- DNA acquisition
- Remains identification
- Search and recovery
- Scene documentation
- Medical/psychological support
- Embalming/casketing
- Family assistance center
- Antemortem data collection
- Postmortem data collection
- Records data entry
- Database administration
- Personal effects processing
- Coordination of release of remains
- Provide a liaison to United States Public Health Service (USPHS)
- Provide communications equipment
- Safety officers and specialists

Critical Incident Stress Management

The psychological impact of a mass casualty event cannot be overestimated. When the event is deliberate, such as with a terrorist event, the impact is event greater. A common goal of terrorist activity is to threaten the psychological cohesion and well-being of a community. Terrorism is psychological warfare. The psychological casualties of an event will far outweigh the physical casualties by design (Everly, 2003). Persons involved in the incident itself, health care workers, rescuers, as well as the general population will all be affected. Efforts to mitigate the adverse psychological effects of terrorism include providing training and education before incidents occur, providing crisis intervention at the time of the event, and supplying the community with information and assistance following an incident (Everly, 2003).

Stress

Stress is the physical and psychological arousal and response to a perceived or real threat, challenge, or change. When the environment changes, people change (Mitchell & Bray, 1980).

Common Signs of Stress

Common signs of stress are divided into emotional, behavioral, cognitive, and physical indicators. Examples of emotional signs of stress include numbness, anger, grief, depression, feeling overwhelmed, hopelessness, and being overly worried. Behavioral signs include changes in one's ordinary pattern of behavior, changes in eating, decreased personal hygiene, a change in smoking pattern, a change in alcohol use pattern, withdrawal, prolonged silences, and sudden gregariousness not in keeping with one's personality. Cognitive changes include confusion in thinking, difficulty making decisions, disorientation, and memory problems. Physical signs include excessive sweating, dizzy spells, increased heart rate, elevated blood pressure, rapid breathing, tremor, and gastrointestinal disturbances (Everly & Mitchell, 1998a, 1998b; Mitchell & Bray, 1980; Mitchell, Sakraida, & Kameg, 2003). Health care workers must be aware of these signs and look for them in themselves and others. Refer to Chapter 12 🌐 for more about stress and adaptation to it.

Another common reaction to stress is the use of "gallows" or "dark" or "black" humor, especially in the rescuer community. Research has shown that this style is not disrespectful of the injured, the deceased, or their survivors (Maxwell, 2003).

Critical Incident

The stressor, which caused the stress, becomes a **critical incident** when it is an abnormal occurrence that is so markedly distressing and powerful that it overcomes a person's normal feeling of control and coping ability. Critical incident stress is the normal response to an abnormal occurrence. It is the occurrence that is abnormal, not the response (Burns & Rosenberg, 2001; Everly & Mitchell, 1998a,1998b; Mitchell & Bray, 1980; Mitchell et al., 2003). These incidents disrupt people's lives with strong emotional reactions that have the potential to interfere with their ability to function either at the scene or later. The severity of the reaction is influenced by many things, including any previous exposure to incidents, length of time of exposure, the severity of the exposure (relative horror), perceptions of the events, preexisting coping strategies, other current stressors, well-being at the time of the event, and the available social support (Everly & Mitchell, 1998b; Mitchell et al., 2003).

For health care workers, the critical incident can be further categorized as the incident itself, the professional's performance, and/or the professional's reaction to the event. For health care workers in the aftermath of a WMD incident, the event itself and all the work that follows have the potential to act as a catalyst for a critical incident stress response (Burns & Rosenberg, 2001; Everly & Mitchell, 1998a, 1998b; Mitchell & Bray, 1980; Mitchell et al., 2003).

Crisis Intervention and Critical Incident Stress Management

Crisis intervention is essentially first aid for those in crisis. The goals of crisis intervention are to stabilize and mitigate the signs and symptoms of stress and dysfunction, and to facilitate a return to functioning (Everly, 2000; Everly & Mitchell, 1998a). **Critical incident stress management** is a comprehensive approach to the management of stress and critical incidents. The goal is to reduce and control the harmful effects of stress, maintain health and productivity, and speed recovery from the stressful event. The approach has seven components: preincident preparation, group information briefings (demobilization), defusings, critical incident stress debriefing, individual intervention, family critical incident stress management, and follow-up and referral (Everly & Mitchell, 1998b). The point of all of these interventions is to prevent the development of post-traumatic stress disorder (PTSD), which has been found to be present in roughly 9% of all of those exposed to critical incidents in recent years (Everly & Mitchell, 1998a, 1998b; Mitchell & Bray, 1980; Mitchell et al., 2003).

Health Care Workers

Health care workers usually have a "rescuer" personality. Those who are unable to help with a major effort such as a WMD event,

especially in the early stages, often will feel greater stress. There is a need to do "something," anything (Everly & Mitchell, 1998b; Levenson & Acosta, 2001; Mitchell & Bray, 1980). As time wears on, cumulative stress also becomes a problem for health care workers due to the overwhelming nature of the situation they face each day. For health care workers and other emergency services personnel, there are three common, formalized ways of assisting to increase knowledge and decrease the perceived stress: demobilization, critical incident defusing, and critical incident stress debriefing. It is important to note that these processes are not psychotherapy but rather sessions for information, education, and ventilation (Everly & Mitchell, 1998b; Mitchell et al., 2003).

Demobilization

Demobilization is also called group information briefings and crisis management briefings. These usually occur during rest breaks, at the end of a shift, or in the middle of the event as the event dictates. This provides information and resources to a group that has been affected by an incident. It brings people together, provides rumor control, and addresses possible reactions and self-help guidelines, usually in the form of a little handout. These are typically only a few minutes long (Everly & Mitchell, 1998b).

Critical Incident Defusing

Critical incident defusings are formal sessions that occur within 8 hours of the event. They typically last 20 to 45 minutes. They are done in small groups of 6 to 8 people of similar job descriptions. There is no record made of the proceedings. Often a defusing will negate the need for a formal debriefing. The facilitators introduce themselves and state the ground rules including strict confidentiality. The event, experiences, and reactions are reviewed. Reassurance is given and an assessment is made for the need for more help. The last phase normalizes the experience and teaches some basic stress survival skills (Everly & Mitchell, 1998b).

Critical Incident Stress Debriefing

Critical incident stress debriefing (CISD) is a formal event run by trained counselors. It is held within 72 hours of the event and typically lasts 2 to 3 hours. Again, no record is made of the proceedings and strict confidentiality is enforced. There are seven phases to a CISD.

In the first phase, the interventional team members and facilitators are introduced along with an explanation of the process and expectations. In the fact phase, each participant describes the event from his perspective on a cognitive level. Each describes his role and location during the event. The thought phase allows the participants to describe their cognitive reactions (thoughts) regarding the events and transitions into the emotional reactions. The fourth phase, the reaction phase, tend to be the most powerful and emotional part of the process. Participants describe the most traumatic part for them and their emotional reactions. In the symptom phase, the participants are guided back from a highly charged emotional state to a more cognitive level by being asked to describe some symptoms of stress they have experienced such as insomnia or tremors. The teaching phase is run more by the facilitators, and it serves as a cognitive anchor. Here the facilitators discuss normal stress reactions and provide some stress survival and management tips. This phase continues until the concerns of the group are exhausted. The seventh and last phase is the reentry phase. The session is summarized and any questions are answered. Handouts with stress management information, such as signs of stress and tips for self-care, and community re-ferrals are given to the participants. There is usually a short social time with refreshments, which allows anyone with an individual question for the facilitators to ask the question outside the group. This technique has been employed in hundreds of large and small events worldwide (Chart 72–12) (Everly & Mitchell, 1998b; Mitchell et al., 2003).

Community

Crisis intervention for a community revolves around providing information, education, and direction. After an event, coordina-tion of services for survivors, families, and communities, along with a centralized list of mental health volunteers, is needed. This should be part of the community's disaster plan with advanced coordination as to who responds and when. Within 24 hours, rep-resentatives for all the organizations and agencies, such as the state or county department of mental health, critical incident stress management teams, professional organizations, universities, and clergy, need to have a meeting to identify needs, resources, and re-sponsibilities. With its extensive experience in handling disasters, its name recognition, and trust, the American Red Cross makes the ideal organization for handling mental health coordination for the community, as the state and county departments are often overwhelmed with delivery of services (Bowenkamp, 2003).

Considerations in planning and delivering mental health care to the community include assessing school needs, screening of volunteer workers, including any licensure issues, and making assignments based on skills and needs. Clergy may be teamed with mental health professionals and function independently depending on the need. The community may need assistance with day care including pediatric counseling. There needs to be defined support for families when notified of a death. The de-fusing and debriefing of each of the teams of volunteers and other mental health workers at the end of their shift is a key component of maintaining the workforce. Teams may also be needed to respond to families or persons unable to go to centers for assistance (Bowenkamp, 2003).

Community "town meetings," either in person or through the media, and frequent news bulletins provide relevant opera-tions updates, stress management, and education. These help to provide rumor control and build and aid in community cohe-sion. These meetings foster personal and community empower-ment (Everly, 2003).

Ottenstein (2003) has proposed a protocol for a guided group discussion that could be used in a community group or in a tel-evised group for the community. Participants are encouraged to take notes. The stated goal during the introduction phase is "to help people share each other's fears and coping strategies so that we can learn a new way of coping with those threats and fears." The point is to help the group members understand what they can do to support themselves, their families, and each other.

Discussion topics include how each person attempts to gain control or to eliminate the threat, how people are using coping strategies to deal with the threat, and the use of unhealthy cop-ing strategies such as increased smoking and drinking when un-der extreme stress. The new safety and security procedures and coping with the frustrations they produce are discussed. Ac-knowledge that spiritual beliefs can be powerful coping tools for difficult times. The concept of constructive ventilation is ex-plained. Time is then given to allow for the constructive ventila-tion of feelings and emotions by the participants. Chart 72–13 summarizes self-care tips for stress management. The discussion is then summarized and the leaders teach additional coping strategies based on the ideas and feelings expressed. This proto-col was implemented following the September 11, 2001, attacks, the anthrax attacks on the postal system, and the sniper attacks in Maryland and Virginia in 2002.

CHART 72–12 **Stages in Critical Incident Stress Debriefing**

1. **Introduction.** Introduce intervention team members (facilitators), explain the process, and set expectations. Strict confidentiality is emphasized.

2. **Fact.** Describe on a cognitive level the event from each participant's view.

3. **Thought.** Describe cognitive reactions and transition to emotional reactions.

4. **Reaction.** Identify emotional reactions to the most traumatic aspect.

5. **Symptom.** Identify personal symptoms of distress and transition back to cognitive level.

6. **Teaching.** Provide cognitive anchor. Educate regarding normal reactions and adaptive coping mechanisms.

7. **Reentry.** Clarify and prepare for termination.

CHART 72–13 **Self-Care Tips for Stress Management**

EXPECT EMOTIONAL REACTIONS

Emotions will vary day to day. They may reemerge weeks to months later.

Do not fight the feelings; they are part of the healing process and will diminish over time.

TAKE CARE OF YOURSELF EMOTIONALLY

Be gentle with yourself and others.

Tell and retell what happened.

Reach out to others for help and support.

Plan extra time to do tasks.

Do not try to make major life decisions at this time.

Try to maintain a normal schedule.

TAKE CARE OF YOURSELF PHYSICALLY

Eat regular meals of nutritious food. Decrease or cut out caffeine, as this will help with decreasing nervousness.

Get regular exercise.

Do activities relaxing for you.

Take rest breaks.

Go to bed for 8 hours each night.

Be wary of alcohol and other drugs, including tobacco. Alcohol is a depressant and interrupts normal sleep cycles.

Give yourself time to heal. If the symptoms do not gradually decrease or they cause you distress, call for assistance.

Source: Adapted from class handouts Critical Incident Stress Management Course # 26128327 May 26 and 27, 2000.

Summary

Regardless whether a disaster is weather related or a terrorist attack, hospitals, cities, counties, states, and the nation must be as prepared as possible. Nurses should know the disaster plan within their facility and where to find information quickly regarding possible substances that the patients may have been exposed to.

NCLEX® REVIEW

1. The student nurse inquires about an example "international" terrorism. The most appropriate response by the nurse would be:
   1. "When an act of terror or violence is generated toward the United States government by a group or an individual from Puerto Rico."
   2. "When a group such as the Ku Klux Klan or the Black Panthers performs terrorist activity against citizens of our own country."
   3. "When the group responsible for committing the violence has connection to a foreign country like al Queda in the Middle East."
   4. "When an individual like Timothy McVeigh uses an unlawful act of violence to destroy or intimidate individuals or the government."

2. The nurse attends a seminar on the use of various biological, chemical, radiological, and explosive agents throughout history. Which of the following statements by the nurse would indicate the need for further instruction?
   1. "The outbreak of an intentionally caused food-borne illness in Oregon during the early 1980s was attributed to *Shigella sonnei*."
   2. "There were never any documented adverse health effects following the Three Mile Island nuclear power leak in the U.S."
   3. "The largest peace-time incident involving a nerve agent occurred when sarin gas was released into the Tokyo subway system."
   4. "One of the earliest documented examples of biologic weapons use occurred in the 6th century B.C. with the Assyrian use of rye ergot."

3. The nurse is caring for the patient with a possible exposure to a biologic agent several days ago. The assessment reveals HR 142, BP 80/53, RR 34 and labored, T 103.2°F with chills, and diaphoresis. The patient complains of headache and chest pain, and chest x-ray reveals a wide mediastinum. Based on these findings, the nurse suspects the patient has contracted:
   1. Septicemic plague.
   2. Undulant fever.
   3. Typhoidal tularemia.
   4. Inhalation anthrax.

4. Which of the following nursing diagnoses would be the priority when caring for the patient with recent known nerve agent exposure?
   1. Ineffective airway clearance related to copious secretions and ineffective cough.
   2. High risk for altered cardiac output related to electrical conduction abnormalities.
   3. Increased risk for fluid and electrolyte imbalance related to vomiting and diarrhea.
   4. Ineffective individual coping related to perceived and actual threat from situation.

5. Approximately 30 minutes after exposure to a radiological leak at an industrial facility, several patients arrive at the emergency department. Upon their arrival at the hospital, the patients are all experiencing nausea, vomiting, diarrhea, fatigue, and hypotension. The nurse understands the patients are in which phase of Acute Radiation Syndrome?
   1. Latent phase
   2. Prodromal phase
   3. Recovery phase
   4. Illness phase

6. Which of the following statements is true regarding the use of the Hospital Incident Command System (HICS)?
   1. The Incident Commander is in charge of all four areas of operations—planning, logistics, safety, and public information.
   2. The plan outlines clearly defined responsibilities and positions that must remain independent of one another and individually run.
   3. This flexible plan allows for only necessary positions and functions to be activated on an as needed basis during the incident.
   4. Media utilization is limited in order to decrease mass hysteria and unwarranted overwhelming of communications.

7. With regard to the Strategic National Stockpile (SNS) the nurse understands that:
   1. It helps augment the local and state resources so as to help decrease the morbidity and mortality in the civilian population following a large-scale disaster.
   2. This program is organized using a four-tiered approach to include medical supplies and equipment, pharmaceutical agents, vaccines, and technical assistance.
   3. The 12-hour push pack is designed to be used to provide pharmaceuticals and medical supplies for treatment of a known agent or for smaller scale events.
   4. A team of logistical and operational experts called the National Disaster Response Unit may be required to assist state and local authorities with supply distribution.

8. Which of the following statements indicates the nurse has a clear understanding of Critical Incident Stress Management as it relates to health care workers?
   1. "Critical Incident Stress Debriefings (CISD) are formal sessions run by trained counselors that are held within 8 hours of a critical event."
   2. "Demobilizations are group briefings that increase knowledge and decrease stress by having each participant describe their cognitive level."
   3. "Group information briefings bring people together in an informal setting to give mutual reassurance and assess the need for more help."
   4. "Critical incident defusings are formal, confidential group sessions where the stressful event and its experiences and reactions are reviewed."

Answers for review questions appear in Appendix D

KEY TERMS

acute radiation syndrome (ARS) *p.2403*
asphyxiates *p.2395*
biologic agent *p.2383*
blister agent *p.2391*
bubo *p.2398*
CBRNE *p.2384*
chemical agent *p.2390*
choking agent *p.2395*
critical incident *p.2410*
critical incident stress debriefing
    (CISD) *p.2410*

critical incident stress management *p.2410*
decontamination *p.2389*
DMAT *p.2408*
DMORT *p.2409*
incapacitating agent *p.2396*
incident command system (ICS) *p.2405*
INCMCE *p.2384*
irritants *p.2396*
nerve agents *p.2391*
persistent *p.2390*
PPE *p.2387*

radiologic agents *p.2401*
RDD *p.2387*
riot control agent *p.2396*
Strategic National Stockpile (SNS) *p.2407*
terrorism *p.2382*
toxin *p.2400*
vesicant *p.2391*
vomiting agent *p.2396*
WMD *p.2384*
zones: cold zone, hot zone, warm
    zone *p.2389*

PEARSON

EXPLORE mynursingkit™

MyNursingKit is your one stop for online chapter review materials and resources. Prepare for success with additional NCLEX®-style practice questions, interactive assignments and activities, web links, animations and videos, and more!

Register your access code from the front of your book at
www.mynursingkit.com

REFERENCES

Abramowicz, M. (Ed.). (2002). Prevention and treatment of injury from chemical warfare agents. *The Medical Letter on Drugs and Therapeutics, 44*(1121), 1–4.

Agency for Toxic Substances and Disease Registry (ATSDR). (2001a). *Managing hazardous materials incidents: Vol. I. Emergency medical services: A planning guide for the management of contaminated patients.* Atlanta, GA: U.S. Department of Health and Human Services.

Agency for Toxic Substances and Disease Registry (ATSDR). (2001b). *Managing hazardous materials incidents: Vol. III. Medical management guidelines for acute chemical exposures.* Atlanta, GA: U.S. Department of Health and Human Services.

Agency for Toxic Substances and Disease Registry (ATSDR). (2001c). *Managing hazardous materials incidents: Vol. II. Hospital emergency departments: A planning guide for the management of contaminated patients.* Atlanta, GA: U.S. Department of Health and Human Services.

Agency for Toxic Substances and Disease Registry (ATSDR). (2004, September). *ATSDR Ammonia CAS # 7664-41-7.* Retrieved December 12, 2006, from http://www.atsdr.cdc.gov/tfacts126.pdf

Agency for Toxic Substances and Disease Registry (ATSDR). (2008). *Medical management guidelines for nerve agents: Tabun (GA); sarin (GB); soman (GD); and VX.* Retrieved September 22, 2008, from http://www.MHMI/mmg166.html

Arnon, S. S., Schechter, R., Inglesby, T. V., Henderson, D. A., Bartlett, J. G., Ascher, M. S., et al. (2001). Botulinum toxin as a biological weapon: Medical and public health management. *Journal of the American Medical Association, 285*(8), 1059–1070.

Auf der Heide, E. (2006). The importance of evidence-based disaster planning. *Annals of Emergency Medicine, 47*(1), 34–49.

Barrueto, F., & Hoffman, R. S. (2002). Biological agents: Botulinum, plague, and tularemia. *Resident and Staff Physician, 48*(4), 34–40.

Borio, L., Inglesby, T., Peters, C. J., Schmaljohn, A. L., Hughes, J. M., Jarling, P. B., et al. (2002). Hemorrhagic fever viruses as biological weapons: Medical and public health management. *Journal of the American Medical Association, 287*(18), 2391–2405.

Bowenkamp, C. (2003). Coordination of mental health and community agencies in disaster response. *International Journal of Emergency Mental Health, 2*(3), 159–165.

British Broadcasting Company (BBC). (2003). *ETA suspects held near Pamplona.* Retrieved October 4, 2008, from http://news.bbc.co.uk/2/hi/europe/3068149.stm

British Broadcasting Company (BBC). (2007). *Timeline: Litvinenko death case.* Retrieved October 4, 2008, from http://news.bbc.co.uk/1/hi/uk/6179074.stm

Burns, C., & Rosenberg, L. (2001). Redefining incidents: A preliminary report. *International Journal of Emergency Mental Health, 3*(1), 17–24.

Bush, G. W. (2002, December). *National strategy to combat weapons of mass destruction.* Retrieved October 31, 2003, from http://www.whitehouse.gov/news/releases/2002/12/WMDStrategy.pdf

Bush, G. W. (2003, February 28). *Homeland Security presidential directive/HSPD-5.* Retrieved December 1, 2006, from http://www.whitehouse.gov/news/releases/2003/02/20030228-9.html

Cable News Network (CNN). (1996, July 28). *Games go on after day of shock, grief.* Retrieved December 14, 2006, from http://www.cnn.com/US/9607/27/bomb.probe.pm

California Emergency Medical Services Authority (EMSA). (2006, August). *Hospital incident command system guidebook.* Retrieved December 14, 2006, from http://www.emsa.ca.gov/HICS/files/Guidebook_Glossary.pdf

Centers for Disease Control and Prevention (CDC). (2004, January 27). *Facts about cyanide.* Retrieved December 12, 2006, from http://www.bt.cdc.gov/agent/cyanide/basics/facts.asp

Centers for Disease Control and Prevention (CDC). (2005, April 14). *Strategic national stockpile.* Retrieved December 13, 2006, from http://www.bt.cdc.gov/stockpile/index.asp

Centers for Disease Control and Prevention (CDC). (2006a). *Bioterrorism agents/diseases.* Retrieved December 12, 2006, from http://www.bt.cdc.gov/agent/agentlist-category.asp

Centers for Disease Control and Prevention (CDC). (2006b, February 22). *Facts about lewisite.* Retrieved December 12, 2006, from http://www.bt.cdc.gov/agent/lewisite/basics/facts.asp

Centers for Disease Control and Prevention (CDC). (2006c, February 22). *Facts about phosgene.* Retrieved December 12, 2006, from http://emergency.cdc.gov/agent/phosgene/basics/facts.asp

Centers for Disease Control and Prevention (CDC). (2006d, February 22). *Facts about phosgene oxime.* Retrieved December 12, 2006, from http://www.bt.cdc.gov/agent/phosgene-oxime/basics/facts.asp

Centers for Disease Control and Prevention (CDC). (2006e, February 22). *Facts about sarin.* Retrieved December 12, 2006, from http://www.bt.cdc.gov/agent/sarin/basics/facts.asp

Centers for Disease Control and Prevention (CDC). (2006f, February 22). *Facts about soman.* Retrieved December 12, 2006, from http://www.bt.cdc.gov/agent/soman/basics/facts.asp

Centers for Disease Control and Prevention (CDC). (2006g, February 22). *Facts about sulfur mustard.* Retrieved December 12, 2006, from http://www.bt.cdc.gov/agent/sulfurmustard/basics/facts.asp

Centers for Disease Control and Prevention (CDC). (2006h, February 22). *Facts about tabun.* Retrieved December 12, 2006, from http://www.bt.cdc.gov/agent/tabun/basics/facts.asp

Centers for Disease Control and Prevention (CDC). (2006i, February 22). *Facts about VX.* Retrieved December 12, 2006, from http://www.bt.cdc.gov/agent/vx/basics/facts.asp

Centers for Disease Control and Prevention (CDC). (2006j, February 22). *Fact sheet: Anthrax information for health care providers.* Retrieved December 10, 2006, from http://www.bt.cdc.gov/agent/anthrax/anthrax-hcp-factsheet.asp

Centers for Disease Control and Prevention (CDC). (2006k, April 19). *Botulism facts for health care providers.* Retrieved December 7, 2006, from http://www.bt.cdc.gov/agent/botulism/hcpfacts.asp

Centers for Disease Control and Prevention (CDC). (2006l, May 10). *Prussian blue.* Retrieved December 7, 2006, from http://www.bt.cdc.gov/radiation/prussianblue.asp

Centers for Disease Control and Prevention (CDC). (2006m, June 14). *Explosions and blast injuries: A primer for clinicians.* Retrieved December 12, 2006, from http://www.bt.cdc.gov/masscasualties/explosions.asp

Centers for Disease Control and Prevention (CDC). (2006n, October 11). *Potassium iodide (KI).* Retrieved December 7, 2006, from http://www.bt.cdc.gov/radiation/ki.asp

Centers for Disease Control and Prevention (CDC). (2008, March 5). *Facts about ricin.* Retrieved September 22, 2008, from http://www.bt.cdc.gov/agent/ricin/facts.asp

Chertoff, M. (2006, June 16). *Nationwide plan review phase 2 report.* Retrieved June 20, 2006, from http://www.dhs.gov/xlibrary/assets/Prep_NationwidePlanReview.pdf

Christopher, G. W., Cieslak, J., Pavlin, J. A., & Eitzen, E. M. (1997). Biological warfare: A historical perspective. *Journal of the American Medical Association, 278*(5), 412–417.

Community Emergency Response Team–Los Angeles (CERT-LA). (2003, March 26). *CERT Los Angeles simple triage and rapid treatment.* Retrieved December 1, 2006, from http://www.cert-la.com/triage/start.htm

Community Research Associates (CRA). (2003). *Emergency response to terrorism: Instructor's guide.* Washington, DC: Office for Domestic Preparedness.

Compton, D., Stewart-Craig, E., & Doak, M. (Eds.). (1999). *SBCCOM domestic preparedness training program.* Washington, DC: Science Applications International Corporation.

Computer Sciences Corporation (CSC). (2008). *Department of Defense Joint Vaccine Acquisition Program (U.S.): CSC's DVC edges one step closer to plague vaccine.* Retrieved September 28, 2008, from http://www.csc.com/industries/government/casestudies/1710.shtml

Dang, C., Kare, J., Schneiderman, A., & Dang, A. B. (2002). Chemical warfare agents. *Topics in Emergency Medicine, 24*(2), 25–39.

Dayton Disaster Medical Assistance Team (DMAT). (2008). *Team basics.* Retrieved October 5, 2008, from http://www.daytondmat.com/dmat/dmatinfo.html

Dennis, D. T., Inglesby, T. V., Henderson, D. A., Bartlett, J. G., Ascher, M. S., Eitzen, E., et al. (2001). Tularemia as a biological weapon: Medical and public health management. *Journal of the American Medical Association, 285*(21), 2763–2773.

Disaster Management Systems (DMS). (2005). *All Risk triage tags.* Retrieved December 14, 2006, from http://www.triagetags.com

Durham, B. (2002). The background and history of manmade disasters. *Topics in Emergency Medicine, 24*(2), 1–14.

Esbitt, D. (2003, July–September). The Strategic National Stockpile. *Disaster Management and Response,* 68–70.

Everly, G. S. (2000). The role of pastoral crisis intervention in disasters, terrorism, violence, and other community crises. *International Journal of Emergency Mental Health, 2,* 139–142.

Everly, G. S. (2003). Psychological counterterrorism. *International Journal of Emergency Mental Health, 5*(2), 57–59.

Everly, G. S., & Mitchell, J. T. (1998a). *Assisting individuals in crisis.* Ellicott City, MD: International Critical Incident Stress Foundation.

Everly, G. S., & Mitchell, J. T. (1998b). *Critical incident stress management: The basic course workbook.* Ellicott City, MD: International Critical Incident Stress Foundation.

Federal Bureau of Investigation–Denver (FBI). (2006). *Terrorism.* Retrieved December 12, 2006, from http://denver.fbi.gov/nfip.htm

Fell-Carlson, D. (2003, January 30). Terrorist danger: Nurses must be ready for radiological threat. *Nurseweek,* 22–23.

Follow-up of deaths among U.S. postal service workers potentially exposed to *Bacillus anthracis*—District of Columbia, 2001–2002. (2003). *Morbidity and Mortality Weekly Report, 52*(39), 937–938.

Franz, D. R., Jarling, P. B., Friedlander, A. M., McClain, D. J., Hoover, D. L., Bryne, W. R., et al. (1997). Clinical recognition and management of patients exposed to biological warfare agents. *Journal of the American Medical Association, 278*(5), 399–411.

Gebbie, K. M., & Qureshi, K. (2002). Emergency and disaster preparedness: Core competencies for nurses. *American Journal of Nursing, 1*(102), 46–51.

Hagler, D. A. (2004). Nursing assessment: Respiratory system. In M. K. Lewis, M. M. Heitkemper, & S. R. Dirksen (Eds.), *Medical surgical nursing: Assessment of clinical problems* (pp. 542–565). St. Louis: Mosby.

Hardin, E. (2002). Biologic casualties: Treatment and management. *Topics in Emergency Medicine, 24*(2), 15–24.

Henderson, D. A., Inglesby, T. V., Bartlett, J. G., Ascher, M. S., Eitzen, E., Jarling, P. B., et al. (1999). Smallpox as a biological weapon: Medical and public health management. *Journal of the American Medical Association, 281*(22), 2127–2137.

Hick, J. L., Hanfling, D., Burstein, J. L., Markham, J., Macintyre, A. G., & Barbera, J. A. (2003). Protective equipment for health care facility decontamination personnel: Regulations, risks, and recommendations. *Annals of Emergency Medicine, 42*(3), 370–380.

House, H., Graber, M. A., & Scheckel, S. S. (2003, October). Is your emergency department ready for a terrorist attack? *Emergency Medicine,* 46–51.

Inglesby, T. V., Dennis, D. T., Henderson, D. A., Bartlett, J. G., Ascher, M. S., Eitzen, E., et al. (2000). Plague as a biologic weapon: Medical and public health management. *Journal of the American Medical Association, 283*(17), 2281–2290.

Inglesby, T. V., O'Toole, T., Henderson, D. A., Bartlett, J. G., Ascher, M. S., Eitzen, E., et al. (2002). Anthrax as a biological weapon, 2002: Updated recommendations for management. *Journal of the American Medical Association, 287*(17), 2236–2253.

International Nursing Coalition for Mass Casualty Education (INCMCE). (2003, July). *Educational competencies for registered nurses responding to mass casualty incidents.* Retrieved December 12, 2006, from http://www.incmce.org/competenciespage.html

Jacocks, J. (Ed.). (2003). *Medical management of radiological casualties* (2nd ed.). Bethesda, MD: Armed Forces Radiobiology Research Institute.

Kortepeter, M. (Ed.). (2001). *USAMRIID's medical management of biological casualties handbook* (4th ed.). Fort Detrick, MD: U.S. Army Medical Research Institute of Infectious Diseases.

Lee, E. C. (2003). Clinical manifestations of sarin nerve gas exposure. *Journal of the American Medical Association, 290*(5), 659–662.

Lehmann, J. (2002, September). Considerations for selecting personal protective equipment for hazardous material decontamination. *Disaster Management and Response,* 21–25.

Lenzer, J. (2003). Preparing your emergency department for a disaster: Whether it's bioterrorism or a natural disaster, make sure you're ready. *ACEP 2003 Reference & Resource Guide,* 10–15.

Levenson, R. L., & Acosta, J. K. (2001). Observations from ground zero at the World Trade Center in New York City: Part I. *International Journal of Emergency Mental Health, 3*(4), 241–244.

Martin, C. O. (2002, July). Cyanide toxins. *Emergency Medicine,* 11–13.

Maxwell, W. (2003). The use of gallows humor and dark humor during crisis situations. *International Journal of Emergency Mental Health, 5*(2), 93–98.

McKee, C. B., Collins, L., Keetley, J., Bausum, H., Besch, T., Moss, C., et al. (2000, May). *USACHPPM tech guide 244: The medical NBC battlebook.* Washington, DC: U.S. Army Center for Health Promotion and Preventative Medicine.

Medical Center of Louisiana at New Orleans (MCLNO). (2003, June). *Medical Center of Louisiana, Hazmat decon training: An operations level course. Student handbook.* New Orleans: Author.

Merck Manuals. (2005, November). *Radiation injury.* Retrieved December 7, 2006, from http://www.merck.com/mmpe/print/sec21/ch317/ch317a.html

Mitchell, A. M., Sakraida, T. J., & Kameg, K. (2003). Critical incident stress debriefing: Implications for best practice. *Disaster Management and Response, 1*(2), 46–51.

Mitchell, J. T., & Bray, G. P. (1980). *Emergency services stress.* Upper Saddle River, NJ: Brady/Prentice-Hall.

National Institute of Justice, Office of Justice Programs. (2003, April). *The effectiveness and safety of pepper spray.* Retrieved December 6, 2006, from http://www.ncjrs.org/pdffiles1/nij/195739.pdf

Neff, J. M., Lane, J. M., Fulginiti, V. A., & Henderson, D. A. (2002). Contact vaccinia—Transmission of vaccinia from smallpox vaccination. *Journal of the American Medical Association, 288*(15), 1901–1905.

Occupational Safety and Health Administration. (2005, January). *OSHA best practices for hospital-based first receivers of victims from mass casualty incidents involving the release of hazardous substances.* Retrieved February 1, 2005, from http://www.osha.gov/dts/osta/bestpractices/html/hospital_firstreceivers.html

Ottenstein, R. J. (2003). Coping with threats of terrorism: A protocol for group intervention. *International Journal of Emergency Mental Health, 5*(1), 39–42.

Plague vaccine. (1982, June 11). *Morbidity and Mortality Weekly Report, 31*(22), 301–304. Retrieved December 12, 2006, from http://www.cdc.gov/MMWR/preview/mmwrhtml/00041848.htm (page converted August 5, 1998, last reviewed May 2, 2001)

Raso, J. (1999, March 1). Three Mile Island: A 20th anniversary remembrance. *American Council on Science and Health.* Retrieved December 12, 2006, from http://www.acsh.org/publications/pubID.867/pub_detail.asp

Ridge, T. (2004, March 1). *National Incident Management System.* Retrieved December 1, 2004, from http://fema.gov/pdf/emergency/nims/nims_doc_full.pdf

Riley, D., Clark, M., & Wong, T. (2002). World Trade Center terror: Explosion trauma-blast, burns, and crush injury. *Topics in Emergency Medicine, 24*(2), 47–59.

Riley, J. M. (2003, July–September). Providing nursing care with federal disaster relief teams. *Disaster Management and Response,* 76–79.

Romig, L. (2008). *The JumpSTART pediatric MCI triage tool.* Retrieved September 22, 2008, from http://www.jumpstarttriage.com/JumpSTART_and_MCI_Triage.php

Scharoun, K., Van Caulil, K., & Liberman, A. (2002). Bioterrorism vs. health security: Crafting a plan of preparedness. *Health Care Manager, 21*(1), 74–92.

Seed, T. M. (2002). Prevention and treatments: Summary statement. In Proceedings of the International Conference on Low-Level Radiation Injury and Medical Countermeasures. Supplement *to International Journal of AMSUS, 167*(2), 87–93.

Sidell, F. R., Patrick, W. C., Dashiell, T. R., Alibel, K., & Layne, S. (Eds.). (2002). *Jane's chem-bio book* (2nd ed.). Alexandria, VA: Jane's Information Group.

Smith, C. (2003, September 11). *Disaster mortuary operations response team.* Presentation at National Healthcare Profession Preparedness Consortium Health Care Leadership Course, Nobles Training Center, Anniston, AL.

Texas Engineering Extension Service, National Emergency Response and Rescue Training Center (TEEX). (2003). *Emergency medical services (EMS): Operations and planning for WMD incidents. Student manual.* Washington, DC: Office of Preparedness and Emergency Operations.

Thomas, R. J. (2002). Acute pulmonary effects from o-Chlorobenzylidenemalonitrile "tear gas": A unique exposure outcome unmasked by strenuous exercise after a military training event. *Military Medicine, 167*(2), 136–139.

3M. (2002, March). *Technical Data Bulletin #151: PAPR management and planning for first responders.* St. Paul, MN: Author.

Torok, T. J, Tauxe, R. V., Wise, R. P., Livengood, J. R., Sokolow, R., Mauvais, S., et al. (1997). A large community outbreak of salmonellosis caused by intentional contamination of restaurant salad bars. *Journal of the American Medical Association, 278*(5), 389–395.

Truab, S. J., & Hoffman, R. S. (2002). Agents of chemical warfare: I. Vesicant and irritant gases. *Resident and Staff Physician, 48*(6), 22–28.

Udeani, J. C., & Aguilera, P. (2002). Management of nuclear casualties. *Topics in Emergency Medicine, 24*(2), 40–46.

U.S. Army Medical Research Institute of Chemical Defense (USAMRICD). (2000). *Medical management of chemical casualties handbook* (3rd ed.). Aberdeen Proving Ground, MD: Author.

U.S. Department of Health and Human Services (DHHS). (2008a). *National disaster medical systems (NDMS).* Retrieved October 5, 2008, from http://www.hhs.gov/aspr/opeo/ndms/index.html

U.S. Department of Health and Human Services (DHHS). (2008b). *National disaster medical systems (NDMS) response teams.* Retrieved October 5, 2008, from http://www.hhs.gov/aspr/opeo/ndms/teams/index.html

U.S. Department of Transportation (DOT). (2008). *2008 Emergency response guidebook.* Washington, DC: U.S. Government Printing Office. Retrieved September 22, 2008, from http://hazmat.dot.gov/pubs/erg/guidebook.htm

U.S. General Accounting Office (GAO). (2003, August). *Report to congressional committees, hospital preparedness.* Washington, DC: Author.

Veenema, T. G., & Karam, P. A. (2003). Radiation: Clinical responses to radiologic incidents and emergencies. *American Journal of Nursing, 103*(5), 32–40.

WashingtonPost.com. (1998). *Oklahoma bombing chronology.* Retrieved December 12, 2006, from http://www.washingtonpost.com/wp-srv/national/longterm/oklahoma/stories/chron.htm

Williams, W. (2002, November 14). *CDC logistician.* Presentation at National Healthcare Profession Preparedness Consortium Health Care Leadership Course, Nobles Training Center, Anniston, AL.

World Nuclear Association. (2008). *Chernobyl accident.* Retrieved October 4, 2008, from http://www.world-nuclear.org/info/chernobyl/inf07.html

Caring for the Patient in the Emergency Department

Renee Semonin-Holleran

Outcome-Based Learning Objectives

After studying this chapter, the learner will be able to:

1. Explain the practice of emergency nursing.
2. Differentiate among the various components of the triage process and determine each component's relevance.
3. Compare and contrast patient priority categories.
4. Explain the legal issues related to the practice of emergency nursing.
5. Describe preparation for emergency nursing practice.

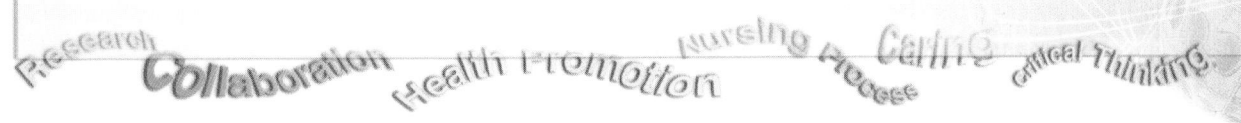

Emergency nursing is described as the care of individuals of all ages who have perceived or actual physical or emotional alterations of health that have not been diagnosed or require further interventions. Emergency nursing care is episodic, may involve primary as well as secondary and tertiary care, and is usually acute or critical in nature (Bonalumi & King, 2007; MacPhail, 2003). Emergency nursing involves care in a variety of areas including the prehospital and hospital environments.

The Emergency Nurses Association (ENA) states that emergency nursing provides care that ranges from birth to death. Emergency nursing also includes injury prevention, women's health, disease management, and providing care aimed at managing life- and limb-threatening emergencies. Unique to emergency nursing practice is the application of the nursing process to patients of all ages who require stabilization and/or resuscitation for a variety of illnesses and injuries (ENA, 1999).

History

Florence Nightingale has long been associated with the origins of emergency nursing when she took nurses out to the field to provide care to wounded soldiers. The care she and her fellow nurses provided on the battlefields demonstrated the value of rapid management of acute patients. As hospitals developed, care that had generally been done by health care providers,

nurses, or even family members in patients' homes was redirected to the hospital.

Emergency nursing and emergency medicine have developed into a specialty during the past 50 years. Care provided to soldiers during the Korean and Vietnam wars demonstrated that rapid and acute care could make a difference in patient outcomes. However, the departments in hospitals that were dedicated to the emergent care of patients were limited. Oftentimes, the emergency department was one room staffed by a nurse who was generally called down from another floor or by the hospital nursing supervisor.

When emergency medicine was recognized as a specialty in the late 1970s, it quickly became one of the fastest growing medical fields. The Emergency Department Nurses Association was established in 1970 by Anita Dorr (Buffalo, New York) and Judith Kelleher (Downey, California). The association's name was later changed to the Emergency Nurses Association. Initially, ENA and the American College of Emergency Physicians shared the same offices. As both associations grew, so did issues between the two groups (Schriver, Talmadge, Chuong, & Hedges, 2003). However, the important issues that face both emergency nurses and health care providers have brought both organizations together. Today emergency medicine and emergency nursing both have specific curricula and clinical requirements. Each also has specialized examinations. For emergency nursing that is the Certified Emergency

Nurse exam or the CEN. For information regarding the exam, go to the Emergency Nurses Association website.

The Role of the Emergency Department

In 2006, more than 119 million visits were made to emergency departments in the United States (National Center for Health Statistics, 2007). Emergency department visits continue to grow, yet emergency departments are closing, initiating ambulance diversions, increasing waiting times, and boarding patients who are critically ill and injured. This overcrowding in emergency departments is occurring because of decreasing numbers of doctors and nurses and limited hospital beds (Institute of Medicine [IOM], 2006; Reeder & Garrison, 2001).

Emergency departments have become the source of care for many types of patients, but particularly for patients who are poor and uninsured. Emergency departments are open 24 hours a day, 7 days a week. Additionally, because of the Emergency Medical Transport and Active Labor Act (discussed later in this chapter), emergency departments cannot refuse to provide a medical screening examination and stabilizing care when patients present for care. The increase in uninsured patients, the open access, and the ability to provide 24-hour-a-day care have stressed the capacity of emergency departments.

Emergency departments must also deal with the challenges of providing care to a more and more diverse patient population. Examples of the types of patients who utilize the emergency department to supply their primary care include illegal immigrants, prisoners, and homeless and underinsured patients. Additionally, the population has become more diverse culturally and care of these patients requires that emergency nurses and health care providers be culturally competent (see the Cultural Considerations box).

In the United States, the emergency department has become the single point of universal access to health care. This will continue to be an important challenge in the practice of emergency nursing, and one for which nursing will need to provide a leadership role in order to solve.

IOM Report and the Future of Emergency Care

In June 2006, the Institute of Medicine released a report on the state of emergency care in the United States. The IOM report recognized many of the challenges that are being faced today by the emergency medical system and its nurses and health care providers. Overcrowding, ambulance diversions, shortage of on-call specialists, lack of emergency preparedness, and deficiencies in pediatric emergency care are some of the issues that were identified. The recommendations summarized in the National Guidelines box have been made to improve emergency care systems in the United States using a multifaceted, multiorganizational approach. The IOM study and these proposals will provide a framework for the delivery of emergency care in the years to come.

Emergency Nursing Roles

The role of the emergency nurse is many and varied. Emergency nursing can be practiced both inside and outside of the hospital. In addition, emergency nurses may be involved in numerous functions within the emergency department including education, prevention, and research. Chart 73–1 summarizes some of the roles of emergency nurses.

Specialty Roles in Emergency Nursing

Emergency care requires a team approach and involves basic and advanced providers. As emergency nursing has evolved, both specialty and advanced practice roles have developed. Many of these roles are governed by specific agencies (e.g., state boards of nursing practice) or national associations (e.g., Sexual Assault Nurse Examiners). Chart 73–2 provides a summary of some of these specialty roles.

Triage

The word *triage* is derived from a French word that means "to sort." In emergency care, **triage** is a process that is used to determine the severity of a patient's illness or injury.

Medical triage evolved during war where battles resulted in lots of casualties and resources were limited. Napoleon's surgeon, Dominique Jean Larrey, has been credited with initiating this concept on the battlefield. Florence Nightingale used the triage concept during the Crimean War. She went out after the daily fighting and sorted out those who might or might not survive and provided much needed care (Thomas, Bernardo, & Herman, 2003).

During the 20th century, battlefield triage consisted of a primary assessment and the performance of critical interventions such as control of bleeding and then rapid transport to MASH units. During the Korean and Vietnam wars, helicopter transport was introduced to enhance the rapidity of patient care (Bracken, 2003).

In the 1960s, as emergency department censuses began to grow, the need for triage was recognized. Initially triage was performed by a physician or nurse physician team. Today, triage is generally performed by experienced emergency department nurses (Gilboy, Travers, & Wuerz, 1999).

Triage is performed in both the prehospital and hospital environments. Triage is a fluid process and is based on the number of patients, the amount of resources available, and the care that is available. Triage is an important component of emergency nursing practice as patient censuses continue to increase and more has to be provided with less.

CULTURAL CONSIDERATIONS for Emergency Care Providers

The cultural competence of emergency care providers should include an awareness of existing racial and ethnic health disparities and recognition of the incidence and prevalence of health problems among diverse populations that may present to the emergency department for care. A culturally competent emergency care provider also possesses the skills to identify and manage racial and ethnic differences in health values, beliefs, and behaviors, incorporating these so that patients receive the best care in the emergency department (Cone, Richardson, Todd, Betancourt, & Lowe, 2003; Lipson & Dibble, 2007).

NATIONAL GUIDELINES Summary of IOM Recommendations for Emergency Care in the United States

Recommendation	Actions
Improve hospital efficiency and patient flow through the emergency department.	Use tools from other disciplines such as engineering and operations research to improve patient flow.
	Establish clinical decision units or 24-hour observation units to hopefully prevent unnecessary admissions.
	Increase use of informational technologies to track and coordinate patient flow.
	Develop standards through accreditation bodies for crowding, boarding, and diversion.
Create a coordinated, regionalized, accountable emergency care system.	Develop regionalized systems that include hospitals, emergency medical services (EMS), and other agencies working together.
	Patients should be taken to the care center that can provide the optimal care, for example, to trauma or stroke centers.
	Develop well-defined standards and performance improvement measures.
Increase funding for emergency care systems.	Fund research to identify best practices.
	Request reimbursement for care of all patients who are treated in the emergency department.
	Acquire funding for disaster preparedness.
Improving pediatric emergency care.	Develop triage and transport protocols designed to provide children with the most appropriate care.
	Educate and train emergency care providers to care for children.
	Include pediatric concerns as part of disaster plans.
	Hire pediatric coordinators in EDs and EMS agencies to ensure that appropriate equipment, training, and services are provided to children.

Source: Institute of Medicine. (2006). *Hospital-based emergency care at the breaking point.* Washington, DC: National Academy of Sciences.

CHART 73–1   Emergency Nursing Roles

Role	Description
Urgent care center nursing	Nurses provide care in free-standing facilities that provide urgent care for minor illnesses and injuries.
Prehospital nursing	Nurses provide care in the prehospital care environment. These nurses are prepared through additional education that is generally regulated by the states in which they practice. For example, some states require nurses to take a prehospital nursing course or become emergency medical technicians (EMTs) or EMT-paramedics.
Transport nursing	Nurses accompany air or ground transport patients. Even though many nurses who perform transport may have emergency nursing experience, transport nurses may also have critical care nursing experience.
Military nurses	Nurses provide care as part of their military service.
Industrial nursing and occupational health nursing	Nurses provide care to specific industries or companies. Basic life support and ACLS are additional responsibilities of many of these nurses.
Correctional nursing	Nurses provide care in prisons and jails.

CHART 73–2   Specialty Roles in Emergency Nursing

Role	Description
Nurse educator	This is a nurse who is responsible for the educational needs of the emergency department. This role may also include patient and community education.
Emergency nurse practitioner (ENP)	ENPs are nurse practitioners who specialize in providing advanced nursing practice. There is no specific certification for emergency nursing, however, many ENPs hold certifications as family nurse practitioners, acute care nurse practitioners, pediatric nurse practitioners, or adult nurse practitioners.
Emergency clinical nurse specialist (ECNS)	A clinical nurse specialist is prepared at either the master's or doctoral level as an expert in emergency nursing. An ECNS may provide direct patient care, provide education, develop and perform research, and serve as a role model and change agent in the emergency department.
Case manager	An emergency case manager can provide care to a single patient or a group of patients. Case managers interact with many departments and outside agencies to assist the patient, families, and emergency department staff with care issues such as home health, drug dependence, and psychiatric problems so that the best and most cost-effective care is given to the patient.

The goals of triage include:

- Early and brief patient assessment
- Determination of the patient's urgency for care
- Documentation of findings
- Control of patient flow through the emergency department
- Assignment of patients to the appropriate care area
- Initiation of diagnostic measures
- Initiation of limited therapeutic interventions
- Infection control
- Promotion of public relations
- Health education for patients and families.

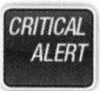 **CRITICAL ALERT** *An important part of triage is the "intuitiveness" that the emergency nurse may have about the patient. The triage nurse recognizes that there is something wrong. Oftentimes, few data are available to validate these "feelings." However, experienced emergency department nurses are good resources to alert new nurses about how to identify the less obvious indicators that a patient may be in trouble.*

Types of Triage

The type of triage that is used in an emergency department is dependent on several things including patient census, department layout, and number and type of staff. As previously stated, triage is usually performed by an experienced registered nurse. However, other types of triage models are summarized in Chart 73–3.

Components of Triage

Triage begins with an "across the room assessment." This involves what the triage nurse sees, smells, or sometimes even feels when first evaluating the patient. For example:

- Is the patient's airway open or is he drooling?
- Is the patient breathing and, if so, is the breathing effective?
- What is the patient's skin color: normal, pale, flushed?
- Are there any obvious signs of illness or injury?

A minimal amount of information should be gathered about why the patient has presented to the emergency department. Several mnemonics can be used to gather data depending on the

patient's chief complaint or reason why she came to the emergency department. Charts 73–4, 73–5, and 73–6 contain mnemonics that can assist with collecting historical data in triage. Even though the CIAMPEDS mnemonic is directed more at collecting data for a pediatric patient, it can easily be adapted for the adult patient as well (ENA, 2004).

A brief, but focused physical assessment should be performed. Objective data can be collected by using a primary assessment that includes airway, breathing, circulation, and disability. The components of the primary assessment are discussed in detail in Chapter 74 ☻.

A secondary assessment may be required in some cases to better differentiate the severity of a patient's condition. The secondary assessment should include exposure with environmental control, a full set of vital signs and family presence, provision of comfort, additional history, and a head-to-toe assessment as needed using inspection, palpation, and auscultation. The components of the secondary survey are discussed in detail in the Chapter 74 ☻.

CHART 73–4 **CIAMPEDS Mnemonic**

C	Chief complaint
I	Immunizations
I	Isolation: exposed to a disease or hazardous material that may put the rest of the department in danger
A	Allergies
M	Medications
P	Parents' or caregivers' impression about the patient
E	Events surrounding the illness or injury
D	Diet
D	Diapers or output
S	Symptoms associated with the chief complaint, for example, fever, nausea, and vomiting

---

CHART 73–3 **Types of Triage**

Type of Triage	Components
Traffic director	*Nonprofessional (hospital registrar)* Writes down chief complaint.
Spot check	*Nurse/health care provider* Evaluates patient. Assigns an urgency category.
Comprehensive triage	*Registered nurse* Evaluates patient. Assigns an urgency category. Implements interventions (e.g., ordering a radiograph). Administers pain medication.

CHART 73–5 **MVIT Mnemonic**

M	Mechanism of injury
V	Vital signs
I	Injury
T	Treatment

CHART 73–6 **AMPLE History Mnemonic**

A	Allergies
M	Medications
P	Past medical history
L	Last meal
E	Everything that is related to the chief complaint

Gerontological Considerations

With the aging population, it is important for the emergency department (ED) nurse to be familiar with the unique aspects of elderly assessment and planning of care. At a hospital in Canada that received 51,000 ED visits annually, adults who were 70 years of age or older used approximately 70% of the total bed days, and in 2005, those 75 years of age and older had an ED admit rate of approximately 37%, compared to an average admit rate for all ages of 15% (Sendecki, 2007). For this reason the hospital in Canada developed a course that applied geriatric/geropsychiatric knowledge, skills, and abilities the ED nurse can implement into their daily practice. An example is the need to assess falls as a symptom that requires investigation of root causes, treatment plan follow-up, and risk reduction to prevent another fall. They also assigned a position in the ED for a geriatric emergency nurse (GEN). The focus of the GEN is to identify needs and start a proactive care plan that is used during the patient's admission. The GEN also alerts community care to anticipated needs upon discharge. At the end of a 4-month trial they found that the GEN had seen approximately 25% of all patients who were 75 years of age or older; of those, 50% were admitted to the hospital; and the average length of stay of those who had been assessed by the GEN was 11.5 days, compared with 15.4 for those of the same age group not seen by the GEN (Sendecki, 2007). The ENA has also focused on ED care for elderly patients, as outlined in the Gerontological Considerations box. Chapter 10 provides detailed information regarding the aging patient.

Triage Urgency Categories

Once an initial evaluation has been made related to the patient's physical condition and chief complaint, the triage nurse will assign the patient an urgency category. Urgency categories rate patient acuity and assist in prioritizing care. Generally, an emergent patient is one who has an immediate life-threatening problem, for example, an airway obstruction. An urgent patient can wait a little longer, but would need to be seen as soon as possible. An example is a patient with chest pain, cardiac risk factors, and stable vital signs. Finally, a nonurgent patient can wait for care.

GERONTOLOGICAL CONSIDERATIONS in the Emergency Department

The Emergency Nurses Association has developed an online course entitled Geriatric Emergency Nursing Education (GENE). The course covers best practices that can be used to deliver optimal care and respond to the special needs of older adults. The course covers these topics:

- Attitudes and ageism
- Physical and psychological changes
- Atypical presentation of illness
- Triage
- Pain management
- Abuse and neglect
- Palliative care
- Discharge planning.

Many emergency departments use a three-level urgency category, but the continued increase in emergency department censuses, the augmented acuity of patients who are being cared for in the emergency department, and the numbers of patients who use the emergency department for primary care have prompted the use of additional levels of urgency. Charts 73–7 and 73–8, respectively, summarize four- and five-level triage urgency scales. There are resources available such as the Emergency Severity Index from the Emergency Nurses Association that describes the use of a five-level triage urgency category.

 Even when patients have been assigned a triage category, their condition may change, so patients who must wait for care must be reassessed at specific intervals. Triage policies and procedures should reflect when this must be done and documented. Unfortunately, patients have suffered significant harm and even death while waiting to be seen!

Disaster Triage

When a disaster occurs (earthquake, tornado, terrorist event), triage is directed at rapidly identifying patient urgency, assigning a category, and rapidly deploying to the most appropriate area for care. However, in a disaster, there may not be enough personnel or resources to care for everyone. In such a case, care may be withheld so that limited resources are used for those who will survive (Delaney & Drummond, 2002).

During a disaster, many emergency departments and community disaster programs use the START (simple triage and rapid treatment) system. This system evaluates respirations, perfusion, and mental status in order to determine who needs immediate transport, who can wait, or who may be unsalvageable. Color codes are used as a method of identification and communication. For example, green may mean that the patient can walk to an area for care (Super, Groth, & Hook, 1994). Refer to Chapter 72 for a detailed description of the START triage system.

Each emergency department and community should have a disaster plan that describes the manner of triage that should be employed during a disaster. The roles of the emergency nurse and other staff members should be practiced on a regularly

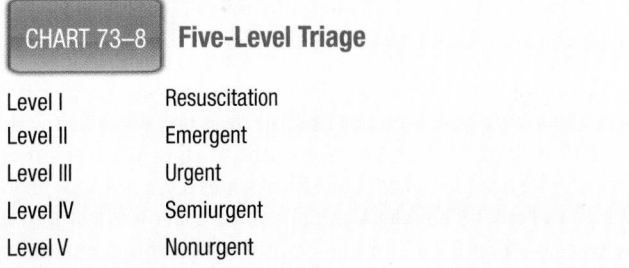

CHART 73–7 Four-Level Triage

Level I	Resuscitation
Level II	Emergent
Level III	Urgent
Level IV	Nonurgent

CHART 73–8 Five-Level Triage

Level I	Resuscitation
Level II	Emergent
Level III	Urgent
Level IV	Semiurgent
Level V	Nonurgent

scheduled basis. Additional information about disaster management is provided in Chapter 72 ⊚.

Legal Issues

The practice of emergency nursing requires comprehension and understanding of some of the legal issues that impact the emergency department. Three of these issues are discussed here: the Emergency Medical Treatment and Active Labor Act, consent, and evidence collection.

Emergency Medical Treatment and Active Labor Act

The **Emergency Medical Treatment and Active Labor Act (EMTALA)** is a part of the 1986 COBRA laws and the 1990 OBRA amendment that defines the legal responsibilities of Medicare-participating hospitals in treating individuals who present with emergency medical conditions (*Federal Register*, 2003). In summary, EMTALA provides that:

- A hospital is required to perform a medical screening exam to determine if there is an emergency when a patient presents to the emergency department.
- If it is determined that an emergency condition exists, the hospital must provide for further medical examination and treatment as required to stabilize the patient.
- If the hospital does not have the capabilities to provide the care needed, the patient may be transferred.
- An appropriate transfer is one in which the medical benefits outweigh the risk of transport or the patient makes an informed consent for transfer.
- The patient must be transferred with an appropriate level of care provided during the transport process.
- A hospital may never delay an appropriate medical screening examination or further examination or treatment to inquire about the patient's payment method or insurance status.

Also under EMTALA, hospitals that receive patients who may have been inappropriately transferred need to report this; signs must be posted in the emergency department that explain a person's rights to emergency treatment (most emergency departments have these posted in multiple languages); and hospitals must maintain patients records, a health care providers on-call list, and emergency department logs. Failure to adhere to these regulations can result in both institutional and individual fines and loss of federal funding.

In summary, EMTALA provides that all patients who seek treatment in the emergency department have a medical screening and treatment as deemed appropriate based on their emergency. No patient can be turned away for financial reasons.

Consent

Consent is defined as "giving permission to do something." However, the nature of emergency practice does not always allow the patient or family the ability to consent to all of the treatments that may be needed to save a life. Most states recognize this problem in the emergency department and have allowed consent to be waived when there is a life- or limb-threatening emergency (Lee, 2003).

The emergency nurse will generally encounter three types of consent. These include a *general (blanket) consent*, which is usually obtained at registration. This type of consent form will allow for evaluation and treatment, such as radiographs, laboratory tests, and medications. If more invasive tests are needed or the patient must undergo a specific procedure such as a fracture reduction that requires conscious sedation, informed consent should be obtained. *Informed consent* involves the patient stating by signing that he has a full understanding of the procedure, including its risks, and is competent to give consent. Even though the emergency nurse should check to see that a consent form has been signed, it is the health care providers responsibility to obtain informed consent. Finally, *implied consent* allows treatment in an emergency situation based on the presumption that if the patient were able to, she would give permission for treatment (Lee, 2003).

Each state dictates ages of consent, situations that may allow for legal consent despite age (pregnant underaged females), and other interesting nuances related to consent. It is imperative that the emergency nurse be familiar with the applicable state laws and hospital policies related to consent. When in doubt, always safely err on the side of the patient and when possible consult hospital risk management personnel before acting. It is also important to document why decisions were made to prevent any "legal" second-guessing.

Evidence Collection and Preservation

Unfortunately, a major part of emergency nursing practice is caring for the victims of violence. Sexual assault, domestic assault, and motor vehicle crashes are only a few of the examples of the types of patients who may require that the emergency nurse collect and preserve evidence. **Forensic evidence** is something that is legally submitted to a court of law as a means of determining the truth related to an alleged crime (Doyle, 2001). Examples of evidence include clothing, body fluids, bite marks, and photographs of injuries.

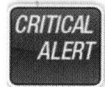 *Every emergency department should have a policy and procedure for the collection and preservation of evidence. Improper collection and preservation could lead to erroneous interpretation of the evidence.*

Evidence must be collected using a specific protocol and procedure that includes how to label the evidence, preserve it, and maintain the chain of custody. Some evidence collection protocols are directed by specific legal agencies or even state agencies. Chart 73–9 contains a summary of procedural steps for evidence collection and preservation in the emergency department (Semonin-Holleran, 2004).

Preparation for Practice

Preparation for practice in the emergency department for new graduates or nurses without emergency experience can be demanding. Nursing care in the emergency department includes learning to manage the care of four or five patients simultaneously; starting all of the patient care, for example, inserting intravenous lines and drawing blood for evaluation; limited and focused patient assessment, oftentimes with little or no patient information; discharge teaching and planning; and care of populations and patient problems not frequently encountered in admitted patients such as acute psychosis, sexual assault, and

CHART 73–9 Collection and Preservation of Evidence and Chain of Custody

1. Identify the indications for evidence collection and consult authorities to ensure that the appropriate evidence is collected and preserved.

2. Obtain and use the appropriate evidence collection kit.

3. Obtain patient consent according to hospital policy and procedure. In some cases consent may not be necessary, for example, in a homicide investigation. Consult appropriate authorities.

4. When collecting evidence, change gloves frequently to prevent cross-contamination.

5. Try not to perform any wound care until photographs have been taken.

6. Place evidence in individual labeled containers.

7. Wet evidence should always be dried before packaging.

8. Always place evidence in a paper bag.

9. Label all evidence with this information:
   a. Patient's name
   b. Source of collection
   c. Date
   d. Time
   e. Person collecting the evidence.

10. Evidence should be sealed with evidence tape. Never lick evidence envelopes.

11. Photographs may be taken by an emergency nurse. They must be labeled and stored in a secured area. Only take photographs if experienced in how to do it properly.

12. Document the evidence collection procedure. Use checklists when available.

13. Place evidence in a secure, locked area until it is released to the appropriate authorities.

14. Maintain the chain of custody, who collected the evidence, anyone who touches or secures it and what is done with the evidence until it is given to law enforcement, for all evidence.

15. Complete the chart and document what was given to authorities and who received the evidence.

---

homelessness. It also requires familiarity with diverse patient populations, varied age groups, and social problems that may never be solved (Proehl, 2002).

Additional education for new orientees to the emergency department should include:

- Advanced Cardiac Life Support (ACLS)
- Trauma Nursing Core Course (TNCC)
- Emergency Nursing Pediatric Course (ENPC).

Nursing care for patients or conditions not frequently encountered by new orientees with their limited experience (e.g., obstetrics and gynecology; eye, ear, nose, and throat; pediatric and psychiatric emergencies) should also be included.

Discharge Priorities

The majority of patients seen in the emergency department are sent home rather than admitted to the hospital. An important part of discharge planning is providing information about how to manage the problem that brought the patient to the emergency department and where the patient should obtain further care.

Discharge instructions should be clear and use terminology that the patient understands. Most educators recommend that discharge instructions be written at a fifth- or sixth-grade level. When possible, they should be translated into a language that the patient or family understands or at a minimum an interpreter should be present when the instructions are given. Illustrations of what is expected (e.g., how to wrap an elastic bandage on an injured extremity) may be of assistance. Instructions must also be age appropriate. This is especially important when medications are being prescribed.

Many commercial programs that provide discharge instructions are available. These instructions can be printed and sent with the patient or, in some cases, they can be accessed online from the patient's home.

Discharge instructions should include information about follow-up care. In some emergency departments, patients may be asked to return; in other EDs, patients may be referred to a health care provider, advanced practitioner, or clinic. It is important to ensure that the patient or family members understand the information that is provided. Asking the patient questions or to do a return demonstration may assist in determining the level of understanding. Some emergency departments have instituted follow-up calls to not only find out about follow-up care, but to check on the patient's status. It is important to allow the patient or family the opportunity to ask questions and feel as comfortable as possible with the prescribed care for their illness or injury.

Health Promotion

Emergency nurses not only play a key role in the management of ill or injured patients, but also in injury and disease prevention. One primary example is through Emergency Nurses CARE (ENCARE). ENCARE was started by two emergency nurses in the 1980s who had become involved in trying to prevent injuries and death from alcohol-related emergencies (ENA Injury Prevention Institute/ENCARE, 2008). Emergency Nurses CARE has now become the Injury Prevention Institute/ENCARE of the Emergency Nurses Association.

ENCARE provides training for volunteer nurses and emergency medical technicians related to specific issues such as injury prevention and public health issues. Currently ENCARE provides five primary education and prevention programs:

- Alcohol Awareness Program
- Bike and Helmet Safety
- Child Passenger Safety
- Gun Safety: It's No Accident
- Healthy Aging: Take Care.

Through the efforts of its many volunteers, ENCARE has reached hundreds of thousands of people throughout the United States.

Much research has been done and is ongoing regarding injury prevention and the best ways to educate communities. Other research opportunities for emergency nursing are included in the Research Opportunities and Clinical Impact feature.

Summary

The practice of emergency nursing involves the care of diverse patient populations in many types of situations. It requires skills that include the ability to identify critically ill and injured patients and start their care from the beginning and patience with difficult societal problems such as caring for the homeless. It also involves ethical challenges as described in the Ethical Issues feature, and the practice of emergency nursing should be evidenced based. The Evidence-Based Practice feature gives an example of evidence-based nursing practice in the emergency department.

Emergency nursing encompasses all aspects of care from pediatric to geriatric, medical to surgical, and to a very diverse popu-

ETHICAL ISSUES Regarding Pain Management in the Emergency Department

Pain is the most common complaint seen in the emergency department. Despite this, only 40% to 60% of the patients are treated for pain. Many patients face **oligoanalgesia**, in which no interventions are provided for pain relief despite patient complaints of pain when they come to the emergency department. Many reasons are cited for this, including fear of "masking" symptoms and concern about the physiological effects of pain medications. Other studies have demonstrated that women and minorities do not receive appropriate pain management. Emergency nurses need to be patient advocates and ensure that a patient's pain is assessed, documented, and managed. Pain management requires a collaborative approach including protocols so that analgesic agents can be administered as soon as possible. All patients should receive pain care (Knox et al., 2007).

lation of patients both culturally and economically. It requires excellent assessment and critical thinking skills as well as procedural proficiency. Emergency nursing is a rewarding way to "nurse."

EVIDENCE-BASED PRACTICE

Family Presence During Resuscitation in the Emergency Department

Clinical Problem

Should the family be allowed to be present during resuscitation in the emergency department?

Research Findings

In 1982, the Foote Hospital in Michigan surveyed 13 surviving relatives about whether they would have liked to be present during the resuscitation of their family members. Seventy-two percent said that they would have liked to have been present. A program was developed to allow selected "accompanied" family members to be allowed to be present during resuscitation. Seventy family members and 21 physicians, nurses, and others were surveyed after the event. Seventy-six percent of the family members felt that being present assisted them in their grieving process. They also felt that the patient did not die alone and emergency care providers did everything that they could. Staff members, however, felt hampered in their resuscitation efforts and reported increased stress because the patients became more "human" in the presence of family members. No family member interfered with the resuscitation efforts (Doyle et al., 1987).

This landmark study opened the "floodgates" to consider the role of the family in resuscitation. Since 1987, more than 60 papers have been published that address this issue. Families have expressed that they are not concerned about what they may see or hear in the resuscitation area—they just want to be with their family member. More than half of the families felt they had a right to be present and, again, felt that their grieving process was aided. The staff's perspective includes fear of interference from the family and the need to display more professional behaviors during the resuscitation process. Interestingly, physicians are more opposed to family presence than are nurses.

Implications for Nursing Practice

When implementing family presence in the ED during resuscitation, a policy needs to be in place that addresses when it can and cannot be

allowed; all staff need to be prepared and trained; well-qualified and trained staff should always accompany the patient; and resources must be available to the staff to help them cope with any issues that may arise (Walker, 2006).

Critical Thinking Questions

1. What should be in place in the emergency department to allow family presence?
   a. A clergy member to provide spiritual care for the patient and family
   b. A policy and procedure that describes how to implement the process
   c. Staff who object to the presence of a family member during resuscitation
   d. Security or police so that the family is kept away during resuscitation

2. Which of the following fears have staff members expressed when allowing a family member to be with a patient during resuscitation?
   a. Fear that the family member may interfere with the resuscitation
   b. Fear that they must see the patient as a human being during the resuscitation
   c. Fear that they must act more professionally during the resuscitation
   d. All of the above

Answers to Critical Thinking Questions appear in Appendix D.

References

Doyle, C., Post, H., Burney, R., Maino, J., Keefe, M., et al. (1987). Family participation during resuscitation: An option. *Annals of Emergency Medicine, 16,* 673–675.

Walker, W. (2006). Witnessed resuscitation: A concept analysis. *International Journal of Nursing Studies, 43,* 377–387.

RESEARCH OPPORTUNITIES AND CLINICAL IMPACT RELATED TO EMERGENCY NURSING

Research Area	Clinical Impact
Physiological Research	
The management of acute and chronic pain in the emergency department	Many patients do not have their pain appropriately managed and frequently present to the emergency department for pain medication.
Use of alternative methods to manage pain in the emergency department	Alternative methods of pain management such as acupuncture, acupressure, and massage could be used by nurses to manage pain in the emergency department.
Development of guidelines to manage shock in the emergency department	Innovative assessment and monitoring methods and treatment therapies would emerge for the management of the patient in shock.
Psychosocial, Ethical, and Legal Research	
Effectiveness of family presence during invasive procedures and resuscitation	Identify how to include the family in the care of their critically ill or injured family member. Assist in end-of-life decision making.
Problem of overcrowding in emergency departments and ambulance diversion by EDs	Learn to manage the limited resources of emergency departments, including nursing staff, in order to meet the needs of all patients, particularly the uninsured and underinsured patients who use the emergency department for their health care.
Effectiveness of follow-up phone calls within 24 hours of a patient visit	Decrease return visits and get patients into the appropriate health care systems, thereby decreasing costs.

NCLEX® REVIEW

1. As it relates to the practice of emergency nursing, the nurse understands that:
   1. It always involves episodic patient care that is usually chronic or critical in nature.
   2. It can describe patient care for perceived, actual, or undiagnosed health problems.
   3. It has long been associated with Judith Kelleher and her care of wounded soldiers.
   4. It is challenged to become culturally competent as the patients become analogous.

2. You are the emergency department nurse responsible for triage. All of the following patients present simultaneously for care. With your triage assessment complete, which patient should be treated first?
   1. A patient complaining of chest pain and shortness of breath with pale, clammy skin, nausea and diaphoresis
   2. A patient with a three centimeter laceration to the right forearm with normal sensation and minimal bleeding
   3. A patient having a possible allergic reaction with facial edema, drooling, stridor, and severe urticaria with pruritis
   4. A patient experiencing increasingly more severe problems urinating and has a large palpable bladder

3. The patient presents to the emergency department with a complaint of nontraumatic back pain for four months that has previously been evaluated by his or her primary care provider. The patient states, "I ran out of my pain medicine last night, and my doctor refuses to call in another prescription." Objective findings are unremarkable. Vital signs are HR 89, BP 130/60, RR 18, T 98.9°F, SpO_2 99%, and pain 5 on a 0–10 scale. Based on the four-level system, how should this patient be categorized at triage?

   1. Level I – Resuscitative
   2. Level II – Emergent
   3. Level III – Urgent
   4. Level IV – Nonurgent

4. The patient presents to the emergency department with a left shoulder dislocation that must be reduced quickly as the radial pulse on the affected side is no longer palpable. The injury occurred 30 minutes prior to arrival, and the patient states he or she is experiencing severe pain. The emergency nurse understands that which of the following consents must be obtained prior to this patient's treatment?
   1. General consent and informed consent
   2. Informed consent and implied consent
   3. Implied consent and blood product consent
   4. Blood product consent and general consent

5. You are orienting a new nurse graduate to the emergency department. Which of the following statements made by the new nurse regarding preparation for emergency nursing would indicate the need for further instruction?
   1. "I am planning on taking additional training to help prepare myself to deal with any potential psychiatric emergencies."
   2. "I am glad that emergency nurses do not have to deal with obstetrical issues because they can call the labor and delivery nurses."
   3. "I will take the Trauma Nursing Core Course soon because I know I need more experience with trauma assessment."
   4. "I now feel more confident in my time management skills when it comes to caring for multiple patients simultaneously."

Answers for review questions appear in Appendix D

KEY TERMS

emergency nursing *p.2415*
Emergency Medical Treatment and Active
   Labor Act (EMTALA) *p.2420*

forensic evidence *p.2420*
oligoanalgesia *p.2422*

triage *p.2416*

PEARSON
EXPLORE mynursingkit™

MyNursingKit is your one stop for online chapter review materials and resources. Prepare for success with additional NCLEX®-style practice questions, interactive assignments and activities, web links, animations and videos, and more!

Register your access code from the front of your book at
www.mynursingkit.com

REFERENCES

Bonalumi, N., & King, D. (2007). Professionalism and leadership. In S. Hoyt and J. Selfridge-Thomas (Eds.), *Emergency nursing core curriculum* (6th ed.). Philadelphia: W. B. Saunders.

Bracken, J. (2003). Triage. In L. Newberry (Ed.), *Sheehy's emergency nursing: Principles and practice* (5th ed.). St. Louis: Mosby.

Cone, D. C., Richardson, L. D., Todd, K., Betancourt, J., & Lowe, R. (2003). Health care disparities in emergency medicine. *Academic Emergency Medicine, 10*(11), 1176–1183.

Delaney, J., & Drummond, R. (2002). Mass casualties and triage at a sporting event. *British Journal of Sports Medicine, 36*, 85–88.

Doyle, C., Post, H., Burney, R., Maino, J., Keefe, M., et al. (1987). Family participation during resuscitation: An option. *Annals of Emergency Medicine, 16*, 673–675.

Doyle, J. S. (2001). *Evidence collection handbook from the Kentucky State Police.* Retrieved October 10, 2008, from http://firearmsid.com/ KSP%20Evidence%20Manual/KSP%20Manual%20Main.htm

Emergency Nurses Association. (1999). *Emergency Nurses Association scope of emergency nursing practice.* Des Plaines, IL: Author.

Emergency Nurses Association. (2004). *Emergency nursing pediatric course.* Des Plaines, IL: Author.

ENA Injury Prevention Institute/ENCARE. (2008). *History and background.* Retrieved October 10, 2008, from http://www.ena.org/ipinstitute/ history

Federal Register. (2003). Department of Health and Human Services 42 CFR Parts 413,482, and 489 Medicare programs; Clarifying policies related to the responsibilities of Medicare-participating hospitals in treating individuals with emergency medical conditions. Final rule September 9, 2003.

Gilboy, N., Travers, D., & Wuerz, R. (1999). Re-evaluating triage in the new millennium: A comprehensive look at the need for standardization and quality. *Journal of Emergency Nursing, 25*(6), 463–473.

Institute of Medicine. (2006). *Hospital-based emergency care at the breaking point.* Washington, DC: National Academy of Sciences.

Knox, T., Ducharme, J., Choiniere, M., Crandall, C., Fosnocht, D., Homel, P., et al. (2007). Pain in the emergency department: Results of the Pain and Emergency Department Initiative (PEMI) multicenter study. *Journal of Pain, 8*(6), 460–466.

Lee, G. (2003). Legal and regulatory constructs. In L. Newberry (Ed.), *Sheehy's emergency nursing: Principles and practice* (5th ed.). St. Louis: Mosby.

Lipson, J. G., & Dibble, S. L. (Eds.). (2007). *Culture and clinical care.* San Francisco: UCSF Nursing Press.

MacPhail, E. (2003). Overview of emergency nursing. In L. Newberry (Ed.), *Sheehy's emergency nursing: Principles and practice* (5th ed., pp. 1–5). St. Louis: Mosby.

National Center for Health Statistics. (2007). *Emergency department visits.* Retrieved September 10, 2007, from http://www.cdc.gov/ nchs/fastats/ervisits.htm

Proehl, J. (2002). Developing emergency nursing competence. *Nursing Clinics of North America, 37*(1), 89–96.

Reeder, T. J., & Garrison, H. G. (2001). When the safety net is unsafe: Real-time assessment of the overcrowded emergency department. *Academic Emergency Medicine, 8*(11), 1070–1073.

Schriver, J., Talmadge, R., Chuong, R., & Hedges, J. (2003). Emergency nursing. *Journal of Emergency Nursing, 29*(5), 431–439.

Semonin-Holleran, R. (2004). Preservation of evidence. In J. Proehl (Ed.), *Emergency nursing procedures.* Philadelphia: W. B. Saunders.

Sendecki, C. (2007). Care of the acutely ill elderly in ER: Growth of the role of geriatric ER nurses. *Outlook* (Fall 2007).

Super, G., Groth, S., & Hook, R. (1994). *START: Simple triage and rapid treatment plan.* Newport Beach, CA: Hoag Memorial Hospital.

Thomas, D. O., Bernardo, L. M., & Herman, B. (2003). *Core curriculum for pediatric emergency nursing.* Boston: Jones and Bartlett Publishers.

Walker, W. (2006). Witnessed resuscitation: A concept analysis. *International Journal of Nursing Studies, 43*, 377–387.

Caring for the Patient with Multisystem Trauma

Cheryl Wraa

Outcome-Based Learning Objectives

After studying this chapter, the learner will be able to:

1. Discuss the correlation between mechanism of injury with patient assessment based on an understanding of the kinematics of trauma.
2. List the priorities of the primary and secondary surveys.
3. Explain the rationale for the tertiary survey.
4. Compare and contrast special considerations experienced during the initial resuscitation.

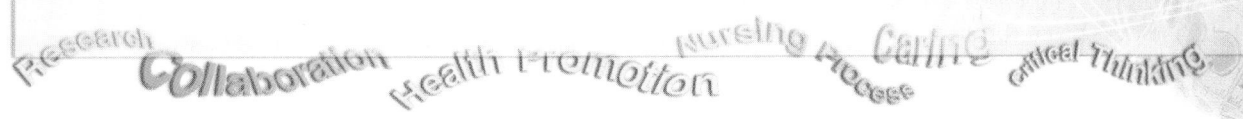

Research Collaboration Health Promotion Nursing Process Caring Critical Thinking

TRAUMATIC INJURY is a major public health problem. It is currently recognized as one of the most important threats to public health and safety in the United States with regard to years of productive life lost, permanent disability, and cost (American College of Surgeons, Committee on Trauma, 2006). In the United States, injury is a leading cause of death regardless of age, race, gender, or economic status (Centers for Disease Control and Prevention [CDC], 2007b). In high-income nations such as the United States, injury is the leading cause of death in the first four decades of life; in low- and middle-income nations it is second only to infectious diseases (Sommers, 2006).

Although traumatic injury is a leading cause of death, many patients survive their injuries but may experience a permanent disability, chronic pain, and a permanent change in their quality of life. The National Trauma Data Bank (NTDB) contains the largest aggregation of data reported from the trauma registries of hospital trauma centers. Their 2006 report reviews combined data from 2001 through 2005. The data show that the majority of injuries are unintentional, with the greatest percentage (41.3%) related to motor vehicle traffic incidents followed by falls (27.2%) (NTDB, 2007). It is important to note that the word *unintentional* is used rather than *accidental*. Throughout the years it has been recognized that the cause of most unintentional injury is the result of poor choices or behaviors, and that these in-

juries may have been preventable. An example of a poor choice is to consume alcohol and then attempt to drive. Alcohol alters a person's judgment and coordination. The following statistics are part of the Emergency Nurses Association (ENA) Injury Prevention Institute/ENCARE *Alcohol Awareness Fact Sheet* (2006a):

- Alcohol-related motor vehicle crashes kill someone every 31 minutes and nonfatally injure someone every 2 minutes.
- Twenty-one-year-olds to 24-year-olds have the highest rate of alcohol impaired driving and the highest percentage of fatal alcohol-related crashes.
- A systematic review of 65 studies on fatal nontraffic injuries, found that intoxication occurred in 31.5% of homicide cases, 31% of unintentional injury deaths, and 22.7% of suicide cases.

Alcohol consumption is also a major factor in family violence, suicides, homicides, and altercations.

Because unintentional injuries are a major source of morbidity and mortality, injury prevention has become a major public health goal. The U.S. Department of Health and Human Services and Public Health Service have developed the *Healthy People 2010: National Health Promotion and Disease Prevention Objectives*. The objectives that pertain to injury and violence prevention are listed in the National Guidelines box (p. 2426).

NATIONAL GUIDELINES *Healthy People 2010*

Goal: Reduce injuries, disabilities, and deaths due to unintentional injuries and violence.

Objectives:

1. Injury prevention to reduce:
   - Nonfatal head injuries
   - Nonfatal spinal cord injuries
   - Firearm-related deaths
   - Nonfatal firearm-related injuries
   - Child fatality
   - Nonfatal poisonings
   - Deaths from poisoning
   - Deaths from suffocation

2. Unintentional injury prevention to:
   - Reduce deaths from unintentional injuries
   - Reduce nonfatal unintentional injuries
   - Reduce deaths from motor vehicle crashes
   - Reduce pedestrian deaths
   - Reduce nonfatal motor vehicle injuries
   - Reduce nonfatal pedestrian injuries
   - Increase use of safety belts
   - Increase use of child restraints

- Increase motorcycle helmet use
- Establish graduated driver licensing
- Increase bicycle helmet use
- Establish bicycle helmet laws
- Reduce residential fire deaths
- Increase functioning smoke alarms in residences
- Reduce deaths from falls
- Reduce hip fractures
- Reduce drowning
- Reduce dog bite injuries
- Increase injury protection in school sports

3. Violence and abuse prevention to:
   - Reduce homicides
   - Reduce maltreatment and maltreatment fatalities of children
   - Reduce physical assault by intimate partners
   - Reduce rape or attempted rape
   - Reduce sexual assault other than rape
   - Reduce physical assaults
   - Reduce physical fighting among adolescents
   - Reduce weapon carrying by adolescents on school property

---

Kinematics of Injury

Imperative in the care of the trauma patient is the ability to identify and treat all life-threatening injuries quickly. Traumatic injury occurs when a source of energy makes contact with the body and the body cannot tolerate the exposure to that energy. The extent of injury depends on the type and amount of energy force and the tissue response to the force. Newton's first law of motion states that a body at rest remains at rest, and a body in motion remains in motion until acted on by an outside force (Feliciano, Mattox, & Moore, 2008). Force is the result of energy transference. Energy is neither created nor destroyed—it is transferred; and different factors influence the amount of energy the human body absorbs, including:

- The amount of energy absorbed by objects that are struck first (the body of the vehicle for example)

- The amount of energy absorbed by protective devices such as helmets, padded dashboards, and air bags.

The slower the energy force is applied, the less energy transference and degree of destruction.

Injury patterns have been identified through the evaluation of the type of trauma that occurred and the amount of force that was generated. These known patterns assist health care providers to be anticipatory when caring for trauma patients. The predictive patterns of injuries are referred to as **kinematics**.

Motor Vehicle Collisions

As stated, motor vehicle collisions cause some of the most commonly seen injuries. When a patient is admitted due to a motor vehicle crash it is important to try to ascertain the speed the vehicle was traveling and where it impacted an object or was impacted by another vehicle. This will enable the nurse to better

understand the amount of energy that was dispersed. Other indicators of the force energy are the amount of damage noted to the vehicle, the amount of intrusion into the passenger compartment, and the amount of damage from the occupant striking parts of the interior such as the steering wheel, dashboard, or windshield.

Frontal Impact

When a vehicle impacts an object or another vehicle head-on, energy is transferred to the vehicle. The front stops and the rear of the automobile continues to move forward until all energy is dispersed. The same principle occurs with the passenger in the vehicle. When the front of the vehicle stops, the body continues to move forward. If the passenger is restrained properly, then the seat belts will absorb most of the energy and prevent the body from colliding with immovable objects such as the windshield. This is also true if the air bag is deployed. A seat belt can impose a load that is 20 to 50 times as great as the weight of the body. The portion of the body that has the ability to receive this load is the pelvis. If the passenger has the belt over the abdomen rather than the pelvis, compression injury may occur to the abdominal organs. Abrasions and/or ecchymosis from the seat belt are important indicators of possible underlying injury (Figure 74–1 ■).

If the passenger is not restrained and the air bag does not deploy, then the body might travel down and under the steering wheel or up and over the steering wheel, incurring injury at the body's point of impact with the vehicle (Figure 74–2 ■). Patterns of injury that are anticipated are:

- Cervical spine fracture
- Traumatic brain injury
- Anterior flail chest
- Myocardial contusion

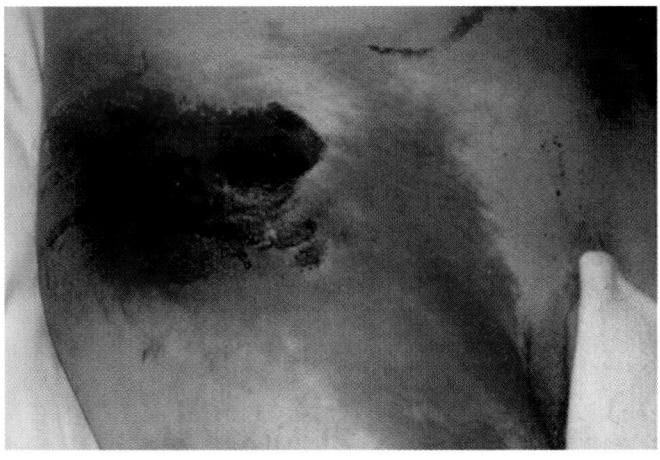
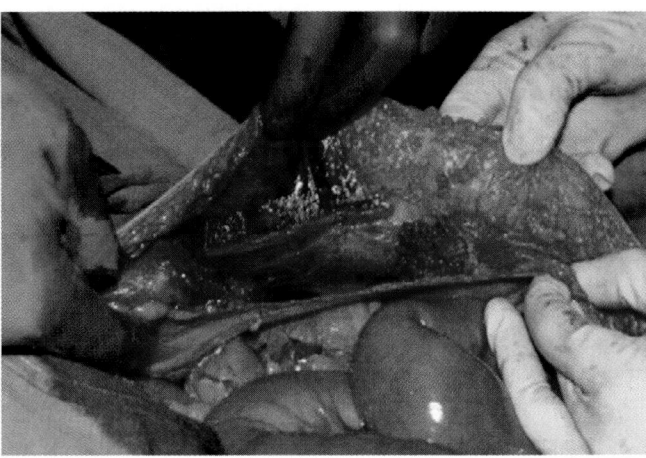

FIGURE 74–1 ■ Sealtbelt injury.
Source: Cheryl Wraa

- Pneumothorax
- Traumatic aortic disruption
- Fractured spleen or liver
- Posterior fracture/dislocation of the hip, knee, and/or ankle (American College of Surgeons [ACS], 2004; Feliciano, Mattox, & Moore, 2008).

Side Impact

As many as 31% of fatalities from motor vehicle crashes are a result of side impact (ACS, 2004). Most injuries from side impact are dependent on whether the vehicle remains in place or moves away from the point of impact. If the vehicle remains in place,

then the amount of damage to the vehicle and intrusion into the passenger compartment signifies the amount of energy that the body may have absorbed. Passengers generally receive most injuries on the same side of the body as the vehicle impact. Patterns of injury that are anticipated are:

- Contralateral neck sprain
- Cervical spine fracture
- Brachial plexus injury
- Lateral flail chest
- Pneumothorax
- Traumatic aortic disruption

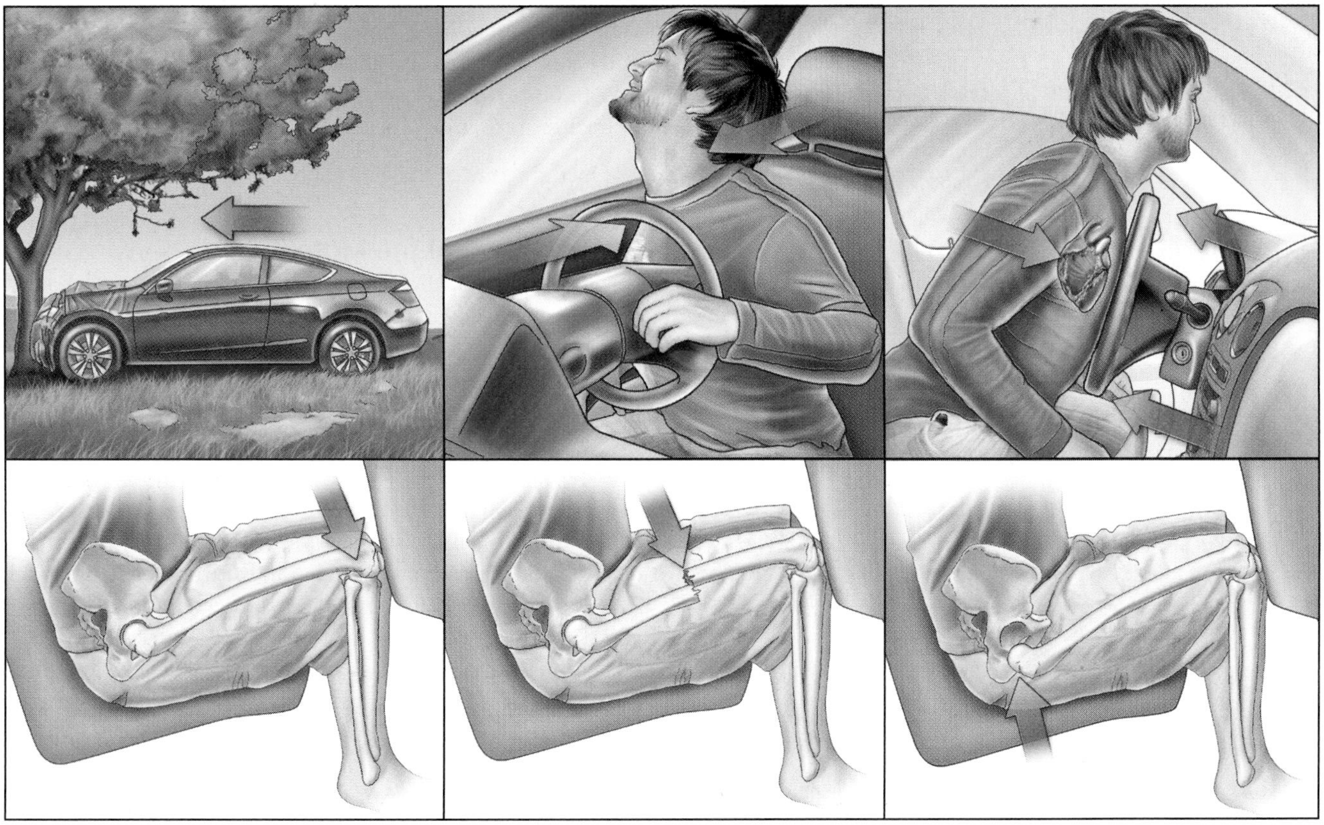

FIGURE 74–2 ■ Unrestrained frontal impact.

- Diaphragmatic rupture
- Fractured spleen/liver and/or kidney depending on the side of impact
- Fractured pelvis or acetabulum (ACS, 2004).

Rear Impact

When a vehicle is struck from behind, the initial impact accelerates the stationary vehicle and may force the vehicle into a frontal collision. If the headrests in the vehicle are not properly positioned, the sudden acceleration may cause hyperextension of the neck. If the vehicle that is hit then stops suddenly from a frontal impact or the driver applying the brakes suddenly, then rapid forward deceleration occurs (Figure 74–3 ■). This increases the chance for passenger injury. Patterns of injury that are anticipated are:

- Cervical spine injury
- Soft tissue injury to the neck (ACS, 2004).

Vehicle Rollover

When a vehicle rolls over it can be difficult to predict the pattern of injury. Injury occurs at the points where the body contacts the vehicle. Generally, this type of mechanism produces more severe injury than other types of crashes because of violent, multiple motions during the rollover. It is important to assess these pa-

Whiplash

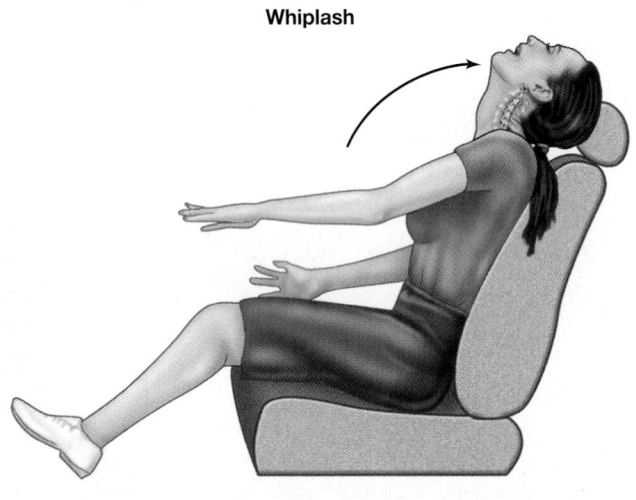

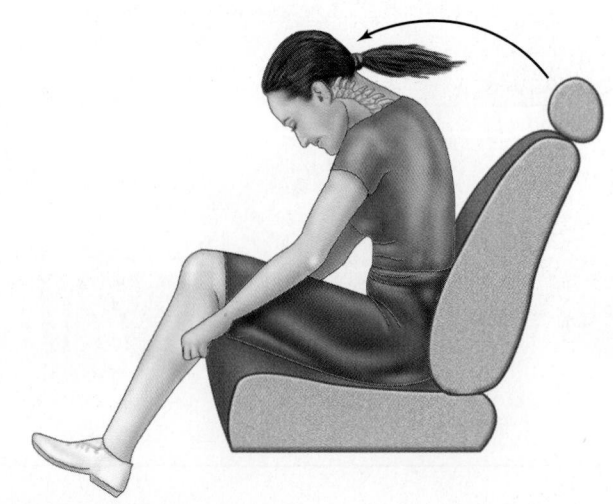

FIGURE 74–3 ■ Rear impact.

tients carefully because they have the potential for multiple-system injuries.

Ejection

When a person is ejected from a vehicle, his chance of severe injury increases by more than 300% (ACS, 2004). Ejection occurs when the passenger is thrown from the vehicle, and injury occurs at the body's point of impact. Ejection places the patient at risk for all injury mechanisms and mortality is significantly increased (ACS, 2004).

Motorcycle Crashes

Motorcycle crashes are also common causes of traumatic injuries. Motorcycles do not have the surface area to absorb energy from impacts, therefore, energy is directly absorbed by the rider and injuries are substantially more severe than in vehicle crashes.

Frontal Impact

A motorcycle's center of gravity is located in front of the driver's seat. When a frontal impact occurs, the back of the motorcycle tips upward from the weight under the handlebars. The driver is propelled over the handlebars, but may not be totally ejected due to the back tipping forward. If there is a passenger behind the driver, this person is often catapulted over the driver and fully ejected. Patterns of injury include:

- Fractured femurs, tibias, and fibulas (from the driver's body hitting the handlebars)
- Chest and abdominal injuries (from compression against the handlebars)
- Traumatic brain and cervical spine injury (ACS, 2004).

Side Impact

When a motorcyclist is impacted from the side, that side of the body is unprotected and absorbs all of the energy. The exposed leg can be crushed between the motorcycle and the second object. Patterns of injury include:

- Open fracture of the femur, tibia/fibula, and malleolus (ACS, 2004).

Laying Down of the Motorcycle

If a motorcyclist anticipates a collision, she may use the technique of laying down the bike and sliding off to the side. The energy transference occurs as the body slides away from the bike. Without sufficient protective clothing, abrasions will occur with pieces of asphalt becoming embedded in the abrasions.

Pedestrian Injuries

More than 7,000 people die in the United States each year after being struck by a motor vehicle (ACS, 2004). Injury patterns can be predicted depending on the age and size of the victim and the size of the vehicle. Children tend to freeze and face the vehicle and, therefore, end up with more frontal injuries than adults. Depending on the height of the child and the vehicle bumper, the impact occurs on the chest or the femurs and then the child is thrown backward with the upper back or head impacting the ground. A very small child may be knocked down and under the vehicle due to his center of gravity, size, and weight. Multiple-system trauma should be suspected on any child hit by a vehicle.

Adults usually try to escape being hit and turn away from the vehicle, thus sustaining lateral injuries on the side impacted by

RISK FACTORS for Youth Violence

Individual Risk Factors

- History of violent victimization or involvement
- Attention deficits, hyperactivity, or learning disorders
- History of early aggressive behavior
- Involvement with drugs, alcohol, or tobacco
- Low IQ
- Poor behavioral control
- Deficits in social-cognitive or information processing abilities
- High emotional distress
- History of treatment for emotional problems
- Antisocial beliefs and attitudes
- Exposure to violence and conflict in the family

Family Risk Factors

- Authoritarian childrearing attitudes
- Harsh, lax, or inconsistent disciplinary practices
- Low parental involvement
- Low emotional attachment to parents or caregivers
- Low parental education and income

- Parental substance abuse or criminality
- Poor family functioning
- Poor monitoring and supervision of children

Peer/School Risk Factors

- Association with delinquent peers
- Involvement in gangs
- Social rejection by peers
- Lack of involvement in conventional activities
- Poor academic performance
- Low commitment to school and school failure

Community Risk Factors

- Diminished economic opportunities
- High concentrations of poor residents
- High level of transiency
- High level of family disruption
- Low levels of community participation
- Socially disorganized neighborhoods

Source: Centers for Disease Control and Prevention. (2007b). *Injury and violence.* Retrieved April 14, 2007, from http://www.cdc.gov/node.do/id/0900f3ec8000e539.

the vehicle. Approximately 80% of adults hit by a vehicle will have injuries to the lower extremities (Feliciano et al., 2008). Injury patterns include:

- Lower extremity fractures above and below the point of impact
- Fractured pelvis (pedestrian hits the hood of the vehicle or point of impact)
- Head injury (pedestrian falls off hood of vehicle to the ground) (ACS, 2004).

Falls

Falls are the leading cause of death for Americans 65 years of age and older (CDC, 2007a) and will be discussed in detail later in the chapter. The injury from a fall is similar to that of a motor vehicle crash in that it is caused by an abrupt change in velocity. The roof line of a one-story house is usually 15 feet. With falls greater than 15 feet, adults usually land on their feet. If the fall is less than 15 feet, adults will land in the same position at which they fell. Small children have larger heads in proportion to their bodies and therefore, no matter the distance of the fall, they tend to land headfirst.

The severity of the injury also depends on the give of the surface on which the person lands. A soft surface, such as sand, will absorb more energy than cement. Patterns of injury include:

- Calcaneus fractures
- Compression fractures to T_{12}–L_1
- Bilateral wrist fractures (as the body falls forward after the first impact)
- Traumatic brain injury (ACS, 2004).

Penetrating Injuries

Violence is an important public health problem. According to the CDC, in 2004, more than 750,000 persons ages 10 to 24 were

treated in emergency departments for injuries due to violence. During that same year, a nationwide survey of high school students revealed that 33% reported being in a fight one or more times during the preceding year and that 17% of students reported carrying a weapon during the month preceding the survey (CDC, 2007b). The CDC also reported that research on youth violence has shown certain risk factors to be associated with youth violence, as listed in the Risk Factors box.

The severity of injury in penetrating trauma depends on the velocity or speed of the penetrating object. Energy created by the object is dissipated into the surrounding tissues much like a shock wave. Consider the shock wave going through human tissue that is elastic in nature (Figure 74–4 ■). The stress that is imparted to the tissue is dependent on the velocity, or speed, of the object entering the body, the velocity of the waves in the tissue, and the mass or density of the object that entered the body. The larger and faster the article, the more damage to the tissues (ACS, 2004).

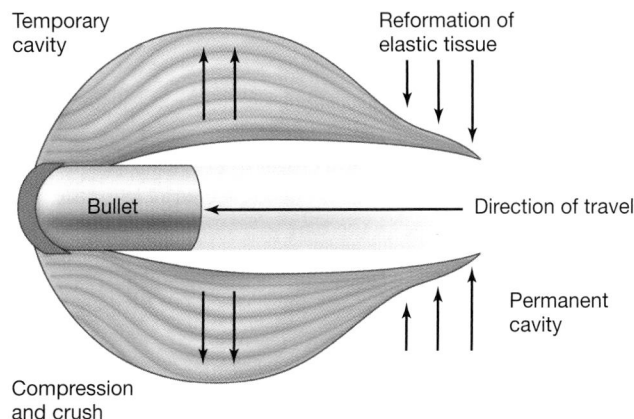

FIGURE 74–4 ■ Cavitation.

Stab Wounds

Stab wounds are low velocity and produce their injury directly as the object penetrates tissue. Knowing the length of the object and how far it entered the body helps the nurse to anticipate what organs might be injured. Also, knowing the position of the attacker and victim can help identify the path of the weapon. Knowing the gender of the attacker may also assist in determining the path of the weapon. Men tend to stab upward and women tend to stab overhand or downward.

Although tissue damage is usually isolated to the area of penetration, a single stab wound may penetrate several body cavities depending on the pathway. During expiration the dome of the diaphragm reaches as high as the fifth rib. Stab wounds to the chest at or below the level of the nipple should be suspect for abdominal injury as well. Also, an attacker may stab the victim only once but move the weapon around causing extensive internal damage to the surrounding structures.

Gunshot Wounds

Every year more than 30,000 Americans are killed with firearms. In the United States, unintentional firearm deaths of children nearly all occur in or around the home. Firearm injuries peak in the 19-year-old age group and then decrease after the age of 22. Serious injuries from a firearm, such as traumatic brain injury, can require a lifetime of care and rehabilitative services that can cost upwards of $1,000,000 over the victim's lifetime (Emergency Nurses Association, Injury Prevention Institute, 2006b; NTDB, 2007).

The severity of the damage caused by a bullet depends on the amount of energy transferred from the bullet to the body. Handguns and some small-caliber rifles are considered medium energy; hunting and assault rifles are considered high energy and, therefore, capable of transferring more energy to the tissue than smaller guns. The degree of deformation of the bullet also influences the degree of tissue damage. Bullets that are constructed of soft lead and flatten on impact, or have a hollow point that "mushrooms" on impact, cause more tissue damage than a full metal jacket bullet due to the increased diameter.

It is important to assess the patient for the number of wounds that are present. It is difficult to determine whether a wound is an entrance or exit wound so the nurse should never assume that the bullet is not still in the body if two wounds are present. Bullets will follow the path of least resistance once they enter the body, so it is almost impossible to truly know the path the bullet has taken from just the external exam.

Blast Injuries

Terrorist activity has increased the chance of blast injury in the United States. In a blast, explosives are detonated and changed to gases. When the gas expands, equal volumes of air are displaced and travel after the blast wave. The energy from the blast wave can cause massive tissue damage. When the blast occurs, the casing that held the explosive ruptures and its pieces become high-velocity projectiles that can cause penetrating injury. Blast injury can occur in three phases:

1. The concussive effects of the pressure wave can cause central nervous system (CNS) injury, rupture of air-containing organs, and tearing of membranes and small vessels.

2. Fragments of glass, rock, and metal debris become high-velocity projectiles that can cause penetrating injury.

3. The victim may be thrown through the air and sustain injury similar to that sustained when ejected from a vehicle or when a person has fallen from a height.

Adequate care of the trauma patient depends on the health care team's ability to quickly identify life-threatening injury and intervene. Understanding kinematics and the subsequent patterns of injury helps the caregivers to be anticipatory and less likely to miss an injury.

◼ Initial Assessment of the Trauma Patient

It is important to develop a systematic approach to the trauma patient. Deaths from trauma occur in a trimodal distribution. The first peak of deaths from trauma occurs prior to definitive care at the scene or en route to the medical facility and results from nonsurvivable injuries such as aortic disruption; the second peak occurs within the first few hours after injury and is most commonly due to hemorrhage or severe traumatic brain injury; the third wave occurs days to weeks after the injury and is a result of complications, including infection or multiple organ dysfunction. A systematic, thorough initial assessment and resuscitation will decrease the number of deaths that occur during the second and third peaks by quickly identifying injury and beginning definitive care.

Initial nursing management follows a systematic approach to care and includes a rapid primary survey, resuscitation of vital functions, a detailed secondary survey, and initiation of definitive care. During the initial assessment the health care team must identify injuries, intervene when life-threatening injuries are present, and prioritize care. It is critical for all members of the trauma team to prepare for the arrival of trauma patients and know their role during the initial resuscitation (Figure 74–5 ◼). As one member of the team completes the primary and secondary survey, many procedures are done simultaneously such as accessing veins, obtaining blood for tests, and inserting a Foley catheter and gastric tube.

It is important to have one team member who is overseeing the resuscitation and directing the team. This person is usually a trauma surgeon and does not provide direct care unless necessary. Instead, this person observes the resuscitation efforts and correlates all data being obtained to direct the plan of care. The nurse should be familiar with the resuscitation area and the equipment available. We discuss the initial steps of trauma care next.

Primary Survey

The primary survey follows a specific sequence:

A Airway maintenance with cervical spine immobilization

B Breathing and ventilation

C Circulation and hemorrhage control

D Disability (neurological status)

E Exposure/environmental control (e.g., remove all clothing but prevent hypothermia by placing warm blankets on the patient or using ambient warmers).

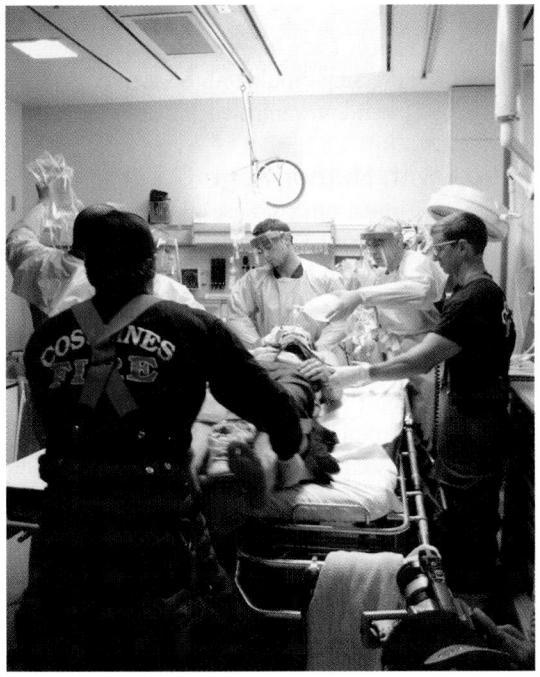

FIGURE 74–5 ■   Trauma team.
Source: Cheryl Wraa

Airway Maintenance

A secure and patent airway is the first priority for the trauma patient. While the airway is assessed, the patient's cervical spine should be maintained in a midline position and not moved (Figure 74–6 ■). The patient's airway should first be assessed for patency. Look for signs of airway obstruction from blood or foreign bodies, facial/mandibular fractures, or tracheal/laryngeal injury that may occlude the airway. If the patient's level of consciousness is such that she would not be able to protect her airway if she began to vomit, then an endotracheal tube should be inserted to protect the airway. Whenever a trauma patient is intubated, it is important to protect the cervical spine by maintaining in-line stabilization during the procedure. All multiple-system trauma patients, particularly with an altered level of consciousness or blunt injury above the clavicle, should be treated as if they have a cervical spine injury until proven otherwise.

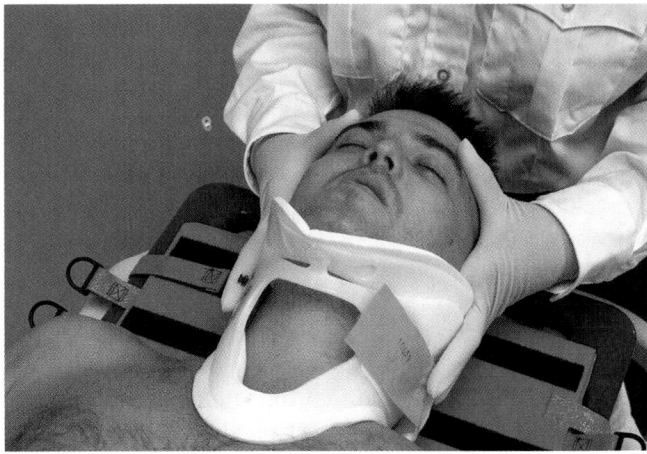

FIGURE 74–6 ■   Cervical stabilization.

 CRITICAL ALERT   *Reevaluation of the patient's airway should be done frequently.*

Breathing and Ventilation

Adequate function of the lungs, chest wall, and diaphragm is necessary for adequate ventilation. Expose the chest to visualize and assess chest wall excursion. Listen to breath sounds to identify a pneumothorax or hemothorax. Palpate the chest wall to identify injuries that might compromise ventilation. Injuries that can impair ventilation acutely include **flail chest**, which occurs when two or more ribs are fractured in two or more places and are no longer attached to the thoracic cage, resulting in a free-floating segment. The free-floating segment moves independently from the rest of the chest resulting in paradoxical chest wall movement (Figure 74–7 ■). This can be observed during inspection of the chest. The impaired movement of the chest wall results in decreased tidal volume, vital capacity, and impaired cough leading to hypoventilation and atelectasis.

The amount of energy exerted on the body to cause a flail chest usually will damage the underlying lung tissue, resulting in a **pulmonary contusion**. Pulmonary contusion is initially a hemorrhage followed by alveolar and interstitial edema. The

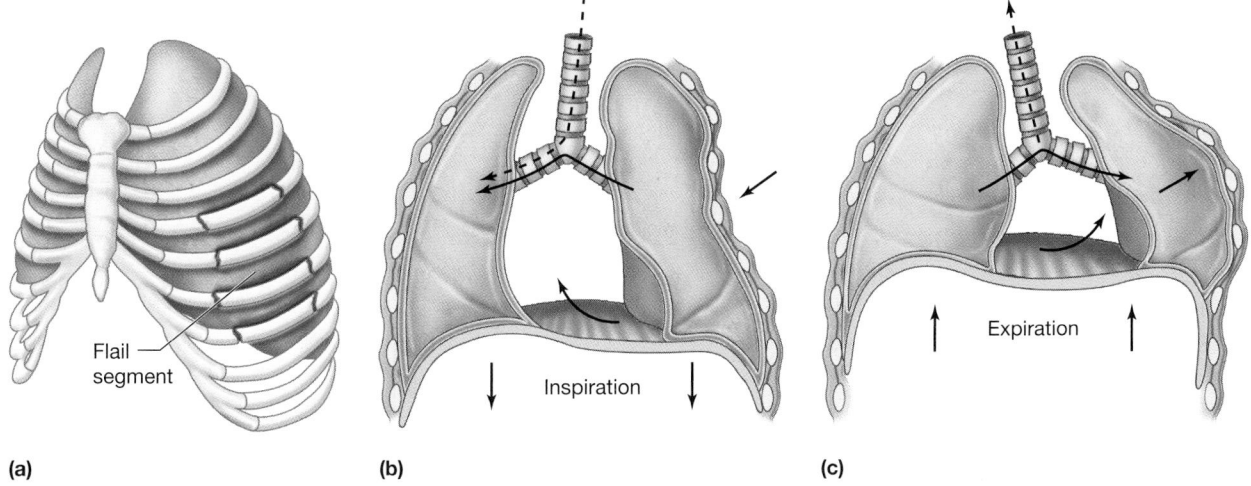

(a)   (b)   (c)

FIGURE 74–7 ■   Flail chest.

edema affects the alveolar-capillary units in the area of the contusion. If the edema increases it can cause decreased compliance and increased pulmonary vascular resistance and can affect pulmonary blood flow. Clinical manifestations may develop over 24 to 48 hours and include moist crackles in the contused lung, cough with blood-tinged sputum, and pulmonary infiltrate on chest radiograph. Pulmonary contusion is the most common, potentially lethal chest injury (Urden, Stacy, & Lough, 2006).

Tension pneumothorax occurs when an injury perforates the chest or pleural space. During inspiration air enters the pleural space and becomes trapped. As more air is trapped, the pressure in the pleural space increases collapsing the lung and causing the mediastinum to shift to the opposite side (Figure 74–8 ). This pressure exerts pressure on the heart and vascular structures in the chest, resulting in decreased cardiac output and venous return. A tension pneumothorax is diagnosed by clinical assessment, and the pressure must be released immediately by venting the chest on the affected side with a large-bore needle or chest tube or the patient will die. Symptoms include severe dyspnea, tachycardia, and hypotension.

A **massive hemothorax** is an accumulation of 1,500 mL or more of blood in the thoracic cavity. This amount of hemorrhage can result from injury to intercostal or internal mammary arteries, lung tissue, the heart, or the great vessels. The patient will present with signs and symptoms of hypovolemic shock with breath sounds diminished or absent over the affected lung. An **open pneumothorax** is an open communication between the atmosphere and intrathoracic pressure and is usually caused by penetrating trauma. This communication with the atmosphere causes an immediate collapse of the lung on the affected side. The patient will present with respiratory distress and as he inspires a sucking sound may be heard as the air moves in and out of the hole in the

chest. An occlusive dressing can be placed over the wound to prevent air from being sucked into the pleural cavity until a chest tube can be placed. The dressing should only be secured on three sides to allow air to escape and prevent a tension pneumothorax.

Circulation with Hemorrhage Control

Hemorrhage is the predominant cause of preventable death in the injured patient (ACS, 2004). During the primary survey, hypotension should be considered hypovolemic in origin until proven otherwise. Elements of the primary survey that provide important information to the nurse regarding the patient's circulatory status are level of consciousness, skin color, and pulse. If the patient's circulating blood volume is reduced, the cerebral perfusion may be impaired, resulting in an altered level of consciousness. As blood volume decreases, the body compensates by shunting blood away from the skin to vital organs. This shunting causes the skin to become pale and cool. Pulses should be assessed bilaterally for quality, rate, and regularity. A weak, thready pulse may be a sign of hypovolemia, but may have other causes as well. The absence of central pulses (femoral and carotid pulses) signifies the need for immediate resuscitative measures to restore depleted blood volume and maintain effective cardiac output.

If external hemorrhage is identified, measures to control the bleeding should be taken immediately. The easiest way to do this is to apply direct manual pressure on the wound.

CRITICAL ALERT *Tourniquets should not be used to control bleeding except in unusual circumstances (e.g., traumatic amputation). Tourniquets crush tissues and cause distal ischemia.*

The major sources of occult blood loss are hemorrhage into the chest or abdominal cavities, into the soft tissue surrounding a major long bone fracture, or into the retroperitoneal space

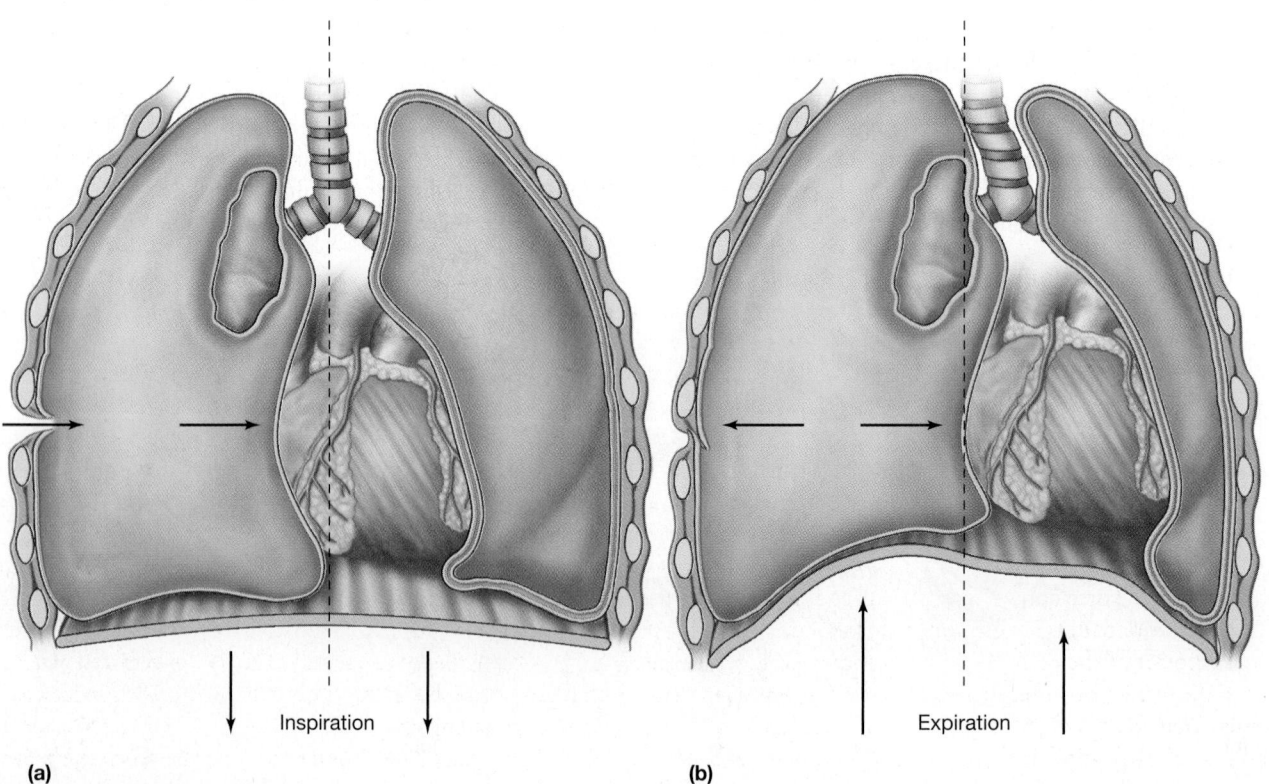

(a) Inspiration

(b) Expiration

FIGURE 74–8 ■ Tension pneumothorax.

from a pelvic fracture. Control of bleeding may require immediate operative intervention.

Treatment of hemorrhage consists of administration of fluids, blood, and blood products. Hypovolemic shock is a life-threatening emergency and affects all organ systems of the body by depriving tissue of adequate oxygen and nutrients. For a detailed discussion of shock, refer to Chapter 61 🔗. The initial response of the body to acute blood loss is to decrease circulation to less vital organs such as the kidneys, gastrointestinal tract, and skin in order to preserve circulation to vital organs such as the heart, brain, and lungs. This response is triggered by the decrease in cardiac output and subsequent change in pulse pressure that is sensed by baroreceptors in the aortic arch and atrium of the heart. Neural reflexes then begin a sympathetic outflow to the heart and other organs, which respond by increasing heart rate and initiating vasoconstriction. The activation of the rennin system leads to vasoconstriction and the retention of sodium and water to help replete the vascular volume. The pituitary and the adrenal medulla are stimulated to release adrenocorticotropic hormone, norepinephrine, and epinephrine to enhance the compensatory mechanisms.

The decrease in oxygen and nutrients to the cells causes the body's metabolism to change from aerobic to anaerobic, releasing lactic acid and causing metabolic acidosis. If the blood loss continues, the compensatory mechanisms will fail and damage occurs throughout the body in all systems. Myocardial hypoperfusion and lactic acidosis cause cardiac dysfunction that, in turn, perpetuates the entire process. Hypoperfusion of the brain causes cardiac and respiratory depression and failure of the sympathetic nervous system. As a result of this failure, vasodilation occurs that leads to venous pooling and increased capillary permeability, which causes the leakage of fluid into the interstitial space (third spacing) and the total body edema (anasarca) noted in trauma patients. Irreversible damage at the cellular level occurs because the cell membrane loses integrity. This is primarily due to free radicals, especially reactive oxygen species and reactive nitrogen species. These free radicals lead to oxidation of DNA molecules, fatty acids, and amino acids advancing cell degradation. Because the electrical gradient is lost, the cell swells, the endoplasmic reticulum and mitochondria are damaged, and utilization of oxygen becomes dysfunctional. Ruptured lysosomes release enzymes that digest other cellular structures and cell death occurs, which further enhances the impact of the initial hemorrhage.

Respiratory distress syndrome may result from the increased permeability of the pulmonary capillary membrane, microemboli formation, and pulmonary vasoconstriction. Hypoperfusion and vasoconstriction to the gastrointestinal system cause decreased peristalsis and functioning of the gut. Renal vasoconstriction and hypoperfusion lead to acute tubular necrosis and, if not reversed, to acute renal failure. Disseminated intravascular coagulation (DIC) develops due to hematologic dysfunction, including acidosis, hypoxemia, hypotension, and cessation of capillary blood flow.

The most abundant type of white blood cells are neutrophils. A large amount of the damage from hemorrhagic shock is the result of the formation of reactive oxygen species (ROSs) in neutrophils. Neutrophils fight infection and use ROSs to fight pathogens as they directly break down microbial pathogens. However, ROSs also signal molecules in programmed cell death (apoptotic) pathways. Although ROSs break down pathogens,

neutrophils overproduce and accumulate ROSs causing **apoptosis** (programmed cell death in a multicellular organism), which would be expressed in the clinical setting as sepsis.

Recent research into the cellular pathways involved in the inflammatory response to injury and shock is concerned with T-cell proliferation in response to stimulators in the adaptive and innate immune responses. Research has found decreased levels of helper T-cell cytokine production and reduced antibody secretion (Spaniol, Knight, Zebley, Anderson, & Pierce, 2007). The decrease in these specific levels corresponds to the suppressed adaptive immune function that is seen in trauma patients with hemorrhagic shock. Research is focused on which receptors are involved in the reduction of the adaptive immune function and how to activate the receptors to maintain the adaptive immune system function at a level that will prevent infection.

Fluid Resuscitation

Traditionally, the treatment for hemorrhagic shock has been immediate, aggressive infusion of normal saline or Ringer's lactate solution. Current data suggest, however, that although aggressive fluid resuscitation may be useful for patients with isolated extremity, thermal, or head injury, fluid resuscitation should be limited in patients with potentially uncontrollable internal hemorrhage, especially in patients with penetrating truncal injury that will be treated at a trauma center (Pepe, Dutton, & Fowler, 2008). The reason aggressive fluid resuscitation may be harmful is that increasing the mean arterial pressure in a patient who is actively bleeding will lead to increased blood loss. The hemostatic mechanisms of the body are overcome by the artificially elevated blood pressure and formed clots are dislodged. Due to the increased bleeding, more fluids and blood are required and the proinflammatory effects of the products develop. Aggressive infusion of crystalloid in the presence of uncontrolled hemorrhage promotes continued bleeding and increases mortality (Hai, 2004). The amount of initial fluid resuscitation will be determined by the patient's response to fluids. The response should be continually assessed to determine if perfusion is adequate. The nurse must also be aware that many factors including age, comorbidities, and medications can affect a patient's response to fluid resuscitation. The goal is to control the bleeding and promote oxygenation at the cellular level.

There is also an area of concern with the administration of Ringer's lactate solution stimulating apoptosis. A study looking at the initial resuscitation of combat casualties found that the use of Ringer's lactate solution for hemorrhagic shock increased apoptosis in intestinal mucosa, smooth muscle, liver, and lung cells, and caused a severe immunologic response, coagulopathy, and renal failure. This was not observed with the use of plasma, natural colloids, and whole blood during resuscitation (Spaniol et al., 2007).

Blood products are used to restore circulating volume, improve oxygen carrying capacity, and replace coagulation factors. Type-specific blood is preferred, but if needed immediately, type O may be used. Ongoing research indicates that fresh frozen plasma and platelets need to be given early in conjunction with packed red cells to treat coagulopathy (Hess, Holcomb, & Hoyt, 2006; Ketchum, Hess, & Hippala, 2006). Trauma centers are developing guidelines for massive transfusion that reflect this practice. Chart 74–1 (p. 2434) is an example of a guideline for massive transfusion.

CHART 74–1 Massive Transfusion Guideline

Purpose: The Massive Transfusion Guideline (MTG) development was a cooperative effort by the Trauma Multidisciplinary Committee at the University of California, Davis Medical Center to provide a standard for efficient and effective procurement and delivery of blood products to patients exhibiting hemorrhagic shock. The term *massive transfusion* is defined as replacement of at least one blood volume (~5 liters in an adult) within the first 12 hours of resuscitation.

MASSIVE TRANSFUSION GUIDELINE PACK

6 units of packed red blood cells (pRBCs)

3 fresh frozen plasma (FFP) Jumbo units (6 units of FFP)

1 plateletpheresis unit (a 6-pack of platelets)

ACTIVATION

The MTGs can be activated in any of the following hospital locations:

Emergency department

Operating room

Critical care unit

Radiology (interventional radiology)

Labor and delivery

- The health care provider caring for the patient (trauma attending or anesthesiologist or direct designee) first determines that massive transfusion is likely to be necessary and notifies the blood bank.
- An order must be placed in the electronic medical record (EMR) for MTGs.

- A properly labeled blood specimen should be sent STAT (ordered in the EMR as "RBC" (red blood cells) if a new patient or "RBC Add-on" if a specimen is 3 days current). A prothrombin time (PT), partial thromboplastin time (PTT), and fibrinogen or thromboelastography (TEG) should also be sent.
- Transfusion of un-crossmatched RBCs should be ongoing until type specific and/or crossmatch compatible RBCs are available.
- FFP should be started as soon as it is determined that more than 3 units of pRBCs are likely to be necessary.
- Upon initiation of MTGs, blood bank personnel will prepare 6 units of pRBCs, and 3 units of FFP Jumbo will be placed into a cooler and delivered to the patient, along with one plateletpheresis not placed in the cooler and instead kept at room temperature. This will be switched out with another cooler prepared in the same manner as above upon return of the first cooler. Subsequent component orders will be repeated until the health care provider caring for the patient determines that the MTG can be discontinued.
- The health care provider initiating the MTGs or a designee must notify the blood bank as soon as possible when the MTGs are no longer needed.
- All blood products should be given via a Level I rapid infuser/fluid warmer or other blood-warming device to prevent hypothermia.
- The patient's medical record number will be held constant throughout the MTGs.

Sources: Hess, J. R., Holcomb, J. B., & Hoyt, D. B. (2006). Damage control resuscitation: The need for specific blood products to treat the coagulopathy of trauma. *Transfusion, 46,* 685–686; Hirshberg, A., Dugas, M., Banez, E. I., Scott, B. G., Wall, M. J. Jr., & Mattox, K. L. (2003). Minimizing dilutional coagulopathy in exsanguinating hemorrhage: A computer simulation. *Journal of Trauma, 54,* 454–463; Ho, A. M., Dion, P. W., Cheng, C. A., et al. (2005). A mathematical model for fresh frozen plasma transfusion strategies during major trauma resuscitation with ongoing hemorrhage. *Canadian Journal of Surgery, 48,* 470–478; Holcomb, J. B., & Hess, J. R. (2006). Early massive trauma transfusion: Current state of the art. *Journal of Trauma, 60*(Suppl), S1–S9; Ketchum, L., Hess, J. R., & Hippala, S. (2006). Indications for early fresh frozen plasma, cryoprecipitate, and platelet transfusion in trauma. *Journal of Trauma, 60*(Suppl.), S51–S58; Malone, D. L., Hess, J. R., & Fingerhut, A. (2006). Massive transfusion practices around the globe and a suggestion for a common massive transfusion protocol. *Journal of Trauma, 60*(Suppl), S91–S96.

Disability

The primary assessment of disability involves a rapid neurological evaluation to establish the patient's level of consciousness. The Glasgow Coma Scale score (see Chart 32–2, p. 841) should be determined at this time. An altered level of consciousness can be indicative of decreased blood volume with poor perfusion, hypoxia, or a traumatic brain injury. Alcohol and mind-altering drugs may alter the level of consciousness, but should never be considered the cause until all other possibilities have been excluded.

Exposure/Environmental Control

The trauma patient should be completely undressed to facilitate a thorough examination. As trauma patients are being examined they should be covered with warm blankets or an external warming device to prevent hypothermia. Intravenous fluids should be warmed prior to infusion to prevent a decrease in a patient's core temperature with the infusion of large amounts of cold solution. Allowing patients to become cold can be very detrimental to their care, as discussed in the Evidence-Based Practice feature.

Adjuncts to the Primary Survey

Monitoring of the patient's physiological parameters is the best way to assess the effectiveness of resuscitation efforts. The patient should be placed on a cardiac monitor. Dysrhythmias may

indicate blunt cardiac injury. Pulseless electrical activity (PEA) may indicate tension pneumothorax, as described earlier in the chapter; profound hypovolemia; and/or **cardiac tamponade**, which is bleeding into the pericardial sac.

As the accumulation of blood increases, it compresses the atria and ventricles decreasing venous return and filling pressure, which leads to decreased cardiac output, myocardial hypoxia, and cardiac failure. The patient with cardiac tamponade presents with findings termed **Beck's triad**. These findings are neck vein distention caused by the elevated central venous pressure, muffled heart sounds, and hypotension. Immediate treatment is required to remove the accumulated blood and relieve the pressure that is being exerted on the heart. This is accomplished either by pericardiocentesis, which involves aspiration via a large-bore needle placed into the pericardial sac, or an emergency surgical thoracotomy to visualize the heart, relieve the accumulated blood, and locate and control the source of bleeding.

Pulse oximetry measures the oxygen saturation of hemoglobin, but does not measure ventilation. Adequacy of ventilation should be monitored by the ventilatory rate and arterial blood gases (ABGs).

Bedside screening radiographs are usually accomplished at this time. As the patient is logrolled off the backboard and

Hypothermia in Trauma Patients

Clinical Problem

Allowing a trauma patient to become cold will contribute to the development of coagulopathy.

Research Findings

Hemorrhage is one of the leading causes of death following trauma. Trauma patients are susceptible to early development of coagulopathy, and patients who are severely injured are coagulopathic on hospital admission. Hypothermia, acidosis, and dilution from standard resuscitation with crystalloid can worsen the presenting coagulopathy and perpetuate bleeding. Rapid diagnosis of coagulopathy, followed by prevention or correction of hypothermia and acidosis should be a priority during the initial assessment and resuscitation (Tieu, Holcomb, & Schreiber, 2007).

Coagulopathy of trauma is a syndrome of bleeding from mucosal lesions, serosal surfaces, and wound and vascular access sites. It is associated with serious injury, hypothermia, acidosis, hemodilution, and occasionally with DIC. The coagulopathy can be largely explained by the effects of cold on platelet function, the effect of pH on coagulation factor activity, and the dilutional effects of resuscitative fluids (Hess & Lawson, 2006).

Hardy, de Moerloose, and Samama (2006) conducted a Medline search for articles on *massive transfusion, transfusion, trauma, surgery, coagulopathy,* and *hemostatic defects.* Experts reviewed the literature. Their principal findings were that coagulopathy results from hemodilution, hypothermia, the use of fractionated blood products, and DIC. In trauma patients, tissue trauma, shock, tissue anoxia, and hypothermia contribute to the development of DIC and microvascular bleeding. Hardy and colleagues compared the clinical significance of the effects of different therapies and stated that maintaining a normal body temperature is a first-line, effective strategy to improve hemostasis during massive transfusion.

The U.S. Army Institute of Surgical Research conducted a study (Martini, Pusateri, Uscilowicz, Delgado, & Holcomb, 2005) to identify the independent contributions of hypothermia and acidosis to coagulopathy in swine. They found that hypothermia caused a delay in the onset of thrombin generation, and acidosis primarily caused a decrease in thrombin generation rates. The results confirmed the need to prevent or correct hypothermia and acidosis.

Implications for Nursing Practice

With the organization of trauma systems, improvements in prehospital care, the development of trauma centers, and the standardization of methods of resuscitation, aggressive resuscitation of patients in extremis has improved over time. Severely traumatized patients may now be in the ICU or operating room before they reach the physiological limit defined as the onset of the triad: hypothermia, acidosis, and coagulopathy. It is important for nurses to understand the triad and the consequences. As stated before, maintaining a normal body temperature is a first-line, effective strategy to improve hemostasis and prevent worsening coagulopathy.

Critical Thinking Questions

1. Which of the following nursing measures would decrease the risk of coagulopathy?
   a. Administering warm intravenous fluids
   b. Covering the patient with a sheet
   c. Administering room temperature intravenous fluids
   d. Covering the patient with warm blankets
   e. a and d
   f. All of the above

2. The nurse understands that prevention of hypothermia is important because:
   a. It increases cardiac output.
   b. It decreases the risk of coagulopathy.
   c. It preserves neurological function.
   d. It increases renal function.

Answers to Critical Thinking Questions appear in Appendix D.

References

Hardy, J. F., de Moerloose, P., & Samama, C. M. (2006). Massive transfusion and coagulopathy: Pathophysiology and implications for clinical management. *Canadian Journal of Anaesthesia, 53*(6 Suppl.), S40–S58.

Hess, J. R., & Lawson, J. H. (2006). The coagulopathy of trauma versus disseminated intravascular coagulation. *Journal of Trauma, 60*(6), S12–S19.

Martini, W. Z., Pusateri, A. E., Uscilowicz, J. M., Delgado, A. V., & Holcomb, J. B. (2005). Independent contributions of hypothermia and acidosis to coagulopathy in swine. *Journal of Trauma, 58*(5), 1002–1009.

Tieu, B. H., Holcomb, J. B., & Schreiber, M. A. (2007). Coagulopathy: Its pathophysiology and treatment in the injured patient. *World Journal of Surgery, 31*(5), 1055–1065.

EVIDENCE-BASED PRACTICE

---

the back is examined, plates may be placed to do chest and abdominal/pelvic radiographs.

Placement of an indwelling urinary catheter and a gastric catheter should be accomplished as part of the resuscitation. Urinary output is an important indicator of the patient's volume status and her response to resuscitation. The placement of an indwelling urinary catheter is contraindicated in patients suspected of having a urethral injury. Signs of possible urethral injury include blood at the urethral meatus, perineal ecchymosis, blood in the scrotum, and a high-riding or nonpalpable prostate, which is identified by manual rectal exam. Placement of a gastric catheter reduces stomach distention and the risk of vomiting and aspiration. If the patient has multiple facial fractures, it may be necessary to place an oral gastric catheter.

 **CRITICAL ALERT**   *Never insert a urinary catheter before the genitalia and rectum have been examined.*

The patient's blood pressure should be monitored frequently to observe for changes and/or trends. Remember, blood pressure may be a poor measure of actual tissue perfusion. Return to an adequate hemodynamic state requires more than a normal blood pressure.

If the patient arrived at a nontrauma center, this is the time to consider initiating the transfer process to a designated trauma center for definitive care (ACS, 2004).

Secondary Survey

Following the primary survey and intervention of resuscitative measures with adequate patient response, the secondary survey should be completed. The secondary survey consists of a detailed head-to-toe evaluation of the patient with reassessment of all vital signs and should ideally be performed in 5 to 10 minutes. As with the primary survey, the secondary survey is done in a systematic fashion to reveal all injuries the patient has sustained.

Head and Face

The nurse palpates through the scalp to identify lacerations and possible depressed skull fractures. Observe the face for the development of **Battle's sign**, which is ecchymosis over the mastoid area and is indicative of a basilar skull fracture. Palpate the face for fractures and midface stability. If the midface is unstable, the patient will have difficulty maintaining a patent airway. When the patient lies supine, the midface collapses and occludes the airway.

Eyes

If the patient is responsive, gross visual acuity should be checked along with pupillary size and reactivity to light. Assess for **raccoon eyes**, which are ecchymoses over the orbit of the eyes and are indicative of a basilar skull fracture. Inspect the eye for any foreign bodies, globe injury, or **hyphema**, a collection of blood in the anterior chamber of the eye. The blood is visible and can block vision. If the nurse notes that the patient is wearing contact lenses, these should be removed at this time.

Ears

The ears should be inspected for blood, cerebrospinal fluid (CSF), or brain matter. Remove and save hearing aids.

Nose

Inspect the nose for blood or a CSF leak. An easy way to test for a CSF leak is to use gauze to absorb the bloody fluid. If CSF is mixed with the blood, it will create a gold-colored ring around the blood. This is commonly referred to as the "halo effect." Palpate for crepitus or deformity.

Mouth

Inspect the mouth for loose or broken teeth, tongue lacerations, or expanding intraoral hematomas. Remove dentures at this time.

Neck

While maintaining cervical spine stabilization, the neck should be palpated for spinous process deformity or crepitance. Inspect the anterior neck carefully for expanding hematomas that may compress the trachea. How to evaluate patients with suspected cervical spine trauma is a controversial topic in medicine. The controversy surrounds which patients require radiographs, how much imaging is necessary, and exactly what sort of imaging should be done. The American College of Radiology's (ACR's) expert panel on musculoskeletal imaging has issued recommendations for imaging of patients with suspected cervical spine trauma (ACR, 2007). In summary, the expert panel recommends that patients who are alert, have no loss of consciousness, are not under the influence of drugs or alcohol, have no distracting injuries, have no cervical tenderness, and have no neurological findings do not need imaging. All others should have a

computed tomography (CT) scan of the cervical spine that includes sagittal and coronal reconstruction.

The ACR's expert panel also recommend that patients who have symptoms referable to the upper cervical spine and have a negative CT scan, should have a single lateral radiograph to evaluate C_2. This is especially important for patients over the age of 65 because such patients have a higher incidence of C_2 fractures. The guidelines recommend that magnetic resonance imaging (MRI) be reserved for patients who have clinical evidence of spinal cord injury, those suspected of ligamentous instability, and to "clear" patients who remain unconscious after 48 hours.

Chest

Inspect the chest for paradoxical chest movement from a flail segment. Palpate for subcutaneous emphysema and bony tenderness. Auscultate for absent or asymmetric breath sounds.

Abdomen

Inspect the abdomen for ecchymoses and distention. Palpate for tenderness. Many centers now use ultrasound for the **FAST examination**, which refers to *focused assessment with sonography for trauma*. Within minutes the FAST exam can confirm the presence of free fluid within the chest or abdomen, which signifies bleeding and the need for rapid intervention.

Pelvis

The pelvis should be assessed for stability by gently compressing the iliac wings and symphysis pubis. If a caregiver has assessed for stability and states that the pelvis feels unstable, then no one else should compress the pelvis because it may cause more damage to the vessels and tissue. A patient with a major pelvic fracture is at risk for retroperitoneal hemorrhage. A prefabricated pelvic stabilization device or a sheet should be applied to an unstable pelvic fracture that may contribute to hemodynamic instability. This will help to decrease the bleeding and prevent further damage until the pelvic bones can be surgically stabilized (Isenhour & Marx, 2007).

Genitalia

In the male patient, inspect the scrotum for ecchymoses or hematomas and the penile meatus for blood. Assess female patients for vaginal bleeding and obtain a history regarding last menstruation and the chance of pregnancy. A pregnancy test should be performed for any woman of childbearing age.

Extremities

Each extremity should be inspected for deformity and swelling. Palpate for tenderness, crepitus, limited joint movement, and pulses. Whenever an injury is suspected, it is important to assess for circulation, sensation, and motor response distal to the injury. Refer to Chapter 56 ↺ for an in-depth review of musculoskeletal trauma.

 CRITICAL ALERT *If an injured extremity is found to be pulseless, notify the trauma team immediately.*

Laboratory and Diagnostic Procedures

Trauma patients are monitored closely during the first 24 hours post injury as not to miss an injury. Diagnostic tests that may be utilized are presented in the Diagnostic Tests feature.

DIAGNOSTIC TESTS for Trauma

Test	Expected Abnormality	Rationale for Abnormality
Hematocrit	Decrease	Initially should obtain a baseline to look for trends downward, signifying ongoing bleeding. Patients requiring crystalloid resuscitation for hemorrhagic shock benefit from serial hematocrit measurement in order to determine the degree of hemodilution and the need for blood transfusion.
White blood cell (WBC) count	Increased	Initially the WBC count will be elevated as part of the body's normal response to trauma. Detection of neutrophilia based on serial evaluations may indicate an inflammatory process in the peritoneal cavity. During the critical care and intermediate phases of care, an elevation in the WBC count can be indicative of a wound infection, pulmonary infection, or sepsis.
Glucose	Decrease or increase	Decrease: used to rule out hypoglycemia in patients with decreased level of consciousness. Increase: stress response from traumatic injury.
Lipase	Increase	Progressive elevation increases suspicion of pancreatic, liver, or bowel injuries.
Arterial blood gases	Metabolic acidosis	Metabolic acidosis is strongly associated with hypoperfusion.
Coagulation studies: International Normalized Ratio (INR) Activated partial thromboplastin time (APT) Partial thromboplastin time (PTT)	Increased	May identify if the patient was on long-term anticoagulation at home. Severe TBI causes the release of tissue thromboplastin, which increases INR. Patients receiving massive blood transfusions require frequent monitoring of clotting factors. Packed RBCs do not contain clotting factors and platelets, so the patient may require FFP to prevent coagulopathy.
Urinalysis	Positive for occult blood Toxicology screening	Signifies injury to urinary tract. A positive toxicology report may help to explain altered mental status. On all female patients of childbearing age, a bedside urine pregnancy test should be performed.
Blood alcohol level and toxicology screening	Elevated blood alcohol and positive toxicology screen	May help to explain altered mental status.
Imaging: Cervical spine Chest Abdomen Pelvis Thoracic spine Lumbosacral spine Injured extremities	Fractures and/or dislocations Pneumothoraxes Hemothoraxes	Helps identify life- or limb-threatening injuries.

■ Nursing Management

During the initial resuscitation, the health care providers present work as a team to evaluate and intervene where necessary. After the initial resuscitation, the nurse has the most consistent contact with the patient and is the team member who will quickly identify trends and changes in the patient condition. The Nursing Process: Patient Care Plan (p. 2438) presents a detailed patient care plan for the trauma patient.

Tertiary Survey

Many trauma patients are unresponsive or confused when they are first evaluated and are unable to furnish valuable medical history data that may affect their care. As thorough as the trauma team may be in evaluating the patient, not all injuries are detected by the primary and secondary survey. For this reason a tertiary trauma survey (TTS) is increasingly being implemented (Petersen, 2004). The TTS is completed within 24 hours of admission as a patient evaluation that identifies and catalogs all injuries after the initial resuscitation and operative intervention. The TTS is repeated when the patient is awake, responsive, and able to communicate and includes a comprehensive review of the medical record, repetition of the primary and secondary surveys, review of all laboratory data, and review of all radiographic studies with an attending radiologist.

Continued reevaluation of the multiple-system trauma patient is key to prevent missed injury and preventable death. A

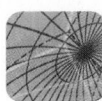

NURSING PROCESS: Patient Care Plan for Trauma

Assessment of Circulation and Perfusion

Subjective Data:
Where are your injuries?
Do you have any other preexisting health problems?
Do you take any medications that may affect your blood pressure?
Do you take any medications that "thin your blood"?

Objective Data:
Assess:
Level of consciousness
Oxygen saturation
Work of breathing
Peripheral and central pulses: rate and quality
Blood pressure
Respiratory rate
Temperature
Skin color and temperature
Urine output

Nursing Assessment and Diagnoses	Outcomes and Evaluation Parameters	Planning and Interventions with *Rationales*
Nursing Diagnosis: *Tissue Perfusion, Ineffective* related to hypovolemia; interruption of flow: arterial and/or venous	**Outcome:** Patient will maintain adequate tissue perfusion. ***Evaluation Parameters:*** Vital signs within normal limits. Level of consciousness: awake, alert, and appropriate. Skin: good color, warm and dry. Peripheral pulses strong and equal Urine output of 1 mL kg^{-1} hr^{-1}.	**Interventions and *Rationales:*** Cannulate two veins with large-bore catheters and regulate fluids at appropriate rates. *Adequate fluid and blood administration help maintain perfusion of vital organs.* Apply direct pressure to obvious external bleeding *to slow the loss of blood.* Notify the health care provider immediately of significant drop in blood pressure, urine output, or increased heart rate. *Patient may have a missed injury that requires surgical intervention.*

Assessment of Airway

Subjective Data:
Are you feeling short of breath?
Are you having difficulty breathing?
Is it painful when you take a deep breath or cough?

Objective Data:
Assess breath sounds.
Assess respiratory rate, rhythm, depth, and symmetry.
Monitor oxygen saturation.
Monitor arterial blood gas values.

Nursing Assessment and Diagnoses	Outcomes and Evaluation Parameters	Planning and Interventions with *Rationales*
Nursing Diagnosis: *Airway Clearance, Ineffective* related to edema of the airway, laryngeal spasm, altered level of consciousness, direct trauma, obstruction by secretions, or aspiration of foreign matter	**Outcome:** Patient will maintain a patent airway. ***Evaluation Parameters:*** Regular rate, depth, and pattern of breathing. Bilateral chest expansion. Effective cough and gag reflex. Absence of stridor or hoarse voice.	**Interventions and *Rationales:*** Open and clear airway. Patient may have debris or blood in mouth from the trauma. Insert oro- or nasopharyngeal airway. Patient may have adequate respiratory drive but needs support to keep airway open. *Prepare to assist with endotracheal intubation. Level of consciousness too low to protect and maintain airway.*

Assessment of Ventilation

Subjective Data:
Are you feeling short of breath?
Are you having difficulty breathing?

Objective Data:
Observe patient for:
Altered chest excursion
Shallow respirations
Nasal flaring
Use of accessory muscles
Increased or decreased respiratory rate

Nursing Assessment and Diagnoses	Outcomes and Evaluation Parameters	Planning and Interventions with *Rationales*
Nursing Diagnosis: *Breathing Pattern, Ineffective* related to chest wall deformity, decreased energy, musculoskeletal impairment, neuromuscular dysfunction, pain	**Outcome:** Patient will demonstrate effective breathing patterns. ***Evaluation Parameters:*** Uncompromised respiratory status as evidenced by depth of inspiration and ease of breathing; chest expansion symmetric; accessory muscle use not present; adventitious breath sounds not present.	**Interventions and *Rationales:*** Control pain *to allow for optimal chest expansion.* Teach patient how to use the incentive spirometer *to help prevent atelectasis.* Suction as needed *to remove secretions and encourage coughing.* Have patient turn, cough, and deep breathe at least every 2 hours *to mobilize secretions and prevent atelectasis.* Administer oxygen as ordered *to maintain adequate PaO$_2$.*

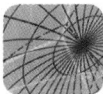

NURSING PROCESS: Patient Care Plan for Trauma—*Continued*

Assessment of Pain

Subjective Data:
On a scale of 1 to 10 with 1 being a little pain and 10 being the worst pain you have ever felt, at what level is your pain?
Do you routinely take pain medication at home? If yes, what is the name of the medication and why do you take it?
Are you allergic to any medications?

Objective Data:
Monitor patient for:
Facial grimacing
Change in breathing pattern
Change in blood pressure and/or pulse rate
Diaphoresis
Agitation

Nursing Assessment and Diagnoses	Outcomes and Evaluation Parameters	Planning and Interventions with *Rationales*
Nursing Diagnosis: *Pain*	**Outcome:** Pain level will be tolerable. *Evaluation Parameters:* Diminished or absent level of pain through patient's self-report. Absence of physiological indicators of pain.	**Interventions and *Rationales*:** **Nonpharmacologic** Reduce lighting and noise. Cultural and spiritual factors such as prayer, ritual, and music can also increase the patient's comfort. *Promotes relaxation and comfort.* **Pharmacologic** Administer intravenous opioid analgesics as prescribed. Assess response. *Intravenous administration is necessary if there is altered tissue perfusion from volume deficit.*

Assessment of Anxiety

Subjective Data:
Ask patient to verbalize thoughts and feelings about the traumatic event.
How do you feel about being in the hospital?

Objective Data:
Observe patient for:
Restlessness
Poor eye contact
Irritability
Hand tremors
Anorexia
Difficulty concentrating

Nursing Assessment and Diagnoses	Outcomes and Evaluation Parameters	Planning and Interventions with *Rationales*
Nursing Diagnoses: *Anxiety and Fear* related to unfamiliar environment, invasive procedures, possible disfigurement, scarring, threat to health status, role functions, or self-concept, loss of control, pain	**Outcome:** Patient will experience decreased anxiety and fear. *Evaluation Parameters:* Ability to verbalize concerns and ask questions. Use of effective coping skills. Decreased fear-related behaviors.	**Interventions and *Rationales*:** Explain all procedures in clear terms. *Increases patient's understanding and alleviates fear of the unknown.* Maintain adequate pain relief. *Pain increases anxiety.* Administer prescribed antianxiety medication *to decrease physiological responses.* Spend therapeutic time with the patient to answer questions. *Anxiety may interfere with understanding of complex explanations.*

Assessment of Nutrition

Subjective Data:
Ask the patient about their appetite and how much of their meal they have eaten.

Objective Data:
24-hour caloric intake
Daily weight
Presence of bowel sounds, nausea and vomiting, or flatus

Nursing Assessment and Diagnoses	Outcomes and Evaluation Parameters	Planning and Interventions with *Rationales*
Nursing Diagnosis: *Nutrition Imbalanced, Risk for Less than Body Requirements* related to decreased appetite secondary to treatments, fatigue, environment, and increased protein and vitamin requirements for healing	**Outcome:** Patient will ingest daily nutritional requirements for activity level and metabolic needs. *Evaluation Parameters:* Maintains adequate weight. Maintains adequate caloric intake.	**Interventions and *Rationales*:** Communicate the need for adequate caloric intake of carbohydrates, fats, protein, vitamins, minerals, and fluids. *Adequate nutrition can reduce the risk of complications and promote healing.* Consult with the nutritionist to establish appropriate daily caloric requirements *to ensure optimal intake.* Offer small frequent meals *to help prevent gastric distention.* Determine the patient's food preferences and arrange to have those foods provided. Encourage family to bring allowed foods from home. Eliminate any offensive odors. Control pain and nausea. Provide a relaxed atmosphere during meals. *Can improve appetite and lead to increased intake.*

study conducted at Harborview Medical Center, University of Washington, Seattle, identified patterns of errors that contributed to inpatient trauma deaths. The study showed important error patterns that included a failure to successfully intubate, secure, or protect the airway; delayed operative or angiographic control of acute abdominal/pelvic hemorrhage; delayed intervention for ongoing intrathoracic hemorrhage; inadequate deep venous thrombosis or gastrointestinal prophylaxis; lengthy initial operative procedures rather than damage control surgery in unstable patients; overresuscitation with fluids; and complications of feeding tubes (Gruen, Jurkovich, McIntyre, Foy, & Maier, 2006). Although preventable deaths will occur, continued reassessment of the multiple-system trauma patient will help to minimize these errors.

Discharge Priorities

Discharge priorities for the trauma patient can be multifactorial depending on the extent of the injuries. When caring for the multiple-system trauma patient, refer to the chapters that concentrate on the specific injury. For example, for multiple extremity fractures refer to the chapter on musculoskeletal injuries (Chapter 55).

◼ Special Considerations

There are clinical situations or conditions that affect the delivery of trauma care. It is important for the nurse to be aware of these special considerations in order to give optimum care to the trauma patient.

End-of-Life Considerations

Trauma care has always focused on curing patients and returning individuals to a quality lifestyle. Unfortunately, trauma patients do die and they and their families may not receive end-of-life care that results in a death that reflects the best interests of the patient and family. One reason this occurs is because the trauma team has been so focused on curative care that it is difficult for them to change to palliative care. It is also a difficult conversation to have with the family because death from injury is usually a sudden event and is emotionally hard to process. According to the American Trauma Society (2003), "Death due to trauma needs to be managed in a manner that is sensitive, caring, and respectful to the patient, the family, and the medical caregivers. For patients with no likelihood of survival, implementation of aggressive resuscitation efforts and transport to a trauma center are empirically and morally questionable. For hospitalized patients, the failure to recognize that curative care is no longer effective and that palliative care needs to be initiated results in less than optimal care for the patient and family and may delay care of other patients who need intensive care to recover" (p. 1).

The need to integrate palliative care into trauma care is an essential part of providing excellent trauma care for all patients and families. To assist nurses caring for trauma patients throughout the continuum of care including end-of-life situations, policies should be in place that assist the trauma team in making the decision to shift from curative to comfort care and that address the changes in the focus of care for dying patients. For an in-depth discussion of end-of-life care, refer to Chapter 17 . The Ethical Issues box further discusses end-of-life care.

ETHICAL ISSUES Related to Trauma Patients and Their Families

One very difficult issue for nurses occurs when a nurse believes that the aggressive curative care being given to a trauma patient is futile or not in the best interest of the patient. The patient may have expressed to his family prior to the trauma that he did not want heroic measures taken if his quality of life would be severely affected. As the nurse it is important to advocate for the patient's wishes. Several steps can be taken by the nurse to clarify the issue. Request a multidisciplinary meeting with the health care team to identify concerns and clarify goals and expected outcomes for the patient. If the team cannot agree on the goals for the patient, an ethics committee consultation can be requested. The nurse can also facilitate a multidisciplinary family conference if there seems to be a conflict between the goals of the team and the expectations of the family. Be respectful of cultural conversational norms, listen to identify concerns, and attempt to match expressed needs with services the nurse can provide or facilitate.

Traumatic Brain Injury

Multiple-system trauma patients who sustain traumatic brain injury (TBI) can be difficult to assess due to their decreased level of consciousness. The patient must be carefully evaluated for injury that may cause hemorrhage because a decrease in the blood pressure is detrimental to cerebral perfusion. Refer to Chapter 29 for an in-depth review of brain injury.

Spinal Cord Injury

Any multiple-system trauma patient must be considered to have a vertebral column injury even if the patient does not have a neurological deficit. If the trauma patient is unconscious, it will be difficult to assess neurological function. For trauma patients, approximately 55% of spinal injuries occur in the cervical region, 15% in the thoracic region, 15% at the thoracolumbar junction, and 15% in the lumbosacral area (ACS, 2004).

It is very important to protect the spine from excessive manipulation. If the patient's spine is protected, a rigid cervical collar is properly placed and manual stabilization is maintained while the patient is logrolled. Then, evaluation of the spine and exclusion of spine injury can be deferred in the presence of systemic instability. If a patient is known to have a neurological deficit and is hypotensive, it should not be assumed that the drop in blood pressure is due to neurogenic shock. All sources of bleeding must be ruled out so as not to miss an injury. Refer to Chapter 32 for an in-depth review of spinal cord injuries.

Trauma in Pregnancy

For any female trauma patient between the ages of 10 and 50, potential for pregnancy should be considered. Because of the significant physiological changes during pregnancy, patterns of injury may be affected. Anatomically, the uterus remains in the pelvis until approximately the 12th week. By 20 weeks gestation, the uterus is at the umbilicus, and it rises to the costal margin at 34 to 36 weeks. As the uterus enlarges the bowel is pushed upward and lies mostly in the upper abdomen. In later pregnancy the bowel is somewhat protected from blunt trauma, but the uterus, placenta, and fetus are at risk. During the third trimester of pregnancy, the uterus is large and thin walled.

In the vertex position the fetal head sits within the pelvis. If the mother sustains a pelvic fracture, the fetus could sustain significant head injury. The placenta has little elasticity, so shearing forces from deceleration (such as a frontal impact crash) could lead to abruption of the placenta from the uteroplacental interface causing bleeding within the uterus. Also, placental vasculature is maximally dilated throughout pregnancy but is very sensitive to catecholamine stimulation. The mother's response to the traumatic injury may cause constriction of the vasculature. Also, an abrupt decrease in the mother's intravascular volume may result in a profound constriction of the uterine vasculature, thus reducing fetal oxygenation even if the mother is exhibiting reasonably normal vital signs.

During pregnancy, plasma volume increases with a smaller increase in red blood cell volume, resulting in a physiological anemia. However, because of the increased plasma volume, a healthy pregnant patient may lose 1,200 to 1,500 mL of blood volume before exhibiting signs of hypovolemia such as tachycardia or hypotension. As stated before, this amount of blood loss can cause fetal distress as evidenced by an abnormal fetal heart rate.

Oxygen consumption is increased during pregnancy. The pregnant trauma patient should always receive supplemental oxygen and be monitored to ensure adequate oxygenation during resuscitation efforts.

Gastric emptying time is prolonged during pregnancy so it should always be assumed that the pregnant woman has a full stomach. To protect the patient from vomiting and possibly aspirating, it is important to place a nasogastric tube early to decompress the stomach.

The pregnant uterus may compress the vena cava and reduce venous return to the heart when the mother is lying supine. Therefore, the mother should be placed on her left side and the uterus displaced manually to the left side to relieve the pressure. If a spinal injury is suspected, the mother can be logrolled 4 to 6 inches to her left and supported with bolstering devices to displace the uterus.

The most important thing to remember when caring for a pregnant trauma patient is that the best treatment for the fetus is the provision of optimum resuscitation of the mother and early assessment and monitoring of the fetus.

Intimate Partner Violence

Statistics regarding intimate partner violence (IPV) are difficult to obtain because the various data sources define IPV differently. Some sources include threats and some only include physical and sexual violence. Also, many incidents are not reported to the police. The CDC (2007c) states that approximately 20% of IPV rapes or sexual assaults, 25% of physical assaults, and 50% of stalkings directed toward women are reported. Even fewer incidents against men are reported. Therefore, available statistics are felt to greatly underestimate the magnitude of the problem. Following are some statistics reported by the CDC (2007c):

- Nearly 5.3 million incidents of IPV occur each year among U.S. women ages 18 and older, and 3.2 million occur among men. Most assaults are relatively minor and consist of pushing, grabbing, shoving, slapping, and hitting.

- In the United States every year, about 1.5 million women and more than 800,000 men are raped or physically assaulted by an intimate partner. This translates into about 47 IPV assaults per 1,000 women and 32 assaults per 1,000 men.

- IPV results in nearly 2 million injuries and 1,300 deaths nationwide every year.

- One study found that 44% of women murdered by an intimate partner had visited an emergency department within 2 years of the homicide. Of these women, 93% had at least one injury visit (Crandall, Nathens, Kernic, Holt, & Rivara, 2004).

- Between 4% and 8% of pregnant women are abused at least once during the pregnancy.

Intimate partner violence can result in death and disability. This type of injury also represents an increasing number of emergency department visits. Aside from sexual violence, physical violence may include the following: scratching, throwing, grabbing, biting, choking, shaking, slapping, punching, burning, use of restraints, and use of a weapon. Indicators that may suggest the presence of domestic violence include:

- Self-blame for injuries
- Injuries inconsistent with stated history
- Frequent emergency department or office visits
- Symptoms suggestive of substance abuse
- Low self-esteem, depression, suicide attempts
- Self-abuse
- Partner insists on being present for interview and examination. May answer questions for patient.

Nutritional Support

The Eastern Association for the Surgery of Trauma (EAST) formed a work group to develop evidence-based guidelines for practice. Understanding the importance of nutrition with regard to healing, the guidelines shown in the National Guidelines for Nutritional Support box (p. 2442) were developed for nutritional support of the trauma patient. The guidelines contain three levels of recommendations:

- **Level I**—The recommendation is convincingly justifiable based on the available scientific information alone.
- **Level II**—The recommendation is reasonably justifiable by available scientific evidence and strongly supported by expert opinion.
- **Level III**—The recommendation is supported by available data but adequate scientific evidence is lacking. The recommendation is useful for educational purposes and in guiding future clinical research.

Gerontological Considerations

Trauma is the seventh leading cause of death in patients 65 years of age or older and accounts for 25% of all injury fatalities (ACS, 2004). Many studies have shown that elderly trauma patients have a higher level of injury-related mortality (Feliciano et al., 2008). This increased risk of death is attributed to preexisting medical conditions that make it difficult for the elderly patient to tolerate changes in their normal physiological parameters during the acute stress of trauma or major surgery. The three leading causes of death in

NATIONAL GUIDELINES for Nutritional Support

Route of Nutritional Support

Level I Recommendations:
- Patients with blunt and penetrating abdominal injuries sustain fewer septic complications when fed enterally rather than parenterally.
- Patients with severe head injuries have similar outcomes whether fed enterally or parenterally.

Early versus delayed feedings

Patients with penetrating and blunt injuries to the abdomen who have small bowel access: Enteral feeding can be started in most after resuscitation is complete and hemodynamic stability has been achieved. Gastrointestinal injury below the site of access may slow advancement of tube feedings but is not a contraindication to direct small bowel feedings.

Level I Recommendation:
- Intragastric feedings should be started in burn patients as soon after admission as possible since delayed enteral feeding (>18 hours) results in a high rate of gastroparesis.

Level II Recommendation:
- Patients with severe head injury who do not tolerate gastric feedings within 48 hours of injury should be changed to postpyloric feedings if feasible and safe for the patient.

Level III Recommendations:
- Patients who are incompletely resuscitated should not have direct small bowel feedings instituted due to the risk of gastrointestinal intolerance and possible internal necrosis.
- For patients undergoing laparotomy, direct small bowel access should be obtained and enteral feedings begun, if not contraindicated, within 12 to 24 hours of injury.

Standard versus enhanced nutritional support

Enhanced enteral formulations are defined by the addition of omega 3 fatty acids, nucleotides, arginine, beta carotene, and/or glutamine when adequate calorie/protein requirements are met early in the course of treatment.

Level I Recommendation:
- Use of enhanced enteral nutrition in severely injured patients is beneficial to the trauma patient when given in conjunction with early feeding and adequate protein/calorie support. Level I evidence shows reduced incidence of multisystem organ dysfunction, infectious complications, and overall length of hospital stay.

Source: EAST Practice Management Guidelines Workgroup. (2003). *Practice management guidelines for nutritional support of the trauma patient.* Retrieved October 18, 2008 from http://www.east.org/tpg/nutrition.pdf.

---

the elderly are falls, motor vehicle crashes, and burns (ACS, 2004). Elder abuse also occurs, as discussed in the Gerontological Considerations box.

Key differences between the elderly and younger people include the following:

- Increased incidence of subdural hematoma because of increased dural vein fragility and less elasticity with age. Elderly patients with head injury have a poorer prognosis than younger patients.

- The thorax is less compliant and therefore more susceptible to injury. A simple fall can cause a flail chest.

- Reduced pulmonary reserve occurs with the aging process. Elderly patients will have progressive pulmonary compromise with multiple rib fractures since splinting often leads to ventilatory failure and pneumonia.

- Elderly patients are less able to increase cardiac output on demand due to decreased compliance and a limited degree of compensatory ability. Elderly patients are also more likely to be taking beta-blockers which will blunt the sympathetic nervous system response and not allow the heart rate to increase.

- The aorta of the elder patient is relatively inelastic and more vulnerable to injury.

- Signs of peritoneal irritation are more subtle.

- The elderly are far more susceptible to postoperative complications due to comorbidities.

GERONTOLOGICAL CONSIDERATIONS
Elder Abuse and Neglect

Elder abuse is underreported by patients due to a fear of abandonment and also failure of health care workers to inquire. When screening for suspected abuse, general questions that could be asked are:

- Do you feel safe?
- Are you able to take care of yourself or do you need help?
- Do you live by yourself or with others?
- Who maintains your checkbook?
- Who prepares your meals?

Clinical evidence of abuse/neglect includes:

- Injuries of varying age (as in child abuse)
- Dehydration and malnutrition
- Poor personal hygiene
- Decubitus ulcers
- Unexplained medication overdoses or lack of compliance with medication regimen
- Unexplained venereal disease or genital infection.

Intervention with suspected elder abuse or neglect requires a multidisciplinary team approach. The different disciplines are better able to assess the multifactorial aspects of the situation including physical and mental status, competency, financial status, assistance, and protection with referrals to community agencies for continual monitoring of the situation.

- Osteoporotic bones are more vulnerable to fracture and elderly patients have decreased pain perception, meaning that subtle fractures may be missed.
- Artificial pacemakers and medications such as beta-blockers and calcium channel blockers blunt the usual chronotropic response to hemorrhage.

Falls

According to the CDC (2007a) falls are the leading cause of injuries that result in death among older adults. Falls are also the most common cause of nonfatal injuries. For those that fall, 20% to 30% sustain moderate to severe injuries that decrease their mobility, make it difficult to live alone, and increase the chance of early death. In 2003, approximately 1.8 million people ages 65 and older were treated in emergency departments for nonfatal injuries from falls. For the elderly patient, falls are the most common cause of TBIs (CDC, 2007a).

Prevention efforts are now moving toward fall assessments for elderly patients, which include physical assessment for fall risk and a survey of the patient's home surroundings for hazards. Older patients can take several steps to reduce their risk of falling:

- Exercise regularly to increase strength and improve balance. Research findings have demonstrated the efficacy of t'ai chi exercise to improve balance and decrease falls among older adults (CDC, 2007a).
- Review medications, both prescription and over-the-counter, to reduce side effects and interactions. This should be done by a health care provider.
- Check vision annually.
- Establish adequate lighting throughout the elderly person's residence.
- Reduce hazards in the home that can lead to falls such as throw rugs on which elderly persons could trip.

The National Fire Protection Agency and the CDC have developed a fire and fall prevention program for elders called Remembering When (NFPA, 2003). The program is available in twenty languages and is available on the NFPA website.

Elderly Drivers

Elderly drivers ages 65 and older have a higher crash death rate per mile driven than all others except teen drivers. This age group is the fastest growing segment of the population: By 2020 more than 40 million elderly adults will be licensed to drive (CDC, 2007d). Changes with aging that put the elderly driver at risk are decreases in vision, hearing, cognitive functions, and physical impairments. Research is being conducted to develop risk assessment tools and prevention programs to increase awareness and assist elderly people to be safe drivers.

▄ Trauma Rehabilitation

Rehabilitation is the multidisciplinary plan of care that maximizes an impaired individual's function by minimizing the deficits to achieve the highest quality of life possible. Rehabilitation of the trauma patient begins the moment health care services are provided. As the patient stabilizes from the initial resuscitation, the focus changes to recovery and adaptation. Depending on the extent of injury to the patient, the rehabilitation team may consist of many disciplines including health care providers, nurses, social workers, physical therapists, occupational therapists, speech therapists, vocational counselors, and financial counselors, as well as family members. It is important for the patient's goals to be developed by the team because this approach assists with consistency and communication among all team members. The primary nursing objectives during this phase of care are to assist the patient in overcoming or adapting to disabilities. This adaptation involves dealing with psychological as well as physical needs regardless of whether the disability is temporary or permanent.

Health Promotion

One-third to one-half of trauma deaths occur in the prehospital setting before any possibility of treatment (Feliciano et al., 2008). These deaths can only be decreased by prevention efforts. Injury prevention is the key to reducing death caused by trauma and decreasing the severity of injuries and the disability that can arise from a traumatic injury.

Strategies and educational programs to decrease traumatic injury and death include safety-related vehicle design and occupant protection; speed limits; laws and education regarding the use of helmets; laws and education regarding driving under the influence of alcohol or drugs; graduated driver's licensing systems; laws and education regarding smoke detectors; education regarding water temperatures and scald burns; laws regarding the use of flame retardants in children's sleepwear; gun laws; and laws and education regarding domestic violence, child abuse, and elder abuse. Injury prevention programs should be multidisciplinary and reach all members of the community. Many prevention programs are available through national organizations such as the CDC, American Trauma Society, Emergency Nurses Association, and the National Fire Protection Association.

In the United States, one of the most significant improvements in the care of injured patients has been the development of trauma systems (Feliciano et al., 2008). The elements of a trauma system are prehospital care, access to care, hospital care, and rehabilitation, along with prevention, disaster planning, patient education, research, and financial planning. Of great importance for a system's success is having prehospital communications, a transport system, trained personnel, and trained trauma care personnel for all phases of care. It is well known that patients who are severely injured benefit from receiving care at a trauma center due to the rapid response of surgeons and trained health care team members who can evaluate, resuscitate, and operate if necessary.

It has also been shown that patients who have not incurred immediate life-threatening problems also benefit from receiving care at a trauma center. Helling, Nelson, Moore, Kintigh, and Lainhart (2005) completed a retrospective study of 1,592 consecutive trauma patients admitted to the trauma service of an urban trauma center. They found that a large proportion of the patients initially thought to have minor injuries required resources that were available at the trauma center, including specialty care, and intensive care unit, and operating room accessibility. The study revealed that more than one-third of the patients had multiple-system injuries and nearly 20% were considered to have major trauma that required the prioritization of care abilities and expertise ideally found in a trauma center environment.

Statewide trauma system planning can enhance community health through an organized system of injury prevention, acute care, and rehabilitation that is integrated into the public health system throughout a state. The goal of the system is to enhance community health by identifying risk factors in the community and creating solutions to decrease the incidence of injury, to provide access to timely, definitive care for the injured patient, and to decrease overall injury-related morbidity, mortality, and years of life lost through rehabilitation. The U.S. Department of Health and Human Services released the Model Trauma Care System Plan in February 2003 under the Trauma System Agenda for the Future (Cooper, 2008). It was established as a framework for measuring progress in trauma system development and set the standard for systems of trauma care.

 Research

Traumatic injury is a major health care and economic issue in the United States. Many trauma patients experience long-term

disabilities. Nurses have a responsibility to promote prevention, education, and research that will result in positive patient outcomes. Some examples of needed research are described in the Research Opportunities and Clinical Impact box.

 Summary

Improvements in the care of the trauma patient are only a partial solution to this health care issue. Support for aggressive trauma prevention programs is essential to reduce not only the loss of life, but also the economic and emotional effects of traumatic injury. The goal of significantly reducing morbidity and mortality from trauma will be achieved through the influence of prevention campaigns.

RESEARCH OPPORTUNITIES AND CLINICAL IMPACT RELATED TO TRAUMA

Research Opportunities	Clinical Impact
Describe the psychological experiences of trauma patients and families.	Help to define the psychosocial impact of the event and identify the needs.
Many research opportunities involve the nutritional needs of trauma patients:	
Energy prediction equations need to be validated, and standard language and definitions determined.	Nutritional needs could be consistently and accurately defined in multiple settings using objective criteria.
Obese patients have more complications from traumatic injury. Are there specific metabolic or nutritional interventions that might improve prognosis?	Decrease morbidity and mortality in the obese trauma patient population.
Identify physiological parameters to assess pain intensity in comatose patients.	Ensure that adequate pain relief is being accomplished.
Should relatives be present and witness trauma resuscitation?	Allowing relatives to see what is happening, even for a short time, may help to prevent anxiety or terrible imagery.

Clinical Preparation

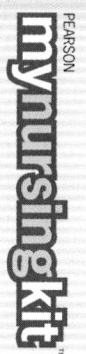

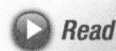 **Read**

- History of Current Illness
- Past Medical History
- Physical Exam
- Admitting Medical Orders
- Laboratory Study Results

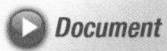 **Document**

- Summary of Hospitalization
- Pathophysiology Form
- Laboratory Values
- Laboratory Results Explanation

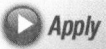 **Apply**

- List of Potential Nursing Diagnoses
- Concept Map
- Critical Thinking Questions

Log on to MyNursingKit.com to download forms you will need and to complete further steps in the Clinical Preparation assignment.

HISTORY OF PRESENT ILLNESS

The patient is an 18-year-old male who was brought into the emergency department by ambulance as a trauma activation. He was in full C-spine precautions including board and collar. The patient was a restrained driver of a vehicle that ran into a tree head-on at approximately 65 miles per hour. There was positive air bag deployment. The patient self-extricated but was unable to ambulate at the scene secondary to left leg pain. A left leg deformity was noted in the field and was splinted. He is amnestic to the event with a Glasgow Coma Scale (GCS) score of 14. He denies abdominal pain, headache, or neck pain. He does complain of severe left leg pain.

Medical–Surgical History

The patient denies any health problems, takes no medications, and states he has no allergies.

Social History

The patient is a freshman at the local college. He does not smoke cigarettes; he drinks beer on the weekends and occasionally smokes marijuana.

Physical Exam

Vital signs on arrival: blood pressure 132/80, heart rate 96, respiratory rate 18, and temperature 36°C. His left thigh, left knee, and left lower leg are tender to palpation with apparent soft tissue swelling. Distal pulses are intact. The left lower extremity is slightly shortened and rotated. Radiographs revealed a left femur and left tibial fracture. A Steinman pin was placed by the orthopedic service for reduction of the femur fracture. C-spine, chest, and pelvic radiographs are normal. CT scan of the abdomen is normal. The patient is admitted to the trauma unit to rule out intra-abdominal injury and will go to the operating room for ORIF of the fractured femur.

Admitting Medical Orders

Service: trauma

Diagnosis: blunt-force trauma, concussion, left femur fracture, left tibial fracture, rule out intra-abdominal injury

Allergies: no known allergies

Vital signs: every 4 hours including oxygen saturation; GCS scale and neurovascular checks to left lower extremity; 20 lb skeletal traction to left lower extremity

Call house officer: temp > 38.5°C, HR > 130 or < 60, RR > 30 or < 12, BP sys > 160 or < 90, O₂ sat < 92%, urine output < 120 mL in 4 hours, change in neurovascular exam to left lower extremity, any Hct result that is 5 less than the baseline ED Hct

Activity: bed rest

Diet: nothing by mouth

IV: D5/0.45NS with 20 mEq KCl at 125 mL/hr

Foley catheter to gravity drainage

I&O: every 4 hours

Respiratory care: use incentive spirometer every hour when awake

DVT prophylaxis: sequential compression device to right lower extremity

Scheduled Medications

Hydromorphine PCA 0.2 mg/mL, incremental dose 0.4 mg, lockout 6 minutes

Docusate 100 mg po twice daily

PRN Medications

Diphenhydramine 25–50 mg IV every 6 hours if needed for itching

Morphine 1–4 mg IV every 3 hours as needed for severe pain

Magnesium hydroxide liquid 30 mL po every 12 hours as needed

Ondansetron 4 mg IV every 12 hours as needed for nausea

Ordered Laboratory Studies

Complete blood count every morning

Hemoglobin and hematocrit every 4 hours

Chemistry panel every other day

LABORATORY STUDY RESULTS

HD1	1030	1245	1510	2200	0400
Hgb	16.4 g/dL	15.4 g/dL	14.7 g/dL	14.4 g/dL	12.6 g/dL
Hct	48.4%	44.9%	43.3%	42.5%	36.8%
WBC	18.1/mm³	21.4/mm³	20.0/mm³	19.2/mm³	13.4/mm³
RBC	5.49/mm³	5.08/mm³	4.93/mm³	4.81/mm³	4.19/mm³
PTT	23.9 seconds				
INR	0.97				
Na	138 mEq/L				
K	3.8 mEq/L				
Cl	102 mEq/L				
CO₂	25 mEq/L				
Glucose	145 mg/dL				
CA	8.9 mg/dL				
Lipase	29 U/dL				

CRITICAL THINKING QUESTIONS

1. What is the main purpose of the primary survey?
2. Having heard the history of the incident, what injury patterns would you anticipate?
3. The CT of the abdomen was normal. Does this rule out intra-abdominal injury?
4. What is the importance of warming the patient?

Answers to Critical Thinking Questions appear in Appendix D.

NCLEX® REVIEW

1. A patient comes into the emergency department after sustaining injuries from a rear impact motor vehicle crash. Which of the following injuries is this patient most likely experiencing?
   1. Pelvis
   2. Tibia
   3. Chest
   4. Spinal

2. A patient comes into the emergency department as a victim of an assault. The patient has multiple bleeding head and facial lacerations with draining coming from the right ear. The patient's speech is slurred and he admits to recent alcohol consumption. Which of the following should be the first priority when treating this patient?
   1. Apply direct pressure to the wounds to control the bleeding.
   2. Perform a full neurologic exam and check for "halo effect."
   3. Utilize a rigid cervical collar to stabilize the cervical spine.
   4. Transport the patient to radiology for a CT scan of the head.

3. The nurse is providing care to a trauma patient. When conducting the tertiary trauma survey, the nurse understands that:
   1. It will include a comprehensive medical record review to help ensure all injuries and treatments for the patient with trauma have been properly addressed.
   2. A work group will develop evidence-based guidelines for practice regarding the best and most important nutritional recommendations for the patient with trauma.
   3. This systematic approach to initial trauma assessment helps the health care team identify injuries, provide appropriate interventions, and prioritize patient care.
   4. The multidisciplinary plan of care developed will help increase the patient's quality of life and maximize the impaired patient's function by minimizing any deficits.

4. A patient who has sustained multiple trauma has a low blood pressure with minimal bleeding from skin lacerations. Which of the following should the nurse do?
   1. Insert an indwelling urinary catheter.
   2. Ensure adequate oxygenation.
   3. Assess for bleeding into the chest, abdomen, pelvis, or around long bones.
   4. Ensure adequate cervical spine support precautions.

Answers for review questions appear in Appendix D

KEY TERMS

apoptosis *p.2433*
Battle's sign *p.2436*
Beck's triad *p.2434*
cardiac tamponade *p.2434*
FAST examination *p.2436*

flail chest *p.2431*
hyphema *p.2436*
kinematics *p.2426*
massive hemothorax *p.2432*
open pneumothorax *p.2432*

pulmonary contusion *p.2431*
tension pneumothorax *p.2432*
raccoon eyes *p.2436*
rehabilitation *p.2443*

EXPLORE PEARSON **mynursingkit**™

MyNursingKit is your one stop for online chapter review materials and resources. Prepare for success with additional NCLEX®-style practice questions, interactive assignments and activities, web links, animations and videos, and more!

Register your access code from the front of your book at
www.mynursingkit.com

REFERENCES

American College of Surgeons. (2004). *Advanced trauma life support for doctors* (7th ed.). Chicago: Author.

American College of Surgeons, Committee on Trauma. (2006). *Resources for optimal care of the injured patient.* Chicago: American College of Surgeons.

American Trauma Society. (2003). *End-of-life issues: Quality, availability, and ethics.* Upper Marlboro, MD: Author.

Centers for Disease Control and Prevention. (2007a). *Falls among older adults.* Retrieved April 14, 2007, from http://www.cdc.gov/ncipc/factsheets/adultfalls.htm

Centers for Disease Control and Prevention. (2007b). *Injury and violence.* Retrieved April 14, 2007, from http://www.cdc.gov/node.do/id/0900f3ec8000e539

Centers for Disease Control and Prevention. (2007c). *Intimate partner violence.* Retrieved April 14, 2007, from http://www.cdc.gov/ncipc/factsheets/older.htm

Centers for Disease Control and Prevention. (2007d). *Older adult drivers.* Retrieved April 14, 2007, from http://www.cdc.gov/ncipc/factsheets/older.htm

Cooper, G. (2008). *HRSA model trauma systems planning and evaluation.* Retrieved on October 17, 2008, from http://www.emsa.ca.gov/systems/files/trauma/ModelTraumaPlan.ppt#256,1,HRSA Model Trauma Systems Planning & Evaluation.

Crandall, M., Nathens, A. B., Kernic, M. A., Holt, V. L., & Rivara, F. P. (2004). Predicting future injury among women in abusive relationships. *Journal of Trauma: Injury, Infection, and Critical Care, 56*(4), 906–912.

Daffner, R. H., Hackno, D. B., Dalinka, M. K., Davis, P. C., Rosnick, C. S., Rubin, D. A., et al. (2007). Expert panel on musculoskeletal and neurologic imaging. Suspected spine truma. Renton, VA. American College of Radiology (ACR). Retrieved June 26, 2008, from http://www.guidelines.gov/summary/summary.aspx?doc_id=11597&nbr=006010-strong=recommendations+AND+imaging+AND+

patients+AND+s-suspected+AND+cervical+AND+Spine+AND+trauma.

Emergency Nurses Association, Injury Prevention Institute. (2006a). *Alcohol awareness fact sheet.* Retrieved June 26, 2008, from http://www.ena.org/ipinstitute/fact/ENAIPFactSheet-Alcohol.pdf

Emergency Nurses Association, Injury Prevention Institute. (2006b). *Gun safety.* Retrieved June 26, 2008, from http://www.ena.org/ipinstitute/fact/ENAIPFactSheet-GunSafety.pdf

Feliciano, D. V., Mattox, K. L., & Moore, E. E. (2008). *Trauma* (6th ed.). New York: McGraw-Hill Medical.

Gruen, R. L., Jurkovich, G. J., McIntyre, L. K., Foy, H. M., & Maier, R. V. (2006). Patterns of errors contributing to trauma mortality: Lessons learned from 2,594 deaths. *Annals of Surgery, 244*(3), 371–380.

Hai, S. A. (2004). Permissive hypotensive resuscitation: An evolving concept in trauma. *Journal of the Pakistan Medical Association, 54*(4), 434–436.

Hardy, J. F., de Moerloose, P., & Samama, C. M. (2006). Massive transfusion and coagulopathy: Pathophysiology and implications for clinical management. *Canadian Journal of Anaesthesia, 53*(6 Suppl.), S40–S58.

Helling, T. S., Nelson, P. W., Moore, B. T., Kintigh, D., & Lainhart, K. (2005). Is trauma center care helpful for less severely injured patients? *Injury, 36*, 1293–1297.

Hess, J. R., Holcomb, J. B., & Hoyt, D. B. (2006). Damage control resuscitation: The need for specific blood products to treat the coagulopathy of trauma. *Transfusion, 46*, 685–686.

Hess, J. R., & Lawson, J. H. (2006). The coagulopathy of trauma versus disseminated intravascular coagulation. *Journal of Trauma, 60*(6), S12–S19.

Isenhour, J., & Marx, J. (2007). *General approach to blunt abdominal trauma in adults.* Retrieved April 14, 2007, from http://www.UpToDate.com

Ketchum, L., Hess, J. R., & Hippala, S. (2006). Indications for early fresh frozen plasma, cryoprecipitate, and platelet transfusion in trauma. *Journal of Trauma, 60*(Suppl.), S51–S58.

Martini, W. Z., Pusateri, A. E., Uscilowicz, J. M., Delgado, A. V., & Holcomb, J. B. (2005). Independent contributions of hypothermia and acidosis to coagulopathy in swine. *Journal of Trauma, 58*(5), 1002–1009.

National Fire Protection Agency (NFPA). (2003). *Remembering when: a fire and fall prevention program for older adults.* Retrieved October 17, 2008, from http://www.nfpa.org/assets/files/PDF/RememberingWhen.ppt#256

National Trauma Data Bank. (2007). *National Trauma Data Bank report 2006.* Chicago: American College of Surgeons.

Pepe, P. E., Dutton, R. P., & Fowler, R. L. (2008). Preoperative resuscitation of the trauma patient. *Current Opinion in Anaesthesiology, 21*(2), 216–221.

Petersen, V. (2004). *Trauma tertiary surveys what, why, when, how, and who: Detecting missed injuries in the multiply-injured patient.* Retrieved July 22, 2004, from http://www.trauma.org/nurse/tertiarysurvey.html

Sommers, M. S. (2006). Injury is a global phenomenon of concern in nursing science. *Journal of Nursing Scholarship, 38*(4), 314–320.

Spaniol, J. R., Knight, A. R., Zebley, J. L., Anderson, D., & Pierce, J. D. (2007). Fluid resuscitation therapy for hemorrhagic shock. *Journal of Trauma Nursing, 14*(3), 152–160.

Tieu, B. H., Holcomb, J. B., & Schreiber, M. A. (2007). Coagulopathy: Its pathophysiology and treatment in the injured patient. *World Journal of Surgery, 31*(5), 1055–1065.

Urden, L. D., Stacy, K. M., & Lough, M. E. (2006). *Thelan's critical care nursing.* St. Louis: Mosby.

APPENDIX A   2009–2011 NANDA-APPROVED NURSING DIAGNOSES

Activity Intolerance

Activity Intolerance, Risk for

Activity Planning, Ineffective

Airway Clearance, Ineffective

Anxiety

Anxiety, Death

Aspiration, Risk for

Attachment, Parent/Infant/Child, Risk for Impaired

Autonomic Dysreflexia

Autonomic Dysreflexia, Risk for

Bleeding, Risk for

Blood Glucose, Risk for Unstable

Body Image, Disturbed

Body Temperature: Imbalanced, Risk for

Bowel Incontinence

Breastfeeding, Effective

Breastfeeding, Ineffective

Breastfeeding, Interrupted

Breathing Pattern, Ineffective

Cardiac Output, Decreased

Caregiver Role Strain

Caregiver Role Strain, Risk for

Childbearing Process, Readiness for Enhanced

Comfort, Impaired

Comfort, Readiness for Enhanced

Communication: Impaired, Verbal

Communication, Readiness for Enhanced

Confusion, Acute

Confusion, Acute, Risk for

Confusion, Chronic

Constipation

Constipation, Perceived

Constipation, Risk for

Contamination

Contamination, Risk for

Coping: Community, Ineffective

Coping: Community, Readiness for Enhanced

Coping, Defensive

Coping: Family, Compromised

Coping: Family, Disabled

Coping: Family, Readiness for Enhanced

Coping (Individual), Readiness for Enhanced

Coping, Ineffective

Decisional Conflict

Decision Making, Readiness for Enhanced

Denial, Ineffective

Dentition, Impaired

Development: Delayed, Risk for

Diarrhea

Disuse Syndrome, Risk for

Diversional Activity, Deficient

Electrolyte Imbalance, Risk for

Energy Field, Disturbed

Environmental Interpretation Syndrome, Impaired

Failure to Thrive, Adult

Falls, Risk for

Family Processes, Dysfunctional: Alcoholism

Family Processes, Interrupted

Family Processes, Readiness for Enhanced

Fatigue

Fear

Fluid Balance, Readiness for Enhanced

Fluid Volume, Deficient

Fluid Volume, Deficient, Risk for

Fluid Volume, Excess

Fluid Volume, Imbalanced, Risk for

Gas Exchange, Impaired

Grieving

Grieving, Complicated

Grieving, Risk for Complicated

Growth, Disproportionate, Risk for

Growth and Development, Delayed

Health Behavior, Risk-Prone

Health Maintenance, Ineffective

Health Management, Ineffective Self

Health-Seeking Behaviors (Specify)

Home Maintenance, Impaired

Hope, Readiness for Enhanced

Hopelessness

Human Dignity, Risk for Compromised

Hyperthermia

Hypothermia

Identity, Disturbed Personal

Immunization Status, Readiness for Enhanced

Infant Behavior, Disorganized

Infant Behavior: Disorganized, Risk for

Infant Behavior: Organized, Readiness for Enhanced

Infant Feeding Pattern, Ineffective

Infection, Risk for

Injury, Risk for

Insomnia

Intracranial Adaptive Capacity, Decreased

Knowledge, Deficient (Specify)

Knowledge (Specify), Readiness for Enhanced

Latex Allergy Response

Latex Allergy Response, Risk for

Liver Function, Impaired, Risk for

Loneliness, Risk for

Maternal/Fetal Dyad, Risk for Disturbed

Memory, Impaired

Mobility: Bed, Impaired

Mobility: Physical, Impaired

Mobility: Wheelchair, Impaired

Moral Distress

Motility, Dysfunctional Gastrointestinal

Motility, Risk for Dysfunctional Gastrointestinal

Nausea

Neonatal Jaundice

Neurovascular Dysfunction: Peripheral, Risk for

Noncompliance (Specify)

Nutrition, Imbalanced: Less than Body Requirements

Nutrition, Imbalanced: More than Body Requirements

Nutrition, Imbalanced: More than Body Requirements, Risk for

Nutrition, Readiness for Enhanced

Oral Mucous Membrane, Impaired

Pain, Acute

Pain, Chronic

Parenting, Impaired

Parenting, Readiness for Enhanced

Parenting, Risk for Impaired

Perfusion, Ineffective Peripheral Tissue

Perfusion, Risk for Decreased Cardiac

Perfusion, Risk for Impaired Renal

Perfusion, Risk for Ineffective Cerebral Tissue

Perfusion, Risk for Ineffective Gastrointestinal Tissue

Perioperative Positioning Injury, Risk for

Personal Identity, Disturbed

Poisoning, Risk for

Post-Trauma Syndrome

Post-Trauma Syndrome, Risk for

Power, Readiness for Enhanced

Powerlessness

Powerlessness, Risk for

Protection, Ineffective

Rape-Trauma Syndrome

Relationship, Readiness for Enhanced

Religiosity, Impaired

Religiosity, Readiness for Enhanced

Religiosity, Risk for Impaired

Relocation Stress Syndrome

Relocation Stress Syndrome, Risk for

Resilience, Impaired Individual

Resilience, Readiness for Enhanced

Resilience, Risk for Compromised

Role Conflict, Parental

Role Performance, Ineffective

Sedentary Lifestyle

Self-Care, Readiness for Enhanced

Self-Care Deficit: Bathing/Hygiene

Self-Care Deficit: Dressing/Grooming

Self-Care Deficit: Feeding

Self-Care Deficit: Toileting

Self-Concept, Readiness for Enhanced

Self-Esteem, Chronic Low

Self-Esteem, Situational Low

Self-Esteem, Risk for Situational Low

Self-Mutilation

Self-Mutilation, Risk for

Self Neglect

Sensory Perception, Disturbed (Specify: Auditory, Gustatory, Kinesthetic, Olfactory, Tactile, Visual)

Sexual Dysfunction

Sexuality Pattern, Ineffective

Shock, Risk for

Skin Integrity, Impaired

Skin Integrity, Risk for Impaired

Sleep Deprivation

Sleep Pattern, Disturbed

Sleep, Readiness for Enhanced

Social Interaction, Impaired

Social Isolation

Sorrow, Chronic

Spiritual Distress

Spiritual Distress, Risk for

Spiritual Well-Being, Readiness for Enhanced

Spontaneous Ventilation, Impaired

Stress, Overload

Sudden Infant Death Syndrome, Risk for

Suffocation, Risk for

Suicide, Risk for

Surgical Recovery, Delayed

Swallowing, Impaired

Therapeutic Regimen Management: Family, Ineffective

Therapeutic Regimen Management, Ineffective

Therapeutic Regimen Management, Readiness for Enhanced

Thermoregulation, Ineffective

Tissue Integrity, Impaired

Tissue Perfusion, Ineffective (Specify: Cerebral, Cardiopulmonary, Gastrointestinal, Renal)

Tissue Perfusion, Ineffective, Peripheral

Transfer Ability, Impaired

Trauma, Risk for

Trauma, Risk for Vascular

Unilateral Neglect

Urinary Elimination, Impaired

Urinary Elimination, Readiness for Enhanced

Urinary Incontinence, Functional

Urinary Incontinence, Overflow

Urinary Incontinence, Reflex

Urinary Incontinence, Stress

Urinary Incontinence, Urge

Urinary Incontinence, Risk for Urge

Urinary Retention

Ventilatory Weaning Response, Dysfunctional

Violence: Other-Directed, Risk for

Violence: Self-Directed, Risk for

Walking, Impaired

Wandering

Source: NANDA Nursing Diagnoses: Definitions and Classification, 2007–2008. Philadelphia: North American Nursing Diagnosis Association. Used with permission.

Standard precautions are designed to reduce the risk of transmission of microorganisms from both recognized and unrecognized sources of infection. They are the primary strategies for preventing nosocomial infections within institutions, and are important to protect health care workers as well. Standard precautions apply to (1) blood; (2) all body fluids, secretions, and excretions except sweat, regardless of whether or not they contain visible blood; (3) nonintact skin; and (4) mucous membranes. Standard precautions are applied to all patients receiving care in hospitals, regardless of their diagnosis or presumed infection status. These precautions are specifically designed for hospitals; however, they also may be implemented in extended and long-term care facilities, and to a more limited extent in providing home care or in other community-based care settings.

Hand Washing

- Wash your hands (a) after touching blood, body fluids, secretions, excretions, and contaminated items, whether or not gloves are worn; (b) immediately after removing gloves, even if gloves appear to be intact; (c) between contacts with patients; and (d) when otherwise indicated to prevent transfer of organisms to other patients. You may need to wash your hands between tasks and procedures on the same patient to prevent cross-contaminating different body sites.
- Use soap and warm water for hand washing when hands are visibly dirty or contaminated with blood or other body fluids.
- If hands are not visibly soiled, use an alcohol-based hand rub for routinely decontaminating hands in all other situations.

Gloves

- Wear clean, nonsterile gloves when touching blood, body fluids, secretions, excretions, and contaminated items.
- Put on clean gloves just before touching mucous membranes and nonintact skin.
- Change your gloves between tasks and procedures on the same patient after contacting material that may contain a high concentration of microorganisms.
- Wear gloves for all invasive procedures such as performing venipuncture or other vascular or surgical procedures.
- Wear gloves if you have cuts, scratches, or other breaks in the skin.
- Remove gloves promptly after use, before touching noncontaminated items and surfaces, and before going to another patient; wash hands immediately after removing gloves.

Mask, Eye Protection, Face Shield

Wear a mask and eye protection or a face shield to protect mucous membranes of your eyes, nose, and mouth during procedures and patient care activities that are likely to generate splashes or sprays of blood, body fluids, secretions, or excretions.

Gown

Wear a gown (clean, disposable) to protect your skin and prevent soiling of clothing during procedures and patient care activities that are likely to generate splashes or sprays of blood, body fluids, secretions, or excretions. Remove soiled gowns promptly, washing your hands immediately after gown removal.

Equipment

Handle used patient care equipment that is soiled with blood, body fluids, secretions, and excretions in a way that prevents exposing your skin and mucous membranes, contaminating your clothing, and transferring microorganisms to other patients or environments. Ensure that reusable equipment is cleaned and appropriately reprocessed before using for the care of another patient.

Environmental Control

Follow hospital procedures for routine care, cleaning, and disinfecting environmental surfaces, beds, bed rails, bedside equipment, and other frequently touched surfaces.

Linen

Handle and transport linens soiled with blood, body fluids, secretions, and excretions in a manner that prevents exposing your skin and mucous membranes, contaminating your clothing, and transferring microorganisms to other patients and environments. Place soiled linen in leakage-resistant bags at the location where it is used.

Occupational Health and Bloodborne Pathogens

- Take care to prevent injuries when using needles, scalpels, and other sharps; when handling sharp instruments after procedures; when cleaning used instruments; and when disposing of used needles.
- Never recap used needles, manipulate them using both hands, or handle them in a manner that directs the point of a needle toward any part of your body. If it is necessary to protect the needle prior to disposal, use a one-handed "scoop" technique or mechanical device to hold the needle sheath.
- Do not remove used needles from disposable syringes by hand; do not bend, break, or otherwise manipulate used needles by hand.
- Place used disposable syringes and needles, scalpel blades, and other sharp items in appropriate puncture-resistant containers located as close as practical to the area in which the items were used.
- Place reusable syringes and needles in a puncture-resistant container for transport to the reprocessing area.

• Use mouthpieces, resuscitation bags, or other ventilation devices as an alternative to mouth-to-mouth resuscitation methods whenever possible.

Patient Placement

Place patients who contaminate the environment or who do not (or are not expected to) assist in maintaining appropriate hygiene or environmental control (e.g., an ambulatory, confused patient with fecal incontinence) in a private room.

Sources: Centers for Disease Control and Prevention. (2002). Guidelines for hand hygiene in health-care settings: Recommendations of the Healthcare Infection Control Practices Advisory Committee and the HICPAC/SHEA/APIC/IDSA Hand Hygiene Taskforce. *MMWR, 51*(RR-16), 1–56; Hospital Infection Control Practices Advisory Committee. (1997). Part II. Recommendations for isolation precautions in hospitals. Atlanta: Public Health Service, U.S. Department of Health and Human Services, Centers for Disease Control and Prevention.

APPENDIX C   Units of Measurement in Metric and Household Systems

ABBREVIATIONS

Volume

Metric		Household	
milliliter	mL	microdrop	mcgtt
liter	L	drop	gtt
cubic centimeter	cc	teaspoon	t or tsp
		tablespoon	T or tbs
		fluid ounce	oz
		pint	pt
		quart	qt

Weight

Metric		Household	
microgram	mcg	ounce	oz
milligram	mg	pound	lb
gram	g		
kilogram	kg		

Length

Metric		Household	
centimeter	cm	inch	in
meter	m	foot	ft

Area

Metric	
square meter	m^2

Evidence-Based Practice Boxes

Chapter 10
Evidence-Based Practice #1 Answers
1. In this scenario, the nurse will need to perform a digital rectal exam to assess for hardened stool in the rectal vault. If the patient is uncooperative, a provider's order for any abdominal x-ray to assess for fecal impaction would be indicated.
2. Because narcotics can cause a slowing of the intestine, with constipation as a result, the nurse will need to consider adding a stool softener or laxative to the patient's medication regimen.
3. Yes, patients often have fecal impaction of stool in the rectum but have small amounts of liquid stool that are expelled around the impaction. The nurse will need to facilitate removal of the hardened stool through the use of either a suppository or an enema or via manual disimpaction, if needed.

Evidence-Based Practice #2 Answers
1. Ask the daughter why she feels her mother should have a mammogram now, when she has refused them in the past. This allows the daughter to verbalize her concerns about her mother, which may reflect the daughter's greater concerns as to her mother's overall medical condition.
2. If the daughter is the patient's appointed spokesperson, share with her your findings. She may already know about the mass and have decided to take no further action, or it may be new information to her. Either way, notify the patient's provider with your findings for further action, if indicated.
3. Call the breast imaging center in advance to determine whether it has the equipment available to accommodate this patient. If the patient is frail, the breast imaging center may want to schedule a longer appointment than usual to give the patient extra time to complete the mammogram.

Evidence-Based Practice #3 Answers
1. The nurse should diplomatically remind the health care provider that Darvocet (propoxyphene) can cause adverse central nervous system effects in the elderly, with little analgesic advantage over acetaminophen. The nurse can suggest a medication more appropriate in this population, such as acetaminophen with a short-acting opiate if necessary for pain control. It is also helpful to know what is available in your facility's emergency medication kit so that you will be able to give a medication without having to order it from the pharmacy and wait for delivery.
2. Diphenhydramine can cause urinary retention, especially in elderly males who may have a baseline prostate hypertrophy. Diphenhydramine should not be used as a sleeping agent; safer alternatives exist. The nurse should notify the health care provider of the patient's symptoms and then discuss a plan of treatment, including addressing the patient's urinary retention as well as insomnia.
3. Her health care provider needs to know about her diazepam use because this medication should be avoided in the elderly due to its extremely long half-life. The nurse needs to discuss with both the patient and the health care provider a plan of care to address the patient's "nerves." Obtaining medications from multiple providers is a dangerous practice, especially for the aging patient.

Chapter 12
1. The perception and chronicity of stress causes a cellular response and an increase in oxidative stress. The cellular response includes a reduction in the number of telomeres and telomerase, a decrease in the ability of the cells to divide, and a decrease in the DNA component, which precipitates genetic damage and eventually cell death. Over time, the tissues comprising the affected cells also die, producing the effects of aging: muscles weaken; skin wrinkles; hair grays; eyesight; hearing; and organs fail; and thinking abilities diminish.
2. Young adults have higher telomerase levels and a greater ability for the enzyme to repair the cell by regenerating telomeres. The telomerase levels decrease with normal aging. This process is accelerated with high levels of chronic psychological stress, thus precipitating premature aging. It is important to know this information to assist in the assessment process. Understanding the age differentiation helps the nurse to know which type of patient is the most vulnerable candidate for cellular response to chronic perceived stress.
3. a. Sleep.
   b. Social connections.
   c. Exercise.
   d. Quiet time alone.
   e. Rest and relaxation.
   f. Meditation/contemplation.
   g. Hobbies.
   h. Nutrition.
   i. Journaling.
   j. Yoga.

Chapter 14
1. Postpyloric placement of a feeding tube into the small bowel can be useful to minimize the risk of high gastric residuals. If it is not contraindicated, elevation of the head of the bed to a 45-degree angle may decrease risk of aspiration.
2. Feedings should not be held until there are two or more consecutive gastric residual volumes greater than 250 mL.

Chapter 15
1. Is this new onset pain?
   What is the patient's perception of discomfort?
   Has this type of pain occurred before?

What has been effective in the past for pain relief?

Drug allergies or unwanted side effects such and nausea and vomiting.

2. Facial grimacing.

   Increased movement.

   Increased heart rate and blood pressure.

   Ask family members and caregivers what the usual response to pain is.

Chapter 17

1. Ask and identify open-ended questions to clarify how they are feeling.
2. Listen carefully to what they are saying. Let them know that you are available to answer questions. Advocate for the patient and family by contacting other members of the health care team as needed.

Chapter 20

1. a. Ensure an adequate diet with vitamins A and C, iron, and zinc.
   b. Avoid exposure to others with infection.
   c. Instruct the patient to wash hands after toileting and before eating.
   d. Report to the surgeon all medications taken.
2. a. Check color; redness may indicate infection.
   b. Check temperature; warmth may indicate infection.
   c. Check for swelling.
   d. Check for drainage from the wound. If present, check the color and amount of drainage.
3. a. Wash hands before and after touching the patient.
   b. Wear gloves when providing wound care.
   c. Keep the patient well hydrated and provide foods that are high in protein.
4. a. Instruct patients to take their prescriptions as directed, including the prescribed frequency and duration.
   b. Educate patients on when antibiotics are appropriate and not appropriate.

Chapter 21

1. Ask the patient an open-ended question to describe what insights have become apparent during the interview.
2. Listen carefully to the story of the patient. Use nonverbal cues to support the patient.

Chapter 23

1. f. b & c
2. a. Slow the transfusion.
   b. Take vital signs and oxygen saturation.
   c. Call the health care provider.

Chapter 25

1. These questions are designed to get one to think about issues that may influence the generalizability of research findings and the need to replicate research studies using subjects of both genders, varying ages, and multiple ethnicities and cultures. In thinking about this study, one might wonder how culture, specifically the Chinese culture, might influence things such as attitudes toward pain and pain expression as well as attitudes toward taking pain medication or using nonpharmacologic therapies for pain control. Culture may also play a role in how the subjects respond to being part of a research study. One needs to know more fully about Chinese culture to theorize about how these research results will generalize to a Western culture. Similarly, it is helpful to know about national health insurance in China. The economics of health care in a country influence aspects of care, such as what kind of preoperative teaching is available, what pain medications are used, how medications are administered, and what nonpharmacologic approaches are covered by the insurance. These may, in turn, influence attitudes.

2. Pain is a subjective experience, and the use of a visual analog scale is a valid and reliable measure of a person's pain experience. The researchers could include objective indices of pain or of physiological stress, with physiological stress serving as a marker for pain. Examples of objective measures might include blood pressure (elevation or changes correlating with pain ratings), heart rate (elevation or correlation with pain rating), respiratory rate (elevation), and plasma cortisol levels (elevation). Objective markers have limitations because they are nonspecific; nevertheless, they could contribute to the discussion of pain reduction. The authors could also use functional performance as indirect markers of pain reduction. Physical performances that often improve with pain relief include ability and distance of ambulation, amount of time spent out of bed, and ability and frequency of deep breathing or ability to perform coughing exercises.

Chapter 26

1. a. Communication with surgical team for timing of antibiotic administration and to maintain surgical asepsis guidelines.
   b. Institute measures to maintain normothermia throughout surgery and postanesthesia care unit.
   c. Develop policies that ensure that standards regarding warning procedures are used by all members of the surgical team.

Chapter 27

1. It is not known which aspects of the protocol accounted for the change in the patient outcomes. One could explain, using Maslow's hierarchy of needs, that the protocol was effective because it helped patients to meet basic needs of comfort: toileting, repositioning, and pain management. These needs were met on a regular basis without the patient having to ask. The protocol also increased patients' sense of personal control over their environment by ensuring that important objects were close by and by giving information about care schedules. Perhaps the consistency of the schedule met higher levels of human need by allowing patients to feel safe and cared for. Several nursing theories can be used to explain the outcomes of this study. Hildegard Peplau's interpersonal relationships theory that puts the nurse–patient relationship at the center of nursing practice or Jean Watson's theory of caring are both appropriate, as are many

nursing theories. Katherine Kolcaba's theory of comfort is particularly relevant to the protocol of nursing rounds. In her theory, enhanced comfort is an immediate and desirable outcome of nursing interventions.

2. It seems as if any number of patient outcomes might be influenced by a nursing round protocol (the protocol used in the study or one that is tailored for specific nursing units). Examples of specific patient outcomes include reduction in urinary or bowel incontinence, reduction in the incidence of decubiti, improved pain management, increased mobility, and increased oral fluid intake.

3. The study could be replicated using a larger number of nursing units and varied types of units (medical, cardiac, oncology, neurology, surgical specialties, etc.). The protocol could be lengthened from the 4 weeks that was used. The nursing rounds protocol could be adapted for specific patient populations (e.g., it could include a reminder to use the incentive spirometry on a surgical unit).

Chapter 29

1. a. Difficulty with concentration.
   b. Family observations of irritability.
   c. Memory impairment.
2. a. A recent motor vehicle accident, with or without loss of consciousness.
   b. Participation in sporting events.
   c. Difficulty in school or work environment.
3. a. Consults for therapies, such as speech and occupational therapies.
   b. Family teaching and support.

Chapter 30

1. The elderly, any patient with uncontrolled hypertension, any patient on Coumadin.
2. Severe headache, difficulty with speech, decreased motor function of either side of the body, sudden loss of consciousness.
3. Close control of blood glucose, careful monitoring of blood pressure, vigilant neurological assessment.

Chapter 31

1. a. Disease process.
   b. Disease and symptom management.
   c. Community resources for assistance at home.
2. a. Verbalize instructions back to the nurse.
   b. Demonstrate the skill back to the nurse.
3. a. Get regular medical checkups.
   b. Get regular physical activity, such as walking.
   c. Use stress management techniques such as pleasurable activities, praying, or meditating.

Chapter 32

1. a. Immobility due to paralysis and spinal precautions.
   b. Ineffective cough.
   c. Use of a cervical orthosis.
   d. Abnormalities in the mechanics of swallowing.
2. a. Frequent coughing with oral intake.
   b. Wet vocal quality.

c. Difficulty managing oral secretions.
3. a. Sitting patient in an upright position for meals once cleared for activity.
   b. Avoid talking while eating.
   c. Avoidance of large boluses of food at one time.
   d. Monitor patient to ensure that food is cleared from the oropharynx.

Chapter 35

1. a. Most people spend 90% of their time indoors.
2. a. Tobacco smoke must be eliminated from the indoor environment.
3. a. Reducing the exposure to indoor allergens and pollutants will reduce exacerbation of respiratory illness.

Chapter 36

1. c. Confused and not able to cooperate.
2. b. COPD.

Chapter 38

1. a. Has anyone in your family, including parents, grandparents, siblings, aunts, and uncles, ever been diagnosed with AF?
   b. Have you ever been diagnosed with any cardiac disorder, such as heart failure, valve disease, heart attack, or rheumatic fever?
   c. Do you smoke, drink caffeine, or drink alcohol, and if so, in what quantity?
   d. Are you diabetic?
2. a. Report light-headedness, dizziness, shortness of breath, or chest pain to your health care provider as soon as they occur.
   b. Stop smoking and drinking alcohol and caffeine.
   c. Consistently take prescribed medications.
   d. Have family members tested if the AF is genetically induced.

Chapter 40

1. a. Use of interpreters.
   b. Instructions written in native languages.
   c. Use of family or friends who can assist with interpretation.
2. a. Are you noticing any changes in your energy level when performing your daily activities?
   b. Is there a change in the number of hours of sleep needed to feel rested?
   c. Has the need to rest during the day increased recently?
3. a. Statistics about the prevalence of heart disease in women.
   b. The types of clinical symptoms that women experience compared to those experienced by men.
   c. Lifestyle changes that would prevent or slow the progress of heart disease.

Chapter 41

1. a. Understand when it is important to seek medical help for the tachycardia.
   b. How to avoid activities that bring on the tachycardia.

    c. How to slow the heart rate when tachycardia occurs.

    d. List of ideas and activities that would be safe.

2. a. Education about the relationship between tachycardic episodes and the progression of the disease.

    b. Providing alternative activities that interest the young person to decrease the frustration associated with the limitations of the disease.

    c. Evaluate the presence of social support and educate these significant individuals about the need for activity restriction.

3. a. Space activities to allow for periods of rest.

    b. Medicate with antianxiety per orders when necessary.

    c. Control the environment and visitors to diminish stress.

    d. Evaluate current measures and the need for further intervention when necessary.

Chapter 42

1. a. Notify the patient's health care provider.

    b. Ask to talk to another member of the family to see if it is possible to get the patient his medications.

    c. Have the patient explore the possibility of having the medications delivered by the pharmacy.

    d. Ask the patient if he can afford to have a taxi deliver the medications.

2. a. Ask the patient specific questions about her diet, in terms of food types and amounts.

    b. Ask the patient to keep track of the amount of fluids consumed each day.

    c. Discuss with the patient/family the implications associated with failure to comply with therapy.

    d. Ascertain the patient/family understanding of failure to comply with medical management.

    e. Report clinical manifestations to the health care provider.

3. a. Ask the patient about diet, fluid intake, and compliance with medications.

    b. Ask the patient about support system and availability of help with cooking and procurement of medications.

    c. Assess patient motivation with compliance with treatment plan.

    d. Assess patient/family understanding of treatment needs and ability to comply.

Chapter 43

1. Assessment of other risk factors for the development of DVT. Reporting homocysteine and risk factors to the health care provider. Instating health care provider orders to prevent DVT. Assessment for the effectiveness of the interventions.

2. Active and passive range of motion. Foot and ankle exercises. Graduated stocking, pneumatic compression devices.

3. Prevent venous pooling of blood.

Chapter 45

1. A, C, E, F

2. Visual inspection of the oral mucosa.

3. When assessing the oral cavity, the nurse should note any subjective complaints, such as soreness or pain of the lips

or gums, reports of increased salivation, toothache, or earache. The objective assessment findings of concern would include indurations or painless ulcer on the lips, ulcerations, areas of thickening, increased salivation, leukoplakia, erythroplakia, rough areas, slurred speech, dysphagia, or difficulty chewing or speaking.

Chapter 46

1. Most medications are metabolized by the liver. Decreased hepatic blood flow and shunting of blood slows the metabolism of medications and creates a higher bioavailability. Also, the shifts in body fluids that occur with decreased serum albumin will change the volume of distribution for the medications.

2. The nurse should check the medication information to see if the pharmacologic half-life is affected by liver failure. Because the metabolism of morphine is greatly affected, the nurse should review the dosage and frequency with the health care team to ensure the safety of the patient.

Chapter 47

1. Nonadherence with fluid restrictions may cause fluid overload with symptoms of shortness of breath, muscle cramping, dizziness, anxiety, panic, pulmonary edema, and hypertension. Nonadherence with dietary restrictions and medication regimens may result in chronically elevated serum levels of phosphate, which contribute to the development of coronary artery disease and the development of secondary hyperparathyroidism.

2. Implement adherence-enhancing interventions with the goal of improving the clinical outcome.

Chapter 49

1. c

2. a

3. a

Chapter 50

1. Meeting the needs of the spouse will improve the quality of life for both the patient and the spouse.

2. d. Involve spouses in medical decision making along with the patient.

Chapter 53

1. The best answer would be "b." This is an adolescent who is not focused so much on the future as on his current lifestyle. It is important to look at what is going on around him to try to find the reason why he is not checking his blood glucose. There may be a variety of reasons as to why he does not test his glucose, including feeling self-conscious about his diabetes. At this point, the nurse can help to explore practical ways to integrate glucose testing into his lifestyle, regardless of whether he really understands the long-term complications or not.

2. The best answer would be "a." The point that you want to emphasize is that regardless of the type of diabetes, the relationship between glucose control and the development of

complications is a primary mediator of complications (chronically elevated blood glucose levels are associated with the development of diabetes-related complications). The nurse may also want to explore whether there are financial or other concerns that are influencing one's ability to check blood glucose levels.

3. Of the two responses, the second is the best. This is because it involves a systematic approach to the problem while recognizing that if the patient and family decide to continue multiple daily injections, the plan will be in place to recognize and prevent hypoglycemia.

Chapter 55

1. Identifying high-risk individuals allows the health care team, patient, and family to develop a plan and implement preventive measures to decrease the chance of a fall and subsequent fracture.
2. Moderate exercise such as walking, swimming, or riding a stationary bike helps to strengthen muscles, slows the loss of calcium from the bone, and helps to maintain balance. Exercise such as yoga helps to strengthen core muscles, which helps with maintenance of balance and flexibility.

Chapter 56

1. The pin site will become infected. Skeletal traction pins are exposed to the environment where they protrude through the skin, and bacteria can travel down to the bone. Moisture creates an area for bacteria, always present at the pin–skin interface, to accumulate and grow.
2. Signs and symptoms of infection include pain, redness, edema, and drainage from the site.

Chapter 57

1. Early control of pain is more effective in controlling pain than is medication administered after pain becomes severe. With amputation, pain normally begins to diminish in intensity 3 or 4 days after surgery.
2. Phantom limb pain is the sensation of pain in the amputated body part. The cause of the phenomenon is unknown, but the perception of pain can interfere with the patient's rehabilitation.

Chapter 58
Critical Thinking Application #1 Answers
1. a. Have the patient take the medication with food.
   b. Encourage small frequent meals.
   c. Drink milk when taking medication.
2. a. Xanthine oxidase inhibitors.
   b. Nonsteroidal anti-inflammatory drugs.
   c. Steroids.
   d. Uricosuric agents.

Critical Thinking Application #2 Answers
1. a. Compliance with multiple treatments, such as medication and lifestyle changes.
   b. What impact can the nursing profession make on improving patient care with gout?

   c. Providing an understanding of the risks and pathophysiology of the disease process.
   d. Teaching the patient ways to improve lifestyle choices and reduce gout attacks.
   e. Educating the patient on medication therapy.

Chapter 60
1. b. Ease of availability and financial resources.
2. a. Diminished or absent diarrhea.
   c. Absence of candidiasis.
   d. No painful swallowing.

Chapter 61
1. a. Hypotension after infusion of 2 liters of isotonic crystalloid infusion.
2. b. Infusing 7 liters of crystalloid solution through a central line.
3. 1. Suctioning blood from the patient's airway.
   2. Initiating a large-caliber IV for fluid resuscitation.
   3. Stabilizing the patient's pelvis with a sheet.
   4. Applying 100% oxygen by mask to the patient.

Chapter 63
Evidence-Based Practice #1 Answers
1. Pain, short duration of inspiration, and frustration.
2. a. Provide patient education regarding the relationship between lung inspiration, oxygenation, and pulmonary complications.
   b. Provide instruction on proper use of IS, including length of inspiration, volume goals, and frequency.
   c. Recruit family to encourage patient.
   d. Provide adequate pain management.
   e. Provide frequent encouragement and progress assessments/reports to patient.
3. a. Lung sounds.
   b. Chest expansion.
   c. Pain level with inspiration.
   d. Oxygenation status.
   e. Incentive spirometry volume and frequency of use.

Evidence-Based Practice #2 Answers
1. a. Assessment.
   b. Regular flushing.
   c. Solution based on clinical assessment.
2. Benefits include prevention of clot formation. However, risks are increased HIT.

Chapter 64
1. a. Understanding at what point during the course of treatment there is a potential to develop fatigue.
   b. Explanation of how the patient may feel as he or she becomes fatigued.
   c. A list of strategies to reduce energy consumption.
   d. Dietary suggestions to optimize nutrition during and after treatment.
2. a. Report presence of fatigue to health care team so that recommendations can be offered.

b. Encourage the patient and family to discuss the impact of fatigue on their daily lives.

c. Referral to social services or psychiatry as needed.

d. Acknowledge the potential for fatigue to alter sexuality.

3. a. Provide information about interventions available to treat fatigue.

b. Accurate assessment and prompt treatment for fatigue.

c. Encourage patients to maintain adequate activity to increase energy stores.

Chapter 67

1. e. All of the above.

2. a. It would combine to form the compound silver chloride and the silver would no longer be bioavailable to perform its function because ionic silver is the element that is effective against bacteria.

3. e. All of the above.

Chapter 68

1. a. Obtain immediate medical care when injuries occur.

b. Understand that there is an increased risk for complications and prolonged hospitalization.

c. Daily foot inspection for breakdown.

d. Avoidance of extreme temperatures when bathing.

e. No exposure to heaters to help keep feet warm.

2. a. Fireplaces.

b. Poorly controlled heaters.

c. Living alone.

d. Confusion and poor memory.

e. Little to no social support.

f. Inadequate nutrition.

g. Inadequate blood sugar control.

3. a. Blood sugar control.

b. Adequate nutritional support.

c. Strict aseptic technique for wound care.

d. Reporting of the first signs of infections.

Chapter 70
Evidence-Based Practice #1 Answers

1. Know which noises can cause damage (those above 85 decibels). Wear earplugs or other hearing protection devices when involved in a loud activity. Be alert to hazardous noise in the environment. Protect children who are too young to protect themselves. Make family, friends, and colleagues aware of the hazards of noise. Have a medical examination by an otolaryngologist, a physician who specializes in diseases of the ears, nose, throat, head, and neck, and a hearing test by an audiologist, a health professional trained to identify and measure hearing loss and to rehabilitate persons with hearing impairments.

2. Everyone is exposed to hazardous sound levels at one time or on a regular basis—individuals of all ages, including children, adolescents, young adults, and older people. Exposure occurs in the workplace, in recreational settings, and at home.

3. A variety of activities can predispose an individual to NIHL. It may occur from only a one-time exposure to loud sound as well as from repeated exposure to sounds at various loudness levels over an extended period of time. Examples of activities are listening to loud iPods, radios, or TV. Examples of workplace noises are jackhammers and explosive sounds. Participation in recreational activities, such as flying loud model airplanes, snowmobiling, go-carting, woodworking, target shooting, and hunting, may even be a factor.

Evidence-Based Practice #2 Answers

1. Culturally deaf adults are at risk for health-related behaviors that address nutrition, psychological well-being, stress management, physical activity and exercise, activities of daily living, and responsible health care practices.

2. Culturally deaf adults may use a variety of interventions to help them adjust to their environments. The following is just a small list of such activities: learning sign language; having communities provide street warning signs for adults with hearing impairments; using devices that help with communication, such as flashing lights for doorbells or visual readings for telephone communication; and participating in educational activities that will inform society of ways to prevent hazards that cause hearing impairment or hearing loss.

3. School nurses not only are helpful in identifying those adolescents with hearing problems through screening programs, but they may act as advocates for educational activities that inform adolescents of hazardous activities that may lead to NIHL.

Chapter 71

1. a. Inform the patient as to what AMD is and how it impacts the vision and general well-being of the patient, with a return demonstration of gained knowledge.

b. Advise patient about possible ways to decrease the advancement of AMD with prevention.

c. Teach the patient about when it is important to seek medical direction for vision changes from AMD, with a return demonstration of information gained.

d. List the problem stages of treatment or management of AMD.

2. a. Educating about the relationship of possible aging, genetics, ultraviolet light, air pollution, smoking, comorbidities, blood thinners, zinc, luteins, antioxidants, and VEGF toward the advancement of AMD.

b. Providing alternative activities that interest older adults to decrease the frustration associated with the limitations of vision with AMD and general well-being.

c. Incorporating a significant other in the relationship and care, depending on the degree of visual impairment, to prevent social isolation.

d. Providing possible activities that would be beneficial and safe in adding to the prevention or stabilization of visual impairment from AMD.

3. a. Educate on maintaining good general health and avoiding comorbidities that may affect or advance a decline in vision health.

b. Educate on self-vision testing, for example, Amsler grid, and coping with vision loss and maintaining quality of life.

c. Control the environment by adding more independence activities with visual impairment.

d. Evaluate current measures and the need for further intervention as needs present.

Chapter 73

1. b. A policy and procedure should be present to assist in the implementation of family presence. Staff members need education and support.

2. d. All of the above.

Chapter 74

1. f. All of the above.

2. b. It decreases the risk of coagulopathy.

Clinical Preparation Boxes

Chapter 14

1. a. Obesity (BMI 33).
   b. Obesity, family history, hypercholesterolemia, hypertension, hyperglycemia, decreased serum HDL cholesterol, sedentary activity level.

2. a. Assess readiness to lose body weight.
   b. Educate on health benefits of losing weight.
   c. Assist in development of short-term goals toward losing 1 to 2 pounds/week:
      • Increase physical activity. Begin with sitting for fewer hours in the day and gradually add activity.
      • Decrease intake by 500 to 100 kcal/day; assist patient with identifying ways to do this, such as decreased intake of alcohol and empty calories (e.g., change cream in coffee to fat-free half and half, snack on fruit instead of chips).
   d. Educate about the DASH diet for hypertension (reduced sodium, saturated fat, and cholesterol; moderate alcohol; adequate dairy; ample fruits, vegetables, and whole grains).
   e. Refer to registered dietitian.

3. a. Fat intake.
   b. Alcohol intake.
   c. Caffeine intake.
   d. Large meals.
   e. Eating large meals late in the evening, close to bedtime (lying flat with increased gastric pressure).
   f. Overweight/obese.

4. Reduced intake of fat, moderating alcohol intake, weight loss.

Chapter 15

1. Sensory, affective, cognitive, and behavioral.

2. Discuss concerns about pain management and discuss reasons for behavior when wife is present.

3. PCA demand doses attempted/given, medication side effects, renal function, patient's current and acceptable level of pain.

Chapter 19

1. This patient has a respiratory acidosis—the $PaCO_2$ is increased and the pH is acid. The HCO_3^- is higher than normal, with a base excess of $+5$.

2. Age, 50 pack/year smoking history, emphysema, history of coronary artery disease.

3. Emphysema and pneumonia.

4. Coughing and deep-breathing exercises. Up in chair and walking at regular intervals.

Chapter 20

1. Room 122—apparent best immune system.

2. Yes—open draining leg wound that is positive for *S. aureus*.

3. Diabetes, living in the woods, age, and smoking.

4. *Body Image, Disturbed.*
   Fatigue.
   Mobility: Physical, Impaired.
   Pain, Acute.
   High Risk for Self-Care Deficit: Toileting.
   Skin Integrity, Impaired.
   Tissue Perfusion, Ineffective, Risk for.

Chapter 21
Part 1

1. *Assessment:* The nurse's initial assessment of Ms. Bell began at the time of her first visit to the health care center. The nurse began to collect the database concerning the characteristics that Ms. Bell was demonstrating. The subjective database suggested depression and distortion of reality concerning her health and work problems. The objective database was anger, agitation, and intolerance for the environment and the reporting of psychosomatic symptoms.

   Related Factors: Ms. Bell has highly ambivalent feelings concerning her family and the loss of employment.

   Nursing Diagnosis: Coping: Family Disabled (Wilkinson, 2005, p. 117).

   Alternative Diagnosis: Management of Therapeutic Regimen: Families/Individual, Ineffective (Wilkinson, 2005, p. 118).

   NOC Outcomes (Wilkinson, 2005):
   • Aggression control.
   • Depression control.
   • Neglect recovery.

   Goals/Evaluation Criteria:
   • Ms. Bell will use *Disabled Family Coping* as demonstrated by satisfactory status in aggression control, depression control, and neglect of recovery.
   • *Family and Individual Coping* with:
     Demonstrates role flexibility.
     Manages problems.
     Receives care and cares for the needs of family members.
     Secures financial stability.
     Asks for assistance when appropriate (Wilkinson, 2005, p. 119).

   NIC Interventions:
   • Coping enhancement: Assist Ms. Bell to adapt to the real and perceived stress and changes that were interfering with her life goals.

- Normalization promotion: Assist Ms. Bell with adaptation to a chronic disease, diabetes mellitus. Encourage her to accept that her life experience is a reality (Wilkinson, 2005).

Nursing Activities:
- Obtain a history of the family's patterns of behavior and changes that have occurred.
- Assess the interaction between Ms. Bell and her family.
- Determine the physical, emotional, educational, and spiritual resources of Ms. Bell.
- Assess Ms. Bell's motivation for resolving the crisis.
- Discuss with Ms. Bell the most effective ways to assist her with becoming familiar with her multiple health needs. Ms. Bell needs referrals to other agencies such as social services, nutrition counseling, support groups, and the Council on Aging.

Part 2

The strategies essential to controlling Ms. Bell's hypertension were an adequate knowledge base of what the disease is, how it may be controlled, the use of lifestyle changes, and weight control. Ms. Bell was encouraged to participate in the plan of care, and her questions can be answered through the use of the office hotline.

Part 3

If Ms. Bell relapses into noncompliance, the nurse will assess the problems interfering with Ms. Bell's following through with her plan of care. With this information, the plan of care can be modified by removing the element that was keeping her from following through. At times, the patient may not understand how and why a particular segment of the plan was important to the management and control of the disease. The use of totally illustrated brochures and conferences within the location may assist in the understanding of hypertension. In addition, the teaching appointments can be recorded on audio tape for the patient's review at home.

2. • Acceptance of the diagnosis of high blood pressure.
   • Enabling Ms. Bell in seeking information about high blood pressure and how the diagnosis is made.
   • Partnership with the nurse as the treatment plan is established, maintained, and revised.
   • Use of the plan and the ability to negotiate changes in the treatment plan as the physiological situation need modification.
   • Understands the reason for keeping appointments with the health care provider. Ms. Bell will report self-screening results at each visit.
   • Ms. Bell monitors herself for the treatment response.
   • Ms. Bell performs self-screening tests such as blood pressure, weight, and glucose monitoring.
   • Ms. Bell seeks to reinforce her lifestyle changes.
3. When the nurse listens to Ms. Bell in a therapeutic manner, the nurse will engage in an assessment of the patterns of communication and as a self-interpreting person. This means listening to the individual for his or her interpretation and the embedded meaning of the situation. This activity, the process of active listening, is "attending to and

attaching significance to a patient's verbal and nonverbal messages" (Wilkinson, 2005, p. 82).

4.

Nursing Assessment of Loss

Nursing Assessment and Diagnoses	Outcomes and Evaluation Parameters	Planning and Interventions with Rationale
Subjective: "I'm standing under a very dark cloud." "How much more can or must I tolerate?"	**Outcome:** Practice effective coping strategies. **Evaluation Parameters:** Documented improvements in self-reports. States reasons for changes in lifestyle and coping styles.	**Interventions and Rationales** Discusses importance of participating in the high blood pressure support group in the community. Discusses changing role in her home, community, and church. Reviews changes in lifestyle. *Lifestyle changes and modification of role within family, community, and church have positive value in fostering effective coping strategies.*
Objective: Death of husband of 35 years Loss of employment due to downsizing Daughter lives 250 miles away		
Nursing Diagnosis: Chronic Losses related to chronic illness and Ineffective Coping with lifestyle related to chronic illness		

Chapter 23

1. ASA and Celebrex.
2. Rehydration, undetected bleeding.
3. Transfusion reactions, lung sounds. Identification of patient, vital signs, and signs and symptoms of transfusion reactions.
4. Fluid overload due to his age and cardiac history.
5. History of taking Lopressor, a beta-blocker that decreases heart rate.
6. The Na and Cl levels are elevated (concentrated blood solutes). The BUN is elevated, but the creatinine is normal. Values return to normal after rehydration.
7. To rule out pancreatitis, which can cause GI bleed.
8. Vitamin K absorption by the intestine is decreased in GI bleed, and vitamin K is needed for clotting. Vitamin K affects the part of the clotting cascade that is measured by the PT and INR.

Chapter 27

1. *Pain:* Abdominal incisions are painful, and Mr. Landry's pain ratings show that he is not getting adequate pain relief. Pain is a likely factor in his reluctance to ambulate and to use the incentive spirometer.
   Impaired Gas Exchange: Mr. Landry is on 4 liters of oxygen but has only marginal oxygen saturation. He is not

performing deep breathing or coughing as needed to open the airways and alveoli and to clear respiratory secretions.

Fluid Volume, Deficient: Mr. Landry is losing fluid through the NGT and because he has a fever. The low urine output, tachycardia, dry skin, thirst, and vertigo when standing suggest that he is dehydrated.

Anxiety: Mr. Landry demonstrates anxious behaviors and he reports feeling anxious. Anxiety is an uncomfortable state, and it can influence all aspects of his care and recovery.

Activity Intolerance: Mr. Landry has vertigo, tachycardia, and tachypnea with activity.

2. Pain: Evidenced by high pain ratings and reluctance to do IS, cough, and ambulate.

Atelectasis: Evidenced by fever, crackles, shallow breathing.

Dehydration: Evidenced by tachycardia, low urine output, warm skin, thirst.

Orthostatic hypotension: Likely, given his complaints of vertigo on standing.

Ileus: Evidenced by no passing of flatus (expected finding for the first several days postop following surgery on colon).

Nausea: Evidenced by complaints of nausea.

Anemia: Evidenced by a low hematocrit and hemoglobin.

Vital Signs: Part of routine nursing care. The data are used to monitor for a variety of postoperative complications, including fever, bleeding, dehydration, abnormal cardiac rhythm.

NPO: To prevent abdominal distention and nausea and vomiting.

NGT to low continuous suction: Used to decompress the stomach. Prevents abdominal distention until peristalsis returns to the bowel. Abdominal distention would place tension on the sutures.

IS: A mechanism used to encourage deep breathing. Deep breathing increases lung volumes and stimulates surfactant. This intervention is used to treat hypoxia and to prevent atelectasis and pneumonia.

Foley: Used to get an accurate, hourly measurement of urine output.

I&O: Used to estimate fluid balance. Many patients are slightly dehydrated at the end of surgery. In this case, Mr. Landry is continuing to lose fluid as a result of a fever and drainage from the NGT.

Pneumatic compression boots: Increase venous return from the legs, helping to prevent deep venous thrombus (DVT).

Ambulate: Ambulation is the single most important intervention to prevent postoperative complications. Ambulation increases respiratory rate, minute ventilation, tidal volume, and inspiratory flow rates, helping to prevent atelectasis and pneumonia. Ambulation increases blood flow to organs and tissues, helping with wound healing, restoring peristalsis, and preventing venous stasis and DVT.

Cardiac telemetry: Used to monitor for bradycardia and dysrhythmia because Mr. Landry is receiving Metoprolol intravenously.

Dextrose 5% and 0.45 sodium chloride with 20 mEq KCl: This is an isotonic solution used to replace routine fluid loss and to cover fluid loss through the NGT. Mr. Landry requires potassium replacement because he is NPO and unable to replace routine loss of potassium in the urine and additional potassium losses from gastric drainage.

3. The most pressing nursing activities are the treatment of Mr. Landry's pain and nausea. Until pain and nausea are controlled, Mr. Landry will be unable to concentrate on learning to use incentive spirometry or participate in morning care. The nurse should first change the syringe in the PCA pump (this activity is entirely within the nurse's control) to make sure that Mr. Landry has uninterrupted pain medication. Second, the nurse should empty and record urine output and then call the surgeon for the antiemetic. Calling for the antinausea medication is important, but Mr. Landry has been having a low urine output that, if it continues, will require intervention (calling the surgeon and administration of a fluid bolus), and measuring urine output will only take a minute. Third, the nurse calls the surgeon for an antiemetic order (and reports the urine output if low). Once Mr. Landry is comfortable, he should receive teaching on use of the incentive spirometry. A.M. care is important to helping patients feel better, but most patients will decline morning care if they are uncomfortable with either pain or nausea.

4. Treatment for cancer, including colon cancer, depends on the stage of the cancer. Although surgery is a treatment for colon cancer, it is also part of the staging process because the tissue and lymph nodes removed will be examined for evidence of cancer cells. Mr. Landry may need adjunctive treatment (chemotherapy or radiation) once the stage of the cancer is determined. The nurse's best response in this situation is to explore with Mr. Landry his understanding of his disease and the treatment plan. The nurse can help clarify information provided by the surgeon and encourage Mr. Landry to ask the surgeon about questions he has regarding further treatment. The nurse can also help clarify for Mr. Landry the roles of the various people who are or will be involved in his care (e.g., the surgeon, the oncologist, the primary health care provider). The nurse should encourage Mr. Landry to keep the appointment with the oncologist.

Chapter 29

1. An injury to the left temporal area may result in speech difficulties, motor and/or sensory deficits to the right side of the body, and/or confusion.

2. The first sign that Jose's neurological status had changed was when he became restless and agitated and tried to climb over the rails. Though a subtle sign, restlessness and/or agitation may be the first sign that the level of consciousness has deteriorated.

3. The significance of this subtle neurological change is the probability that the size of the subdural hematoma may

be expanding. Subdural hematomas are space-occupying lesions; therefore, an expanding lesion has the potential to increase ICP, with neurological deterioration to follow.

4. With a decrease in the patient's neurological assessment, the nurse might expect the size of the subdural hematoma to have increased, causing more mass effect and increasing ICP.

5. Although the change in the patient's level of consciousness is usually the first sign of neurological deterioration, Jose had other signs to support his decrease in status. His severe headache and projectile vomiting were signs of increasing ICP. He also was more confused than on prior examination. The nurse could expect to see further signs of deterioration if the hematoma is not evacuated. If the hematoma continues to increase in size, without treatment, further deterioration of this patient's neurological condition might occur. An increase in the size of the hematoma would result in increased mass effect and cerebral edema. Clinical manifestations of increasing ICP were discussed earlier in this chapter and include further depression of the level of consciousness, continuing through stupor, lethargy, coma, and possibly death from herniation.

Chapter 30

1. The rupture of an aneurysm with hemorrhage into the subarachnoid space produces severe pain. The complaint of "worst headache of my life" is a hallmark complaint of subarachnoid hemorrhage.

2. Motor and speech deficits in a right-handed person usually indicate a left side lesion; hemiparesis of both upper and lower extremities indicates that the middle cerebral artery probably is affected.

3. The patient showed several signs of decreased neurological function. She was agitated, indicating increased ICP. She also had a decrease in her speech function, indicating decreased blood flow to the left middle cerebral artery territory.

4. Resume triple H therapy: Increase IV fluids; raise blood pressure, including the use of vasopressors, if necessary, for the treatment of vasospasm. Hyponatremia is often seen in the presence of vasospasm and must be corrected. The addition of supplemental salt tablets and hypertonic saline should be administered judiciously to increase serum sodium to a normal level.

Chapter 31

1. Stroke, seizure, CSF leak, infection, and prevention of venous thrombotic events (rate is higher in cases >4 hours).

2. Motor status, for improvement of symptoms—tremor, rigidity, bradykinesia. Also complications from overstimulation of dopaminergic neurons: dyskinesia, dystonia, confusion, hallucination.

3. Depression, anxiety, body image.

4. Orthostatic blood pressures; history of nausea with administration; orders for antiemetic other than prochlorperazine; motor status and mental status.

Chapter 32

1. History of smoking, history of submersion, dyspnea, tachypnea, hypoxia on ABGs. Also, patient has a lower cervical spinal cord injury, which may affect the ability to use respiratory accessory muscles.

2. An order should be obtained for prophylactic anticoagulation therapy such as low-molecular-weight heparin. Antiembolic stockings and pneumatic compression devices should be worn by the patient. Mobilization of the patient should be instituted as soon as the patient is medically stable.

3. Ileus, stress ulcer, constipation, bowel incontinence.

4. Lack of social support, refusal to open eyes, poor interaction with staff, diagnosis of a complete cervical spinal cord injury.

5. Severe hypertension, bradycardia, patient complaint of pounding headache, blurred vision, skin flushing, piloerection, and nasal congestion. Sit the patient upright and place lower extremities in a dependent position. Find and eliminate the cause. Common causes include bladder distention, stool impaction, and pressure ulcer formation. If blood pressure remains elevated, an order for a quick-acting antihypertensive may be needed.

Chapter 34

1. The nurse is responsible for recognizing the frustration and concern that this may cause the patient. The nurse also is responsible for assisting the patient in finding ways to communicate. This may take several forms: having the patient use a chalk board to write on, pantomiming, using signs and symbols that the patient can point to, and assisting the patient in lip reading. If the tracheostomy still is in place, a speaking (flutter) valve may be used to assist the patient in speaking.

2. Maintaining an open airway is the first priority for the nurse and patient. The nurse should instruct the patient on keeping the airway open through suctioning and wound care. It is important to instruct the patient on how to keep the stoma clean and free of crusts. It also is important to reassure the patient that he or she can maintain an open airway and adequate oxygenation by following the instructions for keeping the stoma clean and free of crusts. Normal oxygenation is evidenced by normal oxygen saturation levels, lungs that are clear to auscultation, and unlabored breathing. The patient can be taught to assess these critical elements and take appropriate or emergency action if adequate oxygenation is not present.

It is helpful to remember that the patient has made a difficult decision in opting to have the total larynx removed. The nurse's attitude and approach to helping the patient speak should be one of caring and compassion.

3. The patient is dealing with a major change in self-image and, in all probability, a major change in lifestyle, including recreational activities, at least for the present. The nurse, through his or her attitude and approach to the patient, or demeanor, should convey understanding of the

patient's situation and feelings. For example, if the patient reacts with anger or by withdrawing, the nurse should recognize these symptoms as ones of depression and adjustment to the changes the patient is experiencing; they are not directed at the nurse or other health care providers.

If the patient and/or family members can express their feelings, it is helpful for the nurse to listen, to not pass judgment, and to offer resources that may be available to help the patient adjust. Specifically, relative to comportment, the nurse should assume an interested, unhurried approach to patient care, with the nurse's posture and demeanor communicating interest and concern.

Chapter 35

1. The nurse evaluates the spirometry values when available as a measure of lung function and continues to evaluate all lab values daily. Physical assessments with a focus on respiratory status are done twice a shift. The nurse obtains information related to the home environment, such as the presence of stairs or safety hazards and dust or environmental pollutants, average daily exercise and activities of daily living, support systems, family or significant others, the patient's understanding of the disease and treatments, use of oxygen and use and cleaning of oxygen equipment at home, and financial status and insurance. This information will be needed to individualize the discharge plan and identify teaching needs.

2. A barrel chest is one in which the anterior-posterior (A-P) diameter is twice that of the transverse diameter. The normal chest has an A-P diameter of half of the transverse diameter. This manifestation is caused by inflation of alveoli due to emphysema.

3. Solu-Medrol alleviates symptoms of inflammation and may relieve wheezing and chest tightness. Because it is a glucocorticoid, it raises serum blood sugar. It may also cause retention of sodium, with a lowering of potassium. It causes gastric irritation, so it should be taken with an antacid or food. It also depresses the immune response, so the patient is more prone to infections. In some patients it may cause mood swings.

4. Mr. H and his wife should be given plenty of written material to reinforce teaching content. Blood sugars should be checked at least twice a day with a glucometer. The patient and/or spouse should demonstrate this to the nurse before discharge. Usually, if the glucose reading is consistently above 200 g/dL, the health care provider should be notified. Because prednisone depresses the immune system, the patient should avoid crowds and/or individuals with infections. He should be observed using an inhaler and taught to rinse his mouth after using each medication to prevent thrush. If he experiences side effects such as "feeling hyper," palpitations, or a fast heart rate after using Atovent, he should call his health care provider. He should be taught to take his blood pressure and should be given the acceptable range. This should be 100/70 to 140/80. If he experiences dizziness, weakness, or headache, he should call his provider. In addition, the patient should describe reasons for taking an antibiotic and possible side effects, such as gastrointestinal disorders. A representative from the oxygen company should meet Mr. H in the hospital if possible for an introductory information session on his oxygen prescription and needed equipment and follow-up on teaching at home after discharge.

5. Mr. H should receive a balanced diet and high-protein, high-potassium foods. If he is retaining sodium, this will be restricted in the diet to 1 to 4 grams daily. He must adhere to his diabetic meal plan as well. He should drink 8 to 10 glasses of water daily. Dairy products should be used in moderation because they may interfere with mobilization of secretions. He should use his supplemental oxygen during meals because eating requires energy, and this will support his additional oxygen needs at mealtime. While at home, he should continue this routine. Prednisone and any potential exacerbation of his condition are likely to raise his glucose level, so his general physical condition, diet, exercise, fluid intake, and glucose levels should be continually monitored.

6. Use of continuous therapy can prevent the development of cor pulmonale and pulmonary hypertension. This increases the survival rate and general quality of life because the patient is able to lead a more normal, active life without the onset of these cardiopulmonary complications of COPD.

Chapter 36

1. a. Inability to maintain adequate oxygen levels for normal tissue perfusion.
   b. Increased risk of aspiration.
   c. Two other common complications of NPPV include facial trauma related to the tight-fitting mask and abdominal distention. Chart 36-19 outlines the contraindications for NPPV.

2. a. CPAP mask: Holds airways open in order to increase resistance and increase oxygenation.
   b. BiPAP mask: Has IPAO for inspiratory positive airway pressure and EPAP or expiratory airway pressure. Numerous full masks and nasal masks.
   c. Patients who are on NPPV can communicate and eat and require very little, if any, sedation.
   d. The benefit of NPPV is that Mr. A does not have an endotracheal tube in his throat and the further mortality and morbidity associated with intubation and ventilator-associated pneumonia (VAP) are absent.
   e. Patient comfort and prevention of skin breakdown are the indications for selection.

3. a. The nurse should be aware that the most serious potentially fatal complication of NPPV is aspiration. Therefore, the airway must have frequent assessments.
   b. Continuous heart rate, pulse oximetry (SpO_2), and specially trained nurses and respiratory therapists who are experienced with NPPV are essential for these patients.
   c. An NG tube might be considered to empty his stomach and decrease the risk of gastric distention and aspiration of gastric contents.

Chapter 39

1. Hypertension, non–insulin-dependent diabetes, hyperlipidemia, current smoker.
2. Urgent PCI in the setting of AMI is the treatment of choice in eligible patients who can be transported to an appropriate hospital in a timely manner.
3. To inhibit platelet activation resulting from the AMI.
4. Impending cardiogenic shock from the AMI.

Chapter 40

1. Because this patient had a drug-eluting stent placed, it is imperative to have adequate antiplatelet therapy to prevent subacute stent thrombosis, which will then cause a subsequent heart attack, as well as to prevent restenosis.
2. This patient had a STEMI, so it is crucial to follow his cardiac enzymes to know the extent of damage as well as to measure against possible reinfarction.
3. ReoPro will provide maximal protection against platelet activation and aggregation to prevent additional thrombus burden after stent placement. This drug is in the classification of GPIIB/IIIA inhibitors and blocks the final common pathway of the clotting cascade.
4. V_1–V_4.
5. Do a 12-lead ECG, apply oxygen, give nitroglycerin sublingual, and call the doctor. Anticipate changes on the ECG that would be similar to his initial ECG and reflect changes in leads V_1–V_4 representing his left anterior descending artery.

Chapter 41

1. To diagnose problems with heart structure and function in the presence of cardiomegaly in a young person. He has a questionable history of a heart murmur, and he reportedly uses cocaine and drinks alcohol, both of which have an adverse effect on the cardiac structure and function. He will most likely have four-chamber dilation.
2. The patient is complaining of clinical manifestations similar to those of a myocardial infarction; therefore, the enzyme tests are done to rule out a myocardial infarction.
3. To rule out coronary artery disease and any other possible reason for cardiomyopathy.
4. Cardiac dysrhythmias are also frequently associated with cardiomyopathy. Lasix is potassium depleting, thus further increasing the risk of cardiac dysrhythmias.
5. Stop cocaine or alcohol intake due to the increased risk of myocardial ischemia caused by these two substances. Diet and fluid intake changes, medication schedule, and activity restriction. Referral to Alcoholics Anonymous and Narcotics Anonymous; this patient needs to understand that if lifestyle changes do not occur, life expectancy is about 5 years.
6. Forward blood flow and improved pump function as a result of the ACE inhibitors, nitropaste, and Lasix therapy. Decreased preload and afterload will result in decreased cardiac workload and decreased stretch on the myocardial fibers.

Chapter 42

1. • Vital signs every 4 hours, including blood pressure, heart rate, oxygenation saturation, temperature.
   • Medications: simvastatin 20 mg po qhs, levothyroxine 0.125 mg po daily, glipizide 500 mg po bid, furosemide 80 mg po bid, potassium 40 mEq po bid, lisinopril 2.5 mg po daily.
   • Low sodium (<2,000 mg/day), fluid-restricted (<2 liters/day) diet.
   • Intake and output tracking.
   • Blood sugars ac and at bed time.
   • Daily A.M. weights.
2. To assess for an objective measure of fluid volume loss with weight changes in response to diuretic therapy.
3. Day 2 serum potassium.
4. Hypotension, worsened renal function, hyperkalemia.
5. Because the patient is fluid volume overloaded and therefore at risk of further congestion if initiated.

Chapter 43

1. Improved pain management, improved sleep and rest patterns, maintaining skin integrity, preventing injury/infection, improving control of blood sugar, preventing complications of immobility, and emotional and spiritual support.
2. Additional information that would be helpful would include an ankle-brachial index measurement, arterial duplex ultrasonography, and aortic angiogram with run-off.
3. Cigarette smoking is a significant risk factor for developing PAD. Avoiding all nicotine products is essential for the patient with PAD to decrease the risk of complications of vasospasm and poor healing.
4. Angiography of the aorta and lower extremities is performed to visualize anatomy and locate areas of stenosis and/or occlusion. It is an invasive procedure, requiring arterial access and contrast administration.
5. Preventing bleeding from the access site, monitoring for complications, maintaining hydration, providing pain management, accessing neurovascular status of the affected extremity, vital signs, and keeping the affected extremity straight for 4–6 hours.

Chapter 45

1. Aspirin inhibits prostaglandin E_2, which is part of the mucosal barrier that protects the gastric mucosa from the digestive actions of the gastric secretion.
2. Proton pump inhibitors effectively inhibit acid secretion and promote healing of the gastric ulcer.
3. Acute hemorrhage will decrease the hemoglobin, hematocrit, and RBCs and will cause an increase in the release of immature RBCs, as indicated by the increase in the reticulocyte count.

Chapter 46

1. Confusion, irritability, asterixis, and hyperactive reflexes.
2. Continuous damage and regeneration of liver tissue leads to fibrosis and scarring, which can affect liver function and cause structural changes in the liver so that blood and bile

flow is impeded/obstructed, leading to esophageal varices (blood flow) and jaundice (bile). Because the liver function is impaired, the serum albumin may be decreased, contributing to the formation of ascites. The liver converts ammonia to urea and when this function is impaired, ammonia levels increase, leading to neurological symptoms such as irritability, confusion, and asterixis.

3. Ammonia is a by-product of protein metabolism and the liver is unable to convert ammonia to urea, so the diet should provide less protein so that there is less ammonia.

4. Lactulose changes the acidity of the stool, which converts ammonia to ammonium ion, which is not absorbable. It also decreases the number of ammonia-forming bacteria.

Chapter 47

1. The patient was underresuscitated, causing decreased fluid volume. This reduced the perfusion to the kidneys, causing ischemic injury to the tubular epithelium and preventing normal concentration of urine, filtration of waste products, and regulation of acid–base balance, electrolyte hemostasis, and fluid balance.

2. Due to the impaired filtration, the nurse would expect to see elevated serum creatinine, blood urea nitrogen (BUN), potassium, and phosphate.

Chapter 49

1. Donning gloves and assessing the site where the blood is coming from. Observe the site for the amount of drainage, the suture line, and any disrupted sutures or signs of dehiscence. Take a full set of vital signs, including oxygen saturation and temperature, and notify the health care provider if medical intervention is needed. Apply pressure to the oozing incision site with sterile gauze until the oozing has stopped, and then apply a reinforcing dressing to the incision. Maintain very close observation.

   If the nurse chooses to remove the abdominal dressing as top priority, that is an error: The occlusive dressing is adding pressure to the oozing incision and should remain in place.

   If the nurse chooses to leave the patient's bedside, that is an error: Leaving the patient's bedside when vital signs are bordering on shock and she appears very tired, with a bleeding incision, would not be advised.

2. Asking for the health care provider to be notified using the patient call light is a correct action.

   Continue holding pressure on the dressing site.

   Ask another nurse to monitor vital signs and oxygen saturation.

   Apply oxygen to the patient who is hypotensive, tachycardic, or tachypneic.

   Put the head of the bed flat.

   Stay with the patient until the health care provider arrives.

3. **Indicates priorities.

   The incision has just been assessed, so the nurse can wait 30 minutes for the next assessment.

   **The patient has lost a reasonable amount of blood and needs the increased fluids from the IV.

**Oxygen should be applied because the oxygen-carrying capacity has been decreased secondary to drop in hemoglobin and hematocrit.

**The patient is in pain, 7/10, and needs analgesics.

The Unasyn will need to be prepared, so there is leeway before having to give it.

Vital signs are ordered every 4 hours and were done just prior to the retention sutures being inserted.

**CBC is essential due to blood loss.

Calling laboratory results to the health care provider will occur when results received.

**Educating the patient on safety is an important consideration to prevent injury.

**Changing the linens is important because the patient has blood on her sheets, which is unsightly, can increase emotional discomfort, and can cause skin breakdown from the wetness against the patient.

The increased IV rate will take care of fluids temporarily, and the diet change can be implemented at the next meal.

Chapter 50

1. Pain.

2. If the catheter is occluded in any way, the patient will experience increased pain.

3. There is no significance as to the drainage itself because urine often seeps around a suprapubic catheter. There is significance in respect to potential damage to skin tissues from a wet dressing.

4. Low hemoglobin provides decreased oxygen to the patient for healing and it decreases the patient's overall energy level, which can decrease the patient's desire to ambulate and to eat. Oxygen, nutrition, and ambulation contribute to the patient's healing and recovery. The diabetes can alter wound healing, and glucose levels should be kept in good control to increase the ability of the body to heal. Nurses should also track hemoglobin trends to detect internal bleeding. This hemoglobin level is trending downward, and the cause of it needs to be sought.

5. It is not unusual to see a low-grade fever within 24 hours of a significant surgical event. The fever is the body's response to trauma. If the temperature is above 100.4°F or is elevated after 24 hours, it is more indicative of an infection.

Chapter 52

1. Prevailing symptoms include weight gain, constant fatigue, cold intolerance, dry skin, thinning hair, and difficulty concentrating. The patient also expresses that she does not feel as alert as usual and is experiencing a decline in work performance and task completion. These symptoms are indicative of low thyroxine levels and circulating hormone levels and hypothyroidism.

2. A high level of TSH is caused by the pituitary responding to an underproduction of thyroid hormone that, in turn, results in lower thyroxine (T_4). Measurement of the T_4 serum level reflects the amount of unbound thyroxine in the blood and is considered the best clinical measure of thyroxine levels. Low levels of T_4 in the presence of high

levels of TSH indicate that the problem is due to disease of the thyroid gland.

3. The main focus of the plan of care should be symptom management. This includes the following key elements:
   - Instruction in hormone replacement therapy. It is important to understand the prescribed medication and to take it precisely according to directions in order to return the patient to a euthyroid or normal thyroid state.
   - Assessment of fatigue and activity tolerance to determine ability to provide self-care.
   - Assessment of skin, nails, and hair condition because patient is at risk for impaired skin integrity and alopecia.
   - Assessment of bowel function because patient is at risk for constipation and abdominal pain due to the reduced activity (lethargy) and hypometabolic state.
   - Assessment of body temperature and ability to tolerate ambient temperatures. Patient may be prone to hypothermia due to hypometabolic state.
   - Assessment of cognition and thought processes because patient may experience disturbed thought processes due to hypothyroidism. Is patient oriented to time, place, person, and circumstances?

Chapter 53

1. The major biochemical deficits include (1) hyperglycemia, (2) metabolic acidosis, and (3) fluid and (4) electrolyte imbalance.

2. Polyuria, polydipsia, weight loss, and fatigue primarily result from hyperglycemia. The poor skin turgor, dry mucous membranes, and sinus tachycardia primarily result from the fluid imbalance (dehydration). The increasing lethargy, facial flushing, deep rapid breathing, and fruity odor of breath result from the metabolic acidosis (ketosis). The nausea and vomiting are thought to result from the metabolic acidosis (ketosis). The patient's sodium is low and his potassium is high; however, he appears to have no symptoms related to hyponatremia or hyperkalemia.

3. The nursing interventions derived from these treatments include (1) general assessment of patient's response to therapy, (2) evaluation of the patient's response to insulin therapy (e.g., monitoring for changes in blood glucose level; monitoring for signs and symptoms of hypoglycemia; monitoring for correction of metabolic acidosis [ketosis]), (3) evaluating patient's response to fluid replacement, and (4) evaluating the patient's response to electrolyte replacement therapy.

4. Severe DKA is a medical emergency. In terms of clinical signs and symptoms, the most significant difference is that the patient with severe DKA is more likely to present in an obtunded or comatose state. In terms of laboratory values, the most significant differences in the laboratory values between mild and severe DKA are related to the degree of metabolic acidosis: arterial pH < 7.0; serum bicarbonate < 10; anion gap > 12. Although the basic fluid and electrolyte treatments would be the same, the patient may present with more pronounced fluid and electrolyte imbalances (e.g., hyperkalemia, hyperosmolality). The fluid and electrolyte imbalances may reflect renal insufficiency

and/or renal failure. As such, the fluid and electrolyte treatment of severe DKA may become highly individualized.

5. The general discharge plan for this patient includes (1) general teaching about the pathophysiology of type 1 diabetes; (2) basic dietary instruction; (3) instruction on insulin injection techniques; (4) instruction on signs and symptoms of hypoglycemia; (5) instruction on blood glucose monitoring—patients should be provided with a meter or provisions should be made to purchase a blood glucose monitor at discharge; and (6) follow-up appointment with health care provider—patient should be given phone number of person to contact for questions prior to appointment.

Chapter 55

1. Other questions may include these: (1) Is there a history of past fractures? (2) How did her accident occur? (3) What type of activities does she participate in at home? (4) Has she had a bone density study? (5) Has she ever taken hormones?

2. This patient is an older adult, which would lead to suspicion of osteoporosis. This patient's risk factors include the following: (1) age, (2) postmenopausal, and (3) family history of fractures. These risk factors would warrant further investigation.

3. Alkaline phosphate is found in the bone, liver, vascular endothelium, lung, kidney, and intestinal mucosa. Increased levels may be a warning sign and indicate the need for further investigation. An elevated alkaline phosphate can be observed when the body attempts to form new bone (i.e., metastatic cancer) (Corbett, 2004).

4. Serum calcium and phosphate.

5. The goal is to restore function and independence. In the acute phase, the goal of medical management would be to align and stabilize the hip fracture. This is achieved through surgical intervention. Older patients are at a greater risk for postop complications (i.e., infection, pulmonary complications, and thrombophlebitis). Following surgery, medical management would direct treatment in the prevention of postop complications and restoring function.

6. Nursing diagnoses:
   a. *Pain* related to edema and inflammatory response.
   b. *Risk for Impaired Skin Integrity* related to immobility.
   c. *Risk for Infection* related to invasive procedure.
   d. *Deficient Knowledge* related to unfamiliarity with surgical procedure.

7. In the postoperative phase it will be important for the nurse to know the patient's past medical–surgical history. It will be important for the patient to understand that her past medical–surgical history may help the team anticipate and prevent problems. Postoperative teaching should focus on reviewing strategies for preventing postop complications. She should be instructed regarding pain medication and the importance of progressively increasing her activity. Physical therapy is critical to her recovery, so reviewing some of the expectations might be helpful. The patient will need to understand that the Foley catheter may remain in her bladder until she is able to ambulate to the bathroom.

Other topics might include the use of TED, sequential decompression devices, incentive spirometry, and an abduction pillow.

Chapter 56

1. Postoperative complications can include hypovolemic shock, compartment syndrome, and rhabdomyolysis. The nurse should complete a neurovascular exam of the injured extremity that consists of assessing the color, temperature, capillary refill, pulses, edema, sensory and motor function, and pain level.
2. The right leg should be elevated and supported in correct anatomic position.

Chapter 57

1. Compartment syndrome pain is not relieved by narcotic pain medication, and the affected part is swollen and tense. Normal postoperative incisional pain is located only in the surgical site and is relieved by administration of pain medication.
2. Immediately upon admission to the nursing unit, the nurse should assess the patient for airway patency, breathing effectiveness, and evidence of bleeding at the surgical site and perform a neurovascular assessment of structures distal to the surgical site.
3. The type of surgical approach impacts the type of precautions necessary after hip replacement surgery. In the posterior approach, body positions that cause backward action or actions that cause the hip joint to swivel inward will stress the prosthesis and increase the potential for dislocation. Posterior hip precautions include not bending forward greater than 90 degrees and not moving the operative leg across the body midline. Anterior hip precautions include not moving the hip backward and not turning the leg and foot outward.
4. Postoperative pulmonary complications are prevented by early ambulation and use of pulmonary exercises such as coughing and deep breathing and use of incentive spirometry every 2 hours while awake.
5. The nurse must determine whether the patient is exhibiting confusion related to hypoxia, pain, infection, or hypotension or as an adverse effect of medications. The nurse should assess the patient's respiratory status, vital signs, and oxygen saturation. If these are within normal parameters, the nurse should determine whether the patient is in pain and medicate the patient if indicated. Medications can contribute to delirium, and the nurse should assess the medications ordered for the postoperative elderly person for their potential to contribute to confusion.

Chapter 58

1. Weight and pain in the toe.
2. Food with increased purines. Foods that should be avoided are organ meats, meat extracts, anchovies, sardines, herring, mackerel, scallops, game meats, and gravy. Patients should consume a moderate amount of protein and limit meat, fish, and poultry to 4 to 6 ounces per day. Diet should include low-fat dairy products, tofu, and eggs. Alcohol consumption should be limited to one drink three times a week, although beer ingestion should be completely discontinued because it has a high purine count and increases gout risks regardless of amount.
3. Excruciating pain in his right great toe. Stress. Weight.
4. With gouty arthritis, there is an imbalance with purine metabolism. Instead of the uric acid crystals being excreted through the kidneys, they accumulate in the joints. These crystals are needle-like, causing excruciating pain, usually in the joints of the elbows, wrists, fingers, knees, ankles, and toes, with 75% of patients affected in the great toe.

Chapter 60

1. Mr. B is relatively young and has symptoms consistent with significant immune insufficiency evidenced by oral and esophageal candidiasis. Mr. B also has HIV risk factors: history of sexually transmitted infection, indicating unprotected sex, multiple partners, and IV drug use. He currently uses alcohol and tobacco, which are gateway drugs for other forms of illegal substance abuse.
2. HIV testing is often very frightening and overwhelming to a patient. Therapeutic communication includes expressing feelings of caring, empathy, and understanding that HIV testing is frightening because the potential diagnosis is very serious. This should be balanced with calm and direct provision of information on the process of testing. Testing information should include information on consent for testing, confidentiality of test results, process of drawing blood and confirming any positive test with a second blood test, importance of testing to enable diagnosis, and appropriate treatment and the availability of antiretroviral medications that can help control the progression of HIV if the test is positive.
3. The CD4 receptor is the small protein found on T-helper cells and other cells that allows the HIV virus into the cell. Because the receptor was first isolated on T-helper cells and is found there in abundance, T-helper cells are also called CD4. HIV infection results in a progressive decline in the number of CD4 T-helper cells. The role of these CD4 cells in the immune response is critical because they initiate and regulate the process of stimulating other cells to initiate the immune response and attack an invading antigen such as virus or bacteria. They also stimulate B cells to make antibodies. Additionally, T-helper 1 cells (CD4) are responsible for the initiation of a response to a tumor or mutant cells. Therefore, when CD4 cells decline with HIV infection, the patient is at great risk of developing opportunistic infections and some cancers, such as lymphoma.
4. Yes, a CD4 count < 200/mL is a category C3 AIDS defining CD4 count according to CDC Guidelines described in Chapter 59, Chart 59–10.
5. Triple antiretroviral therapy, possibly including zidovudine + lamivudine (Combivir) and indinavir (Crixivan). Triple therapy interferes with HIV replication at different points in the replication process, thus more effectively controlling HIV replication and decreasing viral load levels. Additionally, triple therapy has a lower incidence of viral resistance than monotherapy.

Chapter 61

1. David should be assessed for hyperthermia from infection, seizure activity that may result from meningeal irritation, hypotension and hypoxia, and the development of hypotension that will lead to an altered mental status because of altered circulation. This hypotension can result from the sepsis and the body's inflammatory response.
2. Meningitis can be transmitted from droplet contamination from respiratory exposure. Respiratory isolation should be instituted. The nurse and anyone who has contact with David should wash their hands before and after leaving his room. Chemoprophylaxis may be recommended for any close contacts that David may have had. The local health department and college campus should be notified about David's infection in order to ensure that appropriate precautions are taken to prevent further spread of the disease. Some health care providers recommend a prophylactic vaccination of all college students.
3. Toxins from the bacteria causing David's meningitis will cause vasodilation and hypotension. Levophed has been found to be very beneficial in the early management of sepsis to maintain an adequate blood pressure and end-organ perfusion.

Chapter 63

1. Anemia and thrombocytopenia.
2. The low level of reticulocytes shows that erythropoiesis has not accelerated.
3. Petechiae, conjunctival hemorrhage, GI bleeding, positive guaiac.
4. Shortness of breath, pallor, activity intolerance.
5. Bleeding precautions, ambulation with assistance, reinforcement of patient education to prevent additional injury and falls.

Chapter 64

1. Infection, nutritional status, pain, and coping.
2. Calculate the ANC: 1,050.
3. Perform hand hygiene, assess invasive devices for redness and drainage, assess urine for sign of infection, assess for worsening respiratory status, instruct visitors to avoid contact with patient if they are ill, provide private room.
4. Listen attentively, demonstrate compassion and caring, offer resources as needed, collaborate with health care provider to determine further medical interventions.

Chapter 66

1. Hypotension, decreased level of consciousness, increased wound size, fever, renal failure.
2. Spread through breaks in the skin and contaminated hands. Contact isolation, strict aseptic technique.
3. There will be some scarring, but the goal is to return the leg to normal function, and the extent of the injury is still being determined.

Chapter 68

1. Grief, circulation, gas exchange.
2. Increase circulation distal to the burn injury. Loss of circulation and possible loss of limb.

3. Delays wound healing.
4. Fluid resuscitation will decrease these values.

Chapter 70

1. The nurse can contact environmental services/housekeeping to obtain a device that can be attached to the patient's bed to control the volume on the television. The nurse can instruct Mrs. M to place this device close to her best hearing ear so as to hear the television and not disturb the roommate.
2. Mrs. M most likely is experiencing hearing loss from the ototoxic medication streptomycin, which she took in 1955 for tuberculosis treatment. In addition, she was given the diagnosis of presbycusis. The first course of treatment for her hearing disturbance would be a hearing aid.
3. A hearing aid would be the first step to correcting Mrs. M's hearing disturbance. Because she also has some degree of nerve damage, a cochlear implant might be suggested if the hearing aid proves to be nonbeneficial to restoring her hearing.
4. Four specific discharge instructions for the family with regard to Mrs. M's hearing disorder include:
   a. Face Mrs. M when speaking.
   b. Do not shout.
   c. Drop the pitch of the voice.
   d. Speak slowly and enunciate, avoid slurring, avoid speaking rapidly.

Chapter 71

1. Vitreous hemorrhage, proliferative diabetic retinopathy, diabetic retinopathy with macula edema, retinal detachment.
2. Cholesterol, BUN, perfusion time.
3. Blood sugar under control, blood pressure under control, laser photocoagulation, vitrectomy.
4. Insulin dependent, blood sugar control, weight control, blood pressure control, regular eye examination referrals, and regular exercise.
5. Regular dilated eye examinations once a year if there are no vision problems and more often if there are problems, blood sugar and blood pressure controls, diet, exercise, and staying healthy.

Chapter 74

1. To identify and intervene with life-threatening injuries.
2. Patterns of injury that are anticipated are as follows:
   - Cervical spine fracture
   - Traumatic brain injury
   - Anterior flail chest
   - Myocardial contusion
   - Pneumothorax
   - Traumatic aortic disruption
   - Fractured spleen or liver
   - Posterior fracture/dislocation of the hip, knee, and/or ankle.
3. No, the CT will reveal solid organ injury but may not identify bowel injury.
4. Decreased core temperature with an inflammatory response leads to increased coagulopathy.

End-of-Chapter NCLEX-Style Review Questions

Chapter 1

1. Answer: 1. Health promotion and maintenance

   Rationale: Health promotion and maintenance are emphasized in nursing education. Advocacy is a characteristic of the role in which the nurse acts on behalf of patients in order to protect their rights and assist in obtaining information and services. Complementary therapies are strategies used in conjunction with traditional treatment. Physiological adaptation is the management and provision of care to patients with acute, chronic, or life-threatening physical health conditions.

   Congnitive Level: Analysis

   Nursing process: Implementing

   Client needs: Health Promotion and Maintenance

2. Answer: 2. Psychological and spiritual

   Rationale: Adding the aspects of caring enables nursing to meet psychological and spiritual needs. Without caring, nursing is a scientific and technical profession. The physiological needs will be met without the aspects of caring through the utilization of the technical body of knowledge. Ethical and moral needs are personal values.

   Cognitive level: Application

   Nursing process: Assessment

   Client needs: Psychosocial Integrity

3. Answer: 4. Total patient care nursing

   Rationale: Total patient care refers to a delivery model in which the nurse assumes total responsibility for meeting the needs of assigned patients during their time on duty. Functional nursing is an adaptation of the industrial model and is work assignment based on functions and tasks to be completed within a specific time frame. Modular nursing is the utilization of mini teams who stay near the bedside; it involves assigning a wider range of responsibilities. Primary care nursing has a professional nurse assigned to plan and coordinate care from admission to discharge.

   Cognitive level: Application

   Nursing process: Implementation

   Client needs: Safe, Effective Care Environment

4. Answer: 3. Variety of patient diagnoses and complexities of patient care

   Rationale: A variety of patient diagnoses and complexities of patient care require that the staff nurse incorporate organization and coordination into the practice role. The need to support the achievement of practice standards is a nursing administration level responsibility. Patient advocacy would require coordination but not necessarily organization as an inherent role. The nurse manager has 24-hour accountability for the unit.

   Cognitive level: Application

   Nursing process: Implementation

   Client needs: Safe, Effective Care Environment

5. Answer: 1. Cultural encounters

   Rationale: Cultural encounters are the fourth component of Campinha-Bacote's model. Cultural study is a process that would increase cultural knowledge. Cultural diversity refers to the variations among groups of people with respect to habits, values, preferences, beliefs, taboos, behaviors, and social interaction. Culture refers to a complex of learned patterns of behavior, beliefs, and values that can be attributed to a particular group of people.

   Cognitive level: Application

   Nursing process: Evaluation

   Client needs: Psychosocial Integrity

Chapter 2

1. Answer: 2. Advanced beginner

   Rationale: The novice stage begins in the first year of education to become a nurse. The advanced beginner is a new graduate. There is a level of trust in the environment and legitimacy of coworkers' knowledge. There is freedom with learning, mainly because of no responsibility for situations with which they have no experience. Competency is evidenced by exhilaration with good personal performance as opposed to remorse when performance could have been more precise or effective. Proficiency is evidenced by a change in the perspective of a situation or being able to read and respond to a patient's needs. This nurse was functioning at the level of advanced beginner.

   Cognitive level: Analysis

   Nursing process: Evaluation

   Client needs: Physiological Integrity: Physiological Adaptation

2. Answer: 4. The patient's hemoglobin and hematocrit levels are low.

   Rationale: There is a difference between practical knowledge and theoretical knowledge. With practical knowledge, practice is shaped by one's knowledge of the discipline, the science and technology relevant to the situation at hand. Theoretical knowledge is scientific, formal knowledge that is needed prior to the development of practical knowledge. This patient's hemoglobin and hematocrit levels were low, which could mean bleeding. A reduction in hemoglobin means a lesser amount of oxygen will reach the body organs. This patient's condition is changing, even though the vital signs are not yet reflecting the change.

   Cognitive level: Analysis

   Nursing process: Implementation

   Client needs: Physiological Integrity: Physiological Adaptation

3. Answer: 2. Return the patient to the bed.

   Rationale: Clinical knowledge is knowledge necessary to perform proficiently in the clinical setting. Clinical judgment is clinical reasoning, across time, about a particular patient. Techne is something that can be standardized and replicated. Even though the care map states a day 2 total knee replacement patient should be transferred from the bed to a chair with minimal weight bearing, the sudden onset of bright red bleeding would indicate that this patient be immediately returned to bed and be prepared for further intervention. The care map, or standardized care, should not be followed in the best interest of the patient.

Cognitive level: Application

Nursing process: Implementation

Client needs: Physiological Integrity: Physiological Adaptation

4. Answer: 2. Repeat the questions to evaluate the patient's hearing.

Rationale: Phronesis is a form of rationality and skill-based character. It is similar to clinical judgment, which is clinical reasoning across time about a patient. The nurse should determine if the patient understands the health-related questions before assuming the patient is in acute distress or has a worsening condition.

Cognitive level: Analysis

Nursing process: Implementation

Client needs: Physiological Integrity: Reduction of Risk Potential

5. Answer: 3. Further explore the patient's breathlessness.

Rationale: To make good clinical judgments, the nurse must be skillful in moral and clinical perception. Even though conceptual knowledge is needed, it is not sufficient to ensure the nurse will notice and correctly identify a change in a patient's condition even though the nurse may know conceptually what the formal characteristic of the patient condition is in principle. The most important thing for the nurse to do to help this patient is to further explore the patient's breathlessness. Culturing the leg wounds and elevating the legs could theoretically wait until a later time. The patient should not be ambulated to the bathroom but rather should be provided with a bedpan.

Cognitive level: Analysis

Nursing process: Evaluation

Client needs: Physiological Integrity: Physiological Adaptation

Chapter 3

1. Answer: 2. It is a proven process that produces consistent, high-quality results.

Rationale: Best practices are defined as proven processes that produce consistent, high-quality results. Evidence-based practice can be described as an approach that integrates current research evidence with clinical expertise and patient's needs. Benchmarking offers qualitative or quantitative measurement of specific data related to reported outcome information. The Leapfrog Group focuses on collecting data about medical errors and setting standards that will reduce errors.

Cognitive level: Analysis

Nursing process: Planning

Client needs: Safe, Effective Care Environment: Management of Care

2. Answer: 4. Volume

Rationale: Volume for hospitals overall is based on units of services. The overall hospital generally looks at patient days, and departments look at relative statistics for the type of work they do. Volume is a component of the revenue category. Salaries/wages is a component of controllable operating expenses. Supplies is a component of operating expenses. Overhead is considered an operating expense.

Cognitive level: Application

Nursing process: Planning

Client needs: Safe, Effective Care Environment: Management of Care

3. Answer: 2. Select supplies that can be used over a period of time for less cost.

Rationale: It is important for nurses to take an active role in containing costs through judicial use of supplies. The nurse should select supplies that can be used over a period of time for less cost. Using supplies already charged to another patient is unethical and can lead to contamination issues. Selecting too many supplies or stocking supplies in a patient's room for future use is not a judicial use of supplies.

Cognitive level: Application

Nursing process: Planning

Client needs: Safe, Effective Care Environment: Management of Care

4. Answer: 2. The Joint Commission

Rationale: The Joint Commission conducts accreditation surveys every 3 years. Beginning in 2004 the "tracer" methodology process was implemented that monitors a specific patient through his or her hospitalization and evaluates policies along with the patient's interactions and experience with all services. Effective in 2005, the Commission started making unannounced survey visits. The Occupational Safety and Health Administration (OSHA) is an agency that oversees environmental safety and works through federal and state partnerships to inspect and enforce safety standards in the workplace. The Centers for Disease Control and Prevention (CDC) is an agency that focuses on protecting the health and safety of people within and outside of a health care environment by development and application of disease prevention and control, promotion of environmental health, and education. The state board of nursing is an agency that oversees the practice of professionally licensed care providers by setting specific requirements for initial licensure, ongoing or continuing education hours and courses, the scope of practice for the particular discipline, and the disciplinary action processes.

Cognitive level: Application

Nursing process: Evaluation

Client needs: Safe, Effective Care Environment: Safety and Infection Control

5. Answer: 3. Health care power of attorney

Rationale: A health care power of attorney is a legal document that establishes a surrogate decision maker to make medical treatment decisions for an individual should that individual become incapacitated. A living will is a formal written document that communicates the wishes of the individual about life-sustaining medical treatments should he become terminally ill. An advance directive is instructions about future health care if the patient cannot speak for herself. An oral advance directive includes instructions given to a health care provider during the course of treatment, illness, or stay in the hospital. This directive is documented in the patient's medical record. A written advance directive is a witnessed document, which requires the individual's signature and those of the witnesses.

Cognitive level: Application

Nursing process: Evaluation

Client needs: Safe, Effective Care Environment: Management of Care

Chapter 4

1. Answer: 2. Principlism

   Rationale: Principlism is an emerging theory that incorporates existing ethical principles and attempts to resolve conflicts by applying one or more of the ethical principles. Four principles form the basis for decision making: respect for autonomy, nonmaleficence, beneficence, and justice. In deontology, a sense of duty consists of rational respect for the fulfilling of one's obligations to other human beings, rather than looking at the rewards of one's actions. Rule utilitarianism seeks the greatest happiness for all; it appeals to public agreement as a basis for objective judgment about the nature of happiness. Act utilitarianism tries to determine in a particular situation which course of action will bring about the greatest happiness, or the least harm and suffering, to a single person.

   Cognitive level: Analysis

   Nursing process: Evaluation

   Client needs: Safe, Effective Care Environment: Management of Care

2. Answer: 3. Options

   Rationale: The M stands for massage or identify the issues and all of the people involved. The O stands for examining options. The R stands for resolving the dilemma. The A stands for act by applying the chosen option. And the L stands for look back and evaluate the success of achieving desired outcomes.

   Cognitive level: Application

   Nursing process: Planning

   Client needs: Safe, Effective Care Environment: Management of Care

3. Answer: 2. Social justice model

   Rationale: The social justice model considers broad social issues that may arise within an institution and within this model; many ethics committees hold ethical grand rounds. The autonomy model facilitates decision making for the competent patient. The patient benefit model uses substituted judgment and facilitates decision making for the incompetent patient. Fidelity model does not exist.

   Cognitive level: Application

   Nursing process: Planning

   Client needs: Safe, Effective Care Environment: Management of Care

4. Answer: 1. Read the state nurse practice act.

   Rationale: The state nurse practice act sets educational and examination requirements, provides for licensing by individuals who have met these requirements, defines the functions of each category of nurse, and may include a section on mandatory continuing education hours for renewal of licenses. Reading the organization's standards of patient care and contacting the school in which she earned her nursing education would not be appropriate for the nurse to do. Assuming she can provide all aspects of care is also something this nurse should not do.

   Cognitive level: Analysis

   Nursing process: Assessment

   Client needs: Safe, Effective Care Environment: Management of Care

5. Answer: 4. Tort

   Rationale: Tort law is defined as a wrongful act committed against another person or the person's property. Common law is based on justice, reason, and common sense. It represents law made by judges through decisions in specific cases; these case-by-case decisions are used again and again in similar cases and, thereby, become customary or common to all people living under the authority of the court of law. Civil law starts with abstract rules, which judges must then apply to the various cases before them. Contracts are promises that the law will enforce. Contract law is that which governs the formation of these promises or agreements between two or more parties, in relation to a particular subject.

   Cognitive level: Application

   Nursing process: Planning

   Client needs: Safe, Effective Care Environment: Management of Care

Chapter 5

1. Answer: 1. Case method

   Rationale: The case method of nursing care is one in which the registered nurse is responsible for the patient and has total care responsibility for the patient during the shift worked. Functional nursing is task oriented and nurses perform assigned tasks but are not given a patient assignment. In team nursing, patients are assigned to a team that is led by a registered nurse. In primary nursing, each patient is assigned to a nurse who has 24-hour responsibility for the nursing care provided to a particular patient.

   Cognitive level: Analysis

   Nursing process: Assessment

   Client needs: Safe, Effective Care Environment: Management of Care

2. Answer: 4. Intentional fragmentation of care

   Rationale: The functional nursing model of care is an industrial efficiency model that intentionally fragments care because of the increased number of personnel performing specific tasks for individual patients. Holistic and comprehensive care are characteristics of the case method of care delivery. Maximum use of individual caregivers' strengths for a large number of patients is a characteristic of the team nursing care delivery system. Better care outcomes and greater nurse satisfaction are characteristics of the primary nursing care delivery system.

Cognitive level: Analysis

Nursing process: Assessment

Client needs: Safe, Effective Care Environment: Management of Care

3. Answer: 2. Team

Rationale: Responsibility for the delegation of tasks within team nursing is the same as in the functional nursing care delivery system. In the case method care delivery system, the entire caregiving staff consists of registered nurses. Unlicensed assistive personnel are not used. Within primary nursing, other caregivers are considered associate caregivers and the primary nurse is responsible for delegating responsibilities to these caregivers. Primary care is relationship-based care and is a blend of primary nursing with a professional nursing practice environment.

Cognitive level: Application

Nursing process: Implementation

Client needs: Safe, Effective Care Environment: Management of Care

4. Answer: 1. Highest quality for lowest cost

Rationale: The cost-effective measurement of nursing care delivery systems is difficult to achieve. Identifying the best care for the lowest cost may be deemed a cost-effective choice. The characteristics of job autonomy and nurse accountability are measurements of nurse job satisfaction. Patient acuity is the measurement of patient severity of illness and the amount of nursing care required to care for the patient.

Cognitive level: Analysis

Nursing process: Evaluation

Client needs: Safe, Effective Care Environment: Management of Care

5. Answer: 2. Functional

Rationale: Organizations that follow a functional approach to patient care avoid high labor costs by using lower paid workers and will not change the system to improve coordination and increase costs by adding advanced practice nurses or case managers. In the case method of care delivery, advanced practice nurses and case managers aid in the coordination of care. Advanced practice nurses and case managers are used as consultants within the team nursing care delivery system. Advanced practice nurses are used in the primary nursing care delivery system to add clinical expertise and education; however, the use of case managers is redundant in this model of care delivery.

Cognitive level: Application

Nursing process: Planning

Client needs: Safe, Effective Care Environment: Management of Care

Chapter 6

1. Answer: 3. The Joint Commission

Rationale: Each year the Joint Commission publishes patient safety goals that need to be addressed by health care facilities to improve patient care. They are listed on the Joint Commission website for the current and subsequent years. Medicare and Medicaid do not publish annual patient safety goals but expect organizations to comply with the Joint Commission's goals and standards. State boards of nursing control the practice of nursing by development of state nursing practice acts that establish guidelines to ensure safe practice. The standards set by the practice acts are based on the nursing process, which is a systematic method of planning and providing care to the patient, and requires compliance as evidenced in documentation.

Cognitive level: Analysis

Nursing process: Planning

Client needs: Safe, Effective Care Environment: Management of Care

2. Answer: 2. Draw a single line through the entry, write the word *error,* date, time, and sign the entry.

Rationale: When a documentation error occurs, correct it immediately by drawing a single line through the entry, identify it as an error with the date and time, and sign it. Never try to obliterate the error with ink or correction fluid because this can appear as if the documenter is trying to hide something.

Cognitive level: Application

Nursing process: Implementation

Client needs: Safe, Effective Care Environment: Management of Care

3. Answer: 4. There is a tendency to document everything.

Rationale: A disadvantage to narrative documentation is the tendency to chart everything that happens. The disadvantage of the CBE system is the time it takes to develop the guidelines and standards of care. Listing problems in chronological order is a disadvantage to the problem-oriented system. Having to evaluate each problem once per shift is a disadvantage of the PIE system.

Cognitive level: Application

Nursing process: Implementation

Client needs: Safe, Effective Care Environment: Management of Care

4. Answer: 2. Concept Map

Rationale: The concept map assists the learner in the development of the nursing plan of care using the nursing process. The Kardex contains information regarding the patient's name, age, religion, medical diagnoses, past medical history, surgeries and major procedures since admission, current medications, treatments, diet, intravenous therapy, and diagnostic tests and procedures. The medication administration record includes the usual dose, route, frequency, class, and action of the drug, rationale for administration, side effects with nursing implications, and assessment data that indicate effectiveness. The past medical history is data found within the Kardex.

Cognitive level: Analysis

Nursing process: Planning

Client needs: Safe, Effective Care Environment: Management of Care

Chapter 7

1. Answer: 1. Assessing the wound
   Rationale: Independent activities are those that nurses perform, prescribe, and or delegate based on their education and skills. Examples are assessing, analyzing and diagnosing, planning, implementing, and evaluating. Interdependent activities are those activities that overlap with other health team members, physicians, social workers, pharmacist, nutritionist, and therapists (physical, speech, occupational) and require coordination and planning with these various health team members. Dependent activities are those that are prescribed by the physician and carried out by the nurse. They include implementing the physician's orders to administer medications or treatments.
   Cognitive level: Analysis
   Nursing process: Evaluation
   Client needs: Safe, Effective Care Environment: Management of Care

2. Answer: 1. Assessment
   Rationale: A definition of assessment as it relates to nursing is "the act of reviewing a situation for the purpose of diagnosing the patient's problems." Planning is done after the formulation of nursing diagnoses and is prioritized according to the patient's needs. Implementation is the "doing" or intervening phase of the nursing process. It involves organization and actual delivery of nursing care, which leads to achievement of stated goals and objectives. Evaluation focuses on the patient's behavioral changes and compares them with the criteria stated in the objectives. It consists of both the patient's status and the effectiveness of the nursing care.
   Cognitive level: Application
   Nursing process: Implementation
   Client needs: Health Promotion and Maintenance: Prevention/Early Detection of Health Problems

3. Answer: 3. Psychomotor
   Rationale: To conduct a comprehensive nursing assessment, the nurse must utilize cognitive, affective, and psychomotor skills. Conducting a fingerstick to assess a blood glucose level is utilizing the psychomotor skill. There is no psychosocial skill level utilized to conduct a comprehensive nursing assessment.
   Cognitive level: Analysis
   Nursing process: Implementation
   Client needs: Health Promotion and Maintenance: Prevention/Early Detection of Health Problems

4. Answer: 4. Determining a nursing diagnosis
   Rationale: Goal setting is done during the planning phase of the nursing process. Planning of interventions is done during the planning phase of the nursing process. Nursing diagnoses are clinical judgments about an individual, family, or community response to actual or potential health problems and life processes. Nursing diagnoses are different from collaborative problems such as medical diagnoses because nurses' accountability differs for nursing diagnoses and collaborative problems. Nurses ultimately are accountable

for formulating nursing diagnoses and intervening appropriately.
   Cognitive level: Application
   Nursing process: Evaluation
   Client needs: Health Promotion and Maintenance: Prevention/Early Detection of Health Problems

5. Answer: 2. Planning
   Rationale: The use of critical thinking with the nursing process enhances the validity, reliability, and effectiveness of outcomes to patients. It is essential in nursing when the nurse is assessing, diagnosing, implementing, and evaluating the patient and developing the care plan. Getting a better understanding of something or someone else is part of the assessment phase of the nursing process. Reducing the risk of getting undesirable results is part of the implementation phase of the nursing process. Increasing the likelihood of achieving beneficial results is part of the evaluation phase of the nursing process. Making decisions about an action is part of the planning phase of the nursing process.
   Cognitive level: Analysis
   Nursing process: Evaluation
   Client needs: Health Promotion and Maintenance: Prevention/Early Detection of Health Problems

Chapter 8

1. Answer: 3. The effectiveness of a type of wound dressing
   Rationale: Basic research is done to extend the knowledge base in a discipline or to formulate or refine a theory. This would include studying how Orem's theory can be applied to the nursing process. Applied research focuses on finding solutions to existing problems such as wound dressings, side effects of medications, or outcomes of teaching.
   Cognitive level: Analysis
   Nursing process: Planning
   Client needs: Safe, Effective Care Environment: Management of Care

2. Answer: 3. Collect numerical values within a controlled situation.
   Rationale: Quantitative research is characterized by the collection of numerical values, under a controlled situation, that yield data, which can be generalized. Qualitative research describes events as they occur naturally. It is a systematic, subjective approach used to describe life experiences and give them meaning. This type of research uses methods that are more subjective, a smaller sample size, and fewer research controls. The design of the qualitative study tends to evolve over time during the study. Qualitative studies do not follow the same linear progression of quantitative studies; instead, the process tends to resemble a circle more than a line.
   Cognitive level: Analysis
   Nursing process: Implementation
   Client needs: Safe, Effective Care Environment: Management of Care

3. Answer: 4. In a laboratory
   Rationale: Quantitative designs typically are descriptive, correlational, quasi-experimental, and experimental. An

experimental design is used to find the effects of an intervention, is highly controlled, and most often occurs in a laboratory setting.

Cognitive level: Application

Nursing process: Planning

Client needs: Safe, Effective Care Environment: Management of Care

4. Answer: 2. Identify the problem to be studied.

Rationale: The first step in any research process is to identify a researchable problem. A researchable problem is a situation in need of a solution, alteration, or improvement. It is an area of concern for a particular population that requires investigation and that is derived from a topical area. Determining the patients who will participate in the study, assigning data collection roles, and setting the time frame for the study are all steps involved in research but occur later in the process.

Cognitive level: Analysis

Nursing process: Planning

Client needs: Safe, Effective Care Environment: Management of Care

5. Answer: 4. Write out the research problem or question.

Rationale: The research design is the overall plan for the study and should be described in detail. The research design includes data collection methods and methods to analyze the data. It doesn't matter if the research is quantitative or qualitative. The research question or problem statement is the primary guide for the design of the study.

Cognitive level: Application

Nursing process: Planning

Client needs: Safe, Effective Care Environment: Management of Care

Chapter 9

1. Answer: 2. Data about the patient's physical, social, cultural, environmental, and emotional statuses

Rationale: Assessment, the first step of the nursing process, is when the nurse gathers initial data. It is a systematic process that assists the nurse in identifying current health status, actual and potential problems, and areas that need health promotion. It also provides a baseline on which future comparisons can be made. The assessment includes data about the physical, emotional, mental, spiritual, and cultural factors that impact health. It consists of both objective and subjective data.

Cognitive level: Application

Nursing process: Assessment

Client needs: Health Promotion and Maintenance: Prevention/Early Detection of Health Problems

2. Answer: 4. Address the patient including the surname.

Rationale: When beginning the interview, nurses should address patients using their surnames and then introduce themselves and their role in the agency. They should state if they are students. Finally, nurses should tell patients the purpose for the interview.

Cognitive level: Application

Nursing process: Planning

Client needs: Health Promotion and Maintenance: Prevention/Early Detection of Health Problems

3. Answer: 2. What makes you think that you have cancer?

Rationale: The nurse should ask more probing questions in efforts to have the patient explain his or her fears of cancer. Responses that are nonproductive and should be avoided by the nurse include providing false reassurance, using authoritarian language, giving unwanted advice and not allowing patients to make their own decisions, talking too much, using professional jargon that the patient will not understand, and using avoidance language or euphemisms to avoid reality.

Cognitive level: Application

Nursing process: Implementation

Client needs: Health Promotion and Maintenance: Prevention/Early Detection of Health Problems

4. Answer: 3. Inspection

Rationale: Inspection is the deliberate, systematic examination of the patient using both sight and smell. It begins with the first encounter and continues during the entire time the nurse is with the patient. The nurse observes gait, mannerisms, stature, and other physical attributes. The inspection begins by assessing the patient's appearance and comparing the right and left side of the body for symmetry. Palpation uses touch in order to collect data to determine specific characteristics of the body. Such characteristics as temperature, texture, moisture, tenderness, pain, vibrations, and edema are assessed using palpation. Percussion is the creation of sound vibrations by pushing, tapping, or using a device to generate a vibration. The vibrations produced will help in determining position of organ structures. Auscultation is the technique of listening to body sounds. The nurse must use both the unassisted sense of hearing and, where needed, a stethoscope.

Cognitive level: Analysis

Nursing process: Assessment

Client needs: Health Promotion and Maintenance: Prevention/Early Detection of Health Problems

5. Answer: 1. Analysis of the situation

Rationale: The five components of critical thinking related to health assessment include collection of information, analysis of the situation, generation of alternatives, selection of alternatives, and evaluation. Collection of information begins with the interview and continues throughout the entire health assessment. The second skill is analysis of the situation. During this phase the nurse must distinguish normal from abnormal. The patient's age, gender, genetic background, and culture affect the analysis. The nurse must utilize laboratory findings, diagnostic tests, charts, and measures related to development and aging. Generation of alternatives includes identifying options and establishing priorities. It begins with identification of options and then the nurse and patient work together to establish the priorities. The next step is the selection of alternatives. The critical thinking skills needed for this step are the ability to develop outcomes and plans. The outcome is the final result of what the patient will attain, and the plan is the activities that will lead to that outcome. The last step in critical thinking is evaluation. Evaluation requires the nurse to determine if the expected outcomes have been achieved.

Cognitive level: Analysis

Nursing process: Assessment

Client needs: Health Promotion and Maintenance: Prevention/Early Detection of Health Problems

Chapter 10

1. Answer: 3. Point of maximal impulse may be at the sixth left intercostal space, midclavicular line.

   Rationale: Inspiration tends to be shallower in the elderly patient, but accessory muscle use is often noted during expiration. Thus, vital capacity is decreased while residual capacity is increased. The taste sensation is decreased due to the atrophy of papillae on the outer edges of the tongue. Peristalsis decreases in the elderly client, and a decreased thirst sensation may lead to decreased fluid intake. Enlargement or decreased rigidity of the heart muscle may cause displacement of the point of maximal impulse at the fifth or sixth left intercostal space at the midclavicular line.

   Cognitive level: Analysis

   Nursing process: Assessment

   Client needs: Health Promotion and Maintenance; Physiological Integrity

2. Answer: 2. Elderly patients who are hospitalized may be immunized according to the recommendations, as this can decrease both pneumonia and its resultant death rates.

   Rationale: The United States Preventive Services Task Force guidelines do not address the specific needs for the frail patient, those with functional decline, or those with limited life expectancy. The pneumococcal and influenza vaccines may be given at the same time in separate arms because there is no decreased antibody response or increased reaction severity when given together. Doses of the varicella-zoster virus vaccine should be 14 times greater than the vaccine for the varicella virus in order to boost immunity against shingles and its sequelae, such as post-herpetic neuralgia. When elderly patients are already hospitalized, this may provide an opportunity to update them on their immunizations. Studies have shown that vaccinations for older adults are 50% to 60% effective in preventing hospitalizations from pneumonia and 80% effective in preventing death.

   Cognitive level: Analysis

   Nursing process: Assessment

   Client needs: Safe, Effective Care Environment; Health Promotion and Maintenance; Physiological Integrity

3. Answer: 4. As an adjunct for researchers to evaluate the quality of drug prescribing, utilization, and education in the nursing home

   Rationale: The Beers criteria were initially developed to aid researchers in evaluating the quality of prescribing, utilization, and education related to medications in the

nursing home setting, but now it includes the identification of medications or medication classes that may be either ineffective or potentially harmful among elderly patients, even in home or community settings. Approximately 5% to 15% of hospital admissions among elderly patients may be linked to adverse drug reactions or toxic drug effects. Polypharmacy includes the administration of excessive amounts of medications or numbers of medications together. Polypharmacy is best prevented by a thorough assessment of medication history. The United States Preventive Services Task Force is a panel of independent preventive and primary care specialists whose purposes include making recommendations about preventive services to be included in routine primary care and documenting evidence for the effectiveness and outcomes of screening, counseling, and preventive medications.

Cognitive level: Analysis

Nursing process: Assessment

Client needs: Safe, Effective Care Environment; Health Promotion and Maintenance; Physiological Integrity

4. Answer: 2. Ensure confidentiality and inquire directly about the contusion.

   Rationale: This scenario suggests possible elder abuse. With any abuse situation, the patient should be ensured confidentiality. It is possible that the incident requires reporting to law enforcement or some other appropriate agency, and nurses should be aware of laws regarding mandatory reporting. The patient is a victim and should not be blamed or accused of causing the event, and a questionable situation of abuse or neglect should never be ignored. It is not the nurse's job to contact the news media or make implications or allegations regarding abuse or neglect cases.

   Cognitive level: Application

   Nursing process: Implementation

   Client needs: Safe, Effective Care Environment; Health Promotion and Maintenance; Physiological Integrity

5. Answer: 3. Residential Care Facility.

   Rationale: Residential care facilities can be covered by some long-term care policies and offer assistance with ADLs and medications. These facilities are not usually medically focused. Skilled nursing care facilities provide long-term intermediate or skilled nursing care and are usually covered by insurance for short periods of time. The types of clients who require 24-hour-a-day supervision, special diets or moderate assistance with ADLs need this type of residence. Adult day care programs may not be covered by insurance and offer few to no health services. Senior supported housing is not covered by insurance and includes low-income housing for seniors that may also include social activities and help with meals and laundry. They offer no health services.

   Nursing process: Analysis

   Category of client need: Safe, effective care environment/ Health promotion and maintenance/Psychosocial integrity

Chapter 11

1. Answer: 4. Patients who know they are heterozygous for coronary artery disease can initiate medications and lifestyle changes to help lower cholesterol.

   Rationale: Although legislation to protect patients with genetic disorders is pending, sometimes insurance and employer discrimination exists. Sometimes patients are afraid that being diagnosed as having or carrying the trait for a disease or disorder will make it more difficult, not easier, to find health coverage or employment. The nurse should be able to counsel the parents who are carriers of phenylketonuria that the disease is autosomal recessive and, thus, the chance of having offspring with the disease is 25%, not 50%. Again, the nurse should be able to counsel the parents of a patient with Turner syndrome, but the nurse should inform them about the monosomy cause. Patients who are heterozygous for coronary artery disease can reduce cholesterol levels by means of appropriate medication and lifestyle regimens.

   Cognitive level: Analysis

   Nursing process: Assessment

   Client needs: Health Promotion and Maintenance; Psychosocial Integrity; Physiological Integrity

2. Answer: 2. "There is always either an abundance or deficiency of genes within the chromosome."

   Rationale: The nurse should always remain professional and never give a nonchalant answer to a patient. It is the nurse's responsibility to appropriately educate the patient. A variation in genes, in combination with environmental factors, causes complex disorders; and gene mutation results from a change in the DNA sequence of an individual gene. Chromosomal disorders are caused by an abundance or deficiency of genes in the chromosome, but there is no abnormality with an individual gene.

   Cognitive level: Analysis

   Nursing process: Implementation

   Client needs: Health Promotion and Maintenance

3. Answer: 1. "The primary function of introns is to code for proteins using transcription and translation."

   Rationale: The upregulation, or increased transcription, of mRNA causes a subsequent increase in activity and production of more proteins. A codon codes for a single amino acid. Through transcription and translation, the amino acid will form a protein. The double-helix shape of DNA is formed by the alignment of purines and pyrimidines that forms two polynucleotide chains. Introns are noncoding regions within the gene. The exons code for proteins using transcription and translation.

   Cognitive level: Analysis

   Nursing process: Implementation

   Client needs: Health Promotion and Maintenance

4. Answer: 2. Cystic fibrosis

   Rationale: A mutant gene located on an autosome instead of the X chromosome is an autosomal disorder. The fact that two copies of the mutation are required for expression instead of one makes the disorder recessive. Marfan syndrome is an autosomal dominant disorder where only one copy of the mutation is required for expression of the disorder or disease. Color blindness is not autosomal at all, but rather it is X-linked. However, the disorder is recessive. Leigh disease follows an atypical pattern of inheritance, in which a defect in mtDNA is inherited maternally. Cystic fibrosis is the only disorder included that is both autosomal and recessive.

   Cognitive level: Analysis

   Nursing process: Assessment

   Client needs: Health Promotion and Maintenance

5. Answer: 3. To assist in identifying disease risk and developing a customized prevention program for some conditions

   Rationale: Carrier genetic tests are done to determine if unaffected or healthy individuals are carriers of disease-causing genes that could be passed to offspring. Genotype is the genetic makeup of the individual and not visible by outward signs. Genomic imprinting is caused by a chromatin alteration that affects gene expression but not DNA sequence. Differences in gene expression between maternal and paternal alleles are often caused by genomic imprinting. Core genetic conditions are screened for in newborns, and prenatal genetic testing is often done when the child is at risk for a genetic disorder. Pedigrees are used by health care professionals such as nurses, physicians, and genetic counselors to help identify disease risk and develop a personalized prevention and treatment program for certain genetic conditions.

   Cognitive level: Application

   Nursing process: Planning

   Client needs: Safe, Effective Care Environment; Health Promotion and Maintenance; Physiological Integrity

Chapter 12

1. Answer: 3. Long commute to work each day

   Rationale: Stress may be caused by internal and external sources. Internal stressors originate within a person. They include lifestyle choices, such as the use of caffeine; an overloaded schedule; negative self-talk, such as self-criticism and overanalyzing; and stressful personality traits, such as being a perfectionist, workaholic, or pleaser. External stressors originate outside the body. They are precipitated by changes in the external environment. They may be triggered by the actual physical environment, the social environment, the organizational environment, major life events, or other catastrophic events such as hurricanes, floods, and fires. Daily hassles, such as commuting long distances, misplacing keys, and experiencing mechanical breakdowns, also act as external stressors.

   Cognitive level: Analysis

   Nursing process: Assessment

   Client needs: Psychosocial Integrity: Coping and Adaptation

2. Answer: 2. Attributed to hardiness

   Rationale: According to the stimulus-based theory of stress, stress is defined as a stimulus, a life event, or a set of circumstances that arouses physiological and/or psychological reactions that result in a disrupted response that may increase the individual's vulnerability to illness. The patient is not demonstrating this response to the stressors. Daily hassles are experiences and conditions of daily living that have been appraised as relevant and harmful or threatening to an individual's well-being. Uplifts, the counterpart to hassles, are defined as positive experiences that are likely to occur in everyday life. This patient is demonstrating hardiness. Some individuals who experience high scores in terms of life-event changes do not experience illness. The hardy person has a clear sense of personal values and goals, a strong tendency toward interaction with the environment, a sense of meaningfulness, and an internal rather than an external locus of control.

Cognitive level: Analysis

Nursing process: Assessment

Client needs: Psychosocial Integrity: Coping and Adaptation

3. Answer: 1. Elevated blood pressure

Rationale: The general adaptation syndrome has three phases: alarm, resistance, and exhaustion. Physical signs and symptoms of the alarm reaction generally are those of the sympathetic nervous system stimulation. They include increased blood pressure, increased heart and respiratory rate, decreased gastrointestinal motility, pupil dilation, and increased perspiration. The patient also may complain of such symptoms as increased anxiety, nausea, fatigue, anorexia, and weight loss. There are fewer signs and symptoms of the resistance stage. The bodily symptoms of the alarm reaction disappear, and resistance rises above normal. Instead of continuing to lose weight, such as occurred in the alarm phase, the person returns to a "normal" weight. In the exhaustion phase, physical symptoms of the alarm reaction may reappear briefly in a final attempt by the body to survive. This is exemplified by a terminally ill person whose vital signs become stronger just before death. The individual in the stage of exhaustion usually becomes ill and may die if assistance from outside sources is not available.

Cognitive level: Analysis

Nursing process: Assessment

Client needs: Psychosocial Integrity: Coping and Adaptation

4. Answer: 3. The additional stresses of daily life add more stress hormones to the body, which can lead to disease.

Rationale: In our modern society with stressful daily events, hassles, and relationships, stress does not always let up. The stress hormones continue to wash through the system at high levels, never leaving the blood and tissues. Long-term activation of the stress system can have hazardous effects on the body, increasing the risk of obesity, heart disease, depression, and a variety of other illnesses. Repressed stressful emotions can predispose to a variety of diseases, from rheumatoid arthritis to cancer.

Cognitive level: Analysis

Nursing process: Evaluation

Client needs: Physiological Integrity: Physiological Adaptation

5. Answer: 4. Improve nutritional intake including foods containing vitamin E

Rationale: Oxidative stress is a physiological response to both internal and external stressors. Although it is not a disease, it is a condition that can lead to or accelerate disease development. Oxidative stress occurs when the available supply of the body's antioxidants is insufficient to handle and neutralize free radicals of different types. Free radicals have useful functions in the body under controlled conditions and it is not wise to strive to remove all free radicals from the body. Water-based foods have not been linked to the formation of free radicals. Ingesting high doses of vitamin C has not proven to effect free-radical production. Oxygen free radicals are neutralized by antioxidants such as vitamin E. Poor nutrition contributes to oxidative stress.

Cognitive level: Application

Nursing process: Planning

Client needs: Physiological Integrity: Physiological Adaptation

6. Answer: 1. Increased heart rate and blood pressure

Rationale: The physiological effects of stressors include increased heart rate, increased blood pressure, loss of appetite, sweating, and dilated pupils. Additional signs are pale skin, increased rate and depth of respirations, decreased urine output, dry mouth, and decreased intestinal peristalsis.

Cognitive level: Analysis

Nursing process: Assessment

Client needs: Physiological Integrity: Physiological Adaptation

Chapter 13

1. Answer: 2. Freud

Rationale: This patient is demonstrating the concept of denial, which is considered an ego defense mechanism within Freud's psychoanalytical theory. Erikson's theory addresses how persons develop across the life span. Maslow's theory focuses on the hierarchy of human needs. Piaget's theory focuses on the cognitive development of children.

Cognitive level: Analysis

Nursing process: Assessment

Client needs: Psychosocial Integrity: Psychosocial Adaptation

2. Answer: 3. Asking the patient if more information is needed to help in the decision-making process

Rationale: Certain actions foster the nurse–patient relationship. Conveying respect for the person's uniqueness, being nonjudgmental, showing attentiveness, and being empathic all create the building blocks of a therapeutic nurse–patient relationship. Patients need to feel safe, secure, and understood. Also pivotal is that the nurse is perceived as knowledgeable, trustworthy, sensitive, and unambiguous. There is also an emphasis on problem solving and a mandatory duty to accountability, responsibility, and confidentiality. Integral to the nurse–patient relationship is the concept of empowerment. When we empower persons, we assist them in developing the resources they need in which to make informed decisions about their health care based on their own priorities. The nurse should ask the patient if more information is needed to help in the decision-making process.

Cognitive level: Analysis

Nursing process: Assessment

Client needs: Psychosocial Integrity: Coping and Adaptation

3. Answer: 2. Sit with the patient and encourage him to explain to the best of his ability.

Rationale: Cultural competence is defined as the nurse continually striving to provide culturally appropriate care to patients and families. Nurses must convey empathy, show respect, build trust, establish rapport, listen actively, provide appropriate feedback, and demonstrate genuine interest. Barriers to effective transcultural communication include nurses' lack of knowledge, bias, ethnocentrism, prejudice, and stereotyping. Language differences, differences in the understanding of terminology, and differences in perceptions and expectations also create barriers.

Cognitive level: Analysis

Nursing process: Implementation

Client needs: Psychosocial Integrity: Coping and Adaptation

4. Answer: 1. I will do my best to learn how to do this. I have to.

Rationale: The nurse must assess the emotional and experiential readiness of the patient or family to learn. The following factors are to be considered when assessing the readiness to learn: level of emotional health, motivation to learn, self-concept and body image, social and economic stability, past experiences with learning, and attitude toward learning. The response that best identifies this patient's readiness to learn is the one that positively shows the patient's willingness to learn the skill.

Cognitive level: Analysis

Nursing process: Assessment

Client needs: Safe, Effective Care Environment: Management of Care

5. Answer: 1. Sit with the patient and be prepared to answer any questions.

Rationale: Nurses are often in contact with individuals and families when they are vulnerable or in crisis and, therefore, nurses become a valuable resource. Early intervention is essential to reduce the effects of the crisis. Providing information and resources sometimes serves to prevent a full-blown crisis from occurring. Rapport needs to be established quickly. It is important to understand the meaning the event has for the patient and, further, to allow for free expression of feelings, which can be cathartic. Once these things are accomplished, the nurse can then help the patient clarify the events of the crisis.

Cognitive level: Application

Nursing process: Implementation

Client needs: Psychosocial Integrity: Coping and Adaptation

Chapter 14

1. Answer: 1. Body mass index (BMI), weight, and waist circumference

Rationale: Anthropometric measurements are physical measurements that include height, weight, BMI, waist circumference, body composition, and measurement of fat and muscle. Food diaries provide valuable information, but are not anthropometric measurements. Blood pressure and pulse are measures of cardiovascular status.

Cognitive level: Application

Nursing process: Implementation

Client needs: Health Promotion and Maintenance

2. Answer: 4. Explain importance of adhering to scheduled mealtimes.

Rationale: The nurse should focus on interventions that will help to interrupt the binge–purge cycle. Regular mealtimes help to establish a pattern and avoid hunger that is brought on by long periods without eating. Finger foods should be avoided because portion control is difficult. Avoiding hunger should be stressed since this can lead to overeating. Regular exercise is encouraged, but excessive exercise may prompt the bulimic patient to view the exercise as a compensation for binging.

Cognitive level: Application

Nursing process: Implementation

Client needs: Physiological Integrity: Reduction of Risk Potential

3. Answer: 3. Maintain your carbohydrate intake by eating noodles, toast, and sports drinks.

Rationale: During periods of illness the need for insulin continues, so the patient should try to maintain a carbohydrate intake of 150 to 200 g/day. Some suggested types of carbohydrates that are easy to digest include ginger ale, cranberry and apple juice, sports drinks, toast, noodles, chicken noodle soup, gelatin, and pudding. Carbohydrates should not be restricted or be sugar free. Insulin is still needed during illness; doses may be adjusted but not stopped.

Cognitive level: Application

Nursing process: Implementation

Client needs: Physiological Integrity: Reduction of Risk Potential

4. Answer: 2. The wound drains large amounts of exudates.

Rationale: A large wound draining large amounts of exudates, which are rich in protein, will contribute to further protein losses. Antibiotic therapy should contribute to protein losses. Dairy products are often high in protein and could help to restore protein levels. A need for surgical debridement indicates there is necrotic tissue in the wound.

Cognitive level: Analysis

Nursing process: Diagnosis

Client needs: Physiological Integrity: Physiological Adaptation

5. Answer: 1. Burn injuries

Rationale: Patients recovering from burn injuries have a high caloric requirement that often necessitates intermittent enteral feedings, either in addition to oral feedings or as the sole source of nutrition. The other conditions should not require the need for enteral feedings.

Cognitive level: Application

Nursing process: Assessment

Client needs: Physiological Integrity

Chapter 15

1. Answer: 1. Is a common symptom to most illnesses, disease processes, and traumatic injuries

Rationale: Although pain is recognized by all cultures, the expression and response to that pain can vary greatly among different cultures. Today's health care system can be very unfriendly at times to patients experiencing pain. Many health care providers lack the knowledge to or are unwilling to treat pain. Also, because of the widespread and undertreated nature of pain today, many patients experience significant personal, social, or economic distress. Pain is, however, a common symptom to most illnesses, disease processes, and traumatic injuries.

Cognitive level: Analysis

Nursing process: Assessment

Client needs: Safe, Effective Care Environment

2. Answer: 3. Recognize the fundamental responsibility of all nurses to help alleviate patient suffering and relieve pain.

Rationale: Chronic nonmalignant pain is not usually proportional to objective disease severity. A ban on opiate use in chronic nonmalignant pain is not ethically acceptable, even when patients are being assessed and treated for concurrent psychiatric disorders. A psychiatric disorder does not mean that these patients are not entitled to pain relief. Patients, their families, and even health care providers may have concerns about dependence or addiction associated with chronic opiate use, and disciplinary actions do exist for some nurses who administer inappropriate amounts of pain-controlling medications. However, being prescribed and receiving opiates for pain control does not subject patients to potential legal sanctions. Nurses do have the legal and ethical responsibility to help alleviate patient pain and suffering.

Cognitive level: Analysis

Nursing process: Implementation

Client needs: Safe, Effective Care Environment

3. Answer: 4. "My pain may last for months, years, or for my whole life."

Rationale: Pain of short duration with complete resolution is known as transient pain, whereas pain associated with a recent event, such as surgery, illness, or trauma, is acute pain. Recurrent pain is short in duration but recurs after a pain-free period. Chronic pain usually lasts in excess of 3 to 6 months but may last for years or even a lifetime.

Cognitive level: Analysis

Nursing process: Evaluation

Client needs: Health Promotion and Maintenance

4. Answer: 2. The McGill Pain Questionnaire and the patient interview.

Rationale: The patient's self-report of pain intensity, behavioral assessment, numeric rating system, simple verbal descriptive scale, Critical-Care Pain Observation Tool, and visual analog scale are all examples of unidimensional pain assessment methods. Within the choices given, only the McGill Pain Questionnaire and patient interview are credited with assessing the multidimensional pain experience.

Cognitive level: Application

Nursing process: Assessment

Client needs: Health Promotion and Maintenance

Chapter 16

1. Answer: 2. "There is a potential for the baby to have birth defects."

Rationale: According to genetic theories, each partner contributes on the genetic level and drug use impacts the sperm and egg health. The husband's cocaine use may impact fetal development; birth defects are more commonly linked to paternal DNA damage than maternal DNA damage. Telling the mother the infant should be fine provides false reassurance. It will not help to use barrier contraception at this point because the fetus has already formed. Sociocultural and environmental factors do have an influence on substance abuse, but the biologic and genetic influence also play a large role and at this point in the pregnancy have the greatest influence.

Cognitive level: Application

Nursing process: Implementation

Client needs: Physiological Integrity

2. Answer: 4. Impulsive and extroverted

Rationale: A number of personality traits are associated with disruptive substance abuse, including extroversion, impulsivity, social conformism, anxiousness, tenseness, and being less satisfied with present life situation. Being gregarious, quiet, studious, independent, and loyal are not characteristics usually associated with substance abuse.

Cognitive level: Application

Nursing process: Assessment

Client needs: Psychosocial Integrity

3. Answer: 3. Diaphoresis

Rationale: Symptoms associated with alcohol withdrawal usually develop around 62 hours after the last drink and include elevated temperature, severe diaphoresis, hypertension, and tachycardia. Behavioral symptoms include confusion, agitation and tremors, and altered sensory perception.

Cognitive level: Analysis

Nursing process: Assessment

Client needs: Physiological Integrity

4. Answer: 1. Cardiac arrhythmias

Rationale: Inhalants and solvents can cause life-threatening arrhythmias, such as ventricular fibrillation. Withdrawal of some amphetamines may cause severe depression and suicidal tendencies. Methamphetamine withdrawal may produce outbursts of rage. Hallucinations can occur with the use of hallucinogens and alcohol withdrawal.

Cognitive level: Application
Nursing process: Implementation
Client needs: Physiological Integrity

5. Answer: 3. Diazepam, Valium
   Rationale: Treatment of PCP intoxication includes the use of diazepam to treat the seizures, muscle spasms, and agitation that occur. Naloxone is the antidote for opiate overdoses. Prochlorperazine is a phenothiazine and would be contraindicated because PCP is an anticholinergic. Amitriptyline, a tricyclic antidepressant, is often used to help a patient withdrawing from cocaine because such patients often experience depression.

   Cognitive level: Application
   Nursing process: Planning
   Client needs: Physiological Integrity

Chapter 17

1. Answer: 1. Integrating the goals and expertise of many different disciplines encourages the development of the most comprehensive plan of care.
   Rationale: Patients and their families may receive conflicting information with increasing numbers of medical teams. Advance directives may provide civil and criminal immunity for health care personnel meeting certain conditions, but solely being part of or using an interdisciplinary approach to palliative care does not. Also, the patient's goals of care should guide the utilization of technology in end-of-life care, not vice versa. An interdisciplinary approach does, however, offer the patient the most comprehensive plan of care because of the variety of experience and expertise it brings.

   Cognitive level: Application
   Nursing process: Implementation
   Client needs: Safe, Effective Care Environment; Psychosocial Integrity

2. Answer: 4. "The family usually finds it easier to withdraw life-sustaining treatments than to withhold them."
   Rationale: End-of-life, palliative care is always focused on symptomatology rather than cure. All patients have the rights of autonomy, privacy, and decision making regarding their own health care. However, it is often more emotionally difficult for a family to withdraw life-sustaining treatments once they have been initiated than to withhold them.

   Cognitive level: Application
   Nursing process: Evaluation
   Client needs: Safe, Effective Care Environment; Psychosocial Integrity

3. Answer: 2. "By signing the advance directive my appointed family member will have the ability to make health care decisions for me if I become ill."
   Rationale: An advance directive directs the health care team in the decision-making process for the incapacitated patient, and the patient's own wishes regarding treatment are followed. The living will, a type of advance

directive, also describes the patient's desires for any life-prolonging treatments. Signing the advance directive does not grant proxy for a friend or family member to make health care decisions. Only by signing a medical durable power of attorney may decision-making rights be granted to the person of the patient's choosing.

Cognitive level: Application
Nursing process: Evaluation
Client needs: Safe, Effective Care Environment

4. Answer: 1. "We will continue to increase the pain medication until the symptoms are relieved."
   Rationale: Efforts to control pain in the hospice patient are of great importance. Nonpharmacologic methods such as providing room for the patient's family and reducing excess light and noise may help make the patient more comfortable, and concerns surrounding physical or psychological dependencies related to increased opiate or benzodiazepine use are inappropriate. Conversely, when being titrated for pain control in the hospice patient, opiates have no maximum dose. Dosages are continuously titrated to achieve symptom relief.

   Cognitive level: Application
   Nursing process: Implementation
   Client needs: Physiological Integrity

5. Answer: 2. "Some Russians may make their elderly family members a DNR so they will die comfortably and without life-sustaining treatments."
   Rationale: Followers of Judaism believe the dying person should not be left alone. Baha'i law forbids the body from being cremated, but in Buddhism organ donation is encouraged and cremation is common. People from South Asia tend to express grief openly, whereas American Indians grieve privately. Russians do tend to encourage DNR orders to promote a comfortable death and prevent artificial life support.

   Cognitive level: Analysis
   Nursing process: Evaluation
   Client needs: Psychosocial Integrity

Chapter 18

1. Answer: 3. Extracellular fluid volume deficit
   Rationale: The intracellular fluids (ICFs) are fluids that exist within the cell cytoplasm and nucleus. The extracellular fluids (ECFs) are fluids that exist outside the cell, such as interstitial fluid between cells, fluid in the bloodstream (serum), cerebrospinal fluid (CSF) in the central nervous system, gastrointestinal secretions, sweat, and urine. Two-thirds of the body's water is ICF and one-third is ECF.

   Cognitive level: Analysis
   Nursing process: Assessment
   Client needs: Physiological Adaptation: Physiological Integrity

2. Answer: 2. Prepare to administer a hypotonic intravenous solution.
   Rationale: This patient is dehydrated as evidenced by the elevated hemoglobin and serum sodium and potassium levels. A hypertonic solution would exacerbate the

dehydration and would not be indicated. The nurse should prepare to administer a hypotonic solution, which has a lower osmolality to hydrate the patient. An isotonic intravenous solution has the osmolality of blood and would most likely not serve to rehydrate the patient very effectively. This patient is dehydrated and a sodium and fluid restriction would be detrimental to this patient's care.
Cognitive level: Analysis
Nursing process: Planning
Client needs: Physiological Integrity: Physiological Adaptation

3. Answer: 1. Na+: 115 mEq/L
Rationale: Of the four electrolytes presented, the Na+ of 115 is out of range because normal values for sodium are 135 to 145 milliequivalents/liter (mEq/L). Ninety-eight percent of potassium is found within cells. Small amounts are found in blood (3.5 to 5.0 millimoles/liter [mmol/L]) and bone. Ninety-eight percent of calcium in the body is found in the bones and teeth. Two percent is in the blood serum (8.5 to 10.5 mg/dL; 50% ionized and 45% bound to albumin). More than 50% of body magnesium is stored in muscle and bone, and only 1% is in the blood (1.4 to 2.1 mg/dL).
Cognitive level: Analysis
Nursing process: Assessment
Client needs: Physiological Adaptation: Reduction of Risk Potential

4. Answer: 1. Hypokalemia
Rationale: Diarrhea may increase excretion of potassium to 200 mEq/day. Vomiting and/or nasogastric suction can increase loss through GI fluids removed. Typical circumstances leading to hypocalcemia include primary hyperparathyroidism, bone malignancy, and drug toxicity. Hypermagnesemia is often associated with renal failure. Hypophosphatemia causes include vitamin D deficiency, bowel disorders that lead to malabsorption, excessive use of phosphate-binding antacids, alcoholism, or diabetic ketoacidosis.
Cognitive level: Analysis
Nursing process: Assessment
Client needs: Physiological Integrity: Physiological Adaptation

5. Answer: 1. Dependent edema
Rationale: With fluid volume excess, the patient would likely show dependent edema, increased blood pressure, decreased urine output, shortness of breath, and adventitious breath sounds. An example of this condition is a patient with congestive heart failure.
Cognitive level: Analysis
Nursing process: Assessment
Client needs: Physiological Integrity: Physiological Adaptation

6. Answer: 4. Obtain an electrocardiogram
Rationale: Obtaining an ECG is a priority because serum potassium levels greater than 6.0 mEq/L can be life threatening due to the decreased ability of the heart to repolarize as evidenced by the tented T wave, loss of the P wave, and a wide, bizarre QRS with a depressed ST segment. Evaluating the level of consciousness would be associated with hyponatremia; measuring urine output hourly would be fruitless for a patient with renal failure; and the ABGs, although likely abnormal, would not serve as a priority intervention.
Cognitive level: Analysis
Nursing process: Implementation
Client needs: Physiological Integrity: Physiological Adaptation

7. Answer: 3. Eat a balanced diet including tomato juice and potatoes.
Rationale: Discharge teaching of patient/family with regard to hypokalemia includes properly taking potassium supplements such as K-Dur. In addition, increasing potassium-rich foods in the diet and recognizing/reporting increased muscle weakness are critical teaching points. Kayexalate enemas are used for hyperkalemia and, therefore, would not be an appropriate measure.
Cognitive level: Application
Nursing process: Planning
Client needs: Physiological Integrity: Physiological Adaptation

Chapter 19

1. Answer: 1. Increasing
Rationale: Because it is a negative log, as the hydrogen ion concentration increases, the pH decreases. Conversely, as the hydrogen ion concentration goes down, pH goes up. The hydrogen ion is the smallest ionic particle and it is extremely reactive. The hydrogen ion combines with alkali/bases or other negatively charged ions at low concentrations.
Cognitive level: Analysis
Nursing process: Assessment
Client needs: Physiological Integrity: Physiological Adaptation

2. Answer: 3. Increase the secretion of hydrogen ions.
Rationale: The main metabolic acids are lactic acid, pyruvic acid, ketoacids seen in diabetic acidosis, acetoacetic acid, and beta-hydroxybutyric acid. These acids are eliminated by the kidneys or they are metabolized by the liver. The capacity for elimination of these metabolic acids is much less than that of the lungs. In respiratory acidosis and most cases of metabolic acidosis, the kidneys excrete hydrogen ion and conserve bicarbonate to correct the pH.
Cognitive level: Analysis
Nursing process: Assessment
Client needs: Physiological Integrity: Physiological Adaptation

3. Answer: 4. 10 L/min
Rationale: The amount of ventilation is generally quantified by how much air the lungs move in 1 minute, referred to as the minute ventilation. Minute ventilation is the product of respiratory rate and depth, referred to as the tidal volume. Normal resting respiratory rate is about 12 breaths per minute. Normal resting depth tidal volume is about 500 mL. This yields a normal minute ventilation of

6 L/min: 12 breaths/min $\times$ 500 mL = 6,000 mL or 6 L. This patient's respiratory rate is 20 breaths per minute. The minute ventilation would be 10 L/min.

Cognitive level: Application

Nursing process: Assessment

Client needs: Physiological Integrity: Physiological Adaptation

4. Answer: 2. Deep rapid respirations

Rationale: In a state of metabolic acidosis, such as that which exists during diabetic ketoacidosis, the medullary centers will stimulate the lungs to increase the minute ventilation to blow off CO_2, even if that level is normal. These rapid, deep respirations, referred to as Kussmaul's respirations, are an attempt to correct the arterial pH by decreasing respiratory acid. This process is referred to as compensation.

Cognitive level: Analysis

Nursing process: Assessment

Client needs: Physiological Integrity: Physiological Adaptation

5. Answer: 1. Ammonia

Rationale: In the face of a high load of metabolic acids, the kidneys also increase their production of the urinary buffer, ammonia. Under normal circumstances, ammonia excretion is about 30 mmol/day, or about 0.5 mmol/kg. This excretion can increase to about 280 mmol/day, but this response takes several days to be completed.

Cognitive level: Analysis

Nursing process: Assessment

Client needs: Physiological Integrity: Physiological Adaptation

6. Answer: 4. pH

Rationale: The steps to analyze an arterial blood gas results are as follows: Step 1: Assess the pH; Step 2: Assess the $PaCO_2$; Step 3: Assess the bicarbonate and the base excess; Step 4: Evaluate compensation.

Cognitive level: Application

Nursing process: Assessment

Client needs: Physiological Integrity: Physiological Adaptation

7. Answer: 3. Place the patient in high Fowler's position.

Rationale: The patient is in respiratory acidosis. The main treatment for respiratory acidosis is correction of the underlying disorder that led to its development. For a patient with pneumonia, this would include antibiotic therapy, improving oxygenation, and management of fever. Placing the patient in high Fowler's position will improve air flow. Breathing into a paper bag and/or giving a sedative are indications of respiratory alkalosis. Sodium bicarbonate administered intravenously is a controversial treatment for metabolic acidosis.

Cognitive level: Analysis

Nursing process: Implementation

Client needs: Physiological Integrity: Physiological Adaptation

8. Answer: 3. Slow, shallow respirations

Rationale: Whenever excretion of CO_2 via the lungs fails to keep up with the body's CO_2 production, respiratory acidosis will occur such as with a drug overdose. Kussmaul's respirations (rapid, deep breaths) occur with metabolic acidosis, seizures are associated with respiratory alkalosis, and hyperreflexia is a symptom of metabolic alkalosis.

Cognitive level: Analysis

Nursing process: Assessment

Client needs: Physiological Integrity: Physiological Adaptation

9. Answer: 3. "I will take a stress management class or seek counseling."

Rationale: Respiratory alkalosis is characterized by a lower than normal $PaCO_2$ accompanied by an elevated pH. Respiratory rate is a major determinant of the $PaCO_2$ level. Excessively fast or deep ventilation "blows off" the carbon dioxide, decreasing the level and increasing the pH, causing alkalosis. Psychological conditions such as anxiety and panic or severe pain can also cause overventilation. Patients with psychological hyperventilation syndromes should benefit from reassurance and methods to decrease stress.

Cognitive level: Application

Nursing process: Evaluation

Client needs: Physiological Adaptation: Reduction of Risk Potential

Chapter 20

1. Answer: 1. Response of white blood cells to the cellular injury

Rationale: The inflammatory process involves a vascular phase and a cellular phase. The cellular phase includes the responses and actions of the white blood cells. Neutrophils then die, releasing proteolytic enzymes that liquefy the dead cells and bacteria, resulting in the formation of pus. The vascular phase would include such responses as temporary vasoconstriction followed by vasodilation and leakage of fluid into the interstitial space.

Cognitive level: Analysis

Nursing process: Assessment

Client needs: Physiological Integrity: Physiological Adaptation

2. Answer: 1. Inadequate nutrition

Rationale: A balanced diet helps the body maintain an effective immune system by providing the nutrients needed for growth of new, healthy tissue. With age, the immune system weakens as a result of decreasing thymus gland function and some lymphocytes become less responsive in the elderly, while others function normally. A personality disorder or urban living would not necessarily increase risk for infection.

Cognitive level: Application

Nursing process: Assessment

Client needs: Health Promotion and Maintenance: Prevention/Early Detection of Health Problems

3. Answer: 2. Airborne

Rationale: Tuberculosis is spread by airborne transmission, which occurs when the organism is expelled from the infected person and remains suspended in the air in tiny droplets no larger than 5 microns. Contact transmission can occur by direct contact or indirect contact, such as with sneezing or coughing. Vehicle transmission occurs when the organism's life is maintained on something outside the reservoir until it is passed to the susceptible host. Vector-borne transmission occurs when a disease-producing organism is carried by a living intermediate host that transfers the organism to a susceptible host.

Cognitive level: Analysis

Nursing process: Assessment

Client needs: Physiological Integrity: Physiological Adaptation

4. Answer: 4. Wash for at least 15 seconds covering all surfaces.

Rationale: Guidelines for hand washing include the following: Vigorously rub hands together for 15 seconds, generating friction on all surfaces including between the fingers and under fingernails. Wet hands under running water using tepid, not hot, water. Artificial nails are not to be worn due to high risk for microorganism growth. Avoid the use of petroleum-based moisturizers because they can lead to a deterioration of latex gloves.

Cognitive level: Application

Nursing process: Implementation

Client needs: Safe, Effective Care Environment: Safety and Infection Control

5. Answer: 4. *Staphylococcus epidermidis*

Rationale: *Staphylococcus epidermidis* is found commonly on the skin, nasopharynx, and lower GU tract. Infection occurs with indwelling devices that are inserted through the skin, such as catheters. Group A beta-hemolytic streptococci are found in the nose and throat, respiratory secretions, and the hands. This bacteria is the cause of acute pharyngitis, cutaneous impetigo, and systemic infection. *Staphylococcus aureus* is found in the nasopharynx, skin, and clothing. This bacteria can be found in subcutaneous and cutaneous abscesses, and foreign devices such as IVs. *Neisseria meningitidis* is found in the nasopharynx and transported through the respiratory tract; it causes meningitis.

Cognitive level: Analysis

Nursing process: Assessment

Client needs: Physiological Integrity: Physiological Adaptation

6. Answer: 3. Injecting already formed antibodies into the body

Rationale: Active immunization involves the introduction of live, killed, or attenuated toxin of a disease organism into the body. The immune system responds by producing antibodies. Active immunization provides long-term and possibly lifelong immunity. Some vaccines require boosters to maintain the immunity. Examples of active immunizations include measles, mumps, hepatitis B, and hepatitis A. Passive immunity provides immunity for a short period of time, usually around 6 to 12 weeks. This involves already formed antibodies injected into the body. The individual may still have the disease but it will be a less severe case. An example of this type of immunity is immunoglobulin injections given to people exposed to hepatitis A.

Cognitive level: Analysis

Nursing process: Assessment

Client needs: Health Promotion and Maintenance: Prevention/Early Detection of Health Problems

7. Answer: 2. Increase the proportion of all tuberculosis patients who complete curative therapy within 12 months.

Rationale: Increasing compliance with medication treatment for tuberculosis is an actual *Healthy People 2010* goal. Eradication of the disease is not realistic. No immunization for health care workers is currently available. The rural population is not targeted for focus with avoidance of tuberculosis spread; an overcrowded condition such as that found in urban living is a risk factor however.

Cognitive level: Analysis

Nursing process: Planning

Client needs: Health Promotion and Maintenance: Prevention/Early Detection of Health Problems

8. Answer: 3. Have you received chemotherapy for cancer, psoriasis, or rheumatoid arthritis?

Rationale: The patient should be asked about any preexisting conditions that might affect the immune system such as the use of steroids, chemotherapy, transplants, or other chronic illnesses. Employment history, recreational activities, and exercise routine would not generate information about infectious diseases.

Cognitive level: Analysis

Nursing process: Assessment

Client needs: Health Promotion and Maintenance: Prevention/Early Detection of Health Problems

Chapter 21

1. Answer: 2. Prehypertension

Rationale: The term *prehypertension* describes those individuals with a blood pressure finding on two or more office visits of 130–139/80–89 mmHg as being at twice the risk to develop hypertension as those with lower values. Hypertension stage I is a BP of 140–159 mmHg systolic or 90–99 mmHg diastolic, whereas stage II would be multiple measurements of a systolic pressure greater than 160 mmHg or a diastolic pressure exceeding 100 mmHg.

Cognitive level: Analysis

Nursing process: Diagnosis

Client needs: Physiological Integrity

2. Answers:
   1. Cardiac output
   2. Peripheral vascular resistance
   3. Baroreceptors
   4. Chemoreceptors
   5. Body fluid volume

Rationale: Cardiac output × peripheral vascular resistance equals blood pressure (CO × PVR = BP). Baroreceptors, located in carotid sinuses and the wall of the left ventricle, monitor arterial BP and counteract rising pressure by vasodilation through stimulation of the vagus nerve. Chemoreceptors regulate ventilation and communicate with the brainstem and cardiovascular centers to cause widespread vasoconstriction. Fluid balance is essential to maintaining normal blood pressure. When hypovolemia and hypervolemia occur, it is reflected in the systemic blood pressure. Adrenocorticotropic hormone (ACTH) functions as an aid to growth and development, not affecting blood pressure.

Cognitive level: Analysis
Nursing process: Evaluation
Client needs: Physiological Integrity

3. Answer: 3. 56-year-old male, African American, insulin-dependent diabetic

Rationale: Age (older than 55 for men and 65 for women) is considered a risk factor for hypertension along with being of male gender. African American individuals have two times greater possibility of developing high blood pressure than Caucasian Americans. Environmental factors such as obesity, cigarette smoking, sedentary lifestyle, use of illegal drugs, and excessive alcohol consumption create risk. Stress such as job stresses, economic position, losses and/or gains of any kind, and many other issues of life are risk factors for hypertension.

Cognitive level: Analysis
Nursing process: Assessment
Client needs: Health Promotion and Maintenance

4. Answer: 3. Not crush, break in half, or chew the extended release form of the drug

Rationale: Instruct the patient taking a sustained-action capsule or tablet, such as nifedipine (Procardia XL), a calcium channel blocker, that it cannot be crushed, broken up, or chewed. Adding potassium would be necessary with a loop diuretic; dry cough is most associated with angiotensin-converting enzyme inhibitors. Beta-adrenergic blocking agents require teaching blood pressure and pulse taking prior to medication. If pulse is below 60, inform the health care provider prior to taking the medication.

Cognitive level: Application
Nursing process: Implementation
Client needs: Safe, Effective Care Environment

5. Answers:
   1. Asian populations undergoing Westernization will have significant increases in high blood pressure.
   2. Individuals living in the southeastern region of the United States have a higher percentage of high blood pressure.

Rationale: African Americans have a 3 to 4 times higher risk of angioedema and cough attributed to ACE inhibitors than Caucasians. American Indian and Asian populations undergoing Westernization will have significant increases in high blood pressure. Individuals living in the southeastern region (sometimes called the Salt Belt) of the United States have a higher percentage of high blood pressure. Compliance with the DASH diet and exercise to prevent/control hypertension is not culture dependent.

Cognitive level: Application
Nursing process: Evaluation
Client needs: Health Promotion and Maintenance

6. Answers:
   1. Developing a diet plan that is low in saturated fats and sodium
   2. Eliminating or reducing alcohol consumption to one ounce a day

Rationale: A diet rich in fruits, vegetables, and whole grains and low in sodium and saturated fats is recommended with all stages of hypertension. Alcohol consumption will elevate arterial blood pressure and adds "empty" calories to the patient's diet. A sedentary lifestyle is avoided; aerobic exercise 3 to 5 times per week reduces stress and blood pressure. Smoking cessation is encouraged, not reduction of nicotine. Coping with stress-producing situations is the goal, because total avoidance is not possible. A realistic weight loss goal is 1 to 2 pounds per week.

Cognitive level: Analysis
Nursing process: Planning
Client needs: Health Promotion and Maintenance

7. Answer: 2. Verbalizing the warning signs and symptoms of cerebral vascular accident

Rationale: High blood pressure, referred to as the "silent killer," often goes undetected until signs and symptoms of other organ involvement are present. High blood pressure is the leading contributing cause of cerebral vascular accident; therefore, knowing the warning signs is the priority outcome. Generic brands of antihypertensive drugs are acceptable and a cost-saving method for long-term use. Positive personal relationships help with stress reduction, but are not the priority. Stage II hypertension warrants monitoring of blood pressure more often than once a month.

Cognitive level: Application
Nursing process: Planning
Client needs: Health Promotion and Maintenance

Chapter 22

1. Answer: 3. A midline catheter

Rationale: A midline catheter is the best peripheral vascular access device for parenteral therapy up to 4 weeks. A peripheral short catheter is for infusions that last between 72 and 96 hours. A winged steel infusion set is for infusions of less than 4 hours in duration. A PICC line is a central venous access device and not a peripheral vascular access device.

Cognitive level: Application
Nursing process: Planning
Client needs: Physiological Integrity: Pharmacological and Parenteral Therapies

2. Answer: 4. Secondary administration set

Rationale: A stop cock and extension set are add-on devices that might not be necessary for the infusion of the medication. An elastomeric balloon is a one-time-use device seen most frequently in home care. The secondary administration set is the device used to administer an intravenous medication when the patient is already receiving parenteral therapy. This administration set is piggybacked into the main infusion line.

Cognitive level: Application

Nursing process: Implementation

Client needs: Physiological Integrity: Pharmacologic and Parenteral Therapies

3. Answer: 2. Preserve the patient's right to safe quality care and protect the nurse who administers infusion therapy.

Rationale: The primary goal of the Infusion Nursing Standards of Practice is to preserve the patient's right to safe quality care and protect the nurse who administers infusion therapy. Even though it is important for nurses to follow Standard Precautions, be in compliance with all regulatory agencies, and have adequate skill levels, these are not Standards of Practice of the Infusion Nursing organization.

Cognitive level: Application

Nursing process: Planning

Client needs: Physiological Integrity; Pharmacologic and Parenteral Therapies

4. Answer: 4. Review the procedure with the patient and obtain consent.

Rationale: The first thing the nurse should do is review the procedure with the patient or conduct education. Obtain the patient's consent to have the access device inserted. Once this has been done, the nurse can then gather equipment and prepare flushes all using standard precautions.

Cognitive level: Application

Nursing process: Planning

Client needs: Physiological Integrity: Pharmacologic and Parenteral Therapies

5. Answer: 2. Stop the infusion and remove the catheter.

Rationale: This patient is complaining of an infiltration of the parenteral fluids. The nurse should discontinue the infusion immediately and remove the catheter. The nurse should then elevate the affected extremity to relieve patient discomfort and assist in absorption of excess fluids and improving circulation. The nurse should not take the time to check for a blood return, reposition the catheter, or change the dressing and observe the site.

Cognitive level: Application

Nursing process: Evaluation

Client needs: Physiological Integrity: Pharmacologic and Parenteral Therapies

Chapter 23

1. Answer: 1. Increase plasma colloidal osmotic pressure and plasma volume.

Rationale: Albumin will increase colloidal osmotic pressure and plasma volume. Albumin does not impact platelets or coagulation and does not include red blood cells.

Cognitive level: Analysis

Nursing process: Planning

Client needs: Physiological Integrity: Pharmacologic and Parenteral Therapies

2. Answer: 2. The youngest age for a blood donor is 17.

Rationale: There are specific guidelines for being a blood donor. Vital signs need to be within normal limits. Blood pressure needs to be less than 180/100 mmHg.

Blood count or hemoglobin needs to be greater than 12.4 mg/dL for a female. A blood donor needs to be between the ages of 17 and 65. There are no guidelines or restrictions about family members donating to other family members.

Cognitive level: Application

Nursing process: Implementation

Client needs: Physiological Integrity: Pharmacologic and Parenteral Therapies

3. Answer: 4. Patient provides informed consent for the transfusion.

Rationale: A history of blood transfusion reactions and the patient's circulatory and respiratory status are included in the assessment phase of blood administration. Assembling appropriate equipment is part of the implementation phase of blood administration. The patient providing informed consent for the transfusion is part of the planning phase of blood administration.

Cognitive level: Application

Nursing process: Planning

Client needs: Physiological Integrity: Pharmacologic and Parenteral Therapies

4. Answer: 1. Stop the blood transfusion.

Rationale: Circulatory overload can occur with transfusions when the blood is infused too rapidly or in too large a quantity, causing hypervolemia. High-risk patients include the elderly and those individuals who already have increased circulatory volume or who have a history of heart failure. Clinical manifestations of circulatory overload include dyspnea, tachycardia, distended neck veins, crackles in the lungs, and a rise in blood pressure. If the transfusion is not slowed down or stopped, pulmonary edema will result. Administering an antipyretic or epinephrine and flushing the access device are inappropriate actions.

Cognitive level: Planning

Nursing process: Implementation

Client needs: Physiological Integrity: Pharmacologic and Parenteral Therapies

5. Answer: 2. Stop the transfusion, call for help, and begin life-supporting measures.

Rationale: The sudden onset of chest pain is seen in an acute hemolytic reaction. This is a life-threatening situation. Slowing the transfusion rate and administering epinephrine or antipyretics are not appropriate actions for this level of transfusion reaction.

Cognitive level: Application

Nursing process: Implementation

Client needs: Physiological Integrity: Pharmacologic and Parenteral Therapies

Chapter 24

1. Answer: 2. Help with diagnosis, treatment, and evaluation of care.

Rationale: The three purposes of hemodynamic monitoring are aiding in the diagnosis of various disorders, assisting in guiding therapies to minimize or correct dysfunction, and evaluating the patient's response to therapy. There are noninvasive ways to ensure a correct blood pressure reading. The use of hemodynamic monitoring does not reduce the amount of patient care required. Although hemodynamic monitoring will provide information about the patient's status, it is not used individually to determine if a patient is stable enough for transfer.

Cognitive level: Application

Nursing process: Planning

Client needs: Physiological Integrity: Physiological Adaptation

2. Answer: 3. Find out if the correct type of tubing was used.

Rationale: High-pressure tubing instead of flexible intravenous tubing is necessary to withstand the external pressure exerted by the sleeve and to decrease the distortion of the waveform. The nurse should find out which type of tubing was used.

Cognitive level: Analysis

Nursing process: Assessment

Client needs: Physiological Integrity: Physiological Adaptation

3. Answer: 4. Advance the catheter into the pulmonary artery.

Rationale: This patient is having a pulmonary artery catheter placed. As the pulmonary artery catheter passes through the right ventricle, the tip of the catheter can irritate the ventricle. Patients may exhibit premature ventricular contractions. This rhythm usually ceases when the catheter is advanced into the pulmonary artery or withdrawn from the right ventricle.

Cognitive level: Analysis

Nursing process: Implementation

Client needs: Physiological Integrity: Physiological Adaptation

4. Answer: 4. Compare the result with other measurements.

Rationale: A venous pressure of 2 to 6 mmHg is adequate; however, patients may be hemodynamically stable or unstable with lower or higher pressures. Monitoring the trend in pressure readings, either increasing or decreasing, is of more importance than one observed value. The findings should also be correlated with a patient assessment.

Cognitive level: Application

Nursing process: Assessment

Client needs: Physiological Integrity: Physiological Adaptation

5. Answer: 2. Eliminate any values that differ by 10%.

Rationale: When using the thermodilution method of obtaining a cardiac output, a specified amount of solution, typically 5 to 10 mL, is injected through the proximal injectate port of the PA catheter. This process is commonly referred to as "shooting" a cardiac output. The injectate should be at room temperature when it enters the right atrium and mixes with blood. The cardiac output computer calculates the time required for the solution of a different temperature to reach the thermistor, located at the end of the catheter in the pulmonary artery. The change of temperature occurs over time to produce a cardiac output curve. Hesitation or starting

and stopping during a CO injection would yield an invalid curve. The injectate should be injected smoothly and in less than 4 seconds. Injecting less than or greater than the recommended amount of injectate invalidates the measurement. Any cardiac output value that is questionable based on the curve or two CO measurements that differ by 10% should be discarded.

Cognitive level: Analysis

Nursing process: Evaluation

Client needs: Physiological Integrity: Physiological Adaptation

6. Answer: 1. Fluid volume overload or ventricular failure

Rationale: Excess preload may indicate hypervolemia or ventricular failure. Excessive circulating volume strains the heart and compromises adequate tissue oxygenation. Excess preload increases the workload of the heart and increases myocardial oxygen demands. Diuretics and venodilators are ordered if the cause is hypervolemia. If patients do not respond to diuretic therapy or renal failure is diagnosed, then continuous renal replacement therapy utilizing ultrafiltration or dialysis may be considered. If ventricular failure is determined to be the cause, inotropic medications are prescribed.

Cognitive level: Analysis

Nursing process: Assessment

Client needs: Physiological Integrity: Physiological Adaptation

7. Answer: 4. Closure of the pulmonic valve

Rationale: As the pulmonary artery catheter enters the right atrium, the waveform appears similar to a central venous pressure waveform: the *a* wave correlates with the P wave or atrial contraction (systole); the *c* wave may not be visible on the tracing and reflects retrograde swelling of the tricuspid valve into the right atrium, which occurs during ventricular contraction; and the *v* wave represents atrial diastole and the increased pressure against the closed tricuspid valve in early diastole. As the catheter enters the pulmonary artery, the waveform resembles an arterial pressure waveform with not only systolic and diastolic pressures but also a dicrotic notch. The dicrotic notch represents closure of the pulmonic valve.

Cognitive level: Analysis

Nursing process: Assessment

Client needs: Physiological Integrity: Physiological Adaptation

Chapter 25

1. Answer: 1. Reduce allergic reactions to medications or to latex.

Rationale: Allergies and allergic reactions to medications, chemicals, and foods must always be identified and prominently displayed on the patient's wristband, in the chart, and in the medication record. Patients with histories of allergic reactions have a greater risk of hypersensitivity to anesthesia, so the type of allergic reaction is very important. They also are much more likely to develop latex allergies.

Cognitive level: Application

Nursing process: Planning

Client needs: Physiological Integrity: Reduction of Risk Potential

2. Answer: 3. Antibiotic prophylaxis

Rationale: Patients with valvular disorders may require antibiotic prophylaxis to reduce the risk of bacterial endocarditis. Monitoring fluid and electrolyte status and a BNP level would be indicated for a patient with heart failure.

Cognitive level: Application

Nursing process: Planning

Client needs: Physiological Integrity: Reduction of Risk Potential

3. Answer: 2. Stop all NSAIDs 2 weeks before the scheduled surgery.

Rationale: NSAIDs increase the risk of intraoperative and postoperative bleeding. Aspirin inhibits platelet aggregation and the effect lasts the duration of the thrombocyte life span, 7 to 10 days. Preoperative arterial blood gas and recent hemoglobin A1c level are not indicated for this patient. Routine preoperative electrocardiograms are needed for patients over the age of 55.

Cognitive level: Analysis

Nursing process: Planning

Client needs: Physiological Integrity: Reduction of Risk Potential

4. Answer: 1. Encourage deep breathing and coughing

Rationale: To reduce the risk of pulmonary complications, the patient should be instructed and encouraged to breathe deeply and to cough. Monitoring of oxygen saturation levels would be indicated for a cardiovascular complication. Monitoring intake and output would be indicated for cardiovascular and genitourinary complications. Aspiration precautions would be indicated for a gastrointestinal complication.

Cognitive level: Analysis

Nursing process: Planning

Client needs: Physiological Integrity: Reduction of Risk Potential

5. Answer: 2. Can you explain to me what you mean by cauterized?

Rationale: Preoperative teaching is best accomplished in a calm, quiet, and private environment that facilitates discussion and questions and reduces the patient's anxiety or embarrassment. The nurse needs to be sensitive to the patient's level of anxiety, the patient's ability to understand instructions and express himself, and to cultural issues. Written instructions are important for reinforcing teaching and serving as a reference. When written instructions are given to patients, they should avoid medical jargon, be written at a level that is easy to understand, and be available in various languages. The nurse assesses whether or not a patient is literate in English or in another language before giving written instructions.

Cognitive level: Application

Nursing process: Implementation

Client needs: Physiological Integrity: Basic Care and Comfort

6. Answer: 2. Assess the patient's understanding of the procedure to supplement any areas not reviewed through the Internet.

Rationale: The use of the Internet has altered the amount and focus of preoperative teaching. It may also affect the type and amount of information desired. The best approach for the nurse to take would be to assess the patient's understanding of the procedure and to supplement any areas not reviewed through the Internet. Documenting that the patient had preoperative teaching through the Internet might be appropriate, however the nurse should do more. The nurse should not end the preoperative teaching session or leave the patient with instructions to call the nurse in case of questions.

Cognitive level: Analysis

Nursing process: Implementation

Client needs: Physiological Integrity: Reduction of Risk Potential

Chapter 26

1. Answer: 3. Conduct an interview.

Rationale: Preoperative holding is a semirestricted area usually just inside of the surgical area. This area provides a quiet, calm transition area for the patient to wait immediately before surgery. It provides a shield from the sights and sounds of the busy surgical suite and allows personnel to interview the patient and verify the documentation. Inspecting and ensuring the correct operation of surgical instruments is done in the surgical suite. Inserting an indwelling urinary catheter would be done after anesthesia has been provided to the patient, within the surgical suite.

Cognitive level: Application

Nursing process: Implementation

Client needs: Physiological Integrity: Reduction of Risk Potential

2. Answer: 4. Collaborating with the surgeon and suturing the wound closed

Rationale: The RNFA collaborates with the surgeon and performs the role of first assistant during the operation. This role includes handling tissue, providing exposure, using instruments, suturing the wound closed, and providing hemostasis. The anesthesia care provider administers anesthetic agents. Serving as the patient advocate is the role of the circulating nurse. Providing the surgeon with instruments is a role of the scrub nurse.

Cognitive level: Analysis

Nursing process: Implementation

Client needs: Physiological Integrity: Physiological Adaptation

3. Answer: 2. Anesthesiologist

Rationale: The anesthesiologist is the health care provider who is responsible for maintaining the patient's airway; monitoring and ensuring gas exchanges, respiration, and circulation; estimating and replacing blood and fluid losses; administering medications to maintain hemodynamic stability; managing care in the event of a physiological crisis; and constantly communicating with the surgical and nursing team.

Cognitive level: Application

Nursing process: Implementation

Client needs: Physiological Integrity: Physiological Adaptation

4. Answer: 4. Stop all preparations until it can be verified which knee is the site of surgery.

Rationale: According to the AORN and American College of Surgeons guidelines, if any verification process fails to identify the correct site, all activities should be halted until verification is accurate.

Cognitive level: Application

Nursing process: Planning

Client needs: Physiological Integrity: Reduction of Risk Potential

5. Answer: 2. Examine the leg for possible injury or extent of injury and document the event.

Rationale: The most important role of the perioperative nurse is that of patient advocate. Protecting patients from harm is the essence of the advocacy role of nurses, and it is a critical component for patients whose family members are not readily accessible and whose only possible advocate is the nurse. The essence of the advocacy in the perioperative role is defined as protection, giving a voice, providing comfort, and caring. The nurse should examine the leg for injury and document the event.

Cognitive level: Analysis

Nursing process: Implementation

Client needs: Physiological Integrity: Reduction of Risk Potential

6. Answer: 2. Stop the surgery or deepen the anesthesia.

Rationale: Malignant hyperthermia is an emergency. The surgery should be stopped or the anesthesia deepened. The agent responsible for the hyperthermia should be stopped. Once stabilized, the patient should be transferred to the ICU for postoperative care. Calcium channel blockers should not be administered. One hundred percent oxygen should be delivered to the patient.

Cognitive level: Analysis

Nursing process: Implementation

Client needs: Physiological Integrity: Physiological Adaptation

7. Answer: 4. Respiratory therapist

Rationale: The anesthesiologist heads the anesthesia team and might be assisted by a respiratory therapist, by an anesthesia resident or fellow in a university teaching hospital, or by a certified registered nurse anesthetist (CRNA). The CRNA is an advance practice nurse, educated with a master's degree from an accredited nurse anesthesia educational program. CRNAs administer anesthesia and anesthesia-related care and work under the supervision of the anesthesiologist. The scrub nurse would not be working with the patient's oxygen. The RN first assistant would be assisting the surgeon.

Cognitive level: Analysis

Nursing process: Implementation

Client needs: Physiological Integrity: Reduction of Risk Potential

Chapter 27

1. Answer: 1. Bleeding

Rationale: In the patient who is bleeding postoperatively, initially the heart rate increases in an attempt to maintain a normal cardiac output and blood pressure; thus, it is an early sign of bleeding.

Cognitive level: Analysis

Nursing process: Assessment

Client needs: Physiological Integrity: Physiological Adaptation

2. Answer: 2. Easily arousable and moving all four extremities

Rationale: These activities support the second phase of postanesthesia, which begins when the patient is more alert and functional. The use of an oral airway to maintain an airway would not indicate the patient is ready to be discharged to another inpatient care area. Reduced or lack of motor response of the lower extremities after spinal anesthesia would indicate that the patient has not yet recovered from the anesthesia and should not be transferred to another care area at this time. It would be best to help control the vomiting before transferring the patient to another care area.

Cognitive level: Analysis

Nursing process: Planning

Client needs: Physiological Integrity: Reduction of Risk Potential

3. Answer: 3. Ambulate three times a day.

Rationale: Abdominal distention or a postoperative ileus is common with bowel surgery, anesthesia, narcotics, and decreased mobility. The patient should be kept NPO until flatus returns. If vomiting, the patient should have a nasogastric tube placed and put to suction. The patient should also be ambulated three times a day. The patient should not be given a full diet, should not be placed on a fluid restriction, and should not receive an antiemetic.

Cognitive level: Application

Nursing process: Implementation

Client needs: Physiological Integrity: Physiological Adaptation

4. Answer: 2. Keep the wound open to air and permit the Steri-Strips to fall off on their own.

Rationale: It is theorized that postoperative recovery includes four dimensions: physiological recovery, marked by a return of bodily functions; psychological recovery, a return of well-being; social recovery, a return to social activities and independence; and habitual recovery, a point at which the person returns to a full range of normal activities. Patients need to know that recovery takes time. Staples and sutures are often removed 7 to 10 days after the surgery in a follow-up appointment with the nurse or health care provider. If Steri-Strips cover the wound, they are left in place until they fall off naturally.

Cognitive level: Application

Nursing process: Implementation

Client needs: Physiological Integrity: Reduction of Risk Potential

5. Answer: 3. Nurse's ability to manage postoperative pain

Rationale: A study that looks at nurses' ability to manage postoperative pain would provide a basis for understanding how nurses develop clinical judgment. Factors that influence anxiety levels in the older surgical patient would be a topic of study about the psychological well-being of postoperative patients. Strategies to increase the patient's ability to manage symptoms at home and adjustment of discharge teaching to accommodate cultural differences are both topics of study about how to increase patients' competence in managing their own recovery.

Cognitive level: Analysis

Nursing process: Planning

Client needs: Physiological Integrity: Reduction of Risk Potential

Chapter 28

1. Answer: 1. Central nervous system

Rationale: Neuroglia comprise a major cellular component of the nervous system. Neuroglia do not directly transmit information. There are three main types of neuroglia: oligodendrocytes, astrocytes, and microglia. Oligodendrocytes form the myelin sheath covering many neuronal axons. Multiple sclerosis is a disorder that affects the myelin sheath.

Cognitive level: Analysis

Nursing process: Implementation

Client needs: Physiological Adaptation: Reduction of Risk Potential

2. Answer: 3. Medication history

Rationale: The presenting problem is the reason the individual is seeking care. The presenting problem is followed by the history of the present problem. The nurse should begin with the initial presentation of the symptom and proceed to the present. The medication history should include all medications the patient currently is taking or historically has taken. Herbal, over-the-counter, home remedies, and supplements need to be listed as well as prescribed medications. The past medical history includes major illnesses, including all hospitalizations, surgeries, ambulatory procedures, and both acute and chronic illnesses. In addition, childhood diseases, immunizations, medications, and allergies are explored.

Cognitive level: Application

Nursing process: Assessment

Client needs: Physiological Adaptation: Reduction of Risk Potential

3. Answer: 3. Spinal accessory

Rationale: The spinal accessory nerve has motor function only. This nerve innervates the sternocleidomastoid and trapezius muscles. Damage to this nerve can result in impaired strength in lifting the shoulders, or difficulty in turning the head to either side. The vagus nerve controls swallowing and speaking by innervating the larynx and pharynx. The hypoglossal nerve innervates the tongue. The facial nerve has a sensory and motor function. The facial nerve innervates the sense of taste in the anterior two-thirds of the tongue and the motor functioning of the face.

Cognitive level: Application

Nursing process: Assessment

Client needs: Physiological Adaptation: Reduction of Risk Potential

4. Answer: 1. Level of consciousness

Rationale: The mental status examination assesses the higher cortical functions of thinking and reasoning as well as level of consciousness, orientation, speech and language, memory, attention, fund of knowledge, and abstraction. The Glasgow Coma Scale is the most widely recognized level of consciousness assessment tool and is commonly used in emergency departments, trauma units, and intensive care areas. This tool evaluates three areas: eye opening, verbal response, and best motor response.

Cognitive level: Application

Nursing process: Assessment

Client needs: Physiological Adaptation: Reduction of Risk Potential

5. Answer: 3. Normal

Rationale: Reflexes are graded from 0 to +4. A 0 means there is no muscle reflex response. A +1 indicates a diminished response. A +2 is indicative of a normal reflex response. A +3 is more brisk but can be normal for the patient. A +4 indicates hyperactivity and possibly the presence of disease.

Cognitive level: Analysis

Nursing process: Assessment

Client needs: Physiological Adaptation: Reduction of Risk Potential

6. Answer: 2. Handle of the reflex hammer

Rationale: The Babinski reflex is tested by using a moderately sharp object, such as the handle of a percussion hammer, and stroking the lateral aspect of the sole of the foot from the heel to the ball of the foot, curving medially across the ball. The rubber triangle end of the reflex hammer is used to assess the four major reflex areas. A safety pin is not used to assess reflexes. A cotton swab is used to assess a corneal reflex.

Cognitive level: Application

Nursing process: Planning

Client needs: Physiological Adaptation: Reduction of Risk Potential

7. Answer: 4. Nothing; this can be a normal finding.

Rationale: When assessing cranial nerves III, IV, and VI in an elderly patient, the pupils are generally smaller and reflexes to light and accommodation become slower. This is due to aging changes in the muscles of the pupil sphincter and lens, not neurological changes.

Cognitive level: Analysis

Nursing process: Assessment

Client needs: Physiological Adaptation: Reduction of Risk Potential

Chapter 29

1. Answer: 4. Increasing absorption of CSF
   Rationale: Increased CSF absorption is one mechanism to maintain a constant relationship between the three brain components. Brain tissue does not expand; it is compressed. Autoregulation ensures that the brain receives required sufficient oxygen and glucose to meet metabolic needs; this may be inhibited, but it is not blocked as a normal compensatory mechanism.
   Cognitive level: Application
   Nursing process: Assessment
   Client needs: Physiological Integrity

2. Answer: 3. Complaints of a "different" headache and projectile vomiting
   Rationale: Complaints of a "different" headache and projectile vomiting may be an early indication of increasing ICP. Changes in cranial nerve III, the oculomotor nerve, result in changes in papillary response and are early signs of ICP. Decorticate movements are a late sign. Cushing's triad is a late sign of ICP.
   Cognitive level: Application
   Nursing process: Assessment
   Client needs: Physiological Integrity

3. Answers:
   1. Normocapnia levels ($PaCO_2$ levels of 35–40 mmHg)
   2. Euglycemic levels of 80–120 mg/dL
   3. Normothermia and interventions for body temperatures >99.5°F rectally
   Rationale: Normocapnia levels ($PaCO_2$ levels of 35–40 mmHg) are best for the brain; also good are euglycemic levels of 80–120 mg/dL, because the brain is adversely impacted by both hypoglycemia and hyperglycemia, and normothermia and interventions for body temperatures >99.5°F rectally. Pulse oximetry and supplemental oxygen should be used to maintain saturations of 95% or greater.
   Cognitive level: Analysis
   Nursing process: Assessment
   Client needs: Physiological Integrity

4. Answer: 2. A CAT scan of the head to rule out skull fracture
   Rationale: A CAT scan of the head to rule out skull fracture must be performed before wound closure is undertaken. A complete neurological assessment may indicate symptoms suggestive of a cerebral contusion, but a CAT scan is the diagnostic tool. A cerebral arteriogram is not appropriate in this case because the vessel is outside of the skull. A skull series is used to identify bone placement and continuity and, if a hematoma was suspected, a CAT scan would be the appropriate diagnostic test.
   Cognitive level: Application
   Nursing process: Assessment
   Client needs: Physiological Integrity

5. Answer: 1. In the spinal fluid, protein levels will be high and glucose levels will be low.
   Rationale: With bacterial meningitis, the spinal fluid protein levels will be high and glucose levels will be low. The spinal fluid will be clear in viral meningitis. Option

3 is false. The spinal fluid will be bloody if there has been a bleed within the cranium. If bleeding occurred as a result of the puncture, the fluid would clear.
   Cognitive level: Application
   Nursing process: Application
   Client needs: Physiological Integrity

6. Answer: 3. Benign tumors may be surgically difficult to remove and may compress vital structures.
   Rationale: If the tumor is deep within the brain structure, it may be extremely difficult or impossible to remove surgically. Tumors may not invade surrounding tissue, but their growth will compress them and may interfere with their function. Benign tumors can progress into malignant tumors.
   Cognitive level: Application
   Nursing process: Assessment
   Client needs: Physiological Integrity

7. Answer: 4. A flexible approach due to the changing resistance patterns to specific drugs
   Rationale: Brain tissue has no lymph drainage and this can interfer with clearing drugs and debris. Many chemotherapeutic agents cannot cross the blood–brain barrier. Malignant cells are heterogeneous and their sensitivity to the drugs is variable.
   Cognitive level: Application
   Nursing process: Implementation
   Client needs: Physiological Integrity

8. Answer: 3. Provide answers to questions honestly as they arise, educate them about the treatment plan, and involve them in discussions of the rehabilitation process.
   Rationale: Providing answers to questions honestly as they arise, educating patients and family about the treatment plan, and involving them in discussions of the rehabilitation process is important in keeping families informed and involved and provides as much control as possible and appropriate. The role of the nurse extends beyond teaching about the early detection of cognitive impairment because this would severely limit the family's knowledge and support. The early implementation of rehabilitative therapies does not alter the importance of family teaching. Family teaching should offer encouragement and realistic hope.
   Cognitive level: Application
   Nursing process: Implementation
   Client needs: Physiological Integrity

Chapter 30

1. Answer: 3. The strokes are commonly caused by atherosclerosis.
   Rationale: Eighty percent of all strokes are ischemic in nature and most are caused by atherosclerosis. Hemorrhagic strokes are commonly associated with hypertension. Patients experiencing ischemic strokes are generally older than those experiencing hemorrhagic strokes.
   Cognitive level: Analysis
   Nursing process: Assessment
   Client needs: Physiological Integrity

2. Answers:
   1. Plaque formation that alters the internal diameter of a cerebral artery
   2. Thrombus formation as a result of plaque formation.
   3. Lipohyalinosis, a vascular abnormality, caused by hypertension

   Rationale: Plaque formation that alters the internal diameter in a cerebral artery is a common cause of ischemic stroke. The fragmentation of a clot in the venous system of the leg cannot enter the arterial circulation of the brain unless there is a defect in the heart. The plaque disrupts the integrity of the arterial lining, causing blood to enter the clot and ultimately forming a thrombus. Lipohyalinosis is a process that results in a vascular abnormality in small vessels and is normally associated with hypertension.
   Cognitive level: Application
   Nursing process: Planning
   Client needs: Physiological Integrity

3. Answer: 2. Ischemic cascade further extends the area of infarction.
   Rationale: The ischemic cascade further propagates cerebral edema, cerebral ischemia, cerebral infarction, and cell death. Tissues surrounding the necrotic area have undergone tissue hypoxia and may be viable if perfusion is restored before anoxia occurs. The functional ability of the tissue has not been permanently impaired until cell death occurs. The penumbra is the area surrounding the necrotic core.
   Cognitive level: Application
   Nursing process: Planning
   Client needs: Physiological Integrity

4. Answer: 2. Assessing lung and heart sounds to detect fluid overload
   Rationale: With hypervolemic therapy, plasma expanders may cause pulmonary compromise or congestive heart failure. Cerebral salt wasting is a complication of subarachnoid hemorrhage not associated with vasospasm. The nidus is a concentration of abnormal vessels located at the center of an arteriovenous malformation. Seizures may be generalized or focal depending on the area of the brain involved.
   Cognitive level: Application
   Nursing process: Assessment
   Client needs: Physiological Integrity

5. Answer: 3. Endovascular coiling is associated with the patient being able to return to his activities of normal living and work earlier than patients who had undergone neurosurgical clipping.
   Rationale: Endovascular coiling is associated with a shorter, not longer length of hospital stay. Endovascular coiling, not neurosurgical clipping, is associated with a higher survival and lower morbidity rates 1 year after the procedure. Although the availability of an interventional neuroradiologist is important, if the patient is a candidate for endovascular coiling, this is the option of choice.

Cognitive level: Application
Nursing process: Implementation
Client needs: Physiological Integrity

Chapter 31

1. Answer: 2. Alzheimer's disease
   Rationale: A person with Alzheimer's disease will demonstrate multiple cognitive deficits, including aphasia, apraxia, agnosia, and disturbances with executing functioning. Specific cognitive deficits are not typically seen in multiple sclerosis, Parkinson's disease, or myasthenia gravis.
   Cognitive level: Analysis
   Nursing process: Assessment
   Client needs: Physiological Integrity: Reduction of Risk Potential

2. Answer: 2. Myasthenia gravis
   Rationale: Multiple sclerosis is a neuroimmunologic disease that affects myelin, the protective sheath surrounding nerve fibers. Demyelinating lesions or plaques form along nerve fibers in the brain and spinal cord, producing symptoms related to the location of damage. The brain of a patient with Alzheimer's disease shows a profusion of amyloid plaques and neurofibrillary tangles, which form in the hippocampus and other parts of the brain critical to memory. Myasthenia gravis is a disease of muscle weakness as the result of dysfunction at the neuromuscular junction where the transmission of nerve impulses is blocked. Parkinson's disease is a disease of poor dopamine production, which leads to difficulty with movement, tremor, rigidity, and difficulty maintaining posture.
   Cognitive level: Analysis
   Nursing process: Assessment
   Client needs: Physiological Integrity: Reduction of Risk Potential

3. Answer: 4. Instruct to avoid prolonged exposure to hot temperatures to include showers, baths, and environmental temperatures.
   Rationale: A patient with multiple sclerosis will have episodes of fatigue. Fatigue is exacerbated with exposure to hot temperatures, including showers, baths, and environmental temperatures. The use of assistive devices will decrease fatigue. Voiding patterns will not affect a patient's level of fatigue.
   Cognitive level: Application
   Nursing process: Planning
   Client needs: Physiological Integrity: Reduction of Risk Potential

4. Answer: 2. Increase dietary fiber
   Rationale: Interventions to assist a patient with Parkinson's disease who is experiencing constipation include increasing dietary fluid and fiber and avoiding the use of laxatives. Limiting protein is not recommended to help with constipation. Because protein can interfere with levodopa absorption in a small percentage of patients, patients might be instructed to take levodopa at least 30 minutes before eating or 1 hour after eating.

Cognitive level: Application

Nursing process: Planning

Client needs: Physiological Integrity: Reduction of Risk Potential

5. Answer: 2. Encourage talking about advance directives

Rationale: The physical and mental health of the primary family caregiver is critical to the care of the Alzheimer's patient. One health promotional activity that can optimize both patient and caregiver health is to encourage talking about advance directives for management of advanced stages of AD. Involvement in clinical research studies is often done by patients with Parkinson's disease as a way of advancing science while managing their condition with the latest, most promising treatments. Physical and emotional stress can exacerbate the symptoms of multiple sclerosis, so patients should be instructed to avoid extreme temperatures and exposure to infections. People with ALS do maintain careers and interests; however, referral for psychological and/or spiritual counseling may help the patient and family come to terms with the disease and its prognosis.

Cognitive level: Application

Nursing process: Planning

Client needs: Physiological Integrity: Reduction of Risk Potential

6. Answer: 3. Would you like to talk about things that can help you and your husband?

Rationale: People can live with Parkinson's disease for many years. The chronic and progressive nature of the disease can significantly impact older, spousal caregivers, who may not have the physical strength to handle the weight of a patient with limited mobility. Caregiver stress and burden have been shown to increase as the disease progresses. The nurse should encourage the patient to talk about things that can help both the patient and the husband. Minimizing the patient's concerns would not be an appropriate response. Suggesting the patient discuss the concern with her physician is also not an appropriate response.

Cognitive level: Application

Nursing process: Implementation

Client needs: Physiological Integrity: Reduction of Risk Potential

7. Answer: 4. Impact of meditation and prayer on disease management and experience

Rationale: The impact of meditation and prayer on disease management and experience is a topic that addresses complementary/alternative approaches to neurodegenerative disease processes. Interventions that improve the quality of life focus on quality of life research. Topics about literacy address patient/family education research. Anticipatory grief is a topic within emotional and psychological research.

Cognitive level: Analysis

Nursing process: Planning

Client needs: Physiological Integrity: Basic Care and Comfort

Chapter 32

1. Answer: 4. "A sudden deceleration injury, such as a head-on motor vehicle collision, is frequently the cause of hyperflexion injuries."

Rationale: Hyperextension injuries are caused by a sudden forceful extension of the head and neck, for instance, during a forward fall where the chin or forehead strikes the ground. These injuries can cause spinal ligaments to stretch, can compress the spinal cord, and can fracture the posterior spinous processes, but these injuries usually do not cause dislocations. Axial pressure loaded onto the spine may cause compression injuries, which include vertebral body fractures and spinal cord compression. Rotational injuries are associated with lateral flexion or rotation of the spine, causing posterior ligaments to rupture and facets to dislocate and fracture. Sudden deceleration injury, such as a head-on motor vehicle collision, is often the cause of hyperflexion injuries. These injuries can cause anterior vertebral body fractures and posterior spinal column facet fracture and dislocation.

Cognitive level: Application

Nursing process: Evaluation

Client needs: Safe, Effective Care Environment; Health Promotion and Maintenance; Physiological Integrity

2. Answer: 2. Central cord syndrome

Rationale: Central cord syndrome is often caused by hyperextension injuries, such as a rear-impact motor vehicle collision. This syndrome is caused by central spinal cord damage, which, in turn, causes damage to the more centrally located fibers leading to the upper extremities. The fibers leading to the lower extremities are more laterally located, producing less motor and sensory problems in the lower versus upper extremities. Anterior cord syndrome is caused by direct insult to the anterior portion of the spinal cord. Compression or hyperextension injury may produce this problem, but paralysis and loss of pain and temperature sensations are evident below the level of the injury. Also, light touch, vibration, and proprioception are preserved. Cauda equina syndrome is caused by compression of the lumbar nerve roots below the first lumbar vertebra. The associated signs and symptoms can vary based on the specific nerve root involved, but they often involve motor and sensory loss to the pelvic organs and lower extremities. Brown-Séquard syndrome is usually the result of penetrating trauma that causes hemisection of the spinal cord. The ipsilateral side experiences paralysis and proprioception loss, and the contralateral side experiences pain and temperature sensation loss.

Cognitive level: Analysis

Nursing process: Assessment

Client needs: Physiological Integrity

3. Answer: 3. Use of a reclining wheelchair to gradually progress the patient into an upright position so as not to cause orthostatic hypotension

Rationale: A reclining wheelchair or tilt table gradually places the patient into an upright position, decreasing the development of orthostatic hypotension. The use of an abdominal binder and compression stockings does decrease blood pooling in the peripheral veins, but these interventions are used to help improve venous return to the heart and to prevent orthostatic hypotension as well. A duplex Doppler ultrasound is a highly sensitive screening tool for detecting deep venous thrombosis. It does not dissolve clots. Good nutrition is important is aiding bowel evacuation, but increased caloric, protein, and micronutrient intake is used to aid in wound healing and the promotion of good skin integrity. Increased fiber and fluid intake would help prevent constipation.

Cognitive level: Analysis

Nursing process: Intervention

Client needs: Health Promotion and Maintenance; Physiological Integrity

4. Answer: 1. The patient's family will need ongoing education to help them deal with the stress of any role changes associated with the injury.

Rationale: Role changes within the family are a very real possibility following spinal cord injury, and the family will require ongoing support and education to help deal with this change. Elation and jubilation are not negative emotions; however, patients who experience spinal cord injury often do have negative feelings. They may exhibit denial, anger, grief, hopelessness, and depression. Patients should be encouraged to openly discuss their feelings, but they should also be allowed the opportunity to make their own health care decisions when possible. It is because of the physical challenges caused by the spinal cord injury that the patient usually faces significant psychosocial challenges as well.

Cognitive level: Analysis

Nursing process: Planning

Client needs: Psychosocial integrity

5. Answer: 1. Information regarding support systems that can help the patient and their family adjust to the changes in lifestyle and roles.

Rationale: It is important to put patients and their families in touch with support that can help them cope with the often difficult physical and psychological changes associated with spinal cord injury. Rehabilitative programs that maximize function following spinal cord injury should be multidisciplinary and comprehensive. Infrequent position changes predispose the patient to the development of pressure ulcers, but frequent position changes with good skin care regimens can help with pressure ulcer prevention. Suppository medications, digital bowel stimulation, and disimpaction of stool can aid in the prevention of hyperreflexia.

Cognitive level: Application

Nursing process: Planning

Client needs: Psychosocial Integrity

6. Answer: 4. Ineffective airway clearance related to the loss of spinal innervation of the respiratory and accessory muscles.

Rationale: Airway (with cervical spine immobilization in trauma situations) is always the first priority for any patient. When compared with the other nursing diagnoses listed for this patient, ineffective airway clearance would be the primary diagnosis. *Anxiety* is important and should be attended to, but airway issues should be dealt with first. *Risk for Imbalanced Nutrition* and *Risk for Ineffective Peripheral Tissue Perfusion* are potential problems, and actual problems, such as ineffective airway clearance, should be treated before these other diagnoses are addressed.

Cognitive level: Application

Nursing process: Planning

Client needs: Safe, Effective Care Environment

Chapter 33

1. Answer: 2. Crackles

Rationale: Crackles are sounds caused by fluid in the airways. They are described as intermittent or discontinuous, nonmusical, or popping sounds. They are caused by fluid, inflammation, infection, or secretions. The term *rales* is no longer used to describe fluid effects in the airways. Crackles occur when closed airways snap open during inspiration. Wheezes are high-pitched musical sounds caused by air flowing across strands of mucous, swollen pulmonary tissue that narrows the airway, or from bronchospasm. The term *rhonchi* is no longer used to describe harsh sounds caused by secretions in the airways.

Cognitive level: Application

Nursing process: Assessment

Client needs: Health Promotion and Maintenance: Prevention/Early Detection of Health Problems

2. Answer: 3. It might help to know if there are any recent outbreaks of pulmonary disorders in the area of travel.

Rationale: Area of recent travel may become an important aspect of the history in diagnosing potential respiratory problems. In previous years, the severe acute respiratory syndrome outbreak demonstrated to the world that viral pulmonary disease could be traced to a specific location. Recent travel and area of residence have been demonstrated to be an important factor in the history of respiratory symptoms and should be included in the interview process. The other options would not help in figuring out where the patient might have been exposed to an upper respiratory infection.

Cognitive level: Analysis

Nursing process: Assessment

Client needs: Health Promotion and Maintenance: Prevention/Early Detection of Health Problems

3. Answer: 2. Have you been to any activities or functions around other people with respiratory problems?

Rationale: The social history includes information about the patient's lifestyle and habits that may be relevant to his or her current state of health. Patients who smoke have increased risk for pulmonary disease and patients who have allergies and engage in social activities in the out-of-doors such as golfing may have exacerbations of symptoms after participating in these activities. Also, if patients frequent social events where they may be exposed to people with upper respiratory infections or poor hygienic conditions, they may be predisposed to the development of pulmonary infections. The other choices focus on either the patient's health history, family history, or history of immunizations.

Cognitive level: Application

Nursing process: Assessment

Client needs: Health Promotion and Maintenance: Prevention/Early Detection of Health Problems

4. Answer: 3. Edema indicates heart failure, a common finding in a patient with COPD.

Rationale: Edema of the lower extremities is generally related to right heart or congestive heart failure. Right heart failure and combined left- and right-sided failure are common in patients with COPD. Right-sided failure is caused by pulmonary hypertension. Chronic distention of the lower airways makes forward blood flow more difficult. The right heart hypertrophies in an attempt to increase force of blood through the pulmonary tree. The right heart fails and fluid unable to be accommodated is sequestered in dependent interstitial spaces and causes edema.

Cognitive level: Analysis

Nursing process: Assessment

Client needs: Health Promotion and Maintenance: Prevention/Early Detection of Health Problems

5. Answer: 3. Have an arterial blood gas analysis done to compare the readings.

Rationale: The oxygen saturation measured by infrared technology does not necessarily provide the same values obtained from the calculated oxygen saturation obtained from an ABG. Normal infrared oxygen saturation and ABG saturations range from 95% to 100%. Pulse oximetry probes should not be placed on extremities with automated blood pressure cuffs, hemodialysis fistulas, or arterial lines because these interfere with blood flow. Shock and hypovolemia also cause low-flow states that contribute to inaccurate pulse oximetry readings. Patient movement, ambient light, and venous pulsations may also cause inaccurate readings. If ambient light is interfering with readings (producing results higher than suspected), cover the probe with a towel to see if the result is different. Pulse oximetry does not distinguish methemoglobin or carboxyhemoglobin from oxygen-saturated hemoglobin. Fifty percent carboxyhemoglobin reads as 95%. Patients who have suspected thiocyanate toxicity or inhalation injury should have an ABG analysis to determine respiratory status and oxygen saturation.

Cognitive level: Analysis

Nursing process: Assessment

Client needs: Physiological Integrity: Physiological Adaptation

Chapter 34

1. Answer: 2. Once stable, instruct in the use of a water pik.

Rationale: With mandibular fractures, good oral care is essential for healthy healing and prevention of dental complications. Patient education should include use of the water pik and dietary requirements. The use of systemic antibiotics to prevent meningitis is indicated in the management of temporal bone fractures. The use of eye protection is indicated in the patient with a temporal bone fracture. Facial nerve injury is seen in temporal bone fractures.

Cognitive level: Application

Nursing process: Planning

Client needs: Physiological Integrity: Reduction of Risk Potential

2. Answer: 2. Administer antibiotics as prescribed.

Rationale: Nursing care of the patient relies heavily on assessment of signs and symptoms, which, in turn, is dependent on obtaining a thorough patient history. The history must include the onset and duration of the symptoms including site of pain or discomfort, redness of eyes, flushing of face across the nose, fever, weakness or fatigue, cough, congestion, sore throat, muscle ache, and sore teeth. It also is important to know if any particular event or incident triggered the patient's symptoms. There is no reason to restrict fluids, maintain on bed rest, or consult with a dentist.

Cognitive level: Application

Nursing process: Planning

Client needs: Physiological Integrity: Reduction of Risk Potential

3. Answer: 4. Avoid exposure to strong perfumes, smoke, and rapid changes in temperature.

Rationale: With allergy injections, the dose is gradually increased to a maintenance concentration, which takes about 5 to 6 months. Patients may receive allergy injections for 3 to 5 years, depending on symptoms. The patient should be instructed to stay away from allergens that create a reaction. This means limiting outdoor exposure. Excessive humidity should be reduced and standing water should be removed. The patient should be instructed to eliminate exposure to smoke, strong perfumes and scents, fumes, rapid changes in temperature, and outdoor pollution for patients with nonspecific triggers.

Cognitive level: Application

Nursing process: Planning

Client needs: Health Promotion and Maintenance: Prevention/Early Detection of Health Problems

4. Answer: 1. Presence of smoke detectors in the home and the type of cooking appliances used

Rationale: Caution should be taken to ensure safety around the home. Smoke detectors and electric appliances rather than gas appliances should be used as should technologies that detect the presence of gas fumes in the home.

Cognitive level: Analysis

Nursing process: Assessment

Client needs: Health Promotion and Maintenance: Prevention/Early Detection of Health Problems

5. Answer: 2. Assess the type of difficulty and provide recommendations accordingly.

Rationale: The nursing process guides the management of patients with sleep apnea. The nurse should first assess the patient's description of "difficulty" and then make suggestions accordingly. The nurse should not alter the patient's prescribed treatment without health care provider involvement and should not recommend changing the use of the CPAP machine or not using the device.

Cognitive level: Application

Nursing process: Implementation

Client needs: Health Promotion and Maintenance: Prevention/Early Detection of Health Problems

6. Answer: 2. Smoking is only one cause for the disease. Others include chronic mouth lesions and poor nutrition.

Rationale: A variety of risk factors are associated with head and neck cancer, although some patients do not have any known risk factors; therefore, it is not possible to know for sure how much they contributed to causing the cancer. Some risk factors include alcohol intake, ultraviolet light exposure, tobacco use, mouth irritation, poor nutrition, HPV infection, immune system suppression, male gender, and exposure to Epstein–Barr virus if a first-generation Asian.

Cognitive level: Application

Nursing process: Implementation

Client needs: Psychosocial Integrity: Coping and Adaptation

7. Answer: 4. Secure the tube ties laterally to the chest with suspended ties.

Rationale: Nursing interventions include securing the airway with the appropriate ties in order to prevent the possibility of the tube being dislodged or accidentally removed. The tracheostomy tube ties should be secured to the chest laterally with suspended ties. Circumferential ties can place pressure on the incision lines or reconstruction flaps or grafts. The ties should be changed every day or when soiled to decrease the possibility of infection. The tracheostomy site should be cleaned on a regular basis such as every 8 hours and more frequently as needed to remove crusts and secretions that could obstruct the airway. If the tracheostomy tube has an inner cannula, it should be changed if disposable or cleaned when every tie tracheostomy care procedure is done.

Cognitive level: Application

Nursing process: Implementation

Client needs: Physiological Integrity: Physiological Adaptation

Chapter 35

1. Answer: 2. An acute asthma attack

Rationale: Asthma is a chronic inflammatory disorder of the airways in which many cells and cellular elements play a role, in particular, mast cells, eosinophils, T lymphocytes, macrophages, neutrophils, and epithelial cells. In susceptible individuals, this inflammation causes recurrent episodes of wheezing, breathlessness, chest tightness, and coughing, particularly at night or in the early morning. These episodes usually are associated with widespread but variable airflow obstruction that is often reversible, either spontaneously or with treatment. The inflammation also causes airway hyperresponsiveness or bronchospasm related to a variety of stimuli.

Cognitive level: Analysis

Nursing process: Assessment

Client needs: Physiological Integrity: Physiological Adaptation

2. Answer: 3. Avoid smoking or environments with smoke.

Rationale: The incidence of community-acquired pneumonia is highest in winter months with smoking being an important risk factor. The nurse should emphasize the importance of rest and a gradual increase in activity to avoid fatigue. Instructions should include ways to maintain resistance to infection with proper nutrition and adequate fluid intake. The patient should also be taught about all medications that will be continued at home.

Cognitive level: Application

Nursing process: Planning

Client needs: Physiological Integrity: Physiological Adaptation

3. Answer: 3. Magnesium sulfate

Rationale: Magnesium sulfate is thought to produce bronchodilation through counteraction of calcium-mediated smooth muscle constriction in the patient with COPD. This is given intravenously. Pancreatic enzymes are provided to the patient with cystic fibrosis because of failure of the pancreas to produce these enzymes. Ibuprofen is often used to reduce inflammation in the patient with cystic fibrosis. Pulmozyme decreases sputum viscosity in cystic fibrosis. Its use also has been shown to improve FEV_1 and decrease incidence of exacerbations.

Cognitive level: Application

Nursing process: Planning

Client needs: Physiological Integrity: Physiological Adaptation

4. Answer: 1. Pain management

Rationale: Rib fractures are treated by controlling the patient's pain. Sedation and pain management allow the patient to begin deep breathing and coughing in order to prevent the development of atelectasis, pneumonitis, and hypoxemia. A chest binder may decrease pain on movement. Usually the pain diminishes by the fifth to the seventh day, and healing occurs in 3 to 6 weeks. The nurse emphasizes pain management and gives specific instructions regarding medications for pain until the pain diminishes.

Cognitive level: Analysis

Nursing process: Planning

Client needs: Physiological Integrity: Physiological Adaptation

5. Answer: 4. Pain associated with the primary diagnosis

Rationale: The patient with lung cancer may complain of hoarseness, dysphagia, or vague complaints that have persisted longer than normally expected. Chest pain, tightness, or an ill-defined sensation of fullness may be experienced. This may be accompanied by pleuritic pain on inspiration or a subscapular pain radiating to the arm.

Cognitive level: Analysis

Nursing process: Assessment

Client needs: Physiological Integrity: Physiological Adaptation

6. Answer: 3. Place of employment 10 to 20 years prior to current admission

Rationale: There is a considerable latency period of about 10 to 20 years for asbestosis between exposure and the development of symptomatology. Those at high risk for this disease are asbestos miners, millers, and those employed in the building trade and shipyards, such as loggers, insulation workers, pipe fitters and steamfitters, sheet metal workers, and welders. Working within the roofing materials industry is linked to silicosis.

Cognitive level: Application

Nursing process: Assessment

Client needs: Physiological Integrity: Reduction of Risk Potential

Chapter 36

1. Answer: 1. Oxygen 2 liters nasal cannula

Rationale: Acute respiratory failure results in a failure of oxygenation or ventilation or both. A failure of oxygenation produces hypoxemia, which is defined as a decreased arterial oxygen tension or pressure in the blood below normal range. The administration of oxygen would be the most effective in treating this type of patient. The patient's arterial saturation of oxygen level of less than 90 while breathing room air is representative of hypoxemic respiratory failure. Correcting and treating hypoxia is always a primary goal. Presenting symptoms in acute respiratory failure are shortness of breath, dyspnea, and increased work of breathing with hypoxemia and should always be addressed initially. Educating the patient and family is always important, but addressing the airway is always a priority.

Cognitive level: Application

Nursing process: Implementation

Client needs: Physiological Integrity: Physiological Adaptation

2. Answer: 3. Pulmonary edema

Rationale: The classic clinical presentation of acute pulmonary edema includes rapidly worsening dyspnea, shortness of breath, tachypnea, agitation, increased crackles, and possibly coarse rhonchi in all lung fields. Pink, frothy sputum may also be present. The other clinical signs are hypertension, tachycardia, and possibly S_3 or S_4 heart sounds. The pathophysiology of acute pulmonary edema and the signs and symptoms of this dysfunction are related to the accumulation of fluid, which prevents adequate gas exchange across the alveolar-capillary membrane. Cardiogenic pulmonary edema is pulmonary edema that results from increased hydrostatic pressures in the pulmonary capillary bed secondary to increased pulmonary venous pressure. Noncardiogenic pulmonary edema is related to injury of the alveolar-capillary membrane from numerous causes. Among the most important causes are sepsis, inflammation, inhaled toxins, and drugs. Usually in noncardiogenic pulmonary edema there is no primary cardiac dysfunction.

Cognitive level: Analysis

Nursing process: Assessment

Client needs: Physiological Integrity: Physiological Adaptation

3. Answer: 4. PCWP > 30 mmHg

Rationale: The patient with noncardiogenic pulmonary edema will develop tachycardia, hypertension, bounding pulses, and a drop in PCWP. If the patient's PCWP increases, the health care provider should be notified because this could indicate the development of cardiogenic pulmonary edema where the PCPW > 18 mmHg.

Cognitive level: Application

Nursing process: Assessment

Client needs: Physiological Integrity: Physiological Adaptation

4. Answer: 3. Arterial blood gases showing respiratory acidosis

Rationale: The hypoxemia of a patient with ARDS quickly becomes refractory to standard oxygen therapies, and the patient will require intubation and mechanical ventilation to maintain oxygenation and ventilation. The arterial blood gases frequently demonstrate respiratory acidosis. The chest x-ray exhibits the bilateral patchy infiltrates that are characteristic of the disease instead of the absence of infiltrates. This "white-out" observed on the chest x-ray can cover the entire lung field as the disease progresses. The vital signs are within normal range and will not usually be noted with a patient who has ARDS.

Cognitive level: Application

Nursing process: Assessment

Client needs: Physiological Integrity: Physiological Adaptation

5. Answer: 2. Remove the patient from the ventilator and use the Ambu bag with 100% oxygen.

Rationale: When the patient is experiencing hypoxia, it is imperative that the nurse remove the patient from the mechanical ventilator and administer 100% oxygen until the problem can be detected. Once the oxygenation returns to an acceptable range, the nurse should continue the assessment process. It is also important for the nurse to listen anteriorly and posteriorly in all lung fields. The importance of this exam cannot be overemphasized. When listening, the nurse should compare the right against the left lung and never listen through clothing or other material. The clinician should listen laterally in order to appreciate certain lung segments that can be heard in this position.

Cognitive level: Application

Nursing process: Implementation

Client needs: Physiological Integrity: Physiological Adaptation

6. Answer: 4. When the patient is removed from the ventilator and the Ambu is used it causes overinflation from the Ambu aggressive rates.

Rationale: Most ventilated patients should have PEEP of at least 5 cm of H_2O to prevent the pressure in the alveoli from dropping to zero at the end of expiration. The nurse can cause auto-PEEP with overaggressive rates with an air-mask-bag unit. The patient is removed from the ventilator for transport or for suctioning. Rapid rates are used to bag the patient instead of the rate that was set on the ventilator. The patient might become hypotensive. Treatment would involve disconnecting the patient from the Ambu or ventilator for a few seconds; this would allow the excess pressure to dissipate. PEEP does not have any correlation with hypovolemia.

Cognitive level: Implementation

Nursing process: Assessment

Client needs: Physiological Integrity: Physiological Adaptation

7. Answer: 1. Auscultate lungs for bilateral breath sounds.

Rationale: The nurse as well as other members of the health care team should verify proper placement of the ET tube. The importance of this exam cannot be overemphasized. When listening, the nurse should compare the right against the left lung and never listen through clothing or other material. The clinician should listen laterally in order to appreciate certain lung segments that can be heard in this position. The endotracheal tube being advanced down the right main stem bronchus preventing air form entering the left lung also could cause the absence of lung sounds on the left, so accurate assessment is very important. Securing the ET tube, assessing oxygen saturation, and obtaining a chest x-ray are all important steps that need to be performed after the initial auscultation of breath sounds.

Cognitive level: Application

Nursing process: Implementation

Client needs: Physiological Integrity: Physiological Adaptation

8. Answer: 4. Applying suction when passing the catheter into the patient's tracheostomy

Rationale: To perform tracheostomy suctioning, the nurse or caregiver should use sterile gloves in order to prevent nosocomial infections. The patient should be oxygenated prior to suctioning and the patient's head should be elevated. The patient should always be pre-oxygenated to prevent hypoxemia as well. The nurse/caregiver should never suction going into the tracheostomy, only when withdrawing the catheter.

Cognitive level: Application

Nursing process: Evaluation

Client needs: Physiological Integrity: Physiological Adaptation

9. Answer: 2. A patient with a chest tube on the right side with bubbling in the water seal chamber

Rationale: The nurse should initially see the patient with the chest tube. A pleural tube is inserted in the pleural space in order to evacuate the air or blood and allow the lung to reexpand. The pleural tube re-creates the negative pressure in the chest that has been violated by trauma or surgery. A pleural chest tube should not bubble in the water seal chamber.

Cognitive level: Application

Nursing process: Assessment

Client needs: Physiological Integrity

Chapter 37

1. Answer: 2. Waist circumference is 110 cm.

Rationale: The patient already has two of the criteria for the metabolic syndrome: hypertension and hypertriglyceridemia. The third factor is a waist circumference of greater than 102 cm in males and 88 cm in females. The fasting blood sugar would need to be greater than or equal to 110 mg/dL. The HDL would need to be less than 40 mg/dL in males. Random blood sugars are not part of the criteria for metabolic syndrome.

Cognitive level: Application

Nursing process: Assessment

Client needs: Physiological Integrity: Physiological Adaptation

2. Answer: 4. Decongestants

Rationale: Decongestants cause vasoconstriction and can contribute to hypertension and cardiac arrhythmias. The other medications would not present a cardiac risk.

Cognitive level: Application

Nursing process: Assessment

Client needs: Physiological Integrity: Physiological Adaptation

3. Answer: 2. "How many pillows do you sleep on?"

Rationale: The degree of orthopnea is best measured by the number of pillows that are needed to help the patient breathe comfortably. Frequency of waking up could be caused by many factors and is not specific to orthopnea. Palpitations can occur for many reasons or even be normal and do not correlate with orthopnea. Nocturia may indicate congestive heart failure, but does not correlate with a diagnosis of orthopnea.

Cognitive level: Application

Nursing process: Assessment

Client needs: Physiological Integrity: Physiological Adaptation

4. Answer: 2. Systolic dysfunction

Rationale: S_3 sounds are a marker of systolic dysfunction. They are heard early during diastole and are associated with ventricular dysfunction. S_4 sounds are indicative of diastolic dysfunction. Conduction defects are not heard as heart sounds. Alterations in the mitral valve are heard as abnormal S_1 sounds.

Cognitive level: Application

Nursing process: Assessment

Client needs: Physiological Integrity: Physiological Adaptation

Chapter 38

1. Answer: 2. QRS complex 0.10 second

Rationale: The following criteria must be present to be a normal electrocardiogram: P wave has a normal and

consistent shape and appears before every QRS complex; there is a 1:1 ratio of P wave to QRS complex; PR interval is between 0.12 and 0.20 second; QRS complex is between 0.06 and 0.12 second; QT interval is between 0.34 and 0.43 second; atrial and ventricular rate is between 60 and 100 beats per minute; and atrial and ventricular rhythm is regular.
Cognitive level: Analysis
Nursing process: Assessment
Client needs: Physiological Integrity: Reduction of Risk Potential

2. Answer: 3. 0.12 second
Rationale: Each "small box" is 0.04 second. This patient's QRS complex should be documented as being 0.12 second.
Cognitive level: Application
Nursing process: Assessment
Client needs: Physiological Integrity: Reduction of Risk Potential

3. Answer: 2. Observe and treat the patient for anxiety.
Rationale: This patient is demonstrating premature atrial contractions (PACs) that started after learning of a stressful and/or anxiety-producing event. This patient should be observed for the frequency of the PACs and the anxiety should be treated. Cardioversion is a treatment for atrial flutter. Calcium channel blockers are used with atrial fibrillation. Carotid artery massage is a treatment used for supraventricular tachycardia.
Cognitive level: Analysis
Nursing process: Planning
Client needs: Physiological Integrity: Physiological Adaptation

4. Answer: 1. Have a serum digoxin level drawn.
Rationale: Because some prescribed medications, such as digoxin, cause significant dysrhythmias, the patient's medical history should be reviewed to determine if the dysrhythmia is medication related. Serum drug levels should be ordered as indicated. ACLS protocols would be indicated in some cases of ventricular dysrhythmias. Magnesium is the treatment of choice for torsade de pointes. Lidocaine is used in the treatment of premature ventricular contractions.
Cognitive level: Analysis
Nursing process: Planning
Client needs: Physiological Integrity: Physiological Adaptation

Chapter 39

1. Answer: 4. False positive
Rationale: Sensitivity describes the ability of a test to identify patients with disease. It may be calculated by dividing the number of true positive tests by the sum of true positives plus false negatives. For example, positive tests in subjects with coronary disease are "true positives," whereas negative tests are "false negatives." Similarly, negative tests in patients who are free of disease are "true negatives," and positive tests in patients without disease are "false positives."

Cognitive level: Application
Nursing process: Implementation
Client needs: Health Promotion and Maintenance: Prevention/Early Detection of Health Problems

2. Answer: 4. Echocardiogram
Rationale: With an echocardiogram, hemodynamic data include the amount and speed of blood flow through the valves, enabling the noninvasive detection and follow-up of stenotic or regurgitant heart valves. TEE is frequently used to detect and assess endocarditis, aortic dissection, intracardiac masses such as thrombi or tumors, valvular pathology, and congenital disorders in both children and adults. MRI can be used to evaluate patients with presumed congenital heart diseases, such as coarctation of the aorta or atrial septal defects. PET scan is the current "gold standard" for assessment of myocardial viability.
Cognitive level: Application
Nursing process: Planning
Client needs: Health Promotion and Maintenance: Prevention/Early Detection of Health Problems

3. Answer: 2. Provide intravenous normal saline prior to the procedure.
Rationale: Patients with preexisting renal failure and a history of anaphylactic reaction to contrast dye must be pretreated before the catheterization. Pretreatment for the patient with a history of anaphylactic reaction to contrast dye includes antihistamines and steroids. In the laboratory the patient will usually be given a mild sedative. Patients with renal failure (serum creatinine ≤1.5 mg/dL) should receive intravenous normal saline for several hours before the procedure.
Cognitive level: Application
Nursing process: Planning
Client needs: Physiological Integrity: Reduction of Risk Potential

4. Answer: 4. Stress test
Rationale: A stress test is contraindicated for myocardial infarction within 2 days, unstable angina, aortic stenosis, uncontrolled dysrhythmias, symptomatic heart failure, active endocarditis, uncontrolled hypertension, any acute disorder that may affect exercise, and the inability to obtain informed consent. The ECG is helpful in determining the overall electrical functioning of the patient's heart. The echocardiogram is useful to determining the patient's ejection fraction in addition to the functioning of other cardiac structures. The PCI can be done to prevent further myocardial damage.
Cognitive level: Analysis
Nursing process: Planning
Client needs: Physiological Integrity: Reduction of Risk Potential

5. Answer: 3. Assess the femoral site.
Rationale: All patients must have a complete nursing assessment, with special emphasis on the cardiovascular system including peripheral pulses and the vascular access site. This assessment includes vital signs, ECG monitoring, and assessment of the vascular access site

and pulses distal to the puncture site. Evaluation of the access site includes inspection for any signs of bleeding or swelling and palpation for any tenderness. Diagnosis of suspected arterial injuries is made through a careful physical assessment, and confirmed through noninvasive vascular studies or arteriography. Physical examination of the femoral site is performed assessing for the presence of localized tenderness, bruits, or a pulsatile mass. Hematomas are identified by swelling at the site of the arterial puncture. Large hematomas may need to be assessed by ultrasound to rule out the presence of pseudoaneurysms or arteriovenous fistulas.

Cognitive level: Application

Nursing process: Assessment

Client needs: Physiological Integrity: Reduction of Risk Potential

Chapter 40

1. Answer: 4. "My father died of a heart attack at age 70."

   Rationale: Genetics, sex, and age are nonmodifiable risk factors, or those that cannot be changed. Smoking, hypertension, diabetes, obesity, and a sedentary lifestyle are modifiable risk factors. The patient's smoking and high blood sugars reflect modifiable risk factors. Walking provides exercise to modify the risk factor of a sedentary lifestyle.

   Cognitive level: Application

   Nursing process: Assessment

   Client needs: Physiological Integrity: Reduction of Risk Potential

2. Answer: 3. "Was your pain precipitated by activity?"

   Rationale: Stable angina is frequently precipitated by activity, emotional stress, cold weather, or large meals. Pain lasting 15 minutes would be indicative of a myocardial infarction; angina pain usually lasts 5 to 10 minutes. Anginal pain radiates to the jaw, but not always.

   Cognitive level: Application

   Nursing process: Implementation

   Client needs: Physiological Integrity: Physiological Adaptation

3. Answer: 1. The pain was relieved by taking nitroglycerin.

   Rationale: The three key characteristics of typical angina include pain, pressure, tightness, or heaviness that is substernal, central chest, or in the left arm that is provoked by exertion or emotional stress and that is relieved by nitroglycerin. Angina may be precipitated by eating a large meal, but relief with nitroglycerin provides stronger support for a diagnosis of typical angina. Angina may also cause anxiety and dizziness, but again, these do not provide the best support.

   Cognitive level: Application

   Nursing process: Assessment

   Client needs: Physiological Integrity: Physiological Adaptation

4. Answer: 4. Transmural ischemia

   Rationale: When ischemia traverses the entire width of cardiac muscle, it is called transmural and the ST segment is elevated. The more leads in which the ST segment is elevated indicate greater damage. Mild ischemia of subendocardial injury would be reflected as ST segment depression. Past myocardial infarction damage is diagnosed by the presence of a Q wave.

   Cognitive level: Analysis

   Nursing process: Assessment

   Client needs: Physiological Integrity: Physiological Adaptation

5. Answer: 1. Occurrence of an old myocardial infarction

   Rationale: An old MI is diagnosed when a Q wave is present in the absence of ST elevation, patient symptoms, and blood markers. The Q-wave changes are due to necrosis and are irreversible, so they allow for identification of MIs. They cannot determine how long ago the necrosis occurred, so it would not be safe to conclude the damage was recent. Q waves do not reflect pacemaker function or ventricular hypertrophy.

   Cognitive level: Analysis

   Nursing process: Assessment

   Client needs: Physiological Integrity: Physiological Adaptation

6. Answer: 1. Troponin 1 levels

   Rationale: Troponin 1 levels are specific to cardiac muscle and are released from the myocardial cell within 3 to 12 hours of cellular injury and may stay elevated for 5 to 14 days. Myoglobin levels are not a specific indicator of heart damage and only stay elevated for 24 hours. C-reactive protein is also not specific to cardiac muscle. CK-MB levels are specific to myocardial tissue, but return to normal within 72 hours.

   Cognitive level: Application

   Nursing process: Assessment

   Client needs: Physiological Integrity: Physiological Adaptation

7. Answer: 2. Cardiogenic shock

   Rationale: Cardiogenic shock is an acute condition that must be detected and treated immediately to improve survival. An infarction of greater than 40% of the left ventricle and three-vessel disease place the patient at greater risk to develop cardiogenic shock. Pericarditis is associated with large infarctions and low ejection fractions but is not the highest priority. Dressler's syndrome is indicative of pericarditis that occurs 2 to 12 weeks following an MI. PVCs can occur following any cardiac ischemic event, but are not the highest priority.

   Cognitive level: Analysis

   Nursing process: Planning

   Client needs: Physiological Integrity: Physiological Adaptation

8. Answer: 3. Significant stenosis of the left anterior descending, LAD, and circumflex artery

   Rationale: Class I recommendations indicate a CABG is indicated when the patient has significant stenosis of the proximal LAD and left circumflex artery even though the patient is asymptomatic. A 50% occlusion of the circumflex artery is not part of the criteria. Recent history of angina and heart failure are also not qualifying criteria.

Cognitive level: Application
Nursing process: Assessment
Client needs: Physiological Integrity: Physiological Adaptation

9. Answer: 4. Report the findings to the primary care provider.

Rationale: An output of greater than 100 mL/hr reflects postoperative bleeding and should be reported. Output should continued to be monitored but is not the first priority. Having the patient cough and deep breathe does not address the problem of bleeding. Although the chest tube dressing should be checked, the chest tube output reflects internal bleeding and must be reported immediately.

Cognitive level: Analysis
Nursing process: Implementation
Client needs: Physiological Integrity: Physiological Adaptation

Chapter 41

1. Answer: 3. Mitral stenosis

Rationale: Rheumatic fever produces an inflammatory process that often causes valvular heart damage, leading to stenosis of heart valves. Pericarditis and endocarditis may be experienced during the initial inflammatory process, but should not persist after treatment is done. Pulmonary fibrosis is not caused by rheumatic fever.

Cognitive level: Application
Nursing process: Planning
Client needs: Physiological Integrity: Physiological Adaptation

2. Answer: 2. "I had rheumatic heart disease when I was a child."

Rationale: Aortic stenosis is often caused by rheumatic heart disease, which destroys valve leaflets with calcification and fibrosis, which leads to the stenosis. As the narrowing of the valve increases, clinical manifestations are exhibited; dyspnea is the most frequent complaint and is often accompanied by angina and exertional syncope. Having had a CABG or having a dysrhythmia are not contributing factors for aortic stenosis. Palpitations are associated with mitral valve prolapse and stenosis or aortic regurgitation.

Cognitive level: Application
Nursing process: Assessment
Client needs: Physiological Integrity: Physiological Adaptation

3. Answer: 2. Plan for rest periods throughout the day.

Rationale: Excessive exercise and exertion place demands for increased circulation and oxygen to the heart. Allowing time for rest reduces the workload and therefore oxygen demands on the heart. The valve may not need to be replaced; the patient should be taught to take prophylactic antibiotics before dental work, but not to avoid dental work. An elevated temperature could be a sign of endocarditis, but it is not necessary to take the temperature daily. A diet high in fatty foods should be avoided, but it is not necessary to keep a food diet.

Cognitive level: Application

Nursing process: Implementation
Client needs: Physiological Integrity: Physiological Adaptation

4. Answer: 3. The valve will be repaired, but not replaced.

Rationale: An open procedure involves surgical repair under general anesthesia and cardiopulmonary bypass. Valvuloplasty involves repair of the torn or damaged leaflets, chordae tendineae, or papillary muscle, but the valve is not replaced. Anticoagulation therapy will be needed in the postoperative period to prevent thrombus formation at the surgical site. A valvuloplasty does not guarantee that future repairs or valve replacement will not be necessary.

Cognitive level: Application
Nursing process: Implementation
Client needs: Physiological Integrity: Physiological Adaptation

5. Answer: 4. Supportive therapy with medications

Rationale: Because the prognosis for this type of cardiomyopathy is poor, management is focused at reducing the workload of the heart and diminishing heart failure with use of diuretics, calcium channel blockers, beta-blockers, and antiarrhythmic medications. Alcohol ablation and ICDs are sometimes used in the treatment of hypertrophic cardiomyopathy. Aortic valve repair is not indicated for treatment.

Cognitive level: Application
Nursing process: Planning
Client needs: Physiological Integrity: Physiological Adaptation

6. Answer: 3. "Does the pain become worse if you take a deep breath?"

Rationale: Chest pain associated with pericarditis is often described as sharp and gets worse with deep breathing; it is relieved by sitting up. Anginal pain is not associated with position changes or deep breathing. It is relieved by sitting up, not lying flat. Pericarditis does not occur at any particular time of day and is not associated with palpitations.

Cognitive level: Application
Nursing process: Implementation
Client needs: Physiological Integrity: Physiological Adaptation

Chapter 42

1. Answer: 3. Aortic stenosis

Rationale: Risk factors for heart failure include a history of hypertension, coronary heart disease, obesity, diabetes, and structural and valvular disorders, such as aortic stenosis. Pancreatitis, chronic fatigue syndrome, and pleural effusions are not risk factors for heart failure.

Cognitive level: Application
Nursing process: Assessment
Client needs: Physiological Integrity: Physiological Adaptation

2. Answer: 1. Decreased cardiac output

Rationale: Systolic dysfunction occurs when the ventricle is unable to contract forcefully during systole and often hypertrophies in an effort to compensate. As a result, the percentage of blood ejected from the heart is decreased. Aortic stenosis and mitral regurgitation may contribute to the development of heart failure and may be manifested by the presence of a murmur. Systolic dysfunction primarily affects cardiac output, not heart rate.

Cognitive level: Application

Nursing process: Assessment

Client needs: Physiological Integrity: Physiological Adaptation

3. Answer: 1. Activation of the sympathetic nervous system, SNS

Rationale: Activation of the SNS and RAS systems occurs when cardiac output falls, in an effort to increase blood volume and rate of heart contractility. The parasympathetic system is not activated because this would further decrease the heart rate. Cytokines are also released, not suppressed.

Cognitive level: Application

Nursing process: Assessment

Client needs: Physiological Integrity: Physiological Adaptation

4. Answer: 3. Dyspnea

Rationale: Dyspnea is seen secondary to pulmonary congestion, which occurs most with left-sided heart failure. Fluid accumulates in the pulmonary bed as it backs up from the left ventricle. Right-sided failure causes venous congestion with fluid accumulation in the interstitial spaces, manifested by weight gain, anorexia, nausea, and peripheral edema.

Cognitive level: Application

Nursing process: Assessment

Client needs: Physiological Integrity: Physiological Adaptation

5. Answer: 1. A diagnosis of heart failure can be excluded.

Rationale: The BNP is very useful in ruling out a diagnosis of heart failure if the level is normal. Elevated levels correlate with heart failure, increased risk of mortality, acute MI, PE, and renal failure. Because they are not elevated, the patient does not have long-standing heart failure, cardiac ischemia. Pulmonary tissue damage would not be diagnosed with BNP levels.

Cognitive level: Application

Nursing process: Evaluation

Client needs: Physiological Integrity: Physiological Adaptation

6. Answer: 1. ACE inhibitors and beta-blockers

Rationale: Treatment of stage B heart failure is aimed at reduction afterload with ACE inhibitors and reduction of workload on the heart with beta-blockers, as well as antihypertensives and diuretics. Insertion of a defibrillator may be done for stage C heart failure. A patient with stage D heart failure may need hospice referral.

Cognitive level: Analysis

Nursing process: Application

Client needs: Physiological Integrity: Physiological Adaptation

7. Answer: 2. Medications, activity, weight, diet, and symptoms

Rationale: The most important key concepts that patients with heart failure should learn to incorporate into their daily lives follow the acronym MAWDS: medication, activity, weight, diet, and symptoms. Although finances, psychosocial concerns, social support, and spirituality are also important, they are not the key issues.

Cognitive level: Application

Nursing process: Implementation

Client needs: Physiological Integrity: Physiological Adaptation

8. Answer: 3. Depression and anemia

Rationale: Depression, anemia, renal insufficiency, hypertension, coronary heart disease, and sleep apnea have all been shown to worsen the prognosis of patients with heart failure. Patients with heart failure usually experience hypertension, not hypovolemic shock. Liver failure and DVTs are not identified as factors that will increase mortality of heart failure.

Cognitive level: Application

Nursing process: Assessment

Client needs: Physiological Integrity: Physiological Adaptation

9. Answer: 2. Plans for treatment in the final stages of heart failure

Rationale: Discussion about the level of care should occur ahead of time, not at the time of crisis. The nurse needs to address issues of patient comfort and dignity during the terminal stage of heart failure. In end-stage disease, a heart transplant and surgical interventions are not options. Long-term home care management may not be an option for the family and patient.

Cognitive level: Application

Nursing process: Planning

Client needs: Physiological Integrity: Physiological Adaptation

Chapter 43

1. Answer: 1. Intermittent claudication

Rationale: The risk factors, similar to those of heart disease and stroke, include cigarette smoking, diabetes, hyperlipidemia, hypertension, elevated C-reactive protein, and hyperhomocysteinemia. Intermittent claudication, or exercise-induced leg pain, is the most common symptom of peripheral arterial disease. This pain can occur in the buttocks, hip, thigh, or calf, depending on the portion of the arterial tree affected by atherosclerotic disease. With exercise, such as walking, metabolic demands are increased, and the diseased arteries are unable to deliver the needed oxygen to the muscles or to dispose of the metabolic by-product lactic acid. The buildup of lactic acid causes pain in the affected muscle group of the leg. When the walking ceases, or shortly afterward, the pain resolves and exercise may resume.

Cognitive level: Application

Nursing process: Assessment

Client needs: Physiological Integrity: Physiological Adaptation

2. Answer: 3. Teach importance of regular and structured ambulation.

Rationale: The patient with impaired mobility would benefit from being taught the importance of regular and structured ambulation to enhance circulation and promote collateral development. The use of moist heat would aid in comfort for a venous occlusion. Legs should be kept in the dependent position to enhance arterial perfusion. Cool skin to the touch is one of the six Ps of arterial ischemia and should be reported to a health care professional immediately.

Cognitive level: Application

Nursing process: Planning

Client needs: Physiological Integrity: Physiological Adaptation

3. Answer: 2. Dress warmly in cold weather and limit alcohol intake.

Rationale: Nonpharmacologic management of Raynaud's disease is directed toward avoiding known stressors; controlling exposure to extremes in climate; dressing warmly in cold weather; and limiting tobacco, caffeine, and alcohol intake. Some patients may benefit from learning relaxation techniques. Regular physical exercise is important because it improves circulation and warms the body temperature. Some medications, such as beta-blockers, ergot alkaloids, and hormones, can precipitate episodes of vasospasm. There is no cure for Buerger's disease. The primary treatment is directed toward smoking cessation and avoidance of secondhand smoke.

Cognitive level: Application

Nursing process: Planning

Client needs: Physiological Integrity: Physiological Adaptation

4. Answer: 4. Renal impairment due to alterations in blood flow

Rationale: Interruption in blood flow may occur with the endovascular stent or the open approach and the nurse would monitor urine output and BUN and serum creatinine levels. If an embolus were to follow this procedure, the legs are the most common site for perfusion problems. The insertion site for the stent is through a femoral stick and not through an abdominal incision. The hospital stay for this procedure is shorter than for the traditional surgical approach.

Cognitive level: Application

Nursing process: Assessment

Client needs: Physiological Integrity: Physiological Adaptation

5. Answer: 1. The need for early ambulation, use of compression stockings, and range-of-motion exercises

Rationale: Early ambulation, use of compression stockings, and performance of range-of-motion exercises are important nursing processes for this patient. Patients with a deep venous thrombosis with arterial involvement may still use carefully applied compression stockings. Patients benefit from early ambulation.

Cognitive level: Application

Nursing process: Implementation

Client needs: Physiological Integrity: Physiological Adaptation

6. Answer: 2. The signs and symptoms of bleeding

Rationale: Avoiding foods high in vitamin K is indicated for warfarin sodium therapy. Having an INR drawn is indicated for warfarin sodium therapy. Unfractionated heparin is preferred for patients with kidney failure. When low molecular weight heparin is being administered, the patient should be instructed on signs and symptoms of bleeding.

Cognitive level: Application

Nursing process: Implementation

Client needs: Physiological Integrity: Pharmacologic and Parenteral Therapies

7. Answer: 2. Compression stockings will be worn to decrease venous stasis.

Rationale: Bed rest is recommended for the first 24 hours following surgery. The patient may shower the next day following the procedure. Anticoagulants are not a part of the treatment for varicose veins unless there is a condition that warrants these medications.

Cognitive level: Application

Nursing process: Planning

Client needs: Physiological Integrity; Physiological Adaptation

8. Answer: 1. If an aortic aneurysm is diagnosed that is larger than 6 centimeters, surgery will be performed.

Rationale: The physician will monitor the growth of an AAA and will surgically correct when it has reached 5.5 centimeters. If a patient is on steroids, they are discontinued if possible in the medical management of this patient. The infrarenal area is the most common site for the development of an AAA and is repaired with either the surgical or endovascular option.

Cognitive level: Analysis

Nursing process: Assessment

Client needs: Physiological Integrity: Physiological Adaptation

Chapter 44

1. Answer: 4. Diverticulitis

Rationale: This pain pattern in the adult is suggestive of diverticulitis. The pain of acute appendicitis is predominantly in the right lower quadrant. Intussusception and pyloric stenosis are not seen in the adult.

Cognitive level: Analysis

Nursing process: Assessment

Client needs: Physiological Integrity: Reduction of Risk Potential

2. Answer: 1. Inspection

Rationale: The correct order for examination is inspection, auscultation, percussion, and palpation. Bowel sounds should be auscultated prior to percussion to avoid changing the frequency or rate. Light palpation in all quadrants precedes deep palpation.

Cognitive level: Application

Nursing process: Assessment

Client needs: Health Promotion and Maintenance: Prevention/Early Detection of Health Problems

3. Answer: 4. A full bladder
   Rationale: Percussing the abdomen will elicit different sounds. There should be a hollow sound, similar to that of tapping on a watermelon, over the epigastric area and sometimes over the bowels. If this hollow sound is throughout the entire abdomen, it is called tympany and is indicative of an obstruction or distention of the abdomen. This sound is produced by air in the intestine. The liver and a full bladder give off a dull sound, similar to that when percussing a piece of meat.
   Cognitive level: Application
   Nursing process: Assessment
   Client needs: Health Promotion and Maintenance: Prevention/Early Detection of Health Problems

4. Answer: 3. Inflammatory process in the abdomen
   Rationale: Rebound tenderness describes pain that is more prominent when pressure is released and is indicative of an inflammatory process in the abdomen. A negative obturator's sign is a normal finding and further testing may be warranted depending on the initial complaint. A positive Murphy's sign is seen in inflammation of the gallbladder.
   Cognitive level: Application
   Nursing process: Assessment
   Client needs: Health Promotion and Maintenance: Prevention/Early Detection of Health Problems

5. Answer: 2. Ask the patient what caused the abdominal scar.
   Rationale: When obtaining a medical history from patients with gastrointestinal symptoms, past surgeries play a major role. It is also important to correlate this information with the physical exam. At times, patients will forget a surgery, especially if it was many years ago. Therefore, correlating the history with the scars on the abdomen is a helpful tool. When doing the abdominal examination, confirm which operation relates to which scar. This can also trigger more information from the patient. Pay particular attention to the area around the umbilicus, because laparoscopic scars are small and can be very faint.
   Cognitive level: Application
   Nursing process: Assessment
   Client needs: Physiological Integrity: Reduction of Risk Potential

Chapter 45

1. Answer: 1. Increased salivation and bad breath
   Rationale: Vincent's stomatitis, also known as acute necrotizing stomatitis or trench mouth, is a bacterial infection characterized by erythematous ulceration and necrosis of the gingival margins, red gingival papilla, a purulent gray exudate, increased salivation, bad breath, bleeding gums, and pain. Painful red maculae with erythematous halos are seen in the early stage of contact stomatitis, and ulcers covered with a grayish membrane develop in the ulcerative phase of contact stomatitis. Curd-like patches on the tongue and cheek are characteristic of oral candidiasis.
   Cognitive level: Application

Nursing process: Assessment
Client needs: Physiological Integrity: Physiological Adaptation

2. Answer: 1. Premalignant tissue in the esophagus
   Rationale: With repeated exposure of erosive stomach contents, an inflammatory response is initiated. When the inflammation becomes chronic, normal squamous epithelial cells are replaced with columnar epithelium. This new epithelium is called Barrett's epithelium and is a premalignant tissue that increases the risk of esophageal cancer. Esophageal strictures and fine tears may occur with achalasia. Ulcers and inflamed tissue are associated with exacerbations of GERD.
   Cognitive level: Application
   Nursing process: Assessment
   Client needs: Physiological Integrity: Physiological Adaptation

3. Answer: 4. Biopsy of the small intestine
   Rationale: A biopsy of the small intestine is considered the gold standard and currently the most definitive test to diagnose celiac disease. Stools are not Gram stained. The antigliadin antibody is a new test being used, but still not the most definitive. Gastric pH analysis is done when diagnosing GERD.
   Cognitive level: Analysis
   Nursing process: Implementation
   Client needs: Physiological Integrity: Physiological Adaptation

4. Answer: 3. Malabsorption of nutrients often occurs.
   Rationale: Malabsorption of nutrients is more specific to Crohn's. The inflamed tissue occurs most frequently in the jejunum and ileum, which impairs absorption of nutrients. In ulcerative colitis the inflammation occurs in the rectum and sigmoid colon. The loss of exudates from ulcerated tissues in Crohn's further leads to protein losses. Loose watery stools can occur with both disorders. Abdominal pain is usually present in both conditions. Rectal urgency and incontinence can also occur with both conditions.
   Cognitive level: Application
   Nursing process: Planning
   Client needs: Physiological Integrity: Physiological Adaptation

5. Answer: 3. Drinks citrus juice with meals
   Rationale: Foods with a high acidic content or that are spicy will reduce the lower esophageal sphincter tone, causing reflux of acidic stomach contents into the esophagus. A BMI of 21 is normal; obesity can contribute to reflux. Patients who are lactose intolerant often experience abdominal cramping and bloating after eating, not heartburn. Eating high-fiber foods does not cause GERD.
   Cognitive level: Application
   Nursing process: Assessment
   Client needs: Physiological Integrity: Physiological Adaptation

6. Answers:
   1. Daily alcohol intake
   2. A history of irritable bowel disease (IBD)

Rationale: Recent research indicates that daily alcohol consumption increases the risk for colon cancer. IBD causes a chronic inflammation of the bowel, leading to local tissue injury and cancer. A high-fat diet, not low-fat, causes increased deposition of fatty acids within cell membranes and increases intestinal prostaglandins, which stimulate cell proliferation, contributing to cancer. Intake of folic acid, selenium, vitamin D, and calcium reduce the risk for colon cancer. Daily use of NSAIDs helps to reduce inflammation, which in turn reduces cancer risk.

Cognitive level: Application

Nursing process: Planning

Client needs: Physiological Integrity: Reduction of Risk Potential

7. Answer: 4. Place the tube at the shoulder level of patient.

Rationale: Placing the tube at shoulder level reduces the pull of gravity and fluid into the port. The port should be open and patent to allow for air inflow. The port should never be irrigated or plugged. Placing the patient in a high Fowler's position will not correct the problem if the tube is also not positioned higher.

Cognitive level: Application

Nursing process: Implementation

Client needs: Physiological Integrity: Reduction of Risk Potential

8. Answer: 1. Check for signs of hypoglycemia 2 hours after a meal.

Rationale: When the hyperosmolar load of a meal is dumped into the jejunum, there is a rapid rise in blood sugar followed by a release of excessive amounts of insulin. The insulin then causes a secondary hypoglycemia about 2 to 3 hours after eating. Patients with dumping syndrome should rest or even lie down if tolerated for 30 minutes after a meal; ambulation would not be encouraged. Liquids should be taken between meals to reduce the load entering the jejunum. The diet should be low in simple carbohydrates; protein and fats will help to slow transit time and reduce symptoms.

Cognitive level: Analysis

Nursing process: Implementation

Client needs: Physiological Integrity: Physiological Adaptation

9. Answer: 1. Beefy red and moist

Rationale: A stoma should be pink or beefy red and moist without obvious cyanosis or bleeding. It should extend about 2 to 3 cm from the abdominal wall. A slightly purple or pale pink color could be indicative of impaired circulation to the stoma.

Cognitive level: Application

Nursing process: Planning

Client needs: Physiological Integrity: Physiological Adaptation

Chapter 46

1. Answer: 3. "Have you ever had a tattoo?"

Rationale: Hepatitis C is found predominantly in blood, blood products, and transplanted tissue and it has been transmitted by percutaneous exposures, such as tattooing, body piercing, barbering, and folk medicine practices. Traveling in areas where hepatitis A is endemic and eating uncooked shellfish are risks for exposure to hepatitis A. Sharing utensils with a person infected with hepatitis A put the person at risk for hepatitis A, not hepatitis C.

Cognitive level: Application

Nursing process: Implementation

Client needs: Physiological Integrity: Physiological Adaptation

2. Answer: 4. Constant epigastric pain

Rationale: The prodromal phase of hepatitis occurs between exposure to the virus and appearance of jaundice. Symptoms are often vague and include anorexia, nausea, vomiting, malaise, arthralgias, and mild, but constant abdominal, RUQ or epigastric pain. Hyperthermia, not hypothermia, would occur. Appetite is decreased, not increased. Dark-colored urine would be seen during the icteric phase, as serum bilirubin levels rise.

Cognitive level: Application

Nursing process: Assessment

Client needs: Physiological Integrity: Physiological Adaptation

3. Answer: 1. Peripheral edema

Rationale: An albumin level of 2.5 g/dL reflects hypoalbuminemia, which causes a decrease in colloidal osmotic pressure, leading to leakage of fluid into the tissues and is manifested as ascites or peripheral edema in cirrhosis. Lack of vitamin K and prothrombin production by the liver would cause prolonged blood coagulation. The liver's inability to conjugate bilirubin properly would lead to jaundice. Vitamin A may not be absorbed when bile is not produced or released into the duodenum, which may be seen with gallbladder disease or advanced cirrhosis.

Cognitive level: Application

Nursing process: Assessment

Client needs: Physiological Integrity: Physiological Adaptation

4. Answer: 2. Oxazepam, Serax

Rationale: Serax is a benzodiazepine that is not metabolized by the liver, but is still used cautiously to treat agitation. Lactulose is an osmotic laxative and is given to treat elevated ammonia levels and constipation. Protonix is a proton pump inhibitor given to reduce gastric acidity. Vitamin K is stored in the liver and is given to aid in blood clotting since it may be deficient in the patient with cirrhosis.

Cognitive level: Application

Nursing process: Implementation

Client needs: Physiological Integrity: Physiological Adaptation

5. Answer: 1. Provide supportive and comfort measures to the patient and family.

Rationale: An elevated AFP level is indicative of advanced hepatocellular carcinoma and rapid tumor growth.

Survival rates are short term and so quality of life should be provided with supportive and comfort measures. A TIPS is done to treat portal hypertension and ascites that has been refractory to treatment. Liver transplants are only indicated for small tumors without evidence of spread. Protein restriction is sometimes ordered to treat hepatic encephalopathy associated with cirrhosis, and salt restriction is indicated when ascites is present.

Cognitive level: Application

Nursing process: Implementation

Client needs: Physiological Integrity: Physiological Adaptation

6. Answer: 3. The patient has had rapid weight loss secondary to crash dieting.

Rationale: Risk factors for developing gallstones include obesity, high estrogen states, diabetes, hyperlipidemia, cirrhosis, Crohn's disease, rapid weight loss, and bariatric surgery. A high-fiber diet helps to utilize bile and cholesterol and would not predispose the patient to stones. Some drugs, such as oral contraceptives, clofibrate, and hormone replacement therapy can increase the risk of gallstones, but not aminoglycosides. Native American people have a higher risk; people of northern European descent are at greater risk for osteoporosis.

Cognitive level: Application

Nursing process: Assessment

Client needs: Physiological Integrity: Reduction of Risk Potential

7. Answer: 3. Examine abdomen for rigidity and tenderness.

Rationale: Increasing abdominal pain and tenderness may be a sign of intra-abdominal leak of bile or blood so the patient should first be assessed for abdominal tenderness and rigidity, since the opioid analgesia should have been effective in relieving postoperative pain. Administering a second dose of analgesia without first further assessing the pain could mask the cause of the pain. Ambulating the patient could be done after it has been determined the cause of pain is not peritonitis. A side-lying fetal position is helpful for patients with acute pancreatitis.

Cognitive level: Analysis

Nursing process: Implementation

Client needs: Physiological Integrity: Reduction of Risk Potential

8. Answer: 2. Amylase level is normal.

Rationale: In chronic pancreatitis, amylase levels are not always elevated, whereas amylase is usually always elevated with acute pancreatitis. Stools may be clay colored and the abdomen would be tender in both acute and chronic pancreatitis. The blood sugar would most likely be elevated in chronic pancreatitis due to loss of endocrine function with progressive destruction of the gland.

Cognitive level: Analysis

Nursing process: Assessment

Client needs: Physiological Integrity: Reduction of Risk Potential

9. Answer: 2. Clay-colored stools

Rationale: Jaundice occurs in patients with pancreatic cancer when the bile duct becomes blocked from the tumor.

The bilirubin pigment does not enter the duodenum to be changed and excreted in the stool and so the stools are clay colored. The urine becomes dark, not pale, from the pigment. Patients with pancreatic cancer usually lose, not gain, weight. Easy bruising is seen more with liver cirrhosis and cancer.

Cognitive level: Application

Nursing process: Assessment

Client needs: Physiological Integrity: Physiological Adaptation

10. Answer: 2. Eat a diet low in fat.

Rationale: A low-fat diet is indicated because the pancreas is unable to produce the pancreatic enzyme lipase, which is needed for the breakdown of fats. A replacement enzyme such as Viokase may be prescribed. It is not necessary to avoid all analgesics; acetaminophen may be used, but aspirin is usually contraindicated since it may produce gastric irritation. Abstinence from alcohol is mandatory to prevent future attacks of pancreatitis. Eating utensils can be shared.

Cognitive level: Application

Nursing process: Planning

Client needs: Physiological Integrity: Reduction of Risk Potential

Chapter 47

1. Answer: 3. Sodium level is 152 mg/dL.

Rationale: The elevated sodium level would best substantiate a diagnosis of acute renal failure. In acute renal failure the kidneys are unable to excrete electrolytes properly, resulting in the elevated sodium level. A BUN level of 16 is WNL. A calcium level of 8.7 mg/dL is slightly low. A potassium level of 4.8 is WNL and it would be expected to be elevated in ARF.

Cognitive level: Analysis

Nursing process: Assessment

Client needs: Physiological Integrity: Physiological Adaptation

2. Answer: 3. Casts in the urine

Rationale: Pyelonephritis is a sudden inflammation of the kidney and renal pelvis caused by bacteria. Expected abnormalities in the urine include a low specific gravity, high leukocyte count, and casts in the urine. Counts of 100,000 bacteria or greater are often found. A finding of protein in the urine is associated with hydronephritis and glomerulonephritis.

Cognitive level: Application

Nursing process: Assessment

Client needs: Physiological Integrity: Physiological Adaptation

3. Answer: 3. Congestive heart failure

Rationale: Congestive heart failure causes a decrease in cardiac output, which leads to poor renal perfusion, or blood flow coming into the kidney. Contrast dyes can cause acute tubular necrosis, an intrarenal or intrinsic cause of renal failure. Crushing injuries cause breakdown of muscle cells, which can also cause acute tubular necrosis within the kidney. Urinary calculi are a cause of postrenal failure.

Cognitive level: Application

Nursing process: Assessment

Client needs: Physiological Integrity: Physiological Adaptation

4. Answer: 4. Restrict fluid and salt intake.

Rationale: In chronic renal failure (CRF) the kidneys are unable to excrete sodium and water, leading to fluid retention, which contributes to hypertension and increases the workload of the heart. Applying lotion will help to relieve the dry skin and pruritus associated with CRF, but is not specific to the cardiovascular system. A low-fat, low-sodium diet is indicated. Ankles should be evaluated for edema to identify if fluid is being retained, but this is not the best measure to prevent cardiovascular problems.

Cognitive level: Application

Nursing process: Implementation

Client needs: Physiological Integrity: Physiological Adaptation

5. Answer: 3. Self-catheterization

Rationale: A neobladder is formed by creating an internal urine collection reservoir formed from the small intestine and connected to the urethra. Because the neobladder does not empty fully, self-catheterization should be done twice daily. Kegel exercises are taught as part of bladder training to strengthen the muscles when incontinence is a problem. Crede's method is a done to aid in bladder evacuation by applying manual pressure over the lower abdomen. A stoma wafer change would be necessary if the patient had an ileoconduit done.

Cognitive level: Application

Nursing process: Planning

Client needs: Physiological Integrity: Physiological Adaptation

6. Answer: 3. The leg cramps are because of the extra water and salt that is being removed.

Rationale: One complication of hemodialysis is the onset of muscle cramps, which result from the rapid removal of water and sodium. The muscle cramps are not associated with blood transfusions, infections, or amount of protein ingested.

Cognitive level: Analysis

Nursing process: Implementation

Client needs: Physiological Integrity: Physiological Adaptation

Chapter 48

1. Answer: 2. The uterine lining becomes thicker because of estrogen.

Rationale: The menstrual cycle is a complex physiological process that involves the hypothalamus, pituitary gland, ovaries, and endometrium. The cycle begins with the first day of menses. Menses, or vaginal bleeding, occurs when the thickened endometrial lining that was constructed during the previous cycle is sloughed off or shed. As this occurs, the hypothalamus recognizes a need to secrete gonadotropin-releasing hormone. This hormone stimulates the anterior pituitary to release follicle-stimulating

hormone (FSH), which in turn stimulates a few of the follicles that exist on the ovary. From the follicles that first respond to the FSH, one becomes dominant. This growing follicle produces and secretes estrogen. When estrogen peaks, it signals the anterior pituitary to release luteinizing hormone. When LH peaks, ovulation occurs. The dominant follicle extrudes the ovum. The ovum travels to the fallopian tube and into the uterus. Under the influence of estrogen, the uterine lining has been thickening before ovulation. After ovulation, the lining begins to proliferate, that is, it gets thicker.

Cognitive level: Application

Nursing process: Implementation

Client needs: Health Promotion and Maintenance: Growth and Development Through the Life Span

2. Answer: 1. Any other chronic illnesses such as diabetes

Rationale: Medical comorbidities that may impact the reproductive system would include diabetes, hypertension, hepatitis, and HIV. The male with diabetes or hypertension treated with certain antihypertensive drugs may experience impotence. The childhood disease of concern for men is mumps. This viral illness has the potential to affect the testicles, causing sterility. Sexually transmitted infections do not typically cause impotence. The date of first sexual experience would not contribute to the assessment of the patient's current health concern.

Cognitive level: Application

Nursing process: Assessment

Client needs: Health Promotion and Maintenance: Prevention/Early Detection of Health Problems

3. Answer: 2. Occupations and hobbies

Rationale: There is evidence from cohort and case-control research that cigarette smoking and secondhand smoke increase the risks for cervical cancer. Occupations or hobbies where patients have been exposed to hazardous materials increase the risks of male and female infertility. Ask the patient if she has worked around hazardous materials such as excessive heat, radiation, heavy metals, or organic solvents and how she protects herself. There is no evidence to suggest that the amount of exercise or rest/sleep has an impact on fertility.

Cognitive level: Application

Nursing process: Assessment

Client needs: Health Promotion and Maintenance: Growth and Development Through the Life Span

4. Answer: 1. Smegma, a normal finding

Rationale: The examination of the male external genitalia is completed by inspection followed by palpation. If the male is not circumcised, ask the patient to retract the foreskin so that the glans can be inspected. Lesions that may be seen include chancres or ulcers of syphilis, abnormal contour of the scrotum, cancer, warts, herpetic vesicles, or infestation by lice or other insects in the pubic hair. Smegma or a white, cheesy material is a normal finding under the foreskin. Inflammation of the glans is called balanitis. If the patient has reported discharge, but it is not visible, he

should be asked to strip the penis to bring discharge to the meatus for culture.
Cognitive level: Analysis
Nursing process: Assessment
Client needs: Health Promotion and Maintenance: Prevention/Early Detection of Health Problems

5. Answer: 2. Hair loss over the mons and vulva is a normal part of the aging process.
Rationale: Over time, decreased estrogen levels in females will contribute to the loss of muscle mass and bone, and increased fat on the abdomen. The breasts will atrophy as the glandular tissue is replaced by fat. The vulva will lose fat and the mons and vulva will lose hair. There may also be graying of the pubic hair.
Cognitive level: Application
Nursing process: Assessment
Client needs: Health Promotion and Maintenance: Growth and Development Through the Life Span

6. Answer: 2. Routine screening for prostate cancer can lead to unnecessary anxiety.
Rationale: For older men, the United States Preventive Services Task Force has found that there is insufficient evidence to recommend for or against routine screening for prostate cancer with serum levels of prostate specific antigen and digital rectal examination of the prostate. Routine screening has been shown to cause unnecessary anxiety, biopsies, and treatments with severe side effects for a cancer that may never have affected the patient. In addition, there continue to be many false-positive PSAs.
Cognitive level: Analysis
Nursing process: Assessment
Client needs: Psychosocial Integrity; Coping and Adaptation

Chapter 49

1. Answer: 3. Doryx
Rationale: Penicillin G is used to treat syphilis. Flagyl is used to treat trichomoniasis. Cleocin is used to treat bacterial vaginosis. Doryx and Zithromax are both used to treat a chlamydia infection.
Cognitive level: Application
Nursing process: Planning
Client needs: Physiological Integrity: Pharmacologic and Parenteral Therapies

2. Answer: 4. Have children before the age of 30
Rationale: Modifiable risk factors for the development of breast cancer include having no children or having children after the age of 30, both of which will increase the risk. The use of underarm antiperspirants and dietary fat intake are considered uncertain, controversial, or unproven risk factors for the development of the disease.
Cognitive level: Application
Nursing process: Implementation
Client needs: Health Promotion and Maintenance: Prevention/Early Detection of Health Problems

3. Answer: 2. Use a mirror to examine the shape and size of each breast.
Rationale: The nurse should instruct the patient to establish a regular schedule of examining and not just at any time during the month. The patient should use a mirror to examine the shape and size of each breast. The breasts should be examined standing (in front of a mirror and in the shower) and lying down on a flat surface. The nurse should include that many lumps are benign and that early detection increases the survival rate.
Cognitive level: Application
Nursing process: Implementation
Client needs: Health Promotion and Maintenance: Prevention/Early Detection of Health Problems

4. Answer: 2. Decreased estrogen production
Rationale: Fibroid tumors of the uterus, also known as leiomyomas and myomas, occur in more than 30% of women 40 to 60 years of age but are almost always benign. The lesions are growths arising from the tissue of the uterine muscle for unknown reasons. They develop slowly in women ages 25 through 40, and tend to enlarge during pregnancy and after menopause; fibroids often decrease on their own, due to decreased estrogen production. Fibroids often cause no symptoms, so many are undiscovered unless the patient has dysfunctional uterine bleeding, pelvic pain, and infertility or pregnancy loss.
Cognitive level: Analysis
Nursing process: Assessment
Client needs: Physiological Integrity: Reduction of Risk Potential

5. Answer: 2. Methotrexate
Rationale: A pessary is a device that, when inserted into the vagina, will help support the vaginal walls, reducing the bulging into the vagina. It is used for management of pelvic support defects such as cystocele, rectocele, and uterine prolapse. Cystoceles and rectoceles are repaired using a procedure called a colporrhaphy. Medical treatment of ectopic pregnancy is preferred over surgical treatment. Methotrexate, a drug often used in cancer treatment, is the current drug of choice and will act on the ectopic cells as it does in cancer treatment: to destroy the cells. It is given if the ectopic pregnancy is unruptured and the patient is in stable condition. It is given intramuscularly and often as an outpatient procedure. Successful treatment may require more than one dose of methotrexate. If surgery is indicated with a ruptured ectopic pregnancy, it consists of repair of the tube if future pregnancies are desired. Removal of the tube may be necessary if repair is not possible or may be desired if future pregnancies are not planned.
Cognitive level: Analysis
Nursing process: Planning
Client needs: Physiological Integrity: Physiological Adaptation

6. Answer: 1. Type 1 diabetes mellitus
Rationale: Female-related causes of infertility are most commonly related to ovulatory dysfunction. Other

causes may include hormone imbalance, ovarian cysts, or pelvic infections. Age has also been associated with fertility difficulties. The woman reaches peak fertility in her early 20s, and the likelihood of conceiving after age 35 or 40 is less than 10% per month. In addition to age-related factors, couples at risk for infertility include those with multiple sexual partners, those with a sexually transmitted infection, endometriosis, men with a history of orchitis or a history of undescended testicles, a past history of diethylstilbestrol exposure for both men and women, and those with chronic diseases such as diabetes or thyroid disorders.

Cognitive level: Analysis

Nursing process: Assessment

Client needs: Health Promotion and Maintenance: Growth and Development Through the Life Span

7. Answer: 2. Ambulate

Rationale: An exploratory laparoscopy is a minimally invasive procedure that involves a small incision through which a laparoscope is inserted that allows visualization of the internal organs and structures to assess for disease processes. Carbon dioxide is instilled into the abdomen to elevate the abdominal wall and create a larger work area. After the procedure, the incision is sutured to secure the edges for healing. The patient may experience shoulder pain as the carbon dioxide dissipates from the abdomen. Instruct the patient to sit up and walk to promote gas diffusion and reduce pain.

Cognitive level: Application

Nursing process: Implementation

Client needs: Physiological Integrity: Physiological Adaptation

8. Answer: 4. Locate a SANE immediately.

Rationale: Readily available rape advocates, specially trained law enforcement personnel, and sexual assault nurse examiners (SANEs) should be involved with the patient from the very beginning of the patient's presentation. The importance of careful and meticulous evidence collection is the second priority after ensuring the patient's safety and treatment of injuries. The victim of a sexual assault must consent to the collection of evidence in total or in part. No unnecessary personnel should be involved in handling evidence.

Cognitive level: Application

Nursing process: Implementation

Client needs: Psychosocial Integrity; Psychosocial Adaptation

Chapter 50

1. Answer: 3. Sexually transmitted infections

Rationale: Infection of the epididymis in men younger than 35 years is more likely to be the result of gonococcal, chlamydial, or ureaplasma organisms. A sports injury does not contribute to this condition, mumps can lead to orchitis, and in older men, infection is more likely to be the result of prostatitis, instrumentation of the urinary system, or a structural lesion such as carcinoma of the testis.

Cognitive level: Application

Nursing process: Assessment

Client needs: Physiologic Integrity: Reduction of Risk Potential

2. Answer: 2. Testicular

Rationale: Cancer that forms in the tissue of the testis usually occurs in men between the ages of 20 and 39. It is the most common form of cancer in white men between the ages of 15 and 34.

Cognitive level: Analysis

Nursing process: Assessment

Client needs: Health Promotion and Maintenance: Prevention/Early Detection of Health Problems

3. Answer: 4. Quantifying the symptoms of benign prostatic hypertrophy

Rationale: The American Urological Association (AUA) has developed a symptom index tool that can be used to quantify the symptoms of benign prostatic hypertrophy (BPH) for each patient. The AUA Symptom Score is used both in diagnosing and monitoring therapeutic response. It is a seven-question exploration of symptoms that the patient can answer while waiting to be seen. The score allows the doctor to match treatment options with the severity of the symptoms for each patient. It would focus on sexual dysfunction, urinary tract malignancy, or incontinence.

Cognitive level: Application

Nursing process: Assessment

Client needs: Physiologic Integrity: Reduction of Risk Potential

4. Answer: 4. Checking the drainage tubing for kinks on a regular basis

Rationale: Postsurgical care following a TURP will include maintenance of continuous bladder irrigation to decrease clot formation and bleeding. A three-way catheter is placed after surgery and a steady flow of saline is used to flush the bladder; the amount is determined by the color of outflow and presence of clots. The nurse should be sure that the catheter is secured to the patient's thigh, rather than the bed rail, with a Velcro strap to prevent injury to the urethra and bladder neck. The irrigation and drainage tubing should be checked often for kinks that would block flow. Clot formation will cause obstruction and fluid retention. If a clot should occlude the catheter, the system can be opened and direct irrigation with saline can be done, but this should be a sterile procedure and avoided unless absolutely necessary.

Cognitive level: Application

Nursing process: Planning

Client needs: Physiological Integrity: Reduction of Risk Potential

5. Answer: 3. *Disturbed Body Image*

Rationale: With orchiectomy, the surgery is quick and recovery usually goes well. The loss of the testicles, however, may have a profound effect on the patient. The loss of masculinity can mean depression due to disturbed body image and function with an empty scrotal sac.

Therefore, risk for infection is minimal, mobility should not be affected, nor would impaired urinary elimination be expected.

Cognitive level: Analysis

Nursing process: Planning

Client needs: Psychosocial Integrity: Coping and Adaptation

6. Answer: 1. Encourage to receive a DRE and PSA test annually.

Rationale: It has been recommended that men older than age 50 receive DRE and PSA tests every year. Testicular self-exam should be primarily focused for males under the age of 40. A man's lifetime risk for prostate cancer is 1 in 6, making this disease the most common cancer in men in the United States and the second leading cause of death.

Cognitive level: Application

Nursing process: Implementation

Client needs: Health Promotion and Maintenance: Prevention/Early Detection of Health Problems

Chapter 51

1. Answer: 4. Insulin is a hormone and works through the bloodstream.

Rationale: Because glands are ductless, hormones are released directly into the circulation. The hormone then travels through the bloodstream where it will exert its action on target cells or receptors. A feedback system is a regulatory system that keeps certain activities of body function within a prescribed range to sustain homeostasis. Feedback systems can be positive or negative. In negative feedback, alterations in hormone levels stimulate a series of changes to return the level to normal.

Cognitive level: Application

Nursing process: Implementation

Client needs: Physiological Integrity: Pharmacologic and Parenteral Therapies

2. Answer: 3. Autocrine functioning

Rationale: The endocrine system's functioning is intimately connected to that of the nervous system. Together, they provide a mechanism for communication between cells and organs. This connection is referred to as neuroendocrine regulation. Hormones also function in other ways. If hormones affect cells within the vicinity of their release, it is known as paracrine functioning. Hormones are said to have autocrine functioning when the hormones produced act on the cells that created them. In basal hormone release, small amounts of hormones are released continuously.

Cognitive level: Application

Nursing process: Implementation

Client needs: Health Promotion and Maintenance: Growth and Development Through the Life Span

3. Answer: 3. Epinephrine

Rationale: The adrenal glands have two distinct layers with specialized functions. The outer layer is known as the adrenal medulla. The adrenal medulla produces the catecholamines epinephrine and norepinephrine, substances that play an important role in the body's physiological response to stress. The adrenal cortex secretes corticosteroids of which there are two types, mineralocorticoids and glucocorticoids.

Cognitive level: Analysis

Nursing process: Assessment

Client needs: Physiological Integrity: Physiological Adaptation

4. Answer: 4. Does anyone in your family have diabetes?

Rationale: Exploration of the patient's history is essential. Questioning should seek to assess the onset, characteristics, and severity of symptoms. Along with a review of the entire medical history, family, occupational, and social histories are evaluated. Disorders of the endocrine system tend to occur in a familial pattern. There is a high correlation of diabetes, thyroid disorders, and obesity among families. Knowing this information should assist the interviewer in targeting a more focused assessment. Dietary patterns and involuntary weight losses and gains should be explored. Exposure to chemicals, use of drugs and alcohol, smoking, coping with stress, and behavioral patterns are all areas to be explored.

Cognitive level: Application

Nursing process: Assessment

Client needs: Physiological Integrity: Physiological Adaptation

5. Answer: 3. It checks for ovarian function and might indicate if you are approaching menopause.

Rationale: FSH controls the growth and maturation of ovarian follicles in women and the production of sperm in men. An increased level is seen in ovarian failure of menopause. Blood tests used for adrenal functioning include ACTH stimulation, serum adrenocorticotropic hormone level, serum cortisol level, and urinary cortisol level. The hormones produced from the thyroid include thyroxine, triiodothyronine, and calcitonin. Growth hormone, from the anterior pituitary gland is responsible for the metabolism of carbohydrates, fats, and protein.

Cognitive level: Application

Nursing process: Implementation

Client needs: Physiological Integrity: Physiological Adaptation

Chapter 52

1. Answer: 2. Enterogastrone

Rationale: Enterogastrone is a hormone produced in the gastrointestinal tract. This hormone inhibits secretion and motility. Progesterone is a hormone produced by the placenta and is responsible for gestational support. Angiotensinogen is a hormone produced by the liver that supports the constriction of blood vessels and raises blood pressure. Calcitriol is a hormone produced by the kidney that stimulates calcium absorption from the gastrointestinal tract.

Cognitive level: Analysis

Nursing process: Assessment

Client needs: Physiological Integrity: Reduction of Risk Potential

2. Answer: 1. Giantism

Rationale: Growth hormone is produced by the anterior pituitary gland. An excessive amount of this hormone can lead to giantism in children and adolescents. Acromegaly is the outcome of an excessive amount of growth hormone in adults. Sheehan's syndrome and infertility are seen when there is an underproduction of growth hormone.

Cognitive level: Analysis

Nursing process: Assessment

Client needs: Physiological Integrity: Physiological Adaptation

3. Answer: 2. Take the medication first thing in the morning on an empty stomach.

Rationale: To ensure maximum absorption of the hormone, it is advised that levothyroxine be taken in the early morning on an empty stomach. Synthetic thyroid hormone can be taken safely concurrently with some medications, but patients taking medications such as anticoagulants, beta-blockers, cholesterol-lowering drugs, or seizure control drugs should check with the pharmacist for potential drug interactions. Although administration of levothyroxine will bring thyroid hormone levels within normal limits, it may suppress TSH, which increases the risk of osteoporosis, a side effect that can be avoided by the ingestion of calcium carbonate. However, if the two preparations are taken together, the calcium can interfere with absorption of thyroid hormone. Patients should be advised to take any over-the-counter vitamins, minerals, and antacids at least 4 hours earlier or later than thyroid hormone. Patients also need to be advised that they will be taking thyroid replacement hormone for life. Symptoms of hypothyroidism gradually fade over a period of 3 to 6 weeks as therapy is initiated.

Cognitive level: Application

Nursing process: Implementation

Client needs: Physiological Integrity: Pharmacologic and Parenteral Therapies

4. Answer: 2. Hyperthyroidism

Rationale: Neurological effects of hyperthyroidism include insomnia, jitteriness, shaking, nervousness, irritability, hand tremors, muscle weakness, myalgia, and muscle cramps. Neurological effects of hypothyroidism include drowsiness, fatigue, mental lethargy, forgetfulness, depression, muscular weakness, emotional lability, and paranoia. Patients with pheochromocytoma may experience hypertension, headache, tachycardia, and palpitations. Diabetes insipidus (DI) is characterized by polyuria and polydipsia. Patients with DI present with dry mucous membranes, poor skin turgor, and other signs of dehydration.

Cognitive level: Analysis

Nursing process: Assessment

Client needs: Physiological Integrity: Physiological Adaptation

5. Answer: 2. Strategies to have access to fluids at all times

Rationale: Discharge priorities focus on patient instruction regarding the nature of the disease and the importance of hydration and strategies to ensure the availability of fluid at all times. Medic alert jewelry and a medical identification card should always be carried by the patient so that the patient's condition is known and in emergency situations the treatment is efficient. Patients should be made aware of community resources, including organizations that promote education and research on diabetes insipidus.

Cognitive level: Application

Nursing process: Planning

Client needs: Physiological Integrity: Physiological Adaptation

6. Answer: 3. Consider the onset of myxedema coma and contact the physician.

Rationale: Hypothyroidism is seen clinically at an increasing rate in women over age 50. Clinical manifestations, unless severe, may be too subtle to easily recognize, thus making diagnosis and intervention more difficult. In rare cases, myxedema coma, a rare life-threatening complication in which there is overwhelming cardiopulmonary failure, may be seen in elderly patients, usually precipitated by some untoward event such as infection, trauma, surgery, or neurological disorder. Patients present with all the usual, but exacerbated and serious symptoms of hypothyroidism, and they typically have body temperatures below normal as well. Hypothermia, with body temperature lower than $35°C$ ($95°F$), is a key sign that myxedema coma may be impending.

Cognitive level: Analysis

Nursing process: Implementation

Client needs: Physiological Integrity: Physiological Adaptation

7. Answer: 1. What part of your life is terrible?

Rationale: Improvement in clinical management of endocrine diseases is another important frontier in research. Although medical and surgical interventions, as well as hormone replacement therapy, have reaped big rewards in patient management and outcomes, some patients report decreased quality of life despite treatment. This suggests that although hormone levels may appear to be normal after therapy is initiated in endocrine disease, other complex physiological and psychological factors are at play in restoring patients to optimal health. Nurses in ambulatory clinics could play a role in investigating quality of life issues for patients with endocrine disease.

Cognitive level: Application

Nursing process: Assessment

Client needs: Psychosocial Integrity; Coping and Adaptation

Chapter 53

1. Answer: 2. Approximately 20% of Americans over age 60 have diabetes.

Rationale: Approximately 20.9% of the U.S. population over the age of 60 has diabetes. Type 1 accounts for 5% to 10% of diabetes, with type 2 being the most common form. Native Americans, Mexican Americans, and Native Alaskans have a higher incidence of diabetes than

Caucasians, and the highest incidence worldwide occurs in India and China.

Cognitive level: Analysis

Nursing process: Assessment

Client needs: Health Promotion and Maintenance

2. Answer: 3. Fasting blood sugar (FBS) level is 130 mg/dL.

   Rationale: Pre-diabetes is determined in two ways: an FBS above normal (80 to 110 mg/dL) or abnormal results of an oral glucose tolerance test. Diabetes is no longer classified by age or treatment regimens. A patient on an oral hypoglycemic agent is classified as having type 2 diabetes. Gestational diabetes does not ensure the patient has pre-diabetes, but it does place her at an increased risk to develop type 2 diabetes later in life.

   Cognitive level: Analysis

   Nursing process: Assessment

   Client needs: Physiological Integrity: Physiological Adaptation

3. Answer: 3. A toddler with a monozygotic twin who has type 1 diabetes.

   Rationale: Type 1 diabetes is frequently diagnosed before the age of 20 and it has many genetic, viral, and autoimmune risk factors. There is a 25% to 50% incidence of type 1 diabetes in monozygotic twins, but only a 6% incidence among dizygotic twins. There is an epidemiologic association between viral infections, such as mumps and rubella, and the development of type 1 diabetes, but not bacterial infections. The offspring of a mother with type 1 diabetes has a 3% risk of developing diabetes.

   Cognitive level: Analysis

   Nursing process: Assessment

   Client needs: Physiological Integrity: Reduction of Risk Potential

4. Answer: 2. Abdominal obesity and decreased HDL level

   Rationale: The primary abnormalities associated with metabolic syndrome include central or abdominal obesity, insulin resistance, glucose intolerance (which is often manifested as elevated blood sugar levels), increased triglycerides, decreased HDL cholesterol, and hypertension.

   Cognitive level: Application

   Nursing process: Evaluation

   Client needs: Physiological Integrity: Physiological Adaptation

5. Answer: 2. "Avoid doing any isometric exercises."

   Rationale: Isometric exercises can raise intraocular pressure and worsen the proliferative retinopathy, so they should be avoided. A dilated eye exam should be done yearly. Protein does not need to be restricted with retinopathy, but may be restricted if renal impairment is present. An ideal target for blood sugar is 80 to 110 mg/dL.

   Cognitive level: Application

   Nursing process: Implementation

   Client needs: Physiological Integrity: Reduction of Risk Potential

6. Answer: 4. Instruct patient to eat within 20 minutes of taking the medication.

   Rationale: Patients should eat within 20 minutes of taking a meglitinide to prevent hypoglycemia. They cause a rapid release of insulin, which can lead to hypoglycemia. They should be given before a meal. It is not necessary to check for sulfa allergies; patients taking sulfonylureas should be checked for sulfa allergies.

   Cognitive level: Application

   Nursing process: Implementation

   Client needs: Physiological Integrity: Pharmacologic and Parenteral Therapies

7. Answer: 3. "Exercise may lower your blood sugar for several hours after completing the activity."

   Rationale: During exercise, glucose is transported into the muscle for energy use. Patients taking oral hypoglycemic agents and insulin are at increased risk for hypoglycemia following exercise and this may last for several hours. If the blood sugar is 100 mg/dL or less before starting exercise, the patient should consume carbohydrates. If hypoglycemia occurs, the patient should eat complex carbohydrates that will provide a longer supply of energy.

   Cognitive level: Application

   Nursing process: Implementation

   Client needs: Physiological Integrity: Reduction of Risk Potential

8. Answer: 1. Abdominal bloating and diarrhea

   Rationale: Alpha glucosidase inhibitors delay the absorption of carbohydrates in the small intestine, which helps to prevent the normal sharp rise in postprandial blood sugar. They cause a number of gastrointestinal side effects, such as diarrhea, flatulence, bloating, and softer stools. They do not cause an elevated temperature. Tremors, palpitations, and fatigue are associated with hypoglycemia, which is seen more with sulfonylureas and meglitinides.

   Cognitive level: Application

   Nursing process: Evaluation

   Client needs: Physiological Integrity: Pharmacologic and Parenteral Therapies

9. Answer: 1. Face is flushed and red.

   Rationale: Patients experiencing DKA often have Kussmaul respirations to help correct the acidotic state; the increased levels of $PaCO_2$ have a vasodilating effect, which causes a red, flushed face. Inelastic skin turgor, lethargy, and hypotension can be seen with both DKA and HHS.

   Cognitive level: Analysis

   Nursing process: Assessment

   Client needs: Physiological Integrity: Physiological Adaptation

10. Answer: 3. A male patient with chronic renal failure (CRF).

    Rationale: Factors that have been associated with an increased risk for lower extremity ulcers and amputation include patients who have had diabetes for more than 10 years, male gender, poor glucose control, and the presence of cardiovascular, retinal, or renal complications. According to these risk factors, the male patient with CRF is more at risk than a female with cardiovascular disease. The elderly female has fairly well controlled blood sugar and the patient just diagnosed 2 years ago does not meet these criteria.

Cognitive level: Application

Nursing process: Assessment

Client needs: Physiological Integrity: Reduction of Risk Potential

Chapter 54

1. Answer: 3. Flat

   Rationale: The long bones of the body include the femur, tibia, fibula, humerus, radius, ulna, clavicle, metacarpals, metatarsals, and phalanges. The short and irregular bones include those within the vertebral column and the carpal and tarsal bones. The flat bones include the ribs, scapula, sternum, and the ilium.

   Cognitive level: Analysis

   Nursing process: Assessment

   Client needs: Physiological Integrity: Reduction of Risk Potential

2. Answer: 2. Social

   Rationale: A social history provides additional information about the patient's lifestyle that may affect his or her potential disorder or complaint. The nurse should consider a variety of questions including "Do you use an assistive device such as a cane, walker, or brace?" Characteristics, lengths, exacerbation or diminishment of symptoms, and what is wrong or feared by the patient define the chief complaint. Demographic data may be helpful in determining causes of injury. Biographical data should include age, gender, culture, and educational background.

   Cognitive level: Application

   Nursing process: Assessment

   Client needs: Physiological Integrity: Reduction of Risk Potential

3. Answer: 3. Inspection

   Rationale: When inspecting compare corresponding paired joints for symmetry. The nurse should observe for skin color, scars, shape of the site, deformities, muscle atrophy, masses, or swelling. Palpation is used to determine skin temperature, the presence of any nodules, or muscle or joint tenderness and swelling. The assessment technique of percussion is not used for the musculoskeletal status. Range of motion is used to determine the functionality of joints.

   Cognitive level: Application

   Nursing process: Assessment

   Client needs: Health Promotion and Maintenance: Prevention/Early Detection of Health Problems

4. Answer: 2. Shoulder

   Rationale: The nurse should explain that testing the range of motion of the shoulders involves having the patient perform seven movements, one of which is testing for adduction by asking the patient to raise the arms above the head with the palms facing each other. The elbow is not assessed by having the patient raise the arms above the head. The wrist and hands are not assessed by ask-

ing the patient to raise the arms above the head with the palms facing each other.

   Cognitive level: Application

   Nursing process: Assessment

   Client needs: Health Promotion and Maintenance: Prevention/Early Detection of Health Problems

5. Answer: 4. Toes pointing inward

   Rationale: A normal finding when assessing the feet would be the toes pointing straight and in alignment with the feet, though some may point slightly inward or slightly outward. Abnormal findings include a great toe that is deviated medially and abducted to the first metatarsal with an inflamed bursa or bunion on the medial side or a hallux valgus; an abnormally high arch or a cavus foot; or a wart located over the thick skin of the sole of the foot or a verruca vulgaris.

   Cognitive level: Analysis

   Nursing process: Assessment

   Client needs: Health Promotion and Maintenance: Prevention/Early Detection of Health Problems

6. Answer: 3. External rotation 45 degrees

   Rationale: A normal finding is that the patient is able to externally rotate the hip to 45 degrees. Additional normal findings on assessment of the range of motion of the hip include ability to raise the legs to at least 90 degrees of flexion with the knee straight and 120 degrees of flexion with the knee flexed; adduct leg to 20 to 30 degrees and abduct 45 to 50 degrees; internally rotate to 40 degrees and externally rotate to 45 degrees; hyperextend the leg at least 15 degrees; move the extremities against resistance.

   Cognitive level: Analysis

   Nursing process: Assessment

   Client needs: Health Promotion and Maintenance: Prevention/Early Detection of Health Problems

Chapter 55

1. Answer: 3. Stress and strain

   Rationale: Two concepts are important to remember: stress and strain. First, stress results when mechanical force is applied to a stretched or compressed bone. Compressive stressors are those of the body weight pushing the bone down, and tensile stresses are from the muscles pulling the bones away from each other. Strain, the second concept, is expressed in length/original length and results as a force that is applied, causing an amount of deformation in the bone relative to its original length.

   Cognitive level: Analysis

   Nursing process: Assessment

   Client needs: Health Promotion and Maintenance

2. Answer: 2. Diet low in calcium and vitamin D

   Rationale: A diet low in calcium and vitamin D is a risk factor for both men and women. Low body weight and low body mass index, along with a history of maternal hip fracture, are risk factors affecting men. Anorexia applies to females only.

   Cognitive level: Application

   Nursing process: Assessment

   Client needs: Health Promotion and Maintenance

3. Answer: 1. "Living at my own home increases my chance of a fracture."

Rationale: In addition to gender (being a female), another factor that increases the risk of hip fracture is living in institutional care, rather than one's own home. Other factors include significant cognitive impairment, certain medications (e.g., anticonvulsants, corticosteroids), personal history and lifestyle factors, certain medical conditions (e.g., type 2 diabetes in women) and low bone mineral density.

Cognitive level: Application

Nursing process: Assessment

Client needs: Safe, Effective Care Environment

4. Answer: 3. Muscle membranes have a protein deficiency or absence of dystrophin.

Rationale: Muscular dystrophies are a group of genetic myopathies caused by a protein deficiency in muscle membranes. In other words, a person's DNA is not producing a particular protein named dystrophin that is required by muscles and muscle membranes to function properly. Cardiomyopathy leads to heart failure, which is a major cause of death in patients with muscular dystrophy or respiratory failure. The course of Duchenne muscular dystrophy is progressive and usually fatal in the teens or early 20s. The child/adolescent generally has a normal IQ for age with Becker's dystrophy.

Cognitive level: Analysis

Nursing process: Evaluation

Client needs: Health Promotion and Maintenance

5. Answer: 1. Hypokalemic

Rationale: Hypokalemic myopathy is common in the elderly and is due to a low serum potassium level caused by long-term diuretic use. Other causes of hypokalemic myopathy include potassium deficiency in the diet, excessive alcohol consumption, aldosteronism, intestinal wasting of potassium (malabsorption), and licorice intoxication.

Cognitive level: Analysis

Nursing process: Evaluation

Client needs: Health Promotion and Maintenance

6. Answer: 4. Subjective symptoms

Rationale: The diagnosis of fibromyalgia is based on the patient's subjective symptoms, as well as a medical and surgical history. Patients with fibromyalgia do not have any other associated musculoskeletal disorder; therefore, arthritis, inflammations, and bursitis should be ruled out. Depression is not uncommon. Family tendency is not used as a diagnostic tool.

Cognitive level: Application

Nursing process: Assessment

Client needs: Health Promotion and Maintenance

Chapter 56

1. Answer: 2. Prevention of injuries

Rationale: Prevention is the only method to decrease the effects of injuries to the muscles, tendons, ligaments, and bones. Half of all sports-related injuries are preventable. Education and awareness surrounding protective equipment, safer playing environments, and rules designed to prevent injury are important in reducing the frequency and severity of sports injuries. Stretching, warm-up exercises, and strengthening and balance training regimens are key in preventing sports injuries.

Cognitive level: Application

Nursing process: Planning

Client needs: Health Promotion and Maintenance: Prevention/Early Detection of Health Problems

2. Answer: 4. Ossification

Rationale: A fracture or break in the bone causes a healing cascade beginning with the blood that leaks out at the fracture site. This hematoma is rich in osteoblasts, which make bone. Clotting factors that remain due to the hematoma initiate the formation of a fibrin meshwork that serves as a framework for the fibroblasts and new capillary buds. During cellular proliferation and callus formation, the osteoblasts, or bone-forming cells, multiply and differentiate into the fibrocartilaginous callus. This process begins distal to the fracture where there is greater blood supply. Within a few days a cartilage "collar" is evident around the fracture site. Initially the callus is soft but within the third to fourth week of fracture healing, the bone calcifies as mineral salts are deposited. Ossification is the final lying down of bone after the fracture has been bridged and the fragments are united. Mature bone replaces the callus, and the fracture site feels firm and appears united on radiograph. It is at this point that a cast may be removed.

Cognitive level: Analysis

Nursing process: Assessment

Client needs: Physiological Integrity: Physiological Adaptation

3. Answer: 3. Decrease the potential for contamination.

Rationale: The important concept is that all open fractures have the potential to be contaminated and this increases the morbidity and mortality of the injury. The time frames vary by institution but many consider 6 to 8 hours to be the maximum time that a contaminated fracture can wait to be taken to the operating room and be "washed out," often referred to as an I&D (i.e., inspection and debridement). Pain relief, assessing, treating injury to surrounding tissue, and casting of the fracture would follow this goal.

Cognitive level: Analysis

Nursing process: Planning

Client needs: Physiological Integrity: Physiological Adaptation

4. Answer: 1. Monitoring hemodynamic status

Rationale: The nurse should monitor the patient for signs that would indicate the onset of hypovolemic shock and the need for resuscitative measures. An orthopedic trauma patient who has experienced fractures of the pelvis or long bones is at risk for significant bleeding. The nurse should monitor the patient's hemodynamic status including vital signs and laboratory values. A patient may lose as much as 20% of his or her blood volume before exhibiting signs and symptoms of shock. The nurse should monitor the vital signs for an increase in heart rate, decrease in blood pressure, increase in respiratory rate, and a decrease in urine output. Laboratory results will show a decrease in the hemoglobin and hematocrit. Arranging for traction can be delegated, and explaining care is important, however, this is a psychosocial need that should follow hemodynamic stability. Most patients will require intravenous narcotics, such as a patient-controlled analgesic pump.

Cognitive level: Application

Nursing process: Planning

Client needs: Physiological Integrity: Physiological Adaptation

5. Answer: 2. Dark-colored urine

Rationale: Complications associated with rhabdomyolysis include acute renal failure. This occurs due to renal tubular obstruction from the filtration of the released myoglobin. The patient may also exhibit respiratory distress due to muscle weakness and fluid and electrolyte imbalances. Signs and symptoms of rhabdomyolysis may include pain, tenderness, swelling, bruising, and weakness within the affected muscles. Upon assessment the muscles involved may feel soft and flabby. The patient's urine will also become dark in color, referred to as myoglobinuria, as the renal system attempts to filter the myoglobin. They may also develop systemic symptoms including general malaise, fever, nausea and vomiting, confusion, agitation, and anuria as the acute renal failure progresses.

Cognitive level: Analysis

Nursing process: Assessment

Client needs: Physiological Integrity: Physiological Adaptation

6. Answer: 2. You are experiencing something called phantom sensations.

Rationale: There are as many physical/mobility issues to deal with as there are emotional for the patient with an amputation. The patient may have trouble just looking at it, or may have bizarre sensations such as feeling that the foot is cold or itchy when it is not even there. These are called phantom limb sensations and are not caused by narcotic use. The other responses do not acknowledge the patient's concerns or provide a reason.

Cognitive level: Application

Nursing process: Implementation

Client needs: Psychosocial Integrity; Coping and Adaptation

Chapter 57

1. Answers:
   1. Pain level
   2. Pulse quality
   3. Sensation and movement
   4. Color of extremity
   5. Use of muscles

Rationale: The neurovascular assessment should be performed bilaterally so that the affected extremity can be compared to the unaffected extremity. The neurovascu-

lar assessment includes assessment of the five "Ps": pain, pulse, paresthesia, paralysis, and pallor. A complete assessment of circulation and motor and sensory function must be performed. Neurovascular compromise or deterioration should be reported to the surgeon immediately. The nurse should anticipate performing the neurovascular assessment in conjunction with vital signs. Level of consciousness is part of a neurological assessment.

Cognitive level: Application

Nursing process: Assessment

Client needs: Health Promotion and Maintenance

2. Answer: 4. Use an elevated toilet seat in the main bathroom at home.

Rationale: Discharge teaching should include precautions to avoid adduction, flexion, or any movement that may dislocate the hip prosthesis. Precautions include use of an elevated toilet seat, use of a hip abductor pillow while in bed, not bending the hip greater than 90 degrees, not sitting in low chairs, not twisting or turning the body toward the operative side, not turning the leg or foot inward, and keeping the operative leg straight when getting up using arms to push.

Cognitive level: Application

Nursing process: Planning

Client needs: Physiological Integrity: Reduction of Risk Potential

3. Answer: 1. Ace bandages to wrap around the bivalved cast

Rationale: Treatment of compartment syndrome requires release of the constriction to accommodate swelling. If a cast is causing the restriction, it should be bivalved (cut down both sides) with ace wraps or wide tape placed around it to hold it in place. If the constriction is at the fascia level, the patient will require surgery. If the nurse suspects compartment syndrome is present, the surgeon should be notified immediately to prevent permanent disability or loss of limb. If compartment syndrome in an extremity is suspected, the extremity should not be elevated, but should be maintained at the level of the heart to improve perfusion. As edema and engorgement increase, pain increases and is unrelieved by narcotic pain medication administration.

Cognitive level: Application

Nursing process: Implementation

Client needs: Physiological Integrity: Reduction of Risk Potential

4. Answer: 2. A "reacher" tool

Rationale: It is important for the patient not to bend over or flex the affected extremity. A "reacher" tool can be very helpful for picking up an item off the floor, or overhead to avoid standing on a step stool, which requires flexion. A heel lift boot is used to offset development of pressure ulcers for an immobilized patient and the CPM would be indicated following a total knee replacement. Generally, after hip replacement, the patient would use a walker or cane to assist ambulation and avoid flexion by prolonged sitting rather than a wheelchair.

Cognitive level: Application

Nursing process: Assessment

Client needs: Physiological Integrity: Reduction of Risk Potential

5. Answer: 2. "Every hour 2 mg of morphine is delivered continuously."

Rationale: Patient-controlled analgesia (PCA) or around-the-clock pain medication is often utilized in the early postoperative period. The PCA can be set to deliver a constant or basal rate; in addition, the patient is able to self-administer a preset dose at prescribed intervals to achieve pain control. In this scenario, the patient would receive 2 mg of morphine every hour regardless of intermittent use of the pump.

Cognitive level: Analysis

Nursing process: Evaluation

Client needs: Physiological Integrity: Basic Care and Comfort

Chapter 58

1. Answer: 3. It's a common connective tissue disorder.

Rationale: Common connective tissue disorders include lupus erythematosus, gout, and Lyme disease. A term used to describe rheumatic disease is arthritis. A chronic inflammatory process that affects joints is rheumatoid arthritis. An inflammation associated with psoriasis is psoriatic arthritis.

Cognitive level: Application

Nursing process: Implementation

Client needs: Physiological Integrity: Physiological Adaptation

2. Answer: 4. Prevent deformities

Rationale: During the planning stage, goals for a patient with rheumatoid arthritis include prevention of contractures and deformities and provision of health teaching.

Cognitive level: Application

Nursing process: Planning

Client needs: Physiological Integrity: Physiological Adaptation

3. Answer: 1. Reactive arthritis

Rationale: Reactive arthritis is caused by a reaction to an infection somewhere else in the body. Reactive arthritis most commonly causes secondary conditions such as arthritis, uveitis, and urethritis. Other symptoms that may occur are dactylitis, inflammation of the neck and low back, and painless skin lesions termed circinate balanitis.

Cognitive level: Analysis

Nursing process: Assessment

Client needs: Physiological Integrity: Physiological Adaptation

4. Answer: 3. *Imbalanced Nutrition: More than Body Requirements*

Rationale: For the patient with osteoarthritis, priority nursing diagnoses include *Chronic Pain, Impaired Physical Mobility, Risk for Falls, Disturbed Body Image, Readiness for Enhanced Self-Care, Imbalanced Nutrition: More than Body Requirements,* and *Powerlessness*.

Cognitive level: Application

Nursing process: Planning

Client needs: Physiological Integrity: Physiological Adaptation

5. Answer: 2. Gravies

Rationale: Because gouty arthritis is caused by indulging in foods high in purines, it can be controlled by eating a well-balanced, low-calorie, low-purine diet and by reducing alcohol consumption. Foods to be avoided are alcohol, organ meats, and rich foods such as gravies, dried legumes, and anchovies. These foods will increase uric acid in the blood and can lead to uric acid crystal buildup, most often resulting in uric acid crystals located in the joint of the great toe.

Cognitive level: Application

Nursing process: Implementation

Client needs: Physiological Integrity: Physiological Adaptation

6. Answer: 3. Dermatomyositis

Rationale: Myositis may be triggered by an injury, infection, or an autoimmune disease. Polymyositis consists of muscle weakness. Dermatomyositis has the same symptoms as polymyositis except for a distinctive rash over the face, shoulders, arms, and bony prominences. This purplish blue rash can also appear on the eyelids, bridge of the nose, neck, elbows, knees, knuckles, and upper chest.

Cognitive level: Analysis

Nursing process: Assessment

Client needs: Physiological Integrity: Physiological Adaptation

Chapter 59

1. Answer: 3. Bone marrow

Rationale: Deficiencies in functional bone marrow and stem cells can lead to immune deficiency disorders. Lymph nodes and lymph tissue filter debris from the breakdown of cells, bacteria, virus, and fungal antigens. Adenoids are consolidated lymph tissue located in the throat. They function to remove and filter debris, bacteria, and viruses from the upper airways and mouth. The spleen plays a significant role in immune function as part of the lymphatic system. It is comprised of white and red pulp and is involved in hematologic filtration, sequestering of red and white cells, and immune response.

Cognitive level: Analysis

Nursing process: Assessment

Client needs: Physiological Integrity: Physiological Adaptation

2. Answer: 1. The body reacting to self receptors as an antigen

Rationale: Immune tolerance is defined as the ability of the immune system to tolerate all self antigens while retaining the ability to mount an immune response to non-self antigens. Immune tolerance begins during embryonic development of the immune system. Lymphocytes that react with self antigens are selectively eliminated as the immune system develops. This leaves the newborn with B-cell and T-cell lines that do not attack self antigens. Self antigens include HLAs and MHC, as well as several other antigenic particles that are often cell receptors. When the body reacts to self receptors or other cell parts as an antigen, autoimmune disease may result.

Cognitive level: Analysis
Nursing process: Assessment
Client needs: Physiological Integrity: Physiological Adaptation

3. Answer: 1. Produce antibodies in response to exposure to an antigen

Rationale: Plasma cells are differentiated B cells that are found in the plasma and are responsible for production of specific antibodies. Plasma cells produce the antibodies in response to a primary or initial exposure to an antigen. The most common groups of antibodies, also known as immunoglobulins, include immunoglobulin G (IgG), immunoglobulin A (IgA), immunoglobulin M (IgM), immunoglobulin D (IgD), and immunoglobulin E (IgE). Suppressor T cells, also called CD8 cells, slow or stop the immune response. This downregulation is the primary role of suppressor T cells, and is an important part of regulation of the immune system because the ability to stop the production of antibodies and cell destruction is important once the threat of infection has been overcome. Natural killer cells, also referred to as "null cells," are types of T cells that lack CD4 or CD8 external receptors, but are able to directly kill cells or send cytokine messages to start the process of programmed cell death. T-helper 1 cells help regulate immune activity and produce chemicals called cytokines that stimulate cytotoxic cells to destroy mutant and cancer cells.

Cognitive level: Analysis
Nursing process: Assessment
Client needs: Physiological Integrity: Physiological Adaptation

4. Answer: 3. Complement

Rationale: Complement is a group of small proteins made in the liver and present in blood that can interact with cells and each other for a variety of functions. Complement proteins are important in the inflammatory and immune responses. Tumor necrosis factor is a small peptide that is produced by a variety of cells, including granulocytes and lymphocytes. Interferons are proteins made and released by T cells when the invading organism is a virus. Interleukins are lymphokines, chemical mediators released by lymphocytes, that enable the cells of the immune system to communicate and coordinate the immune response.

Cognitive level: Analysis
Nursing process: Assessment
Client needs: Physiological Integrity: Physiological Adaptation

5. Answer: 2. The vaccine is made from killed flu organisms.

Rationale: Acquired immunity involves lymphocyte cells and chemicals that can confer long-term permanent

protection against the disease for which the antibodies have been produced. Immunization is a term often used interchangeably with vaccination or inoculation and involves the process of stimulating the immune system to create active immunity for protection against a disease. A vaccine, a preparation that contains an infectious agent or its components, is administered to stimulate the production of antibodies that can prevent infection or create resistance to infection from that agent. Antigens used in vaccines to stimulate an immune response may be inactivated (whole-killed microorganisms or purified products derived from them), live-attenuated (live virus weakened through chemical or physical processes), or recombinant (artificially manufactured from segments of DNA from different sources). Vaccines against influenza, diphtheria, and tetanus use inactivated antigens. Attenuated vaccines include vaccines for measles, mumps, rubella, polio, yellow fever, and varicella. Vaccines are most commonly administered by needle injections, but also can be given by mouth and by aerosol.

Cognitive level: Application
Nursing process: Implementation
Client needs: Health Promotion and Maintenance: Prevention/Early Detection of Health Problems

6. Answer: 2. Antigen presentation

Rationale: B cells must be activated or told to make specific antibodies; this is accomplished through the mechanism of antigen presentation. When a foreign antigen enters a host, the macrophages found in tissue, or monocytes found in blood, ingest the bacterium or virus and then digest the antigen. The macrophage expresses a portion of the digested antigen on its cell surface in the form of a small protein receptor with a part of the bacterial wall attached. T cells are often found near macrophages and can chemically bind to the receptor and accept the antigen onto their surface. T cells then present the antigen to the B cells that have a receptor to match the shape of the antigen. Linking of the T cell and B cell at the site of the antigen activates the B cell to make the appropriately shaped antibody to attach to the antigens.

Cognitive level: Analysis
Nursing process: Assessment
Client needs: Physiological Integrity: Physiological Adaptation

7. Answer: 2. Decreased primary and secondary production of antibodies

Rationale: The effects of aging on the immune system include decreased percentage of suppressor T cells, which means the body cannot downregulate the immune system as quickly; decreased primary and secondary production of antibodies, which means the body has a reduced response to infectious organisms leading to more severe infection; increased auto-antibody production, which means the body shows evidence of more exacerbations of autoimmune disease; and a delayed hypersensitivity response, which means the body has a decreased allergic response.

Cognitive level: Application

Nursing process: Assessment

Client needs: Physiological Integrity: Physiological Adaptation

8. Answer: 4. The patient is at risk for malnutrition.

Rationale: Fatigue and weight loss may be associated with chronic disease processes. Inadequate nutrition affects the ability of the immune cells to function normally and causes immunosuppression. Rapid and significant weight loss that is unintentional is a serious concern because it is a symptom of malignancy. An unintentional weight loss of 10 pounds or more in a month is also an indicator of a need for a nutritional consult. Lymphedema, or nonpitting edema at the site of lymph nodes, indicates inadequate drainage from lymphatic vessels and excessive accumulation of fluid in the interstitial spaces around the lymph vessels. Percussion is helpful in determining if there is inappropriate fluid or a mass in an organ, indicating disease. Symptoms of infection include redness, inflammation, streaking lines, edema, or drainage. Signs of rash or petechiae indicate an allergic response or infection.

Cognitive level: Analysis

Nursing process: Assessment

Client needs: Physiological Integrity; Basic Care and Comfort

9. Answer: 1. Erythrocyte sedimentation rate

Rationale: The erythrocyte sedimentation rate is a serum test that is used to diagnose acute and chronic inflammation, as well as rheumatoid and autoimmune diseases. In the presence of inflammatory mediators, blood proteins are altered and red blood cells stick together and then fall out of solution when the blood sample is spun. This results in an elevated sedimentation rate. This test is ordered when an autoimmune disease is suspected such as rheumatoid arthritis. A protein called rheumatoid factor is often present in the serum of patient's with rheumatoid disease in greater quantities than individuals without autoimmune diseases. Antinuclear antibodies are immunoglobulins (IgG, IgM, IgA) that react with the nuclear portion of leukocytes, forming auto-antibodies against the host's DNA and ribonucleic acid. The presence of these antibodies is indicative of systemic lupus erythematosus. The enzyme-linked immunosorbent assay and the Western blot tests detect the presence of antibodies created in response to infection with the HIV antigen.

Cognitive level: Analysis

Nursing process: Assessment

Client needs: Physiological Integrity: Reduction of Risk Potential

Chapter 60

1. Answer: 2. Hypersensitive reactions are determined by the type of antigen, the time sequence of the reaction, and the immunological response.

Rationale: When the immune system loses self-tolerance, immune hypersensitivity reactions result. The primary

mechanism of an immune deficiency is a genetic disorder that occurred during the embryonic development of the immune system. Immune deficiency is associated with opportunistic infections.

Cognitive level: Analysis

Nursing process: Assessment

Client needs: Physiological Integrity: Physiological Adaptation

2. Answer: 3. The trigger for an autoimmune response is a self-antigen.

Rationale: The primary trigger for a hypersensitive reaction is an environmental antigen. An alloimmune reaction is triggered by antigens from another individual. The symptoms of different categories of hypersensitive responses vary according to the origin of the antigen.

Cognitive level: Analysis

Nursing process: Assessment

Client needs: Physiological Integrity: Physiological Adaptation

3. Answers:
   1. AIDS is a syndrome of opportunistic infections that occurs as a final stage in patients infected with HIV.
   2. HIV transmission is limited to contact with infected body fluids that have lymphocytes that can harbor HIV.

Rationale: A syndrome of opportunistic infections, AIDS occurs as a final stage in patients infected with HIV. Transmission of HIV is limited to contact with infected body fluids that have lymphocytes that can harbor HIV. AIDS is the end disease manifestation of HIV. HIV precedes AIDS and is associated with the virus's entry into the host's lymphocytes.

Cognitive level: Analysis

Nursing process: Assessment

Client needs: Physiological Integrity, Physiological Adaptation

4. Answers:
   1. Subjective assessment to promote the early detection of infection from any body region.
   2. Health care providers and family members wash hands before and after patient contact to reduce the risk of opportunistic infection cross-contamination.
   3. Encourage hydration and maintenance of weight to support the immune system.

Rationale: Cultures should be obtained prior to starting antibiotics to ensure the appropriate therapy is initiated in a timely manner.

Cognitive level: Application

Nursing process: Assessment

Client needs: Physiological Integrity: Physiological Adaptation

Chapter 61

1. Answer: 2. Anaphylactic

Rationale: Anaphylactic shock is most likely caused by insect bites, medication allergies, food allergies, latex allergies, and idiopathic reactions. Cardiogenic shock is most often caused by myocardial infarction/contusion, ruptured ventricles or papillary muscles, and cardiomyopathy. Neurogenic shock is most often caused by spinal cord or medulla trauma, anesthetic agents, severe emotional stress, or severe pain. Septic shock is most often caused by bacterial or viral infections, immunosuppression, technological causes, or antibiotic misuse.

Cognitive level: Analysis

Nursing process: Assessment

Client needs: Physiological Integrity: Physiological Adaptation

2. Answer: 1. The stress response

Rationale: Glucose metabolism is impaired in a manner similar to that of oxygen metabolism. The result of this impaired metabolism is insulin resistance. This phenomenon has been observed in patients with sepsis and those who are critically ill or injured. The stress response that is initiated by an illness or injury triggers gluconeogenesis to supply glucose energy to heal. The liver and kidneys produce more glucose in response to epinephrine, norepinephrine, glucagons, and cortisol, which are part of the body's stress response. Insulin resistance is unresponsiveness of anabolic processes to the normal effects of insulin and possibly tissue insensitivity to insulin.

Cognitive level: Analysis

Nursing process: Assessment

Client needs: Physiological Integrity: Physiological Adaptation

3. Answer: 2. Low circulating blood volume or hypoglycemia

Rationale: The brain is dependent on both oxygen and glucose. When either of these is not sufficient, an alteration in cerebral perfusion occurs. The patient will suffer an altered mental status, which will eventually lead to coma and even death.

Cognitive level: Analysis

Nursing process: Assessment

Client needs: Physiological Integrity: Physiological Adaptation

4. Answer: 2. 86-year-old female with abdominal injuries

Rationale: Patient risk factors such as significant injuries, catastrophic illness, age, and allergies must be quickly acknowledged. It is interesting that both the very young and aged share similar risk factors for developing shock including compromised immune systems due to age, fluid shifts, and an integumentary system that may not afford needed protection.

Cognitive level: Analysis

Nursing process: Assessment

Client needs: Physiological Integrity: Physiological Adaptation

5. Answer: 1. Normal saline

Rationale: Fluids that are used for resuscitation include lactated Ringer's solution or normal saline. The type of fluid used will depend on the provider's preference, because at present the research has not clearly defined one more favorably over the other. The initial amount of fluid will range from 2 to 3 liters for an adult if the cause

of the shock is unknown. If the patient has sustained blood loss, then administration of blood and blood products will be needed; however, patients who have sustained blood loss greater than 2 liters should not receive excessive fluid resuscitation from either colloids or crystalloids until surgical management of bleeding has been initiated because it dilutes the existing volume and further diminishes oxygen-carrying capacity.

Cognitive level: Application

Nursing process: Implementation

Client needs: Physiological Integrity: Physiological Adaptation

6. Answer: 2. Nitroprusside sodium

Rationale: Dopamine and dobutamine hydrochloride improve cardiac contractility. Nitroprusside sodium and nitrates decrease afterload. Epinephrine and norepinephrine bitartrate increase afterload.

Cognitive level: Application

Nursing process: Planning

Client needs: Physiological Integrity: Physiological Adaptation

7. Answer: 1. Systemic inflammatory response syndrome

Rationale: Systemic inflammatory response syndrome (SIRS) is an organized immune response that can be triggered by infectious or noninfectious clinical insults including burns, pancreatitis, acute respiratory distress syndrome, surgery, and trauma. Sepsis is a clinical syndrome defined as the presence of SIRS associated with a confirmed infectious process. Septic shock is a state of acute circulatory failure characterized by persistent hypotension unexplained by other causes, for example, despite the fact that adequate fluids have been administered. Severe sepsis is defined as sepsis or the presence of a confirmed infection and a systemic inflammatory response, and single or multiple organ failure. The patient is hypotensive, which causes hypoperfusion abnormalities such as arterial hypoxemia, acute oliguria, and coagulation abnormalities.

Cognitive level: Analysis

Nursing process: Assessment

Client needs: Physiological Integrity: Physiological Adaptation

8. Answer: 4. Central venous pressure 10 mmHg

Rationale: Fluid resuscitation should be directed to achieve a central venous pressure reading of 8 to 12 mmHg, a mean arterial pressure of greater than or equal to 65 mmHg, a urine output of greater than or equal to 0.5 mL/kg, and a central venous or mixed venous oxygen saturation of greater than or equal to 70%.

Cognitive level: Analysis

Nursing process: Evaluation

Client needs: Physiological Integrity: Physiological Adaptation

9. Answer: 1. MODS

Rationale: Reperfusion injury, which results from the reestablishment of blood flow after ischemia, causes conversion of the enzyme xanthine dehydrogenase to xanthine oxidase to form oxygen free radicals with oxygen when hypoperfused tissues are reperfused. These oxygen radicals attack already damaged tissues and can lead to MODS.

Cognitive level: Analysis

Nursing process: Assessment

Client needs: Physiological Integrity: Physiological Adaptation

10. Answer: 4. Frequent assessment of vital signs and clinical status

Rationale: Frequent monitoring and assessment to trend changes in vital signs and clinical manifestations will provide the most reliable information about early signs of MODS. Nursing care needs to be focused on decreasing oxygen demand, which includes pain and anxiety management as well as spacing activity to allow for long periods of rest. The nurse should assess for signs of pain and anxiety and medicate as needed. Tachycardia related to pain and anxiety increases oxygen consumption due to the stress imposed on the body by pain. Positioning of the patient is important to prevent the complications that occur with immobility such as skin breakdown, pulmonary congestion, and pooling of blood and secretions. Hypermetabolism causes loss of muscle, so it is important to prevent additional loss of movement. Patients should receive active and passive ROM exercises to retain strength and joint motion.

Cognitive level: Application

Nursing process: Planning

Client needs: Physiological Integrity: Physiological Adaptation

Chapter 62

1. Answer: 1. The stem cell is a primitive cell located in the bone marrow that is the precursor of red blood cells, white blood cells, and platelets.

Rationale: Stem cells are primitive cells located in the bone marrow that are the precursor to all blood lines. When stimulated these cells undergo a series of cell divisions and differentiations to become the appropriate respective cell in a process known as hematopoiesis. However, when the bone marrow has been destroyed, as with certain diseases or medications, the liver and spleen can produce blood cells in a process known as extramedullary hematopoiesis. Although the blood is considered to be a type of connective tissue, it has two important functions. The first is to transport oxygen, nutrition, secretory products, and waste products, but the second is to house and transport the immunologic products that are critical to the body's defense against infections. The proportion of red bone marrow diminishes and is replaced by yellow bone marrow as the patient ages. However, in the healthy individual the active red bone marrow can replace the fatty yellow bone marrow if an increase in blood cell production is required.

Cognitive level: Analysis

Nursing process: Assessment

Client needs: Health Promotion and Maintenance; Physiological Integrity

2. Answer: 3. "The cells of the reticuloendothelial system facilitate blood clotting and initiate the inflammatory and immune responses."

Rationale: White blood cells are only found in small amounts in the blood unless they are needed. Instead, they can be found in the bone marrow, lungs, liver, spleen, and lymph nodes as developing and mature cells. Reticulocytes are small, immature red blood cells that are released whenever there is an increased demand for red cells. The red blood cells, or erythrocytes, are responsible for transporting, maintaining the chemical integrity of, and distributing oxygen-carrying hemoglobin to the body's tissues. One function of the reticuloendothelial system is to provide phagocytic cells for the inflammatory and immune responses, but these cells do not facilitate blood clotting.

Cognitive level: Application

Nursing process: Evaluation

Client needs: Physiological Integrity; Physiological Adaptation

3. Answer: 4. MCH, MCV, MCHC

Rationale: The PT (prothrombin time) and aPTT (activated partial thromboplastin time) are useful coagulation studies, and the PLT determines the numbers of platelets. The HGB (hemoglobin) and HCT (hematocrit) can be reduced with anemia, but this does not help classify the type of anemia. The ANC (absolute neutrophil count) is helpful when measuring the proportion of white blood cells that are available for an initial immune response. Red blood cell (RBC) count alone is not a reliable indicator of RBC function or adequacy. The RDW (red blood cell distribution width) measures the consistency of RBC size, and the white blood cell (WBC) count determines the number of leukocytes. The MCH (mean corpuscular hemoglobin), MCV (mean corpuscular volume), and MCHC (mean corpuscular hemoglobin concentration) are used primarily for the classification of anemia and delineating the likely cause.

Cognitive level: Application

Nursing process: Planning

Client needs: Physiological Integrity

4. Answer: 1. HCT 28%

Rationale: A HCT level of 28% is dangerously low for any patient and should immediately be reported to the health care provider. The other values, PLT 400,000/μL, WBC 10,000/μL, and MCH 30 pg/dL, are all within normal limits for either a male or female patient.

Cognitive level: Application

Nursing process: Analysis

Client needs: Health Promotion and Maintenance; Physiological Integrity

5. Answer: 2. An increase in the total white blood cell count because of the proliferation of juvenile band and immature blast cells

Rationale: A shift to the left indicates that the total white blood cell count has increased because of the proliferation of juvenile band and immature blast cells. This phenomenon is the result of bone marrow stimulation to release large amounts of leukocytes, usually in response to severe infection. The absolute neutrophil count (ANC) measures the proportion of white blood cells that are available for use in a first response immune reaction. The mean corpuscular hemoglobin (MCH) and mean corpuscular hemoglobin concentration (MCHC) measure the hemoglobin proportion in an erythrocyte, indicating the efficacy of interaction between the hemoglobin molecule and the red cell. Numerous clotting studies are used to indicate problems within the clotting cascade, and these are not related to a shift to the left.

Cognitive level: Analysis
Nursing process: Assessment
Client needs: Physiological Integrity

6. Answer: 2. Vascular contraction, intrinsic adenosine diphosphate release, prothrombin conversion into thrombin, fibrinogen conversion into fibrin

Rationale: The first step in primary hemostasis is vascular contraction, followed by platelet adhesion and formation of a soft aggregate plug, respectively. The initial platelets that respond to the site of insult release intrinsic adenosine diphosphate, which causes more platelets to aggregate together. Once the short-lived primary hemostasis has occurred, secondary hemostasis begins through either the intrinsic or extrinsic pathway. During these mechanisms Factor XII activates Factor XI; active Factor VII and active Factor XI start a cascade of events that eventually activate Factor X; and active Factor X, along with Factor III, Factor V, Ca^{2+}, and platelet thromboplastic factor, activates prothrombin activator. Also, prothrombin activator converts prothrombin into thrombin, and thrombin converts fibrinogen into fibrin.

Cognitive level: Analysis
Nursing process: Assessment
Client needs: Physiological Integrity

7. Answer: 3. "What medications are you currently taking?"

Rationale: Medications that are myelosuppressive in nature or those that affect bleeding times, such as aspirin, can suppress or alter blood cell production or function, respectively. The patient's allergies to shellfish or IV contrast material are irrelevant to hematologic function. Cholecystectomy, assuming minimal blood loss or complications, is also unrelated to hematologic function. A widened pulse pressure or tachycardia may indicate compensatory mechanisms during states of hypoxia, such as with anemia, but heart disease is not known to cause or be caused by a primary hematologic issue.

Cognitive level: Application
Nursing process: Assessment
Client needs: Health Promotion and Maintenance

Chapter 63

1. Answer: 3. Reduction in hematopoietic stem cells

Rationale: Hematopoietic stem cells (HSCs) reside largely in the spongy bone marrow of the femurs, hips, ribs, sternum, and other long bones, while a small volume of HSCs circulates in the peripheral blood. HSCs may be thought of as the common ancestor cell of all of the blood cell lines. Although HSCs eventually give rise to mature red blood cells, platelets, and white cells, they themselves do not possess the full capabilities of oxygen transportation, clotting, or immune response associated with their more mature progeny, the erythrocytes, platelets, and leukocytes.

Cognitive level: Analysis
Nursing process: Assessment
Client needs: Physiological Integrity: Reduction of Risk Potential

2. Answer: 1. Reduced red blood cell production

Rationale: Dietary elements play a key role in red blood cell production. Deficiencies in any of these elements can negatively affect erythropoiesis. This blood cell development is highly dependent on sufficient quantities of metals such as iron, cobalt, and manganese, vitamins B_{12}, B_6, C, E, folate, riboflavin, pantothenic acid, and thiamin, amino acids, and carbohydrates. Although cellular growth requires all of these elements, vitamin B_{12}, folate, and iron play particularly pivotal roles in erythropoiesis. Folate and vitamin B_{12} are required for the extensive DNA synthesis that occurs with erythropoiesis. All proliferating cells require iron, but the iron requirements of erythroid cells in the late basophilic erythroblast through reticulocyte stages, when hemoglobin is synthesized and accumulates, are much greater than for all other cell types. Disease such as megaloblastic anemia and iron deficiency anemia result when sufficient supplies do not exist to support erythropoiesis.

Cognitive level: Analysis
Nursing process: Assessment
Client needs: Physiological Integrity: Reduction of Risk Potential

3. Answer: 4. Glossitis

Rationale: Because the highly efficient iron storage system provides a rich reservoir for active metabolic needs, early iron deficiency anemia often does not produce bothersome symptoms. As with all anemia, the severity of the symptoms correlates with the degree of hemoglobin deficiency, which in turn correlates with the volume of total iron body stores. As erythropoiesis becomes increasingly hampered, the patient may present with the general manifestations of anemia such as fatigue, pallor, shortness of breath, cold intolerance, headache, and activity intolerance. When iron stores fall critically low as to impact epithelial cell production, the patient may present with symptoms uniquely indicative of iron deficiency anemia including pica or clay eating, glossitis or tongue inflammation, gastric atrophy, stomatitis, ice eating or pagophagia, and leg cramping.

Cognitive level: Application
Nursing process: Assessment
Client needs: Physiological Integrity: Physiological Adaptation

4. Answer: 2. RBC mass being lost at the same rate as total blood volume

Rationale: For sudden blood loss, hematocrit values may not accurately indicate the severity of the problem because RBC mass is lost at the same rate as total blood volume, thus the percentage of RBCs in the blood is unaffected. After 2 to 3 days when then body is able to initiate the compensatory mechanism of increasing plasma volume, RBCs become diluted as reflected by decreasing erythrocyte, hemoglobin, and hematocrit values.

Cognitive level: Analysis

Nursing process: Assessment

Client needs: Physiological Integrity: Physiological Adaptation

5. Answer: 4. Frequent skin and oral mucosa assessment

Rationale: Nursing interventions for a patient with thrombocytopenia should focus on reducing the risk for bleeding. This would include assessing the color and presence of blood in the urine and stool. Additional interventions would include frequent vital signs, breath sounds, and abdominal and neurological assessments.

Cognitive level: Application

Nursing process: Planning

Client needs: Physiological Integrity: Physiological Adaptation

6. Answer: 3. Persistent and last for days or weeks

Rationale: The hallmark clinical presentation of hemophilia is prolonged bleeding and inability to form clots in response to injury, both of which can appear and persist for days to weeks. For patients with severe disease completely lacking any Factor VIII or Factor IX, such bleeding can have serious life-threatening consequences. Distinguished from the disease of primary hemostasis, which causes increased bruising and superficial hemorrhages in the integumentary, people with hemophilia typically suffer from bleeding deep in the tissues. Typically, bleeding sites include joints and organs. If left uncontrolled the internal bleeding can cause severe pressure on closed compartments. Serious consequences of internal bleeding into closed spaces include increased intracranial pressure, hemiarthrosis leading to compartment syndrome, and oropharyngeal bleeding. The eventual sequelae following each of these situations can cause lifetime disability. Increased intracranial pressure can cause ischemia and brain tissue damage. Bleeding into the joints predisposes the patient to arthritis, synovial tissue damage, and joint malformation. Oropharyngeal bleeding may occlude the airway so severely as to require intubation.

Cognitive level: Analysis

Nursing process: Planning

Client needs: Physiological Integrity: Physiological Adaptation

Chapter 64

1. Answer: 2. Instruct in the avoidance of tobacco, excessive alcohol, and a high-fat diet.

Rationale: The risk factors for the development of cancer can be divided into endogenous and exogenous causes. Endogenous causes include increasing incidence with age, an occasional genetic link, and the need for immunocompetence to identify antigens. Exogenous causes include exposure to drugs, chemicals, and tobacco smoke; a diet high in fat and low in fiber; multiple sex partners; large consumption of ethyl alcohol; exposure to ultraviolet and ionizing radiation; and exposure to viruses that have been linked to cancer. The effects of psychosocial stress have yet to be linked specifically to the development of cancer.

Cognitive level: Application

Nursing process: Implementation

Client needs: Health Promotion and Maintenance: Reduction of Risk Potential

2. Answer: 3. Angiogenesis

Rationale: Mechanisms of metastasis include angiogenesis, migration, cell attachment, cell invasion, and growth factors. Angiogenesis is the creation of new blood vessels due to migration and proliferation of endothelial cells from existing blood vessels. New blood vessels provide nutrients, protein growth factors, and oxygen to the tumor mass.

Cognitive level: Application

Nursing process: Implementation

Client needs: Physiological Integrity: Physiological Adaptation

3. Answer: 2. Prostate

Rationale: The treatment for prostate cancer includes surgery or a radical prostatectomy, radiotherapy to include external beam or brachytherapy, cryotherapy, chemotherapy, and expectant management or "watchful waiting."

Cognitive level: Analysis

Nursing process: Assessment

Client needs: Physiological Integrity: Physiological Adaptation

4. Answer: 3. Use strict aseptic technique when caring for venous access devices.

Rationale: The patient with cancer is at risk for the development of an infection. Care for this patient should include the avoidance of rectal procedures, including taking rectal temperatures. Foods that could harbor bacteria should be avoided such as raw meat and fresh fruits and vegetables. Intramuscular injections should be avoided. Strict aseptic technique should be used at all times when caring for venous access devices, urinary catheters, and other monitoring devices.

Cognitive level: Application

Nursing process: Planning

Client needs: Physiological Integrity: Reduction of Risk Potential

5. Answer: 1. Cluster care activities to increase rest periods.

Rationale: Many patients who receive radiotherapy experience fatigue. The exact causative mechanism is unknown, although it is thought to be due to the result of tumor breakdown, which releases by-products into the bloodstream. Another explanation for the development of fatigue is the increase in basal metabolic rate consuming the body's energy stores. Fatigue typically begins during the third or fourth week of treatment and will gradually wane once the treatment is over. The loss of energy and feeling of tiredness tend to be cumulative and have a significant impact on patients' quality of life. Patient education regarding the side effects of radiation begins before treatment and needs to continue once it is over. Teaching patients that side effects should be expected may decrease their fear that treatment is ineffective. Nursing care needs to be designed with energy conservation in mind. Clustering patient care activities together will allow for prolonged periods of rest for patients who are experiencing fatigue. Teaching patients and their caregivers these principles will assist the patient in coping with the tiredness experienced with fatigue while at home.

Cognitive level: Application
Nursing process: Implementation
Client needs: Physiological Integrity: Physiological Adaptation

6. Answer: 3. Alter the immunologic relationship between the tumor and the patient.
Rationale: Biotherapy is known as treatment with agents whose origin, mostly mammal, is from biologic sources and/or affecting biologic responses. Biotherapy has emerged since the 1980s as another treatment option for patients with cancer who are receiving high-dose chemotherapy and transplantation. Nurses caring for patients receiving biotherapy need to possess an understanding of the immune system before they can begin to comprehend the rationale behind this unique treatment modality and the primary agents currently used. Although the mechanism of action varies with each type of biologic response modifier, the goal is the same: to destroy or halt the malignant growth of a tumor. A therapeutic effect is accomplished by altering the immunologic relationship between the tumor and the patient.

Cognitive level: Analysis
Nursing process: Planning
Client needs: Physiological Integrity: Physiological Adaptation

Chapter 65

1. Answer: 4. Vitamin D deficiency
Rationale: Functions of the skin include retarding the loss of body heat and fluids, assisting in the control of body temperature, functioning as an excretory organ, and functioning as a synthesizer of vitamin D when sunlight reacts with cholesterol.

Cognitive level: Analysis
Nursing process: Assessment
Client needs: Health Promotion and Maintenance: Prevention/Early Detection of Health Problems

2. Answer: 3. Biographic and demographic data
Rationale: Biographic and demographic data include data such as the patient's name, address, telephone number, Social Security number, contact person, age, gender, race or ethnic origin, marital status, birthplace, occupation, level of education, and religious affiliation. Examples of biographic and demographic data that may be significant to assessment of the skin include travel to different environments such as when camping or travel to rural areas of the world. The patient's current issue or the reason for seeking health care is referred to as the chief complaint. The reason for obtaining information about the past medical history is to identify the patient's entire past relevant health problems. Past illnesses could possibly have some effect on the patient's current health. The nursing assessment includes questions about major illnesses such as diabetes, cardiovascular disease, and infectious diseases. Patients with diabetes are prone to skin breakdown and delayed wound healing. Patients with cardiovascular disease may have clubbed nail beds. Infectious diseases such as cellulitis have skin manifestations, which assist with the diagnosis.

Cognitive level: Application
Nursing process: Assessment
Client needs: Health Promotion and Maintenance: Prevention/Early Detection of Health Problems

3. Answer: 4. Social history
Rationale: Social history includes use of alcohol or street drugs that can have adverse effects on the condition of the patient's skin. The presence of certain cutaneous lesions in a patient should prompt an investigation into the patient's drinking and drug habits. If drug use is suspected due to the presence of a cutaneous lesion, the nurse needs to inquire about skin popping. Skin popping is a technique used by individuals to administer illicit drugs. Skin popping is a significant risk factor in skin and soft tissue infections, which are common among injection drug users.

Cognitive level: Application
Nursing process: Assessment
Client needs: Physiological Integrity: Physiological Adaptation

4. Answer: 3. Inspect and palpate the skin at the same time.
Rationale: The assessment should proceed in an orderly fashion, beginning with an examination of the most frequently exposed areas such as the face, hands, arms, legs, and feet. The nurse inspects the skin while the patient is in a sitting or lying position with all clothes removed except an examination or hospital gown. The nurse will inspect and palpate simultaneously.

Cognitive level: Application
Nursing process: Assessment
Client needs: Health Promotion and Maintenance: Prevention/Early Detection of Health Problems

5. Answer: 4. Normal findings
Rationale: The nail surface is normally slightly curved with the posterior and lateral folds smooth and rounded. The nail edges should be smooth, rounded, and clean. The normal nail bed angle is 160 degrees. The nail base is firm to palpation. A nail bed with greater than a 160-degree angle suggests a clubbed nail. Clubbing of nails indicates a state of chronic hypoxia and is often seen with congenital and adult heart disease and chronic obstructive pulmonary disease. The surface of the nail should be smooth and nonbrittle, with no splitting. Pits, transverse grooves, or

lines may indicate a nutritional deficiency. Patients with arterial insufficiency may have thickened, ridged nails.

Cognitive level: Application

Nursing process: Assessment

Client needs: Health Promotion and Maintenance: Prevention/Early Detection of Health Problems

6. Answer: 3. Keloid

Rationale: A fissure is a linear crack or break from the epidermis to the dermis. A scale is an abundance of dry or oily keratinized cells. A keloid results from the overproduction of scar tissue that extends laterally beyond the initial wound; it is usually raised and smooth in appearance. A cherry angioma is a distinct benign vascular lesion.

Cognitive level: Analysis

Nursing process: Assessment

Client needs: Physiological Integrity: Reduction of Risk Potential

7. Answer: 4. Vitiligo

Rationale: Jaundice is a yellowish discoloration of the skin, sclera, and mucous membranes that is often associated with increased amounts of bilirubin in the blood. Pallor is paleness of the skin that occurs when the red-pink tones from the oxygenated hemoglobin in the blood are lost. Petechiae are pinpoint purpuric lesions of the skin. Vitiligo is the absence of pigmentation in a circumscribed area.

Cognitive level: Analysis

Nursing process: Assessment

Client needs: Physiological Integrity: Reduction of Risk Potential

Chapter 66

1. Answer: 1. Atopic dermatitis

Rationale: Atopic dermatitis is characterized by severe itching. Treatment involves controlling the aggravating factors and treating the rash. It is important to moisturize the skin to maintain the skin barrier. Bathing should be held to a minimum; however, when bathing, the patient should use tepid water and mild, unscented soap such as Cetaphil or Dove.

Cognitive level: Analysis

Nursing process: Implementation

Client needs: Physiological Integrity: Basic Care and Comfort

2. Answer: 2. Eat foods high in vitamin C, iron, and zinc.

Rationale: The nurse should instruct the patient to maintain a high-calorie, high-protein, well-balanced diet. Include vitamin C, iron, and zinc in the diet. Avoid foods that cause hypersensitivity reactions.

Cognitive level: Application

Nursing process: Implementation

Client needs: Physiological Integrity: Physiological Adaptation

3. Answer: 4. Instruct in the use of sunscreen.

Rationale: The sun, along with other pollutants in the air, can irritate and damage the skin, with most of the damage occurring before the age of 18. Nearly 80% of this damage can be prevented if sunscreen is applied properly in those first 18 years of life.

Cognitive level: Application

Nursing process: Implementation

Client needs: Health Promotion and Maintenance: Prevention/Early Detection of Health Problems

4. Answer: 1. Rub the medication into wet skin thoroughly.

Rationale: Topical corticosteroids should be applied in a thin layer and rubbed in thoroughly on wet skin. Retinoic acid can be irritating to the skin and produce phototoxicity. Systemic antihistamines can cause drowsiness.

Cognitive level: Application

Nursing process: Implementation

Client needs: Physiological Integrity: Pharmacologic and Parenteral Therapies

5. Answer: 1. Signs of infection

Rationale: The focus of nursing care is to prevent problems or recognize complications early so they can be successfully treated. The nurse must assess the patient frequently, noting changes in skin color, texture, wound size, drainage, and temperature. Analysis of the data collected during assessment will provide a basis for determining a treatment plan and assessing response to treatment. Patients with skin disorders may develop problems with hydration, fluid balance, or nutrition. Fluid loss through wounds leads to dehydration and electrolyte imbalances. The skin also provides protection against infection, so when its barrier is broken, infection becomes more likely. It is very important to assess for signs of infection both in the wound and systemically. Clinical manifestations of infection include fever, increased redness or drainage, increased pain, changes in odor or color of drainage, increased white blood cell count, and increased tissue erosion. If the infecting organism is contagious, such as occurs with staphylococcus, isolation procedures may be needed.

Cognitive level: Application

Nursing process: Assessment

Client needs: Physiological Integrity: Reduction of Risk Potential

6. Answer: 3. There are light materials that you could wear to protect your arms while still enjoying the summer activities.

Rationale: Psychological assessment needs to be uppermost in the mind of the nurse as care is given to patients with skin disorders. The appearance of the skin affects self-esteem and body image. Skin disorders can cause the patient to withdraw from social situations. Society can be unkind to people who have scars or rashes with an unpleasant appearance. Some individuals may withdraw from the patient, fearing the disorder is contagious. Patients should be provided with an open, supportive environment in which they are comfortable voicing their concerns.

Cognitive level: Application

Nursing process: Implementation

Client needs: Psychosocial Integrity: Coping and Adaptation

7. Answer: 2. This is a normal part of aging.

Rationale: Many anatomic changes occur during the aging process: Skin loses elasticity and water content; the texture and turgor of the skin change; the retaining ligaments of the soft tissue of the face weaken; the face loses volume as a result of decreased subcutaneous adipose stores and muscle mass; facial bones undergo resorption; the eye orbit changes shape, allowing for positional changes of the eye globe; the face becomes elongated and flattened; and smoking, genetics, and sun exposure contribute to the loss of skin elasticity and wrinkle formation.

Cognitive level: Application

Nursing process: Implementation

Client needs: Health Promotion and Maintenance: Growth and Development Through the Life Span

Chapter 67

1. Answer: 3. Proliferation

Rationale: Homeostasis is the tendency of the human body to maintain stability, and maintaining stability is the first reaction when a wound occurs. The inflammatory phase of wound healing begins at the time of the injury or surgery. The purpose of this critical phase is to prepare the site for growth of new tissue. The proliferative phase is the next phase in the healing process. Reconstruction occurs at this phase. It can last up to 3 weeks after the inflammatory phase in a normal, healthy person. Growth factors originating from injured vessels stimulate the formation of vascular buds and regrowth of vascular loops. Stimulated endothelial cells multiply and form tubular structures, differentiating into arterioles or venules, a process referred to as angiogenesis. These new blood vessels can begin to form in a wound within 3 days of injury, provided there is sufficient blood circulation to the wound bed. Remodeling, the third and final phase of wound healing, occurs after the wound is closed. It begins about 3 weeks after the injury and can still be in progress from 6 months to 2 years later.

Cognitive level: Analysis

Nursing process: Assessment

Client needs: Health Promotion and Maintenance: Prevention/Early Detection of Health Problems

2. Answer: 3. Using the clock face method

Rationale: A sinus tract is an area, sometimes referred to as a tunnel, where there is nonhealed detached tissue under intact skin. Sinus tracts are measured in centimeters. Referring to location, the area of tunneling is defined on a clock face with 12 o'clock being the head of the body. For example, if a wound located on the anterior aspect of the leg has tunneling on the medial side of the left leg, the measurement would be x amount of centimeters at the 9 o'clock position. There is also a measurement for undermining. Undermining is like a cliff without tissue below and more broad than a sinus tract. It is measured from each point or side using the clock face method. The surface area of the wound is the length multiplied by the width in centimeters squared (cm^2). The volume is the length multiplied by the width and the depth in centimeters cubed (cm^3).

Cognitive level: Application

Nursing process: Assessment

Client needs: Physiological Integrity: Physiological Adaptation

3. Answer: 2. Use the rule of 30 to reposition the patient every two hours.

Rationale: Positioning is important in the prevention of pressure ulcers. The goal is to get the patient mobile and active as soon as possible; however, when mobility is physically impossible, the patient's position should be changed a minimum of every 2 hours. A sufficient number of people should be available to move the patient so that shearing and friction during movement can be avoided. Assistive devices such as transfer boards or mechanical lifts may be helpful to minimize tissue injury during movement. The "rule of 30" is used for positioning. This rule states that the head of the bed should be elevated 30 degrees or less and the body placed in a 30-degree laterally inclined position when placed on either side. These positions avoid pressure directly over the trochanter and promote improved circulation to the skin over the sacrum and ischial tuberosities. Pillows or foam wedges may be used to keep the patient properly positioned. The prone position may also be used if the patient is able to tolerate it. Attention should be focused on maintaining proper alignment so that functional ability can be maintained.

Cognitive level: Application

Nursing process: Planning

Client needs: Physiological Integrity: Reduction of Risk Potential

4. Answer: 3. Apply a moisture barrier and secure with gauze.

Rationale: Compression is used for venous wounds. Surgery is indicated for arterial wounds. Debridement is appropriate for wounds with eschar. Appropriate care for a skin tear wound includes avoiding the use of adhesive dressings or tapes, applying a moisture barrier, wrapping a gauze bandage around the extremity, using hydrogel sheet dressings or foam, and/or using zinc-impregnated gauze and cotton.

Cognitive level: Application

Nursing process: Implementation

Client needs: Physiological Integrity: Physiological Adaptation

5. Answer: 1. Autolytic debridement

Rationale: Autolytic debridement allows the body to utilize its phagocytes to destroy the necrotic tissue. This is often a preferred method of debridement for those persons for whom daily or more frequent dressing changes would be a hardship; that is, patients who are critically ill and cannot be turned. Autolytic debridement is a slow and nonaggressive treatment. Sharp debridement is done with a scalpel, scissors, or nippers. Anesthetics or the operating room may be required depending on wound size and depth. Mechanical debridement is the

dislodging of necrotic tissue, which is accomplished by wet-to-dry dressings, the whirlpool, or pulse lavage. Enzymatic debridement is chemically induced by prescriptive ointments that contain papain-urea or collagenase, which penetrates the slough and eschar causing them to soften and "melt down." Once softened, the slough and eschar are mechanically debrided.
Cognitive level: Analysis
Nursing process: Planning
Client needs: Physiological Integrity: Physiological Adaptation

6. Answer: 2. Tell me why you think the wound is ugly.
Rationale: Depression can occur when a patient has a wound. It may affect the way she sees herself or the way she perceives that others see her, especially if the wound is easily visible. Not only does the patient have an emotional response to her wound, but almost everyone the patient encounters has an emotional response to her wound. Wounds are perceived as unpleasant, disgusting, scary, and a nuisance. Depression may affect the patient's ability to perform the daily activities she desires to do, and it may limit patient independence. It can be very costly for the treatments and medications. The patient may have to wear some special type of shoe or device that makes her self-conscious. The nurse needs to assess the patient for her feelings about her wound and associated treatment. Empathize with the patient, and try to devise a plan that is least intrusive and yet realistic.
Cognitive level: Application
Nursing process: Assessment
Client needs: Psychosocial Integrity: Coping and Adaptation

7. Answer: 2. Healing rate
Rationale: Poor nutrition will negatively impact the healing rate of a wound. Wound dressings impact the risk of infection. Mechanisms to preventing scar formation impact wound appearance. Appropriate pain management impacts the patient's comfort level.
Cognitive level: Analysis
Nursing process: Evaluation
Client needs: Physiological Integrity: Physiological Adaptation

Chapter 68

1. Answer: 3. Major burn injury
Rationale: This patient has experienced a major burn injury. The classifications are minor, moderate, and major, not medium. Electrical burns and burns involving the feet are always considered major injuries, even though the dermal injuries only appeared as 2% or less.
Cognitive level: Application
Nursing process: Assessment
Client needs: Physiological Integrity

2. Answer: 4. "Liquid at 140°F requires five minutes to cause a full-thickness burn."
Rationale: Liquids at 120°F require 5 minutes to cause a full-thickness burn. At 140°F liquids can cause a burn

injury in 5 seconds or less. Sunscreens help prevent radiation burns from the sun and help decrease the risk of skin cancers. Children's sleepwear should be made from fire retardant materials, and every home should have smoke alarms that are clean and in working order.
Cognitive level: Application
Nursing process: Evaluation
Client needs: Safe and Effective Care Environment

3. Answer: 1. "With bacterial translocation the gastrointestinal mucosal atrophy that occurs causes intraluminal bacteria to migrate to extraluminal sites."
Rationale: Paralytic ileus and gastrointestinal mucosal atrophy are not uncommon with severe burn injuries. This allows opportunity for the intraluminal bacteria to migrate to extraluminal sources in a process called bacterial translocation. Decreased cardiac output can occur early after a burn injury because of the vasoconstriction caused by the sympathetic nervous system. When damaged erythrocytes and muscle tissue cause the release of excess hemoglobin and myoglobin, respectively, the liver is unable to handle this increased load. Therefore, these substances must be excreted through the urine and can clog the renal tubules, causing renal failure. Leukocytes are not transfused, although their stores may be depleted within 48 hours following a burn. Decreased circulating iron causes a resultant low red blood cell count, and it is not uncommon to replace red blood cells or platelets in patients with major burns.
Cognitive level: Application
Nursing process: Assessment
Client needs: Physiological Integrity

4. Answer: 2. The acute care period
Rationale: The emergency and resuscitative periods are the same and include the initial treatment with airway and hemodynamic stabilization with fluid resuscitation. The rehabilitative period begins when the open burn wound size is less than 20% and the patient is at his or her highest level of functioning since admission. This phase focuses on physical and psychological restoration, including increased strength, function, flexibility, and cosmetic restoration. The acute care period begins once the patient is hemodynamically stable. The focus is on wound care, prevention of infection and other complications, and pain control.
Cognitive level: Analysis
Nursing process: Implementation
Client needs: Physiological Integrity

5. Answer: 1. A 35-year-old with a history of migraines and 40% TBSA full-thickness thermal burns to the neck, left upper extremity, and circumferentially around the chest. Vital signs are HR 116, BP 90/68, RR 26 and shallow, SpO$_2$ 90%.
Rationale: The 35-year-old patient has a major burn injury. The size and location of the burn, as well as the circumferential nature of the wound, have the potential to cause increased morbidity and mortality in this patient. The vital signs reflect possible cardiopulmonary

compromise. The 70-year-old patient is older and has a chronic medical condition, but partial-thickness wounds of less than 15% and full-thickness wounds of less than 1% are considered minor. Also, the burns do not involve the head, neck, chest, hands, feet, or perineum nor are the vital signs abnormal. The 12-year-old patient is younger, but not an infant or young child. A partial-thickness burn of 20% is moderate, and it is important to note that while the injury to the foot is significant, it is not full thickness nor would it take precedence over an injury that could compromise airway, breathing, or circulation. The history of astigmatism is unremarkable to the emergent burn treatment, and the vital signs are normal. The 44-year-old patient does have a significant chronic medical condition, as exemplified by the blood pressure reading. However, an 8% full-thickness injury and 15% partial-thickness injury are moderate injuries. It is also important to note that none of the burns are classified as circumferential.
Cognitive level: Analysis
Nursing process: Planning
Client needs: Physiological Integrity

6. Answer: 2. Fluid volume deficit related to increased capillary permeability
Rationale: After airway and breathing, the priority during emergency care is cardiovascular assessment with fluid resuscitation. Therefore, of the choices given, fluid volume deficit would be the priority nursing diagnosis during the emergency phase. Altered skin integrity is addressed during the emergency phase, but it is the basis for care during the acute care phase. Acute pain should certainly be addressed, but it will not take precedence over fluid volume deficit. A potential problem, such as high risk for infection, will also be attended to after actual problems.
Cognitive level: Application
Nursing process: Planning
Client needs: Physiological Integrity

7. Answer: 4. "My pressure garments should be removed one to four times a day to allow for adequate circulation."
Rationale: Exercise programs for burned patients should be progressive in nature so as to improve strength and endurance. These programs may also include stretching exercises to elongate shortened tissues. These exercises are providing adequate stretch when the burn scar blanches. Also beneficial to helping healed burn wounds is scar massage. The massage should be performed daily, from one to four times a day. The massage helps improve the cosmetic appearance and hypertrophy of the scar, as well as increase circulation and possibly range of motion. Pressure garments should be worn continuously for 23 hours a day, not removed several times to promote circulation.
Cognitive level: Analysis
Nursing process: Evaluation
Client needs: Physiological Integrity

8. Answer: 3. Heart rate 114
Rationale: The heart rate is tachycardic, indicating possible hypovolemia. The blood pressure appears normal, but this is a poor early indicator because the increased systemic vascular resistance that occurs causes the blood pressure to be maintained regardless of volume status. A central venous pressure of 6 indicates adequate fluid volume, as does a urine output of 30 mL/hr.
Cognitive level: Analysis
Nursing process: Assessment
Client needs: Physiological Integrity

Chapter 69

1. Answer: 2. Normal
Rationale: The inside of the ear is inspected with an otoscope. An otoscopic examination includes inspection of the auditory canal and tympanic membrane. Look for inflammation, exudates, lesions, and foreign bodies. Check for narrowing of the ear canal, nodules, redness, scales, edema, drainage, and foreign objects. Normally the eardrum is slightly conical, shiny, smooth, and pearl gray. Cerumen should be moist and may vary in color from brown to white, but hardened, dry, or foul-smelling cerumen may indicate infection. In a majority of Asians and Native Americans, cerumen is dry, white, and flaky. In African Americans and Caucasians, cerumen is brown, wet, and sticky.
Cognitive level: Analysis
Nursing process: Assessment
Client needs: Health Promotion and Maintenance: Prevention/Early Detection of Health Problems

2. Answer: 4. Do you think that there is something in the room causing you to sneeze?
Rationale: The nurse needs to inquire about a history of upper respiratory infection. Sneezing, particularly at specific times of the year or under specific environmental circumstances, should be investigated for the possibility of allergies or respiratory infection. Allergic rhinitis is an inflammation of the nasal mucosa caused by an allergic substance, for example, hay fever or pollen. The nurse needs to inquire if the allergies are related to a specific time of year. Does the patient regularly take medications for allergic rhinitis, sinus infections, stuffy nose, or frequent respiratory infections? Some nasal sprays and decongestants may cause rebound nasal swelling. Over-the-counter oral decongestants may have an adverse effect on patients with diabetes, hypertension, hyperthyroidism, and cardiac illnesses.
Cognitive level: Analysis
Nursing process: Assessment
Client needs: Health Promotion and Maintenance: Prevention/Early Detection of Health Problems

3. Answer: 2. Even though you have dentures, seeing a dentist regularly is necessary for good oral health.
Rationale: Poorly fitting dentures or orthotic appliances and inadequate dentition can cause difficulty chewing,

nutritional problems, and mouth sores. To maintain good oral health, the patient should see the dentist at regular intervals and use good oral hygiene measures.

Cognitive level: Analysis

Nursing process: Assessment

Client needs: Health Promotion and Maintenance: Prevention/Early Detection of Health Problems

4. Answer: 3. Social isolation because of hearing loss

Rationale: Age impacts hearing ability. For example, presbycusis, hearing loss in the high-frequency range, is the most common sensorineural hearing loss in older people. The patient experiencing the gradual hearing loss of aging may limit social interactions as it becomes so difficult to understand the spoken word. During the assessment the nurse should inquire about functional ability and social interactions. Loss of hearing also can be perceived as mental status changes. Nurses need to be more aware of the impact of hearing loss on the elderly.

Cognitive level: Analysis

Nursing process: Assessment

Client needs: Psychosocial Integrity: Coping and Adaptation

5. Answer: 1. Normal

Rationale: With the voice whisper test the examiner stands approximately 1 to 2 feet in back of the patient and whispers several words near each ear. The patient should be able to hear bilaterally and equally.

Cognitive level: Analysis

Nursing process: Assessment

Client needs: Health Promotion and Maintenance: Prevention/Early Detection of Health Problems

Chapter 70

1. Answer: 3. Sound transmission

Rationale: The tympanic membrane or eardrum, comprised of tissue that makes up the ear canal, is the final structure within this portion of the outer ear anatomy. It is this structure that transmits sounds from the outer to the middle ear. The cochlea is responsible for hearing, whereas the vestibular system is responsible for balance. Within the inner ear are found the semicircular canals, specifically the horizontal, anterior, and posterior canals, which help with balance and movement. The acoustic nerve consists of two separate parts, the vestibular and cochlear branches. This eighth cranial nerve controls hearing and equilibrium.

Cognitive level: Analysis

Nursing process: Assessment

Client needs: Health Promotion and Maintenance: Prevention/Early Detection of Health Problems

2. Answer: 2. Air conduction

Rationale: There are actually two mechanisms involved with hearing: bone conduction and air conduction. Bone conduction is the conduction of sound to the inner ear through the bones of the skull. Air conduction begins the process when noise enters the external ear and travels to the middle ear. Once inside the middle

ear, the sound is transmitted through the three auditory bones, the malleus, incus, and stapes. Once the sound or noise reaches the stapes, it is then transmitted to the inner ear where it reaches the acoustic nerve and is transmitted to the brain for interpretation. Hearing disorders can be caused by an alteration anywhere within the auditory structures.

Cognitive level: Analysis

Nursing process: Assessment

Client needs: Health Promotion and Maintenance: Prevention/Early Detection of Health Problems

3. Answer: 3. Conductive

Rationale: In conductive hearing loss, sound waves cannot reach the inner ear for processing and interpretation. With sensorineural hearing loss, the cause is damage to the auditory nerve or possibly damage to the small hair cells within the inner ear. Mixed hearing loss refers to both conductive and sensorineural hearing loss caused by a dysfunction of both air and bone conduction processes. Acoustic hearing loss would refer to a damaged acoustic nerve.

Cognitive level: Analysis

Nursing process: Assessment

Client needs: Health Promotion and Maintenance: Prevention/Early Detection of Health Problems

4. Answer: 3. The baby should be tested now.

Rationale: Within the *Healthy People 2010* "Objectives for Reducing Hearing Loss," it is recommended that newborns should have a first hearing examination by 1 month of age. Babies with a hearing loss should have additional testing by 3 months of age. And if hearing loss continues, the baby should be enrolled in a rehabilitative program by 6 months of age. Hearing loss in the newborn can be linked to birth trauma, toxicity, infection, fetal anoxia during delivery, premature or low birth weight, genetics, or an elevated serum bilirubin level. In addition, deafness upon birth has been seen in those women who have been exposed to highly communicable diseases such as rubella and syphilis or who have ingested known ototoxic medications while pregnant. The presence of hearing can be assessed as early as 2 to 3 days of life. Hearing loss is one of the most common developmental abnormalities present at birth. If left undiagnosed, it will impede speech, language, and cognitive developments. Individuals with hearing impairment at this early age will face a lifetime of challenges. Learning how to communicate with sign language and lip reading are just two ways to aid the person born without the sense of hearing.

Cognitive level: Analysis

Nursing process: Assessment

Client needs: Health Promotion and Maintenance: Prevention/Early Detection of Health Problems

5. Answer: 1. Mechanical

Rationale: The causes of hearing impairment or loss can be categorized as mechanical, inflammatory, or an obstructive disorder. One mechanical cause of hearing loss is due to otosclerosis or a primary bone dyscrasia that leads to conductive hearing loss. Otosclerosis is a condition in which the structures of the ear begin to harden. Seen as a common cause of conductive hearing loss, treatment options are limited to a stapedectomy.

Cognitive level: Analysis

Nursing process: Assessment

Client needs: Physiological Integrity: Physiological Adaptation

6. Answer: 3. Mechanism to ensure a visual alert in the event of a home fire

Rationale: The home needs to have services or mechanisms that make the environment safer; for instance, visual fire safety provisions and access to alerting and telephone services, and TVs with teletext ability.

Cognitive level: Application

Nursing process: Planning

Client needs: Health Promotion and Maintenance: Prevention/Early Detection of Health Problems

7. Answer: 2. Drop the tone of the voice when talking.

Rationale: When providing care to an elderly patient with a hearing deficit or balance disorder, the nurse needs to include specific items in the assessment process. First the method of communication must be determined. A loud voice does not ensure successful hearing or comprehension. Depending on the cause and degree of hearing loss, the nurse might simply drop the tone of the voice to be successful with vocal communication with an elderly patient who has a hearing impairment because the loss of high-frequency sounds occurs first.

Cognitive level: Application

Nursing process: Implementation

Client needs: Physiological Integrity: Reduction of Risk Potential

8. Answer: 1. Assure the patient that the call light will be answered as soon as possible.

Rationale: The nurse should implement strategies to reduce the patient's anxiety such as responding to the call light as soon as possible, answering questions, teaching about medications/treatments, and providing emotional support to the patient having difficulty coping with the new sensory deficit.

Cognitive level: Application

Nursing process: Implementation

Client needs: Psychosocial Integrity: Coping and Adaptation

Chapter 71

1. Answer: 3. Floaters

Rationale: The vitreous body is the largest chamber of the eye that maintains the shape of the eyeball. The vitreous gel is made up mainly of water with a collagen framework, which includes collagen, hyaluronic acid, proteins, and solutes. Due to aging, the collagen network can be aggregated by vitreous collapse that forms vitreous opacities, which cast shadows on the retina. These shadows are referred to as floaters.

Cognitive level: Analysis

Nursing process: Assessment

Client needs: Health Promotion and Maintenance: Prevention/Early Detection of Health Problems

2. Answer: 2. The uncovered eye is fixated outward.

Rationale: When conducting the cover–uncover test for tropia, the patient is to wear his own corrective lenses, if he has them. Have the patient fixate on a target about 20 feet away for far and 16 inches for near; it can be a visual acuity chart, picture chart, E chart, or toy. The tester is to sit in front of the patient, but does not block target view. Note the eye that is fixating cover that eye with an occluder, and note what the fellow eye does. If the uncovered eye moves to pick up fixation, note the direction it moves: If toward the nose, then it was fixated outward, so it is exo; if toward the ear, then it was fixated inward, so it is eso. If the uncovered eye does not move and has steady fixation, no strabismus exists. The eye would move up and down to indicate vertical tropia.

Cognitive level: Analysis

Nursing process: Assessment

Client needs: Health Promotion and Maintenance: Prevention/Early Detection of Health Problems

3. Answer: 4. Eye muscle surgery

Rationale: Adult strabismus may be treated with eye muscle exercises, eyeglasses containing prisms, botulinum toxin (Botox) injections, and eye surgery. Eye muscle exercise usually is used when treating a form of adult strabismus, called convergence insufficiency, in which eyes cannot align themselves for close work or reading. These exercises can retrain eyes to focus inward together. Prism eyeglasses can be used to correct the mild double vision associated with adult strabismus. Botox injections are an effective treatment when overactive eye muscles are causing strabismus. Eye muscle surgery is the most common treatment; it is used to loosen or tighten the muscles around the eye in order to correct the misalignment.

Cognitive level: Analysis

Nursing process: Planning

Client needs: Psychosocial Integrity: Coping and Adaptation

4. Answer: 2. The correct use of eyedrops

Rationale: Nursing assessment and education include patient compliance with regular use of eyedrops and follow-up, which is one of the main goals in treating glaucoma. The major reason for the cause of blindness from glaucoma, besides not knowing one has glaucoma, is noncompliance in using eyedrops and not considering glaucoma to be a serious disease. It is imperative that patients understand that the long-term goal of treatment is to lower intraocular pressure to prevent optic nerve damage, and only with continued use of drops can this goal be reached. Patient education includes information on risk factors for glaucoma such as family history, myopia, previous eye trauma, low blood pressure, African ancestry, diabetes, longtime exposure to steroids, and aging. The patient is taught how to instill eyedrops properly for the full benefit of treatment.

Cognitive level: Application

Nursing process: Planning

Client needs: Physiological Integrity: Physiological Adaptation

5. Answer: 2. Explain that whatever decision they make, they have freedom of choice.

Rationale: The decision to donate corneal tissue for transplantation can have ethical considerations. It is important for the family that is being asked to donate a cornea for the benefit of someone else's vision that the decision be a well-informed one, one that is freely chosen, and one that is compatible with the ethical beliefs of the individuals concerned. It is important for the family members to know that whatever decision they make, to donate or not to donate, they have freedom of choice. Under the circumstances of facing the loss of a loved one, any decision they make is the right decision for them. Usually the decision is one of three choices: Donate all organs, donate only the cornea, or do not donate at all. The two most common reasons not to donate are (1) the fear of something being done before the person is dead, and (2) the fear that the health care provider may hasten the death to benefit another. Thoughts that the family should consider include these: Donation is an ethical decision to benefit another person; with treatment of the body after death, respect is the greatest issue, especially for psychological, religious, spiritual, moral, and cultural reasons; donation is the last giving act the person donor does to reflect his life; and the family knows that the loved one still lives on in another person.

Cognitive level: Application

Nursing process: Implementation

Client needs: Psychosocial Integrity: Coping and Adaptation

Chapter 72

1. Answer: 3. "When the group responsible for committing the violence has connection to a foreign country like al Queda in the Middle East."

Rationale: Terrorist acts use force, destruction, and violence to coerce and intimidate and cause disruption, terror, and panic. When the group or individual is operating independently from within the United States or Puerto Rico with acts of terrorism that are directed at the U.S. government or its population, then it is said to be an act of "domestic" terrorism. Terrorist acts committed across international boundaries or by groups with foreign ties are said to be acts of "international" terrorism.

Cognitive level: Analysis

Nursing process: Assessment

Client needs: Safe and Effective Care Environment

2. Answer: 1. "The outbreak of an intentionally caused food-borne illness in Oregon during the early 1980s was attributed to *Shigella sonnei*."

Rationale: In 1979 the nuclear power plant at Three Mile Island in the United States did experience an accidental radiation leak. However, there were never any effects on physical health reported. In both 1994 and 1995, sarin gas was released into the Tokyo subway system by the Aum Shinrikyo cult, making the resultant disaster the largest peace-time event involving nerve gas. Rye ergot was used in the 6th century B.C. by the Assyrians who would use it to poison the water wells of their enemies. In 1984, in The Dalles, Oregon, a religious group known as the Rajneeshees intentionally contaminated a salad bar at a local restaurant with *Salmonella typhimurium*.

Cognitive level: Analysis

Nursing process: Evaluation

Client needs: Safe and Effective Care Environment

3. Answer: 4. Inhalation anthrax

Rationale: Although the patient clearly has an infectious process manifesting with signs of shock, tachypnea, dyspnea, and fever with chills, the complaint of chest pain with radiologic confirmation of a widened mediastinum several days following possible biologic agent exposure are classic for inhalation anthrax. Septicemic plague may also present with signs of sepsis or septic shock, but it also usually includes gastrointestinal symptoms such as vomiting and diarrhea. Also known as the "Black Death," septicemic plague causes purpuric lesions, distal gangrene, and disseminated intravascular coagulopathy. Undulant fever is also called brucellosis. It presents much like the flu, with generalized body aches, fever, headache, and malaise. Patients may also have gastrointestinal symptoms. The onset of typhoidal tularemia is abrupt and progressive. Patients may experience fever, chills, and chest pain, but they usually also have severe body aches, low back pain, sore throat, and pneumonia. They may also have nausea, vomiting, diarrhea, and weight loss.

Cognitive level: Analysis

Nursing process: Assessment

Client needs: Physiological Integrity

4. Answer: 1. Ineffective airway clearance related to copious secretions and ineffective cough

Rationale: Although all of the nursing diagnoses are appropriate for the patient with known nerve agent exposure, the priority for any patient is airway. Nursing diagnoses that relate to actual problems would always take precedence over potential problems, such as increased risk for altered cardiac output or for fluid and electrolyte imbalance. Also, physiological issues should be addressed prior to any psychosocial problems this patient may be experiencing.

Cognitive level: Application

Nursing process: Planning

Client needs: Physiological Integrity

5. Answer: 2. Prodromal phase

Rationale: The prodromal phase is the initial phase after exposure and has an onset of minutes to hours and lasts from hours to days. In this phase the onset of symptoms is rapid and may include nausea, vomiting, and fatigue. Fever, hypotension, and diarrhea may occur with high-level exposure. The rapid onset in this case, within half an hour, is bleak. The latent phase follows the prodromal phase, and during this time, the patient is relatively symptom free. Once the patient has recovered from an exposure, the acute symptoms should not occur. The illness phase is marked by overt illness. Signs and symptoms may be more systemic, involving the hematopoietic, gastrointestinal, central nervous, and dermatologic systems in any combination.

Cognitive level: Analysis

Nursing process: Assessment

Client needs: Safe, Effective Care Environment/Physiological Integrity

6. Answer: 3. This flexible plan allows for only necessary positions and functions to be activated on an as-needed basis during the incident.

Rationale: The Incident Commander is in charge of four areas: operations, planning, logistics, and finance. Although the HICS plan does outline a clear chain of command and responsibilities for each position involved, the positions do not have to have a sole commander nor must they remain independent of other positions. If needed, the positions may be combined under the leadership of one individual. Media use is very helpful if the HICS is activated. Its utilization can decrease mass hysteria by increasing public awareness of the situation. The plan is flexible, allowing for only necessary positions and functions to be activated on an as-needed basis during the incident.

Cognitive level: Analysis

Nursing process: Planning

Client needs: Safe and Effective Care Environment

7. Answer: 1. It helps augment the local and state resources so as to help decrease the morbidity and mortality in the civilian population following a large-scale disaster.

Rationale: The SNS maintains a national repository of pharmaceutical agents, vaccines, and medical supplies and equipment to be delivered to an area after a large-scale disaster. It helps augment the local and state resources so as to help decrease morbidity and mortality in the civilian population. This program is organized with a five-tiered approach that includes 12-hour Push Packs, vendor-managed inventory (VMI), storage of and rapid vaccine deployment, buying power with surge capacity, and technical assistance. The 12-hour Push Packs can be shipped within 12 hours of the decision to do so. They contain critical supplies and pharmaceuticals that might be needed in the event of a large-scale disaster. The VMI is designed to be used to provide pharmaceuticals and medical supplies for treatment of a known agent or for smaller scale events. The Technical Advisory Response Unit is a group of logistical, public health, communications, operations, and emergency preparedness experts who assist state and local authorities with supply receiving, distribution, dispensing, and replenishing.

Cognitive level: Analysis

Nursing process: Planning

Client needs: Physiological Integrity

8. Answer: 4. "Critical incident defusings are formal, confidential group sessions where the stressful event and its experiences and reactions are reviewed."

Rationale: Critical incident stress debriefings are formal sessions run by trained counselors that are held within 72 hours of a critical event. Group information briefings are also called demobilizations. This is a short informal meeting that helps with rumor control, possible reactions, and self-help guidelines. The fact phase of CISD allows for each participant to describe the stressful event from his or her own perspective on a cognitive level. Critical incident defusings give mutual reassurance and assess the need for more help. Critical incident defusings are formal, confidential group sessions where the event and its experiences and reactions are reviewed. Each session consists of six to eight people with similar job descriptions, and each session lasts 20 to 45 minutes.

Cognitive level: Analysis

Nursing process: Evaluation

Client needs: Safe and Effective Care Environment

Chapter 73

1. Answer: 2. It can describe patient care for perceived, actual, or undiagnosed health problems.

Rationale: Emergency nursing does involve episodic patient care, but the care is usually acute or critical in nature. Florence Nightingale has long been associated with the origins of emergency nursing because of her care of wounded soldiers out in the field. Judith Kelleher and Anita Dorr are credited with establishing the Emergency Department Nurses Association in 1970. The patients seeking emergency care are becoming increasingly diverse in culture and ethnicity. Thus, it is important for emergency nurses to also become more educated about, sensitive to, and competent in these diversities and how they affect patient care. Emergency nursing is patient care for perceived, actual, or undiagnosed physical and mental health conditions.

Cognitive level: Analysis

Nursing process: Assessment

Client needs: Safe and Effective Care Environment

2. Answer: 3. A patient having a possible allergic reaction with facial edema, drooling, stridor, and severe urticaria with pruritus

Rationale: Patients requiring immediate airway or cervical spine intervention are always identified and treated first in the emergency department. The patient having an allergic reaction is demonstrating signs of possible airway obstruction (i.e., facial edema, drooling, and stridor). This patient should be treated first among the other patients listed. The patient with chest pain and shortness of breath has signs of a possible cardiac or respiratory event that would require urgent intervention without delay in care, but issues pertaining to airway or cervical spine would be treated emergently. The patients with the urinary condition and the laceration also need intervention, but they are not experiencing life-threatening issues at this time and would be treated after the patients with the airway problem and the cardiopulmonary event, respectively.

Cognitive level: Application

Nursing process: Planning

Client needs: Physiological Integrity

3. Answer: 4. Level IV – Nonurgent

Rationale: The patient's complaint is nontraumatic and chronic, having been an issue for 4 months. Also, the patient has sought previous medical treatment from his or her primary care provider, who now refuses to give the patient access to more prescription analgesics, and the triage assessment is benign. Because the patient's condition does not require immediate resuscitative efforts nor is the patient unstable, categorizing him or her as a Level I or Level II, respectively, would be inappropriate. The Level III category would also be incorrect in this case, because the patient does not have an urgent problem that requires timely intervention. Level IV, nonurgent, is the best choice for this patient in the four-level triage system.

Cognitive level: Application

Nursing process: Evaluation

Client needs: Physiological Integrity

4. Answer: 1. General consent and informed consent.

Rationale: Both general and informed consents should be obtained prior to this patient's treatment. The general consent would be for any treatment, such as evaluation by the staff, and noninvasive procedures, such as radiographs. The informed consent would be for the procedures of conscious sedation and reduction of the dislocation. This consent states that the patient has been fully informed about these procedures and their risks. Implied consent is used only in emergency situations when it is presumed that the patient would give permission for treatment if she or he were able. Blood product consent would be used prior to administration of any blood or blood products.

Cognitive level: Application

Nursing process: Implementation

Client needs: Physiological Integrity

5. Answer: 2. "I am glad that emergency nurses do not have to deal with obstetrical issues because they can call the labor and delivery nurses."

Rationale: Emergency nurses must be prepared for all types of emergencies, including obstetrical issues. Additional preparation for new graduates or nurses who are new to the field of emergency nursing should include instruction in psychiatric emergencies and trauma assessment. The Trauma Nursing Core Course is just one course that is recommended for these nurses. Time management and the ability to care for multiple patients simultaneously are also learned skills that are imperative to emergency nursing.

Cognitive level: Analysis

Nursing process: Evaluation

Client needs: Safe and Effective Care Environment

Chapter 74

1. Answer: 4. Spinal

Rationale: Spinal cord injury is commonly noted in patients following rear-impact motor vehicle crashes.

Cognitive level: Analysis

Nursing process: Assessment

Client needs: Physiological Integrity: Physiological Adaptation

2. Answer: 3. Utilize a rigid cervical collar to stabilize the cervical spine.

Rationale: When assessing and treating patients with trauma, the priorities of the primary survey must be recognized. The first priority is airway with simultaneous cervical spine immobilization. A rigid cervical collar is one way to stabilize the cervical spine in an emergent situation. Controlling bleeding should be performed during the circulation portion of the primary survey. This falls after the priority of airway and cervical spine treatment. A neurological exam would come after dealing with airway, cervical spine, and circulation. Although the patient may need a CT scan to determine if there is a head injury, this is not a priority initially. This intervention would be a portion of the secondary survey that is performed after the primary survey is complete.

Cognitive level: Application

Nursing process: Assessment

Client needs: Health Promotion and Maintenance: Prevention/Early Detection of Health Problems

3. Answer: 1. It will include a comprehensive medical record review to help ensure all injuries and treatments for the patient with trauma have been properly addressed.

Rationale: The tertiary trauma survey includes a comprehensive medical record review, repetition of the primary and secondary surveys, and reviews of all lab and radiologic results to help ensure that all injuries and treatments for the patient with trauma have been properly addressed. It is done within 24 hours of admission and repeated once the patient is awake, responsive, and able to communicate and helps to make certain that all injuries have been properly identified, catalogued, and treated. The Eastern Association for the Surgery of Trauma formed a work group to develop evidence-based guidelines for practice regarding the best and most important nutritional recommendations for the patient with trauma. The primary and secondary surveys provide a systematic approach to initial trauma assessment, helping the health care team identify injuries, provide appropriate interventions, and prioritize patient care. Trauma rehabilitation is a multidisciplinary plan of care developed to help increase the patient's quality of life and maximize the impaired patient's function by minimizing any deficits.

Cognitive level: Analysis

Nursing process: Planning

Client needs: Health Promotion and Maintenance: Prevention/Early Detection of Health Problems

4. Answer: 3. Assess for bleeding into the chest, abdomen, pelvis, or around long bones.

   Rationale: Hemorrhage is the predominant cause of preventable death in the injured patient. During the primary survey, hypotension should be considered hypovolemic in origin until proven otherwise. If external hemorrhage is identified, measures to control the bleeding should be taken immediately. The easiest way to do this is to apply direct manual pressure on the wound. The major sources of occult blood loss are hemorrhage into the chest or abdominal cavities, into the soft tissue surrounding a major long bone fracture, or into the retroperitoneal space from a pelvic fracture. Control of bleeding may require immediate operative intervention.

   Cognitive level: Application

   Nursing process: Assessment

   Client needs: Physiological Integrity: Physiological Adaptation

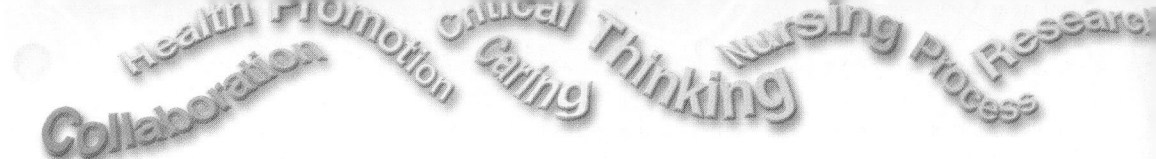

GLOSSARY

12-lead ECG Standard surface ECG with 12 leads, 3 bipolar and 9 unipolar.

2,3-diphosphoglycerate (2,3-DPG) Substance produced by red blood cells during hypoxic states that sustains the deoxyhemoglobin configuration.

abdominojugular reflux An indicator of jugular venous distention that becomes visible as a result of the displacement of excess blood volume when the upper abdominal region is compressed.

abduction Movement of a body part away from the midline (center) of the body.

aberration Deviation from the normal.

ablation Destruction of a specific area of the myocardium through localized delivery of chemicals or electrical energy.

abortion The ending of a pregnancy before the age of fetal viability.

absolute iron deficiency Physiological state indicating insufficient amounts of total body iron.

absolute neutrophil count (ANC) A useful measurement that reveals that proportion of the white blood cells that can be utilized in first-response immune interactions; the most accurate measurement of circulating neutrophils within white blood cells.

absolute refractory period Period of time during which a cardiac cell is unable to respond to any stimulus and cannot spontaneously depolarize. Corresponds with the beginning of the QRS complex and ends at the peak of the T wave on an ECG tracing.

absorption The process by which a medication leaves the site of administration to cross membranes as it journeys to the site of action.

academic nurse educator A nurse who is responsible for designing, implementing, evaluating, and revising academic and continuing education programs for nurses.

accessory muscles The sternocleidomastoid, scalene, and trapezius muscles, which are normally not necessary to respiration, but are utilized by patients who require extra effort to move air in and out of the lungs.

accommodation (1) Process a child goes through to modify existing schema because the incorporation of new knowledge does not fit into existing schema. (2) The ability of the lens to focus up-close or near; to focus a clear image on the retina.

accreditation Process of evaluating an organization against performance standards.

acculturative stress Job-related stress that is exacerbated by cultural differences such as diverse assumptions, values, and beliefs among the participants.

acetylcholine A neurotransmitter critical to the process of memory formation.

achalasia A motor disorder of the esophagus that is characterized by failure of the lower esophageal sphincter to relax properly and by impaired peristalsis.

achlorhydria Lack of hydrochloric acid in the stomach.

acids Compounds in solution that have a pH of less than 7.40. They form hydrogen ion in solution and are proton donors.

acne vulgaris A chronic skin disorder with an increased production of sebum from the sebaceous glands and the formation of comedones that plug the pores.

acoustic neuroma A benign tumor of the eighth cranial (acoustic) nerve.

acquired immunity Type of immunity that occurs after birth and includes antibodies, immune-competent T cells and B cells, and cytokines that act to remove antigens that are considered non-self.

acquired immunodeficiency syndrome (AIDS) The disease resulting from infection by the human immunodeficiency virus; manifested by loss of T cells and opportunistic infections.

acromegaly A hypermetabolic condition of the pituitary gland, characterized by enlargement of the extremities, particularly the hands, feet, and other body parts such as the face, in which excess pituitary hormones (somatotropin and growth hormone) are secreted.

actinic keratosis A skin disorder caused by the sun that leads to proliferation of abnormal, dystrophic cells.

action potential Response of the resting membrane potential to a stimulus that exceeds the membrane threshold value. Carries signals along the muscle cell and conveys information from one cell to another, resulting in cardiac muscle depolarization.

active acquired immunity Type of immunity that involves the production of antibodies by the immune system in response to specific foreign antigens, such as bacteria. This immunity is considered acquired because the body develops the ability to regulate the immune system and produce antibodies after birth and after exposure to antigens in the environment, such as bacteria or viruses.

active immunization Immunization that involves the introduction of a live, killed, or attenuated toxin of a disease organism into the body. The immune system responds by producing antibodies.

activity theory of aging Theory of aging based on the premise that decreased activity later in life leads to meaninglessness and life dissatisfaction, and maintaining activity tends to increase life satisfaction.

acuity The measurement of severity of illness in a patient and the amount of nursing care required to care for the patient.

acute angle-closure glaucoma (AACG) Disorder characterized by the angle in the anterior chamber closing suddenly as a result of iris blockage; prevents aqueous flow through the trabecular meshwork, causing the intraocular pressure to rise suddenly, usually to greater than 40 mmHg.

acute bronchitis Inflammation of the tracheobronchial tree, usually in association with a respiratory infection.

acute care nurse A nurse who works with patients experiencing sudden illness or trauma, usually in the prehospital, hospital, or emergency department.

acute coronary syndrome (ACS) Syndrome collectively described by unstable angina, non–ST segment elevation myocardial infarction (MI), and ST segment elevation MI.

acute graft rejection A type IV cell-mediated immune response that occurs between 2 weeks and 1 month after transplant. This occurs when a recipient's T cells are activated against unmatched HLA antigens in the transplanted tissue.

acute lung injury (ALI) Sometimes used when referring to acute respiratory distress syndrome, but is less severe.

acute pain Pain of relatively short duration that coincides with injury, surgery, or illness.

acute pulmonary edema An abnormal accumulation of fluid in the lungs.

acute radiation syndrome An acute illness caused by irradiation of the whole body. The phases of the illness are prodromal, latent, illness, and recovery or death.

acute respiratory distress syndrome (ARDS) A progressive form of respiratory failure that leads to alveolar capillary inflammation and damage.

acute respiratory failure (ARF) A condition defined as a failure of gas exchange.

acute retroviral syndrome A group of generalized symptoms seen in some individuals during the period of primary infection with the human immunodeficiency virus (1 to 3 months). Symptoms include fever, malaise, lymphadenopathy, and skin rash.

acute stress A reaction to an immediate threat; commonly triggers the fight-or-flight response.

acute stressor One that is brief and involves a tangible threat that is readily identified as a stress.

acute wounds Recent wounds that are either traumatic or iatrogenic in etiology that progress through the stages of wound healing normally.

adaptation A reaction to stress that signifies that the person is able to cope with the stressor or change.

adapter Portion of a catheter that is used to affix infusion equipment to a vascular access device. Also known as the *hub*.

Addisonian crisis (adrenal crisis) A rare, life-threatening disease in which a deficiency of adrenal hormones is exacerbated by stress or trauma.

Addison's disease A rare condition caused by severe or total deficiency of hormones produced by the adrenal cortex.

add-on devices Any extra equipment such as filters, stopcocks, extensions, connectors, and injection ports or caps added to the primary intervenous set.

adduction Movement of a body part toward the midline (center) of the body.

adenomatous polyps Polyps that result from a mutation on chromosome 5. They are long thin projections of tissue arising from the mucosal epithelium and are considered premalignant tissue. Most colorectal cancers develop from this type of polyp.

adjuvant medications Medications that are not primarily indicated for treatment of pain, but are used to augment pain relief medications.

administration set Infusion-specific tubing that delivers parenteral fluid via a sterile pathway from its container to the patient via a vascular access device.

adrenal insufficiency Condition in which the body fails to produce an adequate amount of adrenal hormones.

advanced practice nurse (APRN) A nurse who has been trained to practice beyond the scope defined for a registered nurse by the state nurse practice act. Advanced practice nurses are qualified through postgraduate education and practice through the use of standardized procedures or by indirect supervision of a physician.

advanced practice nursing Specialized type of nursing practice in which nurses diagnose and treat illnesses and provide health care. Most advanced practice nurses are also certified to prescribe medication.

adventitious breath sounds Abnormal lung sound indicating a pathologic process.

adverse drug event (ADE) Noxious and unintended patient event caused by a drug accompanied by various symptoms, signs, and laboratory abnormalities.

adverse drug reaction (ADR) *See* adverse drug event (ADE).

aerophagia The swallowing of air; may lead to intestinal bloating.

affective dimension of pain Describes the emotions patients assign to their pain.

affective learning Involves changes in attitudes, values, and feelings.

afferent Ability to transport toward a center; for example, a sensory nerve that carries impulses from the peripheral nervous system to the central nervous system.

afterload The amount of pressure or resistance the ventricles must overcome to eject blood during systole.

agglutination The surrounding and attaching of antibodies to an antigen, causing the antigens to clump together and stimulate the immune cells to locate the complex and consume it or destroy it.

aging The process of growing old and maturing.

agonist Opioid that is often referred to as morphine-like, or as a mu agonist, because it binds to the mu, kappa, and delta receptors of cells located in the central nervous system, peripheral nervous system, and the gastrointestinal tract.

agonist-antagonist Opioid that is a kappa- or mu-receptor partial agonist; generally considered to be less efficacious than a pure mu agonist.

AIDS indicator conditions Indicates an HIV-infected individual has been diagnosed with opportunistic infections such as *Pneumocystis*

carinii pneumonia or AIDS-defining cancer, such as Kaposi's sarcoma, or that the individual's CD4 count has fallen below 200 mL/µL.

air conduction Process of sound waves reaching the inner ear for interpretation.

air embolism Obstruction of a blood vessel by an air bubble.

air-mask-bag unit (AMBU) A device used to deliver oxygen via a mask when a patient is not adequately ventilating or oxygenating.

airway obstruction Obstruction that occurs most often because medications used in anesthesia cause the muscles to relax.

akinesia Condition characterized by areas of abnormal heart contractility where there is loss of or no muscle movement.

alanine aminotransferase (ALT) An enzyme released from hepatocytes when liver injury occurs.

albumin A commercially prepared product that is derived from the plasma portion of blood.

aldosterone A hormone secreted by the adrenal cortex in response to the conversion of angiotensinogen to angiotensin II. Aldosterone causes sodium reabsorption from the renal tubules and thus causes the body to retain water.

alkaline phosphatase (ALP) An enzyme found mostly in the liver and bone. It is released when liver injury or inflammation occurs and when abnormal osteoblastic activity is present in the bone.

alkalis Compounds in solution that have a pH of greater than 7.40, which is caused by either an increase of base/alkali or a loss of acid. There is more base and less acid, thus raising the 20:1 ratio of bicarbonate to carbonic acid.

allele An alternate or variant form of a gene. On a gene pair, one allele is inherited from the father and the other allele from the mother. The maternal and paternal alleles may be identical or homozygous or they may be different forms of the same gene (heterozygous).

Allen's test Test performed prior to arterial line insertion to test the patency of the palmar arch.

allergen An antigen, or protein, from the external environment. Common allergens include dust, food, pollen, and pet dander.

allergic rhinitis Inflammation of the nasal mucosa caused by an allergic substance such as pollen.

allergy A form of type I hypersensitivity reaction that occurs when an external antigen, or allergen, attaches to IgE antibodies. IgE antibodies attach to mast cells and result in degranulation and release of histamine. Symptoms are the result of the activity of histamine.

allogeneic bone marrow Bone marrow from a histocompatible donor.

allograft Grafting of skin to a wound that was harvested from human cadavers.

allograft valve A valve obtained from human cadaver donations; used primarily to replace the aortic and pulmonic valves. Also called a *homograft valve*.

alloimmune response A hypersensitivity response of the immune system to antigens from another human; usually occurs when tissue is transplanted or grafted.

allopathic medicine Method of treating disease with remedies that produce effects different from those caused by the disease itself.

alopecia Loss of hair, which can be a result of familial patterns of baldness, disease, medications, or a pathologic condition.

alpha-amylase An enzyme mainly in the pancreas; aids in the digestion of carbohydrates.

alternative therapy A therapy used instead of conventional or mainstream therapy. Also called *unconventional therapy*.

alveolar ventilation (V_A) The cumulative gas exchange that takes place within each alveolus.

Alzheimer's disease (AD) A chronic, progressive, irreversible brain disorder found most frequently in adults age 65 and older.

amblyopia Disorder in which a person has an eye with decreased or impaired vision with no obvious anatomic explanation, usually from childhood. Also known by the lay term *lazy eye*.

ametropia A general term used to indicate a refractive error that can usually be corrected with glasses, contact lenses, or possibly refractive surgery.

amputation Surgical removal of an anatomic part.

amyotrophic lateral sclerosis (ALS) A rare, progressive neurological disease characterized by loss of motor neurons.

anal canal The last part of the large intestine situated between the rectum and the anus. It is about 2.5 to 4 cm long.

analog A compound that is structurally similar to another with some slight differences in composition.

analytical preciseness Measure of how findings emerge from the data, how the data collection process is made flexible, and how themes emerge from the data.

anaphylaxis A severe form of type I hypersensitivity response that is systemic. Symptoms can include hives, severe bronchoconstriction, and loss of airway.

anasarca Total body edema.

anatomic dead space Area in the transporting airways or upper airways and bronchi that results when no gas exchange occurs. The amount of the tidal volume taken in that remains in the trachea and bronchi. The amount of anatomic dead space can be estimated as 1 mL per pound of ideal body weight. A person with an ideal body weight of 150 pounds has an anatomic dead space of about 150 mL.

androgenetic alopecia Physiological baldness in which androgen levels are normal; however, there is a genetic predisposition to balding.

androgenic alopecia Loss of hair related to excessive androgen production that causes a decrease in size of the hair follicles, leading to hair loss in central and frontal areas.

andropause A decrease in testosterone associated with aging.

anemia Disorder that results when the total body red blood cell volume is decreased; usually measured by hemoglobin, hematocrit, and red blood cell count.

anemic hypoxia Physiological state of decreased oxygen availability due to decreased concentration of hemoglobin or red blood cells.

anergy Impaired or absent ability to react to common antigens.

aneuploidy Having too many or too few chromosomes in a cell or any number other than 46 chromosomes in somatic or body cells or other than 23 chromosomes in germ cells or the eggs and sperm.

aneurysm Localized diseased segment of an artery that becomes thin and dilated because of degenerative changes in the tunica media layer.

angina pectoris Transient chest pain due to myocardial ischemia.

angiogenesis Process in which stimulated endothelial cells multiply and form tubular structures differentiating into arterioles or venules.

anion A negatively charged ion.

anion gap Represents the concentration of all unmeasured anions in plasma. It is comprised of negatively charged proteins as well as the acid anions produced during metabolism such as lactate. It is calculated by subtracting the sum of the chloride and bicarbonate levels from the sodium level, and its reference range is 8 to 16 mEq.

anisocoria Inequality of the size of the pupils; may be congenital or associated with aneurysms, head trauma, diseases of the nervous system, brain lesion, paresis, or locomotor ataxia.

ankle-brachial index (ABI) Ratio of arterial pressure at the ankle to the pressure at the brachial artery; used to predict the severity of peripheral arterial disease that may be present. A decrease in the ABI result with exercise is a sensitive indicator that significant pulmonary arterial disease is probably present.

ankylosing spondylitis A type of arthritis that affects the spine and the sacroiliac joint.

annuloplasty A surgery done to correct valve regurgitation by repairing the enlarged annulus.

annulus The fibrous ring at the junction of the cardiac valve leaflets and the muscular wall.

anorexia Loss of appetite.

anorgasmia Difficulty reaching orgasm.

anosmia The loss or impairment of the sense of smell.

antagonist Substance that displaces and replaces an opioid at the receptor, reversing the opioid's pharmacologic effect and side effects such as respiratory depression.

anterior circulation Describes the areas of the brain supplied by the right and left carotid arteries and their branches, including circulation in the arteries in the anterior portion of the circle of Willis.

anteriorly Front plane of the body.

anthropometric measurements Any physical measurement of the body.

antibody Proteins made by B cells and found in the plasma that are capable of attaching to antigens and stimulating immune responses.

antidiuretic hormone (ADH) A small peptide molecule released by the pituitary gland at the base of the brain. It has an antidiuretic action that prevents the production of dilute urine.

antigen Any foreign substance (bacterium, virus, protein) that elicits an immune response.

antigen–antibody complex The attachment of the FAB portion of an antibody to an antigen, resulting in the stimulation of a strong immune response; each FAB portion of the antibody is specifically shaped for only one type of antigen. Attracts other phagocytic cells such as neutrophils and macrophages to help eliminate the antigen; stimulates creation of B memory cells for long-term protection.

antigenicity The ability of a pathogen to elicit an immune defense in its host. It affects the ability of the host to develop a long-term immunity.

anti-infectives Drugs that are used to treat infections and include antibiotics, antivirals, and antifungals.

antiplatelet therapy Therapy that inhibits platelet adhesion and aggregation.

antrum Any nearly closed cavity or chamber.

anuria Total loss of urine production.

aortic coarctation Narrowing of the lumen of the aorta.

aortic dissection (AD) Weakening of the layers inside the aorta, which can result in tears in the aortic wall and leakage of blood into the chest or abdomen.

aortic valve regurgitation Incomplete closure of the aortic valve, which causes blood to regurgitate back into the left ventricle through a valve; results from abnormal valve cusps or aortic root.

aortic valve stenosis A narrowing of the aortic valve orifice, which results in an obstruction to blood flow from the left ventricle to the aorta during systole.

apathetic Indifferent; showing a lack of emotion.

aphasia The disorder of speech and language due to cerebral dysfunction. The three primary aphasic deficits are in comprehension of spoken language, expressive language, and naming.

apheresis A technology in which the blood of a donor or patient is passed through a machine that separates out one specific particle and returns the remainder of the blood to circulation.

aphonic Without a voice.

aphthous stomatitis (contact stomatitis) A common ulcerative condition limited to the oral cavity. Also known as *canker sores*.

apnea Cessation of airflow for more than 10 seconds.

apoptosis Programmed cell death in a multicellular organism; process by which cells can self-destruct when infected or mutated.

applied research Research that focuses on finding solutions to existing problems.

apudomas A rare tumor of the islets of Langerhans in the pancreas.

areflexia Loss of reflexive activity.

arrhythmogenic right ventricular cardiomyopathy (ARVC) An electrical disturbance that develops when the muscle tissue in the right ventricle is replaced with fibrous scar and fatty tissues.

arterial line An indwelling catheter inserted into an artery in order to monitor blood pressure.

arterial-venous shunts Shunts placed using surgical anastomosis of venous and arterial structures to facilitate dialysis procedures.

arteriosclerosis Thickening, reduced elasticity, and calcification of arterial walls.

arteriovenous malformation (AVM) A mass of abnormal blood vessels in which arterial blood flows directly into the venous system.

arthrodesis Surgical fusion of bone.

arthroplasty Restoration of a joint either by total joint replacement surgery or by resurfacing bone and removing damaged bone and cartilage.

artifact An ECG pattern from sources outside the heart; creates an abnormal pattern on ECG graph paper. This interference causes the baseline or isoelectric line to become fuzzy; this fuzzy baseline is referred to as 60 cycle.

asbestosis Diffuse lung fibrosis caused by exposure to asbestos.

ascites An abnormal intraperitoneal accumulation of fluid containing large amounts of protein and electrolytes.

aspartate aminotransferase (AST) An enzyme found in the liver, heart, skeletal muscle, and kidneys that is released when cellular injury occurs.

asphyxiates Chemical agents that cause injury, illness, and death by damaging the lungs. Also called *choking agents*.

assault Any action that places another person in apprehension of being touched in a manner that is offensive, insulting, or physically injurious without consent or authority.

assessment The act of evaluating or appraising.

assignment The transfer of a task and the accountability for the outcome.

assimilation Incorporation of new concepts into existing schemas.

assisted living A residential setting in which patients are provided long-term assisted care.

assistive device Device required by a patient to assist with ambulation (e.g., cane, crutches, walker).

associate caregiver An LVN/LPN or unlicensed assistive personnel assigned to provide care to patients according to the plan established by the primary nurse.

associate nurse A registered nurse who assists the primary nurse during off-duty hours and provides care consistent with the plan developed by the primary nurse.

asterixis A flapping tremor of the hands when the arms are outstretched; believed to be caused by the accumulation of substances normally detoxified by the liver.

asthma A disease with multiple precipitating factors resulting in reversible airflow obstruction.

astigmatism An optical defect.

asymmetry Unequal.

asystole Complete termination of ventricular activity with no measurable cardiac electrical activity. Represents cardiac standstill from massive cardiac muscle damage.

ataxia A failure of muscle coordination, resulting in loss of balance and coordination, as well as speech difficulties including dysarthria or slurred and scanning speech.

atelectasis Collapse or airless condition of the alveoli caused by hypoventilation and obstruction of airways by secretions.

atherogenesis The development of atherosclerosis.

atheroma Condition characterized by an accumulation in the inner lining of an artery of a plaque of cholesterol and other constituents.

atherosclerosis A type of arteriosclerosis; the most common etiologic process that causes reduced myocardial blood flow.

atopic dermatitis A chronic inflammatory skin disorder characterized by dry skin related to water loss in the epidermis and decreased skin lipid levels.

atrial dysrhythmia Dysrhythmia that generally results from an irritable focus in the atria that fires off an electrical impulse before the SA node has had a chance to fire in a normal fashion. Results in a P-wave configuration on the ECG that is different from that of a normal P wave; however, the QRS complex is normal.

atrial fibrillation A disorganized, very rapid, and irregular atrial rhythm resulting in an irregular ventricular rhythm. The rhythm is usually described as either course or fine fibrillation.

atrial flutter A rapid, regular atrial rhythm with a rate of about 300 beats per minute. Only a fraction of the impulses are transmitted through the AV node as a protective mechanism. Most of the atrial beats fall during the refractory period of the AV node so they are not conducted.

atrial kick Atrial contraction, which augments the blood supply going to the ventricles and ultimately cardiac output.

atrial natriuretic peptide (ANP) A hormone secreted by the right atrium in response to fluid overload that causes the excretion of sodium, which results in loss of the excess fluid; however, most regulation of excess volume is through decreased aldosterone secretion.

atrioventricular (AV) node Node located on the floor of the right atrium just above the tricuspid valve. The AV node has three regions: the AV junctional tissue between the atria and the node; the nodal area between the junctional tissue and the bundle of His; and the AV junction, the region where the AV node joins the bundle of His.

atrophy A reduction in the size of a cell and tissues or in muscle size.

auscultation Technique of listening to the sounds produced by different body areas.

autoantibodies An antibody produced in response to a self protein. Antinuclear antibodies, antibodies that bind to the nucleus of cells and result in cell destruction, are one example of autoantibodies.

autoantibody tests Tests that measure the amount or presence of antibodies to self proteins. Examples include the antinuclear antibody test and anti-IgG serum test.

autocrine functioning Secretion of cells that act to influence only their own growth.

autograft valve Valve obtained from the patient's own pulmonic valve and pulmonary artery. Also called *autologous valve*.

autografting Grafting of the patient's own skin to somewhere else on the patient's body.

autoimmune diseases Diseases that result from hypersensitivity responses and produce tissue damage and destruction. Examples include Goodpasture's syndrome and systemic lupus erythematosus; in both of these diseases, tissue is damaged by the production of antibodies to self-antigens.

autoimmune hemolytic anemia Red blood cell disorder characterized by destruction of cells by antibodies of the host.

autoimmune response Occurs when the body fails to recognize self cells or proteins and mounts an immune response against the self. Autoantibodies result in immune complexes that stimulate phagocytosis and destruction of cells and tissue.

autologous BMT Procedure in which bone marrow is collected from the patient and frozen. It is then reinfused into the patient following high-dose chemotherapy, with or without radiation.

autologous transfusion The process of collecting and reinfusing a patient's own blood.

automated external defibrillator (AED) A small, lightweight device that can recognize and treat ventricular fibrillation.

automaticity Ability of pacemaker cells to generate their own electrical impulses without depending on nervous system stimulation external to the heart.

autonomic hyperreflexia A syndrome characterized by severe hypertension, bradycardia, vasoconstriction below the level of injury, and vasodilation above the level of injury resulting from unchecked stimulation of the sympathetic nervous system triggered by a noxious stimulus.

autonomy Personal freedom to make choices or decisions.

autoregulation The ability of the brain to change its vessel size to accommodate changes in intracranial pressure.

autosomal dominant inheritance A Mendelian pattern of inheritance in which an affected individual has one copy of a mutant allele and one normal allele. Individuals who have autosomal dominant disorders have a 50–50 chance of passing the mutant allele and disorder to their children. This is in contrast to autosomal recessive disorders in which the individual must have two copies of the mutant allele.

autosomal recessive inheritance A Mendelian pattern of inheritance in which an affected individual receives two copies of a mutant allele, one from each parent, or the phenotype is expressed only when two copies of the mutant allele are present.

autosome A single chromosome from any 1 of 22 pairs of the chromosomes that is not a sex chromosome (XX or XY). Disorders caused by mutation in an autosomal gene or gene pair shows autosomal inheritance.

AV dissociation Independent function of the atria and the ventricles.

avascular necrosis (AVN) Condition in which bone tissue dies due to a temporary or permanent loss of blood supply to the bone.

avulsion fracture Fracture that occurs when a ligament is pulled away from its attachment point at the bone and takes a small piece of the bone with it.

azotemia An increase in blood urea nitrogen (BUN) caused when the kidneys are unable to excrete normally.

B cells White blood cells that are produced in the bone marrow and develop into plasma cells that are responsible for the creation and release of antibodies and development of long-term immune protection.

B lymphocytes Type of white blood cell that make antibodies against antigens, perform the role of antigen in presenting cells, and eventually develop into memory cells after activation by antigen interaction.

Bachmann bundle Part of the electrical conduction system of the heart composed of a group of interatrial fibers contained in the left atrium that conduct electrical impulses from the SA node to the left atrium.

bacterial meningitis Inflammation of the meninges caused by a bacterial pathogen.

bacterial phlebitis Inflammation of a vein associated with an infectious process.

bacterial vaginosis (BV) The most common bacterial infection in women of childbearing age. The cause is not clearly understood.

barium enema Type of enema used to obtain an x-ray of the large intestines. Radiographs are taken after the patient receives barium sulphate through an enema tube.

barotrauma Alveoli damage caused by the increased pressure resulting from use of a ventilator. Physical injury or rupture of tympanic membrane, resulting from changing air pressure.

Barrett's epithelium Columnar epithelial tissue that replaces the normal squamous epithelium in the esophagus after prolonged exposure to gastric juice. It is resistant to gastric acid, supports the healing of the esophagus, and is premalignant.

basal skull fracture A fracture of the skull that extends into the base of the skull.

base excess Part of the blood gas report, this is a calculated value that is based on the bicarbonate and carbon dioxide levels and the hematocrit. It expresses the number of milliequivalents of bicarbonate per liter of extracellular fluid that one has too much of (a base excess) or too little of (a base deficit). It is used as a guide by clinicians as they consider how much bicarbonate to administer to a patient with a severe metabolic acidosis.

basement membrane A thin, acellular layer between the dermis and epidermis that acts as scaffolding for the epidermis. Blood supply and nutrients reach the epidermis by passing through the basement membrane.

bases Compounds that combine with hydrogen ion in solution. A proton acceptor.

basic human needs As defined by Abraham Maslow, needs on the first four rungs of Maslow's hierarchy.

basic research Research undertaken to extend the knowledge base in a discipline or to formulate or refine a theory.

basophil A component of the white blood cell differential; actual function is not well known.

battery Contact with another or with another's immediate "personage" (clothes, car keys, cane, purse, etc.) without consent or authority; the touching of another without permission.

Battle's sign Bogginess of the temporal or postauricular region of the head, which indicates fracture of the basilar area of the skull.

Beck's triad Classic assessment findings for the patient with cardiac tamponade, consisting of decreased blood pressure, muffled heart sounds, and jugular venous distention.

behavioral dimension of pain Includes responses to pain that may be situational, developmental, or learned.

beneficence The ethical duty to do good.

benign Lacking malignant cells.

benign prostatic hyperplasia (BPH) Term applied to age-related benign enlargement of the prostate gland where there is no cancerous growth involved.

berry aneurysm Saccular-shaped aneurysm.

bevel The slanted or angled part of a needle or stylet.

Bier block Process in which an IV catheter is inserted in the extremity at the most distal site possible. A pneumatic tourniquet is applied proximal to the surgical site and inflated higher than the patient's systolic blood pressure. When a local anesthetic (lidocaine) is injected intravenously, the obstruction of blood by the tourniquet prevents it from leaving the surgical area.

bigeminy Premature ventricular contraction that occurs every other beat.

bile A substance produced in the liver containing bile salts, cholesterol, bilirubin, electrolytes, and water. It is concentrated and stored in the gallbladder, where it is released in response to a meal to aid in the emulsification and absorption of dietary fat.

bile canaliculi Small channels adjacent to the hepatocytes that move bile toward the common bile duct.

biliary dyskinesia Motility disorders of the gallbladder.

bilirubin A product in the breakdown of hemoglobin. It is conjugated by the hepatocytes and is excreted in bile.

binge-eating disorder (BED) Disorder characterized by the same type of binge eating as bulimia nervosa, but without the compensatory purging.

bioavailable Pertaining to a molecular form that can be readily used by the body.

bioavailable testosterone Free testosterone and testosterone that is loosely bound to albumin.

biologic agent Viruses, bacteria, and toxins that can be weaponized to cause disease, illness, and/or death.

biologic aging theory General theory of aging comprised of programmed theories and error theories. *See* error theories of aging *and* programmed theory of aging.

biologic dressing Heterografts such as pigskin or allografts obtained from living or deceased humans.

biologic valve Valve obtained from other species, most commonly from pigs (porcine valves), although cow valves (bovine) also are used. Also referred to as *xenografts*.

biopsy A portion of tissue examined for the presence of abnormal cells.

biosynthetic dressing A combination of biologic and synthetic materials that are effective as temporary covering for a variety of wounds.

biotherapy Treatment with agents whose origin, mostly mammal, is from biologic sources and/or affecting biologic responses.

biotransformation The process of changing a medication's structure in preparation for elimination. Metabolism occurs primarily in the liver, but also in the kidneys and, to a very small degree, other organ systems. Once a medication is metabolized, it is no longer the same and effectively discontinues its pharmacologic activity.

BiPAP Stands for *bi-level positive airway pressure*, which is a breathing apparatus that helps people get more air into their lungs. The air is delivered through a mask that can be set at two different pressures, one for inhaling (IPAP or inspiratory positive airway pressure) and another for exhaling (EPAP or expiratory airway pressure).

biphasic defibrillation Defibrillation procedure that delivers a charge in one direction for half of the shock and in the opposite direction for the second half.

bipolar lead ECG leads that have electrodes with opposite polarity, one positive and one negative.

biventricular heart failure A global inability of the heart muscle to pump blood effectively from both ventricles, compromising forward flow leading to right and left heart failure symptoms.

blackouts Amnesia for short-term events; can occur in patients with alcohol abuse problems.

bladder suspension A procedure designed to correct urinary incontinence. It is done to suspend the bladder and correct urinary incontinence that is often caused by weakened ligaments due to childbirth. Also called a *Burch procedure*.

blepharoplasty Surgical procedure to fix ptosis or drooping of the eyelid.

blister agent Chemical agent that can cause redness and irritation of the skin and blistering. Also called a *vesicant*.

blood pressure The pressure created by blood circulating through the arteries and veins and the chambers of the heart.

blood transfusion The process of infusing blood products in order to restore circulating volume and therefore increase oxygen carrying capacity.

blunt percussion Technique of placing the palm of the nondominant hand over a body area (such as the kidney) and striking the palm with the closed fist of the dominant hand.

bone conduction Process of sound vibrations reaching the inner ear for interpretation.

bone marrow transplantation Procedure in which hematopoietic cells from the bone marrow of one person are transferred into another person; used to treat a variety of diseases.

Botox Botulism toxin that has been purified and is injected into the lower esophageal sphincter to relax the muscle.

Bouchard's nodes Hard, painless nodules at the joints of the fingers; may indicate osteoarthritis (progressive loss of cartilage at a joint). Bouchard's nodes are found over the proximal interphalangeal joints.

boutonnière deformity Flexion of the proximal interphalangeal joint.

Bowman's capsule A thin, double-walled capsule encasing the glomerulus.

brachytherapy The use of localized radiation within the coronary artery to increase the size of the lumen of the artery.

bradykinesia Slowed movement; primary symptom of Parkinson's disease.

bradypnea A respiratory rate of less than 12 breaths per minute.

brain abscess A localized infection carried from other sites of the body and extending into the cerebral tissue.

breach of confidentiality Failure to prevent the disclosure of all or parts of a patient's medical record without the proper authority to do so.

breakthrough pain A transitory exacerbation of pain that occurs on a background of otherwise stable pain in a patient receiving chronic opioid therapy.

breast cancer The formation of a malignant glandular tumor, which over time destroys normal breast tissue and can spread to other parts of the body.

Brief Pain Inventory (BPI) Questionnaire that asks multiple questions regarding pain and its impact on patient function and addresses the multidimensionality of the pain experience.

bronchial breath sounds Breath sounds normally heard over the right or left bronchus of the lung.

bronchovesicular breath sounds Breath sounds normally heard between the bronchus and the smaller airways.

bruits The sound heard with a stethoscope of blood flowing through a narrowed blood vessel that is outside of the heart.

bubo Acutely swollen and usually painful lymph node seen in plague near the site of the flea bite.

Buck's boots traction A foam boot used for traction.

buffer A compound that minimizes the change in hydrogen ion concentration (and also the pH) when ions are added to or removed from solution. Think of a buffer as a sponge. When there is too much hydrogen ion, the sponge soaks up the extra. When the level of hydrogen ion is decreased, the sponge can be squeezed out to return hydrogen ions to the blood.

bundle branch block Discontinuity of conduction (complete or incomplete) in one branch of the bundle of His that affects normal transmission of the impulse through the ventricles. When one bundle is blocked, the ventricles depolarize asynchronously. Characterized by a delay of excitation to one ventricle; therefore, an abnormal spread of electrical activity through the ventricles occurs.

bundle of His Part of the conduction system that lies on top of the interventricular septum, between the right and left ventricles; it contains pacemaker cells. Also referred to as the *common bundle*.

bursae Sac containing synovial fluid that cushions joints during movement.

burst fracture Fracture that occurs when an axial load is placed on the spine and vertebrae.

cachexia Wasting of skeletal muscle and adipose.

café-au-lait spot Pigmented macules that are light brown in color.

calciphylaxis A condition during severe serum calcium excess, as in renal failure, in which calcium is deposited into the soft tissues of the body. This can be reflected in irregular purple lesions on the lower extremities that may lead to necrosis and gangrene.

calcium The most abundant cation in the body, primarily found in bones and teeth. Serum calcium plays a role in neuromuscular transmission (including cardiac) and cell membrane permeability. Normal serum levels are 8.5 to 10.5 mg/dL, 50% ionized and 40% bound to albumin.

caloric test Assesses abnormal nystagmus, tinnitus, or hearing loss as a result of vestibular dysfunction from eighth cranial nerve lesions by inserting water into the ear.

cancellous (trabecular) bone Bone with a hard outer casing and an interior that is porous, spongy, and meshwork-like in structure.

cancer Common term for all malignant neoplasms.

cancer pain Pain associated with malignancy; can be acute and chronic in nature.

candidiasis A common fungal infection caused by the *Candida* species of fungus; more commonly known as a yeast infection.

capnography Use of a device to measure exhaled or end-tidal carbon dioxide.

capture Term used to indicate that sufficient voltage has been put out by a pacemaker to make a myocardial contraction occur.

caput medusae A term used to describe the engorged, tortuous, and visible blood vessels radiating from the umbilicus in patients with severe liver disorders. In mythology, Medusa's hair was a tangle of snakes.

carbon dioxide An atmospheric gas composed of one carbon atom and two oxygen atoms. Produced as a by-product of metabolism, carbon dioxide can be thought of as a potential acid because, when it is dissolved in water, it forms carbonic acid.

carbon monoxide poisoning Occurs when an individual breathes carbon monoxide fumes that have built up in an enclosed space.

carbonic acid A weak acid formed by water reacting with carbon dioxide. If carbonic acid loses one proton, it becomes the bicarbonate ion.

carboxypeptidase An enzyme that breaks away the end amino acids on protein molecules.

carbuncle An infection of the skin composed of a cluster of boils caused by *Staphylococcus aureus*.

carcinoembryonic antigen (CEA) A glycoprotein found in embryonic gastrointestinal epithelium, but also found in tumors of the adult gastrointestinal tract. It is used to detect colon cancer, most specifically adenocarcinoma.

carcinogenesis Pertaining to the production of cancer.

carcinoma *in situ* Disorder in which neoplasms have not invaded the basement membrane of the epithelial site, thus the surrounding tissues are left untouched by malignant cells.

cardia The upper orifice of the stomach connecting with the esophagus.

cardiac catheterization A term used to describe a variety of invasive procedures used to identify atherosclerotic disease as well as provide anatomic and hemodynamic information about the heart and great vessels using radiopaque catheters.

cardiac conduction system Conduction system unique to the myocardium that is composed of specialized cells that enable it to generate and transmit action potentials without stimulation from the nervous system. The specialized cells are concentrated in the sinoatrial and atrioventricular nodes, and the Purkinje network.

cardiac depolarization Muscle contraction of the heart resulting from electrolyte exchange in the cardiac cells.

cardiac index (CI) Individualized measurement of cardiac output by taking into account the body surface area.

cardiac output (CO) The amount of blood leaving the left ventricle per minute.

cardiac pacemaker An electronic device that is capable of delivering an electrical stimulus to the heart.

cardiac repolarization Process whereby a depolarized cell is polarized, causing a return to the resting membrane potential. Also referred to as the recovery phase that every cardiac cell must go through in order to be ready to accept another stimulus.

cardiac resynchronization therapy (CRT) Therapy that uses atrial-synchronized biventricular pacemakers.

cardiac risk factors Habits, lifestyles, and/or genetic factors that predispose an individual to the development of coronary artery disease.

cardiac tamponade Bleeding into the pericardial sac. As the accumulation of blood increases, it compresses the atria and ventricles decreasing venous return and filling pressure, which leads to decreased cardiac output, myocardial hypoxia, and cardiac failure.

cardioesophageal Pertaining to the junction of the esophagus and the stomach.

cardiogenic embolism Blood clots from cardiac sources.

cardiogenic pulmonary edema (CPE) An abnormal accumulation of fluid in the lungs caused by cardiac failure; results from increased hydrostatic pressures in the pulmonary capillary bed secondary to increased pulmonary venous pressure.

cardiomegaly Enlargement of the heart.

cardiomyopathies (CMPs) Diseases of the myocardial muscle fibers that result in progressive structural and functional abnormalities of the myocardium.

cardioversion The timed delivery of an electrical current to depolarize cardiac muscle in order to terminate tachyarrhythmias, atrial tachycardia, rapid atrial fibrillation, atrial flutter, and junctional tachycardia.

caring The core of nursing; constitutes the essence of nursing regardless of the level at which nursing is practiced.

carotid endarterectomy (CEA) Surgical procedure to correct carotid stenosis by opening the carotid artery, removing plaque, and restoring blood flow in the lumen.

carpal tunnel syndrome Compression of the median nerve in the carpal tunnel, just below the palm dorsally.

carrier People or animals that do not have symptoms of infection but carry an active pathogenic microorganism.

case management An approach to coordinating care for patients in the hospital or in an outpatient setting.

case manager A person who collaboratively plans, coordinates, and evaluates services for cost effectiveness, but does not provide direct patient care.

case method A nursing care delivery system in which total patient care is delivered by a registered nurse who has shift responsibility for the patient.

cast A rigid circumferential encasement device made of plaster or fiberglass.

cataracts The opacity of the natural crystalline lens.

catheter A device that is introduced through the skin, into the vascular network, for the purpose of infusing parenteral solutions and medications.

catheter embolism Occurs when a piece of catheter is fractured and enters the circulatory system. The catheter may block a major vein, causing loss of circulation, or may travel to the heart, causing cardiac irritability and cardiac arrest.

cation A positively charged ion. Major cations affecting cardiac function are potassium (K), sodium (Na), and calcium (Ca).

cauda equina syndrome The bundle of nerve roots in the lower portion of the spinal canal, below the conus medullaris, which when compressed or inflamed causes symptoms of pain, altered reflexes, decreased strength, and decreased sensation. When extreme, can cause paralysis of the lower extremities, bowel and bladder dysfunction, and loss of the Achilles reflex; most commonly seen with large disk herniations at L_4/L_5, causing mass effect on the nerve roots as they descend through the spinal canal.

cavernous malformation Low-flow, cluster-type nodular lesion, not separated by brain tissue.

CBRNE Acronym suggested for common use by the Department of Justice to describe weapons of mass destruction. The acronym stands for chemical, biologic, radiologic, nuclear, and explosive devices.

CD4+ T cells T lymphocytes with cluster of differentiation 4 (CD4) receptors. The HIV particle can attach and enter T-helper (CD4) cells via the CD4 receptor.

celiac disease An autoimmune disorder involving a sensitivity to gluten, a protein found in wheat, that results in an immune-mediated response that causes a histologic change in the villi of the small intestine, resulting in malabsorption.

celiac sprue A lifelong condition affecting the small intestine in which the villi morphology is damaged because of the presence of gluten in the diet.

cell-mediated immune response Immune responses that are initiated through specific antigen recognition by the T cells; important in identifying and destroying cells that are already infected and providing protection against fungi, and has major involvement in rejection of transplant tissues, tumor immunity, and hypersensitivity reactions.

cellulitis A diffuse inflammatory process of the dermis and subcutaneous tissue layers characterized by erythema, edema, and pain; usually caused by staphylococcus or streptococcus infections.

Centers for Disease Control and Prevention (CDC) Agency under the U.S. Department of Health and Human Services whose function is to protect the health and safety of the public with regard to disease prevention and control.

central retinal artery occlusion (CRAO) Blockage of the central retinal artery, usually by an embolism. Its symptom is sudden, painless, unilateral blindness.

central vascular access device (CVAD) A vascular access device that is inserted into a centrally located vein with the tip residing in the vena cava.

central venous pressure (CVP) Measurement of venous return to the right atrium after insertion of a central venous catheter.

centromere The narrowed portion near the center of a human chromosome where the two sister chromatids or spindle traction fibers attach during mitosis or meiosis.

cerebral aneurysm A balloon-like outpouching, or widening, of an artery.

cerebral blood flow (CBF) The measurement of blood flow in the brain.

cerebral edema An increase in water content of the brain; swelling.

cerebral infarction A condition in which brain tissue dies due to lack of oxygen.

cerebral ischemia A condition in which brain tissue is oxygen deprived.

cerebral perfusion pressure (CPP) The pressure gradient that drives cerebral blood flow.

cerebral salt wasting Electrolyte abnormality characterized by loss of sodium and loss of extracellular fluid volume.

certified nurse midwife (CNM) An advanced practice nurse with postgraduate training and state certification to deliver healthy babies without direct supervision by a physician.

certified registered nurse anesthetist (CRNA) An advanced practice nurse with postgraduate training and state certification to administer anesthesia without direct supervision by a physician.

cerumen Earwax.

chain of infection Consists of a causative agent, reservoir, portal of exit, mode of transmission, portal of entry, and susceptible host.

Chance fracture A fracture through the body and posterior elements of the vertebrae of the spine; caused by forward flexion, causing a distraction injury.

chancres Ulcers of syphilis.

chancroid A bacterial, sexually transmitted infection that is rare outside of the tropics.

chemical agent Chemicals that can be used as weapons to cause injury, illness, and death. They are roughly divided by their mechanism of action into blood agents, blister agents, choking agents, irritants, and nerve agents.

chemical burns Burns that occur when the skin is in contact with caustic chemical compounds such as strong acids, alkalis, or organic compounds.

chemical phlebitis Inflammation of a vein associated with infusates of varying ranges of pH or osmolarities.

chemotaxis The movement of white blood cells to an area of inflammation or infection in response to the release of chemical mediators from neutrophils, macrophages, T cells, and injured tissue.

chief complaint Information about what brought the patient to the health care provider in the patient's own words.

chlamydia Most frequently reported sexually transmitted infection in the United States. It is caused by *Chlamydia trachomatis* and is treatable with antibiotics.

chloride A primary anion in extracellular fluid; its normal serum level is 95 to 108 mEq/L. Chloride is usually found in combination with sodium to create electrical neutrality in the body; it assists in the reabsorption of sodium in the kidneys and combines with hydrogen ion to form hydrochloric acid for digestion.

choking agent Chemicals that cause injury, illness, and death by damaging the lungs. Also called an *asphyxiate*.

cholangiocarcinoma Cancer of the gallbladder.

cholecystectomy Surgical removal of the gallbladder either through an open incision or with a laparoscope.

cholecystitis Inflammation of the gallbladder; most commonly caused by gallstones.

cholecystokinin A hormone secreted by the gastrointestinal mucosa that stimulates the gallbladder to eject bile and the pancreas to secrete alkaline fluid.

choledocholithiasis A gallstone in the common bile duct.

cholelithiasis Disorder in which stones form in the gallbladder that may be composed of cholesterol or calcium.

cholesterol A steroid molecule produced primarily by the liver that is essential for the formation and maintenance of cell membranes.

cholinergic crisis A life-threatening condition associated with myasthenia gravis; results from excess acetylcholine.

chromosomal disorder Condition caused by an abnormal chromosome makeup in which there is duplication, loss, or rearrangement of chromosomal material.

chromosome Threadlike structures in the nucleus of a cell that contain the genes. Chromosomes occur in pairs, with a typical human cell containing 46 chromosomes: 22 pairs of autosomes, and 2 sex chromosomes.

chronic bronchitis Hypersecretion of mucus and chronic productive cough that continues at least 3 months of the year for at least 2 consecutive years.

chronic graft rejection Occurs months to years after graft transplant and involves the slow, progressive failure of a transplanted organ.

chronic lymphocytic thyroiditis An autoimmune condition characterized by high titers of the circulating antibodies thyroid peroxidase and thyroglobulin that destroy thyroid cells and may lead to hypothyroidism. It is the most common thyroid disease in the United States. Also known as *Hashimoto's thyroiditis*.

chronic obstructive pulmonary disease (COPD) A disease state characterized by airflow limitation that is not fully reversible.

chronic pain Pain that does not resolve within the expected time frame, and is persistent beyond 3 to 6 months.

chronic stress Stress that occurs on a daily basis and is the result of an ongoing situation.

chronic wounds Wounds that do not follow the expected sequence of repair in a timely and uncomplicated manner.

Chvostek's sign Spasm of facial muscles; latent tetany, which can be demonstrated by tapping the inferior portion of the zygoma resulting in facial spasms.

chyle Lymphatic system drainage; a milky fluid comprised of serous fluid, white cells, and fatty acids, arising from the interstitial fluid of the gastrointestinal tract. It contains a high proportion of fat and proteins.

chyle leak A disruption in the lymph system into the tissues of the neck and chest.

chymotrypsin An enzyme that aids in the breakdown of large protein molecules by breaking the interior bonds of the amino acids.

circadian rhythm Pertinent to events that occur at approximately 24-hour intervals.

circinate balanitis Inflammation surrounding the circular muscle around the penis.

circulating nurse Nurse in the operating room whose duties are performed outside the sterile field. They encompass responsibilities of nursing care management within the operating room to create and maintain a safe, comfortable environment for surgery.

cirrhosis An inflammatory disease of the liver in which normal structure and function are disrupted.

civil law Rules and regulations that form the bases of legal actions; branch of law that pertains to contracts, torts, patents, and the like.

clinical judgment A complex skill involving several cognitive phases and integrative processes; clinical reasoning across time about a particular patient.

clinical knowledge Knowledge necessary to perform proficiently in the clinical setting, including recognizing signs and symptoms, applying skilled know-how in titrating an intravenous rate, recognizing signs of physiological distress and changes in patient's vital signs, and using clinical judgment.

clinical nurse leader (CNL) An advanced practice nurse with postgraduate training with the responsibility to integrate care among other disciplines and manage care at the bedside.

clinical nurse specialist (CNS) An advanced practice nurse with postgraduate training in a clinical disease specialty. The CNS may schedule clinic visits with patients, provide specialized inpatient or nurse education, or case manage a group of patients.

coal miner pneumoconiosis A chronic lung disease leading to pulmonary fibrosis. It is caused by inhalation of coal dust.

code of ethics A formal statement by a group that expresses the group's ideals, values, and ethical principles, which have been agreed on by the group's members to reflect their moral judgments and serve as a standard for their professional actions.

codon The sequence of three nucleotides in mRNA that specifies a single amino acid.

cognitive dimension of pain Includes the impact of personal beliefs, attitudes, and meanings attached to pain.

cognitive reappraisal The process of allowing for changes in the person's evaluation of an event or a relabeling of the cognitive appraisal.

coiling An endovascular procedure in which an aneurysm is filled with a soft coil. Also referred to as a *GDC (Guglielmi detachable coil)*.

collaborative problems Problems that are identified by other health care workers, such as physicians, in contrast to nursing problems, which are identified by nurses. The nurse is accountable for monitoring for changes in the status of the problem and initiating the appropriate interventions.

collagen synthesis Multistep process in which fibrin proteins form a matrix to support the newly forming tissue.

colon The large intestine from the end of the ileum to the anal canal that surrounds the anus.

colon cancer Disease in which malignant tissue arises from the cells in the colon; it is frequently associated with adenomatous polyps. When there is an allelic deletion on chromosomes 5, 17, or 18, the transformation from normal to malignant colon tissue is promoted.

colonoscopy Visualization of the lower gastrointestinal tract, usually through the insertion of an endoscope through the anus.

colposcopy A test in which the health care provider looks at the cells of the cervix through a special magnifying scope that is placed near the opening of the speculum that is inserted into the vagina.

comminuted skull fracture The fragmented interruption of the skull resulting from multiple linear fractures.

commissure The site where cardiac valve leaflets meet each other.

commissurotomy Surgical procedure used to separate fused heart valve leaflets.

common law System of law derived from principles rather than rules and regulations; consists of principles based on justice, reason, and common sense.

community-acquired infection An infection acquired outside a health care facility.

community-based care A setting for practice outside of acute care institutional walls. Care is directed toward individuals and families within any community setting and is designed to assist patients as they move among health care settings. Also describes a philosophy of care in settings that reflect *how* nursing care is provided, not *where*.

community health nursing Type of nursing practice for registered nurses who work in various health district programs. RNs provide follow-up care, immunizations, health education, and referrals of clients to appropriate agencies for assistance.

compact (cortical) bone Bone that is resistant to compression, is dense, and is laid down in concentric layers.

compartment syndrome An acute problem following injury or surgery caused when pressure within the muscles builds to dangerous levels. The resulting increased pressure within the fascial compartment impairs blood supply.

compensation Correction of the blood pH by the system that is *not* the cause of abnormal levels of carbon dioxide or bicarbonate. For example, when an excess of metabolic acid leads to metabolic acidosis, the lungs increase their ventilation to "blow off" carbon dioxide and reduce its level below normal, thus helping bring the pH back toward normal. Metabolic compensation for a respiratory problem is slower; it takes days to weeks to retain the bicarbonate.

complement A group of proteins in the blood that stimulates the inflammatory response and serves as a primary chemical mediator of the antigen–antibody reactions of the B-cell immune response.

complementary therapy A therapy used in addition to a conventional therapy.

complete spinal cord injury Permanent loss of all neurological function below the level of injury.

comprehensive exam A head-to-toe assessment usually performed on new patients who will be seen on a routine basis by various clinicians.

compression injuries Injuries that occur when pressure is applied to the spinal cord as a result of mass effect from bone fragments, disk herniation, tumor, abscess, or blood clot.

Compromised Family Coping Nursing diagnosis that refers to the inability of a family to function optimally.

concentric When referring to coronary artery stenosis, the term used to describe a lesion that occupies the whole circumference.

concussion A recognized collection of symptoms that result from a mild head injury.

conductive hearing loss Type of hearing loss in which sound waves cannot reach the inner ear for processing and interpretation; caused by diseases such as external ear infections.

conductivity Ability of the cardiac cell to accept and then transmit a stimulus to other cardiac cells.

configuration Refers to the pattern of arrangement or position of lesions.

congenital Present at birth or prenatally.

conjugate gaze Paired or joined eyes moving in tandem in the cardinal fields of gaze.

conscious A mental state that encompasses all things that are easily remembered.

conscious sedation A minimally depressed level of consciousness and satisfactory analgesia that allows the patient to retain the ability to maintain an airway independently and to respond to physical stimulation and verbal commands, obtained through the administration of a combination of pharmacologic agents.

constrictive pericarditis Occurs when the pericardial layers adhere to each other as a result of fibrosis of the pericardial sac.

contact dermatitis An inflammation of the skin related to exposure to an irritant or allergen in the environment.

continent ileostomy (Kock ileostomy or Kock pouch) During ileostomy surgery, the procedure in which the terminal ileum is folded back on itself and the inner wall removed, thereby forming a reservoir and a nipple valve that prevents leakage of fecal contents through the stoma.

continuity theory of aging Theory of aging based on the premise that successful aging is obtained by maintaining values, habits, and behaviors from adult life.

continuous passive motion device Machine into which an extremity is placed to perform continuous passive range of motion.

continuous positive airway pressure (CPAP) Procedure that delivers air into a patient's airway through a specially designed nasal mask or pillows.

continuous subcutaneous infusion (CSI) The uninterrupted infusion of small-volume parenteral medication via the subcutaneous route.

continuous subcutaneous insulin infusion (CSII) A method of exogenous insulin delivery that uses an external "insulin pump," which allows for programmed delivery of insulin into subcutaneous tissue.

contractility A mechanical function that enables the cardiac cells to shorten and cause the muscle to contract in response to an electrical stimulus. Also referred to as *rhythmicity*.

contrast sensitivity (CS) The function of being able to distinguish subtle gradations of grayish patterns between targets and background.

contusion An injury to soft tissue caused by trauma; a bruise.

convalescent phase In viral hepatitis, the phase that occurs approximately 6 to 8 weeks after exposure to the virus and lasts up to 10 weeks when liver function returns to normal. Also called the *recovery phase*.

convenience sampling Type of statistical sampling in which the most available persons or units are selected for inclusion in the study; the researcher has no control over the characteristics of the sample. Also referred to as *accidental sampling*.

coping A compensatory process with physiological and psychological components that allows the individual to adapt to a stressor.

cor pulmonale Enlargement of the right ventricle in response to pulmonary hypoxia; literally means "heart of the lungs."

coronary artery disease (CAD) A progressive atherosclerotic disorder of the coronary arteries that results in narrowing or complete occlusion of the vessel lumen.

correlational research design Research conducted to examine linear relationships between two or more variables.

corticosteroids A class of synthetic steroid hormones that decreases the inflammatory response and suppresses immune activity; used to prevent graft rejection. Examples include Solu-Medrol, Solu-Cortef, hydrocortisone, dexamethasone, and prednisone.

cosmetic surgery Surgery performed for the primary purpose of improving physical appearance.

cotton-wool spots (CWS) Soft exudates that appear as white cotton spots in the nerve fiber layer of the retina; caused by lack of blood supply to the tissue.

counterregulatory hormones Hormones that antagonize the actions of insulin. Examples include glucagon, cortisol, growth hormone, and catecholamines.

crackles When auscultating the lungs, common abnormal, short popping sounds heard on inspiration; caused by the movement of fluid or exudates.

C-reactive protein (CRP) A protein released from the liver in response to local inflammation or tissue injury; useful as a marker for inflammation and colon cancer.

creatinine kinase (CK) An enzyme found in high concentrations in the heart and skeletal muscle and in smaller concentrations in the brain.

cremasteric reflex Condition in which testicles rise in the scrotum to the abdominal cavity when the thigh is stroked or the room is cold.

crepitus Abnormal sounds (grating, snapping, crackling, rattling) emanating from a joint while in movement.

cretinism Condition caused by the congenital absence or atrophy of the thyroid gland, resulting in hypothyroidism and characterized by mental deficiency, large tongue, puffy facial features, and dwarfism.

criminal law Law pertaining to conduct that is offensive or contrary to the public good, such as murder, theft, and rape.

crisis The occurrence of an event or series of events that creates a situation that is perceived as threatening.

critical incident A stressful incident that is so markedly distressing and powerful as to overcome a person's normal feelings of control and coping.

critical incident stress debriefing (CISD) Formal event run by trained counselors to assist those involved in a critical incident to better cope with the incident.

critical incident stress management A comprehensive approach to the management of stress and critical incidents.

critical pathways Comprehensive plans of care for specific patient situations or disease processes. Critical pathways include nursing interventions, medical interventions, and expected timelines for patient outcomes.

critical thinking A purposeful, two-dimensional, goal-directed process that is context bound. Two dimensions are necessary for the development of critical thinking: the cognitive, which is reflective, reasoned thinking, and the affective, which is open-mindedness to divergent perspectives and an inquisitive spirit.

Crohn's disease An inflammatory bowel disease that involves all layers (transmural) of the intestinal wall and can occur anywhere from the mouth to the anus, but commonly affects the ileum.

cross-linking theory of aging Theory of aging based on the premise that the binding of glucose to protein causes various problems. Also referred to as the *glycosylation theory of aging*.

cryoprecipitates Clotting factors used to treat bleeding associated with hemophilia and disorders that cause a depletion of the clotting factors.

cryptorchidism Undescended testicle(s).

cultural competence The ongoing practice of knowing, respecting, and incorporating the values of others; being open to the cultural beliefs and behaviors of others.

cultural diversity Variety and differences in the customs and practices of defined social groups; refers to the variation among groups of people with respect to the habits, values, preferences, beliefs, taboos, and rules determined to be appropriative for individual and social interaction.

culture Learned patterns of behavior, beliefs, and values that can be attributed to a particular group of people.

curative procedures Surgeries performed for the primary purpose of curing a condition.

Cushing's syndrome A hypermetabolic state in which there is a chronic excess of corticosteroid hormones for a variety of reasons.

Cushing's triad Combination of widening pulse pressure, bradycardia, and irregular respiratory patterns; may indicate increasing intracranial pressure.

cyanosis Bluish-tinged skin or mucous membranes due to deoxygenated hemoglobin in blood vessels close to the skin.

cystic fibrosis (CF) A chronic disease in which the process of transportation of salt and water across cell membranes is disturbed, leading to production of unusually thick mucus that blocks bodily passages, particularly in the digestive and respiratory systems. This disorder affects all exocrine glands.

cystocele Occurs when the wall between the bladder and the anterior vagina weakens, often as a result of childbirth, and the bladder protrudes into the vaginal vault.

cytogenetics A specialization of genetics that involves the study of chromosomes.

cytokines Chemical signals released by white blood cells (predominately T cells) that act as messages between cells and instruct immune cells to proliferate, differentiate, or alter activities; more than 100 different cytokines have been identified.

cytotoxic edema The accumulation of intracellular water, causing brain swelling.

dactylitis A uniform swelling of the soft tissues between the metacarpophalangeal and interphalangeal joints.

DASH diet A diet low in saturated fat, cholesterol, and total fat. There are two versions of the DASH plan: Plan 1 limits the patient to 2,000 mg of sodium per day; plan 2 limits the patient to 1,500 mg of sodium per day.

data saturation Sampling to the point at which no new information is obtained and redundancy is achieved.

dawn phenomenon Situation in which a patient has fasting hyperglycemia that is not related to nocturnal hypoglycemia and rebound hyperglycemia.

dead space The portion of the tidal volume that does not reach the alveoli of the lungs or take part in the exchange of oxygen and carbon dioxide.

dead space ventilation (V_D) The portion of the tidal volume that is not participating in gas exchange.

decannulation Term used to refer to the process of weaning a patient toward the goal of removing a tracheotomy tube.

decerebrate posturing The characteristic posture of an individual with decerebrate rigidity. The extremities are stiff and extended, and the head is retracted.

decibel (dB) A measurement of sound. Sounds typically range from 0 to 140 dB or greater.

decontamination The reduction or removal of contaminating agents.

decorticate posturing The characteristic posture of a person with a lesion at or above the upper brainstem. The person is rigidly still with arms flexed, fists clenched, and legs extended.

deep venous thrombosis (DVT) The formation of a blood clot within a deep vein, commonly in the thigh or calf.

defamation of character Publication of anything that is injurious to the good name or reputation of another or that tends to bring another's reputation into question.

defibrillation Basically the same as cardioversion in that electrical voltage is delivered to cause depolarization of the myocardium to terminate unwanted rhythms, except it is done in an emergency situation when sudden cardiac arrest has occurred.

degenerative joint disease Progressive loss of cartilage at a joint.

delayed hypersensitivity reaction Occurs when the immune system responds to an antigen over several hours to days. An example is contact dermatitis.

delegation The assignment of work to others while maintaining accountability for the outcome of the work.

deletion The loss of a chromosome or DNA segment of any length.

delirium A disturbance in consciousness resulting in decreased attention and a change in cognition, or development of a perceptual disturbance that develops over a short period of time and tends to fluctuate throughout the day.

delirium tremens (DTs) Tremor and clouding of consciousness that can accompany physiological withdrawal from alcohol.

dementia A general term for brain dysfunction characterized by a decline in cognition and memory that causes loss of ability to carry out activities of daily living and communicate with others, ultimately resulting in death.

deontological theories In ethics, theories that derive norms and rules from the duties human beings owe one another by virtue of commitments that are made and roles that are assumed.

deoxyhemoglobin Configuration of hemoglobin stimulated by hypoxic states and characterized by rapid release of oxygen to peripheral tissues.

deoxyribonucleic acid (DNA) A complex protein present in the chromosomes of the nuclei of cells that is the basis of heredity and the carrier of genetic information for all organisms except RNA viruses.

dependent activities Activities prescribed by the physician and carried out by the nurse; includes implementing the physician's orders to administer medications or treatments.

depressed skull fracture Displacement of a comminuted skull fracture.

dermabrasion Process of removing the epidermis and upper dermis of the skin so that the skin can regenerate into a smooth surface.

dermatofibromas Common, fibrous, tumor-like nodules of the skin.

dermatomyositis Progressive inflammatory muscle condition that occurs with inflammatory skin changes.

dermatophyte A fungus parasite on the skin.

descriptive research design Type of research question, design, and data analysis that will be applied to a given topic.

descriptive vividness In qualitative research, the practice of describing the site, participants, experience of collecting data, and the thinking of the research so clearly that the reader has a sense of personally experiencing the event.

desensitization The process of introducing small amounts of a triggering allergen to an allergic individual in increasing amounts over time. The goal is to reduce the severity of the allergic response.

desquamation Shedding of the outer layer of epidermis (skin or mucosa).

developmental stressor Stressor that occurs during specific periods of the life span, for examples, as a child, adolescent, young adult, middle adult, or older adult.

Diabetes Control and Complications Trial (DCCT) A landmark research study in the United States and Canada which demonstrated that intensive management of type 1 diabetes (aimed at normal blood glucose levels) resulted in decreased occurrence and progression of development of microvascular complications (i.e., retinopathy, neuropathy, nephropathy).

diabetes insipidus (DI) A hypometabolic disorder of the adrenal gland in which there is excretion of a large volume of dilute urine due to deficiency of antidiuretic hormone (ADH) or an inability of the kidneys to respond to ADH.

Diabetes Prevention Program (DPP) A major clinical research trial of patients with pre-diabetes that clearly demonstrated that lifestyle modification was superior to pharmacologic therapy with metformin (an oral diabetes medication) in preventing diabetes.

diabetic ketoacidosis (DKA) An acute emergent complication of diabetes (usually type 1 diabetes) primarily characterized by hyperglycemia, dehydration, and metabolic acidosis.

diabetic peripheral neuropathy (DPN) A chronic complication of diabetes in which the nerves outside of the spinal cord are damaged. Diabetic peripheral neuropathy is associated with numbness, weakness, burning pain (which often worsens at night), and loss of reflexes in the extremities.

diabetic retinopathy (DR) Disorder characterized by weakened and damaged blood vessels (capillaries) that result in edema from leaking capillaries that hemorrhage.

diagnostic procedures Surgeries performed for the purpose of diagnosing a condition.

dialysis catheter A large-bore vascular access device used as a temporary means to facilitate dialysis procedures; its configuration is similar to that of a pheresis catheter.

diaphysis Shaft of a long bone, between both metaphysis.

diascopy Examination of superficial skin lesions with a diascope.

diastolic A blood pressure reading of the minimum pressure in the arteries, which occurs just prior to the next cycle of ventricular ejection of blood; reflects cardiac relaxation.

diastolic dysfunction Impaired relaxation, preventing the heart from filling appropriately at normal preload pressures.

differentiation Maturation process of blood cells during which cell generations gain increasing specialization; begins with the hematopoietic stem cell and goes to the fully mature peripheral cell.

diffuse axonal injury (DAI) A primary injury of diffuse white matter that results in tearing or shearing of axons and small blood vessels.

diffusion The movement of molecules from an area of high concentration to an area of low concentration in liquids, gases, and solids.

dilated cardiomyopathy A disorder of the myocardium characterized by dilation and impaired contraction of one or more ventricles; the most common form of cardiomyopathy.

diploid The number of chromosomes in most cells except the gametes. The diploid number in humans is 46.

diplopia Seeing double vision, when one object appears as two.

direct inguinal hernia Occurs when abdominal contents herniate through a weak point in the fascia of the abdominal wall and into the inguinal canal.

direct percussion Technique of using gentle tapping to illicit the presence or absence of fluid, which results in a dull sound; used to examine such areas as the sinuses.

direct question Question used to elicit specific information and to clarify specific details; for example, "Is the pain sharp or dull?"

discectomy Surgery to remove a diseased disk.

discrete lesion An individual or separate lesion.

disengagement theory of aging Theory of aging based on the premise that age-related changes bring about a mutual and reciprocal withdrawal of the individual from society.

dislocation Displacement of a bone from its normal position in a joint.

dissecting aortic aneurysm A localized dilation of the aorta that has a longitudinal dissection between the outer and middle layers of the vascular wall.

distribution (1) A description of the lesions on the skin according to location or body region affected. (2) The process of moving a medication into the bloodstream and the extracellular and intracellular compartments, as well as in the compartment that is the site of absorption.

diverticular disease Disease in which abnormal saclike outpouchings (diverticula) of the intestinal wall occur anywhere in the gastrointestinal tract except the rectum, but usually occurring in the distal large intestine.

diverticulitis Inflammation of a diverticulum.

diverticulosis The presence of one or more diverticula.

DMAT Acronym for disaster medical assistance team. A group of volunteer health care professionals and ancillary staff that can provide emergency medical services and relief in times of disaster.

DMORT Acronym for disaster mortuary operations response team. A team of volunteers that can assist with handling mass casualities in time of disaster.

doll's eye reflex *See* oculocephalic reflex.

donor site An area on the body where skin is surgically harvested to use for covering burn wounds.

dopamine A neurotransmitter necessary for ease of movement; loss of dopamine is a key factor in Parkinson's disease.

Dressler's syndrome Condition characterized by fever, pericarditis, chest pain, and pericardial and pleural effusions. Believed to be an autoimmune response, it occurs in 5% to 15% of patients 1 to 4 weeks after a myocardial infarction.

Dreyfus model of skill acquisition A learning model based on determining the level of practice evident in particular situations. It elucidates strengths as well as problems. In this model, situated practice capacities are described rather than traits or talents of the practitioners.

drip factor The number of drops equal to 1 mL of fluid.

drusen Yellowish, round, slightly elevated, different-sized subretinal pigment epithelial deposits in the macula.

dual-channel pump Pole-mounted electronic infusion devices that have multiple channels for infusion within a single device.

dullness A high-pitched tone of short duration that is soft in quality. It is heard over the large organs such as the liver and kidney.

duodenal ulcer An erosion of the duodenal lining resulting from *Helicobacter pylori* infection and hypersecretion of acid and pepsin.

Dupuytren's contracture Difficulty or an inability to extend the ring or fifth finger.

durable power of attorney for health care (DPAHC) A document that allows a patient to appoint a decision maker in the case of future incapacity. The DPAHC specifically states which powers the patient gives to the surrogate. The appointed person responsible for making medical decisions does not need consent from other family members or friends.

dwell The time period during which an infusion catheter remains in place.

dynamic response test A test to assess whether a transducer system is accurately transmitting pressures.

dysconjugate gaze Eyes moving separately from each other in the cardinal fields of gaze.

dyskinesia Involuntary, writhing movements that may involve limbs, trunk, face, and neck; results from overstimulation of dopamine receptors. Condition characterized by areas of abnormal heart contractility where muscle movement is impaired.

dysmenorrhea Painful menstruation.

dyspareunia Painful intercourse; can be a result of several factors such as endometriosis or menopause.

dysphagia Difficulty swallowing.

dysphoria An exaggerated feeling of depression and unrest without apparent cause; a mood of general dissatisfaction, restlessness, anxiety, discomfort, and unhappiness.

dysplasia Change in the appearance of cells after they have been subjected to chronic irritation.

dyspnea Subjective feeling of shortness of breath or difficulty breathing.

dysrhythmia A heartbeat originating from a site other than the primary cardiac pacemaker tissue. The terms *dysrhythmia*, *arrhythmia*, and *ectopic focus* all mean the same thing and are used interchangeably.

eccentric When discussing plaque buildup in a coronary artery, the term used to describe a lesion that occupies part of a vessel wall.

ecchymosis A lesion that is initially dark red or purple, but gradually fades to yellowish green before it disappears.

ECG single photon emission computed tomography (SPECT) A nuclear medicine technique that uses radiopharmaceuticals, a rotating camera, and a computer to produce images representing slices through the body in different planes.

ECG waveform Movement away from the baseline, or the isoelectric line, on an ECG tracing on graph paper.

echocardiography The noninvasive assessment of the structures and function of the heart and great vessels utilizing high-frequency (ultrasound) sound waves.

ectopic Implantation of the products of conception outside the uterine endometrium.

ectopic focus A heartbeat originating from a site other than the primary cardiac pacemaker tissue. Also called *dysrhythmia*.

edema Accumulation of fluid in the intercellular spaces that causes swelling of tissue.

efferent Ability to transport away from a central organ or section; conducts impulses from the brain or spinal cord to the periphery. In the nervous system, efferent nerves are known as motor or effector neurons that carry nerve impulses *away* from the central nervous system to effectors such as muscles or glands.

ego Mediates the drives of the id with a dose of reality.

ego defense mechanisms Utilized to alleviate anxiety by denying, distorting, and misinterpreting reality.

ejection fraction (EF) The amount of blood ejected from the left or right ventricle; calculated by comparing end-diastolic volume to stroke volume.

elastomeric balloon A portable, disposable mechanical infusion device that requires no power source to function.

elective procedures Procedure for which the timing is determined by the patient and the surgeon. A total knee replacement scheduled in advance is an example of an elective surgery.

electrocardiogram Surface recording of the electrical activity of the heart.

electrode An adhesive pad that contains conducting gel and is connected to a cardiac monitor by lead wires. Electrodes serve as sensing devices to detect changes in electrical activity of the heart. Electrodes must be placed in certain positions in order for the ECG machine to have a clear picture of the electrical impulse, and they must have a positive, a negative, and a ground lead.

electrolytes Ionized minerals (calcium, chloride, magnesium, phosphorus, potassium, and sodium) serving as energy transfer mechanisms in combinations of positive charges (cations) or negative charges (anions).

electromyelogram (EMG) A graphic recording that tests the contraction of muscles that have been electrically stimulated.

electron beam computed tomography (EBCT) Procedure that uses an electron gun and a stationary tungsten target to rapidly (about 90 seconds) acquire multiple images of the heart during a single breath hold.

electroneutrality The principle that asserts that the sum of all positive or cationic charges in plasma must equal the sum of all negative or anionic charges. The primary cations measured in venous plasma are sodium and potassium. The main anions are chloride and bicarbonate or serum carbon dioxide.

electronic infusion device (EID) An infusion device that can be portable, or pole mounted; requires a power supply (i.e., batteries or electric current) to function; used to control delivery of parenteral solutions or medications.

electrophysiology study (EPS) An invasive procedure that involves placing multiple multipolar catheter electrodes into the venous and sometimes the arterial side of the heart in order to evaluate the electrical activity of the heart and to identify areas of initiation and propagation of dysrhythmias.

elemental iron Amount of iron in a food substance that is available for absorption from the digestive tract.

elimination The process of excretion from the body that is generally accomplished in the renal system. Elimination can occur after medications are metabolized or medications may be eliminated in their primary form.

emancipated minors Persons under the legal age of adulthood who are no longer under the control and regulation of their parents and who may give valid consent for medical procedures.

embolectomy Mechanical removal of a clot in a blood vessel.

embolization Endovascular procedure in which an aneurysm is obliterated by filling it with a glue-type substance.

emergency doctrine Allows implied consent for treatment to exist in true emergency situations in which an individual is in danger of loss of life or limb.

Emergency Medical Treatment and Active Labor Act (EMTALA) A part of the 1986 COBRA laws and the 1990 OBRA amendment that defines the legal responsibilities of Medicare-participating hospitals in treating individuals who present with emergency medical conditions; ensures that patients have access to emergency services regardless of their ability to pay.

emergency nursing The care of individuals of all ages with perceived or actual physical or emotional alterations of health that are undiagnosed or require further interventions.

emergent (emergency) surgery Surgery that must be performed suddenly without advanced planning.

emmetropia The condition of the normal eye when parallel rays are focused exactly on the retina and vision is perfect. Normal refractive error or vision without any corrective optical devices.

emphysema A disease of the airways that involves destruction of the alveolar walls.

empiric therapy Therapy that is begun before culture results are available; physicians determine if empiric therapy is necessary based on the severity of the infection.

encephalitis Inflammation of brain tissue.

endocrine Glands that secrete directly into the bloodstream.

endoleaks Continued leakage of blood into the aneurysmal sac.

endometriosis Condition in which endometrial-like cells are found outside of the uterus. During the menstrual cycle, these cells respond to hormone production and may swell and bleed. In response, the body will surround these lesions with scar tissue, which can form adhesions on the area of attachment.

end-organ perfusion The blood perfusion of the end organs such as the integumentary system.

endorphins Endogenous, morphine-like substances that reduce or inhibit pain perception in the descending pathways.

endoscopic retrograde cholangiopancreatography (ERCP) Radiograph following injection of a radiopaque material into the papilla of Vater.

endoskeletal Pertaining to the cartilaginous and bony skeleton of the body.

endotoxins Produced by live bacteria and released when the bacteria are killed.

endotracheal tube Tube used to deliver oxygen that is placed in the trachea.

end-stage renal disease (ESRD) A patient is considered to have end-stage renal disease when the loss of filtration ability reaches approximately seven-eighths, at which point the survival of the patient depends on dialysis or, if an acceptable candidate, a kidney transplant.

engraftment Establishment of new bone marrow.

enkephalins Pentapeptides produced in the brain that act as an opiate.

enteral nutrition Use of the gastrointestinal tract for feeding.

enthesitis Upon palpitation, discomfort at the site of the attachment of bone to the tendon.

enzyme immunoassays (EIAs) Laboratory tests of blood to determine whether or not antibodies are present. A specific enzyme is used to link to antibodies, in this case, HIV antibodies. A positive test indicates antibodies are present.

eosinophil Acts as a phagocyte in inflammatory conditions, particularly allergic reactions.

ependymomas Tumors originating from the ependymal cells of the cerebral ventricles.

epididymitis Inflammation of the long, tubular structure that connects and carries sperm from the testicle to the vas deferens.

epidural anesthesia A type of regional anesthesia in which an anesthetic agent is injected in the epidural space.

epidural hematoma (EDH) Bleeding into the space between the skull and the dura.

epiglottitis Infection and inflammation of the epiglottis and surrounding supraglottic structures often resulting in airway obstruction. Usually caused by *Haemophilus influenzae* type B.

epiphysis The end of the bone beyond the physis.

epistaxis Bleeding from the nose.

epithelialization Process by which a wound closes from its margins, covering the defect with a layer of new skin.

erectile dysfunction (ED) The inability to achieve or maintain an erection sufficient to allow intercourse.

error theories of aging Theory of aging based on the premise that environmental factors negatively impact the human body, causing destruction and damage.

erysipelas A form of cellulitis characterized by inflammation and redness of the skin due to group A hemolytic streptococci.

erythrocyte Red blood cell.

erythropoiesis Process of red blood cell development.

erythropoietic stem cell (proerythroblast) The earliest of four stages in development of the normoblast. Ancestor cell giving rise to red blood cells.

erythropoietin Hormone that stimulates the production of red blood cells.

escape Term that applies to the emergence of a pacemaker that is lower in the heart and sustains a heart rate when the SA node fails.

eschar Nonviable burned tissue.

escharotomies Incisions made through burn tissue to relieve the constricting effects of the edema that accompanies circumferential injuries.

esophageal cancer Cancer that occurs anywhere in the esophagus, but more often occurs in the middle and distal portions; is usually squamous cell carcinoma.

esophageal varices Varicose veins in the distal esophagus that result most often from portal hypertension, a complication of cirrhosis of the liver.

esophagus The muscular tube that carries swallowed foods and liquids from the pharynx to the stomach.

esophoria Inward deviation of the eye.

ethical decision making Evaluating the principles and values of all persons involved in a decision before coming to a conclusion.

ethical dilemma A situation that involves two or more unfavorable alternatives to a given situation.

ethics Discipline relating to moral actions and moral values.

ethnography A form of research that focuses on the sociology of meaning through field observation and description of a sociocultural phenomenon.

ethos Notions of what counts as good nursing or good scientific practice.

euphoria An exaggerated feeling of well-being.

eustress Stress associated with positive events.

euthymia Normal, nondepressed, reasonably positive mood.

euthyroid Appearing to function as a normal thyroid gland.

euvolemia Term used when the body is in a state of equal fluid balance, without fluid retention.

evaluation Focuses on a patient's behavioral changes and compares them with criteria stated in predetermined patient outcomes. Evaluation is ongoing through all phases of the nursing process.

evidence-based practice (EBP) A problem-solving approach to clinical decision making that incorporates a search for the best and latest evidence, clinical expertise, and assessment, and a patient's preferences and values within a context of caring. This decision-making approach integrates clinical expertise with the best available evidence from systematic research in contrast to opinion-based health care decision making that is based primarily on values and resources.

excitability Ability of an electrical cell to respond to a stimulus. All cardiac cells possess this property. Also referred to as *irritability*.

exercise testing A cardiovascular stress test combining exercise (either physical or pharmacologic) and electrocardiographic and blood pressure monitoring, typically to evaluate patients with suspected coronary artery disease.

exocrine pancreas The portion of the pancreas that secretes enzymes for digestion into the duodenum.

exon The portion of a gene that contains the code for producing the gene's protein.

exophthalmos Abnormal protrusion of the eyeball; may be due to thyrotoxicosis, tumor of the orbit, orbital cellulitis, leukemia, or aneurysm.

exostosis A condition of the ear canal in which the bony lining under the skin develops a number of lumps that grow into the tube. Also called *surfer's ear*.

exotoxins Proteins released by bacterial cells during growth; they have very specific actions. Exotoxins modify cell enzymes and functions, leading to cell death or dysfunction. They are usually named for the site they affect.

experience An active process of gaining knowledge and skill, not just a passage of time.

experiential learning Requires a turning around of preconceptions, or an adding of nuances to one's understanding. Experiential learning requires openness and responsiveness by the learner to improve practice over time.

experimental research design Type of research in which the researcher attempts to maintain control over all factors that may affect the results of an experiment. In so doing, the researcher attempts to determine or predict what may occur when a hypothesis is tested and conclusions are drawn between independent and dependent variables.

exploratory surgery Surgery performed for the purpose of identifying abnormalities when the diagnosis of a condition is not established beforehand.

expressivity The degree or amount of symptomology to which an individual with a genotype is affected. For example, two individuals may have the same genotype, but one may have all of the symptoms of the disorder, while the second one has relatively few symptoms.

extension set Tubing that adds length and/or access ports to an administration set.

external fixation A treatment in which the bones or bone ends of a fracture are held in place by skeletal pins. The pins are screwed into the bone and attached to a frame worn on the outside of the body.

external locus of control An orientation in which a person believes that events in his or her life are controlled more by fate, luck, and external circumstances.

external stressor Stressor that originates outside the body.

extra-axial tumors Tumors originating from the supporting structures of the brain.

extracellular fluid (ECF) Fluid between the cells (interstitial fluids) and in plasma (serum).

extravasation Inadvertent administration of a vesicant solution or medication into surrounding tissues.

Factor VIII A clotting factor that may be administered intravenously for the treatment of hemophilia A.

false imprisonment The unjustified detention or confinement of a person without legal warrant.

familial intracranial aneurysms The presence of proven aneurysms in two or more family members among first- and second-degree relatives.

fascicles Anterior and posterior pathways that branch off the heart's left bundle branch. The anterior fascicle carries electrical impulses to the anterior wall of the left ventricle. The posterior fascicle spreads electrical impulses to the posterior ventricular wall.

fasciculation Involuntary contraction or twitching of a group of muscles or muscle fibers, visible under the skin.

fasciotomy Incisions made to release skin and muscle coverings.

FAST examination Focused assessment with sonography for trauma.

fast-tracking Term used to describe a situation in which a patient is transferred from the operating room to the postanesthesia care unit (PACU) phase II, bypassing PACU phase I. Fast-tracking is possible when surgical techniques are minimally invasive and anesthesia is of a short duration.

fat embolus Fat that enters the circulatory system after the fracture of a long bone.

ferritin A form of iron in the body acting as a supply reservoir.

fetal alcohol syndrome (FAS) Physical and mental defects found in babies of women who consumed alcohol during pregnancy.

fetid breath Halitosis or foul or putrid breath.

fever of unknown origin (FUO) A fever that lasts 2 weeks or more without identification of the cause.

fibroblasts Small cells that migrate along the fibrin network to produce the connective tissue and collagen fibers.

fibrocystic breast An increase in glandular and fibrous tissues in the breast; characterized by small, nodular cysts that are palpable in the breast.

fibroid tumor Growths arising from the tissue of the uterine muscle; they develop slowly in women ages 25 through 40 years of age.

fibrous cap A dense connective tissue matrix in the inner lining of an artery that is formed when smooth muscle cells secrete collagen, elastin, and glycosaminoglycans.

fidelity In ethics, keeping one's promises or commitments.

fill time Period of time needed for blood to enter the heart between contractions.

filter Add-on device used to screen particulate matter, bacteria, and toxins from the infusion system.

filtration The movement of molecules from an area of higher concentration through permeable membranes to an area of lower concentration as a result of hydrostatic pressure.

first-degree AV block Conduction disturbance in which electrical impulses flow normally from the SA node through the atria, but are delayed at the AV node. This results in a prolongation of conduction rather than an actual block. Due to this delay, the PR interval is greater than 0.20 second, making it abnormal.

Fisher grading scale Grading scale for subarachnoid hemorrhage referring to the amount of blood on a CT scan.

fissure Deep linear crack or furrow in the continuity of the epidermis.

fistula Dehiscent wound that traverses between two different tissue planes; a communication between two areas such as the oral cavity and the skin.

flail chest Occurs when a person sustains two or more rib fractures in two or more places such that the ribs are no longer attached to the thoracic cage, resulting in a free or floating segment of chest wall. As a result, during spontaneous ventilation the floating segment moves in the opposite direction or paradoxically to the chest wall. This condition is almost always associated with pulmonary contusion.

flame-shaped hemorrhages Retinal hemorrhages that occur in the nerve fiber layer.

flare A round area of redness surrounding the wheal of an allergic reaction on the skin.

flashback chamber Small space located after the hub of the catheter and attached to the stylet; used to collect blood.

flashes Sudden bright light noticed by a person; flashes appear as sparks or minuscule strands of light, almost like streaks of lightning across the sky that occur when the vitreous gel bumps, rubs, or tugs against the retina.

flatness A soft, high-pitched tone of short duration. It is heard over muscle and bone.

flexible sigmoidoscopy A sigmoidoscope that uses fiber optics to inspect the sigmoid colon.

floaters Deposits of various size, shape, consistency, refractive index, and motility within the eye's vitreous humor, which is normally transparent.

flow control device Device used to regulate fluid administration.

flushing Procedure performed to maintain device patency and prevent mixing of incompatible solutions or medications.

focused exam An exam performed in emergent or urgent situations that focuses on a specific problem.

folate Naturally occurring, water-soluble form of vitamin B critical for red blood cell formation.

folliculitis Inflammation of the hair follicles.

Folstein Mini-Mental State Exam A common screening tool used by clinicians to evaluate dementia.

foreign body sensation (FBS) A feeling in the eye of a "gritty" feeling, as if something is in the eye.

forensic evidence Something that is legally submitted to a court of law as a means of determining the truth related to an alleged crime.

foreseeability of harm Concept that certain actions are known to cause or create specific outcomes.

for-profit (proprietary) organization Organization that focuses on making a profit from operations and distributing those profits to the owners or investors in the organization.

fraction of inspired oxygen (FiO_2) The amount expressed as a number of oxygen in a gas mixture, 0 (0%) to 1 (100%). For example the FiO_2 of normal room air is 0.21 (21%).

fractures Discontinuities in bone that may be complete or incomplete.

fragment antigen binding (FAB) portion The section of an antibody that is capable of being shaped to receive a specific antigen. DNA within B cells is capable of creating many millions of combinations of FAB portions of antibodies to match an antigen and help protect the body against an invasion by pathogens.

fragment crystalline (FC) portion The section of an antibody that is capable of attaching to the cell membrane of infected or mutant cells or of foreign pathogens (bacteria, viruses) and assisting macrophages to eliminate them.

Frank-Starling law The ability of muscle fibers to stretch to accommodate filling during diastole.

free radical theory of aging Theory of aging that postulates that aging changes are caused by free radical reactions that cause cells and organs to lose function and reserve energy.

fremitus Tactile vibration felt over airways.

frequency The number of sound waves emanating per second; measured in hertz (Hz). Hearing frequencies from 500 to 2,000 Hz are needed to understand everyday speech.

fresh frozen plasma A process in which the plasma portion of blood is separated from the cells and frozen until needed. Units of fresh frozen plasma are used to increase the level of clotting factors in patients with demonstrated deficiency.

friable Easily damaged.

frozen RBCs Red blood cells coated in glycerol prior to freezing and then washed after thawing to remove the glycerol prior to administration. This is a method of storage.

full-thickness injury An injury that extends into the underlying structures and organs.

full-thickness skin graft Grafting of skin that is surgically removed by excising the entire thickness of the donor skin to the level of the subcutaneous tissue, typically 0.025 to 0.30 inch thick.

functional iron deficiency Physiological state characterized by failure to supply enough iron for erythropoiesis despite sufficient quantities.

functional nursing A task-oriented nursing care delivery system in which individual caregivers are not given patient assignments but are expected to perform specific assigned tasks within their capability for all patients in a given area.

furuncle A boil or a walled-off, deep, painful, firm inflammation of the skin that contains pus.

fusiform aneurysms Elliptically shaped aneurysm.

gait Walking.

galactogenesis Formation of breast milk from nutrients available from the bloodstream.

galactorrhea The spontaneous flow of milk in a breast unassociated with childbirth or nursing.

gamete Reproductive cell, ovum or sperm, with the haploid chromosome number.

gamma-glutamyltransferase (GGT) An enzyme found mostly in the liver that is released when cellular damage occurs.

gastric carcinoma Cancer in the stomach, most commonly in the antrum and distal portions; is usually an adenocarcinoma.

gastric outlet obstruction Results from edema, inflammation, or scarring and obstructs the flow of gastric contents from the stomach to the duodenum. Also called *pyloric obstruction*.

gastric ulcer An erosion of the stomach lining that develops most often in the antrum, which is adjacent to the body of the stomach. It is not associated with increased acid secretion, but rather, with a defect in the mucosal barrier to hydrogen ions, allowing the ions to permeate the mucosa.

gastroduodenostomy (Billroth I) A partial gastrectomy in which the lower portion of the stomach is removed and the remainder is anastomosed with the duodenum.

gastroesophageal reflux The backflow of gastric contents into the lower end of the esophagus.

gastroesophageal reflux disease (GERD) A common condition in which acid from the stomach flows back into the esophagus, causing discomfort and, in some cases, damage to the esophageal lining.

gastrojejunostomy (Billroth II) Procedure in which a larger distal portion of the stomach is removed than with the gastroduodenostomy (Billroth I) procedure, and the remainder is anastomosed to the jejunum.

gastroparesis Delayed emptying of food from the stomach into the small bowel.

gate control theory Proposes that the spinal cord has a gating mechanism that either permits or inhibits the transmission of pain information to the brain.

gating Dividing the cardiac cycle into segments so that images viewed in cine mode allow the clinician to evaluate wall motion and systolic thickening in all areas of the left ventricle.

gauge Needle or catheter size.

gene The functional unit of heredity that occupies a certain position on a chromosome and is passed from parent to offspring. Genes consist of DNA and most contain information for making a specific protein.

gene mutations Abnormal genes inherited from parents.

gene therapy Therapy that involves adding a functional gene or group of genes to a cell by gene insertion to correct a hereditary disorder.

general adaptation syndrome (GAS) Physical response to stress as defined by Selye. GAS is composed of three stages: alarm reaction, stage of resistance, and stage of exhaustion.

general anesthesia The production of complete unconsciousness, muscular relaxation, and absence of pain sensation.

genetic variance Variation in genotype that is associated with phenotype.

genital herpes An incurable condition caused primarily by the herpes simplex virus; it can be treated with antiviral drugs.

genital warts Sexually transmitted, cauliflower-like growths in the genital, anal, and vaginal areas. Also called *human papillomavirus*.

genome All of the DNA in an organism or cell to include the 44 autosomes, 2 sex chromosomes, and the mitochondrial DNA.

genomic imprinting Genetic inheritance process in which both maternal and paternal alleles are present, but one allele is expressed and the other remains silent.

genomics The field of genetics concerned with structural and functional studies of the genome.

genotype The genetic makeup of an individual that is not evident as outward or visible characteristics.

germ line cells The sex cell or gamete (egg or spermatozoan).

gerontological nurse practitioner (GNP) A registered nurse with a master's degree from a nurse practitioner program specializing in the care of older adults.

gestational diabetes mellitus (GDM) A specific type of diabetes that occurs during pregnancy in women who had no history of diabetes prior to the pregnancy.

gigantism Condition brought on by overproduction of pituitary growth hormone in youth before the long bones have closed. Characterized by abnormal height.

gingival hyperplasia Excessive proliferation of normal cells of the gingiva.

glaucoma A group of diseases of the optic nerve involving loss of retinal ganglion cells in a characteristic pattern of optic neuropathy. Raised intraocular pressure is a significant risk factor for developing glaucoma (above 22 mmHg).

glomerulus A compact tuft of capillaries in which blood is filtered.

glucagon A hormone produced by the alpha cells of the pancreas. Glucagon has several actions, the most important of which is (along with insulin) maintaining blood glucose levels within a normal range. In diabetes, elevated levels of glucagon contribute to hyperglycemia and ketosis.

gluconeogenesis The formation of glucose from noncarbohydrate organic molecules (i.e., lactate, glycerol, and amino acids); is a function of the liver.

glucose-6-phosphate dehydrogenase (G6PD) deficiency The most common enzyme deficiency contributing to hemolytic anemia. Enzymatic deficiencies in erythrocytes increase the red blood cell's sensitivity and susceptibility to oxidative stress. Deficiencies in the enzyme are genetically encoded and relatively common especially in persons of African American and Mediterranean descent.

glutamate An excitatory neurotransmitter implicated in cell death.

glycated serum proteins (GSPs) A test of short-term blood glucose control (14 to 20 days) obtained by measuring the glycosylation of total serum proteins or glycosylation of albumin. The most widely used method to measure GSPs is the hemoglobin A$_{1c}$ (HbA$_{1c}$) test. A normal HbA$_{1c}$ is less than 6%. This test is also known as glycated hemoglobin or glycosylated hemoglobin, and is frequently is referred to as "A1C."

glycogen A starch polysaccharide that is stored in the liver and muscles of humans and can be hydrolyzed to glucose.

glycogenolysis The conversion of glycogen to glucose.

glycolysis A biochemical pathway that results in the generation of high-energy compounds (e.g., ATP and NADH).

goal A broad statement of purpose that describes the aim of nursing care.

goiter Abnormal enlargement of the thyroid gland.

goitrogen A substance in a food or a drug that inhibits the production of thyroid hormone.

goniometer Used for measuring a patient's range of motion.

gonorrhea A sexually transmitted infection that is caused by the bacterium *Neisseria gonorrhoeae*, which infects the warm moist environment of the reproductive tract, along with any other mucous membranes in the body.

Gottron's sign Reddish raised rash or papules over the knuckles.

gouty arthritis Condition in which there is an imbalance in purine metabolism, which increases uric acid in the joints by the formation of uric acid crystals.

gouty joint Inflammation of the big toe, dorsum, ankles, heels, or elbows.

graduated compression stockings Elastic stockings that apply varying degrees of pressure on the lower leg with the greatest exertion of pressure at the ankle and the lowest pressure at the thigh (or knee in shorter stockings).

graft versus host disease (GVHD) An alloimmune response in which the grafted tissue initiates an immune response against tissue of the host or recipient of the grafted tissue. An example of graft versus host disease is seen in transplanted bone marrow.

granulation tissue Tiny, round granule-like nodules that become beefy, red, and moist because of the dense revascularization process.

granulocyte White blood cell with numerous granules in the cytoplasm; granulocytes are divided into neutrophils, eosinophils, and basophils.

graph paper Paper specifically designed and used to measure various calculations related to the electrical activity of the heart; it is arranged as a series of horizontal and vertical lines and is standardized to allow for consistency in ECG tracing analysis.

Graves' disease A hypermetabolic condition caused by an autoimmune disease in which the thyroid gland produces too much thyroid hormone.

grounded theory The idea that conclusion of a qualitative study should be grounded in the data, that is, based on direct and careful observations of everyday life within the group.

growth factors A group of extracellular polypeptides (secreted by platelets and macrophages) that affect cell growth, reproduction, movement, or function.

growth needs The top levels of Maslow's hierarchy associated with psychological needs.

gynecomastia Male breast enlargement due to a hormonal imbalance.

hairy tongue A condition in which the tongue is covered with hairlike papilla due to the overgrowth of the fungus *Candida albicans* or *Aspergillus niger*.

haploid The number of chromosomes in an egg or sperm cell; it is half the diploid number.

hardiness Condition in which a person has a clear sense of personal values and goals, a strong tendency toward interaction with the environment, a sense of meaningfulness, and an internal rather than an external locus of control. It is a mediating factor in how people respond to stress.

Hashimoto's thyroiditis An autoimmune condition characterized by high titers of the circulating antibodies thyroid peroxidase and thyroglobulin that destroy thyroid cells and may lead to hypothyroidism. It is the most common thyroid disease in the United States. Also known as *chronic lymphocytic hypothyroidism*.

hassles Experiences and conditions of daily living that have been appraised as relevant and harmful or threatening to an individual's well-being.

Haversian canals Canals located in cortical bone; they contain one or two capillaries and nerve fibers that serve as the transport system for nutrients.

health care delivery system System that provides client-centered, comprehensive, interdisciplinary, integrated, and accessible health care that meets the needs of the clients.

Health Insurance Portability and Accountability Act (HIPAA) A federal law designed to improve the portability of health care coverage for people who lose or change employment, to simplify the administrative process through the use of electronic transactions, and to ensure the privacy of membership information.

health maintenance organization (HMO) Organization that provides coverage for medical care and controls costs through utilization review and management and by restricting access to a specific network of providers.

heart failure A complex and debilitating clinical syndrome in which there is loss or dysfunction of the cardiac muscle or an inability of the ventricle to fill or eject blood.

heaves Palpable sustained lifts of the chest wall due to forceful cardiac contractions.

Heberden's nodes Hard, painless nodules at the joints of the fingers; may indicate osteoarthritis. Heberden's nodes are found over the distal interphalangeal joints.

Helicobacter pylori (H. pylori) A bacterium that infects the stomach and duodenum and is associated with peptic ulcers.

hematocrit The ratio of the volume of erythrocytes (red blood cells) to that of the whole blood.

hematology The branch of biology (physiology), pathology, clinical laboratory, internal medicine, and pediatrics that is concerned with the study of blood, the blood-forming organs, and blood diseases.

hematoma An area of swelling or mass of blood confined to an organ, tissue, or space, due to a broken blood vessel.

hematopoiesis The formation and development of blood cells.

hematopoietic stem cell (HSC) Bone marrow cell that is the precursor to all hematologic cell types.

hematuria The presence of blood in the urine.

heme iron Form of dietary iron that is common in red meats and fish.

hemodynamic monitoring The monitoring of pressures and blood flow within the cardiovascular system.

hemoglobin The oxygen carrying pigment of the erythrocytes, formed by the developing erythrocyte in bone marrow.

hemoglobin A$_{1c}$ (HbA$_{1c}$) test Refers to a series of stable minor hemoglobin components formed nonenzymatically from the glycosylation of the hemoglobin molecule. The amount of HbA$_{1c}$ is directly proportional to the ambient glucose concentration, providing an estimation of blood glucose control during the previous 2 to 3 months. Sometimes also referred to as *glycohemoglobin, glycosylated hemoglobin,* or *A1C.*

hemoglobinopathies Red blood disorders characterized by abnormal hemoglobin.

hemolytic anemia Group of diseases characterized by increased red blood cell destruction.

hemophilia Genetic disorder resulting from mutated genes controlling Factors VIII or Factor IX; characterized by uncontrolled bleeding.

hemoptysis Coughing up of blood from the lower respiratory tract.

hemosiderin A form of iron in the body acting as a supply reservoir.

hemosiderin staining Occurs when the heme part of the red blood cell is deposited in the tissues as red blood cells get trapped and accumulate due to venous congestion. As the red blood cell dies, the heme is deposited and a brownish hue staining color results.

hemostasis Cessation of bleeding; a complex process that changes blood from a fluid to a solid state. Hemostasis occurs in two phases: primary and secondary. Primary hemostasis is characterized by vascular contraction, platelet adhesion, and formation of a soft aggregate plug. Secondary hemostasis is responsible for stabilizing the soft clot and maintaining vasoconstriction.

hemothorax Partial or complete collapse of the lung due to blood in the pleural space.

heparin-induced thrombocytopenia (HIT) Drug-induced, immune-mediated thrombocytopenia; caused by exposure to heparin therapy.

hepatic artery catheter A catheter inserted into the hepatic artery for targeted antineoplastic therapies.

hepatic encephalopathy A result of an increased level of circulating neurotoxins. The most abundant neurotoxin is ammonia and is the end product of protein digestion.

hepatic first pass Refers to the reduction of a medication's effect due to partial metabolism in the liver prior to distribution to the ultimate site of action.

hepatitis A virus (HAV) An RNA virus that causes hepatitis and is transmitted mainly through contaminated food and water.

hepatitis B virus (HBV) A DNA virus that causes hepatitis and is transmitted sexually and parenterally.

hepatitis C virus (HCV) An RNA virus that causes hepatitis and is transmitted mainly parenterally. The majority of the cases develop chronic hepatitis.

hepatitis D virus (HDV) An RNA virus that occurs only in the presence of HBV.

hepatitis E virus (HEV) An RNA virus that is transmitted mostly through the fecal–oral route and is endemic in Southeast Asia and parts of Africa.

hepatocellular Pertaining to the cells of the liver.

hepatojugular reflux An increase in jugular venous pressure when pressure is applied over the abdomen; is suggestive of right-sided heart failure.

hepatorenal syndrome Syndrome characterized by azotemia occurring in a patient with liver failure.

hepcidin Hormone produced in the liver that is responsible for iron supply regulation.

hereditary spherocytosis (HS) Hemolytic anemia disorder characterized by insufficient red blood cell membrane proteins.

hernia Protrusion of an anatomic structure through the wall that normally contains it.

herniation The displacement of brain structures under pressure, causing compression and damage of brain tissue.

herpetic stomatitis Inflammation of the oral cavity caused by the herpes simplex virus.

heterografts Biologic dressing made from animals such as pigs.

heterotropic ossification (OS) The development of bone tissue in areas where bone tissue is not normally present.

heterozygous Having two different alleles for a given gene, one inherited from each parent.

heuristic relevance Discovering or revealing a relationship that may lead to additional development along a particular line of research.

hiatal hernia Protrusion of the upper portion of the stomach into the thorax through the esophageal hiatus.

high-altitude pulmonary edema (HAPE) Type of pulmonary edema that develops in persons who rapidly ascend to heights greater than 2,500 to 3,000 meters (8,202 to 9,842 feet).

high density lipoprotein A type of lipoprotein that binds to cholesterol to transport it back to the liver; lipoproteins may actually remove excess cholesterol from plaque in the arteries.

highly active antiretroviral drug therapy (HAART) Combination therapy has the greatest effect in controlling HIV proliferation and minimizing the development of drug resistance. Antiretroviral drugs are grouped according to the mechanism of action against HIV.

hirsutism Abnormal growth of hair, especially in women.

histamine A protein produced by mast and other cells. Release of histamine results in vasodilation and bronchoconstriction. Symptoms associated with histamine release include shortness of breath, wheezing, itching, and hives.

histamine$_2$ (H$_2$)-receptor blockers Drugs that block the H$_2$-receptors located in the gastrointestinal tract and reduce acid secretion.

HIV antibody positive status An individual's status when enough HIV antibodies have been produced in response to infection by the HIV virus to be measured by antibody serology, usually after 3 weeks to 3 months. Symptoms may or may not be present.

hoarseness Condition that occurs when the normal vibration of the vocal cords is disrupted.

holding area A physical space located adjacent to the operating room where patients wait prior to an operation.

holism An idea based on the premise that the whole is more than the sum of its parts.

Holter monitoring Ambulatory electrocardiogram monitoring for an extended period of time.

homeostasis The tendency toward stability within an organism; it is the first reaction toward that stability when a wound occurs.

homograft valve *See* allograft valve.

homologous transfusion The process of collecting blood from a donor for transfusion into other individuals who are in need of blood.

homozygous Having identical alleles at a given location.

honeymoon period A transient period of time when newly diagnosed patients with type 1 diabetes have restoration of insulin production and thus a reduced requirement for exogenous insulin.

horizontal organization model Service structure of hospitals aligned to form a multihospital system; focuses on traditional acute care services.

hospice Palliative care and support services for patients with terminal illnesses and their families.

hospitalist Physician who concentrates her or his practice in the acute care environment.

host versus graft disease (HVGD) A type of alloimmune hypersensitivity response that involves transplanted organs or tissues; occurs when a recipient's immune system reacts against the foreign antigens on the cells of the graft.

human genome The complete DNA sequence that contains the entire genetic information for a human.

Human Genome Project (HGP) An international research project to map each human gene and completely sequence human DNA.

human immunodeficiency virus (HIV) The infective agent responsible for causing AIDS; HIV is a retrovirus that infects CD4 T cells and fatally impairs immune function. Two specific strains of HIV have been identified: HIV type 1 and HIV type 2.

human leukocyte antigens (HLAs) Genetic protein markers on the cell wall of white blood cells that alert the immune system to the appropriateness of a cell belonging to the system. HLAs can differentiate self from non-self. There are six different HLA markers: HLA-A, HLA-B, HLA-C, HLA-D, HLA-DR, and HLA-DQ. Each of these markers is capable of creating multiple different antigen subtype combinations. HLA matching between donor and recipient is key to preventing transplant graft rejection.

human papillomavirus (HPV) *See genital warts.*

humoral immune response Mechanism by which organisms gain immunity to previously encountered substances; involves B lymphocytes and antibody-mediated immunity. The term *humoral* comes from the Greek word "humor," which means body fluids; B cells are in the plasma.

Hunt-Hess classification Grading scale for subarachnoid hemorrhage.

hydrocele Swelling of the scrotum caused by fluid collection.

hydrogen ion A single, charged atomic proton that is not orbited by any electrons. It is the smallest ionic particle and is extremely reactive.

hydronephrosis Collection of urine in the pelvis of the kidney from obstructed outflow.

hydroxyapatite Inorganic hexagonal matrix of bone composed of calcium and phosphorus.

hyperacute rejection Occurs within the first hours after transplant when the recipient has a preexisting antibody to the antigen in the graft tissue. Blanching of the graft is one of the earliest signs of rejection.

hyperbaric oxygen therapy (HBOT) Refers to intermittent treatment of the entire body with 100% oxygen at greater than normal atmospheric pressures.

hypercarbic drive The stimulus for ventilation that occurs when elevated levels of carbon dioxide alter the pH of the blood and cerebrospinal fluid, making them more acid. Central chemoreceptors located in the brainstem react to this change in the pH and stimulate the body to breathe more deeply and more rapidly. It is the strongest stimulus of ventilation.

hypercatabolism Metabolic state in which degradation of protein stores is elevated.

hypercholesterolemia An increased cholesterol level in the blood.

hyperflexion injuries Increased flexion of a joint from trauma.

hyperglycemia Elevated blood glucose levels.

hypergranulation The formation of soft, pink fleshy projections as the body attempts to heal an enlarged wound track.

hyperkalemia An excess of potassium in the blood.

hyperlipidemia An elevated cholesterol and/or triglyceride level in the blood that is a modifiable risk factor for the development of coronary artery disease.

hypermetabolism Metabolic state in which resting energy expenditure is elevated.

hyperopia A defect in vision caused by an imperfection in the eye (often the eyeball is too short).

hyperosmolar hyperglycemic nonketotic syndrome (HHS) An emergent complication of diabetes characterized by serum hyperosmolarity, hyperglycemia, and dehydration.

hyperparathyroidism A hypermetabolic condition in which the parathyroid gland produces an excess of parathyroid hormone.

hyperplasia An increase in the number of new cells in an organ or tissue.

hyperpnea Refers to both the increased rate and depth of respiration associated with metabolic acidosis. It is sometimes referred to as *Kussmaul's breathing*.

hyperreflexia Exaggeration of the deep tendon reflexes.

hyperresonance A loud, low tone of longer duration than resonance. It is heard when air is trapped in a space such as the lungs.

hypertensive crisis A rare, sometimes fatal, occurrence that is characterized by the sudden onset of a diastolic blood pressure reading of 120 to 130; the clinical manifestation indicates target organ vascular damage and the presence of retinal exudates and hemorrhages.

hypertensive encephalopathy A very dangerous state of multifocal cerebral ischemia due to a severe acutely or subacutely elevated blood pressure.

hyperthyroidism A hypermetabolic condition in which the thyroid gland produces and the body responds to an excess production of thyroid hormones.

hypertonic Term used to identify a solution that contains a higher concentration of electrolytes than that found in body cells. If such a solution is allowed to enter the bloodstream, the osmotic pressure difference between the blood and the cells will cause water to flow out of the cells, which will then shrink.

hypertonic formula An enteral or parenteral nutrition formula with an osmolality, or concentration, that is greater than that of the body's plasma.

hypertrophic cardiomyopathy A disorder of the sarcomere, the contractile element of the cardiac muscle; characterized by left ventricular and occasionally right ventricular hypertrophy, with greater hypertrophy occurring in the septum. Also referred to as *idiopathic hypertrophic subaortic stenosis (IHSS)*.

hypertrophic scar Scar tissue that is an overgrowth of dermal tissue that remains within the boundaries of the wound.

hypertrophy An increase in the size of an organ caused by an increase in the size of the cells and tissues rather than the number of cells.

hyperventilation A state that exists when there is a lower than normal level of carbon dioxide in the blood. Also referred to as *hypocapnia*.

hyphema A collection of blood cells in the anterior chamber of the eye.

hypoalbuminemia Refers to low serum albumin, which most often results from liver damage.

hypochromic Term describing red blood cells that are paler in color than normal, suggesting iron deficiencies.

hypodermoclysis Continuous subcutaneous infusion of a large volume of isotonic parenteral fluids for purposes of rehydration.

hypoglycemia Decreased blood glucose levels.

hypoglycemic unawareness Condition that results from altered counterregulation, particularly deficient glucagon and epinephrine responses to hypoglycemia. This results in a loss of autonomic nervous system symptoms; for instance, tachycardia, palpitations, and tremors are absent. Patients are unaware that they are hypoglycemic and, without treatment, can progress rapidly into severe hypoglycemia.

hypokinesia Condition characterized by areas of abnormal heart contractility where muscle movement is hypoactive.

hypokinetic dysarthria Speech difficulty as a result of slowed, rigid muscles of tongue, mouth, and throat; associated with Parkinson's disease.

hypomimia Decreased facial expression due to rigid facial muscles.

hypoparathyroidism A hypometabolic condition in which the parathyroid gland fails to produce adequate parathyroid hormone.

hypophonia Soft, muffled voice.

hypopituitarism A hypometabolic condition in which the secretion of pituitary hormones is inadequate.

hypopnea A reduction but not complete cessation of airflow to less than 50% of normal.

hypopyon White layer of inflammatory cells in the anterior chamber.

hypospadias Opening of the urinary meatus on the ventral or bottom of the penis, between the penis and scrotum.

hypothalamic–pituitary–adrenal (HPA) axis A feedback loop by which signals from the brain trigger the release of hormones needed to respond to stress. Because of its function, the HPA axis also is referred to as the *stress circuit*.

hypothermia A core body temperature of less than 96.8°F (36°C) or a condition, regardless of body temperature, in which a person experiences shivering, peripheral vasoconstriction, piloerection, and feelings of cold.

hypothesis A statement that predicts a certain relationship between two or more variables.

hypothyroidism A metabolic condition in which the thyroid gland fails to produce adequate thyroid hormones.

hypotonia The absence of muscle tone, resulting in flaccidity of the muscles.

hypotonic Term used to identify a solution in which the concentration of electrolyte is below that found in body cells. In this situation osmotic pressure leads to the migration of water into the cells in an attempt to equalize the electrolyte concentration inside and outside the cell walls.

hypoventilation Decreased ventilation, which causes an increased $PaCO_2$; exists when there is a higher than normal level of carbon dioxide in the blood. Also referred to as *hypercapnia*.

hypoxemia Insufficient oxygen content in the blood.

hypoxia Physiological state of decreased blood oxygen levels.

hypoxic drive The stimulus to ventilation that occurs when peripheral chemoreceptors located in the carotid arteries and the aorta sense a decrease in the oxygen concentration in the blood.

hypoxic hypoxia Physiological state of decreased oxygen availability due to cardiac or pulmonary causes.

hysterectomy A surgical procedure to remove the uterus.

iatrogenic wounds Include intravenous puncture sites, incisions, radiation-induced skin damage, and grafts that occurred while a patient was in the hospital.

icteric phase The phase of acute hepatitis in which jaundice occurs, usually 1 to 2 weeks after the prodromal phase.

id Represents all of a person's biological and psychological drives.

IgE antibodies A class of antibodies produced by the B-lymphocyte plasma cells in response to exposure to a foreign antigen or allergen. They create an antibody–antigen complex that connects to receptors on mast cells and causes degranulation of mast cells and release of histamine; they are the major factor in type I hypersensitivity reactions.

ileal pouch anal anastomosis (IPAA) Procedure in which the entire colon, including the rectum, is removed and a pouch formed from the terminal ileum, which is then attached to the anus.

ileostomy Procedure in which a stoma is formed from the ileum. In a permanent ileostomy, the entire colon is removed and fecal material is collected in an external collection bag.

ileus A condition in which peristalsis does not return as expected postoperatively and the bowel remains hypoactive.

iliopsoas Refers to three muscles of the abdomen—psoas major, psoas minor, and iliacus—that pass from the abdomen through the pelvis and are partially responsible for hip flexion.

immediate hypersensitivity reaction An excessive response of the immune system that occurs in seconds to hours after exposure to an antigen. A systemic anaphylaxis is one example of an immediate hypersensitivity reaction response.

immune complex A substance formed when antibodies attach to antigens to destroy them.

immune deficiencies Deficiencies that occur when all or some part of the immune system fails to develop or is damaged through disease processes and, thus, cannot mount an appropriate immune response. There are two types, primary and secondary.

immune hypersensitivity response Occurs when the immune system overresponds to an antigen, either from the environment, from the individual himself, or from another individual. Disorders fall into three broad categories based on the type of triggering antigen, and include allergy, autoimmune, and alloimmune reactions.

immune tolerance The ability of the immune system to differentiate self from non-self and tolerate all self-antigens while retaining the ability to mount an immune response to non-self-antigens.

immunity The protective process of response to a foreign substance.

immunization The process of stimulating the immune system to create active immunity for protection against a disease by injection with a live or killed vaccine. Often used interchangeably with *vaccination* or *inoculation*.

immunoglobulin A diverse group of plasma proteins, made of polypeptide chains; one of the primary mechanisms for protection against diseases.

immunologic theory of aging Theory of aging based on the premise that the aging body is less able to distinguish its own cells from foreign cells.

impaired fasting glucose (IFG) A category of pre-diabetes in which the fasting glucose level is >100 mg/dL but <126 mg/dL.

impaired glucose tolerance (IGT) A category of pre-diabetes in which the blood glucose level following an oral glucose load of 75 grams is >140 mg/dL but <200 mg/dL.

impaired wound healing The disruption of the normal biochemical repair or regeneration process.

impetigo A common, contagious skin infection caused by *Staphylococcus aureus* and/or group A beta-hemolytic streptococcus that is characterized by vesicles that rupture and form yellow crusts.

implantable cardioverter defibrillator (ICD) Device that can automatically terminate the potentially lethal dysrhythmias of ventricular tachycardia and ventricular fibrillation. Currently these devices are incorporated into cardiac pacemakers.

implanted port A surgically placed central vascular access device; a chambered device comprised of a reservoir and an attached catheter; used for long-term or chronic infusion therapies.

implementation The "doing" or intervening phase of the nursing process.

implied consent Permission that is inferred by a person's conduct or by law.

impotence Refers to problems associated with ejaculation or orgasm, in addition to erectile dysfunction.

incapacitating agent Chemical agents that decrease acetylcholine at nerve synapses. They work in the opposite manner of nerve agents.

incidence The number of newly diagnosed cases of cancer in a specific time period in a defined population.

incident command system (ICS) A system of policies and procedures within a framework that allows for safe and effective management during a disaster.

INCMCE Acronym for International Nursing Coalition for Mass Casualty Education.

incomplete spinal cord injury Preservation of some degree of motor and/or sensory function below the level of a spinal injury.

incretin mimetics A class of medications that enhances glucose-dependent insulin secretion from the pancreatic β-cell resulting in a reduction in postprandial glucose levels. The incretins suppress elevated glucagon levels, promoting satiety, decreasing food intake, and slowing gastric emptying.

independent activities Activities that nurses perform, prescribe, and or delegate based on their education and skills. Assessing, analyzing, diagnosing, planning, implementing, and evaluating are independent activities.

independent practice association (IPA) Organization that contracts on the behalf of individuals or groups of physicians to provide health care to members of a health maintenance organization.

indirect calorimetry The measurement of energy expenditure by measuring oxygen intake and carbon dioxide output.

indirect inguinal hernia Occurs when abdominal contents protrude through the deep inguinal ring.

indirect percussion Technique that involves using the hyperextended middle finger of the nondominant hand (pleximeter) and then the finger tip of the middle finger of the dominant hand (plexor) to strike the pleximeter by using a wrist action that will elicit a sound.

Ineffective Coping Nursing diagnosis that refers to an inability to manage internal or environmental stressors appropriately as a result of inadequate physical, psychological, behavioral, or cognitive resources.

infarction An area of dead tissue.

infective endocarditis An infection of the cardiac endocardial layer of the heart, which may include one or more heart valves, the mural endocardium, and/or a septal defect; previously known as bacterial endocarditis.

infectivity The ability of a pathogen to enter a host and then live and grow within that host.

infiltration Inadvertent administration of a nonvesicant solution or medication into surrounding tissues.

inflammation A defensive mechanism of the body that is intended to neutralize, control, or eliminate an offending agent to prepare a site for repair. It is a nonspecific response that is meant to serve a protective function.

inflammatory bowel disease (IBD) An immunologic disease that results in idiopathic intestinal inflammation; includes Crohn's disease and ulcerative colitis.

inflammatory phase A phase of wound healing that begins at the time of the injury or surgery. The purpose of this phase is to prepare the site for growth of new tissue.

influenza A contagious disease that is caused by the influenza virus. Also known as the *flu*.

informatics The theory, science, and practice of the use of computer and informational technologies to store, retrieve, transmit, and manipulate data.

information technology Refers to those systems, including software programs and computer hardware, used to manage and process information.

informed consent Doctrine that mandates that individuals must be fully appraised of the nature, risks, benefits, alternative therapies, and potential consequences of procedures and therapies in health care settings.

infradian rhythm Rhythmic repetition of cycles lasting for more than a 24-hour period; an example is the female menstrual cycle.

infusate Parenteral fluid or medication.

inhalation injury Inhalation of smoke, causing injury to the lungs.

injection port or cap Device that allows entrance to a catheter's fluid pathway.

insensible fluid loss Water lost from the body carried as vapor in exhaled gases and evaporated from the body as sweat.

insomnia Difficulty falling or remaining asleep.

inspection The deliberate, systematic examination of a patient using both sight and smell.

Institute of Medicine (IOM) Organization that provides unbiased, evidence-based, authoritative information on medicine and health to policy makers, professionals, and the public at large in an effort to improve health.

insulin A hormone produced by the beta cells of the pancreas that has multiple effects. Insulin is necessary for glucose transport into insulin-sensitive tissues and storage of carbohydrates, fats, and proteins.

insulin resistance Unresponsiveness of anabolic processes to the normal effects of insulin and possibly tissue insensitivity to insulin.

intentional torts Wrongful conduct that is intentional in nature and designed to cause harm or damage to another.

interdependent activities Activities that overlap with other health care team members, physicians, social workers, pharmacists, nutritionists, and therapists, and require coordination and planning with those various team members.

interface pressure The pressure between a bony prominence and a surface such as a hospital bed or seating surface.

interferon (IFN) Protein made and released by T cells when the invading organism is a virus; functions to protect other cells from viral attack and stimulates the immune response; also inhibits the growth of certain tumor cells.

interleukin (IL) Chemical message produced by lymphocytes that enables the cells of the immune system to communicate and stimulate or slow an immune response. The various types of IL include IL-1 and IL-6, which are pro-inflammatory and stimulate B-cell production, whereas others, such as IL-12 and IL-13, help slow and inhibit the immune and inflammatory responses.

intermittent claudication (IC) Exercise-induced leg pain.

intermittent pneumatic compression devices Devices used to apply intermittent compression of the calf muscle, thereby increasing venous return.

internal locus of control An orientation in which a person believes that events in his or her life are controlled by his or her own actions and decisions.

internal stressor Stressor that originates within a person.

interphalangeal joint Joints between the fingers.

interstitial fluid Fluid between cells, but not in serum.

intervention An action designed to facilitate achievement of desired patient outcomes. It must be purposeful, must be supported by a rationale, and involve organization and actual delivery of nursing care, which ideally leads to achievement of stated patient goals and objectives.

intestinal obstruction The impairment of the forward movement of intestinal contents by mechanical causes (tumors), adhesions, or functional causes (surgery, anesthesia, medications); can occur anywhere from the pylorus to the rectum.

intra-atrial pathways Part of the electrical conduction system of the heart that consists of the internodal pathways and the Bachmann bundle.

intra-axial tumors Tumors originating from glial cells; found mostly in white matter.

intracellular fluid (ICF) Fluid contained within the cells.

intracranial pressure (ICP) The pressure exerted by cerebrospinal fluid within the ventricles.

intramedullary (I-M) rodding A method of fracture fixation that entails sliding a metal rod down the medullary canal of a long bone.

intraoperative During surgery.

intraosseous therapy Administration of parenteral fluids via the bone marrow; used in emergent situations when vascular access is not available.

intraspinal catheter A catheter used to access the intraspinal route.

intrathecal anesthesia A type of anesthesia in which a local anesthetic agent is inserted into the spinal fluid by penetrating the spinal dura.

intrathecal therapy Delivery of parenteral medications into the cerebrospinal fluid.

intrinsic factor (IF) Chemical secreted by the gastric mucosa required for vitamin B_{12} absorption.

intrinsic pathway Also known as the contact activation pathway, describes the clotting cascade branch initiated by the contact between circulating plasma proteins and the negatively charged surface of the injured subendothelial layer.

intron A noncoding segment of DNA that is transcribed into nuclear RNA, but removed in the subsequent processing into mRNA.

intussusception The slipping of one part of an intestine into another part just below it.

invasion of privacy Violation of the right to protection against unreasonable and unwarranted interference with one's solitude.

invasiveness Degree to which an organism can spread through the body.

ion Electrically charged components derived from the molecules of electrolytes. When placed in water the molecules dissociate into charged components or ions, producing positively and negatively charged ions.

iron deficiency anemia (IDA) Most common cause of anemia resulting from insufficient iron in the diet.

irregularly-irregular rhythm Heartbeats that occur when the R-to-R intervals exhibit no regularity in their distance from each other.

irritants Agents that generally cause pain, burning, lacrimation, or discomfort upon exposure to mucous membranes. Also called *riot control agents*.

ischemia Tissue hypoxia resulting from reduced blood flow to the tissues.

ischemia cascade A series of events that occurs as a compensatory mechanism in response to cerebral hypoxia. Also called *ischemic cascade*.

ischemia reperfusion injury A multifactorial process that occurs when anaerobic metabolism is initiated by hypoperfusion and hypoxia that leads to an oxygen deficit in endothelial, parenchymal, or immune competent cells.

ischemic cascade *See* ischemia cascade.

isoelectric line Straight line on the ECG graph paper that marks the beginning and ending point of all waves. Also referred to as the *baseline*.

isotonic Having the same osmolality as blood (275 to 295 mOsm/kg of body weight).

isotonic formula An enteral or parenteral nutrition formula with an osmolality, or concentration, that is approximately equal that of the body's plasma.

J point On an ECG tracing, the point at which the QRS meets the ST segment.

Joint Commission The accrediting body for hospitals and health care organizations; it is an independent, private, not-for-profit organization.

jugular venous distention (JVD) Increased blood pressure in the jugular vein that reflects the volume and pressure of venous blood, when volume overload is present.

jugular venous pressure (JVP) An indication of the hemodynamic events of the right atrium; derived from measurement of the pulsations of the right internal jugular vein.

junctional dysrhythmia Dysrhythmia resulting from an irritable focus in the junctional tissue that fires off before the SA node has had a chance to, or because the SA node has failed to fire. Three typical junctional dysrhythmias are junctional escape rhythm, premature junctional contraction, and junctional tachycardia.

junctional escape rhythm Dysrhythmia that occurs when the SA node fails to produce an impulse, or when the SA node's rate of firing falls below the intrinsic rate of the AV node. When this occurs, the AV node assumes the role of pacemaker.

justice In ethics, states that people should be treated fairly and equally.

Kaposi's sarcoma A malignancy involving the endothelial layer of blood and lymphatic vessels. Kaposi's is the most common cancer associated with AIDS.

karyotype A set of photographed, banded chromosomes of an individual, arranged from largest to smallest.

keloid scar Hypertrophic scar tissue that extends beyond the wound edges.

ketogenesis Condition in which an excessive amount of ketones are produced during diabetic ketoacidosis (DKA); is the cause of metabolic acidosis during DKA.

kinematics The predictive patterns of injuries.

KUB Abbreviation for kidney-ureter-bladder radiograph, and is also known as a "plain film of the abdomen." The radiograph helps to determine position, size, and structure of the kidneys and urinary tract. It is useful in evaluating for the presence of calculi and masses. This is also an excellent test for intestinal obstruction because it shows the air in the colon nicely.

Kupffer cells Cells that line the liver sinusoids and are phagocytic.

Kussmaul's respirations Deep, sighing respirations. Also called *hyperpnea*.

kyphosis Curvature of the spine that creates a stooped-over "humpback" appearance.

L'Hermite's sign Electric shock-like sensation throughout the body, elicited by flexing the neck.

labyrinthectomy Surgical procedure in which the labyrinth is excised to eradicate vertigo; results in complete hearing loss to the ear.

labyrinthitis Organ of balance within the middle ear.

lactase An enzyme that breaks down lactose, a sugar found in milk.

lactation Breast-feeding.

lactic dehydrogenase (LDH) An intracellular enzyme present in many cells, but high concentrations are found in the liver. The enzyme is released in response to liver injury.

lactose intolerance Results from a deficiency of lactase, the enzyme responsible for the breakdown of lactose, at the brush border of the small intestine, resulting in malabsorption.

lacunar stroke Thrombosis of a small penetrating artery, resulting in ischemia and infarction of deep white matter of the brain.

lamellar bone Mature bone.

laminectomy The removal of a vertebral posterior arch intended to remove a lesion or herniated disk.

laryngeal spasm An abnormal reflexive response to a laryngeal insult.

laryngectomy A permanent surgical airway with removal of the larynx, usually for cancer.

laryngitis Inflammation of the larynx and/or vocal cords.

laryngopharyngeal reflux disease (LPRD) Inflammation of the laryngopharynx as a result of gastric reflux into the pharynx and larynx.

laryngospasm Occurs when the muscles of the larynx contract forcefully, causing a closure or partial closure of the airway.

latent autoimmune diabetes in adults (LADA) An autoimmune form of diabetes that affects adults.

law Rules and regulation by which a society is governed.

lead axis Refers to the imaginary line drawn between the positive and negative electrodes.

leading health indicators Ten indicators from *Healthy People 2010* that reflect major public health concerns: (1) physical activity, (2) overweight and obesity, (3) tobacco use, (4) substance abuse, (5) responsible sexual behavior, (6) mental health, (7) injury and violence, (8) environmental quality, (9) immunization, and (10) access to health care.

Leapfrog Group A coalition of public and private organizations that provides health care benefits. The coalition provides public information on medical errors, health care standards, and health care provider quality performance measures.

left-sided heart failure An abnormal cardiac condition characterized by the impairment of the left side of the heart and elevated pressure and congestion in the pulmonary veins and capillaries.

left ventricular ejection fraction (LVEF) The proportion of blood ejected during each ventricular contraction compared with the total ventricular filling volume.

legal blindness The best-corrected visual acuity of 20/200 or a visual field of 20 degrees or less in both eyes.

leukemia Malignancy of the hematopoietic system.

leukocyte White blood cell.

leukocyte-poor RBCs A unit of packed red blood cells that had most of the white blood cells removed as soon as the blood was taken from the donor (i.e., prior to storage).

leveling Positioning of a transducer system in line with the chamber being monitored.

levodopa Precursor to dopamine; key drug used to treat Parkinson's disease.

licensed vocational/practical nurse (LVN/LPN) A nurse with 1 to 2 years of technical training to provide basic care.

licensure Process for approving a health care organization to provide medical care or services. Also refers to the certification process for professionals.

ligament A strong fibrous band of connective tissue.

limits of formalization In philosophy, the inability to make explicit or formal all elements of a social practice.

linear lesion Lesion that forms a line.

linear skull fracture A simple break in the continuity of the skull with no displacement of bone.

lipase An enzyme secreted by the pancreas that hydrolyzes triglycerides, cholesterol, and phospholipids.

lipodystrophy Abnormal deposition of adipose in the body.

lipohyalinosis Coating of the walls of small arteries with a lipid substance, causing narrowing of the arterial lumen.

lipolysis Breakdown of triglycerides to free fatty acids and glycerol.

lipoma Benign tumor consisting of fat cells.

liposuction Common type of cosmetic surgery, the purpose of which is to remove subcutaneous fat.

literature review A search of the latest research articles and scholarly studies.

lithotomy Position in which the patient lies on the back with the legs flexed at the hips and knees and the legs spread widely at the hip.

living wills A form of an advanced directive that describes a patient's preferences in case he or she becomes incapacitated. They usually describe what level of life-prolonging interventions the patient would or would not want and under what circumstances they should be completed, withheld, or withdrawn.

local adaptation syndrome (LAS) A local response to a stressor that proceeds through the same three stages as the general adaptation syndrome: alarm, resistance, and exhaustion.

locus of control The perception a person has about how much control he or she exerts over the events that happen in his or her life.

long-term care insurance Private insurance that covers the expenses of nursing care in a variety of settings, depending on the policy.

lordosis Excessive inward curvature of the spine.

low density lipoproteins A type of lipoprotein that transports cholesterol and triglycerides from the liver to peripheral tissues.

lower esophageal sphincter (LES) An area at the distal end of the esophagus that prevents the movement of gastric juice into the esophagus.

Ludwig's angina A deep neck infection involving the sublingual, submandibular, and submental spaces; usually the result of a dental abscess.

Luer-Lok™ Screw-type locking mechanism used to prevent accidental separation of infusion equipment.

lumen The bore or internal opening of a catheter.

lumpectomy Removal of a cancerous growth and a small amount of surrounding normal tissue.

Lund-Browder formula Formula for determining burn size that divides the body into percentage areas.

lung abscess An area of pulmonary infection with parenchymal necrosis.

Lyme disease A bacterial infection that affects the organs and joints; transmitted by black-legged ticks.

lymph nodes Lymph tissue that filters debris from the breakdown of cells, bacteria, viruses, and fungal antigens located throughout the body.

lymphangitis An acute inflammation of the lymphatic channels.

lymphatic system The circulatory system of the immune system that is comprised of the lymph vessels, lymph nodes, and lymph tissue and functions to drain lymph fluid (chyle) from throughout the body and return it to venous circulation in the chest.

lymphedema Edema due to the obstruction of the lymphatics.

lymphocyte Mature white cell; the two types of lymphocytes are T lymphocytes (T cells) and B lymphocytes (B cells).

lymphogranuloma venereum (LGV) A sexually transmitted infection caused by *Chlamydia trachomatis*. It is a rare condition, with only 200 cases reported each year.

lymphokines Cytokines that are made by lymphocytes; act as chemical messengers between cells and instruct immune cells to proliferate, differentiate, or alter activities. The major lymphokines are interleukins and interferons.

lymphoma Malignancy of the lymphatic system.

macrocephalic Abnormally large head size; found in acromegaly, hydrocephalus, rickets, osteitis deformans, leontiasis ossea, myxedema, leprosy, and pituitary disturbances.

macronutrients Nutritional components such as protein, carbohydrates, and fat that are needed in large quantities by living organisms.

macrovascular Pertaining to the large blood vessels of the arterial and venous system (e.g., coronary arteries).

macular degeneration (MD) The deterioration and mottling of the macula through the course of time.

magnesium An intracellular cation primarily in muscle and bone (only 1% is in the blood; 1.8 to 2.4 mg/dL).

magnet hospital A hospital designated by the American Nurses Credentialing Center as meeting the standards that result in excellence in delivery of nursing services and promoting a professional practice environment.

magnetic resonance cholangiopancreatography (MRCP) A noninvasive imaging test used to detect bile duct stones and pancreatic duct obstruction.

magnetic resonance imaging (MRI) Technique that uses radiofrequency pulses from a large, powerful magnet to temporarily disrupt the normal spin of certain atoms within the body. When the pulses are stopped, the atoms emit small amounts of energy while returning to their original spin; this energy can be imaged and recorded as high-resolution images that allow detailed noninvasive assessment of the both cardiac anatomy and physiology.

malabsorption The failure of the small intestine to absorb nutrients from digested food.

maladaptive coping mechanisms Those responses to stress that are not effective.

maldigestion The failure of chemical processes such as inadequate pancreatic enzymes or bile salts.

malignant Containing cancerous cells.

malignant hyperthermia (MH) A rare but life-threatening metabolic complication of anesthesia that usually occurs during the induction phase but could occur anytime during surgery. Certain people have a genetic predisposition to this illness. Immediate attention is vital to the recovery of the patient, and intensive care monitoring is mandatory following its occurrence.

malnutrition The physical consequences resulting from underconsumption of energy or nutrients compared to recommended amounts.

malpractice Professional misconduct; failure to meet the standards of care that a reasonably prudent member of the profession would employ.

mammography A low-dose x-ray procedure that allows visualization of the internal structure of the breast.

mandatory reporter A person required by law to report allegations and/or suspicions of abuse.

masked facies Immobile, expressionless facial appearance commonly seen in Parkinson's disease.

massive hemothorax An accumulation of 1,500 mL or more of blood in the thoracic cavity.

mastalgia Breast pain.

mastectomy Removal of the entire breast (total) or a modified radical mastectomy, which is removal of the entire breast along with the surrounding lymph nodes.

mastitis Inflammation of the breast tissue; occurs most frequently in breast-feeding women. Microorganisms invade the tissue through some portal of entry, such as a crack, fissure, or duct.

mastoidectomy Surgical procedure in which the mastoid process is excised in the event of infection.

mastoiditis Infection of the mastoid bone.

mature minors Persons under the legal age of adulthood who are legally able to give valid informed consent.

maturity onset diabetes of the young (MODY) Diabetes that has early onset (usually before the age of 25); it is inherited in an autosomal dominant manner and more closely resembles type 2 diabetes rather than type 1.

McGill Pain Questionnaire (MPQ) Assesses pain intensity, character, and location of pain using a body diagram, and also the duration of the pain experience.

mean arterial pressure (MAP) The average pressure in the arteries during one cardiac cycle.

mean corpuscular hemoglobin (MCH) Amount of hemoglobin per red blood cell.

mean corpuscular hemoglobin concentration (MCHC) Concentration of hemoglobin in each red blood cell.

mean corpuscular volume (MCV) Measure of the size of a red blood cell.

mechanical infusion device (MID) Infusion system that does not rely on an external power source.

mechanical phlebitis Inflammation of a vein associated with a catheter, its insertion, and the selected insertion site.

mechanical valves Commercially manufactured heart valves.

Medicaid Federally aided, but state-operated and -administered, program for providing medical care to qualifying low-income individuals.

medical durable power of attorney (MDPA) A document that sets out wishes for health care if an individual becomes too ill to make those decisions; a trusted person is designated to make health care decisions.

medical nutrition therapy (MNT) Meal planning approaches for patients with diabetes that combine clinical evidence, cultural, social, and ethnic approaches, and patient motivation.

medical record The legal document for all information regarding a patient's hospital course and evidence for the extent of care provided and the outcome of that care.

Medicare Federally sponsored health insurance program for people over age 65, some individuals with disabilities who are younger than age 65, and patients with end-stage renal disease. Medicare consists of Part A, hospital insurance, and Part B, general medical insurance and other options. Medicare also administers its own managed care plan.

medication nurse A registered nurse assigned the specific task of giving all patient medications under a functional nursing care delivery system.

medication reconciliation Process of identifying an accurate list of all medications the patient is taking, and using this list to provide correct medications for the patient anywhere in the health care system.

megakaryocytic stem cells Ancestor cells form giving rise to platelets.

megaloblast Large, immature red blood cells.

megaloblastic anemia Anemia resulting from impaired DNA synthesis of the red blood cells' ancestor cells.

melena Black or maroon, sticky, foul-smelling feces resulting from the digestion of blood.

menarche Beginning of menstruation or first menses.

Ménière's disease Inner ear disorder that affects hearing and balance.

meningiomas Tumors originating from the meninges.

meningismus Meningeal irritation.

menorrhagia Heavy bleeding during a menstrual period.

meshed skin graft Procedure of cutting holes in harvested skin, which allows it to be stretched over a greater surface area.

messenger ribonucleic acid (mRNA) RNA containing genetic information that is transcribed from DNA and translated to produce polypeptides.

metabolic equivalent (MET) A measure of oxygen consumption. One MET is the energy requirement for a person at rest while sitting: around 3.5 mL of oxygen per kilogram of body weight per minute.

metabolic syndrome The diagnosis given when a patient has a cluster of cardiac risk factors, including having three out of the five following conditions: abdominal obesity, high triglycerides, low HDL-C, high blood pressure, and high fasting glucose ($\geq$100 mg/dL).

metabolism All energy and material transformations that occur within a living cell.

metacarpophalangeal joints Joints at the knuckles.

metamorphopsia Condition characterized by vision distortion, that is, when straight lines, such as door frames or posts, look crooked or irregular.

metaphysis An area of widening between the diaphysis and physis.

metaplasia Cell transformation in which a highly specialized cell changes into a less specialized cell.

metastasis The spread of cancerous cells beyond the tumor to distant sites.

metastatic tumors Tumors that originate somewhere else in the body and migrate to another organ.

metered-dose inhaler (MDI) A device that helps deliver a specific amount of medication to the lungs, usually by supplying a short burst of aerosolized medicine that is inhaled by the patient. It is commonly used to treat asthma, chronic obstructive pulmonary disease, and other respiratory disorders.

metered-volume chamber set An administration set comprised of tubing, a semirigid metered chamber, and an access spike to be inserted in the fluid container.

methodological congruence Congruence among four dimensions of a research study: documentation rigor, procedural rigor, ethical rigor, and auditability.

metrorrhagia Bleeding between menstrual periods.

microalbuminuria Small amounts of protein (30 to 299 mg/24 hours) in the urine.

microcephalic Abnormal smallness of the head, often seen in mental retardation.

microcytic Term describing red blood cells that are smaller in size than normal.

micrographia Small, cramped handwriting.

micronutrients Nutritional components such as vitamins or minerals that are needed in small quantities by living organisms.

microvascular Pertaining to the small blood vessels of the arterial and venous system.

midline (ML) catheter A flexible catheter measuring not more than 8 inches with the distal tip dwelling in the basilica, cephalic, or brachial veins, level with the axilla and distal to the shoulder.

mild cognitive impairment (MCI) A term used to describe memory loss that appears greater than what is expected for a patient's age.

millivolts A unit of electrical voltage or potential difference equal to one-thousandth of a volt.

minute ventilation (V$_E$) A measurement of how much air the lungs move in 1 minute; it is equal to respiratory rate times tidal volume. A normal resting respiratory rate and a normal resting tidal volume of about 500 mL yield a normal minute ventilation of 6 L/min.

missense mutation A mutation that changes a codon specific for one amino acid to specify a different amino acid.

mitral valve prolapse Occurs when one or more of the valve leaflets bulge or prolapse into the left atrium during systole. This prolapse of the valve results in valve regurgitation.

mitral valve regurgitation An inability of the mitral valve to close due to an abnormality in the structure and function of the valve.

mitral valve stenosis Occurs when the mitral valve assumes an abnormal funnel shape due to thickening and shortening of the valve structures as a result of calcification. Contractures develop between the junctions or commissures (leaflets) of the valve. The stenosis narrows the opening of the valve, which obstructs blood flow from the left atrium to the left ventricle.

mixed hearing loss Type of hearing loss that is both conductive and sensorineural in cause.

mixed venous oxygen saturation Measurement of venous oxygen content in the pulmonary artery; used to assess oxygen consumption and metabolic needs of the tissues.

Mobitz I/Wenckebach One of the two types of second-degree block that occurs in the AV node, a progressive prolongation of the electrical impulse delay in the AV node until there is a complete loss of the QRS complex and, thus, no ventricular contraction. Depicted on an ECG tracing as a progressive lengthening of the PR interval until the P wave does not progress through the conduction system, resulting in a dropped QRS complex.

Mobitz II/second-degree block Periodic blocking of sinus impulses at the AV node, the bundle of His, or bundle branches. Occurs when there is an intermittent interruption in the electrical conduction system near or below the AV node and is a more serious dysrhythmia than either first-degree AV block or Mobitz I/ Wenckebach. This dysrhythmia indicates an increased risk of progression to third-degree, or complete, heart block.

mode of transmission Means by which an organism travels from a reservoir to a susceptible host.

modeling The process by which bone growth occurs and where there is a higher rate of bone formation relative to bone loss.

molecular mimicry A process in which peptides from proteins, such as viruses, become structurally similar to self-peptides and activate T-cell autoimmunity.

molimenal Symptoms of menstruation.

MONA A protocol for empirical treatment of patients with suspected myocardial infarction. Cited in the Advanced Cardiac Life Support guidelines, the mnemonic stands for *m*orphine, *o*xygen, *n*itroglycerin, and *a*spirin.

monocyte The largest of the white blood cells and makes up about 3% to 8% of the total leukocyte count. Monocytes are a part of the reticuloendothelial (or mononuclear phagocytic) system, whose function is to engulf and digest microbes and other foreign substances. Monocytes migrate from the blood to various tissues where they mature into macrophages, working to kill invading antigens.

monophasic defibrillation Traditional means by which electrical voltage is delivered to patients in ventricular tachycardia and fibrillation.

monosomy A chromosomal constitution in which one member of the chromosome pair is missing.

Monro-Kellie doctrine Doctrine that provides the foundation for understanding the implications of increased intracranial pressure. Incompressible structures within the cranial vault are in a state of volume equilibrium, such that any increase of the volumes of one component (i.e., blood, CSF, or brain tissue) must be compensated by a decrease in the volume of another. If this cannot be achieved then pressure will rise and once the expandable reserve of the intracranial space is exhausted then small changes in volume can lead to precipitous increases in pressure.

moral agency The ability to affect and influence situations.

MORAL model An ethical decision-making model based on a series of five steps that represent the acronym MORAL: *m*assage the dilemma; *o*utline the options; *r*esolve the dilemma; *a*ct by applying the chosen option; and *l*ook back and evaluate.

morality A code of conduct held to be authoritative in matters of right and wrong.

morphologic classification Classification of skin lesions in terms of type of lesion (primary, secondary, or vascular), size, shape or configuration, color, texture, elevation or depression, and pedunculation.

mortality The number of deaths from cancer in a specific period of time and within an identified population.

mosaicism Nondisjunction of a pair of chromosomes that occurs in a mitotic division after formation of the zygote, and leads to an individual with at least two cell lines differing in genotype or karyotype, derived from a single zygote.

mucormycosis A fungal infection often seen in the sinuses of patients with diabetes who do not have good glycemic control.

multichannel pump Electronic infusion device often used in critical care areas; used to administer multiple parenteral therapies simultaneously.

multiflow adapter Add-on device used to facilitate multiple administrations of fluids and medications via a single vascular access device.

multiple organ dysfunction syndrome (MODS) Diagnosed when two or more organ systems fail.

multiple sclerosis (MS) Disease in which the immune system attacks the nerve tissues in the central nervous system, causing damage to the neurons, which disrupts the body's ability to send signals and causes symptoms. Believed to be an autoimmune disease.

multislice helical CT Detailed, noninvasive imaging of the heart using 16-slice helical scanners, accompanied by ECG gating and iodinated contrast. This device can scan the entire volume of the heart, proximal great vessels, and the coronary arteries with a single 25-second breath hold.

murmurs Abnormal heart sounds produced by turbulent blood flow.

muscle atrophy Shortening of a muscle attached to a joint.

mutation A permanent structural change in DNA.

myasthenia gravis A chronic autoimmune neuromuscular disorder in which acetylcholine receptors at the neuromuscular junction are destroyed.

myasthenic crisis A life-threatening exacerbation of myasthenia gravis that requires mechanical ventilation.

myelin A soft, white coating that surrounds and protects nerve fibers. Myelin also helps nerve fibers conduct electrical impulses.

myeloid progenitor cell Ancestor cell that gives rise to granulocytes and monocytes.

myelopathy Motor, sensory, and reflex abnormalities due to an abnormality of the spinal cord.

myocardial hibernation Condition in which myocardial tissue undergoes cellular structural changes and progressive apoptosis (cell death) in response to prolonged cardiac ischemia.

myocardial infarction (MI) The loss of myocytes or myocardial cell death as a result of prolonged ischemia.

myocardial perfusion Blood flow to the heart muscle.

myocardial perfusion imaging (MPI) Use of a radioactive tracer and a gamma camera to detect blood flow to the myocardium.

myocardial stunning A temporary dysfunction that occurs in response to artery occlusion of short duration (artery spasm) or transient global hypoperfusion during a limited low-flow state such as shock.

myocardial viability Term applied to areas of the myocardium that appear to have normal functioning as well as areas that appear dysfunctional (hibernating or stunned) that might improve with revascularization.

myocarditis A focal or diffuse inflammation of the myocardium or heart muscle; an uncommon disorder that is frequently associated with pericarditis.

myocutaneous flap A piece of tissue, muscle or skin, used in reconstructive surgery; may be used for reconstructing breasts, large lateral temporal, scalp, or intraoral defects, and defects involving the trunk and chest wall.

myoglobin A heme-containing, oxygen-binding protein that is exclusive to striated and nonstriated muscle. Because of its very small molecular weight, it is released into interstitial fluid as early as 2 hours following damage to muscle tissue.

myopia Individuals see nearby objects clearly, but distant objects appear blurred.

myositis An uncommon disease in which the immune system inflames the body's own healthy muscle tissue.

myringotomy Surgical procedure in which tubes are placed in the ears to facilitate drainage and prevent the buildup of pressure within the inner ear and prevent ear infections.

myxedema A long-term consequence of hypothyroidism in which the facial features are coarsened and changed by puffiness, periorbital edema, and a mask-like appearance.

myxedema coma A rare, life-threatening complication of hypothyroidism.

nadir The point at which the lowest blood count is reached.

nasal polyps Small saclike growths inside the nasal cavity and sinuses.

national standards of care Statements of actions consistent with minimum safe professional conduct under specific medical conditions as determined by professional medical organizations.

natural immunity Type of immunity that is the responsibility of a group of body organs, cells, and chemicals that are present at birth or shortly after.

near drowning Condition that connotes survival for at least 24 hours after submersion.

neck dissection Surgical procedure to remove nodal disease in conjunction with the central part of the cancer surgery.

necrotizing fasciitis (NF) An infection of the superficial fascia or the connective tissue surrounding muscle and subcutaneous tissue leading to necrosis.

needleless system Components of infusion equipment that do not use needles.

negative deflection Any waveform that goes below the isoelectric line on ECG graph paper.

negative feedback A compensatory mechanism by which homeostasis is achieved in which the endocrine glands respond to a decrease in hormone levels, leading to gland stimulation and increased hormone production. When a normal level of hormone is reached, it feeds back to suppress the stimulating hormone and a normal state occurs.

negative pressure pulmonary edema (NPPE) A disorder caused by attempts to ventilate a person with an apparent airway obstruction. Also called *postobstruction pulmonary edema* and *airway obstruction pulmonary edema*.

negligence Failure to exercise the degree of care that a person of ordinary prudence would exercise under the same or similar conditions.

neoantigens Antigens created by the developing fetal immune system while it is in the process of eliminating autoreactive lymphocytes.

neoplasm New growth.

nephron The functional unit of the kidney.

nerve agents Chemicals that inactivate acetylcholinesterase at the receptor site. They cause symptoms of SLUDGE'M (*s*alivation, *l*acrimation, *u*rination, *d*efecation, *g*astric upset, *e*mesis, and *m*iosis).

network sampling Type of sampling in which participants refer other participants to the study. Also referred to as *snowball sampling*.

neurofibromatosis An autosomal dominant inherited disorder characterized by the formation of tumors of the peripheral nerves over the entire body.

neurogenic pulmonary edema (NPE) A rare type of pulmonary edema that develops after a neurological insult to the central nervous system.

neurogenic shock Occurs in spinal cord injuries above T_6 thoracic spine and results in interruption of the sympathetic change, causing bradycardia, hypotension, and vasodilation of the peripheral vascular system.

neuromatrix theory Addresses the brain's role in pain perception as well as other multiple determinants.

neuron A nerve cell; the structural and functional unit of the nervous system.

neuropathic pain Pain resulting from injury or dysfunction in one or more nerves.

neuroprotection Therapies used to arrest the sequence of events that occur during the ischemic cascade.

neutralization Action of antibodies that involves the process of changing the charge or shape of the antigen and blocking its ability to attach to another cell.

neutrophil Primary phagocytic defense; responds to bacteria, inflammation, injury, infection, and foreign objects.

nevi Well-circumscribed malformations of the skin. Also known as *moles*.

New York Heart Association (NYHA) classification system A functional classification system that categorizes cardiac patients' subjective degree of symptoms into NYHA classes I through IV.

nidus Refers to the focus of an arteriovenous malformation.

nits The eggs of a louse.

nociception The process by which tissue damage (noxious stimuli) activates sensory neurons to send a pain message to the central nervous system, resulting in a nociceptive pain response; literally means "pain sense."

nociceptive pain Pain resulting from the process of nociception.

nocturia The need to get up at night to urinate.

nodes (bundles) Special cells and fibers that make up the electrical conduction system of the heart.

nodules Small aggregation of cells formed in response to injury or inflammation.

noise-induced hearing loss (NIHL) Hearing loss caused by noises or sounds at a high decibel level for long periods of time.

noncardiogenic pulmonary edema (NCPE) An abnormal accumulation of fluid in the lungs caused by a noncardiac etiology.

noncoring needle Type of access needle required to access an implanted port or reservoir; used to prevent accidental coring of the port's septum.

nondisjunction The failure of two members of a chromosome pair to separate during meiosis or mitosis, resulting in daughter cells with either a missing or extra chromosome.

nonexperimental research design Research design in which the researcher collects data without introducing an intervention.

nongranulocyte White blood cell that is produced in the bone marrow and develops into a lymphocyte or monocyte; does not contain granules in its cytoplasm.

nonheme iron Form of dietary iron available in vegetables, cereals, and fortified food.

nonintentional torts Actions that result in harm to another, but intent is lacking; often synonymous with carelessness.

noninvasive positive pressure ventilation (NPPV) Procedure for delivering breaths to a patient without placement of an artificial airway, such as an endotracheal or tracheostomy tube.

nonmaleficence The duty to do no harm.

nonprobability sampling Type of sampling in which elements and participants are selected by nonrandom methods.

nonsense mutation A single base substitution in DNA that results in a chain-termination codon.

nontunneled and noncuffed device Type of central vascular access device; inserted by a puncture directly through the skin and to the intended location without passing through subcutaneous tissue.

normal sinus rhythm (NSR) A regular heart rate between 60 and 100 beats per minute that has all of the normal components of one cardiac cycle (PQRST) and normal time intervals between the waveforms.

normoglycemia Normal blood glucose levels.

normothermia A normal body temperature.

nosocomial infection An infection that occurs in a hospitalized patient.

not-for-profit organization Organization that reinvests profits from operations back into the organization.

notifiable disease Any of certain diseases or conditions that must be reported to local, county, or state public health departments.

noxious stimuli Tissue damage that activates sensory neurons to send a pain message to the central nervous system, resulting in a nociceptive pain response.

NSTEMI Non–ST segment elevation myocardial infarction is the result of transient subtotal occlusion of a coronary artery with reduced coronary blood flow resulting from plaque disruption and ensuing pathophysiological processes. Serum blood markers and persistent ECG changes are present with NSTEMI.

numeric rating scale (NRS) A horizontal line marked with the numbers 0 to 10 from left to right with three interval descriptors of pain located along the scale: "no pain," "moderate pain," and "worst pain."

nurse–patient relationship The means for applying the nursing process. It is the mechanism by which the nurse works with the patient.

nurse practice acts State guidelines that define the practice of nursing and give guidance in terms of scope of practice issues; they are designed to ensure safe practice.

nurse practitioner (NP) An advanced practice nurse with postgraduate training who is licensed by the state to provide basic medical care under standardized procedures.

nursing care delivery systems A set of concepts based on principles that involve clinical decision making, work allocation, communication, and management.

nursing diagnosis The end product of the nursing assessment. Describes an actual or potential health problem, based on gathered data, that a nurse can legally manage.

nursing process A thinking/doing approach to patient care that provides the nurse with a systematic means of identifying, preventing, and treating actual and potential health problems.

Nursing's Agenda for the Future The American Nurses Association statement outlining issues related to nursing practice. Issues include an expanded role for registered nurses and advanced practice nurses in the delivery of basic and primary health care, obtaining federal funding for nurse education and training, and helping to change and improve the health care workplace.

nutritional imbalance A deficiency or excess of one or more essential nutrients, resulting from inadequate nutrition or too much nutrition.

nystagmus A constant, involuntary tremor, oscillation, or jerky movement of the eyeball; the movement may be in any direction.

objective data Behaviors, activities, and events that can be observed or measured by another person using the senses of observation, palpation, auscultation, percussion, and smell. Objective data are factual: They can be seen, heard, touched, smelled, or tasted.

obstructive sleep apnea (OSA) Disorder of sleep with habitual snoring characterized by brief periods of breathing cessation or a marked reduction in tidal volume with a minimum of five episodes per hour during sleep with excessive daytime somnolence.

occupational asthma Occurs when a worker experiences asthmatic symptoms upon exposure to substances that trigger an asthma attack.

Occupational Safety and Health Administration (OSHA) Agency under the U.S. Department of Labor whose function is to inspect and enforce safety standards in the workplace.

oculocephalic reflex Reflex eye movement that stabilizes images on the retina during head movement by producing an eye movement in the direction opposite to the head movement that maintains the visual field or a more-or-less steady gaze. Also called *doll's eye reflex*.

oculovestibular reflex Reflex that stabilizes images on the retina during head movement by producing an eye movement in the direction opposite that of the head movement.

odontoid process The toothlike projection of C_2 (cervical spine), which sits behind the anterior portion of the ring of C_1.

oligoanalgesia Results when a patient complains of pain, but no interventions are provided for pain relief.

oliguria Decreased urine output of less than 400 mL in a 24-hour period.

Ommaya reservoir Nonvascular infusion device inserted with the catheter tip residing in the ventricles of the brain; used to deliver targeted therapies (i.e., pain and antineoplastic therapies) or to obtain cerebrospinal fluid.

oncosis Cell swelling as a result of changes in membrane permeability.

oncotic pressure In the circulatory system, the term refers to a form of osmotic pressure exerted by proteins in blood plasma that normally tends to pull water into the circulatory system. Also referred to as *colloid osmotic pressure*.

on–off phenomena Abrupt fluctuations in movement ability associated with Parkinson's disease.

open-ended questions Questions that ask for narrative information by stating a topic in general terms; for example, "What brought you to the hospital?"

open globe An open eyeball with a laceration, penetrating injury, or intraocular foreign body; usually results from blunt trauma or projectile injury.

open pneumothorax An open communication between the atmosphere and intrathoracic pressure; usually caused by penetrating trauma.

open reduction internal fixation (ORIF) A treatment in which a fracture is exposed by an incision in the skin directly over the fracture. Implants such as plates (strips of metal), screws, and wires are placed directly on or in the bone to anatomically stabilize a fracture.

opportunistic infections (OIs) Infections from microorganisms that are not usually considered pathogens, but cause disease if the immune system is impaired.

opsonization A chemical coating of an antigen by cytokines or antibodies that makes that cell more attractive to phagocytes.

oral cancer Cancer that arises from the flat cells that line the oral cavity and is slow growing; most often squamous cell carcinoma.

oral candidiasis An overgrowth of the yeast-like fungus *Candida albicans*.

oral glucose tolerance test (OGTT) A test in which the glycemic response to a prescribed dose of oral glucose is used to determine glucose tolerance status (i.e., normal glucose tolerance, impaired glucose tolerance, or diabetes).

orchiectomy Surgical removal of the testes.

orchiopexy Surgical fixation of a testis.

orchitis Inflammation of one or both testes.

orthopnea Shortness of breath relieved by sitting or standing erect.

osmolality Number of molecules of solute per kilogram of water.

osmosis The movement of water from one compartment of low solute concentration through a semipermeable membrane into a second compartment with high solute concentration.

osmotic diuresis Excessive urination caused by the presence of certain substances (such as glucose) in the renal tubules.

osteitis fibrosa cystica A complication of hypoparathyroidism in which the bone softens and becomes deformed or forms cysts.

osteoarthritis (OA) Chronic condition that accompanies aging, affecting the weight-bearing joints most commonly; is the most common form of arthritis.

osteoblasts Any cells that form bone within the body.

osteoclasts Large cells formed in bone marrow and originating from macrophage-like cells; designed to absorb and remove unwanted bone tissue, causing the bone to be "remodeled" or "destroyed."

osteocytes Mature osteoblasts that maintain the bony matrix and participate in the dynamic task of releasing calcium into the bloodstream.

osteoid Type I collagen and noncollagenous protein osteocalcin.

osteology The study of bones and the bone structure of the human body.

osteolysis Destruction of implanted synthetic or cement components of repaired bone segments.

osteonecrosis The death of bone tissue.

osteoporosis A skeletal disease that is characterized by low bone mass and deterioration of the bone tissue. This continued deterioration results in bone fragility and susceptibility to fractures.

otalgia Ear pain.

otitis externa Inflammation/infection of the external ear canal.

otitis media Inflammation/infection of the middle ear.

otolaryngology (otorhinolaryngology) The study of ear, nose, and throat disorders.

otosclerosis Abnormal bone growth within the middle ear that causes hearing loss.

ototoxic Something that, if ingested, causes damage to the auditory nerve, affecting hearing.

ototoxicity Harmful effect on the eighth cranial nerve or organs of hearing and balance.

outcome Individual, measurable patient objective; measurable criterion that indicates the patient's care objectives have been met; a change in patient behavior that results from nursing interventions.

outcome standards Quality standards that focus on whether the services provided by an organization make any difference to patients or to the health status of the patient population.

overnutrition The physical consequences resulting from overconsumption of energy or nutrients compared to recommended amounts.

over-the-needle peripheral-short catheter A catheter with a stylet needle housed in the catheter lumen.

oxidative stress Stress to the cells caused by a decrease in the removal of or an overproduction of oxygen free radicals, common in physiological disorders of the critically ill; the imbalance between reactive oxygen species and the body's defense system.

oxytocin Peptide hormone produced in the hypothalamus but secreted by the posterior pituitary gland. It causes uterine contraction and stimulates breast milk production.

P wave Part of the cardiac cycle; represents atrial contraction or depolarization on an ECG tracing.

pacemaker cell Cardiac cell found in the electrical conduction system, which lies in the heart wall and septum. It generates and conducts impulses.

pacemaker sensitivity Amount of electrical activity the pacemaker will sense or "hear"; measured in millivolts (mV).

packed RBCs Red blood cells that have had the plasma portion of the blood removed by a centrifuge process.

pain An unpleasant sensory and emotional experience associated with actual or potential tissue damage, or described in terms of such damage.

palliative The alleviation (not curative) of suffering from symptoms.

palliative care Comprehensive care focused on alleviating suffering and promoting the quality of remaining life of patients living with a chronic life-threatening or terminal illness; allows patients and families to guide treatment and set goals for care.

palliative procedures Surgeries performed for the primary purpose of alleviating symptoms rather than affecting a cure.

palpation Technique of using touch to collect data to determine specific characteristics of the body.

palpitations An awareness of the beating of the heart.

pancarditis Inflammation of all three layers of the heart: the endocardium, myocardium, and pericardium.

pancreatic beta cells Cells in the pancreatic islets of Langerhans that produce insulin.

pancreatic insufficiency A deficiency of pancreatic enzymes resulting in malabsorption of nutrients.

pancreatic polypeptide A complex peptide hormone secreted by the pancreatic islet cells whose role is not completely understood.

pancreaticoduodenal (Whipple) resection A radical surgical procedure to treat pancreatic cancer that involves removal of the head of the pancreas, the duodenum, the distal portion of the stomach, part of the jejunum, and the lower half of the common bile duct.

pancreatitis Inflammation of the pancreas.

panendoscopy Surgical procedure to evaluate the upper aerodigestive tract, locate the organ of origin, and obtain a cellular diagnosis.

panhypopituitarism Condition in which there is inadequate secretion of all of the hormones of the anterior pituitary.

paracentesis Removal of ascites fluid from the abdomen.

paracrine functioning Bioregulation of one cell type that influences the activity of an adjacent cell type by secreting chemicals that diffuse into the tissue and act specifically on cells in that area.

paraphimosis Condition in which the foreskin is retracted, but cannot be returned to its normal position covering the glans.

paraplegia Paralysis of the lower half of the body including both lower extremities and loss of bowel and bladder function.

parenteral Term used to describe fluids and medications that are administered via routes other than the alimentary canal.

parenteral nutrition Provision of nutrients and energy by means of intravenous access, without use of the gastrointestinal tract.

paresthesia An abnormal physical sensation such as prickling, tingling, or numbness.

Parkinson's disease (PD) A disease of the basal ganglia characterized by a slowing down in the innervation and executive of movement, increased muscle tone rigidity, tremors at rest, and impaired postural reflexes.

paronychia Inflammation of the folds of tissue surrounding the fingernail.

paroxysmal junctional tachycardia (PJT) An irritable focus in the AV junction that assumes the pacemaker role by discharging impulses more rapidly than the SA node. Begins and ends abruptly.

partial-thickness injury Injury in which the epidermis and part of the dermis are destroyed.

passive immunization Immunization that provides immunity for a short period of time, usually around 6 to 12 weeks; involves the injection of already formed antibodies into the body.

paternalism In ethics, policy that allows one to make decisions for another.

pathogenicity Disease-causing potential of a microorganism, the number of invading microorganisms, and the host defenses.

pathologic dead space A portion of the tidal volume that does reach the alveoli, but does not take place in gas exchange. Various lung pathologies and disease conditions can increase this dead space amount and affect the lungs' ability to oxygenate and ventilate.

pathologic fractures Fractures that occur without trauma due to bone thinning.

patient care plan A documented record of the nursing process, a plan designed to incorporate the patient's identified problems, outcomes, and actions to be implemented by the nurse.

patient-centered care An innovative approach to the planning, delivery, and evaluation of health care that is based on mutually beneficial partnerships among health care patients, families, and providers.

patient-controlled analgesia (PCA) pump A computerized machine that is attached to a patient's intravenous line and allows the patient to control the amount of medication that is administered based on his or her pain level.

pattern theory a group of theories that asserts that pain receptors share nerve pathways with other sensory pathways and that the intensity of the stimulus determines the frequency of firing of the receptor.

pediculosis Infestation with lice.

pedigree A diagram that shows the heredity of a particular trait or genetic disorder through many generations of a family.

pelvic inflammatory disease (PID) An infection of the internal reproductive organs, including the fallopian tubes. It is a very common and a very serious complication of many sexually transmitted infections.

The highest risk for the development of PID is seen in women of childbearing age who are sexually active.

penectomy Removal of part of or the entire penis.

penetrance The proportion of individuals with a genotype known to cause a genetic disorder who have signs and symptoms of the disorder.

peptic ulcer A generic term used for any ulceration in the digestive surfaces of the upper GI tract.

percussion Technique of either pushing, tapping, or using a device to generate a sound vibration. The vibrations produced will help in determining position of organ structures.

percutaneous angioplasty The use of mechanical widening when opening blood vessels other than coronary arteries.

percutaneous coronary intervention (PCI) The use of devices to either remove plaque or alter its morphology in the catheterization laboratory, including atherectomy devices, lasers, and intracoronary stents.

percutaneous transluminal coronary angioplasty (PTCA) Treatment of coronary artery disease (CAD) using expandable balloons to crack (tear or rupture) atherosclerotic plaque, thereby enlarging the lumen of the coronary artery.

percutaneously Passing through the skin.

perfusion The movement of blood carrying oxygen.

pericardial effusion An excess buildup of pericardial fluid that is a threat to normal cardiac function. The fluid buildup is the result of an accumulation of infectious exudates or toxins and/or blood.

pericardial friction rub A grating, scraping, squeaking, or a crunching sound that is the result of friction between the roughened, inflamed layers of the pericardium.

pericardial window An opening in the pericardial sac that allows fluid from effusion and tamponade to drain.

pericardiectomy Removal of the pericardial sac to allow fluid to drain from around the heart.

pericarditis Inflammation of the pericardial sac due to an inflammatory process in which the two layers of the pericardium become inflamed and roughened, causing fluid to build up.

perimenopause The time during which periods may increase, decrease, and become irregular as the function of the ovaries waxes and wanes.

perioperative A broad term that refers to the time period surrounding a surgical procedure. It includes the preoperative, intraoperative, and postoperative time periods.

perioperative blood salvage The process of collecting and reinfusing blood lost during both the intraoperative and early postoperative periods.

periosteum Fibrous membrane that covers bone.

peripheral arterial disease (PAD) Disease that affects the arteries of the extremities.

peripheral blood stem cell (PBSC) transplantation Transplantation of stem cells located in peripherally circulating blood.

peripheral nerve block An anesthesia technique in which a local anesthetic is injected into or around a nerve plexus to produce anesthesia of a selected area without inducing a systemic effect.

peripheral parenteral nutrition (PPN) Provision of nutrition intravenously through a peripheral vein.

peripheral-short catheter Type of vascular access device used for short-term infusion therapies.

peripheral vascular resistance The resistance in the pulmonary vasculature.

peripherally inserted central catheter (PICC) Central vascular access device that is inserted into an extremity, typically in the antecubital fossa, and advanced until the tip is positioned in the vena cava.

peristalsis A progressive wavelike movement that occurs involuntarily in hollow tubes of the body.

peritonsillar abscess A rare complication of tonsillitis in which the infection spreads to the tissue around the tonsillar capsule.

perivascular Situated around a blood vessel.

pernicious anemia Anemia caused by insufficiencies in intrinsic factor.

persistent The ability of a chemical agent to remain in an area. In general, the agent would have a low vapor pressure and a high vapor density.

pessary A device that, when inserted into the vagina, will help support the vaginal walls, reducing the bulging of those walls into the vagina.

Peyronie's disease Condition in which plaque forms on the erectile tissue of the penis, primarily in middle-aged or older men.

pH An indicator of hydrogen ion concentration; the negative logarithm of the hydrogen ion concentration expressed in nanomoles per liter. A normal pH of 7.4 is equivalent to 40 nmol/L of hydrogen ion (or 0.0004 mEq/L).

phagocytes Granulocytes, macrophages, and lymphocytes, which are attracted to an injured site by the complement factors and antigens.

phagocytosis The process by which phagocytes absorb and enzymatically degrade foreign matter and devitalized tissue.

phantom limb pain Pain appearing to come from an amputated limb.

pharmacogenetics Area of biochemical genetics concerned with drug responses and their genetically controlled variations.

pharmacogenomics The application of genomic information or methods to pharmacogenetics problems.

pharyngitis Inflammation of the pharynx caused by upper respiratory infection, which causes a sore throat.

pharyngoesophageal Pertaining to the pharynx and the esophagus.

phenomenology A qualitative research method that describes the meaning of a lived experience through the perspective of the participant.

phenotype Observable characteristics of an organism produced by the organism's genotype interacting with the environment.

pheochromocytoma A tumor (usually benign) that originates from the adrenal medulla.

pheresis catheter Central vascular access device used for plasma exchange therapies.

phimosis The inability to retract the foreskin over the penile glans.

phlebostatic axis Reference point used to level transducers.

phoria A tendency toward a functional deviation or defect that results from a break in visual fusion by covering an eye. Latent deviation meaning that the deviation is not apparent unless fusion of the eyes is broken.

phosphorus An abundant mineral used in all sources of energy (ATP, ADP, and AMP). Eighty percent is found bound to calcium in the bone as calcium phosphate. Normal serum levels are 2.5 to 4.5 mg/dL.

photodermatitis A common, inflammatory adverse reaction to sunlight in which the individual sunburns more easily than usual or develops papular or vesicular lesions with exposure to the sun.

phronesis A form of rationality and skill-based character that is similar to clinical judgment.

physes Growth plates.

physiological stress Metabolic conditions characterized by hypermetabolism and hypercatabolism.

pilosebaceous follicles A sebaceous cyst containing hair follicles.

pilot study A small preliminary study prior to conducting a larger study.

pitch Describes frequency; low pitch is 100 Hz and high pitch is 10,000 Hz.

pitting An indention that remains for a short time after pressing edematous skin with the finger.

planning Determining how expected patient outcomes can be achieved through nursing interventions by establishing priorities of care.

plasma The protein portion of blood that remains when cells have been removed.

plasma cells Differentiated B cells that are found in the plasma and are responsible for production of specific antibodies or immunoglobulins.

plasmapheresis A treatment used in some autoimmune diseases that involves removing blood from the body and filtering antibodies out of the plasma. The red blood cells and fluids are returned to the body. The removal of antibodies decreases immune stimulation and helps control clinical symptoms of some autoimmune diseases.

platelet Thrombocyte of blood that is small and colorless with no nucleus, which assists in blood clotting by adhering to other platelets and to damaged epethelium. Also called *blood platelet, thrombocyte.*

pleasure principle The principle of tension reduction.

pleural effusion Abnormal accumulation of fluid in the pleural space.

pleural friction rubs Harsh leathery sound created from inflamed pleural surfaces rubbing against each other.

pneumatoscope An otoscope with a bulb attachment that can be used to introduce air into the ear canal and middle ear to test for ruptured tympanic membrane.

Pneumocystis carinii **pneumonia (PCP)** An opportunistic fungal respiratory infection that can be seen in severely immune-compromised hosts.

pneumonia An inflammatory process that results in edema of interstitial lung tissue and extravasation of fluid into the alveoli, thus causing hypoxemia.

pneumothorax Partial or complete collapse of the lung.

point mutation A single nucleotide base-pair change in DNA.

polycythemia vera A hematocrit value that is elevated beyond normal values; frequent occurrence in chronic hypoxemia.

polymorphism A common variation in the sequence of DNA among individuals seen in more than 1% of the population.

polypharmacy The administration of many drugs together; also, the administration of excessive medications.

polysomnography Multichannel electrophysiological recording used to detect disturbances of breathing during sleep.

population Entire aggregation of cases in which a researcher is interested.

population-based care Care focused on aggregates and communities. A population is a collection of individuals who have in common one or more personal or environmental characteristics. As an aggregate, the members are defined in terms of geography, special interest, disease state, or other common characteristics.

portal hypertension Increased pressure in the hepatic circulation that is a complication of cirrhosis.

portal of entry The path by which an infective organism enters a susceptible host.

portal of exit Path in the chain of infection that allows a causative agent to escape from a reservoir.

positive deflection Any waveform that goes above the isoelectric line on ECG graph paper.

positive feedback Process by which a deviation from normal is reinforced or accelerated, producing an increased stimulus. For example, uterine contraction stimulates oxytocin secretion, which brings about increased contractions and increased oxytocin.

positive pressure infusion pump Electronic infusion device used to administer parenteral fluids and medications under preset pressures.

postacute withdrawal syndrome (PAWS) An enduring physical remnant of neurotransmitter production and/or receptor site damage. The mood is affected, as are interpersonal interactions and cognitive skills.

postanesthesia care unit (PACU) A physical space located adjacent to the operating room where patients are monitored closely as they recover from anesthesia.

postconcussion syndrome A condition that may follow mild head injury.

posterior circulation Refers to circulation in the arteries in the posterior portion of the circle of Willis.

posteriorly Back plane of the body.

postoperative blood salvage The process of salvaging blood in which blood is obtained from mediastinal and chest tubes, and then reinfused.

It is used following major surgeries, typically cardiovascular, thoracic, and some orthopedic procedures.

post-test probability The likelihood that a disease is actually present in a patient after testing (a positive test indicates disease).

postural instability Diminished postural reflexes, which contribute to difficulty maintaining balance.

potassium An intracellular cation with 98% found within cells. Small amounts are in blood (3.5 to 5.0 mEq/L) and bone. Its function is to maintain intracellular osmolality and participate in cellular depolarization and repolarization.

power analysis A research design's ability to detect relationships that exist among variables.

PPE Acronym for personal protective equipment, which is designed to protect the wearer from various hazards.

PR interval Part of the cardiac cycle; represents time from atrial depolarization to ventricular depolarization on an ECG tracing. Sometimes referred to as the *PRI* or *PR segment.*

practical knowledge Knowledge shaped by one's familiarity with the discipline and practice of the science and technology relevant to the situation at hand.

precipitation One of the actions of antibodies; occurs when an immune complex falls or precipitates out of circulation and is more easily located by neutrophils and monocytes for phagocytosis.

pre-diabetes A condition of glucose intolerance ranging between normal glucose tolerance and overt diabetes.

predictive accuracy Ability of a diagnostic test to predict the presence or absence of disease.

preferred provider organization (PPO) Organization that provides health care coverage through a coordinated plan for medical care that includes a network of contracted providers.

prehypertension A term used to describe those individuals who have a blood pressure finding on two or more office visits of 130 to 139/80 to 89 mmHg. These individuals are at twice the risk of developing hypertension as those with lower values.

preload The volume of blood in the ventricle at the end of diastole.

premature atrial contraction (PAC) An ectopic focus in the atria that occurs early, before the next expected SA impulse, causing depolarization and contraction of the atrial muscle.

premature junctional contraction (PJC) Dysrhythmia that originates in the AV junction. It discharges before the next expected sinus impulse and activates the ventricles in a normal manner. Due to retrograde conduction, the P wave is inverted and may appear before, buried, or after the QRS complex on an ECG tracing.

premature ventricular contraction (PVC) An irritable focus within the ventricle that discharges before the next sinus impulse; thereby, stimulating the ventricle directly and causing a contraction, which is followed by a full compensatory pause. Each contraction is an individual beat, not a rhythm.

premenstrual dysphoric disorder (PMDD) A severe form of premenstrual syndrome that includes five or more symptoms of depression for most of the time during the last week of the luteal phase and begins to remit within a few days after onset of the follicular phase of the menstrual cycle.

premenstrual syndrome (PMS) A complex, often misunderstood condition, involving physical, psychological, and behavioral symptoms associated with the menstrual cycle.

preoperative health evaluation An evaluation done within 30 days of a planned operation and must be documented in the patient's chart per the Joint Commission requirements.

presbycusis Hearing loss caused by changes in the middle and inner ear due to the aging process.

presbyopia Condition where the eye exhibits a progressively diminished ability to focus on near objects with age; also recognized as a symptom of aging.

pressure ulcer A localized injury to the skin and/or underlying tissue usually over a bony prominence, as a result of pressure or pressure in combination with shear and/or friction.

pretest probability The likelihood that a disease is actually present in a patient before testing.

prevalence The measurement of all cancer cases at a designated point in time.

priapism A persistent erection.

PRICE Acronym for *protection* (immobilize and prevent weight bearing), *rest*, *ice*, *compression*, and *elevation*.

primary adrenal insufficiency Condition in which 90% of the adrenal gland has been destroyed, resulting in an absence of adrenal hormones.

primary appraisal The process of evaluating the significance of a transaction as it relates to a person's well-being, based on Lazarus's theory of stress.

primary biliary cirrhosis An autoimmune disease in which there is inflammation and destruction of the intrahepatic biliary system, resulting in fibrosis.

primary immune deficiency Results from genetic abnormalities in immune system development and causes partial or total immune system dysfunction.

primary immune response The first exposure to a specific antigen; results in creation of B memory cells, which provide lifelong protection against the specific antigen.

primary injury Refers to mechanical injury to the brain.

primary intention A wound that is surgically closed or one with smooth, closely aligned margins.

primary lesion Lesion that results from the initial reaction to a pathologic condition.

primary nursing A primary nursing care delivery system is a system in which a registered nurse providing direct care to the patient has 24-hour responsibility for the planning, implementation, and outcomes of patient care.

primary set Infusion set with a single fluid pathway from the fluid container to a vascular access device.

primary tumors Tumors that are at the original site where it first arose. For example, a primary brain tumor is one that arose in the brain as opposed to one that arose elsewhere and metastasized to the brain.

principlism An emerging theory in ethics that incorporates the various ethical principles in attempting to resolve conflicts in clinical settings.

probability sampling Type of sampling that involves random selection when choosing the elements and participants.

process standards Quality standards that focus on whether the activities within an organization are being conducted appropriately.

prodromal phase The phase of acute hepatitis that occurs between exposure to the virus and the appearance of jaundice. It is characterized by fatigue, anorexia, malaise, nausea, vomiting, and a headache; often mistaken for the flu.

progenitor cells In development, a parent cell that gives rise to a distinct cell lineage by a series of cell divisions. Like stem cells, progenitor cells have a capacity to differentiate into a specific type of cell. In contrast to stem cells, however, they are already far more specific: They are pushed to differentiate into their "target" cell.

progesterone Steroid hormone produced by the ovaries and the placenta. It is responsible for uterine changes in the second half of the menstrual cycle.

programmed theory of aging Theory of aging based on the premise that aging follows a biological timetable.

prolactin Peptide hormone produced by the anterior pituitary gland. Stimulates breast development and breast milk during and after pregnancy.

prolapse Condition in which the uterus is unable to remain high in the vaginal canal and begins to protrude into the vagina; can occur if the structures supporting the uterus are weakened during childbirth.

proprioception The awareness of posture, movement, and changes in equilibrium and the knowledge of position, weight, and resistance of objects in relation to the body.

proptosis A downward displacement of the eyeball in exophthalmic goiter or in inflammatory conditions of the orbit.

prostaglandin A long-chain fatty acid that regulates platelet aggregation and controls inflammation.

prostatectomy Removal of the prostate and seminal vesicles.

prostatitis Inflammation of the prostate gland.

protein C A normal component of the coagulation system.

protein-calorie malnutrition Physical state resulting from the underconsumption of energy and protein specifically.

proteinuria The presence of protein in the urine.

proton pump inhibitor (PPI) Drug that blocks the proton pump in the stomach, thus reducing gastric acid secretion.

psoriasis A chronic, noncontagious inflammatory skin disorder; characterized by erythematous papules and plaques with silver-white scales that are sharply demarcated and the result of hyperproliferation of keratinocytes.

psoriatic arthritis An inflammatory process associated with psoriasis.

psychogenic polydipsia Condition in which excessive thirst occurs for psychogenic, rather than organic, reasons.

psychomotor learning Learning that occurs when a physical skill has been acquired.

psychosocial theories of aging Theories of aging that describe the changes that take place emotionally and socially as one enters the later years of life.

ptosis Drooping of the upper eyelid, generally due to paralysis.

pulmonary artery catheter (PAC) A flow-directed, balloon-tipped catheter used to measure intracardiac pressures.

pulmonary artery occlusion pressure (PAOP) Pressure obtained by inflating the balloon on a pulmonary artery catheter at the end of expiration to reflect left ventricular end-diastolic pressure.

pulmonary contusion Occurs when blunt thoracic trauma is applied through the chest wall to the parenchyma, causing disruption of alveolar capillary networks and usually resulting in hypoxemia; initially a hemorrhage into the lung tissue followed by alveolar and interstitial edema.

pulmonary embolism (PE) The presence of a thrombus or blood clot in the pulmonary vessels, which obstructs blood flow and impedes gas exchange.

pulmonic valve regurgitation The inability of the pulmonic valve to completely close, causing blood to regurgitate back into the right ventricle.

pulmonic valve stenosis A narrowing of the cardiac valve orifice that restricts blood flow due to an inability of the valve to completely open, thus, obstructing blood from the right ventricle from flowing into the pulmonary vasculature during systole.

pulse pressure The difference between the systolic and diastolic pressure, which is about 40 mmHg.

pulseless electrical activity (PEA) Absence of a detectable pulse and blood pressure in the presence of electrical activity in the heart as evidenced by some type of ECG rhythm other than ventricular fibrillation or ventricular tachycardia. It is not an actual rhythm, but represents a clinical condition wherein the patient is clinically dead, despite the fact that some type of organized rhythm appears on the ECG monitor.

pulsus paradoxus A greater than 10 mmHg drop in systolic blood pressure during inspiration.

Purkinje network fibers Part of the cardiac conduction system; a network of fibers that carries impulses directly to the ventricular muscle cells. Ventricular contraction is facilitated by the rapid spread of the electrical impulse through the left and right bundle branches, the Purkinje network fibers, and the ventricular muscle.

purposive sampling Type of sampling that implies that certain people or elements are deliberately selected for the study.

pyloric stenosis Narrowing of the pyloric orifice. In adults, frequently results from peptic ulcer disease, malignant compression of the gastric outlet, or pneumatosis intestinalis.

QRS complex Part of the cardiac cycle; represents ventricular contraction or depolarization on an ECG tracing.

QT interval Part of the cardiac cycle; is measured from the Q wave to the end of the T wave. The normal QT interval is 0.34 to 0.43 second.

quadrigeminy Premature ventricular contraction that occurs every fourth beat.

quadriplegia (*Latin*) Paralysis of all four extremities.

qualitative research A systematic, subjective approach used to describe life experiences and give them meaning.

quality Refers to characteristics of and the pursuit of excellence.

quality in fact Conforming to standards and meeting one's own expectations.

quality in perception Meeting the customer's expectations.

quality of care The degree to which health services for individuals and populations increase the likelihood of desired health outcomes and are consistent with current professional knowledge.

quantitative research Research characterized by the collection of numerical values, under a controlled situation, that yield data, which can be generalized.

quasi-experimental research design A study with an intervention, but one in which it is difficult to manipulate or control the setting, subjects, or variables, as is needed for a true experimental study.

quasi-intentional torts Volitional actions that result in harm to another, but intent is lacking.

quota sampling Type of sampling in which participants are selected by a researcher in a nonrandom manner using prespecified characteristics of the sample to increase their representation.

raccoon eyes Ecchymosis over the orbit of the eyes that is indicative of a basilar skull fracture. Also called *raccoon sign*.

radiation Waves and particles of energy. Radiation causes mutation of cells' DNA, which can weaken the cells' defense against a carcinogen or cause cell death.

radiation burns Burns that usually result from overexposure to the sun or are associated with radiation treatment for cancer.

radiologic agents Agents that are a source of alpha, beta, or gamma radiation that can be used as a weapon.

random assignment Subjects are randomly assigned to treatment versus control groups.

range of motion (ROM) Movement of a joint within its normal range.

rate of living theory of aging Considered one of the oldest theories on aging, it is based on the belief that individuals possess a finite amount of some "vital substance." When that substance is consumed, the individual dies.

rationality The ability to reason across time when changes in the patient's condition occurs. It includes noticing subtle changes, not limited to explicit vital signs and may not show up immediately in the vital sign trends.

RDD Acronym for radiation dispersal device, a device that can release radiation into the environment.

reactive arthritis A type of arthritis caused by a reaction to an infection somewhere else in the body. Also called *Reiter's syndrome* or *undifferentiated spondyloarthropathy*.

reactive oxygen species (ROS) Intermediary products, or species, that are produced in the metabolic production of energy; occur when oxygen is used to oxidize molecules and generate energy. A phenomenon that occurs during oxidative stress development and a major contributing factor in diseases in patients who are critically ill.

receptors Structure in a cell membrane or within a cell that combines with a hormone to alter an aspect of the functioning of the cell.

reconstructive surgery Surgery performed for the purpose of rebuilding tissues or body structures to achieve a more normal function and appearance.

rectocele Occurs when the posterior vaginal wall is weakened and the rectum bulges into the vagina.

rectum The lower part of the large intestine between the sigmoid colon and the anal canal.

recurrent pain Acute pain that completely resolves, leaving the patient free from pain for a period of time before the pain reoccurs.

red blood cell (RBC) A type of blood cell that transports oxygen and carbon dioxide. Also called an *erythrocyte*.

red blood cell distribution width (RDW) A direct measurement of the homogeneity (consistency) of red blood cell size.

refeeding syndrome Syndrome consisting of metabolic disturbances that arise from reinstitution of nutrition to patients who are severely malnourished.

refractory period Period of time that ensures the cardiac muscle is totally relaxed before another action potential or depolarization can be initiated.

regional anesthesia The production of insensibility of a part by interrupting the sensory nerve conductivity of any region of the body by local injection of a medication.

regional (locality) rule Existence of a prevailing community standard.

registered nurse (RN) An individual licensed by the state to practice nursing in accordance with the nurse practice act.

rehabilitation The multidisciplinary plan of care that maximizes an impaired individual's function by minimizing the deficits to achieve the highest quality of life possible.

relative refractory period Period when depolarization is almost complete, and corresponds with the top and the downslope of the T wave on an ECG tracing.

remodeling The fourth and final phase of wound healing that begins about 3 weeks after the injury and can still be in progress 6 months to 2 years later.

renal calculi Kidney stones.

renin An enzyme produced in the kidneys that converts angiotensinogen to angiotensin, which is an enzyme that helps elevate blood pressure.

repatriation Return of patients from one health care setting to another appropriate level of care or to a contracted institution.

reperfusion injury Injury to the cells after blood supply to an ischemic area is restored.

research A formal, systematic, and organized method of answering a question, solving a problem, validating and redefining existing knowledge, and developing new knowledge.

research critique A critical appraisal of a piece of completed research.

research design Overall plan or blueprint for a study; guides an investigator in planning and implementing a study.

research problem A situation or circumstance that requires a solution to be described, explained, or predicted.

research process Process of undertaking discrete steps to conduct a research study. Includes identifying a researchable problem, completing a literature review, creating the theoretical/conceptual framework, selecting an appropriate design, and collecting, analyzing, and distributing data/findings.

research purpose A concise, clear statement of the specific goal or aim of the study that is generated from the problem.

research question A research problem stated in an interrogative form.

research utilization (RU) The purposeful application of research findings to the clinical setting to improve patient care.

reservoir A place where an organism can survive and may or may not multiply.

resonance A low-pitched, clear, hollow tone of long duration. It is commonly heard over the lungs.

respect for others In ethics, the highest principle because it incorporates all other principles.

respiratory quotient (RQ) Ratio between carbon dioxide produced and oxygen consumed per molecule of fat, carbohydrate, and protein. Fat has an RQ of 0.7, protein 0.8, and carbohydrate 1.0.

restenosis Accumulation of smooth muscle cells at the site of the original percutaneous coronary intervention that occurs because of an artery's response to injury.

resting membrane potential The difference in electrical charge, or voltage, between the inside and outside of a cardiac cell.

restrictive cardiomyopathy A disorder characterized by endometrial scarring that usually affects one or both ventricles and restricts filling of blood, resulting in systolic dysfunction. The ventricle has normal wall thickness, but the walls are rigid, producing elevated filling pressures and dilated atria.

rete pegs Protrusions in the fifth layer of the epidermis that extend down into the dermis and help anchor the epidermis to the dermis. Also called *epidermal ridges*.

reticular activating system (RAS) Network of neurons that is involved with arousal and consciousness.

reticulocyte A biconcave, immature red blood cell disk without a nucleus.

reticuloendothelial system (RES) Part of the immune system; consists of the phagocytic cells located in reticular connective tissue, primarily monocytes and macrophages.

retinal detachment The separation of the sensory retinal layers from the retinal pigment epithelium, where subretinal fluid collects in the potential space.

retinopathy Degenerative changes in the retina.

retrograde ejaculation Backward ejaculation of semen into the bladder.

retroperitoneal space Area behind the peritoneum and outside the kidney.

reverse transcriptase An enzyme present is some classes of virus, including HIV, that is capable of replicating DNA from RNA, the reverse of normal replication of DNA.

Rh factor A protein substance made up of numerous complex antigens. When it is present on the surface of red blood cells, the person is Rh positive (Rh+); if not present, the person is Rh negative (Rh–). Also called *factor D*.

rheumatic fever A pharyngeal infection caused by Lancefield group A beta-hemolytic streptococci. In 3% of the cases it leads to rheumatic heart disease.

rheumatic heart disease An inflammatory disease of the heart that causes long-term damage, scarring, and malfunction of the heart valves.

rheumatoid arthritis (RA) Chronic inflammatory process that affects the peripheral joints and surrounding muscles, ligaments, tendons, and blood vessels.

rhinitis A collection of symptoms predominantly in the nose and eyes that occur after exposure to airborne particles of dust, dander, or the pollens of certain seasonal plants in people who are allergic to these substances.

rhinoplasty Plastic surgery of the nose.

rhytidectomy Surgical excision of skin to eliminate wrinkles of the face.

right-sided heart failure An abnormal cardiac condition characterized by impairment of the right side of the heart and congestion and elevated pressure in the systemic veins and capillaries.

rigidity Abnormal stiffness or inflexibility associated with Parkinson's disease.

Rinne test A hearing test that measures conduction of sound by bone when placing an activated tuning fork on the right and left mastoid sequentially.

riot control agent Agents that generally cause pain, burning, lacrimation, or discomfort upon exposure to mucous membranes. Also called an *irritant*.

risk management A comprehensive program for identifying and evaluating potential risks to the health care organization. Risks can be illness or injury related as well as financial.

robotics Electromechanical devices that are computer controlled and used to perform surgical tasks.

rolling (paraesophageal) hernia A protrusion of the greater curvature of the stomach through the esophageal hiatus.

Romberg test Assesses inner ear balance, proprioceptive ability, and visual and cerebellar system function by asking the patient to maintain an upright posture when arms are held out in front, with eyes open and eyes closed.

rotational injuries Injuries resulting from extreme lateral flexion or flexion-rotation of the spine, causing disruption of the posterior spinal ligaments and spinal instability.

rule of nines Divides the body into seven areas, which represent 9% or multiples of 9% of the body surface area; used to determine burn size.

S$_3$ (third heart sound) Abnormal third heart sound in the cardiac cycle; often heard when the ventricles are volume overloaded.

S$_4$ (fourth heart sound) Abnormal fourth heart sound heard in the cardiac cycle; often heard with heart failure and hypertension.

salience Having some things stand out as more or less important in a practical situation, it is a form of practical knowledge that is learned from many concrete clinical experiences in which a range of relevant clinical issues stand out as high priority.

same-day admission A hospital process in which the patient is not hospitalized prior to a surgical procedure but instead reports directly to the reception area of the operating room from home.

sample A portion selected from a population and interpreted to represent that population; a subset of the population.

sampling Process of selecting a portion of the population to represent the entire population.

scabies Contagious skin disease caused by a mite; commonly found in underdeveloped countries and places where there is overcrowding and poor hygiene.

scald burns Type of thermal injury that occurs from contact with hot foods or liquids, including steam.

schema Coordinated patterns of recurring actions that are created for the purpose of organizing and interpreting information.

Schilling test Procedure to identify anemia due to malabsorption.

Schwabach test Tests hearing for air and bone conduction by using an activated tuning fork on the mastoid process.

schwannomas Tumors of the Schwann cells (nerve sheath tumor).

sclerosing cholangitis An inflammatory disorder of the biliary tract that leads to fibrosis and strictures in the biliary system.

sclerotherapy A treatment for esophageal varices in which a bleeding vessel is sclerosed with a chemical agent.

scoliosis Lateral curvature of the spine.

scope of practice Refers to legally permissible boundaries of practice for a given health care profession.

scrub nurse Nurse in the operating room who works directly with the surgeon within the sterile field, passing instruments, sponges, and other items needed during the surgical procedure.

seborrheic keratosis A benign epidermal lesion seen predominantly in the middle-aged and elderly populations.

secondary adrenal insufficiency Condition in which the pituitary gland has insufficient secretion of ACTH, resulting in insufficient cortisol production by the adrenal glands.

secondary appraisal The process of evaluating the significance of a transaction between the person and his or her environment as it relates to available coping resources and options.

secondary immune deficiencies Impaired immune responses that result from a nongenetic cause such as aging, malnutrition, malignancies, immunosuppressive drug therapy, and infections such as the human immunodeficiency virus.

secondary immune response Second exposure to a specific antigen that triggers a stronger and quicker immune response than the first exposure, with production of greater amounts of antibodies due to the presence of memory B cells; results in a milder set of clinical symptoms or no observable response to the pathogen because the immune system quickly eliminates the pathogen.

secondary injury The body's response that can result from a primary injury.

secondary intention In the granulation process, healing that occurs when major tissue defects gradually close by epithelialization and contracture formation, and then form scar tissue.

secondary lesion Lesion that results from a change in the primary lesion or external trauma to the primary lesion.

secondary set Infusion set used to administer supplemental infusion therapies via the primary infusion system.

second-impact syndrome A condition characterized by a second concussion that occurs before the brain completely recovers from the first concussion.

secretion The active process of moving substances, such as H⁺ ion, from the blood into the tubular fluid against the concentration gradient.

self-antigen Receptors on cells that are recognized as unique to that individual.

self-sheathing Engineered safety mechanism in which a needle is encased in a protective chamber.

senile purpura A type of hemorrhaging under the skin that occurs most frequently in the elderly because their blood vessels are thinner and more fragile than those of younger people.

sense of coherence (SOC) Refers to how an individual sees the world and one's life in it.

sensitivity Describes the ability of a test to identify patients with disease; calculated by dividing the number of true positive tests by the sum of true positives plus false negatives.

sensitization The process of producing antibodies to an antigen present in the body.

sensorineural hearing loss Type of hearing loss attributed to damage to the eighth cranial nerve.

sensory dimension of pain Includes consideration of the location, intensity, quality, and temporal patterns of pain.

sentinel event Unexpected occurrence that has the potential to, or actually does, result in death or serious physical or psychological injury. Serious injury specifically includes loss of limb or function.

sepsis Clinical syndrome that is defined by the presence of infection and a systemic inflammatory response.

septic arthritis The most destructive form of acute arthritis; can result from trauma, direct inoculation of bacteria during joint surgery, spread of infection from another part of the body (hematogenous), or when an infection from an adjacent bone extends through the cortex into the joint space. Also called *nongonococcal bacterial arthritis*.

septic shock In adults, septic shock refers to a state of acute circulatory failure characterized by persistent hypotension unexplained by other causes. In pediatric patients, septic shock is defined as a tachycardia with signs of decreased perfusion. Hypotension is a late sign in children.

septum Material covering a portal; access point of an implanted port or reservoir, usually made of compressed silicon.

sequelae Residual problems that result from an illness.

seroma A mass caused by the accumulation of serum within a tissue or organ. It is similar to a hematoma except that instead of a collection of blood it is a collection of serous fluid.

serum immunoglobulin G (IgG) An antibody produced by the body that is an indicator of long-term immunity or resolving infection.

serum immunoglobulin M (IgM) An antibody produced by the body in response to an antigen; usually present during the acute phase of an infection.

setting The environment or place (locale) in which research is conducted; may be classified as natural, partially controlled, or highly controlled.

severe sepsis Sepsis with one or more organ system dysfunction.

sex chromosome One of the two chromosomes that determine an individual's genetic sex. The two kinds of sex chromosomes are X and Y. Normal females possess two X chromosomes and normal males one X and one Y.

sheet skin grafts Split-thickness grafts that have not been meshed.

shingles A viral infection that occurs because of the reactivation of latent varicella zoster virus or the virus that causes chickenpox. Also known as *herpes zoster*.

short bowel syndrome Syndrome in which the surface of the small intestine is reduced as a result of surgical resection of the small bowel, typically because of tumors, Crohn's disease, infarction, trauma, or radiation.

shunt A hole or passage that allows movement of fluid from one part of the body to another. Pulmonary shunts exist when there is normal perfusion to an alveolus, but ventilation fails to supply the perfused region.

sick role A set of expectations that people who are ill must meet and which society, including caregivers, expects of them.

sick sinus syndrome (SSS) Term that encompasses a broad range of abnormalities, including disorders of impulse generation and conduction, failure of pacemakers, and a susceptibility to paroxysmal or chronic atrial tachycardia. Also referred to as *sinoatrial disease* and *sinoatrial dysfunction*, a disorder in which the SA node is severely depressed due to heart disease or drugs.

sickle cell anemia Chronic erythrocyte disorder characterized by misshapen "sickle-shaped" red blood cells resulting from malfunctioning hemoglobin molecules.

silicosis Disease that results from exposure to free crystalline silica in mines, foundries, blasting operations, stone, clay, and glass manufacturing.

simple random sampling Type of sampling strategy in which each person in a population has an equal chance of being selected for a study.

simple verbal descriptive scale (SVDS) Scale that uses a horizontal line marked with the numbers 0 to 10 from left to right, but also includes interval descriptors of "no pain," "mild," "discomforting," "distressing," "horrible," or "excruciating pain."

single-gene disorder A disorder due to one or a pair of mutant alleles at a single locus.

sinoatrial (SA) node Part of the electrical conduction of the myocardium; located in the upper posterior portion of the right atrial wall near the opening of the vena cava. The SA node is commonly referred to as the primary pacemaker of the heart.

sinus arrest Momentary cessation of sinus impulse formation, causing a pause in the cardiac rhythm followed by spontaneous resumption of electrical activity. This dysrhythmia may be referred to as sinus pause, and is reflected as an absence of the PQRST complex on an ECG tracing and an absence of cardiac output.

sinus arrhythmia/dysrhythmia Dysrhythmia resembling normal sinus rhythm except for a slight irregularity in the heart rhythm.

sinus bradycardia Situation in which the SA node is firing at a heart rate of less that 60 beats per minute. Often called *sinus brady*.

sinus tachycardia Rapid firing of the sinus node at rates of more than100 beats per minute at rest. There may be a compensatory response to a decreased cardiac output state.

sinusitis Infection or inflammation of the sinuses.

situational stressor Stressor that is unpredictable and may occur at any time during life; such stressors can be positive or negative. The effect of the situational stressor may vary depending on the developmental stage of the individual experiencing the stress.

Sjögren's syndrome An autoimmune disease in which the immune system attacks and destroys the glands that produce tears and saliva.

skeletal traction Treatment that entails placement of a skeletal pin through the bone which is then attached to a weighted cord to maintain proper alignment of the fractured bone.

skills of involvement The skills of perceiving relevant changes or nuances in clinical situations; these skills are experientially learned and form part of a nurse's practical clinical knowledge.

skin testing Introduction of small amounts of various allergens into the skin of an allergic individual through either intradermal injection or a scratch or "prick test" technique to evaluate for a triggering allergen. Individuals sensitive or capable of producing immediate IgE response to allergens will show a wheal and flare when the allergen is introduced in a skin test.

skin traction Treatment that uses straps or foam boots secured to the lower extremity attached to a weighted cord that is pulling no more than 6 pounds to maintain proper alignment of the fractured bone.

sleep apnea A disorder in which a person stops breathing for more than 10 seconds, typically more than 20 to 30 times in an hour. The three main types of sleep apnea are central, obstructive, and a combination of central and obstructive.

sliding (direct) hiatal hernia Occurs when a portion of the fundus of the stomach moves upward through the esophageal hiatus into the thoracic cavity.

sodium Most numerous cation in extracellular fluid (ECF); maintains ECF volume through osmotic pressure, assists acid–base balance, and conducts nerve impulses via sodium channels. Normal blood values are 135 to 145 mEq/L.

sodium bicarbonate A base or alkali that removes hydrogen ion when added to the blood.

solar lentigo Lesions that develop due to a familial tendency and chronic sun exposure in Caucasians older than 60 years of age. They are macules that are darker and larger than freckles and do not fade during winter. Commonly referred to as *age spots* or *liver spots*.

Somogyi effect A response to the use of exogenous insulin, which results in nocturnal hypoglycemia. The hypoglycemia is accompanied by release of counterregulatory hormones; as a result patients awake in the morning with elevated blood glucose levels. This is often referred to as *rebound hyperglycemia*.

specific gravity (SG) An estimate of the solute concentration in a volume of liquid measured with a hydrometer which compares the liquid to an equal amount of distilled water. Normal urine values are 1.016 to 1.022.

specificity Describes the frequency with which a test is normal in subjects who are free of disease; calculated by dividing the number of true negatives in the population by the sum of true negatives plus false positives.

specificity theory Theory asserting that pain is directly related to the degree of injury. Once a noxious stimulus has occurred, the message is carried directly to the pain centers in the brain.

spermatocele Painless, sperm-containing cysts found on the testicle.

spermatogenesis Production of mature male germ cells.

Spetzler-Martin AVM grading scale A scale to grade arteriovenous malformations (AVMs) based on the degree of surgical difficulty in removing them.

spinal anesthesia An anesthesia technique in which a local anesthetic is injected into the subarachnoid space and directly into the cerebrospinal fluid. Also called *intrathecal anesthesia*.

spinal cord injury (SCI) Injury to the spinal cord that results in impairment or loss of motor, sensory, and autonomic functions.

spinal precautions Methods of immobilizing the spine and moving patients to prevent or avoid additional spinal injury. Spinal precautions are initiated at the trauma scene and maintained until spinal injury has been ruled out or appropriate treatment strategies have been implemented.

spinal shock A period of flaccid paralysis and absent reflexes lasting up to 6 weeks after spinal cord injury.

split-thickness skin graft Grafting of a partial layer of skin, including the epidermis and part of the dermis.

spondylitic disease A condition consisting of inflammation and degenerative changes of the spine including formation of osteophytes, calcification and hypertrophy of the ligaments, and degeneration of the intervertebral disks.

sprain An injury to a ligament.

spring-coil container Mechanical infusion device with a combination of a spring coil and collapsable disk; used to deliver small-volume parenteral solutions or medications.

spring-coil syringe Mechanical infusion device that uses a syringe to deliver parenteral solutions or medications.

ST segment Interval between the end of the QRS complex and the beginning of the T wave on an ECG tracing. Represents the time during which the ventricles have been completely depolarized and are beginning ventricular repolarization. Normally is isoelectric on ECG graph paper.

stage 1 hypertension A blood pressure of 140 to 159 mmHg systolic or 90 to 99 mmHg diastolic measured during multiple office visits following the guidelines for obtaining accurate blood pressure measurements.

stage 2 hypertension A blood pressure of greater than 160 mmHg systolic or greater than 100 mmHg diastolic measured during multiple office visits following the guidelines for obtaining accurate blood pressure measurements.

staghorn calculus A calculus or stone that remains in the renal pelvis and becomes so large that it fills the pelvis completely, blocking the flow of urine.

staging The portion of the tumor classification system that describes the extent of the tumor and evidence of metastasis throughout the body.

standards of care General standards of care and guidelines for nursing practice formulated in 1991 by the American Nurses Association.

standards of nursing practice Authoritative statements by which the nursing profession describes the common level of performance or care by which the quality of practice can be determined and responsibilities for which its practitioners are accountable.

standards of professional performance Standards that address the professional nursing role with regard to education, ethics, research, collegiality, and resource utilization.

stapedectomy Removal of the stapes bone and its replacement to restore hearing.

statistical significance A term indicating that the results from an analysis of sample data are unlikely to have been caused by chance, at some specified level of probability.

steady state Dynamic balance of the body's internal environment, even in the presence of change.

steatorrhea Feces that have a high fat content. The stool is typically foul-smelling, greasy, and floats.

stem cell Primitive cell in the bone marrow from which mature blood cells derive.

STEMI Acronym for ST segment elevation myocardial infarction; refers to myocardial injury associated with ST segment elevation on the ECG. ST segment elevation means that myocardial tissue is undergoing severe anoxia and cellular damage, in most cases resulting from complete coronary artery blockage from thrombotic occlusion over an underlying plaque lesion.

stenosis Narrowing of the lumen of a blood vessel.

stent A device used to secure a widened arterial lumen; it is inserted permanently inside the coronary artery, compressing plaque and providing structural support of the vessel. The two general type of stents are bare-metal stents, which do not have a coating, and drug-eluting stents, which are "coated" with medications, including heparin and various immunosuppressant agents, in such a manner that the medications diffuse (elute) into the vessel wall over a period of weeks to months.

Stevens-Johnson syndrome (SJS) A severe, acute, self-limiting skin reaction to infection or to certain medications; affects the epidermal layer of the skin and mucous membranes.

stomatitis Generalized inflammation of the oral mucosa; it is classified according to the etiology.

stopcock Manually operated add-on device used to direct the flow of an infusate.

strabismus A condition in which an individual's eyes do not look at the same object together. Also referred to as *cross-eyed*.

strain An injury to the muscle belly or its tendon attachment to bone.

strategic national stockpile (SNS) A national repository of pharmaceutical agents, vaccines, medical supplies, and equipment that can be delivered to the site of a large-scale disaster to augment local and state resources in order to reduce the morbidity and mortality in the civilian population.

stratified random sampling Type of sampling that gives individuals within designated categories an equal chance of selection. The population is first divided into two or more strata or subpopulations. The goal is to enhance representation.

stress An organism's response to stimulation or change; a state produced by a change in the environment that may be perceived as challenging, threatening, or damaging to the person's dynamic balance or equilibrium. These changes may be real or perceived, and they activate an organism's attempts to cope by means of neural and endocrine mechanisms.

stress perception Recognition of a stressor by the brain.

stress response Activation of physiological fight-or-flight-or-fright systems within the body.

stressor A stimulus that activates a stress response.

stridor A raspy noise heard in the upper airway as a result of air attempting to move through a narrowed opening.

stroke Syndrome characterized by a set of neurological deficits that fit a known vascular region.

stroke volume (SV) The amount of blood leaving a ventricle with each contraction.

structure standards Quality standards that focus on the internal characteristics of an organization and its personnel.

subarachnoid hemorrhage (SAH) A condition characterized by bleeding into the space below the arachnoid space.

subchondral bone The smooth tissue at the ends of bones that is covered with cartilage.

subconscious A mental state that encompasses things that have been forgotten but can easily be brought to consciousness.

subcutaneous emphysema Air that escapes into the subcutaneous tissue.

subcutaneous nodules Small, nontender swellings found over bony prominences on the hands and feet.

subdural hematoma (SDH) Bleeding between the dura and the arachnoid layers of the meninges.

subjective data Data that consists of information the patient or caretaker tells the nurse; information that can be perceived only by the patient and not by the observer.

substance abuse Repeated use of a substance despite significant and repeated negative substance-related consequences.

substance dependence A pattern of substance use that is continued despite significant consequences, usually with physiological tolerance effects and a withdrawal syndrome if the substance is withdrawn.

substance intoxication Reversible substance-specific changes in thinking, emotions, behavior, and/or physiological functions caused by recent substance ingestion.

substance withdrawal A substance-specific mental disorder that follows the cessation or reduced intake of a substance that has regularly been used to induce a state of intoxication.

substance withdrawal syndrome The symptoms that occur when drug use is reduced or discontinued.

substantia nigra Structure located in the midbrain beneath the basal ganglia.

substituted judgment A subjective determination of what a person would have chosen to do had that person been capable of making his or her opinion known.

sudden cardiac death (SCD) Type of cardiac arrest most often associated with abrupt coronary artery occlusion from plaque disruption over severely stenotic lesions in the setting of poorly developed collateral circulation.

superego An extension of the ego that represents an individual's early moral training and ideal values imparted by societal norms.

suppurative Pertaining to the formation of pus.

supraventricular tachycardia (SVT) Tachycardia that is generated somewhere above the ventricles. The term encompasses all fast rhythms with normal QRS complexes and heart rates greater than 100 beats per minute. Rhythms included in this category include sinus tachycardia, premature atrial tachycardia, and paroxysmal junctional tachycardia. This term may be used when it is impossible to identify the source of the tachycardia.

surfactant Surface-active agent that promotes alveolar stability.

surveillance The systematic and continuous assessment of patients for the recognition and management of potentially catastrophic events.

survival Observation of persons with cancer over time and the likelihood of their dying over several time periods; a link between incidence and mortality data.

Swan-Ganz catheter A pulmonary artery catheter that is inserted into the pulmonary artery via the right atrium and ventricle; used to measure cardiac output and pulmonary artery pressure and to infuse fluids.

sympathectomy Excision of a portion of the sympathetic division of the autonomic division of the autonomic nervous system.

synapse The space between the junction of two neurons in a neural pathway where the termination of the axon of one neuron comes into proximity with the cell body or dendrites of another.

syncope Temporary dizziness or loss of consciousness caused by low blood pressure and insufficient blood flow.

syndrome of inappropriate antidiuretic hormone (SIADH) A hypermetabolic state of the adrenal glands in which antidiuretic hormone is produced in excess, leading to the retention of fluid and hyponatremia.

syphilis A sexually transmitted infection (STI) that is caused by the *Treponema pallidum* bacterium; has been called the "great imitator" because its symptoms often mimic those of other STIs.

systemic inflammatory response (SIRS) A systemic response of the immune system that can be triggered by both infectious and noninfectious causes.

systemic lupus erythematosus (SLE) An example of a systemic type III hypersensitivity autoimmune disease characterized by damage to joints and soft organs as a result of the effects of autoantibodies and antibody–antigen activity (immune complex responses).

systemic vascular resistance The arterial systolic pressure; normal SVR is 900 to 1,400 · dyn s/cm^5.

systolic A blood pressure reading of the maximum pressure in the aorta and major arteries, which occurs when the left ventricle contracts and ejects blood onto the central vascular system.

systolic dysfunction Impaired ventricular function with volume overload and decreased contractility.

T cells White blood cells that are vital to initiating and regulating an immune response; produced in the bone marrow and mature and differentiate into various types of T cells in the thymus and other lymphatic tissue such as CD4 (cluster of differentiation, a type of receptor), CD8, T-memory, and T-suppressor cells. They are a crucial part of the immune response because they function as the regulatory cells of the immune system and are responsible for initiating and controlling immune processes such as phagocytosis, cytokine/lymphokine secretion, and activation of B cells.

T lymphocyte Lymphocytes that, when active, divide rapidly and secrete small proteins called cytokines that regulate or assist in the immune response.

T wave Represents ventricular recovery or repolarization in the cardiac cycle; often referred to as the resting phase of the cycle.

tachypnea Rapid respiratory rate.

tau A specialized protein that is a key component of the neurofibrillary tangles associated with Alzheimer's disease.

teaching Any deliberate act that involves the planning, implementation, and evaluation of instructional strategies that meet expected learner outcomes.

team nursing A nursing care delivery system in which a group of RNs, LVNs/LPNs, and unlicensed assistive personnel are assigned shift responsibility for a group of patients, with the RN assuming a leadership role in accordance with the nurse practice act.

techne Something that can be standardized and replicated.

telemedicine Systems or programs that use video or computer-based equipment to link providers or monitor patients electronically.

teleological theories Theories that derive norms or rules for conduct from the consequences of actions; looks merely at consequences to determine the rightness or wrongness of an action.

telomere The tip or end of each chromosome arm.

temporary transvenous pacing Procedure that involves insertion of a pacemaker wire through a major vein, such as the internal jugular, subclavian, or femoral. The pacemaker wire is then advanced into the heart for pacing.

tenosynovitis An infection of the flexor tendon sheaths.

tension pneumothorax Occurs when an injury perforates the chest or pleural space. During inspiration air enters the pleural space and becomes trapped. As more air is trapped, the pressure in the pleural space increases, collapsing the lung and causing the mediastinum to shift to the opposite side.

terrorism An act designed to disrupt daily life and cause terror and panic. The definition according to the FBI is "The unlawful use of force or violence against persons or property to intimidate or coerce a government, the civilian population, or any segment thereof, in furtherance of political or social objectives."

tertiary or third intention Healing that occurs in wounds that have not been sutured in a timely manner or have broken down and been sutured later.

testicular torsion Twisting of the spermatic cord.

tetraplegia (Greek) Paralysis of both upper and lower extremities.

thalassemia Class of hematologic disorders characterized by genetic inheritance of a mutated hemoglobin-coding gene; characterized by increased hemolysis.

T-helper cells A type of T cell that is identified and named by the kind of receptor that is on its surface, a CD4 receptor (cluster of differentiation receptor 4). T-helper cells regulate immune function by stimulating B lymphocytes to produce antibodies and chemically stimulate the cell-mediated response to viral and mutant cells.

theoretical connectedness Requires that the theoretical schema developed for the study be clearly expressed, logically consistent, reflective of the data, and compatible with the practice of nursing.

therapeutic alliance An alliance that involves the nurse and the patient consciously working together to reach mutually agreed-on goals.

therapeutic communication Purposeful communication that is designed to convey openness and caring.

therapeutic lifestyle changes (TLC) Dietary modifications recommended for treatment and prevention of disease.

thermal burns Injury from flames; the most common type of burn injury.

thermistor Thermometer imbedded in a pulmonary artery catheter that is used to detect core temperatures.

third-degree AV block (complete block) Independent excitation and contraction of the atria and ventricles due to the inability of any atrial impulses to reach the ventricles. The top and the bottom of the heart are not communicating; they are each beating independently. This dysrhythmia is referred to as AV dissociation because of the independent function of the atria and the ventricles.

threshold Point at which a stimulus will produce a cell response or depolarization.

thrills Palpable vibratory sensations from turbulent blood flow across cardiac valves due to cardiac murmurs.

thromboangiitis obliterans (TAO) A chronic inflammatory vascular occlusive disease most common in men who smoke. Also known as *Buerger's disease*.

thrombocyte Platelet.

thrombopoietin Hormone produced by the liver and kidneys; responsible for stimulating thrombopoiesis.

thrombus Blood clot that forms in a blood vessel and remains at the site of formation.

through-the-needle peripheral-short catheter Vascular access device in which the catheter is inserted into the vein by threading it through the lumen of an introducer.

thyroid storm A life-threatening, hypermetabolic condition in which excess production of thyroid hormones causes serious cardiac disorders.

thyroidectomy Full or partial surgical removal of the thyroid gland.

thyroiditis Inflammation of the thyroid gland.

thyromegaly Abnormal growth of thyroid tissue.

thyrotoxicosis A critical, hypermetabolic condition in which excess production of thyroid hormones threatens physiological stability and well-being.

tinnitus A buzzing, roaring, or ringing in the ears.

tissue factor (TF) Cytokine that is important in immune function and inflammation; released by a variety of injured tissue cells, macrophages, and platelets; stimulates platelets to stick together and form the beginning of a clot to stop bleeding when injury occurs.

tissue-specific antigens Proteins located in the cell membrane of some tissues such as blood, nerves, lungs, and kidneys that are involved in type II tissue-specific–mediated hypersensitivity reactions.

tolerance Physiological habituation to a substance, resulting in the need for progressively greater amounts to achieve intoxication and/or a diminished effect from continued use of the same amount of the substance.

toll receptors Part of the natural immune response; microcellular receptors on the surface of many types of immune and tissue cells that are able to initiate immune responses when pieces of bacterial cell walls attach to them. Functions include stimulation of a cell to release tumor necrosis factor or start the process of programmed cell death (apoptosis).

tomography Imaging technology that displays images of a single plane (slice) of the heart.

tonsillitis An acute or recurrent infection of the tonsils.

tophi Accumulation of uric acid crystals in the cartilage of the earlobe.

torsade de pointes Form of ventricular tachycardia in which the QRS complexes have varying morphology or shape and width. This dysrhythmia resembles a turning about or twisting motion along the baseline or isoelectric line and tends to recur repeatedly.

tort law A brand of civil law concerning legal wrongs committed by one person against another or against another's property.

total joint replacement A diseased or injured joint that is surgically removed, and replaced with an orthosis.

total parenteral nutrition (TPN) Provision of nutrition intravenously via a central vein.

total patient care Another name for the case method of nursing care delivery.

toxic epidermal necrolysis (TEN) Part of the same syndrome of diseases as Stevens-Johnson syndrome, but it is a more severe form of the disorder and is life threatening with more extensive skin detachment.

toxin Material produced by living organisms that has chemical properties that can cause injury, illness, and death.

tracheal breath sounds Breath sounds auscultated over the trachea; they are normally loud and high pitched.

tracheal deviation Shifting of the tracheal position to the right or left of midline due to the push or pull of thoracic structures.

tracheostomy Refers to the making of a semipermanent or permanent opening into the trachea, and to the opening itself.

tracheotomy A temporary surgical airway into the trachea.

transcription Formation of an RNA molecule on a DNA template in the cell nucleus.

transcutaneous electrical nerve stimulation (TENS) Low-voltage electrical stimulation through the skin; used to relieve pain.

transcutaneous pacing (TCP) Procedure that delivers an electrical stimulus directly through the chest wall.

transduction The transmission of pain from the periphery to the central nervous system.

transection Cutting across.

transesophageal echocardiography (TEE) Echocardiogram performed using a miniaturized transducer advanced down the esophagus. Because the esophagus passes directly behind the posterior surface of the heart, TEE affords excellent views of the posterior structures of the heart and great vessels.

transesophageal ultrasound A diagnostic test that uses an ultrasound device that is passed into the esophagus of a patient to create a clear image of the heart muscle and other parts of the heart.

transferrin Protein concentrated in the small intestine; responsible for transportation of iron from the gut to target cells.

transfusion-related acute lung injury (TRALI) A serious, life-threatening clinical syndrome that is a complication of blood transfusions. It is thought to be caused by the presence of granulocyte antibodies and biologically active lipids in the donor plasma to which the recipient reacts.

transient ischemia attack (TIA) An episode of neurological deficits resulting from temporary ischemia that produces strokelike symptoms but no lasting damage. It occurs when the blood supply to part of the brain is briefly interrupted. Also referred to as a *warning stroke* or *mini-stroke*.

transient pain Acute pain that is brief and then resolves completely such as is the case in a needlestick for phlebotomy or an intramuscular injection.

translation Formation of a polypeptide chain from its mRNA template.

translocation A chromosome aberration that results from a transfer of a segment of one chromosome to another chromosome.

traumatic brain injury (TBI) An acute brain disorder characterized by an injury to the brain secondary to trauma.

traumatic wounds Abrasions, blisters, cuts, bites, stab wounds, gunshot wounds, and first- and second-degree burns.

tremors Involuntary muscle movements of a body part or limb.

triage A process that is used to determine the severity of a patient's illness or injury.

trichomoniasis A sexually transmitted protozoan infection caused by *Trichomonas vaginalis*.

tricuspid valve regurgitation Inability of a heart valve to completely close, resulting in a backflow of blood from the right ventricle to the right atrium.

tricuspid valve stenosis Obstruction of blood flow between the right atrium and the right ventricle due to a narrowed valve orifice.

trigeminy Premature ventricular contraction that is evidenced every third beat.

triglycerides A form of fat derived from fats in food and produced by the body from other sources such as carbohydrates.

triple-H therapy A triad of medical treatments for vasospasm (hemodilution, hypervolemia, and hypertension).

trismus Restricted movement of the jaw.

trisomy The state of having three representatives of a given chromosome instead of the usual pair.

tropia Deviation of an eye from the normal position with respect to the line of vision when the eyes are open.

Trousseau's sign Contraction of the muscles when the nerves are mildly compressed; for example, inflating a blood pressure cuff and keeping it above systolic will induce carpal spasms.

trypsin A pancreatic enzyme that hydrolyzes the interior bonds of large protein molecules.

tumor necrosis factor (TNF) A small peptide produced by a variety of cells, including granulocytes and lymphocytes; critical in the stimulation of the initial inflammatory response, specifically the activity of macrophages and granulocytes; also stimulates cells to initiate programmed apoptosis when mutations occur, which is important in inhibiting tumor development and growth.

tunica adventitia The outer layer of an artery; flexible stratum that consists of fibrous tissue made of collagen and elastic fibers surrounded by collagen bundles.

tunica intima Layer of an artery that consists of a monolayer of connecting endothelial cells and a lamina of connective tissue and smooth muscle cells.

tunica media The middle layer of an artery that consists of multiple layers of smooth muscle cells and connective tissue made up of elastic fibers, collagen, and proteoglycans.

tunneled and cuffed device Long-term central vascular access device whose proximal end is tunneled subcutaneously from the insertion site and the remaining length is brought out through the skin at an exit site.

turgor The elasticity and mobility of the skin; reflects the skin's hydration status.

tympanic membrane Eardrum.

tympanoplasty Surgical repair of the eardrum or bones of the middle ear in an effort to restore hearing.

tympany (1) A high-pitched, drum-like tone of medium duration. It is commonly heard over the air-filled intestines. (2) Abdominal distention with gas.

type 1 diabetes mellitus Type of diabetes characterized by the destruction of pancreatic beta cells.

type 2 diabetes mellitus Type of diabetes characterized by insulin resistance and decreased insulin secretion.

type A blood Blood type for an individual with A antigen.

type AB blood Blood type for an individual with both A and B antigens.

type B blood Blood type for an individual with B antigen.

type I (IgE-mediated) allergic reactions Involve the production of antigen-specific IgE antibodies after exposure to a foreign antigen or allergen; most common of the immune hypersensitivity disorders.

type II (tissue-specific–mediated) hypersensitivity reactions Involve IgG and IgM antibody–antigen immune complexes; tissue-specific antigens on the surface of cells are not recognized as self by the immune system and are attacked and damaged or destroyed. Only tissues with the specific antigens are involved.

type III (immune complex–mediated) hypersensitivity reactions Involve IgG and IgM antibody–antigen immune complexes; differentiated from type II reactions in that such reactions are soluble in plasma and circulate in the blood and are not localized at a tissue-specific surface. The traveling antibody–antigen complexes can deposit in tissue or joints and precipitate phagocytosis and inflammation. Multiple body systems/locations can be involved and a variety of clinical symptoms may be observed.

type IV (cell-mediated) hypersensitivity reactions T-cell–mediated immune response, instead of an antibody response as is the case with type I, II, and III hypersensitivity reactions. Additionally, the response is delayed, with the onset of symptoms 24 to 48 hours after antigen exposure. One example of a type IV hypersensitivity response is poison ivy reaction.

type O blood Blood type for an individual with neither A or B antigens.

type-specific hypersensitivity reactions Four specific mechanisms of overreactive immunologic response (types I, II, III, and IV) to environmental allergens, self-antigens, or antigens from another human.

U wave Follows the T wave in the cardiac cycle and is present only in some people on an ECG tracing.

ulcerative colitis (UC) Disorder that involves chronic inflammation of the mucosal and submucosal layers of the colon and rectum.

unconscious A mental state that encompasses all of those things that cannot be remembered or brought to conscious thought.

undernutrition Synonym for *malnutrition*.

unipolar lead Lead with one positive electrode and one indifferent zero reference point; consists of standard leads and augmented limb leads. The leads provide the five frontal plane leads of a 12-lead ECG.

United Kingdom Prospective Diabetes Study (UKPDS) A large clinical research study in Great Britain of patients with type 2 diabetes which concluded that tight glucose control (i.e., maintaining blood glucose levels close to normal ranges) results in decreased microvascular complications.

unlicensed assistive personnel Health care personnel who are not licensed; they may be technicians or certified nurses' aides or nursing assistants.

Unna's boot A rigid bandage that prevents edema while promoting healing; it is worn for several days at a time. Commonly used to treat venous ulcers.

unstable angina A transitory syndrome falling between stable angina and myocardial infarction wherein thrombus forms in an area of arterial stenosis, but is subsequently fully or partially lysed by endogenous antithrombotic mechanisms.

uplifts Positive experiences that are likely to occur in everyday life.

urgent procedures Surgeries that must be performed sooner rather than later.

urticaria Raised, erythematous, intensely pruritic plaques or wheals that are surrounded by a white halo. Also known as *hives*.

U.S. Preventive Services Task Force (USPSTF) A group of health care experts that makes recommendations for appropriate preventive services and screening exams in adults ages 65 and over.

vaccine A preparation that contains an infectious agent (live or killed) or its components; administered to stimulate the production of antibodies that can prevent infection or create resistance to infection from that agent; a type of acquired artificial immunity.

vaginismus Condition in which the vaginal muscles at the introitus contract very tightly, making vaginal penetration painful.

values Freely chosen beliefs or attitudes about the worth of an individual or object.

valvular regurgitation Inability of a heart valve to completely close, resulting in a backflow of blood through the incompetent valve orifice into the previous chamber.

valvuloplasty A surgical procedure to repair torn or damaged leaflets, chordae tendineae, or papillary muscle.

variables Attributes of a person or object that vary, that is, take on different values. Examples include body temperature, age, and blood pressure.

variant, Prinzmetal, or vasospastic angina Condition characterized by a vasospasm occurring at a single or multiple sites in major coronary arteries and their large branches.

varicocele Varicosities of the veins of the scrotum.

varicose veins Dilated, tortuous, superficial veins most commonly seen in the lower extremities.

vascular access device (VAD) A catheter, tube, or device inserted into the vascular system.

vascular lesion Lesions that appear as red or purple pigmented.

vasectomy Male sterilization surgery.

vasodilator A substance that causes the dilation of blood vessels.

vasodilatory cascade A series of events triggered by hypoxia, resulting in increased intracranial pressure.

vasogenic edema A condition characterized by an alteration in vascular permeability with disruption of the blood–brain barrier.

vasospasm Refers to the transient narrowing of an artery, causing decreased blood flow.

venous thromboembolism (VTE) Includes the disorders of deep venous thrombosis and pulmonary embolism.

ventilated-associated pneumonia (VAP) Pneumonia that develops in mechanically ventilated patients after more than 48 hours of intubation, with no clinical evidence of pneumonia at the time of intubation.

ventilation The movement of air between the atmosphere and the alveoli accomplished by respirations or the ability of the lungs to remove carbon dioxide.

ventilation/perfusion mismatching (V/Q) Usually there is a near equal relationship of ventilation ($\dot{V}$) to perfusion ($\dot{Q}$) in the lungs. The formula $\dot{V}/\dot{Q}$, where ventilation is 4 L/min and perfusion is 5 L/min, explains this relationship. Normal ventilation to perfusion equals 4/5 or 0.8.

ventral hernia A hernia through the abdominal wall.

ventricular dysrhythmia Dysrhythmia that originates in the ventricle and is caused by ectopic or irritable foci in the wall of the ventricle. These are the most serious types of dysrhythmias.

ventricular fibrillation (VF) Dysrhythmia marked by rapid, disorganized depolarization of the ventricles. There are no organized electrical impulses or coordinated atrial or ventricular contractions or palpable pulse.

ventricular tachycardia (VT) Life-threatening excitable ventricular focus arising from the tissue distal to the bifurcation of the bundle of His. It discharges repetitively, acting as the dominant pacemaker. When present, three or more premature ventricular contractions occur in a row at a rate of 130 to 250 beats per minute.

veracity In ethics, truth-telling.

verrucae Viral epidermal eruptions caused by human papilloma virus. Also known as *warts*.

vertically integrated models Organizational service structure of hospitals and related health care services aligned along a continuum of care. This model includes the integration of physician, hospital, and ancillary services. Integrated systems can offer a broad range of services pre- and post-hospitalization from primary care to long-term care.

vertigo Subjective sensation of spinning; dizziness; the illusion of rotational movement, tilting, and swaying with feelings of imbalance during standing or walking; symptom of a balance disorder.

vesicant (1) Chemical agent that can cause redness and irritation of the skin and blistering. Also called a *blistering agent*. (2) Parenteral solution or medication known to cause tissue damage and possible necrosis if infiltrated.

vesicular breath sounds Breath sounds normally heard over most of the chest wall from the movement of air in small airways distal to the bronchioles.

vestibular nerve dissection Surgical procedure to cut the vestibular nerve in the event of constant vertigo or dizziness.

viability The ability of a pathogen to survive outside of its host.

Vincent's stomatitis An acute bacterial infection of the gingiva oral mucous membranes caused most often by the bacteria *Borrelia vincentii*. Also known as *acute necrotizing stomatitis* or *trench mouth*.

viral hepatitis Inflammation of the liver caused by several viruses: HAV, HBV, HCV, HDV, and HEV.

viral load The number of HIV viral particles in a sample of blood, expressed as *copies*. Used to monitor the virulence of HIV infection. Levels of >100,000 copies indicate increased risk of AIDS-related illness.

viral meningitis Inflammation of the meninges due to a viral pathogen.

Virchow's triad The three factors that contribute to thrombosis: damage to the venous wall, a change in flow, and blood hypercoagulability.

virulence Related to the severity of disease a pathogen is capable of causing; virulence can vary depending on the ability of the host to mount an immune response. It is expressed as the number of cases of infection that are serious or produce a disability in all those infected.

visual analog scale (VAS) Does not have numeric intervals; rather it uses "no pain" and "pain as bad as it can possibly be" as descriptors at either end of a horizontal line measuring 10 cm in length.

vital signs Temperature, pulse, respirations, blood pressure, and pain level. Used to monitor patients for infection and hemodynamic changes.

vitamin B$_{12}$ (cobalamin) Essential nutrient found in animal proteins; responsible for the activation of folate iron.

vitiligo Condition leading to a localized loss of melanocytes and, thus, patches of depigmentation.

voice whisper test A hearing test in which the examiner stands 1 to 2 feet in back of the patient and whispers.

volumetric pump Electronic infusion device that calculates the volume of solution delivered based on the amount displaced in the set's reservoir.

volutrauma Similar to barotrauma, but the lung damage is caused by increased volume that causes overdistention of alveoli.

vomiting agent Chemical agents that cause vomiting.

von Willebrand's disease Most common inherited bleeding disorder; characterized by deficiencies in von Willebrand factor.

wandering atrial pacemaker A pacemaker from at least three different sites above the bundle of His. Pacemaker sites may include the SA node, the AV junction, an atrial ectopic site, or any combination of these areas.

washed RBCs Red blood cells that have undergone a washing process that increases the removal of immunoglobulins and proteins that cause reactions. The use of washed RBCs is indicated when previous transfusion reactions have occurred.

wasting syndrome Involves the loss of lean tissue from increased protein metabolism, changes in metabolic rate, and anorexia and diarrhea. It is a hallmark of AIDS-related disease.

wear-and-tear theory of aging Theory of aging based on the premise that exposure to internal and external stressors results in the death of cells.

Weber test A hearing screening test that distinguishes whether hearing loss in an ear is conductive or sensorineural.

Western blot (WB) A specific and sensitive serum test that measures the presence of antibodies to HIV; generally done as a confirmation test when enzyme immunoassay tests for HIV are positive.

wheal A small, round, serous-filled raised blister on the skin that is the result of exposure to an allergen.

wheezes High-pitched musical sounds created by air moving over mucous strands.

white blood cell (WBC) A type of blood cell involved in protecting the body against foreign matter.

white coat phenomenon Phenomenon that occurs when a patient's blood pressure is susceptible to elevation as a result of apprehension and anxiety in a health care provider's office or during any other stressful situation.

whole blood Blood that is obtained from a donor, processed, and infused into a recipient.

wild type A normal allele of a gene or its normal phenotype.

window period The time between actual HIV infection and when HIV tests can detect the presence of the virus or antibodies to the virus in blood; usually 1 to 6 months.

winged steel infusion set A metal needle manufactured with flexible plastic attachments to facilitate insertion technique; used for phlebotomy procedures or for single-dose parenteral administrations and infusions of less than 4 hours duration.

withdrawal Uncomfortable and maladaptive physiological, cognitive, emotional, and behavioral changes associated with lowered blood or tissue concentrations of a substance after an individual has established some tolerance toward it, usually through heavy recent use.

WMD Acronym for weapons of mass destruction, which are agents that can cause massive damage and injury.

Wolff-Parkinson-White (WPW) syndrome AV conduction disorder characterized by two AV conduction pathways. This disorder generates an accessory conduction pathway.

wound dehiscence The separation of sutures or staples along the incision in a previously closed wound.

wound evisceration The protrusion of organs from a wound site.

xerosis A skin condition characterized by dry, pruritic, cracked, or fissured skin with scaling and flaking.

X-linked dominant Disorder in which a trait is dominant if it is phenotypically expressed in heterozygotes due to one or more genes located on the X chromosome.

X-linked recessive Disorder in which a trait is recessive if the trait is expressive only in homozygotes due to one or more genes located on the X chromosome.

Y set Devices used for administration of two or more infusates simultaneously. Access to the multiflow adapter is usually via a cap that maintains sterility of the fluid pathway.

zone of coagulation Area where the amount of injury to the tissue is the greatest.

zone of hyperthermia The outermost portion of an injured area where cell damage is minor.

zone of stasis Area surrounding the zone of coagulation that has potentially viable but injured cells.

zones; hot zone, warm zone, cold zone The hot zone, also called the exclusion or the red zone, is the area of highest contamination in a decontamination area. The warm zone, or yellow zone, is also called the contamination reduction corridor, and this is where actual decontamination takes place. The cold zone, or green zone, is also known as the support zone. No one is allowed in the cold zone without first being decontaminated. Those waiting to be decontaminated would be in the hot zone as well as the triage area.

zygote Fertilized egg.

INDEX

Page numbers followed by *f* indicate figures and those followed by *t* indicate tables, boxes, or special features. The titles of special features (e.g., Nursing Process: Patient Care Plans) are also capitalized. Trade names of drugs are capitalized and cross-referenced to their generic name.

A

AACG (acute angle-closure glaucoma), 2345. *See also* glaucoma
abacavir, 1939*t*
abandonment, of elderly person, 184, 185*t*
abbreviations:
  approved, 99
  banned, 97
abciximab:
  for acute coronary syndrome, 1197, 1201*t*
  for ischemic stroke, 760
abdomen, 1369–70, 1370*f*, 1370*t*
abdominal aortic aneurysm (AAA), 1342. *See also* aortic aneurysm
abdominal hysterectomy, 604*t*
abdominal pain/complaints:
  gerontological considerations, 1379
  history
    biographic and demographic data, 1371
    chief complaint, 1371–72
    cultural considerations, 1371
    duration of symptoms, 1372
    exacerbation or diminishment of symptoms, 1372*t*
    examples of questions, 1373*t*
    family history, 1374
    past medical history, 1372–73
      allergies, 1374
      childhood illnesses and immunizations, 1373
      diagnostic procedures and surgeries, 1373, 1374*t*
      medications, 1374
      previous illnesses and hospitalizations, 1373, 1373*t*
      sexual history, 1373–74
    patient's opinion of cause, 1372
    present symptoms, 1372, 1372*t*
    social history, 1374
      habits, 1374
      recent travel, 1374–75
  invasive procedures
    colonoscopy, 1378
    endoscopic retrograde cholangiopancreatography, 1378–79
    endoscopy, 1378
  laboratory studies, 1379, 1379*t*
  physical examination
    auscultations, 1375–76, 1376*f*
    iliopsoas sign, 1378
    inspection, 1375
    Murphy's sign, 1378
    obturator sign, 1378
    palpation, 1376–77, 1377*f*
    percussion, 1376, 1376*f*
    rebound tenderness, 1377–78
  radiologic examination
    barium enema, 1378
    CT of abdomen and pelvis, 1378

kidney-ureter-bladder, 1378
three-way abdominal films, 1378
ultrasound, 1378
stress and, 232
abdominal reflex, 709*t*
abdominojugular reflex, 1061
abdominoplasty, 2186
abducens nerve (CN VI), 703–4, 711*t*
abduction, 1712*t*, 1715
aberration, 2331
ABG. *See* arterial blood gas
ABI (ankle-brachial index), 1327, 1327*f*, 1328*t*
ablation, 1139
ABO incompatibility, 549*t*, 550
abortion, 1550–56, 1551*t*
above knee amputation (AKA), 1816
abscess, 2143*t*
absence seizure, 747*t*
absolute iron deficiency, 2019. *See also* iron deficiency anemia
absolute neutrophil count (ANC), 2001, 2113
absolute refractory period, 1077, 1077*f*
absorption, 343
abuse, elder, 184–85, 185*t*, 2442*t*
academic nurse educator, 18
Academy of Medical–Surgical Nurses (AMSN), 4–5
acarbose, 1679*t*
accessory muscles, 872
accommodation, 254, 2328
accommodation reflex, 704
accreditation, 58–59
acculturative stress, 240
Accupril. *See* quinapril
Accutane. *See* isotretinoin
ACE inhibitors. *See* angiotensin-converting enzyme (ACE) inhibitors
acetaminophen:
  in acute brain disorders, 733*t*
  in cerebral vascular disorders, 762*t*
  for pain management, 344, 344*t*
  postoperative use, 663
acetic acid solution, 2313*t*
acetylcholine, 794, 820
acetylcholinesterase inhibitors (AChEIs), 794, 795*t*
acetylcysteine, 981*t*
achalasia, 1389
  medical management, 1391, 1392*t*
  nursing management, 1391–92
    assessment, 1392
    interventions, 1392
  pathophysiology, 1389
achlorhydria, 1397
acid–base imbalances:
  in aging patients, 449*t*
  arterial blood gas changes in, 440*t*
  causes, 442*t*
  Clinical Preparation, 453–54*t*
  collaborative management, 449
  complex, 441
  health promotion, 449, 452
  metabolic acidosis. *See* metabolic acidosis
  metabolic alkalosis. *See* metabolic alkalosis
  nursing management, 449
  Nursing Process: Patient Care Plan, 450–51*t*
  Research Opportunities and Clinical Impact, 452*t*
  respiratory acidosis. *See* respiratory acidosis

respiratory alkalosis. *See* respiratory alkalosis
  terminology, 437*t*
acid–base status:
  assessment, 439–41, 440*t*
  buffer systems, 437–38
  homeostasis, 436–37
  imbalances. *See* acid–base imbalances
  kidney's role in, 439
  respiratory system's role in, 438–39
acidemia, 437*t*
acidosis, 433, 437*t*
acids, 436
acinus, 1004
Aciphex. *See* rabeprazole
ACL (anterior cruciate ligament) repair, 1813, 1814*t*
acne vulgaris, 2159–60, 2159*f*
acoustic immittance tests, 2312*t*
acoustic neuroma, 737, 738*t*, 2306*t*, 2307
acoustic reflexes, 2312*t*
acquired immunity, 1865*t*, 1869
  cellular immune response
    complement proteins, 1872, 1873*f*
    cytokines and lymphokines, 1871, 1872*t*
      interferons, 1871
      interleukins, 1871
      tissue factor, 1871–72
      tumor necrosis factor, 1871
    immune cell differentiation, 1870*f*
    T lymphocytes, 1869–70, 1871*t*
      natural killer cells, 1871
      suppressor T cells, 1871
      T-helper cells, 1870–71
  humoral immune response, 1872
    antibodies, 1872. *See also* immunoglobulin(s)
    antigen presentation and recognition, 1874, 1876*f*
    B lymphocytes (B cells), 1872, 1874, 1874*f*
    memory B cells, 1874–76
    plasma cells, 1874
acquired immunodeficiency syndrome (AIDS), 1922, 1927, 1928*t*. *See also* human immunodeficiency virus (HIV) infection
acral lentiginous melanoma, 2163*t*
acromegaly, 1639
  clinical manifestations, 1639, 1640*f*
  medical management, 1640
  pathophysiology, 1639
acromioclavicular joint, 1805
acromion, 1805
ACS. *See* acute coronary syndrome
ACTH. *See* adrenocorticotrophic hormone
Actifed. *See* pseudoephedrine
Actigall. *See* ursodiol
actinic keratosis, 2153, 2369
action potential, 1077, 1077*f*
activated partial thromboplastin time (aPTT), 2002*t*, 2051
activated protein C, 1981*t*, 2042
active acquired immunity, 1869
active immunization, 468
activities of daily living (ADLs), 110, 112*t*
activity theory of aging, 169
Actonel. *See* risedronate
acuity, 86
acupuncture, 375, 1296*t*
acute angle-closure glaucoma (AACG), 2345. *See also* glaucoma

in ventilated patient, 1031
wound healing and, 318
trition assessment:
  Cultural Considerations, 276t
  Gerontological Considerations, 277t
  in HIV infection, 315t
  parameters
    laboratory measurements, 274, 275t
    nutrition history, 274, 276, 276t
    physical assessment, 272–74
  preoperative, 597
  tools, 276
    Mini Nutrition Assessment, 276
    REAP, 276, 278t
    Subjective Global Assessment, 276
    WAVE, 276, 278t
drazid. See isoniazid
stagmus, 704, 2308, 2335
statin, 1383, 1384t, 2181t

A. See osteoarthritis
ASIS (Outcome and Assessment Information
    Set), 57
besity:
  assessment for weight loss intervention,
      281, 282t
  asthma and, 967
  bariatric surgery for. See bariatric surgery
  behavior modification for, 284t
  BMI classifications, 281t
  as cardiac risk factor, 1169
  in diabetes mellitus, 299–300
  genetic component, 201
  Gerontological Considerations, 285t
  medical nutrition therapy, 280–84, 284t
    calorie-saving alternatives, 284t
    healthy diet for, 284t
  National Guidelines for treatment and
      prevention, 1170t
  Nursing Process: Patient Care Plan, 286–89t
    activity level, 288t
    changes to be made in food intake, 287–88t
    current nutritional and dietary intake,
        286–87t
    current nutritional status, 286t
    disease risk factors, 287t
    knowledge regarding surgical methods of
        weight loss, 288–89t
  physical activity and, 282
  respiratory disorders and, 869
  treatment algorithm, 283f
  type 2 diabetes mellitus and, 1665–66
bjective data, 110, 110t
blique fracture, 1783, 1783f
bstructive sleep apnea (OSA), 897, 2294. See also
    sleep apnea
bturator sign, 1378
ccipital lobe ischemia, 2365t
ccupational asthma, 996
ccupational health nurse, 16, 2417t
ccupational lung disorders, 995
  asbestosis, 996
  clinical manifestations, 996
  coal miner pneumoconiosis, 996
  collaborative management, 997
  discharge priorities, 996
  health promotion, 996
  nursing management, 996
  occupational asthma, 996
  silicosis, 996
ccupational rhinitis, 888. See also rhinitis

Occupational Safety and Health Administration
    (OSHA), 58
octreotide, 1447t, 1640, 1641t
ocular hypertension, 2344
ocular migraine, 2365t
oculocephalic reflex, 704
oculomotor nerve (CN III), 703–4, 711t
oculopharyngeal muscular dystrophy, 1755, 1756t.
    See also muscular dystrophies
oculovestibular reflex, 704
odontoid process, 842
ofloxacin, 478t, 981t
OGTT (oral glucose tolerance test), 1610t, 1668
oil-droplet cataract, 2351t
olanzapine, 795t
OLD CARTS mnemonic, 471t, 697t
older adult. See aging patient
olfactory nerve (CN I), 702, 711t
oligoanalgesia, 2422t
oligodendroglioma, 736, 738t
oliguria, 1464
olsalazine, 1414t
–oma, 2066
omega-3 fatty acids, 295
omeprazole:
  in acute brain disorders, 733t
  in cerebral vascular disorders, 762t
  for gastroesophageal reflux, 1390t
  implications for surgery, 595t
  in spinal cord injury, 845t
Ommaya reservoir, 519
oncogene, 2064
Oncology Nursing Society (ONS), 2061
oncosis, 1164
oncotic pressure, 419
ondansetron:
  in acute brain disorders, 733t
  in cerebral vascular disorders, 762t
  for chemotherapy-related vomiting, 1585t
  for postoperative nausea and vomiting, 661t
  preoperative use, 611t
Online Mendelian Inheritance in Man, 197
on–off phenomena, 801
onychomycosis, 2150
oophorectomy, 1555
open-angle glaucoma, 2344. See also glaucoma
open-ended questions, 152
open fracture, 1782, 1783t
open globe, 2362
open pneumothorax, 2432
open reduction internal fixation (ORIF),
    1786, 1786f
operating expenses, in hospital budget, 52t
operating room, 621–22. See also intraoperative care
ophthalmodynamometry, 2333t
opioid antagonists, 733t, 762t
opioids:
  abuse, 378
  in acute brain disorders, 733t
  as anesthesia adjunct, 627–28t
  barriers to effective use, 346
  in cerebral vascular disorders, 762t
  classification, 347
  in end-of-life care, 398–99, 398t
  half-life in liver disease, 1455t
  for lower airway disorders, 981t
  for pain management, 345t, 346
  postoperative use, 662
  preoperative use, 611t
  side effects, 347–48t
  tolerance, dependence, and addiction, 346t
opportunistic infections (OIs), 1922
  in HIV/AIDS, 1928, 1929–31t, 1931–32

oprelvekin, 2103t
OpSite, 2261t
opsonization, 1871
optical coherence tomography, 2333t
optic nerve (CN II), 702–3, 703f, 711t
optic neuropathy, 2365t
oral cancer, 1383
  etiology, 1384–85
  Evidence-Based Practice, 1387t
  health promotion, 1385
  medical management, 1385
  nursing management, 1385
  Nursing Process: Patient Care Plan, 1386t
  pathophysiology, 1384
  risk factors, 1383
  signs and symptoms, 2296t
oral candidiasis, 1382
oral cavity, 2285–86, 2286f. See also mouth; upper
    airway disorders
oral contraceptives, 1057t
oral glucose tolerance test (OGTT), 1610t, 1668
oral route, drug administration, 349, 2110t
oral transmucosal route, drug administration, 349
orbit, 2326
orbital cellulitis:
  clinical manifestations, 2357, 2357f
  discharge priorities and health promotion, 2357
  medical management, 2357
  pathophysiology, 2357
  Patient Teaching & Discharge Priorities,
      2358–60t
orbital tumors, 2370
orchiectomy, 1568
orchiopexy, 1568
orchitis, 1567
  clinical manifestations, 1567
  etiology, 1567
  medical management, 1567
  nursing management, 1567, 1568f
organ of Corti, 2303
organ transplantation. See also specific organs
  alloimmune hypersensitivity response in. See
      alloimmune hypersensitivity response
  medical nutrition therapy, 320–21
  Nursing Process: Patient Care Plan, 1917–20t
    infection, 1917–18t
    knowledge deficit, 1917t
    post-transplant self-care, 1919–20t
    skin and oral mucosa, 1918–19t
orientation, 700
oronasal mask, for noninvasive positive pressure
    ventilation, 1034f
oropharyngeal fistula, 914
oropharyngeal tularemia, 2399
–orraphy, 588
Orthoclone OKT3. See muromonab-CD3
orthopedic surgery:
  anesthetic, 1805
  Clinical Preparation, 1830–31t
  collaborative management, 1829
  complications
    compartment syndrome, 1828
    heterotrophic ossification, 1829
    infection, 1828
    joint dislocation, 1828
    pressure ulcers, 1828
    respiratory insufficiency, 1827
    venous thromboembolism, 1827–28
  health promotion, 1829–30
  Nursing Process: Patient Care Plan, 1822–24t
  postoperative care
    discharge planning, 1826–27
    home environment, 1827

SPECIAL FEATURES

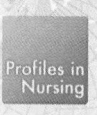
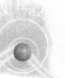

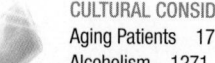

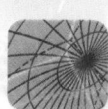

NURSING PROCESS: PATIENT CARE PLAN

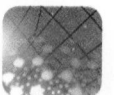

PATIENT TEACHING & DISCHARGE PRIORITIES

RISK FACTORS